Campbell-Walsh UROLOGY

EDITORS

Louis R. Kavoussi, MD

Chairman
The Arthur Smith Institute for Urology
North Shore-Long Island Jewish Health System
Manhasset, New York
Professor of Urology
New York University School of Medicine
New York, New York

Andrew C. Novick, MD

Chairman
Glickman Urological Institute
Cleveland Clinic Foundation
Professor of Surgery
Cleveland Clinic Lerner College of Medicine of
Case Western Reserve University
Cleveland, Ohio

Alan W. Partin, MD, PhD

David Hall McConnell Professor and Director
James Buchanan Brady Urological Institute
Johns Hopkins Medical Institutions
Baltimore, Maryland

Craig A. Peters, MD

John E. Cole Professor of Urology
University of Virginia
Charlottesville, Virginia

Campbell-Walsh
UROLOGY

NINTH EDITION

EDITOR-IN-CHIEF

Alan J. Wein, MD, PhD(Hon)
Professor and Chair
Division of Urology
University of Pennsylvania School of Medicine
Chief of Urology
University of Pennsylvania Medical Center
Philadelphia, Pennsylvania

Volume 1

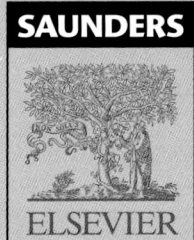

SAUNDERS

ELSEVIER

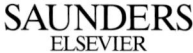

1600 John F. Kennedy Blvd.
Ste 1800
Philadelphia, PA 19103-2899

CAMPBELL-WALSH UROLOGY

ISBN 13: 978-0-7216-0798-6
ISBN 10: 0-7216-0798-5
E-dition ISBN 13: 978-1-4160-2966-3
ISBN 10: 1-4160-2966-4
International Edition ISBN 13: 978-0-8089-2353-4
ISBN 10: 0-8089-2353-6

Notice

Knowledge and best practice in this field are constantly changing. As new research and experience broaden
our knowledge, changes in practice, treatment, and drug therapy may become necessary or appropriate.
Readers are advised to check the most current information provided (i) on procedures featured or (ii) by
the manufacturer of each product to be administered, to verify the recommended dose or formula, the
method and duration of administration, and contraindications. It is the responsibility of the practitioner,
relying on his or her own experience and knowledge of the patient, to make diagnoses, to determine
dosages and the best treatment for each individual patient, and to take all appropriate safety precautions. To
the fullest extent of the law, neither the publisher nor the editors assume any liability for any injury and/or
damage to persons or property arising out of or related to any use of the material contained in this book.

Note that the term ESWL has been trademarked by Dornier MedTech in the United States. The generic
term for extracorporial shock wave lithotripsy is SWL. As the use of ESWL has become part of the
vernacular of urology, some of the authors have elected to use this term in their chapters.

The Publisher

Library of Congress Cataloging-in-Publication Data
Campbell-Walsh urology.—9th ed. / editor-in-chief, Alan J. Wein; editors, Louis R. Kavoussi . . . [et al.].
    p. ; cm.
    Rev. ed. of: Campbell's urology / editor-in-chief, Patrick C. Walsh; editors, Alan B. Retik . . . [et al.]. 8th
ed. ©2002.
    Includes bibliographical references and index.
    ISBN 0-7216-0798-5 (set)
    1. Urology. I. Campbell, Meredith F. (Meredith Fairfax). II. Wein, Alan J. III. Kavoussi,
Louis R. IV. Campbell's urology. V. Title: Urology.
    [DNLM: 1. Urogenital Diseases. 2. Urology—methods. WJ 100 c192 2007]
RC871.C33 2007
616.6—dc22

                                                                            2006041807

Acquisitions Editor: Rebecca Schmidt Gaertner
Developmental Editor: Anne Snyder
Publishing Services Manager: Tina Rebane
Project Manager: Norm Stellander
Design Direction: Ellen Zanolle

Printed in China
Last digit is the print number: 9 8 7 6 5 4 3 2 1

To our families, our teachers, and our residents, all of whom have suffered our behavior in various ways and are responsible for our ability to do what we do.

CONTRIBUTORS

Paul Abrams, MD, FRCS
Professor of Urology,
Bristol Urological Institute,
Southmead Hospital,
Bristol, United Kingdom
Overactive Bladder

Mark C. Adams, MD
Professor, Division of Pediatric Urology,
Vanderbilt Children's Hospital,
Vanderbilt University Medical Center,
Nashville, Tennessee
Urinary Tract Reconstruction in Children

Mohamad E. Allaf, MD
Assistant Professor,
James Buchanan Brady Urological Institute,
Johns Hopkins Medical Institutions,
Baltimore, Maryland
Diagnosis and Staging of Prostate Cancer

J. Kyle Anderson, MD
Assistant Professor,
Department of Urologic Surgery,
Veterans Affairs Medical Center,
University of Minnesota Medical School,
Minneapolis, Minnesota
*Surgical Anatomy of the Retroperitoneum, Adrenals,
Kidneys, and Ureters*

Karl-Erik Andersson, MD, PhD
Professor, Lund University;
Head Physician, Clinical Chemistry and Pharmacology,
Lund University Hospital,
Lund, Sweden
*Pharmacologic Management of Storage and
Emptying Failure*

Kenneth W. Angermeier, MD
Associate Professor,
Prosthetic Surgery and Genitourethral Reconstruction,
Glickman Urological Institute,
Cleveland Clinic Foundation,
Cleveland, Ohio
Surgery of Penile and Urethral Carcinoma

Rodney A. Appell, MD
Professor, Scott Department of Urology,
Baylor College of Medicine;
F. Bantley Scott Chair in Urology,
St. Luke's Episcopal Hospital,
Houston, Texas
Injection Therapy for Urinary Incontinence

Dean G. Assimos, MD
Professor,
Division of Surgical Sciences,
Head, Section of Endourology and Nephrolithasis,
Department of Urology,
Wake Forest University School of Medicine,
Winston-Salem, North Carolina
Pathophysiology of Urinary Tract Obstruction

Anthony Atala, MD
W. Boyce Professor and Chair,
Department of Urology,
Wake Forest University School of Medicine;
Director, Wake Forest Institute for Regenerative Medicine,
Winston-Salem, North Carolina
*Tissue Engineering and Cell Therapy:
Perspectives for Urology*

Darius J. Bägli, MDCM, FRCSC, FAAP, FACS
Associate Professor of Surgery,
Institute of Medical Science,
University of Toronto;
Director of Urology Research,
Research Institute,
The Hospital for Sick Children,
Toronto, Ontario, Canada
Reflux and Megaureter

John M. Barry, MD
Professor of Surgery,
Head, Division of Urology and Renal Transplantation,
The Oregon Health & Science University School
of Medicine;
Staff Surgeon, Doernbecher Children's Hospital,
Portland, Oregon
Renal Transplantation

Georg Bartsch, MD
Professor and Chairman,
Department of Urology,
Medical University of Innsbruck,
Innsbruck, Austria
Surgery of Testicular Tumors

Stuart B. Bauer, MD
Professor of Surgery (Urology),
Harvard Medical School;
Senior Associate in Urology,
Children's Hospital,
Boston, Massachusetts
*Anomalies of the Upper Urinary Tract
Voiding Dysfunction in Children: Non-Neurogenic and
Neurogenic*

Clair J. Beard, MD
Assistant Professor, Harvard Medical School;
Vice-Chair, Division of Radiation Oncology,
Dana-Farber Cancer Institute,
Brigham and Women's Hospital,
Boston, Massachusetts
Radiation Therapy for Prostate Cancer

Arie S. Belldegrun, MD, FACS
Professor of Urology,
Chief, Division of Urologic Oncology,
Roy and Carol Doumani Chair in Urologic Oncology,
David Geffen School of Medicine,
University of California, Los Angeles,
Los Angeles, California
Cryotherapy for Prostate Cancer

Mark F. Bellinger, MD
Professor of Urology,
Children's Hospital of Pittsburgh,
University of Pittsburgh Medical Center,
Pittsburgh, Pennsylvania
*Abnormalities of the Testes and Scrotum and
Their Surgical Management*

Mitchell C. Benson, MD
George F. Cahill Professor and Chairman,
J. Bently Squier Urological Clinic,
Columbia University Medical Center,
New York, New York
Cutaneous Continent Urinary Diversion

Sam B. Bhayani, MD
Assistant Professor of Surgery,
Department of Urology,
Washington University School of Medicine,
St. Louis, Missouri
Urinary Tract Imaging: Basic Principles

Jay T. Bishoff, MD
Associate Clinical Professor of Surgery,
University of Texas Health Science Center,
San Antonio, Texas;
Director,
Endourology Section,
Wilford Hall Medical Center,
Lackland AFB, Texas
Laparoscopic Surgery of the Kidney

Jerry G. Blaivas, MD
Clinical Professor of Urology,
Weill Medical College of Cornell University;
Attending,
New York-Presbyterian Hospital,
Lenox Hill Hospital,
New York, New York
*Urinary Incontinence: Epidemiology, Pathophysiology,
Evaluation, and Management Overview*

Jon D. Blumenfeld, MD
Associate Professor of Medicine,
Weill Medical College of Cornell University;
Director of Hypertension,
Director of The Susan R. Knafel Polycystic Kidney
    Disease Center,
The Rogosin Institute;
Associate Attending Physician,
New York-Presbyterian Hospital,
New York, New York
*Pathophysiology, Evaluation, and Medical Management
of Adrenal Disorders*

Michael L. Blute, MD
Professor of Urology,
Mayo Medical School;
Chairman, Department of Urology,
Mayo Clinic,
Rochester, Minnesota
Surgery of the Adrenal Glands

Joseph G. Borer, MD
Assistant Professor of Surgery,
Department of Urology,
Harvard Medical School;
Assistant in Urology,
Children's Hospital Boston,
Boston, Massachusetts
Hypospadias

George J. Bosl, MD
Chairman, Department of Medicine,
Patrick M. Byrne Chair in Clinical Oncology,
Memorial Sloan-Kettering Cancer Center,
New York, New York
Surgery of Testicular Tumors

Charles B. Brendler, MD
Professor and Chief, Section of Urology,
University of Chicago School of Medicine,
Chicago, Illinois
*Evaluation of the Urologic Patient: History, Physical
Examination, and Urinalysis*

Gregory A. Broderick, MD
Professor of Urology,
Mayo Medical School,
Mayo Clinic,
Jacksonville, Florida
*Evaluation and Nonsurgical Management of Erectile
Dysfunction and Premature Ejaculation*

James D. Brooks, MD
Associate Professor,
Department of Urology,
Stanford University Medical Center,
Stanford, California
Anatomy of the Lower Urinary Tract and Male Genitalia

Ronald M. Bukowski, MD
Professor of Medicine,
Cleveland Clinic Lerner College of Medicine of
    Case Western Reserve University;
Director, Experimental Therapeutics,
Cleveland Clinic Foundation,
Cleveland, Ohio
Renal Tumors

Arthur L. Burnett, MD
Professor of Urology, Cellular and Molecular Biology,
Johns Hopkins University School of Medicine;
Staff Urologist, The Johns Hopkins Hospital,
Baltimore, Maryland
Priapism

Jeffrey A. Cadeddu, MD
Associate Professor,
Clinical Center for Minimally Invasive Urologic
    Cancer Treatment;
Department of Urology,
University of Texas Southwestern Medical Center,
Dallas, Texas
*Surgical Anatomy of the Retroperitoneum, Adrenals,
Kidneys, and Ureters*

Anthony A. Caldamone, MD, MMS, FAAP, FACS
Professor of Surgery and Pediatrics,
Department of Urology,
Brown University School of Medicine;
Head of Pediatric Urology,
Hasbro Children's Hospital,
Providence, Rhode Island
Prune Belly Syndrome

Steven C. Campbell, MD, PhD
Professor of Surgery,
Cleveland Clinic Lerner College of Medicine of
    Case Western Reserve University;
Section of Urological Oncology,
Glickman Urological Institute,
Cleveland Clinic Foundation,
Cleveland, Ohio
Renal Tumors
Non–Muscle-Invasive Bladder Cancer (Ta, T1, and CIS)

Douglas A. Canning, MD
Professor of Urology,
University of Pennsylvania School of Medicine;
Director, Division of Urology,
Children's Hospital of Philadelphia,
Philadelphia, Pennsylvania
Evaluation of the Pediatric Urology Patient

Michael Carducci, MD
Associate Professor of Oncology and Urology,
Johns Hopkins University School of Medicine;
Staff Physician, The Sidney Kimmel Comprehensive Cancer
    Center at Johns Hopkins,
Baltimore, Maryland
Treatment of Hormone-Refractory Prostate Cancer

Michael C. Carr, MD, PhD
Associate Professor of Surgery in Urology,
University of Pennsylvania School of Medicine;
Attending Surgeon, Pediatric Urology,
Children's Hospital of Philadelphia,
Philadelphia, Pennsylvania
*Anomalies and Surgery of the Ureteropelvic Junction in
Children*

Peter R. Carroll, MD
Professor and Chair,
Department of Urology,
University of California, San Francisco, School of Medicine;
Surgeon in Chief, Comprehensive Cancer Center,
University of California, San Francisco, Cancer Center,
San Francisco, California
Treatment of Locally Advanced Prostate Cancer

H. Ballentine Carter, MD
Professor of Urology and Oncology,
James Buchanan Brady Urological Institute,
Johns Hopkins Medical Institutions,
Baltimore, Maryland
Basic Instrumentation and Cystoscopy
Diagnosis and Staging of Prostate Cancer

Anthony J. Casale, MD
Professor and Chairman,
Department of Urology,
University of Louisville;
Chief of Urology,
Kosair Children's Hospital,
Louisville, Kentucky
Posterior Urethral Valves and Other Urethral Anomalies

William J. Catalona, MD
Professor of Urology,
Feinberg School of Medicine,
Northwestern University;
Director, Clinical Prostate Cancer Program,
Robert H. Lurie Comprehensive Cancer Center,
Northwestern Memorial Hospital,
Chicago, Illinois
*Definitive Therapy for Localized Prostate Cancer—
An Overview*

David Y. Chan, MD
Assistant Professor of Urology and Pathology,
Director of Outpatient Urology,
James Buchanan Brady Urological Institute,
Johns Hopkins Medical Institutions,
Baltimore, Maryland
Basic Instrumentation and Cystoscopy

Michael B. Chancellor, MD
Professor of Urology,
McGowan Institute of Regenerative Medicine,
University of Pittsburgh School of Medicine,
Pittsburgh, Pennsylvania
Physiology and Pharmacology of the Bladder and Urethra

C. R. Chapple, BSc, MD, FRCS (Urol)
Professor of Urology (Hon),
Sheffield Hallam University;
Consultant Urological Surgeon,
Royal Hallamshire Hospital,
Sheffield, United Kingdom
*Retropubic Suspension Surgery for Incontinence
in Women*

Robert L. Chevalier, MD
Benjamin Armistead Shepherd Professor and Chair,
Department of Pediatrics,
University of Virginia;
Pediatrician-In-Chief,
University of Virginia Medical School,
Charlottesville, Virginia
*Renal Function in the Fetus, Neonate, and Child
Congenital Urinary Obstruction: Pathophysiology*

Ben H. Chew, MD, MSc, FRCSC
Assistant Professor of Urology,
University of British Columbia,
Vancouver, British Columbia, Canada
Ureteroscopy and Retrograde Ureteral Access

George K. Chow, MD
Assistant Professor,
Department of Urology,
The Mayo Clinic,
Rochester, Minnesota
Surgery of the Adrenal Glands

Ralph V. Clayman, MD
Professor of Urology,
University of California, Irvine, Medical Center;
Chair of the Department of Urology,
University of California, Irvine, School of Medicine,
Orange, California
Basics of Laparoscopic Urologic Surgery

Craig V. Comiter, MD
Associate Professor of Surgery/Urology,
Instructor of Obstetrics and Gynecology,
University of Arizona;
Chief, Section of Urology,
Director, Urology Residency,
University of Arizona Health Sciences Center,
Tucson, Arizona
*Surgical Treatment of Male Sphincteric Urinary
Incontinence: The Male Perineal Sling and Artificial
Urinary Sphincter*

Michael J. Conlin, MD
Associate Professor of Surgery,
Director, Minimally Invasive Urologic Surgery,
Division of Urology and Renal Transplantation,
The Oregon Health & Science University School
of Medicine,
Portland, Oregon
Renal Transplantation

Juanita Crook, MD
Associate Professor of Radiation Oncology,
University of Toronto;
Radiation Oncologist,
University Health Network,
Princess Margaret Hospital,
Toronto, Ontario, Canada
Radiation Therapy for Prostate Cancer

Douglas M. Dahl, MD
Assistant Professor of Surgery,
Department of Urology,
Harvard Medical School;
Assistant in Urology,
Massachusetts General Hospital,
Boston, Massachusetts
Use of Intestinal Segments in Urinary Diversion

Anthony V. D'Amico, MD, PhD
Professor of Radiation Oncology,
Harvard Medical School;
Professor and Chief of Genitourinary Radiation Oncology,
Dana-Farber Cancer Institute,
Brigham and Women's Hospital,
Boston, Massachusetts
Radiation Therapy for Prostate Cancer

John W. Davis, MD
Assistant Professor of Urology,
University of Texas MD Anderson Cancer Center,
Houston, Texas
Tumors of the Penis

John D. Denstedt, MD, FRCSC
Professor of Urology,
Chairman, Department of Surgery,
Schulich School of Medicine and Dentistry,
The University of Western Ontario,
London, Ontario, Canada
Ureteroscopy and Retrograde Ureteral Access

Theodore L. DeWeese, MD, PhD
Professor of Oncology,
Johns Hopkins University School of Medicine;
Radiation Oncologist-in-Chief,
Department of Radiation Oncology and Molecular
    Radiation Science,
Johns Hopkins Medical Institutions,
Baltimore, Maryland
Radiation Therapy for Prostate Cancer

David A. Diamond, MD
Associate Professor of Surgery,
Department of Urology,
Harvard Medical School;
Associate in Urology,
Children's Hospital,
Boston, Massachusetts
Sexual Differentiation: Normal and Abnormal

Roger R. Dmochowski, MD, FACS
Professor,
Department of Urologic Surgery,
Vanderbilt University Medical Center,
Nashville, Tennessee
Tension-Free Vaginal Tape Procedures

Steven G. Docimo, MD
Professor of Urology,
Vice Chairman of Urology,
University of Pittsburgh School of Medicine;
Director of Urology,
Division of Pediatric Urology,
Children's Hospital of Pittsburgh,
Pittsburgh, Pennsylvania
Pediatric Endourology and Laparoscopy

Marcus Drake, DM, MA
Consultant Urological Surgeon,
Bristol Urological Institute,
Southmead Hospital,
Bristol, United Kingdom
Overactive Bladder

James A. Eastham, MD
Associate Professor,
Department of Urology,
Memorial Sloan-Kettering Cancer Center,
New York, New York
Expectant Management of Prostate Cancer

Louis Eichel, MD
Clinical Associate Professor of Urology,
University of Rochester School of
    Medicine and Dentistry;
Director of Minimally Invasive Surgery,
Center for Urology,
Rochester, New York
Basics of Laparoscopic Urologic Surgery

Mario A. Eisenberger, MD
R. Dale Hughes Professor of Oncology and Urology,
The Sidney Kimmel Comprehensive Cancer Center at
    Johns Hopkins,
Johns Hopkins University School of Medicine,
Baltimore, Maryland
Treatment of Hormone-Refractory Prostate Cancer

Alaa El-Ghoneimi, MD, PhD
Professor of Pediatric Surgery,
University of Paris;
Senior Surgeon,
Hospital Robert Debré,
Paris, France
*Anomalies and Surgery of the Ureteropelvic Junction
in Children*

Jack S. Elder, MD
Professor and Vice Chairman,
Department of Urology,
Case Western Reserve University School of Medicine;
Division of Pediatric Urology,
Children's Hospital,
Cleveland, Ohio
*Abnormalities of the Genitalia in Boys and
Their Surgical Management*

Jonathan I. Epstein, MD
Professor of Pathology, Urology, and Oncology,
The Reinhard Professor of Urologic Pathology,
Johns Hopkins University School of Medicine;
Director of Surgical Pathology,
Johns Hopkins Medical Institutions,
Baltimore, Maryland
Pathology of Prostatic Neoplasia

Andrew P. Evan, PhD
Chancellor's Professor,
Department of Anatomy and Cell Biology,
Indiana University School of Medicine,
Indianapolis, Indiana
Surgical Management of Upper Urinary Tract Calculi

Robert L. Fairchild, PhD
Professor of Pathology,
Case Western Reserve University School of Medicine;
Staff, Department of Immunology,
Cleveland Clinic Foundation,
Cleveland, Ohio
Basic Principles of Immunology

Amr Fergany, MD, MB, BCh
Staff, Section of Urologic Oncology,
Section of Laparoscopic Surgery and Robotics,
Glickman Urological Institute,
Cleveland Clinic Foundation,
Cleveland, Ohio
Renovascular Hypertension and Ischemic Nephropathy

James H. Finke, PhD
Professor of Molecular Medicine,
Cleveland Clinic Lerner College of Medicine of
    Case Western Reserve University;
Staff, Department of Immunology,
Cleveland Clinic Foundation,
Cleveland, Ohio
Basic Principles of Immunology

John M. Fitzpatrick, MCh, FRCSI, FRCS(Glas), FRCS
Professor and Chairman,
Department of Surgery,
University College, Dublin;
Professor of Surgery and Consultant Urologist,
Mater Misericordiae University Hospital,
Dublin, Ireland
*Minimally Invasive and Endoscopic Management
of Benign Prostatic Hyperplasia*

Robert C. Flanigan, MD
Albert J. Jr. and Claire R. Speh Professor and Chair,
Department of Urology,
Stritch School of Medicine,
Loyola University;
Chair of the Department of Urology,
Loyola University Medical Center,
Maywood, Illinois
Urothelial Tumors of the Upper Urinary Tract

Stuart M. Flechner, MD
Professor of Urology,
Cleveland Clinic Lerner College of Medicine of
    Case Western Reserve University;
Director of Clinical Research,
Section of Renal Transplantation,
Glickman Urological Institute,
Cleveland Clinic Foundation,
Cleveland, Ohio
Basic Principles of Immunology

Tara Frenkl, MD, MPH
Assistant Professor of Urology,
Director, Female Urology and Reconstructive Surgery,
Robert Wood Johnson Medical School,
The University of Medicine and Dentistry of New Jersey,
New Brunswick, New Jersey
Sexually Transmitted Diseases

Dominic Frimberger, MD
Assistant Professor of Urology,
University of Oklahoma Health Sciences Center;
Pediatric Urologist,
Children's Hospital of Oklahoma,
Oklahoma City, Oklahoma
Bladder Anomalies in Children

John P. Gearhart, MD
Professor of Pediatric Urology,
Johns Hopkins University School of Medicine;
Chief of Pediatric Urology,
The Johns Hopkins Hospital,
Baltimore, Maryland
Exstrophy-Epispadias Complex

Glenn S. Gerber, MD
Associate Professor,
Department of Surgery (Urology),
University of Chicago School of Medicine,
Chicago, Illinois
*Evaluation of the Urologic Patient: History, Physical
Examination, and Urinalysis*

Inderbir S. Gill, MD, MCh
Professor of Surgery,
Head, Section of Laparoscopic and Robotic Urology,
Glickman Urological Institute,
Cleveland Clinic Foundation,
Cleveland, Ohio
Laparoscopic Surgery of the Urinary Bladder

Kenneth I. Glassberg, MD
Professor of Urology,
Columbia University College of Physicians and Surgeons;
Director, Division of Pediatric Urology,
Morgan Stanley Children's Hospital of
    New York-Presbyterian,
New York, New York
Renal Dysgenesis and Cystic Disease of the Kidney

David A. Goldfarb, MD
Head, Section of Renal Transplantation,
Glickman Urological Institute,
Cleveland Clinic Foundation,
Cleveland, Ohio
Etiology, Pathogenesis, and Management of Renal Failure

Irwin Goldstein, MD
Editor-In-Chief,
The Journal of Sexual Medicine,
Milton, Massachusetts
*Urologic Management of Women With
Sexual Health Concerns*

Marc Goldstein, MD, FACS
Professor of Urology and Reproductive Medicine,
Surgeon-In-Chief, Male Reproductive Medicine and Surgery,
Executive Director, Men's Service Center,
Cornell Institute for Reproductive Medicine,
Weill Medical College of Cornell University;
Senior Scientist, Center for Biomedical Research,
The Population Council,
New York, New York
*Male Reproductive Physiology
Surgery of the Scrotum and Seminal Vesicles*

Leonard G. Gomella, MD
Professor and Chairman,
Department of Urology,
Jefferson Medical College;
Director,
Jefferson Prostate Diagnostic Center,
Kimmel Cancer Center,
Thomas Jefferson University Hospital,
Philadelphia, Pennsylvania
Ultrasonography and Biopsy of the Prostate

Mark L. Gonzalgo, MD, PhD
Associate Professor of Urology and Oncology,
Johns Hopkins Medical Center,
Baltimore, Maryland
Management of Invasive and Metastatic Bladder Cancer

Richard W. Grady, MD
Associate Professor of Urology,
The University of Washington School of Medicine;
Director, Clinical Research,
Children's Hospital & Regional Medical Center,
Seattle, Washington
*Surgical Techniques for One-Stage Reconstruction of
the Exstrophy-Epispadias Complex*

Matthew B. Gretzer, MD
Assistant Professor of Clinical Surgery,
Department of Surgery/Urology,
University of Arizona Health Science Center,
Tucson, Arizona
  Prostate Cancer Tumor Markers

Mantu Gupta, MD
Associate Professor,
Columbia University College of Physicians and Surgeons;
Director of Endourology, and Director of
    Kidney Stone Center,
Columbia University Medical Center New York-
    Presbyterian Hospital,
New York, New York
  Percutaneous Management of the Upper Urinary Tract

Ethan J. Halpern, MD
Professor of Radiology and Urology,
Jefferson Prostate Diagnostic Center,
Thomas Jefferson University,
Philadelphia, Pennsylvania
  Ultrasonography and Biopsy of the Prostate

Misop Han, MD, MS
Assistant Professor,
Department of Urology,
James Buchanan Brady Urological Institute,
Johns Hopkins Medical Institutions,
Baltimore, Maryland
  Retropubic and Suprapubic Open Prostatectomy
  Definitive Therapy for Localized Prostate Cancer—
  An Overview

Philip M. Hanno, MD, MPH
Professor of Urology,
University of Pennsylvania School of Medicine;
Medical Director, Department of Clinical Effectiveness
    and Quality Improvement,
University of Pennsylvania Health System,
Philadelphia, Pennsylvania
  Painful Bladder Syndrome/Interstitial Cystitis and
  Related Disorders

Matthew P. Hardy, PhD
Professor, Department of Urology,
Weill Medical College of Cornell University;
Member, Population Council,
The Rockefeller University,
New York, New York
  Male Reproductive Physiology

David M. Hartke, MD
Resident Physician,
Department of Urology,
University Hospitals of Cleveland;
Case Western Reserve University School of Medicine,
Cleveland, Ohio
  Radical Perineal Prostatectomy

Jeremy P. W. Heaton, MD, FRCSC, FACS
Professor of Urology,
Assistant Professor Pharmacology and Toxicology,
Queen's University,
Kingston, Ontario, Canada
  Androgen Deficiency in the Aging Male

Sender Herschorn, BSc, MDCM, FRCSC
Professor and Chairman, Division of Urology,
Martin Barkin Chair in Urological Research,
University of Toronto;
Attending Urologist,
Director, Urodynamics Unit,
Sunnybrook Health Sciences Centre,
Toronto, Ontario, Canada
  Vaginal Reconstructive Surgery for Sphincteric
  Incontinence and Prolapse

Khai-Linh V. Ho, MD
Endourology Fellow,
Mayo Clinic,
Rochester, Minnesota
  Lower Urinary Tract Calculi

Thomas H. S. Hsu, MD
Assistant Professor of Urology,
Director of Laparoscopic and Minimally
    Invasive Surgery,
Department of Urology, Stanford University
    School of Medicine;
Director of Laparoscopic, Robotic, and Minimally
    Invasive Urologic Surgery,
Stanford University Medical Center,
Stanford, California
  Management of Upper Urinary Tract Obstruction

Mark Hurwitz, MD
Assistant Professor,
Harvard Medical School;
Director, Regional Program Development,
Department of Radiation Oncology,
Dana-Farber/Brigham and Women's Cancer Center,
Boston, Massachusetts
  Radiation Therapy for Prostate Cancer

Douglas Husmann, MD
Professor of Urology,
Vice Chairman,
Department of Urology,
Mayo Clinic,
Rochester, Minnesota
  Pediatric Genitourinary Trauma

Jonathan P. Jarow, MD
Professor of Urology,
James Buchanan Brady Urological Institute,
Johns Hopkins Medical Institutions,
Baltimore, Maryland
  Male Infertility

Thomas W. Jarrett, MD
Professor of Urology,
Chairman, Department of Urology,
George Washington University,
Washington, DC
Management of Urothelial Tumors of the Renal Pelvis

Christopher W. Johnson, MD
Clinical Instructor of Urology,
Weill Medical College of Cornell University,
New York, New York;
Assistant Attending,
North Shore-Long Island Jewish Health System,
Manhasset, and St. Francis Hospital, Roslyn, New York
*Tuberculosis and Parasitic and Fungal Infections of
the Genitourinary System*

Warren D. Johnson, Jr., MD
B. H. Kean Professor of Tropical Medicine,
Chief, Division of Internal Medicine and Infectious Diseases,
Weill Medical College of Cornell University;
Attending Physician,
New York-Presbyterian Hospital, Cornell Campus,
New York, New York
*Tuberculosis and Parasitic and Fungal Infections of
the Genitourinary System*

Deborah P. Jones, MD
Associate Professor of Pediatrics,
University of Tennessee Health Science Center;
Attending, Le Bonheur Children's Medical Center,
Children's Foundation Research Center,
Memphis, Tennessee
Renal Disease in Childhood

J. Stephen Jones, MD, FACS
Associate Professor of Surgery (Urology),
Vice Chairman, Glickman Urological Institute,
Cleveland Clinic Lerner College of Medicine of
    Case Western Reserve University,
Cleveland Clinic Foundation,
Cleveland, Ohio
Non–Muscle-Invasive Bladder Cancer (Ta, T1, and CIS)

Gerald H. Jordan, MD, FACS, FAAP
Professor of Urology,
Eastern Virginia Medical School,
Norfolk, Virgina
Peyronie's Disease
Surgery of the Penis and Urethra

Mark L. Jordan, MD
Harris L. Willits Professor and Chief,
Division of Urology,
University of Medicine and Dentistry of New Jersey,
New Jersey Medical School;
Chief of Urology, University Hospital,
Newark, New Jersey
Renal Transplantation

David B. Joseph, MD
Professor of Surgery,
University of Alabama at Birmingham;
Chief of Pediatric Urology,
The Children's Hospital of Alabama,
Birmingham, Alabama
Urinary Tract Reconstruction in Children

John N. Kabalin, MD
Adjunct Assistant Professor of Surgery,
Section of Urologic Surgery,
University of Nebraska College of Medicine,
Omaha, Nebraska;
Regional West Medical Center,
Scottsbluff, Nebraska
*Surgical Anatomy of the Retroperitoneum, Adrenals,
Kidneys, and Ureters*

Martin Kaefer, MD
Associate Professor, Indiana University,
Riley Hospital for Children,
Indianapolis, Indiana
*Surgical Management of Intersexuality, Cloacal
Malformation, and Other Abnormalities of the
Genitalia in Girls*

Irving Kaplan, MD
Assistant Professor of Radiation Oncology,
Harvard Medical School;
Radiation Oncologist,
Beth Israel Deaconess Medical Center,
Boston, Massachusetts
Radiation Therapy for Prostate Cancer

Louis R. Kavoussi, MD
Chairman, The Arthur Smith Institute for Urology,
North Shore-Long Island Jewish Health System,
Manhasset, New York;
Professor of Urology,
New York University School of Medicine,
New York, New York
Laparoscopic Surgery of the Kidney

Mohit Khera, MD, MBA, MPH
Fellow, Division of Male Reproductive Medicine
    and Surgery,
Scott Department of Urology,
Baylor College of Medicine,
Houston, Texas
Surgical Management of Male Infertility

Antoine Khoury, MD, FRCSC, FAAP
Chief of Urology,
Senior Associate Scientist,
The Hospital for Sick Children;
Professor of Surgery,
The University of Toronto,
Toronto, Ontario, Canada
Reflux and Megaureter

Adam S. Kibel, MD
Associate Professor, Division of Urologic Surgery,
Washington University School of Medicine,
St. Louis, Missouri
Molecular Genetics and Cancer Biology

Roger Kirby, MD, FRCS
Professor and Director, The Prostate Centre;
Visiting Professor, St. George's Hospital,
Institute of Urology,
London, United Kingdom
*Evaluation and Nonsurgical Management of Benign
Prostatic Hyperplasia*

Eric A. Klein, MD
Professor of Surgery,
Cleveland Clinic Lerner College of Medicine of
    Case Western Reserve University;
Head, Section of Urologic Oncology,
Glickman Urological Institute,
Cleveland Clinic Foundation,
Cleveland, Ohio
Epidemiology, Etiology, and Prevention of Prostate Cancer

John N. Krieger, MD
Professor of Urology,
University of Washington School of Medicine;
Chief of Surgical Urology,
VA Puget Sound Health Care System,
Seattle, Washington
Urological Implications of AIDS and HIV Infection

Bradley P. Kropp, MD
Professor of Urology,
University of Oklahoma Health Science Center;
Chief, Pediatric Urology,
Children's Hospital of Oklahoma,
Oklahoma City, Oklahoma
Bladder Anomalies in Children

John S. Lam, MD
Clinical Instructor in Urology,
David Geffen School of Medicine,
University of California, Los Angeles;
Attending Urologist,
University of California, Los Angeles, Medical Center,
Los Angeles, California
Cryotherapy for Prostate Cancer

Herbert Lepor, MD
Professor and Martin Spatz Chair,
Department of Urology,
New York University School of Medicine;
Chief of Urology,
New York University Medical Center,
New York, New York
*Evaluation and Nonsurgical Management of Benign
Prostatic Hyperplasia*

Ronald W. Lewis, MD
Witherington Chair in Urology,
Professor of Surgery (Urology) and Physiology,
    and Chief of Urology,
Medical College of Georgia,
Augusta, Georgia
Vascular Surgery for Erectile Dysfunction

James E. Lingeman, MD
Director of Research,
Methodist Hospital Institute for Kidney Stone Disease;
Volunteer Clinical Professor,
Department of Urology,
Indiana University School of Medicine,
Indianapolis, Indiana
Surgical Management of Upper Urinary Tract Calculi

Richard E. Link, MD, PhD
Associate Professor of Urology,
Director, Division of Endourology and Minimally
    Invasive Surgery,
Scott Department of Urology,
Baylor College of Medicine,
Houston, Texas
Cutaneous Diseases of the External Genitalia

Larry I. Lipshultz, MD
Professor of Urology,
Scott Department of Urology,
Lester and Sue Smith Chair in Reproductive Medicine,
Chief, Division of Male Reproductive Medicine
    and Surgery,
Baylor College of Medicine,
Houston, Texas
Surgical Management of Male Infertility

Mark S. Litwin, MD, MPH
Professor of Urology and Health Services,
David Geffen School of Medicine,
University of California, Los Angeles;
University of California, Los Angeles, School of
    Public Health,
Los Angeles, California
Outcomes Research

Yair Lotan, MD
Assistant Professor,
Department of Urology,
University of Texas Southwestern Medical Center;
Attending,
Parkland Health and Hospital Systems,
Zale Lipshy University Medical Center,
Veterans Affairs Medical Center,
Dallas, Texas
*Urinary Lithiasis: Etiology, Epidemiology,
and Pathogenesis*

Tom F. Lue, MD
Professor and Vice Chair,
Emil Tanagho Endowed Chair,
Department of Urology,
University of California School of Medicine, San Francisco,
San Francisco, California
  *Physiology of Penile Erection and Pathophysiology of
  Erectile Dysfunction*
  *Evaluation and Nonsurgical Management of
  Erectile Dysfunction and Premature Ejaculation*

Donald F. Lynch, Jr., MD
Professor and Chairman,
Department of Urology,
Professor of Obstetrics and Gynecology,
Eastern Virginia School of Medicine;
Urologic Oncologist,
Sentara Hospitals;
Consultant Urologist,
Jones Institute for Reproductive Medicine,
Norfolk, Virginia
  Tumors of the Penis

Michael Marberger, MD, FRCS(Ed)
Professor and Chairman,
Department of Urology,
Medical University of Vienna,
Vienna, Austria
  Ablative Therapy of Renal Tumors

Fray F. Marshall, MD
Professor and Chairman,
Department of Urology,
Emory University School of Medicine,
Atlanta, Georgia
  Surgery of Bladder Cancer

Brian R. Matlaga, MD, MPH
Assistant Professor of Urology,
Johns Hopkins University School of Medicine;
Director of Stone Disease,
Johns Hopkins Bayview Medical Center,
Baltimore, Maryland
  Surgical Management of Upper Urinary Tract Calculi

Ranjiv Mathews, MD
Associate Professor of Pediatric Urology,
James Buchanan Brady Urological Institute,
Johns Hopkins Medical Institutions,
Baltimore, Maryland
  Exstrophy-Epispadias Complex

Julian Mauermann, MD
Senior Resident,
Department of Urology,
Medical University of Vienna,
Vienna, Austria
  Ablative Therapy of Renal Tumors

Sarah J. McAleer, MD
Chief Resident, Department of Urology,
Brigham and Women's Hospital,
Boston, Massachusetts
  *Tuberculosis and Parasitic and Fungal Infections of the
  Genitourinary System*

Jack W. McAninch, MD
Professor of Urological Surgery,
Department of Urology,
University of California, San Francisco, School of Medicine;
Chief of Urology, San Francisco General Hospital,
San Francisco, California
  Renal and Ureteral Trauma

John D. McConnell, MD
Professor of Urology, Department of Urology,
Executive Vice-President for Health Systems Affairs,
University of Texas Southwestern Medical Center,
Dallas, Texas
  *Benign Prostatic Hyperplasia: Etiology, Pathophysiology,
  Epidemiology, and Natural History*

W. Scott McDougal, AB, MD, MA(Hon)
Walter S. Kerr, Jr. Professor of Urology,
Harvard Medical School;
Chief of Urology, Massachusetts General Hospital,
Boston, Massachusetts
  Use of Intestinal Segments in Urinary Diversion

Elspeth M. McDougall, MD, FRCSC
Professor of Urology,
Irvine Medical Center,
University of California, Irvine,
Irvine, California
  Basics of Laparoscopic Urologic Surgery
  Percutaneous Management of the Upper Urinary Tract

Edward J. McGuire, MD
Professor, Department of Urology,
University of Michigan,
Ann Arbor, Michigan
  Pubovaginal Sling

James M. McKiernan, MD
Assistant Professor, Department of Urology,
Herbert Irving Comprehensive Cancer Center,
Columbia University;
Assistant Attending Urologist,
New York-Presbyterian Hospital,
New York, New York
  Cutaneous Continent Urinary Diversion

Alan W. McMahon, MD
Associate Professor, Department of Medicine,
Division of Nephrology and Transplant Immunology,
University of Alberta,
Edmonton, Alberta, Canada
  Renal Physiology and Pathophysiology

Maxwell V. Meng, MD
Assistant Professor,
Department of Urology,
University of California, San Francisco,
San Francisco, California
Treatment of Locally Advanced Prostate Cancer

Edward M. Messing, MD
W. W. Scott Professor,
Chairman, Department of Urology,
Professor of Pathology and Oncology,
University of Rochester School of Medicine and Dentistry,
Rochester, New York
Urothelial Tumors of the Bladder

Michael E. Mitchell, MD
Professor and Chief of Pediatric Urology,
University of Washington School of Medicine,
Children's Hospital & Regional Medical Center,
Seattle, Washington
*Surgical Techniques for One-Stage Reconstruction of the
Exstrophy-Epispadias Complex*

Drogo K. Montague, MD
Professor of Surgery,
Cleveland Clinic Lerner College of Medicine of
    Case Western Reserve University;
Head, Section of Prosthetic Surgery and
    Genitourethral Reconstruction,
Glickman Urological Institute,
Cleveland Clinic Foundation,
Cleveland, Ohio
Prosthetic Surgery for Erectile Dysfunction

Alvaro Morales, MD, FRCSC, FACS
Emeritus Professor,
Queen's University;
Director, Center for Advanced Urological Research,
Kingston General Hospital,
Kingston, Ontario, Canada
Androgen Deficiency in the Aging Male

Allen F. Morey, MD
Clinical Associate Professor of Urology,
University of Texas Health Science Center;
Chief, Urology Service,
Brooke Army Medical Center,
San Antonio, Texas
Genital and Lower Urinary Tract Trauma

John Morley, MB, BCh
Dammert Professor of Gerontology,
    and Director of Geriatrics, St. Louis University Medical
    Center;
Director of GRECC, St. Louis Veterans Affairs Hospital,
    St. Louis, Missouri
Androgen Deficiency in the Aging Male

Michael J. Morris, MD
Assistant Member,
Memorial Sloan-Kettering Cancer Center;
Instructor in Medicine,
Weill Medical College of Cornell University;
Assistant Attending Physician,
Memorial Hospital for Cancer and Allied Diseases,
New York, New York
*The Clinical State of the Rising PSA Level after Definitive
Local Therapy: A Practical Approach*

M. Louis Moy, MD
Assistant Professor,
Division of Urology,
University of Pennsylvania Medical School;
University of Pennsylvania Health System,
Philadelphia, Pennsylvania
Additional Therapies for Storage and Emptying Failure

Ricardo Munarriz, MD
Assistant Professor of Urology,
Boston University School of Medicine,
Boston, Massachusetts
Vascular Surgery for Erectile Dysfunction

Stephen Y. Nakada, MD
Professor of Surgery,
University of Wisconsin School of Medicine and
    Public Health;
Chairman of Urology,
University of Wisconsin Hospital and Clinics,
Madison, Wisconsin
Management of Upper Urinary Tract Obstruction

Joseph V. Nally, Jr., MD
Staff, Department of Nephrology and Hypertension,
Cleveland Clinic Foundation,
Cleveland, Ohio
Etiology, Pathogenesis, and Management of Renal Failure

Joel B. Nelson, MD
Frederic N. Schwentker Professor,
Chair, Department of Urology,
University of Pittsburgh School of Medicine;
Chairman of Urology,
University of Pittsburgh Medical Center;
Co-Chair, Prostate and Urological Diseases Program,
University of Pittsburgh Cancer Institute,
Pittsburgh, Pennsylvania
Hormone Therapy for Prostate Cancer

Michael T. Nguyen, MD
Fellow, Pediatric Urology,
The Children's Hospital of Philadelphia,
Philadelphia, Pennsylvania
Evaluation of the Pediatric Urology Patient

J. Curtis Nickel, MD
Professor of Urology, Queen's University;
Staff Urologist, Department of Urology,
Kingston General Hospital,
Kingston, Ontario, Canada
*Inflammatory Conditions of the Male Genitourinary
Tract: Prostatitis and Related Conditions, Orchitis,
and Epididymitis*

Peter T. Nieh, MD
Assistant Professor, Department of Urology,
Emory University School of Medicine,
Atlanta, Georgia
Surgery of Bladder Cancer

Victor W. Nitti, MD
Associate Professor and Vice-Chairman,
Department of Urology,
New York University School of Medicine;
Attending Physician,
New York University Hospitals Center,
New York, New York
*Urinary Incontinence: Epidemiology, Pathophysiology,
Evaluation, and Management Overview*

H. Norman Noe, MD
Professor of Urology,
Chief, Pediatric Urology,
University of Tennessee,
Saint Jude's Children's Research Hospital,
Memphis, Tennessee
Renal Disease in Childhood

Andrew C. Novick, MD
Chairman, Glickman Urological Institute,
Cleveland Clinic Foundation;
Professor of Surgery,
Cleveland Clinic Lerner College of Medicine of
    Case Western Reserve University,
Cleveland, Ohio
*Renovascular Hypertension and Ischemic Nephropathy
Renal Tumors
Open Surgery of the Kidney*

Seung-June Oh, MD, PhD
Associate Professor, Department of Urology,
Seoul National University Hospital,
Seoul National University College of Medicine,
Seoul, Korea
Pubovaginal Sling

Carl A. Olsson, MD
John K. Lattimer Professor and Chairman Emeritus,
Columbia University College of Physicians and Surgeons;
Attending, New York-Presbyterian Hospital,
New York, New York
Cutaneous Continent Urinary Diversion

Michael C. Ost, MD
Fellow, Endourology and Laparoscopy,
Institute of Urology,
North Shore-Long Island Jewish Medical Center,
New Hyde Park, New York
Percutaneous Management of the Upper Urinary Tract

Vernon M. Pais Jr., MD
Assistant Professor,
Department of Surgery,
Division of Urology,
University of Kentucky School of Medicine;
University of Kentucky Medical Center,
Lexington, Kentucky
Pathophysiology of Urinary Tract Obstruction

John M. Park, MD
Associate Professor of Urology,
University of Michigan Medical School;
Chief of Pediatric Urology,
University of Michigan Health System,
Ann Arbor, Michigan
Normal Development of the Urogenital System

Alan W. Partin, MD, PhD
David Hall McConnell Professor and Director,
James Buchanan Brady Urological Institute,
Johns Hopkins Medical Institutions,
Baltimore, Maryland
*Retropubic and Suprapubic Open Prostatectomy
Prostate Cancer Tumor Markers
Diagnosis and Staging of Prostate Cancer
Anatomic Radical Retropubic Prostatectomy*

Christopher K. Payne, MD
Associate Professor of Urology,
Director,
Female Urology and Neurourology,
Stanford University Medical School,
Stanford, California
*Conservative Managment of Urinary Incontinence:
Behavioral and Pelvic Floor Therapy, Urethral and
Pelvic Devices*

Margaret S. Pearle, MD, PhD
Professor of Urology and Internal Medicine,
University of Texas Southwestern Medical Center,
Dallas, Texas
Urinary Lithiasis: Etiology, Epidemiology, and Pathogenesis

Craig A. Peters, MD
John E. Cole Professor of Urology,
University of Virginia,
Charlottesville, Virgina
*Congenital Urinary Obstruction: Pathophysiology
Perinatal Urology
Pediatric Endourology and Laparoscopy*

Andrew C. Peterson, MD, FACS
Assistant Professor of Surgery,
Uniformed Services University of the Health Sciences,
Bethesda, Maryland;
Program Director,
Urology Residency,
Madigan Army Medical Center,
Tacoma, Washington
  Urodynamic and Videourodynamic Evaluation of
  Voiding Dysfunction

Curtis A. Pettaway, MD
Associate Professor of Urology, and
  Associate Professor of Cancer Biology,
Department of Urology,
University of Texas MD Anderson Cancer Center,
Houston, Texas
  Tumors of the Penis

Paul K. Pietrow, MD
Director of Minimally Invasive Surgery,
Hudson Valley Urology,
Poughkeepsie, New York
  Evaluation and Medical Management of Urinary Lithiasis

Louis L. Pisters, MD
Associate Professor of Urology,
Department of Urology,
University of Texas MD Anderson Cancer Center,
Houston, Texas
  Cryotherapy for Prostate Cancer

Elizabeth A. Platz, ScD, MPH
Associate Professor,
Department of Epidemiology,
Johns Hopkins Bloomberg School of Public Health,
Johns Hopkins Medical Institutions,
Baltimore, Maryland
  Epidemiology, Etiology, and Prevention of Prostate Cancer

Jeannette Potts, MD
Senior Clinical Instructor,
Department of Family Medicine,
Cleveland Clinic Lerner College of Medicine of
  Case Western Reserve University;
Staff Physician,
Glickman Urological Institute,
Cleveland Clinic Foundation,
Cleveland, Ohio
  Sexually Transmitted Diseases

Glenn M. Preminger, MD
Professor of Urologic Surgery,
Duke University Medical Center,
Durham, North Carolina
  Evaluation and Medical Management of Urinary Lithiasis

Raymond R. Rackley, MD
Professor of Surgery (Urology),
Cleveland Clinic Lerner College of Medicine of
  Case Western Reserve University,
Co-Head, Section of Female Urology and Voiding
  Dysfunction,
The Glickman Urological Institute,
Cleveland Clinic Foundation,
Cleveland, Ohio
  Electrical Stimulation for Storage and Emptying Disorders

John R. Ramey, MD
Jefferson Prostate Diagnostic Center,
Departments of Urology and Radiology,
Kimmel Cancer Center,
Thomas Jefferson University,
Philadelphia, Pennsylvania
  Ultrasonography and Biopsy of the Prostate

Robert E. Reiter, MD
Professor of Urology,
Member, Molecular Biology Institute,
Associate Director,
Prostate Cancer Program,
Geffen School of Medicine,
University of California, Los Angeles,
Los Angeles, California
  Molecular Genetics and Cancer Biology

Neil M. Resnick, MD
Professor of Medicine,
Chief, Division of Gerontology and Geriatric Medicine,
Director, University of Pittsburgh Institute on Aging,
University of Pittsburgh and University of Pittsburgh
  Medical Center,
Pittsburgh, Pennsylvania
  Geriatric Incontinence and Voiding Dysfunction

Martin I. Resnick, MD
Lester Persky Professor and Chair,
Department of Urology,
Cleveland Clinic Lerner College of Medicine of
  Case Western Reserve University,
Cleveland Clinic Foundation,
Cleveland, Ohio
  Radical Perineal Prostatectomy

Alan B. Retik, MD
Professor of Surgery (Urology),
Harvard Medical School;
Chief, Department of Urology,
Children's Hospital,
Boston, Massachusetts
  Ectopic Ureter, Ureterocele, and Other Anomalies of
  the Ureter
  Hypospadias

Jerome P. Richie, MD
Elliot C. Cutler Professor of Urologic Surgery,
Chairman, Harvard Program in Urology,
Harvard Medical School,
Brigham and Women's Hospital,
Boston, Massachusetts
   Neoplasms of the Testis

Richard Rink, MD
Professor, Indiana University,
Riley Hospital for Children,
Indianapolis, Indiana
   *Surgical Management of Intersexuality, Cloacal
   Malformation, and Other Abnormalities of the
   Genitalia in Girls*

Michael L. Ritchey, MD
Professor of Urology,
Mayo Clinic College of Medicine,
Phoenix, Arizona
   Pediatric Urologic Oncology

Ronald Rodriguez, MD, PhD
Associate Professor of Urology, Medical Oncology, Radiation
   Oncology, Cellular and Molecular Medicine,
Johns Hopkins University School of Medicine,
Baltimore, Maryland
   *Molecular Biology, Endocrinology, and Physiology of the
   Prostate and Seminal Vesicles*

Claus G. Roehrborn, MD
Professor and Chairman, Department of Urology,
University of Texas Southwestern Medical Center,
Dallas, Texas
   *Benign Prostatic Hyperplasia: Etiology, Pathophysiology,
   Epidemiology, and Natural History*

Jonathan A. Roth, MD
Assistant Professor of Urology and Pediatrics,
Temple University Children's Hospital,
Temple University,
Philadelphia, Pennsylvania
   Renal Function in the Fetus, Neonate, and Child

Eric S. Rovner, MD
Associate Professor of Urology,
Department of Urology,
Medical University of South Carolina,
Charleston, South Carolina
   Urinary Tract Fistula
   Bladder and Urethral Diverticula

Thomas A. Rozanski, MD
Professor, Department of Urology,
The University of Texas Health Science Center;
Chief, Medical Operations,
University Hospital,
San Antonio, Texas
   Genital and Lower Urinary Tract Trauma

Arthur I. Sagalowsky, MD
Professor of Urology and Surgery,
Chief of Urologic Oncology,
Dr. Paul Peters Chair in Urology in Memory of Rumsey
   and Louis Strickland,
The University of Texas Health Science Center,
Dallas, Texas
   *Management of Urothelial Tumors of the Renal Pelvis
   and Ureter*

Jay I. Sandlow, MD
Associate Professor and Vice-Chair,
Department of Urology,
Medical College of Wisconsin;
Director of Andrology and Male Infertility,
Froedtert Memorial Lutheran Hospital,
Milwaukee, Wisconsin
   Surgery of the Scrotum and Seminal Vesicles

Richard A. Santucci, MD
Associate Professor and Chief of Urology,
Wayne State University School of Medicine,
Detroit, Michigan
   Renal and Ureteral Trauma

Peter T. Scardino, MD
Chair, Department of Surgery,
Head, Prostate Cancer Program,
Memorial Sloan-Kettering Cancer Center,
New York, New York
   Expectant Management of Prostate Cancer

Harriette Scarpero, MD
Assistant Professor,
Department of Urologic Surgery,
Vanderbilt University Medical Center,
Nashville, Tennessee
   Tension-Free Vaginal Tape Procedures

Anthony J. Schaeffer, MD
Herman L. Kretschmer Professor and Chair,
Department of Urology,
Northwestern University Feinberg School of Medicine;
Chief of Urology,
Northwestern Memorial Hospital,
Chicago, Illinois
   Infections of the Urinary Tract

Edward M. Schaeffer, MD, PhD
Department of Urology,
James Buchanan Brady Urological Institute,
Johns Hopkins Medical Institutions,
Baltimore, Maryland
   Infections of the Urinary Tract

Howard I. Scher, MD
Professor of Medicine,
Weill Medical College of Cornell University;
Member, Department of Medicine,
Memorial Sloan-Kettering Cancer Center;
Attending Physician,
Memorial Hospital for Cancer and Allied Diseases,
New York, New York
*The Clinical State of the Rising PSA Level after Definitive
Local Therapy: A Practical Approach*

Peter N. Schlegel, MD
Professor and Chairman,
Department of Urology,
Professor of Reproductive Medicine,
Weill Medical College of Cornell University;
Staff Scientist, The Population Council;
Urologist-in-Chief, New York-Presbyterian Hospital;
Associate Physician, Rockefeller University Hospital,
New York, New York
Male Reproductive Physiology

Steven M. Schlossberg, MD
Professor, Eastern Virginia Medical School,
Norfolk, Virginia
Surgery of the Penis and Urethra

Richard N. Schlussel, MD
Assistant Professor, Department of Urology,
Columbia University;
Assistant Professor, Division of Pediatric Urology,
Morgan Stanley Children's Hospital of New York-
  Presbyterian,
Columbia University Medical Center,
New York, New York
*Ectopic Ureter, Ureterocele, and Other Anomalies of
the Ureter*

Francis X. Schneck, MD
Associate Professor of Urology,
Children's Hospital of Pittsburgh,
University of Pittsburgh Medical Center,
Pittsburgh, Pennsylvania
*Abnormalities of the Testes and Scrotum and
Their Surgical Management*

Mark P. Schoenberg, MD
Professor of Urology and Oncology,
Director of Urologic Oncology,
James Buchanan Brady Urological Institute,
Johns Hopkins Medical Institutions,
Baltimore, Maryland
Management of Invasive and Metastatic Bladder Cancer

Martin J. Schreiber, Jr., MD
Chairman,
Department of Nephrology and Hypertension,
Cleveland Clinic Foundation,
Cleveland, Ohio
Etiology, Pathogenesis, and Management of Renal Failure

Joseph W. Segura, MD
Consultant in Urology,
Carl Rosen Professor of Urology,
Department of Urology,
The Mayo Clinic,
Rochester, Minnesota
Lower Urinary Tract Calculi

Jay B. Shah, MD
Chief Resident,
Columbia College of Physicians and Surgeons;
Department of Urology,
Columbia University Medical Center,
New York, New York
Percutaneous Management of the Upper Urinary Tract

Robert C. Shamberger, MD
Robert E. Gross Professor of Surgery,
Harvard Medical School;
Chief of Surgery, Children's Hospital,
Boston, Massachusetts
Pediatric Urologic Oncology

David S. Sharp, MD
Fellow, Department of Urology,
Memorial Sloan-Kettering Cancer Center,
New York, New York
Surgery of Penile and Urethral Carcinoma

Joel Sheinfeld, MD
Vice-Chairman, Department of Urology,
Memorial Sloan-Kettering Cancer Center,
New York, New York
Surgery of Testicular Tumors

Linda M. Dairiki Shortliffe, MD
Professor and Chair, Department of Urology,
Stanford University School of Medicine;
Chief of Pediatric Urology,
Stanford Hospital and Clinics,
Lucile Salter Packard Children's Hospital,
Stanford, California
*Infection and Inflammation of the Pediatric
Genitourinary Tract*

Daniel A. Shoskes, MD, FRCSC
Professor of Surgery, Cleveland Clinic Lerner College of
  Medicine of Case Western Reserve University;
Urologist, Glickman Urological Institute,
Cleveland Clinic Foundation,
Cleveland, Ohio
Renal Physiology and Pathophysiology

Cary L. Siegel, MD
Associate Professor of Radiology,
Division of Diagnostic Radiology,
Mallinckrodt Institute of Radiology,
Washington University School of Medicine,
St. Louis, Missouri
Urinary Tract Imaging: Basic Principles

Mark Sigman, MD
Associate Professor of Surgery (Urology),
Brown University,
Providence, Rhode Island
Male Infertility

**Jennifer D.Y. Sihoe, MD, BMBS(Nottm),
FRCSEd(Paed), FHKAM(Surg)**
Specialist in Pediatric Surgery,
Division of Pediatric Surgery and Pediatric Urology,
The Chinese University of Hong Kong,
Prince of Wales Hospital,
Hong Kong, China
*Voiding Dysfunction in Children: Non-Neurogenic and
Neurogenic*

Donald G. Skinner, MD
Professor and Chair,
Department of Urology,
Keck School of Medicine of the University of Southern
    California, Norris Cancer Center,
Los Angeles, California
Orthotopic Urinary Diversion

Arthur D. Smith, MD
Professor, Department of Urology,
Albert Einstein School of Medicine,
New York, New York;
Chairman Emeritus, Department of Urology,
North Shore-Long Island Jewish Medical Center,
New Hyde Park, New York
Percutaneous Management of the Upper Urinary Tract

Joseph A. Smith, Jr., MD
Professor,
Department of Urologic Surgery,
Vanderbilt University School of Medicine,
Vanderbilt University Medical Center,
Nashville, Tennessee
*Laparoscopic and Robotic-Assisted Laparoscopic Radical
Prostatectomy and Pelvic Lymphadenectomy*

Jonathan Starkman, MD
Clinical Instructor,
Department of Urologic Surgery,
Vanderbilt University Medical Center,
Nashville, Tennessee
Tension-Free Vaginal Tape Procedures

David R. Staskin, MD
Director, Section of Voiding Dysfunction,
Female Urology and Urodynamics,
New York Hospital-Cornell;
Associate Professor, Urology and Obstetrics and Gynecology,
Weill Medical College of Cornell University,
New York, New York
*Surgical Treatment of Male Sphincteric Urinary
Incontinence: The Male Perineal Sling and Artificial
Urinary Sphincter*

Graeme S. Steele, MD
Assistant Professor of Surgery,
Harvard Medical School;
Urologist, Brigham and Women's Hospital,
Boston, Massachusetts
Neoplasms of the Testis

John P. Stein, MD
Associate Professor in Urology,
Keck School of Medicine of the University of Southern
    California, Norris Cancer Center,
Los Angeles, California
Orthotopic Urinary Diversion

John T. Stoffel, MD
Assistant Professor of Urology,
Tufts University School of Medicine,
Boston, Massachusetts;
Senior Staff Urologist, Department of Urology,
Lahey Clinic Medical Center,
Burlington, Massachusetts
Pubovaginal Sling

Jack W. Strandhoy, PhD
Professor, Department of Physiology and Pharmacology,
Wake Forest University School of Medicine,
Winston-Salem, North Carolina
Pathophysiology of Urinary Tract Obstruction

Stevan B. Streem, MD (*deceased*)
Head, Section of Stone Disease and Endourology,
Glickman Urological Institute,
Cleveland Clinic Foundation,
Cleveland, Ohio
Management of Upper Urinary Tract Obstruction

Li-Ming Su, MD
Associate Professor of Urology,
Director of Laparoscopic and Robotic Urologic Surgery,
James Buchanan Brady Urological Institute,
Johns Hopkins Medical Institutions,
Baltimore, Maryland
*Laparoscopic and Robotic-Assisted Laparoscopic Radical
Prostatectomy and Pelvic Lymphadenectomy*

Anthony J. Thomas, Jr., MD
Head, Section of Male Infertility,
Glickman Urological Institute,
Cleveland Clinic Foundation,
Cleveland, Ohio
Surgical Management of Male Infertility

Ian M. Thompson, MD
Glenda and Gary Woods Distinguished Chair in
    Genitourinary Oncology,
Henry B. and Edna Smith Dielman Memorial Chair in
    Urologic Science,
The University of Texas Health Science Center,
San Antonio, Texas
Epidemiology, Etiology, and Prevention of Prostate Cancer

Sandip P. Vasavada, MD
Associate Professor of Surgery (Urology),
Cleveland Clinic Lerner College of Medicine of
    Case Western Reserve University;
Co-Head, Section of Female Urology and
    Voiding Dysfunction,
Glickman Urological Institute,
Cleveland Clinic Foundation,
Cleveland, Ohio
    Electrical Stimulation for Storage and Emptying Disorders

E. Darracott Vaughan, Jr., MD
James J. Colt Professor and Chairman Emeritus of Urology,
Weill Medical College of Cornell University,
New York-Presbyterian Hospital,
New York, New York
    *Pathophysiology, Evaluation, and Medical Management of
    Adrenal Disorders*

Robert W. Veltri, PhD
Associate Professor,
Department of Urology
Johns Hopkins University School of Medicine,
Baltimore, Maryland
    *Molecular Biology, Endocrinology, and Physiology of the
    Prostate and Seminal Vesicles*

Patrick C. Walsh, MD
University Distinguished Service Professor of Urology,
James Buchanan Brady Urological Institute,
Johns Hopkins Medical Institutions,
Baltimore, Maryland
    Anatomic Radical Retropubic Prostatectomy

George D. Webster, MD
Professor of Urologic Surgery,
Department of Urology,
Duke University Medical Center,
Durham, North Carolina
    *Urodynamic and Videourodynamic Evaluation of
    Voiding Dysfunction*

Alan J. Wein, MD, PhD(Hon)
Professor and Chair,
Division of Urology,
University of Pennsylvania School of Medicine;
Chief of Urology,
University of Pennsylvania Medical Center,
Philadelphia, Pennsylvania
    *Pathophysiology and Classification of Voiding Dysfunction
    Lower Urinary Tract Dysfunction in Neurologic Injury
    and Disease
    Pharmacologic Management of Storage and
    Emptying Failure
    Additional Therapies for Storage and Emptying Failure*

Robert M. Weiss, MD
Donald Guthrie Professor and Chief,
Section of Urology,
Yale University School of Medicine,
New Haven, Connecticut
    Physiology and Pharmacology of the Renal Pelvis and Ureter

Howard N. Winfield, MD, FRCS
Professor, Department of Urology,
Director, Laparoscopy and Minimally Invasive Surgery,
The University of Iowa Hospitals and Clinics,
University of Iowa,
Iowa City, Iowa
    Surgery of the Scrotum and Seminal Vesicles

J. Christian Winters, MD
Clinical Associate Professor,
Louisiana State University Health Sciences Center;
Vice-Chairman and Director of Female Urology and
    Voiding Dysfunction,
Ochsner Clinic Foundation,
New Orleans, Louisiana
    Injection Therapy for Urinary Incontinence

John R. Woodard, MD
Formerly: Clinical Professor of Urology,
Director of Pediatric Urology,
Emory University School of Medicine;
Formerly: Chief of Urology,
Henrietta Egleston Hospital for Children,
Atlanta, Georgia
    Prune Belly Syndrome

Subbarao V. Yalla, MD
Professor of Surgery (Urology),
Harvard Medical School;
Chief, Urology Division,
Boston Veterans Affairs Medical Center,
Boston, Massachusetts
    Geriatric Incontinence and Voiding Dysfunction

**C. K. Yeung, MBBS, MD, FRCSE, FRCSG, FRACS, FACS,
FHKAM(Surg), DCH(Lond)**
Clinical Professor in Pediatric Surgery and
    Pediatric Urology,
Chinese University of Hong Kong,
Prince of Wales Hospital,
Hong Kong, China
    *Voiding Dysfunction in Children: Non-Neurogenic
    and Neurogenic*

Naoki Yoshimura, MD, PhD
Associate Professor of Urology and Pharmacology,
University of Pittsburgh School of Medicine,
Pittsburgh, Pennsylvania
    Physiology and Pharmacology of the Bladder and Urethra

For each discipline in medicine and surgery, there is generally an acknowledged authoritative text, otherwise known as "the bible." For virtually every urologist in current practice, *Campbell's Urology* has had that distinction. The text, first published in 1954 with Meredith Campbell as its sole editor, has seen the editor-in-chief position pass to J. Hartwell Harrison, and then to Patrick Walsh. Under Dr. Walsh's leadership as editor-in-chief for the past 20 years (4 editions), *Campbell's Urology* has changed as much as the field itself—in virtually every way possible except for its preeminence. The current editorial board felt strongly that Pat's contributions to urologic education through his continuing improvements and innovations to *Campbell's* should be recognized in perpetuity by renaming the text in his honor; thus the new title—*Campbell-Walsh Urology.*

Aside from the name, the 9th edition is quite different from its predecessors, continuing the tradition of a constant evolution paralleling the changing nature of the field and its relevant pertinent information. We have changed the editorial board and increased it by one. Louis Kavoussi, Andrew Novick, Alan Partin, and Craig Peters all have moved up from their associate editor positions. From the standpoint of organization, Volume 1 now covers anatomy; molecular and cellular biology, including tissue engineering; the essentials of clinical decision-making; the basics of instrumentation, endoscopy, and laparoscopy; infection and inflammation; male reproductive function and dysfunction; and sexual function and dysfunction in both men and women. Volume 2 covers all aspects of the upper urinary tract and adrenal, including physiology, obstruction, trauma, stone disease, and neoplasia. Volume 3 includes all topics related to lower urinary tract function and dysfunction, including calculi; trauma, bladder, and prostate disease; and all aspects of urine transport, storage, and emptying. Volume 4 remains a 900-page textbook of pediatric urology. There are 24 totally new chapters; an additional 19 chapters have new authors; and the remaining 89 chapters have all undergone substantial revision. All chapters contain the latest concepts, data, and controversies. Illustrations, algorithms (extensively used), and tables are now in color, as are clinical photographs. Extensive highlighting is utilized, as well as key point boxes. The complete reference list is now online and bound on a CD; a list of suggested key references appears at the end of each chapter. An **e**-dition includes a fully searchable online version with downloadable images (for powerpoint, papers, etc.) and video clips of the key portions of certain procedures, and it will include weekly content updates (summaries of key journal articles in all areas) for the life of the edition. The *Review*, with questions, answers, and explanations, will continue as a separate publication.

Each of us is grateful for the opportunity to be a part of the continuing tradition of *Campbell-Walsh Urology* and wish to express our immense appreciation to all of our superb authors and to those at Elsevier who facilitated our efforts in bringing the 9th edition to publication: Rebecca Schmidt Gaertner, Senior Acquisitions Editor, and Anne Snyder, Senior Developmental Editor.

ALAN J. WEIN, MD, PhD (Hon)
For the Editors

CONTENTS

VOLUME 3

SECTION XIV
URINE TRANSPORT, STORAGE, AND
EMPTYING 1889

VOLUME 4

SECTION XVII
PEDIATRIC UROLOGY 3119

SECTION I

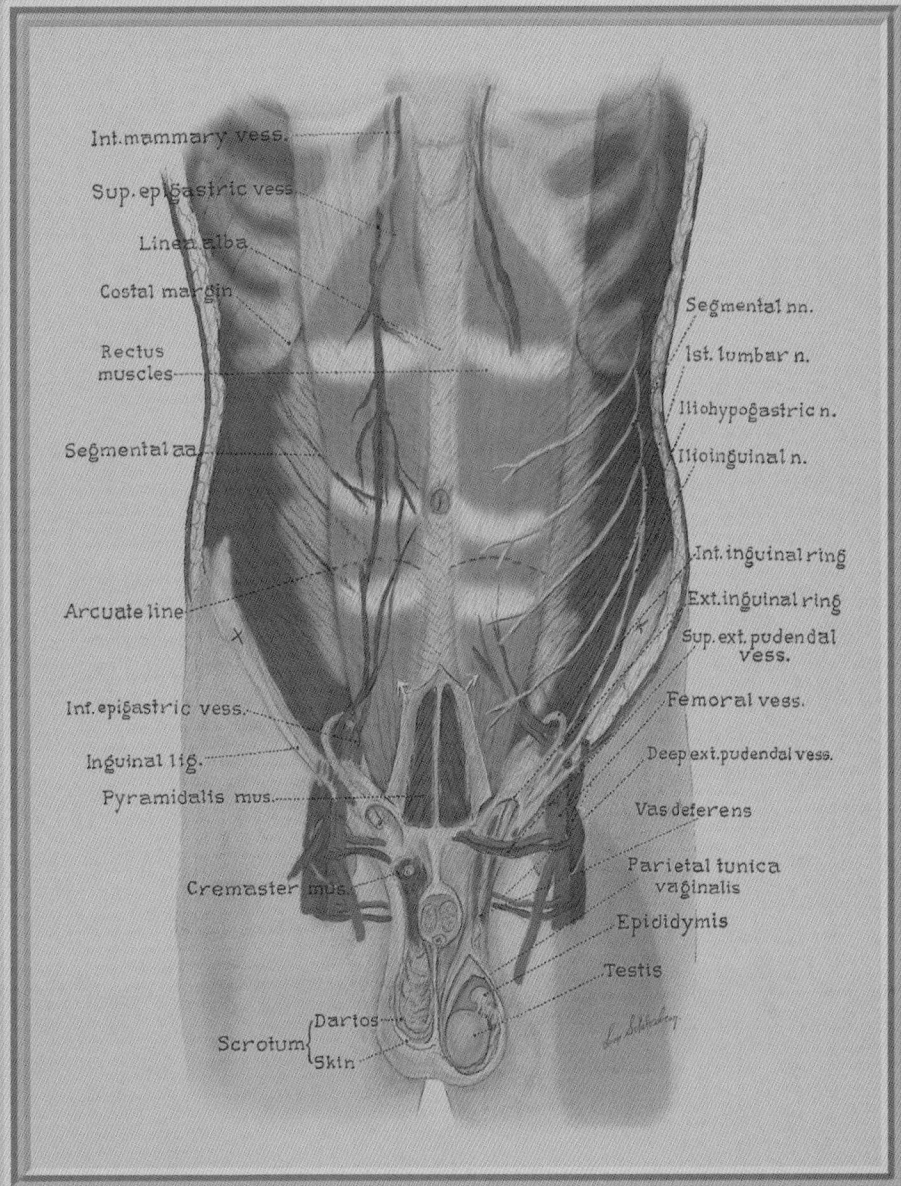

Int.mammary vess.
Sup. epigastric vess.
Linea alba
Costal margin
Rectus muscles
Segmental aa.
Arcuate line
Inf. epigastric vess.
Inguinal lig.
Pyramidalis mus.
Cremaster mus.
Scrotum {Dartos
Skin

Segmental nn.
1st. lumbar n.
Iliohypogastric n.
Ilioinguinal n.
Int. inguinal ring
Ext. inguinal ring
Sup. ext. pudendal vess.
Femoral vess.
Deep ext. pudendal vess.
Vas deferens
Parietal tunica vaginalis
Epididymis
Testis

ANATOMY

1 Surgical Anatomy of the Retroperitoneum, Adrenals, Kidneys, and Ureters

J. KYLE ANDERSON, MD • JOHN N. KABALIN, MD • JEFFREY A. CADEDDU, MD

THE RETROPERITONEUM

THE ADRENAL GLANDS

THE KIDNEYS

THE URETERS

There is no greater aid to surgical expertise than an intimate knowledge of anatomy. For the urologist, the areas of greatest importance are the retroperitoneum and pelvis. In this chapter, retroperitoneal structures important to the practice of urologic surgery are described in detail and clinical correlations are provided where helpful.

THE RETROPERITONEUM (Fig. 1–1)

The retroperitoneum is bounded posteriorly by the abdominal wall, which consists of the lumbodorsal fascia and the enclosed sacrospinalis and quadratus lumborum muscles. Laterally, the retroperitoneum is contiguous with the preperitoneal fat and is bounded laterally by the transversus abdominis musculature of the lateral abdominal wall. The peritoneum is the anterior limit while cranially the diaphragm (Fig. 1–2) limits the retroperitoneum. Caudally the retroperitoneum is contiguous with the extraperitoneal pelvic structures.

Posterior Abdominal Wall

Posterior Musculature and Lumbodorsal Fascia
(Figs. 1–3 to 1–6, Table 1–1)

The lumbodorsal fascia surrounds the sacrospinalis and quadratus lumborum, which together comprise the posterior abdominal wall. The lumbodorsal fascia originates from the

---

KEY POINTS: THE RETROPERITONEUM

- The three layers of the lumbodorsal fascia cover the musculature of the posterior abdominal wall.

- The lower ribs are in intimate contact with the kidneys and adrenal glands. Injury to the lower ribs suggests injury to retroperitoneal structures.

- The renal artery lies posterior to the renal vein, but this relationship is reversed when the aorta and inferior vena cava divide into the common iliac vessels. Here, the common iliac arteries are anterior to the common iliac veins.

- As lymphatic drainage moves within the retroperitoneum from caudal to cranial there is also a predominantly right-to-left flow.

- The nervous system is divided into the autonomic and somatic systems.

- The autonomic system is further divided into sympathetic and parasympathetic innervation. The sympathetics originate from the thoracic and lumbar vertebrae. From the sympathetic chain ganglia preganglionic fibers proceed to autonomic plexuses. From these plexuses postganglionic sympathetic fibers proceed to their targets. The parasympathetics originate from the cranial and sacral vertebrae and again synapse in peripheral plexuses before proceeding to their targets.

- The somatic system provides innervation to the retroperitoneum and lower extremities via the lumbosacral plexus.

---

spinous processes of the lumbar vertebrae and extends anteriorly and cranially. As it progresses upward, it separates into three layers: posterior, middle, and anterior.

The posterior layer provides the posterior covering for the sacrospinalis muscle as well as the origin for the latissimus

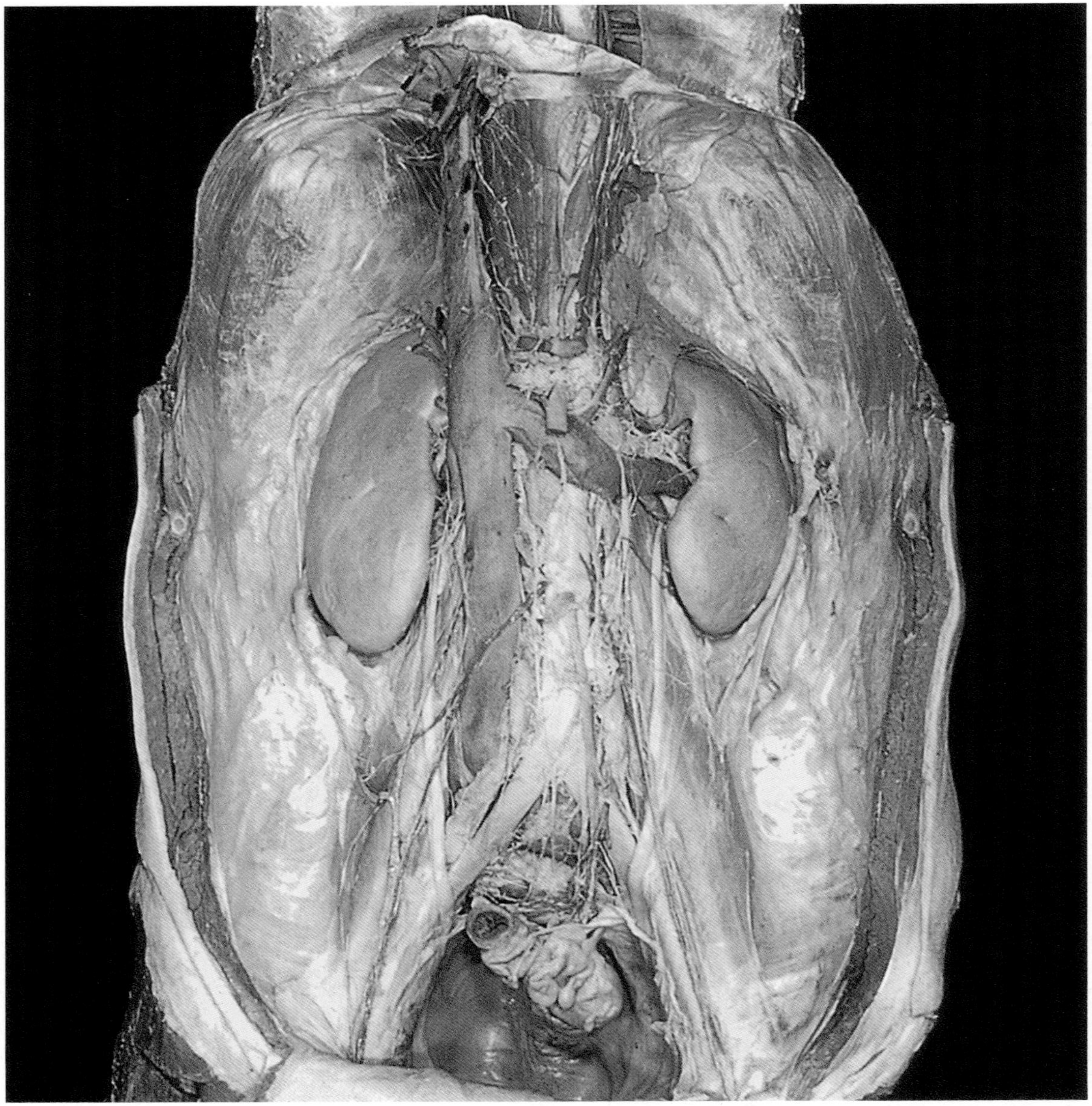

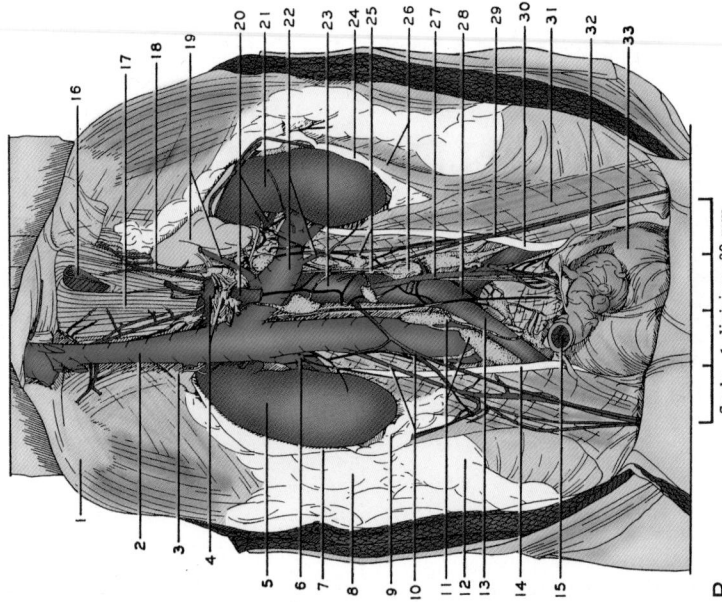

Scale—1 division=30 mm.

B

Figure 1–1. **A**, The retroperitoneum dissected. The anterior perirenal (Gerota's) fascia has been removed. **B**, 1, Diaphragm. 2, Inferior vena cava. 3, Right adrenal gland. 4, *Upper pointer,* celiac artery; *lower pointer,* celiac autonomic nervous plexus. 5, Right kidney. 6, Right renal vein. 7, Gerota's fascia. 8, Pararenal retroperitoneal fat. 9, Perinephric fat. 10, *Upper pointer,* right gonadal vein; *lower pointer,* right gonadal artery. 11, Lumbar lymph nodes. 12, Retroperitoneal fat. 13, Right common iliac artery. 14, Right ureter. 15, Sigmoid colon (cut). 16, Esophagus (cut). 17, Right crus of diaphragm. 18, Left inferior phrenic artery. 19, *Upper pointer,* left adrenal gland; *lower pointer,* left adrenal vein. 20, *Upper pointer,* superior mesenteric artery; *lower pointer,* left renal artery. 21, Left kidney. 22, *Upper pointer,* left renal vein; *lower pointer,* left gonadal vein. 23, Aorta. 24, Perinephric fat. 25, Aortic autonomic nervous plexus. 26, *Upper pointer,* Gerota's fascia; *lower pointer,* inferior mesenteric ganglion. 27, Inferior mesenteric artery. 28, Aortic bifurcation into common iliac arteries. 29, Left gonadal artery and vein. 30, Left ureter. 31, Psoas major muscle covered by psoas sheath. 32, Cut edge of peritoneum. 33, Pelvic cavity.

Continued

A

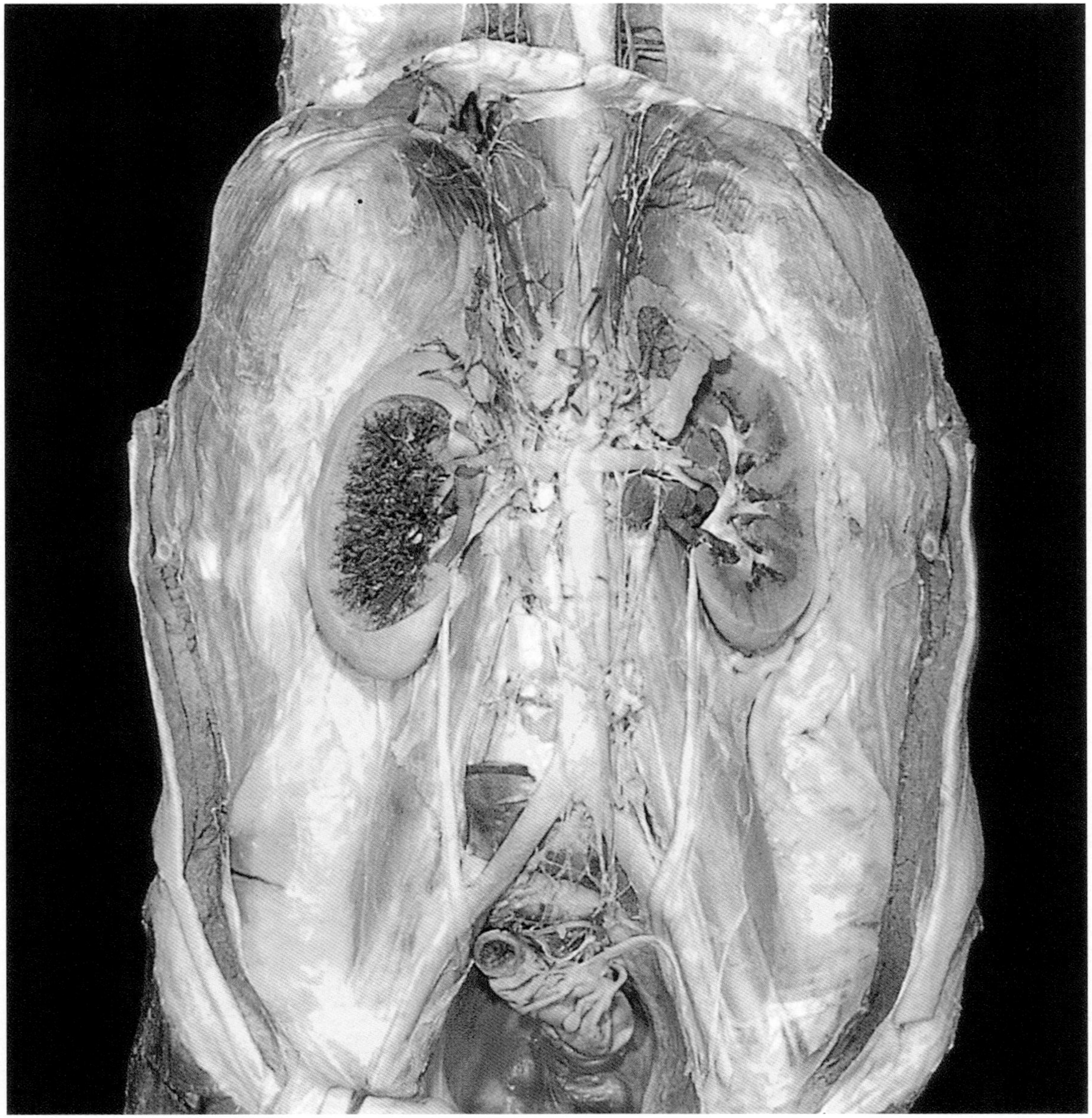

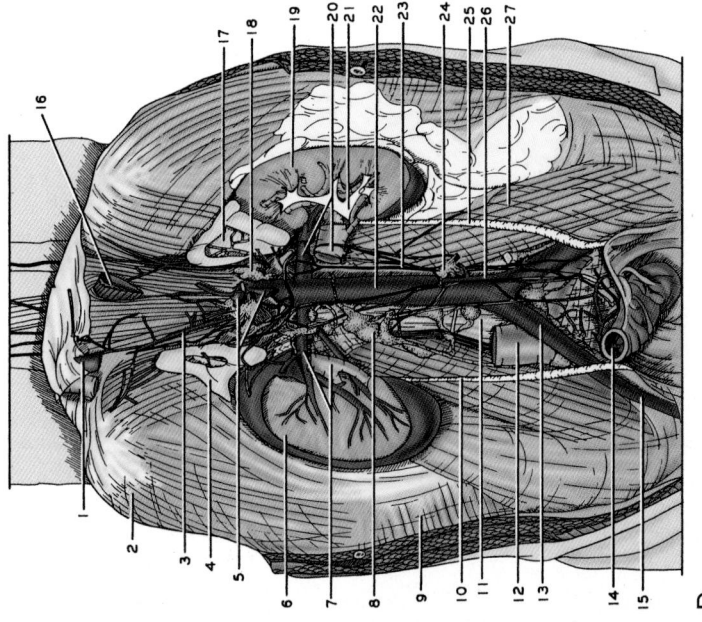

Figure 1–1, cont'd. C, The retroperitoneum dissected. The kidneys and adrenal glands have been sectioned, and the inferior vena cava has been excised over most of its intra-abdominal course. **D,** 1, Inferior vena cava (cut). 2, Diaphragm. 3, Right inferior phrenic artery. 4, Right adrenal gland. 5, *Upper pointer,* celiac artery; *lower pointer,* superior mesenteric artery. 6, Right kidney. 7, *Upper pointer,* right renal artery; *lower pointer,* right renal vein (cut). 8, Lumbar lymph node. 9, Transversus abdominis muscle covered with transversalis fascia. 10, Right ureter. 11, Anterior spinous ligament. 12, Inferior vena cava (cut). 13, Right common iliac artery. 14, Sigmoid colon (cut). 15, Right external iliac artery. 16, Esophagus (cut). 17, Left adrenal gland. 18, Celiac ganglion. 19, Left kidney. 20, *Upper pointer,* left renal artery; *lower pointer,* left renal vein (cut). 21, Left renal pelvis. 22, Aorta. 23, Aortic autonomic nervous plexus. 24, Inferior mesenteric ganglion. 25, Left ureter. 26, Inferior mesenteric artery. 27, Psoas major muscle covered by psoas sheath. **(A** to **D,** Reproduced from the Bassett anatomic collection, with permission granted by Dr. Robert A. Chase.)

C

D

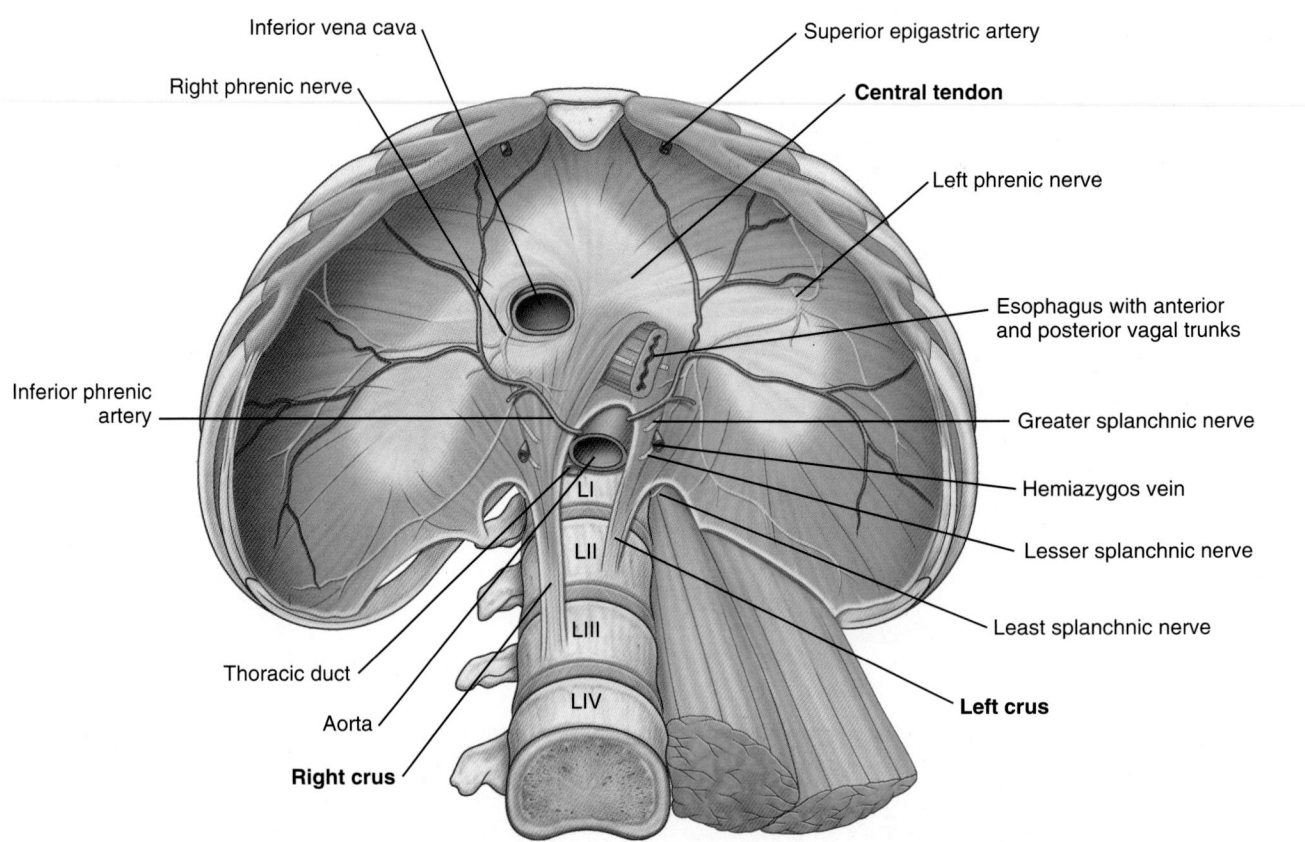

Figure 1–2. The diaphragm: abdominal surface. (From Drake RL, Vogl W, Mitchell AWM: Gray's Anatomy for Students. Philadelphia, Elsevier, 2005, p 317.)

Labels (Figure 1–2):
- Inferior vena cava
- Right phrenic nerve
- Superior epigastric artery
- Central tendon
- Left phrenic nerve
- Esophagus with anterior and posterior vagal trunks
- Inferior phrenic artery
- Greater splanchnic nerve
- Hemiazygos vein
- Lesser splanchnic nerve
- Least splanchnic nerve
- Left crus
- Thoracic duct
- Aorta
- Right crus
- LI
- LII
- LIII
- LIV

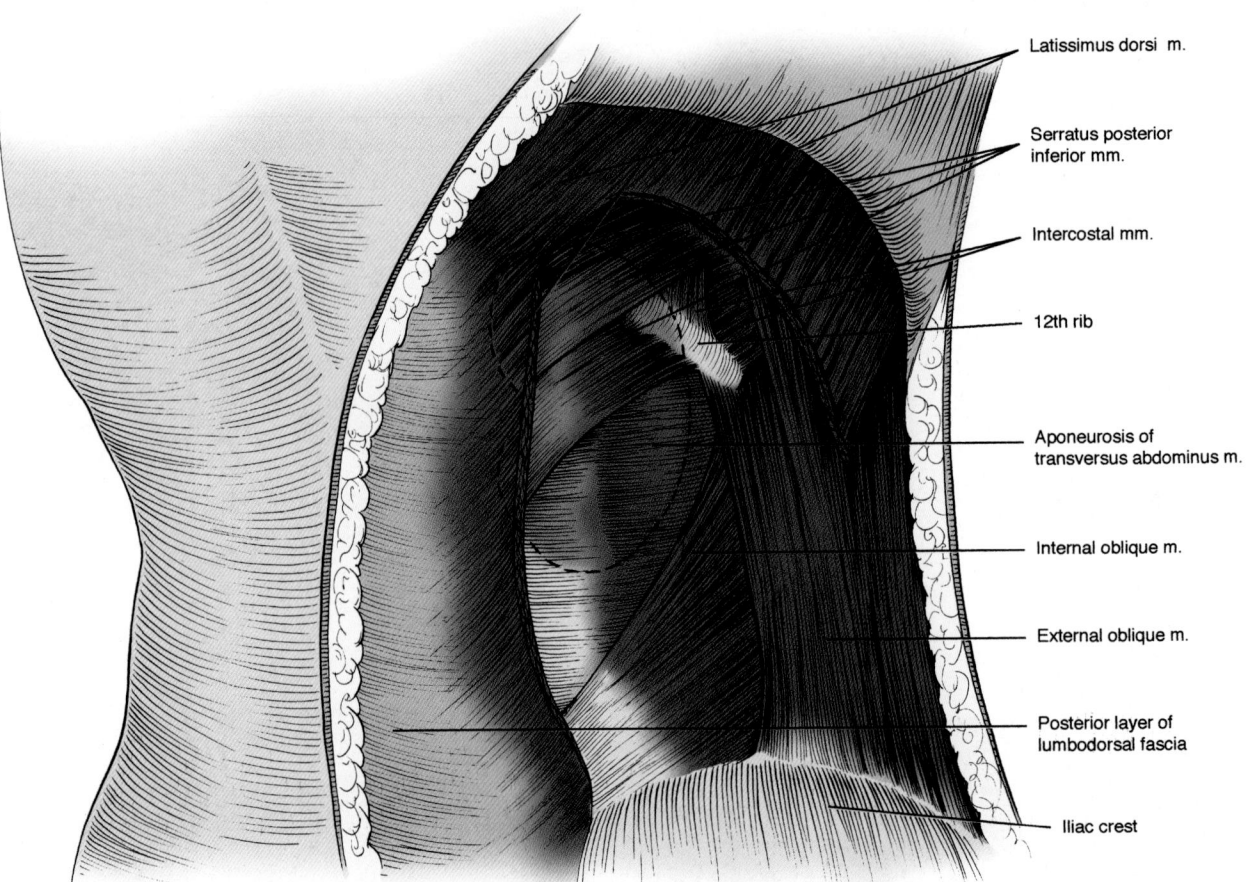

Figure 1–3. Posterior abdominal wall musculature, superficial dissection. A section of the latissimus dorsi muscle has been removed. The location of the right kidney within the retroperitoneum is shown by *dashed outline*.

Labels (Figure 1–3):
- Latissimus dorsi m.
- Serratus posterior inferior mm.
- Intercostal mm.
- 12th rib
- Aponeurosis of transversus abdominus m.
- Internal oblique m.
- External oblique m.
- Posterior layer of lumbodorsal fascia
- Iliac crest

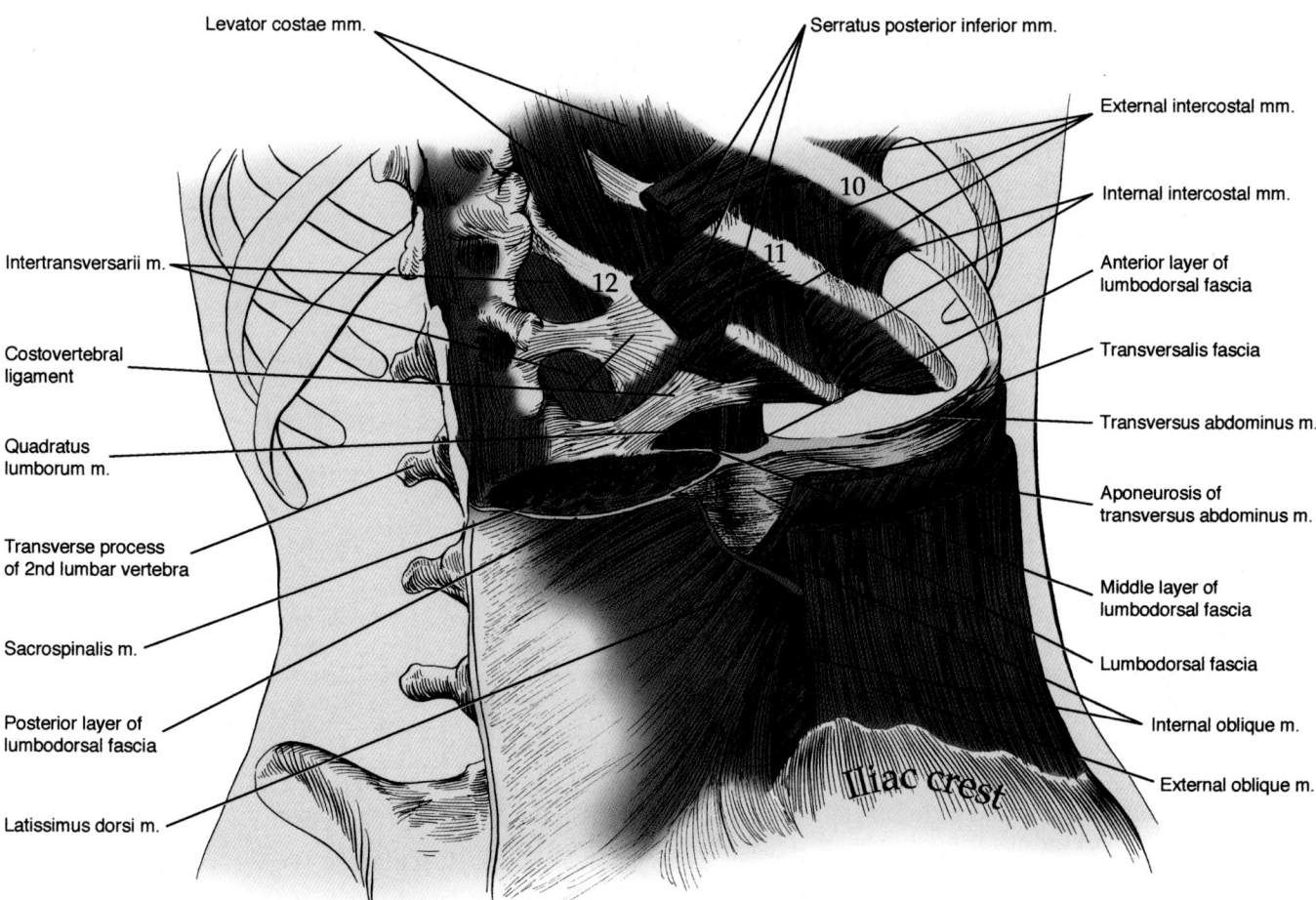

Levator costae mm.

Serratus posterior inferior mm.

External intercostal mm.

Internal intercostal mm.

Anterior layer of
lumbodorsal fascia

Transversalis fascia

Transversus abdominus m.

Aponeurosis of
transversus abdominus m.

Middle layer of
lumbodorsal fascia

Lumbodorsal fascia

Internal oblique m.

External oblique m.

Intertransversarii m.

Costovertebral
ligament

Quadratus
lumborum m.

Transverse process
of 2nd lumbar vertebra

Sacrospinalis m.

Posterior layer of
lumbodorsal fascia

Latissimus dorsi m.

Iliac crest

10

11

12

Figure 1–4. Posterior abdominal wall musculature, intermediate dissection. The sacrospinalis muscle and three anterolateral flank muscle layers are seen in cut section, and the three layers of the lumbodorsal fascia posteriorly can be appreciated.

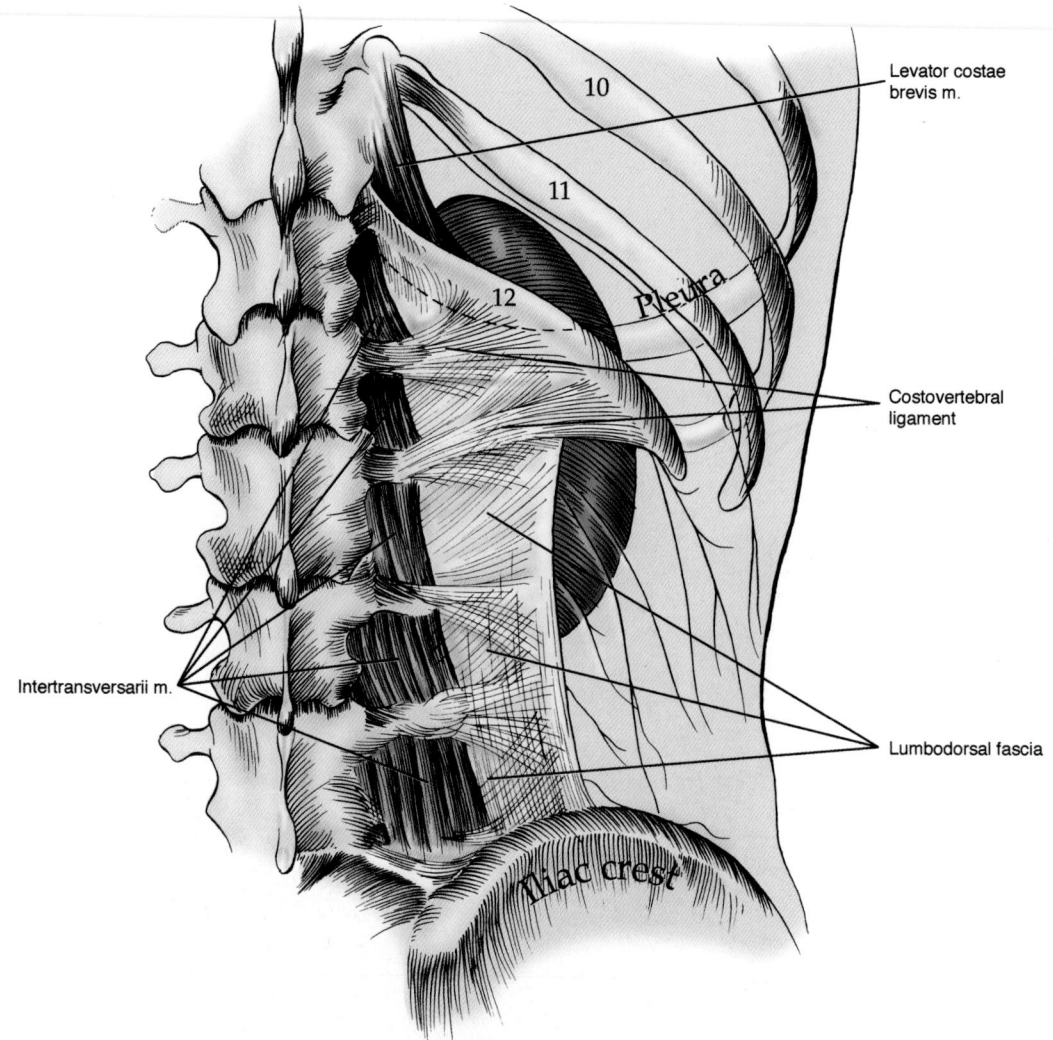

Figure 1–5. Posterior abdominal wall musculature, deep dissection. The lumbodorsal fascia and costovertebral ligament are visualized, arising from the transverse processes of the lumbar vertebrae. The relation of the kidney and pleura is also shown.

dorsi muscle. **The middle layer forms the fascial layer separating the anterior aspect of the sacrospinalis muscle from the posterior aspect of the quadratus lumborum. The anterior layer of the lumbodorsal fascia provides the anterior covering to the quadratus lumborum muscle and forms the posterior margin of the retroperitoneum.** As one moves laterally away from the sacrospinalis and quadratus lumborum muscles, the lumbodorsal fascial layers fuse together and then connect with the transversus abdominis muscle.

The quadratus lumborum and sacrospinalis muscles (Figs. 1–6 and 1–7) **form the muscular portion of the posterior abdominal wall filling the space between the 12th rib, spine, and iliac crest.** The quadratus lumborum serves a number of functions. It supports the 12th rib, thus improving diaphragmatic contraction and inspiration as well as aiding intercostal muscle function during forced expiration. Finally, it controls lateral bending of the trunk. The sacrospinalis also controls movement of the trunk by promoting extension of the spine. These muscular and fascial relationships become important clinically when performing a **dorsal lumbotomy incision.** As seen in Figure 1-7, this is a vertical incision lateral to the border of the sacrospinalis and quadratus lumborum.

This approach allows entrance to the retroperitoneum without the violation of the musculature.

Lateral Flank Musculature (Fig. 1–8; see Table 1–1)

Three muscular layers comprise the lateral flank musculature. From superficial to internal, these are the external oblique, internal oblique, and transversus abdominis muscles. The most superficial structure is the external oblique muscle. This muscle arises from the lower ribs and moves from lateral to medial as it progresses caudally. Final attachment is to the iliac crest caudally and the rectus sheath anteriorly. The posterior border remains free as it terminates before reaching the lumbodorsal fascia. Next is the internal oblique muscle. Again, this muscle arises from the lower rib cage, but the orientation of the fibers is from medial to lateral as they move caudally. Final attachment is to the iliac crest and lumbodorsal fascia. The final structures are the transversus abdominis muscle and transversalis fascia. This muscle arises from the lumbodorsal fascia with fibers running directly transversely until it attaches anteriorly and medially onto the rectus sheath. Immediately deep to the transversus abdominis muscle is the transversalis fascia and then the retroperitoneal

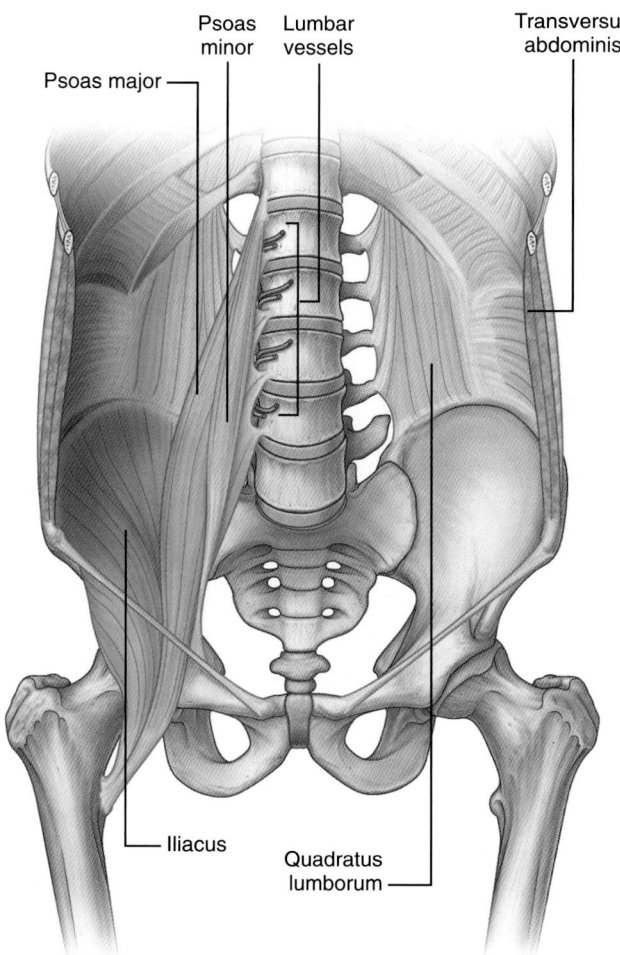

Psoas major — Psoas minor — Lumbar vessels — Transversus abdominis — Iliacus — Quadratus lumborum

Figure 1–6. Muscles of the posterior abdominal wall. (From Drake RL, Vogl W, Mitchell AWM: Gray's Anatomy for Students. Philadelphia, Elsevier, 2005, p 316.)

space. The function of the lateral flank musculature is to compress and stabilize the abdomen and trunk. This provides controlled movement as well as protection for the abdominal organs.

Psoas and Iliacus Muscles (see Fig. 1–6)

The psoas major muscle originates on the 12th thoracic through the 5th lumbar vertebrae. A smaller psoas minor is identifiable in about one half of the population and resides medial to the psoas major. The psoas muscle(s) is covered by the psoas fascia. In close proximity to the psoas muscle is the iliacus muscle, which attaches to the inner aspect of the iliac pelvic wing. As the iliacus progresses caudally it joins with the psoas muscle to form the iliopsoas muscle. This combined muscle then joins to the lesser trochanter of the femur and controls flexion of the hip.

Lower Rib Cage (Fig. 1–9)

In addition to the protection provided by the muscular layers of the posterior and lateral abdominal wall, **the 10th, 11th, and 12th ribs safeguard the upper retroperitoneal space and are intimately related to the adrenal glands and kidneys. Given the close proximity, injury to these ribs can be associated with significant retroperitoneal injury.** While providing protection, the lower ribs and the accompanying pleura and lung limit surgical exposure to the upper retroperitoneum. The limits of the pleura are the 8th rib anteriorly, the 10th rib in the midaxillary line, and the 12th rib posteriorly. Given this location of the pleura, flank incisions at or above the 11th or 12th ribs risk pleural violation.

Great Vessels

The abdominal aorta and inferior vena cava are the great vessels of the abdomen, providing vascular supply to the abdominal organs and lower extremities (Figs. 1–10 and 1–11).

Abdominal Aorta

The aorta enters the abdomen via the aortic hiatus found between the diaphragmatic crura in the posterior diaphragm at the level of the 12th thoracic vertebrae (see Fig. 1–2). It continues caudally to the 4th lumbar vertebrae where it bifurcates into the common iliac arteries. During its course through the abdomen the aorta gives off a number of large branches (Table 1–2). **The paired inferior phrenic arteries are first.** They supply the inferior diaphragm and the superior portion of the adrenal gland (see Fig. 1–2). **Next is the celiac trunk, which is the origin for the common hepatic, left gastric, and splenic arteries that supply the liver, stomach, and spleen, respectively. The paired adrenal arteries follow with an artery going to each adrenal gland.**

Table 1–1. Musculature of the Posterior and Lateral Abdominal Wall

Muscle	Origin	Insertion	Function
Sacrospinalis	Sacrum and lumbar vertebrae	Lower ribs and thoracic vertebrae	Extension of the spine
Quadratus lumborum	5th lumbar vertebra	1st through 4th lumbar vertebrae, 12th rib	Depress and stabilize 12th rib, lateral bending of the trunk
External oblique	Lower eight ribs	Lateral lip of iliac crest, aponeurosis ending in midline raphe	Compress abdominal contents, flexion of the trunk
Internal oblique	Lumbodorsal fascia, iliac crest	Lower four ribs, aponeurosis ending in linea alba	Compress abdominal contents, flexion of the trunk
Transversus abdominis	Lumbodorsal fascia, medial lip of iliac crest	Aponeurosis ending in linea alba	Compress abdominal contents
Psoas	12th thoracic through 5th lumbar vertebrae	Lesser trochanter of femur	Flexion of the hip
Iliacus	Inner aspect of iliac pelvic wing	Lesser trochanter of femur	Flexion of the hip

Adapted from Drake RL, Vogl W, Mitchell AWM: Gray's Anatomy for Students. Philadelphia, Elsevier, 2005, pp 250 and 316.

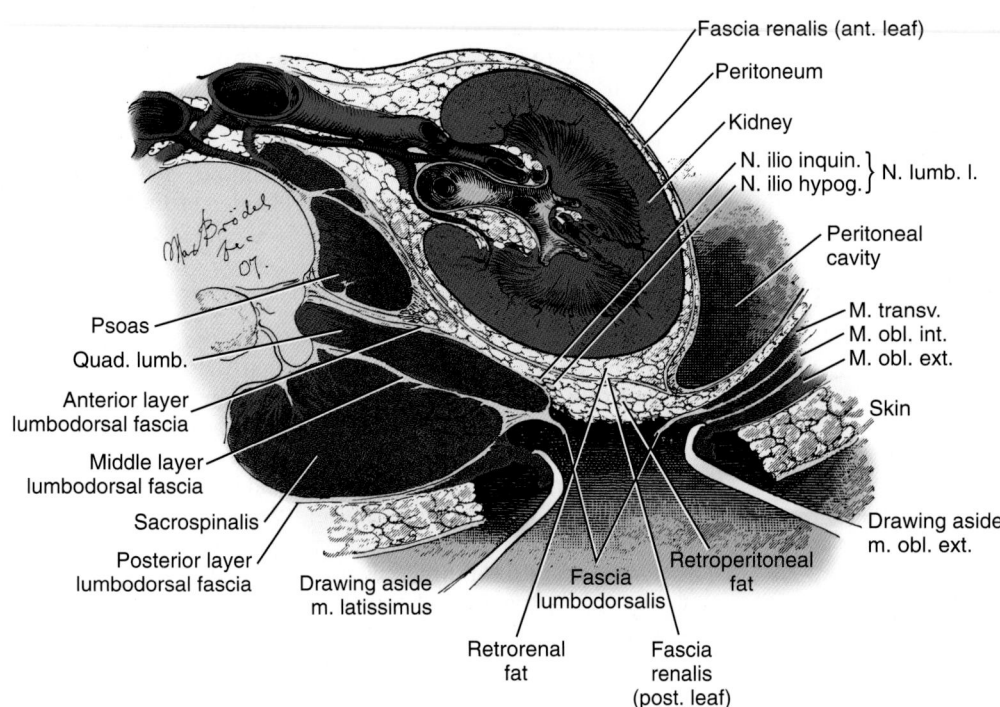

Fascia renalis (ant. leaf)

Peritoneum

Kidney

N. ilio inquin. ⎫
N. ilio hypog. ⎭ N. lumb. l.

Peritoneal cavity

M. transv.
M. obl. int.
M. obl. ext.

Skin

Psoas

Quad. lumb.

Anterior layer lumbodorsal fascia

Middle layer lumbodorsal fascia

Sacrospinalis

Posterior layer lumbodorsal fascia

Drawing aside m. latissimus

Drawing aside m. obl. ext.

Retroperitoneal fat

Fascia lumbodorsalis

Retrorenal fat

Fascia renalis (post. leaf)

Figure 1-7. Transverse section through the kidney and posterior abdominal wall showing the lumbodorsal fascia incised. Note that through such a lumbodorsal incision the kidney can be reached without incising muscle. (After Kelly and Burnam, from McVay C: Anson & McVay Surgical Anatomy, 6th ed. Philadelphia, WB Saunders, 1984.)

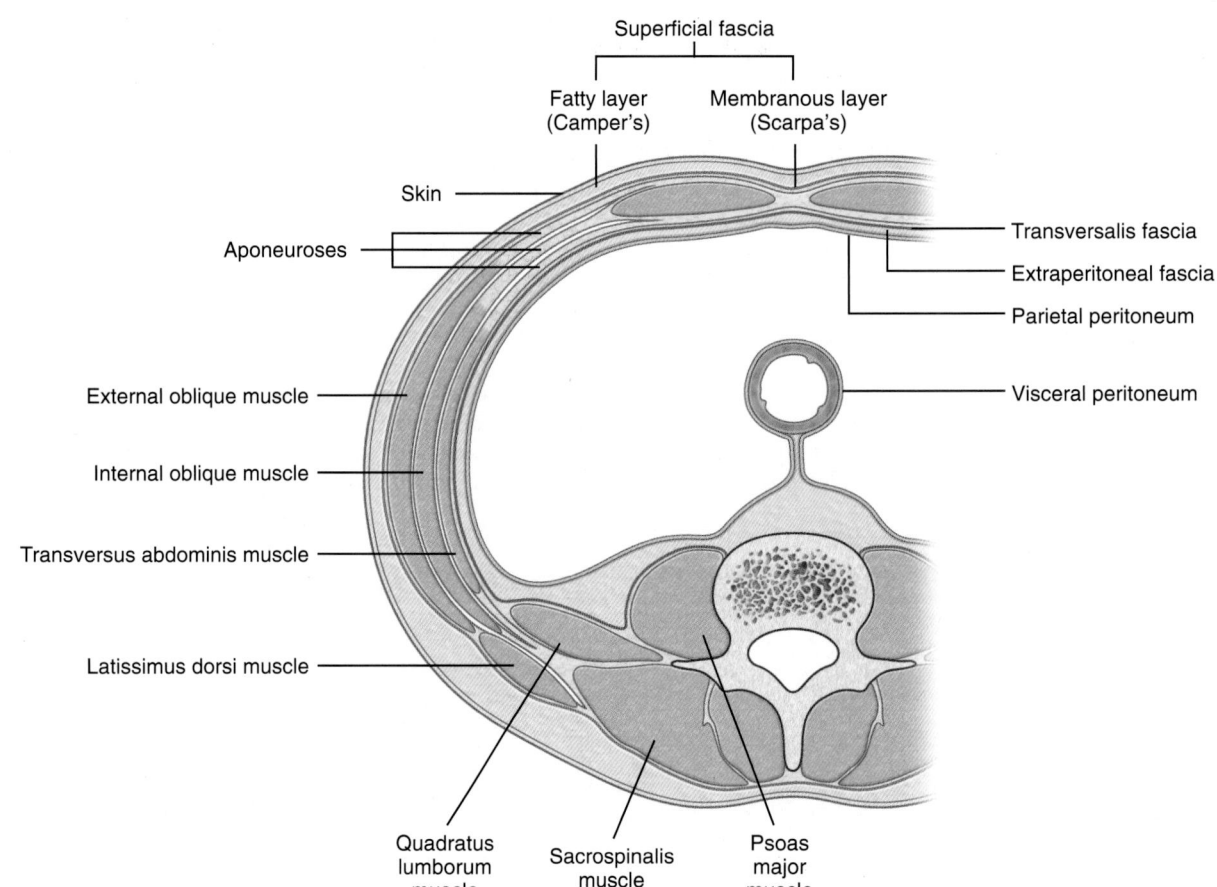

Superficial fascia

Fatty layer (Camper's)

Membranous layer (Scarpa's)

Skin

Aponeuroses

Transversalis fascia

Extraperitoneal fascia

Parietal peritoneum

External oblique muscle

Visceral peritoneum

Internal oblique muscle

Transversus abdominis muscle

Latissimus dorsi muscle

Quadratus lumborum muscle

Sacrospinalis muscle

Psoas major muscle

Figure 1-8. Transverse section showing layers of the lateral flank musculature. (From Drake RL, VoGL W, Mitchell AWM: Drake RL, Vogl W, Mitchell AWM: Gray's Anatomy for Students. Philadelphia, Elsevier, 2005, p 252.)

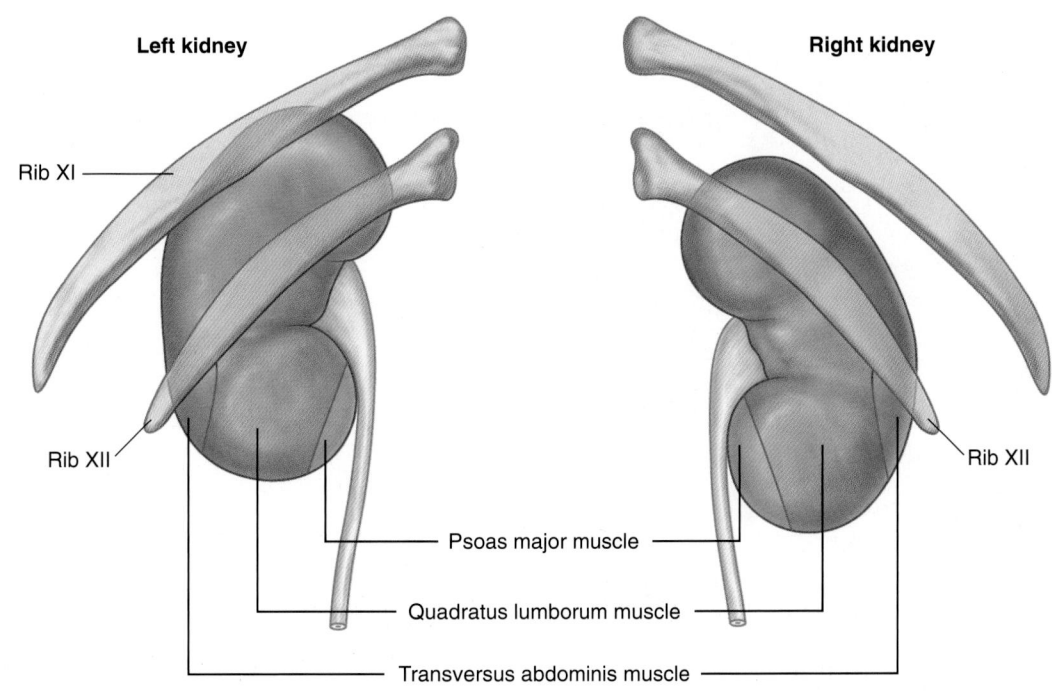

Figure 1–9. Structures related to the posterior surface of the kidney. (From Drake RL, VogL W, Mitchell AWM: Gray's Anatomy for Students. Philadelphia, Elsevier, 2005, p 322.)

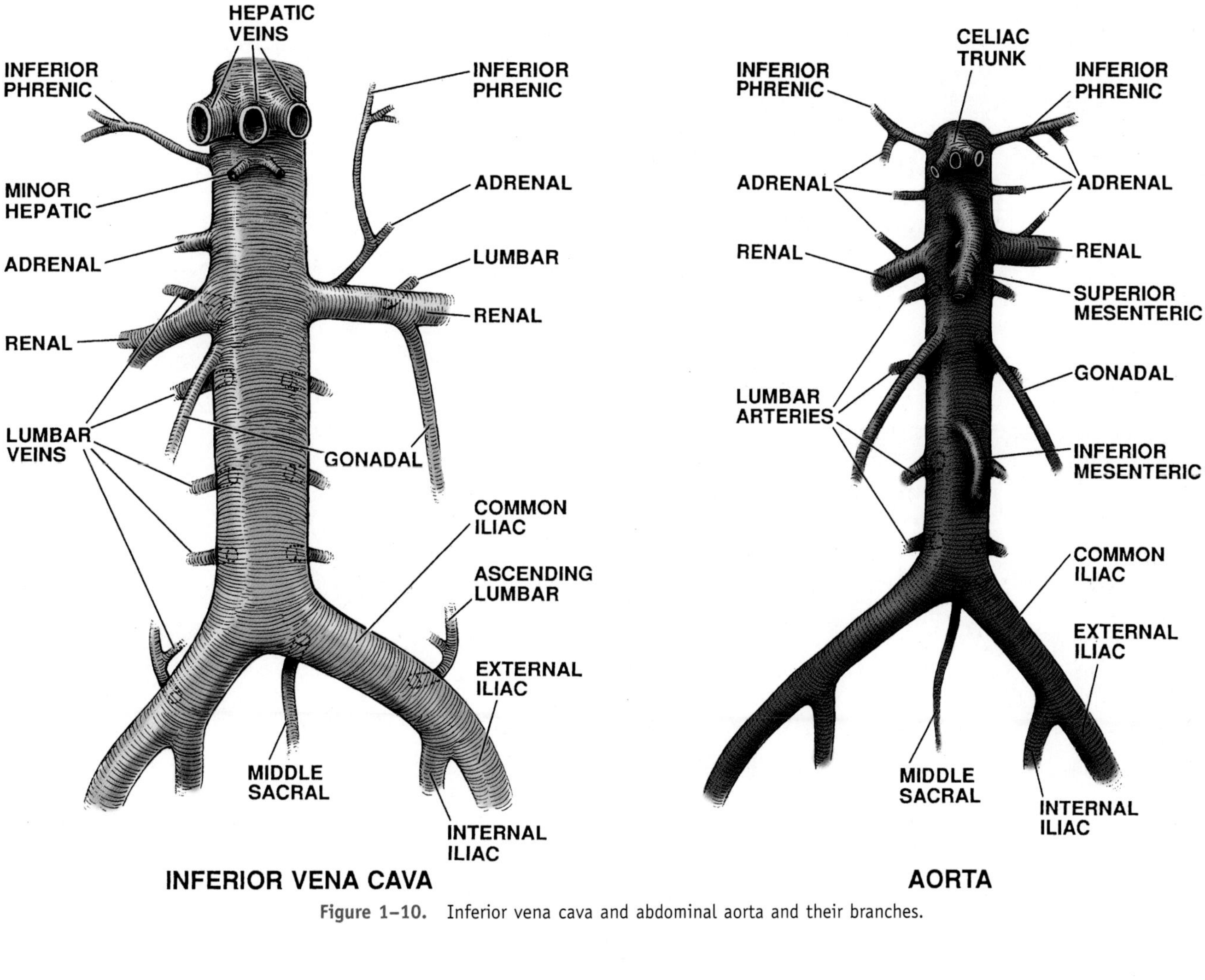

Figure 1–10. Inferior vena cava and abdominal aorta and their branches.

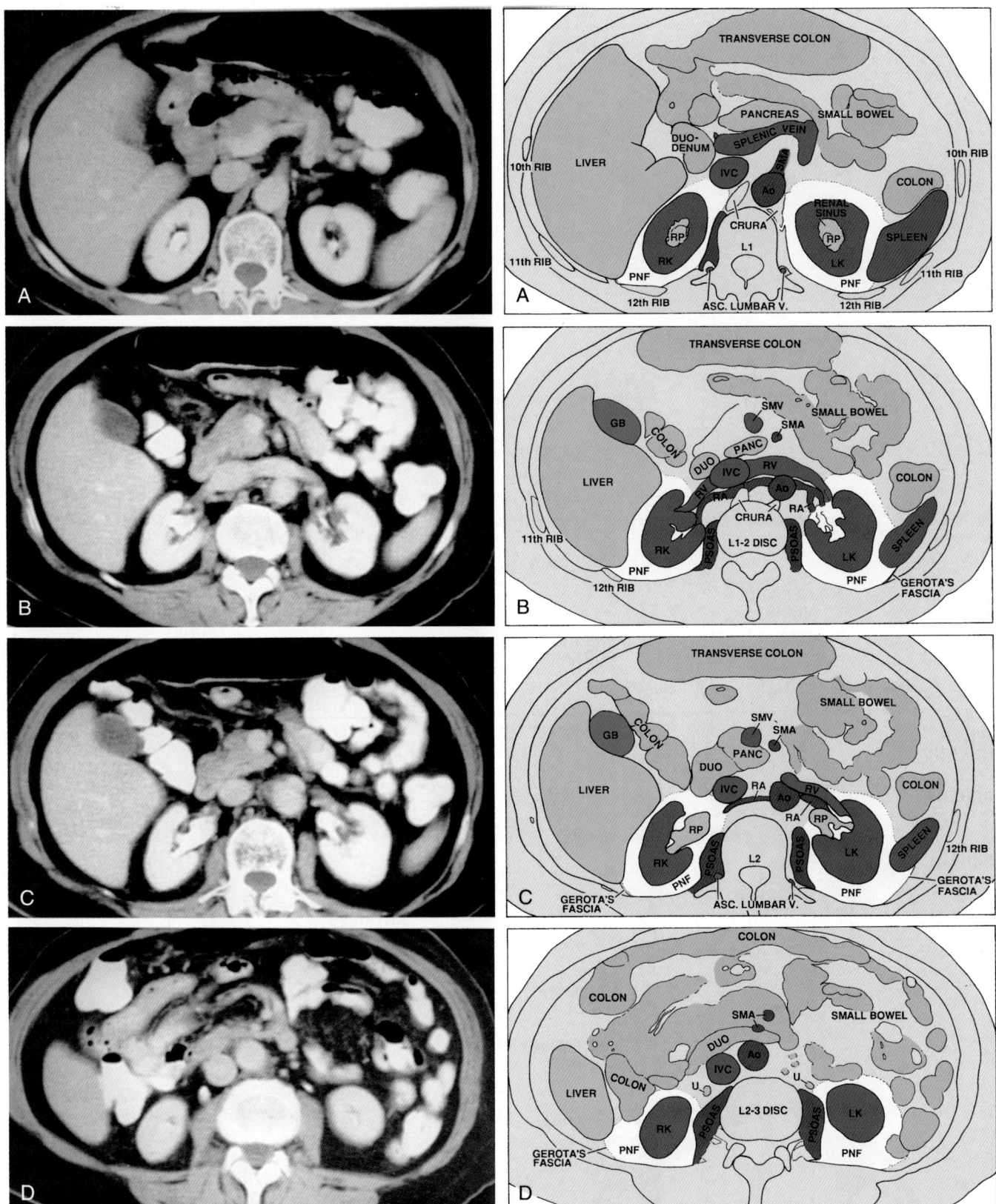

Figure 1–11.   Cross-sectional anatomy of the upper abdomen at the level of the kidneys demonstrated with transverse sections obtained by computed tomography. Sections are arranged from most cephalic to caudal. **A,** Section through the upper poles of the kidneys, superior to the renal vascular pedicles. **B,** Section through the level of the renal arteries and veins. **C,** Slightly more inferior section showing the renal pelves and relation of the duodenum to the right renal hilum. **D,** Section through the lower poles of the kidneys showing the upper ureters. Ao, aorta; DUO, duodenum; GB, gallbladder; IVC, inferior vena cava; LK, left kidney; PANC, pancreas; PNF, perinephric fat; RA, renal artery; RK, right kidney; RP, renal pelvis; RV, renal vein; SMA, superior mesenteric artery; SMV, superior mesenteric vein; U, ureter.

Table 1-2. Branches of the Abdominal Aorta

Artery	Branch	Origin	Parts Supplied
Celiac trunk	Anterior	Immediately inferior to aortic hiatus of diaphragm	Abdominal foregut
Superior mesenteric artery	Anterior	Immediately inferior to celiac trunk	Abdominal midgut
Inferior mesenteric artery	Anterior	Inferior to renal arteries	Abdominal hindgut
Middle adrenal arteries	Lateral	Immediately superior to renal arteries	Adrenal glands
Renal arteries	Lateral	Immediately inferior to superior mesenteric artery	Kidneys
Testicular or ovarian arteries	Paired anterior	Inferior to renal arteries	Testes in male and ovaries in female
Inferior phrenic arteries	Paired	Immediately inferior to aortic hiatus	Diaphragm
Lumbar arteries	Posterior	Usually four pairs	Posterior abdominal wall and spinal cord
Median sacral arteries	Posterior	Just superior to aortic bifurcation, pass inferiorly across lumbar vertebrae, sacrum, and coccyx	
Common iliac arteries	Terminal	Bifurcation usually occurs at the level of L4 vertebra	

From Drake RL, Vogl W, Mitchell AWM: Gray's Anatomy for Students. Philadelphia, Elsevier, 2005, p 331.

The superior mesenteric artery leaves the aorta on the anterior side and supplies the entire small intestine and majority of the large intestine. Also of note, this artery communicates with the celiac trunk vasculature via the pancreaticoduodenal artery. Overlying the 2nd lumbar vertebrae, the paired renal arteries are the next branching point of the aorta. To the urologist, renal artery anatomy is obviously of great importance and is discussed in detail in the kidney section.

Moving distally on the aorta, the paired gonadal arteries are encountered. In the male this artery is also called the testicular artery and in the female it is the ovarian artery. The initial course in both the male and female is similar, with the artery moving caudally and laterally from the aorta, with **the right gonadal artery crossing anterior to the inferior vena cava. In men, the gonadal artery then crosses over the ureter and exits the retroperitoneum at the internal inguinal ring. In women the course is different: instead of exiting the pelvis the artery crosses medially back over the external iliac vessels and enters the pelvis.** It then proceeds via the suspensory ligament to the ovary. The destination of the gonadal artery (the testis in the male and the ovary in the female) has significant collateral sources of arterial blood, from the deferential and cremasteric arteries in the male and the uterine artery in the female. Thus the gonadal artery can generally be ligated during retroperitoneal surgery without detrimental effect.

After the gonadal arteries, **the inferior mesenteric artery is found on the anterior side of the aorta before its bifurcation into the common iliac vessels.** This vessel provides vascular supply to the left third of the transverse colon, descending colon, sigmoid colon, and rectum. In patients without significant vascular disease, this artery can be sacrificed without ill effect because there is collateral circulation to these bowel segments from the superior mesenteric, middle hemorrhoidal, and inferior hemorrhoidal arteries.

In addition to the listed arteries that exit the aorta from its anterior or lateral aspect, there are a number of small branches from the posterior side of the aorta. **Lumbar arterial branches are found at regular intervals along the length of the aorta, with generally four pairs located within the retroperitoneum.** These branches supply the posterior body wall and spine. Again these arteries can generally be ligated

without detrimental effects, although spinal ischemia and paralysis has occurred after ligation at multiple levels. **The final posterior branch from the aorta is the middle sacral artery,** which exits the aorta immediately before the branching of the common iliac arteries and then sends branches to the rectum and anterior sacrum. The common iliac arteries then proceed into the pelvis, thus completing the arterial course through the retroperitoneum.

The Inferior Vena Cava

The inferior vena cava (IVC) arises from the confluence of the common iliac veins at the level of the 5th lumbar vertebra (see Fig. 1–10). **Because the common iliac veins lie medial and posterior to the iliac arteries, the confluence of the iliac veins is posterior and to the right of the aortic bifurcation.** As the IVC progresses cranially through the abdomen, tributaries include the gonadal, renal, adrenal, and hepatic veins. In addition, the middle sacral vein enters the inferior vena cava posteriorly and the lumbar veins enter throughout the length of the abdominal vena cava.

The first tributary encountered along the IVC is the **middle sacral vein,** which enters at the junction of the common iliac veins. Also entering along the posterior aspect of the IVC throughout its course are **lumbar veins.** These veins course anterior to the spinal transverse processes and generally parallel the lumber arteries. In addition to providing vascular drainage, the lumbar veins connect the IVC to the azygous venous system on the right side and hemiazygous venous system on the left side of the thorax. This provides alternate routes of venous drainage within the retroperitoneum (Fig. 1–12).

The next tributaries to the IVC are the gonadal veins, whose course is analogous to the gonadal arteries until approaching the IVC. During the cranial portion of their course these veins are more lateral and closer to the ipsilateral ureter. Of surgical importance is their terminal drainage because **the right gonadal vein drains directly into the IVC and the left empties into the inferior aspect of the left renal vein** (see Fig. 1–10).

After the gonadal veins, the renal veins are encountered. **The renal veins are generally directly anterior to the accompanying renal artery, but it is not unusual for them to be separated by 1 to 2 cm in the craniocaudal direction.** The right

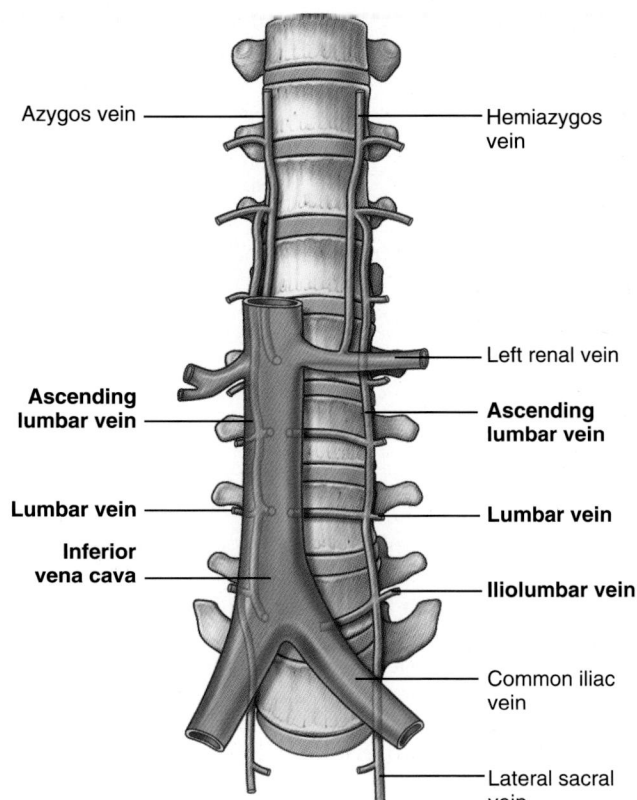

Azygos vein

Hemiazygos vein

Left renal vein

Ascending lumbar vein

Ascending lumbar vein

Lumbar vein

Lumbar vein

Inferior vena cava

Iliolumbar vein

Common iliac vein

Lateral sacral vein

Figure 1–12. Lumbar, azygos, and hemiazygos veins. (From Drake RL, Vogl W, Mitchell AWM: Gray's Anatomy for Students. Philadelphia, Elsevier, 2005, p 332.)

renal vein typically is short and without branches, but in a small minority of patients the right gonadal vein can enter the right renal vein as opposed to the IVC. In a second anatomic variation, a lumbar vein will enter on the posterior aspect of the right renal vein as opposed to entering the IVC directly. The left renal vein is significantly longer than the right and receives additional branches before entering the IVC. Typically after exiting the renal hilum, the left renal vein receives a lumbar vein posteriorly, the left gonadal vein inferiorly, and the adrenal vein superiorly. Next, the left renal vein crosses anterior to the aorta and under the caudal edge of the superior mesenteric artery before draining into the IVC. Rarely the left renal vein crosses the aorta to the IVC in a retroaortic or circumaortic path.

Proceeding cranially, **the posterior aspect of the IVC receives the right adrenal vein.** This short vein is located posteriorly on the IVC, making it challenging to expose during right adrenal or renal surgery. As noted already, the left adrenal vein drains into the left renal vein as opposed to the IVC. **The inferior phrenic vein on the right side enters along the posterior or posterior lateral aspect of the IVC, with the left inferior phrenic vein typically entering the left renal vein.** The final tributaries to the IVC before it leaves the retroperitoneum are the short hepatic veins draining the liver. Inferiorly these veins are small, but superiorly three large hepatic trunks are encountered.

Lymphatics

Lymphatic drainage of the lower extremities, external genitalia, testes, kidneys, and intestines is located in the retroperitoneum (Fig. 1–13). Knowledge of these lymphatic channels is useful not only for urologic oncology (e.g., testis cancer) but also for prevention of complications such as lymphocele. Drainage of the lower extremities, perineum, and external genitalia progresses through the retroperitoneum via common iliac lymph vessels and then forms ascending vertical lumbar lymphatic chains. **There is flow not only cranially but also laterally, predominantly from the right to the left.** Gastrointestinal lymphatic drainage also follows the vascular supply, with the majority of the lymphatics paralleling the inferior mesenteric, superior mesenteric, and celiac arteries. Eventually these lymphatics join posterior to the aorta at the level of the first or second lumbar vertebrae to form the **thoracic duct.** This coalescence is classically marked by a local dilation called **the cisterna chyli,** which tends to lie within the thorax just to the right of the aorta in a retrocrural position.

For the urologist, the lumbar lymphatics are important as the primary lymphatic drainage from two urologic organs: the kidneys and testes. Given the kidney's retroperitoneal location, the lumbar path of its lymphatic drainage is not surprising and is discussed in more depth later in this chapter. Embryologically, the testes develop within the retroperitoneum and maintain both blood flow (testicular arteries) and lymphatic drainage through this area even after they descend into the scrotum. To better describe the lymphatic drainage within the retroperitoneum a practical system has been developed. This system defines three major nodal areas: right paracaval, interaortal caval, and left para-aortic. The right paracaval nodal region extends from the midline of the IVC to the right ureter. The interaortal caval region extends from the midline of the IVC to the midline of the aorta, and the left para-aortic region extends from the midline of the aorta to the left ureter.

Study of lymphatic metastases from testicular tumors have shown that testicular lymphatic drainage is consistent and follows the general scheme of vertical drainage with lateral flow from right to left. Lymphatic metastases from the right testis drain primarily into the interaortal caval nodes with significant drainage to the right paracaval nodes. In addition there is a small amount of drainage to the left para-aortic nodes. On the other hand, the left testis drains primarily to the left para-aortic nodes with significant drainage to the interaortal caval nodes. There is essentially no drainage to the right paracaval nodes from left-sided tumors.

Nervous System Structures

The nervous structures within the retroperitoneum are part of the peripheral nervous system and can be divided into two categories: autonomic and somatic nerves. **The autonomic nerves provide afferent and efferent innervation to organs, blood vessels, glands, and smooth muscles. They are further characterized by the presence of peripheral synapses. Thus there are least two peripheral nerves between the central nervous system and the viscera. The somatic nerves supply afferent and efferent innervation to the skin, skeletal**

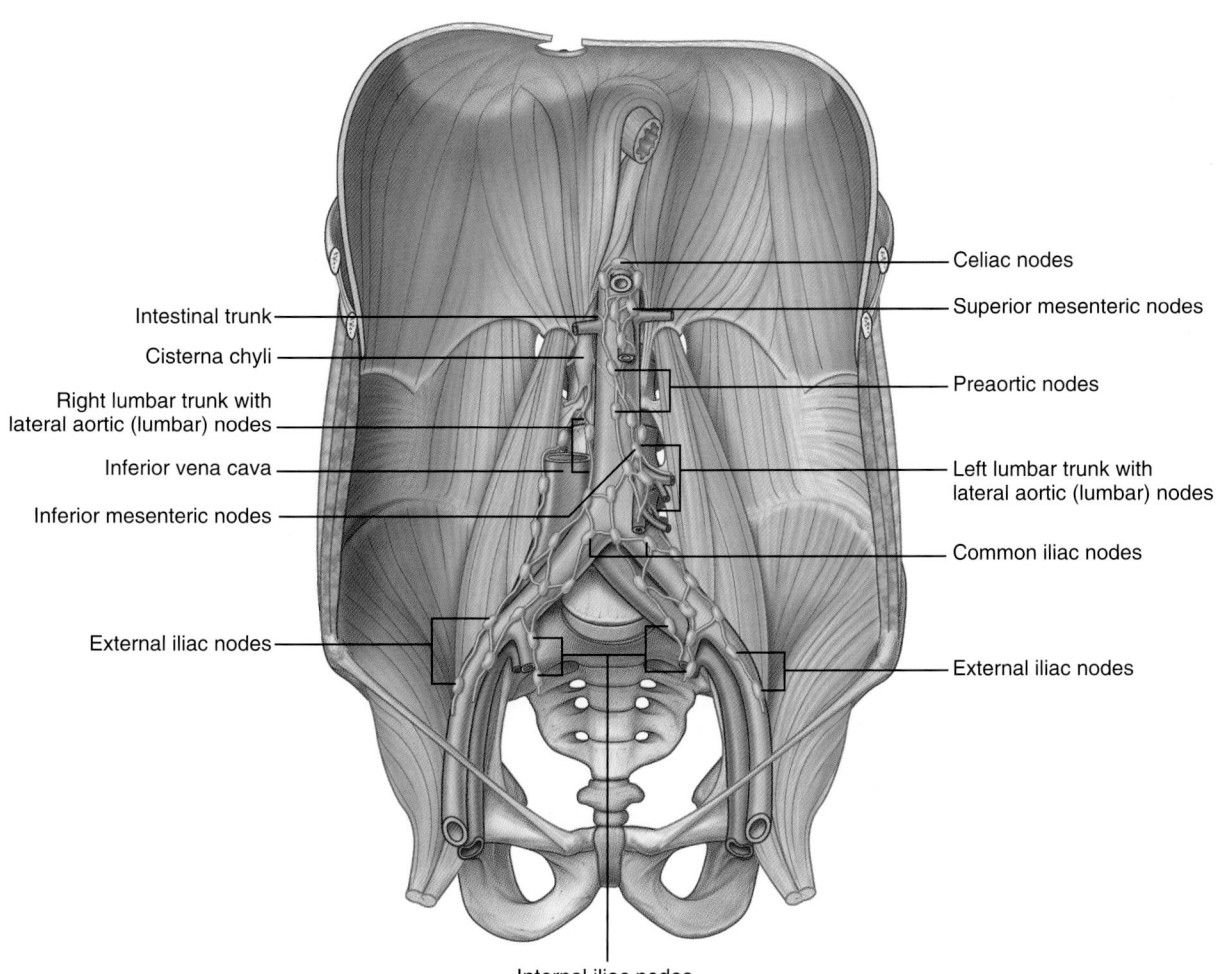

Figure 1–13. Retroperitoneal lymphatics. (From Drake RL, Vogl W, Mitchell AWM: Gray's Anatomy for Students. Philadelphia, Elsevier, 2005, p 335.)

muscles, and joints. Although these two nerve types leave the spinal column within shared spinal nerves, their course and functions quickly diverge.

Autonomic System

The autonomic system is further divided into sympathetic and parasympathetic fibers. The origin of these two nerve types is quite different, with **the sympathetic preganglionic fibers originating from the thoracic and lumbar portions of the spinal column and the parasympathetic preganglionic fibers beginning in the cranial and sacral spinal column segments. Preganglionic sympathetic fibers enter the retroperitoneum through both the paired sympathetic chains and input from the lumbar spinal nerves** (Fig. 1–14). **The lumbar portion of this sympathetic chain then sends preganglionic fibers to autonomic plexuses associated with the major branches of the abdominal aorta. Within these aortic plexuses the preganglionic fibers synapse and postganglionic fibers are then distributed to the various abdominal viscera and organs. Parasympathetic input from the vagus nerve also supplies these ganglia.**

In more detail, the thoracic and lumbar portions of the sympathetic chain originate from preganglionic sympathetic fibers arising from the first thoracic through the third lumbar spinal nerves (see Fig. 1–14). **This chain then courses vertically along the anterolateral aspect of the spine just medial to the psoas muscle.** Within the retroperitoneum lumbar arteries and veins are closely associated with the lumbar sympathetic chain, in some instances even splitting the fibers as they cross the chain perpendicularly. **From this sympathetic chain preganglionic fibers follow one of three courses. First, preganglionic fibers are sent to the various autonomic plexuses (splanchnic nerves). Once in the plexus, the preganglionic fibers synapse within a ganglion to postganglionic fibers, which in turn proceed to the abdominal viscera. Second, preganglionic fibers can synapse within the sympathetic chain ganglia and send postganglionic fibers to the body wall and lower extremities. Finally, preganglionic sympathetic fibers can proceed directly to the adrenal gland without synapsing. Within the adrenal medulla, these preganglionic fibers control release of catecholamines.**

The major autonomic nerve plexuses are associated with the primary branches of the aorta. These plexuses include the **celiac, superior hypogastric,** and **inferior hypogastric plexuses** (Fig. 1–15). These plexuses receive sympathetic input from the sympathetic chains via the greater, lesser, and least thoracic splanchnic nerves originating from the 5th through 12th thoracic spinal nerves. They also receive input

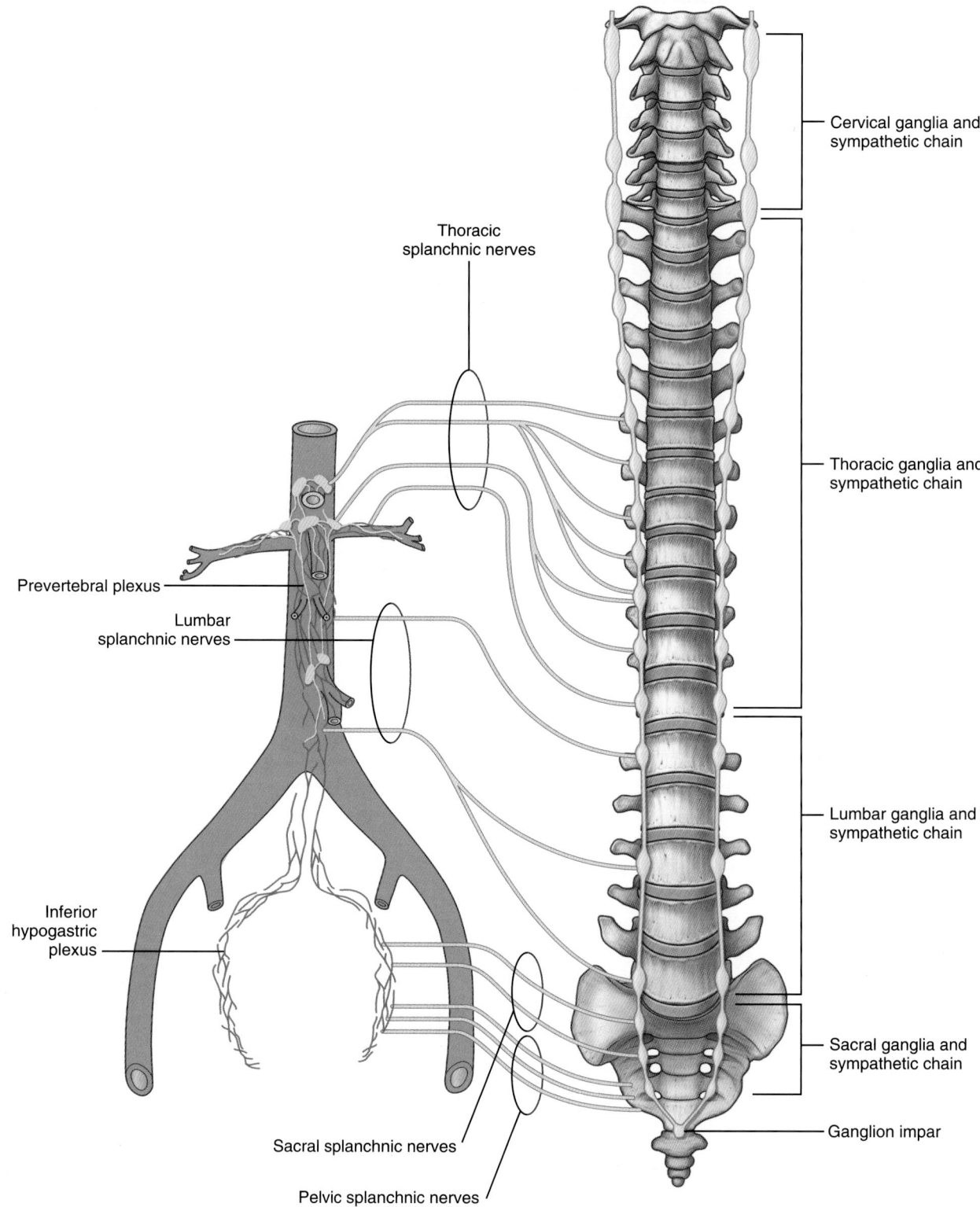

Figure 1–14.   Sympathetic chain and splanchnic nerves. (From Drake RL, Vogl W, Mitchell AWM: Gray's Anatomy for Students. Philadelphia, Elsevier, 2005, p 309.)

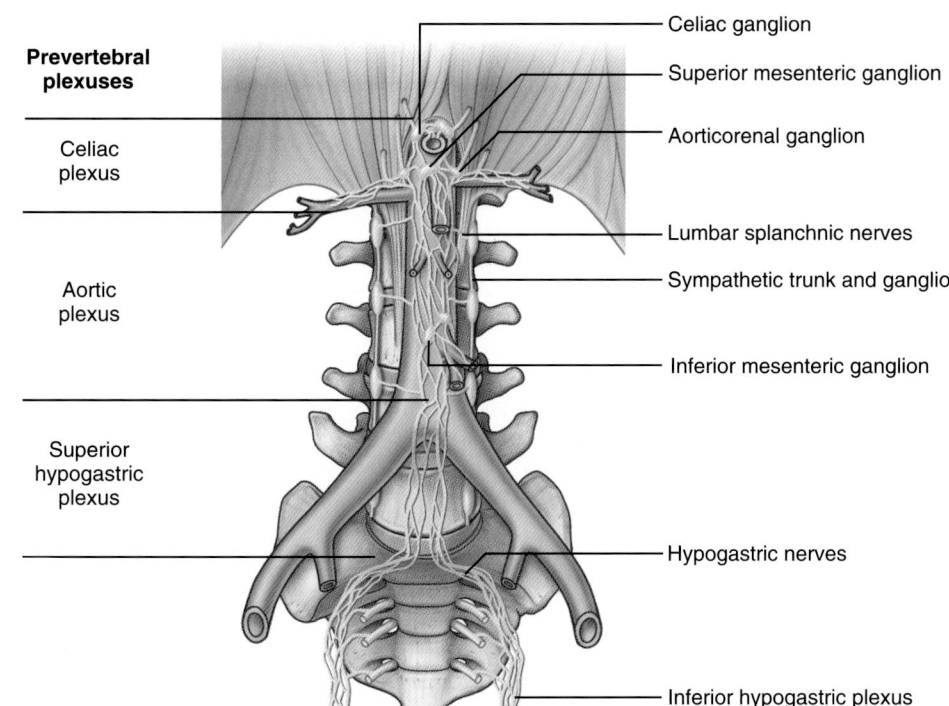

Figure 1–15. Autonomic plexuses associated with branches of the aorta. (From Drake RL, Vogl W, Mitchell AWM: Gray's Anatomy for Students. Philadelphia, Elsevier, 2005, p 337.)

from the lumbar portion of the sympathetic chain via the lumbar splanchnic nerves as well as parasympathetic input via the vagus nerve.

The largest is the celiac plexus and is located to either side of the celiac arterial trunk as a paired structure. It is through this plexus that much or all of the autonomic input to the kidney, adrenal, renal pelvis, and ureter passes. In addition, some of the sympathetic innervation to the testes passes through this ganglion before continuing in parallel with the testicular artery to the testis. A separate aorticorenal ganglion usually exists as an inferior extension of the celiac ganglion, forming part of the renal autonomic plexus. The latter plexus surrounds the renal artery and its branches and is contiguous with the celiac plexus. At the lower extent of the abdominal aorta, **much of the autonomic input to the pelvic urinary organs and genital tract travels through the superior hypogastric plexus.** This plexus lies on the aorta anterior to its bifurcation and extends inferiorly on the anterior surface of the fifth lumbar vertebra. This plexus is contiguous bilaterally with inferior hypogastric plexuses, which extend into the pelvis. **Disruption of the sympathetic nerve fibers that travel through these plexuses during retroperitoneal dissection can cause loss of seminal vesicle emission and/or failure of bladder neck closure, resulting in retrograde ejaculation.**

Somatic

The somatic sensory and motor innervation to the abdomen and lower extremities arises in the retroperitoneum and is called the lumbosacral plexus. The lumbosacral plexus is formed from branches of all lumbar and sacral spinal nerves, with some contribution from the 12th thoracic spinal nerve as well (Fig. 1–16). Superiorly, nerves of this plexus form

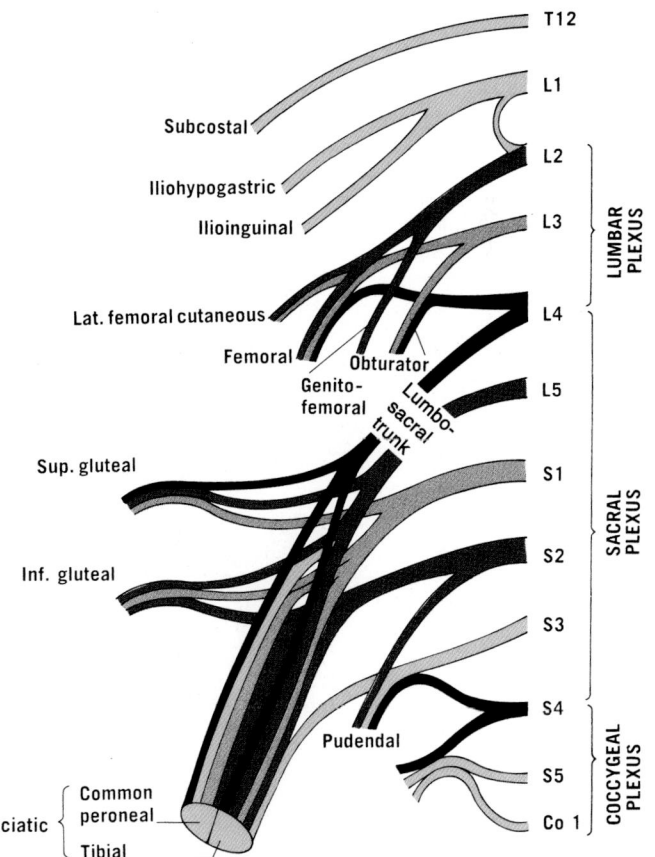

Figure 1–16. Diagrammatic representation of the lumbosacral nervous plexus.

within the body of the psoas muscle and pierce this muscle, with more inferior branches passing medial to the psoas as the pelvis is entered (Fig. 1–17). The origins and functions of these lumbosacral somatic nerves are summarized in Table 1–3.

The subcostal nerve is the anterior extension of the 12th thoracic nerve and extends laterally beneath the 12th rib. As one proceeds inferiorly, the **iliohypogastric nerve** and the **ilioinguinal nerve** originate together as an extension from the first lumbar spinal nerve. These three nerves cross the anterior or inner surface of the quadratus lumborum muscle before piercing the transversus abdominis muscle and continuing their course between this and the internal oblique muscle. Together they provide multiple motor branches to the muscles of the abdominal wall as well as sensory innervation to the skin of the lower abdomen and genitalia. The **lateral**

femoral cutaneous nerve and the **genitofemoral nerve** arise from the first through third lumbar nerves and are primarily sensory nerves to the skin of the upper thigh and genitalia; however, the genital branch of the genitofemoral nerve also supplies the cremaster and dartos muscles in the scrotum. The genitofemoral nerve lies directly atop and parallels the psoas muscle throughout most of its retroperitoneal course and is easily identified in this position.

The **femoral nerve** is a larger structure arising from the second through fourth lumbar spinal nerves and is largely hidden by the body of the psoas muscle before exiting the abdomen just lateral to the femoral artery. This important nervous structure supplies the psoas and iliacus muscles as well as the large muscle groups of the anterior thigh. It also provides sensory innervation of the anteromedial portions of the lower extremity. Intraoperatively, it may be compressed by

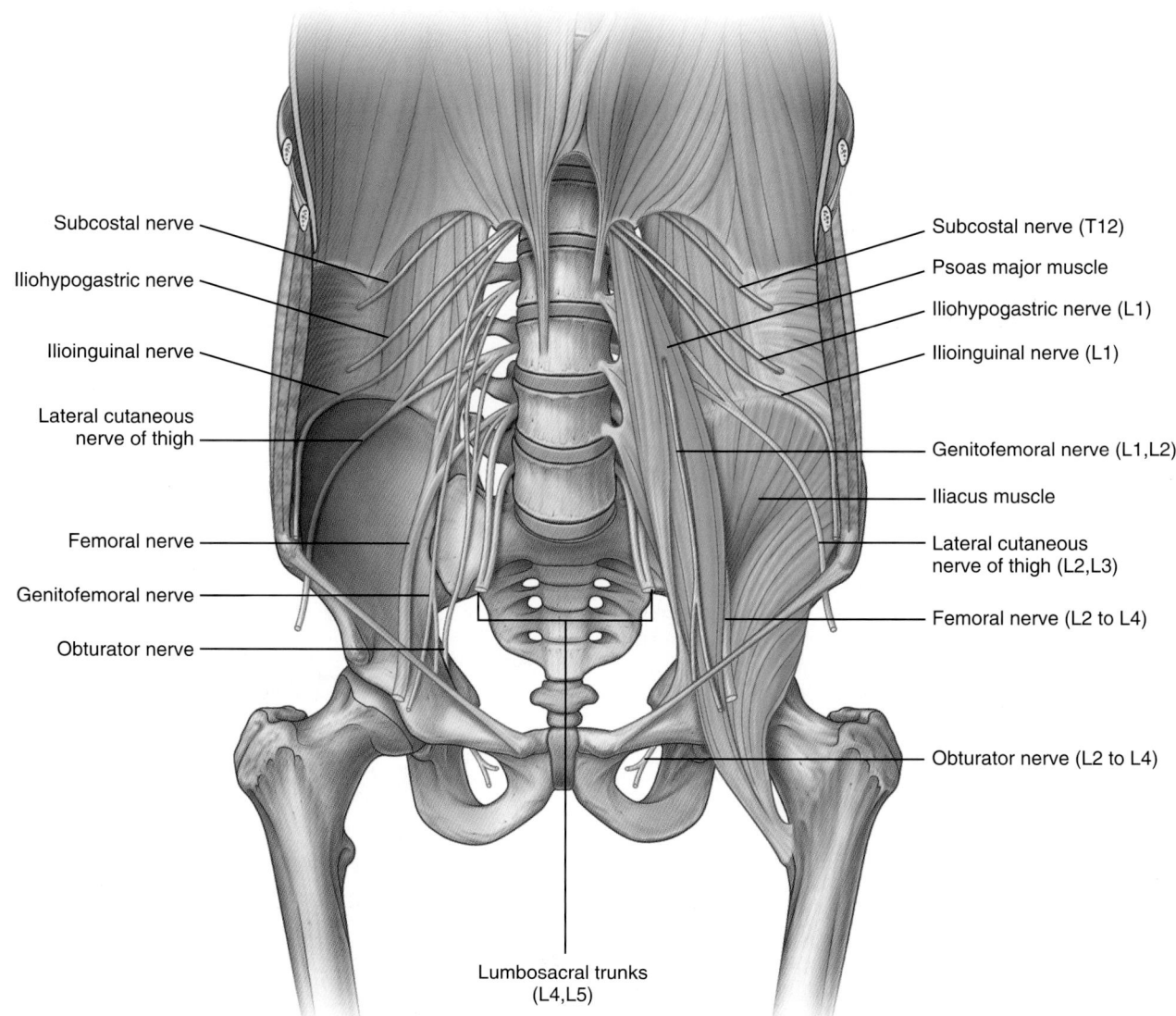

Figure 1–17. Lumbar plexus in the posterior abdominal region. (From Drake RL, Vogl W, Mitchell AWM: Gray's Anatomy for Students. Philadelphia, Elsevier, 2005, p 341.)

From Drake RL, Vogl W, Mitchell AWM: Gray's Anatomy for Students. Philadelphia, Elsevier, 2005, p 340.

Table 1-3. Branches of the Lumbosacral Plexus

Branch	Origin	Spinal Segments	Function: Motor	Function: Sensory
Iliohypogastric	Anterior ramus L1	L1	Internal oblique and transversus abdominis	Posterolateral gluteal skin and skin in pubic region
Ilioinguinal	Anterior ramus L1	L1	Internal oblique and transversus abdominis	Skin in the upper medial thigh, and either the skin over the root of the penis and anterior scrotum or the mons pubis and labium majus
Genitofemoral	Anterior rami L1 and L2	L1, L2	Genital branch—male cremasteric muscle	Genital branch—skin of anterior scrotum or skin of mons pubis and labium majus; femoral branch—skin of upper anterior thigh
Lateral cutaneous nerve of thigh	Anterior rami L2 and L3	L2, L3		Skin on anterior and lateral thigh to the knee
Obturator	Anterior rami L2 to L4	L2 to L4	Obturator externus, pectineus, and muscles in medial compartment of thigh	Skin on medial aspect of the thigh
Femoral	Anterior rami L2 to L4	L2 to L4	Iliacus, pectineus, and muscles in anterior compartment of thigh	Skin on anterior thigh and medial surface of leg

retractor blades placed inferolaterally against the inguinal ligament in lower abdominal incisions, producing a significant motor palsy that prevents active extension of the knee.

The final lumbosacral plexus nerves include the **obturator and sciatic nerves.** The obturator nerve, an important pelvic landmark, arises behind the psoas muscle in the retroperitoneum from the third and fourth lumbar spinal nerves. It then courses inferiorly, where its major function is to supply the adductor muscles of the thigh. The **sciatic nerve** receives input from the fourth lumbar through third sacral spinal nerves, taking final form in the deep posterior pelvis as the body's single largest nerve, supplying the bulk of both sensory and motor innervation to the lower extremity.

Duodenum, Pancreas, Colon (Fig. 1–18)

The duodenum is divided into four anatomic components. The first (ascending) portion is short (5 cm) and intimately related to the gallbladder. **The second (descending portion) is of most importance to the urologist because it lies immediately anterior to the right renal hilum and pelvis.** This portion of the duodenum is frequently mobilized (referred to as a Kocher maneuver) to expose the right kidney, right renal pelvis, and additional upper abdominal structures. The second portion of the duodenum also receives the common bile duct and surrounds the head of the pancreas. The third (horizontal) and fourth (ascending) portions of the duodenum cross from right to left over the IVC and aorta before transitioning into the jejunum.

As noted earlier, the head of the pancreas is on the medial border of the descending duodenum. **The body and tail of the pancreas continue across the IVC and aorta to the left side of the abdomen where the pancreas is closely related to the left adrenal gland and the upper pole of the left kidney.** The splenic artery and vein travel laterally along the posterior aspect of the pancreas, with the artery just superior to the vein. In this position these vascular structures are also closely related to the upper pole of the left kidney.

The final retroperitoneal gastrointestinal structure is the colon, with the ascending and descending portions being retroperitoneal. **Both the ascending colon at the hepatic flexure and descending colon at the splenic flexure overlie the ipsalateral kidney.** In addition, the hepatocolic ligament and splenocolic ligament tether the liver and spleen to the respective portions of the colon. Given the close anatomic relationship to the kidneys, mobilization of the colon and its mesentery is important for transperitoneal exposure of the kidneys and ureters.

THE ADRENAL GLANDS (Fig. 1–19)

KEY POINTS: THE ADRENAL GLANDS

■ Embryologically the adrenals are distinct from the kidney. Developmental abnormalities of one do not affect the other.

■ The adrenal is divided into the medulla and the cortex.

■ The adrenal medulla receives preganglionic sympathetic input that stimulates the release of catecholamines from medullary chromaffin cells.

■ The adrenal cortex is composed of three distinct areas: the zona glomerulosa, zona fasciculata, and zona reticularis.

■ Arterial supply to the adrenal comes from branches of the inferior phrenic artery, aorta, and renal artery.

■ Venous drainage of the adrenal varies by side, with the right adrenal vein directly entering the IVC and the left adrenal vein draining into the left renal vein.

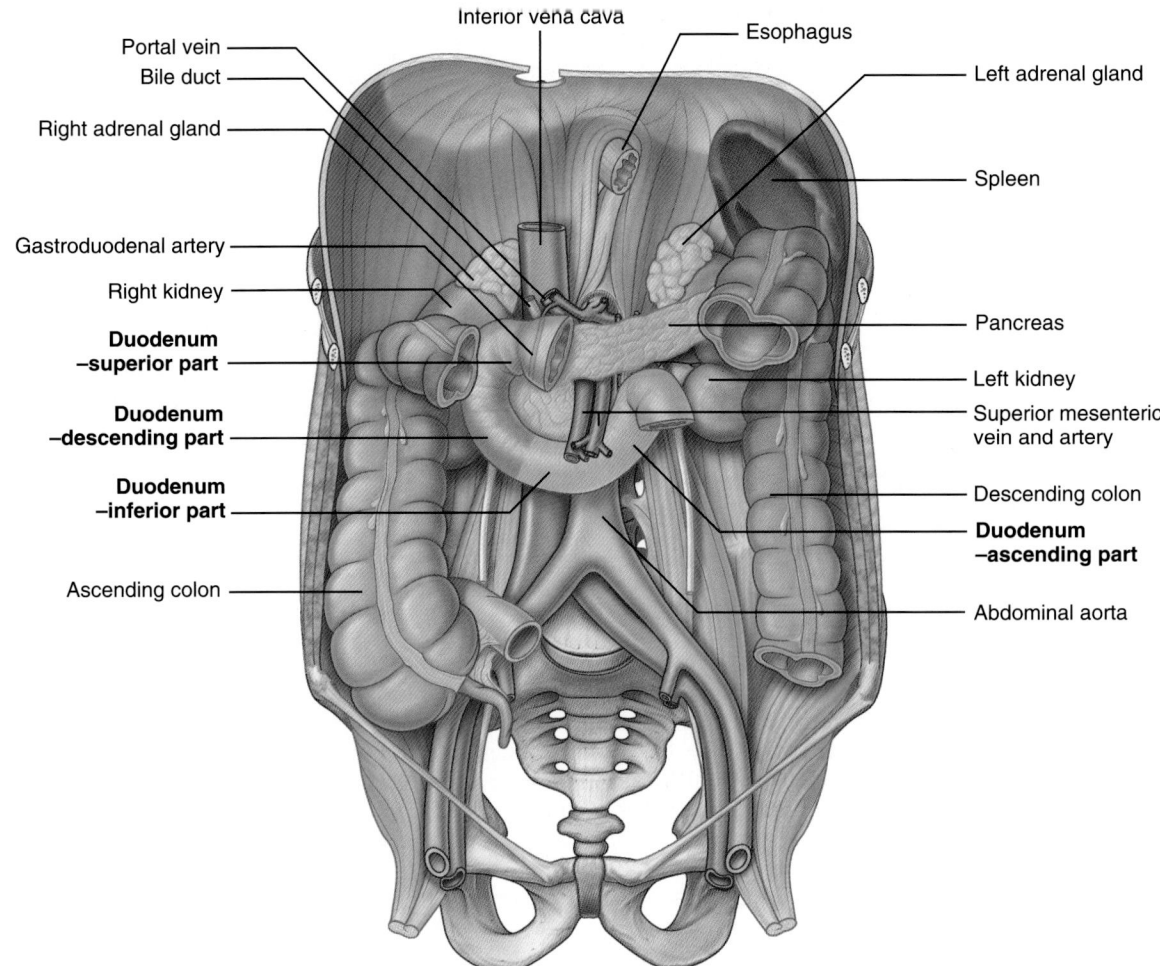

Figure 1–18. Colon, duodenum, and pancreas within the retroperitoneum. (From Drake RL, Vogl W, Mitchell AWM: Gray's Anatomy for Students. Philadelphia, Elsevier, 2005, p 274.)

Anatomic Relationships

The adult adrenal glands are 3 to 5 cm in greatest transverse dimension and weigh approximately 5 g. Grossly, they are yellow-orange and noticeably more orange than the surrounding adipose tissue. The position of this bilateral gland varies from right to left, but both glands are enclosed within the perirenal (Gerota's) fascia and are separated from the upper pole of the kidneys by a layer of connective tissue.

The right gland is more superiorly located in the retroperitoneum and is pyramidal. It is almost directly cranial to the upper pole of the right kidney. Surrounding structures include the liver anterolaterally, the duodenum anteromedially, and the inferior vena cava medially. It is also important to note that there is often a retrocaval extension of one wing. The left gland is more crescenteric and medial to the upper pole of the left kidney. The upper and anterior aspects are related to the stomach, tail of the pancreas, and splenic vessels.

Composition

Embryologically, the adrenal is distinct from the kidney. Thus, in cases of renal ectopia, the adrenal gland is not affected.

Histologically, the adrenal is divided into two components: the centrally located medulla and the peripherally located cortex (Fig. 1–20). The medulla itself is composed of chromaffin cells derived from neural crest origin. These chromaffin cells are innervated directly by presynaptic sympathetic fibers traveling to the adrenal gland from the sympathetic chains. The secretion of neuroactive catecholamines by the adrenal medulla is thus under sympathetic control.

The adrenal cortex is of mesodermal origin and makes up approximately 90% of the adrenal mass. It is composed of three layers, from external to internal, the zona glomerulosa, zona fasciculata, and zona reticularis. Each layer has a different function, with the glomerulosa producing mineralocorticoids (e.g., aldosterone), the fasciculata producing glucocorticoids (e.g., cortisol), and the reticularis synthesizing sex steroids (androgens).

Adrenal Vessels

The arterial supply to the adrenal gland originates from three sources (Fig. 1–21). Superiorly, branches from the inferior phrenic artery feed the adrenal, while middle

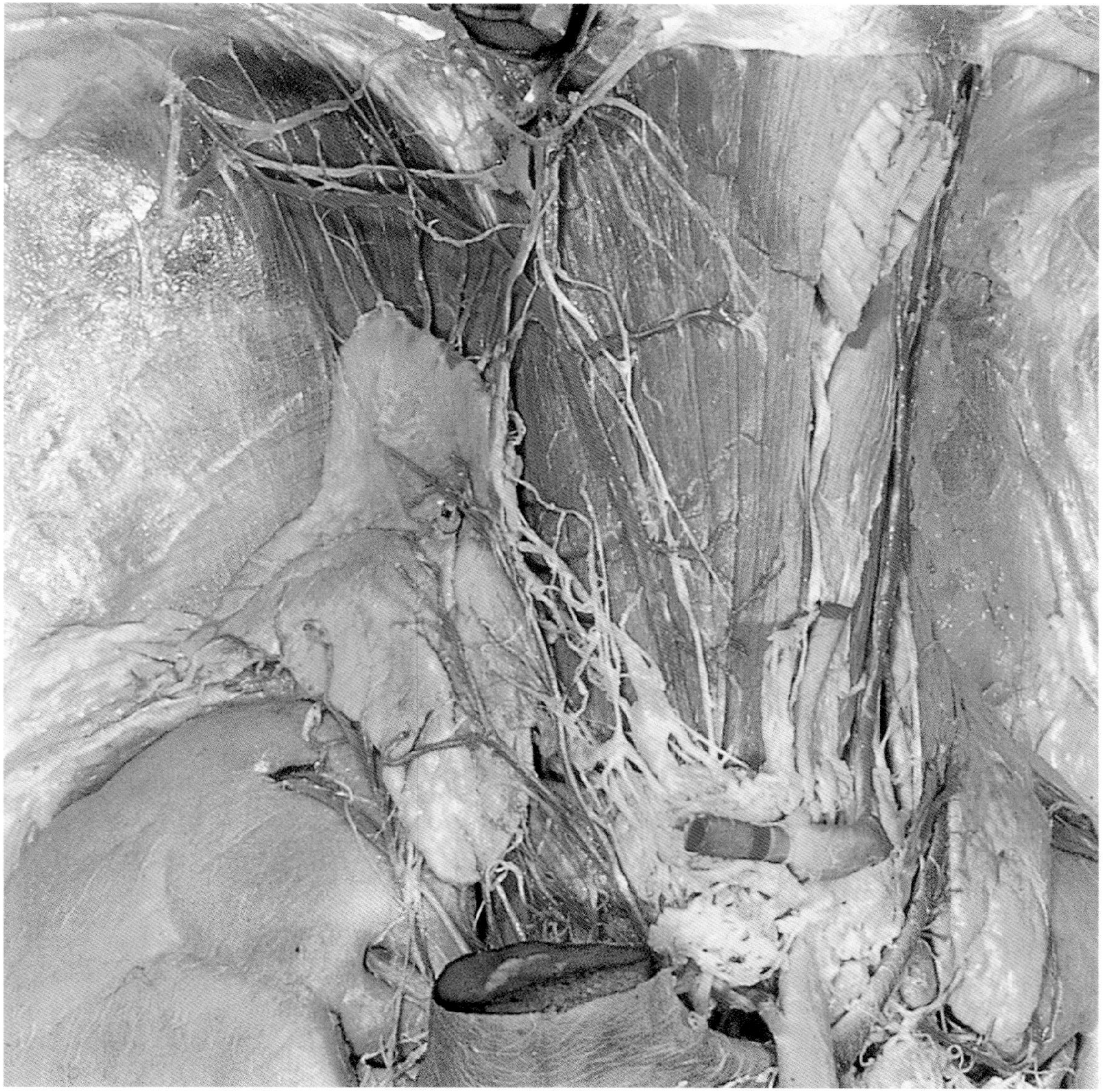

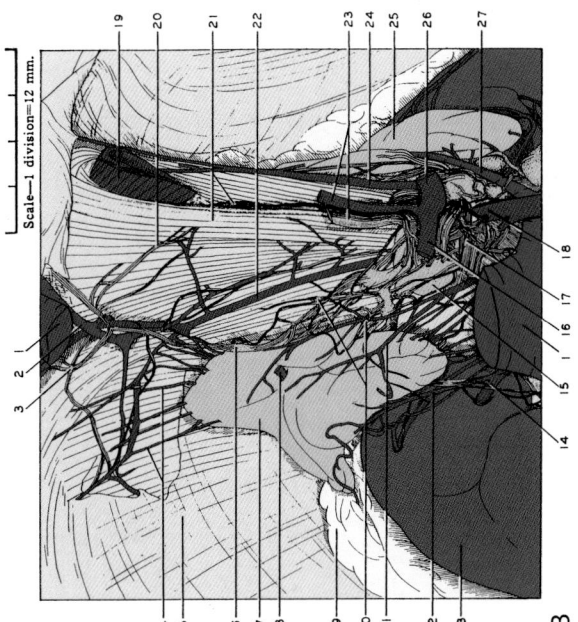

Scale—1 division=12 mm.

B

Figure 1–19. **A,** Right adrenal gland dissected. The inferior vena cava has been excised to fully expose the gland. The celiac arterial trunk, its branches, and associated autonomic nervous plexus are also well demonstrated. **B,** 1, Inferior vena cava (cut). 2, Right inferior phrenic vein. 3, Right phrenic nerve. 4, Superior adrenal arteries (branching from right inferior phrenic artery). 5, Diaphragm. 6, Inferior phrenic ganglion. 7, Right adrenal gland. 8, Right adrenal vein (cut). 9, Pararenal retroperitoneal fat. 10, Autonomic nerves to adrenal gland. 11, Middle adrenal artery (from aorta). 12, Inferior adrenal artery (from renal artery). 13, Right kidney. 14, Branch of right renal artery. 15, Celiac ganglion. 16, Common hepatic artery. 17, Celiac autonomic nervous plexus. 18, Superior mesenteric artery. 19, Esophagus (cut). 20, Branch of phrenic nerve. 21, *Upper pointer,* right crus of diaphragm; *lower pointer,* vagus nerve. 22, Right inferior phrenic artery. 23, *Upper pointer,* left gastric artery; *lower pointer,* superior extension of celiac autonomic nervous plexus. 24, Left inferior phrenic artery. 25, Left adrenal gland. 26, Splenic artery. 27, Left adrenal vein.

Continued

A

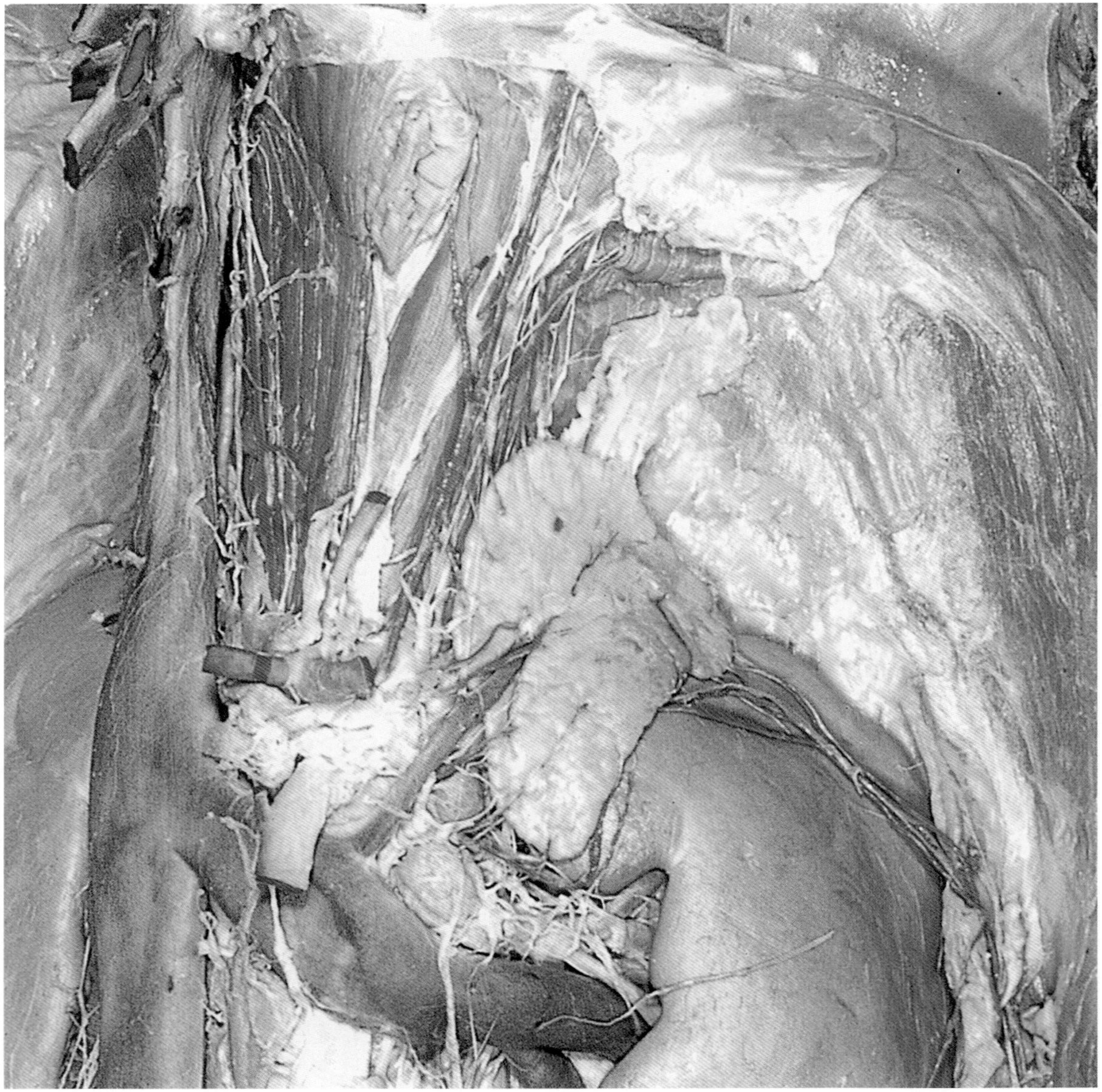

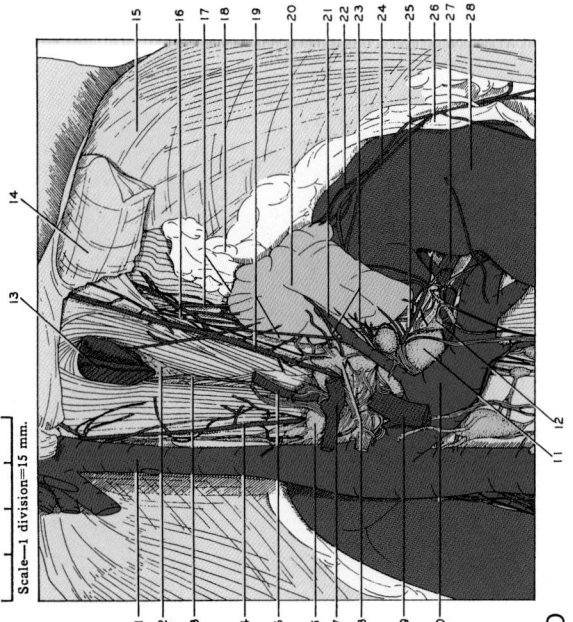

Scale—1 division=15 mm.

D

1
2
3
4
5
6
7
8
9
10

11 12

13 14

15
16
17
18
19
20
21
22
23
24
25
26
27
28

C

Figure 1-19, cont'd. **C,** Left adrenal gland dissected. **D,** 1, Inferior vena cava. 2, Esophageal hiatus. 3, Vagus nerve. 4, Right inferior phrenic artery. 5, Left gastric artery. 6, Right celiac ganglion. 7, Celiac artery. 8, Left celiac ganglion. 9, Superior mesenteric artery. 10, Left renal vein. 11, Renal hilar lymph node. 12, Renal autonomic nervous plexus. 13, Esophagus (cut). 14, Peritoneum (cut). 15, Diaphragm. 16, Phrenic autonomic nervous plexus. 17, *Upper pointer,* superior adrenal arteries (from inferior phrenic artery); *ower pointer,* superior margin of left adrenal gland. 18, Perinephric fat. 19, *Upper pointer,* left inferior phrenic artery; *lower pointer,* medial margin of left adrenal gland. 20, Left adrenal gland. 21, Left adrenal vein. 22, Inferior adrenal artery (in this case branching from perinephric/capsular artery of kidney). 23, Middle adrenal arteries (from aorta). 24, Perinephric blood vessels within Gerota's fascia. 25, Inferior adrenal artery (from renal artery). 26, Perinephric fat. 27, Branch of left renal artery. 28, Left kidney. (**A** to **D,** Reproduced from the Bassett anatomic collection, with permission granted by Dr. Robert A. Chase.)

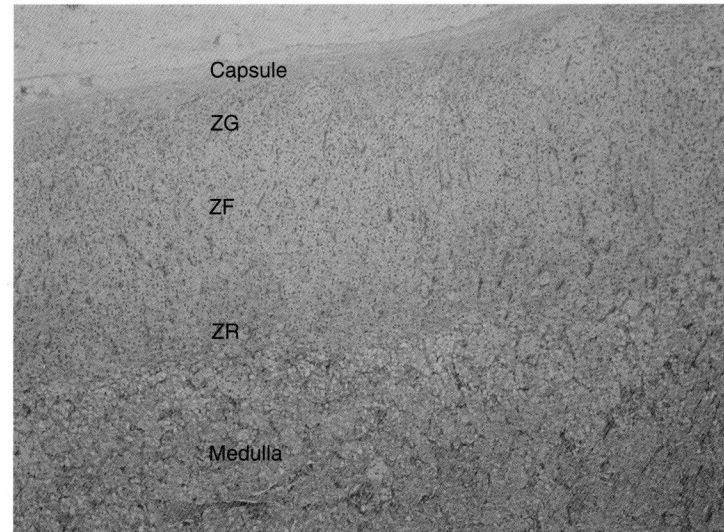

Figure 1–20. Microscopic section of the adrenal gland showing the adrenal medulla and cortex. The three cortical layers are visible: zona glomerulosa (ZG), zona fasciculata (ZF), and zona reticularis (ZR). (Courtesy of Dr. Hossein Saboorian.)

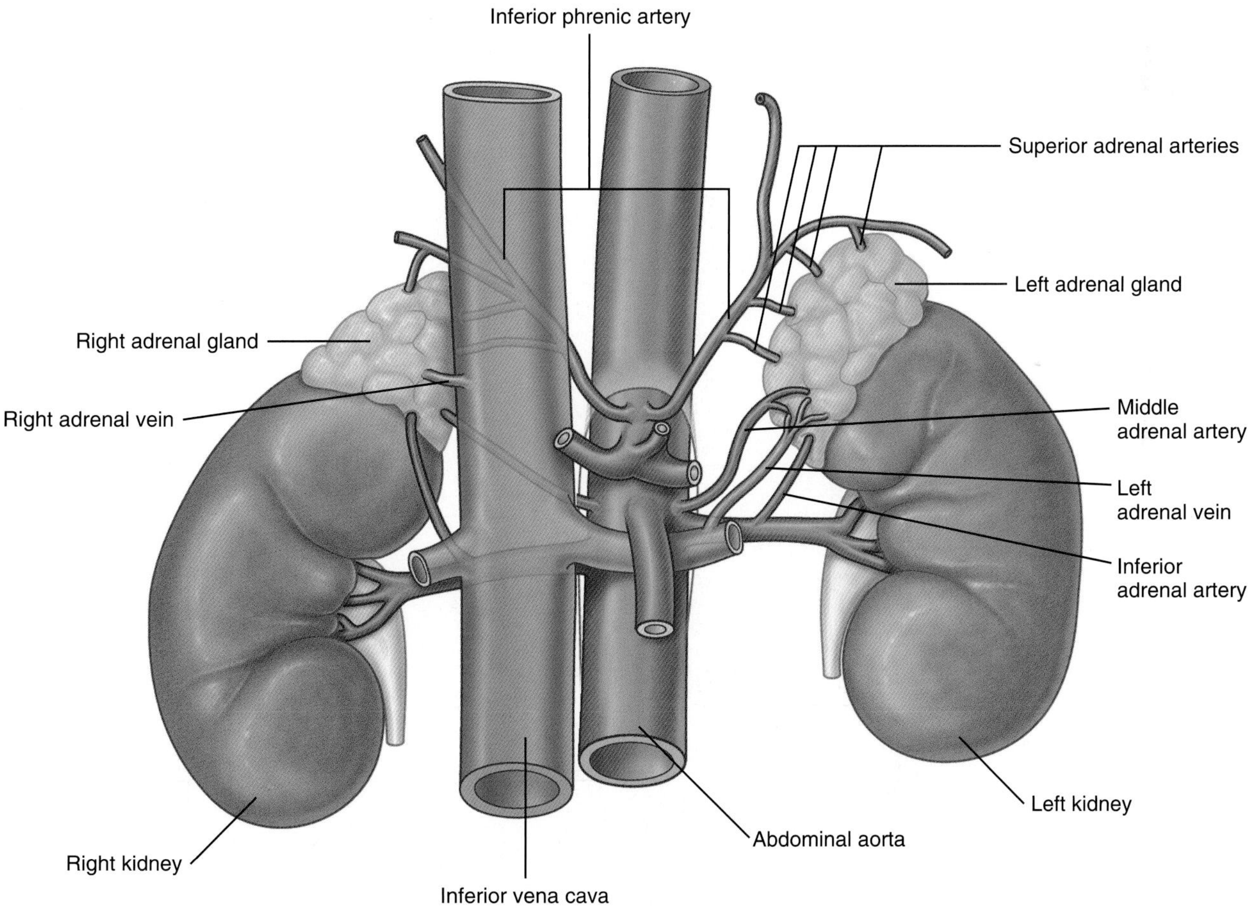

Figure 1–21. Arterial supply to the adrenal glands. (From Drake RL, Vogl W, Mitchell AWM: Gray's Anatomy for Students. Philadelphia, Elsevier, 2005, p 329.)

branches originate directly from the aorta. Finally, branches from the ipsilateral renal artery supply the adrenal gland. The venous drainage varies by side, although both adrenal glands are drained by a single large vein that exits anteromedially. On the left side this vein joins with the inferior phrenic vein and enters the cranial aspect of the left renal vein. On the right side, the adrenal vein enters the IVC directly on its posterolateral aspect. The lymphatic drainage of the adrenals follows the course of these veins and empties into para-aortic lymph nodes.

THE KIDNEYS
Gross and Microscopic Anatomy

The kidneys serve a number of important functions required to maintain normal human physiologic function. They are the primary organ for maintaining fluid and electrolyte balance, and they play a large role in maintaining acid-base balance. They produce renin, which plays a vital role in controlling blood pressure, and erythropoietin, affecting red blood cell production. They affect calcium metabolism, in particular calcium absorption, by converting a precursor of vitamin D to the most active form 1,25-dihydroxyvitamin D.

Grossly, the kidneys are bilaterally paired reddish brown organs (see Figs. 1–1 and 1–22). Typically each kidney weighs 150 g in the male and 135 g in the female. The kidneys generally measure 10 to 12 cm vertically, 5 to 7 cm transversely,

and 3 cm in the anteroposterior dimension. Because of compression by the liver, the right kidney tends to be somewhat shorter and wider. In children, the kidneys are relatively larger and possess more prominent fetal lobations. These lobations are present at birth and generally disappear by the first year of life, although occasionally they persist into adulthood. An additional common feature of the gross renal anatomy is a focal renal parenchymal bulge along the kidney's lateral contour, known as a dromedary hump. This is a normal variation without pathologic significance. It is more common on the left than the right and is believed to be caused by downward pressure from the spleen or liver.

As one proceeds centrally from the peripherally located reddish brown parenchyma of the kidney, the renal sinus is encountered. Here the vascular structures and collecting system coalesce before exiting the kidney medially. These structures are surrounded by yellow sinus fat, which provides an easily recognized landmark during renal procedures such are partial nephrectomy. At its medial border, the renal sinus narrows to form the renal hilum. It is through the hilum that the renal artery, renal vein, and renal pelvis exit the kidney and proceed to their respective destinations.

Both grossly and microscopically there are two distinct components within the renal parenchyma: the medulla and the cortex. **Unlike the adrenal gland, the renal medulla is not a contiguous layer. Instead, the medulla is composed of multiple, distinct, conically shaped areas noticeably darker in color than the cortex** (Fig. 1–22). **These same structures are**

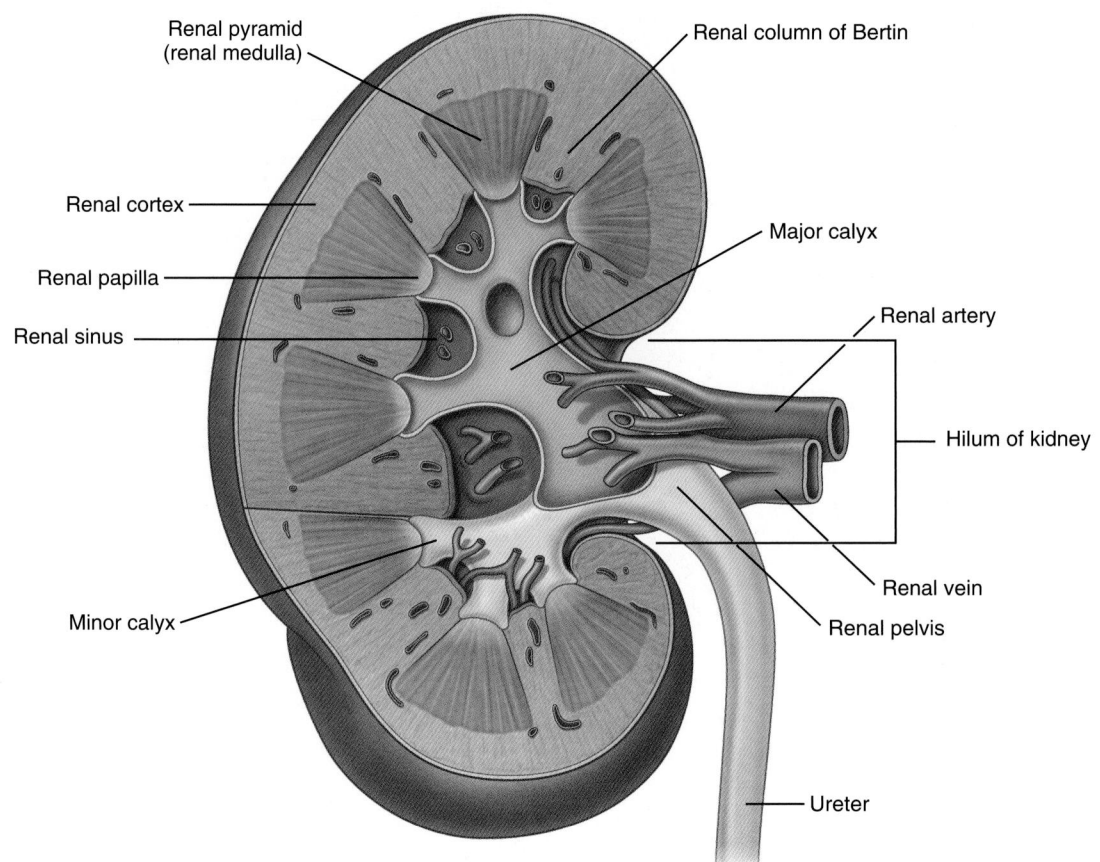

Figure 1–22. Internal structure of the kidney. (From Drake RL, Vogl W, Mitchell AWM: Gray's Anatomy for Students. Philadelphia, Elsevier, 2005, p 323.)

KEY POINTS: THE KIDNEYS

- The kidney is divided into cortex and medulla. The medullary areas are pyramidal, more centrally located, and separated by sections of cortex. These segments of cortex are called the columns of Bertin.

- Orientation of the kidney is greatly affected by the structures around it. Thus the upper poles are situated more medially and posteriorly than the lower poles. Also, the medial aspect of the kidney is more anterior than the lateral aspect.

- Gerota's fascia envelops the kidney on all aspects except inferiorly, where it is not closed but instead remains an open potential space.

- From anterior to posterior, the renal hilar structures are the renal vein, renal artery, and collecting system.

- The renal artery splits into segmental branches. Typically, the first branch is the posterior segmental artery, which passes posterior to the collecting system. There are generally three to four anterior segmental branches that pass anteriorly to supply the anterior kidney.

- The progression of arterial supply to the kidney is as follows: renal artery → segmental artery → interlobar artery → arcuate artery → interlobular artery → afferent artery.

- The venous system anastomoses freely throughout the kidney. The arterial supply does not. Thus, occlusion of a segmental artery leads to parenchymal infarction but occlusion of a segmental vein is not problematic because there are many alternate drainage routes.

- Anatomic variations in the renal vasculature are common, occurring in 25% to 40% of kidneys.

- Each renal pyramid terminates centrally in a papilla. Each papilla is cupped by a minor calyx. A group of minor calyces join to form a major calyx. The major calyces combine to form the renal pelvis. There is great variation in the number of calyces, calyceal size, and renal pelvis size. The only way to determine pathologic from normal is by evidence of dysfunction.

also frequently called **renal pyramids, making the terms** *renal medulla* and *renal pyramid* **synonymous. The apex of the pyramid is the renal papilla, and each papilla is cupped by an individual minor calyx.**

The renal cortex is lighter in color than the medulla and not only covers the renal pyramids peripherally but also extends between the pyramids themselves. The extensions of cortex between the renal pyramids are given a special name: the **columns of Bertin.** These columns are significant surgically because it is through these columns that renal vessels traverse from the renal sinus to the peripheral cortex, decreasing in diameter as the columns move peripherally. It is because of

this anatomy that percutaneous access to the collecting system is made through a renal pyramid into a calyx, thus avoiding the columns of Bertin and the larger vessels present within them.

Relations and Investing Fascia

Anatomic Relationships

The position of the kidney within the retroperitoneum varies greatly by side, degree of inspiration, body position, and presence of anatomic anomalies (Fig. 1–23). The right kidney sits 1 to 2 cm lower than the left in most individuals owing to displacement by the liver. Generally, the right kidney resides in the space between the top of the 1st lumbar vertebra to the bottom of the 3rd lumbar vertebra. The left kidney occupies a more superior space from the body of the 12th thoracic vertebral body to the 3rd lumbar vertebra.

Of surgical importance are the structures surrounding the kidney (see Figs. 1–9 and 1–24). Both kidneys have similar muscular surroundings. Posteriorly, the diaphragm covers the upper third of each kidney, with the 12th rib crossing at the lower extent of the diaphragm. Also important to note for percutaneous renal procedures and flank incisions is that the pleura extends to the level of the 12th rib posteriorly. Medially the lower two thirds of the kidney lie against the psoas muscle, and laterally the quadratus lumborum and aponeu-

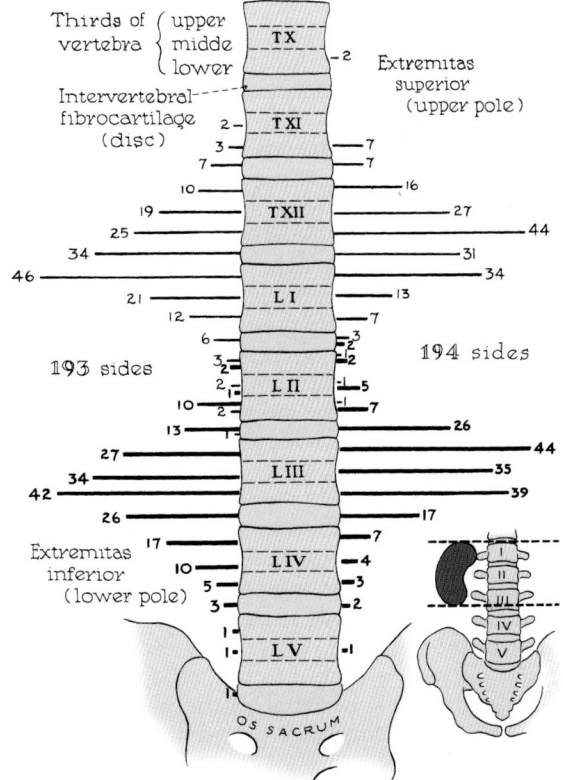

Figure 1–23. Variation between individuals in level of the kidneys relative to the spinal column. *Lighter lateral lines* represent upper poles of kidneys; *darker lateral lines* represent lower poles. (From Anson BJ, Daseler EH: Common variations in renal anatomy, affecting blood supply, form, and topography. Surg Gynecol Obstet 1961;112:439-449.)

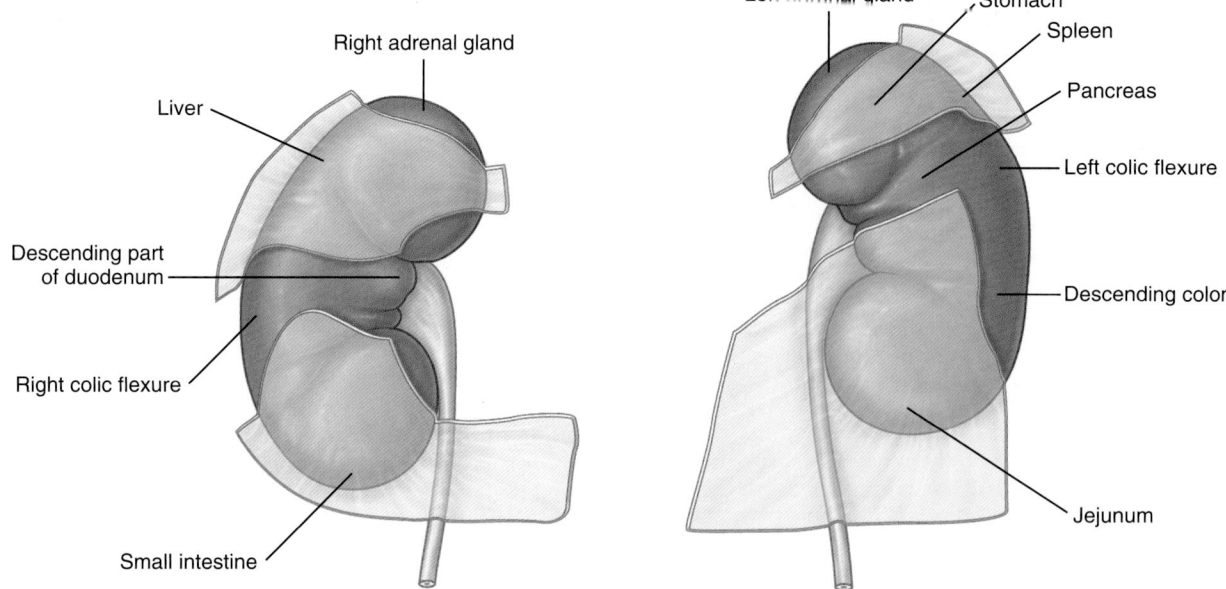

Figure 1–24. Structures related to the anterior surfaces of each kidney. (From Drake RL, Vogl W, Mitchell AWM: Gray's Anatomy for Students. Philadelphia, Elsevier, 2005, p 321.)

rosis of the transversus abdominis muscle are encountered. The effect of the muscular relations on the kidneys is several-fold (Fig. 1–25). First, the lower pole of the kidney lies later-ally and anteriorly relative to the upper pole. Second, the medial aspect of each kidney is rotated anteriorly at an angle of approximately 30 degrees. An understanding of this renal orientation is again of particular interest for percutaneous renal procedures in which kidney orientation influences access site selection.

Anteriorly, the right kidney is bordered by a number of structures (see Fig. 1–24). Cranially, the upper pole lies against the liver and is separated from the liver by the peritoneum except for the liver's posterior bare spot. The hepatorenal lig-ament further attaches the right kidney to the liver because this extension of parietal peritoneum bridges the upper pole of the right kidney to the posterior liver. Also at the upper pole, the right adrenal gland is encountered. On the medial aspect, the descending duodenum is intimately related to the medial aspect of the kidney and hilar structures. Finally, on the anterior aspect of the lower pole lies the hepatic flexure of the colon.

The left kidney is bordered superiorly by the tail of the pan-creas with the splenic vessels adjacent to the hilum and upper pole of the left kidney. Also cranial to the upper pole is the left adrenal gland and further superolaterally, the spleen. The splenorenal ligament attaches the left kidney to the spleen. This attachment can lead to splenic capsular tears if excessive downward pressure is applied to the left kidney. Superior to the pancreatic tail, the posterior gastric wall can overlie the kidney. Caudally, the kidney is covered by the splenic flexure of the colon.

Gerota's Fascia

Interposed between the kidney and its surrounding structures is the perirenal or Gerota's fascia (Figs. 1–26 through 1–28).

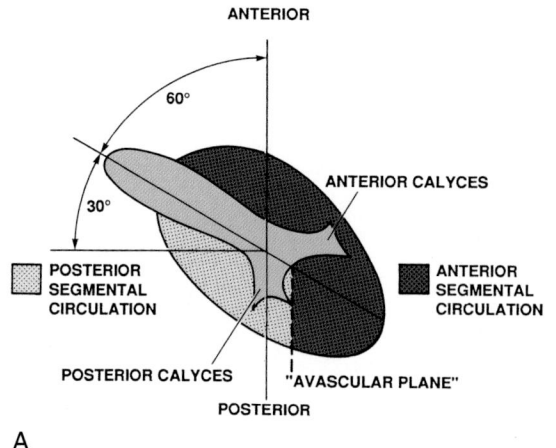

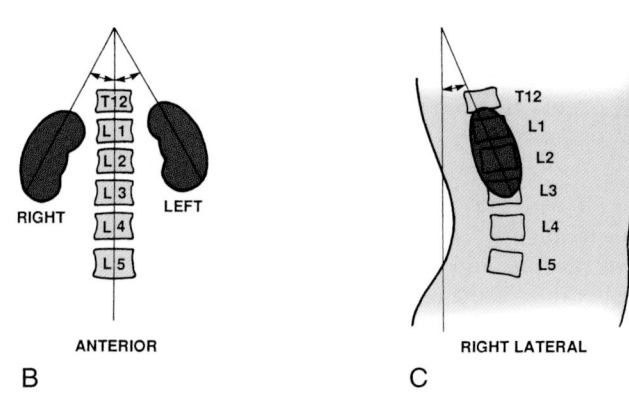

Figure 1–25. Normal rotational axes of the kidney. **A,** Transverse view showing approximate 30-degree anterior rotation of the left kidney from the coronal plane, relative positions of the anterior and posterior rows of calyces, and location of the relatively avascular plane separating the ante-rior and posterior renal circulation. **B,** Coronal section demonstrating slight inward tilt of the upper poles of the kidneys. **C,** Sagittal view showing ante-rior displacement of the lower pole of the right kidney.

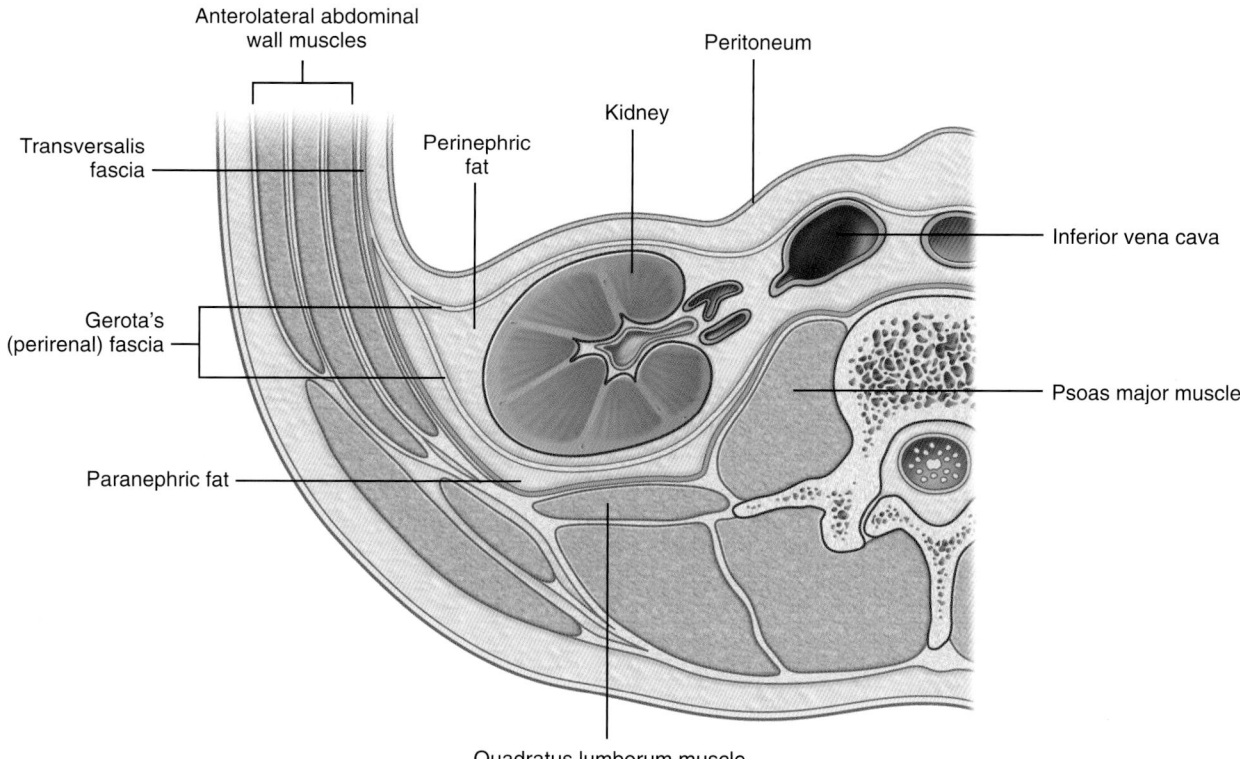

Figure 1–26. Organization of the fat and fascia surrounding the kidney. (From Drake RL, Vogl W, Mitchell AWM: Gray's Anatomy for Students. Philadelphia, Elsevier, 2005, p 322.)

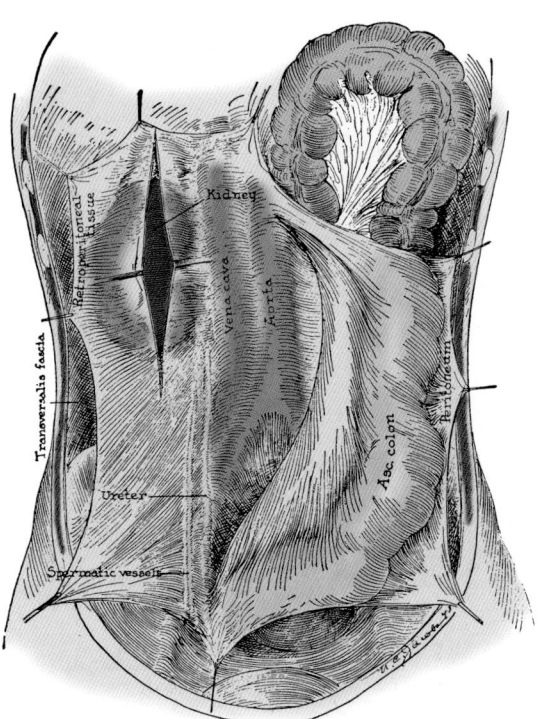

Figure 1–27. Anterior view of Gerota's fascia on the right side, split over the right kidney (which it contains), and showing inferior extension enveloping the ureter and gonadal vessels. The ascending colon and overlying peritoneum have been reflected medially. (From Tobin CE: The renal fascia and its relation to the transversalis fascia. Anat Rec 1944;89:295-311.)

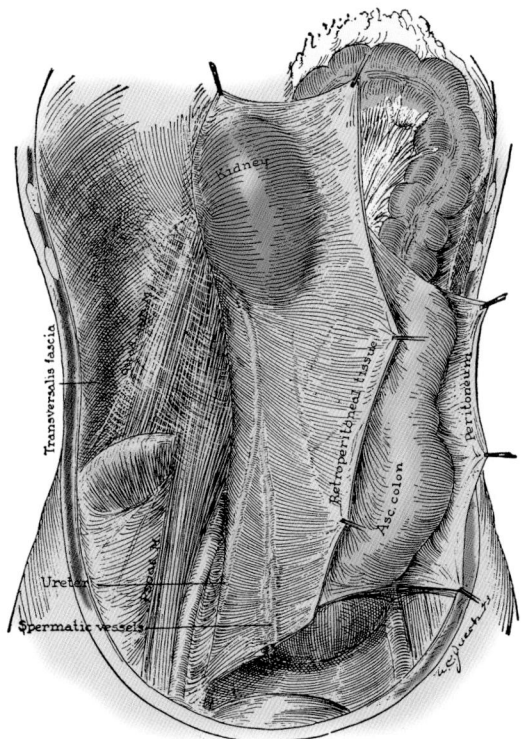

Figure 1–28. Posterior view of Gerota's fascia on the right side, rotated medially with the contained kidney, ureter, and gonadal vessels, exposing the muscular posterior body wall covered by the transversalis fascia. (From Tobin CE: The renal fascia and its relation to the transversalis fascia. Anat Rec 1944;89:295-311.)

This fascial layer encompasses the perirenal fat and kidney and encloses the kidney on three sides: superiorly, medially, and laterally. Superiorly and laterally Gerota's fascia is closed, but medially it extends across the midline to fuse with the contralateral side. Inferiorly, Gerota's fascia is not closed and remains an open potential space. Gerota's fascia serves as an anatomic barrier to the spread of malignancy as well as a means of containing perinephric fluid collections. Thus, perinephric fluid collections can track inferiorly into the pelvis without violating Gerota's fascia.

Renal Vasculature

The renal pedicle classically consists of a single artery and a single vein that enter the kidney via the renal hilum (see Fig. 1–22). These structures branch from the aorta and inferior vena cava just below the superior mesenteric artery at the level of the second lumbar vertebra. **The vein is anterior to the artery. The renal pelvis and ureter are located further posterior to these vascular structures.**

Renal Artery

Specifically, the right renal artery leaves the aorta and progresses with a caudal slope under the IVC toward the right kidney. The left renal artery courses almost directly laterally to the left kidney. Given the rotational axis of the kidney (see Fig. 1–25), both renal arteries move posteriorly as they enter the kidney. Also, both arteries have branches to the respective adrenal gland, renal pelvis, and ureter.

Upon approaching the kidney, the renal artery splits into four or more branches, with five being the most common. These are the renal segmental arteries (Fig. 1–29). **Each seg-**mental artery supplies a distinct portion of the kidney with no collateral circulation between them (Fig. 1–30). **Thus, occlusion or injury to a segmental branch will cause segmental renal infarction.** Generally, the first and most constant branch is the posterior segmental branch, which separates from the renal artery before it enters the renal hilum. There are typically four anterior branches, which from superior to inferior are apical, upper, middle, and lower. The relationship of these segmental arteries is important because the posterior segmental branch will pass posterior to the renal pelvis while the others pass anterior to the renal pelvis. Ureteropelvic junction obstruction caused by a crossing vessel can occur when the posterior segmental branch passes anterior to the ureter causing occlusion. This division between the posterior and anterior segmental arteries has an additional surgical importance in that between these circulations is an avascular plane (see Figs. 1–25 and 1–30). This longitudinal plane lies just posterior to the lateral aspect of the kidney. Incision within this plane results in significantly less blood loss than outside this plane. However, there is significant variation in the location of this plane, requiring delineation before incision. This can be done with either preoperative angiography or intraoperative segmental arterial injection of a dye, such as methylene blue.

Once in the renal sinus, the segmental arteries branch into **lobar arteries,** which further subdivide in the renal parenchyma to form **interlobar** arteries (Fig. 1–31). These interlobar arteries progress peripherally within the cortical columns of Bertin, thus avoiding the renal pyramids but maintaining a close association with the minor calyceal infundibula. At the base (peripheral edge) of the renal pyramids, the interlobar arteries branch into **arcuate arteries.**

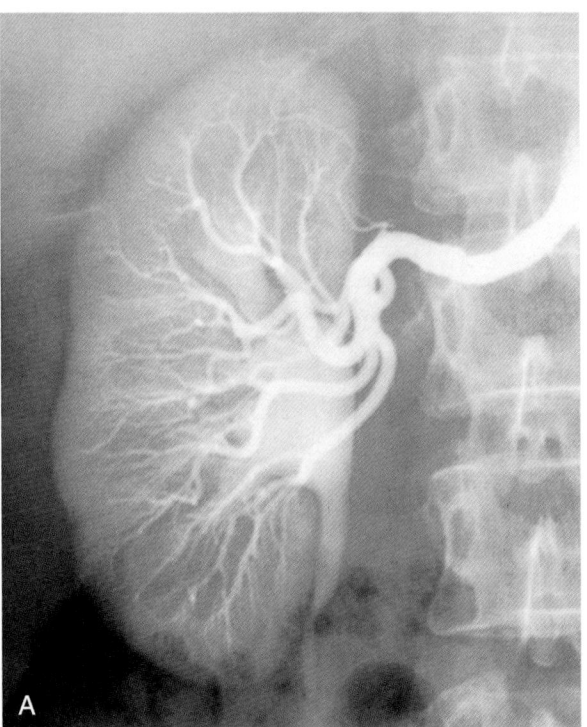

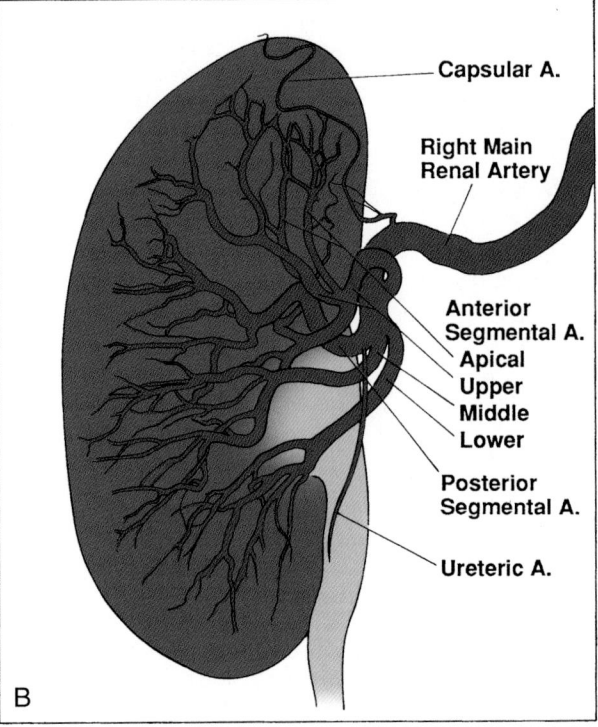

Figure 1-29. **A** and **B,** Segmental branches of the right renal artery demonstrated by renal angiogram.

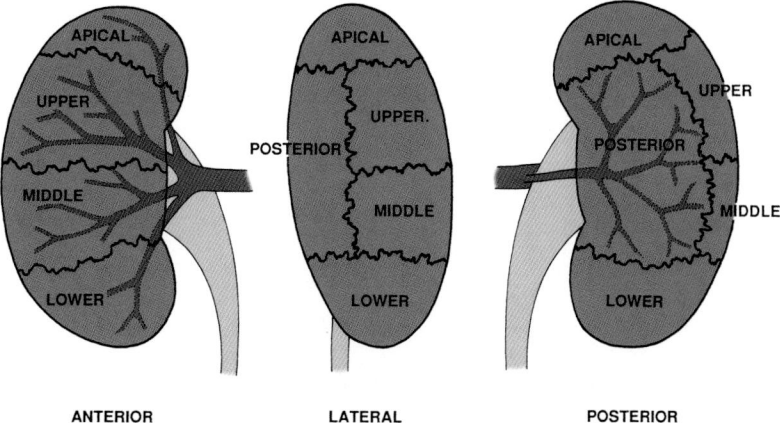

Figure 1–30. Typical segmental circulation of the right kidney, shown diagrammatically. Note that the posterior segmental artery is usually the first branch of the main renal artery and it extends behind the renal pelvis.

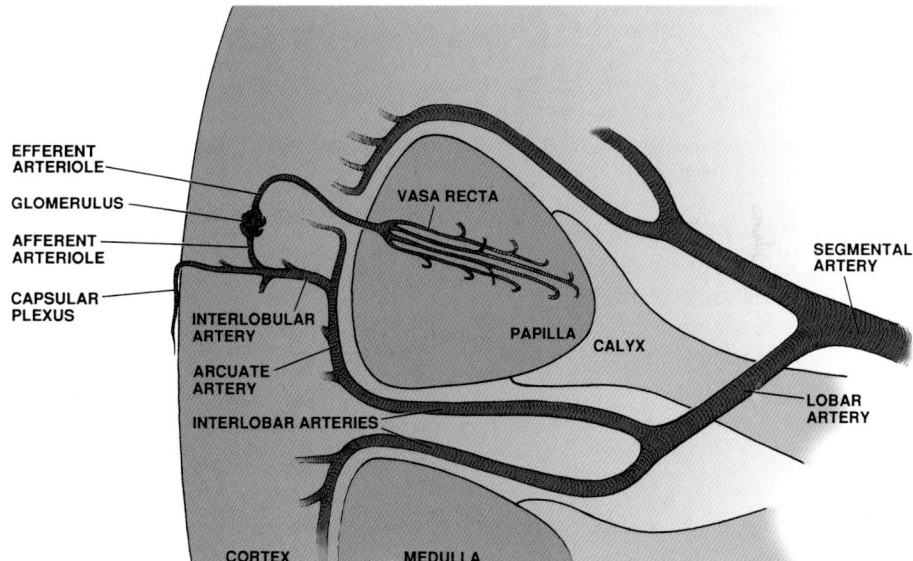

Figure 1–31. Intrarenal arterial anatomy.

Instead of moving peripherally, the arcuate arteries parallel the edge of the corticomedullary junction. **Interlobular arteries** branch off the arcuate arteries and move radially, where they eventually divide to form the **afferent arteries** to the glomeruli.

The 2 million glomeruli within each kidney represent the core of the renal filtration process. Each glomerulus is fed by an afferent arteriole. As blood flows through the glomerular capillaries, the urinary filtrate leaves the arterial system and is collected in the glomerular (Bowman's) capsule. Blood flow leaves the glomerular capillary via the efferent arteriole and continues to one of two locations: secondary capillary networks around the urinary tubules in the cortex or descending into the renal medulla as the vasa recta.

Renal Veins

The renal venous drainage correlates closely with the arterial supply. **The interlobular veins drain the post glomerular capillaries. These veins also communicate freely via a subcapsular venous plexus of stellate veins with veins in the perinephric fat. After the interlobular veins, the venous drainage progresses through the arcuate, interlobar, lobar, and segmental branches, with the course of each of these branches paralleling the respective artery.** After the segmental branches, the venous drainage coalesces into three to five venous trunks that eventually combine to form the renal vein. **Unlike the arterial supply, the venous drainage communicates freely through venous collars around the infundibula, providing for extensive collateral circulation in the venous drainage of the kidney** (Fig. 1–32). **Surgically, this is important, because unlike the arterial supply, occlusion of a segmental venous branch has little effect on venous outflow.**

The renal vein is located directly anterior to the renal artery, although this position can vary up to 1-2 cm cranially or caudally relative to the artery. The right renal vein is generally 2 to 4 cm in length and enters the right lateral to posterolateral edge of the IVC. The left renal vein is typically 6 to 10 cm in length and enters the left lateral aspect of the IVC after passing posterior to the superior mesenteric artery and anterior to the aorta (Fig. 1–33). Compared with the right renal vein, the left renal vein enters the IVC at a slightly more cranial level and a more anterolateral location. **Additionally, the left renal vein receives the left adrenal vein superiorly, lumbar vein posteriorly, and left gonadal vein inferiorly** (see Fig. 1–32). The right renal vein typically does not receive any branches.

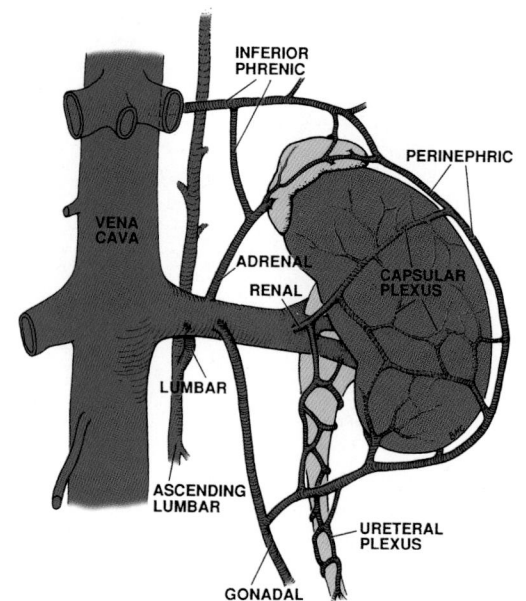

Figure 1–32. Venous drainage of the left kidney showing potentially extensive venous collateral circulation.

Common Anatomic Variants

Anatomic variations in the renal vasculature are common, occurring in 25% to 40% of kidneys. The most common variation is supernumerary renal arteries, with up to five arteries reported. This occurs more often on the left. These additional arteries can enter through the hilum or directly into the parenchyma. **Lower pole arteries on the right tend to cross anterior to the IVC whereas lower pole arteries on either side can cross anterior to the collecting system, causing a ureteropelvic junction obstruction.** When the kidney is ectopic, supernumerary arteries are even more common and their origin even more varied, with the celiac trunk, superior mesenteric artery, or iliac arteries all possible sources of ectopic renal arteries. Supernumerary veins occur as well, but this is a less common entity. The most common example is duplicate renal veins draining the right kidney via the right renal hilum. Polar veins are quite rare. Finally, the left renal vein may course behind the aorta or divide and send one limb anterior and one limb posterior to the aorta, resulting in a collar-type circumaortic formation.

Renal Lymphatics

The renal lymphatics largely follow blood vessels through the columns of Bertin and then form several large lymphatic trunks within the renal sinus. As these lymphatics exit the hilum, branches from the renal capsule, perinephric tissues, renal pelvis, and upper ureter drain into these lymphatics. They then empty into lymph nodes associated with the renal vein near the renal hilum. From here, the lymphatic drainage between the two kidneys varies (Figs. 1–34 and 1–35). **On the left, primary lymphatic drainage is into the left lateral para-aortic lymph nodes including nodes anterior and posterior to the aorta between the inferior mesenteric artery and the**

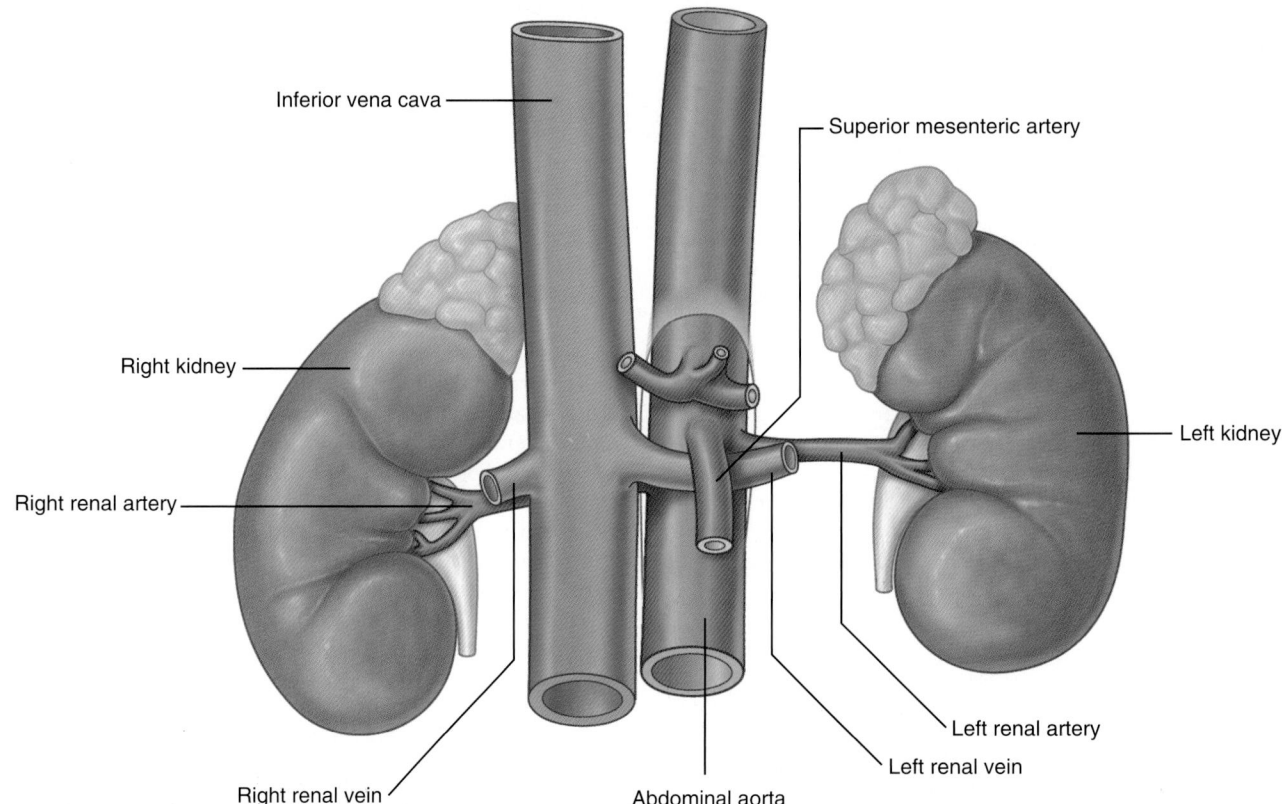

Figure 1–33. Renal vasculature. Note path of left renal vein under the superior mesenteric artery. (From Drake RL, Vogl W, Mitchell AWM: Gray's Anatomy for Students. Philadelphia, Elsevier, 2005, p 324.)

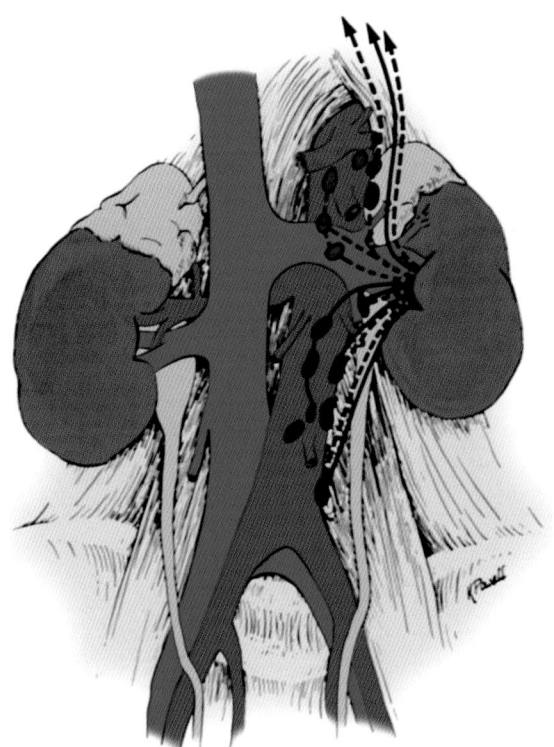

Figure 1–34. Regional lymphatic drainage of the left kidney. *Dark nodes,* anterior; *light nodes,* posterior. *Solid lines,* anterior lymphatic channels; *dashed lines,* posterior lymphatic channels. *Arrows* lead to the thoracic duct.

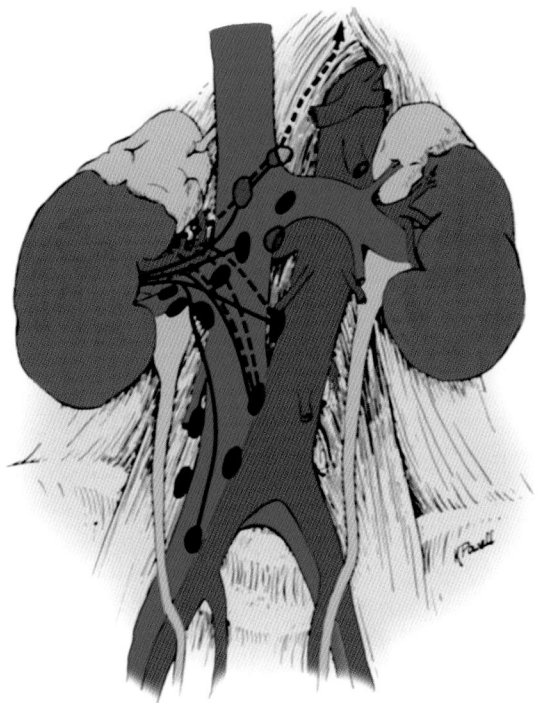

Figure 1–35. Regional lymphatic drainage of the right kidney. *Dark nodes,* anterior; *light nodes,* posterior. *Solid lines,* anterior lymphatic channels; *dashed lines,* posterior lymphatic channels. *Arrow* leads to the thoracic duct.

diaphragm. Occasionally, there will be additional drainage from the left kidney into the retrocrural nodes or directly into the thoracic duct above the diaphragm. On the right, drainage is into the right interaortalcaval and right paracaval lymph nodes, including nodes located anterior and posterior to the vena cava, from the common iliac vessels to the diaphragm. Occasionally, there will be additional drainage from the right kidney into the retrocrural nodes or the left lateral para-aortic lymph nodes.

Renal Collecting System

Microscopic Anatomy from Glomerulus to Collecting System

Microscopically, the renal collecting system originates in the renal cortex at the glomerulus as filtrate enters into Bowman's capsule (Fig. 1–36). Together the glomerular capillary network and Bowman's capsule form the renal corpuscle (malpighian corpuscle) (Fig. 1–37). The glomerular capillary network is covered by specialized epithelial cells called **podocytes** that, along with the capillary epithelium, form a selective barrier across which the urinary filtrate must pass. The filtrate is initially collected in Bowman's capsule and then moves to the proximal convoluted tubule. The **proximal tubule** is composed of a thick cuboidal epithelium covered by dense microvilli. These microvilli greatly increase the surface area of the proximal tubule, allowing a large portion of the urinary filtrate to be reabsorbed in this section of the nephron.

The proximal tubule continues deeper into the cortical tissue where it becomes the **loop of Henle.** The loop of Henle extends variable distances into the renal medulla. Within the renal medulla, the loop of Henle reverses cource and moves back toward the periphery of the kidney. As it ascends out of the medulla the loop thickens and becomes the **distal convoluted tubule.** This tubule eventually returns to a position adjacent to the originating glomerulus and proximal convoluted tubule. Here the distal convoluted tubule turns once again for the interior of the kidney and becomes a collecting tubule. Collecting tubules from multiple nephrons combine into a collecting duct that extends inward through the renal medulla and eventually empties into the apex of the medullary pyramid, the renal papilla.

Renal Papillae, Calyces, and Pelvis

The renal papillae are the tip of a medullary pyramid and constitute the first gross structure of the renal collecting system. Typically, there are 7 to 9 papillae per kidney, but this number is variable, ranging from 4 to 18. The papillae are aligned in two longitudinal rows situated approximately 90 degrees from one another. There is an anterior row that owing to the orientation of the kidney faces in a lateral direction and a posterior row that extends directly posterior (see Figs. 1–25 and 1–38). **Each of these papillae is cupped by a minor calyx** (see Fig. 1–22). At the upper and lower poles, compound calyces are often encountered. These compound calyces are the result of renal pyramid fusion and because of their anatomy are more likely to allow reflux into the renal parenchyma (Fig. 1–39). Clinically, this can result in more severe scarring of the parenchyma overlying compound calyces.

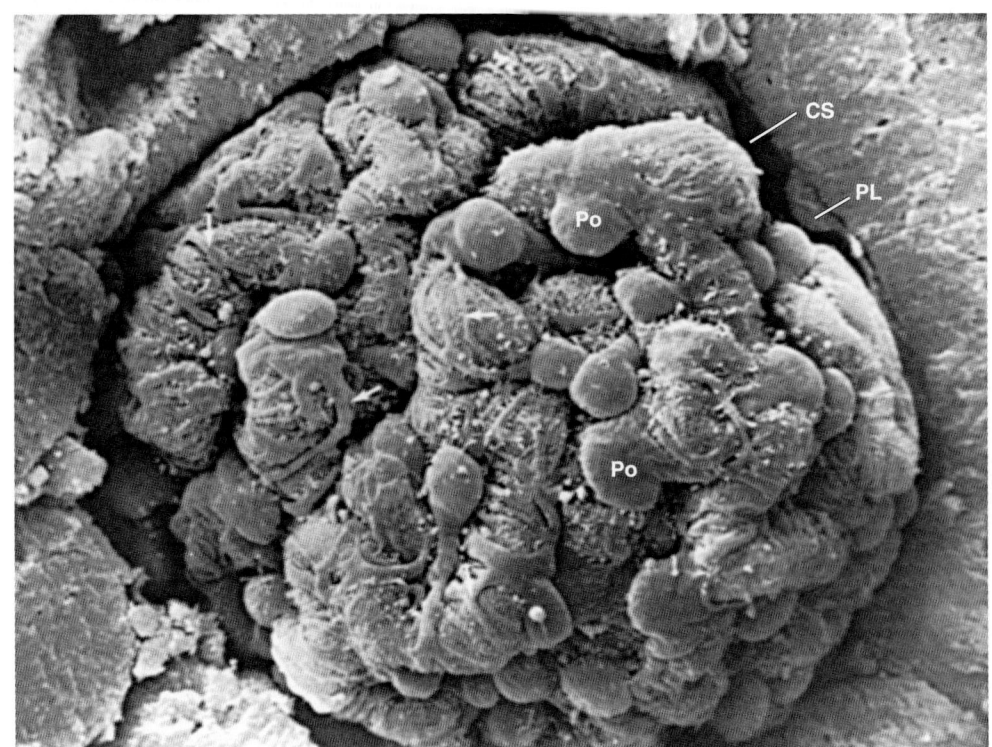

Figure 1–36. Electron micrograph of the renal corpuscle. The glomerular capillary network is enveloped by podocytes and contained within Bowman's capsule. CS, capsular space of Bowman; PL, parietal layer of Bowman's capsule; Po, podocyte. *Arrows* indicate cytoplasmic extensions from podocytes that enwrap the glomerular capillaries. (From Kessel RG, Kardon RH: Tissues and Organs: A Text-Atlas of Scanning Electron Microscopy. Copyright 1979 by WH Freeman and Co.)

After cupping an individual papillae, each minor calyx narrows to an infundibulum. Just as there is frequent variation in the number of calyces, the diameter and length of the infundibula varies greatly. **Infundibuli combine to form two or three major calyceal branches. These are frequently termed the *upper, middle, and lower pole calyces,* and these calyces in turn combine to form the renal pelvis. The renal pelvis itself can vary greatly in size, ranging from a small intrarenal pelvis to a large predominantly extrarenal pelvis.** Eventually the pelvis narrows to form the ureteropelvic junction, marking the beginning of the ureter.

On close examination, it is clear that there is significant variation in the anatomy of the renal collecting system (Figs. 1–40 through 1–42). Number of calyces, diameter of the infundibuli, and size of the renal pelvis all vary significantly between normal individuals. Even in the same individual, the renal collecting systems may be similar but are rarely identical. **Because of this variation, it can be difficult to distinguish pathologic from normal based on anatomy alone. Instead, it is demonstrated dysfunction that is needed to make the diagnosis of a pathologic anatomic formation within the renal collecting system.**

Renal Innervation

Sympathetic preganglionic nerves originate from the eighth thoracic through first lumbar spinal segments and then travel to the celiac and aorticorenal ganglia. From here, postganglionic fibers travel to the kidney via the autonomic plexus surrounding the renal artery. Parasympathetic fibers originate from the vagus nerve and travel with the sympathetic fibers to the autonomic plexus along the renal artery. The primary function of the renal autonomic innervation is vasomotor, with the sympathetics inducing vasoconstriction and the parasympathetics causing vasodilation. Despite this innervation, it is important to realize that the kidney functions well even without this neurologic control, as evidenced by the successful function of transplanted kidneys.

THE URETERS

KEY POINT: THE URETERS

■ The course of the ureter begins posterior to the renal artery and continues along the anterior edge of the psoas muscle. The gonadal vessels cross anterior to the ureter in this region. The ureter next passes over the iliac vessels, generally marking the bifurcation of common iliac into internal and external iliacs.

The ureters are bilateral tubular structures responsible for transporting urine from the renal pelvis to the bladder (see Fig. 1–1). They are generally 22 to 30 cm in length with a wall composed of multiple layers (Fig. 1–43). The inner layer is transitional epithelium. Next is the lamina propria. This is a connective tissue layer that along with the epithelium makes up the mucosal lining. Overlying the lamina propria is a layer of smooth muscle that is contiguous with muscle covering the renal calyces and pelvis, although in the ureter this layer is

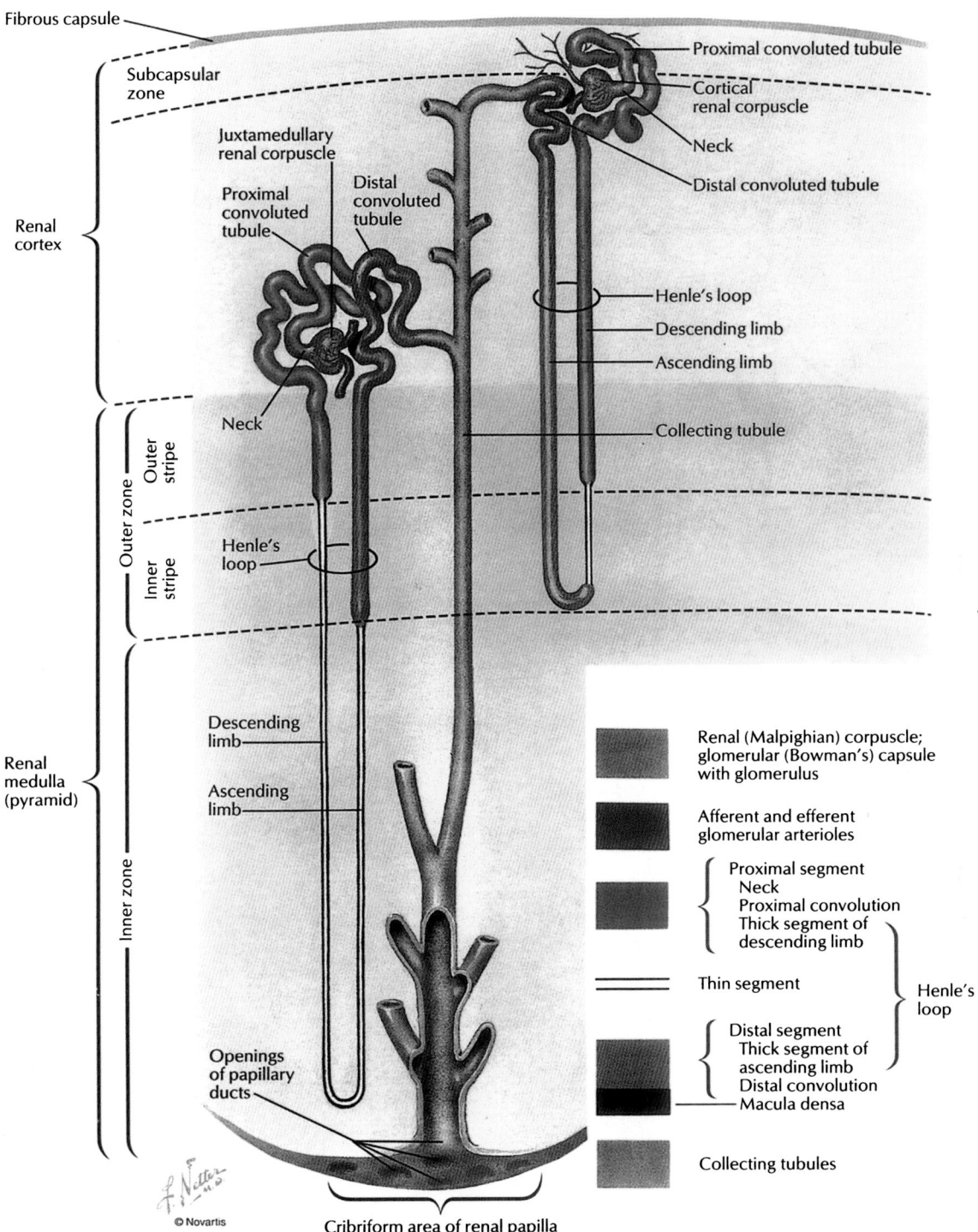

Figure 1–37.   Renal nephron and collecting tubule. (From Netter F: Atlas of Human Anatomy, 2nd ed. Summit, NJ, Novartis Corp., Plate 317.)

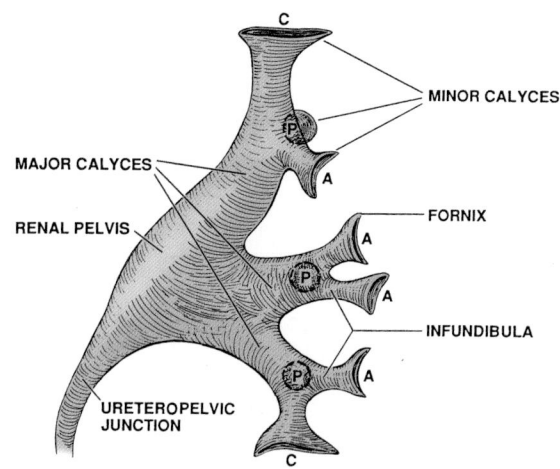

Figure 1–38. The renal collecting system (left kidney) showing major divisions into minor calyces, major calyces, and renal pelvis. A, anterior minor calyces; C, compound calyces at the renal poles; P, posterior minor calyces.

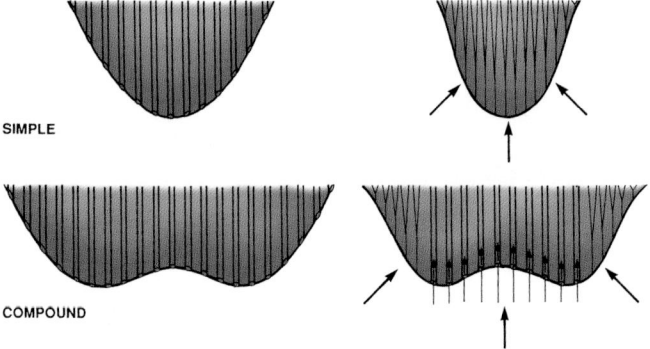

Figure 1–39. Diagram demonstrating structural and functional distinctions between simple and compound renal papillae. Back pressure causes closure of the collecting ducts in a simple papilla, effectively preventing reflux of urine into the renal parenchyma. The structure of the compound papilla allows intrarenal reflux of urine with sufficient back pressure.

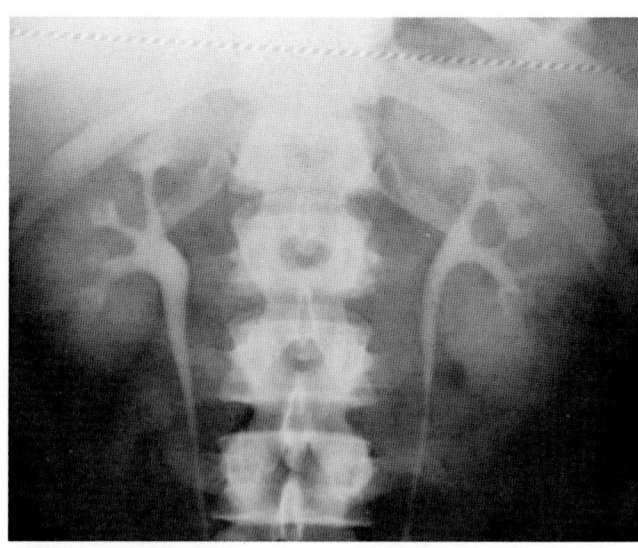

Figure 1–40. Normal bilateral renal collecting systems, demonstrated by excretory urography.

divided into an inner longitudinal and an outer circular layer. Together, these muscular layers provide the peristaltic wave that actively transports urine from the renal collecting system through the ureter to the bladder. The outermost layer is the adventitia. This thin layer surrounds the ureter and encompasses the blood vessels and lymphatics that travel along the ureter.

Anatomic Relationships

Key to many urologic procedures is an understanding of ureteral anatomic relationships. The ureter begins at the ureteropelvic junction, which lies posterior to the renal artery

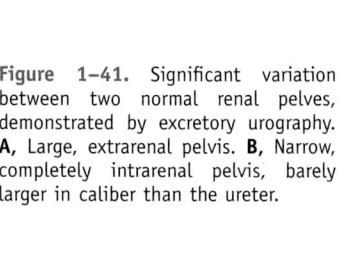

Figure 1–41. Significant variation between two normal renal pelves, demonstrated by excretory urography. **A,** Large, extrarenal pelvis. **B,** Narrow, completely intrarenal pelvis, barely larger in caliber than the ureter.

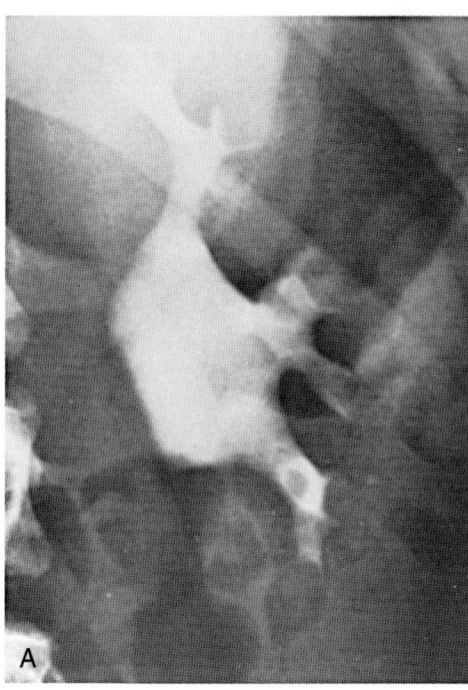

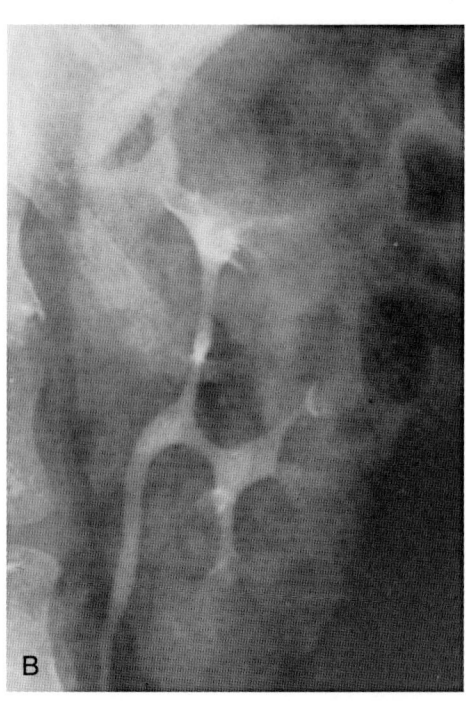

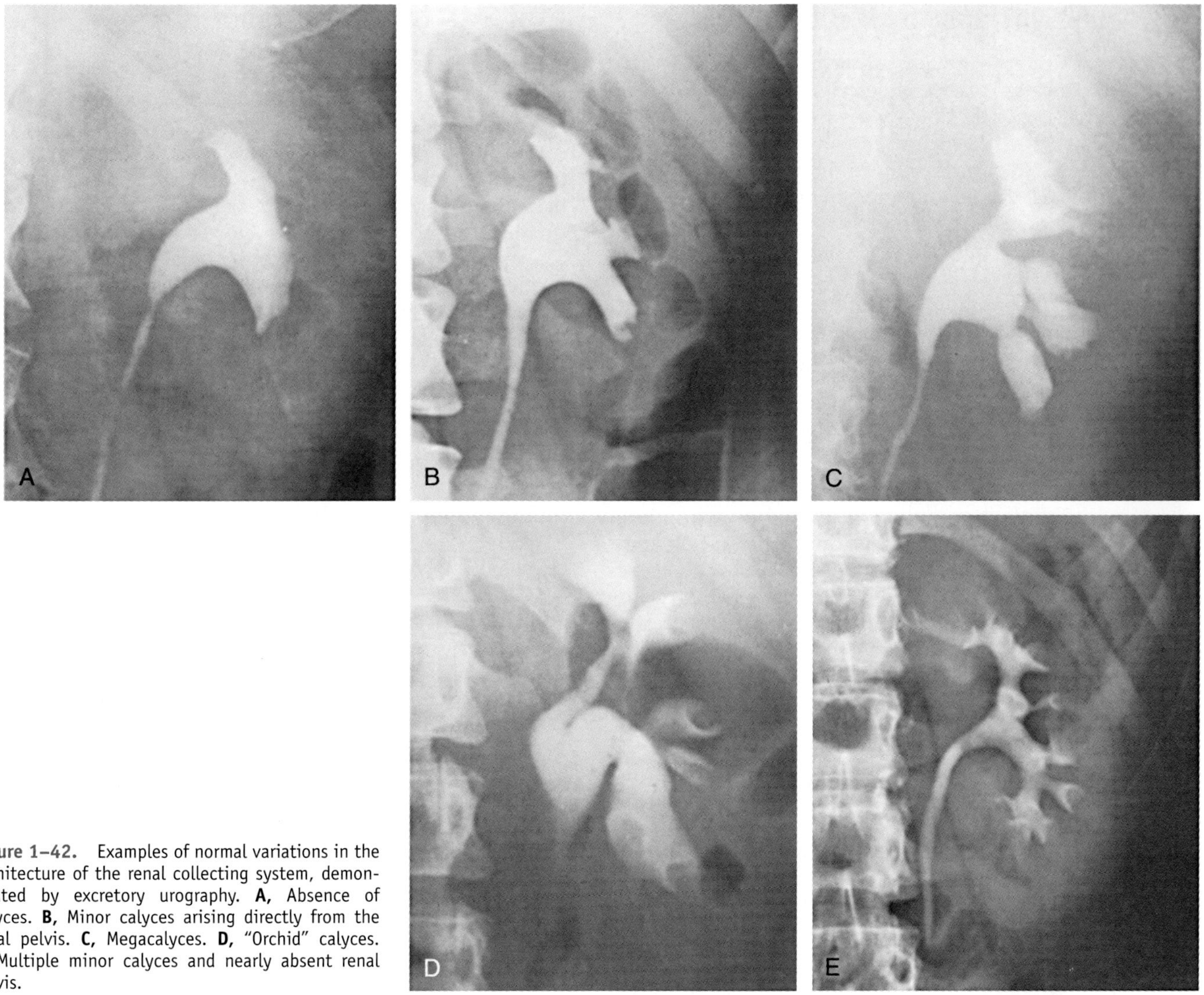

Figure 1–42. Examples of normal variations in the architecture of the renal collecting system, demonstrated by excretory urography. **A,** Absence of calyces. **B,** Minor calyces arising directly from the renal pelvis. **C,** Megacalyces. **D,** "Orchid" calyces. **E,** Multiple minor calyces and nearly absent renal pelvis.

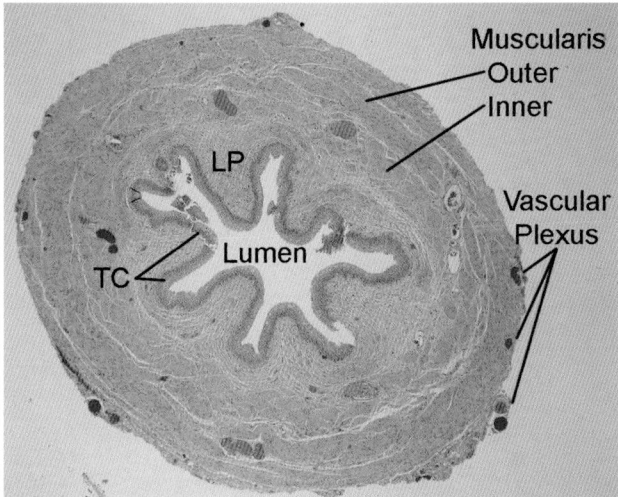

Figure 1–43. Transverse microscopic section through the ureter. Inner longitudinal layer is distinguished from outer circular and oblique muscle fibers. The rich vascular supply of the ureter is also demonstrated. LP, lamina propria; TC, transitional epithelium. (Courtesy of Dr. Hossein Saboorian.)

and vein. It then progresses inferiorly along the anterior edge of the psoas muscle. Anteriorly, the right ureter is related to the ascending colon, cecum, colonic mesentery, and appendix. The left ureter is closely related to the descending and sigmoid colon and their accompanying mesenteries. Approximately a third of the way to the bladder the ureter is crossed anteriorly by the gonadal vessels. As it enters the pelvis the ureter crosses anterior to the iliac vessels. **This crossover point is usually at the bifurcation of the common iliac into the internal and external iliac arteries, thus making this a useful landmark for pelvic procedures.**

Given the proximity of the ureters to several bowel segments, malignant and inflammatory processes of the terminal ileum, appendix, right or left colon, and sigmoid colon may involve the ureter. Effects can range from microhematuria to fistula or total obstruction. Within the female pelvis, the ureters are crossed anteriorly by the uterine arteries and are closely related to the uterine cervix. This location places the ureters at risk during hysterectomy. Pathologic processes of the fallopian tube and ovary may also encroach on the ureter at the pelvic brim.

Normal Variations in Ureteral Caliber

The normal ureter is not of uniform caliber, with three distinct narrowings classically described: the ureteropelvic junction, crossing of the iliac vessels, and the ureterovesical junction (Fig. 1–44). At the ureteropelvic junction, the renal pelvis tapers into the proximal ureter. In many cases, this perceived narrowing may be more apparent than real, with no evidence of obstruction evident on radiographic or endoscopic investigation. The second region of narrowing occurs as the ureter crosses the iliac vessels. This is due to a combination of extrinsic compression of the ureter by the iliac vessels and the necessary anterior angulation of the ureter as it crosses the iliac vessels to enter into the pelvis. There is also no intrinsic change in the ureteral caliber at this location. The third site of narrowing observed in the normal ureter is the ureterovesical junction. There is a true physical restriction of the ureter as it makes the intramural passage through the bladder wall to the ureteral orifice. These three sites of ureteral narrowing are clinically significant because they are common locations for urinary calculi to lodge during passage. In addition, the angulation of the ureter, first anteriorly as it passes over the iliac vessels, then posteromedially as it enters the pelvis and courses behind the bladder, may restrict successful passage of rigid endoscopes. Appreciation of this normal angulation and the three-dimensional course of the ureter is critical for safe and successful ureteral endoscopy.

Ureteral Segmentation and Nomenclature

The ureter is often arbitrarily divided into segments to facilitate ureteral description. The simplest system divides the ureter into the abdominal ureter extending from renal pelvis to the iliac vessels and the pelvic ureter extending from the iliac vessels to the bladder. **Alternatively, the ureter can be divided into upper, middle, and lower segments** (Fig. 1–45). **The upper ureter extends from the renal pelvis to the upper border of the sacrum. The middle ureter comprises the segment from the upper to the lower border of the sacrum. The lower (distal or pelvic) ureter extends from the lower border of the sacrum to the bladder.**

Ureteral Blood Supply and Lymphatic Drainage

The ureter receives its blood supply from multiple arterial branches along its course (Fig. 1–46). **Of greatest importance to the surgeon is that arterial branches to the abdominal ureter approach from a medial direction whereas arterial**

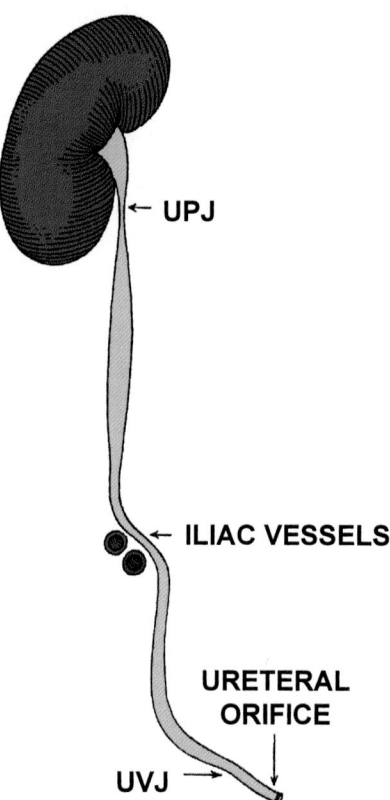

Figure 1–44. The ureter demonstrating sites of normal functional or anatomic narrowing at the ureteropelvic junction (UPJ), the iliac vessels, and the ureterovesical junction (UVJ). Note also the anterior displacement and angulation of the ureter, which occurs over the iliac vessels, as shown here diagrammatically.

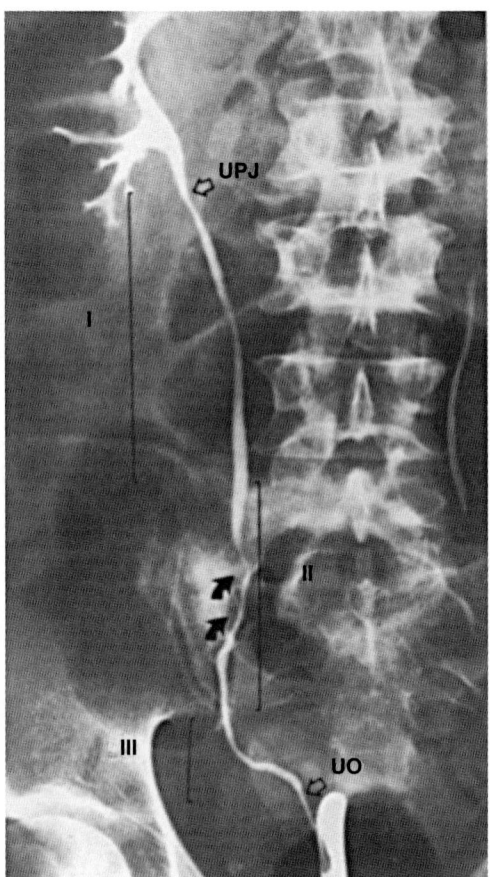

Figure 1–45. The right ureter, illustrated by retrograde injection of contrast material. UO, ureteral orifice in the bladder; UPJ, ureteropelvic junction; I, upper ureter, extending to the upper border of the sacrum; II, middle ureter, extending to the lower border of the sacrum; III, distal or lower ureter, traversing the pelvis to end in the bladder. *Arrows* indicate the course of the common iliac artery and vein.

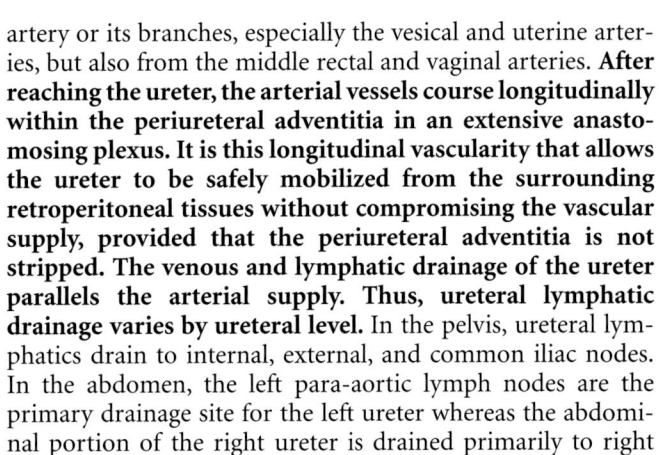

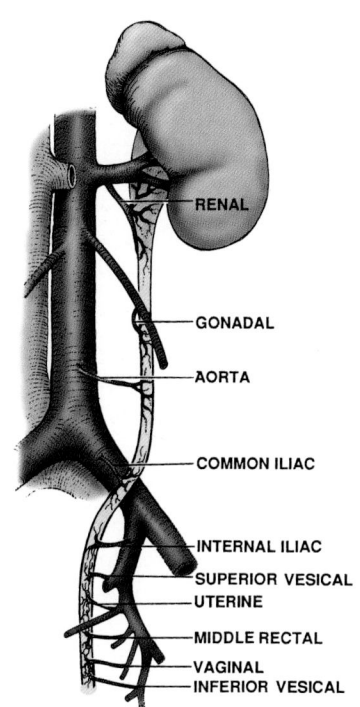

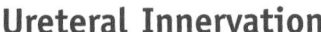

Figure 1–46.   Sources of arterial blood supply to the ureter.

branches to the pelvic ureter approach from a lateral direction. For the upper ureter these branches originate from the renal artery, gonadal artery, abdominal aorta, and common iliac artery. After entering the pelvis, additional small arterial branches to the distal ureter may arise from the internal iliac

artery or its branches, especially the vesical and uterine arteries, but also from the middle rectal and vaginal arteries. **After reaching the ureter, the arterial vessels course longitudinally within the periureteral adventitia in an extensive anastomosing plexus. It is this longitudinal vascularity that allows the ureter to be safely mobilized from the surrounding retroperitoneal tissues without compromising the vascular supply, provided that the periureteral adventitia is not stripped. The venous and lymphatic drainage of the ureter parallels the arterial supply. Thus, ureteral lymphatic drainage varies by ureteral level.** In the pelvis, ureteral lymphatics drain to internal, external, and common iliac nodes. In the abdomen, the left para-aortic lymph nodes are the primary drainage site for the left ureter whereas the abdominal portion of the right ureter is drained primarily to right paracaval and interaortocaval lymph nodes. The lymphatic drainage of the upper ureter and renal pelvis tends to join the renal lymphatics and is identical to that of the ipsilateral kidney.

Ureteral Innervation

The exact role of the ureteral autonomic input is unclear. Normal ureteral peristalsis does not require outside autonomic input but, rather, originates and is propagated from intrinsic smooth muscle pacemaker sites located in the minor calyces of the renal collecting system. The autonomic nervous system may exert some modulating effect on this process, but the exact role is unclear. The ureter receives preganglionic sympathetic input from the 10th thoracic through 2nd lumbar spinal segments. Postganglionic fibers arise from several ganglia in the aorticorenal, superior, and inferior hypogastric autonomic plexuses. Parasympathetic input is received from the 2nd through 4th sacral spinal segments.

Pain Perception and Somatic Referral

Renal pain fibers are stimulated by tension (distention) in the renal capsule, renal collecting system, or ureter. Direct mucosal irritation in the upper urinary tract may also stimulate nociceptors. Signals travel with the sympathetic nerves and result in a visceral-type pain referred to the sympathetic distribution of the kidney and ureter (eighth thoracic through second lumbar). Pain and reflex muscle spasm are typically produced over the distributions of the subcostal, iliohypogastric, ilioinguinal, and/or genitofemoral nerves, resulting in flank, groin, or scrotal (or labial) pain and hyperalgesia, depending on the location of the noxious visceral stimulus (Fig. 1–47).

SUGGESTED READINGS

Sampaio FJB: Renal anatomy: Endourologic considerations. Urol Clin North Am 2000;27:585-607.
Williams PL, Bannister LH, Berry MM, et al: Gray's Anatomy, 38th ed. New York, Churchill Livingstone, 1995.

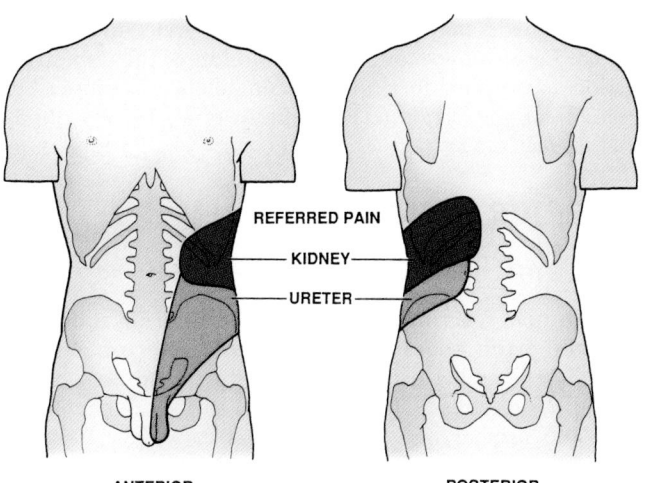

REFERRED PAIN

KIDNEY

URETER

ANTERIOR   POSTERIOR

Figure 1–47.   Patterns of referred somatic pain from the upper urinary tract.

2 Anatomy of the Lower Urinary Tract and Male Genitalia

JAMES D. BROOKS, MD

This chapter provides a general anatomic framework for understanding diseases of the pelvis. The bony, ligamentous, and muscular framework of the pelvis is presented first. Next, the pelvic vessels and nerves and the genital, urinary, and gastrointestinal viscera are discussed. Finally, the perineum and external genitalia are reviewed.

BONY PELVIS

The pelvic bones are the sacrum (the termination of the axial skeleton) and the two innominate bones. The latter are formed by the fusion of the iliac, ischial, and pubic ossification centers at the acetabulum (Fig. 2–1). The ischium and pubis also meet below, in the center of the inferior ramus, to form the obturator foramen. The weight of the upper body is transmitted from the axial skeleton to the innominate bones and lower extremities through the strong sacroiliac (SI) joints. As a whole, the pelvis is divided into a bowl-shaped false pelvis, formed by the iliac fossae and largely in contact with intraperitoneal contents, and the circular true pelvis wherein lie the urogenital organs. At the pelvic inlet, the true and false pelves are separated by the arcuate line, which extends from the sacral promontory to the pectineal line of the pubis. The lumbar lordosis that accompanies erect posture tilts the axis of the pelvic inlet so that it parallels the ground; the pelvic inlet faces anteriorly, and the inferior ischiopubic rami lie

horizontal (Fig. 2–2). When approaching the pelvis through a low midline incision, the surgeon gazes directly into the true pelvis.

The anterior and posterior iliac spines, the iliac crests, the pubic tubercles, and the ischial tuberosities are palpable landmarks that orient the pelvic surgeon (see Fig. 2–1). Cooper's (pectineal) ligament overlies the pectineal line and offers a sure hold for sutures in hernia repairs and urethral suspension procedures (see Fig. 2–7). The ischial spine is palpable transvaginally and attaches to the pelvic diaphragm and the sacrospinous ligament. The sacrospinous ligament separates the greater and lesser sciatic foramina. Together with the sacrotuberous ligament, it stabilizes the SI joint by preventing downward rotation of the sacral promontory. The SI joint, synovial in type, gains additional strength from anterior and posterior ligaments. In pelvic trauma, fractures virtually never involve this joint but they occur adjacent to it. The pubes, the thinnest of the pelvic bones, are nearly always fractured, and their fragments may injure the adjacent bladder, urethra, and vagina. Resection or congenital nonunion of the pubes (e.g., bladder exstrophy) does not affect ambulation because of the strength of the SI joint (Waterhouse et al, 1973; Golimbu et al, 1990).

ANTERIOR ABDOMINAL WALL

Skin and Subcutaneous Fasciae

To minimize scarring, incisions of the anterior abdominal wall and flank should follow Langer's lines of cleavage. These lines parallel dermal collagen fibers and are oriented along lines of stress. They correspond to the segmental thoracic and lumbar nerves. The skin is backed by Camper's fascia, a loose layer of fatty tissue that varies in thickness with the nutritional status of the patient. The superficial circumflex iliac, external pudendal, and superficial inferior epigastric vessels branch from the femoral vessels to run in this layer (Figs. 2–3 and 2–4). The superficial inferior epigastric vessels are encountered during inguinal incisions and can cause troublesome bleeding during placement of pelvic laparoscopic ports.

Scarpa's fascia forms a distinct layer deep to this Camper's fascia, although it may be difficult to discern in older

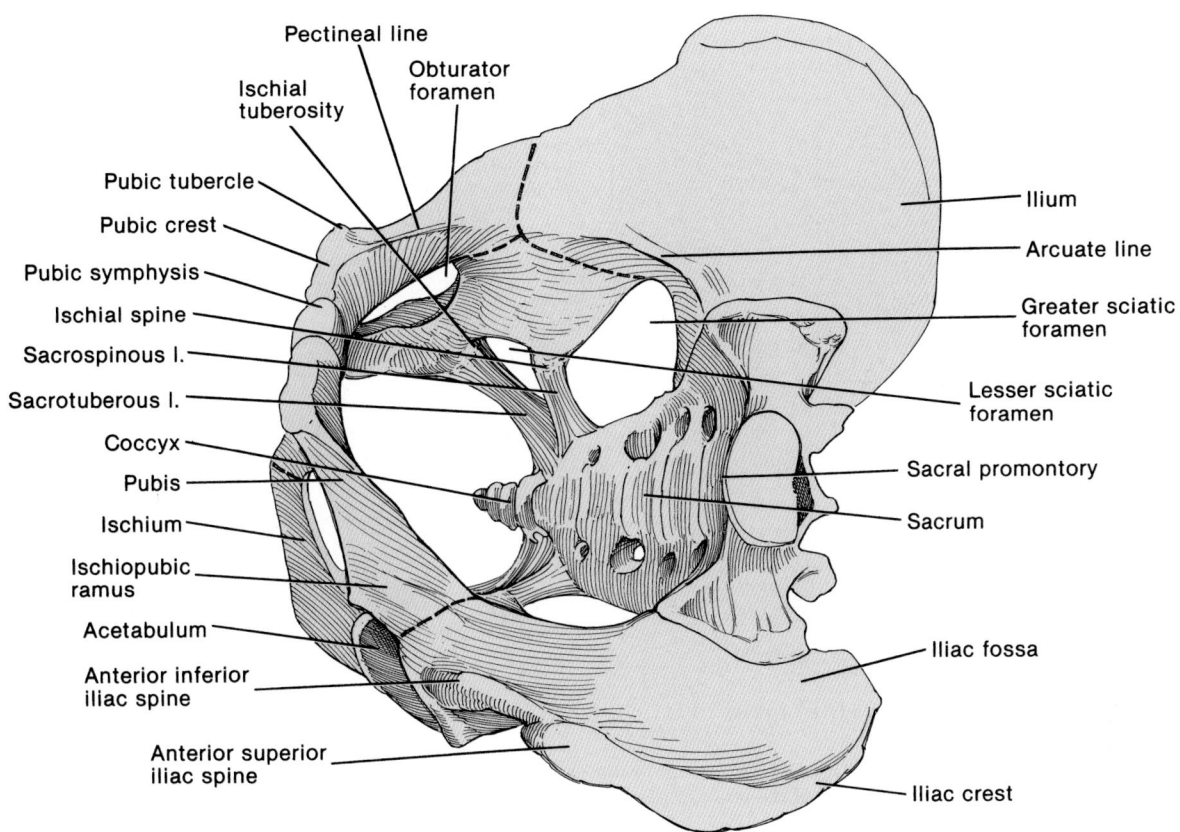

Figure 2–1. The bones and ligaments of the pelvis. (From Hinman F Jr: Atlas of Urosurgical Anatomy. Philadelphia, WB Saunders, 1993, p 196.)

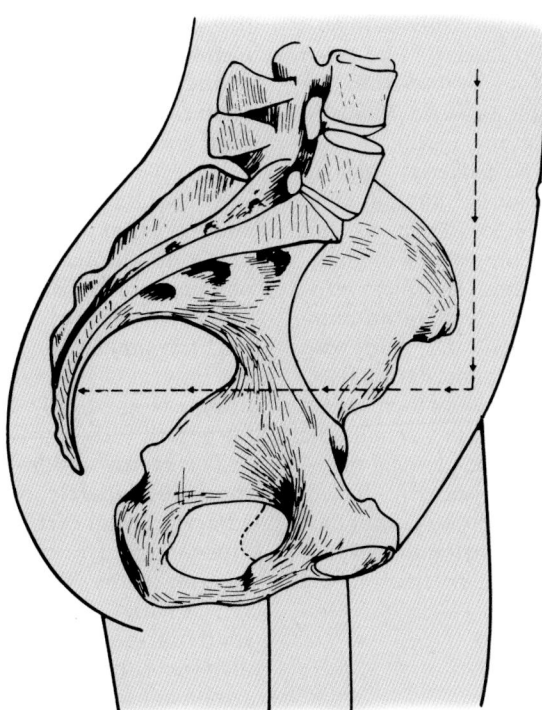

Figure 2–2. Pelvis in standing position. The axis of the pelvic cavity is horizontal because of lumbar lordosis. (From Zacharin RF: Pelvic Floor Anatomy and the Surgery of Pulsion Enterocele. New York, Springer-Verlag, 1985, p 15.)

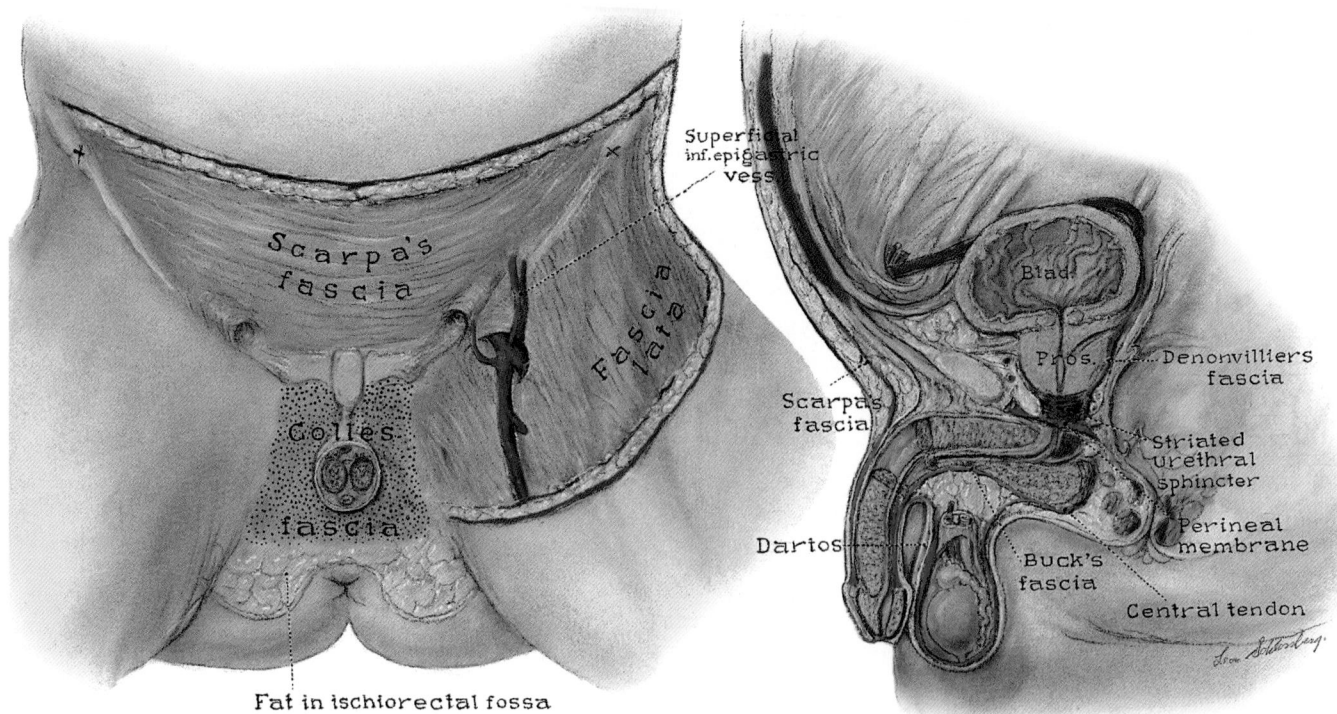

Figure 2–3.   **Left,** Anterior view of the deep fasciae of the abdomen, perineum, and thigh. Note the superficial inferior epigastric artery passing superiorly in Camper's fascia. **Right,** Midline sagittal view of the pelvic fasciae and their attachments.

patients. Superiorly and laterally, it blends with Camper's fascia. Inferiorly, it fuses with the deep fascia of the thigh 1 cm below the inguinal ligament along a line from the anterior superior iliac spine to the pubic tubercle. Medially, it is continuous with Colles' fascia of the perineum (see Fig. 2–3). Colles' fascia attaches to the posterior edge of the urogenital diaphragm and the inferior ischiopubic rami. It is continuous with the dartos fascia of the penis and scrotum. These fasciae can limit both the spread of infection in necrotizing fasciitis of the scrotum (Fournier's gangrene) and the extent of urinary extravasation in an anterior urethral injury. For instance, blood and urine can accumulate in the scrotum and penis deep to the dartos fascia after an anterior urethral injury. In the perineum, their spread is limited by the fusions of Colles' fascia to the ischiopubic rami laterally and to the posterior edge of the perineal membrane; the resulting hematoma is therefore butterfly shaped. They will not extend down the leg or into the buttock, but they can freely travel up the anterior abdominal wall deep to Scarpa's fascia to the clavicles and around the flank to the back.

Abdominal Musculature

The abdominal musculature lies immediately below Scarpa's fascia. The origins of the external oblique, internal oblique, and transversus abdominis muscles and the orientation of their fibers are presented in Chapter 1, Surgical Anatomy of the Retroperitoneum, Kidneys, and Ureters. **These muscles terminate on the anterior abdominal wall as broad, tough aponeurotic sheets that fuse in the midline (linea alba) and form the rectus sheath** (see Fig. 2–4). The linea alba is avascular and is a convenient point of access to the peritoneal and pelvic cavities. In its upper portion, the anterior rectus sheath is formed by the aponeurosis of the external oblique muscle and a portion of the internal oblique muscle (Fig. 2–5). The posterior sheath is derived from the remaining internal oblique aponeurosis and the transversus abdominis aponeurosis. Two thirds of the distance from the pubis to the umbilicus, the arcuate line is formed, as all aponeurotic layers abruptly pass anterior to the rectus abdominis, leaving this muscle clothed only by transversalis fascia and peritoneum posteriorly.

The rectus abdominis arises from the pubis medial to the pubic tubercle and inserts on the xiphoid process and adjacent costal cartilages. The muscle is crossed by three or four tendinous intersections that are firmly attached to the anterior rectus sheath; thus, the muscle can be divided transversely without significant retraction. It is supplied by the last six thoracic segmental nerves that enter it laterally. Paramedian incisions lateral to the rectus divide these nerves, cause atrophy of the rectus, and predispose to ventral hernia. Anterior to the rectus and within its sheath, the triangle-shaped pyramidalis muscle arises from the pubic crest and inserts into the linea alba (see Fig. 2–4). It is supplied by the subcostal nerve (T12).

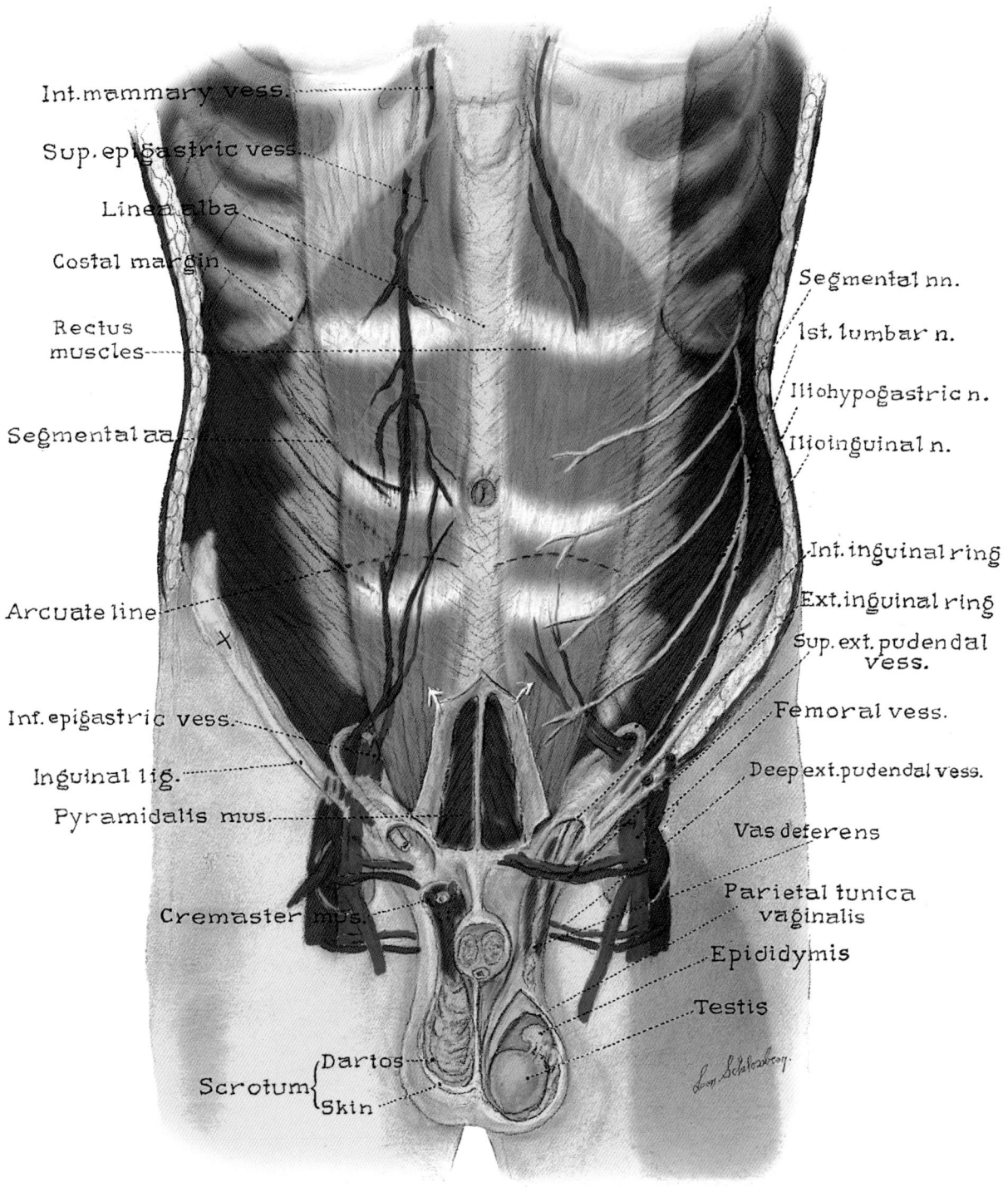

Figure 2–4. Muscles, vessels, and nerves of the anterior abdominal wall. The rectus abdominis muscles are semitransparent to demonstrate the vessels posteriorly.

Abdominal wall anatomy above the arcuate line.

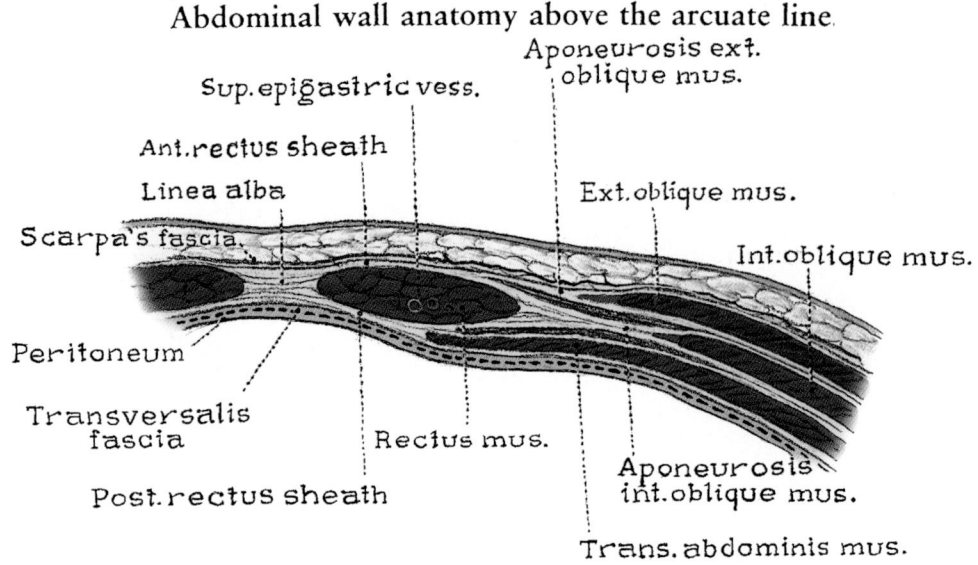

Sup. epigastric vess.

Aponeurosis ext. oblique mus.

Ant. rectus sheath

Linea alba

Scarpa's fascia

Ext. oblique mus.

Int. oblique mus.

Peritoneum

Transversalis fascia

Rectus mus.

Post. rectus sheath

Aponeurosis int. oblique mus.

Trans. abdominis mus.

Abdominal wall anatomy below the arcuate line

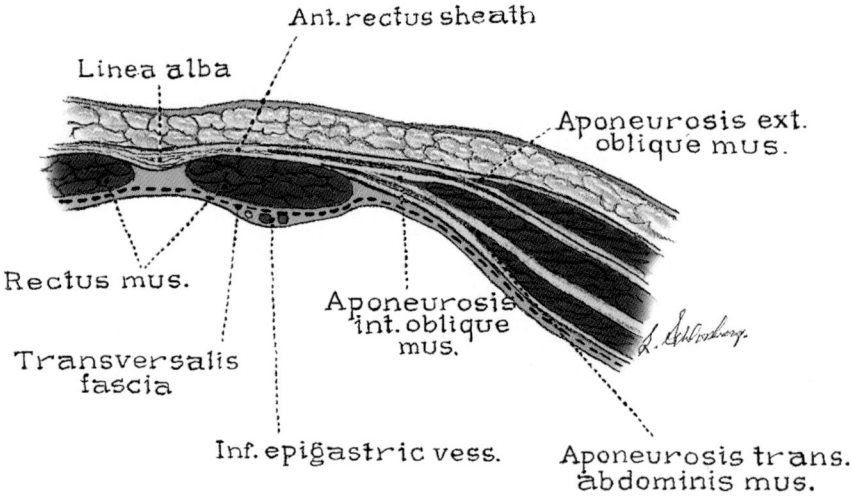

Ant. rectus sheath

Linea alba

Aponeurosis ext. oblique mus.

Rectus mus.

Transversalis fascia

Aponeurosis int. oblique mus.

Inf. epigastric vess.

Aponeurosis trans. abdominis mus.

Figure 2–5. Cross section of the rectus sheath. **Top,** Above the arcuate line, the aponeurosis of the external oblique muscle forms the anterior sheath and the transversus aponeurosis forms the posterior sheath. The internal oblique muscle splits to contribute to both the anterior and the posterior sheaths. **Bottom,** Below the arcuate line, all aponeuroses pass anterior to the rectus.

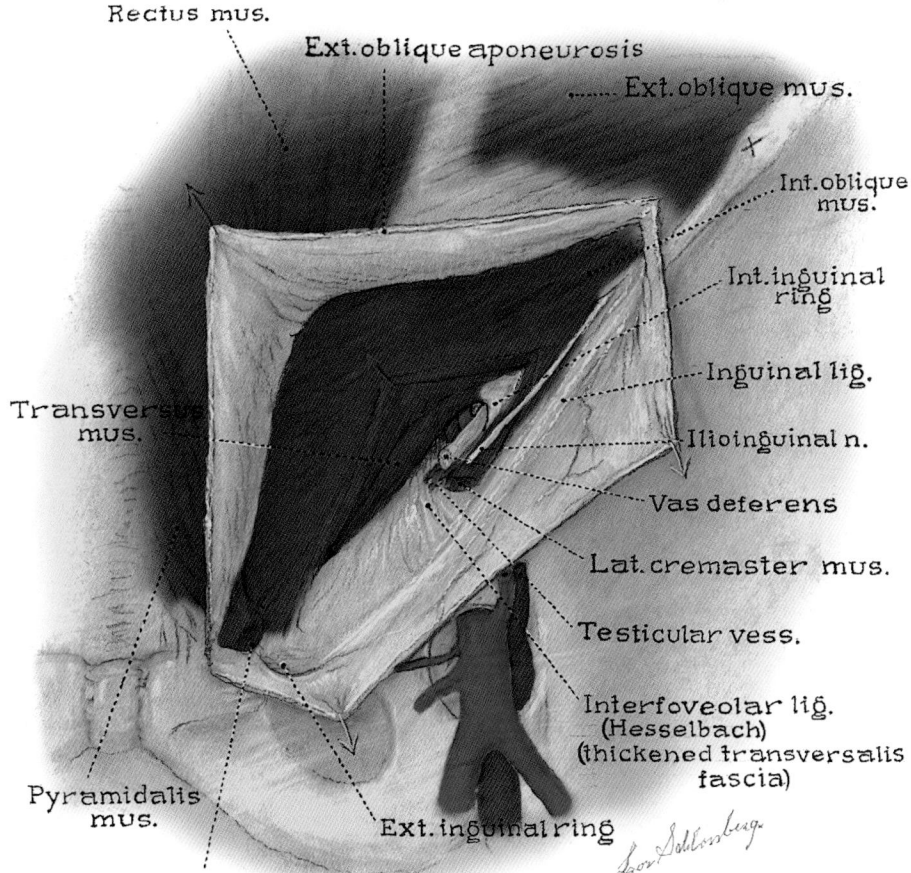

Figure 2–6. Deep structures of the left inguinal canal, viewed from the front.

Labels on figure:
Rectus mus.
Ext. oblique aponeurosis
Ext. oblique mus.
Int. oblique mus.
Int. inguinal ring
Inguinal lig.
Ilioinguinal n.
Vas deferens
Lat. cremaster mus.
Testicular vess.
Interfoveolar lig. (Hesselbach) (thickened transversalis fascia)
Transversus mus.
Pyramidalis mus.
Ext. inguinal ring
Medial cremaster mus.

Inguinal Canal

The inguinal canal transmits the spermatic cord in the male, the round ligament in the female, and the ilioinguinal nerve in both sexes (Fig. 2–6; see also Fig. 2–4). Its anterior wall and floor are formed by the external oblique muscle, which folds over at its inferior edge as the inguinal ligament. Above the pubic tubercle, the fibers of the external oblique aponeurosis split to form the lateral edges (crura) of the external inguinal ring. Transverse (intercrural) fibers bridge the crura to form the superior edge of the external ring. By dividing the intracrural fibers, the external oblique can be separated along its fibers to gain access to the cord. The posterior wall of the canal is formed by transversalis fascia, which lines the inner surface of the abdominal wall. The cord structures pierce this fascia lateral to the inferior epigastric vessels at the internal inguinal ring (Fig. 2–7). The internal inguinal ring lies midway between the anterior superior iliac spine and the pubic tubercle, above the inguinal ligament, and 4 cm lateral to the external ring. Fibers of the internal oblique and transversus abdominis arise from the iliopsoas fascia and inguinal ligament lateral to the internal ring and arch over the canal to form its roof. They fuse as the conjoint tendon, pass posterior to the cord, and insert into the rectus sheath and pubis. The conjoint tendon reinforces the posterior wall of the inguinal canal at the external ring. With contraction of the internal oblique and transversus muscles, the roof of the canal closes against the floor. Hernias into the canal may occur medial (direct) or lateral (indirect) to the inferior epigastric vessels (see Figs. 2–6 and 2–7).

Internal Surface of the Anterior Abdominal Wall

Approached laparoscopically, **three elevations of the peritoneum, referred to as the median, medial, and lateral umbilical folds,** are visible on the anterior abdominal wall below the umbilicus (Fig. 2–8). The median fold overlies the median umbilical ligament (urachus), a fibrous remnant of the cloaca that attaches the bladder to the anterior abdominal wall. The obliterated umbilical artery in the medial umbilical fold serves as an important landmark for the surgeon. It may be traced to its origin from the internal iliac artery to locate the ureter, which lies on its medial side. During transperitoneal laparoscopic pelvic lymph node dissection, the obturator packet is accessed by incising the peritoneum lateral to the obliterated umbilical artery. The lateral umbilical fold contains the inferior epigastric vessels as they ascend to supply the rectus abdominis.

SOFT TISSUES OF THE PELVIS

Pelvic Musculature

Muscles and fascia line the true pelvis and form its floor. **The obturator internus arises from the inner surface of the**

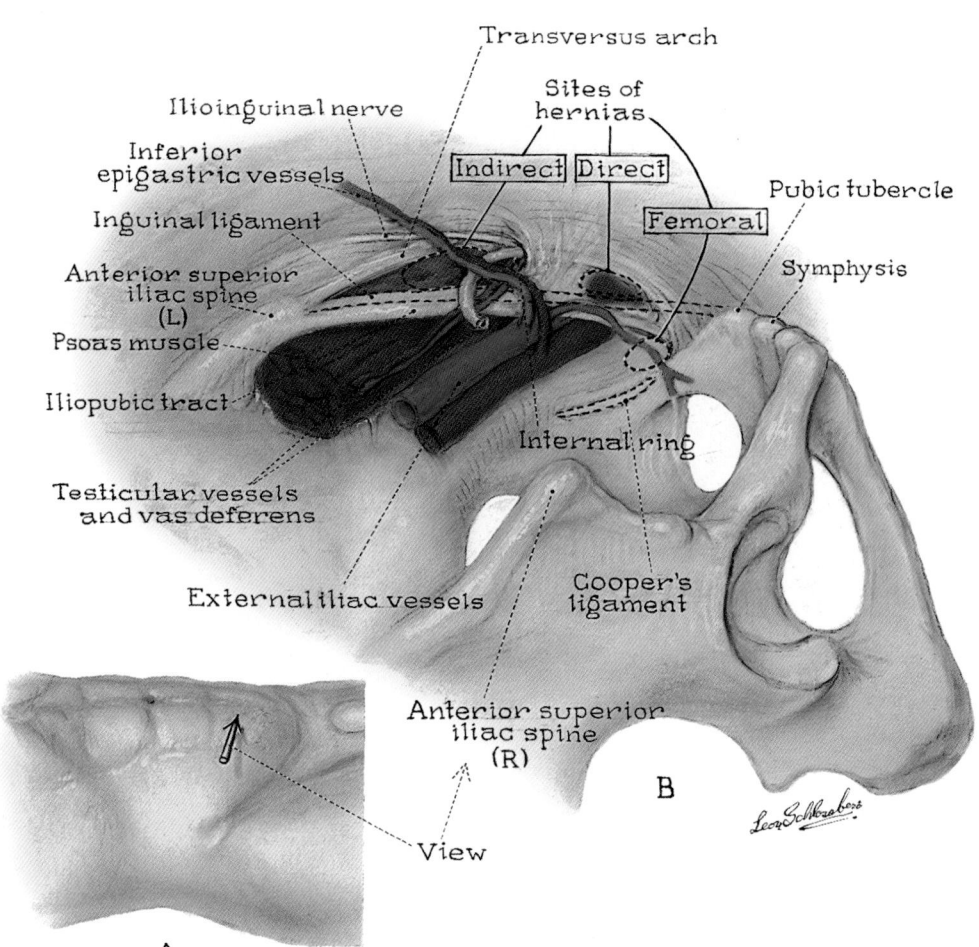

Ilioinguinal nerve

Inferior
epigastric vessels

Inguinal ligament

Anterior superior
iliac spine
(L)

Psoas muscle

Iliopubic tract

Testicular vessels
and vas deferens

External iliac vessels

Transversus arch

Sites of
hernias

Indirect | Direct

Femoral

Pubic tubercle

Symphysis

Internal ring

Cooper's
ligament

Anterior superior
iliac spine
(R)

B

View

A

Leon Schlozzabooz

Figure 2–7. Topography (**A**) and posterior wall (**B**) of the left inguinal canal, viewed from the preperitoneal space. The location of three types of inguinal hernia is demonstrated. (From Schlegel PN, Walsh PC: Simultaneous preperitoneal hernia repair during radical pelvic surgery. J Urol 1987; 137:1180-1183.)

obturator foramen and the obturator membrane and passes **through the lesser sciatic foramen to insert on the femur** (see Fig. 2–8). The fascia on the pelvic surface of this muscle is thickened into a tough line extending from the lower half of the pubis to the ischial spine. This tendinous arc of the levator ani serves as the origin of the muscles of the pelvic diaphragm: pubococcygeus and iliococcygeus (Fig. 2–9). These muscles are not truly separable, and they form a diaphragm that closes the pelvic outlet. Anteriorly, a narrow U-shaped hiatus remains through which the urethra and rectum exit in the male and the urethra, vagina, and rectum exit in the female (Fig. 2–10). The muscle bordering this hiatus has been referred to as *pubovisceral* because it provides a sling for (pubourethralis, puborectalis), inserts directly into (pubovaginalis, puboanalis, levator prostatae), or inserts into a structure intimately associated with the pelvic viscera (Lawson, 1974). The pubovisceral group provides strong fixation and support for the pelvic viscera. The coccygeus muscle extends from the sacrospinous ligament to the lateral border of the sacrum and coccyx to complete the pelvic diaphragm. Muscles of the pelvic diaphragm contain type I (slow-twitch) fibers, which provide tonic support to pelvic structures, and type II (fast-twitch) fibers, for sudden increases in intra-abdominal pressure (Gosling et al, 1981). The piriformis muscle arises from the lateral aspect of the sacrum and passes through and fills the greater sciatic foramen to form the posterolateral wall of the pelvis.

It is important to recognize that the pelvic diaphragm is not flat or bowl shaped, as it is frequently depicted. At the urogenital and anal hiatus, the muscles lie in a near-vertical configuration and are thickened inferiorly (see Fig. 2–10) (Brooks et al, 1998; Myers et al, 1998). Behind the anus, they flatten to form a nearly horizontal diaphragm, referred to as the *levator plate*. In the female, the levator plate provides critical support to the pelvic viscera, as discussed later.

Pelvic Fasciae

The pelvic fasciae are not merely collagenous; they are also rich in elastic tissue and smooth muscle. This suggests that they are active in the support, and possibly the function, of the pelvic viscera. The pelvic fasciae are continuous with the retroperitoneal fasciae and have been categorized somewhat arbitrarily into outer, intermediate, and inner strata. The outer stratum, or endopelvic fascia, lines the inner surface of the pelvic muscles and is continuous with the transversalis layer of the abdomen. It is fixed to the arcuate line of the pelvis, Cooper's ligament, the sacrospinous ligament, the ischial spine, and the tendinous arc of the levator ani. The intermediate stratum embeds the pelvic viscera in a fatty, compressible layer that accommodates their filling and emptying. Its tissues are easily swept aside to reveal the retropubic, paravesical, rectogenital, and retrorectal potential spaces. All pelvic vessels and some pelvic nerves travel in this stratum and

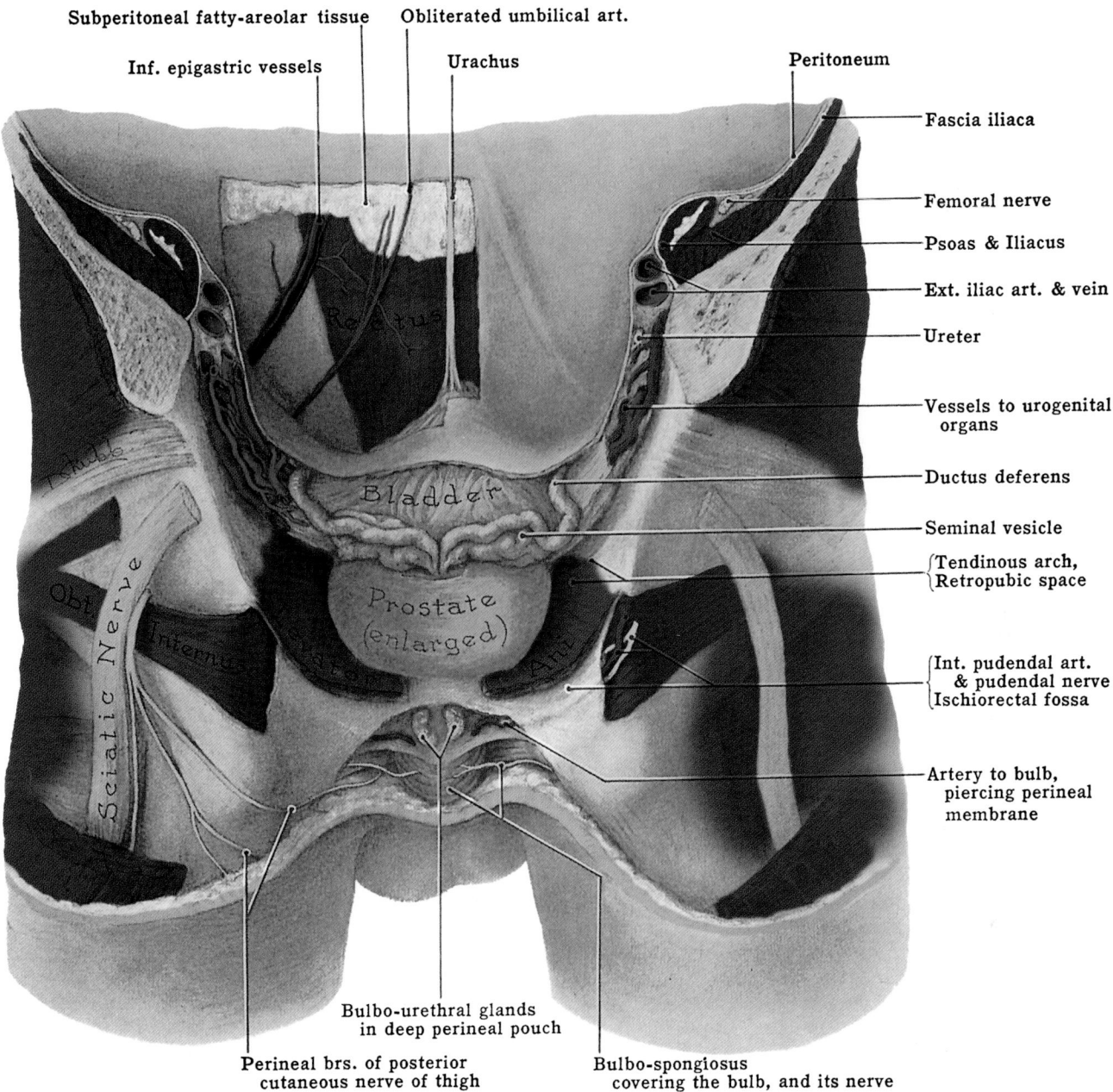

Figure 2–8. Male pelvis and anterior abdominal wall viewed from behind. The sacrum and ilia have been removed. (From Anderson JE: Grant's Atlas of Anatomy, 7th ed. Baltimore, Williams & Wilkins, 1978.)

are subject to injury when these potential spaces are developed at surgery. The intermediate stratum coalesces around vessels and nerves supplying the pelvic organs to form named ligaments (e.g., cardinal, uterosacral, lateral, and posterior vesical) that suspend and tether these organs in the pelvis. This fascia also thickens around the pelvic urogenital organs to form their visceral fascia. These are not true ligaments but are a meshwork of connective tissue and smooth muscle investing the visceral neurovascular pedicles (DeCaro et al, 1998). The inner stratum lies just beneath the peritoneum and is associated with the entire gastrointestinal tract. In the pelvis, it covers the rectum and the dome of the bladder and forms the rectogenital septum (Denonvilliers' fascia). This septum is the developmental remains of the rectogenital pouch of peritoneum

that extended between the rectum and internal genitalia to the pelvic floor.

The pelvic fasciae have been given a confusing array of appellations by anatomists and surgeons interested in female pelvic organ prolapse. To add to the confusion, the strength of pelvic fasciae can differ significantly between individuals and races, and these differences may predispose some individuals to pelvic prolapse (Zacharin, 1985). **There are three important components of the pelvic fasciae:** (1) Anteriorly, the puboprostatic ligaments attach to the lower fifth of the pubis, lateral to the symphysis and to the junction of the prostate and external sphincter (see Fig. 2–40). They are called the pubo-urethral ligaments in the female and insert on the proximal third of the urethra (Fig. 2–11). (2) Laterally, the arcus

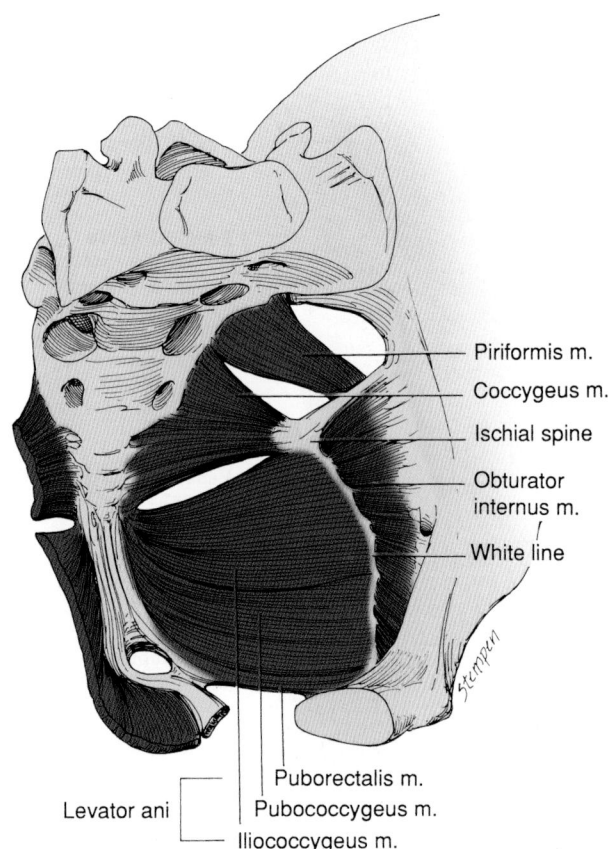

Figure 2–9. Muscles of the true pelvis (three-quarter view).

tendineus fascia pelvis extends from the puboprostatic (pubo-urethral) ligament to the ischial spine (see Fig. 2–11). This fascia forms at the junction of the endopelvic and visceral fasciae. It should not be confused with the arcus tendineus levator ani, which lies above its anterior portion (Fig. 2–12). In the male, the arcus tendineus fascia pelvis is found at the base of a sulcus between the pelvic side wall and the prostate and bladder. In the female, it corresponds to the lateral attachment of the anterior bladder wall to the pelvic side wall. Paravaginal suspension procedures for stress urinary incontinence entail lateral reapproximation of the vaginal wall to this tendinous arc (Richardson et al, 1981). The lateral branches of the dorsal venous complex are directly beneath the arcus tendineus fascia pelvis; thus, the endopelvic fascia should be opened lateral to this landmark. In the female, fascia extending medially from this arch carries a variety of names (pubo-vesical, periurethral, urethropelvic ligament) and provides important support to the urethra and anterior vaginal wall. Damage to this fascia and its attachments has been implicated in urethrocele, cystocele, and stress urinary incontinence. (3) Posterior to the ischial spine, the fascia fans out to either side of the rectum and attaches to the pelvic side wall as the lateral and posterior vesical ligaments. In the female, these are the strong cardinal and uterosacral ligaments. They are not true ligaments; rather, they are condensations of intermediate stratum around visceral neurovascular pedicles. The peritoneum over these ligaments forms discrete folds (rectovesical in the male and rectouterine in the female) that can be appreciated at cystectomy (Fig. 2–13). Taken as a whole, the pelvic fasciae form a Y-shaped scaffolding for the pelvic viscera (see Fig. 2–12).

Fasciae of the Perineum and the Perineal Body

The weakest point in the pelvic floor, the urogenital hiatus, is bridged by the urogenital diaphragm, a structure unique to humans (see Fig. 2–10). The fibrous perineal membrane lies at the center of, and defines, the urogenital diaphragm (see Figs. 2–3, 2–10, and 2–30). It is triangular and spans the inferior ischiopubic rami from the pubis to the ischial tuberosities. Posteriorly, it ends abruptly; the superficial and deep transverse perinei run along its free edge (Fig. 2–14). The external genitalia attach to its inferior surface; superiorly, it supports the urethral sphincter (discussed later). The perineal body represents the point of fusion between the free posterior edge of the urogenital diaphragm and the posterior apex of the urogenital hiatus. This pyramid-shaped structure lies at the hub of pelvic support. Virtually every pelvic muscle (superficial and deep transverse perinei, bulbocavernosus, levator ani, rectourethralis, external anal sphincter, striated urethral sphincter) and fascia (perineal membrane, Denonvilliers', Colles', and endopelvic) insert into the perineal body. At its core are abundant elastin and richly innervated smooth muscle, which suggests that it may have a dynamic role in support. Damage to the perineal body during perineal prostatectomy risks postoperative urinary incontinence.

PELVIC CIRCULATION

Arterial Supply

Major arteries of the pelvis are summarized in Table 2–1. At the bifurcation of the aorta, the **middle sacral artery** arises posteriorly and travels on the pelvic surface of the sacrum to supply branches to the sacral foramina and the rectum. The common iliac arteries arise at the level of the fourth lumbar vertebra, run anterior and lateral to their accompanying veins, and bifurcate into the external and internal iliac arteries at the SI joint (Fig. 2–15). The external iliac artery follows the medial border of the iliopsoas muscle along the arcuate line and leaves the pelvis beneath the inguinal ligament as the femoral artery (Fig. 2–16). Its inferior epigastric artery is given off proximal to the inguinal ligament and ascends medial to the internal inguinal ring to supply the rectus muscle and overlying skin. Because the rectus is richly collateralized from above and laterally, the inferior epigastric arteries may be ligated with impunity. A rectus myocutaneous flap based on this artery has been used to correct major pelvic and perineal tissue defects. Near its origin, the inferior epigastric artery sends a deep circumflex iliac branch laterally and a pubic branch medially. Both vessels travel on the iliopubic tract and may be injured during inguinal hernia repair. Its cremasteric branch joins the spermatic cord at the internal inguinal ring and forms a distal anastomosis with the testicular artery (see Fig. 2–44). In 25% of people, an accessory obturator artery arises from the inferior epigastric artery and runs medial to the femoral vein to

Text continued on p. 51

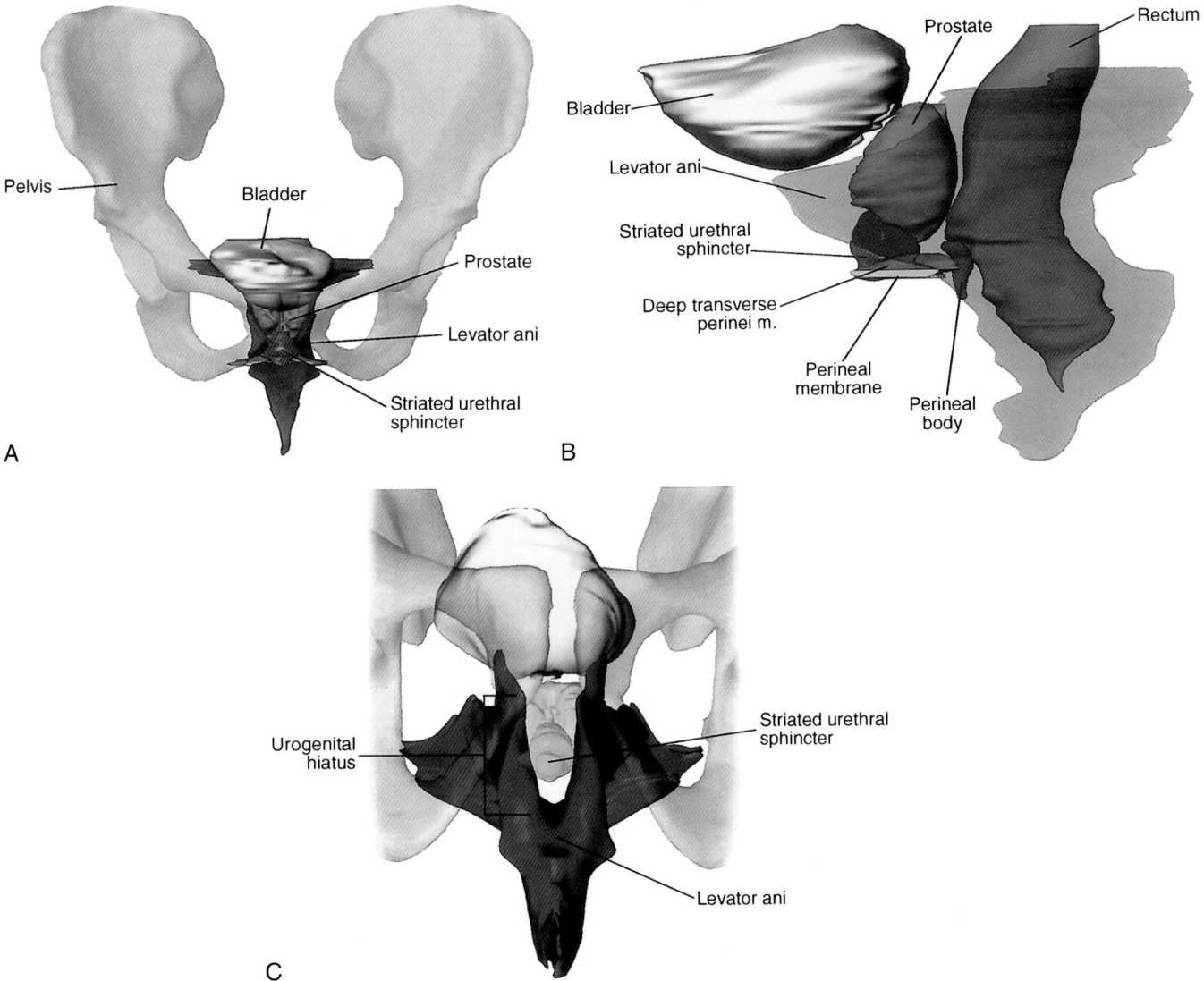

Figure 2–10. Location and contour of the levator ani and pelvic viscera. **A,** Anterior view demonstrating the near-vertical orientation of the lateral walls of the levator ani and the horizontal wings at its posterior superior aspect. **B,** Lateral view in which the levator ani has been made transparent. The perineal membrane bridges the urogenital hiatus, and the urethral sphincter fills much of the hiatus. **C,** View of the levator ani from below showing the urogenital hiatus and the thickened inferior border of the levator ani. The perineal body and related structures are not shown. (From Brooks JD, Chao W-M, Kerr J: Male pelvic anatomy reconstructed from the Visible Human data set. J Urol 1998;159:868-872.)

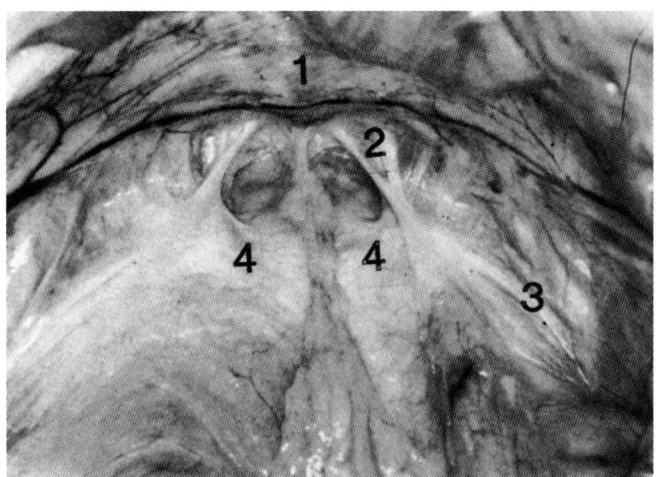

Figure 2–11. Floor of the space of Retzius in a thin, elderly female cadaver. The fat has been removed to show the continuous sheet of endopelvic fascia, and the bladder has been retracted posteriorly. 1, Symphysis pubis; 2, right pubourethral ligament; 3, lateral condensation of endopelvic fascia forming the right arcus tendineus fasciae pelvis; 4, condensation of the endopelvic fascia, which forms a firm, whitish aponeurosis over the proximal urethra and internal vesical orifice. (From Mostwin JL: Current concepts of female pelvic anatomy and physiology. Urol Clin North Am 1991;18:175-195.)

Table 2–1. Arteries of the Pelvis

Artery Name	Origin	Supplies
Middle sacral	Aorta	Sacral nerves and sacrum
External Iliac Branches		
Inferior epigastric	External iliac	Rectus abdominis muscle and overlying skin and fascia
Deep circumflex iliac	Inferior epigastric	Inguinal ligament and surrounding structures laterally
Pubic	Inferior epigastric	Inguinal ligament and surrounding structures medially
Cremasteric	Inferior epigastric	Vas deferens and testis
Internal Iliac Branches		
Superior gluteal	Posterior trunk	Gluteus muscles and overlying skin
Ascending lumbar	Posterior trunk	Psoas and quadratus lumborum muscles and adjacent structures
Lateral sacral	Posterior trunk	Sacral nerves and sacrum
Superior vesical	Anterior trunk	Bladder, ureter, vas deferens, and seminal vesicle
Middle rectal	Anterior trunk	Rectum, ureter, and bladder
Inferior vesicle	Anterior trunk	Bladder, seminal vesicle, prostate, ureter, and the neurovascular bundle
Uterine	Anterior trunk	Uterus, bladder, and ureter
Internal pudendal	Anterior trunk	Rectum, perineum, and external genitalia
Obturator	Anterior trunk	Adductor muscles of the leg and overlying skin
Inferior gluteal	Anterior trunk	Gluteus muscles and overlying skin

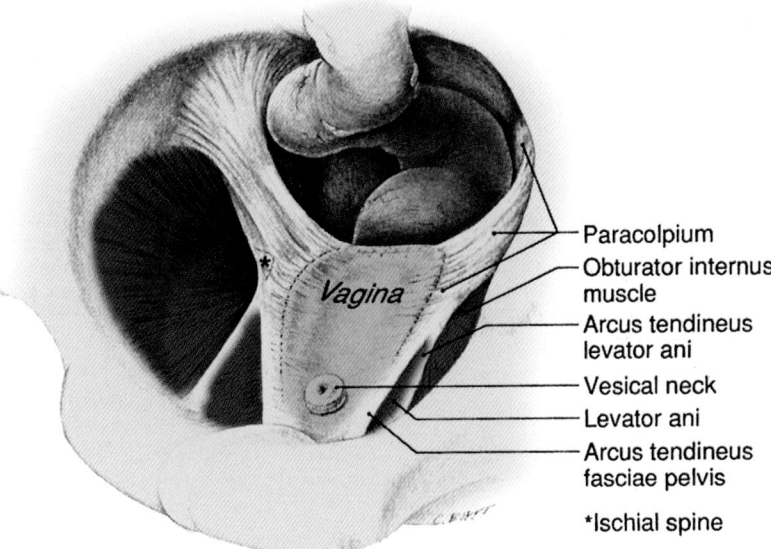

Paracolpium
Obturator internus muscle
Arcus tendineus levator ani
Vesical neck
Levator ani
Arcus tendineus fasciae pelvis
*Ischial spine

Figure 2–12. Vagina and supportive structures after removal of the bladder and uterus. The arcus tendineus fascia pelvis and the cardinal and uterosacral ligaments (paracolpium) form a continuous structure that supports the pelvic viscera. (From DeLancey JO: Structural support of the urethra as it relates to stress urinary incontinence: The hammock hypothesis. Am J Obstet Gynecol 1994;170:1713-1720.)

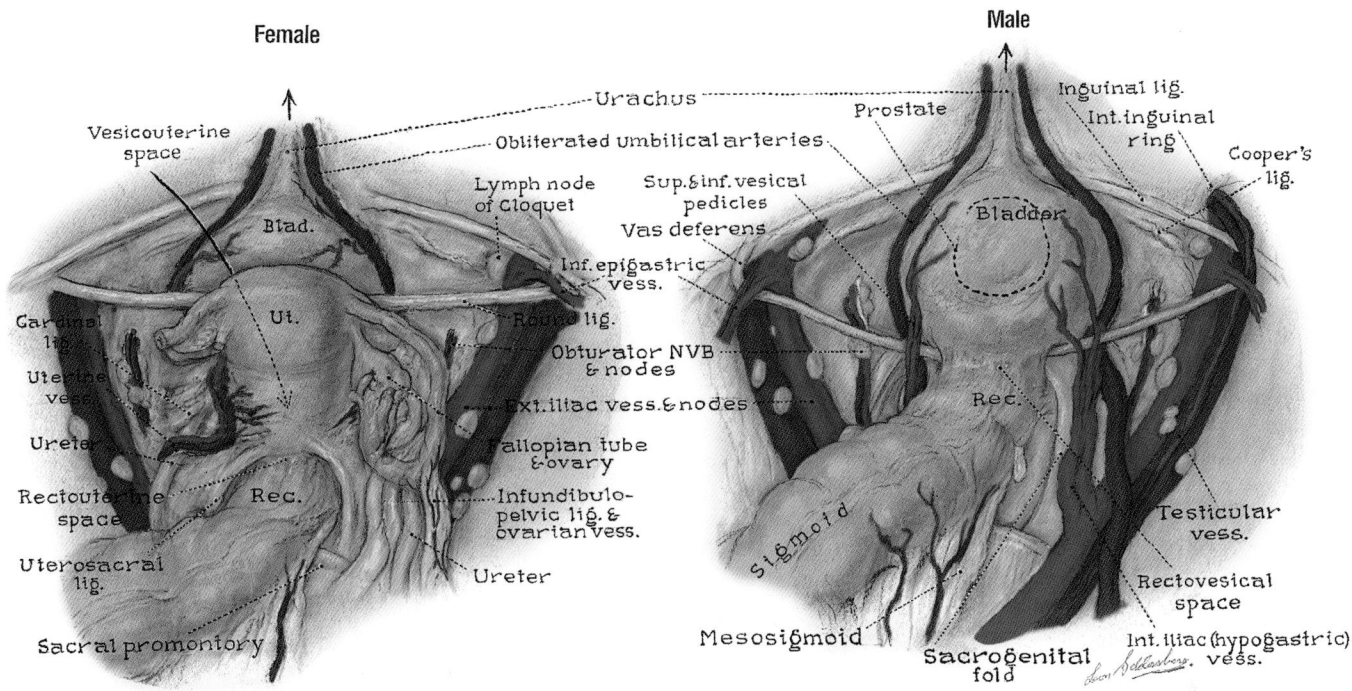

Female

Vesicouterine space

Urachus

Obliterated umbilical arteries

Lymph node of Cloquet

Blad.

Sup.&inf. vesical pedicles

Vas deferens

Ut.

Inf. epigastric vess.

Cardinal lig.

Round lig.

Uterine vess.

Obturator NVB & nodes

Ureter

Ext. iliac vess. & nodes

Rectouterine space

Rec.

Fallopian tube & ovary

Uterosacral lig.

Infundibulo-pelvic lig. & ovarian vess.

Ureter

Sacral promontory

Male

Prostate

Inguinal lig.

Int. inguinal ring

Cooper's lig.

Bladder

Rec.

Testicular vess.

Sigmoid

Rectovesical space

Mesosigmoid

Sacrogenital fold

Int. iliac (hypogastric) vess.

Figure 2–13. Peritoneal surfaces of the female and male pelves. In the female, the ureter passes medial to the ovarian vessels, then deep to the uterine artery within the substance of the cardinal ligament. The sacrogenital and sacrouterine folds represent the posterior portions of pelvic fascial support.

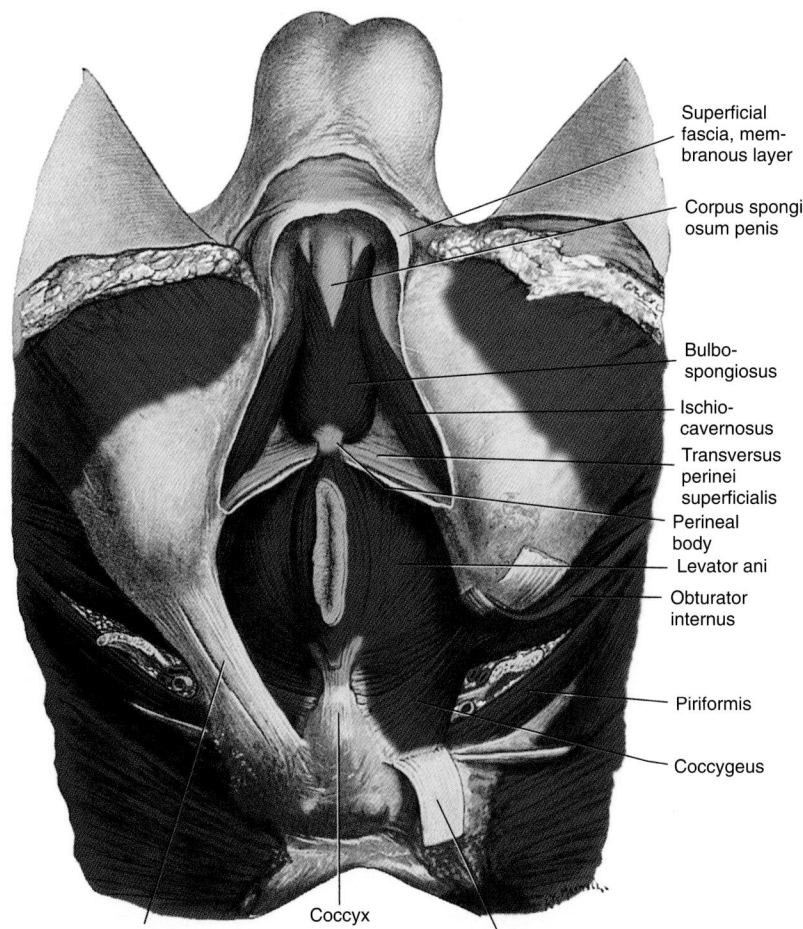

Superficial fascia, membranous layer

Corpus spongiosum penis

Bulbospongiosus

Ischiocavernosus

Transversus perinei superficialis

Perineal body

Levator ani

Obturator internus

Piriformis

Coccygeus

Sacrotuberous ligament

Coccyx

Sacrotuberous ligament

Figure 2–14. Muscles of the male perineum. The transversus perinei and ischiocavernosi frame the urogenital diaphragm. (From Williams PL, Warwick R: Gray's Anatomy, 35th British ed. Philadelphia, WB Saunders, 1973, p 530.)

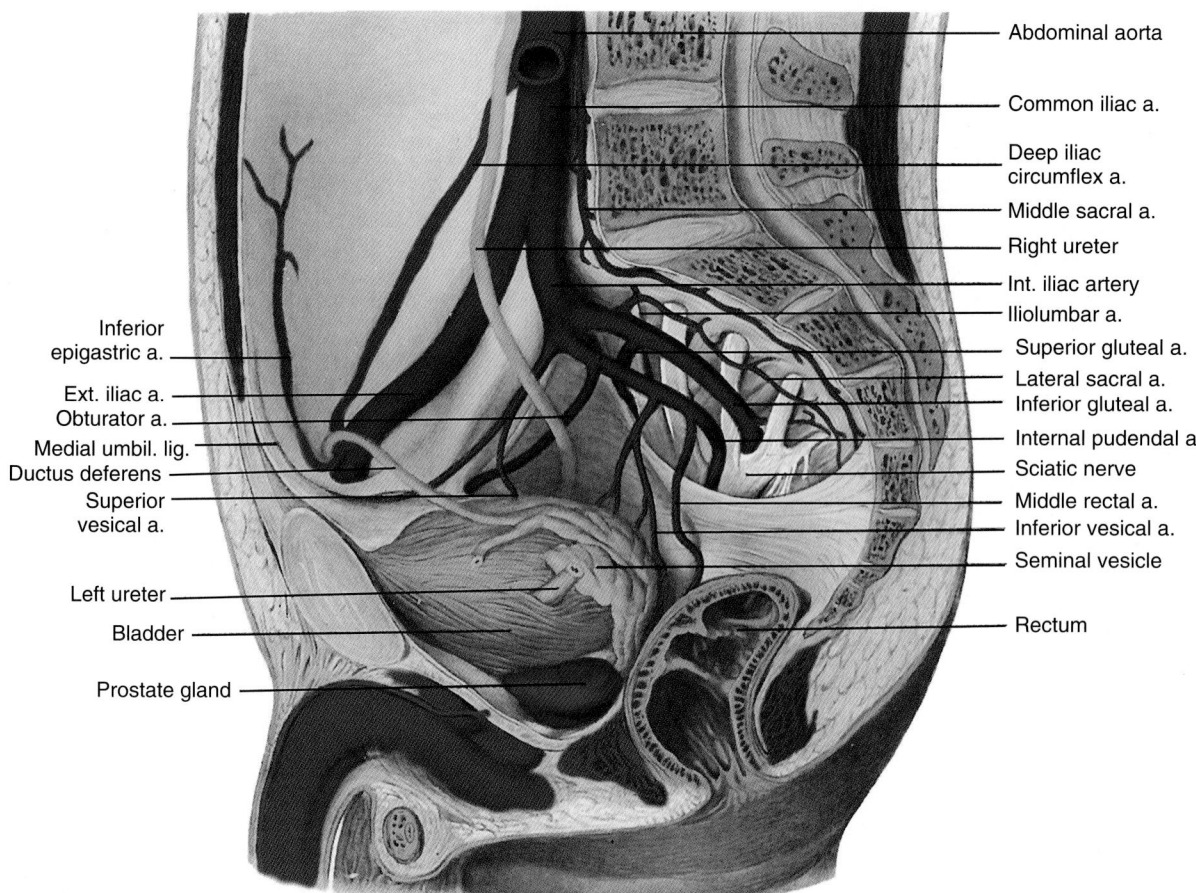

Figure 2–15. Right internal and external iliac arteries. The ureter and vas deferens pass medial to the vessels. (From Clemente CD: Gray's Anatomy, 30th American ed. Philadelphia, Lea & Febiger, 1985, p 750.)

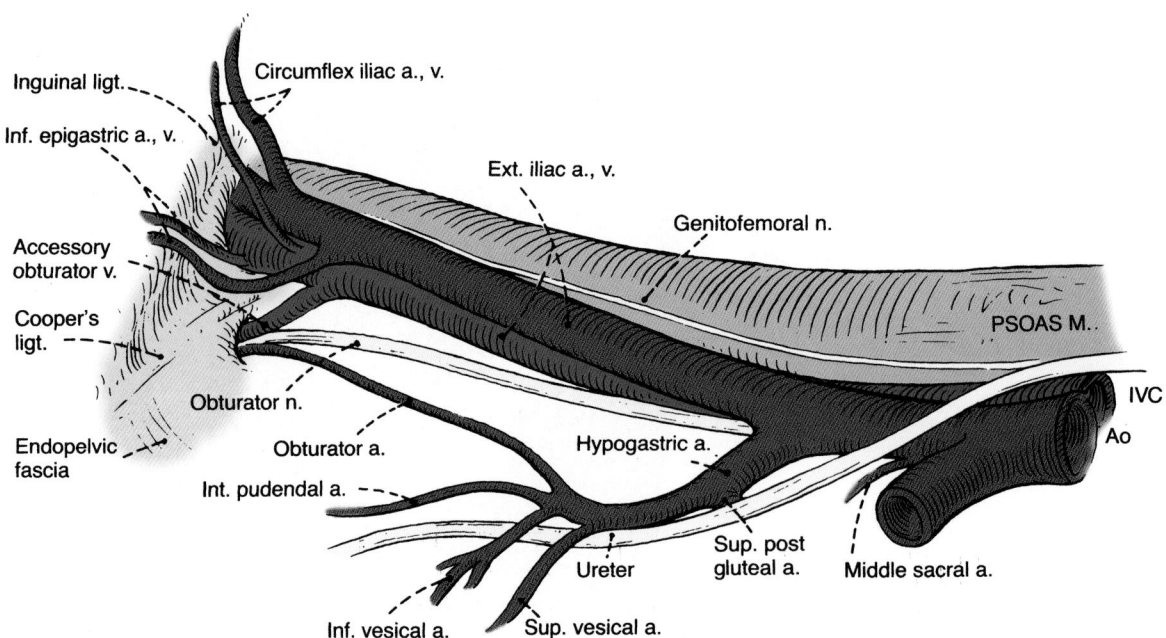

Figure 2–16. Right obturator fossa, showing the iliac vessels and obturator nerve. (From Skinner DG: Pelvic lymphadenectomy. In Glenn JF [ed]: Urological Surgery, 2nd ed. New York, Harper & Row, 1975, p 591.)

reach the obturator canal. This vessel must be avoided during obturator lymph node dissection.

The internal iliac (hypogastric) artery descends in front of the SI joint and divides into an anterior and a posterior trunk (see Fig. 2–15). The posterior trunk gives rise to three parietal branches: (1) the superior gluteal, which exits the greater sciatic foramen; (2) the ascending lumbar, which supplies the posterior abdominal wall; and (3) the lateral sacral, which passes medially to join the middle sacral branches at the sciatic foramina.

The anterior trunk gives off seven parietal and visceral branches: (1) The superior vesical artery arises from the proximal portion of the obliterated umbilical artery and gives off a vesiculodeferential branch to the seminal vesicles and vas deferens. The artery of the vas deferens travels the length of the vas to meet the cremasteric and testicular arteries distally (see Fig. 2–44). Because of these anastomoses, the testicular artery may be sacrificed without compromising the viability of the testis. (2) The middle rectal artery gives small branches to the seminal vesicles and prostate and anastomoses with the inferior and superior rectal arteries in the rectal wall. (3) The inferior vesical branches supply the lower ureter, the bladder base, the prostate, and the seminal vesicles. In the female, they supply the ureter, the bladder base, and the vagina. (4) The uterine artery passes above and in front of the ureter ("water flows under the bridge") to ascend the lateral wall of the uterus and meet the ovarian artery in the lateral portion of the fallopian tube (see Figs. 2–13 and 2–31). The ureter is vulnerable during division of the uterine pedicles. (5) The internal pudendal artery leaves the pelvic cavity through the greater sciatic foramen, passes around the sacrospinous ligament, and enters the lesser sciatic foramen to gain access to the perineum. Its perineal course is discussed later. (6) The obturator artery, variable in origin, travels through the obturator fossa medial and inferior to the obturator nerve and passes through its canal to supply the adductors of the thigh (see Fig. 2–16). (7) The inferior gluteal artery travels through the greater sciatic foramen to supply the buttock and thigh.

The internal iliac artery can be ligated to control severe pelvic hemorrhage. Ligation decreases the pulse pressure, allowing hemostasis to occur more readily. Internal iliac blood flow does not stop but reverses its direction because of critical anastomoses (lumbar segmentals to iliolumbar; median sacral to lateral sacral; and superior rectal and middle rectal). Bilateral ligation almost invariably produces vasculogenic impotence.

Venous Supply

The dorsal vein of the penis passes between the inferior pubic arch and the striated urinary sphincter to reach the pelvis, where it trifurcates into a central superficial branch and two lateral plexuses (Reiner and Walsh, 1979) (Fig. 2–17). To minimize blood loss at radical retropubic prostatectomy, the dorsal vein complex is best divided distally, before its ramification. Part of this complex runs within the anterior and lateral wall of the striated sphincter; thus, care must be taken not to injure the sphincter when securing hemostasis. The superficial branch pierces the visceral endopelvic fascia between the puboprostatic ligaments and drains the retropubic fat, the anterior bladder, and the anterior prostate (see Figs. 2–17 and 2–40).

The lateral plexuses sweep down the sides of the prostate, receiving drainage from it and the rectum, and communicate with the vesical plexuses on the lower part of the bladder. Three to five inferior vesical veins emerge from the vesical plexus laterally and drain into the internal iliac vein. In the female, the dorsal vein of the clitoris bifurcates to empty into the laterally placed vaginal plexuses. These connect with the vesical, uterine, ovarian, and rectal plexuses and drain into the internal iliac veins. Connections between the pelvic plexuses, the emissary veins of the pelvic bones, and the vertebral plexus have been proposed to be routes for the dissemination of infection or tumor from the pelvic viscera to the axial and pelvic skeleton (Batson, 1940).

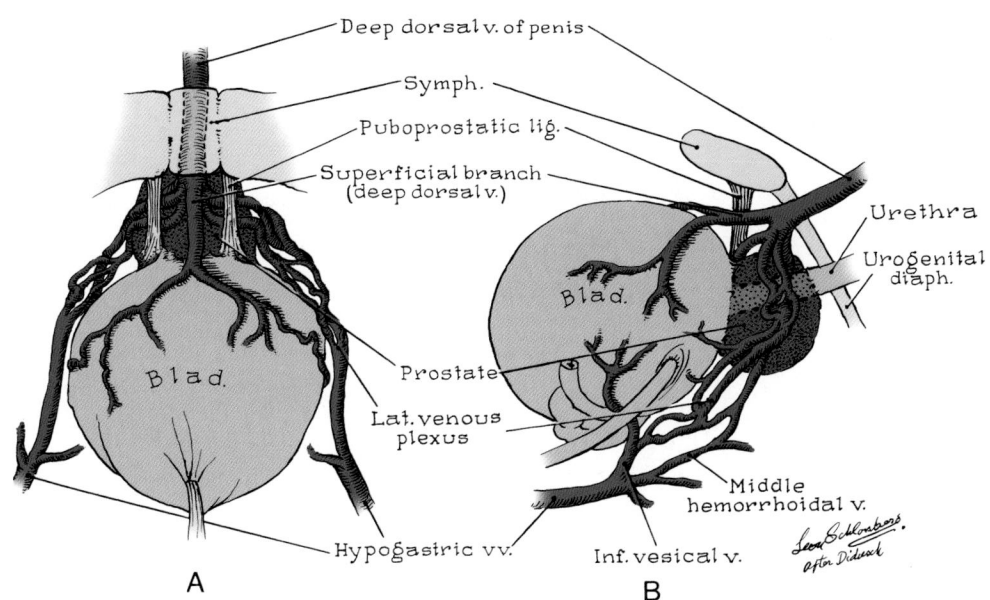

Figure 2–17. Pelvic venous plexus. **A,** Trifurcation of the dorsal vein of the penis, viewed from the retropubic space. The relationship of the venous branches to the puboprostatic ligaments is shown. **B,** Lateral view of the pelvic venous plexus after removal of the lateral pelvic fascia. Normally these structures are difficult to see because they are embedded in pelvic fascia. (From Reiner WG, Walsh PC: An anatomical approach to the surgical management of the dorsal vein and Santorini's plexus during radical retropubic surgery. J Urol 1979;121:198-200.)

The internal iliac vein is joined by tributaries corresponding to the branches of the internal iliac artery and ascends medial and posterior to the artery. This vein is relatively thin walled and at risk for injury during dissection of the artery or the nearby pelvic ureter. The external iliac vein travels medial and inferior to its artery and joins the internal iliac vein behind the internal iliac artery. In half the patients, one or **more accessory obturator veins drain into the underside of the external iliac vein and can be easily torn during lymphadenectomy** (see Fig. 2–16).

Pelvic Lymphatics

The pelvic lymph nodes can be difficult to appreciate on gross examination because they are embedded in the fatty and fibrous tissue of the intermediate stratum. Three major lymph node groups are associated with the pelvic vessels (Fig. 2–18). A substantial portion of pelvic visceral lymphatic drainage passes through the **internal iliac nodes and their tributaries: the presacral, obturator, and internal pudendal nodes.** The external iliac nodes lie lateral, anterior, and medial to the vessels and drain the anterior abdominal wall, urachus, bladder, and, in part, internal genitalia. The external genitalia and perineum drain into the superficial and deep inguinal nodes (see later discussion). The inguinal nodes communicate directly with the internal and external iliac chains. The common iliac nodes receive efferent vessels from the external and internal iliac nodes and the pelvic ureter and drain into the lateral aortic nodes.

PELVIC INNERVATION

Lumbosacral Plexus

The lumbosacral plexus and its rami are well illustrated in Chapter 1, Surgical Anatomy of the Retroperitoneum, Kidneys, and Ureters; only the pelvic courses of its nerves are reviewed here (see Figs. 2–6 and 2–12 and Table 2–2). The **iliohypogastric nerve** (L1) travels between, and supplies, the internal oblique and the transversus muscles and pierces the internal and external oblique muscles 3 cm above the external inguinal ring to supply sensation over the lower anterior abdomen and pubis (see Fig. 2–4). The ilioinguinal nerve (L1) passes through the internal oblique muscle to enter the inguinal canal laterally. It travels anterior to the cord and exits the external ring to provide sensation to the mons pubis and anterior scrotum or labia majora (see Figs. 2–4 and 2–6). The genitofemoral nerve (L1, L2) pierces the psoas muscle to reach its anterior surface in the retroperitoneum and then travels to the pelvis and splits into genital and femoral branches. The latter supplies sensation over the anterior thigh below the inguinal ligament. The genital branch follows the cord through the inguinal canal, supplies the cremaster muscle, and supplies sensation to the anterior scrotum.

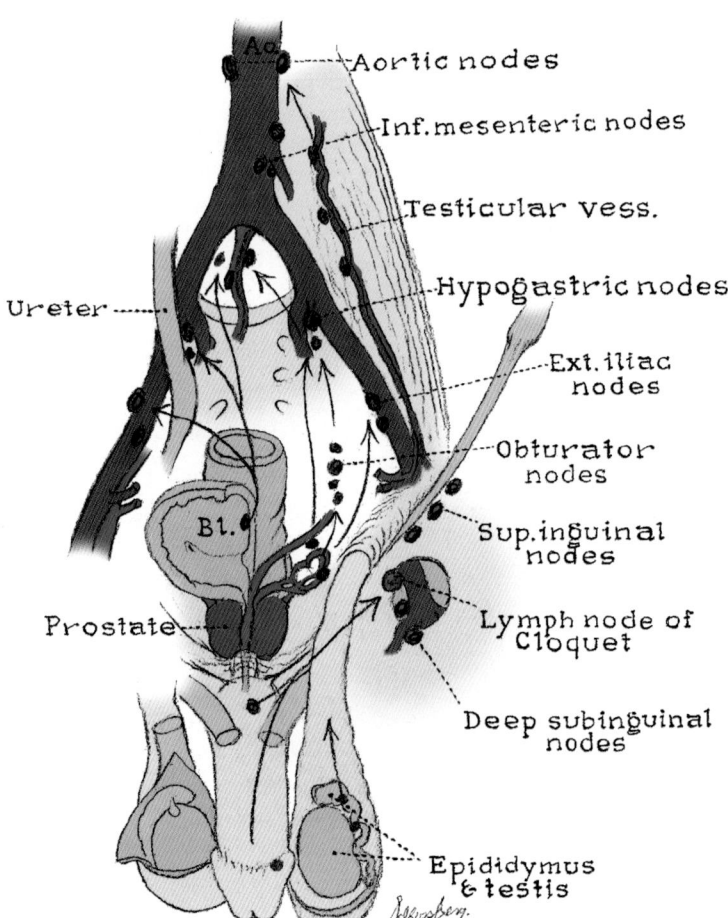

Figure 2–18.   Lymphatic drainage of the male pelvis, perineum, and external genitalia.

Table 2–2. **Somatic Nerves of the Lower Abdomen and Pelvis**		
Nerve Name	*Origin*	*Supplies*
Iliohypogastric	L1	Motor supply to internal oblique, transversus muscles, sensation over lower anterior abdominal wall
Ilioinguinal	L1	Sensation over anterior pubis (mons) and anterior scrotum or labia
Genitofemoral	L1, L2	Genital branch: motor supply to cremaster muscle, sensation to anterior scrotum; femoral branch: sensation to anterior thigh
Femoral	L2, L3, L4	Motor supply to extensors of the knee, sensation to anterior thigh
Obturator	L2, L3, L4	Motor supply to adductors of the thigh, sensation to medial thigh
Lumbosacral trunk	L4, L5	Joins the sacral nerves to form the lumbosacral plexus that supplies motor and sensory innervation to the lower extremities
Posterior femoral cutaneous	S2, S3	Sensation to perineum, posterior scrotum, and posterior thigh
Pudendal	S2, S3, S4	Motor to levator ani, muscles of the urogenital diaphragm, anal and striated urethral sphincter, sensation to the perineum, scrotum, and penis
Pelvic somatic efferents	S2, S3, S4	Motor supply to levator ani and striated urethral sphincter
Nervi erigentes	S2, S3, S4	Parasympathetic fibers from the sacral cord supply the pelvic viscera

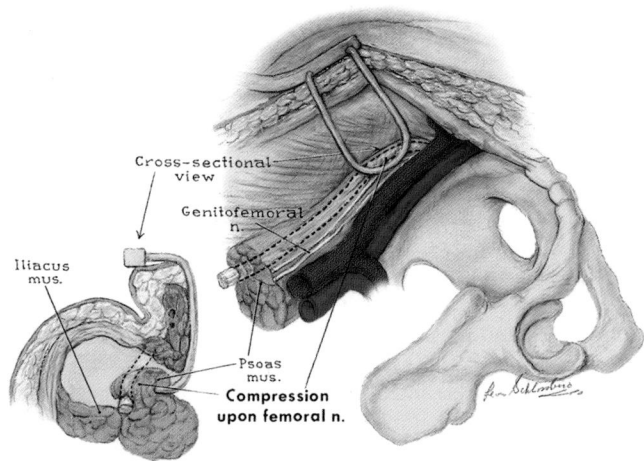

Figure 2–19. Femoral nerve as it relates to the psoas muscle. Retractor blades may compress this nerve to produce a femoral nerve palsy. (From Burnett AL, Brendler CB: Femoral neuropathy following major pelvic surgery: Etiology and prevention. J Urol 1994;151:163-165.)

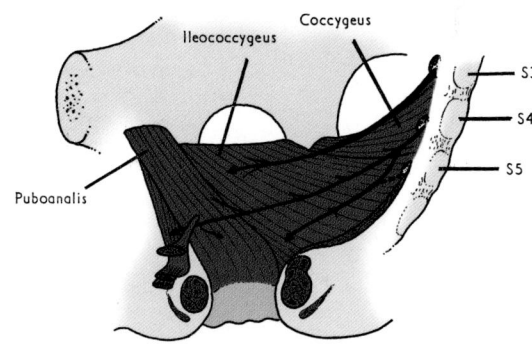

Figure 2–20. Pelvic floor somatic efferent nerves extending anteriorly on the pelvic surface of the levator ani to supply this muscle and the striated urethral sphincter. (From Lawson JON: Pelvic anatomy: Pelvic floor muscles. Ann R Coll Surg Engl 1974;54:244-252.)

For most of its pelvic course, the femoral nerve (L2, L3, L4) travels within the substance of the psoas muscle and then exits its lateral side to pass under the inguinal ligament (Fig. 2–19). It supplies sensation to the anterior thigh and motor innervation to the extensors of the knee. **During a psoas hitch, sutures should be placed in the direction of the nerve (and the psoas muscle fibers) to avoid nerve damage or entrapment. Retractor blades must not rest on the psoas muscle because they can produce a femoral nerve palsy,** a potentially dangerous setback after pelvic surgery. The lateral femoral cutaneous nerve (L2, L3) may be seen lateral to the psoas in the iliacus fascia.

The **obturator nerve** (L2, L3, L4) emerges in the true pelvis from beneath the psoas muscle, lateral to the internal iliac vessels, and passes through the obturator fossa to the obturator canal. In the fossa, it is lateral and superior to the obturator vessels and surrounded by the obturator and internal iliac lymph nodes. Damage to this nerve during pelvic lymphadenectomy weakens the adductors of the thigh.

The lumbosacral trunk (L4, L5) passes into the true pelvis behind the psoas and unites with the ventral rami of the sacral segmental nerves to form the sacral plexus. This plexus lies on the pelvic surface of the piriformis deep to the endopelvic fascia and posterior to the internal iliac vessels (see Fig. 2–15). It leaves the pelvis through the greater sciatic foramen immediately posterior to the sacrospinous ligament (where it may be injured during sacrospinous culposuspen-

sion) and supplies motor and sensory innervation to the posterior thigh and lower leg. An exaggerated lithotomy position may stretch this nerve or place pressure on its peroneal branch at the fibular head to produce footdrop. Pelvic and perineal branches of the sacral plexus include (1) the posterior femoral cutaneous nerve (S2, S3), which, after passing through the greater sciatic foramen, gives an anterior sensory branch to the perineum and posterior scrotum (see Fig. 2–8); (2) the pudendal nerve (S2, S3, S4), which follows the internal pudendal artery to the perineum (to be discussed); (3) the nervi erigentes (S2, S3, S4) to the autonomic plexus; and (4) pelvic somatic efferent nerves from the ventral rami of S2, S3, and S4 (Fig. 2–20). These last nerves travel on the pelvic surface of the levator ani in close association with the rectum and prostate and are separated from the pelvic autonomic plexus by the endopelvic fascia. They supply the levator ani and extend anteriorly to the striated urethral sphincter (Lawson, 1974; Zvara et al, 1994).

Pelvic Autonomic Plexus

The presynaptic sympathetic cell bodies that project to the pelvic autonomic plexus reside in the lateral column of gray matter in the last three thoracic and first two lumbar segments of the spinal cord. They reach the pelvic plexus by two pathways: (1) The **superior hypogastric plexus** is formed by sympathetic fibers from the celiac plexus and the first four lumbar splanchnic nerves (Fig. 2–21). Anterior to the bifurcation of the aorta, it divides into two hypogastric nerves that enter the pelvis medial to the internal iliac vessels, anterior to the sacrum, and deep to the endopelvic fascia. (2) The pelvic continuations of the sympathetic trunks pass deep to the common iliac vessels and medial to the sacral foramina and fuse in front of the coccyx at the ganglion impar (see Fig. 2–21). Each chain comprises four to five ganglia that send branches anterolaterally to participate in the formation of the pelvic plexus.

Presynaptic parasympathetic innervation arises from the intermediolateral cell column of the sacral cord. Fibers emerge from the second, third, and fourth sacral spinal nerves as the pelvic splanchnic nerves (nervi erigentes) to join the hypogastric nerves and branches from the sacral sympathetic ganglia to form the inferior hypogastric (pelvic) plexus (see Fig. 2–21). Some pelvic parasympathetic efferent fibers travel up the hypogastric nerves to the inferior mesenteric plexus, where they provide parasympathetic innervation to the descending and sigmoid colon.

The pelvic plexus is rectangular and is 4 to 5 cm long, and its midpoint is at the tips of the seminal vesicles (Schlegel and Walsh, 1987). It is oriented in the sagittal plane on either side of the rectum and pierced by the numerous vessels going to and from the rectum, bladder, seminal vesicles, and prostate (Fig. 2–22). **Division of these vessels (the so-called lateral pedicles of the bladder and prostate) risks injury to the pelvic plexus with attendant postoperative impotence** (Walsh and Donker, 1982; Walsh et al, 1983). The right and left components of the pelvic plexus communicate behind the rectum and anterior and posterior to the vesical neck.

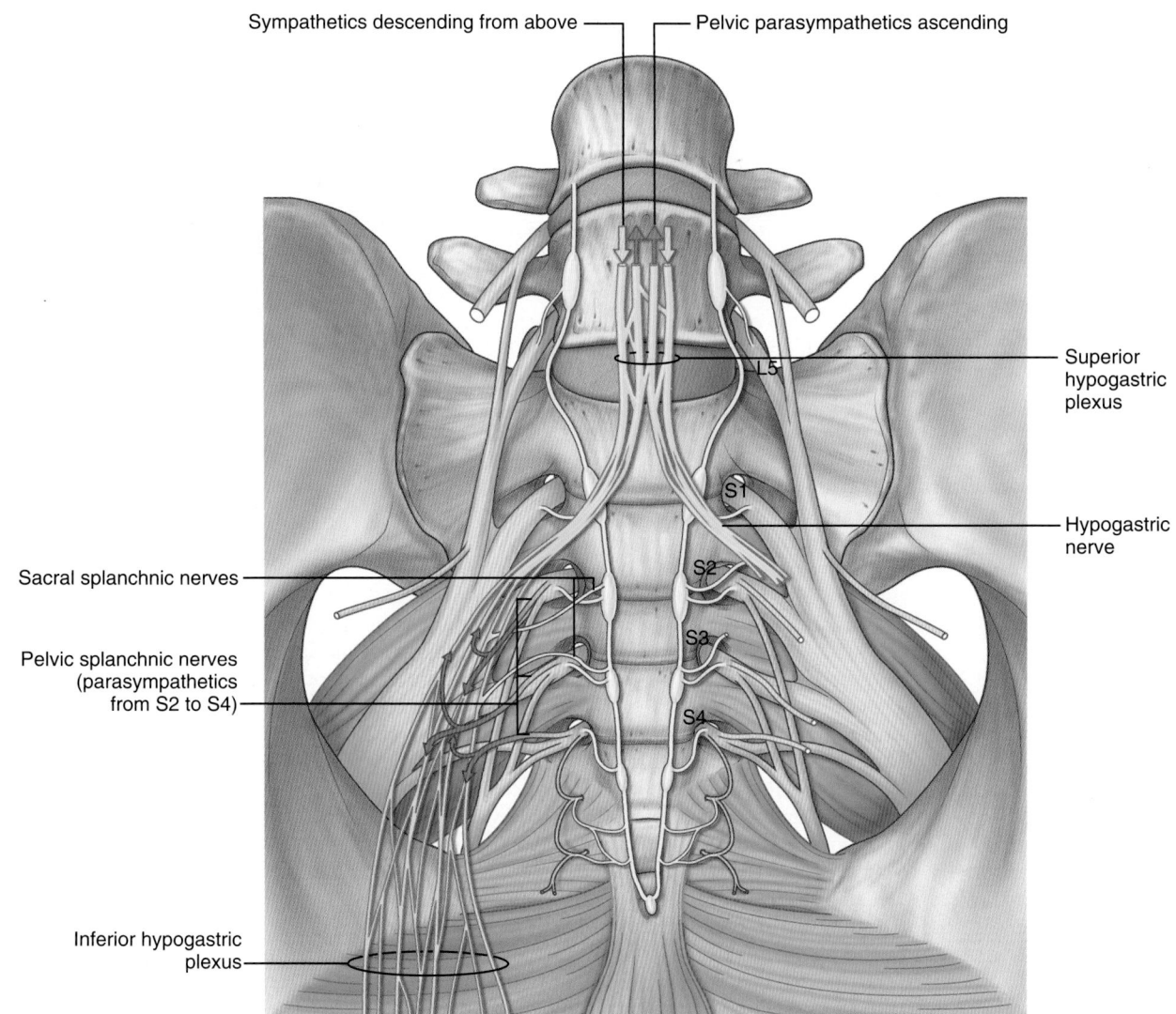

Figure 2–21. Sympathetic and parasympathetic contributions to the pelvic autonomic nervous plexus. (From Drake RL, Vogl W, Mitchell AWM: Gray's Anatomy for Students. Philadelphia, Elsevier, 2005.)

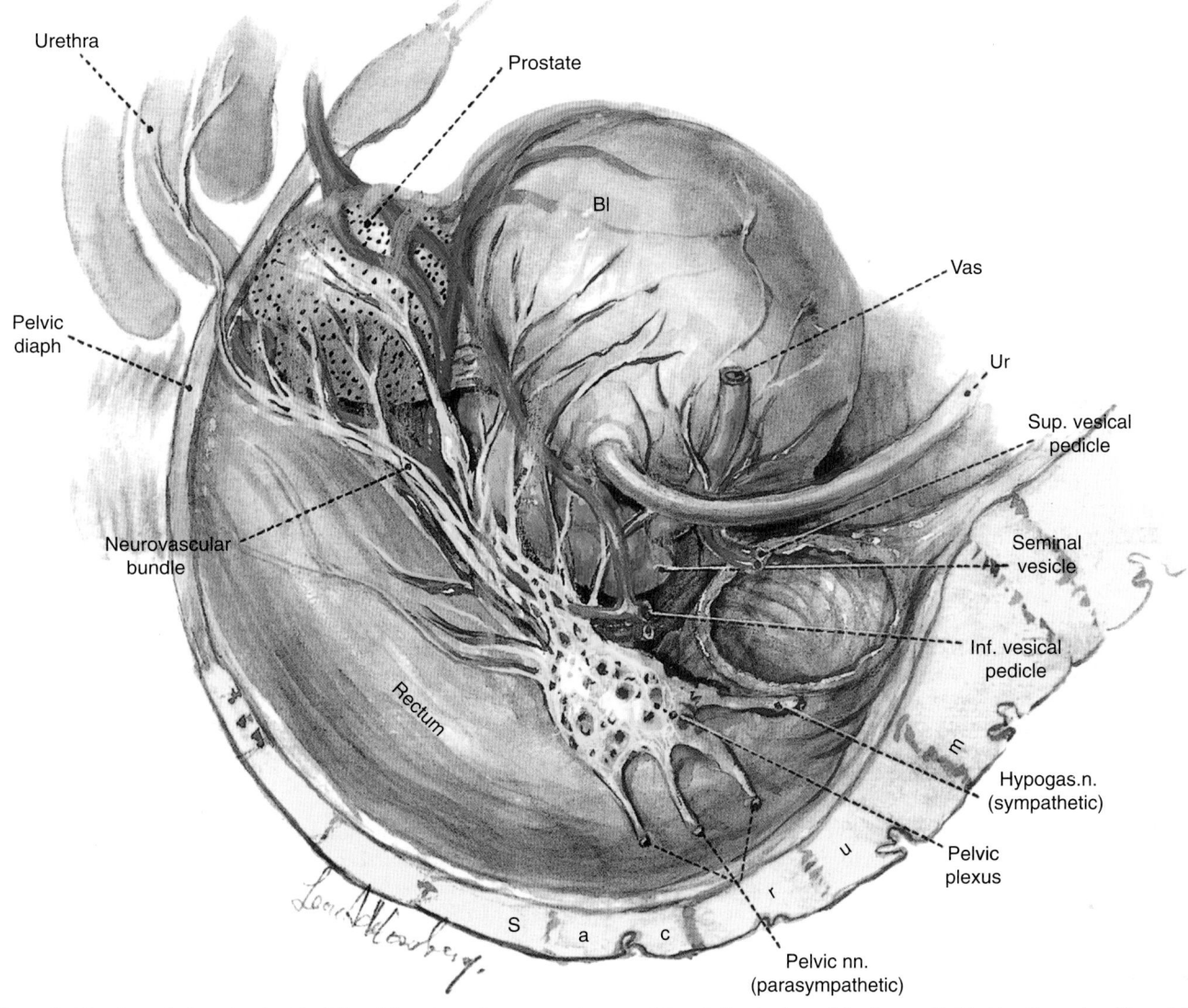

Figure 2–22. Lateral view showing the left pelvic autonomic nervous plexus and its relation to the pelvic viscera. Bl, bladder; Ur, ureter. (From Schlegel PN, Walsh PC: Neuroanatomical approach to radical cystoprostatectomy with preservation of sexual function. J Urol 1987;138:1402-1406.)

Branches of the pelvic plexus follow pelvic blood vessels to reach the pelvic viscera, although nerves to the ureter may join it directly as it passes nearby. Visceral afferent and efferent nerves travel on the vas deferens to reach the testis and epididymis (see later discussion).

The most caudal portion of the pelvic plexus gives rise to the innervation of the prostate and the important cavernosal nerves (Walsh and Donker, 1982). After passing the tips of the seminal vesicles, these nerves lie within leaves of the lateral endopelvic fascia near its juncture with, but outside, Denonvilliers' fascia (Lepor et al, 1985). They travel at the posterolateral border of the prostate on the surface of the rectum and are lateral to the prostatic capsular arteries and veins (see Fig. 2–22). Because the nerves are composed of multiple fibers not visible on gross inspection, these vessels serve as a surgical landmark for the course of these nerves (the neurovascular bundle of Walsh). During radical prostatectomy, the nerves are most vulnerable at the apex of the prostate, where they closely approach the prostatic capsule at the 5- and 7-o'clock positions. On reaching the membranous urethra, the nerves divide into superficial branches, which travel on the lateral surface of the striated urethral sphincter at 3- and 9-o'clock positions, and deep fibers, which penetrate the substance of this muscle and send twigs to the bulbourethral glands. As the nerves reach the hilum of the penis, they join to form one to three discrete bundles, related to the urethra at 1- and 11-o'clock positions, superficial to the cavernous veins, and dorsomedial to the cavernous arteries (see Fig. 2–41) (Lue et al, 1984; Breza et al, 1989). With the arteries, they pierce the corpora cavernosa to supply the erectile tissue (see later discussion). Small fibers also join the dorsal nerves of the penis as they course distally. In the female, the nerves to vestibular bodies and corpora cavernosa of the clitoris travel between the anterior vaginal wall and the bladder in association with the lateral venous plexuses.

PELVIC VISCERA

Rectum

The rectum begins with the disappearance of the sigmoid mesentery opposite the third sacral vertebra. **Peritoneum continues anteriorly over the upper two thirds of the rectum as the rectovesical pouch in males and as the rectouterine pouch (of Douglas) in females** (Fig. 2–23; see also Fig. 2–11). This peritoneal pouch extends inferiorly to the seminal vesicles or to the posterior fornix of the vagina. Inferior to this pouch, the anterior rectum is related to its fascial continuation (the rectogenital or Denonvilliers' fascia) down to the level of the striated urethral sphincter (see Figs. 2–3, 2–23, and 2–33). The rectum describes a gentle curve on the sacrum, coccyx, and levator plate (see Fig. 2–21) and receives innervation from the laterally placed pelvic autonomic plexus and blood supply from the superior (from inferior mesenteric), middle (from internal iliac), and inferior (from internal pudendal) rectal arteries.

The rectal wall is composed of an inner layer of circular smooth muscle and a virtually continuous sheet of outer longitudinal smooth muscle derived from the tenia of the colon. In its lowest part, the rectum dilates to form the rectal ampulla. At the most inferior portion of the ampulla, anterior fibers of the longitudinal muscle leave the rectum to join Denonvilliers' fascia and the posterior striated urethral sphincter in the apex of the perineal body (Brooks et al, 2002). When approached from below, these fibers, **the rectourethralis muscle, are 2 to 10 mm thick and must be divided to gain access to the prostate** (see Fig. 2–36). The apices of the prostate and ampulla are in close proximity, and rectal injuries during radical prostatectomy commonly occur at this location. As the rectourethralis is given off, the rectum makes a right-angle turn posteroinferiorly to exit the pelvis at the anal canal (see Fig. 2–10). The anatomy of the anal canal is considered with the perineum.

Pelvic Ureter

The ureter is divided into abdominal and pelvic portions by the common iliac artery. The structure of the ureter and its abdominal course are reviewed in Chapter 1, Surgical Anatomy of the Retroperitoneum, Kidneys, and Ureters. Intraoperatively, the ureter is identified by its peristaltic waves and is readily found anterior to the bifurcation of the common iliac artery. At ureteroscopy, pulsations of this artery can be seen in the posterior ureteral wall. **The ovarian vessels (infundibulopelvic ligament) cross the iliac vessels anterior and lateral to the ureter, and dissection of the ovarian vessels at the pelvic brim is a common cause of ureteral injury** (see Fig. 2–13) (Daly and Higgins, 1988). Pyeloureterography discloses a narrowing of the ureter at the iliac vessels, and ureteral calculi frequently become lodged at this location. Because the ureter and iliac vessels rest on the arcuate line, the ureter is subject to compression and obstruction by the gravid uterus and by masses within the true pelvis.

The ureters come within 5 cm of each other as they cross the iliac vessels. On entering the pelvis, they diverge widely along the pelvic side walls toward the ischial spines. The ureter travels on the anterior surface of the internal iliac vessels and is related laterally to the branches of the anterior trunk. Near the ischial spine, the ureter turns anteriorly and medially to reach the bladder. In males, the anteromedial surface of the ureter is covered by peritoneum, and the ureter is embedded in retroperitoneal connective tissue, which varies in thickness (see Fig. 2–13). As the ureter courses medially, it is crossed anteriorly by the vas deferens and runs with the inferior vesical arteries, veins, and nerves in the lateral vesical ligaments. Viewed from the peritoneal side, the ureter is just lateral and deep to the rectogenital fold. In females, the ureter first runs posterior to the ovary and then turns medially to run deep to the base of the broad ligament before entering a loose connective tissue tunnel through the substance of the cardinal ligament (see Fig. 2–13). As in the male, the ureter can be found

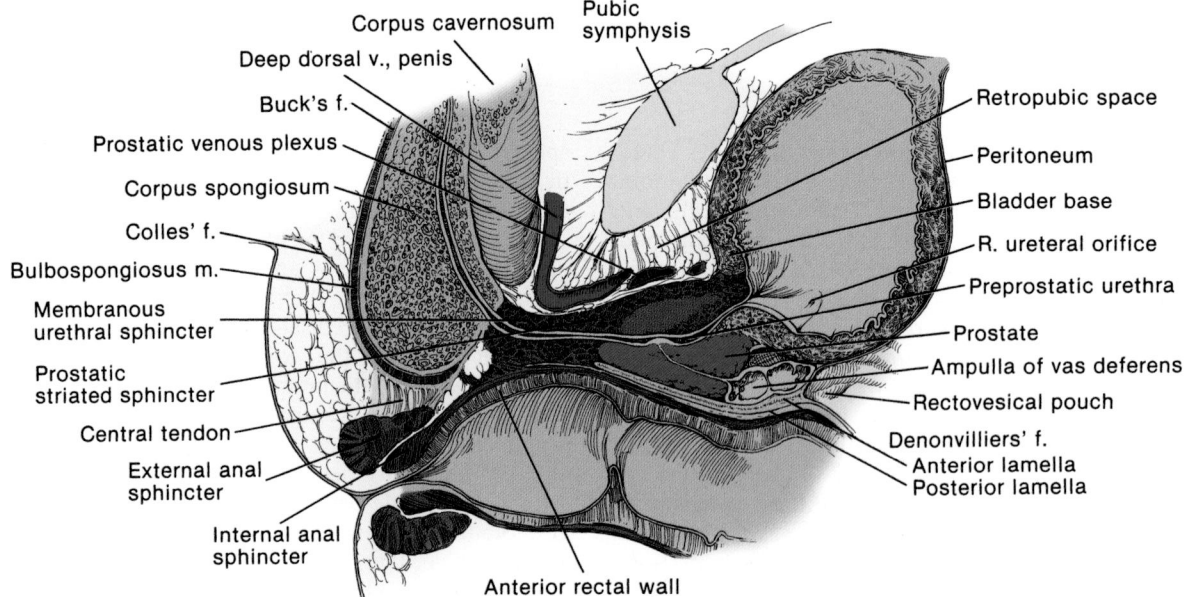

Figure 2–23. Sagittal section through the prostatic and membranous urethra, demonstrating the midline relations of the pelvic structures. (From Hinman F Jr: Atlas of Urosurgical Anatomy. Philadelphia, WB Saunders, 1993, p 356.)

slightly lateral and deep to the rectouterine folds of peritoneum. It is crossed anteriorly by the uterine artery and is therefore subject to injury during hysterectomy. As it passes in front of the vagina, it crosses 1.5 cm anterior and lateral to the uterine cervix. The ureter may be injured at this level during hysterectomy, resulting in a ureterovaginal fistula. The ureter courses 1 to 4 cm on the anterior vaginal wall to reach the bladder. Occasionally, a stone lodged in the distal ureter can be palpated through the anterior vaginal wall. The intramural ureter is discussed in the section on the bladder.

The pelvic ureter receives abundant blood supply from the common iliac artery and most branches of the internal iliac artery. The inferior vesical and uterine arteries usually supply the ureter with its largest pelvic branches. **Blood supply to the pelvic ureter enters laterally; thus, the pelvic peritoneum should be incised only medial to the ureter.** Intramural vessels of the ureter run within the adventitia and generally follow one of two patterns. In approximately 75% of specimens, longitudinal vessels run the length of the ureter and are formed by anastomoses of segmental ureteral vessels. In the remaining ureters, the vessels form a fine interconnecting mesh (plexiform) with less collateral flow (Shafik, 1972). The pelvic ureter appears to have a high preponderance of plexiform vessels, which render it more susceptible to ischemia and less suitable for ureteroureterotomy (Hinman, 1993). Lymphatic drainage of the pelvic ureter is to the external, internal, and common iliac nodes. Pathologic enlargement of the common and internal iliac nodes can encroach on and obstruct the ureter.

The pelvic ureter has rich adrenergic and cholinergic autonomic innervation derived from the pelvic plexus. The functional significance of this innervation is unclear, inasmuch as the ureter continues to contract peristaltically after denervation. Afferent neural fibers travel through the pelvic plexus and account for the visceral quality of referred pain from ureteral irritation or acute obstruction.

Bladder

Anatomic Relationships

When filled, the bladder has a capacity of approximately 500 mL and assumes an ovoid shape. The empty bladder is tetrahedral and is described as having a superior surface with an apex at the urachus, two inferolateral surfaces, and a posteroinferior surface or base with the bladder neck at the lowest point (see Fig. 2–23).

The urachus anchors the bladder to the anterior abdominal wall (see Fig. 2–8). There is a relative paucity of bladder wall muscle at the point of attachment of the urachus, predisposing to formation of diverticula. The urachus is composed of longitudinal smooth muscle bundles derived from the bladder wall. Near the umbilicus, it becomes more fibrous and usually fuses with one of the obliterated umbilical arteries. Urachal vessels run longitudinally, and the ends of the urachus must be ligated when it is divided. An epithelium-lined lumen usually persists throughout life and uncommonly gives rise to aggressive urachal adenocarcinomas (Begg, 1930). In rare instances, luminal continuity with the bladder serves as a bacterial reservoir or results in an umbilical urinary fistula.

The superior surface of the bladder is covered by peritoneum. Anteriorly, the peritoneum sweeps gently onto the anterior abdominal wall (see Fig. 2–13). With distention, the bladder rises out of the true pelvis and separates the peritoneum from the anterior abdominal wall. It is therefore possible to perform a suprapubic cystostomy without risking entry into the peritoneal cavity. Posteriorly, the peritoneum passes to the level of the seminal vesicles and meets the peritoneum on the anterior rectum to form the rectovesical space.

Anteroinferiorly and laterally, **the bladder is cushioned from the pelvic side wall by retropubic and perivesical fat and loose connective tissue.** This potential space (of Retzius) may be entered anteriorly by dividing the transversalis fascia and provides access to the pelvic viscera as far posteriorly as the iliac vessels and ureters (see Fig. 2–11). The bladder base is related to the seminal vesicles, ampullae of the vas deferentia, and terminal ureter. The bladder neck, located at the internal urethral meatus, rests 3 to 4 cm behind the midpoint of the symphysis pubis. It is firmly fixed by the pelvic fasciae (see earlier discussion) and by its continuity with the prostate; its position changes little with varying conditions of the bladder and rectum.

In the female, the peritoneum on the superior surface of the bladder is reflected over the uterus to form the vesicouterine pouch and then continues posteriorly over the uterus as the rectouterine pouch (see Fig. 2–13). The vagina and uterus intervene between the bladder and the rectum, so that the base of the bladder and urethra rest on the anterior vaginal wall. Because the anterior vaginal wall is firmly attached laterally to the levator ani, contraction of the pelvic diaphragm (e.g., during increases in intra-abdominal pressure) elevates the bladder neck and draws it anteriorly. In many women with stress incontinence, the bladder neck drops below the pubic symphysis. In infants, the true pelvis is shallow and the bladder neck is level with the upper border of the symphysis. The bladder is a true intra-abdominal organ that can project above the umbilicus when full. By puberty, the bladder has migrated to the confines of the deepened true pelvis.

Structure

The internal surface of the bladder is lined with transitional epithelium, which appears smooth when the bladder is full but contracts into numerous folds when the bladder empties. This urothelium is usually six cells thick and rests on a thin basement membrane. Deep to this, the lamina propria forms a relatively thick layer of fibroelastic connective tissue that allows considerable distention. This layer is traversed by numerous blood vessels and contains smooth muscle fibers collected into a poorly defined muscularis mucosa. Beneath this layer lies the smooth muscle of the bladder wall. The relatively large muscle fibers form branching, interlacing bundles loosely arranged into inner longitudinal, middle circular, and outer longitudinal layers (Fig. 2–24). However, in the upper aspect of the bladder, these layers are clearly not separable, and any one fiber can travel between each of the layers, change orientation, and branch into longitudinal and circular fibers. This meshwork of detrusor muscle is ideally suited for emptying the spherical bladder.

Near the bladder neck, the detrusor muscle is clearly separable into the three layers described earlier. Here, the

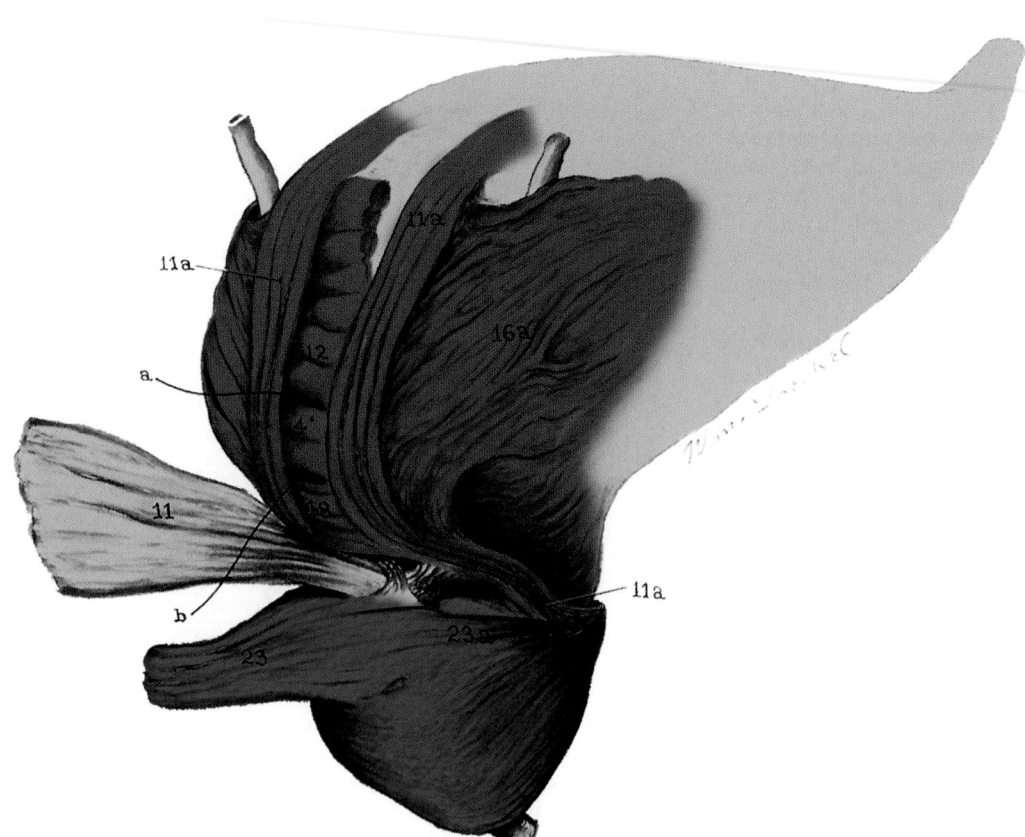

Figure 2–24. Dissection of the male bladder. 11, Posterior outer longitudinal detrusor, which forms the backing of the ureters *(folded back);* 11a, posterolateral portion of the outer longitudinal muscle forming a loop around the anterior bladder neck; 4', 12, and 18, middle circular layer backing the trigone; 23 and 23a, lateral pedicle of the prostate. (From Uhlenhuth E: Problems in the Anatomy of the Pelvis. Philadelphia, JB Lippincott, 1953, p 187.)

smooth muscle is morphologically and pharmacologically distinct from the remainder of the bladder, because the large-diameter muscle fascicles are replaced by much finer fibers. The structure of the bladder neck appears to differ between men and women. In men, radially oriented inner longitudinal fibers pass through the internal meatus to become continuous with the inner longitudinal layer of smooth muscle in the urethra.

The middle layer forms a circular preprostatic sphincter that is responsible for continence at the level of the bladder neck (Fig. 2–25). The bladder wall posterior to the internal urethral meatus and the anterior fibromuscular stroma of the prostate form a continuous ringlike structure at the bladder neck (Brooks et al, 1998). The fact that perfect continence can be maintained in men in whom the striated urethral sphincter is destroyed attests to the efficacy of this sphincter (Waterhouse et al, 1973). This muscle is richly innervated by adrenergic fibers, which, when stimulated, produce closure of the bladder neck (Uhlenhuth, 1953). Damage to the sympathetic nerves to the bladder, as a result of diabetes mellitus or retroperitoneal lymph node dissection for testis cancer, can cause retrograde ejaculation.

The outer longitudinal fibers are thickest posteriorly at the bladder base. In the midline, they insert into the apex of the trigone and intermix with the smooth muscle of the prostate to provide a strong trigonal backing. Laterally, the fibers from this posterior sheet pass anteriorly and fuse to form a loop around the bladder neck (see Fig. 2–24). This loop is thought to participate in continence at the bladder neck. On the lateral and anterior surfaces of the bladder, the longitudi-

nal fibers are not as well developed. Some anterior fibers course forward to join the puboprostatic ligaments in men and the pubourethral ligaments in women. These fibers contribute smooth muscle to these supports and are speculated to contribute to bladder neck opening during micturition (DeLancey, 1989).

At the female bladder neck, the inner longitudinal fibers converge radially to pass downward as the inner longitudinal layer of the urethra, as described earlier. The middle circular layer does not appear to be as robust as that of the male, and several authors have denied its existence altogether (Gosling, 1979, 1985; Williams et al, 1989). Whereas several other investigators have noted an anterior loop of external longitudinal muscle (see Fig. 2–32), the authors just cited deny the existence of this structure as well. They maintain instead that the external fibers pass obliquely and longitudinally down the urethra to participate in forming the inner longitudinal layer of smooth muscle. Regardless, the female bladder neck differs strikingly from the male in possessing little adrenergic innervation. In addition, its sphincteric function is limited; in 50% of continent women, urine enters the proximal urethra during a cough (Versi et al, 1986).

Ureterovesical Junction and the Trigone

As the ureter approaches the bladder, its spirally oriented mural smooth muscle fibers become longitudinal. Two to 3 cm from the bladder, a fibromuscular sheath (of Waldeyer) extends longitudinally over the ureter and follows it to the trigone (Tanagho, 1992). The ureter pierces the bladder wall obliquely, travels 1.5 to 2 cm, and terminates at the ureteral

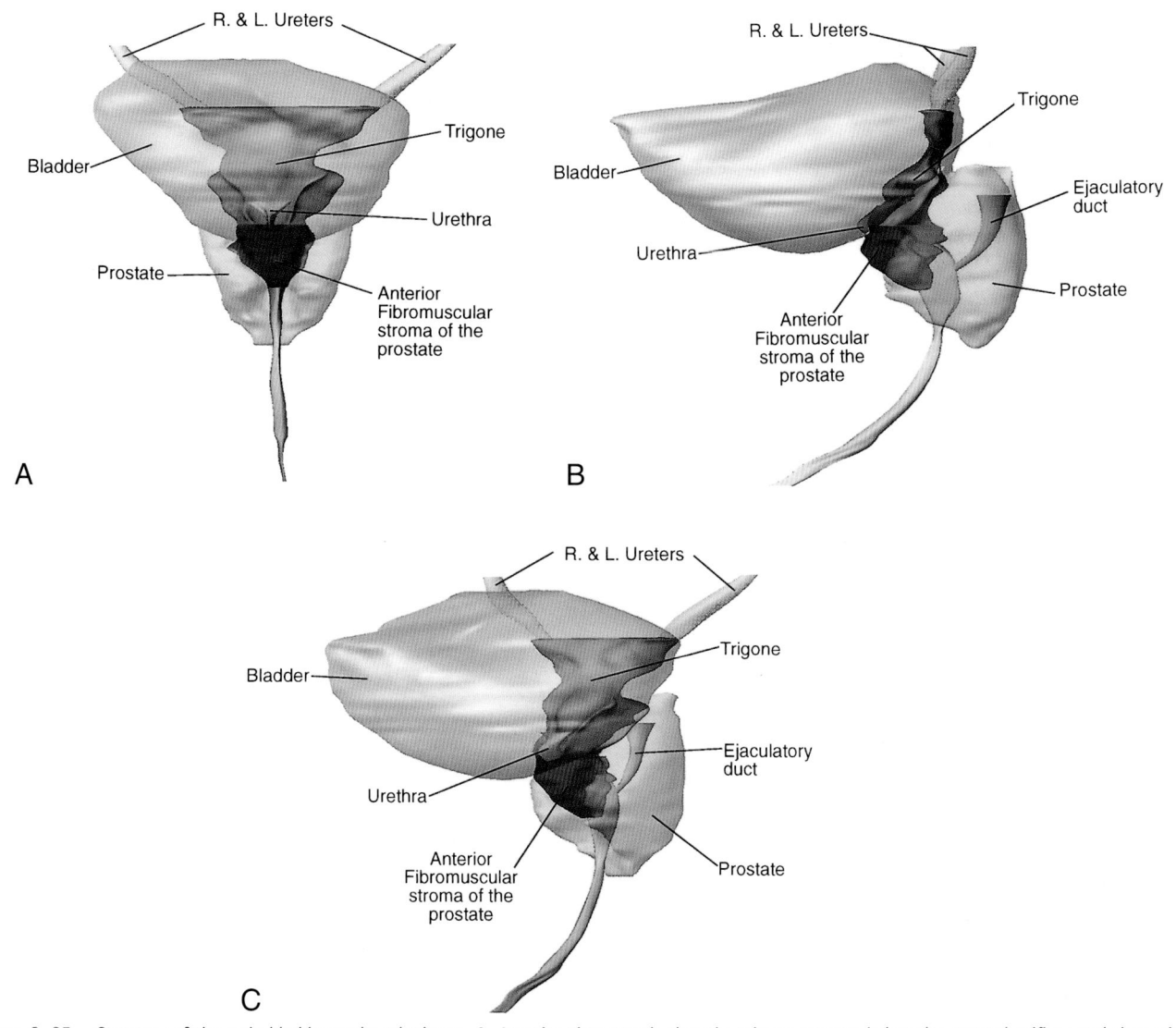

Figure 2-25. Structure of the male bladder neck and trigone. **A,** Anterior view reveals that the trigone narrows below the ureteral orifices and then widens at the bladder neck to become continuous with the anterior fibromuscular stroma of the prostate. **B,** Lateral projection shows that the trigone and anterior fibromuscular stroma are in continuity. The trigone thickens near the bladder neck as it meets the anterior fibromuscular stroma. **C,** Oblique view shows this structure at the bladder neck, where it forms the internal urethral sphincter. (From Brooks JD, Chao W-M, Kerr J: Male pelvic anatomy reconstructed from the Visible Human data set. J Urol 1998;159:868-872.)

orifice (Fig. 2–26). As it passes through a hiatus in the detrusor (intramural ureter), it is compressed and narrows considerably. This is a common site in which ureteral stones become impacted. The intravesical portion of the ureter lies immediately beneath the bladder urothelium and therefore is quite pliant; it is backed by a strong plate of detrusor muscle. With bladder filling, this arrangement is thought to result in passive occlusion of the ureter, like a flap valve. Indeed, reflux does not occur in fresh cadavers when the bladder is filled (Thomson et al, 1994). Vesicoureteral reflux is thought to result from insufficient submucosal ureteral length and poor detrusor backing. Chronic increases in intravesical pressure resulting from bladder outlet obstruction can cause herniation of the bladder mucosa through the weakest point of the hiatus above the ureter and produce a "Hutch diverticulum" and reflux (Hutch et al, 1961).

The triangle of smooth urothelium between the two ureteral orifices and the internal urethral meatus is referred to as the *trigone of the bladder* (see Fig. 2–26). The fine longitudinal smooth muscle fibers from the vesical side of the ureters pass to either side of their respective orifices to join the lateral and posterior ureteral wall fibers and fan out over the base of the bladder. Fibers from each ureter meet to form a triangular sheet of muscle that extends from the two ureteral orifices to the internal urethral meatus. The edges of this muscular sheet are thickened between the ureteral orifices (the interureteric crest or Mercier's bar) and between the ureters and the internal urethral meatus (Bell's muscle).

The muscle of trigone forms three distinct layers: **(1) a superficial layer, derived from the longitudinal muscle of the ureter,** which extends down the urethra to insert at the verumontanum; (2) **a deep layer,** which continues from Waldeyer's

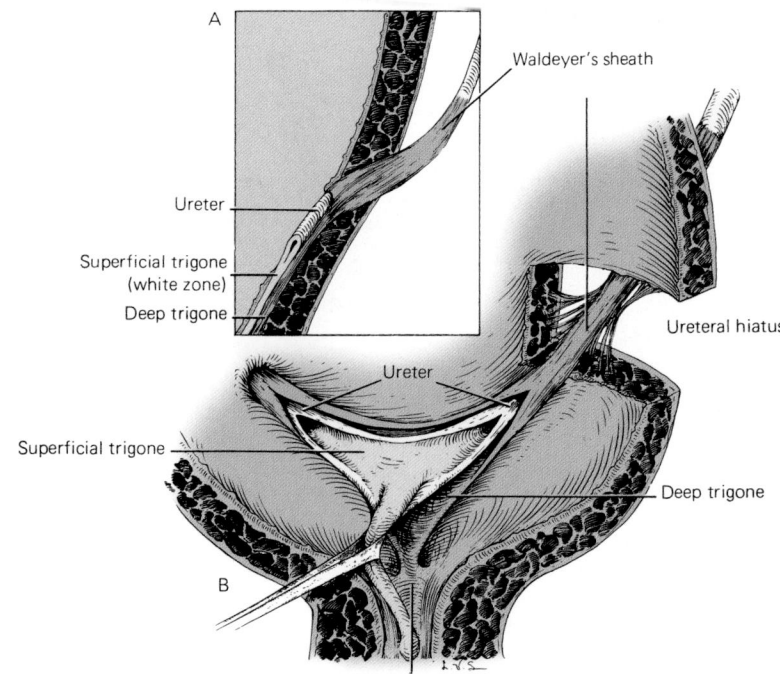

Figure 2–26. Normal ureterovesical junction and trigone. **A,** Section of the bladder wall perpendicular to the ureteral hiatus shows the oblique passage of the ureter through the detrusor and also shows the submucosal ureter with its detrusor backing. Waldeyer's sheath surrounds the prevesical ureter and extends inward to become the deep trigone. **B,** Waldeyer's sheath continues in the bladder as the deep trigone, which is fixed at the bladder neck. Smooth muscle of the ureter forms the superficial trigone and is anchored at the verumontanum. (From Tanagho EA, Pugh RC: The anatomy and function of the ureterovesical junction. Br J Urol 1963;35:151-165.)

sheath and inserts at the bladder neck; and (3) **a detrusor layer,** formed by the outer longitudinal and middle circular smooth muscle layers of the bladder wall. Through its continuity with the ureter, the superficial trigonal muscle anchors the ureter to the bladder. During ureteral reimplantation, this muscle is tented up and divided to gain access to the space between Waldeyer's sheath and the ureter. In this space, only loose fibrous and muscular connections are found. This anatomic arrangement helps prevent reflux during bladder filling by fixing and applying tension to the ureteral orifice. As the bladder fills, its lateral wall telescopes outward on the ureter, thereby increasing intravesical ureteral length (Hutch et al, 1961).

The urothelium overlying the muscular trigone is usually only three cells thick and adheres strongly to the underlying muscle by a dense lamina propria. During filling and emptying of the bladder, this mucosal surface remains smooth.

Bladder Circulation

In addition to the vesical branches, the bladder may be supplied by any adjacent artery arising from the internal iliac artery. For convenience, surgeons refer to the vesical blood supply as the *lateral* **and** *posterior* **pedicles,** which, when the bladder is approached from the rectovesical space, are lateral and posteromedial to the ureters, respectively. These pedicles are the lateral and posterior vesical ligaments in the male and part of cardinal and uterosacral ligaments in the female (see Fig. 2–13). The veins of the bladder coalesce into the vesicle plexus and drain into the internal iliac vein. Lymphatics from the lamina propria and muscularis drain to channels on the bladder surface, which run with the superficial vessels within the thin visceral fascia. Small paravesical lymph nodes can be found along the superficial channels. The bulk of the lymphatic drainage passes to the external iliac lymph nodes (see Fig. 2–18). Some anterior and lateral drainage may go through the obturator and internal iliac nodes, whereas portions of the bladder base and trigone may drain into the internal and common iliac groups.

Bladder Innervation

Autonomic efferent fibers from the anterior portion of the pelvic plexus (the vesical plexus) pass up the lateral and posterior ligaments to innervate the bladder. The bladder wall is richly supplied with parasympathetic cholinergic nerve endings and has abundant postganglionic cell bodies. Sparse sympathetic innervation of the bladder has been proposed to mediate detrusor relaxation but probably lacks functional significance. A separate nonadrenergic, noncholinergic (NANC) component of the autonomic nervous system participates in activating the detrusor, although the neurotransmitter has not been identified (Burnett, 1995). As mentioned, the male bladder neck receives abundant sympathetic innervation and expresses α_1-adrenergic receptors. The female bladder neck has little adrenergic innervation. Nitric oxide synthase–containing neurons have been identified in the detrusor, particularly at the bladder neck, where they may facilitate relaxation during micturition. The trigonal muscle is innervated by adrenergic and nitric oxide synthase–containing neurons. Like the bladder neck, it relaxes during micturition. Afferent innervation from the bladder travels with both sympathetic (via the hypogastric nerves) and parasympathetic nerves to reach cell bodies in the dorsal root ganglia located at thoracolumbar and sacral levels. As a consequence, presacral neurectomy (division of the hypogastric nerves) is ineffective in relieving bladder pain.

Prostate

Anatomic Relationships

The normal prostate weighs 18 g; measures 3 cm in length, 4 cm in width, and 2 cm in depth; and is traversed by the prostatic urethra (see Fig. 2–23). Although ovoid, **the prostate is referred to as having anterior, posterior, and lateral surfaces, with a narrowed apex inferiorly and a broad base superiorly** that is contiguous with the base of the bladder. It is enclosed by a capsule composed of collagen, elastin, and abundant smooth muscle. Posteriorly and laterally, this capsule has an average thickness of 0.5 mm, although it may be partially transgressed by normal glands. Microscopic bands of smooth muscle extend from the posterior surface of the capsule to fuse with Denonvilliers' fascia. Loose areolar tissue defines a thin plane between Denonvilliers' fascia and the rectum. On the anterior and anterolateral surfaces of the prostate, the capsule blends with the visceral continuation of endopelvic fascia. Toward the apex, the puboprostatic ligaments extend anteriorly to fix the prostate to the pubic bone (see Fig. 2–40). The superficial branch of the dorsal vein lies outside this fascia in the retropubic fat and pierces it to drain into the dorsal vein complex.

Laterally, the prostate is cradled by the pubococcygeal portion of levator ani and is directly related to its overlying endopelvic fascia (see Figs. 2–8 and 2–10). Below the juncture of the parietal and visceral endopelvic fascia (arcus tendineus fascia pelvis), the pelvic fascia and prostate capsule separate and the space between them is filled by fatty areolar tissue and the lateral divisions of the dorsal vein complex. During a radical retropubic prostatectomy, the endopelvic fascia should be divided lateral to the arcus tendineus fascia pelvis to avoid injury to the venous complex. In the process, the endopelvic fascia overlying the levator ani is actually peeled off the muscle and displaced medially with the prostate. Although this is truly a parietal endopelvic fascia, it is commonly referred to as the "lateral prostatic fascia" (Myers, 1994). As mentioned earlier, the cavernosal nerves run posterolateral to the prostate in the substance of the parietal pelvic fascia (lateral prostatic fascia). Thus, to preserve these nerves, this fascia must be incised lateral to the prostate and anterior to the neurovascular bundle (Walsh et al, 1983).

The apex of the prostate is continuous with the striated urethral sphincter (see Fig. 2–30). Histologically, normal prostatic glands can be found to extend into the striated muscle with no intervening fibromuscular stroma or "capsule." At the base of the prostate, outer longitudinal fibers of the detrusor fuse and blend with the fibromuscular tissue of the capsule. As mentioned, the middle circular and inner longitudinal muscles extend down the prostatic urethra as a preprostatic sphincter. As with the apex, no true capsule separates the prostate from the bladder. In surgically resected prostate carcinomas, this peculiar anatomic arrangement can make interpretation of these margins difficult and has led some pathologists to propose that the prostate does not possess a true capsule (Epstein, 1989).

Structure

The prostate is composed of approximately 70% glandular elements and 30% fibromuscular stroma. The stroma is continuous with capsule and is composed of collagen and abundant smooth muscle. It encircles and invests the glands of the prostate and contracts during ejaculation to express prostatic secretions into the urethra.

The urethra runs the length of the prostate and is usually closest to its anterior surface. It is lined by transitional epithelium, which may extend into the prostatic ducts. The urothelium is surrounded by an inner longitudinal and an outer circular layer of smooth muscle. A urethral crest projects inward from the posterior midline, runs the length of the prostatic urethra, and disappears at the striated sphincter (Fig. 2–27). To either side of this crest, a groove is formed (prostatic sinuses) into which all glandular elements drain (McNeal, 1972). At its midpoint, the urethra turns approximately 35 degrees anteriorly, but this angulation can vary from 0 to 90 degrees (see Figs. 2–23, 2–25, and 2–28). This angle divides the prostatic urethra into proximal (preprostatic) and distal (prostatic) segments that are functionally and anatomically discrete (McNeal, 1972, 1988). In the proximal segment, the circular smooth muscle is thickened to form the involuntary internal urethral (preprostatic) sphincter described earlier. Small periurethral glands, lacking periglandular smooth muscle, extend between the fibers of the longitudinal smooth muscle to be enclosed by the preprostatic sphincter. Although these glands constitute less than 1% of the secretory elements of the prostate, they can contribute significantly to prostatic volume in older men as one of the sites of origin of benign prostatic hyperplasia.

Beyond to the urethral angle, all major glandular elements of the prostate open into the prostatic urethra. The urethral crest widens and protrudes from the posterior wall as the verumontanum (see Fig. 2–27). The small slitlike orifice of the prostatic utricle is found at the apex of the verumontanum and may be visualized cystoscopically. The utricle is a 6-mm müllerian remnant in the form of a small sac that projects upward and backward into the substance of the prostate. In males with ambiguous genitalia, it may form a large diverticulum that protrudes from the posterior side of the prostate. To either side of the utricular orifice, the two small openings of the ejaculatory ducts may be found. The ejaculatory ducts form at the juncture of the vas deferens and seminal vesicles and enter the prostate base where it fuses with the bladder. They course nearly 2 cm through the prostate in line with the distal prostatic urethra and are surrounded by circular smooth muscle (Fig. 2–28; see also Figs. 2–23 and 2–25).

In general, **the glands of the prostate are tubuloalveolar with relatively simple branching and are lined with simple cuboidal or columnar epithelium. Scattered neuroendocrine cells, of unknown function, are found between the secretory cells. Beneath the epithelial cells, flattened basal cells line each acinus and are believed to be stem cells for the secretory epithelium.** Each acinus is surrounded by a thin layer of stromal smooth muscle and connective tissue.

The glandular elements of the prostate have been divided into discrete zones, distinguished by the location of their ducts in the urethra, by their differing pathologic lesions, and, in some cases, by their embryologic origin (see Fig. 2–28). These zones can be demonstrated clearly with transrectal ultrasonography. **At the angle dividing the preprostatic and prostatic urethra, the ducts of the transition zone arise and pass beneath the preprostatic sphincter to travel on its lateral and posterior sides.** Normally, the transition zone accounts for 5%

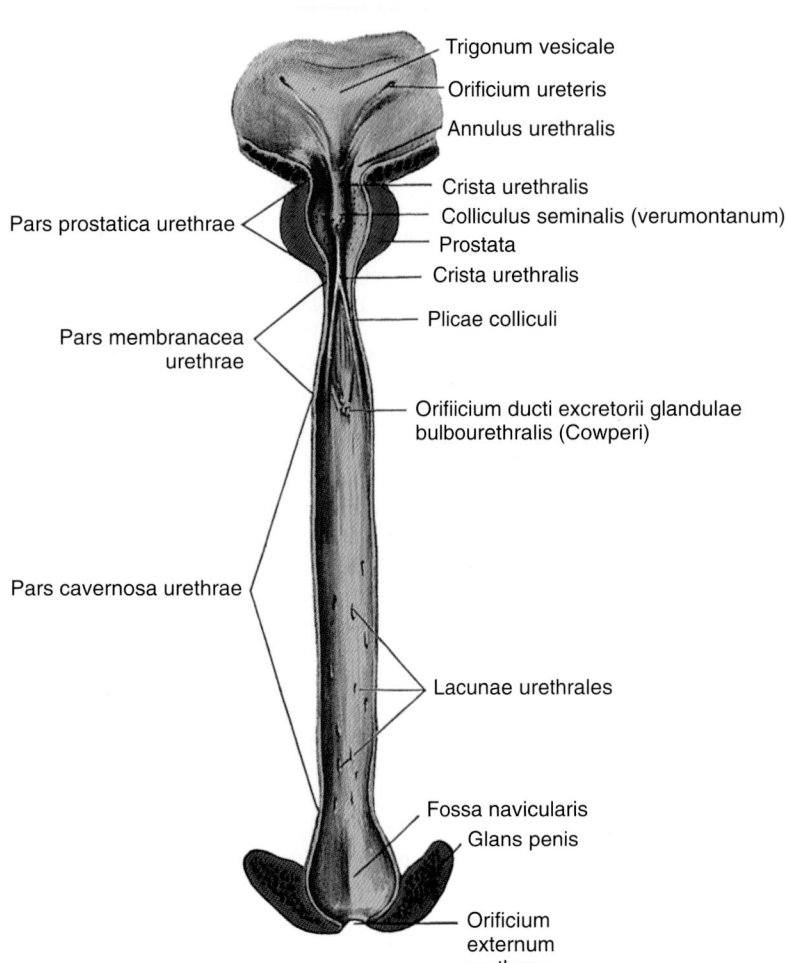

Trigonum vesicale

Orificium ureteris

Annulus urethralis

Pars prostatica urethrae

Crista urethralis

Colliculus seminalis (verumontanum)

Prostata

Crista urethralis

Plicae colliculi

Pars membranacea urethrae

Orifiicium ducti excretorii glandulae bulbourethralis (Cowperi)

Pars cavernosa urethrae

Lacunae urethrales

Fossa navicularis

Glans penis

Orificium externum urethrae

Figure 2–27. Posterior wall of the male urethra. (From Anson BJ, McVay CB: Surgical Anatomy, 6th ed. Philadelphia, WB Saunders, 1984, p 833.)

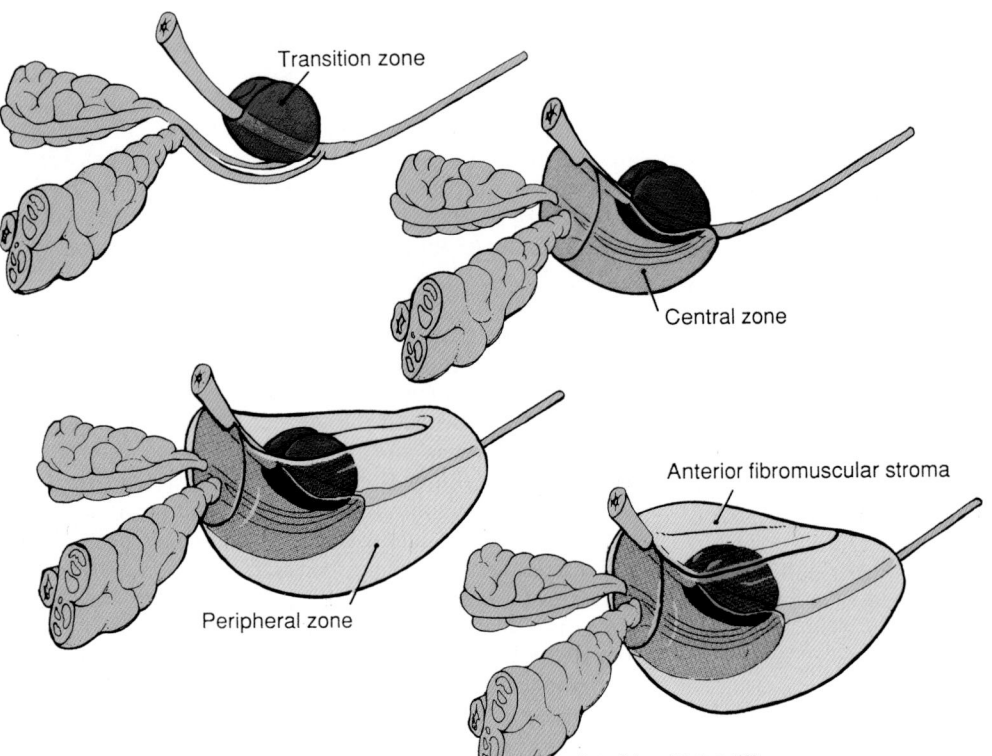

Transition zone

Central zone

Anterior fibromuscular stroma

Peripheral zone

Baylor College of Medicine 1990

Figure 2–28. Zonal anatomy of the prostate as described by J. E. McNeal (Am J Surg Pathol 1988;12:619-633). The transition zone surrounds the urethra proximal to the ejaculatory ducts. The central zone surrounds the ejaculatory ducts and projects under the bladder base. The peripheral zone constitutes the bulk of the apical, posterior, and lateral aspects of the prostate. The anterior fibromuscular stroma extends from the bladder neck to the striated urethral sphincter.

to 10% of the glandular tissue of the prostate. A discrete fibro-muscular band of tissue separates the transition zone from the remaining glandular compartments and may be visualized at transrectal ultrasonography of the prostate. The transition zone commonly gives rise to benign prostatic hypertrophy, which expands to compress the fibromuscular band into a surgical capsule seen at enucleation of an adenoma. It is estimated that 20% of adenocarcinomas of the prostate originate in this zone.

The ducts of the central zone arise circumferentially around the openings of the ejaculatory ducts. This zone constitutes 25% of the glandular tissue of the prostate and expands in a cone shape around the ejaculatory ducts to the base of the bladder. The glands are structurally and immuno-histochemically distinct from the remaining prostatic glands (which branch directly from the urogenital sinus), which has led to the suggestion that they are of wolffian origin (McNeal, 1988). In keeping with this suggestion, only 1% to 5% of adenocarcinomas arise in the central zone, although it may be infiltrated by cancers from adjacent zones.

The peripheral zone makes up the bulk of the prostatic glandular tissue (70%) and covers the posterior and lateral aspects of the gland. Its ducts drain into the prostatic sinus along the entire length of the (postsphincteric) prostatic urethra. Seventy percent of prostatic cancers arise in this zone, and it is the zone most commonly affected by chronic prostatitis.

Up to one third of the prostatic mass may be attributed to the nonglandular **anterior fibromuscular stroma.** This region normally extends from the bladder neck to the striated sphincter, although considerable portions of it may be replaced by glandular tissue in adenomatous enlargement of the prostate. It is directly continuous with the prostatic capsule, anterior visceral fascia, and anterior portion of the preprostatic sphincter and is composed of elastin, collagen, and smooth and striated muscle. It is rarely invaded by carcinoma.

Clinically, the prostate is often spoken of as having two lateral lobes, separated by a central sulcus that is palpable on rectal examination, and a middle lobe, which may project into the bladder in older men. These lobes do not correspond to histologically defined structures in the normal prostate but are usually related to pathologic enlargement of the transition zone laterally and the periurethral glands centrally.

Vascular Supply

Most commonly, **the arterial supply to the prostate arises from the inferior vesical artery.** As it approaches the gland, the artery (often several) divides into two main branches (Fig. 2–29). The urethral arteries penetrate the prostatovesical junction posterolaterally and travel inward, perpendicular to the urethra. They approach the bladder neck in the 1- to 5-o'clock and 7- to 11-o'clock positions, with the largest branches located posteriorly. They then turn caudally, parallel to the urethra, to supply it, the periurethral glands, and the transition zone. Thus, in benign prostatic hypertrophy, these arteries provide the principal blood supply of the adenoma (Flocks, 1937). When these glands are resected or enucleated, the most significant bleeding is commonly encountered at the bladder neck, particularly at the 4- and 8-o'clock positions.

The capsular artery is the second main branch of the prostatic artery. This artery gives off a few small branches that

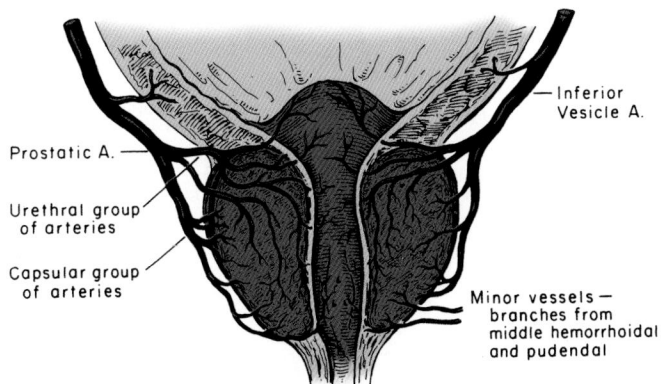

Figure 2–29. Arterial supply of the prostate. (Adapted from Flocks RH: The arterial distribution within the prostate gland: Its role in transurethral prostatic resection. J Urol 1937;37:524-548.)

pass anteriorly to ramify on the prostatic capsule. The bulk of this artery runs posterolateral to the prostate with the cavernous nerves (neurovascular bundles) and ends at the pelvic diaphragm. The capsular branches pierce the prostate at right angles and follow the reticular bands of stroma to supply the glandular tissues. Venous drainage of the prostate is abundant through the periprostatic plexus (see Fig. 2–17).

Lymphatic drainage is primarily to the obturator and internal iliac nodes (see Fig. 2–18). A small portion of drainage may initially pass through the presacral group, or less commonly, the external iliac nodes.

Nerve Supply

Sympathetic and parasympathetic innervation from the pelvic plexus travels to the prostate through the cavernous nerves. Nerves follow branches of the capsular artery to ramify in the glandular and stromal elements. Parasympathetic nerves end at the acini and promote secretion; sympathetic fibers cause contraction of the smooth muscle of the capsule and stroma. α_1-Adrenergic blockade diminishes prostate stromal and preprostatic sphincter tone and improves urinary flow rates in men affected with benign prostatic hypertrophy; this emphasizes that this disease affects both the stroma and the epithelium. Peptidergic and nitric oxide synthase–containing neurons also have been found in the prostate and may affect smooth muscle relaxation (Burnett, 1995). Afferent neurons from the prostate travel through the pelvic plexuses to pelvic and thoracolumbar spinal centers. A prostatic block may be achieved by instilling local anesthetic into the pelvic plexuses.

Membranous Urethra

In its course from the apex of the prostate to the perineal membrane, **the membranous urethra spans on average 2 to 2.5 cm** (range, 1.2 to 5 cm) (Myers, 1991). It is surrounded by the striated (external) urethral sphincter, which is often incorrectly depicted as a flat sheet of muscle sandwiched between two layers of fascia. The striated sphincter is actually signet ring–shaped, broad at its base and narrowing as it passes through the urogenital hiatus of the levator ani to meet the apex of the prostate (Fig. 2–30; see also Figs. 2–10 and 2–23).

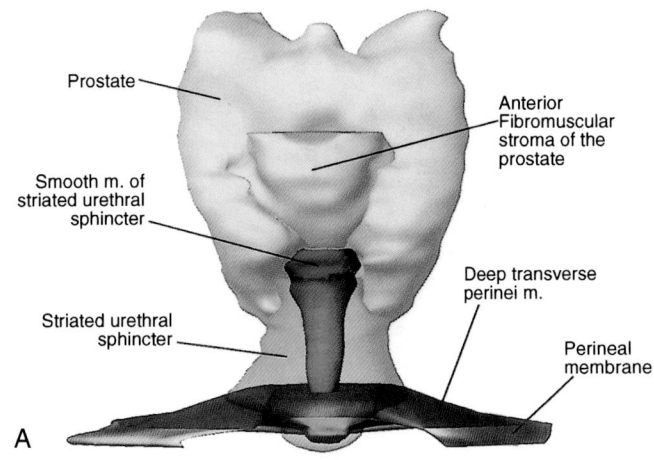

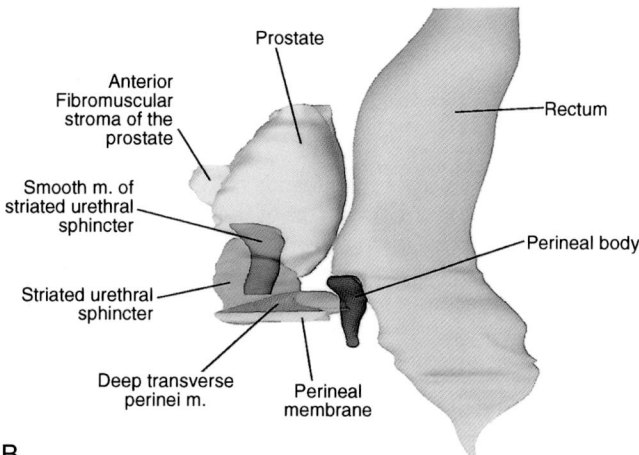

Figure 2–30. Structure of the male striated urethral sphincter. **A,** Anterior projection shows the cone shape of the sphincter and the smooth muscle of the sphincter. **B,** Viewed laterally, the anterior wall of the sphincter is nearly twice the length of the posterior wall, although both are of comparable thickness. (From Brooks JD, Chao W-M, Kerr J: Male pelvic anatomy reconstructed from the Visible Human data set. J Urol 1998;159:868-872.)

In utero, this muscle forms a vertically oriented tube that extends from the perineal membrane to the bladder neck (Oelrich, 1980). As the prostate grows, posterior and lateral portions of this muscle atrophy, although transverse fibers persist on the entire anterior prostate through adulthood. At the apex of the prostate, circular fibers surround the urethra, and they thin posteriorly to insert into a fibrous raphe. Distally, the fibers do not meet posteriorly; rather, they acquire an Ω shape as they fan out laterally over the perineal membrane. Throughout its length, the posterior portion of the striated sphincter inserts into the perineal body. When the sphincter contracts, the walls of the urethra are pulled posteriorly toward the perineal body (Strasser et al, 1998). In contrast to the levator ani, the sphincter consists only of fine, type I (slow-twitch) fibers, rich in acid-stable myosin adenosine triphosphatase, which appear designed for tonic contraction. The myofibrils are surrounded by abundant connective tissue that blends with adjacent supporting structures.

The striated sphincter is related anteriorly to the dorsal vein complex (which may invade its anterior portion with age) and laterally to the levator ani. **Connective tissue from deep within the lateral and anterior walls inserts into the puboprostatic ligaments posteriorly and into the suspensory ligament of the penis anteriorly to form a sling of fibrous tissue that suspends the urethra from the pubis** (Steiner, 1994). A similar suspensory mechanism is found in the female urethra (see later discussion and Fig. 2–34). Two bulbourethral glands lie superior to the perineal membrane and are invested in the broad base of sphincter muscle. During sexual excitement, these glands secrete clear mucus into the bulbous urethra.

The striated sphincter corresponds to the location of peak urethral closing pressure and is responsible for continence after prostatectomy. Components involved in generating this closing pressure are (1) the pseudostratified columnar epithelium, which contracts into radial folds as it meets to occlude the lumen; (2) the submucosa, which is rich with blood vessels and soft connective tissue and contributes to urethral sealing (Raz et al, 1972); (3) the longitudinal and circular urethral smooth muscle (intrinsic component of the external sphincter); (4) the striated sphincter; and (5) the pubourethral component of the levator ani.

Gross dissection and retrograde axonal tracing techniques have confirmed that the striated sphincter is supplied by the pudendal nerve (Tanagho et al, 1982). However, urologists have long been puzzled as to why pudendal nerve sectioning does not ablate sphincter activity. Lawson (1974) and Zvara and colleagues (1994) identified **a second source of somatic innervation to the sphincter: a branch of the sacral plexus that runs on the pelvic surface of the levator ani** (see Fig. 2–20). Injury to this nerve at radical prostatectomy may contribute to postoperative urinary incontinence (Hollabaugh et al, 1997). Autonomic innervation to the intrinsic smooth muscle of the membranous urethra is likely given by the cavernous nerves as they pass nearby, although dividing these nerves does not appear to affect urinary continence significantly (Steiner et al, 1991). Afferent fibers from the striated sphincter have not been defined but are sure to have interesting and important functional roles, because this muscle lacks proprioceptive muscle spindles (Gosling et al, 1981).

Vas Deferens and Seminal Vesicle

As it arises from the tail of the epididymis, the vas (ductus) deferens is somewhat tortuous for 2 to 3 cm (see Fig. 2–43). It runs posterior to the vessels of the cord and through the inguinal canal and emerges in the pelvis lateral to the inferior epigastric vessels (see Fig. 2–7). At the internal ring, it diverges from the testicular vessels and passes medial to all structures of the pelvic side wall to reach the base of the prostate posteriorly (see Figs. 2–7, 2–13, and 2–15). The terminal vas is dilated and tortuous (ampulla) and is capable of storing spermatozoa. The vas has a thick wall of outer longitudinal and inner circular smooth muscle and is lined by pseudostratified columnar epithelium with nonmotile stereocilia.

The seminal vesicle is a lateral outpouching of the vas, approximately 5 cm long, with a capacity of 3 to 4 mL (see Figs. 2–8 and 2–28). Despite its name, it does not store sperm but contributes the largest portion of fluid to the ejaculate. The seminal vesicle comprises a single coiled tube with several outpouchings that is lined by columnar epithelium with goblet cells. The tube is encased in a thin layer of smooth muscle and is held in its coiled configuration by a loose adventitia.

The seminal vesicle and ampulla of the vas lie posterior to the bladder. The ureter enters the bladder medial to the tip of the seminal vesicle. As they join to form the ejaculatory duct, their smooth muscle coats fuse with the prostatic capsule at its base. **Denonvilliers' fascia or, occasionally, the rectovesical pouch of peritoneum separates these structures from the rectum** (see Fig. 2–23). Unless involved by a pathologic process, these structures are not palpable on rectal examination.

The blood supply for both structures comes from the vesiculodeferential artery, a branch of the superior vesical artery. This artery supplies the vas throughout its length and then passes onto the anterior surface of the seminal vesicle near its tip. Additional arterial supply may come from the inferior vesical artery. The pelvic vas and seminal vesicle drain into the pelvic venous plexus. Lymphatic drainage passes to the external and internal iliac nodes (see Fig. 2–18). Innervation arises from the pelvic plexus, with major excitatory efferents contributed by the (sympathetic) hypogastric nerves (Kolbeck and Steers, 1993).

Female Pelvic Viscera

The uterus measures $8 \times 6 \times 4\,cm$ in a normal woman and is composed largely of dense smooth muscle (Fig. 2–31). It has a narrowed neck, the cervix, that opens through the anterior vaginal wall and a broad corpus that is capped by the rounded fundus. As discussed earlier, it lies in front of the rectum and over the dome of bladder; its impression may be appreciated cystoscopically (Figs. 2–32 and 2–33). The fallopian tubes extend laterally from the junction of the corpus and fundus and are draped by leaves of peritoneum called the broad ligaments (see Figs. 2–13 and 2–31). As they extend to the pelvic side walls, the fallopian tubes angle up and backward to open posteromedially. The tubes are divided into four segments: uterine, isthmus, ampulla, and infundibulum, which is crowned by the fimbriae. The ovary rests posterior to the elbow of the tube and is supported by its own peritoneal fold,

the mesovarium. The ureter may be found directly posterior to the ovary, covered by pelvic peritoneum. The infundibulopelvic ligament, mentioned earlier, suspends the ovary and lateral fallopian tube from the pelvic side wall and transmits the ovarian vessels to both structures. The round ligament of the ovary passes medially through the broad ligament to fix the ovary to the lateral wall of the uterus. Beneath its point of attachment, the round ligament of the uterus passes laterally, in the leaves of the broad ligament, to exit through to inguinal canal and attach to the labial fat pad (see Figs. 2–13 and 2–31).

The uterine artery crosses in front of the ureter and runs in the broad and cardinal ligaments to supply the proximal vagina, uterus, and medial two thirds of the fallopian tube (see Fig. 2–31). It is joined by a rich plexus of uterine veins that freely connect with the ovarian veins. Nerves from the pelvic plexus travel to the female pelvic viscera through the cardinal and uterosacral ligaments in the company of the vessels; thus, after hysterectomy, the bladder may become neurogenic.

The vagina extends inward from the vestibule at a 45-degree angle and then turns horizontal over the levator plate (see Fig. 2–33). It is lined by rugate nonkeratinized squamous epithelium backed by a thick, well-vascularized lamina propria. It is surrounded by a smooth muscle coat of inner circular and stronger external longitudinal layers. In cross section, the vagina is H shaped (Fig. 2–34) as a result of firm attachments of its anterior wall to the levator ani at the arcus tendineus fascia pelvis and of its posterior wall to the rectovaginal septum. The anterior vaginal wall is pierced by the cervix proximally. The shallow fossae around the cervix are referred to as the *anterior, lateral,* and *posterior* fornices. Because the apex of the vagina is covered with the peritoneum of the rectouterine pouch, the peritoneal cavity may be accessed through the posterior fornix (see Fig. 2–33).

Immediately in front of the cervix, the base of the bladder rests on the vaginal wall. Smooth muscle fibers tether the posterior bladder wall and base to the uterine cervix and vagina (see Fig. 2–33). Division of these fibers yields posterior access to the vesicovaginal space. This space extends distally to the proximal third of the urethra (where the urethra and vagina fuse) and is limited to each side by the lateral ligaments of the bladder. It may be accessed transvaginally through inci-

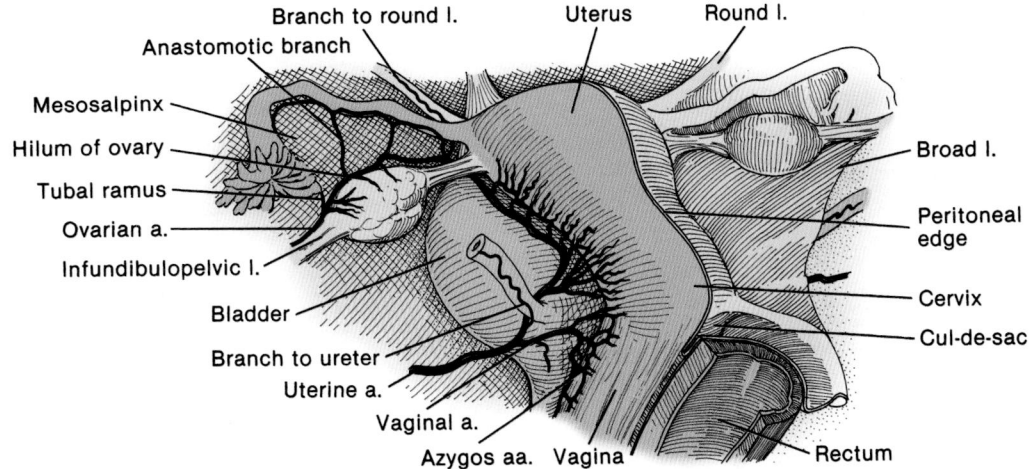

Figure 2–31. Female internal genitalia, from behind. The ureter passes beneath the uterine artery. (From Hinman F Jr: Atlas of Urosurgical Anatomy. Philadelphia, WB Saunders, 1993, p 402.)

Branch to round l.
Anastomotic branch
Mesosalpinx
Hilum of ovary
Tubal ramus
Ovarian a.
Infundibulopelvic l.
Bladder
Branch to ureter
Uterine a.
Vaginal a.
Azygos aa. Vagina
Uterus
Round l.
Broad l.
Peritoneal edge
Cervix
Cul-de-sac
Rectum

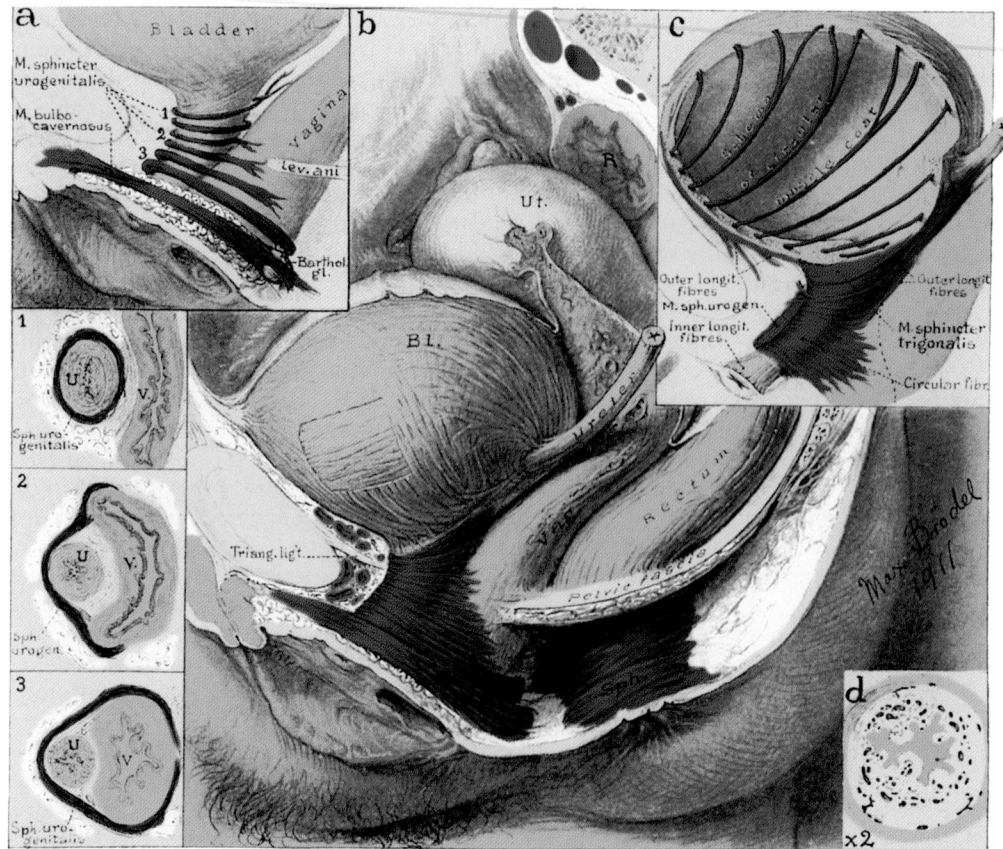

Figure 2–32. Female bladder and striated urethral sphincter. **a,** Diagram of striated urethral sphincter showing disposition of the muscle fibers. 1, The proximal third of the sphincter encircles the urethra entirely. 2, The middle bundles surround the urethra in front and pass off the lateral sides to blend with the vaginal wall (compressor urethrae). 3, The distal portion surrounds the urethra and vagina together and has been called the urethrovaginal sphincter. The bulbocavernosus also acts as a sphincter around the vaginal vestibule. **b,** Urethral sphincter in its entirety. The relationship of the pelvic viscera is shown. Interlacing detrusor fibers are also demonstrated. **c,** Posterolateral outer longitudinal detrusor muscle looping anterior to the bladder neck. Inner longitudinal smooth muscle fibers run the length of the urethra, deep to the striated sphincter. **d,** Cross section of the urethra, showing thick, highly vascularized lamina propria and folded mucosa, which act as a urethral seal. Longitudinal smooth muscle surrounds the lamina propria. (From the Brödel Archives, Johns Hopkins School of Medicine, Baltimore.)

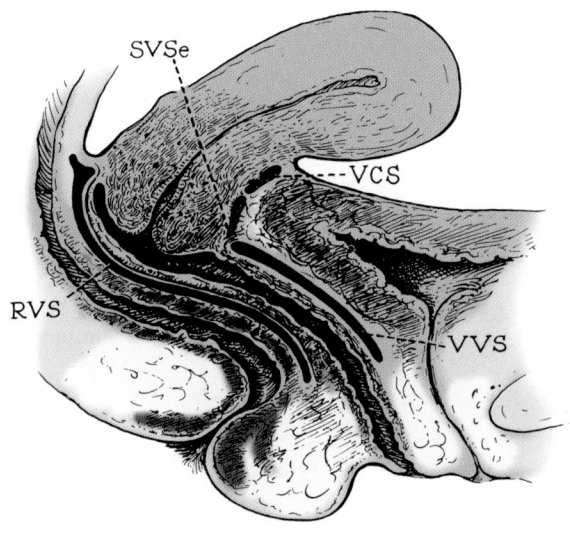

Figure 2–33. Median sagittal section of the female pelvis, showing the potential spaces between the pelvic organs. The posterior two thirds of the vagina lie nearly horizontal and rest with the uterine cervix on the rectum, which is in turn supported by the posterior portion of levator ani (the levator plate, *not shown*). RVS, rectovaginal space, the anterior wall is formed by the rectovaginal (Denonvilliers') fascia; SVSe, supravaginal septum, the fusion between the bladder and cervix; VCS, vesicocervical space; VVS, vesicovaginal space. (From Nichols DH, Randall CL: Vaginal Surgery, 3rd ed. Baltimore, Williams & Wilkins, 1989, p 34.)

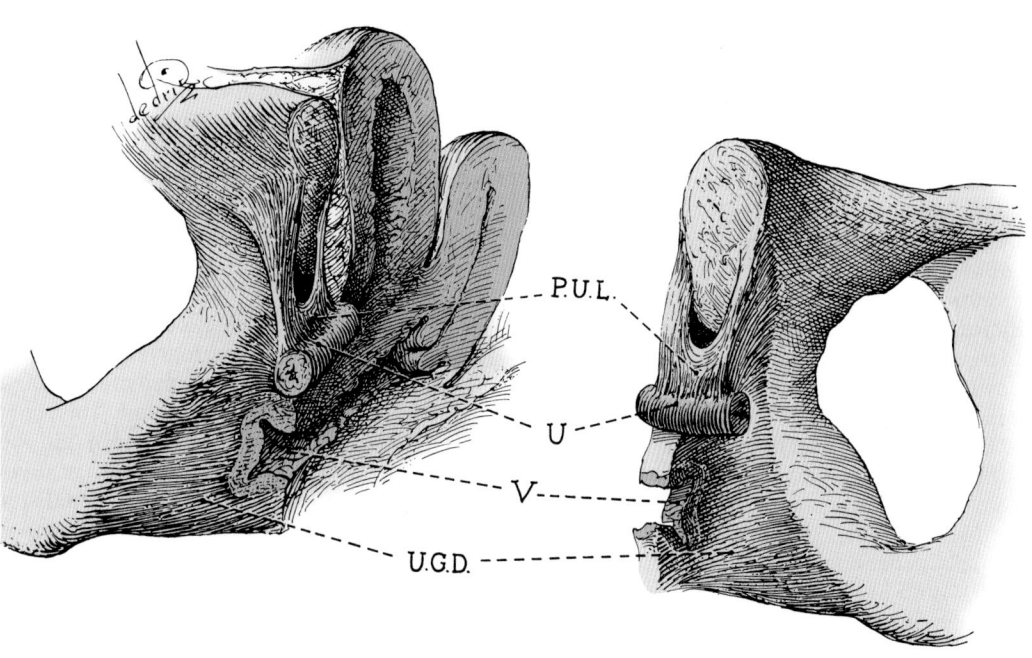

Figure 2–34. Urethral suspensory mechanism. The pubourethral ligament (P.U.L.) is composed of an anterior portion (suspensory ligament of the clitoris), a posterior portion (pubourethral ligament of endopelvic fascia), and an intermediate portion that bridges the other two. U.G.D., urogenital diaphragm; V, vagina; U, urethra. (From Milley PS, Nichols DH: The relationship between the pubourethral ligaments and the urogenital diaphragm in the human female. Anat Rec 1971;170:281-283.)

P.U.L.

U

V

U.G.D.

sion of the anterior vaginal wall in front of the cervix. Incision of the anterior vaginal wall to either side of the urethra leads into the retropubic space (see Fig. 2–12). The tough leaves of visceral endopelvic fascia are felt medially and should be included in all transvaginal urethral suspension procedures (Mostwin, 1991).

The vagina is separated from the rectum by the rectovaginal septum (see Fig. 2–33), and rectoceles result from a loss of integrity of this septum. Deep to this septum lies a second potential space, the rectovaginal space. The bowel may herniate into this space to form an enterocele. On its lateral surfaces, the vagina is related to the levator ani. Near the vestibule, fibers of the levator ani blend and fuse with the vaginal muscularis. The vaginal vessels and nerves lie on the anterolateral surface of the vagina deep to arcus tendineus fascia pelvis.

Female Urethra

On average, the female urethra traverses 4 cm from the bladder neck to the vaginal vestibule. Its lining changes gradually from transitional to nonkeratinized stratified squamous epithelium. Many small mucous glands open into the urethra and can give rise to urethral diverticula. Distally, these glands group together on either side of the urethra (Skene's glands) and empty through two small ducts to either side of the external urethral meatus. A thick, richly vascular submucosa supports the urethral epithelium and glands (see Fig. 2–32). Together, the mucosa and submucosa form a cushion that contributes significantly to urethral closure pressure (Raz et al, 1972). These layers are estrogen dependent; at menopause they may atrophy, resulting in stress incontinence. A relatively thick layer of inner longitudinal smooth muscle continues from the bladder to the external meatus to insert into periurethral fatty and fibrous tissue. In contrast to the male proximal urethra, no circular smooth muscle sphincter can be identified. A rather thin layer of circular smooth muscle

envelops the longitudinal fibers throughout the length of the urethra. It is thought that the longitudinal smooth muscle of the urethra contracts coordinately with the detrusor during micturition to shorten and widen the urethra (Gosling, 1979).

The striated urethral sphincter invests the distal two thirds of the female urethra (Oelrich, 1983). It is composed exclusively of delicate type I (slow-twitch) fibers surrounded by abundant collagen. Proximally, it forms a complete ring around the urethra that corresponds to the zone of highest urethral closure pressure (see Fig. 2–32). Farther down the urethra, the fibers do not meet posteriorly but continue off the lateral sides of the urethra onto the anterior and lateral walls of the vagina. Contraction of these fibers (the compressor urethrae) closes the urethra against the fixed anterior vaginal wall. Near the vestibule, the fibers completely surround the urethra and vagina to form a urethrovaginal sphincter. Contraction of this muscle group, along with bulbospongiosus, tightens the urogenital hiatus.

The suspensory ligament of the clitoris (anterior urethral ligament) and the pubourethral ligaments (posterior urethral ligaments) form a sling that suspends the urethra beneath the pubis (see Figs. 2–12 and 2–34) (Zacharin, 1963). The striated urethral sphincter receives dual somatic innervation, like that in the male, from the pudendal and pelvic somatic nerves (Borirakchanyavat et al, 1997). Little sympathetic innervation is found in the female urethra. Parasympathetic cholinergic fibers are found throughout the smooth muscle. Somatic and autonomic nerves to the urethra travel on the lateral walls of the vagina near the urethra. During transvaginal incontinence surgery, the anterior vaginal wall should be incised laterally to avoid these nerves and prevent type III urinary incontinence (Ball et al, 1997).

Female Pelvic Support

The pelvic muscles and fasciae cooperate to prevent prolapse of the urogenital organs through the hiatus. **Three functional** supportive elements are recognized: (1) the pubovisceral and perineal muscles, which form a sphincter around the urogenital hiatus (see Fig. 2–32); (2) the levator plate, which acts as a horizontal shelf beneath the bladder, uterine cervix, posterior vagina, and rectum (see Fig. 2–33); and (3) the cardinal and uterosacral ligaments, which anchor the pelvic viscera over the levator plate (Zacharin, 1985; Mostwin, 1991; DeLancey, 1993). The pelvic muscles contract tonically to counteract gravitational forces. In response to stress, the levator ani contracts, closing the urogenital hiatus and increasing the anteroposterior length of the levator plate. Increased intra-abdominal pressure forces the pelvic viscera downward against a fixed levator plate, closing the vagina like a flap valve.

Pelvic and perineal muscles play the greatest role in pelvic support. Damage to the perineal body during parturition destroys the urogenital sphincter, enlarges the urogenital hiatus, and erodes the levator plate. Aging and birth trauma partially denervate and weaken the levator ani (Snooks et al, 1985). With loss of muscular support, intra-abdominal forces impinge directly on the pelvic fasciae; over time, these either tear or stretch. Procedures to correct pelvic prolapse or urinary incontinence that rely solely on these fasciae may be successful initially but do not fare well over time (Trockman et al, 1995). Repair of a single pelvic defect—a cystocele for instance—may unmask another (e.g., enterocele, rectocele); therefore, successful repair of pelvic prolapse must address all components of anatomic support (Zacharin, 1985; DeLancey, 1993).

PERINEUM

The perineum lies between the pubis, thighs, and buttocks and is limited superiorly by the levator ani. Viewed from below, the symphysis pubis, ischial tuberosities, and coccyx outline the diamond shape of the perineum; the inferior ischiopubic rami and sacrotuberous ligaments form its bony and ligamentous walls (Figs. 2–35 and 2–36). A line drawn through the ischial tuberosities divides the perineum into an anal and a urogenital triangle.

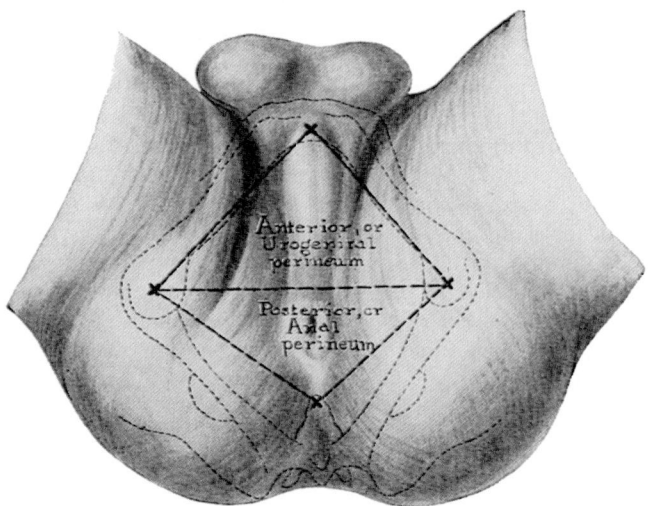

Figure 2–35. Male perineum. (From Anson BJ, McVay CB: Surgical anatomy, 6th ed. Philadelphia, WB Saunders, 1984, p 893.)

Anal Triangle

At the apex of the prostate, the rectum turns approximately 90 degrees posteriorly and inferiorly to become the anus (see Figs. 2-10 and 2-30). It traverses 4 cm to reach the skin near the center of the anal triangle. The subcutaneous fat that surrounds the anus is continuous with that of the urogenital triangle, buttocks, and medial thigh. Laterally, the fat fills the ischiorectal fossa, a space bounded by the levator ani medially, and obturator internus, and the sacrotuberous ligament laterally (see Fig. 2–14). Anteriorly, this space extends into a recess above the urogenital diaphragm; posteriorly, it is continuous with the intermediate stratum of the pelvis through the sciatic foramina. Through this continuity, infections may travel between the perineum and the pelvic cavity.

The anal sphincter is divided into internal and external components. **The internal sphincter represents a thickening of the inner circular smooth muscle layer of the rectum.** The outer longitudinal smooth muscle thins beyond the rectourethralis and blends with the external sphincter, although a few fibers insert in the skin around the anus (corrugator cutis ani) to give it a puckered appearance. The external sphincter surrounds the internal sphincter and is divided into subcutaneous, superficial, and deep portions. The subcutaneous part attaches to the perineal body by collagenous and muscular fibers that are thickest superficially and referred to as the *central tendon of the perineum.* The superficial sphincter attaches to the perineal body and coccyx. At the posterior inflection of the rectum, the deep sphincter blends with the puborectalis sling of levator ani. At this level, a firm band may be felt on rectal examination and corresponds to the internal and external sphincter. Division of this muscular band results in fecal incontinence. The prostate may be accessed anterior to the sphincter, by dividing the central tendon and sphincteric attachments to the perineum (Young's procedure) or by following the anterior rectal wall beneath the external anal sphincter (Belt's procedure).

Male Urogenital Triangle

The entire urogenital triangle is bridged by the urogenital diaphragm. The scrotum is dependent from the anterior aspect of the urogenital triangle; in the posterior aspect, skin and subcutaneous fat overlie Colles' fascia. The perineal membrane and the posterior and lateral attachments of Colles' fascia limit a potential space known as the superficial pouch (see Figs. 2–3, 2–14, and 2–36). In this space, the three erectile bodies of the penis have their bony and fascial attachments (the root of the penis). The paired corpora cavernosa attach to the inferior ischiopubic rami and perineal membrane and are surrounded by the ischiocavernosus muscles. The corpus spongiosum dilates as the bulb of the penis and is fixed to the center of the perineal membrane. It is encompassed by the bulbospongiosus muscles that arise from the perineal body and from a central tendinous raphe and pass around the bulb to attach to the perineal membrane and dorsum of the penis. Contraction of the ischiocavernosus and bulbospongiosus muscles compresses the erectile bodies and potentiates penile erection. The transversus perinei muscles (superficial and deep) run along the posterior edge of the perineal membrane and are thought to stabilize the perineal body. Deep to the

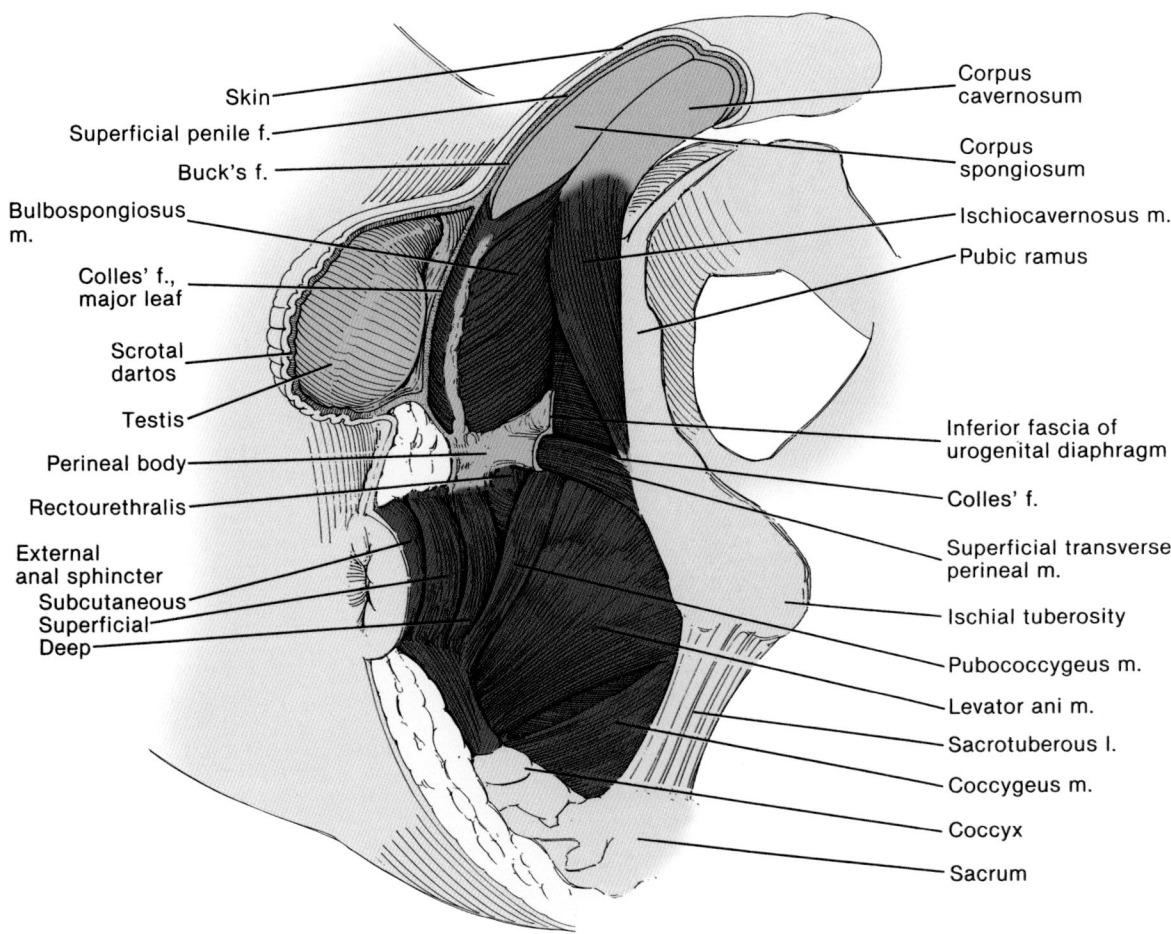

Figure 2–36. Muscles and superficial fasciae of the male perineum. (From Hinman F Jr: Atlas of Urosurgical Anatomy. Philadelphia, WB Saunders, 1993, p 219.)

perineal membrane rests the striated urethral sphincter (discussed earlier).

Blood supply to the anal and urogenital triangles is derived largely from the internal pudendal vessels (Fig. 2–37). After entering the perineum through the lesser sciatic foramen, the artery runs in a fascial sheath on the medial aspect of obturator internus, the pudendal canal (of Alcock). Early in its course, it gives off three or four inferior rectal branches to the anus. Its perineal branch pierces Colles' fascia to supply the muscles of the superficial pouch and continues anteriorly to supply the back of the scrotum. The internal pudendal terminates as the common penile artery (to be discussed).

The internal pudendal veins communicate freely with the dorsal vein complex by piercing the levator ani. These communicating vessels enter the pelvic venous plexus on the lateral surface of the prostate and are a common, often unexpected, source of bleeding during apical dissection of the prostate. The inferior rectal veins anastomose with the middle and superior rectal veins and produce an important connection between the portal and the systemic circulation. Obstruction of the portal or systemic venous system may cause shunting of collateral venous drainage through the portal system, manifested by hemorrhoids.

The pudendal nerve follows the vessels in their course through the perineum (see Fig. 2–37). Its first branch, the dorsal nerve of the penis, travels ventral to the main pudendal trunk in Alcock's canal. Several inferior rectal branches supply the external sphincter muscle and provide sensation to perianal skin. The perineal branches follow the perineal artery into the superficial pouch to supply the ischiocavernosus, bulbospongiosus, and transversus perinei muscles. A few of these branches continue anteriorly to supply sensation to the posterior scrotum. Additional perineal branches pass deep to the perineal membrane to supply the levator ani and striated urethral sphincter.

Penis

As discussed, the root of the penis is fixed to the perineum within the superficial pouch. **The corpora cavernosa join beneath the pubis (penile hilum) to form the major portion of the body of the penis.** They are separated by a septum that becomes pectiniform distally, so that their vascular spaces freely communicate. They are enclosed by the tough tunica albuginea, which is predominantly collagenous (Fig. 2–38). Its outer longitudinal and inner circular fibers form an undulating meshwork when the penis is flaccid and appear tightly

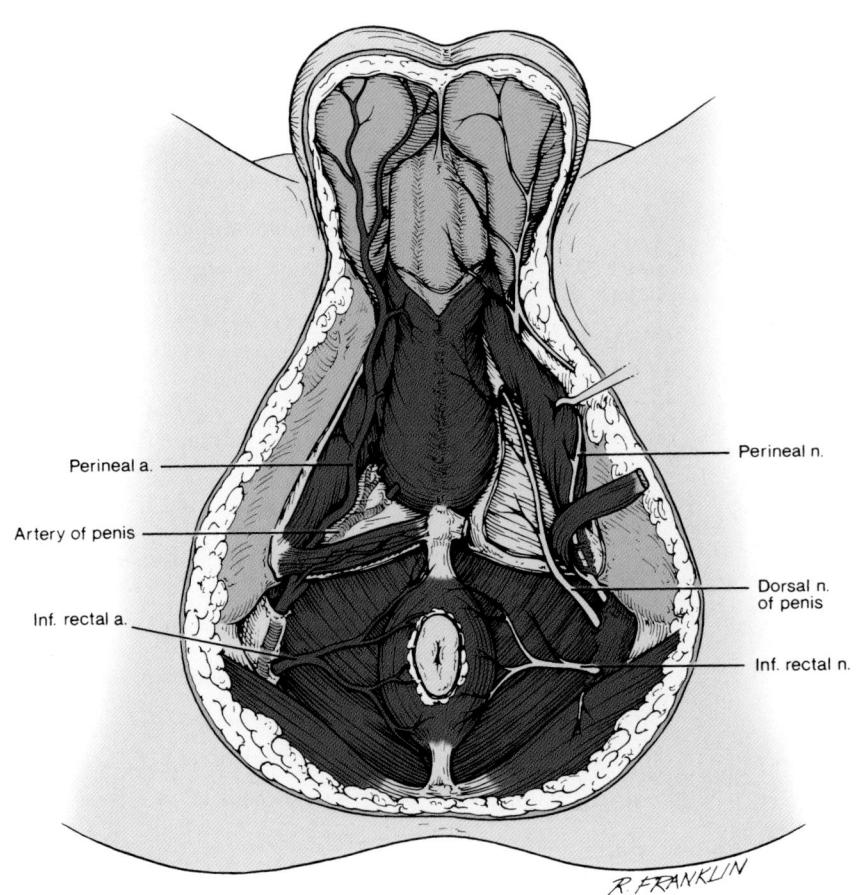

Figure 2–37. Male perineum, illustrating the internal pudendal artery and its branches on the left and the pudendal nerve and its branches on the right.

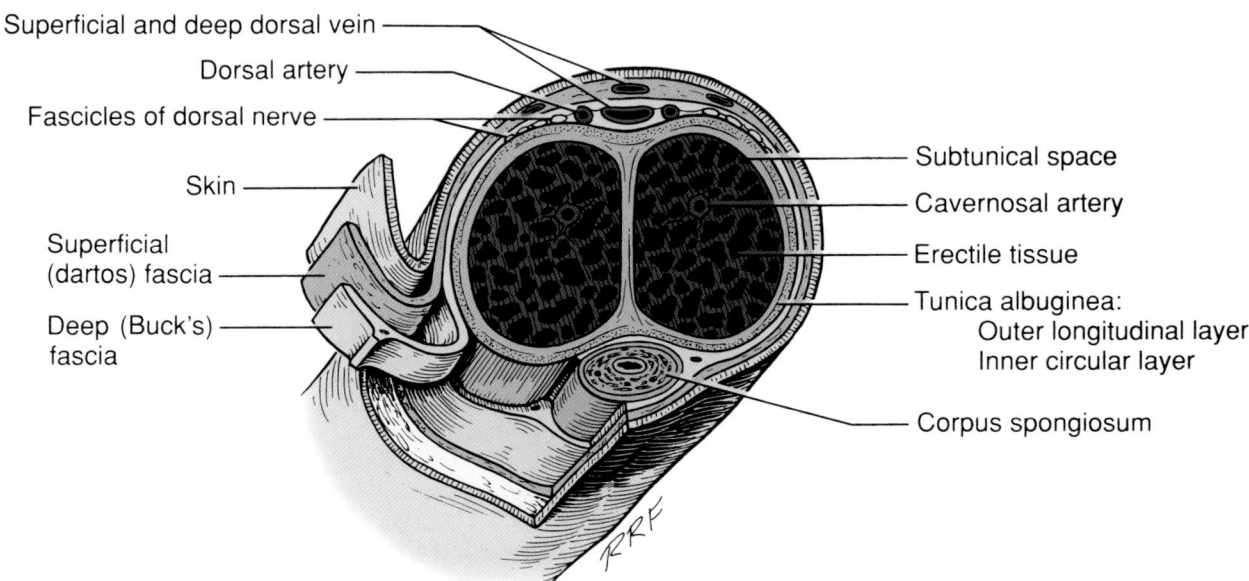

Figure 2–38. Cross section of the penis, demonstrating the relationship between the corporal bodies, penile fascia, vessels, and nerves. (From Devine CJ Jr, Angermeier KW: Anatomy of the penis and male perineum. AUA Update Series 1994;13:10-23.)

stretched with erection (Goldstein et al, 1982). Smooth muscle bundles traverse the erectile bodies to form the endothelium-lined cavernous sinuses. These sinuses give the erectile tissue a spongy appearance on gross examination.

Distal to the bulb, the corpus spongiosum tapers and runs on the underside (ventrum) of the corpora cavernosa and then expands to cap them as the glans penis. The corona separates the base of the glans from the shaft of the penis. The spongiosum is traversed throughout its length by the anterior urethra, which begins at the perineal membrane (see Fig. 2–27). The anterior urethra is dilated in its bulbar and glanular segments (fossa navicularis) and narrowest at the external meatus. Proximally, it is lined by stratified and pseudostratified columnar epithelium, distally by stratified squamous epithelium. The mucus-secreting glands (of Littre) may be seen as small outpouchings of the mucosa.

Buck's fascia surrounds both cavernosal bodies dorsally and splits to surround the spongiosum ventrally (see Fig. 2–38). Elastic and collagenous fibers from the rectus sheath blend with and surround Buck's fascia as the fundiform ligament of the penis. Deeper fibers from the pubis form the suspensory ligament of the penis. In the perineum, Buck's fascia fuses with the tunica albuginea deep to the muscles of the erectile bodies (Uhlenhuth et al, 1949). Distally, it fuses with the base of the glans at the corona. Bleeding from a tear in the corporal bodies (e.g., penile fracture) is usually contained within Buck's fascia, and ecchymosis is limited to the penile shaft.

The skin of the penile shaft is highly elastic and without appendages (hair or glandular elements), except for the smegma-producing glands at the base of the corona. It is devoid of fat and quite mobile because of the loose attachment of its dartos backing to Buck's fascia. Distally, it folds over the glans as the foreskin and attaches firmly below the corona. Its blood supply is independent of the erectile bodies and is derived from the external pudendal branches of the femoral vessels (see Fig. 2–4). These vessels enter the base of the penis to run longitudinally in the dartos fascia as a richly anastomotic network. Thus, penile skin may be mobilized on a vascular pedicle as the ideal tissue for urethral reconstruction. The skin of the glans is immobile as a result of its direct attachment to the underlying thin tunica albuginea.

The common penile artery continues in Alcock's canal, above the perineal membrane, and terminates in three branches to supply the erectile bodies (Fig. 2–39). The bulbourethral artery penetrates the perineal membrane to enter the spongiosum from above at its posterolateral border. This large, short artery can be difficult to isolate and control during urethrectomy. It supplies the urethra, spongiosum, and glans. The cavernosal artery pierces the corporal body in the penile hilum to near the center of its erectile tissue. It gives off straight and helicine arteries that ramify to supply the cavernous sinuses. The dorsal artery of the penis passes between the crus penis and the pubis to reach the dorsal surface of the corporal bodies. It runs between the dorsal vein and the dorsal penile nerve and with them attaches to the underside of Buck's fascia (see Fig. 2–41). As it courses to the glans, it gives off cavernous branches and circumferential branches to the spongiosum and urethra. The rich blood supply to the spongiosum allows safe division of the urethra during stricture repair (Devine and Angermeier, 1994).

The surgeon contemplating penile revascularization must be aware **that the penile arteries are highly variable in their**

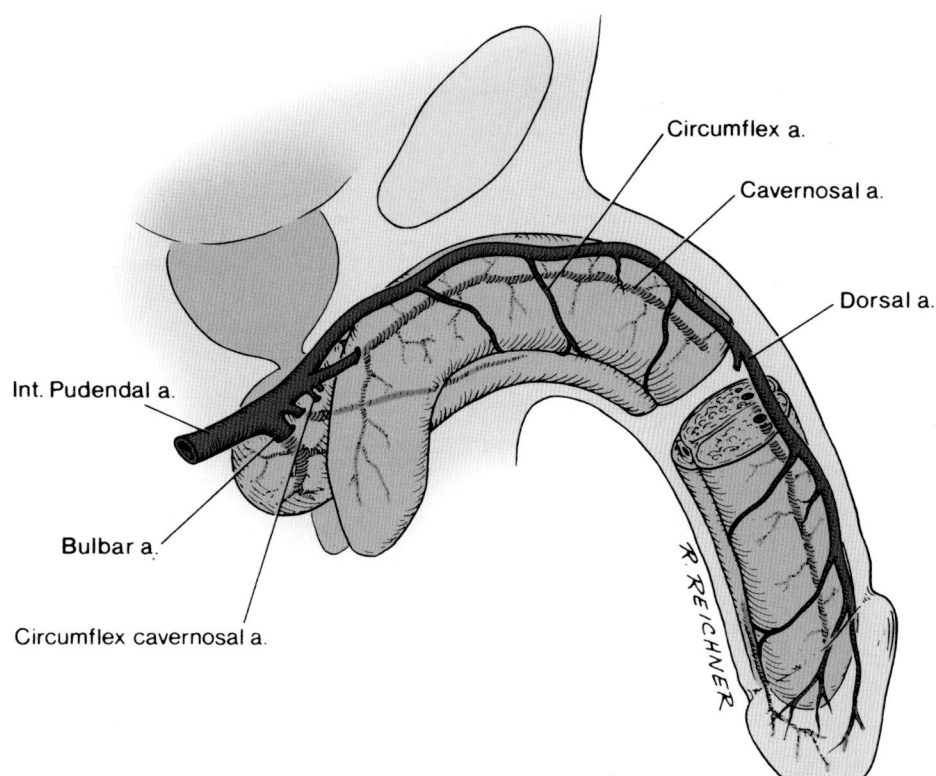

Figure 2–39. Arterial supply of the penis.

Int. Pudendal a.

Bulbar a.

Circumflex cavernosal a.

Circumflex a.

Cavernosal a.

Dorsal a.

R. REICHNER

branching, courses, and anastomoses (Bare et al, 1994). It is not uncommon for a single cavernosal artery to supply both corporal bodies or to be absent altogether. Alternatively, an accessory pudendal artery may supplement or completely replace branches of the common penile artery (Fig. 2–40). This artery usually arises from the obturator or inferior vesical arteries and runs anterolateral to or within the prostate to reach the penis in the company of the dorsal vein. This artery has been identified in 7 of 10 cadaveric specimens (Breza et al, 1989) and noted at 4% of radical prostatectomies (Polascik and Walsh, 1995); its resection at prostatectomy may adversely affect postoperative potency (Droupy et al, 1999).

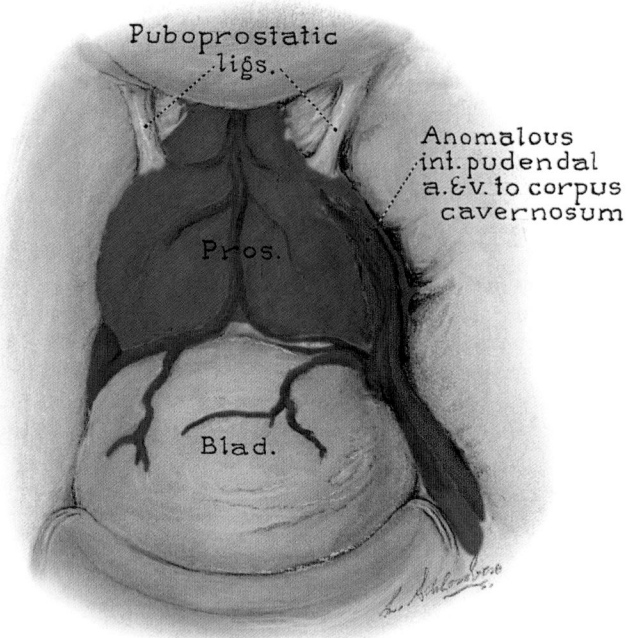

Figure 2–40. Accessory pudendal arteries, as seen in the retropubic space. (From Polascik TJ, Walsh PC: Radical retropubic prostatectomy: The influence of accessory pudendal arteries on the recovery of sexual function. J Urol 1995;153:150-152.)

At the base of the glans, several venous channels coalesce to form the dorsal vein of the penis, which runs in a groove between the corporal bodies and drains into the preprostatic plexus (Fig. 2–41). The circumflex veins originate in the spongiosum and pass around the cavernosa to meet the deep dorsal vein perpendicularly. They are present only in the distal two thirds of the penile shaft and number 3 to 10. Intermediary venules form from the cavernous sinuses to drain into a subtunical capillary plexus. These plexuses give rise to emissary veins, which commonly follow an oblique path between the layers of the tunica and drain into the circumflex veins dorsolaterally. Emissary veins in the proximal third of the penis join on the dorsomedial surface of the cavernous bodies to form two to five cavernous veins. At the hilum of the penis, these vessels pass between the crura and the bulb, receiving branches from each, and join the internal pudendal veins. Valves are found in the emissary, cavernosal, and deep dorsal veins and may thwart attempts to revascularize the penis by arteriovenous anastomosis (Sohn, 1994).

The dorsal nerves provide sensory innervation to the penis. These nerves follow the course of the dorsal arteries and richly supply the glans (see Fig. 2–41). Small branches from the perineal nerve supply the ventrum of the penis near the urethra as far as the glans distally (Uchio et al, 1999). These nerves must be anesthetized when performing a penile block to numb the ventrum of the penis. The route of the cavernous nerves has been described. After piercing the corporal bodies, they ramify in the erectile tissue to supply sympathetic and parasympathetic innervation from the pelvic plexus. Tonic sympathetic tone inhibits erection. Parasympathetic nerves release acetylcholine, nitric oxide, and vasoactive intestinal polypeptide, which cause the cavernosal smooth muscle and arterial relaxation necessary for erection (Burnett, 1995). It is thought that during erection, the subtunical venules are occluded by being compressed against the nondistensible tunica albuginea. Insufficient venous occlusion, particularly in vessels draining into the deep dorsal and cavernosal veins, is thought to cause vasculogenic impotence.

Scrotum

The scrotal skin is pigmented, hair bearing, devoid of fat, and rich in sebaceous and sweat glands. It varies from

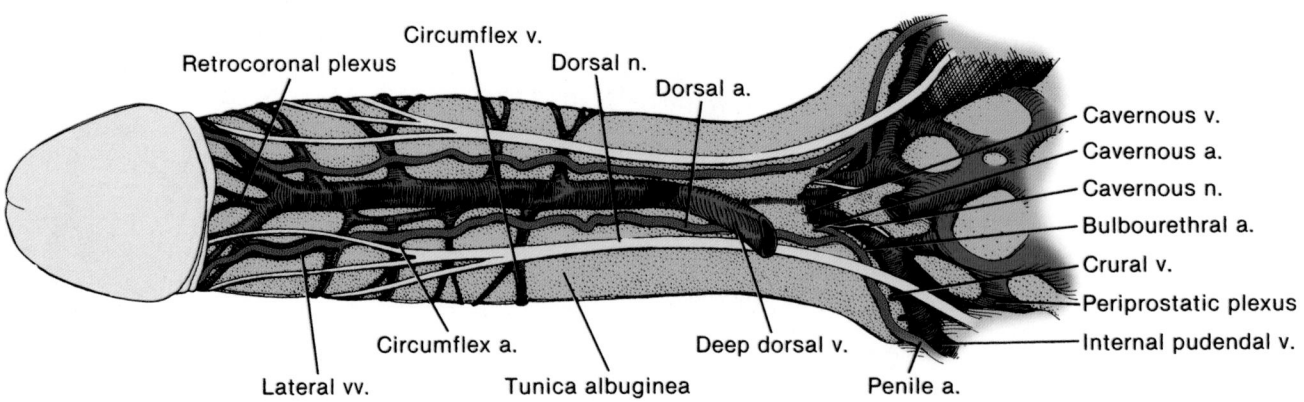

Figure 2–41. Dorsal penile arteries, veins, and nerves. (From Hinman F Jr: Atlas of Urosurgical Anatomy. Philadelphia, WB Saunders, 1993, p 445.)

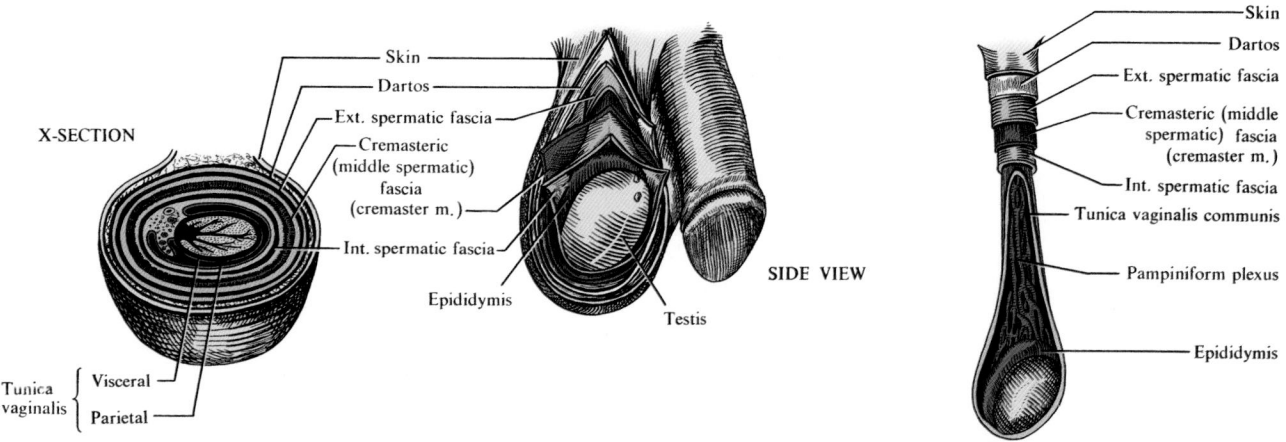

Figure 2–42. Scrotum and its layers. (From Pansky B: Review of Gross Anatomy, 6th ed. New York, McGraw-Hill, 1987, p 483.)

loose and shiny to highly folded with transverse rugae, depending on the tone of its underlying smooth muscle. A midline raphe runs from the urethral meatus to the anus and represents the line of fusion of the genital tubercles. Deep to this raphe, the scrotum is separated into two compartments by a septum.

The dartos layer of smooth muscle is continuous with Colles', Scarpa's, and the dartos fascia of the penis (see Figs. 2–3 and 2–36). The testes are suspended by their cords in the scrotal compartments. As the testes descend, they acquire coverings from the layers of the abdominal wall, known as the *spermatic fascia,* that form part of the scrotal wall (Fig. 2–42). The external spermatic fascia derives from the external oblique fascia and remains firmly attached to the borders of the external ring. The cremasteric muscle and fascia arise from the internal oblique muscle and attach laterally to the inguinal ligament and iliopsoas fascia and medially to the pubic tubercle. The internal spermatic fascia is a continuation of the transversalis fascia. The parietal and visceral tunica vaginalis surround the testis with a mesothelium-lined pouch and are derived from the peritoneum. They are continuous at the posterolateral border of the testis at its mesentery, where it is fixed to the scrotal wall. The testis is also fixed at its lower pole by the gubernaculum. Occasionally, the mesentery and gubernaculum may be deficient, leaving the testis unfixed (bell-clapper deformity) and predisposing to torsion of the cord.

The anterior wall of the scrotum is supplied by the external pudendal vessels and the ilioinguinal and genitofemoral nerves (see Fig. 2–4). The anterior vessels and nerves typically run parallel to the rugae and do not cross the raphe; thus, transverse or midline raphe scrotal incisions are most appropriate. The back of the scrotum is supplied by the posterior scrotal branches of the perineal vessels and nerves (see Fig. 2–37). In addition, the posterior femoral cutaneous nerve (S3) gives a perineal branch to supply the scrotum and perineum (see Fig. 2–8). In accordance with their origin, the spermatic fasciae have a blood supply (cremasteric, vasal, testicular) separate from that of the scrotal wall. Fournier's gangrene usually does not involve these structures, and they may be spared during débridement.

Perineal Lymphatics

The penis, scrotum, and perineum drain into the inguinal lymph nodes. These nodes may be divided into superficial and deep groups, which are separated by the deep fascia of the thigh (fascia lata). In relation to the external pudendal, superficial inferior epigastric, and superficial circumflex iliac vessels, the superficial nodes lie at the saphenofemoral junction. At the saphenous opening (fossa ovalis) in the fascia lata, the greater saphenous vein joins the femoral vein, and the superficial nodes communicate with the deep group. Most of the deep inguinal nodes lie medial to the femoral vein and send their efferents through the femoral ring (beneath the inguinal ligament) to the external iliac and obturator nodes. Just outside the femoral ring, a large node (Cloquet's or Rosenmuller's node) is consistently present.

The scrotal lymphatics do not cross the median raphe and drain into the ipsilateral superficial inguinal lymph nodes. Lymphatics from the shaft of the penis converge on the dorsum and then ramify to both sides of the groin. Those of the glans pass deep to Buck's fascia dorsally and drain to superficial and deep groups in both sides of the groin. Direct lymphatic channels from the glans to the pelvic nodes, which bypass the inguinal nodes, have been proposed by anatomists; however, clinical studies have not confirmed their existence. Other studies have suggested that all penile lymphatic drainage passes through "sentinel nodes," which lie medial to the superficial inferior epigastric veins. Clinical studies have also called this speculation into question (Catalona, 1988). The perineal skin and fasciae drain into superficial nodes; the structures of the superficial pouch likely drain into the superficial and deep groups.

Testes

The testes are 4 to 5 cm long, 3 cm wide, and 2.5 cm deep and have a volume of 30 mL. **They are enclosed in a tough capsule comprising (1) the visceral tunica vaginalis; (2) tunica albuginea, with collagenous and smooth muscle elements; and (3) the tunica vasculosa.** The epididymis attaches to the posterolateral aspect of the testis. Beneath it, the tunica

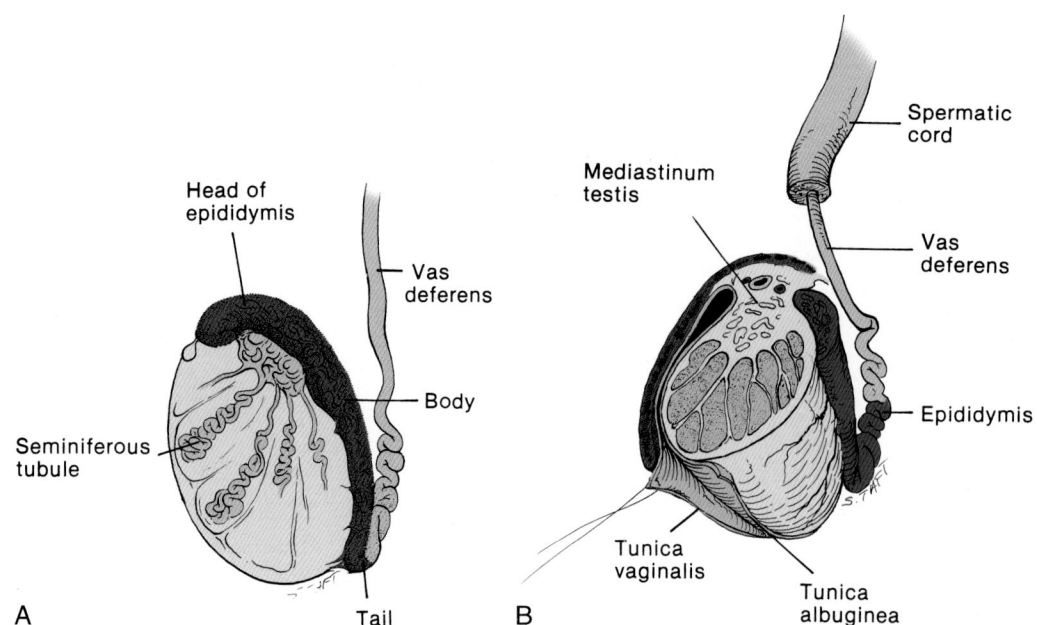

Figure 2–43. Testis and epididymis. **A,** One to three seminiferous tubules fill each compartment and drain into the rete testis in the mediastinum. Twelve to 20 efferent ductules become convoluted in the head of the epididymis and drain into a single coiled duct of the epididymis. The vas is convoluted in its first portion. **B,** Cross section of the testis, showing the mediastinum and septations continuous with the tunica albuginea. The parietal and visceral tunica vaginalis are confluent where the vessels and nerves enter the posterior aspect of the testis.

albuginea projects inward to form the mediastinum testis, the point at which vessels and ducts traverse the testicular capsule (Fig. 2–43). Septa radiate from the mediastinum to attach to the inner surface of the tunica albuginea to form 200 to 300 cone-shaped lobules, each of which contains one or more convoluted seminiferous tubules. Each tubule is U-shaped and has a stretched length of nearly 1 m. Interstitial (Leydig) cells lie in the loose tissue surrounding the tubules and are responsible for testosterone production. Toward the apices of the lobules, the seminiferous tubules become straight (tubuli recti) and enter the mediastinum testis to form an anastomosing network of tubules lined by flattened epithelium. This network, known as the rete testis, forms 12 to 20 efferent ductules and passes into the largest portion of the epididymis, the caput. Here, the efferent ductules enlarge, become more convoluted, and form conical lobules. The duct from each lobule drains into a single epididymal duct, which winds approximately 6 m within the fibrous sheath of the epididymis to form its body and tail. As the duct approaches the tail, it thickens and straightens to become the vas deferens.

The spermatic cord is composed of the vas deferens, testicular vessels, and spermatic fasciae. As discussed in Chapter 1, Surgical Anatomy of the Retroperitoneum, Kidneys, and Ureters, the testicular arteries arise from the aorta and travel in the intermediate stratum of the retroperitoneum to reach the internal inguinal ring. **Lateral to the internal inguinal ring, the attachments of the intermediate stratum form the lateral spermatic fascia.** These attachments may be taken down at orchidopexy to gain cord length. At the internal ring, the vessels are joined by the genital branch of the genitofemoral nerve, the ilioinguinal nerve, the cremasteric artery, and the vas deferens and its artery.

In its course to the testis, the testicular artery branches into an internal artery and an inferior testicular artery and into a capital artery to the head of the epididymis (Fig. 2–44). The level of this branching varies and has been noted to occur within the inguinal canal in 31% to 88% of cases (Beck et al, 1992; Jarow et al, 1992). When performing an inguinal varicocelectomy, the surgeon must remember that there may be two or three arterial branches at this level (Hopps et al, 2003). A rich arterial anastomosis occurs at the head of the epididymis, between the testicular and the capital arteries, and at the tail between the testicular, the epididymal, the cremasteric, and the vasal arteries (see Fig. 2–44). The testicular arteries enter the mediastinum and ramify in the tunica vasculosa, principally in the anterior, medial, and lateral portions of the lower pole and the anterior segment of the upper pole (Fig. 2–45). Thus, placement of a traction suture through the lower pole tunica albuginea risks damaging these important superficial vessels and devascularizing the testis (Jarow, 1991). Testicular biopsy should be carried out in the medial or lateral surface of the upper pole, where the risk of vascular injury is minimal.

The testicular veins form several highly anastomotic channels that surround the testicular artery as the pampiniform plexus. This arrangement allows countercurrent heat exchange, which cools the blood in the testicular artery. At the level of the inguinal canal, the veins join to form two or three channels and then a single vein that drains into the inferior vena cava on the right and the renal vein on the left. The testicular veins may anastomose with the external pudendal, cremasteric, and vasal veins (Fig. 2–46). These connections can allow varicoceles to recur after ablative procedures. Testicular lymphatic vessels drain to the para-aortic and interaortocaval

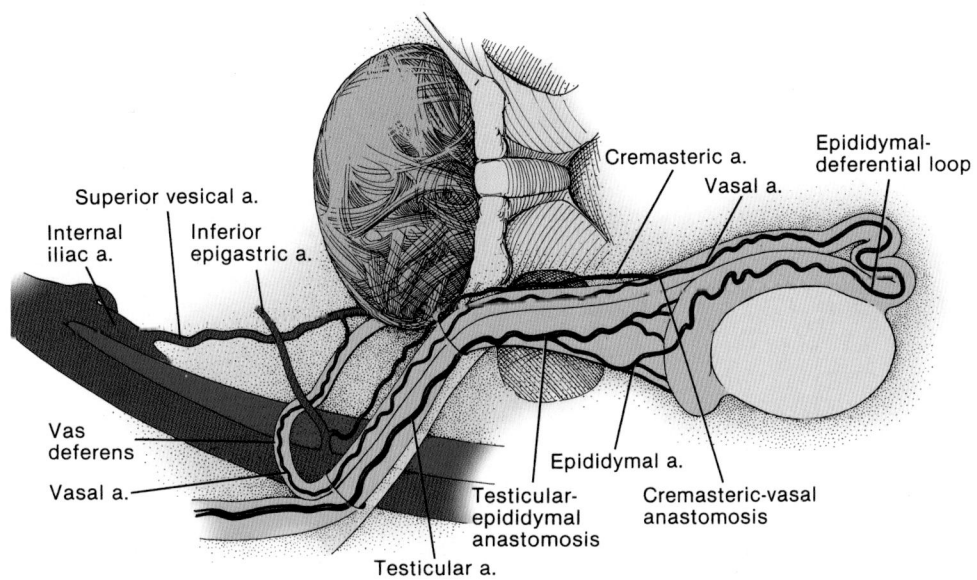

Figure 2–44.   Collateral arterial circulation to the testis. (From Hinman F Jr: Atlas of Urosurgical Anatomy. Philadelphia, WB Saunders, 1993, p 497.)

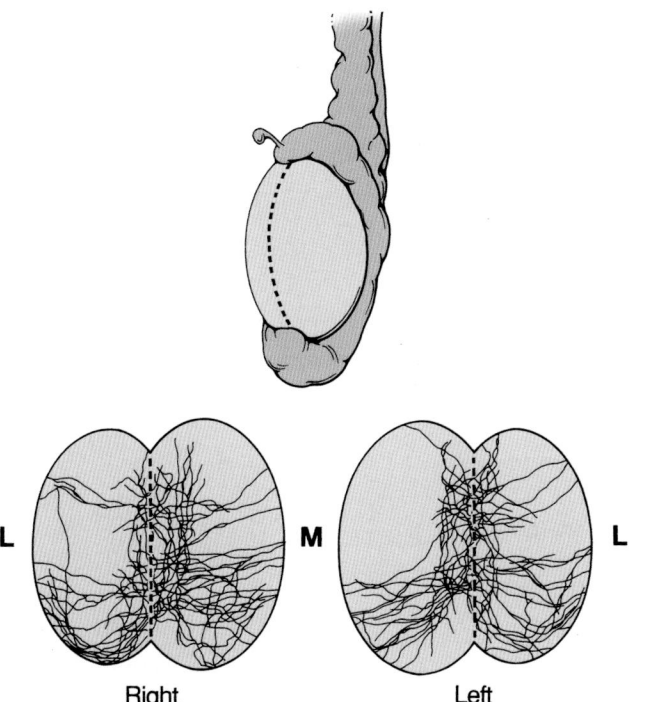

Figure 2-45.   Distribution of subtunical testicular arteries compiled from 27 right and 26 left vascular casts. The highest density of subtunical arteries is found at the anterior upper pole and the entire lower pole. Lateral (L) and medial (M) sides of the upper pole are relatively free of arterial branches. (From Jarow JP: Clinical significance of intratesticular anatomy. J Urol 1991;145:777-779.)

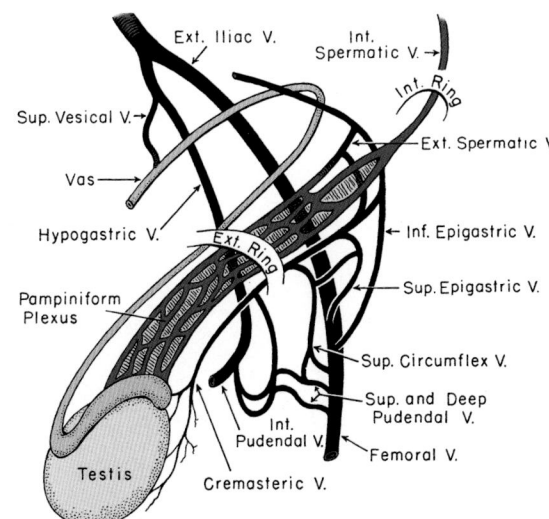

Figure 2–46.   Venous drainage of the testis and epididymis. Note connections between the pampiniform plexus and the saphenous, internal iliac, and external iliac veins.

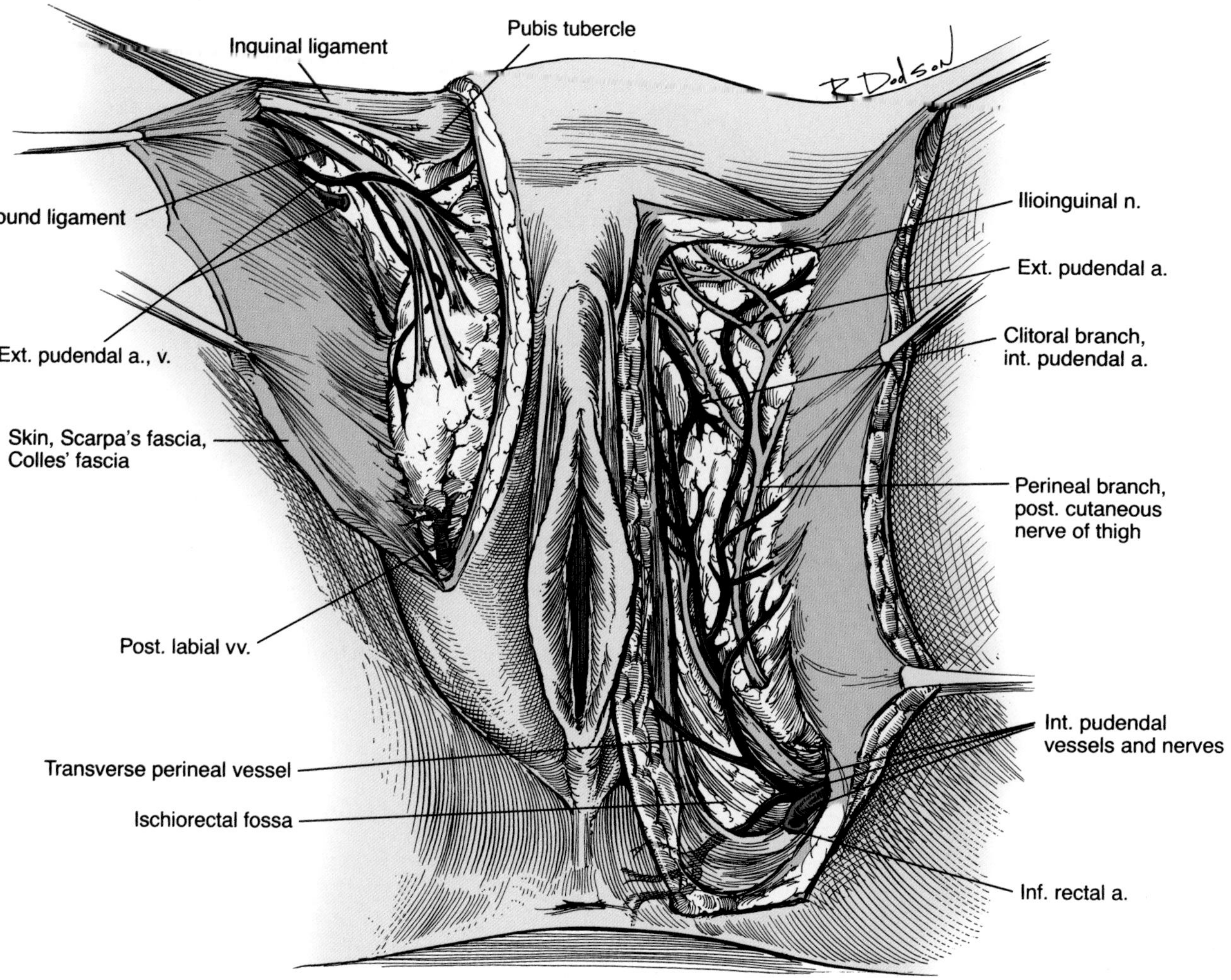

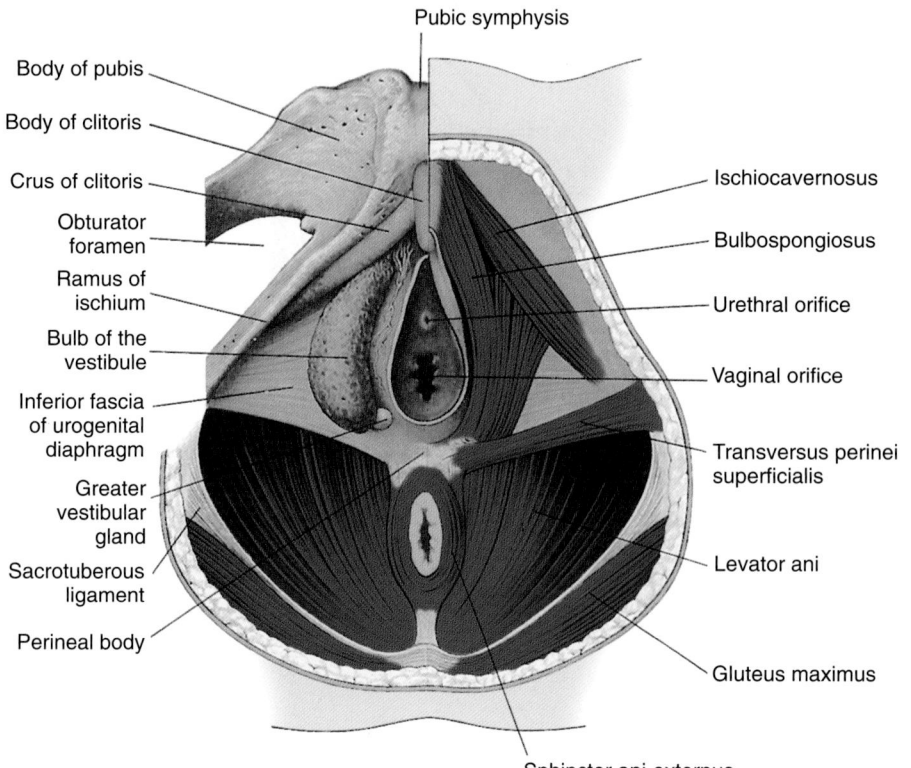

Figure 2-47. Arteries and nerves of the female perineum. (From Doherty MG: Clinical anatomy of the pelvis. In Copeland LJ [ed]: Textbook of Gynecology. Philadelphia, WB Saunders, 1993, p 51.)

Inguinal ligament

Pubis tubercle

Round ligament

Ilioinguinal n.

Ext. pudendal a.

Ext. pudendal a., v.

Clitoral branch, int. pudendal a.

Skin, Scarpa's fascia, Colles' fascia

Perineal branch, post. cutaneous nerve of thigh

Post. labial vv.

Int. pudendal vessels and nerves

Transverse perineal vessel

Ischiorectal fossa

Inf. rectal a.

Pubic symphysis

Body of pubis

Body of clitoris

Crus of clitoris

Ischiocavernosus

Obturator foramen

Bulbospongiosus

Ramus of ischium

Urethral orifice

Bulb of the vestibule

Vaginal orifice

Inferior fascia of urogenital diaphragm

Transversus perinei superficialis

Greater vestibular gland

Levator ani

Sacrotuberous ligament

Perineal body

Gluteus maximus

Sphincter ani externus

Figure 2-48. Female superficial perineal pouch. On the left side, the muscles have been removed to show the vestibular bulb and Bartholin's gland. (From Williams PL, Warwick R: Gray's Anatomy, 35th British ed. Philadelphia, WB Saunders, 1973, p 1364.)

nodes as detailed in Chapter 1, Surgical Anatomy of the Retroperitoneum, Kidneys, and Ureters.

Visceral innervation to the testis and epididymis travels by two routes. A portion arises in the renal and aortic plexuses and travels with the gonadal vessels. Additional gonadal afferent and efferent nerves course from the pelvic plexus in association with the vas deferens (Rauchenwald et al, 1995). Intractable orchialgia may respond to anesthesia of the pelvic plexus (Zorn et al, 1994). Intriguingly, some afferent and efferent nerves cross over to the contralateral pelvic plexus (Taguchi et al, 1999). This neural cross-communication may explain how pathologic processes in one testis (e.g., tumor or varicocele) may affect the function of the contralateral testis. The genital branch of the genitofemoral nerve supplies sensation to the parietal and visceral tunica vaginalis and the overlying scrotum.

Female Urogenital Triangle

The vestibule of the vagina runs vertically throughout the length of the urogenital triangle. The labia majora form its lateral sides and fuse anteriorly as the hood of the clitoris. The subcutaneous fat pad of the mons pubis continues posteriorly in the labia majora to frame the vestibule. The labial fat pads receive blood supply from the external pudendal vessels and may be raised on these vessels as a rotational flap for repair of vesicovaginal or urethrovaginal fistulas (Fig. 2–47). The urethra enters the vestibule between the clitoris and the vagina.

The structure of the superficial pouch is similar to that of the male (Fig. 2–48). The crura of the clitoris attach to the inferior ischiopubic rami, surrounded by the ischiocavernosus muscles, and converge to form the body of the clitoris. The vestibular bulbs lie to either side of the vaginal vestibule, covered by the bulbospongiosus muscles. As homologues of the penile bulb, they are composed of erectile tissue and meet anteriorly to form the glans of the clitoris. The vestibular glands are deep to the vestibular bulbs but, unlike the bulbourethral glands in the male, are superficial to the perineal membrane. Their ducts travel 2 cm to open in the vaginal vestibule on the posteromedial sides of the labia minora. The perineal membrane, pierced in its center by the vagina, is less well developed than that of the male. The innervation, blood supply, and lymphatic drainage of the external genitalia and superficial pouch are similar to those described in the male.

SUGGESTED READINGS

DeLancey JO: Anatomy and biomechanics of genital prolapse. Clin Obstet Gynecol 1993;36:897-909.

Hinman F Jr: Atlas of Urosurgical Anatomy. Philadelphia, WB Saunders, 1993.

Myers RP: Radical prostatectomy: Pertinent surgical anatomy. Atlas Urol Clin North Am 1994;2:1-18.

Uhlenhuth E: Problems in the Anatomy of the Pelvis. Philadelphia, JB Lippincott, 1953.

Williams PL, Warwick R, Dyson M, Bannister LH: Gray's Anatomy, 37th ed. New York, Churchill Livingstone, 1989.

KEY POINTS: LOWER URINARY TRACT AND MALE GENITALIA

- The pelvic cavity is divided into the false pelvis superiorly, and the true pelvis, inferiorly, wherein lie all of the pelvic organs.

- The bony prominences and ligaments of the pelvis and lower abdomen will orient the surgeon during physical examination and in the operating room.

- The pelvic floor is closed off by the levator ani and urogenital diaphragm, and the muscles and fasciae of the pelvic floor provide critical support for the pelvic organs.

- The rectum, bladder, prostate, seminal vesicles, uterus, vagina, penis, and clitoris receive blood supply from the anterior trunk of the internal iliac artery and innervation from the pelvic autonomic plexus.

- The urethra, vagina, and anus exit through the perineum in association with the external genitalia.

- Detailed knowledge of the relationships of the pelvic organs to each other and the bones and muscles of the pelvis, as well as the locations of the blood supply and innervation of all pelvic and perineal structures, is critical for safely performing all pelvic operations.

SECTION II

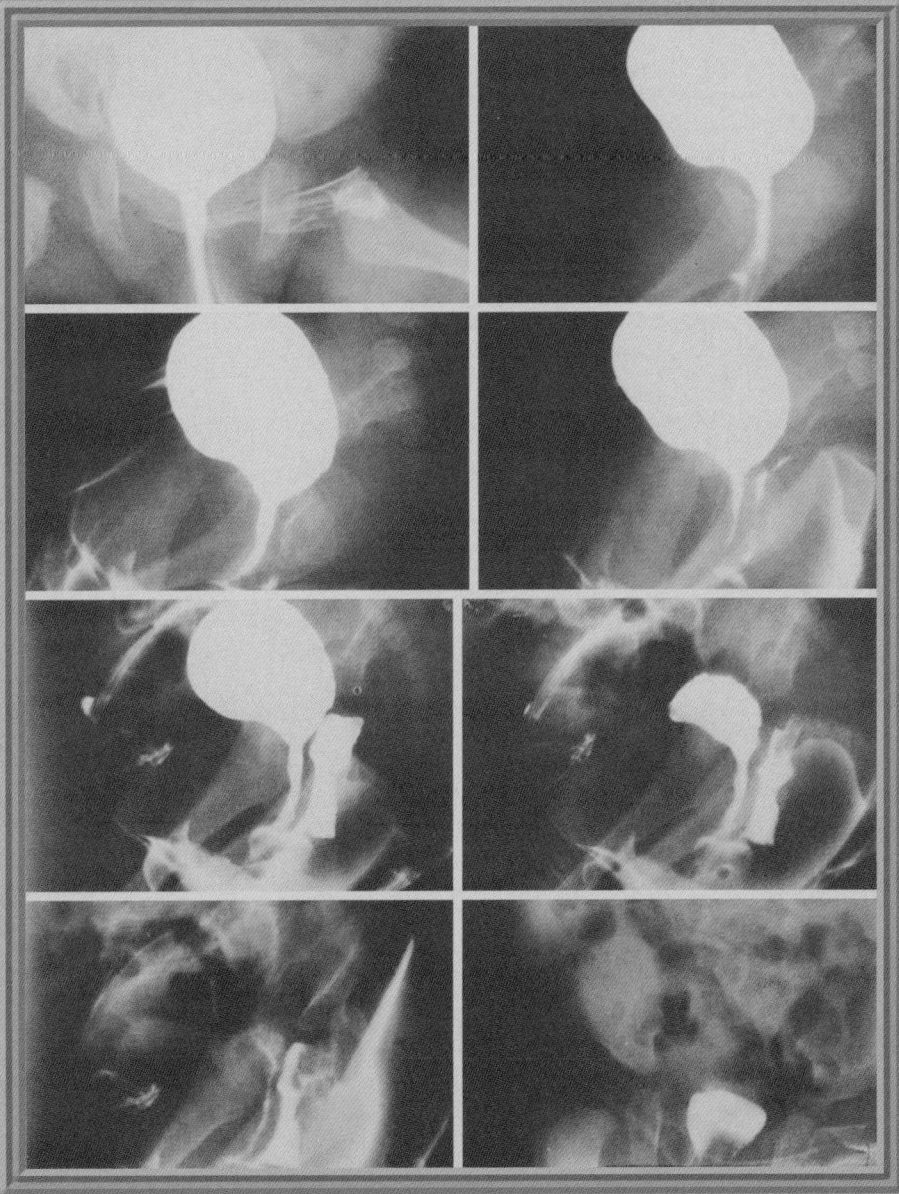

CLINICAL
DECISION-MAKING

3 Evaluation of the Urologic Patient: History, Physical Examination, and Urinalysis

GLENN S. GERBER, MD • CHARLES B. BRENDLER, MD

HISTORY

PHYSICAL EXAMINATION

URINALYSIS

SUMMARY

Urologists have a unique and interesting position in medicine. Their patients encompass all age groups, including prenatal, pediatric, adolescent, adult, and geriatric. Because there is no medical subspecialist with similar interests, **the urologist has the ability to make the initial evaluation and diagnosis and to provide medical and surgical therapy for all diseases of the genitourinary (GU) system.** Historically, the diagnostic armamentarium has included urinalysis, endoscopy, and intravenous pyelography. Recent advances in ultrasonography, computed tomography (CT), magnetic resonance imaging (MRI), and endourology have expanded our diagnostic capabilities. Despite these advances, however, the basic approach to the patient is still dependent on taking a complete history, executing a thorough physical examination, and performing a urinalysis. These basics dictate and guide the subsequent diagnostic evaluation.

HISTORY

Overview

The medical history is the cornerstone of the evaluation of the urologic patient, and a well-taken history will frequently elucidate the probable diagnosis. However, many pitfalls can inhibit the urologist from obtaining an accurate history. The patient may be unable to describe or communicate symptoms because of anxiety, language barrier, or educational background. Therefore, the urologist must be a detective and lead the patient through detailed and appropriate questioning to obtain accurate information. There are practical considerations in the art of history taking that can help to alleviate some of these difficulties. In the initial meeting, an attempt should be made to help the patient feel comfortable. During this time, the physician should project a calm, caring, and competent image that can help foster two-way communication. Impaired hearing, mental capacity, and facility with English can be assessed promptly. These difficulties are frequently overcome by having a family member present during the interview or, alternatively, by having an interpreter present.

Patients need to have sufficient time to express their problems and the reasons for seeking urologic care; the physician, however, should focus the discussion to make it as productive and informative as possible. Direct questioning can then proceed logically. The physician needs to listen carefully without distractions to obtain and interpret the clinical information provided by the patient. **A complete history can be divided into the chief complaint and history of the present illness, the patient's past medical history, and a family history.** Each segment can provide significant positive and negative findings that will contribute to the overall evaluation and treatment of the patient.

Chief Complaint and Present Illness

Most urologic patients identify their symptoms as arising from the urinary tract and frequently present to the urologist for the initial evaluation. For this reason, the urologist frequently has the opportunity to act as both the primary physician and the specialist. The chief complaint must be clearly defined because it provides the initial information and clues to begin formulating the differential diagnosis. Most importantly, **the chief complaint is a constant reminder to the urologist as to why the patient initially sought care.** This issue must be addressed even if subsequent evaluation reveals a more serious or significant condition that requires more urgent attention. In our personal experience, a young woman presented with a chief complaint of recurrent urinary tract infections (UTIs). In the course of her evaluation, she was found to have a right adrenal mass. We subsequently focused on this problem and performed a right adrenalectomy for a benign cortical adenoma. We forgot about the woman's original symptoms until she presented for her subsequent postoperative examination. She reminded us of her original symptoms at that time, and subsequent evaluation revealed that she had a nylon suture that had eroded into the anterior wall of her bladder from a previous abdominal vesicourethropexy performed 2 years earlier for stress urinary incontinence. Her UTIs resolved after surgical removal of the suture.

In obtaining the history of the present illness, **the duration, severity, chronicity, periodicity, and degree of disability are important considerations.** The patient's symptoms need to be clarified for details and quantified for severity. Listed next are a variety of typical initial complaints. Specific questions that focus the differential diagnosis are provided.

Pain

Pain arising from the GU tract may be quite severe and is usually associated with either urinary tract obstruction or inflammation. Urinary calculi cause severe pain when they obstruct the upper urinary tract. Conversely, large, nonobstructing stones may be totally asymptomatic. Thus, a 2-mm-diameter stone lodged at the ureterovesical junction may cause excruciating pain whereas a large staghorn calculus in the renal pelvis or a bladder stone may be totally asymptomatic. Urinary retention from prostatic obstruction is also quite painful, but the diagnosis is usually obvious to the patient.

Inflammation of the GU tract is most severe when it involves the parenchyma of a GU organ. This is due to edema and distention of the capsule surrounding the organ. Thus, pyelonephritis, prostatitis, and epididymitis are typically quite painful. Inflammation of the mucosa of a hollow viscus such as the bladder or urethra usually produces discomfort, but the pain is not nearly as severe.

Tumors in the GU tract usually do not cause pain unless they produce obstruction or extend beyond the primary organ to involve adjacent nerves. Thus, pain associated with GU malignancies is usually a late manifestation and a sign of advanced disease.

Renal Pain. Pain of renal origin is usually located in the ipsilateral costovertebral angle just lateral to the sacrospinalis muscle and beneath the 12th rib. **Pain is usually caused by acute distention of the renal capsule, generally from inflammation or obstruction.** The pain may radiate across the flank anteriorly toward the upper abdomen and umbilicus and may be referred to the testis or labium. A corollary to this observation is that renal or retroperitoneal disease should be considered in the differential diagnosis of any man who complains of testicular discomfort but has a normal scrotal examination. Pain due to inflammation is usually steady,

whereas pain due to obstruction fluctuates in intensity. Thus, the pain produced by ureteral obstruction is typically colicky in nature and intensifies with ureteral peristalsis, at which time the pressure in the renal pelvis rises as the ureter contracts in an attempt to force urine past the point of obstruction.

Pain of renal origin may be associated with gastrointestinal symptoms because of reflex stimulation of the celiac ganglion and because of the proximity of adjacent organs (liver, pancreas, duodenum, gallbladder, and colon). Thus, renal pain may be confused with pain of intraperitoneal origin; it can usually be distinguished, however, by a careful history and physical examination. Pain that is due to a perforated duodenal ulcer or pancreatitis may radiate into the back, but the site of greatest pain and tenderness is in the epigastrium. Pain of intraperitoneal origin is seldom colicky, as with obstructive renal pain. Furthermore, pain of intraperitoneal origin frequently radiates into the shoulder because of irritation of the diaphragm and phrenic nerve; this does not occur with renal pain. Typically, patients with intraperitoneal pathology prefer to lie motionless to minimize pain, whereas patients with renal pain usually are more comfortable moving around and holding the flank.

Renal pain may also be confused with pain resulting from irritation of the costal nerves, most commonly T10-T12. Such pain has a similar distribution from the costovertebral angle across the flank toward the umbilicus. However, the pain is not colicky in nature. Furthermore, the intensity of radicular pain may be altered by changing position; this is not the case with renal pain.

Ureteral Pain. **Ureteral pain is usually acute and secondary to obstruction.** The pain results from acute distention of the ureter and by hyperperistalsis and spasm of the smooth muscle of the ureter as it attempts to relieve the obstruction, usually produced by a stone or blood clot. The site of ureteral obstruction can often be determined by the location of the referred pain. With obstruction of the midureter, pain on the right side is referred to the right lower quadrant of the abdomen (McBurney's point) and thus may simulate appendicitis; pain on the left side is referred over the left lower quadrant and resembles diverticulitis. Also, the pain may be referred to the scrotum in the male or the labium in the female. Lower ureteral obstruction frequently produces symptoms of vesical irritability, including frequency, urgency, and suprapubic discomfort that may radiate along the urethra in men to the tip of the penis. Often, by taking a careful history, the astute clinician can predict the location of the obstruction. Ureteral pathology that arises slowly or produces only mild obstruction rarely causes pain. Therefore, ureteral tumors and stones that cause minimal obstruction are seldom painful.

Vesical Pain. Vesical pain is usually produced either by overdistention of the bladder as a result of acute urinary retention or by inflammation. **Constant suprapubic pain that is unrelated to urinary retention is seldom of urologic origin.** Furthermore, patients with slowly progressive urinary obstruction and bladder distention (e.g., diabetics with a flaccid neurogenic bladder) frequently have no pain at all despite residual urine volumes over 1 L.

Inflammatory conditions of the bladder usually produce intermittent suprapubic discomfort. Thus, the pain in conditions such as bacterial cystitis or interstitial cystitis is usually most severe when the bladder is full and is relieved at least partially by voiding. Patients with cystitis sometimes experience sharp, stabbing suprapubic pain at the end of micturition, and this is termed *strangury*. Furthermore, patients with cystitis frequently experience pain referred to the distal urethra that is associated with irritative voiding symptoms such as urinary frequency and dysuria.

Prostatic Pain. Prostatic pain is usually secondary to inflammation with secondary edema and distention of the prostatic capsule. Pain of prostatic origin is poorly localized, and the patient may complain of lower abdominal, inguinal, perineal, lumbosacral, and/or rectal pain. Prostatic pain is frequently associated with irritative urinary symptoms such as frequency and dysuria, and, in severe cases, marked prostatic edema may produce acute urinary retention.

Penile Pain. Pain in the flaccid penis is usually secondary to inflammation in the bladder or urethra, with referred pain that is experienced maximally at the urethral meatus. Alternatively, penile pain may be produced by *paraphimosis*, a condition in which the uncircumcised penile foreskin is trapped behind the glans penis, resulting in venous obstruction and painful engorgement of the glans penis (see later). Pain in the erect penis is usually due to Peyronie's disease or priapism (see later).

Testicular Pain. Scrotal pain may be either primary or referred. **Primary pain arises from within the scrotum and is usually secondary to acute epididymitis or torsion of the testis or testicular appendices.** Because of the edema and pain associated with both acute epididymitis and testicular torsion, it is frequently difficult to distinguish these two conditions. Alternatively, scrotal pain may result from inflammation of the scrotal wall itself. This may result from a simple infected hair follicle or sebaceous cyst, but it may also be secondary to Fournier's gangrene, a severe, necrotizing infection arising in the scrotum that can rapidly progress and be fatal unless promptly recognized and treated.

Chronic scrotal pain is usually related to noninflammatory conditions such as a hydrocele or a varicocele, and the pain is generally characterized as a dull, heavy sensation that does not radiate. Because the testes arise embryologically in close proximity to the kidneys, pain arising in the kidneys or retroperitoneum may be referred to the testes. Similarly, the dull pain associated with an inguinal hernia may be referred to the scrotum.

Hematuria

Hematuria is the presence of blood in the urine; **greater than three red blood cells per high-power microscopic field (HPF) is significant.** Patients with gross hematuria are usually frightened by the sudden onset of blood in the urine and frequently present to the emergency department for evaluation, fearing that they may be bleeding excessively. Hematuria of any degree should never be ignored and, in adults, should be regarded as a symptom of urologic malignancy until proved otherwise. In evaluating hematuria, several questions should always be asked, and the answers will enable the urologist to target the subsequent diagnostic evaluation efficiently:

Is the hematuria gross or microscopic?
At what time during urination does the hematuria occur (beginning or end of stream or during entire stream)?
Is the hematuria associated with pain?
Is the patient passing clots?
If the patient is passing clots, do the clots have a specific shape?

Gross versus Microscopic Hematuria. The significance of gross versus microscopic hematuria is simply that **the chances of identifying significant pathology increase with the degree of hematuria.** Thus, it is uncommon for patients with gross hematuria not to have identifiable underlying pathology whereas it is quite common for patients with minimal degrees of microscopic hematuria to have a negative urologic evaluation.

Timing of Hematuria. The timing of hematuria during urination frequently indicates the site of origin. **Initial hematuria usually arises from the urethra;** it occurs least commonly and is usually secondary to inflammation. Total hematuria is most common and indicates that the bleeding is most likely coming from the bladder or upper urinary tracts. Terminal hematuria occurs at the end of micturition and is usually secondary to inflammation in the area of the bladder neck or prostatic urethra. It occurs at the end of micturition as the bladder neck contracts, squeezing out the last amount of urine.

Association with Pain. Hematuria, although frightening, is usually not painful unless it is associated with inflammation or obstruction. Thus, patients with cystitis and secondary hematuria may experience painful urinary irritative symptoms but the pain is usually not worsened with passage of clots. More commonly, **pain in association with hematuria usually results from upper urinary tract hematuria with obstruction of the ureters with clots.** Passage of these clots may be associated with severe, colicky flank pain similar to that produced by a ureteral calculus, and this helps identify the source of the hematuria.

Presence of Clots. The presence of clots usually indicates a more significant degree of hematuria, and, accordingly, the probability of identifying significant urologic pathology increases.

Shape of Clots. Usually, if the patient is passing clots, they are amorphous and of bladder or prostatic urethral origin. However, **the presence of vermiform (wormlike) clots, particularly if associated with flank pain, identifies the hematuria as coming from the upper urinary tract** with formation of vermiform clots within the ureter.

It cannot be emphasized strongly enough that **hematuria, particularly in the adult, should be regarded as a symptom of malignancy until proved otherwise and demands immediate urologic examination.** In a patient who presents with gross hematuria, cystoscopy should be performed as soon as possible, because frequently the source of bleeding can be readily identified. Cystoscopy will determine whether the hematuria is coming from the urethra, bladder, or upper urinary tract. In patients with gross hematuria secondary to an upper tract source, it is very easy to see the jet of red urine pulsing from the involved ureteral orifice.

Although inflammatory conditions may result in hematuria, all patients with hematuria, except perhaps young women with acute bacterial hemorrhagic cystitis, should undergo urologic evaluation. Older women and men who present with hematuria and irritative voiding symptoms may have cystitis secondary to infection arising in a necrotic bladder tumor or, more commonly, flat carcinoma in situ of the bladder. **The most common cause of gross hematuria in a patient older than age 50 years is bladder cancer.**

Lower Urinary Tract Symptoms

Irritative Symptoms. *Frequency* is one of the most common urologic symptoms. The normal adult voids five or six times per day, with a volume of approximately 300 mL with each void. **Urinary frequency is due either to increased urinary output (polyuria) or to decreased bladder capacity.** If voiding is noted to occur in large amounts frequently, the patient has polyuria and should be evaluated for diabetes mellitus, diabetes insipidus, or excessive fluid ingestion. Causes of decreased bladder capacity include bladder outlet obstruction with decreased compliance, increased residual urine, and/or decreased functional capacity due to irritation; neurogenic bladder with increased sensitivity and decreased compliance; pressure from extrinsic sources; or anxiety. By separating irritative from obstructive symptoms, the astute clinician should be able to arrive at a proper differential diagnosis.

Nocturia is nocturnal frequency. Normally, adults arise no more than twice at night to void. As with frequency, nocturia may be secondary to increased urine output or decreased bladder capacity. **Frequency during the day without nocturia is usually of psychogenic origin and related to anxiety. Nocturia without frequency may occur in the patient with congestive heart failure and peripheral edema in whom the intravascular volume and urine output increase when the patient is supine. Renal concentrating ability decreases with age; therefore, urine production in the geriatric patient is increased at night, when renal blood flow is increased as a result of recumbency.** In general, nocturia may be attributed to nocturnal polyuria (nocturnal urine overproduction) and/or diminished nocturnal bladder capacity (Weiss and Blaivas, 2000). Nocturia may also occur in people who drink large amounts of liquid in the evening, particularly caffeinated and alcoholic beverages, which have strong diuretic effects. In the absence of these factors, nocturia signifies a problem with bladder function secondary to urinary outlet obstruction and/or decreased bladder compliance.

Dysuria is painful urination that is usually caused by inflammation. **This pain is usually not felt over the bladder but is commonly referred to the urethral meatus.** Pain occurring at the start of urination may indicate urethral pathology, whereas pain occurring at the end of micturition (strangury) is usually of bladder origin. Dysuria is frequently accompanied by frequency and urgency.

Obstructive Symptoms. *Decreased force of urination* is usually secondary to bladder outlet obstruction and commonly results from benign prostatic hyperplasia (BPH) or a urethral stricture. In fact, except for severe degrees of obstruction, **most patients are unaware of a change in the force and caliber of their urinary stream.** These changes usually occur gradually and go generally unrecognized by most patients.

The other obstructive symptoms noted later are more commonly recognized and are usually secondary to bladder outlet obstruction in men due to either BPH or a urethral stricture.

Urinary hesitancy refers to a delay in the start of micturition. Normally, urination begins within a second after relaxing the urinary sphincter, but it may be delayed in men with bladder outlet obstruction.

Intermittency refers to involuntary start-stopping of the urinary stream. It most commonly results from prostatic obstruction with intermittent occlusion of the urinary stream by the lateral prostatic lobes.

Postvoid dribbling refers to the terminal release of drops of urine at the end of micturition. **This is secondary to a small amount of residual urine in either the bulbar or the prostatic urethra that is normally "milked back" into the bladder at the end of micturition** (Stephenson and Farrar, 1977). In men with bladder outlet obstruction, this urine escapes into the bulbar urethra and leaks out at the end of micturition. Men frequently will attempt to avoid wetting their clothing by shaking the penis at the end of micturition. In fact, this is ineffective, and the problem is more readily solved by manual compression of the bulbar urethra in the perineum and blotting the urethral meatus with a tissue. Postvoid dribbling is often an early symptom of urethral obstruction related to BPH, but, in itself, seldom necessitates any further treatment.

Straining refers to the use of abdominal musculature to urinate. Normally, it is unnecessary for a man to perform a Valsalva maneuver except at the end of urination. Increased straining during micturition is a symptom of bladder outlet obstruction.

It is important for the urologist to distinguish irritative from obstructive lower urinary tract symptoms. This most frequently occurs in evaluating men with BPH. Although BPH is primarily obstructive, it produces changes in bladder compliance that result in increased irritative symptoms. In fact, men with BPH more commonly present with irritative than obstructive symptoms, and the most common presenting symptom is nocturia. **The urologist must be careful not to attribute irritative symptoms to BPH unless there is documented evidence of obstruction.** In general, lower urinary tract symptoms are nonspecific and may occur secondary to a wide variety of neurologic conditions as well as to prostatic enlargement (Lepor and Machi, 1993). In this regard, two important examples are mentioned. Patients with high-grade flat carcinoma in situ of the bladder may present with urinary irritative symptoms. The urologist should be particularly aware of the diagnosis of carcinoma in situ in men who present with irritative symptoms, a history of cigarette smoking, and microscopic hematuria. In our personal experience, we cared for a 54-year-old man who presented with this history and was treated for BPH for 2 years before the diagnosis of bladder cancer was established. Once the correct diagnosis was made, the patient had developed muscle-invasive disease and required a cystectomy for cure.

The second important example is irritative symptoms resulting from neurologic disease, such as cerebrovascular accidents, diabetes mellitus, and Parkinson's disease. Most neurologic diseases encountered by the urologist are upper motor neuron in etiology and result in a loss of cortical inhibition of voiding with resultant decreased bladder compliance and irritative voiding symptoms. The urologist must be extremely careful to rule out underlying neurologic disease before performing surgery to relieve bladder outlet obstruction. Such surgery not only may fail to relieve the patient's irritative symptoms but also may result in permanent urinary incontinence.

Since its introduction in 1992, **the American Urological Association (AUA) symptom index has been widely used and validated as an important means of assessing men with lower urinary tract symptoms** (Barry et al, 1992).

The original AUA symptom score is based on the answers to seven questions concerning frequency, nocturia, weak urinary stream, hesitancy, intermittency, incomplete bladder emptying, and urgency. The International Prostate Symptom Score (I-PSS) includes these seven questions, as well as a global quality of life question (Table 3–1). The total symptom score ranges from 0 to 35 with scores of 0 to 7, 8 to 19, and 20 to 35 indicating mild, moderate, and severe lower urinary tract symptoms, respectively. The I-PSS is a helpful

Table 3–1. International Prostate Symptom Score

Patient's Name Date of Birth Date Completed	Not At All	Less Than 1 Time in 5	Less Than Half the Time	About Half the Time	More Than Half the Time	Almost Always	Your Score
1. Incomplete emptying Over the past month, how often have you had a sensation of not emptying your bladder completely after you finished urinating?	0	1	2	3	4	5	
2. Frequency Over the past month, how often have you had to urinate again less than two hours after you finished urinating?	0	1	2	3	4	5	
3. Intermittency Over the past month, how often have you found you stopped and started again several times when you urinated?	0	1	2	3	4	5	
4. Urgency Over the past month, how often have you found it difficult to postpone urination?	0	1	2	3	4	5	
5. Weak stream Over the past month, how often have you had a weak urinary stream?	0	1	2	3	4	5	
6. Straining Over the past month, how often have you had to push or strain to begin urination?	0	1	2	3	4	5	

	None	1 Time	2 Times	3 Times	4 Times	5 Times or More	
7. Nocturia Over the past month, how many times did you most typically get up to urinate from the time you went to bed at night until the time you got up in the morning?	0	1	2	3	4	5	

Total I-PSS Score

Quality of Life Due to Urinary Symptoms	Delighted	Pleased	Mostly Satisfied	Mixed—About Equally Satisfied and Dissatisfied	Mostly Dissatisfied	Unhappy	Terrible
If you were to spend the rest of your life with your urinary condition just the way it is now, how would you feel about that?	0	1	2	3	4	5	6

From Cockett ATK, Aso Y, Denis L, et al: The Second International Consultation on Benign Prostatic Hyperplasia (BPH). In Cockett ATK, Aso Y, Chatelain C, et al (eds): The Second International Consultation on Benign Prostatic Hyperplasia (BPH). Pairs, Scientific Communication International, 1994, p 553.

tool both in the clinical management of men with lower urinary tract symptoms and in research studies regarding the medical and surgical treatment of men with voiding dysfunction.

There are limitations to the use of symptom indices, and it is important for the physician to discuss the patient's responses with him. It has been demonstrated that a grade 6 reading level is necessary to understand the I-PSS, and some patients with neurologic disorders and dementia may also have difficulty completing the symptom score (Mac-Diarmid et al, 1998). In addition, the symptom score, as well as the obstructive and irritative voiding symptoms, is non-specific, and the symptoms may be caused by a variety of conditions other than BPH. Similar symptom scores have been demonstrated to be present in age-matched men and women between 55 and 79 years of age (Lepor and Machi, 1993). **Despite these limitations, the I-PSS is a simple adjunct in assessing men with lower urinary tract symptoms and may be used in the initial evaluation of men with lower urinary tract symptoms as well as in the assessment of treatment response.**

Incontinence. *Urinary incontinence* is the involuntary loss of urine. A careful history of the incontinent patient will often determine the etiology. Urinary incontinence can be subdivided into four categories.

Continuous Incontinence. **Continuous incontinence is most commonly due to a urinary tract fistula that bypasses the urethral sphincter.** The most common type of fistula that results in urinary incontinence is a vesicovaginal fistula usually secondary to gynecologic surgery, radiation, or obstetric trauma. Less commonly, ureterovaginal fistulas may occur from similar causes.

A second major cause of continuous incontinence is an ectopic ureter that enters either the urethra or the female genital tract. An ectopic ureter usually drains a small, dysplastic upper pole segment of kidney, and the amount of urinary leakage may be quite small. Such patients may void most of their urine normally but have a continuous amount of small urinary leakage that may be misdiagnosed for many years as a chronic vaginal discharge. In our experience, we cared for a 30-year-old woman—who had been misdiagnosed with enuresis in childhood and as having a chronic vaginal discharge in adult life—whose urinary leakage was totally corrected by surgical removal of the dysplastic, upper pole segment of her right kidney. Ectopic ureters never produce urinary incontinence in males because they always enter the bladder neck or prostatic urethra proximal to the external urethral sphincter.

Stress Incontinence. Stress incontinence refers to the sudden leakage of urine with coughing, sneezing, exercise, or other activities that increase intra-abdominal pressure. During these activities, intra-abdominal pressure rises transiently above urethral resistance, resulting in a sudden, usually small amount of urinary leakage. Stress incontinence is most common in women after childbearing or menopause and is related to a loss of anterior vaginal support and weakening of pelvic tissues. Stress incontinence is also observed in men after prostatic surgery, most commonly radical prostatectomy, in which there may be injury to the external urethral sphincter. **Stress urinary incontinence is difficult to manage pharma-**cologically, and patients with significant stress incontinence are usually best treated surgically.

Urgency Incontinence. Urgency incontinence is the precipitous loss of urine preceded by a strong urge to void. This symptom is commonly observed in patients with cystitis, neurogenic bladder, and advanced bladder outlet obstruction with secondary loss of bladder compliance. It is important to distinguish urgency incontinence from stress incontinence for two reasons. First, **urgency incontinence may result from a secondary underlying pathologic process, which should be identified;** treatment of this primary problem, such as infection or bladder outlet obstruction, may result in resolution of urgency incontinence. Second, patients with urgency incontinence usually are not amenable to surgical correction but, rather, are more appropriately treated with pharmacologic agents that increase bladder compliance and/or increase urethral resistance.

Overflow Urinary Incontinence. Overflow urinary incontinence, often called paradoxical incontinence, is secondary to advanced urinary retention and high residual urine volumes. In these patients, the bladder is chronically distended and never empties completely. Urine may dribble out in small amounts as the bladder overflows. This is particularly likely to occur at night when the patient is less likely to inhibit urinary leakage. **Overflow incontinence has been termed *paradoxical incontinence* because it can often be cured by relief of bladder outlet obstruction.** It is, however, often difficult to make the diagnosis of overflow incontinence by history and physical examination alone, particularly in the obese patient, in whom percussion of the distended bladder may be difficult. Overflow incontinence usually develops over a considerable length of time, and patients may be totally unaware of incomplete bladder emptying. Thus, any patient with significant incontinence should undergo measurement of postvoid residual urine.

Enuresis. *Enuresis* refers to urinary incontinence that occurs during sleep. It occurs normally in children up to 3 years of age **but persists in about 15% of children at age 5 and about 1% of children at age 15** (Forsythe and Redmond, 1974). Enuresis must be distinguished from continuous incontinence, which occurs in the day as well as night and which, in a young girl, usually indicates the presence of an ectopic ureter. All children older than age 6 years with enuresis should undergo a urologic evaluation, although the vast majority will be found to have no significant urologic abnormality.

Sexual Dysfunction

Male sexual dysfunction is frequently used synonymously with *impotence* or erectile dysfunction, although impotence refers specifically to the inability to achieve and maintain an erection adequate for intercourse. Patients presenting with "impotence" should be questioned carefully to rule out other male sexual disorders, including loss of libido, absence of emission, absence of orgasm, and, most commonly, premature ejaculation. Obviously, it is important to identify the precise problem before proceeding with further evaluation and treatment.

Loss of Libido. Because androgens have a major influence on sexual desire, a decrease in libido may indicate androgen deficiency arising from either pituitary or testicular dysfunction.

This can be evaluated directly by **measurement of serum testosterone that, if abnormal, should be further evaluated by measurement of serum gonadotropins and prolactin.** Because the amount of testosterone required to maintain libido is usually less than that required for full stimulation of the prostate and seminal vesicles, patients with hypogonadism may also note decreased or absent ejaculation. Conversely, if semen volume is normal, it is unlikely that endocrine factors are responsible for loss of libido. A decrease in libido may also result from depression and a variety of medical illnesses that affect general health and well-being.

Impotence. *Impotence* refers specifically to the inability to achieve and maintain an erection sufficient for intercourse. **A careful history will often determine whether the problem is primarily psychogenic or organic.** In men with psychogenic impotence, the condition frequently develops rather quickly secondary to a precipitating event such as marital stress or change or loss of a sexual partner. In men with organic impotence, the condition usually develops more insidiously and frequently can be linked to advancing age or other underlying risk factors.

In evaluating men with impotence, it is important to determine whether the problem exists in all situations. Many men who report impotence may not be able to have intercourse with one partner but will with another. Similarly, it is important to determine whether men are able to achieve normal erections with alternative forms of sexual stimulation (e.g., masturbation, erotic videos). Finally, the patient should be asked whether he ever notes nocturnal or early morning erections. In general, **patients who are able to achieve adequate erections in some situations but not others have primarily psychogenic rather than organic impotence.**

Failure to Ejaculate. **Anejaculation may result from several causes: (1) androgen deficiency, (2) sympathetic denervation, (3) pharmacologic agents, and (4) bladder neck and prostatic surgery.** Androgen deficiency results in decreased secretions from the prostate and seminal vesicles causing a reduction or loss of seminal volume. Sympathectomy or extensive retroperitoneal surgery, most notably retroperitoneal lymphadenectomy for testicular cancer, may interfere with autonomic innervation of the prostate and seminal vesicles, resulting in absence of smooth muscle contraction and absence of seminal emission at time of orgasm. Pharmacologic agents, particularly α-adrenergic antagonists, may interfere with bladder neck closure at time of orgasm and result in retrograde ejaculation. Similarly, previous bladder neck or prostatic urethral surgery, most commonly transurethral resection of the prostate, may interfere with bladder neck closure, resulting in retrograde ejaculation. Finally, retrograde ejaculation may develop spontaneously in diabetic men.

Patients who complain of absence of ejaculation should be questioned regarding loss of libido or other symptoms of androgen deficiency, present medications, diabetes, and previous surgery. A careful history will usually determine the cause of this problem.

Absence of Orgasm. **Anorgasmia is usually psychogenic or caused by certain medications used to treat psychiatric diseases.** Sometimes, however, anorgasmia may be due to decreased penile sensation owing to impaired pudendal nerve function. Most commonly, this occurs in diabetics with peripheral neuropathy. Men who experience anorgasmia in association with decreased penile sensation should undergo vibratory testing of the penis and further neurologic evaluation as indicated.

Premature Ejaculation. Men who complain of premature ejaculation should be questioned carefully because this is obviously a very subjective symptom. It is common for men to ejaculate within 2 minutes after initiation of intercourse, and many men who complain of premature ejaculation in actuality have normal sexual function with abnormal sexual expectations. However, there are men with true premature ejaculation who reach orgasm within less than 1 minute after initiation of intercourse. **This problem is almost always psychogenic** and best treated by a clinical psychologist or psychiatrist who specializes in treatment of this problem and other psychological aspects of male sexual dysfunction. With counseling and appropriate modifications in sexual technique, this problem can usually be overcome. Alternatively, treatment with serotonin reuptake inhibitors, such as sertraline and fluoxetine, have been demonstrated to be helpful in men with premature ejaculation (Murat Basar et al, 1999).

Hematospermia

Hematospermia refers to the presence of blood in the seminal fluid. **It almost always results from nonspecific inflammation of the prostate and/or seminal vesicles and resolves spontaneously, usually within several weeks.** It frequently occurs after a prolonged period of sexual abstinence, and we have observed it several times in men whose wives are in the final weeks of pregnancy. Patients with hematospermia that persists beyond several weeks should undergo further urologic evaluation, because, rarely, an underlying etiology will be identified. A genital and rectal examination should be done to exclude the presence of tuberculosis, a prostate-specific antigen (PSA) and a rectal examination done to exclude prostatic carcinoma, and a urinary cytology done to exclude the possibility of transitional cell carcinoma of the prostate. It should be emphasized, however, that hematospermia almost always resolves spontaneously and rarely is associated with any significant urologic pathology.

Pneumaturia

Pneumaturia is the passage of gas in the urine. In patients who have not recently had urinary tract instrumentation or a urethral catheter placed, this is almost always **due to a fistula between the intestine and the bladder. Common causes include diverticulitis, carcinoma of the sigmoid colon, and regional enteritis (Crohn's disease).** In rare instances, patients with diabetes mellitus may have gas-forming infections, with carbon dioxide formation from the fermentation of high concentrations of sugar in the urine.

Urethral Discharge

Urethral discharge is the most common symptom of venereal infection. A purulent discharge that is thick, profuse, and yellow to gray is typical of gonococcal urethritis; the discharge in patients with nonspecific urethritis is usually scant and watery. A bloody discharge is suggestive of carcinoma of the urethra.

Fever and Chills

Fever and chills may occur with infection anywhere in the GU tract but are most commonly observed in patients with pyelonephritis, prostatitis, or epididymitis. **When associated with urinary obstruction, fever and chills may portend septicemia and necessitate emergency treatment to relieve obstruction.**

Medical History

The past medical history is extremely important because it frequently provides clues to the patient's current diagnosis. The past medical history should be obtained in an orderly and sequential manner.

Previous Medical Illnesses with Urologic Sequelae

There are obviously many diseases that may affect the GU system, and it is important to listen and record the patient's previous medical illnesses. **Patients with diabetes mellitus frequently develop autonomic dysfunction that may result in impaired urinary and sexual function.** A previous history of tuberculosis may be important in a patient presenting with impaired renal function, ureteral obstruction, or chronic, unexplained UTIs. Patients with hypertension have an increased risk of sexual dysfunction because they are more likely to have peripheral vascular disease and because many of the medications that are used to treat hypertension frequently cause impotence. Patients with neurologic diseases such as multiple sclerosis are also more likely to develop urinary and sexual dysfunction. In fact, 5% of patients with previously undiagnosed multiple sclerosis present with urinary symptoms as the first manifestation of the disease (Blaivas and Kaplan, 1988). As mentioned earlier, in men with bladder outlet obstruction, it is important to be aware of preexisting neurologic conditions. Surgical treatment of bladder outlet obstruction in the presence of detrusor hyperreflexia may result in increased urinary incontinence postoperatively. Finally, patients with sickle cell anemia are prone to a number of urologic conditions, including papillary necrosis and erectile dysfunction secondary to recurrent priapism. There are obviously many other diseases with urologic sequelae, and it is important for the urologist to take a careful history in this regard.

Family History

It is similarly important to obtain a detailed family history because many diseases are genetic and/or familial. Examples of genetic diseases include adult polycystic kidney disease, tuberous sclerosis, von Hippel-Lindau disease, renal tubular acidosis, and cystinuria; these are but a few common and well-recognized examples.

In addition to these diseases of known genetic predisposition, there are other conditions in which the precise pattern of inheritance has not been elucidated but that clearly have a familial tendency. It is well known that individuals with a family history of urolithiasis are at increased risk for stone formation. More recently, it has been recognized that **8% to 10% of men with prostate cancer have a familial form of the disease that tends to develop about a decade earlier than the more common type of prostate cancer** (Bratt, 2000). There are other familial conditions that are mentioned elsewhere in the text, but suffice it to state again that obtaining a careful history of previous illnesses and a family history of urologic disease can be extremely valuable in establishing the correct diagnosis.

Medications

It is similarly important to obtain an accurate and complete list of present medications because many drugs interfere with urinary and sexual function. For example, **most of the anti-hypertensive medications interfere with erectile function, and changing antihypertensive medications can sometimes improve sexual function.** Similarly, many of the psychotropic agents interfere with emission and orgasm. In our own recent experience, we cared for a man who presented with anorgasmia. He had been to several physicians without improvement in this problem. When we obtained his past medical history, he mentioned that he had been taking a psychotropic agent for transient depression for several years, and his anorgasmia resolved when this no longer needed medication was discontinued. The list of medications affecting urinary and sexual function is exhaustive, but, once again, each medication should be recorded and its side effects investigated to be sure that the patient's problem is not drug related. A listing of common medications that may cause urologic side effects is presented in Table 3–2.

Previous Surgical Procedures

It is important to be aware of previous operations, particularly in a patient in whom surgery is intended. Obviously, previous operations may make subsequent ones more difficult. If the previous surgery was in a similar anatomic region, it is worthwhile to try to obtain the previous operative report. In our own experience, this small additional effort has been rewarded on numerous occasions by providing a clear explanation of the patient's previous surgery that greatly simplified the subsequent operation. In general, **it is worthwhile obtaining as much information as possible** *before* **any intended surgery** because most surprises that occur in the operating room are unhappy ones.

Smoking and Alcohol Use

Cigarette smoking and consumption of alcohol are clearly linked to a number of urologic conditions. **Cigarette smoking is associated with an increased risk of urothelial carcinoma, most notably bladder cancer, and it is also associated with increased peripheral vascular disease and erectile dysfunction. Chronic alcoholism may result in autonomic and peripheral neuropathy with resultant impaired urinary and sexual function. Chronic alcoholism may also impair hepatic metabolism of estrogens, resulting in decreased serum testosterone, testicular atrophy, and decreased libido.**

In addition to the direct urologic effects of cigarette smoking and alcohol consumption, patients who are actively smoking or drinking at the time of surgery are at increased risk for perioperative complications. Smokers are at increased risk for both pulmonary and cardiac complications. If possible, they should **discontinue smoking at least 8 weeks before surgery to optimize their pulmonary function** (Warner et al, 1989). If they are unable to do this, they should at least quit

Table 3-2. Drugs Associated with Urologic Side Effects

Urologic Side Effects	Class of Drugs	Specific Examples
Decreased libido Erectile dysfunction	Antihypertensives	Hydrochlorothiazide Propranolol
	Psychotropic drugs	Benzodiazepines
Ejaculatory dysfunction	α-Adrenergic antagonists	Prazosin Tamsulosin α-Methyldopa
	Psychotropic drugs	Phenothiazines Antidepressants
Priapism	Antipsychotics	Phenothiazines
	Antidepressants	Trazodone
	Antihypertensives	Hydralazine Prazosin
Decreased spermatogenesis	Chemotherapeutic agents	Alkylating agents
	Drugs with abuse potential	Marijuana Alcohol Nicotine
	Drugs affecting endocrine function	Antiandrogens Prostaglandins
Incontinence or impaired voiding	Direct smooth muscle stimulants	Histamine Vasopressin
	Others	Furosemide Valproic acid
	Smooth muscle relaxants	Diazepam
	Striated muscle relaxants	Baclofen
Urinary retention or obstructive voiding symptoms	Anticholinergic agents or musculotropic relaxants	Oxybutynin Diazepam Flavoxate
	Calcium channel blockers	Nifedipine
	Antiparkinsonian drugs	Carbidopa Levodopa
	α-Adrenergic agonists	Pseudoephedrine Phenylephrine
	Antihistamines	Loratadine Diphenhydramine
Acute renal failure	Antimicrobials	Aminoglycosides Penicillins Cephalosporins Amphotericin
	Chemotherapeutic drugs	Cisplatin
	Others	Nonsteroidal anti-inflammatory drugs Phenytoin
Gynecomastia	Antihypertensives	Verapamil
	Cardiac drugs	Digoxin
	Gastrointestinal drugs	Cimetidine Metoclopramide
	Psychotropic drugs	Phenothiazines
	Tricyclic antidepressants	Amitriptyline Imipramine

smoking for 48 hours before surgery, because this will result in a significant improvement in cardiovascular function. Similarly, chronic alcoholics are at increased risk for hepatic toxicity and subsequent coagulation problems postoperatively. Furthermore, alcoholics who continue drinking up to the time of surgery may experience acute alcohol withdrawal during the postoperative period that can be life threatening. Prophy-lactic administration of lorazepam (Ativan) greatly reduces the potential risk of this significant complication.

Allergies

Finally, medicinal allergies should be questioned because, obviously, these medications should be avoided in future treatment of the patient. **All medicinal allergies should be marked boldly on the front of the patient's chart** to avoid potential complications from inadvertent exposure to the same medications.

In summary, a careful and thorough medical history, including the chief complaint and history of present illness, past medical history, and family history, should be obtained in every patient. Unfortunately, time constraints often make it difficult for the physician to spend the necessary time to obtain a full history. A reasonable substitute is to have a trained nurse or other health professional see the patient first. By using a standard history form, much of the information discussed previously can be obtained in a preliminary interview. It then remains for the urologist to only fill in the blanks, have the patient elaborate on potentially relevant aspects of the past medical history, and then perform a complete physical examination.

PHYSICAL EXAMINATION

KEY POINTS: EVALUATION OF THE UROLOGIC PATIENT

- The urologist can undertake the initial evaluation and establish a diagnosis for almost all patients with diseases of the GU system.

- A complete history and appropriate physical examination is critical in the assessment of urologic patients.

- A complete urinalysis including chemical and microscopic analyses should be performed because this may provide important information critical to the diagnosis and treatment of urologic patients.

A complete and thorough physical examination is an essential component of the evaluation of patients who present with urologic disease. Although it is tempting to become dependent on results of laboratory and radiologic tests, **the physical examination often simplifies the process and allows the urologist to select the most appropriate diagnostic studies.** Along with the history, the physical examination remains a key component of the diagnostic evaluation and should be performed conscientiously.

General Observations

The visual inspection of the patient provides a general overview. The skin should be inspected for evidence of jaundice or pallor. The nutritional status of the patient should be noted. **Cachexia is a frequent sign of malignancy, and obesity may be a sign of underlying endocrinologic abnor-**

malities. In this instance, one should search for the presence of truncal obesity, a "buffalo hump," and abdominal skin striae, which are stigmata of hyperadrenocorticism. In contrast, debility and hyperpigmentation may be signs of hypoadrenocorticism. Gynecomastia may be a sign of endocrinologic disease as well as a possible indicator of alcoholism or previous hormonal therapy for prostate cancer. Edema of the genitalia and lower extremities may be associated with cardiac decompensation, renal failure, nephrotic syndrome, or pelvic and/or retroperitoneal lymphatic obstruction. Supraclavicular lymphadenopathy may be seen with any GU neoplasm, most commonly prostate and testis cancer; inguinal lymphadenopathy may occur secondary to carcinoma of the penis or urethra.

Kidneys

The kidneys are fist-sized organs located high in the retroperitoneum bilaterally. In the adult, the kidneys are normally difficult to palpate because of their position under the diaphragm and ribs with abundant musculature both anteriorly and posteriorly. Because of the position of the liver, the right kidney is somewhat lower than the left. **In children and thin women, it may be possible to palpate the lower pole of the right kidney with deep inspiration.** However, it is usually not possible to palpate either kidney in men, and the left kidney is almost always impalpable unless it is abnormally enlarged.

The best way to palpate the kidneys is with the patient in the supine position. **The kidney is lifted from behind with one hand in the costovertebral angle** (Fig. 3–1). On deep inspiration, the examiner's hand is advanced firmly into the anterior abdomen just below the costal margin. At the point of maximal inspiration, the kidney may be felt as it moves downward with the diaphragm. With each inspiration, the examiner's hand may be advanced deeper into the abdomen. Once again, it is more difficult to palpate kidneys in men because the kidneys tend to move downward less with inspiration and because they are surrounded with thicker muscular layers. In children, it is easier to palpate the kidneys because

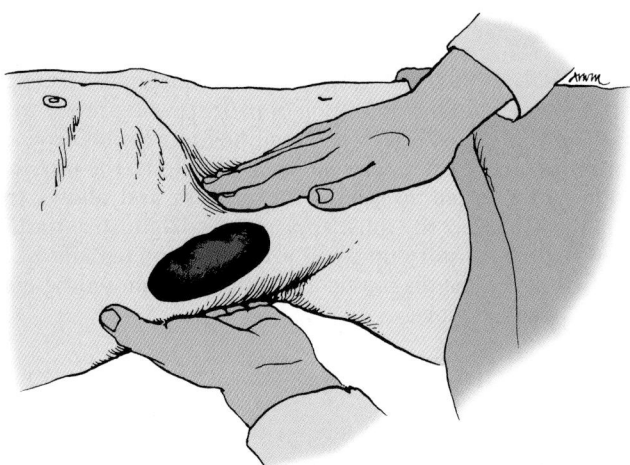

Figure 3–1. Bimanual examination of the kidney. (From Judge RD, Zuidema GD, Fitzgerald FT [eds]: Clinical Diagnosis, 5th ed. Boston, Little, Brown, 1989, p 370.)

of decreased body thickness. In neonates, the kidneys can be felt quite easily by palpating the flank between the thumb anteriorly and the fingers over the costovertebral angle posteriorly.

Transillumination of the kidneys may be helpful in children younger than 1 year of age with a palpable flank mass. Such masses frequently are of renal origin. A flashlight or fiberoptic light source is positioned posteriorly against the costovertebral angle. Fluid-filled masses such as cysts or hydronephrosis produce a dull reddish glow in the anterior abdomen. Solid masses such as tumors do not transilluminate. Other diagnostic maneuvers that may be helpful in examining the kidneys are percussion and auscultation. Although renal inflammation may cause pain that is poorly localized, percussion of the costovertebral angle posteriorly more often localizes the pain and tenderness more accurately. Percussion should be done gently, because in a patient with significant renal inflammation this may be quite painful. Auscultation of the upper abdomen during deep inspiration may occasionally reveal a systolic bruit associated with renal artery stenosis or an aneurysm. A bruit may also be detected in association with a large renal arteriovenous fistula.

Every patient with flank pain should also be examined for possible nerve root irritation. The ribs should be palpated carefully to rule out a bone spur or other skeletal abnormality and to determine the point of maximal tenderness. Unlike renal pain, radiculitis usually causes hyperesthesia of the overlying skin innervated by the irritated peripheral nerve. This hypersensitivity can be elicited with a pin or by pinching the skin and fat overlying the involved area. Finally, the pain experienced during the pre-eruptive phase of herpes zoster involving any of the segments between T11 and L2 may also simulate pain of renal origin.

Abnormal Findings. The most common abnormality detected on examination of the kidneys is a mass. In adult patients, particularly those who are obese, renal masses may be difficult to palpate unless these masses are very large. In most cases, palpable renal masses are either benign cysts or malignant renal tumors, and this distinction generally cannot be made based on physical examination. In children, renal masses are frequently easier to palpate than in adults and may be either cystic (multicystic kidney, polycystic kidney, hydronephrosis) or malignant (Wilms' tumor, neuroblastoma). **In neonates and younger children, the distinction between cystic, benign, and solid malignant masses can often be made by transillumination.**

Bladder

A normal bladder in the adult cannot be palpated or percussed until there is at least 150 mL of urine in it. At a volume of about 500 mL, the distended bladder becomes visible in thin patients as a lower midline abdominal mass.

Percussion is better than palpation for diagnosing a distended bladder. The examiner begins by percussing immediately above the symphysis pubis and continuing cephalad until there is a change in pitch from dull to resonant. Alternatively, it may be possible in thin patients and in children to palpate the bladder by lifting the lumbar spine with one hand and pressing the other hand into the midline of the lower abdomen.

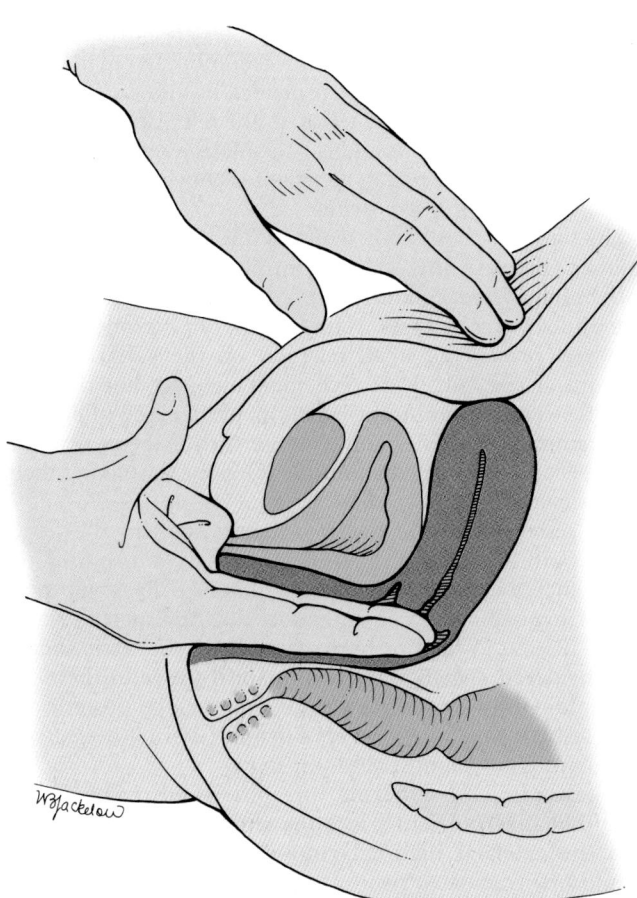

Figure 3–2. Bimanual examination of the bladder in the female. (From Swartz MH: Textbook of Physical Diagnosis. Philadelphia, WB Saunders, 1989, p 405.)

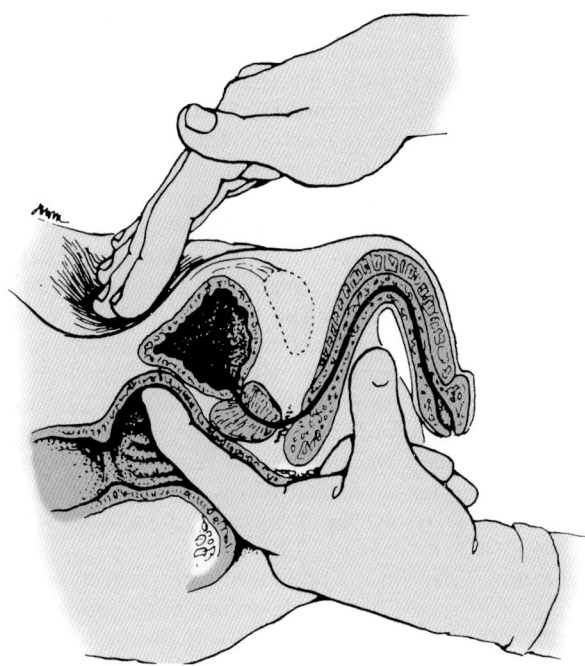

Figure 3–3. Bimanual examination of the bladder in the male. (From Judge RD, Zuidema GD, Fitzgerald FT [eds]: Clinical Diagnosis, 5th ed. Boston, Little, Brown, 1989, p 376.)

A careful bimanual examination, best done with the patient under anesthesia, is invaluable in assessing the regional extent of a bladder tumor or other pelvic mass. The bladder is palpated between the abdomen and the vagina in the female (Fig. 3–2) or the rectum in the male (Fig. 3–3). In addition to defining areas of induration, the bimanual examination allows the examiner to assess the mobility of the bladder; such information cannot be obtained by radiologic techniques such as CT and MRI, which convey static images.

Abnormal Findings. The most common palpable abnormality involving the urinary bladder is a full bladder resulting from overdistention. This may occur in men with bladder outlet or urethral obstruction due to BPH or urethral stricture disease. In addition, a variety of neurologic conditions may lead to poor bladder emptying in men or women. Large bladder tumors or calculi may also be palpable in some patients, particularly on bimanual examination under anesthesia. Tenderness over the suprapubic area may indicate cystitis.

Penis

If the patient has not been circumcised, the foreskin should be retracted to examine for tumor or balanoposthitis (inflammation of the prepuce and glans penis). **Most penile cancers occur in uncircumcised men and arise on the prepuce or glans penis.** Therefore, in a patient with a bloody penile discharge in whom the foreskin cannot be withdrawn, a dorsal slit or circumcision must be performed to adequately evaluate the glans penis and urethra.

The position of the urethral meatus should be noted. It may be located proximal to the tip of the glans on the ventral surface (hypospadias) or, much less commonly, on the dorsal surface (epispadias). The penile skin should be examined for the presence of superficial vesicles compatible with herpes simplex and for ulcers that may indicate either venereal infection or tumor. The presence of venereal warts (condylomata acuminata), which appear as irregular, papillary, velvety lesions on the male genitalia, should also be noted.

The urethral meatus should be separated between the thumb and the forefinger to inspect for neoplastic or inflammatory lesions within the fossa navicularis. The dorsal shaft of the penis should be palpated for the presence of fibrotic plaques or ridges typical of Peyronie's disease. Tenderness along the ventral aspect of the penis is suggestive of periurethritis, often secondary to a urethral stricture.

Abnormal Findings

Phimosis. Phimosis is a condition in which the foreskin cannot be retracted behind the glans penis. **In males younger than 4 years old it is normal for the foreskin to be unretractable;** in older boys and adults, however, the foreskin usually can be easily withdrawn to the corona (Oster, 1968). Phimosis is usually not painful, but it may produce urinary obstruction with ballooning of the foreskin and may lead to chronic inflammation and carcinoma.

Paraphimosis. Paraphimosis is a condition in which the foreskin has been retracted and left behind the glans penis, constricting the glans and causing painful vascular engorgement and edema. **Paraphimosis is often iatrogenic and frequently occurs after a well-meaning health care professional has examined the penis or inserted a urethral catheter and forgotten to replace the foreskin in its natural position.** Paraphimosis can result in marked swelling of the glans penis such that the foreskin can no longer be drawn forward, necessitating an emergency dorsal slit or circumcision.

Peyronie's Disease. Peyronie's disease is a common condition that results in **fibrosis of the tunica albuginea,** the elastic membrane that surrounds each corpus cavernosum, producing curvature of the penis during erection. Peyronie's disease may be difficult to diagnose in the flaccid state; however, the patient's history of curvature with erection establishes the diagnosis. Physical examination reveals fibrous plaques or ridges along the shaft of the penis. Peyronie's disease can be alarming to patients who may fear it represents malignancy. They should be reassured that this is always a benign condition that may resolve or stabilize spontaneously without treatment.

Priapism. Priapism is a prolonged painful erection that is not related to sexual activity. **It occurs most commonly in patients with sickle cell disease but can also occur in those with advanced malignancy, coagulation disorders, and pulmonary disease and in many patients without an obvious etiology.** The patient usually presents with a painful, spontaneous erection of several hours' duration. Physical examination reveals the penis to be rigid and mildly tender; the glans penis, however, is usually flaccid.

Hypospadias. Hypospadias is a congenital abnormality in which the urethral meatus is positioned either along the ventral shaft of the penis or on the scrotum or perineum instead of being located at the tip of the penis. **This is a relatively common condition, occurring in about 1 in 300 live male births** (Avellan, 1975). In the more common, less severe forms of hypospadias, the urethra is located at or distal to the corona of the penis; these conditions frequently do not necessitate treatment except for cosmetic purposes. The less common but more severe forms of hypospadias, in which the meatus is located on the penile shaft or in the perineum, may interfere with normal urination in the usual male standing position and may, in adult life, interfere with fertility, because the semen is deposited in the distal vagina rather than at the cervix. Such cases are best corrected early in childhood to avoid social embarrassment and psychological trauma. Neonates with hypospadias and bilateral cryptorchidism (undescended testes) should be evaluated for the possibility of intersex, of which the most common cause is adrenogenital syndrome.

Carcinoma. Carcinoma of the penis usually presents as a velvety, raised lesion arising on the glans penis or inner surface of the prepuce. Alternatively, it may present as an ulcerative lesion. Carcinoma of the penis occurs almost exclusively in uncircumcised men. It is more common in underdeveloped nations where there is poor hygiene. Penile carcinoma is most commonly a squamous cell tumor and is frequently associated with palpable inguinal lymphadenopathy.

Scrotum and Contents

The scrotum is a loose sac containing the testes and spermatic cord structures. The scrotal wall is made up of skin and an underlying thin muscular layer. The testes are normally oval, firm, and smooth; in adults, they measure about 6 cm in length and 4 cm in width. They are suspended in the scrotum, with the right testis normally anterior to the left. The epididymis lies posterior to the testis and is palpable as a distinct ridge of tissue. The vas deferens can be palpated above each testis and feels like a piece of heavy twine.

The scrotum should be examined for dermatologic abnormalities. **Because the scrotum, unlike the penis, contains both hair and sweat glands, it is a frequent site of local infection and sebaceous cysts.** Hair follicles can become infected and may present as small pustules on the surface of the scrotum. These usually resolve spontaneously, but they can give rise to more significant infection, particularly in patients with reduced immunity and in those with diabetes. Patients often become concerned about these lesions, mistaking them for testicular tumors.

The testes should be palpated gently between the finger tips of both hands. The testes normally have a firm, rubbery consistency with a smooth surface. Abnormally small testes suggest hypogonadism or an endocrinopathy such as Klinefelter's disease. **A firm or hard area within the testis should be considered a malignant tumor until proved otherwise.** The epididymis should be palpable as a ridge posterior to each testis. Masses in the epididymis (spermatocele, cyst, epididymitis) are almost always benign.

To examine for a hernia, the physician's index finger should be inserted gently into the scrotum and invaginated into the external inguinal ring (Fig. 3–4). The scrotum should be invaginated in front of the testis, and care should be taken not to elevate the testis itself, which is quite painful.

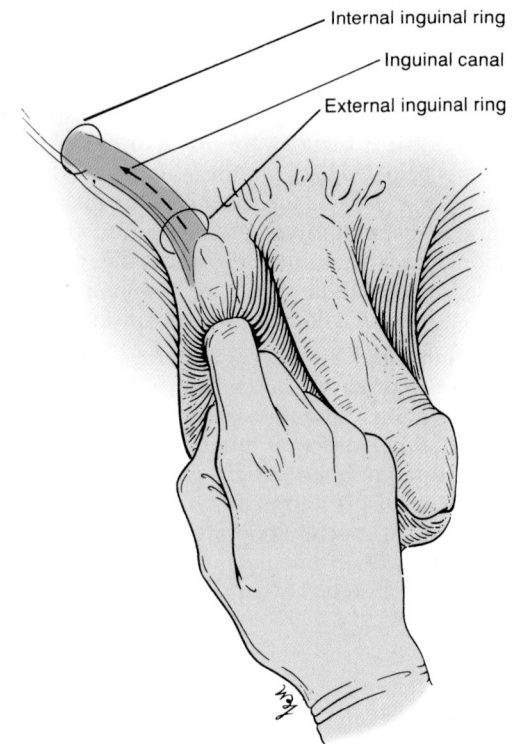

Figure 3–4. Examination of the inguinal canal. (From Swartz MH: Textbook of Physical Diagnosis. Philadelphia, WB Saunders, 1989, p 376.)

Once the external ring has been located, the physician should place the fingertips of his or her other hand over the internal inguinal ring and ask the patient to bear down (Valsalva's maneuver). A hernia will be felt as a distinct bulge that descends against the tip of the index finger in the external inguinal ring as the patient bears down. Although it may be possible to distinguish a direct inguinal hernia arising through the floor of the inguinal canal from an indirect inguinal hernia prolapsing through the internal inguinal ring, this is seldom possible and of little clinical significance because the surgical approach is essentially identical for both conditions.

The spermatic cord is also examined with the patient in the standing position. A varicocele is a dilated, tortuous spermatic vein that becomes more obvious as the patient performs a Valsalva maneuver. The epididymis can again be palpated as a ridge of tissue running longitudinally, posterior to each testis. The testis should be palpated again between the fingers of both hands, once again taking care not to exert any pressure on the testis itself so as to avoid pain.

Transillumination is helpful in determining whether scrotal masses are solid (tumor) or cystic (hydrocele, spermatocele). A small flashlight or fiberoptic light cord is placed behind the mass. A cystic mass transilluminates easily, whereas light is not transmitted through a solid tumor.

Abnormal Findings

Testicular Cancer. The most common physical finding in the testis is a mass. **A useful guideline is that most masses arising from the testis are malignant, whereas almost all masses arising from the spermatic cord structures are benign.** Thus, it is very important to distinguish the testis and epididymis during the physical examination. Testicular tumors usually present as painless, firm, irregular masses on the surface of the testis. They are usually discovered incidentally by the patient when showering or during self-examination. Testicular tumors can be readily distinguished from benign masses arising from the spermatic cord by transillumination and scrotal ultrasound.

Torsion. Torsion is the twisting of the testis on the spermatic cord, resulting in strangulation of the blood supply and infarction of the testis. **Torsion occurs most commonly between the ages of 12 and 20 years, although it does occur less frequently during the first year of life.** The patient usually presents with the sudden onset of pain and swelling of the involved testis. The pain may radiate into the groin and lower abdomen; thus, it may be confused with appendicitis unless the physician examines the genitalia carefully. On physical examination, it is difficult to distinguish the testis from the epididymis because of localized swelling. For this reason, the condition is frequently misdiagnosed as epididymitis. Age is the most useful criterion in distinguishing torsion from epididymitis, because torsion usually occurs around puberty whereas epididymitis more often occurs in sexually active males, usually after age 20 years.

Hydrocele. A hydrocele is a collection of fluid between the tunica vaginalis and the testis. The patient presents with progressive swelling and local discomfort on the involved side of the scrotum. Physical examination reveals smooth, symmetrical enlargement of one side of the scrotum in which it is very difficult to feel the testis. The diagnosis is made by transillumination of the scrotum. However, **because about 10% of testicular tumors present as an associated reactive hydrocele,** it is important to be sure that the hydrocele transilluminates completely and, if there is any doubt, to confirm the diagnosis with a subsequent scrotal ultrasound.

Varicocele. A varicocele is an enlarged, tortuous spermatic vein above the testis that almost always occurs on the left side. The patient presents with a soft mass or swelling above the testis noted when he stands or strains. This has been described as a "bag of worms." Varicoceles typically decrease in size and may disappear when the patient is supine. **Patients with the sudden onset of a varicocele, a right-sided varicocele, or a varicocele that does not reduce in size in the supine position should be suspected of having a retroperitoneal neoplasm** with obstruction of the spermatic vein where it enters either the renal vein on the left or the inferior vena cava on the right. Such patients should undergo ultrasonography or CT to rule out malignancy before receiving treatment for the varicocele.

Rectal and Prostate Examination in the Male

Digital rectal examination (DRE) should be performed in every male after age 40 years and in men of any age who present for urologic evaluation. Prostate cancer is the second most common cause of male cancer deaths after age 55 years and the most common cause of cancer deaths in men older than 70 years. Many prostate cancers can be detected in an early curable stage by DRE, and about 25% of colorectal cancers can be detected by DRE in combination with a stool guaiac test.

DRE should be performed at the end of the physical examination. It is done best with the patient standing and bent over the examining table or with the patient in the knee-chest position. In the standing position, the patient should stand with his thighs close to the examining table. The feet should be about 18 inches apart, with the knees flexed slightly. The patient should bend at the waist 90 degrees until his chest is resting on his forearms. The physician should give the patient adequate time to get in the proper position and relax as much as possible. A few reassuring words before the examination are helpful. The physician should place a glove on the examining hand and should lubricate the index finger thoroughly.

Before performing the DRE, the physician should place the palm of his other hand against the patient's lower abdomen. This provides subtle reassurance to the patient by allowing the physician to make gentle contact with the patient before touching the anus. It also allows the physician to steady the patient and provide gentle counterpressure if the patient tries to move away as the DRE is being performed. The DRE itself begins by separating the buttocks and inspecting the anus for pathology, usually hemorrhoids, but, occasionally, an anal carcinoma or melanoma may be detected. The gloved, lubricated index finger is then inserted gently into the anus. Only one phalanx should be inserted initially to give the anus time to relax and to easily accommodate the finger. Estimation of anal sphincter tone is of great importance; a flaccid or spastic anal sphincter suggests similar changes in the urinary sphincter and may be a clue to the diagnosis of neurogenic disease. If the physician waits only a few seconds, the anal sphincter will normally relax to the degree that the finger can be advanced to the knuckle without causing pain. The index finger then sweeps over the prostate; the entire posterior surface of the gland can usually be examined if the patient is in the proper position. **Normally, the prostate is about the size of a chestnut and has a consistency similar to that of the contracted thenar eminence of the thumb (with the thumb opposed to the little finger).**

The index finger is extended as far as possible into the rectum, and the entire circumference is examined to detect an early rectal carcinoma. The index finger is then withdrawn gently, and the stool on the glove is transferred to a guaiac-impregnated (Hemoccult) card for determination of occult blood. Although there may be a significant incidence of false-positive and false-negative results associated with fecal occult blood testing, particularly without dietary and drug restrictions, **the guaiac test is simple and inexpensive and may lead to the detection of significant gastrointestinal abnormalities** (Bond, 1999). Adequate tissues, soap, and towels should be available for the patient to cleanse himself after the examination. The physician should then leave the room and allow the patient adequate time to wash and dress before concluding the consultation.

Abnormal Findings

Acute Prostatitis. **Acute prostatitis most commonly occurs in sexually active men between the ages of 20 and 40 years.** Symptoms include fever, malaise, perineal and rectal discomfort, urinary frequency, urgency, dysuria, and sometimes urinary retention. When acute prostatitis is suspected, rectal examination should be performed carefully. Examination reveals the prostate to be warm, tender, and sometimes fluctuant or boggy in consistency. A localized fluctuant, tender region within the prostate may indicate a prostatic abscess for which surgical drainage is required. The prostate should never be massaged for secretions in men with acute prostatitis. Massage of the acutely infected prostate is not only unnecessary but also extremely uncomfortable for the patient. In addition, massage may disseminate bacteria through the vas deferens, causing secondary epididymitis or, more significantly, may disseminate bacteria into the bloodstream, producing gram-negative septicemia.

Benign Prostatic Hyperplasia. The physical findings in BPH are usually limited to the prostate. In BPH, the prostate remains rubbery in consistency, but may be variably enlarged from normal chestnut size to the size of a lemon, or, occasionally, even as large as an orange. There is only a general correlation between prostatic size and degree of symptoms.

Because BPH affects almost all men older than age 50 years, the finding of an enlarged prostate on physical examination is not a reason per se to initiate further urologic evaluation. The severity of the disease and the need for treatment are best determined by the patient's symptoms as well as the results of further urologic testing, such as measurement of a urinary flow rate and postvoid residual urine.

Carcinoma of the Prostate. Prostate cancer usually arises in the posterior peripheral region of the prostate and, therefore, is frequently palpable in its early stages on rectal examination. On physical examination, **prostatic carcinomas are palpable as firm, indurated nodules or regions within the prostate.** These areas of induration are characterized by

having a woodlike consistency. As prostatic carcinomas progress, the entire gland becomes firmer than usual. Eventually, these tumors may progress beyond the capsule of the prostate, extending cephalad into the seminal vesicles and laterally toward the pelvic side wall.

It should be emphasized that **men with early, localized carcinoma of the prostate are almost always asymptomatic.** Therefore, a patient should never be allowed to dissuade the urologist from performing a rectal examination simply because he is asymptomatic. Urinary obstructive symptoms and skeletal pain are symptoms of advanced, incurable disease.

Detection of early prostatic carcinoma on rectal examination takes practice and has been greatly facilitated by the discovery of PSA. An elevated PSA value should raise the suspicion of prostatic carcinoma, regardless of the findings on rectal examination. Conversely, a normal PSA test does not exclude the possibility of early prostate cancer, and, in fact, **30% of men with early prostate cancer will have a normal serum PSA test** (Partin et al, 1993).

A prostatic biopsy should be performed for any palpable lesion within the prostate. In one study, the detection rate of prostate cancer was 18% among men with an abnormal DRE and a PSA less than 4.0 ng/mL (Crawford et al, 1999). In contrast, 56% of men with palpable abnormalities and a PSA greater than 4.0 ng/mL were found to have malignancy. Other causes of prostatic induration besides cancer include calculi (which are typically harder than tumors), inflammation, fibrous BPH, and infarction. Biopsies are now done easily using topical anesthesia under transrectal ultrasound guidance. **There is no excuse for delaying a prostatic biopsy in an otherwise healthy younger man with either an abnormal DRE or an elevated PSA level.** It serves no purpose to have the patient return in 6 months for a repeat examination to see whether the nodule has changed, because prostate cancers usually grow very slowly; the fact that a nodule does not change appreciably with time is of no clinical significance.

Pelvic Examination in the Female

Male urologists should always perform the female pelvic examination with a female nurse or other health care professional present. The patient should be allowed to undress in privacy and be fully draped for the procedure before the physician enters the room. The examination itself should be performed in standard lithotomy position with the patient's legs abducted. Initially, the external genitalia and introitus should be examined, with particular attention paid to atrophic changes, erosions, ulcers, discharge, or warts, all of which may cause dysuria and pelvic discomfort. The urethral meatus should be inspected for caruncles, mucosal hyperplasia, cysts, and mucosal prolapse. The patient is then asked to perform a Valsalva maneuver and is carefully examined for a cystocele (prolapse of the bladder) or rectocele (prolapse of the rectum). The patient is then asked to cough, which may precipitate stress urinary incontinence. Palpation of the urethra is done to detect induration, which may be a sign of chronic inflammation or malignancy. Palpation may also disclose a urethral diverticulum, and palpation of a diverticulum may cause a purulent discharge from the urethra. Bimanual examination of the bladder, uterus, and adnexa should then be performed with two fingers in the vagina and the other hand on the lower abdomen (see Fig. 3–3). Any abnormality of the pelvic organs should be evaluated further with a pelvic ultrasound or CT scan.

Abnormal Findings. A careful bimanual examination of the female pelvis may reveal a variety of abnormalities of the uterus, ovaries, and cervix, including benign and malignant masses and inflammatory lesions. Various forms of pelvic prolapse, such as cystocele, rectocele, and enterocele, may also be detected. Inspection of the urethral meatus and vaginal introitus may also be helpful in identifying condylomata, urethral lesions, and other abnormalities.

Neurologic Examination

There are a variety of clinical situations in which the neurologic examination may be helpful in evaluating urologic patients. In some cases, the level of neurologic abnormalities can be localized by the pattern of sensory deficit noted during physical examination using a dermatome map (Fig. 3–5). Sensory deficits in the penis, labia, scrotum, vagina, and perianal area generally indicate damage or injury to sacral roots or nerves. In addition to sensory examination, testing of reflexes in the genital area may also be performed. The most important of these is the bulbocavernosus reflex (BCR), which is a reflex contraction of the striated muscle of the pelvic floor that occurs in response to a variety of stimuli in the perineum or genitalia. This reflex is most commonly tested by placing a finger in the rectum and then squeezing the glans penis or clitoris. If a Foley catheter is in place, the BCR can also be elicited by gently pulling on the catheter. If the BCR is intact, tightening of the anal sphincter should be felt and/or observed. The BCR tests the integrity of the spinal cord mediated reflex arc involving S2-S4 and may be absent in the presence of sacral cord or peripheral nerve abnormalities.

The cremasteric reflex can be elicited by lightly stroking the superior and medial thigh in a downward direction. The normal response in males is contraction of the cremasteric muscle that results in immediate elevation of the ipsilateral scrotum and testis. There is limited clinical utility for testing superficial reflexes such as the cremasteric when investigating neurologic dysfunction. However, there may be a role for testing this reflex when assessing patients with suspected testicular torsion or epididymitis. Finally, an overly active cremasteric reflex in children can lead to the mistaken diagnosis of an undescended testis in some cases.

URINALYSIS

The urinalysis is a fundamental test that should be performed in all urologic patients. Although, in many instances, a simple dipstick urinalysis will provide the necessary information, **a complete urinalysis includes both chemical and microscopic analyses.**

Collection of Urinary Specimens

Males

In the male patient, a midstream urine sample is obtained. The uncircumcised male should retract the foreskin, cleanse the glans penis with antiseptic solution, and continue to retract the foreskin during voiding. The male patient begins

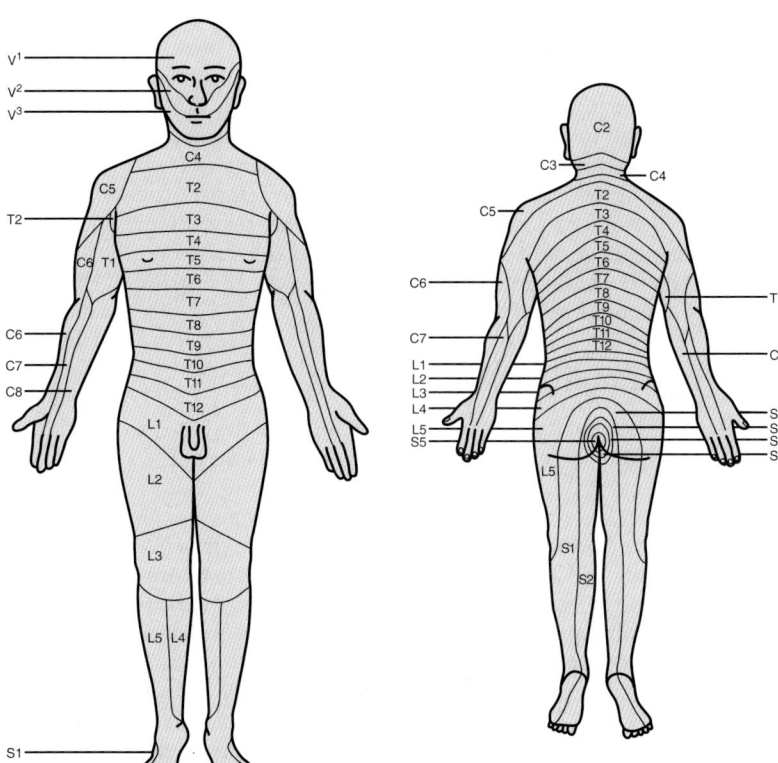

Figure 3–5. Sensory dermatome maps used to help localize the level of neurologic deficit.

urinating into the toilet, and then places a wide-mouth sterile container under his penis to collect a midstream sample. This avoids contamination of the urine specimen with skin and urethral organisms.

In men with chronic UTIs, four aliquots of urine are obtained. **These aliquots have been designated Voided Bladder 1, Voided Bladder 2, Expressed Prostatic Secretions, and Voided Bladder 3 (VB1, VB2, EPS, and VB3).** The VB1 is the initial 5 to 10 mL of urine voided, whereas the VB2 is the midstream urine. The EPS is the secretions obtained after gentle prostatic massage, and the VB3 specimen is the initial 2 to 3 mL of urine obtained after prostatic massage. The value of these cultures for localization of UTIs is that the VB1 sample represents urethral flora; the VB2, bladder flora; and the EPS and VB3 samples, prostatic flora. The VB3 sample is particularly helpful when there is little or no prostatic fluid obtained by massage. To better obtain prostatic secretions, patients should be instructed to attempt to void during prostatic massage and to avoid tightening the anal sphincter and pelvic floor muscles. The four-part urine sample is particularly useful in evaluating men with suspected bacterial prostatitis (Meares and Stamey, 1968).

Females

In the female, it is more difficult to obtain a clean-catch midstream specimen. The female patient should cleanse the vulva, separate the labia, and collect a midstream specimen as described for the male patient. If infection is suspected, however, the midstream specimen is unreliable and should never be sent for culture and sensitivity. **To evaluate for a possible infection in a female, a catheterized urine sample should always be obtained.**

Neonates and Infants

The usual way to obtain a urine sample in a neonate or infant is to place a sterile plastic bag with an adhesive collar over the infant's genitalia. Obviously, however, these devices may not be able to distinguish contamination from true UTI. Whenever possible, **all urine samples should be examined within 1 hour of collection and plated for culture and sensitivity if indicated.** If urine is allowed to stand at room temperature for longer periods of time, bacterial overgrowth may occur, the pH may change, and red and white blood cell casts may disintegrate. If it is not possible to examine the urine promptly, it should be refrigerated at 5°C.

Physical Examination of Urine

The physical examination of the urine includes an evaluation of color, turbidity, specific gravity and osmolality, and pH.

Color

The normal pale yellow color of urine is due to the presence of the pigment urochrome. **Urine color varies most commonly because of concentration, but many foods, medications, metabolic products, and infection may produce abnormal urine color.** This is important, because many patients will seek consultation primarily because of a change in their urine color. Thus, it is important for the urologist to be aware of the common causes of abnormal urine color, and these are listed in Table 3-3.

Table 3-3.   Common Causes of Abnormal Urine Color

Colorless	Very dilute urine
	Overhydration
Cloudy/milky	Phosphaturia
	Pyuria
	Chyluria
Red	Hematuria
	Hemoglobinuria/myoglobinuria
	Anthrocyanin in beets and blackberries
	Chronic lead and mercury poisoning
	Phenolphthalein (in bowel evacuants)
	Phenothiazines (e.g., Compazine)
	Rifampin
Orange	Dehydration
	Phenazopyridine (Pyridium)
	Sulfasalazine (Azulfidine)
Yellow	Normal
	Phenacetin
	Riboflavin
Green-blue	Biliverdin
	Indicanuria (tryptophan indole metabolites)
	Amitriptyline (Elavil)
	Indigo carmine
	Methylene blue
	Phenols (e.g., IV cimetidine [Tagamet], IV promethazine [Phenergan])
	Resorcinol
	Triamterene (Dyrenium)
Brown	Urobilinogen
	Porphyria
	Aloe, fava beans, and rhubarb
	Chloroquine and primaquine
	Furazolidone (Furoxone)
	Metronidazole (Flagyl)
	Nitrofurantoin (Furadantin)
Brown-black	Alcaptonuria (homogentisic acid)
	Hemorrhage
	Melanin
	Tyrosinosis (hydroxyphenylpyruvic acid)
	Cascara, senna (laxatives)
	Methocarbamol (Robaxin)
	Methyldopa (Aldomet)
	Sorbitol

From Hanno PM, Wein AJ: A Clinical Manual of Urology. Norwalk, CT, Appleton-Century-Crofts, 1987, p 67.

Turbidity

Freshly voided urine is clear. **Cloudy urine is most commonly due to phosphaturia,** a benign process in which excess phosphate crystals precipitate in an alkaline urine. Phosphaturia is intermittent and usually occurs after meals or ingestion of a large quantity of milk. Patients are otherwise asymptomatic. The diagnosis of phosphaturia can be accomplished either by acidifying the urine with acetic acid, which will result in immediate clearing, or by performing a microscopic analysis, which will reveal large amounts of amorphous phosphate crystals.

Pyuria, usually associated with a UTI, is another common cause of cloudy urine. The large numbers of white blood cells cause the urine to become turbid. **Pyuria is readily distinguished from phosphaturia either by smelling the urine** (infected urine has a characteristic pungent odor) or by microscopic examination, which readily distinguishes amorphous phosphate crystals from leukocytes.

Rare causes of cloudy urine include chyluria (in which there is an abnormal communication between the lymphatic system and the urinary tract resulting in lymph fluid being mixed with urine), lipiduria, hyperoxaluria, and hyperuricosuria.

Specific Gravity and Osmolality

Specific gravity of urine is easily determined from a urinary dipstick and usually varies from 1.001 to 1.035. Specific gravity usually reflects the patient's state of hydration but may also be affected by abnormal renal function, the amount of material dissolved in the urine, and a variety of other causes mentioned later. A specific gravity less than 1.008 is regarded as dilute, and a specific gravity greater than 1.020 is considered concentrated. A fixed specific gravity of 1.010 is a sign of renal insufficiency, either acute or chronic.

In general, specific gravity reflects the state of hydration but also affords some idea of renal concentrating ability. Conditions that decrease specific gravity include (1) increased fluid intake, (2) diuretics, (3) decreased renal concentrating ability, and (4) diabetes insipidus. Conditions that increase specific gravity include (1) decreased fluid intake; (2) dehydration owing to fever, sweating, vomiting, and diarrhea; (3) diabetes mellitus (glucosuria); and (4) inappropriate secretion of antidiuretic hormone. Specific gravity will also be increased above 1.035 after intravenous injection of iodinated contrast and in patients taking dextran.

Osmolality is a measure of the amount of material dissolved in the urine and usually varies between 50 and 1200 mOsm/L. Urine osmolality most commonly varies with hydration, and the same factors that affect specific gravity will also affect osmolality. Urine osmolality is a better indicator of renal function, but it cannot be measured from a dipstick and must be determined using standard laboratory techniques.

pH

Urinary pH is measured with a dipstick test strip that incorporates two colorimetric indicators, methyl red and bromothymol blue, which yield clearly distinguishable colors over the pH range from 5 to 9. Urinary pH may vary from 4.5 to 8; the average pH varies between 5.5 and 6.5. A urinary pH between 4.5 and 5.5 is considered acidic, whereas a pH between 6.5 and 8 is considered alkaline.

In general, the urinary pH reflects the pH in the serum. In patients with metabolic or respiratory acidosis, the urine is usually acidic; conversely, in patients with metabolic or respiratory alkalosis, the urine is alkaline. Renal tubular acidosis (RTA) presents an exception to this rule. In patients with both type I and II RTA, the serum is acidemic, but the urine is alkalotic because of continued loss of bicarbonate in the urine. In severe metabolic acidosis in type II RTA, the urine may become acidic; but in type I RTA, the urine is always alkaline, even with severe metabolic acidosis (Morris and Ives, 1991). Urinary pH determination is used to establish the diagnosis of RTA; inability to acidify the urine below a pH of 5.5 after administration of an acid load is diagnostic of RTA.

Urine pH determinations are also useful in the diagnosis and treatment of UTIs and urinary calculus disease. **In patients with a presumed UTI, an alkaline urine with a pH greater than 7.5 suggests infection with a urea-splitting organism, most commonly *Proteus*.** Urease-producing bacteria convert ammonia to ammonium ions, markedly elevating the urinary pH and causing precipitation of calcium magnesium ammonium phosphate crystals. The massive amount of crystallization may result in staghorn calculi.

Urinary pH is usually acidic in patients with uric acid and cystine lithiasis. Alkalinization of the urine is an important feature of therapy in both of these conditions, and frequent monitoring of urinary pH is necessary to ascertain adequacy of therapy.

Chemical Examination of Urine

Urine Dipsticks

Urine dipsticks provide a quick and inexpensive method for detecting abnormal substances within the urine. Dipsticks are short, plastic strips with small marker pads that are impregnated with different chemical reagents that react with abnormal substances in the urine to produce a colorimetric change. **The abnormal substances commonly tested for with a dipstick include (1) blood, (2) protein, (3) glucose, (4) ketones, (5) urobilinogen and bilirubin, and (6) white blood cells.**

Substances listed in Table 3–3 that produce an abnormal urine color may interfere with appropriate color development on the dipstick. In our experience, this most commonly occurs in patients taking phenazopyridine (Pyridium) for a UTI. Phenazopyridine turns the urine bright orange and makes dipstick evaluation of the urine unreliable.

Appropriate technique must be used to obtain an accurate dipstick determination. The reagent areas on the dipstick must be completely immersed in a fresh uncentrifuged urine specimen and then must be withdrawn immediately to prevent dissolution of the reagents into the urine. As the dipstick is removed from the urine specimen container, the edge of the dipstick is drawn along the rim of the container to remove excess urine. The dipstick should be held horizontally until the appropriate time for reading and then compared with the color chart. **Excess urine on the dipstick or holding the dipstick in a vertical position will allow mixing of chemicals from adjacent reagent pads on the dipstick, resulting in a faulty diagnosis.** False-negative results for glucose and bilirubin may be seen in the presence of elevated ascorbic acid concentrations in the urine. However, increased levels of ascorbic acid in the urine do not interfere with dipstick testing for hematuria. Highly buffered alkaline urine may cause falsely low readings for specific gravity and may lead to false-positive results for urinary protein. Other common causes of false results with dipstick testing are outdated test strips and exposure of the sticks, leading to damage to the reagents. In general, when the sticks are damaged, there will be color changes on the pads before their immersion in urine. If such color changes are noted, results with the dipstick may be inaccurate.

Hematuria

Normal urine should contain less than three red blood cells per HPF. A positive dipstick for blood in the urine indicates either hematuria, hemoglobinuria, or myoglobinuria. **The chemical detection of blood in the urine is based on the peroxidase-like activity of hemoglobin.** When in contact with an organic peroxidase substrate, hemoglobin catalyzes the reaction and causes subsequent oxidation of a chromogen indicator, which changes color according to the degree and amount of oxidation. The degree of color change is directly related to the amount of hemoglobin present in the urine specimen. Dipsticks frequently demonstrate both colored dots and field color change. If present, free hemoglobin and myoglobin in the urine are absorbed into the reagent pad and catalyze the reaction within the test paper, thereby producing a field change effect in color. Intact erythrocytes in the urine undergo hemolysis when they come in contact with the reagent test pad, and the localized free hemoglobin on the pad produces a corresponding dot of color change. Obviously, the greater the number of intact erythrocytes in the urine specimen, the greater the number of dots that will appear on the test paper, and a coalescence of the dots occurs when there are more than 250 erythrocytes/mL.

Hematuria can be distinguished from hemoglobinuria and myoglobinuria by microscopic examination of the centrifuged urine; the presence of a large number of erythrocytes establishes the diagnosis of hematuria. If erythrocytes are absent, examination of the serum will distinguish hemoglobinuria and myoglobinuria. A sample of blood is obtained and centrifuged. In hemoglobinuria, the supernatant will be pink. This is because free hemoglobin in the serum binds to haptoglobin, which is water insoluble and has a high molecular weight. This complex remains in the serum, causing a pink color. Free hemoglobin will appear in the urine only when all of the haptoglobin-binding sites have been saturated. In myoglobinuria, the myoglobin released from muscle is of low molecular weight and water soluble. It does not bind to haptoglobin and is therefore excreted immediately into the urine. Therefore, in myoglobinuria the serum remains clear.

The sensitivity of urinary dipsticks in identifying hematuria, defined as greater than 3 erythrocytes/HPF of centrifuged sediment examined microscopically, is over 90%. Conversely, the specificity of the dipstick for hematuria compared with microscopy is somewhat lower, reflecting a higher false-positive rate with the dipstick (Shaw et al, 1985).

False-positive dipstick readings most often are due to contamination of the urine specimen with menstrual blood. Dehydration with resultant urine of high specific gravity can also yield false-positive results owing to the increased concentration of erythrocytes and hemoglobin. The normal individual excretes about 1000 erythrocytes/mL of urine, with the upper limits of normal varying from 5000 to 8000 erythrocytes/mL (Kincaid-Smith, 1982). Therefore, examining urine of high specific gravity, such as the first morning voided specimen, increases the likelihood of a false-positive result. In addition to dehydration, another cause of false-positive results is exercise, which can increase the number of erythrocytes in the urine.

The efficacy of hematuria screening using the dipstick to identify patients with significant urologic disease is somewhat controversial. Studies in children and young adults have shown a very low rate of significant disease (Woolhandler et al, 1989). In older adults, one study from the Mayo Clinic of 2000 patients with asymptomatic hematuria showed that only 0.5% had a urologic malignancy and only 1.8% developed other serious urologic diseases within 3 years after identification of the hematuria (Mohr et al, 1986). Conversely, investigators at the University of Wisconsin found that 26% of adults who had at least one positive dipstick reading for hematuria were subsequently found to have

significant urologic pathology (Messing et al, 1987). Obviously, the age of the population, the completeness of the subsequent urologic evaluation, and the definition of significant disease all influence the disease rate in the group of patients with asymptomatic hematuria identified by dipstick screening. It is important to remember that, before proceeding to more complicated studies, the dipstick result should be confirmed with a microscopic examination of the centrifuged urinary sediment.

Differential Diagnosis and Evaluation of Hematuria. Hematuria may reflect either significant nephrologic or urologic disease. **Hematuria of nephrologic origin is frequently associated with casts in the urine and almost always associated with significant proteinuria. Even significant hematuria of urologic origin will not elevate the protein concentration in the urine into the 100 to 300 mg/dL or 2+ to 3+ range on dipstick,** and proteinuria of this magnitude almost always indicates glomerular or tubulointerstitial renal disease.

Morphologic evaluation of erythrocytes in the centrifuged urinary sediment also helps localize their site of origin. **Erythrocytes arising from glomerular disease are typically dysmorphic and show a wide range of morphologic alterations. Conversely, erythrocytes arising from tubulointerstitial renal disease and of urologic origin have a uniformly round shape;** these erythrocytes may or may not retain their hemoglobin ("ghost cells"), but the individual cell shape is consistently round. In individuals without significant pathology with minimal amounts of hematuria, the erythrocytes are characteristically dysmorphic but the number of cells observed is far fewer than that observed in patients with nephrologic disease. Erythrocyte morphology is more easily determined using phase contrast microscopy, but with practice this can be accomplished using a conventional light microscope (Schramek et al, 1989).

Glomerular Hematuria. Glomerular hematuria is suggested by the presence of dysmorphic erythrocytes, red blood cell casts, and proteinuria. Of those patients with glomerulonephritis proven by renal biopsy, however, about 20% will have hematuria alone without red blood cell casts or proteinuria (Fassett et al, 1982).

The glomerular disorders associated with hematuria are listed in Table 3–4. Further evaluation of patients with glomerular hematuria should begin with a thorough history. Hematuria in children and young adults, usually males, associated with low-grade fever and an erythematous rash suggests a diagnosis of immunoglobulin A (IgA) nephropathy (Berger's disease). A family history of renal disease and deafness suggests familial nephritis or Alport's syndrome. Hemoptysis and abnormal bleeding associated with microcytic anemia are characteristic of Goodpasture's syndrome, and the presence of a rash and arthritis suggest systemic lupus erythematosus. Finally, poststreptococcal glomerulonephritis should be suspected in a child with a recent streptococcal upper respiratory tract or skin infection.

Further laboratory evaluation should include measurement of serum creatinine, creatinine clearance, and, when proteinuria in the urine is 2+ or greater, a 24-hour urine protein determination. Although these tests will quantitate the specific degree of renal dysfunction, further tests are usually required

Table 3–4. **Glomerular Disorders in Patients with Glomerular Hematuria**	
Disorder	**Patients**
IgA nephropathy (Berger's disease)	30
Mesangioproliferative GN	14
Focal segmental proliferative GN	13
Familial nephritis (e.g., Alport's syndrome)	11
Membranous GN	7
Mesangiocapillary GN	6
Focal segmental sclerosis	4
Unclassifiable	4
Systemic lupus erythematosus	3
Postinfectious GN	2
Subacute bacterial endocarditis	2
Others	4
Total	100

GN, glomerulonephritis; IgA, immunoglobulin A.
Adapted from Fassett RG, Horgan BA, Mathew TH: Detection of glomerular bleeding by phase-contrast microscopy. Lancet 1982;1:1432.

to establish the specific diagnosis and particularly to determine whether the disease is due to an immune or a nonimmune etiology. **Frequently, a renal biopsy is necessary to establish the precise diagnosis, and biopsies are particularly important if the result will influence subsequent treatment of the patient.** Renal biopsies are extremely informative when examined by an experienced pathologist using light, immunofluorescent, and electron microscopy.

An algorithm for the evaluation of glomerular hematuria is provided in Figure 3–6.

IgA Nephropathy (Berger's Disease). IgA nephropathy, or Berger's disease, is the most common cause of glomerular hematuria, accounting for about 30% of cases (Fassett et al,

1982). Therefore, it is described in greater detail in this section. IgA nephropathy occurs most commonly in children and young adults, with a male predominance (Berger and Hinglais, 1968). Patients typically present with hematuria after an upper respiratory tract infection or exercise. Hematuria may be associated with a low-grade fever or rash, but most patients have no associated systemic symptoms. Gross hematuria occurs intermittently, but microscopic hematuria is a constant finding in some patients. The disease is chronic, but the prognosis in most patients is excellent. Renal function remains normal in the majority, but about 25% will subsequently develop renal insufficiency. An older age at onset, initial abnormal renal function, consistent proteinuria, and hypertension are indicators of a poor prognosis (D'Amico, 1988).

The pathologic findings in Berger's disease are limited to either focal glomeruli or lobular segments of a glomerulus. The changes are proliferative and usually confined to mesangial cells (Berger and Hinglais, 1968). Renal biopsy reveals deposits of IgA, IgG, and β_{1c}-globulin, although IgA and IgG mesangial deposits are found in other forms of glomerulonephritis as well. The role of IgA in the disease remains uncertain, although the deposits may trigger an inflammatory reaction within the glomerulus (van den Wall Bake et al, 1989). Because gross hematuria frequently follows an upper respiratory tract infection, a viral etiology has been suspected but not established. The frequent association between hematuria and exercise in this condition remains unexplained.

The clinical presentation of IgA glomerulonephritis is alarming and similar to certain systemic diseases, including Schönlein-Henoch purpura, systemic lupus erythematosus, bacterial endocarditis, and Goodpasture's syndrome. Therefore, a careful clinical and laboratory evaluation is indicated

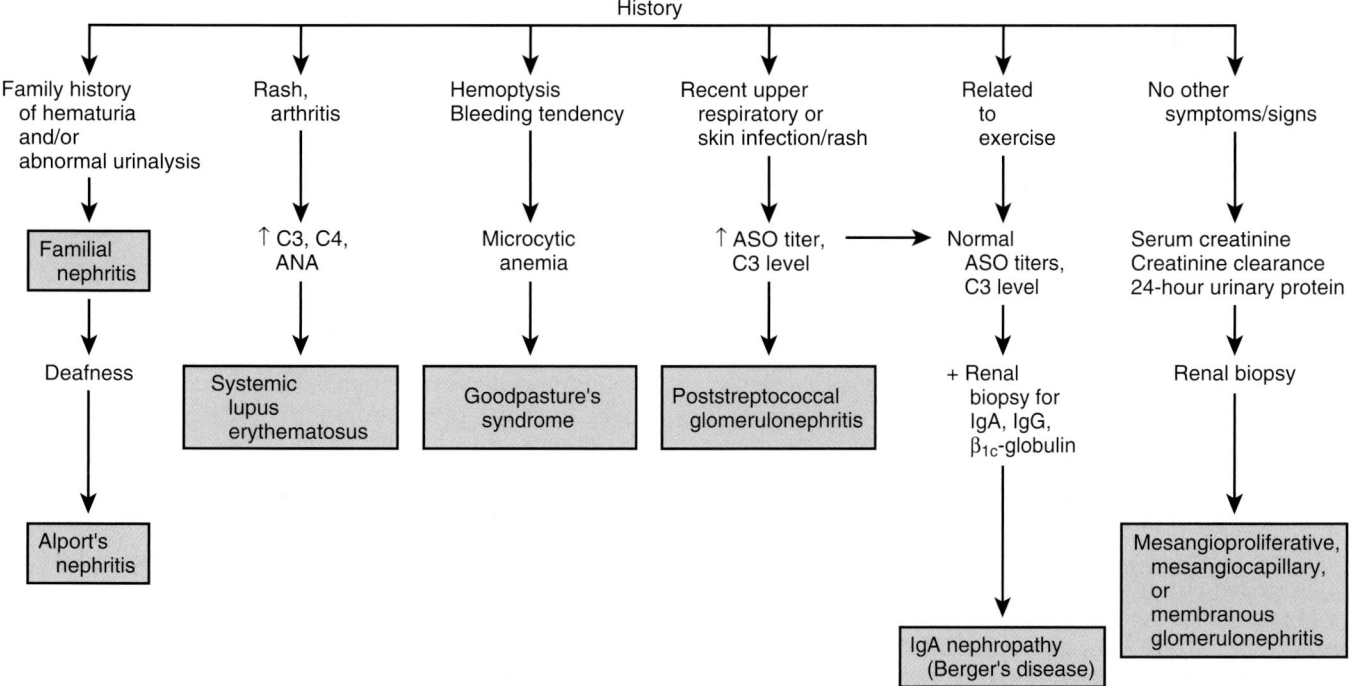

Figure 3–6. Evaluation of glomerular hematuria (dysmorphic erythrocytes, erythrocyte casts, and proteinuria). ANA, antinuclear antibody; ASO, antistreptolysin O; Ig, immunoglobulin.

to establish the correct diagnosis. The presence of red blood cell casts establishes the glomerular origin of the hematuria. In the absence of casts, a urologic evaluation is indicated to exclude the urinary tract as a source of bleeding and to confirm that the hematuria is arising from both kidneys. The diagnosis of IgA nephropathy is confirmed by renal biopsy demonstrating the classic deposits of immunoglobulins in mesangial cells, as described previously. Once the diagnosis has been established, repeat evaluations for hematuria are generally not indicated. Although there is no effective treatment for this condition, renal function remains stable in most patients and there are no other known long-term complications.

Nonglomerular Hematuria

Medical. Except for renal tumors, nonglomerular hematuria of renal origin is secondary to either tubulointerstitial, renovascular, or systemic disorders. **The urinalysis in nonglomerular hematuria is distinguished from that of glomerular hematuria by the presence of circular erythrocytes and the absence of erythrocyte casts.** Like glomerular hematuria, nonglomerular hematuria of renal origin is frequently associated with significant proteinuria, which distinguishes these nephrologic diseases from urologic diseases in which the degree of proteinuria is usually minimal, even with heavy bleeding.

As with glomerular hematuria, a careful history frequently helps establish the diagnosis. A family history of hematuria or bleeding tendency suggests the diagnosis of a blood dyscrasia, which should be investigated further. A family history of urolithiasis associated with intermittent hematuria may indicate stone disease, which should be investigated with serum and urine measurements of calcium and uric acid. A family history of renal cystic disease should prompt further radiologic evaluation for medullary sponge kidney and adult polycystic kidney disease. **Papillary necrosis as a cause of hematuria should be considered in diabetics, African Americans (secondary to sickle cell disease or trait), and suspected analgesic abusers.**

Medications may induce hematuria, particularly anticoagulants. **Anticoagulation at normal therapeutic levels, however, does not predispose patients to hematuria.** In one study, the prevalence of hematuria was 3.2% in anticoagulated patients versus 4.8% in a control group. Urologic disease was identified in 81% of patients with more than one episode of microscopic hematuria, and the cause of hematuria did not vary between groups (Culclasure et al, 1994). Thus, anticoagulant therapy per se does not appear to increase the risk of hematuria unless the patient is excessively anticoagulated.

Exercise-induced hematuria is being observed with increasing frequency. It typically occurs in long-distance runners (>10 km), is usually noted at the conclusion of the run, and rapidly disappears with rest. The hematuria may be of renal or bladder origin. An increased number of dysmorphic erythrocytes have been noted in some patients, suggesting a glomerular origin. Exercise-induced hematuria may be the first sign of underlying glomerular disease such as IgA nephropathy. Conversely, cystoscopy in patients with exercise-induced hematuria frequently reveals punctate hemorrhagic lesions in the bladder, suggesting that the hematuria is of bladder origin.

Vascular disease may also result in nonglomerular hematuria. Renal artery embolism and thrombosis, arteriovenous fistulas, and renal vein thrombosis may all result in hematuria. Physical examination may reveal severe hypertension, a flank or abdominal bruit, or atrial fibrillation. In such patients, further evaluation for renal vascular disease should be undertaken.

An algorithm for the evaluation of nonglomerular hematuria is provided in Figure 3–7.

Surgical. Nonglomerular hematuria or essential hematuria includes primarily urologic rather than nephrologic diseases. Common causes of essential hematuria include urologic tumors, stones, and UTIs.

The urinalysis in both nonglomerular medical and surgical hematuria is similar in that both are characterized by circular erythrocytes and the absence of erythrocyte casts. Essential hematuria is suggested, however, by the absence of significant proteinuria usually found in nonglomerular hematuria of renal parenchymal origin. It should be remembered, however, that proteinuria is not always present in glomerular or nonglomerular renal disease.

The American Urological Association (AUA) Best Practice Policy Panel on Microscopic Hematuria has formulated practice recommendations for the detection and evaluation of asymptomatic microscopic hematuria (Grossfeld et al, 2001a, 2001b). The panel concluded that, due to the lack of specificity of urinary dipstick examination, as well as the risk and expense of evaluation, patients with a positive dipstick test should only undergo complete evaluation for hematuria if this is confirmed by the finding of 3 or more RBC/HPF on subsequent microscopic evaluation. The mainstays of evaluation, according to the panel, are voided urinary cytology, cystoscopy, and urinary tract imaging using ultrasonography, CT, and/or intravenous urography (IVU). The use of these tests in an individual patient should be based in most cases on the relative risk of significant urinary tract pathology.

An algorithm for the evaluation of essential hematuria is provided in Figure 3–8.

Proteinuria

Although healthy adults excrete 80 to 150 mg of protein in the urine daily, the qualitative detection of proteinuria in the urinalysis should raise the suspicion of underlying renal disease. **Proteinuria may be the first indication of renovascular, glomerular, or tubulointerstitial renal disease, or it may represent the overflow of abnormal proteins into the urine in conditions such as multiple myeloma.** Proteinuria also can occur secondary to nonrenal disorders and in response to various physiologic conditions such as strenuous exercise.

The protein concentration in the urine obviously depends on the state of hydration, but it seldom exceeds 20 mg/dL. In patients with dilute urine, however, significant proteinuria may be present at concentrations less than 20 mg/dL. **Normally, urine protein is about 30% albumin, 30% serum globulins, and 40% tissue proteins, of which the major component is Tamm-Horsfall protein.** This profile may be altered by conditions that affect glomerular filtration, tubular reabsorption, or excretion of urine protein, and determination of the urine protein profile by such techniques as protein electrophoresis may help determine the etiology of proteinuria.

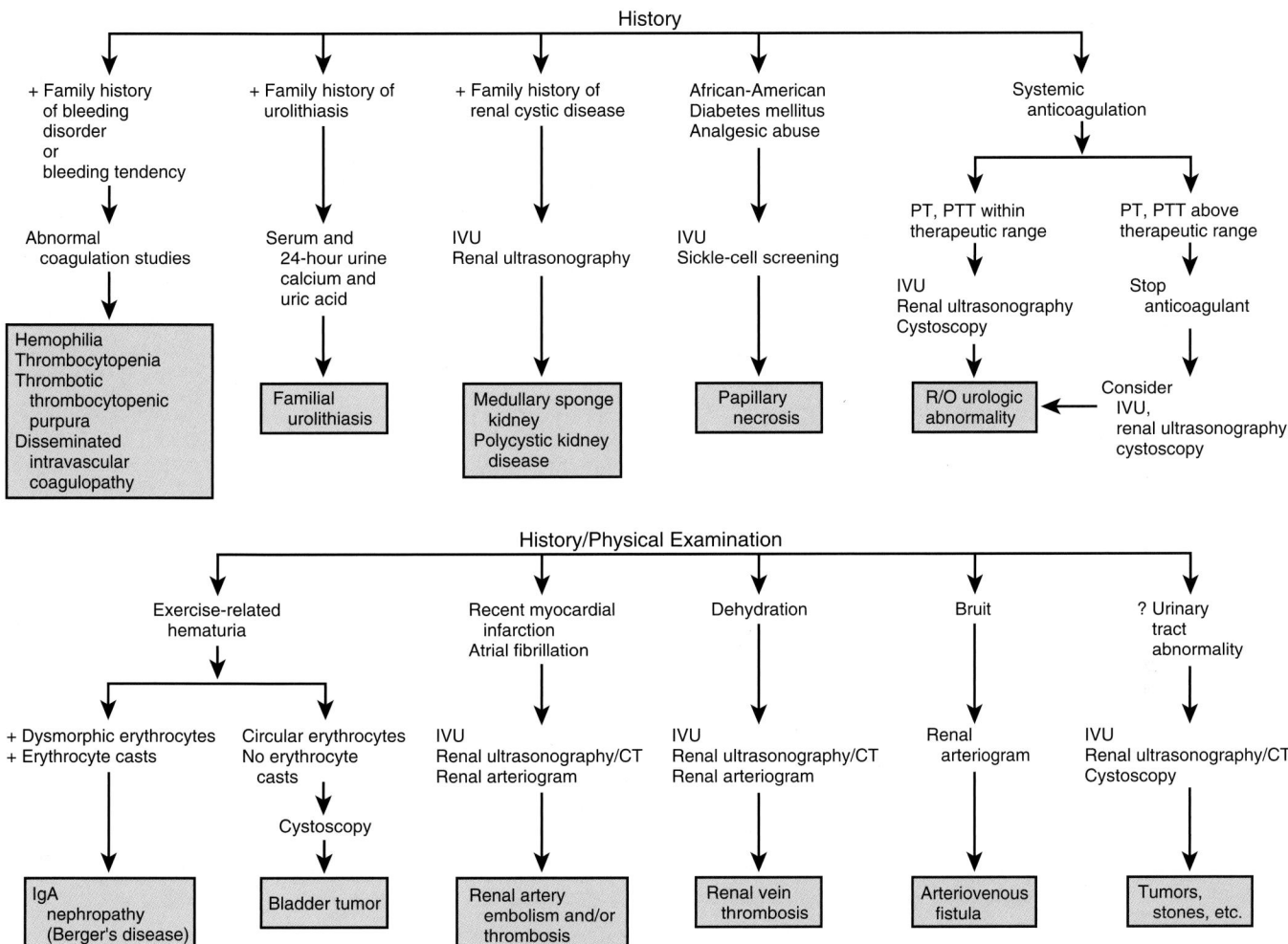

Figure 3–7. Evaluation of nonglomerular renal hematuria (circular erythrocytes, no erythrocyte casts, and proteinuria). CT, computed tomography; IgA, immunoglobulin A; IVU, intravenous urography; PT, prothrombin time; PTT, partial thromboplastin time; R/O, rule out.

Pathophysiology. Most causes of proteinuria can be categorized into one of three categories: glomerular, tubular, or overflow. Glomerular proteinuria is the most common type of proteinuria and results from increased glomerular capillary permeability to protein, especially albumin. Glomerular proteinuria occurs in any of the primary glomerular diseases such as IgA nephropathy or in glomerulopathy associated with systemic illness such as diabetes mellitus. Glomerular disease should be suspected when the 24-hour urine protein excretion exceeds 1 g and is almost certain to exist when the total protein excretion exceeds 3 g.

Tubular proteinuria results from failure to reabsorb normally filtered proteins of low molecular weight such as immunoglobulins. In tubular proteinuria, the 24-hour urine protein loss seldom exceeds 2 to 3 g and the excreted proteins are of low molecular weight rather than albumin. Disorders that lead to tubular proteinuria are commonly associated with other defects of proximal tubular function, such as glucosuria, aminoaciduria, phosphaturia, and uricosuria (Fanconi's syndrome).

Overflow proteinuria occurs in the absence of any underlying renal disease and is due to an increased plasma concentration of abnormal immunoglobulins and other low-molecular-weight proteins. The increased serum levels of abnormal proteins result in excess glomerular filtration that exceeds tubular reabsorptive capacity. The most common cause of overflow proteinuria is multiple myeloma, in which large amounts of immunoglobulin light chains are produced and appear in the urine (Bence Jones protein).

Detection. Qualitative detection of abnormal proteinuria is most easily accomplished with a dipstick impregnated with tetrabromophenol blue dye. The color of the dye changes in response to a pH shift related to the protein content of the urine, mainly albumin, leading to the development of a blue color. Because the background of the dipstick is yellow, various shades of green will develop, and the darker the green, the greater the concentration of protein in the urine. The minimal detectable protein concentration by this method is 20 to 30 mg/dL. **False-negative results can occur in alkaline urine, dilute urine, or when the primary protein present is not albumin.** Nephrotic range proteinuria in excess of 1 g/24 hr, however, is seldom missed on qualitative screening. Precipitation of urinary proteins with strong acids such as 3%

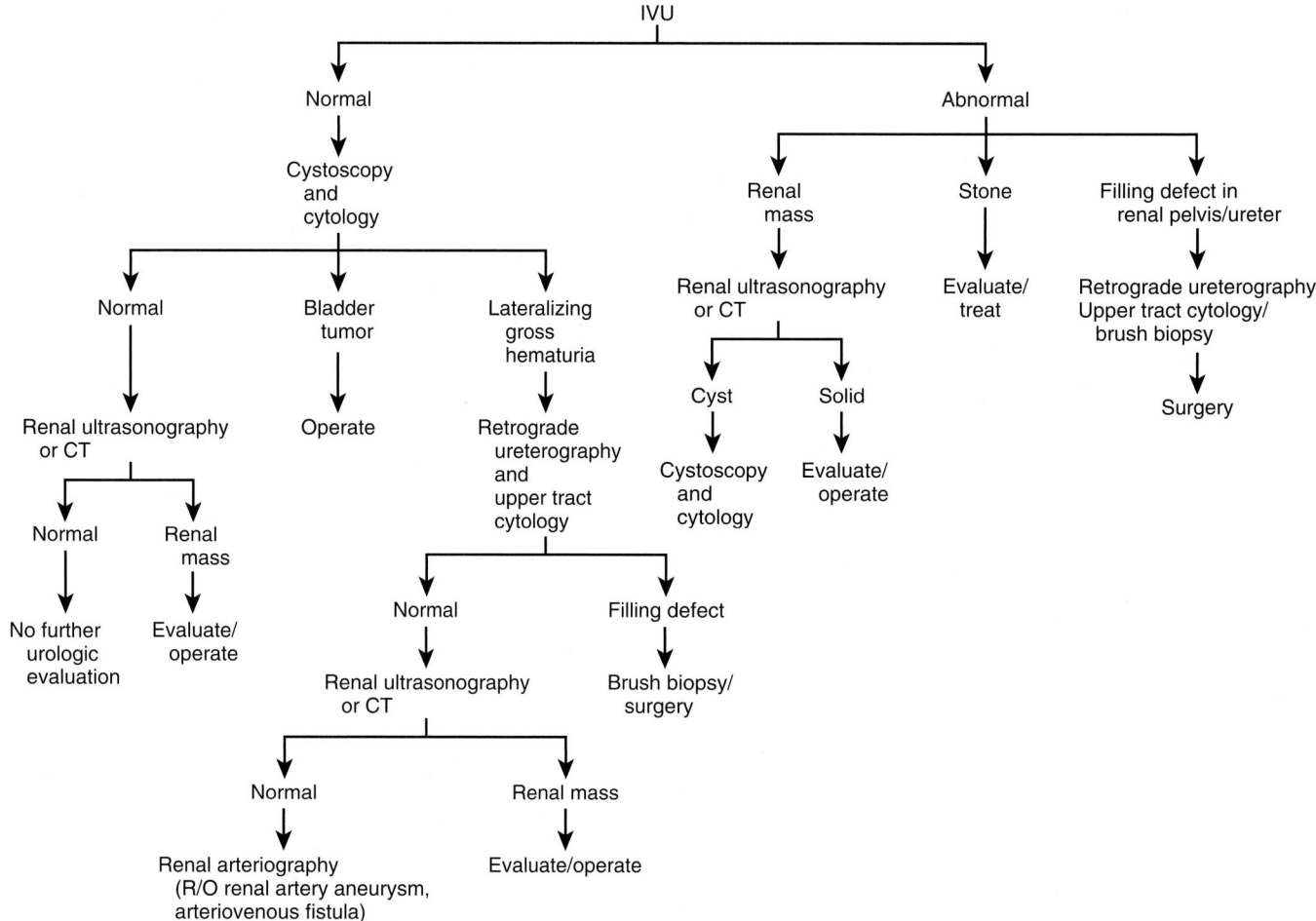

Figure 3–8. Evaluation of essential hematuria (circular erythrocytes, no erythrocyte casts, no significant proteinuria). CT, computed tomography; IVU, intravenous urography; R/O, rule out.

sulfosalicylic acid will detect proteinuria at concentrations as low as 15 mg/dL and is more sensitive at detecting other proteins as well as albumin. Patients whose urine is negative on dipstick but strongly positive with sulfosalicylic acid should be suspected of having multiple myeloma, and the urine should be tested further for Bence Jones protein.

If qualitative testing reveals proteinuria, this should be quantitated with a 24-hour urinary collection. Further qualitative assessment of abnormal urinary proteins can be accomplished by either protein electrophoresis or immunoassay for specific proteins. **Protein electrophoresis is particularly helpful in distinguishing glomerular from tubular proteinuria. In glomerular proteinuria, albumin makes up about 70% of the total protein excreted, whereas in tubular proteinuria, the major proteins excreted are immunoglobulins with albumin making up only 10% to 20%. Immunoassay is the method of choice for detecting specific proteins such as Bence Jones protein in multiple myeloma.**

Evaluation. Proteinuria should first be classified by its timing into transient, intermittent, or persistent. Transient proteinuria occurs commonly, especially in the pediatric population, and usually resolves spontaneously within a few days (Wagner et al, 1968). It may result from fever, exercise, or emotional stress. In older patients, transient proteinuria may be due to congestive heart failure. If a nonrenal cause is identified and a subsequent urinalysis is negative, no further evaluation is necessary. Obviously, if proteinuria persists, it should be evaluated further.

Proteinuria may also occur intermittently, and this is frequently related to postural change (Robinson, 1985). Proteinuria that occurs only in the upright position is a frequent cause of mild, intermittent proteinuria in young males. Total daily protein excretion seldom exceeds 1 g, and urinary protein excretion returns to normal when the patient is recumbent. Orthostatic proteinuria is thought to be secondary to increased pressure on the renal vein while standing. It resolves spontaneously in about 50% of patients and is not associated with any morbidity. Therefore, if renal function is normal in patients with orthostatic proteinuria, no further evaluation is indicated.

Persistent proteinuria requires further evaluation, and most cases have a glomerular etiology. A quantitative measurement of urinary protein should be obtained through a 24-hour urine collection, and a qualitative evaluation should be obtained to determine the major proteins excreted. The findings of greater than 2 g of protein excreted per 24 hours, of which the major components are high-molecular-weight proteins such as albumin, establishes the diagnosis of glomerular proteinuria. Glomerular proteinuria is the most common cause of abnormal proteinuria, especially in patients presenting with persistent proteinuria. If glomerular proteinuria is associated with hematuria characterized by dysmorphic erythrocytes and erythrocyte casts, the patient should be evaluated as outlined previously for glomerular hematuria (see Fig. 3–6). Patients with glomerular proteinuria who have no or little associated hematuria should be evaluated for other conditions, of which the most common is diabetes mellitus. Other possibilities include amyloidosis and arteriolar nephrosclerosis.

In patients in whom total protein excretion is 300 to 2000 mg/day, of which the major components are low-molecular-weight globulins, further qualitative evaluation with immunoelectrophoresis is indicated. This will determine whether the excess proteins are normal or abnormal. Identification of normal proteins establishes a diagnosis of tubular proteinuria, and further evaluation for a specific cause of tubular dysfunction is indicated.

If qualitative evaluation reveals abnormal proteins in the urine, this establishes a diagnosis of overflow proteinuria. Further evaluation should be directed to identify the specific protein abnormality. The finding of large quantities of light-chain immunoglobulins or Bence Jones protein establishes a diagnosis of multiple myeloma. Similarly, the finding of large amounts of hemoglobin or myoglobin establishes the diagnosis of hemoglobinuria or myoglobinuria.

An algorithm for the evaluation of proteinuria is provided in Figure 3–9.

Glucose and Ketones

Urine testing for glucose and ketones is useful in screening patients for diabetes mellitus. Normally, almost all the glucose filtered by the glomeruli is reabsorbed in the proximal tubules. Although very small amounts of glucose may normally be excreted in the urine, these amounts are not clinically significant and are below the level of detectability with the dipstick. If, however, the amount of glucose filtered exceeds the capacity of tubular reabsorption, glucose will be excreted in the urine and detected on the dipstick. **This so-called renal threshold corresponds to a serum glucose of about 180 mg/dL; above this level, glucose will be detected in the urine.**

Glucose detection with the urinary dipstick is based on a double sequential enzymatic reaction yielding a colorimetric change. In the first reaction, glucose in the urine reacts with glucose oxidase on the dipstick to form gluconic acid and hydrogen peroxide. In the second reaction, hydrogen peroxide reacts with peroxidase, causing oxidation of the chromogen on the dipstick, producing a color change. **This double-oxidative reaction is specific for glucose, and there is no cross-reactivity with other sugars.** The dipstick test becomes

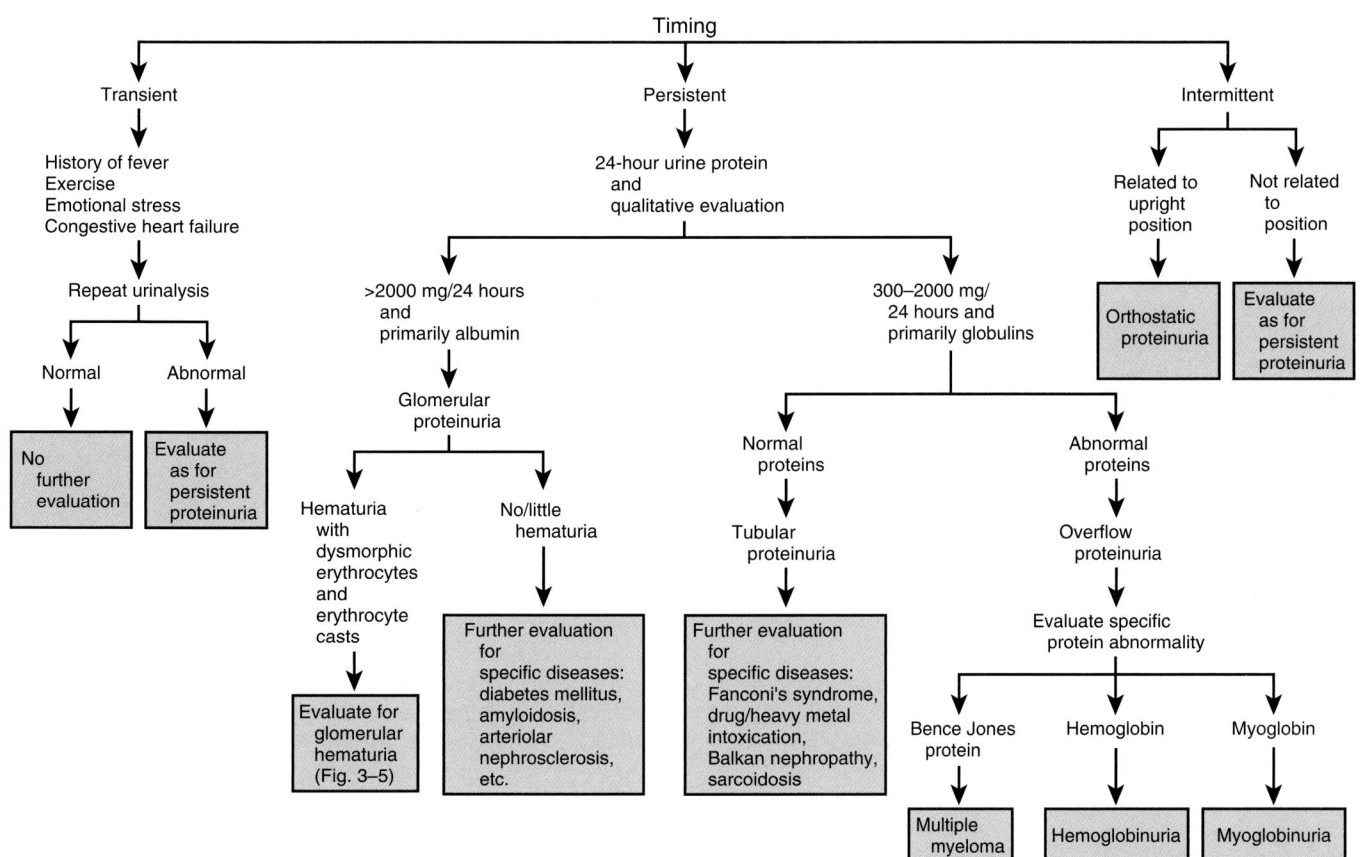

Figure 3–9. Evaluation of proteinuria.

less sensitive as the urine increases in specific gravity and temperature.

Ketones are not normally found in the urine but will appear when the carbohydrate supplies in the body are depleted and body fat breakdown occurs. This happens most commonly in diabetic ketoacidosis but may also occur during pregnancy and after periods of starvation or rapid weight reduction. **Ketones excreted include acetoacetic acid, acetone, and β-hydroxybutyric acid. With abnormal fat breakdown, ketones will appear in the urine before the serum.**

Dipstick testing for ketones involves a colorimetric reaction: sodium nitroprusside on the dipstick reacts with acetoacetic acid to produce a purple color. **Dipstick testing will identify acetoacetic acid at concentrations of 5 to 10 mg/dL but will not detect acetone or β-hydroxybutyric acid.** Obviously, a dipstick that tests positively for glucose should also be tested for ketones, and diabetes mellitus is suggested. False-positive results, however, can occur in very acidic urine of high specific gravity, in abnormally colored urine, and in urine containing levodopa metabolites, 2-mercaptoethane sulfonate sodium, and other sulfhydryl-containing compounds (Csako, 1987).

Bilirubin and Urobilinogen

Normal urine contains no bilirubin and only very small amounts of urobilinogen. There are two types of bilirubin, direct (conjugated) and indirect. Direct bilirubin is made in the hepatocyte, where bilirubin is conjugated with glucuronic acid. **Conjugated bilirubin has a low molecular weight, is water soluble, and normally passes from the liver into the small intestine through the bile ducts, where it is converted to urobilinogen. Therefore, conjugated bilirubin does not appear in the urine except in pathologic conditions in which there is intrinsic hepatic disease or obstruction of the bile ducts.**

Indirect bilirubin is of high molecular weight and bound in the serum to albumin. It is water insoluble and, therefore, does not appear in the urine even in pathologic conditions.

Urobilinogen is the end product of conjugated bilirubin metabolism. Conjugated bilirubin passes through the bile ducts, where it is metabolized by normal intestinal bacteria to urobilinogen. Normally, about 50% of the urobilinogen is excreted in the stool and 50% reabsorbed into the enterohepatic circulation. A small amount of absorbed urobilinogen, about 1 to 4 mg/day, will escape hepatic uptake and be excreted in the urine. Hemolysis and hepatocellular diseases that lead to increased bile pigments can result in increased urinary urobilinogen. Conversely, obstruction of the bile duct or antibiotic usage that alters intestinal flora, thereby interfering with the conversion of conjugated bilirubin to urobilinogen, will decrease urobilinogen levels in the urine. In these conditions, obviously, serum levels of conjugated bilirubin rise.

There are different dipstick reagents and methods to test for both bilirubin and urobilinogen, but the basic physiologic principle involves the binding of bilirubin or urobilinogen to a diazonium salt to produce a colorimetric reaction. False-negative results can occur in the presence of ascorbic acid, which decreases the sensitivity for detection of bilirubin. False-positive results can occur in the presence of phenazopyridine because it colors the urine orange and, similar to the colorimetric reaction for bilirubin, turns red in an acid medium.

Leukocyte Esterase and Nitrite Tests

Leukocyte esterase activity indicates the presence of white blood cells in the urine. The presence of nitrites in the urine is strongly suggestive of bacteriuria. Thus, both of these tests have been used to screen patients for UTIs. Although these tests may have application in nonurologic medical practice, the most accurate method to diagnose infection is by microscopic examination of the urinary sediment to identify pyuria and subsequent urine culture. All urologists should be capable of performing and interpreting the microscopic examination of the urinary sediment. Therefore, leukocyte esterase and nitrite testing are less important in a urologic practice. For purposes of completion, however, both techniques are described briefly herein.

Leukocyte esterase and nitrite testing are performed using the Chemstrip LN dipstick. Leukocyte esterase is produced by neutrophils and catalyzes the hydrolysis of an indoxyl carbonic acid ester to indoxyl (Gillenwater, 1981). The indoxyl formed oxidizes a diazonium salt chromogen on the dipstick to produce a color change. It is recommended that leukocyte esterase testing be done 5 minutes after the dipstick is immersed in the urine to allow adequate incubation (Shaw et al, 1985). The sensitivity of this test subsequently decreases with time because of lysis of the leukocytes. Leukocyte esterase testing may also be negative in the presence of infection, because not all patients with bacteriuria will have significant pyuria. Therefore, if one uses leukocyte esterase testing to screen patients for UTI, it should always be done in conjunction with nitrite testing for bacteriuria (Pels et al, 1989).

Other causes of false-negative results with leukocyte esterase testing include increased urinary specific gravity, glycosuria, presence of urobilinogen, medications that alter urine color, and ingestion of large amounts of ascorbic acid. **The major cause of false-positive leukocyte esterase tests is specimen contamination.**

Nitrites are not normally found in the urine, but many species of gram-negative bacteria can convert nitrates to nitrites. Nitrites can readily be detected in the urine because they react with the reagents on the dipstick and undergo diazotization to form a red azo dye. The specificity of the nitrite dipstick for detecting bacteriuria is over 90% (Pels et al, 1989). The sensitivity of the test, however, is considerably less, varying from 35% to 85%. The nitrite test is less accurate in urine specimens containing fewer than 10^5 organisms/mL (Kellog et al, 1987). As with leukocyte esterase testing, the major cause of false-positive nitrite testing is contamination.

It remains controversial whether dipstick testing for leukocyte esterase and nitrites can replace microscopy in screening for significant UTIs. This issue is less important to urologists, who usually have access to a microscope and who should be trained and encouraged to examine the urinary sediment. **A protocol combining the visual appearance of the urine with leukocyte esterase and nitrite testing has been proposed** (Fig. 3–10) that reportedly detects 95% of infected urine specimens and decreases the need for microscopy by as much as 30% (Flanagan et al, 1989). Other studies, however, have shown that dipstick testing is not an adequate replacement for microscopy (Propp et al, 1989). In summary, it has not been

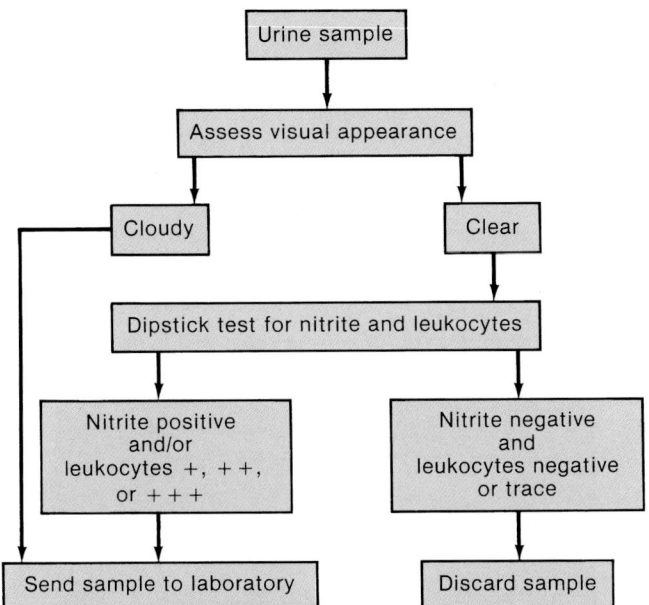

Figure 3–10. Protocol for determining the need for urine sediment microscopy in an asymptomatic population. (From Flanagan PG, Rooney PG, Davies EA, Stout RW: Evaluation of four screening tests for bacteriuria in elderly people. Lancet 1989;1:1117. © by The Lancet Ltd., 1989.)

demonstrated conclusively that dipstick testing for UTI can replace microscopic examination of the urinary sediment. In our personal experience, we always examine the urinary sediment whenever we suspect a UTI and subsequently culture the urine when pyuria is identified.

Urinary Sediment

Obtaining and Preparing the Specimen

A clean-catch midstream urine specimen should be obtained. As described earlier, uncircumcised men should retract the prepuce and cleanse the glans penis before voiding. It is more difficult to obtain a reliable clean-catch specimen in females because of contamination with introital leukocytes and bacteria. If there is any suspicion of a UTI in a female, a catheterized urine sample should be obtained for culture and sensitivity.

If possible, **the first morning urine specimen is the specimen of choice and should be examined within 1 hour.** A standard procedure for preparation of the urine for microscopic examination has been described (Cushner and Copley, 1989). Ten to 15 milliliters of urine should be centrifuged for 5 minutes at 3000 rpm. The supernatant is then poured off, and the sediment is resuspended in the centrifuge tube by gently tapping the bottom of the tube. Although the remaining small amount of fluid can be poured onto a microscope slide, this usually results in excess fluid on the slide. It is better to use a small pipette to withdraw the residual fluid from the centrifuge tube and to place it directly on the microscope slide. This usually results in an ideal volume of between 0.01 and 0.02 mL of fluid deposited on the slide. The slide is then covered with a coverslip. The edge of the coverslip should be placed on the slide first to allow the drop of fluid to ascend onto the coverslip by capillary action. The coverslip is then

gently placed over the drop of fluid, and this technique allows for most of the air between the drop of fluid and the coverslip to be expelled. If one simply drops the coverslip over the urine, the urine will disperse over the slide and there will be a considerable number of air bubbles that may distort the subsequent microscopic examination.

Microscopy Technique

Microscopic analysis of the urinary sediment should be performed with both low-power (×100 magnification) and high-power (×400 magnification) lenses. The use of an oil immersion lens for higher magnification is seldom, if ever, necessary. Under low power, the entire area under the coverslip should be scanned. **Particular attention should be given to the edges of the coverslip, where casts and other elements tend to be concentrated.** Low-power magnification is sufficient to identify erythrocytes, leukocytes, casts, cystine crystals, oval fat macrophages, and parasites such as *Trichomonas vaginalis* and *Schistosoma hematobium*.

High-power magnification is necessary to distinguish circular from dysmorphic erythrocytes, to identify other types of crystals, and, particularly, to identify bacteria and yeast. In summary, **the urinary sediment should be examined microscopically for (1) cells, (2) casts, (3) crystals, (4) bacteria, (5) yeast, and (6) parasites.**

Cells

Erythrocyte morphology may be determined under high-power magnification. Although phase contrast microscopy has been used for this purpose, circular (nonglomerular) erythrocytes can generally be distinguished from dysmorphic (glomerular) erythrocytes under routine brightfield high-power magnification (Figs. 3–11 to 3–15). **This is facilitated by adjusting the microscope condenser to its lowest aperture, thus reducing the intensity of background light. This allows one to see fine detail not evident otherwise and also creates the effect of phase microscopy because cell membranes and other sedimentary components stand out against the darkened background.**

Circular erythrocytes generally have an even distribution of hemoglobin with either a round or a crenated contour, whereas dysmorphic erythrocytes are irregularly shaped with minimal hemoglobin and irregular distribution of cytoplasm. Automated techniques for performing microscopic analysis to

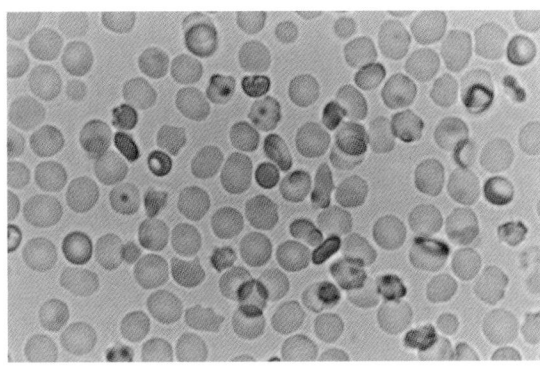

Figure 3–11.   Red blood cells, both smoothly rounded and mildly crenated, typical of epithelial erythrocytes.

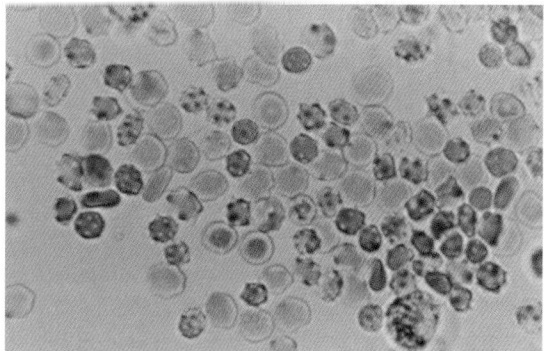

Figure 3–12. Red blood cells from a patient with a bladder tumor.

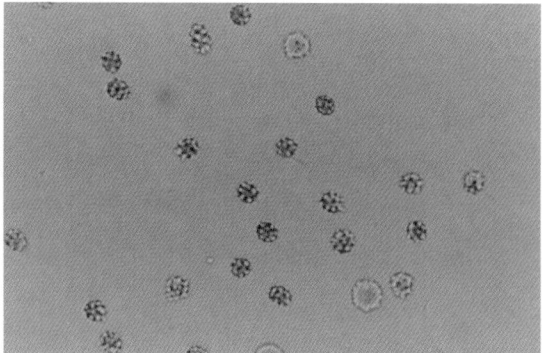

Figure 3–13. Red blood cells from a patient with interstitial cystitis. Cells were collected at cystoscopy.

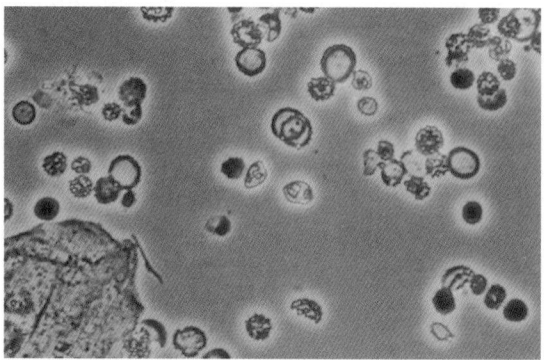

Figure 3–14. Red blood cells from a patient with Berger's disease. Note variations in membranes characteristic of dysmorphic red blood cells.

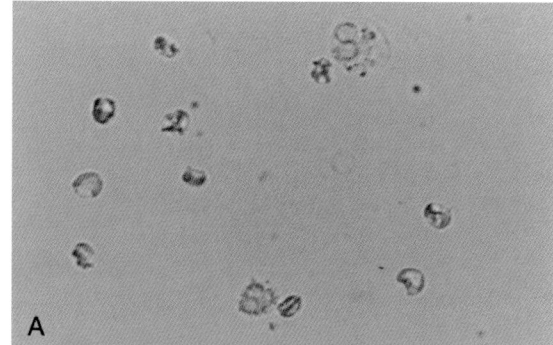

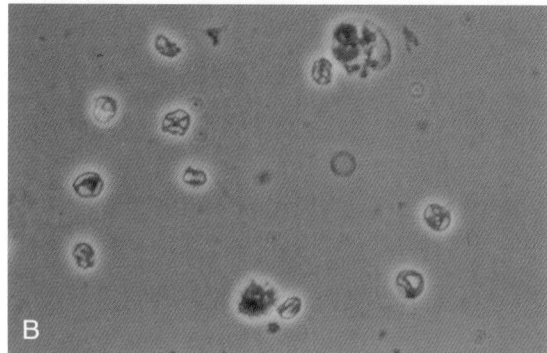

Figure 3–15. Dysmorphic red blood cells from a patient with Wegener's granulomatosis. **A,** Brightfield illumination. **B,** Phase illumination. Note irregular deposits of dense cytoplasmic material around the cell membrane.

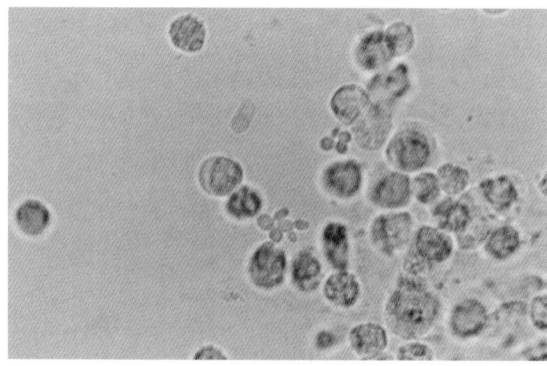

Figure 3–16. *Candida albicans.* Budding forms surrounded by leukocytes.

distinguish the two types of erythrocytes have been investigated but have not yet been accepted into general urologic practice and are probably unnecessary. In one study using a standard Coulter counter, microscopic analysis was found to be 97% accurate in differentiating between the two types of erythrocytes (Sayer et al, 1990). **Erythrocytes may be confused with yeast or fat droplets** (Fig. 3–16). Erythrocytes can be distinguished, however, because yeast will show budding and oil droplets are highly refractile.

Leukocytes can generally be identified under low power and definitively diagnosed under high-power magnification (Figs. 3–17 and 3–18; see also Fig. 3–16). It is normal to find 1 or 2 leukocytes/HPF in men and up to 5/HPF in women in whom the urine sample may be contaminated with vaginal secretions. A greater number of leukocytes generally indicates infection or inflammation in the urinary tract. It may be possible to distinguish **old leukocytes, which have a characteristic small and wrinkled appearance** and which are commonly found in the vaginal secretions of normal women, from fresh leukocytes, which are generally indicative of urinary tract pathology. Fresh leukocytes are generally larger and rounder, and, when the specific gravity is less than 1.019, the granules in the cytoplasm demonstrate glitter-like movement, so-called glitter cells.

Epithelial cells are commonly observed in the urinary sediment. Squamous cells are frequently detected in female urine specimens and are derived from the lower portion of the urethra, the trigone of postpubertal females, and the vagina. **Squamous epithelial cells are large, have a central small**

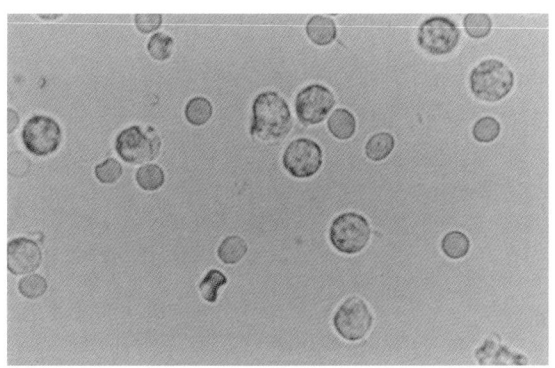

Figure 3–17. Old leukocytes. Staghorn calculi with *Proteus* infection.

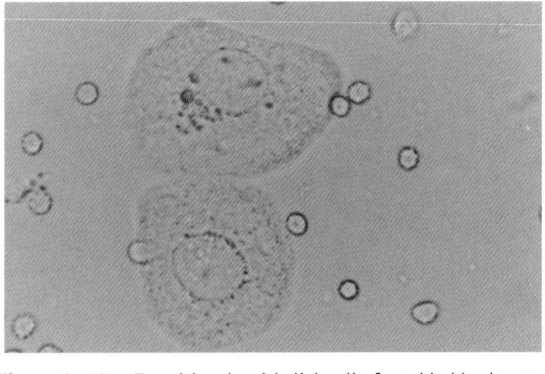

Figure 3–19. Transitional epithelial cells from bladder lavage.

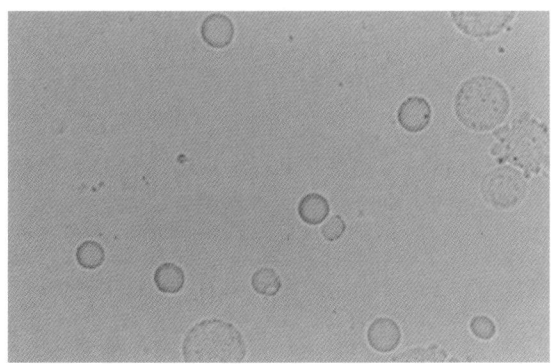

Figure 3–18. Fresh "glitter cells" with erythrocytes in background.

Casts

A cast is a protein coagulum that is formed in the renal tubule and traps any tubular luminal contents within the matrix. **Tamm-Horsfall mucoprotein is the basic matrix of all renal casts; it originates from tubular epithelial cells and is always present in the urine.** When the casts contain only mucoproteins, they are called hyaline casts and may not have any pathologic significance. Hyaline casts may be seen in the urine after exercise or heat exposure but may also be observed in pyelonephritis or chronic renal disease.

Red blood cell casts contain entrapped erythrocytes and are diagnostic of glomerular bleeding, most likely secondary to glomerulonephritis (Figs. 3–20 and 3–21). White blood cell casts are observed in acute glomerulonephritis, acute pyelonephritis, and acute tubulointerstitial nephritis. Casts with other cellular elements, usually sloughed renal tubular epithelial cells, are indicative of nonspecific renal damage (Fig. 3–22). Granular and waxy casts result from further degeneration of cellular elements. Fatty casts are seen in nephrotic syndrome, lipiduria, and hypothyroidism.

Crystals

Identification of crystals in the urine is particularly important in patients with stone disease, because it may help determine the etiology (Fig. 3–23). Although other types of crystals may be seen in normal patients, **the identification of cystine crystals establishes the diagnosis of cystinuria.** Crystals precipitated in acidic urine include calcium oxalate, uric acid, and cystine. Crystals precipitated in an alkaline urine include calcium phosphate and triple-phosphate (struvite) crystals.

nucleus about the size of an erythrocyte, and have an irregular cytoplasm with fine granularity.

Transitional epithelial cells may arise from the remainder of the urinary tract (Fig. 3–19). Transitional cells are smaller than squamous cells, have a larger nucleus, and demonstrate prominent cytoplasmic granules near the nucleus. Malignant transitional cells have altered nuclear size and morphology and can be identified with either routine Papanicolaou staining or automated flow cytometry.

Renal tubular cells are the least commonly observed epithelial cells in the urine but are most significant, because their presence in the urine is always indicative of renal pathology. Renal tubular cells may be difficult to distinguish from leukocytes, but they are slightly larger.

Figure 3–20. Red blood cell cast. **A,** Low-power view demonstrates distinct border of hyaline matrix. **B,** High-power view demonstrates the sharply defined red blood cell membranes *(arrow)*. Berger's disease.

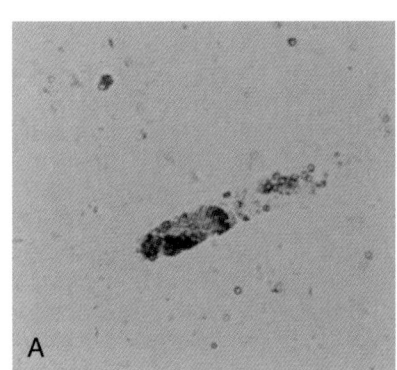

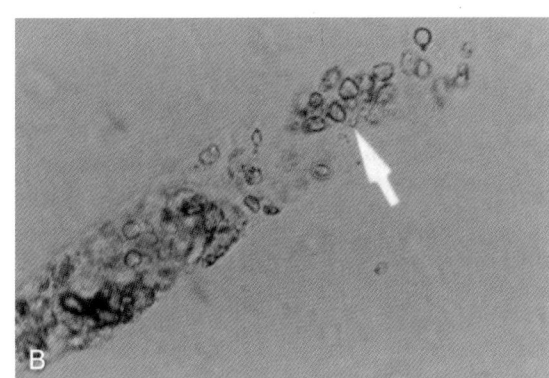

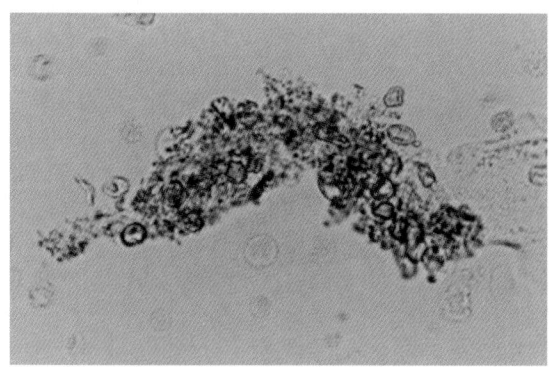

Figure 3–21.   Red blood cell cast.

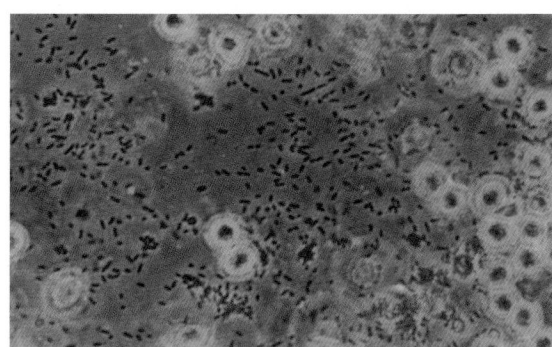

Figure 3–24.   Gram-negative bacilli. Phase microscopy of *Escherichia coli*.

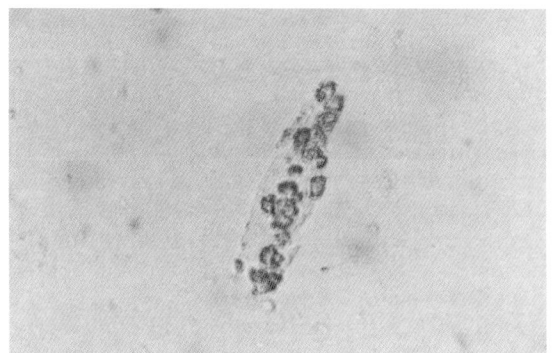

Figure 3–22.   Cellular cast. Cells entrapped in a hyaline matrix.

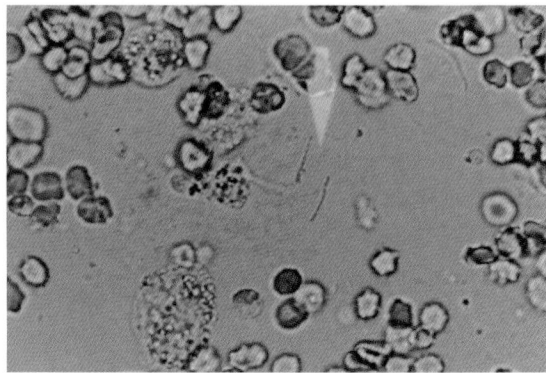

Figure 3–25.   Streptococcal urinary tract infection with typical chain formation *(arrow)*.

Crystals

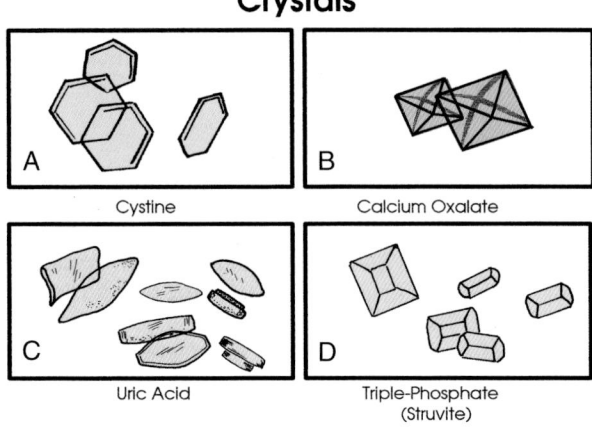

Figure 3–23.   Urinary crystals. **A,** Cystine. **B,** Calcium oxalate. **C,** Uric acid. **D,** Triple phosphate (struvite).

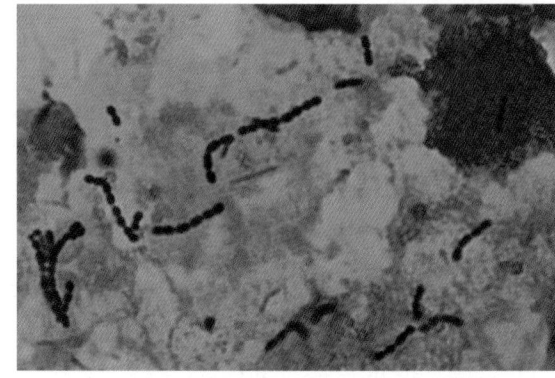

Figure 3–26.   Streptococcal urinary tract infection (Gram's stain).

Cholesterol crystals are rarely seen in the urine and are not related to urinary pH. They occur in lipiduria and remain in droplet form.

Bacteria

Normal urine should not contain bacteria; and in a fresh uncontaminated specimen, the finding of bacteria is indicative of a UTI. Because each HPF views between 1/20,000 and 1/50,000 mL, each bacterium seen per HPF signifies a bacterial count of more than 20,000/mL. Therefore, **5 bacteria/HPF reflects colony counts of about 100,000/mL.** This is the stan-

dard concentration used to establish the diagnosis of a UTI in a clean-catch specimen. This level should apply only to women, however, in whom a clean-catch specimen is frequently contaminated. The finding of any bacteria in a properly collected midstream specimen from a male should be further evaluated with a urine culture.

Under high power, it is possible to distinguish various bacteria. Gram-negative rods have a characteristic bacillary shape (Fig. 3–24), whereas streptococci can be identified by their characteristic beaded chains (Figs. 3–25 and 3–26) and staphylococci can be identified when the organisms are found in clumps (Fig. 3–27).

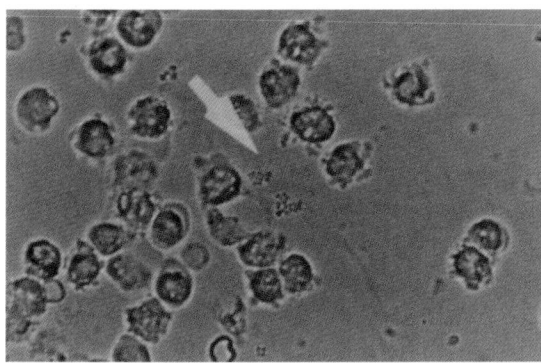

Figure 3–27. *Staphylococcus aureus* in typical clumps *(arrow).*

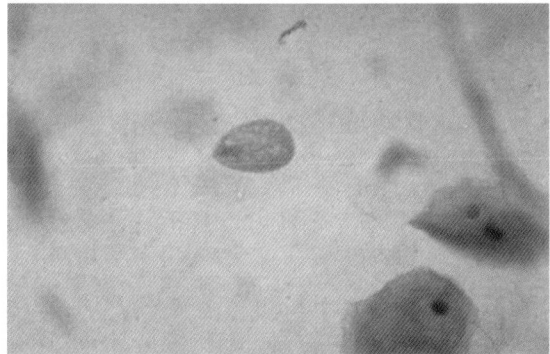

Figure 3–28. Trichomonad with ovoid shape and motile flagella.

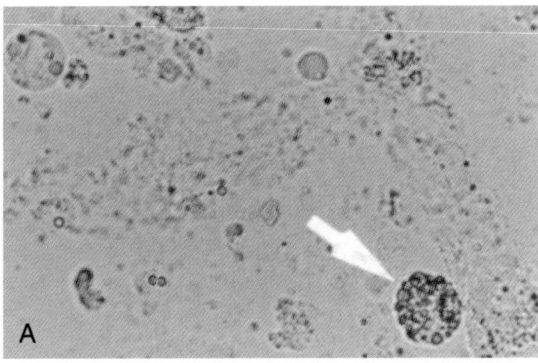

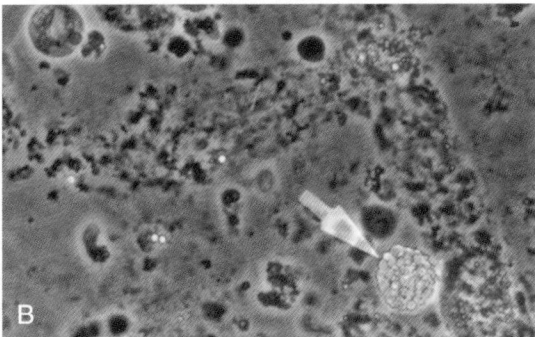

Figure 3–29. Oval fat macrophage. **A,** High-power view showing doubly refractile fat particles *(arrow).* B, Phase microscopy of the same specimen *(arrow).*

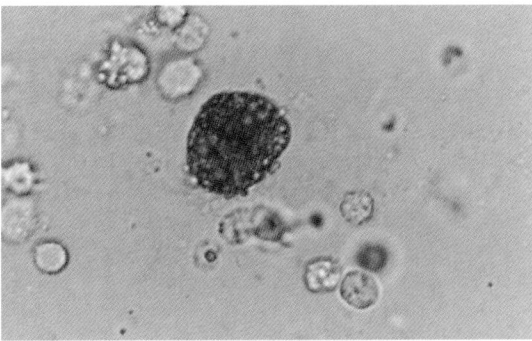

Figure 3–30. Oval fat microphage, high-power view. Note the fine secretory granules in the prostatic fluid.

Yeast

The most common yeast cells found in urine are *Candida albicans.* The biconcave oval shape of yeast can be confused with erythrocytes and calcium oxalate crystals, but **yeasts can be distinguished by their characteristic budding and hyphae** (see Fig. 3–16). Yeasts are most commonly seen in the urine of patients with diabetes mellitus or as contaminants in women with vaginal candidiasis.

Parasites

Trichomonas vaginalis **is a frequent cause of vaginitis in women and occasionally of urethritis in men.** Trichomonads can be readily identified in a clean-catch specimen under low power (Fig. 3–28). Trichomonads are large cells with rapidly moving flagella that quickly propel the organism across the microscopic field.

Schistosoma hematobium **is a urinary tract pathogen that is not found in the United States but is extremely common in countries of the Middle East and North Africa.** Examination of the urine shows the characteristic parasitic ova with a terminal spike.

Expressed Prostatic Secretions

Although not strictly a component of the urinary sediment, the expressed prostatic secretions should be examined in any man suspected of having prostatitis. Normal prostatic fluid should contain few, if any, leukocytes, and the presence of a larger number or clumps of leukocytes is indicative of prostatitis. **Oval fat macrophages are found in postinfection prostatic fluid** (Figs. 3–29 and 3-30). Normal prostatic fluid

contains numerous secretory granules that resemble but can be distinguished from leukocytes under high power because they do not have nuclei.

SUMMARY

This chapter has detailed the basic evaluation of the urologic patient, which should include a careful history, physical examination, and urinalysis. These three basic components form the cornerstone of the urologic evaluation and should precede any subsequent diagnostic procedures. After completion of the history, physical examination, and urinalysis, the urologist should be able to establish at least a differential, if not specific, diagnosis that will allow the subsequent diagnostic evaluation and treatment to be carried out in a direct and efficient manner.

SUGGESTED READINGS

Barry MJ, Fowler FJ Jr, O'Leary MP, et al: The American Urological Association symptom index for benign prostatic hyperplasia. J Urol 1992;148:1549.

Grossfeld GD, Litwin MS, Wolf JS Jr, et al: Evaluation of asymptomatic microscopic hematuria in adults: The American Urological Association Best Practice Policy—Part I: Definition, Prevalence and Etiology. Urology 2001a;57:599.

Grossfeld GD, Litwin MS, Wolf JS Jr, et al: Evaluation of asymptomatic microscopic hematuria in adults: The American Urological Association Best Practice Policy—Part II: Patient evaluation, cytology, voided markers, imaging, cystoscopy, nephrology evaluation and follow-up. Urology 2001b;57:604.

Mohr DN, Offord KP, Owen RA, Melton LJ 3rd: Asymptomatic microhematuria and urologic disease. A population-based study. JAMA 1986;256:224.

Pels RJ, Bor DH, Woolhandler S, et al: Dipstick urinalysis screening of asymptomatic adults for urinary tract disorders: II. Bacteriuria. JAMA 1989; 262:1221.

Schramek P, Schuster FX, Georgopoulos M, et al: Value of urinary erythrocyte morphology in assessment of symptomless microhematuria. Lancet 1989;2:1316.

4 Urinary Tract Imaging: Basic Principles

SAM B. BHAYANI, MD • CARY L. SIEGEL, MD

CONVENTIONAL RADIOGRAPHY

ULTRASOUND

COMPUTED TOMOGRAPHY

MAGNETIC RESONANCE IMAGING

NUCLEAR SCINTIGRAPHY

Imaging of the urinary tract is an essential aspect of the diagnosis and treatment of urologic disease. Imaging may provide anatomic, functional, and physiologic information. Newer techniques, such as positron emission tomography (PET), magnetic resonance urography and angiography (MRU and MRA), and three-dimensional computed tomography (CT) have evolved into routine diagnostic studies. Nevertheless, imaging techniques such as intravenous urography and ultrasonography continue to be valuable in the diagnosis of urologic pathology. In this chapter we outline the foundations of urinary tract imaging. Indications, limitations, and alternatives to the imaging techniques are discussed. Findings germane to specific pathologic processes are presented in later chapters.

CONVENTIONAL RADIOGRAPHY

Although the field of uroradiology has brought increasingly complex studies to the armamentarium of the practitioner, conventional radiography has a role in the diagnosis and management of urologic disease. Conventional radiography includes abdominal plain radiography, intravenous urography, cystography, loopography, and retrograde urethrography. All of these techniques may be obtained in a fluoroscopy suite or in the operating room if clinically indicated.

Abdominal Plain Radiography

Abdominal plain radiography allows a conventional view of the skeletal and intra-abdominal structures. The radiograph may be used as a scout film, to which contrast studies may be compared, or as a primary survey to assess urologic or abdominal pathologic processes. The typical field of view includes the kidneys at the superior extent and the bladder inferiorly. Other structures included in the field of view will be the lower ribs, liver, bowel, spleen, lumbar spine, sacrum, and bony pelvis. In larger patients two films may be required to encompass these areas.

The anatomic landmarks that are readily apparent include several skeletal and visceral structures. Differing radiographic densities of air (black), calcification (white), and soft tissue (gray) allow outlining and differentiation of intra-abdominal structures. Calcifications may be seen near the expected location of the kidneys, ureter, or bladder (Fig. 4–1). Vascular calcifications, bowel opacities, and phleboliths also may be viewed (Fig. 4–2). Uric acid calculi may not be seen, and calcifications over the bony structures may be difficult to visualize (Fig. 4–3).

Strengths and Limitations. The abdominal radiograph has been superseded by more complex imaging techniques, and it is not an ideal diagnostic test. Nevertheless, it is useful in the detection of urolithiasis and may be an economical technique to follow known stones. **False-negative results are possible, particularly if the stone lies over the sacrum and iliac wings or if it is radiolucent.** False-positive results may occur with vascular calcifications and phleboliths. The abdominal radiograph is particularly valuable before shockwave lithotripsy, because if the stone cannot be visualized, treatment with another modality may be necessary. The radiograph is of use in the evaluation of foreign bodies in the urinary tract, and it is also valuable to assess position or placement of ureteral catheters, stents, and drains. A kidney-ureter-bladder (KUB) view is indicated before contrast studies to obtain a scout film by which postcontrast studies may be compared. Furthermore, it may reveal residual contrast media in the visceral structures, thus altering interpretation of the study.

The abdominal plain radiograph has a limited role in the diagnosis of complex urologic pathology. Although the film may suggest abnormalities in the regions of the kidney, ureters, or bladder, such suggestions are further evaluated with cross-sectional imaging techniques or ultrasound, which offer better differentiation of visceral structures.

Contrast Media

Conventional imaging techniques may rely on the use of contrast media to opacify urinary tract. Iodinated contrast agents

111

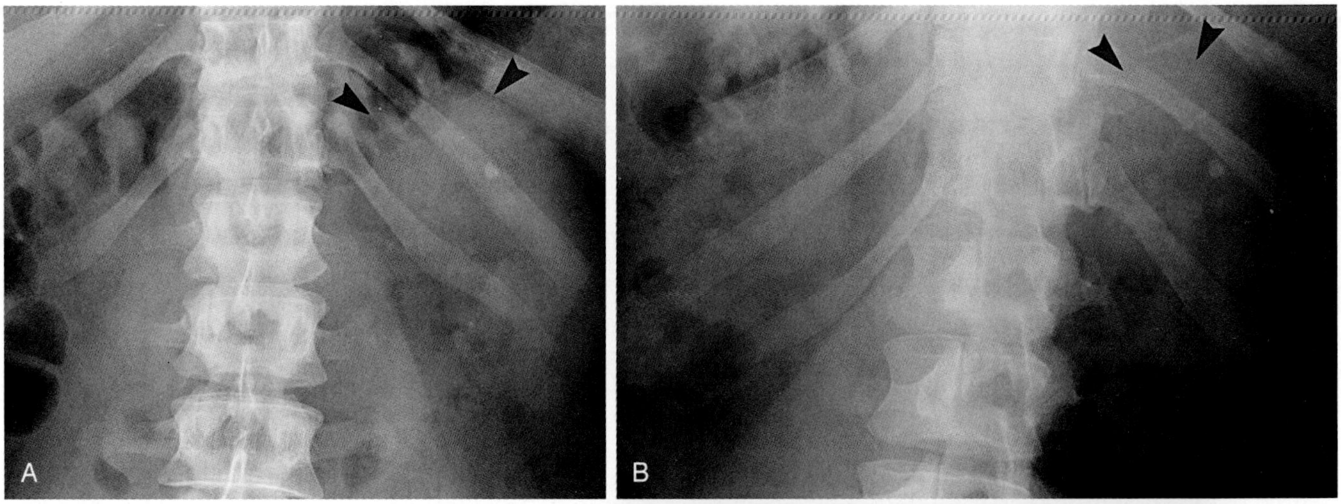

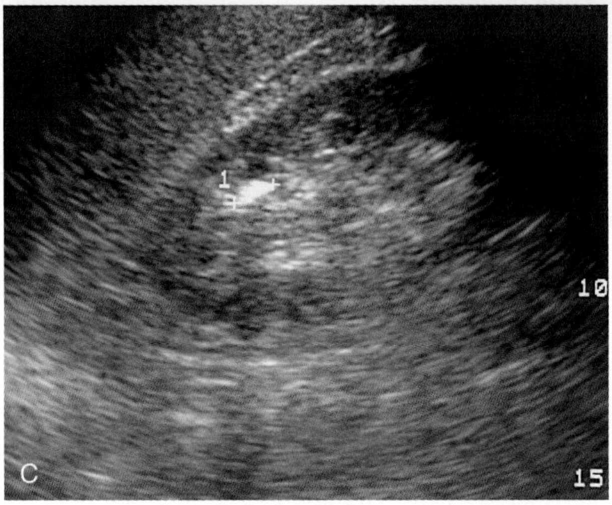

Figure 4–1. Renal calculus. **A,** Abdominal radiograph demonstrating a small calculus in the upper pole of the left kidney superimposed over the 11th rib. **B,** An oblique film confirms the intrarenal location of the stone (*arrowheads* outline the upper pole of the left kidney). **C,** Renal ultrasound also demonstrates an echogenic focus with acoustical shadowing in the upper pole of the left kidney. (Reprinted from Ramchandani P: Radiological evaluation of renal calculous disease. In Pollack HM, McClennan BL, Dyer R, Kenney PJ [eds]: Clinical Urography, 2nd ed. Philadelphia, WB Saunders, 2000.)

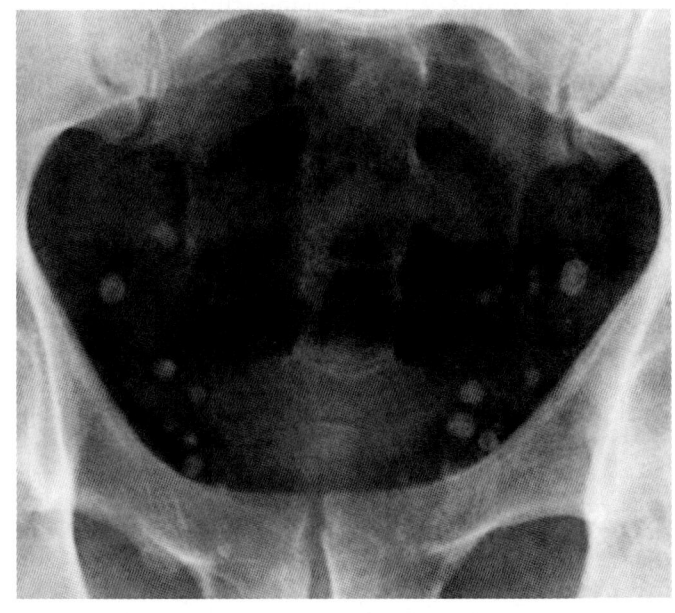

Figure 4–2. Typical radiographic picture of multiple pelvic phleboliths. The phleboliths are steered to either side of the pelvis and arranged in the distribution of the pelvic veins. Phleboliths tend to be round and fairly opaque, and they commonly measure 2 to 6 mm in diameter, although numerous exceptions occur. (Reprinted from Barbaric ZL, Pollack HM: Abdominal plain radiography. In Pollack HM, McClennan BL, Dyer R, Kenney PJ [eds]: Clinical Urography, 2nd ed. Philadelphia, WB Saunders, 2000.)

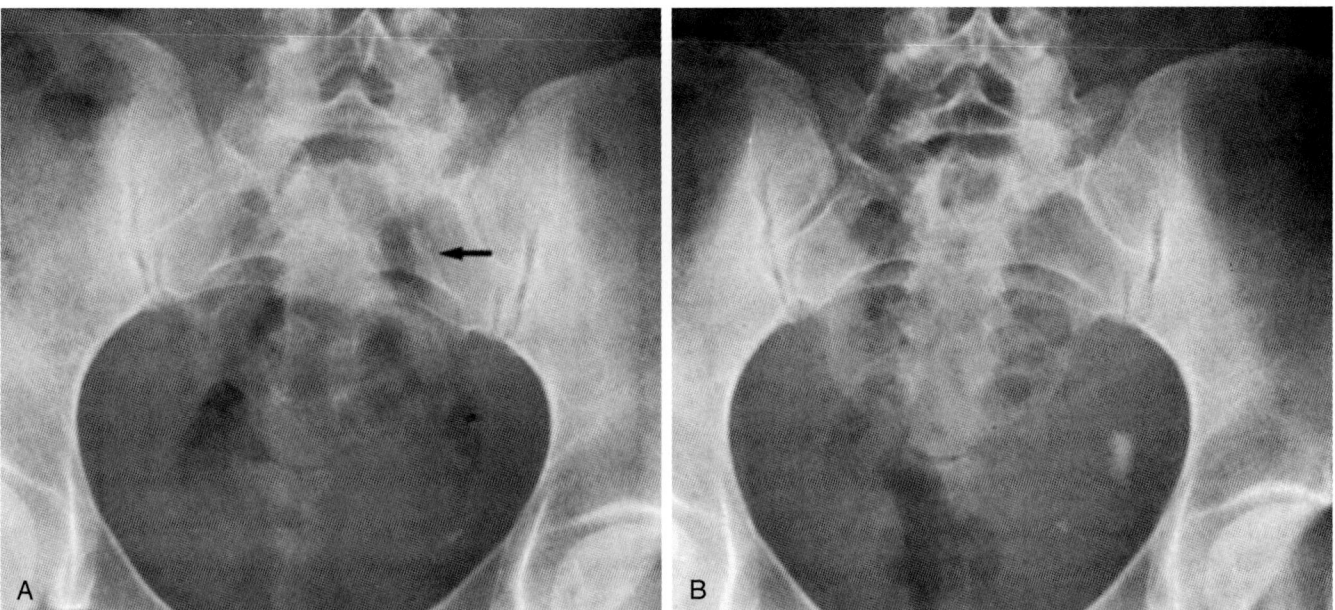

Figure 4–3. Unapparent ureteral calculus. **A,** A plain abdominal radiograph reveals a barely perceptible opacity superimposed on the sacrum *(arrow)*. The patient was complaining of left flank pain and was initially told that there was "no evidence of a stone." In retrospect, a calculus was identified. **B,** A film exposed 10 weeks later now reveals a calculus in the distal end of the left ureter. The opacity over the sacrum is no longer seen. In such cases, oblique films usually clarify the issue. (Reprinted from Barbaric ZL, Pollack HM: Abdominal plain radiography. In Pollack HM, McClennan BL, Dyer R, Kenney PJ [eds]: Clinical Urography, 2nd ed. Philadelphia, WB Saunders, 2000.)

were developed in the 1950s (Robbins et al, 1951; Hoppe et al, 1956), and derivatives are used in intravenous urography, retrograde pyelography, antegrade studies, and cystography. Although contrast media offer advantages of urinary tract visualization, potential adverse reactions are possible (Wolf et al, 1989; Barrett et al, 1992).

Iodinated contrast media are required to perform several urologic imaging techniques. Iodinated contrast agents are rapidly concentrated by the kidneys and opacify the urinary tract. **Various formulations of iodinated contrast media have been developed, but all derive from a 2,4,6-triiodinated benzene ring, with a carboxyl group at the 1-position.** Differing side chains at the 3- and 5-positions represent different brands. Additionally, low osmolar nonionic forms of contrast media (LOCM) have been developed that eliminate the carboxyl group but add hydrophilic hydroxyl groups at the organic side chain positions. Because LOCM do not ionize in solution, the relative osmotic load of the agents is approximately 50% less than that of high osmolar contrast media (HOCM). **The osmotic load of the HOCM has been associated with an increased risk of complications.**

Contrast media reactions may be dose dependent or idiosyncratic. The major toxicities include allergic reactions, cardiovascular alterations, and renal toxicities. Idiosyncratic reactions are often described as anaphylactoid, owing to their similarity to allergic reactions. The incidence of complications after the administration of ionic contrast media is as high as 12% (Katayama et al, 1990). Most reactions are mild and include nausea, vomiting, urticaria, and facial edema. These may be treated with an antihistamine. Bronchospasm can be treated with a β-adrenergic agonist or epinephrine if respiratory distress is noted (Thomsen and Bush, 1998). Severe reactions, including profound shock, are rare but have been

reported. Hospitalization is recommended in severe cases, and epinephrine may be administered. Nonionic (LOCM) media has an improved safety profile over HOCM, with adverse reactions occurring in up to 3% of patients.

Cardiovascular Toxicity. Transient cardiovascular alterations occur with contrast medium injection (Popio et al, 1978; Katzberg et al, 1983). A wide variety of minor electrocardiographic changes may occur but are often minimized when bolus injection is avoided. Depression of myocardial contractility and the electrical activity of the sinoatrial and atrioventricular nodes is possible. In rare cases, arrhythmia and ischemia may occur. Reactions are also limited with the use of LOCM.

Renal Toxicity. Contrast media may result in acute renal toxicity (Lautin et al, 1991; Barrett and Carlisle, 1993). Patients with existing renal insufficiency are at greater risk for contrast nephrotoxicity. **LOCM have decreased risk for such reaction compared with HOCM.** The risk of renal insufficiency in patients with normal renal function is likely less than 1%. The pathogenesis of the renal dysfunction is not completely known and may be multifactorial. Direct toxicity to renal tubules, ischemia, alterations in circulation, and precipitation of uric acid may all contribute to the dysfunction. Patients at risk for contrast nephropathy should be well hydrated, LOCM should be used, and large contrast media loads should be avoided.

Intravenous Urography

Intravenous excretory urography (IVU) has been a mainstay of urologic imaging for several years. The indications for performing an IVU are numerous. IVU allows imaging of the renal parenchyma, collecting system, and ureter. It can be used in the evaluation of urothelial abnormalities in evaluation of hematuria or in the evaluation of urolithiasis. As a parenchymal imaging technique, it may detect gross abnormalities, but it has been superseded by cross-sectional imaging methods (Lang et al, 2003). IVU had been a core study in urologic imaging, but recently the number of examinations has declined, likely secondary to the increased use of CT (Chen and Zagoria, 1999).

Patient Preparation. Although a minor bowel preparation may allow for improved visualization of the collecting system, an emergent examination should not be delayed for a preparation. A pregnancy test may be indicated before the examination if clinical suspicion arises. Some institutions recommend a formal bowel preparation before examination, although routine use is controversial. A typical bowel preparation consists of clear liquids for 24 hours before examination and a cathartic agent or enema. **Randomized studies have not shown a clear advantage in visualization of the urinary tract with bowel preparation,** but prepared groups do have fewer feces in their colon, which may have a subjective impact on IVU efficacy (Bailey et al, 1991; George et al, 1993). Bowel preparation should be considered in patients with chronic constipation, such as patients with neurologic deficits.

Dehydration may improve imaging quality but has risks (Dunbar et al, 1960). Similar to bowel preparation, the necessity of dehydration is controversial. Dehydration induces an increase in antidiuretic hormone, thus increasing tubular water resorption and subsequent concentration of the contrast medium (Talner, 1972). Caution, however, is advised in patients with renal insufficiency, because dehydration may exacerbate nephrotoxicity. Overhydration should be avoided, because poor visualization of the collecting system may necessitate reexamination. In practice, withholding fluids after midnight before examination is sufficient to allow adequate imaging.

Technique. First a scout radiograph is taken in the supine position. This radiograph, which encompasses the field from the renal outlines to the pubic symphysis, is essential in revealing renal outlines, calcifications, residual contrast media, and positioning. For larger patients, two films may be necessary to fully image the field. Oblique views may be taken if necessary to allow better distinction of calcifications from bony structures.

Contrast medium injection may be given as a bolus or drip infusion, with bolus being the predominant technique. Fifty to 100 mL of contrast medium is given through an 18- or 19-gauge needle. Immediately after injection and in the first few minutes after injection the nephrographic phase produces images of the renal parenchyma. Several tomograms may be taken to adequately document the parenchymal outlines. By 5 minutes the collecting system should opacify, and imaging of the pyelographic phase commences. A compression device may be attached, which distends the collecting system and allows better visualization of the pelvis and ureters. After the 5-minute films, further imaging is individualized to the patient, and subsequent images should document the entire length of the ureter for filling abnormalities. Ureteral peristalsis may be viewed, and images may be taken after peristal-

sis for better visualization. A normal intravenous urogram is shown in Figure 4-4.

Certain accessory radiographs may be taken to document special circumstances. Oblique views may better visualize the calyceal system or can allow clarification of filling defects that may overlap in the routine anteroposterior views. **Prone images place the ureter in a dependent position and may be useful in distending and imaging the ureter** (Fig. 4–5). Upright films can document renal ptosis or layering of contrast media in severely hydronephrotic systems. The postvoid film may be useful in evaluating bladder outlet obstruction, diverticula, or filling defects within the bladder (DeFilippo et al, 1984).

Loopography

Loopography generally implies imaging of a urinary conduit or diversion. The most common urinary diversion is the ileal conduit, but any bowel segment may be used. Additionally, complex continent diversions and neobladders may also require imaging, and the urologist and radiologist should be familiar with the details of the surgical reconstruction.

Indications. Loopography may be performed for a wide variety of indications. A critical point is whether the imaging study is ordered to evaluate the loop or the ureters. If ureteral imaging is desired, IVU may suffice. However, if contraindications to intravenous contrast media exist (e.g., renal insufficiency, hypersensitivity), a loopogram may be used as an alternate method to perform ureteral imaging (Hudson et al, 1981). Imaging of the ureters via loopography requires reflux of contrast media into the upper urinary tract. Although most methods of ureteral-ileal implantation do allow reflux, some surgical techniques produce a nonrefluxing anastomosis. A loopogram in the presence of a nonrefluxing anastomosis may not allow ureteral imaging, and an alternate method may be necessary, such as IVU, antegrade nephrostography, or cross-sectional (CT or MR) urography. If the imaging study is performed to evaluate the loop itself, then a standard loopogram can allow a complete radiographic evaluation of the conduit segment.

Loopography is indicated to evaluate for a pathologic process related to the conduit or for evaluation of the upper urinary tract. Typical indications include evaluation of hematuria, stones, stoma stenosis, loop ischemia, urinary fistulas, urinary leak, ureteroenteric anastomosis stricture, hydronephrosis, and surveillance for transitional cell carcinoma.

Patient Preparation. A loopogram is a contrast study. A sensitivity to contrast media should be documented but is not necessarily a contraindication because intravenous use is not necessary for this test. Bowel preparation is usually not indicated, unless residual contrast media from a previous study obscures the images. A negative urine culture is ideal but rarely encountered in the setting of an ileal conduit. Thus, a broad-spectrum antibiotic or genitourinary irrigant may be used to limit potential infection. An appropriate catheter should be available to intubate the conduit for contrast medium instillation. Patients with spinal cord lesions above T7 should be treated cautiously because of the possibility for autonomic dysreflexia and severe hypertension.

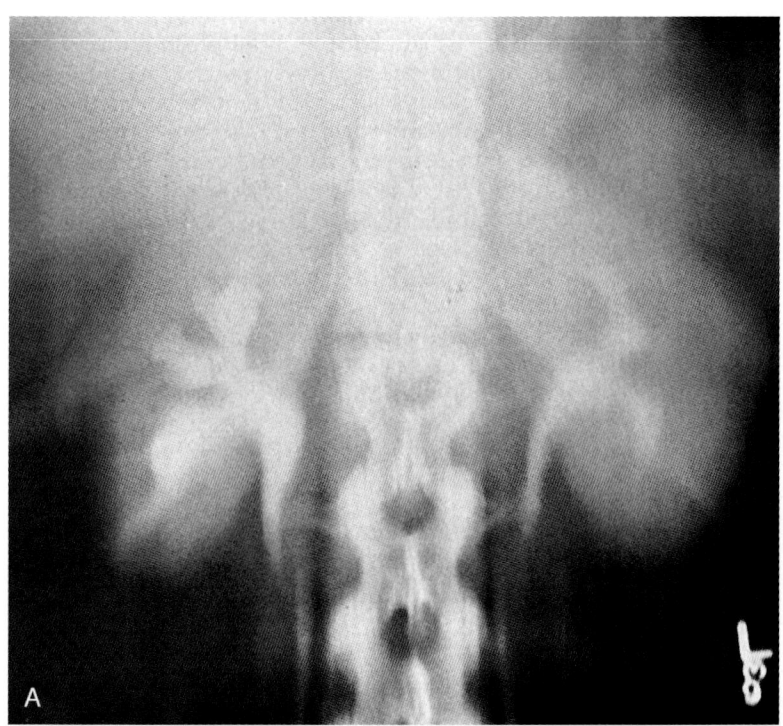

Figure 4–4. Normal excretory urogram. **A,** A tomogram at 3 minutes shows distention of the collecting systems from ureteral compression. Visualization of the nephrograms is good. **B,** A 10-minute film with compression maintained shows excellent visualization of the collecting systems and proximal two thirds of the ureters above the area of compression. Note the symmetrically placed, fully inflated compression balloons overlying the pelvic portions of the ureters. **C,** A 30-minute supine film. After release of compression, the calyces are slightly less dilated and the ureters not as well filled, which is indicative of satisfactory drainage. The bladder is fully distended. (Reprinted from Friedenberg RM, Harris RD: Excretory urography. In Pollack HM, McClennan BL, Dyer R, Kenney PJ [eds]: Clinical Urography, 2nd ed. Philadelphia, WB Saunders, 2000.)

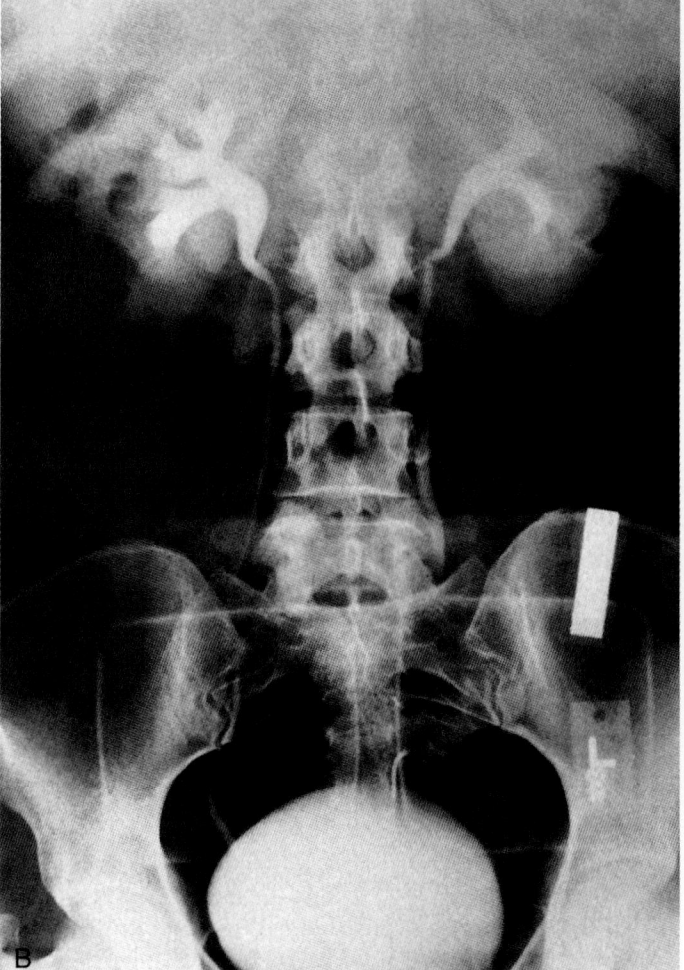

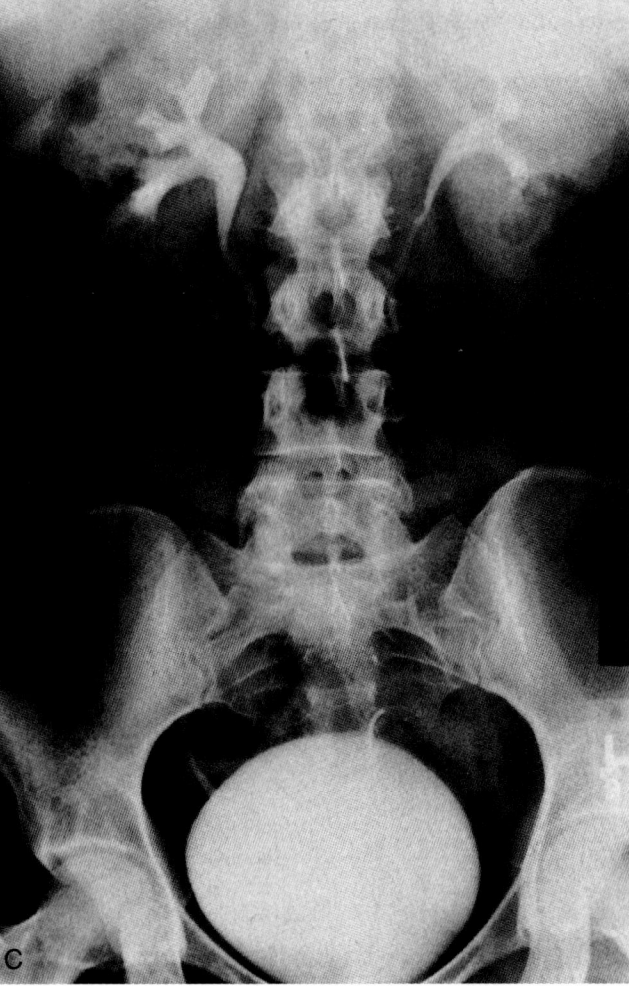

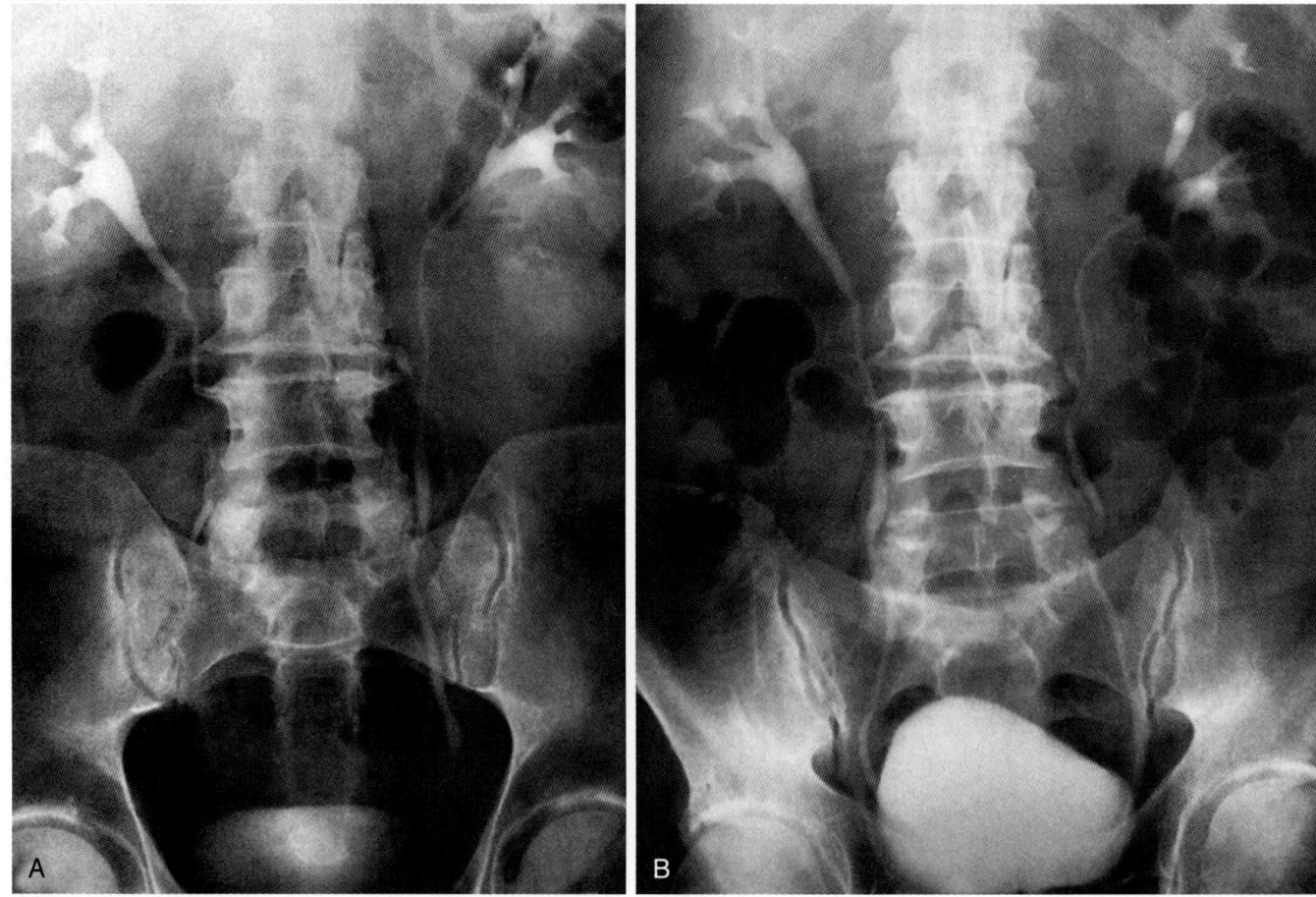

Figure 4–5. Value of the prone film. **A,** Supine 10-minute film from a urogram with poor visualization of the distal end of the right ureter. **B,** A prone film shows complete visualization of both ureters. (Reprinted from Friedenberg RM, Harris RD: Excretory urography. In Pollack HM, McClennan BL, Dyer R, Kenney PJ [eds]: Clinical Urography, 2nd ed. Philadelphia, WB Saunders, 2000.)

Technique. The patient is placed in the supine position in the radiology suite. A scout radiograph is taken. Next, via a catheter in the conduit, contrast medium is injected into the conduit until distention of the conduit occurs. Reflux may be seen, and contrast media may be administered to distend the ureters and collecting system (Fig. 4–6). Care should be taken not to exert high pressures. Films are taken depending on the area of interest when the structure in question is opacified. Drainage films may be taken to evaluate for obstruction.

Cystourethrography

Cystourethrography is performed for evaluation of pathology in the lower urinary tract. The three major studies that may be performed are static cystography, voiding cystourethrography, and retrograde urethrography. The examinations potentially allow evaluation of both anatomic defects and functional anomalies.

Static Cystography

Indications. Retrograde cystography is performed to evaluate bladder lesions, rupture, or leakage. It is commonly used in the postsurgical patient or the trauma patient to evaluate the integrity of the bladder or any urinary anastomosis

(Leibovitch et al, 1995). It can also be used to evaluate for urinary fistulas.

Technique. A scout film is obtained first to evaluate for calcifications and residual contrast media and to establish the field of view. Then, via a catheter, the bladder is filled with contrast medium up to 200 to 400 mL, depending on bladder capacity and patient comfort. Films are taken with anteroposterior (Fig. 4–7) and oblique views so extravasation posterior to the bladder is visualized. A postdrainage film is obtained to allow complete evaluation of bladder pathology. In the presence of a fresh anastomosis or suspected bladder rupture, contrast media may be instilled with gravity, and complete bladder distention is often unnecessary to demonstrate extravasation. Oblique and drainage films should still be obtained for complete evaluation of extravasation.

Voiding Cystourethrography

Indications. The voiding cystourethrogram (VCUG) allows both functional and anatomic evaluation of the bladder. It is most commonly performed in children and is used in the evaluation of recurrent urinary tract infection. It is a critical examination in the evaluation of the posterior urethra. A variety of pediatric urologic pathologic processes may be seen, including reflux, urethral valves, ureterocele, and

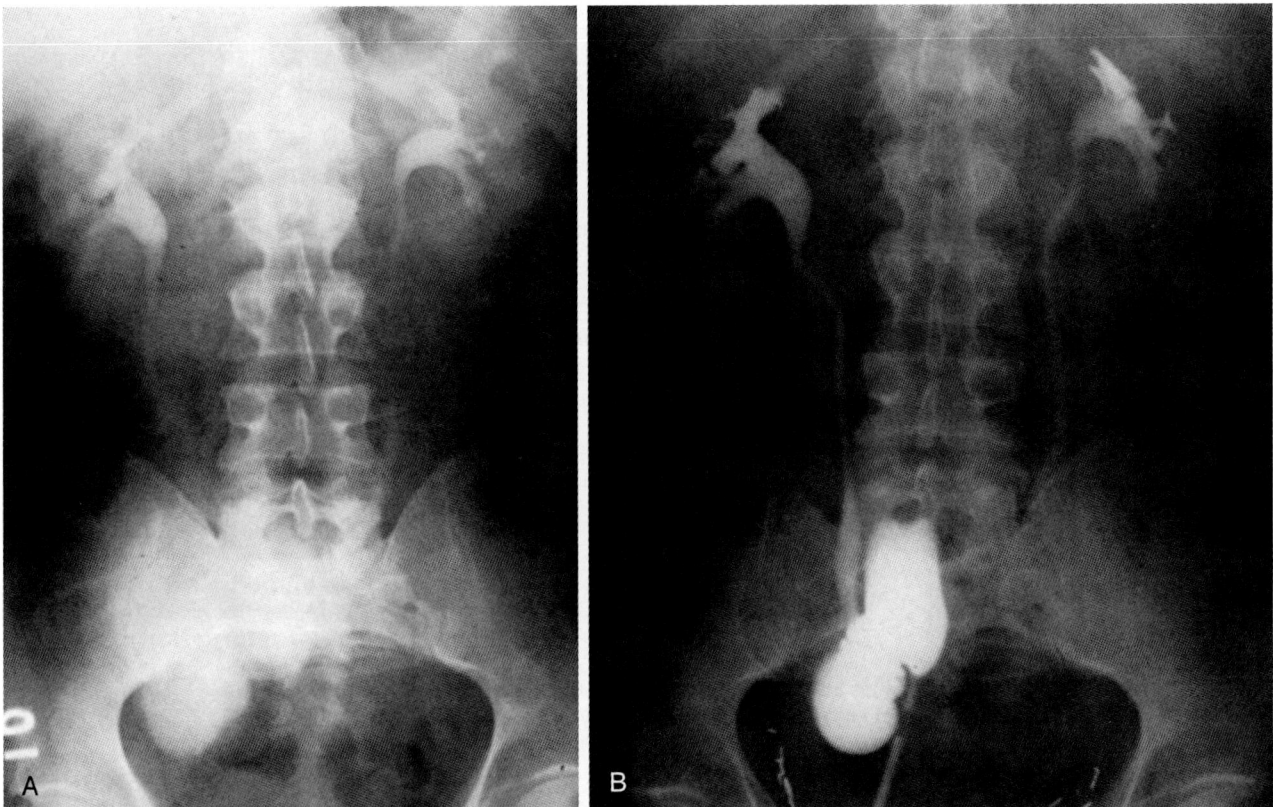

Figure 4-6. Ureteroileal cutaneous anastomosis (ileal loop). **A,** An excretory urogram shows normal upper tracts, but the loop, which overlies the sacrum, is difficult to see clearly. Oblique films are particularly helpful. **B,** A retrograde "loopogram" shows the distal ureteroileal anastomoses at their points of entry into the ileal loop. One normally expects to identify bilateral reflux of contrast-laden urine into the ureters and renal pelves. Note the atypical near-midline location of the stoma. (Reprinted from Spring DB, Deshon GE: Radiology of vesical and supravesical urinary diversions and orthotopic bladder replacements. In Pollack HM, McClennan BL, Dyer R, Kenney PJ [eds]: Clinical Urography, 2nd ed. Philadelphia, WB Saunders, 2000.)

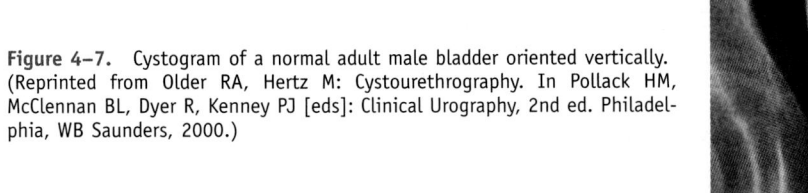

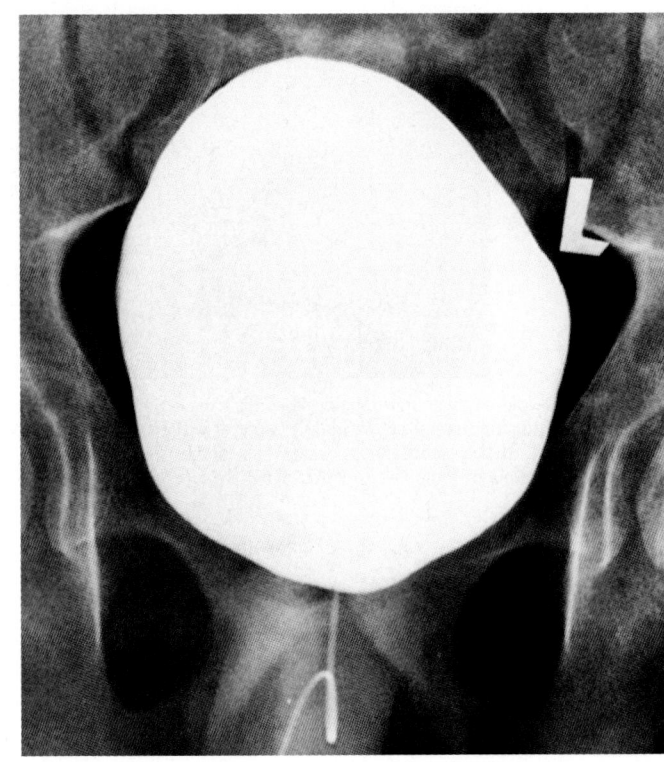

Figure 4-7. Cystogram of a normal adult male bladder oriented vertically. (Reprinted from Older RA, Hertz M: Cystourethrography. In Pollack HM, McClennan BL, Dyer R, Kenney PJ [eds]: Clinical Urography, 2nd ed. Philadelphia, WB Saunders, 2000.)

SECTION II

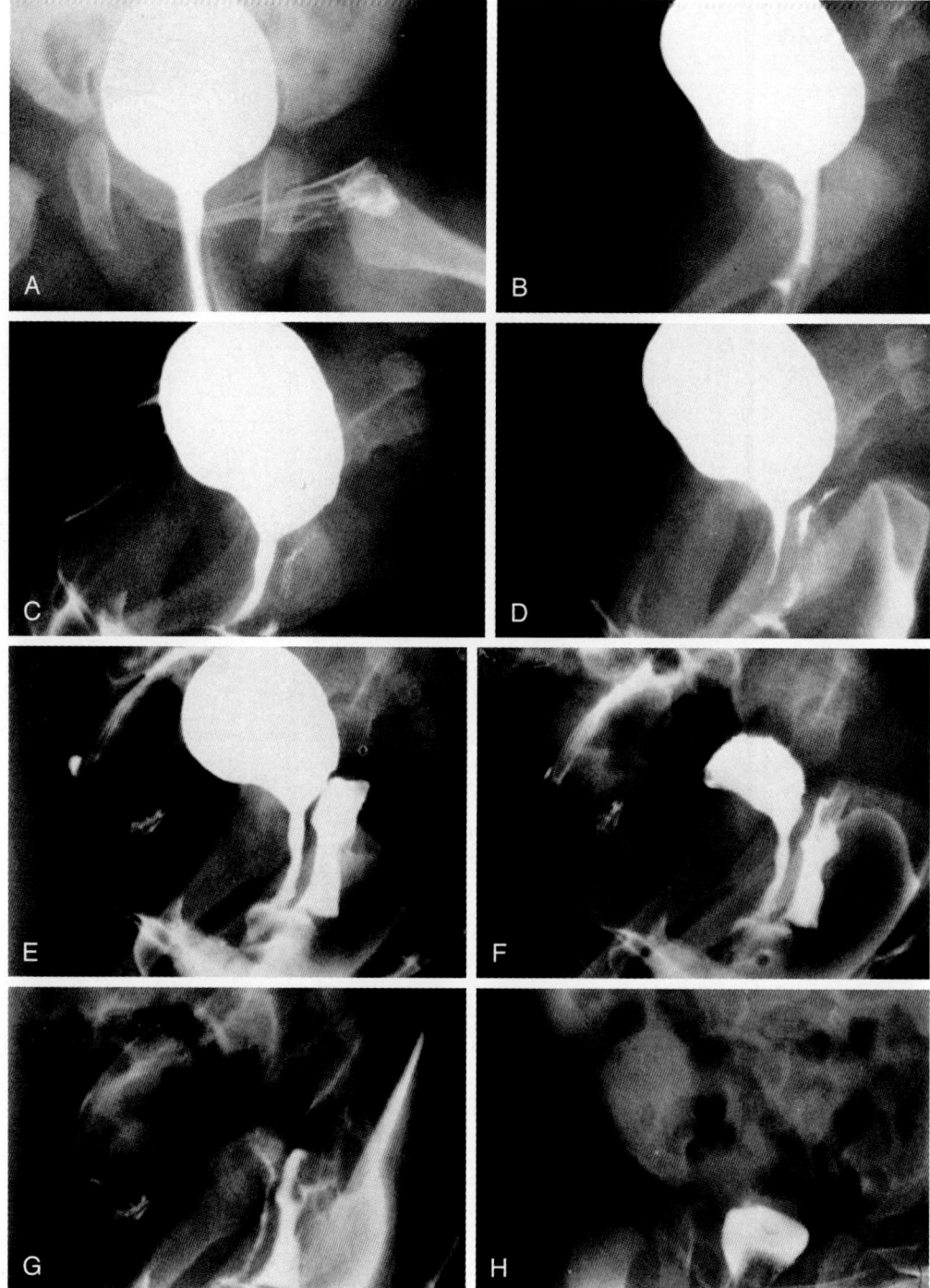

Figure 4–8. Voiding cystourethrogram demonstrating a voiding sequence in an infant girl. **A,** Cystogram, frontal projection. The catheter is still in the urethra. **B,** Cystogram, lateral projection. **C,** Catheter withdrawn; voiding starts. The trigonal canal is formed, and the vagina starts to fill. **D** to **G,** The vagina continues to fill as the bladder empties. **H,** Film in the frontal projection. The bladder is empty whereas the vagina remains filled. (Reprinted from Older RA, Hertz M: Cystourethrography. In Pollack HM, McClennan BL, Dyer R, Kenney PJ [eds]: Clinical Urography, 2nd ed. Philadelphia, WB Saunders, 2000.)

dysfunctional voiding patterns. In adult populations, the indications for VCUG are not well established, but it may be utilized in the evaluation of urethral stricture or bladder or urethral diverticula or to rule out vesicourethral reflux.

Technique. As in most conventional radiographic studies, a scout film is taken first. In the pediatric population, a 5 French or 8 French feeding tube is placed and the bladder is filled with contrast media. Generally, a volume (mL) of (age [years] + 2) × 30 is appropriate for instillation, but this may vary widely based on patient comfort (Berger et al, 1983; Koff, 1983). In the adult population a standard catheter can be used. Films are taken during filling to document bladder pathology and early reflux. Then the patient voids and films are taken during the voiding sequence to document potential reflux and urethral abnormalities (Figs. 4–8 and 4–9). Oblique films are often used to evaluate for grade 1 reflux, which may not be visible on an anteroposterior view. Oblique films are also necessary in evaluation of the male urethra. A postvoid film is also taken.

Retrograde Urethrography

Indications. A retrograde urethrogram (RUG) is used to evaluate the anterior and posterior urethra. It is commonly used to evaluate for urethral stricture and urethral trauma. The study is only rarely performed in the female.

Technique. A Foley catheter (8 to 16 French) is inserted into the fossa navicularis, and the balloon is inflated with 1 to 2 mL. Thirty to 50 percent aqueous contrast solution is gently injected while films are obtained. The patient is typically positioned obliquely, to allow visualization of the entire urethra. Some resistance may be encountered as contrast distends the membranous urethra at the sphincter. A normal male RUG is shown in Figure 4-10.

Retrograde Pyelography

The retrograde pyelogram (RP) is an often-used study to evaluate the renal collecting system and the ureters. It is a unique study in that the operating urologist, as opposed to the radiologist, is intimately involved in the imaging process. The study allows superb visualization of the urothelium of the upper urinary tract but is limited by the need for operating room facilities, anesthesia, and expense.

Indications. The indications for an RP are extensive. Commonly, it is employed in evaluation of hematuria, in lieu of IVU. Patients who possess renal insufficiency, contrast medium sensitivity, or suboptimal IVU imaging are candidates for an RP. Despite the low risk in patients with contrast medium sensitivity, rare anaphylactoid reactions have been described (Johenning, 1980; Weese et al, 1993). Additionally, if the patient is undergoing cystoscopy in the operating suite, many urologists will perform an RP instead of a separate IVU. Retrograde pyelography is also often performed in conjunction with a retrograde or antegrade endourologic procedure, as an anatomic guide to the collecting systems.

Technique. Because the procedure is invasive, a sterile urine culture is preferred. The patient usually requires at least intravenous sedation, and the procedure is usually performed in conjunction with an anesthesiologist in the operating suite. A scout radiograph is taken to evaluate for residual contrast medium and to assess positioning and landmarks. Care should be taken to remove all radiopaque items from the patient's gown, operating room drapes, and table. Light cords for the cystoscope should be positioned out of the field. Typically the procedure is performed with a rigid cystoscope, which is introduced into the bladder and positioned near the ureteral orifice. An injection catheter is introduced into the distal orifice, and contrast medium is injected under real-time fluoroscopy to generate images of the ureter and collecting system (Fig. 4–11). A variety of catheters may be used, which differ in size, length, and end effector. A drainage film may be obtained after 5 to 10 minutes to evaluate clearance of the contrast medium. Generally, contrast media should be diluted to less than 50% to allow adequate opacification without obscuring small filling defects.

Backflow. Backflow occurs when the contrast media extravasates into surrounding tissues (Fig. 4–12) and usually results from relatively high injection pressures (Green et al, 1969). A variety of patterns may be seen, depending on the area of extravasation. Intrarenal backflow occurs when contrast medium enters the collecting ducts. Striations are seen emanating from the calyces when this phenomenon occurs (Thomsen, 1983). Pyelosinus backflow occurs when small tears in the collecting system allow contrast medium to enter the renal sinus (Thomsen et al, 1981). Pyelolymphatic and pyelovenous backflow occurs when extravasated media enter the lymphatic system or the venous system (Bidgood et al, 1981).

Antegrade Urography (Nephrostography)

Antegrade urography is an examination in which contrast medium is injected into the collecting system via an existing nephrostomy tube. The indications for this procedure are limited and highly specialized (Fritzsche, 1986). It may be used in a postsurgical patient to evaluate for urine leak. After percutaneous nephrolithotomy, residual stones can be assessed with this study. It may also be used to evaluate the site of urinary obstruction after a nephrostomy tube has been placed. Ureteral fistulas may be diagnosed with this technique (Ferrie, 1985). The study is performed by injecting contrast medium via an existing nephrostomy tube, and images are taken both of the collecting system and the ureter. A sterile urine culture or antibiotic use is preferred.

ULTRASOUND

Ultrasound is a commonly used modality to image the urinary tract. It has several advantages, including the lack of invasiveness, cost, resolution, and lack of nephrotoxic contrast agent administration. It is also relatively easy to perform in the pediatric population, unlike other cross-sectional techniques, because it does not require the child to be immobilized. Grayscale ultrasound in the current era offers excellent detail and resolution, and the advent of Doppler examinations allows assessment of vascular flow. Although it possesses limitations and is ultimately operator dependent, ultrasound is considered an excellent tool to image selected areas of the urinary tract.

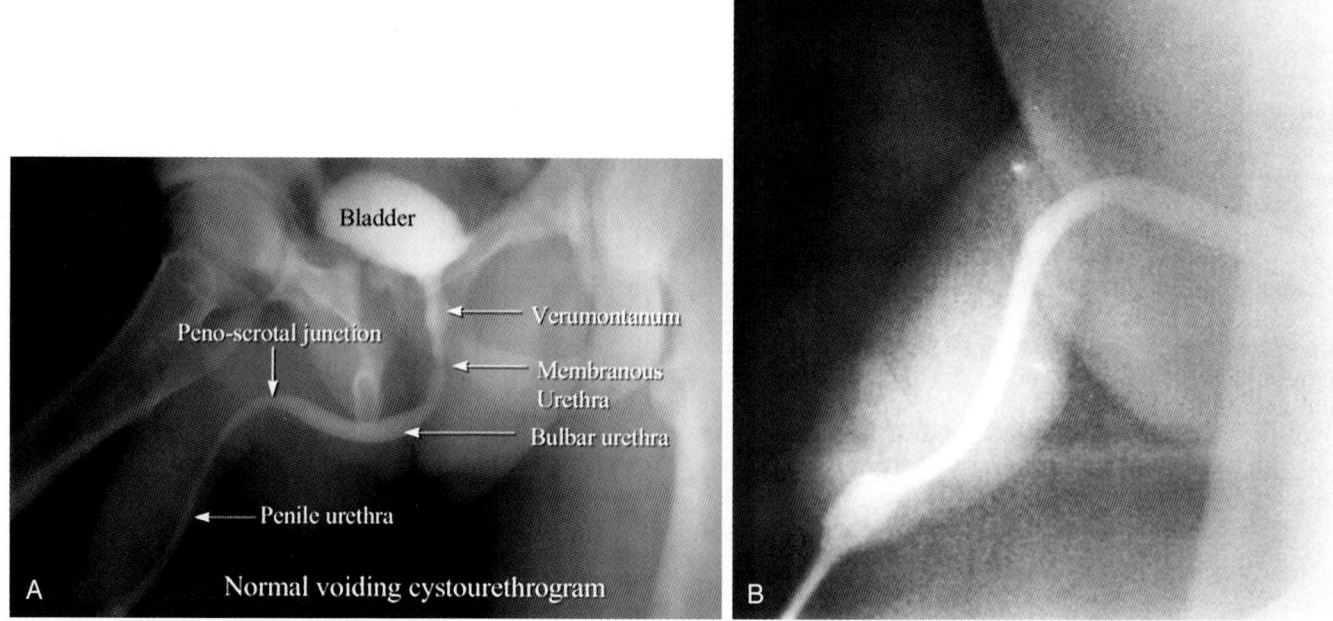

Figure 4-9. **A,** Labeled voiding cystourethrogram (VCU). **B,** VCU in a normal adult male. The most distal part of the urethra shows typical widening of the fossa navicularis. (Reprinted from Older RA, Hertz M: Cystourethrography. In Pollack HM, McClennan BL, Dyer R, Kenney PJ (eds). Clinical Urography, 2nd ed. WB Saunders, Philadelphia, 2000.)

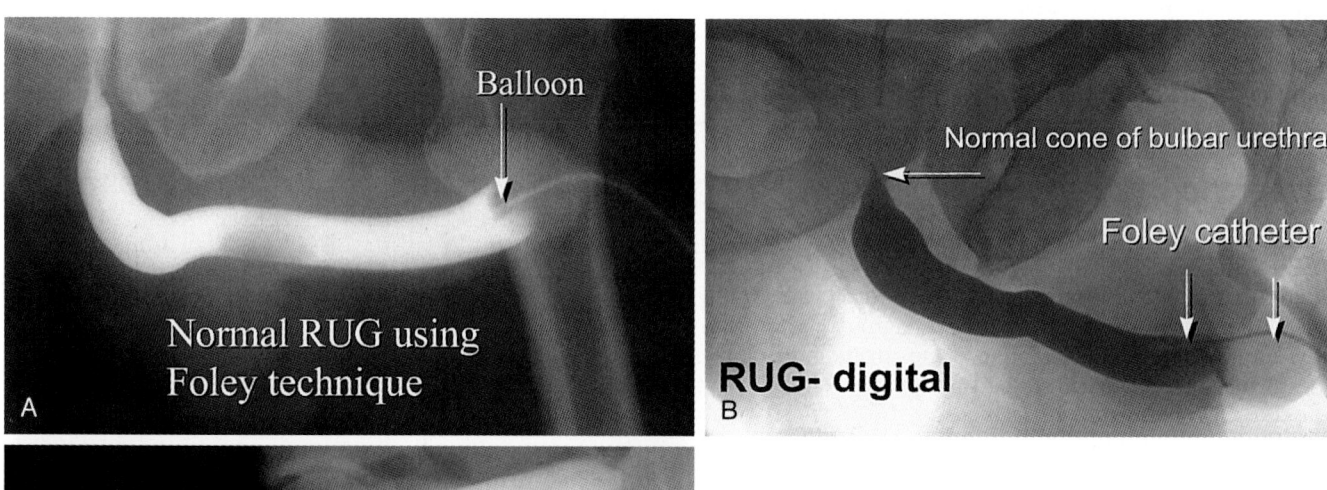

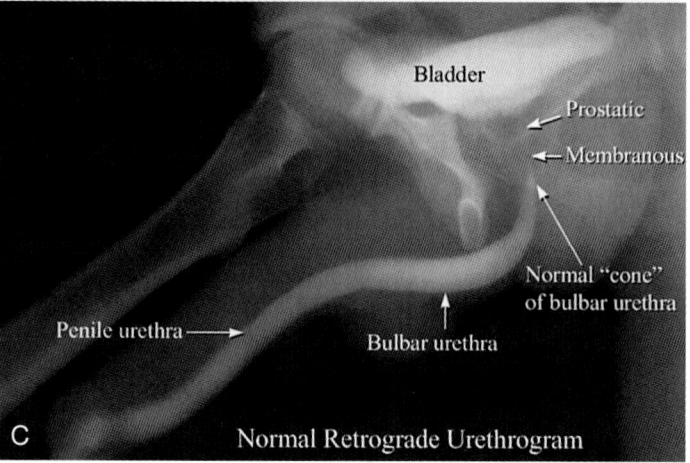

Figure 4-10. **A,** Normal retrograde urethrogram (RUG) using a Foley catheter technique with the Foley balloon in the fossa navicularis. Note the air bubble in the penile urethra (conventional radiographic technique). **B,** Digital retrograde urethrogram using the Foley catheter technique. **C,** Labeled normal retrograde urethrogram. (Reprinted from Older RA, Hertz M: Cystourethrography. In Pollack HM, McClennan BL, Dyer R, Kenney PJ [eds]: Clinical Urography, 2nd ed. Philadelphia, WB Saunders, 2000.)

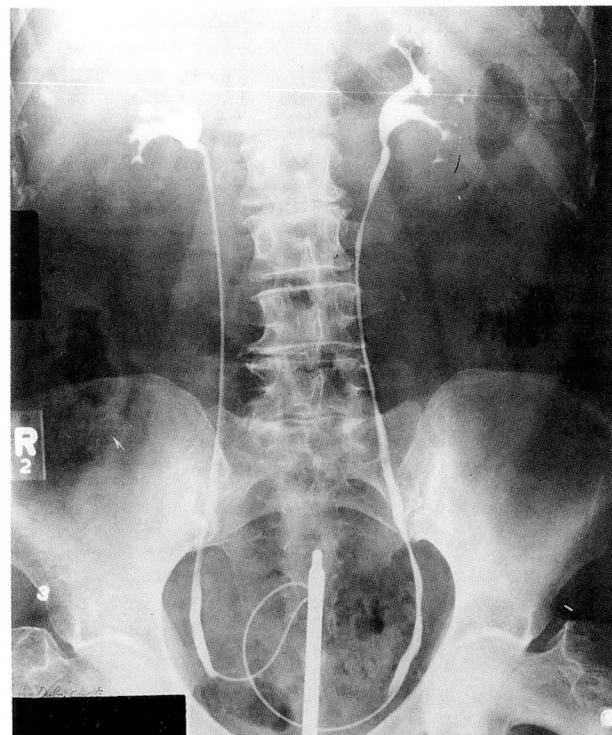

Figure 4–11. Normal retrograde pyelogram. The film demonstrates visualization of the pyelocalyceal system and ureters.

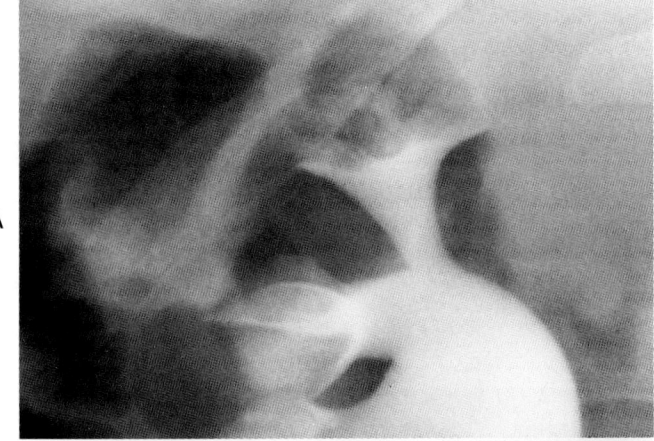

A

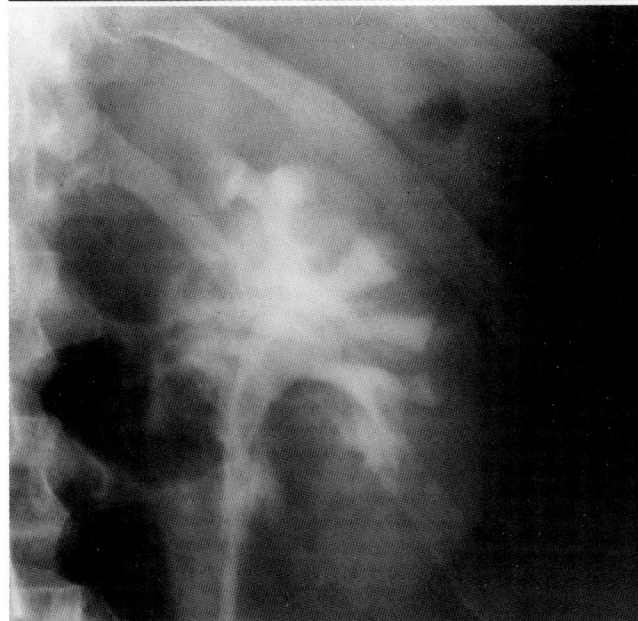

B

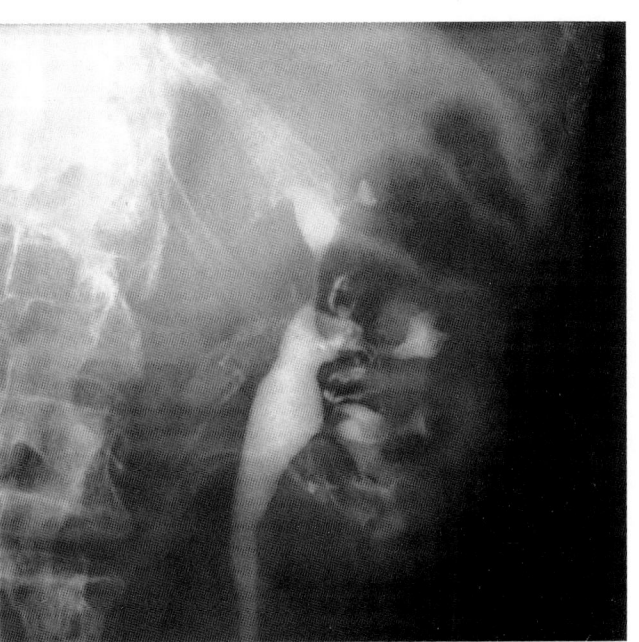

C

Figure 4–12. **A,** Pyelotubular backflow. **B,** Pyelosinus backflow. **C,** Pyelolymphatic backflow.

Ultrasound waves are generated by crystals in the transducer, which are projected into the patient's body. As the sound waves encounter various tissues or interfaces they are reflected back to the transducer. The transducer and ultrasound unit convert this information into a visible picture of the tissues. **As the frequency of the transducer increases, resolution increases but depth of penetration decreases.** Doppler ultrasound relies on the changes in sound waves in relation to moving objects, most notably blood flow. When sound waves encounter moving blood cells, they are reflected back at differing frequencies, thus allowing an assessment of vascular flow.

Renal Ultrasound

Ultrasound of the kidney is an excellent test to evaluate for renal parenchymal abnormalities, differentiate solid from cystic structures, and evaluate hydronephrosis.

It is often used in conjunction with IVP for evaluation of hematuria. It is also useful in assessing renal allografts and congenital renal anomalies. Stones may be identified from their hyperechoic appearance and their acoustical shadow.

The ultrasound anatomy of the kidney derives from the changes in echogenicity of the various tissues within the organ. The renal outline is readily apparent because the echogenicity of the capsule differs from the surrounding fat. Thus, renal size can be accurately assessed with this technique. The central renal sinus fat is highly echogenic, and this area also contains the renal pelvis and branches of the arterial, venous, and lymphatic systems (Fig. 4–13). **The cortex and medulla also can be differentiated, because the medullary pyramids typically are less echogenic than the cortex and they abut the sinus fat.** This corticomedullary differentiation is usually more apparent in children than adults. Doppler evaluation can be used to study the renal vasculature to assess anomalies of flow and location of renal vessels (Fig. 4–14).

Renal ultrasound is often used to differentiate between solid and cystic lesions of the renal parenchyma (Balfe et al, 1982). Simple renal cysts are round, are well defined, are without echogenic foci, and have enhanced through-transmission (Fig. 4–15). Doppler studies can be used to assess for renal artery stenosis and renovascular hypertension (Hansen et al, 1990; Johansson et al, 2000).

Adrenal Ultrasound

Cross-sectional imaging techniques such as CT and magnetic resonance imaging (MRI) are the procedures of choice in imaging the adult adrenal gland. In the pediatric population ultrasound is useful, particularly because of the lack of retroperitoneal fat. The adrenal gland may be assessed for nodules, cysts, hemorrhage, location, and tumors. The right adrenal gland may be easier to image than the left (Yeh, 1980), secondary to the acoustic window provided by the liver; the left adrenal gland may be obscured by the colon or stomach. The adrenal cortex is usually hypoechoic (Gunther et al, 1984), and the adrenal medulla is echogenic (Fig. 4–16); however, this differentiation is difficult to ascertain in adults.

Bladder Ultrasound

Bladder sonography is often combined with renal sonography. It can be used as a technique to examine the bladder wall or intravesical lesions. Although cystoscopy is the accepted standard with which to examine the bladder for mucosal abnormalities, ultrasound may prompt cystoscopic evaluation. In the pediatric population, ultrasound can be used to diagnose congenital anomalies, such as ectopic ureterocele. Ultrasound of the bladder may be performed via a transabdominal, transvaginal, or transrectal approach. The transabdominal approach is the most often used technique. Visualization is

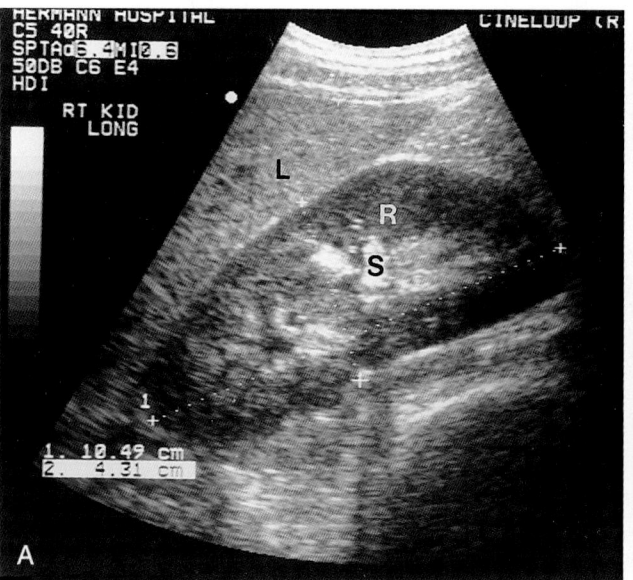 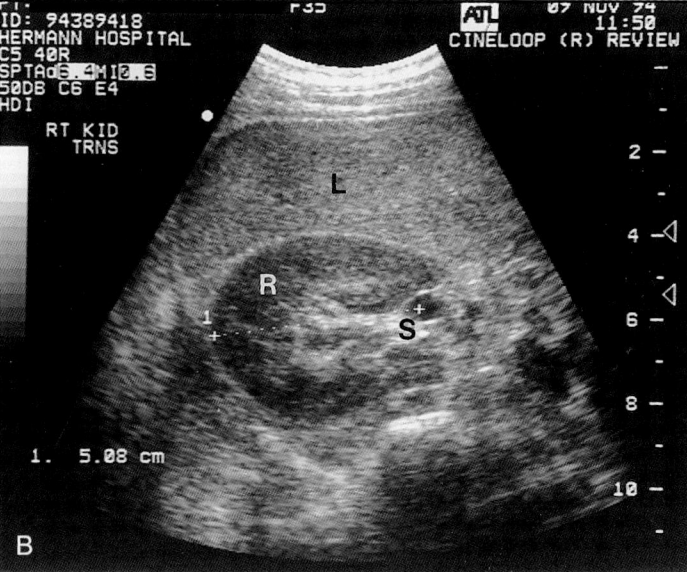

Figure 4–13. Gray-scale ultrasonography of the normal kidney. Longitudinal **(A)** and transverse **(B)** ultrasound views outline the contour of the right kidney (R), the parenchyma of which is hypoechoic relative to the liver (L). The renal sinus fat (S) appears echogenic.

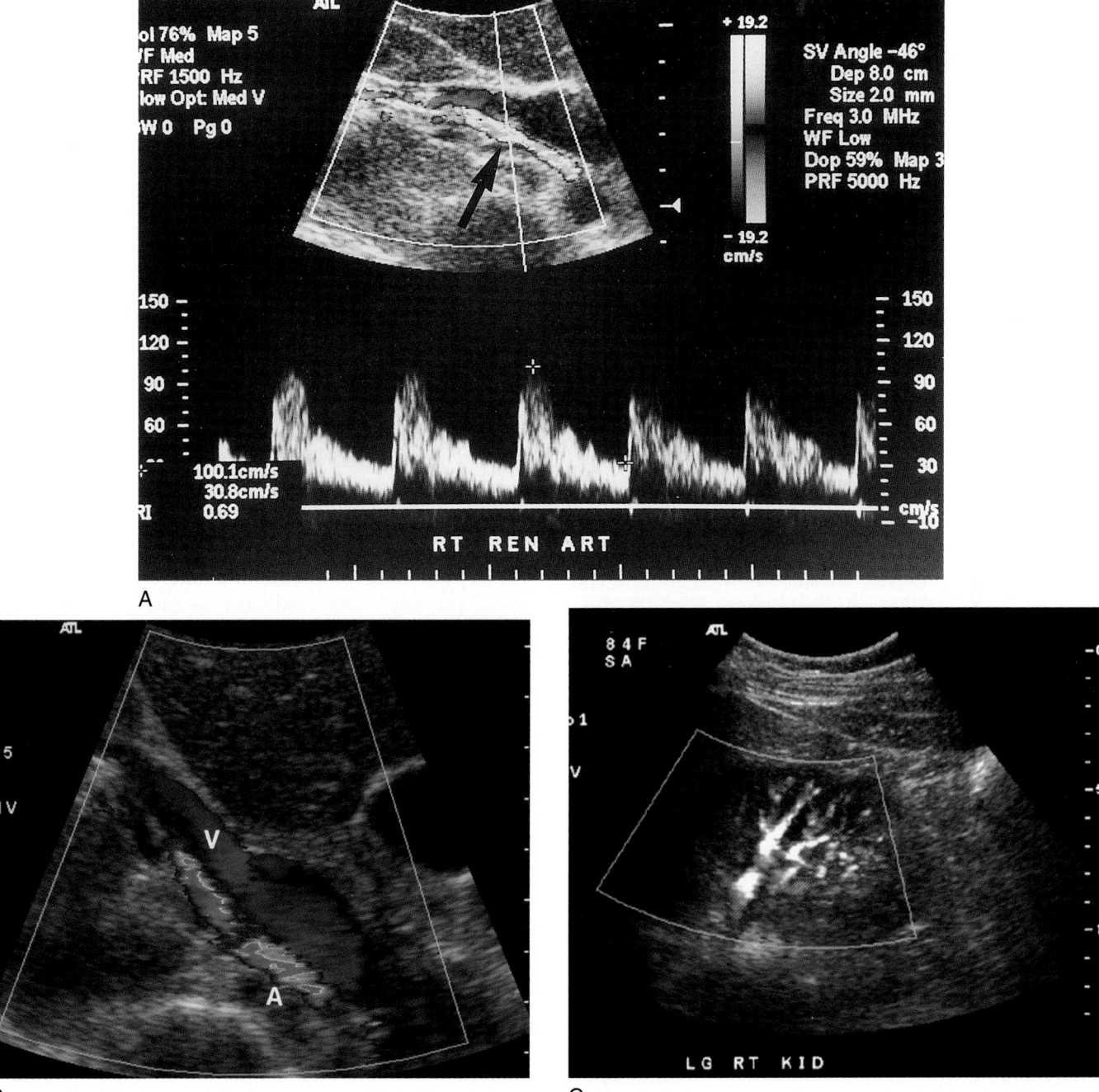

Figure 4–14.   A, Duplex Doppler ultrasonography of the proximal main renal artery. The Doppler gate is positioned over the right main renal artery *(arrow).* The resulting waveform is displayed below the gray scale. The resistive index of the right renal artery measured 0.69 (peak systolic velocity divided by end-diastolic velocity), which is within the normal range. **B,** Color-mode Doppler ultrasonography of the main renal artery. Color-mode Doppler imaging of the right main renal artery uses a color map to display information based on the detection of frequency shifts from moving targets. The right main renal artery (A) is encoded in shades of red, representing blood flow toward the transducer, whereas the right renal vein (V) is displayed in blue, indicative of blood flow away from the transducer. **C,** Power-mode Doppler imaging of the intrarenal arteries. A long view of a power-mode Doppler imaging of the right kidney reveals the detailed detection of blood flow. The color sensitivity of power-mode Doppler ultrasonography is superior to that of conventional color Doppler ultrasonography in depicting flow in the intrarenal arteries. However, power-mode Doppler imaging does not provide any information about velocity or the direction of blood flow. (**C,** courtesy of P. Chen, University of Texas-Houston Medical School, Houston.)

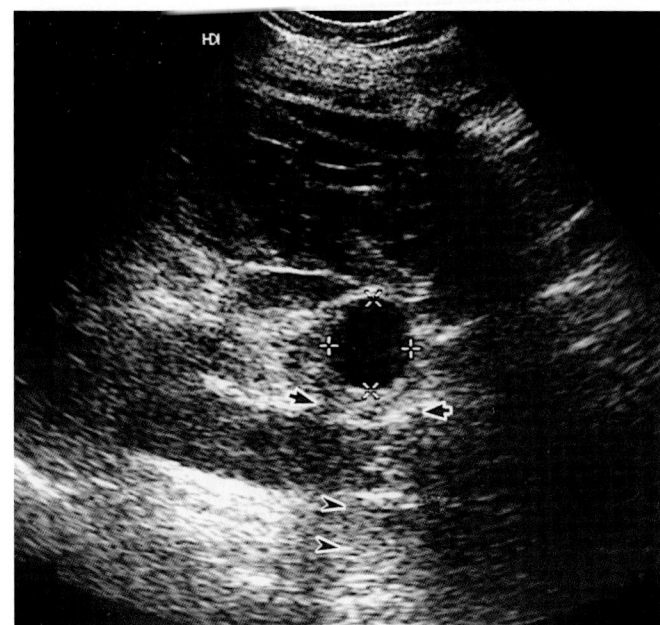

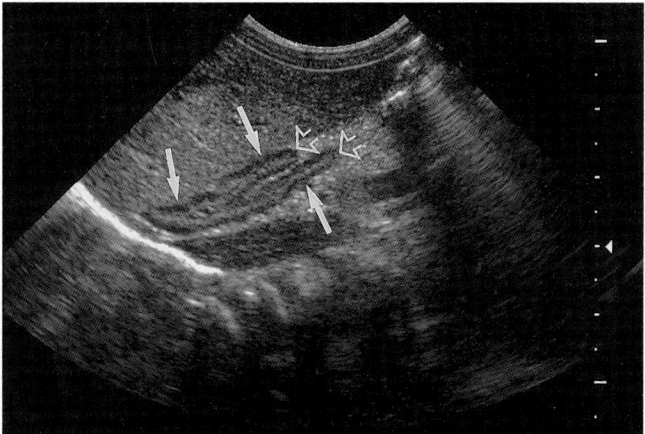

Figure 4–16. Normal adrenal gland in a neonate. A longitudinal ultrasound view of the right adrenal gland *(solid arrows)* demonstrates a thin echogenic medulla with a rim of the hypoechoic cortex. The caudal right adrenal gland has two limbs *(open arrows)*.

Figure 4–15. A simple renal cyst *(calipers)* is completely anechoic. Edge refraction-linear black posterior shadowing from the lateral edges of the cyst *(small arrows)* and increased through-transmission and increased brightness posterior to the cyst *(arrowheads)* are also noted. (From Scoutt LM, et al: Ultrasound evaluation of the urinary tract. In Pollack HM, McClennan BL, Dyer R, Kenney PJ [eds]: Clinical Urography, 2nd ed. Philadelphia, WB Saunders, 2000.)

enhanced with a distended bladder, and the patient is instructed to postpone voiding and maintain hydration before imaging.

The normal anatomy of the bladder may vary. The shape is ideally symmetrical, and fluid in the bladder lacks internal echoes (Fig. 4–17). The normal bladder wall is less than or equal to 6 mm thick. The bladder wall may have some thickening secondary to outlet obstruction, but asymmetry in wall thickness may indicate a mucosal or infiltrative abnormality (Fig. 4–18). Debris, foreign bodies, or infection may render a degree of echogenicity to the fluid within the bladder. Postvoid residual urine and bladder volume may be addressed.

Ureteral jets may also be seen with the use of Doppler ultrasound in a well-hydrated patient (Fig. 4–19). Importantly, a ureteral jet may be seen with a partial ureteral obstruction. The bladder must be partially distended and visualization occurs at the bladder base. **A ureteral jet should appear within 15 minutes of observation, unless some degree of obstruction exists** (Burge et al, 1991). The imaging of ureteral jets, however, is highly user dependent, and difficulty with visualization may be limited by a variety of technical and physiologic factors (Baker and Middleton, 1992).

Prostate Ultrasound

The prostate is best imaged sonographically via a transrectal approach. This approach also offers access for prostate biopsy. Ultrasound of the prostate is discussed in detail in Chapter 92, Ultrasonography and Biopsy of the Prostate.

Scrotal Ultrasound

Ultrasound is the procedure of choice in diagnosing and evaluating intrascrotal pathology. A variety of testicular and extratesticular lesions may be visualized. Color Doppler imaging can be used to assess vascular flow, which is crucial in diagnosing some intrascrotal diseases. Because the scrotal contents are superficial in location, high-frequency ultrasound probes (up to 10 MHz) may be utilized, producing excellent resolution. Although MRI, CT, and nuclear scintigraphy are occasionally used to image the scrotum, ultrasound offers superb imaging at a reasonable cost. Scrotal ultrasound may be used to identify testicular and extratesticular masses. Other indications include the evaluation of testicular pain, assessment for testicular torsion, identification of orchitis or epididymitis, and evaluation of hydroceles, hernias, and varicoceles.

Scrotal ultrasound is best performed in a slightly warm room with the patient in the supine position. Acoustic gel is necessary as an interface, and direct examination of the testes at the time of ultrasound can guide the examination. The testis has a granular sonographic appearance and measures approximately 4 cm in length and 3 cm in width (Fig. 4–20). A small amount of fluid is normally present in the tunica vaginalis, but this compartment may be more prominent when a hydrocele is present. The normal appendix testis is not usually visible under routine ultrasound examination. The epididymis is isoechoic or slightly hyperechoic to the testis. **Veins larger than 2 mm may be seen when a varicocele is present but often require evaluation in the erect position and/or with the Valsalva maneuver.** Doppler evaluation can show alterations in vascular flow, which may be helpful in the diagnosis of scrotal pathology (Figs. 4–21 and 4–22).

Urethral Ultrasound

Ultrasound of the male urethra can be useful in the evaluation of urethral stricture. A transducer could be placed longitudinally along the phallus, or intraluminal ultrasound can be

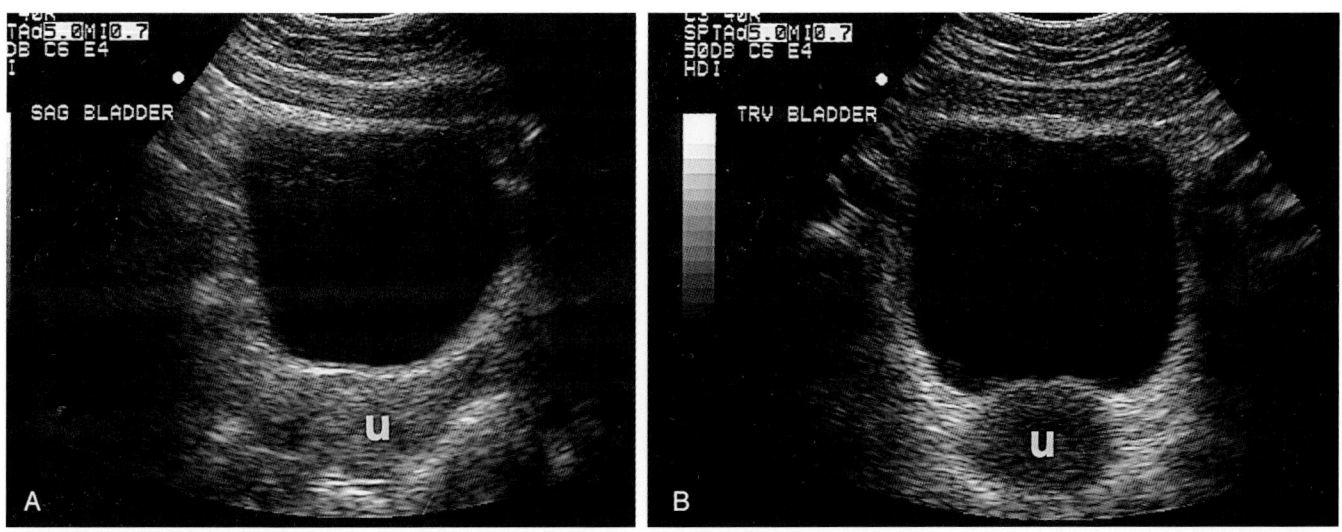

Figure 4–17. Sagittal **(A)** and transverse **(B)** transabdominal images of the distended urinary bladder anterior to the uterus (U). Note that the bladder wall is thin, smooth, and regular. (From Scoutt LM, et al: Ultrasound evaluation of the urinary tract. In Pollack HM, McClennan BL, Dyer R, Kenney PJ [eds]: Clinical Urography, 2nd ed. Philadelphia, WB Saunders, 2000.)

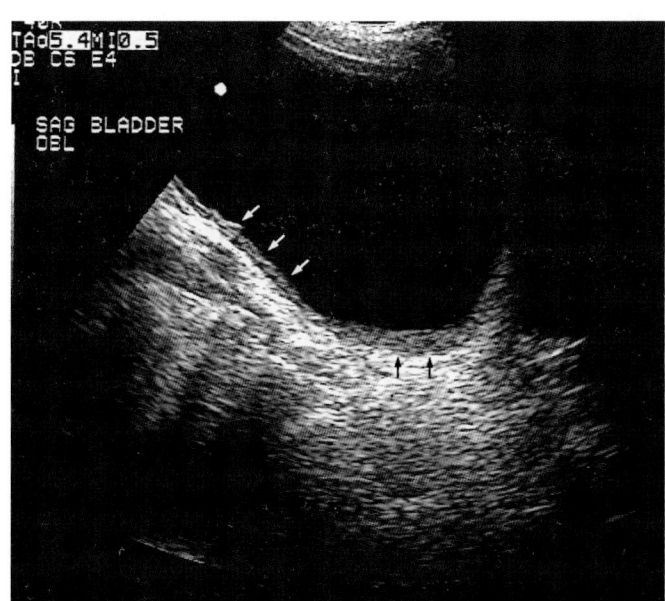

Figure 4–18. A sagittal image of the bladder from a patient with recurrent cystitis reveals irregular thickening of the bladder wall *(white arrows)* and dependent layering debris *(black arrows)*. (From Scoutt LM, et al: Ultrasound evaluation of the urinary tract. In Pollack HM, McClennan BL, Dyer R, Kenney PJ [eds]: Clinical Urography, 2nd ed. Philadelphia, WB Saunders, 2000.)

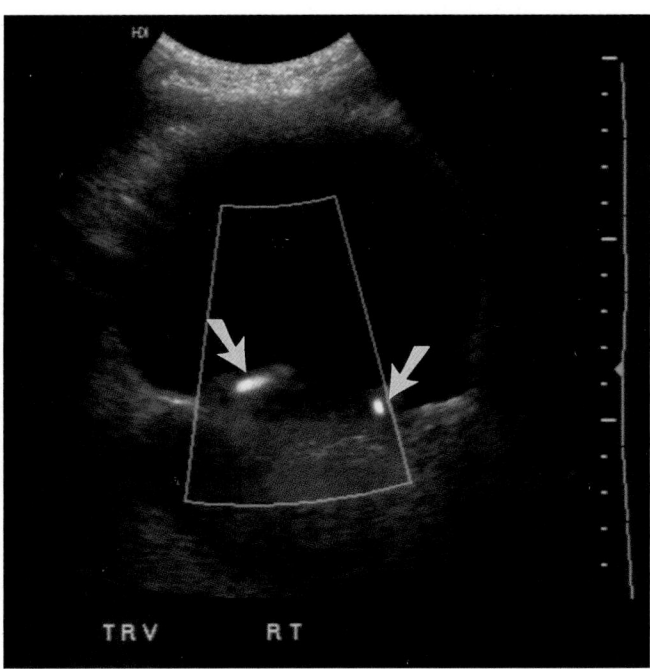

Figure 4–19. Ureteral jet phenomena. A transverse view of a power-mode Doppler ultrasonogram of the lower bladder reveals a urine jet from the orifice of the ureter bilaterally *(arrows)*, indicative of ureteral orifice patency. (Courtesy of U.M. Hamper, Johns Hopkins University, Baltimore.)

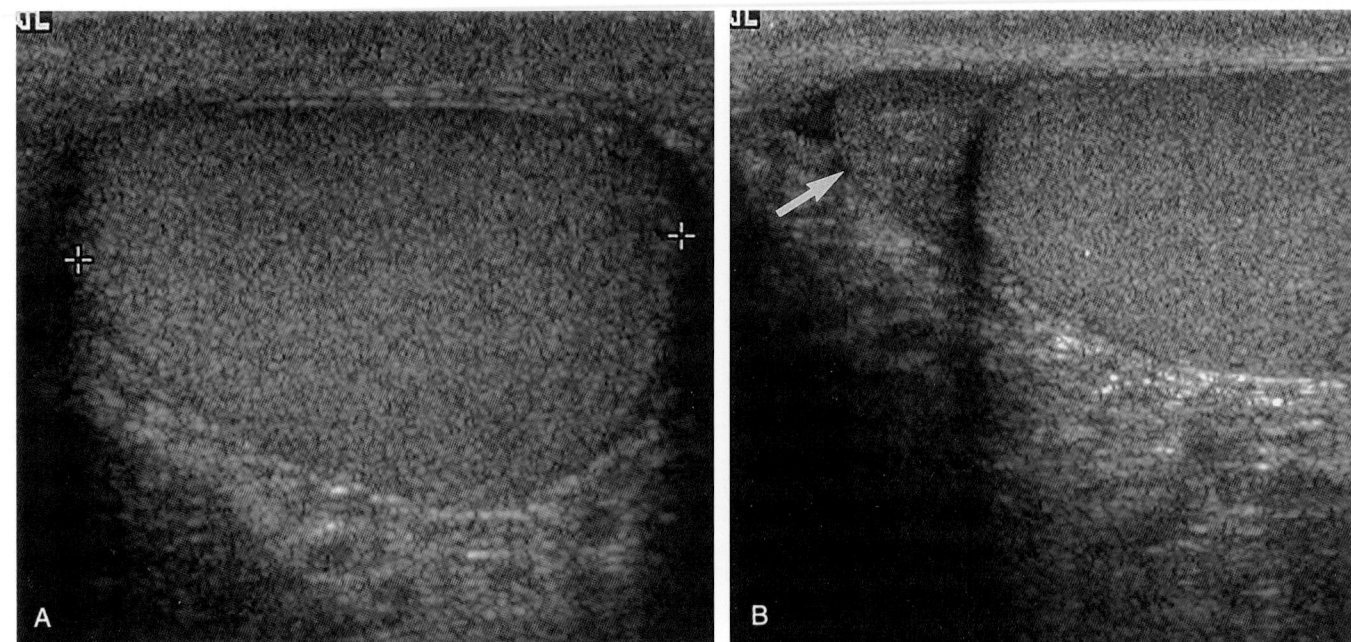

Figure 4–20. Normal testis and epididymal head. **A,** Longitudinal view of a scrotal ultrasonogram reveals the homogeneous texture of the right testis. The mediastinum of the testis *(not shown)* appears as an elongated echogenic structure extending craniocaudally on the posterolateral side of the testis. **B,** Longitudinal view demonstrates a normal head of the epididymis *(arrow)*.

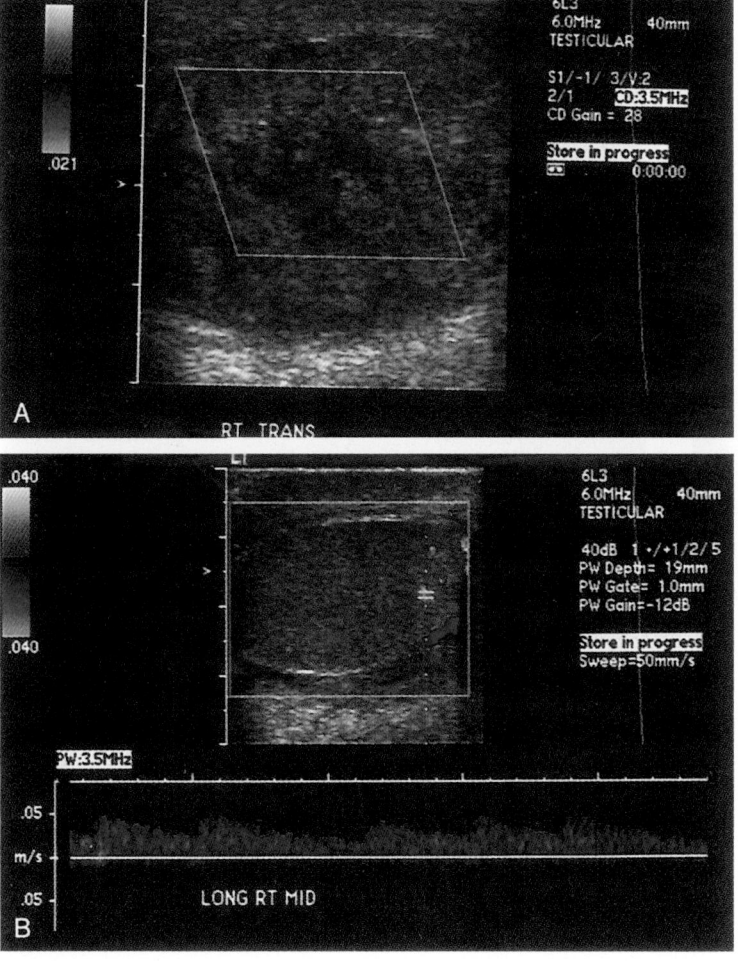

Figure 4–21. A transverse image **(A)** of the right testis in a patient with acute right testicular pain reveals no blood flow on color Doppler interrogation *(box)*. In this clinical setting these findings are diagnostic of testicular infarction. For comparison, a longitudinal image **(B)** of the right testis in an asymptomatic patient reveals normal testicular blood flow. (From Scoutt LM, et al: Ultrasound evaluation of the urinary tract. In Pollack HM, McClennan BL, Dyer R, Kenney PJ [eds]: Clinical Urography, 2nd ed. Philadelphia, WB Saunders, 2000.)

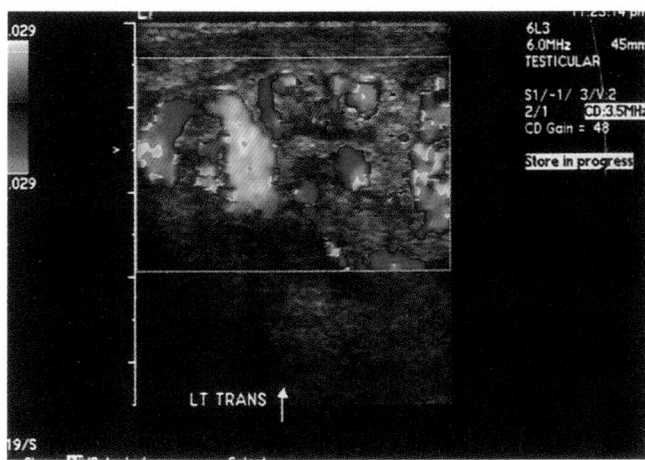

Figure 4–22. Color Doppler evaluation of a patient with acute left testicular pain and fever revealed diffuse increased vascularity in the left testis consistent with orchitis. (From Scoutt LM, et al: Ultrasound evaluation of the urinary tract. In Pollack HM, McClennan BL, Dyer R, Kenney PJ [eds]: Clinical Urography, 2nd ed. Philadelphia, WB Saunders, 2000.)

performed via a transurethral transducer. The technique may be valuable in assessing stricture length and possibly the degree and depth of fibrosis (Fig. 4–23) (McAninch et al, 1988; Pavlica et al, 2003). In the female patient, urethral ultrasound is highly useful in the diagnosis and evaluation of urethral diverticulum (Siegel et al, 1998).

COMPUTED TOMOGRAPHY

CT is rapidly becoming a mainstay of imaging of the urinary tract. It is particularly useful when imaging the kidneys and adrenal glands and is also beneficial in the evaluation of urolithiasis. CT has certain advantages over the IVU: it offers

better visualization of the renal parenchyma and it may delineate nonurologic issues. Modern CT scanners are helical or spiral scanners (Fielding et al, 1999; Schreyer et al, 2002). With prior generation scanners, a sectional film would be taken at defined slices as the patient was moved along the table. Current helical scanners allow a constant image to be generated as the patient is moved rapidly along the scanner. In addition to the time savings of such an approach, a number of images can be generated and reconstructed depending on the needs of the study. Three-dimensional reconstruction can also be performed (Leder and Nelson, 2001).

A variety of protocols may be used depending on the imaging feature that is needed, and an exhaustive review of these protocols is beyond the reach of this chapter. Generally, noncontrast images are useful to evaluate for urolithiasis and gross renal abnormalities. Contrast images are useful to evaluate the renal parenchyma and adrenal lesions. Three-dimensional reconstructions and CT angiography may be useful to view fine aspects of the vascular system. Figure 4–24 demonstrates normal CT images of the genitourinary tract.

Contrast Media

Oral contrast media are not typically needed for evaluation of most urologic issues, but opacification of the bowel loops may aid in distinguishing them from genitourinary structures. An oral contrast agent is given at a defined time interval before scanning to allow the agent to travel to the distal intestines. Oral contrast media may make visualization of the ureters more difficult, particularly if the contrast agent is evident near a suspected stone.

Intravenous contrast media are very helpful in visualization of the kidneys, adrenal glands, and the vasculature. A variety of protocols to image these structures exist. Most commonly, 100 to 150 mL of contrast agent is given as a bolus injection. Precontrast images and a series of postcontrast images are

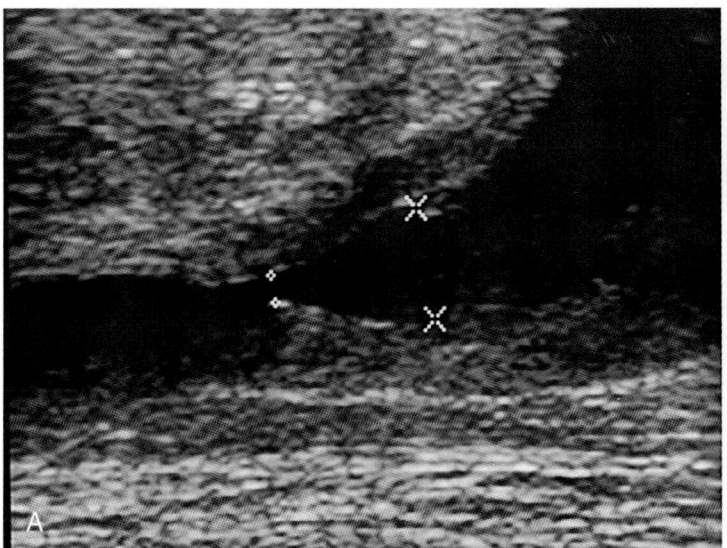

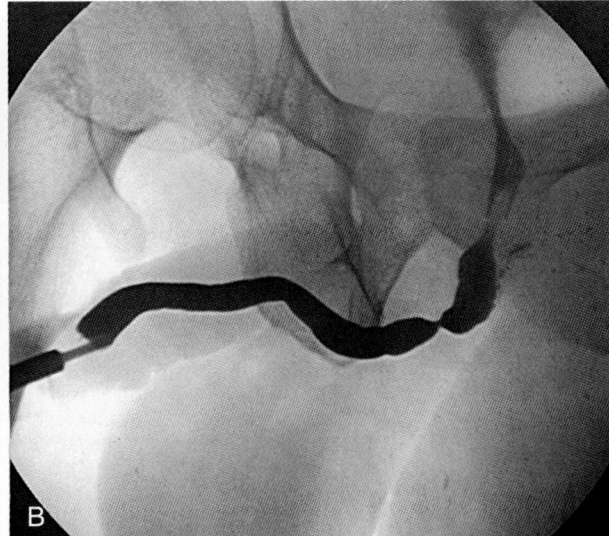

Figure 4–23. Urethral stricture in an adult male patient. Sonographic evaluation shows the urethral caliber (X) in detail. Scar tissue and the extent of stricture are well defined. Retrograde urethrography using a vacuum suction cannula reveals a midbulbar stricture. Also note reflux into Cowper's gland and good definition of the verumontanum. (Courtesy of Cary Lynn Siegel, MD, Mallinckrodt Institute of Radiology.)

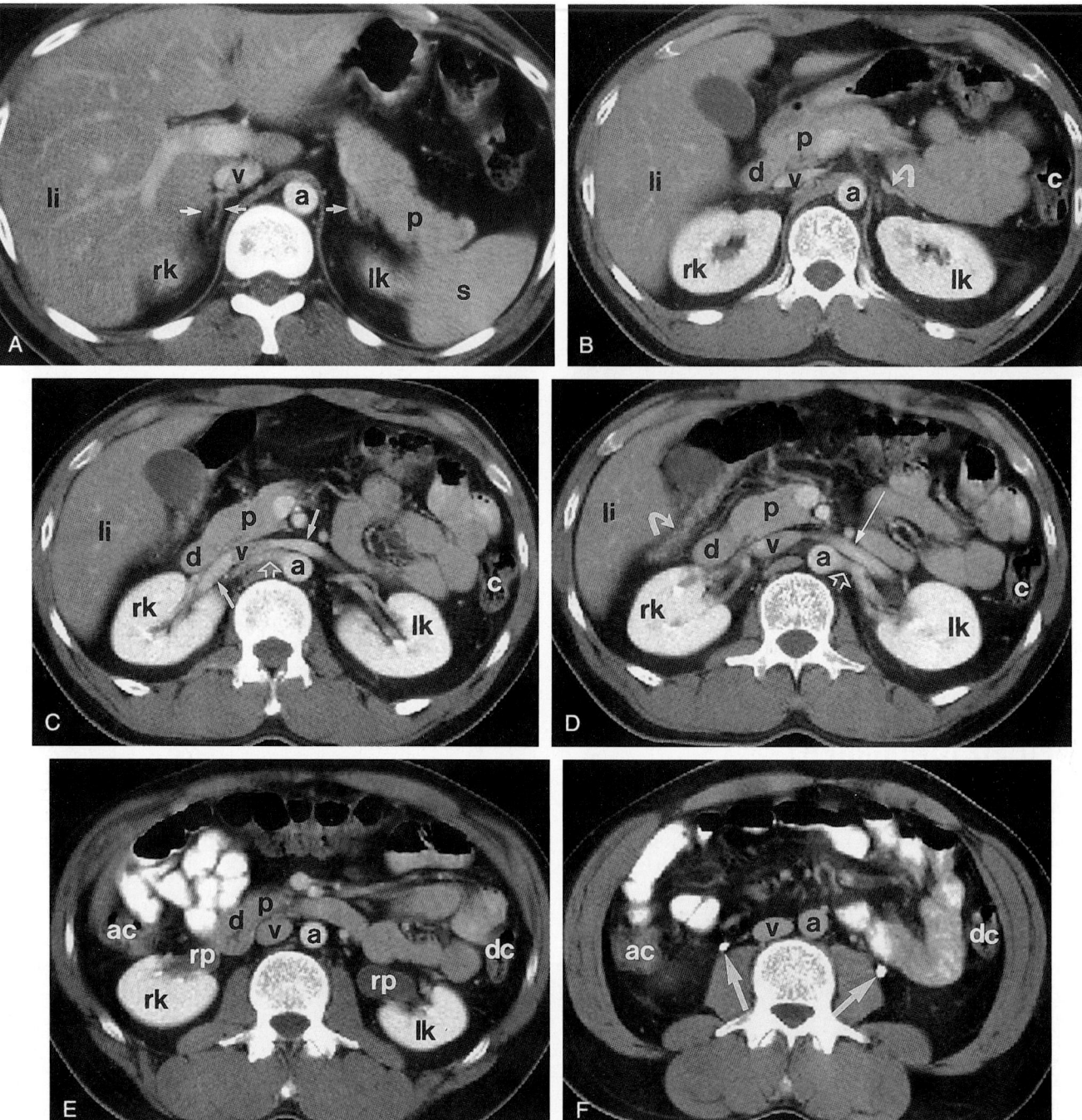

Figure 4–24. Normal anatomy of the genitourinary tract. **A,** The adrenal glands are indicated with *arrows*. The upper pole of the right and left kidneys is indicated with rk and lk, respectively. a, aorta; li, liver; p, pancreas; s, spleen; v, inferior vena cava. **B,** Scan through the upper pole of the kidneys. The left adrenal gland is indicated with an *arrow*. a, aorta; c, colon; d, duodenum; li, liver; lk, left kidney; p, pancreas; rk, right kidney; v, inferior vena cava. **C,** Scan through the hilum of the kidneys. The main renal veins are indicated with *solid arrows,* and the right main renal artery is indicated with an *open arrow.* a, aorta; c, colon; d, duodenum; li, liver; lk, left kidney; p, pancreas; rk, right kidney; v, inferior vena cava. **D,** Scan through the hilum of the kidneys slightly caudal to **C.** The left main renal vein is indicated with a *solid straight arrow,* and the left main renal artery is indicated with an *open arrow.* The hepatic flexure of the colon is indicated with a *curved arrow.* a, aorta; c, colon; d, duodenum; li, liver; lk, left kidney; p, pancreas; rk, right kidney; v, inferior vena cava. **E,** Scan through the mid to lower polar region of the kidneys. a, aorta; ac, ascending colon; d, duodenum; dc, descending colon; lk, left kidney; p, pancreas; rk, right kidney; rp, renal pelvis; v, inferior vena cava. **F,** CT scan obtained below the kidneys reveals filling of the upper ureters *(arrows).* The wall of the normal ureter is usually paper thin or not visible on CT. a, aorta; ac, ascending colon; dc, descending colon; v, inferior vena cava.

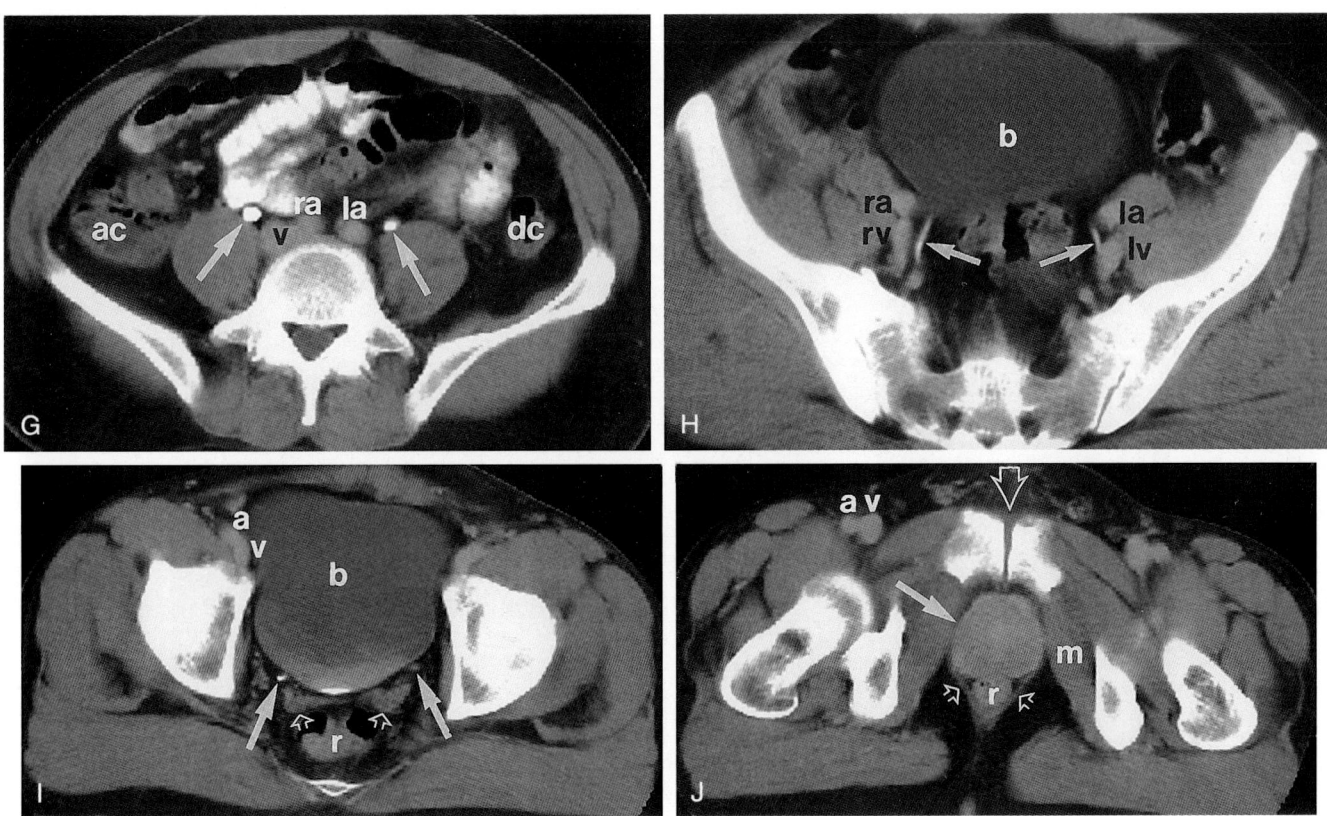

Figure 4–24—Cont'd G, Contrast filling of the midureters *(arrows)* on a scan obtained at the level of the iliac crest and below the aortic bifurcation. ac, ascending colon; dc, descending colon; la, left common iliac artery; ra, right common iliac artery; v, inferior vena cava. **H,** The distal ureters *(arrows)* course medial to the iliac vessels on a scan obtained below the promontory of the sacrum. b, urinary bladder; la, left external iliac artery; lv, left external iliac vein; ra, right external iliac artery; rv, right external iliac vein. **I,** Scan through the roof of the acetabulum reveals distal ureters *(solid arrows)* near the ureterovesical junction. The bladder (b) is filled with urine and partially opacified with contrast material. The normal seminal vesicle *(open arrows)* usually has a paired bow-tie structure with slightly lobulated contour. a, right external iliac artery; r, rectum; v, right external iliac vein. **J,** Scan at the level of the pubic symphysis *(open arrow)* reveals the prostate gland *(solid arrow)*. a, right external iliac artery; m, obturator internus muscle; r, rectum; v, right external iliac vein.

taken to evaluate all phases of enhancement. Delayed views are useful to generate a CT urogram.

Evaluation of Urolithiasis

Unenhanced CT has become the imaging modality of choice for evaluation of urolithiasis (Fig. 4–25) (Fielding et al, 1998; Chen and Zagoria, 1999; Sourtzis et al, 1999). Although IVU was historically used, the immediate availability of CT, combined with the lack of need for contrast medium enhancement, the rapid acquisition of images, and the high sensitivity have been major reasons for CT supplanting IVU. CT also allows assessment of coincident pathology such as hydronephrosis and periureteral and perinephric inflammation, which may be useful if a stone has passed. Furthermore, in the patient with flank pain, CT may identify nonurologic causes if a stone is not present. A further evaluation of CT for diagnosis of urolithiasis is presented in Chapter 43, Evaluation and Medical Management of Urinary Lithiasis.

Renal CT

Enhanced CT of the kidneys is useful in addressing the renal mass. Because renal lesions may not appear on certain phases,

a multiphase imaging protocol is needed. Imaging of the kidneys during an unenhanced (precontrast) phase, corticomedullary phase, nephrographic phase, and pyelographic phase allows broad visualization and maximizes the ability to detect renal pathology (Yuh and Cohan, 1999). The unenhanced phase allows assessment of possible urolithiasis, visualization of parenchymal and vascular calcifications, and a general view of renal contour. The corticomedullary phase, which occurs approximately 30 seconds after contrast agent injection, shows distinction between the cortex and medulla. At approximately 100 seconds, the nephrographic phase is entered, which shows uniform enhancement of the parenchyma (Fig. 4–26). Renal masses are more easily detected in this phase (Fig. 4–27) (Cohan et al, 1995; Birnbaum et al, 1996). The pyelographic, or excretory phase, is entered when contrast medium fills the collecting system.

CT produces excellent anatomic detail of the normal kidney. The kidneys are surrounded by perinephric fat, which appears dark. The renal capsule cannot be delineated from the renal parenchyma. The renal parenchyma appears homogeneous on unenhanced and later phase– enhanced CT. During the corticomedullary phase, the cortex and medulla can be distinguished. The renal veins are readily visualized; the left renal vein can be seen coursing anterior to the aorta and

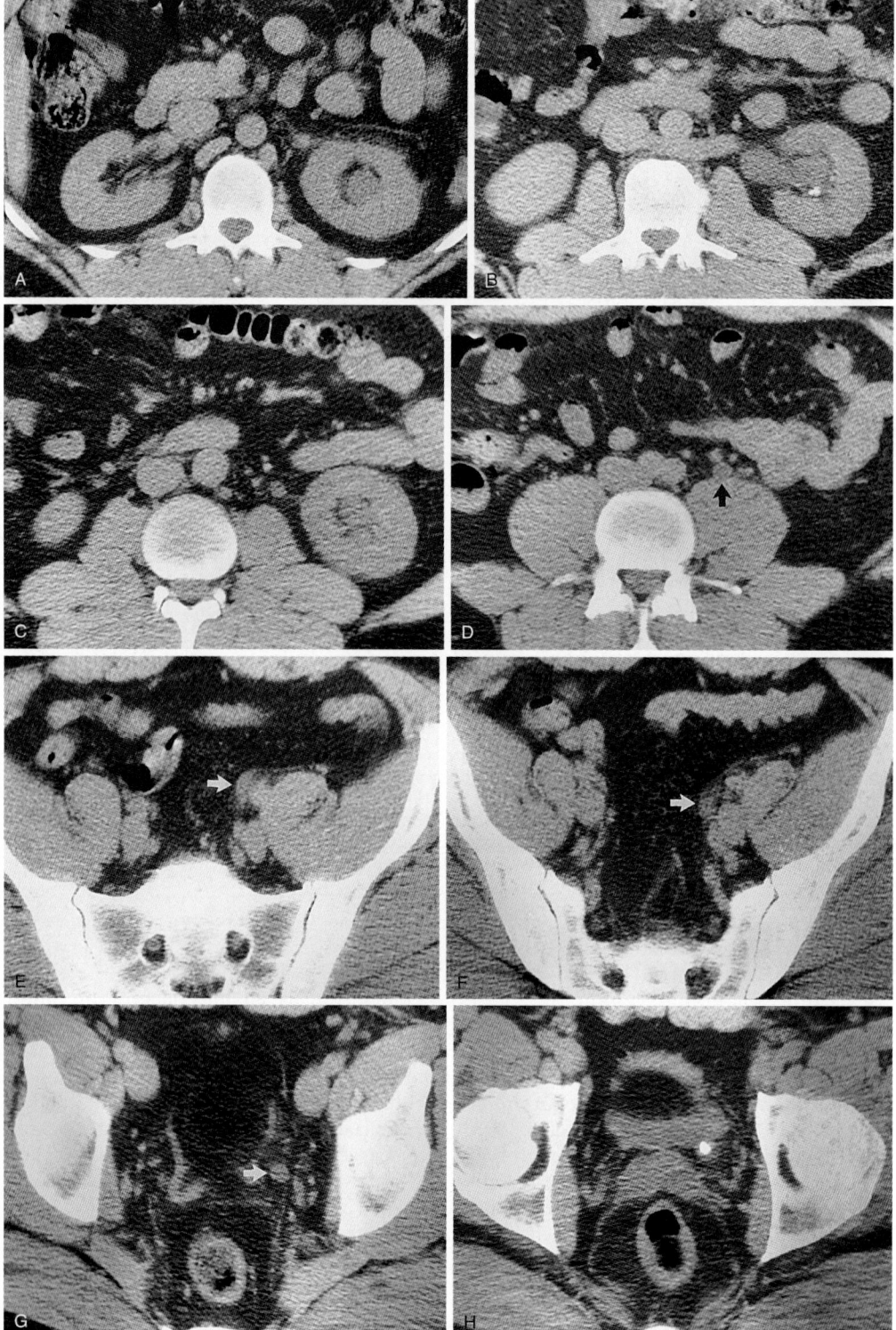

Figure 4–25. Typical findings on helical, non–contrast-enhanced CT in a patient with an obstructing ureterovesical junction (UVJ) stone. Follow the left ureter on axial images. **A,** Level of the left upper pole. Mild renal enlargement, caliectasis, and perinephric stranding are apparent. **B,** Level of the left renal hilum. Left pyelectasis with a dependent stone, mild peripelvic and perinephric stranding, and a retroaortic left renal vein are shown. **C,** Level of the left lower pole. Left caliectasis, proximal ureterectasis, and mild periureteral stranding are present. **D,** Level of the aortic bifurcation. The dilated left ureter *(arrow)* has lower attenuation than do nearby vessels. **E,** Level of the upper portion of the sacrum. A dilated left ureter *(arrow)* crosses anteromedial to the common iliac artery. **F,** Level of the mid sacrum. A dilated left ureter *(arrow)* is accompanied by periureteral stranding. **G,** Level of the top of the acetabulum showing a dilated pelvic portion of the left ureter *(arrow)*. **H,** Level of the UVJ. The impacted stone with a "cuff" or "tissue rim" sign that represents the edematous wall of the ureter. (Reprinted from Talner LB, O'Reilly PH, Wasserman NF: Specific causes of obstruction. In Pollack HM, McClennan BL, Dyer R, Kenney PJ [eds]: Clinical Urography, 2nd ed. Philadelphia, WB Saunders, 2000.)

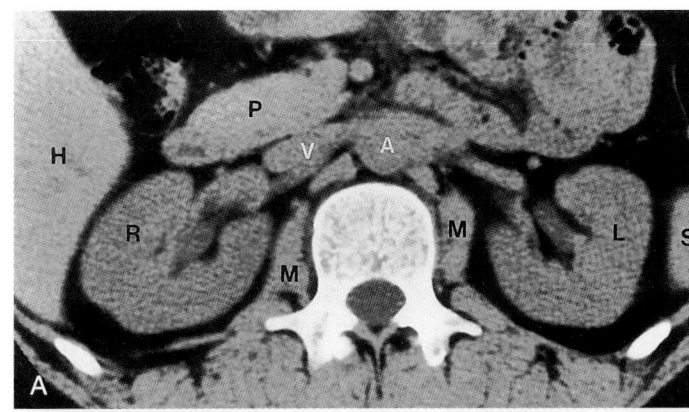

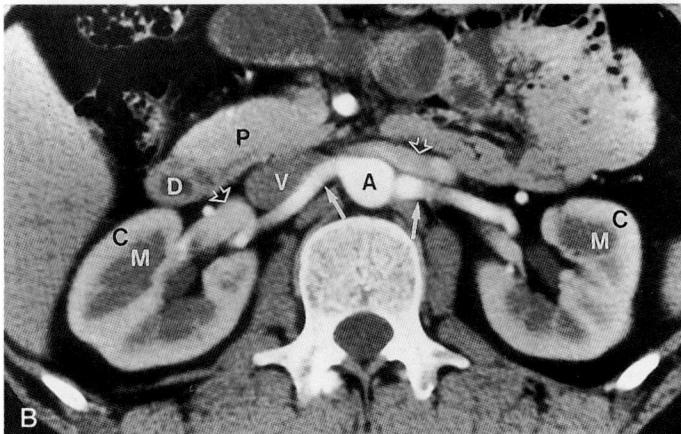

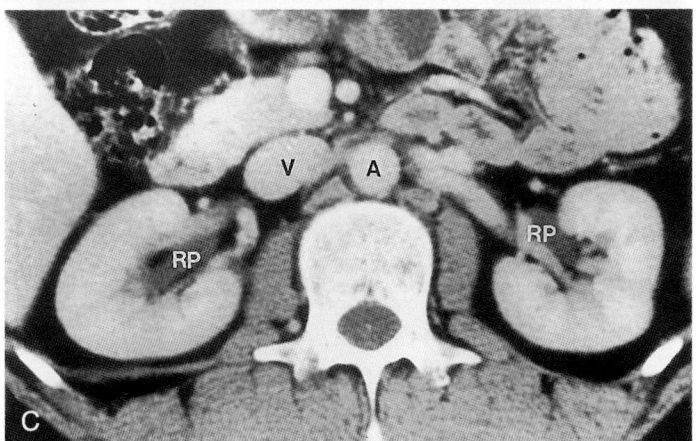

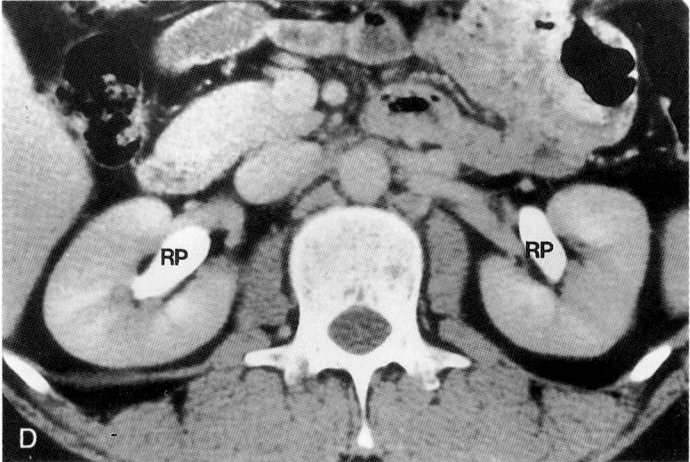

Figure 4–26. Normal nephrographic progression. **A,** Unenhanced CT scan obtained at the level of the renal hilum shows right (R) and left (L) kidneys of CT attenuation values slightly less than those of the liver (H) and pancreas (P). A, abdominal aorta; M, psoas muscle; S, spleen; V, inferior vena cava. **B,** Enhanced CT scan obtained during a cortical nephrographic phase, generally 25 to 80 seconds after contrast medium injection, reveals increased enhancement of the renal cortex (C) relative to the medulla (M). The main renal artery is indicated with *solid arrows* bilaterally. Main renal veins *(open arrows)* are less opacified with respect to the aorta (A) and arteries. D, duodenum; P, pancreas; V, inferior vena cava. **C,** CT scan obtained during the homogeneous nephrographic phase, generally between 85 and 120 seconds after contrast medium administration, reveals a homogeneous, uniform, increased attenuation of the renal parenchyma. The wall of the normal renal pelvis (RP) is paper thin or not visible on the CT scan. A, abdominal aorta; V, inferior vena cava. **D,** CT scan obtained during the excretory phase shows contrast medium in the renal pelvis (RP) bilaterally; this starts to appear approximately 3 minutes after contrast medium administration.

SECTION II

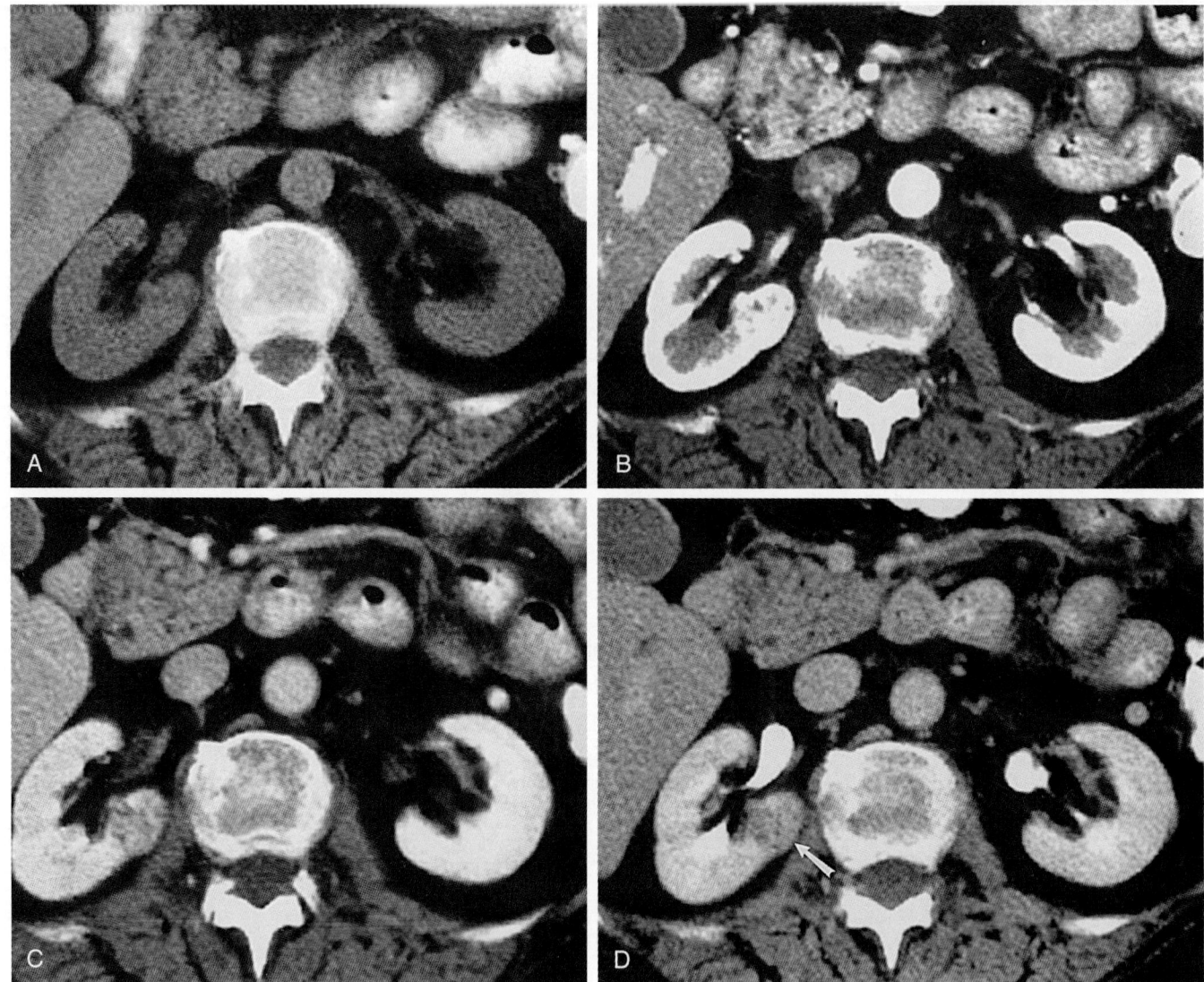

Figure 4–27. Small renal cell carcinoma in the infrahilar lip of the right kidney is poorly visualized on unenhanced image **(A)**. On corticomedullary phase image **(B)**, the lesion is subtly visible as a hyperenhancing focus within the renal medulla. On nephrographic **(C)** and pyelographic phase **(D)** images, the full extent of the lesion *(arrow)* within the medulla and cortex is depicted. (Reprinted from Brink JA, Siegel CL: Computed tomography of the upper urinary tract. In Pollack HM, McClennan BL, Dyer R, Kenney PJ [eds]: Clinical Urography, 2nd ed. Philadelphia, WB Saunders, 2000.)

directly inferior and posterior to the superior mesenteric artery. The right renal vein can be seen extending posterolaterally from the inferior vena cava. The renal arteries may be more difficult to identify secondary to their smaller size but usually are located posterior to the renal veins. Other structures abutting the right kidney include the liver, duodenum, ascending colon, gallbladder, and pancreatic head. The left kidney lies in close proximity to the tail of the pancreas, spleen, and descending colon.

Adrenal CT

CT often detects incidental adrenal lesions. It is also useful to image the gland when a suspected adrenal lesion may be present. The adrenal gland may harbor a variety of pathologic conditions, including primary malignancy, metastases, and functional adenomas. **If the density of an adrenal mass is less than 0 Hounsfield units on unenhanced CT, it may be con-sidered an adenoma.** Indeterminate lesions and lesions with density greater than 20 HU may represent metastases, and a percutaneous biopsy should be considered. Although CT is an excellent modality to evaluate adrenal lesions, MRI is the study of choice in suspected pheochromocytoma (Goldstein et al, 2004; Hussain and Korobkon, 2004).

The normal right adrenal gland is located anteromedial and extends superior to the right kidney (Fig. 4–28). It is located in close proximity to the vena cava and may seem to be extending posterior to the vena cava. It often appears to have two to three limbs. The left adrenal gland is medial to the kidney and often is adjacent to the superior aspect of the renal hilum. It also may appear branched, with two to three limbs.

Bladder CT

The appearance of the bladder is markedly dependent on the amount of fluid within it. A distended bladder may reach the

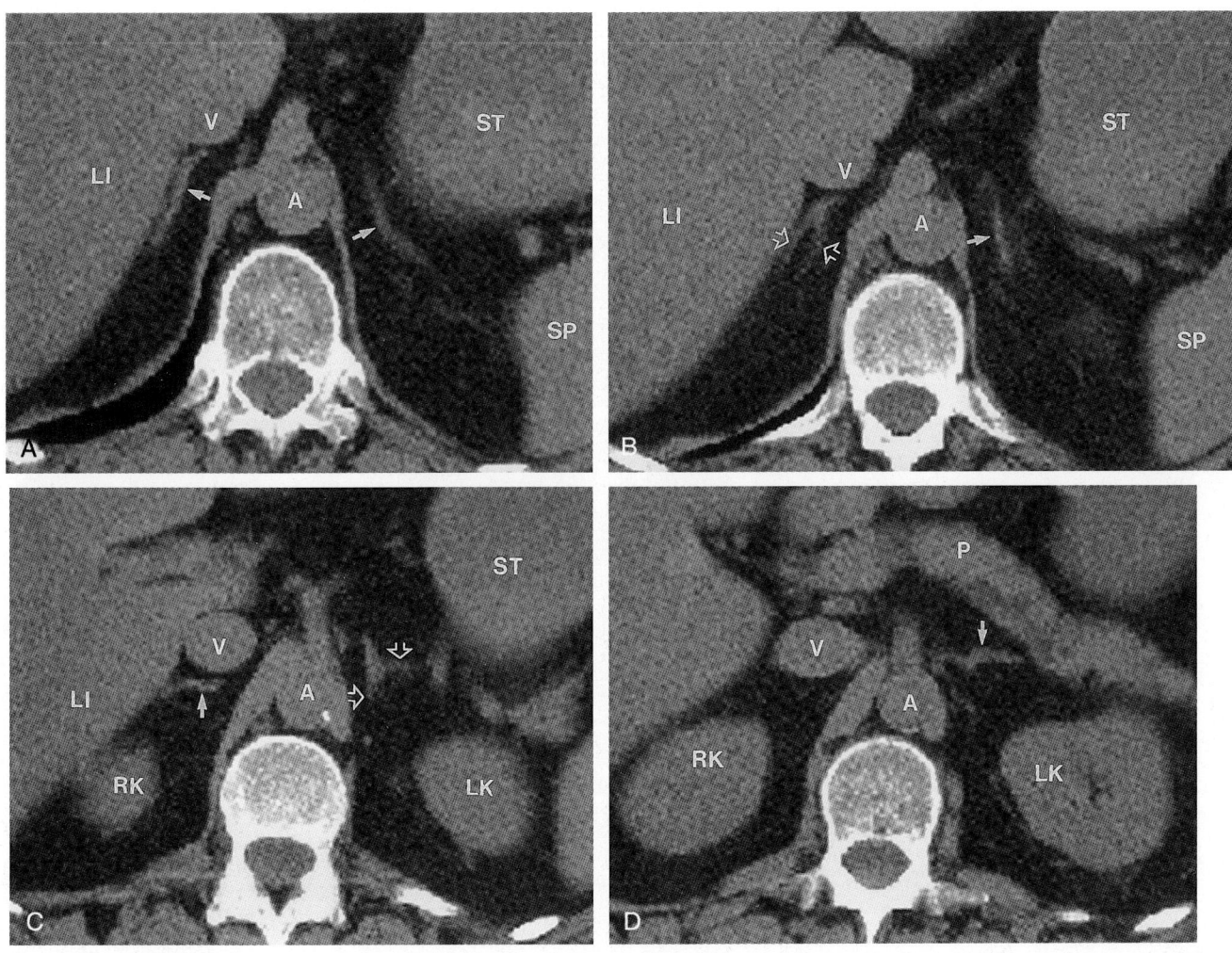

Figure 4-28. Normal adrenal gland. The adrenal glands are outlined by the retroperitoneal fat without discrete nodularity on unenhanced multidetector helical CT scan at 2.5-mm slice thickness. **A,** The cephalad portion of the gland appears linear bilaterally *(arrows)*. A, abdominal aorta; LI, liver; SP, spleen; ST, stomach; V, inferior vena cava. **B,** The right adrenal gland is located behind the inferior vena cava (V) and appears as an inverted Y (the medial and lateral limbs are indicated with *open arrows*). The upper aspect of the left adrenal gland *(solid arrow)* appears linear. A, abdominal aorta; LI, liver; SP, spleen; ST, stomach. **C,** More caudally, the left adrenal gland has an inverted Y shape (the medial and lateral limbs are indicated with *open arrows*). The caudate aspect of the right adrenal gland *(straight arrow)* is shown to be posterior to the inferior vena cava (V). A, abdominal aorta; LI, liver; LK, left kidney; RK, right kidney; ST, stomach. **D,** The caudate aspect of the left adrenal gland *(arrow)* is located posterior to the pancreas (P). The right adrenal gland does not appear. A, abdominal aorta; LK, left kidney; RK, right kidney; V, inferior vena cava.

pelvic sidewalls laterally and superiorly may displace the peritoneal contents. An empty bladder may be collapsed around a Foley catheter balloon, with little anatomic detail visualized. The bladder may contain contrast agent, which may alter the ability to detect mucosal lesions. The posterior aspect of the bladder is in contact with the uterus, sigmoid colon, and/or rectum.

Prostate and Seminal Vesicle CT

CT is rarely used as a primary study to evaluate the prostate, with the exception of the detection of abscesses or cysts of the gland. The prostate lies inferior to the bladder but may appear to extend into the bladder when a prominent median lobe is detected. The rectum lies directly posterior to the prostate and can be identified by air in its lumen. Fat surrounds the prostate and demarcates it from the pelvic floor musculature.

CT Urography

CT is often used to image the ureters, most commonly as an unenhanced scan to evaluate for urolithiasis. An enhanced CT may also detect ureteral anomalies but may obscure ureteral stones. The ureters generally course medial to the kidney and anterior to the psoas muscle. When the ureters enter the pelvis, they cross anterior to the iliac vessels and travel posteromedially behind the bladder until they enter the caudal aspect of the bladder at the trigone.

With CT becoming an increasingly important alternative to IVU in evaluation of hematuria, an enhanced view of the ureters is necessary. CT urography allows a contrast medium–enhanced reconstructed view of the ureters (Fig. 4–29). This technology is dependent on the imaging and processing capabilities of the scanner and workstation, and most modern scanners have the capability of producing excellent images. The technique involves capturing

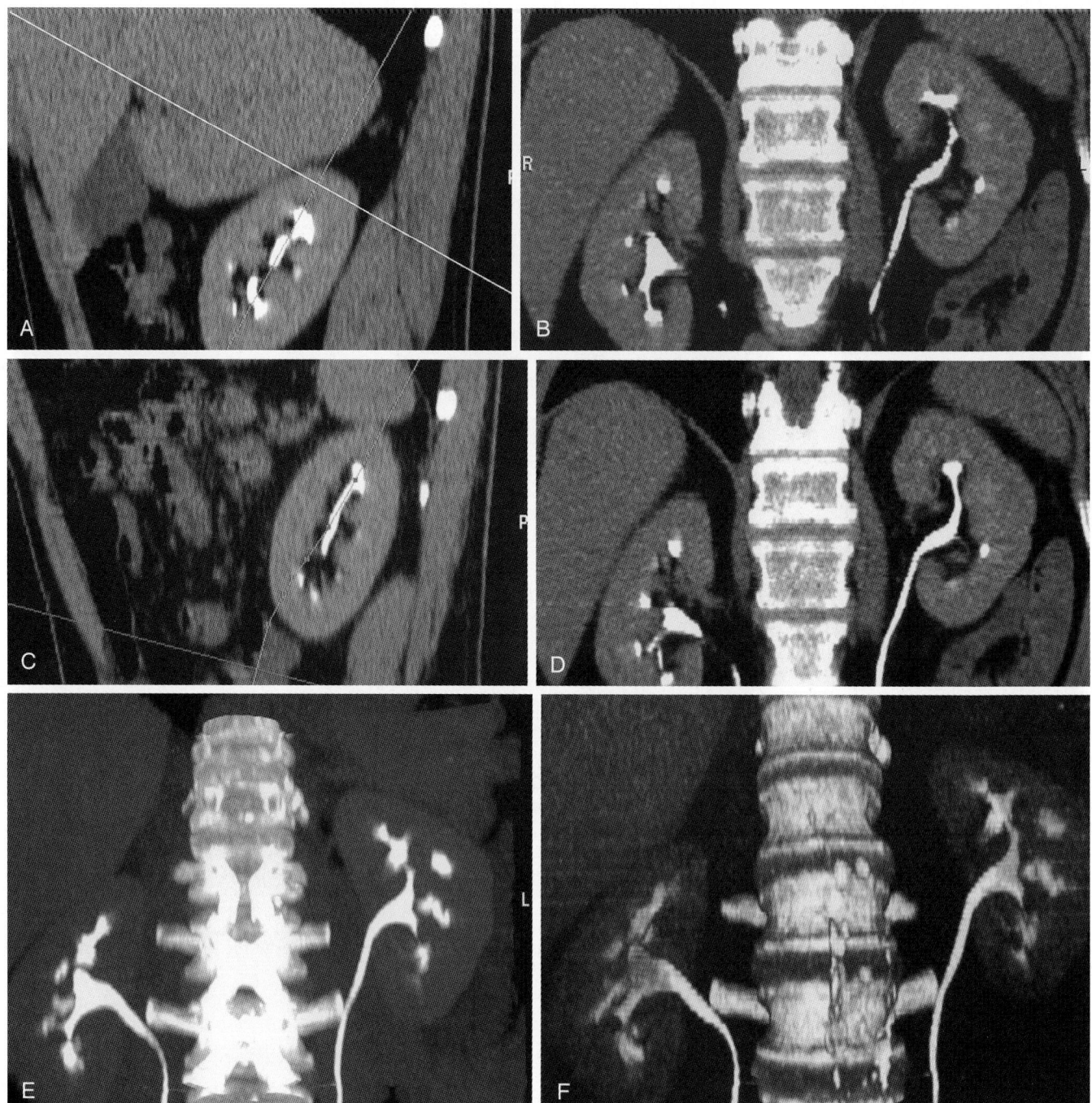

Figure 4–29. CT urography technique. Using a sagittal re-formation through the right kidney **(A)**, a paracoronal re-formation is generated **(B)** along the cut line depicted in **A.** Such standard re-formations do not permit depiction of the entire proximal ureter. By describing a curved cut line through the left kidney and proximal ureter on a similar sagittal re-formation **(C)**, a curved planar re-formation **(D)** is generated, revealing the entire left renal pelvis and proximal ureter. Conversely, three-dimensional techniques, such as maximum intensity projection **(E)** and volume rendering **(F)**, depict the collecting system and proximal ureters with great clarity. (Reprinted from Brink JA, Siegel CL: Computed tomography of the upper urinary tract. In Pollack HM, McClennan BL, Dyer R, Kenney PJ [eds]: Clinical Urography, 2nd ed. Philadelphia, WB Saunders, 2000.)

traditional cross-sectional images from the helical scanner during the late excretory phase. The images are reconstructed into a CT urogram with a similar gross appearance from that of IVU. The reconstruction combined with the routine cross-sectional images are an alternative to IVU and ultrasound in evaluation of hematuria (Joffe et al, 2003; Kawashima et al, 2003).

CT Angiography

CT angiography is a minimally invasive method to image the vasculature without the morbidity of direct large vessel vascular access. A rapid injection rate of contrast agent is given, and a helical scan is performed during the arterial phase. Oral administration of contrast agent is usually avoided. After

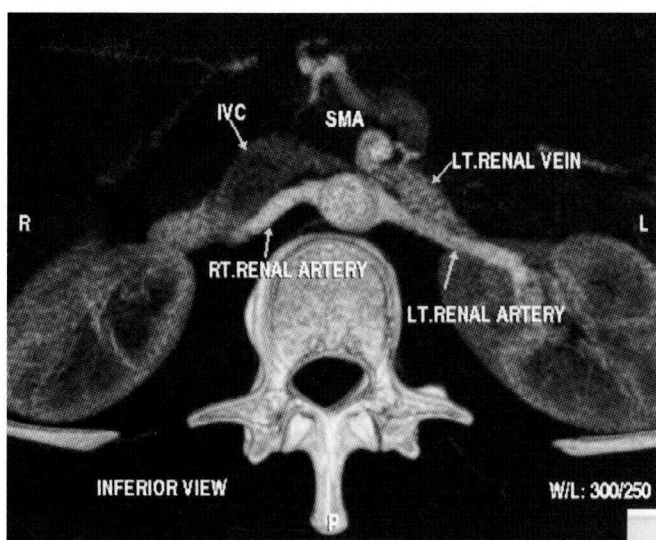

Figure 4–30. Volume-rendered image from CT angiogram of a potential living-related renal donor. Single, normal-appearing renal arteries are seen bilaterally. (Reprinted from Brink JA, Siegel CL: Computed tomography of the upper urinary tract. In Pollack HM, McClennan BL, Dyer R, Kenney PJ [eds]: Clinical Urography, 2nd ed. Philadelphia, WB Saunders, 2000.)

image acquisition, a workstation eliminates soft tissues and bone from the scan (Fig. 4–30). Three-dimensional reconstruction is then performed and images are then interpreted by the physician. **Indications include assessment of the renal vasculature in preparation for donor nephrectomy** (Del Pizzo et al, 1999; Lewis et al, 2004) **or for identification of extra vessels in evaluation of ureteropelvic junction obstruction** (Quillin et al, 1996). The technique may also be used to assess for renal artery stenosis (Beregi et al, 1996; Prokop, 1999).

MAGNETIC RESONANCE IMAGING

MRI is a tomographic technique that relies on alterations of magnetic properties in the imaging field. Unlike CT, it does not require ionizing radiation, and images can be obtained in multiple planes. **Additionally, iodinated contrast media is not used, which allows the technique to be safe in patients with renal insufficiency.** Moreover, soft tissue resolution with MRI is superior to that of CT. Certain contraindications may exist, such as when the patient has implants that could be affected by the magnetic field (Shellock and Curtis, 1991). In particular, patients with pacemakers, aneurysmal clips, retained foreign bodies, and other metallic prostheses should be counseled before MRI because the magnetic field may cause object deflection.

The physics of MRI are complex, and the number of protocols is astounding (Kressel et al, 2000). In a very basic sense, images are created by alignment of protons in response to an external magnet. Then, radiofrequency energy applied to the tissue causes differences in their energy. This is detected by the scanner, and images are generated. The T1-weighted images are generated by the time to return to equilibrium in the z-axis. The T2-weighted images are generated by the time required to return to equilibrium in the xy-axis. **Generally, on T1-weighted images fluid is dark and fat is bright. On T2-**weighted images, fluid is bright and fat is dark.** This simplified representation of MRI physics does not explain the complex imaging protocols that can be used to address specific clinical concerns.

Renal MRI

Indications to perform MRI of the kidneys include any situation in which cross-sectional imaging is needed but renal insufficiency prevents the use of enhanced CT. MRI, however, is not a useful method to evaluate for urolithiasis. MRI may be used to image the kidneys for evaluation of renal masses or cysts. Often, because MRI is more expensive than CT or ultrasound, it is used to clarify a renal lesion after a primary imaging test. MRI may also be used when there is a sensitivity to iodinated contrast media. MRI is highly accurate in determining the extent of tumor thrombus in the inferior vena cava (Hockley et al, 1990; Aslam et al, 2002).

In the normal MRI anatomy of the kidney, the cortex and medulla can be differentiated, with the cortex appearing brighter on T1-weighted images (Fig. 4–31). Gadolinium-enhanced images exhibit a phasic pattern depending on the time of imaging after the administration of the contrast agent.

Adrenal MRI

MRI is commonly used to image the adrenal glands. Benign adenomas generally contain a large amount of lipid compared with carcinomas or pheochromocytomas, and modern MRI imaging techniques may exploit this difference to lead to differences in imaging. Opposed phase imaging and fat-saturated imaging can aid in the diagnosis of adrenal lesions. MRI is often used as a secondary examination to further characterize an incidentally discovered adrenal lesion or may be used as a primary examination to rule out an adrenal mass. MRI is particularly useful in the diagnosis of a pheochromocytoma, in which the lesion will appear bright on T2-weighted images.

On T1-weighted images, the adrenal glands are easily visualized, secondary to the bright fat surrounding the gland. On T2-weighted images, the adrenals appear isointense with the liver. Fat-saturated imaging of the adrenals leads to a bright image (Fig. 4–32).

Bladder MRI

The main indication to image the bladder with MRI is for assessment of invasion of the bladder wall with transitional cell carcinoma. MRI may also be used to assess bladder invasion from other pelvic neoplasms. The normal bladder wall is difficult to visualize on T1-weighted images, because urine in the bladder exhibits similar signal intensity. On T2-weighted images, urine has a relatively high signal intensity and the bladder wall is distinguishable from the luminal fluid (Fig. 4–33). If a bladder mass is present, muscle invasion may be assessed with T2-weighted MRI.

Prostate MRI

Prostate MRI is usually performed for evaluation of prostate cancer. The gland can be well visualized with endorectal coils

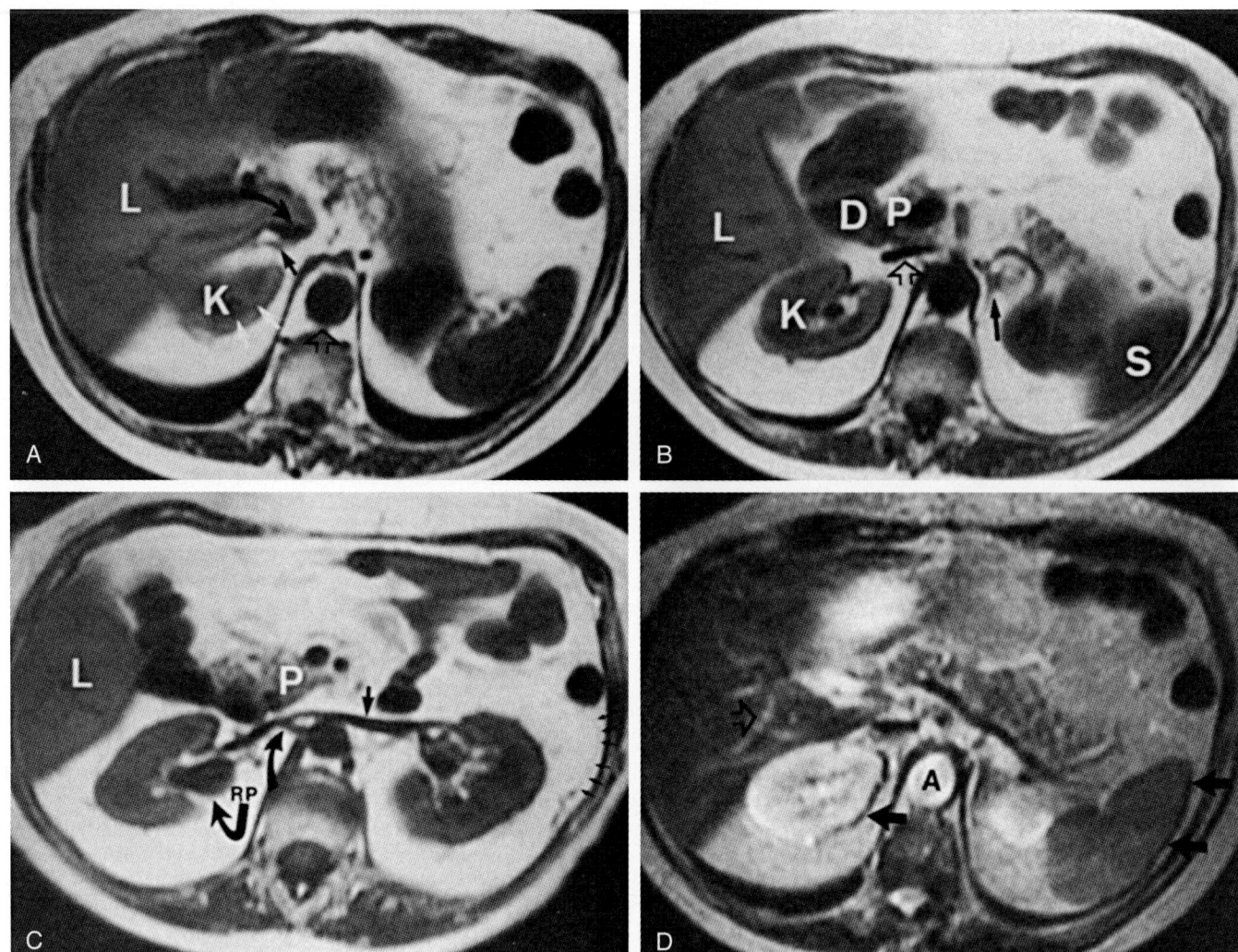

Figure 4–31. MR image of the upper abdomen and kidneys, 1.5 T. **A,** Short TR/TE (TR = 400 ms, TE = 20 ms) axial MRI (T1-weighted) was taken through the level of the upper pole of the left kidney (K). The renal medulla is of lower signal intensity *(white arrows)* than the cortex, and it appears darker. The right adrenal gland *(arrow)* is identified with an inverted-V configuration, immediately posterior to the inferior vena cava *(curved arrow)*. The inferior vena cava and the aorta *(open short arrow)* demonstrate the flow void phenomenon and appear low in signal intensity. **B,** T1-weighted, short TR/TE (TR = 400 ms, TE = 20 ms) scan performed 1.5 cm below that shown in **A**. The left adrenal gland is now identified *(black arrow)*. The liver (L), kidney (K), spleen (S), duodenum (D), pancreas (P), and inferior vena cava *(open arrow)* are also noted. **C,** T1-weighted, short TR/TE (TR = 400 ms, TE = 20 ms) scan through the renal hilum is shown. The left renal vein is identified *(short arrow)* as it traverses anterior to the aorta and enters the inferior vena cava. The right renal artery *(upper curved arrow)* is identified posterior to the inferior vena cava. The somewhat diluted extrarenal pelvis (RP) is identified as a structure of low signal intensity arising in the hilum. A minimal amount of renal sinus fat is identified as a high-signal region surrounding the renal pelvis. Gerota's fascia is visualized faintly *(short arrows)* on the left. Also identified are the liver (L) and the pancreas (P). **D,** T2-weighted image in the midabdomen. The kidney is of higher signal intensity than the liver or spleen. Chemical shift artifact is demonstrated *(arrows)*. The aorta (A) and intrahepatic vessels *(open arrow)* are of high signal intensity owing to the gradient moment nulling techniques that have been employed to minimize motion artifacts in this patient. (Reprinted from Kressel HY, Chen Q, Prasad P, Hatabu H: Magnetic resonance imaging. In Pollack HM, McClennan BL, Dyer R, Kenney PJ [eds]: Clinical Urography, 2nd ed. Philadelphia, WB Saunders, 2000.)

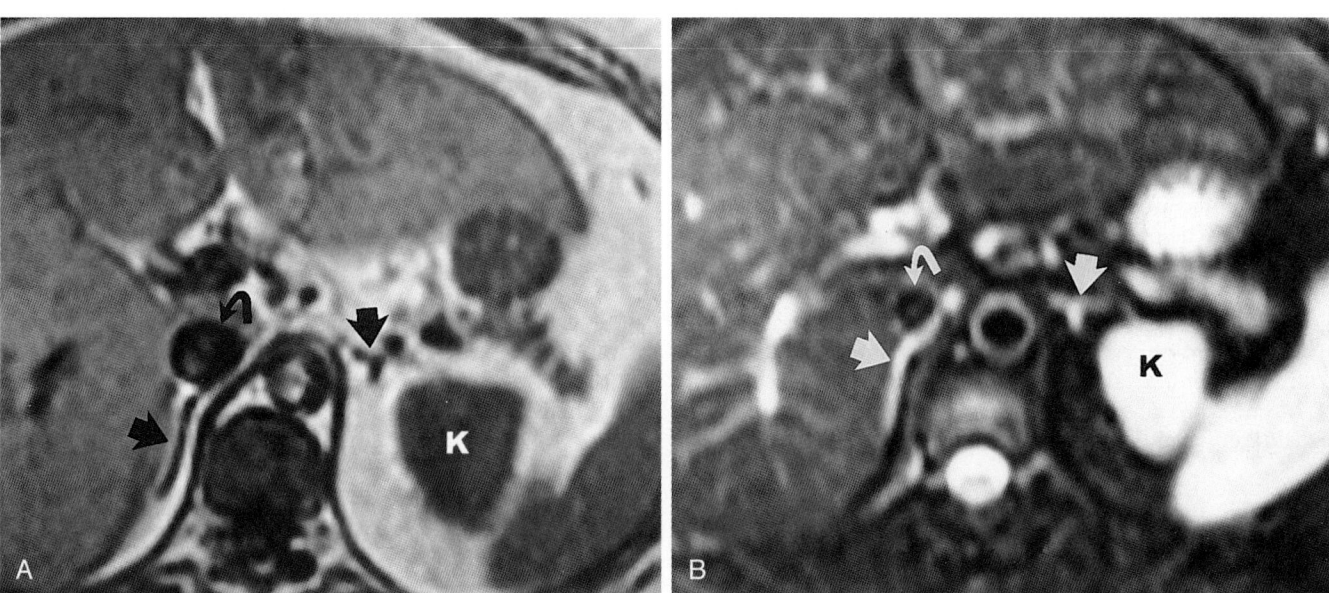

Figure 4–32. Magnetic resonance imaging of normal adrenals. **A,** Axial T1-weighted image (two-dimensional flash, TR = 130 ms, TE = 4 ms) shows the normal adrenals *(straight arrows)*. Note the vena cava *(curved arrow)* and the left kidney (K). **B,** Axial T2-weighted image (TR = 2000 ms/TE = 100 ms) with fat suppression of the same patient. The adrenals appear relatively hyperintense. (Reprinted from Mitty H, Parsons RB: Adrenal embryology, anatomy, and imaging techniques. In Pollack HM, McClennan BL, Dyer R, Kenney PJ [eds]: Clinical Urography, 2nd ed. Philadelphia, WB Saunders, 2000.)

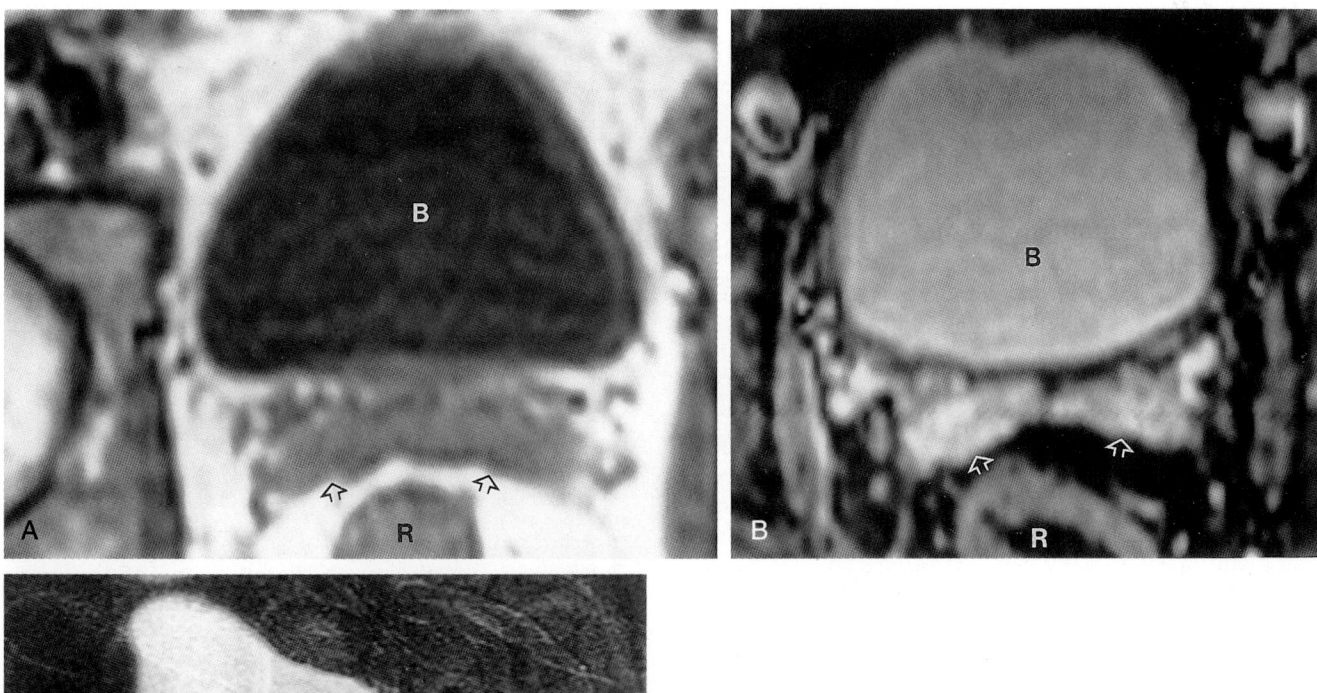

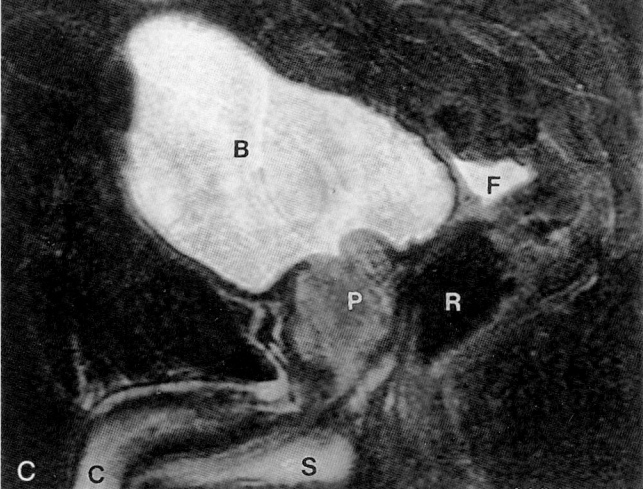

Figure 4–33. Normal bladder. Urine in the bladder (B) is low in signal intensity on the axial T1-weighted spin-echo image **(A)** and markedly high in signal intensity on the T2-weighted fast spin-echo image **(B)**. The seminal vesicles *(open arrows)* are intermediate in signal intensity on the T1-weighted image and markedly bright on the T2-weighted image. R, rectum. **C,** Sagittal T2-weighted fast spin-echo image shows the relation of the bladder (B) to the prostate (P). There is a minimal amount of fluid in the rectovesical recess (F). C, corpora cavernosa; R, rectum; S, corpora spongiosa.

and can be evaluated for intraprostatic lesions or capsular penetration of prostate carcinoma. On T1-weighted images the prostate has an intermediate signal intensity, similar to muscle, and it may be distinguished from the surrounding fat, which appears bright (Fig. 4–34). Very little intraprostatic detail is possible on the T1-weighted images.

T2-weighted images offer excellent prostatic visualization (Fig. 4–35). The peripheral zone has high signal intensity, and the central zone is intermediate in intensity. The neurovascular bundles can be visualized, which appear bright on T2-weighted images. The dorsal venous complex is also well visualized and appears bright on T2-weighted images. The seminal vesicles are also well visualized by MRI. They appear of intermediate intensity on T1-weighted images and of high signal intensity on T2-weighted images.

Urethra MRI

An intraluminal coil can be used in the male or female urethra to evaluate for stricture or diverticulum, respectively. MRI of the male urethra is a tertiary examination, because most cases may be evaluated with ultrasound or retrograde urethrography. The female urethra, however, is difficult to image with traditional techniques, and diverticulum of the female urethra can be a difficult clinical diagnosis. In these cases, MRI of the female urethra is indicated (Kim et al, 1993; Blander et al, 2001). MRI may also be useful in the evaluation of local extension of urethral carcinoma.

MR Urography

MRU is a technique that seeks to image the ureters and collecting system (Rothpearl et al, 1995; Tang et al, 1996; Nolte et al, 2003). It is useful in patients with renal insufficiency or iodinated contrast sensitivity or in pregnant women. Although it may be a substitute for IVP or CT urography, MRU may have some difficulty in the direct imaging of urolithiasis. Stones generally cannot be distinguished from tumors or blood clots. Additionally, all lesions less than 4 mm may be difficult to image. Nevertheless, hydroureteronephrosis and obstruction can be visualized with the technique. Rapid acquisition T2-weighted sequences are used, in which fluid appears bright and other tissues appear dark (Fig. 4–36).

MR Angiography

MRA is a useful alternative to CT angiography or traditional angiography (Ho and Corse, 2003; Zhang and Prince, 2004).

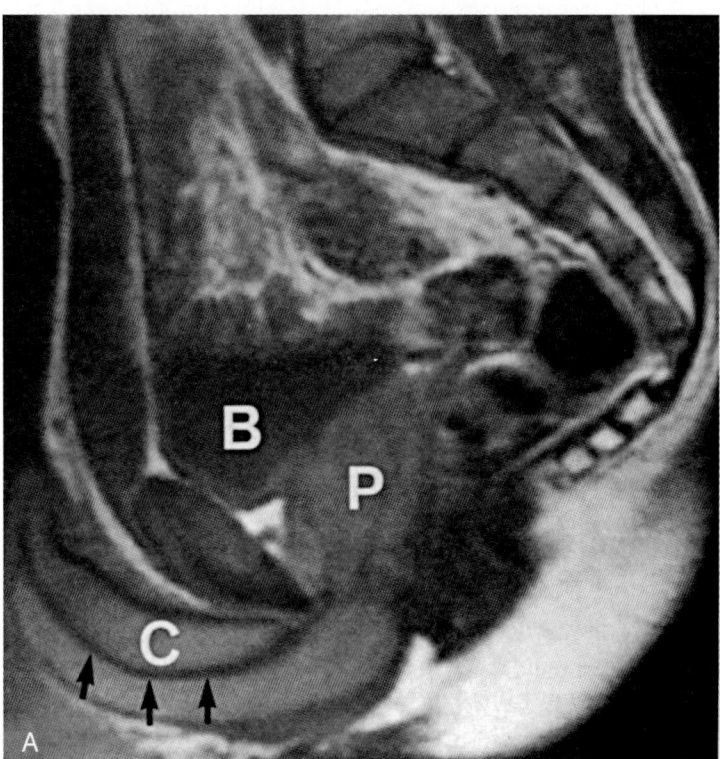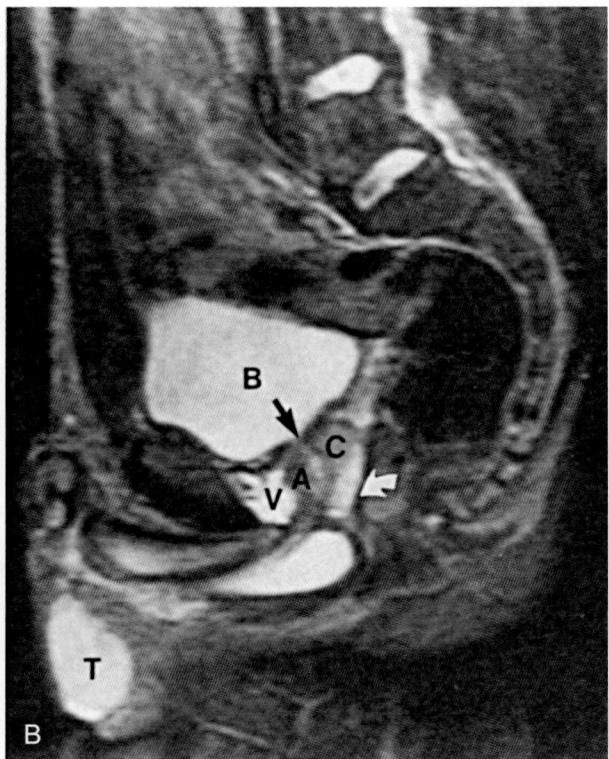

Figure 4-34. Prostatic anatomy, sagittal view, 1.5 T. **A,** T1-weighted (short TR/TE) sagittal scan through the mid pelvis. The prostate (P) is a structure of intermediate signal intensity identified posterior to the bladder (B). Little intraprostatic parenchymal detail is identified on this image. The corpus cavernosum (C) is of intermediate signal intensity and is surrounded by the lower-signal tunica albuginea *(arrows)*. **B,** Midsagittal T2-weighted (long TR/TE image) shows high-signal urine in the bladder (B). The intraprostatic urethra is identified *(arrow)*. Considerable intraprostatic parenchymal detail is present. The lower-signal anterior fibromuscular stroma (A) is noted anterior to the intraprostatic urethra. Posteriorly, the high-signal peripheral zone *(white arrow)* is identified. The central glandular portion (C) is posterior to the intraprostatic urethra and anterior to the peripheral zone. The anterior venous plexus (V) is noted outside the prostate margins. It is of high signal intensity in view of the slow flow in these venous structures. The normal high-signal testes (T) are also noted on the parasagittal images. The corpora cavernosa are increased in signal compared with **A.** Note how the intervertebral disks have also become high signal intensity structures, owing to the water content. (Reprinted from Kressel HY, Chen Q, Prasad P, Hatabu H: Magnetic resonance imaging. In Pollack HM, McClennan BL, Dyer R, Kenney PJ [eds]: Clinical Urography, 2nd ed. Philadelphia, WB Saunders, 2000.)

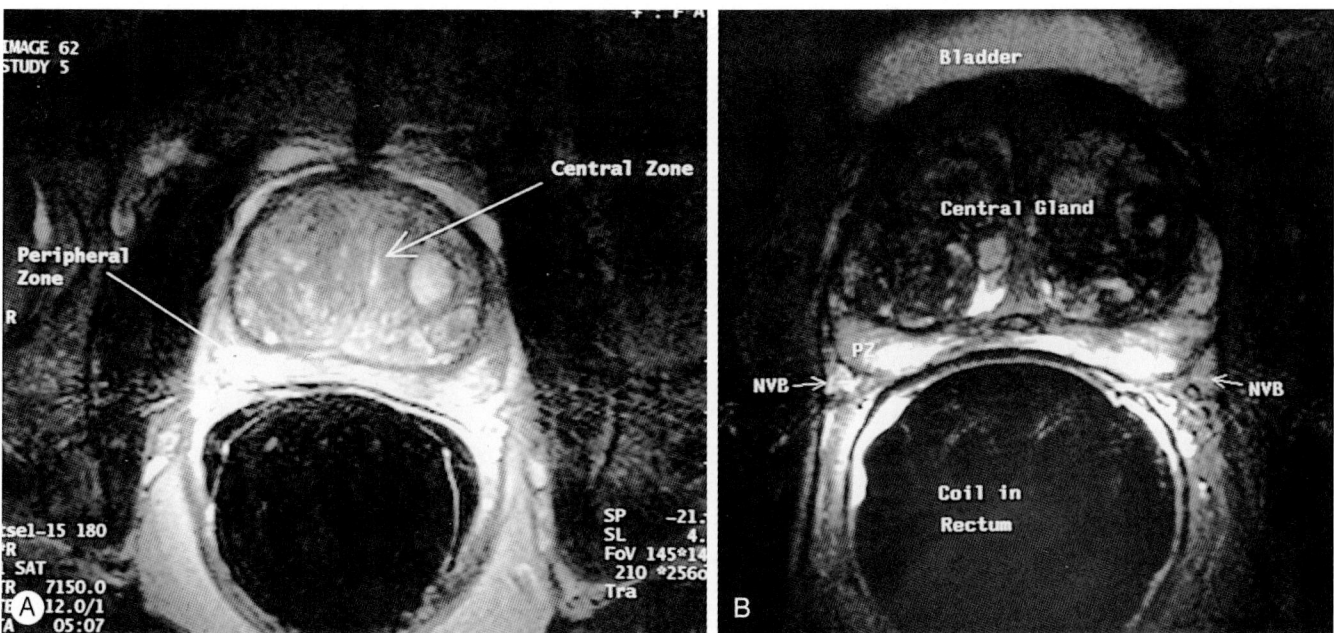

Figure 4–35. Normal prostate images obtained with an endorectal surface coil. **A,** Axial T2-weighted image. Note the high-signal peripheral zone and the intermediate signal central zone. **B,** Axial T2-weighted image through the base of the prostate gland. Note the peripheral zone. (Reprinted from Kressel HY, Chen Q, Prasad P, Hatabu H: In Pollack HM, McClennan BL, Dyer R, Kenney PJ [eds]: Clinical Urography, 2nd ed. Philadelphia, WB Saunders, 2000.)

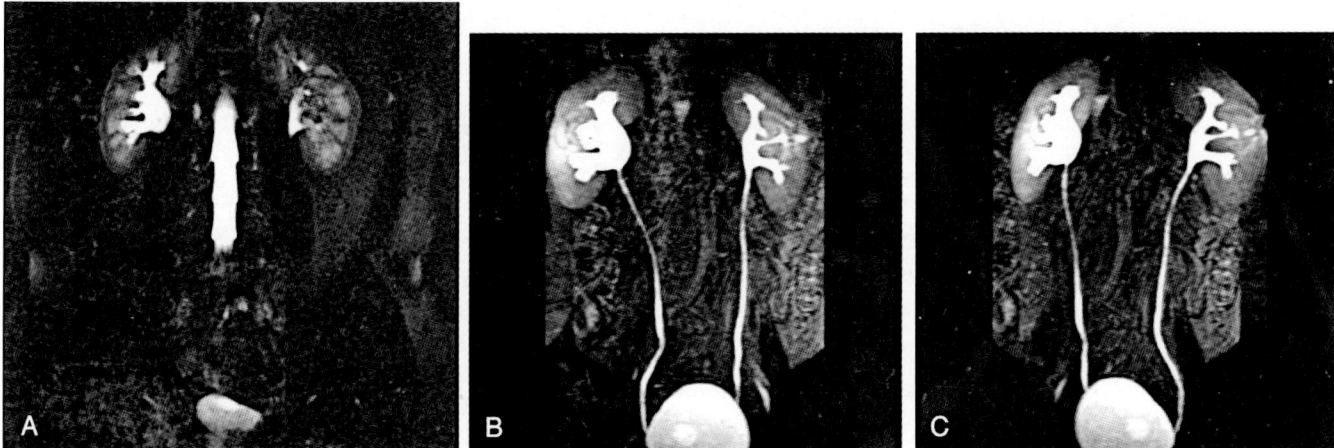

Figure 4–36. **A,** Maximum intensity projection (MIP) of nine slices of 4 mm each of HASTE MRU (TR/TE effective = 4.3/285 ms) shows the renal pelves and bladder. However, the anatomic coverage is not complete owing to the limited number of slices that were acquired. **B** and **C,** MIPs of contrast medium–enhanced MRU obtained with three-dimensional sequence (TR/TE/FA = 3.5/1.4 ms/25 degrees; 56 slices of L8 mm each) show complete coverage of the renal pelves, ureters, and bladder. Also, by projecting the three-dimensional data set at different angles, the UP and UV junctions can be clearly visualized on either side. (Reprinted from Kressel HY, Chen Q, Prasad P, Hatabu H: Magnetic resonance imaging. In Pollack HM, McClennan BL, Dyer R, Kenney PJ [eds]: Clinical Urography, 2nd ed. Philadelphia, WB Saunders, 2000.)

The main advantage is the lack of iodinated contrast media, which makes the technique suitable in patients with renal insufficiency or contrast agent hypersensitivity. The best resolution is obtained with gadolinium-enhanced sequences with three-dimensional volumetric data sets. Image acquisition is rapid, and breath-hold techniques may be used with timed contrast agent administration to deliver images with excellent resolution. The study is often used for evaluation of the abdominal aorta, renal artery stenosis, and pre-donor nephrectomy.

NUCLEAR SCINTIGRAPHY

Radionuclide evaluation of the genitourinary system offers physiologic and anatomic details that may not be apparent with other radiologic imaging modalities. Absorbed radiation with these techniques is minimal, and valuable functional information may be obtained. Rotating gamma scintillation cameras and complex digital workstations have refined the examinations.

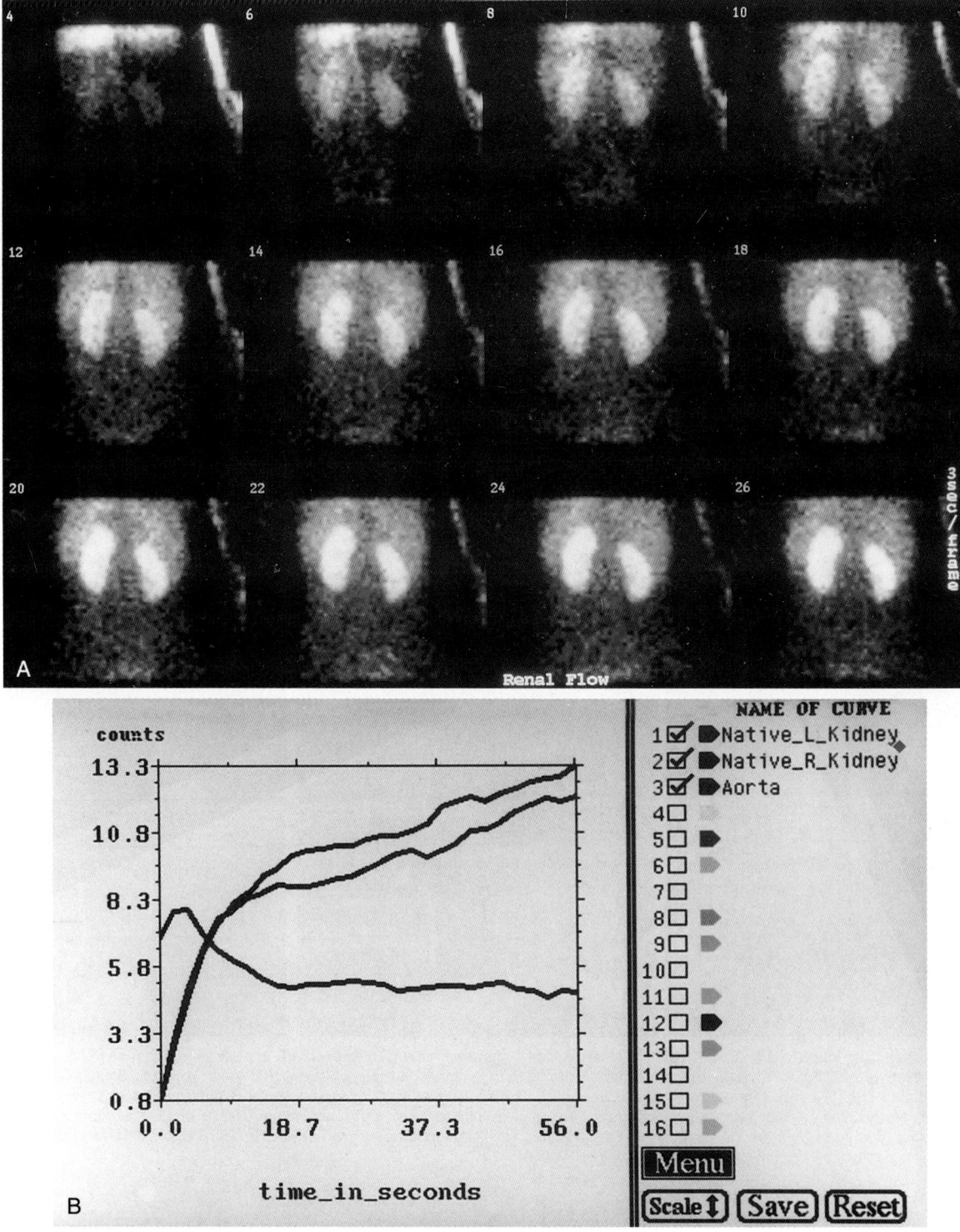

Figure 4–37. Technetium Tc99m mercaptoacetyltriglycine (^{99m}Tc-MAG3). **A,** ^{99m}Tc-MAG3 perfusion images demonstrating prompt blood flow to the kidneys. Note that there is no early peaking of activity as with the ^{99m}Tc-DTPA flow study. There is a gradual increase of radioactivity. This is due to the greater retention of MAG3. Each frame is 3 seconds. **B,** Perfusion time-activity curves demonstrating essentially symmetrical flow to both kidneys. Note the rising curve typical of ^{99m}Tc-MAG3 flow studies, as explained in **A.**

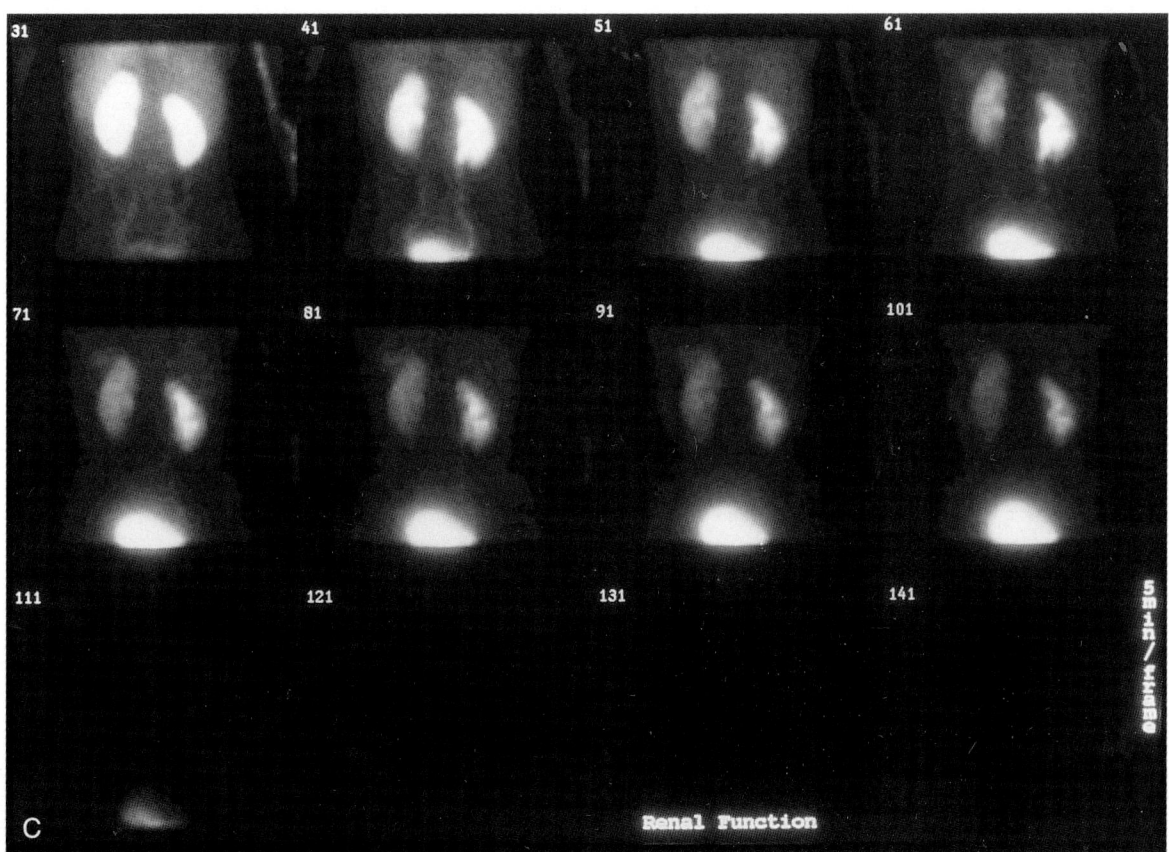

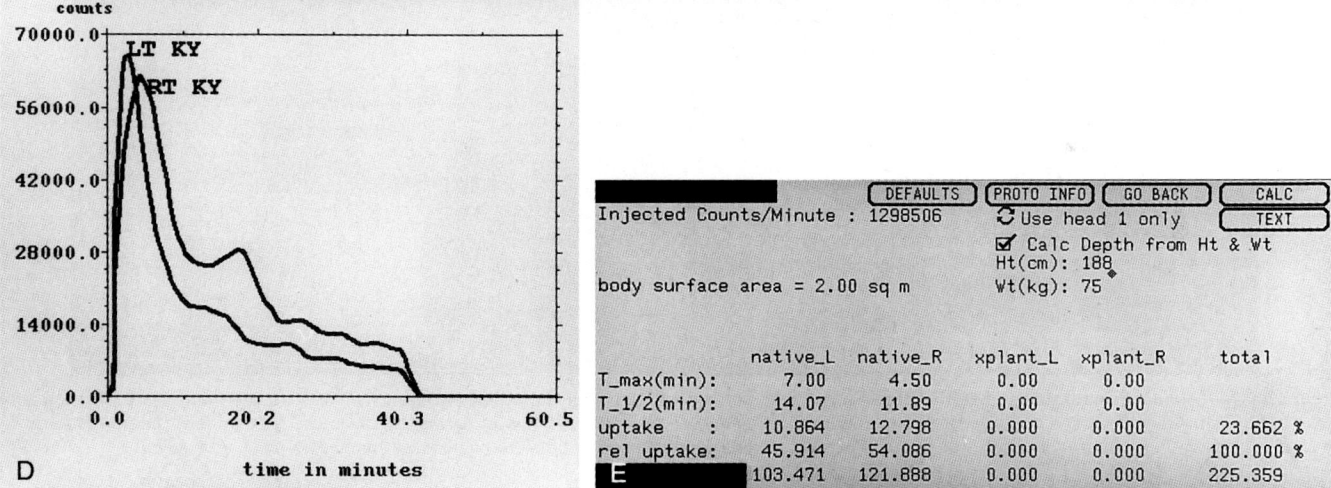

Figure 4–37—Cont'd **C,** Dynamic function images over 40 minutes demonstrate good uptake of tracer by both kidneys and prompt visualization of the collecting systems. A slight relative delay in clearance from the right kidney is noted. **D,** Function time-activity curve or renogram over each kidney. This renogram demonstrates prompt peaking of activity in both kidneys, slightly later on the right. Normally, peak activity is between 3 and 5 minutes for ^{99m}Tc-MAG3. The upslope represents a combination of perfusion and tubular function. The downslope represents prompt drainage of activity from the kidneys. The normal half-life for drainage is less than 17 minutes when ^{99m}Tc-MAG3 is used. **E,** Printout of quantitative data showing the time to minimal renal activity; half-life of the renogram differential contribution of left and right kidneys; and MAG3 clearance, which totals 225 mL/min in this case.

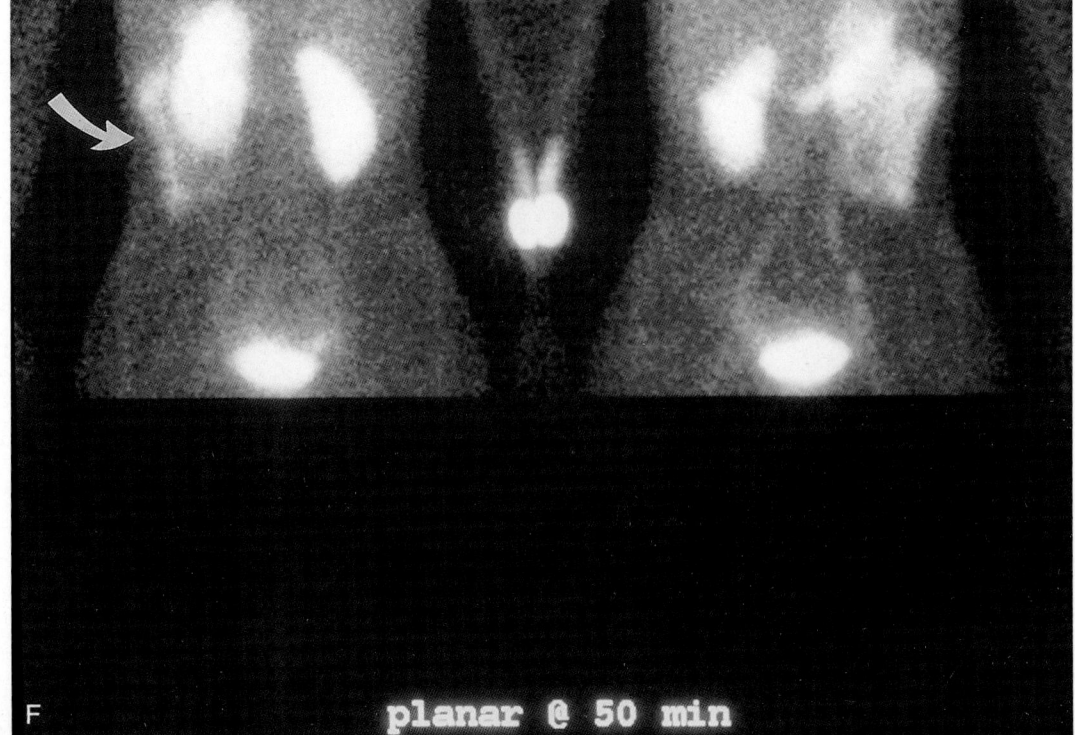

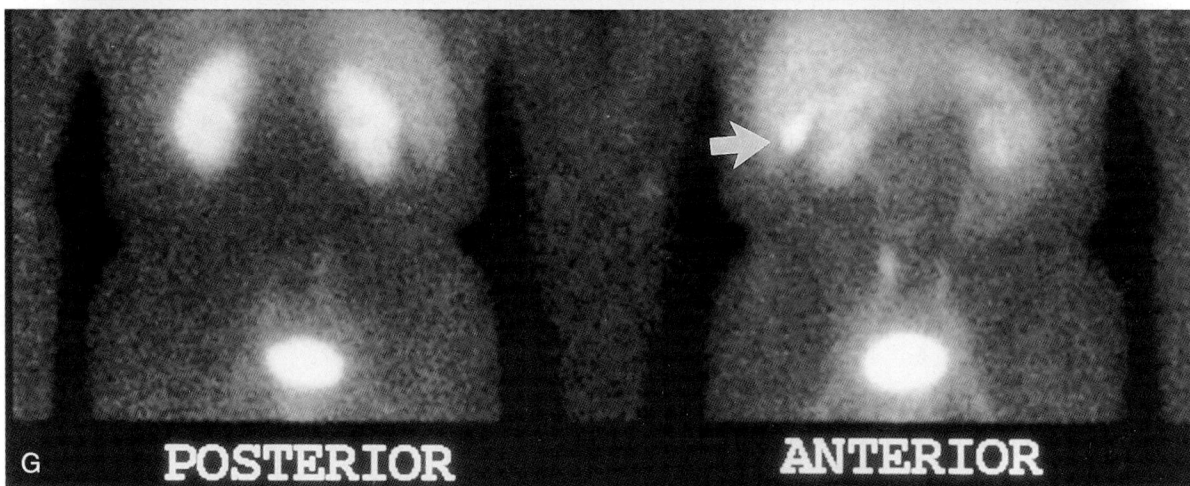

Figure 4–37—Cont'd **F** and **G,** Delayed static images in the posterior and anterior projections demonstrate gallbladder activity (*arrow* in **F**) and intestinal activity (*arrow* in **G**), reflecting a normal mode of excretion of ^{99m}Tc-MAG3. Gallbladder activity, in particular, can cause false-positive interpretation when it overlies activity in the renal collecting system. Liver activity is variable and tends to be more pronounced in children or in renal failure.

In the past, iodine-131 (^{131}I) was used as the primary tracer to evaluate the urinary tract. ^{131}I-Orthoiodohippurate was used to evaluate effective renal plasma flow, excretion, and obstruction. ^{131}I tracers, however, have been supplanted by technetium-99m (^{99m}Tc) tracers, which have a shorter half life (6 hours vs. 8 days) and offer better images. The main tracers used in evaluation of the kidney are diethylenetriaminepentaacetic acid (DTPA), mercaptoacetyltriglycine (MAG3), and dimercaptosuccinic acid (DMSA).

^{99m}Tc-MAG3 is cleared by tubular secretion, and no glomerular filtration occurs (Eshima et al, 1990; Itoh, 2001). The tracer is well suited for evaluation of renal function and diuretic scintigraphy. Also, it is an excellent tracer to evaluate renal plasma flow. ^{99m}Tc-DTPA is primarily a glomerular fil-

tration agent (Peters, 1998; Gates, 2004). It is also useful for evaluation of obstruction and renal function. It is less useful in patients with renal failure. ^{99m}Tc-DMSA is cleared by both filtration and secretion, but the clearance is relatively complex and it does bind to parenchymal tissues. It is useful as a renal cortical imaging agent.

Diuretic Scintigraphy

Hydronephrosis may not necessarily indicate renal obstruction, which must be identified and quantified because corrective surgery can be used to relieve the obstruction. Renal obstruction can be evaluated with IVU, Whitaker test, or washout films from a retrograde pyelogram. Diuretic scinitig-

Figure 4–38. Chronic pyelonephritis. **A,** Renal sonogram shows a small left kidney *(calipers)*. **B,** Posterior image of the kidneys obtained 3 hours after administration of ^{99m}Tc-DMSA shows that the left kidney is decreased in size, has globally decreased activity in comparison with the right kidney, and contains several focal cortical defects, most notably at both poles. The findings are consistent with cortical scarring and reduced function of the kidney. (Reprinted from Siegel MJ: Pediatric urinary tract infection. In Pollack HM, McClennan BL, Dyer R, Kenney PJ [eds]: Clinical Urography, 2nd ed. Philadelphia, WB Saunders, 2000.)

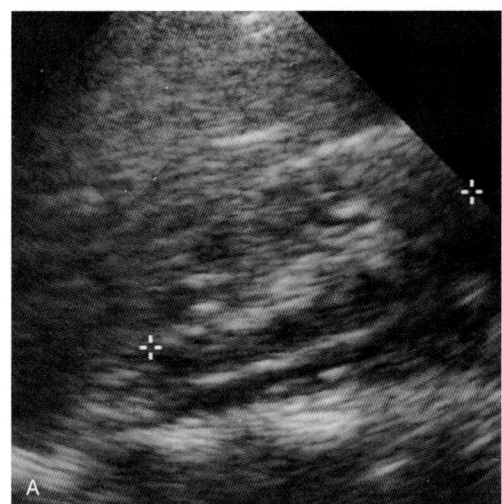
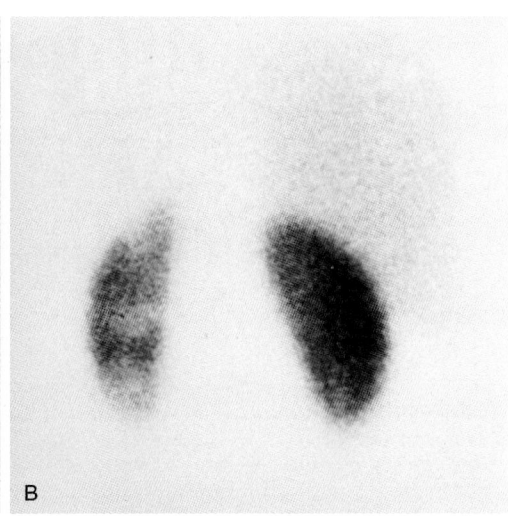

raphy, however, offers a quantitative assessment of obstruction and does not require an invasive procedure, intravenous iodinated contrast medium, or anesthesia.

Diuretic scintigraphy is performed with DTPA or MAG3. MAG3 is more useful in patients with renal insufficiency, but DTPA is more economical. After a bolus injection of the tracer, images are obtained that can be used to estimate relative renal function. When the tracer reaches the collecting system, a diuretic is given and half-life is calculated based on the slope of the curve in response to the diuretic (Fig. 4–37).

Renal Cortical Scintigraphy

Renal cortical scintigraphy with ^{99m}Tc-DMSA is used to evaluate for cortical scars or pyelonephritis (Fig. 4–38). The test may be indicated to detect a history of pyelonephritis and may guide the urologist in correcting an underlying pathologic condition (e.g., vesicoureteral reflux). Importantly, acute infection can produce abnormalities in the scan; and if the test is being performed to evaluate for cortical scarring, it should be done at least 3 months after an acute infection (Rosenberg et al, 1992).

SUGGESTED READINGS

Barrett BJ, Parfrey PS, Vavasour HM, et al: A comparison of nonionic, low osmolality radiocontrast agents with ionic, high osmolality agents during cardiac catheterization. N Engl J Med 1992;326:431

Burge HJ, Middleton WD, McClennan BL, et al: Ureteral jets in healthy subjects and in patients with unilateral ureteral calculi. Radiology 1991;180:437.

Cohan RH, Sherman LS, Korobkin M, et al: Renal masses: Assessment of corticomedullary phase and nephrographic phase CT scans. Radiology 1995;196:445-451.

Fielding JR, Silverman SG, Samuel S, et al: Unenhanced helical CT of ureteral stones: A replacement for excretory urography in planning treatment. AJR Am J Roentgenol 1998;171:1051-1053.

Kressel HY, Chen Q, Prasad P, Hatabu H: Magnetic resonance imaging. In Pollack HM, McClennan BL, Dyer R, Kenney PJ (eds): Clinical Urography, 2nd ed. Philadelphia, WB Saunders, 2000, pp 525-555.

Lang EK, Macchia RJ, Thomas R, et al: Improved detection of renal pathologic features on multiphasic helical CT compared to IVU in patients with microscopic hematuria. Urology 2003;61:528-532.

Peters AM: Scintigraphic imaging of renal function. Exp Nephrol 1998;6:391-397.

KEY POINTS: URINARY TRACT IMAGING

- High osmolar contrast media are associated with an increased risk of complications compared with low osmolar media.

- Ultrasound is the procedure of choice in evaluating scrotal pathology.

- CT has supplanted IVU for the evaluation of urolithiasis.

- Multiphase-enhanced CT is necessary to evaluate for the renal mass.

- MRI is a useful modality in imaging patients with renal insufficiency, because the contrast media are generally not nephrotoxic.

- MRI can be used to assess muscle invasion from bladder cancer.

- Renal scintigraphy with ^{99m}Tc-DMSA is useful to assess renal cortical pathology.

5 Outcomes Research

MARK S. LITWIN, MD, MPH

ACCESS TO CARE

COSTS OF CARE

QUALITY OF CARE

HEALTH-RELATED QUALITY OF LIFE

FUTURE IMPLICATIONS

KEY POINTS: FACTORS DETERMINING USE OF MEDICAL SERVICES

- Predisposing factors (e.g., health beliefs and attitudes)
- Enabling factors (e.g., health insurance and geographic proximity)
- Need factors (e.g., the presence of symptoms or diseases)

The discipline of health services research, often loosely referred to as outcomes research, is primarily focused on the study of access to care, costs of care, and quality of care.

ACCESS TO CARE

Access to care includes the "actual use of personal health services and everything that facilitates or impedes their use. **It is the link between health services systems and the populations they serve**" (Andersen and Davidson, 2001). Andersen presented a behavioral model for considering health care access in which three categories of factors determine how and whether individuals utilize medical services. These include predisposing factors (e.g., health beliefs and attitudes), enabling factors (e.g., health insurance and geographic proximity), and need factors (e.g., the presence of symptoms or diseases) (Aday and Andersen, 1981; Andersen, 1995). Barriers to health care access often result from financial determinants such as the lack of health insurance or adequate income; logistical challenges in coordinating child care, public transportation, and work schedules; clinic waiting times; and difficulties with the geographic proximity of clinics and hospitals (Griffiths et al, 2004). Barriers to access may also result from more subtle factors, such as fear of the health care system, ethnic disparities, cultural norms, embarrassment, perceived health status (Fitzpatrick et al, 1998), lack of self-efficacy, or special social circumstances. Even in health care systems that are considered to provide "equal access," such as the U.S. Veterans Affairs hospitals, different patient groups utilize outpatient and inpatient care at markedly different rates, leading to variations in outcomes. Differences in access to care have been cited as a fundamental reason for disparities in health status among various populations (Kelley et al, 2005a, 2005b).

COSTS OF CARE

The cost of medical care may be measured in many ways. Although it is difficult to put a price tag on the toll of human suffering, physicians today are asked to reduce costs, improve quality, and provide services for greater numbers of patients in an increasingly austere environment. This often requires rationing of resources, although it is seldom explicitly labeled as such. In the present era of sweeping change in health care financing and health services delivery, increasing emphasis has been placed on efficiency in the allocation of scarce medical resources. The field of medical economics is well beyond its nascence, and broad public interest has emerged in studying the costs of medical and surgical therapies. As we spend more administrative dollars on cost-containment, scrutiny is reaching all potential areas for conservation, including oncology, a province once considered sacred and off-limits to cost-cutting efforts.

Urologists have long been attentive to issues of cost in managing health care. In his autobiography, Hugh Hampton Young, the father of American urology, described a patient on whom he agreed to perform a prostatectomy in the 1920s for a fixed fee of $500 with a promise of only 3 weeks in the hospital. Because the patient suffered complications and remained hospitalized for much longer than planned, Young had to spend his entire professional fee plus an additional $350 to pay off the hospital bill (Young, 1940).

Health policy decisions today are based not only on biomedical research but also on sound evaluations of health care costs. The introduction of oral erectogenics, beginning in the late 1990s, has provided a perfect illustration of the tension between therapeutic advances and economic forces. The scientific discoveries that led to the advent of sildenafil and similar agents were rewarded with a Nobel Prize (Rajfer et al, 1992), yet insurers initially fervently resisted paying for them

(Lee, 1999). As such, as a surgical subspecialty with large numbers of Medicare patients, urology is a discipline in which cost-saving maneuvers may have tremendous financial impact.

KEY POINT: COSTS OF CARE

- Health policy decisions today are based not only on biomedical research but also on sound evaluations of health care costs.

Terms and Methods of Analysis

In its purist form, **research on health care costs involves counting the amount of money that is expended on facilities, equipment, supplies, and personnel during the provision of medical care.** But many costs are hidden. A more extensive approach would also include the opportunity cost of the time patients spend receiving care. For example, when estimating the cost of an interval cystoscopy after resection of a bladder tumor, a thorough assessment would include not only the cost of overhead, supplies, lidocaine jelly, urine cytology, and professional fees but also the cost to the patient in lost wages—or to his or her employer in lost productivity—during the time away from work for the procedure, travel, or any complications. This component is not insignificant. Employee absence from work has been estimated to cost U.S. businesses tens of millions of dollars annually (Walsh et al, 1989; Luz and Green, 1997; Stewart et al, 2003).

Because true costs are difficult to quantify at the individual, institutional, or population level, researchers instead often report data on charges. *Charges* **represent the amount that is billed for a service, whereas** *costs* **reflect what the provider expended to supply that service.** Most of the available administrative databases in health care are based either on financial discharge abstracts from hospitals or on claims data from large payers, insurance companies, or government agencies such as the Center for Medicare and Medicaid Services. These data sets primarily include information on charges and payments but not costs. The major advantage of using charge data is that they are much easier to obtain. The primary disadvantage is that they may not accurately reflect the true underlying costs of individual medical services. For example, a hospital that is losing money on intravenous pyelograms may make up the deficit by increasing its charges for urine cytologic studies. This practice may help balance the annual budget, but it corrupts the quality of the charge data. An economic analysis using charges for bladder cancer follow-up in this hospital will err by incorporating the inflated amounts charged for interval urine cytologic studies. Some analysts attempt to circumvent this problem by calculating a ratio of costs to charges for entire facilities, individual medical services, or diagnosis-based categories of care. Although imperfect, charges are frequently used to estimate the amount of money spent on health care.

To avoid the inherent problems in calculating costs and charges, some researchers instead measure *resource utilization* in terms of duration, frequency, and intensity of services (Munoz et al, 1988b). One of the most commonly reported units of comparative analysis is length of stay (LOS). Since 1983 when the prospective payment system was instituted to reimburse hospitals a predetermined amount of money based on the diagnosis-related group (DRG) into which each Medicare inpatient is classified (Munoz et al, 1988a, 1990a, 1990b, 1990c; Kahn et al, 1990), attention to LOS as an outcome variable in cost analyses has greatly increased.

In addition, **cost of care may be measured as intensity or numbers of services provided.** For example, rather than calculating the costs or charges for a 4-day hospitalization for radical nephrectomy, analysis may be based on the total number of complete blood cell counts, chest radiographs, bags of intravenous fluid, doses of antibiotic, and doses of narcotic ordered on any given day of the hospital stay or during the entire 4 days. By examining duration or frequency of medical services when studying costs, researchers can avoid the biases involved in using financial data.

Cost-effectiveness analysis is another popular technique used to evaluate new or established medical therapies. A cost-effectiveness analysis is performed by developing a probability model of the possible medical outcomes of different interventions (or a nonintervention such as watchful waiting for benign prostatic hyperplasia), identifying the expenses associated with each outcome, and comparing the results, typically reported as cost per year of life saved (Shepard and Thompson, 1979; Henriksson and Edhag, 1987; Chandhoke and DeAntoni, 1998; Manca et al, 2003). **Years of life saved, or** *life-years (LYs)*, **are calculated for a population, not for individuals.** Ten life-years might represent 2 patients, each of whom survives for 5 additional years or 120 patients, each of whom survives for 1 additional month (Smith et al., 1993). LYs are usually adjusted to account for different health states that may result from various treatments. These are called *quality-adjusted life-years (QALYs)*. For example, when comparing two treatments for localized prostate cancer, if both options are determined to cost $10,000 per year of life saved, then the two may seem equivalent. However, if one treatment yields years that are compromised by bothersome sexual dysfunction while the other yields years that are free of such problems, then the difference in quality of the years saved must be factored into the equation. Analyses that rely on estimations of QALYs are facilitated by the estimation of patient utilities, or preferences, for various health states (Nease and Owens, 1994; Albertsen et al, 1998; Saigal et al, 2001, 2002). If patients appraise an impotent year as being worth less than a potent year, then quality adjustments may make the first treatment more expensive per QALY saved. *Cost-benefit analysis* differs by including not only the costs but also the equivalent monetary value of any benefits garnered during the extra years of life. Often, this refers to wages earned or income accrued during that time. In more sophisticated analyses, future income and expenses related to a particular health state are discounted to present value by incorporating projected interest and inflation rates over time.

KEY POINT: TERMS AND METHODS OF ANALYSIS

- Analyses that rely on estimations of quality-adjusted life years are facilitated by the estimation of patient utilities, or preferences, for various health states.

Patterns of Care

Much of the current research into the cost of treating urologic conditions is predicated on the observation that patterns of care differ substantially for certain conditions. Physician demographics as well as patient age have been found to affect practice patterns (Bennett et al, 1991; O'Leary et al, 2000; Bird et al, 2003; Joudi et al, 2003; Fallon et al, 2005). Despite the relative scarcity of cost analyses in urology, significant variations in length of stay and charges have been reported for many nonurologic medical and surgical hospitalizations (Fisher et al, 2003a, 2003b; Weinstein, 2004; Wennberg, 2004). Cost savings can be achieved by identifying variations in urologists' practice habits and targeting them for reduction in intensity and duration (Sage et al, 1988; Kramolowsky et al, 1995a, 1995b). These changes in urologic practice have been shown to result in equivalent medical outcomes (Cleary et al, 1991), despite the finding that patients tend to dislike shorter postoperative hospital stays (Litwin et al, 1997; Durieux et al, 2004). Overall, studies have been mixed. Some have described the successful use of cost-control mechanisms in urology (Cuckow 1992a, 1992b), whereas others have failed to show sustained results (Forrest et al, 1981).

Analysis of both medical and surgical DRGs indicates that consistent patterns of resource utilization are identifiable during the course of hospitalizations, suggesting that elements of utilization may be managed more effectively to yield cost savings (Carter and Melnick, 1990). This is particularly true in treatments for genitourinary conditions, such as hematuria or incontinence, many of which may be standardized. Urology is a fertile area for economic analysis because so little is known about the cost-effectiveness of screening and treatment interventions for even the most common genitourinary conditions (Perlman et al, 1996; Grossfeld and Carroll, 1998; Benoit et al, 2001; Mor et al, 2001; Shaw, 2004).

The advent of managed care has greatly facilitated the study of practice patterns and medical outcomes. **Most researchers agree that health maintenance organizations (HMOs) improve access to medical services and cost-efficiency of care without compromising quality** (Holtgrewe 1998a, 1998b; Haffer and Bowen, 2004). However, contrary evidence suggests that cancer patients may wait longer for treatment in HMOs than in fee-for-service plans (Greenwald, 1987). Among men newly diagnosed with prostate cancer, those cared for in HMOs are almost 1.5 times more likely to receive radiation than surgery for clinically localized tumors. This appears consistent with the general HMO emphasis on outpatient care. In this study, HMO patients had a lower overall mortality rate than did non-HMO patients. Interestingly, low income men treated in HMOs enjoyed survival times that were significantly greater than for middle or high income men in HMOs or fee-for-service plans (Greenwald and Henke, 1992).

The National Institute of Diabetes and Digestive and Kidney Diseases recently conducted the Urologic Diseases in America project (accessible at www.uda.niddk.nih.gov) that began to define the burden of urologic disease on the American public by quantifying trends in resource utilization, practice patterns, costs, outcomes, and epidemiology across the spectrum of urologic conditions (Litwin et al, 2005; Williams, 2005). Documenting these trends has broad

implications for quality of health care, access to care, and the equitable allocation of scarce resources, both in terms of medical services and research budgets.

Case Mix

When studying patterns of care or medical costs, it is critical to adjust for case mix. *Case mix refers to the severity of illness and degree of comorbidity in a group of patients* (Iezzoni, 1996; Iezzoni et al, 1996). These patient characteristics may influence treatment outcomes. For example, older patients are more likely to experience complications after surgery. If this fact is not considered when comparing surgical complication rates across hospitals, evaluators may erroneously conclude that a hospital with an older patient population is providing poorer quality care. To use outcomes to measure quality of care, we need to adjust for these other factors, including baseline patient characteristics and intervening treatments. This adjustment (referred to as case-mix adjustment or risk adjustment) can be extremely complex, and the selection of factors must be carried out carefully so that outcomes can be interpreted accurately. For a variety of reasons, sicker patients cost more, and it is important to control for this difference in comparative analyses. When examining the factors that lead to higher hospital charges for more ill patients, two forces must be considered: duration and intensity of care. **Duration is usually quantified as inpatient LOS, whereas intensity of care may be assessed as numbers of services or charges per day.** Patients with greater comorbidity may remain hospitalized longer even if they do not receive more intense care during their stays. Duration and not intensity appears to be the primary force driving up hospital charges for sicker urology patients (Litwin et al, 1993).

Various comorbidity measures (Kaplan and Feinstein, 1974; Charlson et al, 1987; Greenfield et al, 1993, 1995; Crabtree et al, 2000; Di Gangi Herms et al, 2003) have been used by researchers to adjust for case mix and predict mortality from competing causes in clinical studies. Although all perform reasonably well in the research setting, most are based on diagnoses from retrospective chart review and are difficult to apply clinically (Albertsen et al, 1996).

Physicians have been largely successful at attenuating the increases in hospital costs by eliminating unnecessary hospital days, but maximal savings may have been reaped from this strategy (Bodenheimer, 2005). Nevertheless, continued tailoring of the intensity and duration of service to patient burden of illness may still be shown to reduce costs. Urology has played a central role in the ongoing struggle to balance the competing priorities of minimizing costs and maximizing quality in health care (Loughlin, 2003). The most recent government strategy adopted in pursuit of this goal is Medicare's pay-for-performance initiative, in which providers are differentially reimbursed based on their adherence to various condition-specific quality indicators (Corrigan and Ryan, 2004).

KEY POINT: CASE MIX

■ Physicians have been largely successful at attenuating the increases in hospital costs by eliminating unnecessary hospital days, but maximal savings may have been reaped from this strategy.

QUALITY OF CARE

As detailed in a prostate cancer quality infrastructure proposed by Rand Corporation researchers (Litwin et al, 2000; Spencer et al, 2003), **quality of care research evaluates "the degree to which health services for individuals and populations increase the likelihood of desired health outcomes and are consistent with current professional knowledge"** (Lohr 1990; Lohr et al, 1992). Several initiatives are underway to collect and disseminate performance information about medical care. For example, the National Committee on Quality Assurance (www.ncqa.org) provides information to health care purchasers about the comparative performance of health plans in the U.S. The Joint Commission on the Accreditation of Healthcare Organizations (www.jcaho.org) applies outcomes-based quality measures to accredit hospitals. The Foundation for Accountability (www.facct.org), a consumer organization, "creates tools that help people understand and use quality information, develops consumer-focused quality measures, supports efforts to gather and provide quality information, and encourages health policy to empower and inform consumers." More than 200 performance indicators have been collected in the National Library of Healthcare Indicators.

The conceptual framework for the measurement of quality of care in medicine was established 40 years ago by Donabedian (1966). In this model, quality of care measures are categorized into three domains: structure, process, and outcome. Structure of care includes the equipment, resources, and provider experience necessary to provide care. Examples include volume of cases and board certification of providers. Process of care refers to technical and interpersonal elements of care that transpire between doctor and patient, such as the extent of the history and physical examination, documentation of the workup, and ordering of diagnostic and laboratory tests. Process measures are often considered to be the best measure of quality (Brook et al, 1996, 2000). Outcomes of care include survival rates, complications, and patient-reported outcomes (PROs), such as health-related quality of life. As underscored in his exposition on quality of care, Blumenthal argues that the most important new development in our current understanding of medical outcomes was the recognition that it is patients who define which outcomes are most important and whether or not they have been achieved (Blumenthal 1996a, 1996b; Blumenthal and Epstein, 1996).

Hence, we have seen the advent of patient-reported outcomes as primary endpoints in clinical trials and the primary focus of much attention in evidence-based medicine.

KEY POINTS: QUALITY OF CARE

■ Quality of care measures are categorized into three domains: structure, process, and outcome.

■ Structure of care includes the equipment, resources, and provider experience necessary to provide care (e.g., volume of cases and board certification of providers).

■ Process of care refers to technical and interpersonal elements of care that transpire between doctor and patient (e.g., the extent of the history and physical examination, documentation of the workup, and ordering of diagnostic and laboratory tests).

■ Process measures are often considered to be the best measure of quality.

■ Outcomes of care include survival rates, complications, and patient-reported outcomes (e.g., health-related quality of life).

Structure of Care

Structure encompasses the human, technical, and financial resources needed to provide medical care. Organizations such the Joint Commission on the Accreditation of Healthcare Organizations and the American College of Surgeons have generally relied on structural measures in their accreditation procedures. Important structural attributes for quality of care may include clinician characteristics (e.g., percentage of physicians who have board certification, average years of experience, distribution of specialties), organizational characteristics (e.g., staffing patterns, reimbursement method), patient characteristics (e.g., insurance type, illness profile), and community characteristics (e.g., per capita hospital beds, transportation system, environmental risks). Structural measures specific to prostate cancer quality could include the presence of a multidisciplinary cancer center or psychological support services.

Although certain structural characteristics may be necessary to provide good care, they are usually insufficient to ensure quality of care. Therefore, the best structural measures are those that can be shown to have a positive influence on the process of care and on patient outcomes, although this relationship has not been confirmed (Brook et al, 1990). One structural measure that is positively associated with outcomes is the volume or number or cases treated by a particular physician or institution (Joshi and Miller, 2004; Katz et al, 2004; Lee et al, 2004; Nuttall et al, 2004; Dibra et al, 2005; Killeen et al, 2005; Lyman et al, 2005; Vitale et al, 2005). Patients treated at facilities or by surgeons who performed fewer radical prostatectomies experience more surgical complications than those treated by higher volume providers (Lu-Yao et al, 1996; Ellison et al, 2000; Begg et al, 2002; Hu et al, 2003). It is not clear what characteristics of providers performing many surgeries contribute to better outcomes; however, high volume appears to be an important predictor of good quality care.

Process of Care

Process of care is the set of activities that goes on between patients and practitioners and is often divided into interpersonal process and technical process. *Interpersonal process* refers to the way that the clinician relates to the patient and includes issues such as whether the clinician supplied sufficient information in a clear enough manner for the patient to make an informed choice regarding his or her treatment. Patient survey data are generally used to assess quality of interpersonal process.

Technical process **refers to whether the medically appropriate decisions are made when diagnosing and treating the patient and whether care is provided in an effective and skillful manner.** One way to evaluate the appropriateness of medical treatment is to determine if the care provided is consistent with current medical knowledge and adheres to the professional standard. This assessment can be done by developing *quality indicators* that describe a process of care that should occur for a particular type of patient in a specific clinical circumstance. To be valid, these quality indicators should be based on the evidence in the medical literature and on current professional standards of care. Determining the latter often requires an expert panel to achieve consensus. The performance of physicians and health plans is then assessed by calculating rates of adherence to the indicators for a sample of patients.

Using quality indicators to evaluate appropriateness of care is relatively straightforward. However, assessing the effectiveness or skill of technical process of care is much more difficult. Indeed, direct observation may be necessary to assess quality of technical process of care. Alternatively, we may have to rely on measuring outcomes to evaluate whether care was provided in a skillful manner. For example, measurement of surgical blood loss or number of specimens with positive margins, both surgical outcomes, may be indicators of the quality of surgical technical process. Conversely, operative time may represent the surgeon's manual dexterity or the technical complexity of a case. Hence, celerity is not generally considered an accurate indicator of operative quality.

Outcomes of Care

Outcomes include changes in patients' current and future health status, including health-related quality of life, as well as their satisfaction. Cancer researchers generally use survival or progression-free survival as the main outcome measure in clinical studies. Sometimes proxy measures (also called surrogate endpoints or intermediate outcomes) are used that do not measure the outcome directly but are thought to be correlated with it. When a proxy measure is used as a quality indicator, there must be evidence that the proxy measure is truly a substitute for the outcome of interest. For example, rapid increase in prostate-specific antigen (PSA) level after treatment of localized prostate cancer appears to be associated with cause-specific mortality (Patel et al, 1997; D'Amico et al, 2005), so PSA doubling time may be a reasonable proxy outcome. For proxy measures to be useful as quality measures, intervention

should affect both the measure and the underlying disease (Schatzkin et al, 1996).

The most important patient-reported outcome is health-related quality of life, a multidimensional construct that includes somatic symptoms, functional ability, emotional well-being, social functioning, body image, as well as overall well-being (Guyatt et al, 1986, 1997; Cella and Bonomi, 1995). Quality of life assessment provides a comprehensive evaluation of how the illness and its treatment affect patients.

Another patient-reported outcome commonly measured is patient satisfaction (Strasser et al, 1993), which refers to patients' perceptions of the quality of care they received. Patient satisfaction is also usually assessed by patient survey. One limitation of satisfaction ratings is that patients are not generally able to evaluate the technical quality of their care. In fact, studies have found no consistent relationship between patient satisfaction and technical quality of care (Cleary and McNeil, 1988; Hayward et al, 1993). That is, a physician who interacts with patients in a warm and open way may provide care that is technically poor (Aharony and Strasser, 1993). In addition, patients' satisfaction ratings may vary with their expectations. Nonetheless, when used in conjunction with other measures, data about patient satisfaction can provide useful information about overall quality of care.

KEY POINT: OUTCOMES OF CARE

- The most important patient-reported outcome is health-related quality of life, a multidimensional construct that includes somatic symptoms, functional ability, emotional well-being, social functioning, body image, as well as overall well-being.

Challenges to Using Outcomes to Evaluate Quality of Care

Adverse outcomes may be uncommon events, so large samples of patients may be needed when using outcome measures to detect differences in quality among health systems or hospitals. For example, to detect a two percentage point difference in the rate of postoperative wound infections between two hospitals (e.g., 5% for one and 7% for the other), each hospital would need to have at least 1900 patients who had the surgery.

In addition, a single outcome may be affected by many different factors, making it difficult to establish accountability. When comparing differences in surgical outcomes across hospitals, one does not know if the differences in outcomes are related to the skill of the surgeon, the competence of the surgical team, the postoperative care, or the case mix. And the more time that elapses between the intervention and the outcome, the more difficult this problem becomes. For example, when comparing 10-year outcomes in women treated for incontinence at different facilities, what is more important, the quality of the initial treatment or the quality of care for recurrent symptoms?

Outcomes can also be measured for more than one purpose. Although we are interested in developing outcome measures for evaluating the quality of care received by patients with urologic diseases, outcomes are also used clinically to track a patient's progress and, in clinical trials, to measure the efficacy or effectiveness of a new drug or intervention (Williams et al, 2004). The same measures can sometimes be used for both purposes, but certain measures are better suited for one purpose or the other. For example, 5-year survival rates are a standard measure used in studies of new cancer treatments. However, when measuring quality of care for purposes of accountability or quality improvement, we generally need a shorter time horizon than 5 years. If we compared the 5-year survival of men with early-stage prostate cancer at two institutions, we might indeed find that one institution had higher survival rates, suggesting that it had better quality of care. However, during those 5 years, staff changes, revamped procedures, or new technology may have improved or weakened the quality of care at the hospitals, thereby making the comparison of only historical relevance.

Other Quality Measurement Approaches

In addition to the Donabedian model, other approaches to measuring quality of care rely on implicit review or assessment without explicit criteria. This typically involves having an acknowledged expert carry out a formal evaluation of the episode of care by reviewing the medical chart without the establishment of specific criteria for quality. The evaluator makes an implicit judgment of whether the care rendered was of high quality. This approach is de facto qualitative and may not yield results that are as valid and reproducible.

HEALTH-RELATED QUALITY OF LIFE

Health-related quality of life (HRQOL) is one of several variables commonly studied in the field of medical outcomes research. HRQOL encompasses a wide range of human experience, including the daily necessities of life, such as food and shelter, intrapersonal and interpersonal responses to illness, and activities associated with professional fulfillment and personal happiness (Patrick and Erickson, 1993). Contemporary interpretations of HRQOL are based on the World Health Organization's (1948) long-standing definition of health as a "state of complete physical, mental, and social well-being and not merely the absence of disease." Because illness may affect both quantity and quality of life, all constituents of well-being must be addressed when treating patients with urologic diseases. Perhaps most importantly, HRQOL involves patients' own perceptions of their health and ability to function in life. Indeed, patient perceptions of physical function have prognostic value in predicting survival (Fossa, 1994). In light of evidence that survival and clinical outcomes may be similar across treatments for many conditions, quality of life considerations may be the critical factor in medical decision-making for some instances.

Whereas quantity of life is relatively easy to assess in terms of survival, the measurement of quality of life presents more challenges, primarily because it is less familiar to most clinicians (Litwin, 1994). To quantify these qualitative phenomena, the principles of psychometric test theory are applied. This

KEY POINT: WORLD HEALTH ORGANIZATION DEFINITION OF HEALTH

■ Health is not merely the absence of disease but a state of complete physical, mental, and social well-being.

discipline provides the theoretical underpinnings for the science of survey research (Tulsky, 1990; Aaronson, 1991; Deyo et al, 1991; McSweeny and Creer, 1995; Testa and Simonson, 1996; Guyatt et al, 1997). Data are collected with HRQOL surveys, called instruments. Instruments typically contain questions, or items, that are organized into scales. Each scale measures a different aspect, or domain, of HRQOL. For example, items on a particular instrument may address a patient's ability to have an erection and his satisfaction with ejaculation, both of which might be included in a sexual domain.

Some scales comprise dozens of items, whereas others may include only one or two items. Each item contains a stem (which may be a question or a statement) and a response set. Most response sets are one of the following types: (1) Likert scale, in which the respondent selects from a list of degrees of agreement or disagreement with the stem; (2) Likert-type scale, in which the respondent chooses from a list of text responses; (3) visual analog scale, in which the respondent marks a point on a line that is anchored on both ends by descriptors; and (4) numerical rating scale, in which the respondent chooses a number, usually between 0 and 10. Other response sets and approaches have been developed for children, people of low literacy, and various other populations (Nelson et al, 1990; Adler et al, 2000; Finlay and Lyons, 2001).

It is axiomatic that HRQOL assessments capture patients' own perceptions of their health and ability to function in life. Instruments are best when they are self-administered by the patient, but if interviewer assistance is required it must be from a neutral third party in a standardized fashion. Some studies have demonstrated that physicians typically underestimate the symptom burden experienced by prostate cancer patients, perhaps because their queries are not sensitive enough or because patients tend to understate their problems when speaking directly with the primary caregiver (Slevin et al, 1988; Fossa et al, 1990; Litwin et al, 1998b). Other studies, however, suggest that physicians tend to overestimate the impact of the disease and its treatment on patients' psychosocial functioning and sense of well-being (Fossa et al, 1996; Lampic et al, 1996; Sneeuw et al, 1997). Conversely, spouses may overstate some domains and understate others when compared with patient assessments (Sprangers and Aaronson, 1992). Kornblith and colleagues (1994) presented results from a large sample of patients and spouses, both of whom were administered several validated HRQOL measures. Spouses reported greater psychological distress but fewer sexual problems than did the patients. In a study of perspectives on HRQOL during antihypertensive therapy, Testa (1993) demonstrated that physicians were less sensitive to the impact of side effects, reporting less than 15% of the symptoms reported by patients. Spousal reports were more sensitive than patient self-assessments, particularly in the area of sexual function.

HRQOL Instruments

HRQOL instruments may be general or disease specific. General HRQOL domains address the components of overall well-being, and disease-specific domains focus on the impact of particular organic dysfunctions that may affect HRQOL. General HRQOL instruments typically address general health perceptions, sense of overall well-being, and function in the physical, emotional, and social domains. Disease-specific HRQOL instruments focus on special and/or more directly relevant domains, such as anxiety about cancer recurrence, dizziness from antihypertensive medications, or suicidal thoughts during depression therapy (Patrick and Deyo, 1989). **Disease-specific and general HRQOL domains often impact each other, leading to important interactions that must be considered in the interpretation of HRQOL data** (Fossa et al, 1997). Further research is needed in urology to explore how much of the variation in overall HRQOL is explained by variation in the disease-specific domains.

In some conditions, such as chronic renal failure, cirrhosis with ascites, and stroke, general HRQOL may be so profoundly impacted that disease-specific HRQOL assessment is unnecessary. In many indolent conditions, however, the treatments may alter bodily functions that are not fully appreciated by assessing only the broader domains of general HRQOL. Conversely, in patients with advanced cancer, HRQOL may be affected predominantly by pain, fatigue, and other constitutional symptoms that are well captured by general HRQOL instruments.

There are numerous HRQOL instruments validated for use in urologic and other conditions; Table 5–1 presents several examples. Many psychologists, sociologists, and statisticians devote their entire professional careers to the activity of developing and validating these instruments. At least one medical journal, *Quality of Life Research,* is dedicated exclusively to presenting this research. Hence, an abundance of literature exists on general HRQOL, and a significant body of work has been published on HRQOL in patients with various conditions (McDowell and Ewell, 1987; Patrick and Erickson, 1993). In urology, most HRQOL research has focused on individuals with prostate cancer, urinary incontinence, benign prostatic hyperplasia, end-stage renal disease, and bladder cancer (Edgell et al, 1996; Blaivas, 1998; Eton and Lepore, 2002; Botteman et al, 2003; Penson et al, 2003; Matza et al, 2004). The National Cancer Institute has been particularly active in establishing interest in outcomes measurement for patients with malignant disease (www.outcomes.cancer.gov). A comprehensive resource for validated HRQOL instruments is available on the Internet at www.proqolid.org.

General HRQOL Instruments

General quality of life instruments have been extensively studied and validated in many types of patients, sick and well. Examples include the RAND Medical Outcomes Study 36-Item Health Survey, also known as the SF-36 (Ware and Sherbourne, 1992; Ware et al, 1994; Gandek et al, 1998b), the Quality of Well-Being scale (QWB) (Kaplan et al, 1976, 1997, 1998; Kaplan and Bush, 1982; Kaplan and Anderson, 1988;

Anderson et al, 1989), the Sickness Impact Profile (SIP) (Bergner et al, 1976, 1981), and the Nottingham Health Profile (NHP) (Martini and McDowell, 1976; McDowell et al, 1978; Hunt et al, 1985). Each assesses various components of HRQOL, including physical and emotional functioning, social functioning, and symptoms. Each has been thoroughly validated and tested.

The RAND Medical Outcomes Study 36-Item Health Survey (SF-36) is one of the most commonly used instruments and is regarded by some as a "gold standard" measure of general HRQOL. It is a 36-item, self-administered instrument that takes less than 10 minutes to complete and quantifies HRQOL in multi-item scales that address eight different health concepts: physical function, role limitation due to physical problems, bodily pain, general health perceptions, social function, emotional well-being, role limitation due to emotional problems, and energy/fatigue. The SF-36 may also be scored in two summary domains: physical and mental. Recently, a shorter 12-item version, the SF-12, has been developed for use in studies requiring greater efficiency. It provides a somewhat narrower view of overall health status and is usually scored only in the two summary domains (Ware et al, 1995, 1996; Gandek et al, 1998a).

The QWB summarizes three aspects of health status—mobility, physical activity, and social activity—in terms of QALYs, quantifying HRQOL as a single number that may range from death to complete well-being. The original QWB contains only 18 items, but it requires a trained interviewer. A newer self-administered version of the QWB is now available and has been shown to produce scores that are equivalent to the interviewer-administered version and are stable over time (Kaplan et al, 1997). The SIP measures health status by assessing the impact of sickness on changing daily activities and behavior. It is self-administered but contains 136 items and can take 30 minutes or longer to complete. The NHP covers six types of experience that may be affected by illness—pain, physical mobility, sleep, emotional reactions, energy, and social isolation—by using a series of weighted "yes" or "no" items. It contains 38 self-administered items and can be completed fairly quickly. Mental health is often measured with the Profile of Mood States (POMS) (Jacobson et al, 1978; Norcross et al, 1984; Cella et al, 1987; Albrecht and Ewing, 1989), a 65-item self-administered instrument that measures dimensions of affect or mood in six domains, including anxiety, depression, anger, vigor, fatigue, and confusion. A validated short form is also available (Baker et al, 2002).

Cancer-Specific HRQOL Instruments

Because of the well-documented impact of malignancies and their treatment on HRQOL, cancer-specific quality of life also has been investigated extensively. Numerous instruments have been developed and tested that measure the special impact of cancer (regardless of primary site) on patients' routine activities. Examples include the European Organization for the Research and Treatment of Cancer Quality of Life Questionnaire (EORTC QLQ-C30) (Aaronson et al, 1993), the Functional Assessment of Cancer Therapy (FACT) (Cella et al, 1993), and the Cancer Rehabilitation Evaluation System (CARES) and its short form (CARES-SF) (Schag and Heinrich, 1990; Schag et al, 1991, 1994). Each has been validated and tested in patients with various types of cancer.

Table 5-1. Examples of Instruments for Quality of Life and Symptom Assessment in Urology

Name	Length	Reference
General		
MOS 36-Item Health Survey (SF-36)	36	Ware and Sherbourne, 1992
MOS 12-Item Health Survey (SF-12)	12	Ware et al, 1996
Quality of Well Being Scale (QWB)	18	Kaplan et al, 1976
Sickness Impact Profile (SIP)	136	Bergner et al, 1981
Nottingham Health Profile (NHP)	38	Hunt et al, 1985
Profile of Mood States (POMS)	65	Norcross et al, 1984
McGill-Melzack Pain Questionnaire	21	Meissner, 1980
Benign Prostatic Hyperplasia		
American Urological Association Symptom Index	7	Barry et al, 1992
BPH Impact Index	4	Barry et al, 1995a
BPH Symptom Problem Index	7	Barry et al, 1995b
Cancer		
European Organization for the Research and Treatment of Cancer (EORTC) QLQ-C30	30	Aaronson et al, 1993
Functional Assessment of Cancer Therapy (FACT)	28	Cella et al, 1993
Cancer Rehabilitation Evaluation System Short Form (CARES-SF)	59	Schag et al, 1991
Rotterdam Symptom Checklist	27	de Haes et al, 1990
University of California, Los Angeles Prostate Cancer Index (UCLA-PCI)	20	Litwin et al, 1998b
UCLA-PCI Short Form (UCLA-PCI-SF)	15	Litwin and McGuigan, 1999
Expanded Prostate Cancer Index Composite	50	Wei et al, 2000
Functional Assessment of Cancer Therapy—Prostate (FACT-P)	12	Esper et al, 1997
Prostate Cancer Treatment Outcome Questionnaire (PCTO-Q)	41	Shrader-Bogen et al, 1997
European Organization for the Research and Treatment of Cancer QLQ-PR25	25	Borghede and Sullivan, 1996
Prostate Cancer–Specific Quality-of-Life Instrument (PROSQOLI)	10	Stockler et al, 1998
Functional Assessment of Cancer Therapy—Bladder (FACT-Bl)	12	Mansson et al, 2002
Incontinence		
King's Health Questionnaire (KHQ)	21	Kelleher et al, 1997
Incontinence Impact Questionnaire (IIQ)	30	Shumaker et al, 1994
Incontinence Impact Questionnaire (IIQ) Short Form	7	Uebersax et al, 1995
Urological Distress Inventory (UDI)	19	Shumaker et al, 1994
Urological Distress Inventory (UDI) Short Form	6	Uebersax et al, 1995
Symptom Severity Index and Symptom Impact Index	8	Black et al, 1996
Stress and Urge Incontinence and Quality of Life Questionnaire	9	Kulseng-Hanssen and Borstad, 2003
SEAPI-QMM Quality of Life Index	15	Stothers, 2004
International Consultation on Incontinence Questionnaire (ICIQ)	4	Avery et al, 2004
Overactive Bladder Questionnaire (OAB-q)	33	Coyne et al, 2002
Other		
NIH Chronic Prostatitis Symptom Index	9	Litwin et al, 1999
International Index of Erectile Function	15	Rosen et al, 1997
Brief Male Sexual Function Inventory	11	O'Leary et al, 1995
Erectile Dysfunction Inventory of Treatment Satisfaction (EDITS)	11+5	Althof et al, 1999
Kidney Disease Quality of Life instrument	134	Hays et al, 1994
Dialysis Symptom Index	30	Weisbord et al, 2004

Readers are directed to the Quality of Life Instruments Database (www.proqolid.org) for guidance when selecting an instrument for quality of life measurement in studies of prostate or other cancers.

The EORTC QLQ-C30 was designed to measure cancer-specific HRQOL in patients with a variety of malignancies. Its 30 items address domains that are common to all cancer patients. The questionnaire includes five functional scales (physical, role, emotional, cognitive, and social functioning), a global health scale, three symptom scales (fatigue, nausea/vomiting, and pain), and six single items concerning dyspnea, insomnia, appetite loss, constipation, diarrhea, and financial difficulties due to disease. The EORTC QLQ-C30 has performed well in populations with urologic malignancies (Curran et al, 1997). Disease-specific modules for cancers of the prostate (Aaronson and van Andel, 2001), breast (Sprangers et al, 1996), lung (Bergman et al, 1994), head and

neck (Bjordal et al, 1994), and other sites have been developed according to methodologically rigorous techniques. Additional disease-specific modules are being developed.

The FACT is usually applied as a two-part instrument that includes a general item set pertaining to all cancer patients (FACT-G) and one of several item sets containing special questions for patients with specific tumors (see later). Each item is a statement that a patient may agree or disagree with across a five-point range. The FACT-G domains include well-being in five main areas: physical, social/family, relationship with doctor, emotional, and functional. The FACT-G includes 28 items and is easily self-administered. Disease-specific modules are available for numerous patient tumor groups, including prostate (Esper et al, 1997), bladder, colorectal (Ward et al, 1999), breast (Brady et al, 1997), ovary (Basen-Engquist et al, 2001), and other cancers. Modules are also available for issues specific to bone marrow transplantation

(McQuellon et al, 1997), anemia, and fatigue (Cella, 1997; Yellen et al, 1997).

The CARES Short Form (CARES-SF) is a 59-item, self-administered instrument that measures cancer-related quality of life with five multi-item scales: physical, psychosocial, medical interaction, marital interaction, and sexual function. A large and valuable database of patients with many different tumors, including urologic tumors, has been collected by the instrument's authors (Schag et al, 1994). These data are helpful when comparing the experience of prostate cancer patients with that of patients with other types of cancer.

Selecting a Quality of Life Instrument

Investigators or clinicians considering measuring HRQOL in a clinical study or in clinical practice should choose an instrument (or instruments) depending on the particular population being studied and the clinical questions being asked. Using previously validated instruments, to the extent they are applicable and appropriate, obviates the need for an arduous process of instrument development and validation. A general and a disease-specific module in combination are suitable for most studies. However, if a particular domain (e.g., pain) is the focus of the study, specific, expanded questionnaires should be sought focusing on the area of interest. Respondent burden needs to be considered, particularly for longitudinal studies where subjects will complete the same instruments multiple times. Pretesting instruments that will be used in clinical studies is advisable.

Psychometric Validation of New HRQOL Instruments

The development and validation of new instruments and scales is a long and arduous process. It is not undertaken lightly. Simply drawing up a list of questions that seem appropriate is fraught with potential traps and pitfalls. For this reason, it is always preferable to use established, validated HRQOL instruments (Guyatt et al, 1992).

When scales and instruments are developed, they are first pilot tested to ensure that the target population can understand and complete them with ease. Pilot testing is usually preceded by focus groups to refine the wording of items and

to ensure comprehensive coverage of concepts and domains deemed important by respondents. Pilot testing of an instrument should also include formal cognitive testing. This process is typically led by behavioral scientists who specialize in developing and assessing the wording and ordering of questionnaire items to ensure that they can be easily understood by respondents and that the answers that respondents provide are what investigators hope to learn from their study. Cognitive testing is usually performed on a very small number of respondents, usually 5 to 10 volunteers, who are asked to "think aloud" during the process of questionnaire completion. After cognitive testing, a larger pilot test is then performed on a somewhat larger sample, using the exact planned enrollment procedures and materials that are intended for the full study. Pilot testing can reveal problems that might otherwise go unrecognized by researchers. For example, many terms that are commonly used by medical professionals are poorly understood by patients. This may result in missing data if patients leave questions blank. Furthermore, because many patients with urologic malignancy are older and may have poor eyesight, pilot testing often identifies easily corrected visual barriers, such as type size and page layout. In addition, self-administered instruments with complicated skip patterns (e.g., "If you answered yes to item 16b, continue with item 16c; if you answered no to item 16b, skip to item 19a") may be too confusing for even the most competent patients to follow. This, too, can result in missing data and introduce difficulties in the analysis. Pilot testing is a necessary and valuable part of instrument development. It serves as a reality check on those developing the scales.

Scales and instruments are also evaluated for the two fundamental statistical properties, reliability and validity (Litwin, 2002).

Reliability

Reliability (Table 5–2) **refers to how free the scale is of measurement error,** that is, what proportion of a patient's test score is true and what proportion is due to chance variation. Two of the most commonly used metrics are test-retest and internal consistency reliability.

Test-retest reliability is the most commonly used indicator of survey instrument reliability. It is measured by having the same respondents complete a survey at two different points in

Type of Reliability	Characteristics	Comments
Test-retest	Measures the stability of responses over time, typically in the same group of respondents	Requires administration of survey to a sample at 2 different and appropriate points in time. Time points that are too far apart may produce diminished reliability estimates that reflect actual change over time in the variable of interest.
Intra-observer	Measures the stability of responses over time, in the same individual respondent	Requires completion of a survey by an individual at 2 different and appropriate points in time. Time points that are too far apart may produce diminished reliability estimates that reflect actual change over time in the variable of interest.
Alternate-form	Uses differently worded stems or response sets to obtain the same information about a specific topic	Requires 2 items in which the wording is different but aimed at the same specific variable and at the same vocabulary level
Internal consistency	Measures how well several items in a scale vary together in a sample	Usually requires a computer and statistician to carry out calculations
Inter-observer	Measures how well 2 or more different respondents rate the same phenomenon	May be used to demonstrate reliability of a survey or may itself be the variable of interest in a study

Table 5–2. Reliability Assessments for Health-Related Quality of Life Instruments

time to see how stable their responses are. It is a measure of how reproducible a set of results is. Correlation coefficients are then calculated to compare the two sets of responses. These correlation coefficients are collectively referred to as the survey instrument's test-retest reliability. In general, the correlation coefficients are considered good if they are at least 0.70. This implies that the survey responses are reasonably consistent from one point in time to another. When measuring test-retest reliability, one must be careful not to select items or scales that measure variables likely to change over short periods of time. Variables that are likely to change over a given period of time will produce low test-retest reliability in measurement instruments. This does not mean that the survey instrument is performing poorly but simply that the attribute itself has changed. One can certainly measure characteristics that tend to change over time. In fact, this is often the purpose of HRQOL research. But test-retest reliability must be documented over shorter periods to decrease the degree of measurement error attributable to the survey itself.

When measuring test-retest reliability, one must also consider that individuals may become familiar with the items and answer partly based on their memory of what they answered the last time. Called the *practice effect,* this presents a challenging problem to address in measures of test-retest reliability over short periods of time. As a result of the practice effect, test-retest reliability figures can be falsely inflated.

Alternate-form reliability provides one way to escape the problem of the practice effect. It involves using differently worded items to measure the same attribute. Questions and responses are reworded or their order is changed to produce two items that are similar but not identical. One must be careful to create items that address the same exact aspect of behavior with the same vocabulary level and the same level of difficulty. Items must differ only in their wording. Items or scales are administered to the same population at different time points, and correlation coefficients are again calculated. If these are high, the survey instrument or item is said to have good alternate-form reliability. One common way to test alternate-form reliability is to change the order of the response set. Changing the order of the response set is most effective when the two time points are close together. This approach forces the respondent to read the items and response sets very carefully, thereby decreasing the practice effect. Another way to test alternate-form reliability is to change the wording of the response sets without changing the meaning (Fig. 5–1). Another common method to test alternate-form reliability is to change the actual wording of the items themselves. Again, one must be careful to design items that are truly equivalent to each other. Items that are worded with different degrees of reading difficulty do not measure the same attribute. They are more likely to measure the reading comprehension or cognitive function of the respondent.

Item 1: Circle one number in each response set

During the last week, how often did you usually empty your bladder?	
1 to 2 times per day	1
3 to 4 times per day	2
5 to 8 times per day	3
12 times per day	4
More than 12 times per day	5
During the last week, how often did you usually empty your bladder?	
Every 12 to 24 hours	1
Every 6 to 8 hours	2
Every 3 to 5 hours	3
Every 2 hours	4
More than every 2 hours	5

Figure 5–1. Alternate-form reliability. Equivalent but differently worded response sets to 2 items on urinary function are presented. The response sets for each item are differently worded but functionally equivalent. This makes them good candidates for use in a test of alternate-form reliability.

Item 2: Circle one number in each response set

During the last 4 weeks, how much did you leak urine?	
Never	1
A little bit	2
A moderate amount	3
A lot	4
Constantly	5
During the last 4 weeks, how much did you leak urine?	
I used no pads in my underwear	1
I used 1 pad per day	2
I used 2 to 3 pads per day	3
I used 4 to 6 pads per day	4
I used 7 or more pads per day	5

Sometimes data are not collected from a group of subjects but are recorded by a single observer. In this case, test-retest reliability is assessed by having that individual make two separate measurements. Both data sets from the same observer are then compared with each other. The correlation between two data sets from the same individual is commonly known as *intra-observer reliability*. It measures the stability of responses from the same respondent and is a form of test-retest reliability.

Inter-observer (inter-rater) reliability provides a measure of how well two or more evaluators agree in their assessment of a variable. It is usually reported as a correlation coefficient between different data collectors. When survey instruments are self-administered and designed to measure the respondent's own behaviors or attitudes, inter-observer reliability is not used. However, whenever there is a subjective component in the measurement of an external variable, it is important to calculate this statistic. Sometimes inter-observer reliability is used as a psychometric property of a survey instrument, whereas other times it is itself the variable of interest. Inter-observer reliability is often used when the measurement process is less quantitative than the variable being measured.

Internal consistency reliability is a measure of the similarity of an individual's responses across several items, indicating the homogeneity of a scale (Tulsky, 1990). It is applied not to single items but to groups of items that are thought to measure different aspects of the same concept. Internal consistency is an indicator of how well the different items measure the same issue. This is important because a group of items that purports to measure one variable should indeed be clearly focused on that variable. Although single items may be quicker and less expensive to administer, the data set is richer and more reliable if several different items are used to gain information about a particular behavior or topic. The statistic most often used to quantify this unidimensionality or internal consistency of a scale is called Cronbach's coefficient alpha (Cronbach, 1951). Internal consistency can be reported for any scale with more than one item, whereas test-retest reliability requires the scale to be administered to some patients twice within a short interval, preferably less than 1 month.

Validity

Validity (Table 5–3) **refers to how well the item, scale, or instrument measures the attribute it is intended to measure.** An item designed to measure pain should measure pain and not some related variable such as anxiety. A scale meant to measure emotional quality of life should not measure depression, which is a related but different variable. When an instrument has validity, it is said to measure the truth. Validity provides evidence to support drawing inferences about quality of life from the scale scores. Validity has three general forms: content, criterion, and construct.

Content validity, sometimes casually referred to as face validity, involves a subjective assessment of the scope and completeness of a scale and is usually measured in the early stages of an instrument's development from experts and patient focus groups. The assessment of content validity typically involves an organized review of an instrument's contents to ensure that it includes everything it should and does not

Table 5–3. Validity Assessments for Health-Related Quality of Life Instruments

Type of Validity	Characteristics	Comments
Content	Formal expert review of how good an item or series of items appear	Usually assessed by individuals with expertise in some aspect of the subject under study
Criterion: Concurrent	Measures how well the item or scale correlates with gold-standard measures of the same variable	Requires the identification of an established generally accepted gold standard
Criterion: Predictive	Measures how well the item or scale predicts expected future observations	Used to predict outcomes or events of significance that the item or scale might subsequently be used to predict
Construct	A theoretical measure of how meaningful a survey instrument is, usually after years of experience by numerous investigators	Not easily quantifiable

include anything it should not. Patients should be involved in this assessment. Clinicians may be unaware of the subtle nuances experienced by patients who live day to day with a given condition. Families also may provide helpful insights into dimensions that might otherwise be overlooked by experts. This said, it remains important for clinicians to review the items for relevance to and focus on the variables of interest. Content validity is not quantified with statistics. Rather, it is presented as an overall opinion of a group of trained judges. Nevertheless, it provides a good foundation on which to build a methodologically rigorous assessment of a survey instrument's validity.

Criterion validity is a more quantitative approach to assessing the performance of scales and instruments. It requires the correlation of scales scores with results from other established tests (concurrent validity) or with future measurable outcomes (predictive validity). For example, concurrent validity of a new sexual function scale might be correlated with objective performance on infusion cavernosometry. Likewise, the predictive validity of a new quality of life scale for physical function might be correlated with the number of subsequent physician visits or hospitalizations.

Concurrent validity requires that the survey instrument in question be judged against some other method that is acknowledged as a gold standard for assessing the same variable. It may be a published psychometric index, a scientific measurement of some factor, or another generally accepted test. The fundamental requirement is that it be regarded as a good way to measure the same concept. The statistic is calculated as a correlation coefficient with that test. A high correlation suggests good concurrent validity. Alternatively, a test may be selected for comparison that is expected to measure an attribute or behavior that is opposite to the dimension of interest. In this case, a low correlation indicates good concurrent validity. The reason one would not simply use the established gold standard as your measure of choice is that it may be too cumbersome, expensive, or invasive to apply.

Predictive validity is the ability of a survey instrument to forecast future events, behaviors, attitudes, or outcomes. It may be used during the course of a study to predict response to a stimulus, success of an intervention, or time to a medical endpoint. Over a brief interval, predictive validity is similar to concurrent validity in that it involves correlating the results of one test with the results of another test administered around the same time. If the time frame is longer and the second test occurs much later, then the assessment is of predictive validity. Like concurrent validity, predictive validity is calculated as a correlation coefficient between the initial test and the secondary outcome.

Construct validity is the most valuable yet most difficult way of assessing a survey instrument. Often determined only after years of experience with an instrument, it is a measure of how meaningful the scale or survey instrument is when in practical use. It is typically not calculated as a statistic but as a gestalt of how well a survey instrument performs in a multitude of settings and populations over a number of years. Construct validity implies that the instrument of interest yields results that are similar to (convergent validity) or different from (divergent validity) several other methods for obtaining the same information about a given trait or concept.

Responsiveness

Responsiveness of an HRQOL instrument refers to how sensitive the scales are to change over time (Deyo et al, 1991; Stockler et al, 1998). That is, a survey may be reliable and valid when used at a single point in time but in some circumstances it must also be able to detect meaningful improvements or decrements in quality of life during longitudinal studies. The instrument must "react" in a time frame that is relevant for patients over time. Because HRQOL may change over time, longitudinal measurement of these outcomes is important (Olschewski and Schumacher, 1990; Zwinderman, 1990). Different domains may become more or less prominent over time as the course of disease and recovery evolves. While their perception of cure waxes and wanes with time since treatment or the latest PSA level, patients may feel more or less impacted by their HRQOL impairments.

To make useful inferences regarding absolute scores or change scores over time, it is important to determine what meaning different numerical values have (Samsa et al, 1999). For example, the minimally important difference of the American Urological Association Symptom Index (Barry et al, 1992) has been measured at about 3 points (Barry et al, 1995b). When no such thresholds have been established, one can roughly approximate the smallest difference that is important to the patient as one third to one half of a standard deviation (Norman et al, 2003; Sloan and Dueck, 2004). A more quantitative approach involves calculating an effect size, or Guyatt statistic, typically expressed as the ratio of the raw change in score among those who change to the standard deviation of the change among those who did not change (Guyatt et al, 1987, 2002).

Over time, patients' perceptions of quality of life impairments may change. This phenomenon, known as response shift, must be considered when evaluating longitudinal patterns in HRQOL outcomes (Breetvelt and Van Dam, 1991; Sprangers, 1996).

Responsiveness and minimally important differences may be ascertained by correlation with a self-administered global response assessment (GRA) item that measures improvement or worsening over time on a Likert-type scale such as markedly, moderately, or minimally worse, unchanged, or minimally, moderately, or markedly better.

Comparison Groups

Prospective, longitudinal data collection beginning at baseline before treatment is always best, because this approach may reveal time-dependent evolution of HRQOL domains (Talcott et al, 1998). Patients may then serve as their own controls. Assessing HRQOL at baseline before treatment allows for the inclusion of baseline age- or comorbidity-related changes that should not be attributed to treatment. This approach facilitates the stratification of discriminants from determinants of HRQOL.

However, investigators often use methodologies in which HRQOL is assessed cross-sectionally, rather than longitudinally. In cross-sectional surveys, patients cannot serve as their own temporal controls because recall of pre-treatment HRQOL is notoriously inaccurate (Aseltine et al, 1995; Herrmann, 1995). Hence, studies must rely on appropriate comparison groups. Selecting the best comparison group is an important step in conducting a meaningful analysis of HRQOL outcomes. If "normal" is defined as the absence of any dysfunction, then treatment groups may be held to too high a standard. For example, to interpret the HRQOL effects of prostate cancer treatment meaningfully, a valid context is provided by assessing HRQOL in older men without prostate cancer (Litwin, 1999; Litwin et al, 1995) or in prostate cancer patients on watchful waiting. Hence, in comparisons of the effect of treatment efficacy on HRQOL, longitudinal studies starting before treatment provide the most compelling results. In cross-sectional studies, a suitable comparison group is critical.

Cultural Issues and Translations

When designing new HRQOL instruments or applying established ones in populations of different ethnicity or nationality, one must make sure that the items translate well into both the language and the culture of the target audience. Although the items may have been linguistically translated into a new language, they may not measure the same dimension in that culture (Herdman et al, 1997). This is particularly relevant when studying social attitudes and health behaviors, for example as related to pain, sexual function, or urinary incontinence. Different cultures have very different concepts of health, well-being, illness, and disease. A well-developed concept in one culture may not even exist in another. Failing to be attentive to multicultural issues may result in significant bias when collecting data. For example, when classifying ethnicities, survey researchers often categorize all Asians together. For some projects this may be acceptable, however, many attitudes and behaviors vary markedly among Chinese, Japanese, Filipino, Korean, Indian, and other cultures within Asia. By lumping them all into one class, researchers may overlook differences that are important to the conclusions.

When translating an HRQOL instrument into a new language, one must also consider issues of linguistics. Specific methodologies have been developed for cross-validating HRQOL instruments in other languages (Vela Navarrete et al, 1994; Boyle, 1997). One begins by having two to three bilingual individuals perform independent "forward translations" into the new language. Next, these translators reconcile any differences in word choice in the new language. Next, two to three different bilingual individuals perform independent "back translations," in which the reconciled translation is converted back into the primary language. Then, translators independently review the forward, reconciled, and back-translated versions to resolve any language differences in the translation and agree on a final wording in the new language. Finally, after pilot testing the instrument with bilingual subjects, a larger-scale validation must be conducted to establish reliability and validity in the new language. This process has been accomplished for a variety of instruments used in the assessment of patients with urologic diseases (Sagnier et al, 1994, 1996; Arocho et al, 1995; Boyle, 1997; Krongrad et al, 1997; Badia et al, 1998; Gandek et al, 1998; Collins et al, 2001; Hochreiter et al, 2001; Kakehi et al, 2002; Duarte, et al, 2005).

During a recent linguistic translation of an instrument to measure symptoms in men with chronic prostatitis, researchers collected data from many Spanish-speaking patients, including subjects from Argentina, Mexico, Spain, and the United States. The translation had high overall reliability, but respondents expressed difficulty in distinguishing the response categories "a menudo" ("often") from "normalmente" ("usually") in one of the items. Hence, the researchers revised "a menudo" to "muchas veces" ("much of the time") and "normalmente" to "casi siempre" ("almost always") to improve the distinctiveness of response categories.

In addition to varying cultural perspectives on disease and health, international differences in health systems may also have a substantial impact on the way patients view their quality of life. For example, in countries where patients are required to pay all or most of the treatment costs, spending a lot of money for marginally better survival rates may have a larger effect on quality of life than the disease or its treatments. Furthermore, in cultures where the patient's relatives are compelled to absorb the costs of care, the quality of life of the entire family unit should also be considered.

KEY POINT: CULTURAL ISSUES AND TRANSLATIONS

■ When designing new HRQOL instruments or applying established ones in populations of different ethnicity or nationality, one must make sure that the items translate well into both the language and the culture of the target audience.

Caveats on the Collection of HRQOL Data

Although there are some single instruments that are multidimensional, many quality of life researchers have endorsed a "battery approach," in which the various components of

HRQOL are measured with different scales to ensure that each domain receives adequate attention. Longer instruments can provide greater precision, but they also increase the chance that patients will tire of the exercise and not provide reliable or valid answers. This is particularly true in the multicenter clinical trial setting. Hence, shorter instruments are generally preferable when obtaining HRQOL measurements under such circumstances. In general, it is easier and more efficient to use established instruments that have already undergone psychometric validation. HRQOL data collected using published instruments allow the researcher to compare the study results to data from other samples or diverse populations with various chronic diseases. Nevertheless, sometimes it is necessary to develop new questionnaire items to ensure that a particular concept is adequately evaluated. Under such circumstances new scales can be tested for reliability and validity during the course of data collection.

Once an instrument is thoroughly pilot tested and found to be reliable and valid, it must be administered in a manner that minimizes bias. Quality of life data cannot and should not be collected from patients directly by the treating health care provider. Patients often provide socially desirable responses under such circumstances (Tannock, 1990). This introduces measurement error. No matter how objective the treating clinician may claim to be, it is impossible for him or her to collect objective and unbiased outcomes data through direct questioning. Variations in phrasing, inflection, eye contact, rapport, mood, and other factors are difficult or impossible to eliminate. Data must be gathered by disinterested third parties using established psychometric scales and instruments.

KEY POINT: CAVEATS ON HRQOL DATA COLLECTION

■ Once an instrument is thoroughly pilot tested and found to be reliable and valid, it must be administered in a manner that minimizes bias.

FUTURE IMPLICATIONS

HRQOL research questions begin with the need for basic descriptive analysis of quality of life in patients treated for urologic diseases. Depiction of the fundamental elements in quality of life for these individuals requires study of their health perceptions and how their daily activities are affected by both their general health and their cancer. Physical and emotional well-being form the cornerstone of this approach, but research must also extend to other issues that can affect a patient's quality of life and satisfaction, such as eating and sleeping habits, anxiety and fatigue, depression, rapport with the physician, presence of a spouse or partner, and social interactions. Characterization of all domains must address not only the actual functions but also the relative importance of these issues to patients.

Beyond simple descriptive analysis, HRQOL outcomes must be compared between patients undergoing different modes of therapy. General and disease-specific HRQOL must be measured to facilitate comparison with patients treated for diabetes, heart disease, arthritis, and other common chronic

Table 5-4. Quality of Life Objectives in Research and Practice

- To assess overall treatment efficacy, including subjective morbidity
- To help determine whether the goals of treatment have been met
- To educate patients and clinicians about the full spectrum of treatment outcomes
- To facilitate medical decision-making
- To provide the defining issue if treatments are otherwise equivalent

conditions. Quality of life outcomes may be correlated with medical variables, such as comorbidity, or sociodemographic variables, such as age, race, education, income, insurance status, geographic region, and access to health care. In this context, HRQOL may be linked with many factors other than the traditional medical ones.

All clinical trials and observational cohort studies in patients with benign or malignant urologic disease should include an HRQOL component. One example of a cohort study that has been particularly fruitful with regard to quality of life analyses is the Cancer of the Prostate Strategic Urologic Research Endeavor (CAPSURE), an industry-funded longitudinal disease registry for men with prostate cancer (Lubeck et al, 1996, 1997; Cooperberg et al, 2004). Resources are scarce in any clinical trial, but clinical trials provide the best setting for prospective outcomes measurement and contribute to the thoughtful interpretation of more clinical endpoints (Steineck et al, 2002). Nonetheless, HRQOL data collections are labor intensive; hence, when planning clinical trial budgets investigators must be aware that they are expensive to include. The more instruments that are selected, the richer the potential database, but it is important to remain parsimonious in instrument selection, choosing only the relevant domains of HRQOL.

The ultimate goal of quality of life research is to improve medical care and assist in medical decision-making (Table 5-4). Individual patients who incorporate quality of life con-

siderations into their decision equations tend to feel better about their treatment choices, are more satisfied overall with their care, and experience less regret (Cassileth et al, 1989). Hence, patient education provides a potent impetus for studying and reporting quality of life. With accurate measurement of quality of life outcomes, we can better assess whether the specific and overall goals of therapy have been met. This allows individuals and societies to balance the competing health care priorities of optimizing survival, quality of life, and resource utilization. Furthermore, the evaluation of patient-perceived HRQOL permits assessment of low-grade subjective morbidity that, although not typically life threatening, may present considerable distress for the patient. Such minor morbidity is often overlooked during the busy daily routine of patient care.

KEY POINT: FUTURE IMPLICATIONS

- The ultimate goal of quality of life research is to improve medical care and assist in medical decision-making.

SUGGESTED READINGS

Coons SJ, Rao S, Keininger DL, et al: A comparative review of generic quality-of-life instruments. Pharmacoeconomics 2000;17:13-35.

Guyatt GH, Kirshner B, Jaeschke R: Measuring health status: What are the necessary measurement properties? J Clin Epidemiol 1992;45:1341-1345.

Litwin MS, Hays RD, Fink A, et al: Quality-of-life outcomes in men treated for localized prostate cancer. JAMA 1995;273:129-135.

Marquis P, Chassany O, Abetz L: A comprehensive strategy for the interpretation of quality-of-life data based on existing methods. Value Health 2004;7:93-104.

Slevin ML, Plant H, Lynch D, et al: Who should measure quality of life, the doctor or the patient? Br J Cancer 1988;57:109-112.

Ware JE Jr, Sherbourne CD: The MOS 36-item short-form health survey (SF-36): I. Conceptual framework and item selection. Med Care 1992;30:473-483.

SECTION III

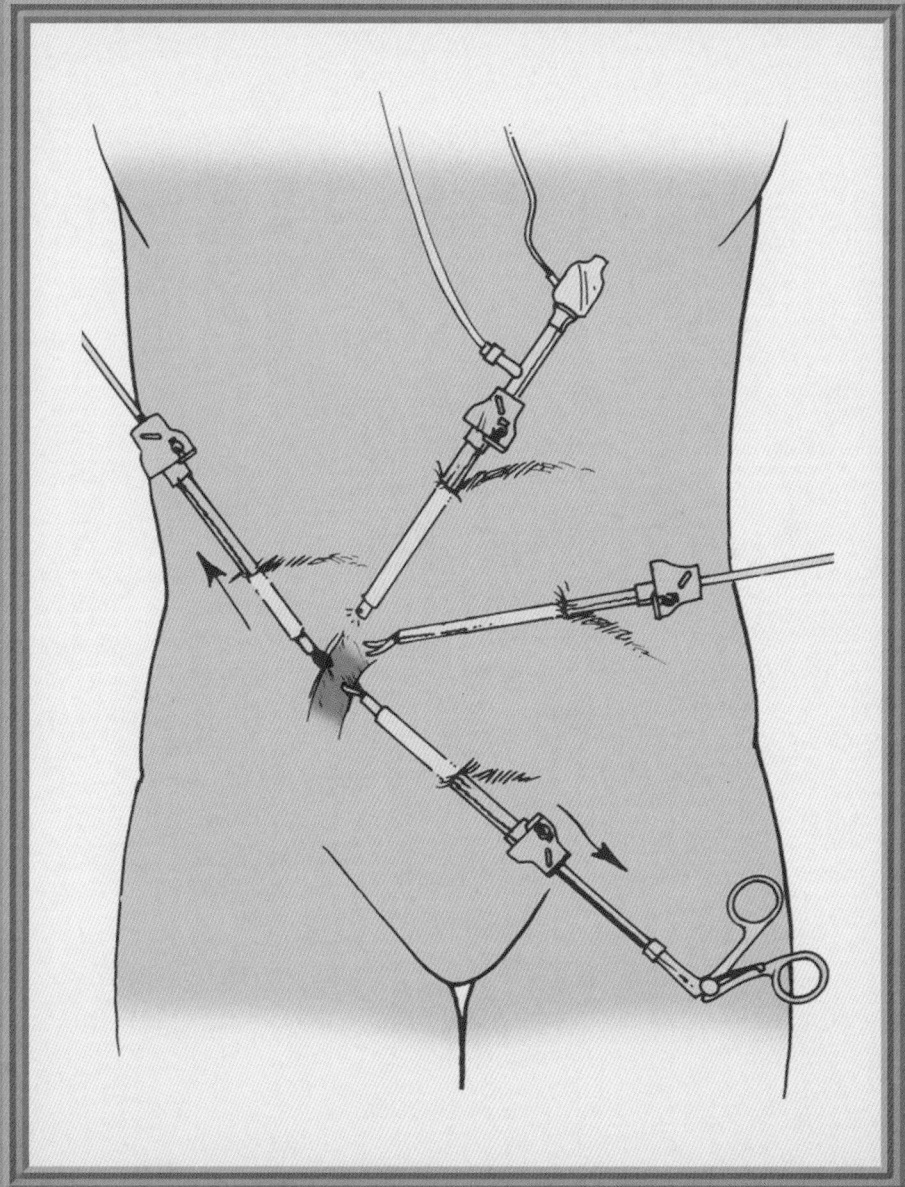

BASICS OF UROLOGIC SURGERY

6 Basic Instrumentation and Cystoscopy

H. BALLENTINE CARTER, MD • DAVID Y. CHAN, MD

Instrumentation and endoscopy of the lower urinary tract are performed routinely for the diagnosis and treatment of urologic diseases. A basic understanding of lower urinary tract anatomy and available instruments is essential for safe and successful manipulation of the lower urinary tract. In this chapter we address basic techniques that are used in the office practice of urology. Ureteroscopy and other endoscopic techniques are addressed in Chapter 45, Ureteroscopy and Retrograde Ureteral Access.

URETHRAL CATHETERIZATION

Indications

Urethral catheterization is performed for diagnosis and treatment of urologic disease. Many types of catheters are available for urethral catheterization, and the choice of a specific type of catheter depends on the reason for catheterization.

With respect to diagnosis, catheterization is often performed in females for collection of urine for culture to avoid contamination by skin flora. This practice is usually not necessary in males because clean-catch specimens can be obtained without contamination by skin flora. Measurement of the postvoid residual urine can be performed less invasively with ultrasonography; however, catheterization can be performed for this purpose if ultrasound equipment is not available. Instillation of contrast agents into the bladder and urethra for cystourethrography along with urodynamic studies to assess bladder and urethral function necessitates urethral catheterization. Administration of intravesical therapy such as with bacillus Calmette-Guérin (BCG) or mitomycin-C for bladder cancer also requires temporary catheterization.

Relief of infravesical obstruction is one of the most common therapeutic indications for urethral catheterization. Infravesical obstruction can occur as a result of prostatic enlargement, blood clots within the bladder, postsurgical strictures, and urethral inflammatory processes. In these instances, a specialized catheter may be required to relieve the obstruction. Urethral catheters are also used to drain the bladder after surgical procedures involving the lower urinary tract and in both medical and surgical fields to accurately monitor urinary output. Clean intermittent catheterization performed by the patient or an assistant is a common means of managing neurogenic bladder dysfunction when the bladder functions as a storage organ but no longer empties normally. Although many institutionalized patients are left with indwelling catheters because of urinary incontinence, it is preferable to manage these patients with clean intermittent catheterization or a condom device for urine collection, if possible, because of the risk of infection with long-term indwelling urethral catheters. Finally, in urologic practice, urethral catheters are often used as stents after surgery to allow healing of an anastomosis or incision involving the bladder neck or urethra.

Types of Catheters (Fig. 6–1)

Catheter size is usually referred to using the French (Fr) scale (circumference is in millimeters), in which 1 Fr = 0.33 mm in diameter. For conversion from one scale to the other, it is easier to remember that each millimeter in diameter is approximately 3 Fr; thus, a No. 18 Fr catheter is about 6 mm in diameter. Catheter sizes refer to the outside circumference of the catheter, not the luminal diameter. Thus, a No. 20 Fr catheter may have a different luminal size for urinary drainage, depending on the type of material used for construction and the number of lumens within the catheter (see later discussion).

Straight rubber or latex catheters (see Fig. 6–1A to C), often referred to as Robinson catheters, are most commonly used for one-time catheterizations (straight catheterization). These catheters are also available with multiple eyes, making them ideal for irrigating the bladder free of clots. Although these catheters can be left in place for bladder drainage by taping them to the penis, they are not as well tolerated as other catheter materials (e.g., silicone) because they have a tendency

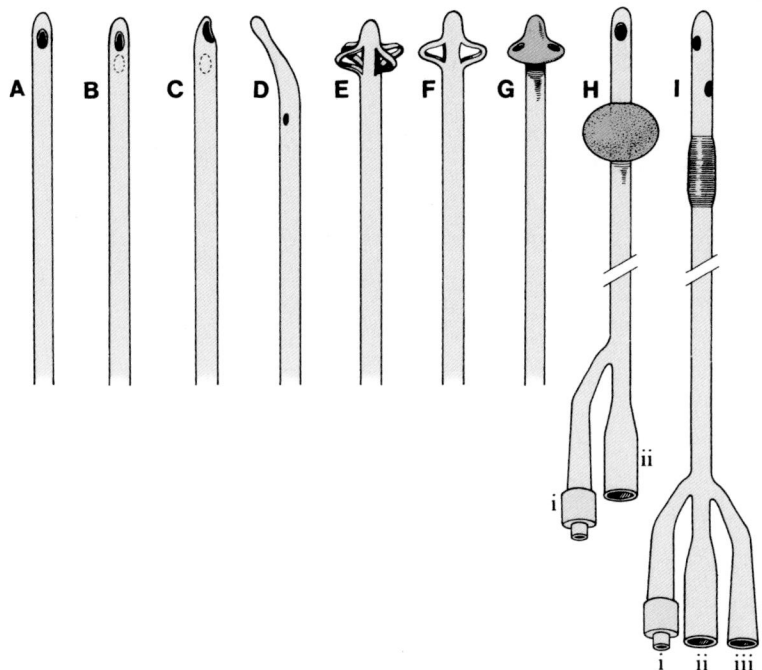

Figure 6–1. Types of large-diameter catheters. **A,** Conical tip urethral catheter, one eye. **B,** Robinson urethral catheter. **C,** Whistle-tip urethral catheter. **D,** Coudé hollow olive-tip catheter. **E,** Malecot self-retaining, four-wing urethral catheter. **F,** Malecot self-retaining, two-wing catheter. **G,** Pezzer self-retaining drain, open-end head, used for cystotomy drainage. **H,** Foley-type balloon catheter, one limb of distal end for balloon inflation (i), one for drainage (ii). **I,** Foley-type, three-way balloon catheter, one limb of distal end for balloon inflation (i), one for drainage (ii), and one to infuse irrigating solution to prevent clot retention within the bladder (iii).

to become encrusted with urinary precipitates. Shorter, straight catheters are available for female patients.

Catheters with a curved tip (e.g., coudé catheters, see Fig. 6–1D) are specifically designed to help bypass areas of the male urethra that are difficult to negotiate with a straight catheter. The normal S-shaped male bulbar urethra and the prostatic urethra associated with an enlarged prostate can be difficult to bypass with a straight catheter because of the urethral angle associated with the former and bladder neck elevation associated with the latter. Curved-tip catheters with balloons on the end (see description of Foley catheters) are available if it is necessary to leave the catheter indwelling after successfully passing a coudé catheter. In addition, coudé catheters can be used to irrigate out bladder clots by cutting additional holes in the end of the catheter if a straight catheter cannot be passed into the bladder.

Self-retaining catheters (see Fig. 6–1E to G), such as the Pezzer and Malecot catheters, are shaped in such a way that after placement at open surgery the catheter configuration maintains the catheter within a hollow viscus. For insertion, the wings of the catheter (i.e., retention mechanism) are flattened by stretching the catheter with a wire placed inside the catheter or stretching the catheter from outside with a clamp. The advantages of these catheters include the excellent urinary drainage afforded by the single lumen (no balloon mechanism) and the tip design, which make them ideal for use as cystostomy or nephrostomy tubes.

Foley-type catheters (see Fig. 6–1H and I) are most often used for long-term urethral catheterization. As such, they have a balloon mechanism at the distal end that, when inflated, keeps the catheter from sliding past the bladder neck. Two-way (see Fig. 6–1H) and three-way (see Fig. 6–1I) Foley catheters are available in multiple sizes. Two-way catheters have a small lumen for inflating the balloon mechanism and a larger lumen for urinary drainage. Three-way catheters have a small lumen for inflating the balloon mechanism, a lumen

for instilling irrigant, and a larger lumen for bladder drainage. Two-way catheters are used when an indwelling catheter for urinary drainage is indicated. Three-way catheters are used when bladder irrigation and drainage are necessary, as, for example, in a patient with bladder hemorrhage at risk for forming clots within the bladder that may lead to obstruction of the bladder outlet. It should be remembered that **catheters without a lumen for balloon inflation (e.g., Malecot) have a larger luminal size for bladder drainage than do Foley catheters of the same outer circumference. Likewise, for a given outer circumference, two-way catheters (with a balloon port) have a larger luminal size for urinary drainage than three-way catheters (with a balloon port and fluid instillation port).**

Patient Preparation

As with all procedures, the patient should be informed of the reason for catheterization and what to expect in terms of discomfort. Because catheterization is the instrumentation of a potentially sterile tract, it is essential to prepare and drape the urethra and surrounding area as for a surgical procedure. In the male, retrograde injection of 10 to 15 mL of a water-soluble lubricant-anesthetic (e.g., 2% lidocaine hydrochloride jelly) and placement of a urethral clamp for 5 to 10 minutes to allow the anesthetic to contact the mucosal surfaces are recommended before any urethral instrumentation. In the female, the lubricant-anesthetic can be placed directly on the catheter or a cotton-tipped applicator coated with lubricant-anesthetic can be placed in the urethra before catheterization.

Technique

In the male patient, the penis is placed on stretch perpendicular to the body (pointing slightly toward the umbilicus) without compressing the urethra and then the catheter is placed in the urethral meatus by holding the catheter at the tip. Gentle advancement of the catheter causes the least amount of discomfort, and, with experience, one can feel the natural resistance offered as the catheter traverses the external sphincter. As one approaches the bulbomembranous urethra (i.e., level of external sphincter), asking the patient to take slow, deep breaths will help relax the patient and often allow easier catheter passage. If resistance is met, one should not attempt forceful catheter insertion but should apply continuous, gentle pressure and ascertain at what level the potential obstruction exists.

In the female patient, shorter catheters are available for one-time catheterizations. After spreading the labia, one can usually identify the urethral meatus easily, and the catheter is placed gently into the bladder. **If long-term catheterization is anticipated** (>1 wk), it is advisable to use a Foley catheter made of the most biocompatible material. Catheters made of silicone are, in general, better tolerated over the long-term than those made of materials such as latex and polyurethane. In addition, one should choose the smallest urethral catheter that will accomplish the purpose of catheterization, because

urethral secretions drain more easily around smaller catheters. Allowing egress of urethral secretions lessens the chance of a clinically significant urethral inflammatory response. In the adult, catheters of No. 16 to 18 Fr are most often chosen for routine bladder drainage; in the pediatric age group, it is often necessary to use feeding tubes of No. 3 to 5 Fr.

Difficult Catheterizations

Difficulty in catheterizing the male patient can result from a variety of causes. Inability to pass the S-shaped bulbar urethra and resistance to catheter passage at the bulbomembranous urethra with tightening of the external sphincter are common. These problems are usually easily overcome with a coudé catheter to negotiate the bulb or with slow, gentle pressure to bypass the external sphincter.

Urethral strictures, prostatic enlargement, and postsurgical bladder neck contractures can make urethral catheterization difficult. If one encounters difficulty passing a catheter, it is wise to have a logical stepwise plan to maximize the chances of success in overcoming the difficulty (Fig. 6–2). Often, the

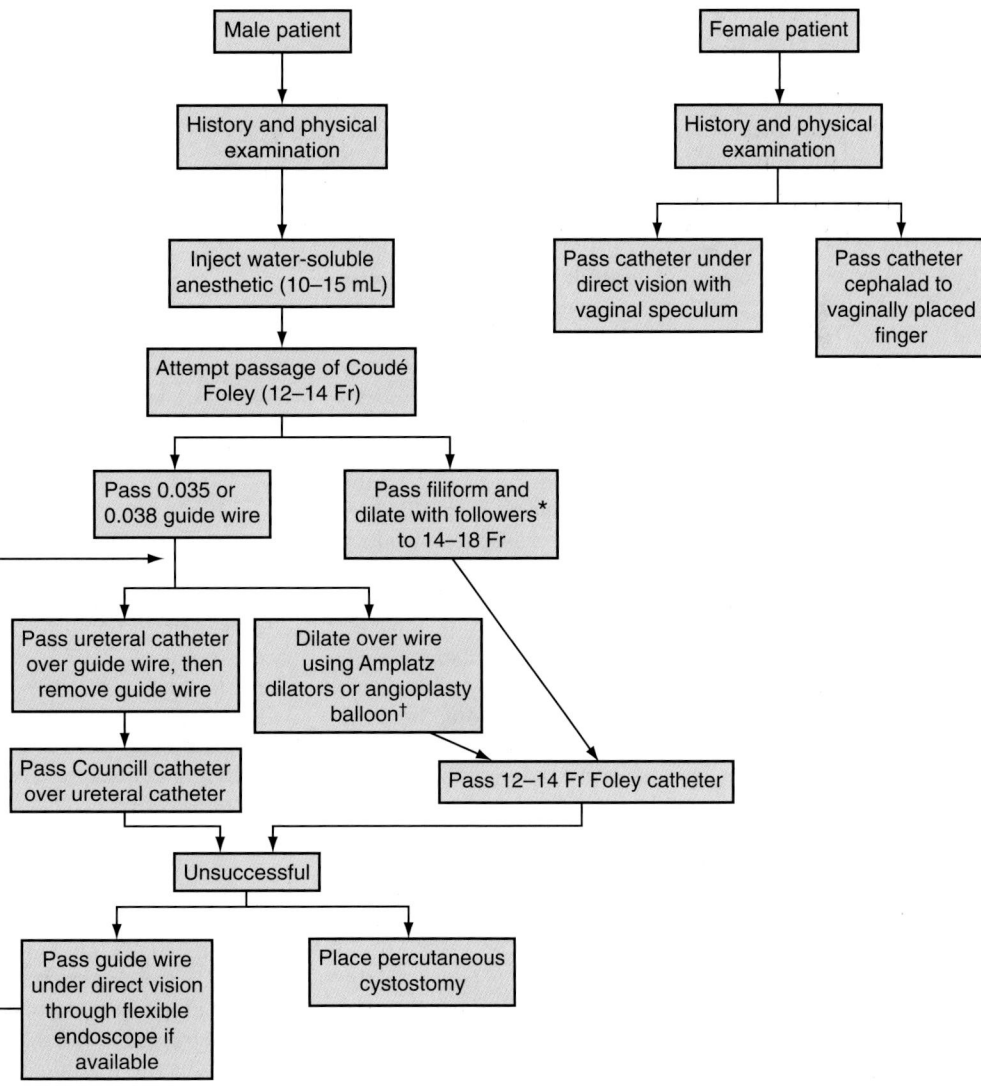

Figure 6–2. Suggested algorithm for approaching the difficult-to-catheterize patient. *Arrows* indicate the next reasonable step; *horizontal lines* indicate that either option is reasonable. (*See Fig. 6–4 and text for explanation of filiform and follower; †see Chapter 46, Percutaneous Approaches to the Upper Urinary Tract, for further explanation of Amplatz dilators.)

urologic history will give a clue to the most likely problem preventing catheterization. For example, the patient with a history of gonococcal urethritis in whom catheterization presents a problem is likely to have a pendulous urethral stricture whereas the patient who has undergone an open prostatectomy may have a bladder neck contracture. The history, together with the clinical observations from the initial unsuccessful urethral manipulation, should give the physician a clue to the problem.

If difficulty in initial catheterization is encountered, it is advisable to inject in a retrograde manner 10 to 15 mL of a water-soluble lubricant-anesthetic into the urethra. If the catheter is believed to have passed the bulbomembranous urethra and the problem is thought to be a bladder neck contracture, it is helpful to use a latex coudé catheter starting at No. 12 Fr, which will often bypass the obstruction. The coudé tip may allow negotiation of the lip, which is sometimes present at the 6 o'clock bladder neck position in men with bladder neck contractures. The curved tip of the catheter must be maintained in the same position during catheter passage, with the 12 o'clock position (curved tip pointing up) marked at the connector end of the catheter.

If coudé catheterization is not successful, it is sometimes possible to pass a guide wire with a floppy tip into the bladder. Next, an open-ended ureteral catheter is passed over the guide wire, and then a urethral catheter with an end hole (Councill catheter) can be passed over the guide wire and ureteral catheter (Fig. 6–3) (a No. 6 Fr ureteral catheter will pass over a 0.038-inch guide wire; a No. 5 Fr will pass over a 0.035-inch guide wire). Any catheter can be used as a Councill catheter if a hole punch is available so that an opening can be made in the catheter tip for insertion of the guide wire (see Fig. 6–3). A filiform catheter (Fig. 6–4) may negotiate the bladder neck if guide wire placement is unsuccessful. The filiform catheter can then be followed gently with a small follower screwed to the filiform (see section on "Urethral Dilatation"). If more than gentle pressure is necessary when attempting to pass any instrument into the bladder, the procedure should be aborted before urethral trauma occurs.

If available, a flexible cystoscope (see sections on "Urethral Dilatation" and "Cystourethroscopy") can be passed to the level of obstruction and a guide wire placed in the bladder under direct vision. The guide wire can be used to introduce a ureteral catheter, as described previously, or to guide passage of Amplatz semirigid dilators for dilatation of a urethral stricture (see section on "Urethral Dilatation").

When it is not possible to gently bypass a bladder neck contracture using the approaches previously described, placement of a cystostomy tube is preferable, because continued attempts at catheterization will cause urethral trauma. At a later time, investigation (radiographic and/or endoscopic) can be performed to define the nature of the obstruction. Percutaneous cystostomy kits are available with catheter and obturator (Fig. 6–5A). Percutaneous puncture of the bladder is accomplished with the obturator and catheter assembled; withdrawal of the obturator leaves the catheter indwelling within the bladder.

In preparation for percutaneous cystostomy placement, the suprapubic area is prepared and draped, with the patient in the supine position. The percutaneous tract, 3 to 4 cm above the symphysis pubis in the midline, should be anesthetized.

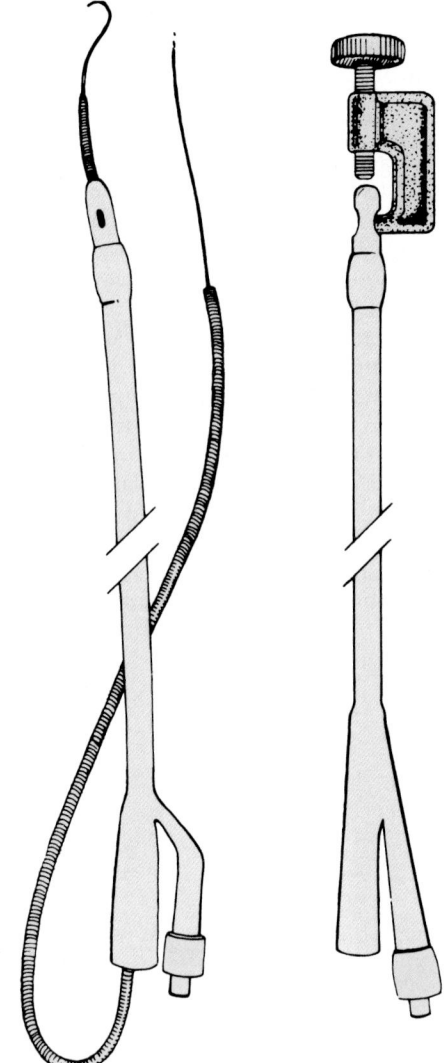

Figure 6–3. **Left,** Councill catheter—with end hole—passed over a guide wire and ureteral catheter. **Right,** Creation of an end hole in a Foley-type catheter with a hole punch.

Next, a spinal needle with a 10-mL syringe on the end is placed perpendicular to the skin and advanced while withdrawing on the syringe (see Fig. 6–5B). Correct placement of the needle is documented by withdrawal of urine into the syringe. The cystostomy catheter and obturator assembly is then placed in the same manner as the spinal needle, and the obturator is withdrawn, leaving the cystostomy catheter in place. The catheter is secured to the abdominal wall with suture material. Before considering percutaneous cystostomy placement, if there has been prior abdominal or pelvic surgery, or if the bladder is not full, one should consider using ultrasound for bladder localization, because the bowel may be in close proximity to the percutaneous tract.

Difficulty in catheterization of the female urethra is uncommon and usually results from extreme obesity and inability to locate the urethral meatus. Placement of a vaginal speculum can aid in localization of the urethra. Also, a catheter can be directed cephalad into the urethra by using the vaginally placed finger as a guide (see the algorithm in Figure 6-2).

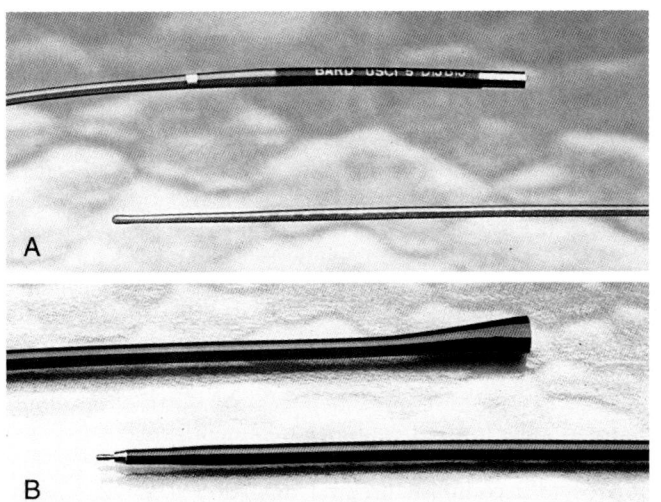

Figure 6–4. **A,** Filiform with grooved metal end to accept follower. **B,** Follower with metal tip designed to screw onto filiform. (**A** and **B,** Courtesy of CR Bard, Inc., Covington, GA.)

URETHRAL DILATATION
Indications

Urethral dilatation in the male is most commonly performed in preparation for placement of an endoscope or as therapy for a urethral stricture or bladder neck contracture. It is not uncommon for the outer circumference of the instruments used in transurethral surgery (No. 24 to 28 Fr) to exceed the diameter of the urethra, especially the urethral meatus and fossa navicularis. In such a case, it is necessary to dilate the urethra gently before passing the endoscope.

Dilatation for urethral stricture disease and bladder neck contractures is a therapeutic option. However, repeated dilatation can result in urethral trauma, which may ultimately increase the inflammatory process and worsen the stricture disease. True urethral strictures in the female are uncommon without a history of prior urethral or bladder neck surgery. Although dilatation of the female urethra as treatment for voiding dysfunction and recurrent infections was once a common practice, there are no objective data to support this form of treatment over other forms (e.g., medication). Occa-

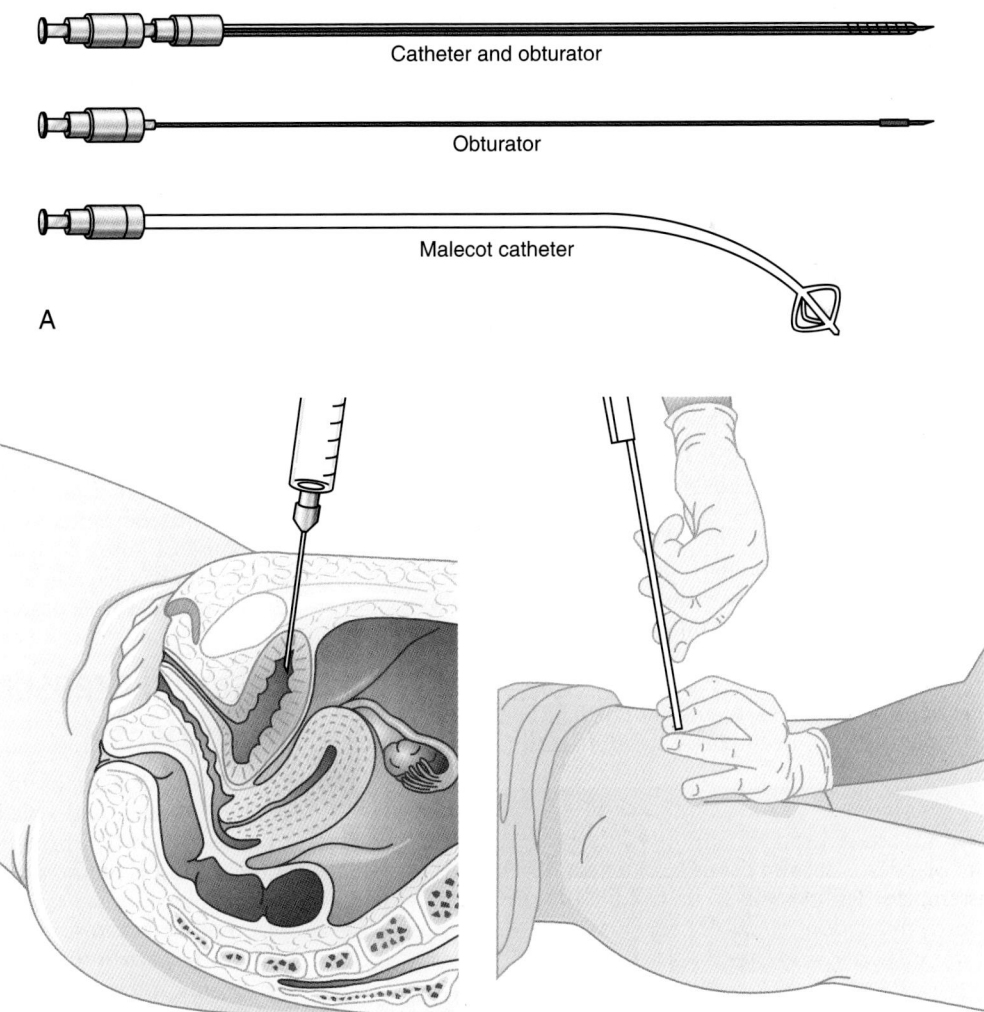

Figure 6–5. **A,** Stamey percutaneous cystostomy set with obturator and catheter. **B,** Localization of the bladder with a spinal needle placed percutaneously above the pubic bone. **C,** Placement of a percutaneous cystostomy catheter with obturator (right).

sionally, it is necessary to dilate the female urethra gently before introducing a larger endoscope.

Patient Preparation

When urethral dilatation is required before a transurethral procedure, no specific preparation is necessary because the patient has already been prepared and draped for surgery. Before urethral dilatation is begun in an outpatient setting, it is mandatory to ensure sterility and obtain adequate local anesthesia, as described previously for urethral catheterization. If the patient has a urinary tract infection, it must be treated effectively before elective instrumentation.

Technique

Urethral dilatation can be accomplished with metal sounds or bougies, urethral catheters of increasing size, filiforms and followers, Amplatz dilators, or balloon expansion. Metal sounds with curved tips (Fig. 6–6) are useful for dilating the male urethra before endoscopy if the endoscope is too large to easily pass transurethrally. The urethra is generally dilated to 1 Fr size greater than the endoscopic instrument to be used. In males, this is accomplished by holding the penis on stretch and rotating the sound while raising the penis cephalad as the sound approaches the bulbar urethra so that the curve of the sound conforms to the curve of the bulbar urethra. Care should be exercised in passing metal sounds; if resistance is met, it is unwise to exert force, because this can result in severe urethral trauma. In the short female urethra, the passage of short straight metal sounds, like that of catheters, is straightforward.

Urethral catheters of increasing size can be used for urethral dilatation and are passed as previously described. Patients can be taught self-dilatation to help prevent strictures from re-forming after treatment. This approach is more appropriate for older patients with strictures that are easily bypassed by urethral catheters after surgical incision of the stricture.

Filiforms are small-caliber, straight or spiral tip (No. 5 Fr or smaller) catheters without a lumen, onto which a larger catheter (follower) with a lumen can be attached (see Fig. 6–4). The filiform tip is passed without the follower first and maintains access to the bladder once it has been passed by coiling in the bladder. The follower is then screwed onto the filiform and is used to dilate the obstruction by gentle passage behind the filiform. On withdrawal of the follower, a larger follower can be placed on the filiform and the catheterization repeated.

Filiforms and followers are useful for bypassing and dilating urethral strictures. A single filiform (straight or spiral tip) can occasionally negotiate a tight stricture; however, more commonly, the filiform will pass into a false passage associated with the stricture. One can often continue gently passing multiple filiforms into the urethra and eventually occlude the false passage, allowing one of the filiforms to pass through the strictured area into the bladder. This is most often successful by "loading" the false passage with straight filiforms and using a spiral tip filiform to pass into the bladder. Placement of 5 to 10 filiforms may be required to bypass a difficult urethral obstruction. Filiforms and followers can be used for initial dilatation of a urethral stricture to allow passage of a catheter, as described previously. However, repeated dilatations with filiforms and followers are not recommended for the treatment of urethral strictures. Patients with strictures that require repeated passage of filiforms to bypass the obstruction should undergo some form of definitive treatment.

An angioplasty balloon can be placed over a wire and inflated to accomplish urethral dilatation if a wire can be negotiated into the bladder. This method of urethral dilatation requires fluoroscopy for proper placement of the balloon and may cause less trauma than other forms of urethral dilatation.

If available, flexible cystoscopy (see section on "Cystourethroscopy") can be used in the emergency department or on the patient floor to directly visualize the area of obstruction. Once visualized, a guide wire can usually be placed through the endoscope into the bladder. The endoscope can then be removed, leaving the guide wire in place to allow access for dilatation of strictures. Dilatation can be accomplished using an angioplasty balloon, as described previously, or semirigid Amplatz dilators of increasing diameter.

The Amplatz dilator system was developed by Kurt Amplatz in 1982 initially to dilate nephrostomy tracts. This system can also be used to dilate urethral strictures. It consists of a No. 8 Fr polytef catheter that is tapered to fit over a 0.038-inch guide wire. Under endoscopic guidance, a guide wire is passed beyond the urethral stricture. A No. 8 Fr polytef catheter is passed over the guide wire beyond the stricture. A series of progressively larger catheters are then passed over the 8 Fr polytef catheter and guide wire to dilate the obstructing lesion until the desired opening is achieved. The dilating catheters range in diameter from 12 to 30 Fr in increments of 2 Fr (Fig. 6–7). The No. 8 Fr polytef catheter remains during the entire dilation process as it allows larger dilators to slide over it and avoid risk of false passage. If there is significant resistance or angulation of the catheters, the procedure should be discontinued to avoid false passage or perforation into the rectum.

CYSTOURETHROSCOPY
Indications

Direct visualization of the anterior and posterior urethra, bladder neck, and bladder is accomplished by cystourethroscopy. The primary indication for cystourethroscopy is the diagnosis of lower urinary tract disease. However, access to the upper urinary tract for diagnosis and treatment can be accomplished cystoscopically.

With respect to the diagnosis of lower urinary tract disorders, signs and symptoms that may be related to the urinary tract are evaluated using cystourethroscopy to directly visualize lower urinary tract anatomy and macroscopic pathology,

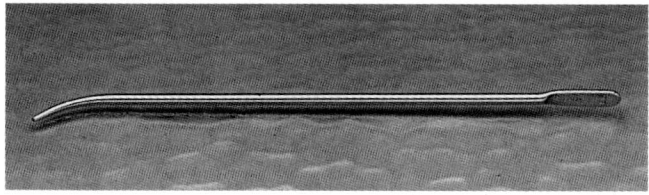

Figure 6–6. Metal sound with a curved tip designed for negotiating the male urethra and commonly used for urethral dilatation. (Courtesy of CR Bard, Inc., Covington, GA.)

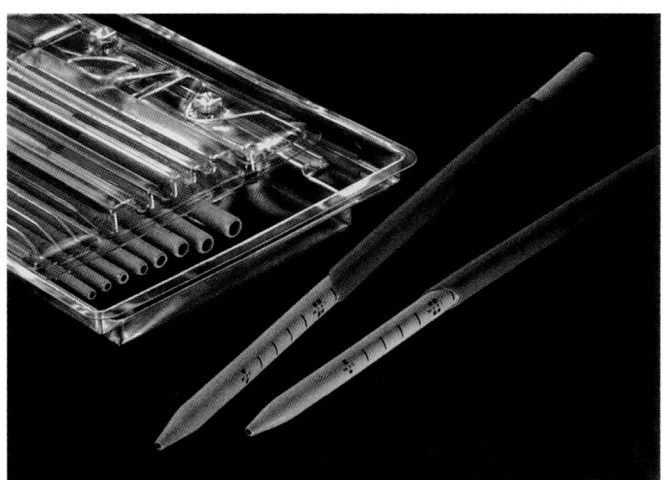

Figure 6–7. Amplatz dilator and sheath set.

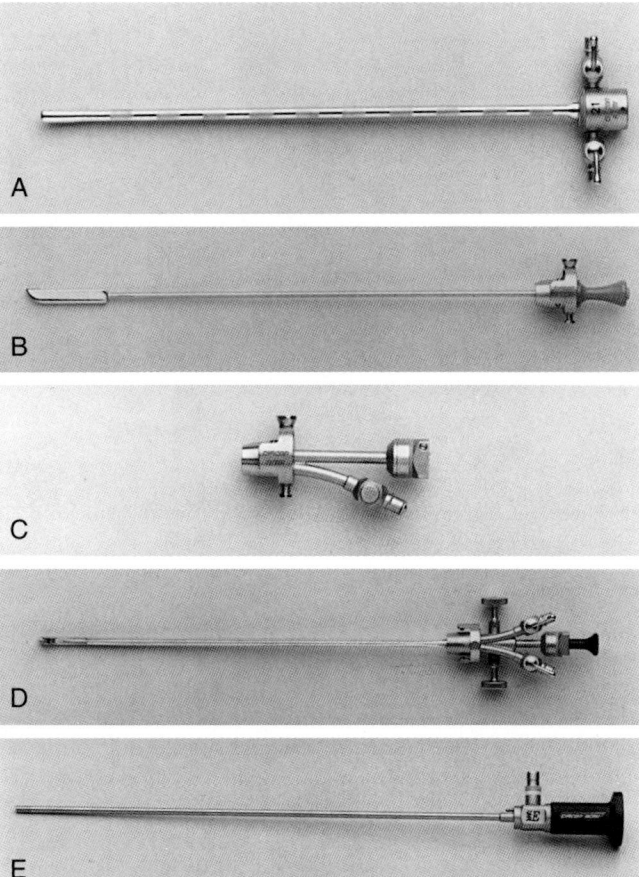

Figure 6–8. Rigid cystoscope consists of metal sheath to which a water source is attached (**A**); obturator (**B**); bridge (**C**); deflector system (Albarran lever) (**D**); and lens to which a light source is attached (**E**). (**A** to **E**, Courtesy of Circon Corp., Santa Barbara, CA.)

which may be responsible for the clinical picture under evaluation. In addition, material for both cytologic and histologic examination can be obtained using cystourethroscopic techniques. One of the most common indications for cystourethroscopy is in the evaluation of microscopic and gross hematuria. By combining radiographic and endoscopic techniques, one can usually determine the source of bleeding in the upper or lower urinary tract (see section on "Retrograde Pyelography"). Other indications for cystourethroscopy include evaluation of voiding symptoms (obstructive and irritative), which may be the result of neurologic, inflammatory, neoplastic, or congenital abnormalities.

Access to the upper urinary tract can be obtained cystoscopically. Diagnostic contrast examination of the entire upper urinary tract is accomplished by retrograde injection of contrast agents through small catheters passed cystoscopically (see section on "Retrograde Pyelography"). Ureteral stents to bypass or prevent ureteral obstruction as well as ureteral catheters and brushes can be passed cystoscopically to obtain material for cytologic and histologic examination from the upper urinary tract. In most cases, fluoroscopy is used in conjunction with these diagnostic and therapeutic procedures of the upper urinary tract.

Patient Preparation

It is important to ensure that the patient does not have an active urinary tract infection before cystourethroscopy, because of the possibility of exacerbating the infection by instrumentation of the urinary tract. After the patient has been counseled regarding the purpose of the procedure, the preparation is the same in the male as for urethral catheterization. In the female, 5 to 10 mL of lubricant-anesthetic jelly should be instilled into the urethra before the procedure. It is important to ensure sterility and obtain adequate urethral anesthesia for diagnostic cystourethroscopy. Using local urethral anesthesia, one can accomplish fulguration of the bladder and obtain small-cup biopsy specimens of the urethral and bladder mucosa cystoscopically. In addition, upper urinary tract instrumentation can be performed. More extensive endoscopic procedures should be performed with the patient under general or regional anesthesia.

Endoscopic Equipment

Cystourethroscopy can be performed with either rigid (Fig. 6–8) or flexible (Fig. 6–9) endoscopes. There are many advantages to the use of the rigid endoscope for cystourethroscopy: (1) better optics because of the use of a rod-lens system in rigid instruments in contrast to the fiberoptic system in flexible instruments; (2) a larger working channel that allows the urologist greater versatility in passage of accessory instruments; (3) a larger lumen for water flow, thus improving visualization; and (4) ease of manipulation and maintaining orientation during inspection within the bladder. The advantages of flexible endoscopes for cystourethroscopy include (1) greater comfort for the patient; (2) the ability to perform the procedure with the patient in the supine position; (3) the ease of passing the instrument over an elevated bladder neck; and (4) the ability to inspect at any angle with deflection of the tip of the instrument.

The size of cystourethroscopes is usually given using the French scale and refers to the outside circumference of the instrument in millimeters. Instruments of different sizes are available to accommodate pediatric patients (No. 8 to 12 Fr) and adults (No. 16 to 25 Fr).

Modern rigid cystourethroscopes consist of a sheath, obturator, bridge, and telescopes (see Fig. 6–8). The telescopic lens

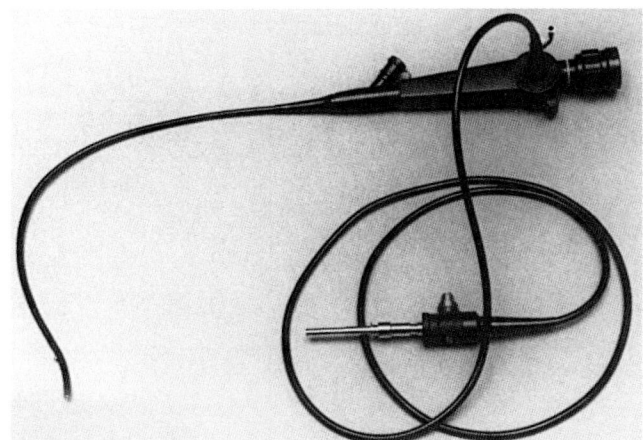

Figure 6–9. Flexible cystoscope with an attached light source and a deflectable tip. (From Denstedt JD: Cystoscopy: Rigid and flexible. In Krane RJ, Siroky MB, Fitzpatrick JM [eds]: Clinical Urology. Philadelphia, JB Lippincott, 1994, p 529.)

is placed through the sheath by attaching a bridge to the sheath. The bridge allows both passage of the telescope and access to the working channel of the sheath for passage of accessory instruments. A deflector system (Albarran lever) can be placed through the sheath to allow passage and controlled deflection of catheters through the working channel. The irrigant fluid is connected to the sheath, and the fiberoptic light source connects directly to the telescope. Obturators can be placed through the sheath to provide a smooth, blunt tip for easy passage, and obturators through which a telescope can be passed (visual obturators) provide a method of easy direct visual passage of the endoscope.

Telescopes consist of illuminating and imaging systems. Modern telescopes use fiberoptic illumination and a rod-lens imaging system. The objective lens at the tip of the instrument collects the light of the image and transmits the image to the eyepiece through the rod-lens system. Telescopes are available with different angles of view for urethroscopy and bladder inspection. A 0-degree lens, which is focused to view straight ahead, is usually used for urethroscopy. A 30-degree lens best affords visualization of the base and anterolateral aspect of the bladder, and a 70- to 90-degree lens is used to view the bladder dome. Retrograde lenses with an angle of view greater than 90 degrees can be used to visualize the anterior bladder neck.

Flexible cystourethroscopes (see Fig. 6–9) contain fiberoptic bundles within a flexible shaft for illumination and visualization. The shaft has an irrigating channel and a working channel for passage of accessory instruments. The tip of a flexible endoscope can be deflected 180 to 220 degrees by a thumb control located near the eyepiece. Flexible cystoscopes that are completely digital are also available, eliminating the need for fiber bundles and the honeycomb pattern of the image.

The image from a rigid or flexible endoscope can be transmitted to a TV monitor with the use of a video-camera (video-cystourethroscopy) (Fig. 6–10). Modern video-cameras may contain an optical device that divides the light into two paths (beam-splitter) to provide simultaneous video-monitor projection and direct viewing through the endoscope. Endoscopic images can be transferred to a video-recording device and

taped, allowing documentation and review of a procedure. A video-cystoscopic unit consists of the endoscope, video-camera head and controller, light source, TV monitor, and video-recording device for storage of images on tape (see Fig. 6–10). With a video-cystoscopic unit, the endoscopist can perform the procedure using the image on the TV monitor to guide movement of the endoscope instead of looking through the eyepiece of the endoscope. The advantages of this approach include (1) avoidance of contact with body fluids; (2) documentation of the procedure using a video-recorder; (3) use of a TV monitor for teaching purposes; and (4) patient education.

Technique

Any urologic irrigant can be used for cystourethroscopy; most often, sterile water or saline solution is used. **If electrocoagulation is planned, it is necessary to avoid solutions containing electrolytes.**

In general, the choice of an endoscope with respect to size should be the same as for catheter size—the smallest outer circumference that will accomplish the task. If diagnostic cystourethroscopy is being performed, a small instrument (No. 16 to 17 Fr) is adequate. If a larger working channel is needed for accessory equipment (e.g., biopsy device), a larger endoscope is chosen.

Systematic inspection of the entire urethra and bladder should be performed during cystourethroscopy. Before insertion of the instrument, the urethral meatus should be inspected if this has not already been accomplished. If the meatal size appears inadequate to accept the endoscope, it can be dilated with metal sounds (see section on "Urethral Dilatation"). After the sheath of the cystourethroscope is generously lubricated with a water-soluble anesthetic-lubricant, the endoscope can be passed under direct vision with a 0- to 30-degree lens, remembering the urethral anatomy.

In the male, the penis should be grasped and straightened so that it forms almost a right angle to the abdominal wall. The endoscope is passed through the fossa navicularis, and the anterior urethra is inspected as the instrument is gently passed. Any mucosal abnormality should be noted, and the diameter of the urethra should be evaluated. If there is resistance to the passage of the endoscope, a smaller instrument should be used or the urethra should be dilated. As the instrument is advanced and enters the bulbar urethra with its greater diameter, the endoscope and penis are lowered while the instrument is passed until the penis is parallel with the floor. This allows passage of the instrument through the membranous urethra. The external sphincter is easily identifiable at the level of the membranous urethra by the mucosal folds radiating from a narrow lumen ahead of the endoscope. Gentle pressure facilitates passage of the endoscope through this area. When the instrument passes into the prostatic urethra, the verumontanum is noted. The prostatic urethra is inspected, and the size of the prostatic lobes is evaluated together with the length of the prostatic urethra, which can be elongated with prostatic hyperplasia. At the level of the bladder neck, it may be necessary to depress the endoscope gently to pass the instrument into the bladder over the bladder neck. An alternative technique is to pass the rigid endoscope "blindly" into the bladder as one would pass a metal dilator,

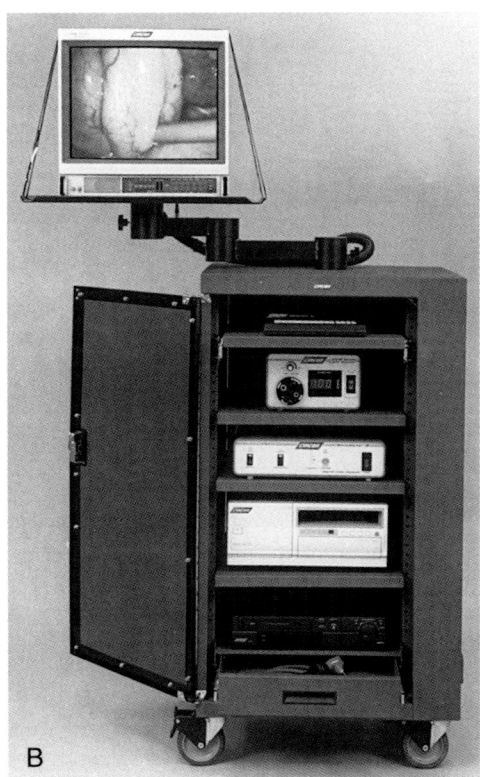

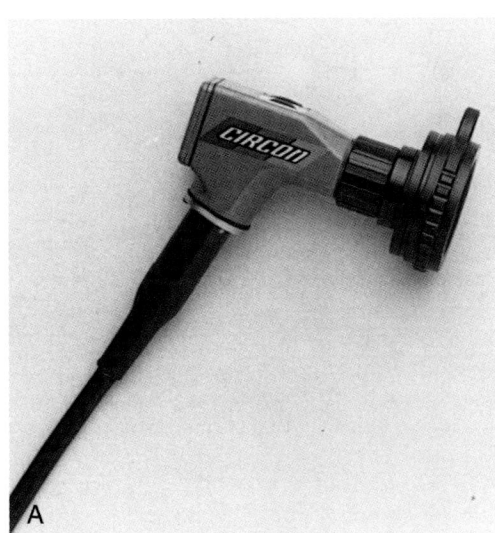

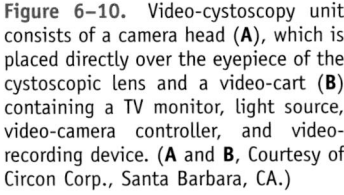

Figure 6–10. Video-cystoscopy unit consists of a camera head (**A**), which is placed directly over the eyepiece of the cystoscopic lens and a video-cart (**B**) containing a TV monitor, light source, video-camera controller, and video-recording device. (**A** and **B**, Courtesy of Circon Corp., Santa Barbara, CA.)

with inspection of the urethra on withdrawal of the endoscope.

Inspection of the female urethra is easily performed by inserting the endoscope under direct vision into the urethral meatus and by directing the instrument cephalad toward the umbilicus. Once the endoscope is inside the bladder, a systematic evaluation of the entire bladder surface is performed. Using the 30-degree lens with the bladder only slightly filled, one can identify the interureteric ridge just inside the bladder neck along the trigone. Next, the ureteral orifices are visually located several centimeters lateral from the center of the interureteric ridge and should be observed to efflux clear urine bilaterally. The floor of the bladder behind the trigone and posterior bladder wall are inspected. By using the 70- to 90-degree lens, one can systematically inspect the lateral walls of the bladder by moving the endoscope from anterior to posterior and back as the bladder fills slowly. Finally, the dome and anterior bladder wall are evaluated with the 70- to 90-degree lens, with the bladder air bubble instilled at the time of instrumentation as a landmark on the dome of the bladder. The anterior bladder wall just behind the bladder neck is best seen with the bladder only partially filled and with one hand exerting suprapubic pressure to depress the anterior bladder wall. After complete inspection of the urethra and bladder has been accomplished, the bladder is drained and the instrument is gently removed.

It is important to document the procedure in a systematic fashion as it was performed. The urologist should have a systematic method of performing cystourethroscopy that allows careful inspection of the entire lower urinary tract from the urethral meatus to the bladder that at the same time causes minimal discomfort for the patient.

RETROGRADE PYELOGRAPHY

Retrograde pyelography is a technique of radiographically demonstrating the ureter and renal collecting system (pelves, infundibula, and calyces) by injecting a radiopaque contrast agent under pressure into the ureter. With increasing use of, and improvements in, other imaging modalities, retrograde pyelography is used less often than in the past. However, specific indications remain for the use of this technique in urologic practice.

Indications

The primary reason for performing retrograde pyelography is to visualize radiographically the ureter or renal collecting system as part of a urologic workup in which the intravenous urogram has provided inadequate radiographic visualization. Better definition of the upper urinary tract by retrograde pyelography is sometimes required during the evaluation of hematuria, persistent filling defects of the ureter or renal collecting system, an unexplained positive urinary cytology collected from the upper urinary tract, and fistulas or obstructions involving the ureter. With the advent of nonionic contrast agents, retrograde pyelography is rarely indicated for visualization of the ureter and renal collecting system in a patient who is allergic to intravenous contrast agents.

Retrograde injection of contrast media can result, albeit rarely, in allergic reactions because absorption of contrast agents can occur during retrograde pyelography. In addition, retrograde pyelography can result in urinary sepsis from increased intrapelvic pressures, with extravasation of bacteria into the venous or lymphatic system. This occurs when patients with an unrecognized urinary tract infection undergo retrograde studies. Less acute but significant urinary tract infections can be precipitated by introduction of bacteria during retrograde injection above an upper tract obstruction. Consideration should be given to decompression of the urinary tract by retrograde ureteral stent placement or nephrostomy tube placement in the patient with an obstructed upper urinary tract who has undergone retrograde pyelography and in whom poor drainage of contrast material is demonstrated on delayed films.

Patient Preparation

Retrograde pyelography is a cystoscopic procedure that can be performed with local intraurethral anesthesia, as previously described. Patient preparation is the same as for cystoscopy. Care should be exercised in ensuring that the urinary tract is sterile before retrograde injection and that patients with poorly draining upper urinary tracts receive preprocedural antibiotics. The patient with sterile urine and a normally draining upper urinary tract does not routinely require preprocedural antibiotics.

Technique

Prior to retrograde pyelography, cystourethroscopy should be routinely performed. Several types of ureteral catheters (Fig. 6–11) are available for performing retrograde pyelography, and the choice depends on the preference of the urologist and the purpose of the study. Whistle, olive, spiral, and cone tip catheters can be used for retrograde injection of contrast media. The No. 4 to 6 Fr whistle, olive, or spiral tip catheters and the No. 8 to 12 Fr cone tip catheters are used most often. The cone tip catheter is designed to occlude the ureteral orifice as contrast material is injected retrogradely, thus filling the ureter and renal collecting system at the same time. The whistle, olive, and spiral tip catheters are placed into the upper tract before injection of contrast material, and the renal collecting system and ureter are filled on separate films.

Regardless of the type of catheter chosen, several important points should be kept in mind. A scout film should be routinely performed before injection of contrast material, as with intravenous urography (see discussion on urography). The ureteral catheter should be placed gently without force to prevent submucosal undermining and possible perforation of the ureter. If the study is being performed for evaluation of a possible transitional cell cancer of the upper tract and collection of urine for cytologic analysis from the upper tract is being considered, it is important to collect the cytologic specimen before retrograde injection of contrast material. Hyperosmolar contrast agents can result in poorly preserved cytologic specimens, thus making interpretation difficult.

After cystoscopic examination, the ureteral orifice is catheterized with the ureteral catheter after making certain that any air bubbles have been flushed out of the catheter. An additional film is often performed at this point to document the location of the ureteral catheter before injection of contrast material, especially if the catheter has been passed into the renal pelvis. Ureteral catheters designed for passage into

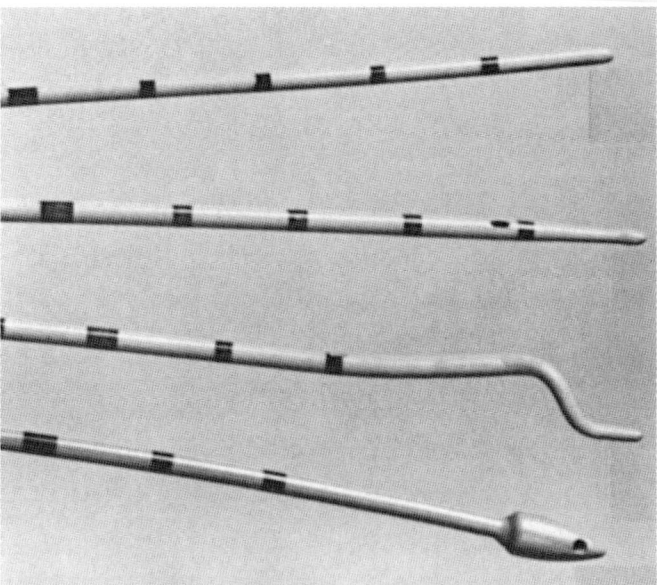

Figure 6–11. Commonly used ureteral catheters, from *top* to *bottom*, have round, olive, spiral, and conical or "bulb" tips. (From Imray TJ, Lieberman RP: Retrograde pyelography. In Pollack HM [ed]: Clinical Urography. Philadelphia, WB Saunders. 1990, p 245.)

the renal pelvis have markings on the catheter that can be seen cystoscopically in such a manner that one can ascertain how far the catheter has been passed. The distance from the ureteral orifice to the ureteropelvic junction is between 20 and 25 cm. A syringe filled with contrast material is attached to the ureteral catheter with a needle or adapter. Five to 10 mL of a 50% solution of any routinely used urographic contrast agent is injected slowly and gently into the ureter (cone tip) or renal pelvis (whistle, olive, spiral tip)—unless the upper tract is known to be dilated, in which case, additional contrast material may be needed. After contrast material injection, anteroposterior and oblique films are developed as needed to visualize the ureter and collecting system with respect to any abnormality. If fluoroscopy is available, the study can be monitored and the need for additional contrast material to completely fill the collecting system will be evident during injection.

If a whistle, olive, or spiral tip catheter has been passed into the collecting system for contrast agent injection, once the renal collecting system has been visualized, a ureterogram is performed. This is accomplished by injecting several additional milliliters of contrast agent into the renal pelvis and continuing injection as the catheter is slowly withdrawn (as in a withdrawal ureterogram). A film is developed immediately as the catheter is withdrawn from the ureteral orifice. Alternatively, one can use a cone tip catheter to obstruct the ureteral orifice and fill the ureter with contrast material. Once the ureter and renal collecting system have been visualized, a delayed film can be helpful in evaluating upper tract drainage. The patient is instructed to sit or stand for approximately 15 minutes, and an additional film is developed. Retention of contrast material in the upper urinary tract on delayed films is abnormal and suggestive of obstruction.

7 Basics of Laparoscopic Urologic Surgery

LOUIS EICHEL, MD • ELSPETH M. McDOUGALL, MD •
RALPH V. CLAYMAN, MD

HISTORY OF LAPAROSCOPY IN UROLOGIC SURGERY

Transperitoneal, Standard, and Hand-Assisted Approach

The foundation of modern laparoscopy was laid in 1805 when Bozzini developed the first self-contained endoscope (Bozzini, 1806). Although his concept of direct visual inspection of the urethra was fiercely rejected by his peers, other investigators pursued his original concept; among them was Nitze (1877), who was the first to introduce glass optics for magnification (Nitze, 1879).

The shift toward laparoscopy was initiated by Kelling (1901), a surgeon who was the first to apply Nitze's cystoscope, introduced through a trocar, in a closed-cavity endoscopic examination of a living dog. During the initial step of this procedure, Kelling insufflated the peritoneal cavity with air using a needle to observe changes to the intra-abdominal organs at pneumoperitoneum pressures sufficient to stop intra-abdominal hemorrhage (i.e., up to 50 to 60 mm Hg).

Jacobaeus (1910), an internist in Stockholm, is credited with transforming Kelling's concept into a clinical diagnostic technique, which he named *koelioskopie*. Jacobaeus used a trocar with a trapdoor as a single port of entry, thus allowing for simultaneous insufflation and endoscopy of the abdominal cavity. In the United States, Bernheim (1911) performed a visual inspection of the peritoneal cavity with a proctoscope, a procedure he termed *organoscopy*, at Johns Hopkins University.

In the early 1900s, a major problem for all endoscopic procedures was the attainment of a clear, bright image. The problem was twofold, in that the endoscopist needed both a high-power light source and high-quality optics. Improvements in the former area were made by French and English investigators in the early 1950s, resulting in an external high-power light source that was efficient and cold, thereby precluding potential intra-abdominal thermal damage. Major advances in endoscope resolution and contrast were subsequently achieved by Hopkins, who introduced large, rod-shaped quartz lenses to transmit light in the early 1960s (Harrison, 1976).

Parallel to the development of light sources and improved optical instruments, inventions and changes in the areas of insufflation techniques and trocars occurred. After Kelling reported his use of air filtered through sterile cotton to insufflate the peritoneum with a needle, Zollikofer of Switzerland introduced the use of carbon dioxide (CO_2) in 1924. The insufflating needle was modified in 1918 by Goetze, who developed a needle with an automatic spring for gas insufflation (Gaskin et al, 1991). In 1938, Veress, a Hungarian internist, reported on his experience with a spring-loaded needle to insufflate the pleural space to create a pneumothorax; this needle subsequently became the standard for closed insufflation of the abdomen (Veress, 1938). Subsequently, major contributions in the development of automatic insufflation and monitoring of intracavitary pressure were made (Palmer, 1947; Eisenburg, 1966). In 1974, Hasson reported on his concept of gaining open access to the peritoneal cavity before introduction of the first trocar, thereby reducing the incidence of potential complications.

The early application of laparoscopy was largely limited to diagnostic purposes and became a technique generally practiced by internists and in particular by gastroenterologists.

Indeed, one of the largest series in the United States of laparoscopic procedures for examining the liver was reported by Ruddock (1957). In the surgical arena, it was gynecologists who pushed laparoscopy into the realm of therapeutic procedures (e.g., tubal ligation, therapeutic abortion). Semm, a German gynecologist, is recognized as the "father" of modern-day laparoscopy owing to his broad development of laparoscopic operative techniques and instruments (Gunning, 1974; Semm, 1987). Indeed, he was the first to perform a laparoscopic appendectomy (Semm, 1983). However, it was not until the mid 1980s that laparoscopy moved from gynecology into the realm of general surgery. With the advent of laparoscopic cholecystectomy, initiated by the French investigators Filipi and Mouret, the old world order of incisional surgery started to crumble. In 1985, Filipi performed the first laparoscopic cholecystectomy on an animal (Davis and Filipi, 1995). In 1987, Mouret of Lyon, France, performed the first clinical laparoscopic cholecystectomy. He never published his case but did report it at a meeting. Subsequently, Dubois performed his first clinical cases in 1988 (Dubois et al, 1989). Meanwhile, Reddick and Olsen (1989) served as early pioneers in popularizing laparoscopic cholecystectomy in the United States. By the mid 1990s, laparoscopic cholecystectomy was the procedure of choice for most indications for surgical removal of the gallbladder.

The development of laparoscopy in urology paralleled, to a large extent, the changes in general surgery. Up until the late 1980s, laparoscopy had limited applications in urology. Indeed, aside from Cortesi and colleagues' (1976) report of using the laparoscope in pediatric patients to explore for undescended testes (Silber et al, 1980) and Smith's report in 1985 of using the laparoscope to aid in the percutaneous removal of a stone from a pelvic kidney, laparoscopy remained a technique in search of a broad application (Eshghi et al, 1985). This situation drastically changed over 24 months, from 1989 through 1990. First, Schuessler and colleagues (1991) reported their initial experience with laparoscopic staging pelvic obturator lymphadenectomy for prostate cancer after having performed the first case in 1989. Then in 1990, after extensive laboratory trials, including the development of the basic concepts of organ entrapment and tissue morcellation, Clayman and coworkers (1991b) performed the first clinical laparoscopic nephrectomy. Also in 1990, Sanchez-de-Badajoz and colleagues (1990) reported the first laparoscopic varicocelectomy, a feat rapidly corroborated independently by Donovan and Winfield (1992) and Hagood and associates (1992). As in general surgery, laparoscopy took urology by storm. Numerous courses, books, and articles soon appeared on the scene to guide urologists into the laparoscopic realm.

A new era in operative urology had begun. Soon, a steady stream of newly developed laparoscopic procedures started to challenge their conventional open surgical counterparts. Initial emphasis was on ablative procedures: lymphadenectomy, varicocelectomy, transperitoneal and retroperitoneal nephrectomy for benign and malignant disease, nephroureterectomy, partial nephrectomy, adrenalectomy, cyst decortication, lymphocele drainage, cystectomy for benign disease, bladder diverticulectomy, retroperitoneal lymphadenectomy, and orchiectomy (Sanchez-de-Badajoz E, 1990; Clayman et al, 1991; McCullough et al, 1991; Schuessler et al, 1991; Das, 1992; Donovan and Winfield, 1992; Gagner

et al, 1992; Hagood et al, 1992; Hulbert and Fraley, 1992; Morgan and Rader, 1992; Parra et al, 1992; Suzuki et al, 1992; Thomas et al, 1992; Winfield et al, 1992; Kerbl et al, 1993; McDougall et al, 1993; Nadler et al, 1995). In 1995, Kavoussi and associates performed the first clinical donor nephrectomy (Ratner et al, 1995). Over the next 5 years, the technique became more refined, and it has since spread throughout the world. At many centers, laparoscopic donor nephrectomy is the standard of care. As urologists became more skilled, they expanded their laparoscopic procedures into the realm of more difficult ablative surgery.

Hand-assisted laparoscopy was originally developed as a supportive technique to laparoscopic splenectomy (Kusminsky et al, 1995). Subsequently, hand-assisted laparoscopy was also embraced by urologic surgeons (Saadeh et al, 1995; Tschada et al, 1995). Developments in commercially available devices: the Gelport (Applied Medical, Rancho Santa Margarita, CA), the Omniport (Advanced Surgical Concepts, Wicklow, Ireland), and the LapDisc (Ethicon Endosurgery, Cincinnati, OH) have further spurred this approach. The first report on the use of the PneumoSleeve in laparoscopic nephrectomy was published in 1997 by Nakada and coworkers. In the meantime, hand-assisted techniques have been successfully applied to a variety of other laparoscopic procedures, among them nephroureterectomy, colectomy, Roux-en-Y gastric bypass, complex hysterectomy, distal pancreatectomy, rectopexy, and fundoplication (Bemelman et al, 1996; Gorey and Bonadio, 1997; Klingler et al, 1998; Pelosi and Pelosi, 1999; Schweitzer et al, 1999). The hand-assist approach opened the door for more urologists to enter the arena of laparoscopic ablative renal surgery.

The most challenging aspect of laparoscopy is reconstructive surgery. Urologists began to develop skills in this area and thus expanded the indications for laparoscopic surgery into other areas. By using laparoscopic techniques for suturing and intracorporeal knot tying, the following procedures were successfully completed laparoscopically: reimplantation of the ureter, ureteroureterostomy, pyeloplasty, bladder neck suspension, Fowler-Stephens orchidopexy, transperitoneal and extraperitoneal bladder autoaugmentation, and nephropexy (Bloom, 1991; Nezhat et al, 1992; Ehrlich and Gershman, 1993; Schuessler et al, 1993; Urban et al, 1993; McDougall et al, 1995; Vallancien et al, 2002). In some new laparoscopic procedures, the technical steps and surgical feasibility were established at one academic institution, with subsequent clinical applications performed elsewhere (Urban et al, 1992; Atala et al, 1993; Gill et al, 1994).

In the mid 1990s, interest in laparoscopy waned as the need for pelvic lymph node dissection dropped precipitously owing to advances in nonoperative staging of prostate cancer. Indeed, with the combination of Gleason grade, physical examination, and prostate-specific antigen level, the need for pelvic lymph node dissection was eliminated in upward of 95% of patients presenting with potentially surgically curable prostate cancer. Also, data revealed that laparoscopic varicocelectomy and bladder neck suspension, although feasible, were not as cost effective as, or better for the patient than, alternative, well-established surgical methods. These developments, combined with the complexity of renal and ureteral laparoscopic procedures, caused a major decrease in laparoscopic interest in the urologic community.

However, as more data were published on the beneficial aspects of laparoscopic renal and ureteral surgery, and as donor nephrectomy became accepted worldwide, more urologists grew to embrace laparoscopy as the technique of choice for these procedures. This was further spurred by the pioneering work of Vallancien and Guillonneau in the realm of radical prostatectomy; although the initial report by Schuessler was of interest, it was the development and dissemination of this procedure at L'Institut Mutualiste Montsouris that re-ignited interest among urologists in laparoscopy. Additional procedures soon followed, including **cystectomy, gastrocystoplasty, enterocystoplasty, and ileal ureter** (Parra et al, 1992; Docimo et al, 1995; Raboy et al, 1997; Schuessler et al, 1997; Abbou et al, 2000; Gill, et al, 2000, 2000c; Guillonneau et al, 2000). Raising the bar even higher, Gill and associates (2000) reported on laparoscopic radical cystoprostatectomy, bilateral pelvic lymphadenectomy, and ileal conduit urinary diversion in patients with muscle-invasive bladder cancer, with the entire procedure being performed intracorporeally. In addition. laparoscopy is being used more and more in the area of retroperitoneal lymph node dissection (RPLND) for testicular cancer. Although still somewhat controversial, several centers offer laparoscopic RPLND and have shown that the outcomes can be equal to open surgery (Allaf et al, 2005).

With an increasing number of multi-institutional studies emerging in which laparoscopic procedures are compared with their open surgical counterparts, it becomes clear that, owing to equivalent efficacy combined with distinct advantages in postoperative pain, cosmesis, recovery, and length of hospital stay, laparoscopy has moved into the mainstream of urologic surgery. Indeed, it is becoming increasingly clear that the objectives of almost all aspects of open retroperitoneal surgery, be it of the kidney, ureter, adrenal gland, or lymph nodes, can now be achieved laparoscopically with far less patient injury and suffering. Minimally invasive surgery is superseding open surgery at major medical centers throughout the world. In this new millennium, the old craft of open surgery has an ever-diminishing role in the treatment of urologic disease. The sage musings of Osler at the inception of the 20th century continue to stimulate surgeons to further refine their craft: "Diseases that harm require treatments that harm less."

Retroperitoneal and Extraperitoneal Approach

Wittmoser first explored the *retroperitoneoscopic* approach for performing lumbar sympathetectomy in 1973. The initial application of retroperitoneoscopy in urology was by Wickham in 1979 for percutaneous ureterolithotomy. In 1991, Figenshau and colleagues described the initial retroperitoneoscopic nephrectomy. Similar to the early experiences with pelvic extraperitoneoscopy, difficulty was encountered in obtaining an adequate working space, as well as in achieving satisfactory pneumoretroperitoneum. Gaur's seminal description of creating an adequate working space in the retroperitoneum by atraumatic balloon dilation revolutionized this form of laparoscopy and promoted its application at other centers (Gaur, 1992). Directed balloon dilation rapidly and

atraumatically converts the preperitoneal space into a capacious working area, facilitating the performance of simple and advanced laparoscopic maneuvers.

The history of endoscopic manipulation of the *extraperitoneal* space dates back to Bartel's initial description, in 1969, of the use of a 19-inch mediastinoscope for minimally invasive access to the pelvic extraperitoneal space. Hald and Rasmussen successfully used this technique of pelvioscopy for sampling pelvic lymph nodes in 1980. Ferzli and associates described the initial extraperitoneoscopic pelvic lymphadenectomy in 1992, employing digital dissection to create a working extraperitoneal space before port placement. However, inadequacy of the created working space limited the widespread use of these techniques. More recently, the extraperitoneal approach has been reborn with the advent of interest in laparoscopic radical prostatectomy. At many centers this is the approach of choice for radical prostatectomy (Gettman et al, 2003; Wolfram et al, 2003; Erdogru et al, 2004; Hoznek et al, 2004; Stolzenburg et al, 2004; Tobias-Machado et al, 2004).

Robotics

The first robotic-assisted surgery was described by Kwoh and colleagues in 1985; they used a modified light-duty industrial robotic arm to guide a laser for stereotactic brain surgery. Four years later the first robotic-assisted procedure on soft tissue was described by Davies and coworkers (1991) when they used a modified industrial robotic arm to perform transurethral resection of the prostate in humans. The first commercially available robotic system, RoboDoc, was described in 1992. This was a robotic arm designed to precisely core out femoral shafts for hip prostheses.

The first commercial robotic system used specifically for laparoscopic applications was the Automated Endoscopic System for Optimal Positioning (AESOP). The AESOP is a table-mounted robotic arm that precisely manipulates a standard laparoscope or instrument. This system was initially designed using seed money from the U.S. military but later went into commercial production by Computer Motion Inc. This was the first U.S. Food and Drug Administration (FDA)-approved surgical robotic system (1993) and remains one of the most widely used systems today.

The AESOP was not the only project of this nature initially supported by the U.S. military and ultimately licensed by private industry. The predecessor to the three-armed da Vinci system (Intuitive Surgical, Sunnyvale, CA) was first conceptualized by researchers at the National Aeronautics and Space Administration (NASA) and later the Pentagon (Satava, 2002) . This system was originally intended to allow surgeons in a Mobile Advanced Surgical Hospital (MASH) to operate on wounded soldiers who had been transported to the back of a Bradley Fighting Vehicle equipped with a robotic surgical system. This concept of remote telemanipulation has remained a central theme in modern surgical robotic systems.

The da Vinci system provided an array of instruments with 6 degrees of freedom (Endowrist), greatly enhancing the laparoscopic capabilities of the surgeon. Shortly after, the ZEUS system (Computer Motion Inc., Santa Barbara, CA) came onto the market in 1998. This system combined an AESOP system with an additional two table-mounted robotic arms. At the time the ZEUS system came with instruments with 4 degrees of freedom (like standard laparoscopic instruments), but in 2002 their MicroWrist instruments gained FDA approval. In 2003, Intuitive Surgical and Computer Motion Inc., the two leaders in robotic surgical technology, merged. As a result, the ZEUS system has been phased out. The current cost for a da Vinci system is $1.09 million for a three-arm system and $1.285 million for a four-arm system. Service is free for the first year and costs $109,000 to $125,000 per year thereafter. Instruments cost $180 per case multiplied by how many are used per case. The da Vinci does not yet have force feedback (haptic feedback). Currently the da Vinci is the only commercially available telesurgical system.

The da Vinci system was first used clinically for laparoscopic cholecystectomy in 1997 and gained FDA approval the same year. Following swiftly on the pathway forged by traditional laparoscopic surgeons robotic assisted laparoscopic radical prostatectomy was born. Capitalizing on the steady three-dimensional (3-D) vision and improved dexterity provided by the da Vinci system, the original technique was described by Abbou and associates (2001); and, more recently, other surgeons such as Ahlering and Menon and their associates have matured the procedure into a viable alternative to open prostatectomy (Ahlering et al, 2003, 2004; Menon et al, 2002; Tewari et al, 2003). As of 2005, the da Vinci Surgical System has been used to perform almost every laparoscopic urologic procedure from adrenalectomy to vesicovaginal fistula repair, although the machine is most useful for reconstructive procedures.

PREOPERATIVE PATIENT MANAGEMENT
Patient Selection and Contraindications

Careful patient selection and identification of possible relative and absolute contraindications are vital to a successful outcome of laparoscopic procedures. To this end, a meticulous past history, focusing on prior abdominal or renal/ureteral surgery, and physical examination, detailing the location and extent of all abdominal scars, are the initial steps in patient evaluation for possible laparoscopic surgery. Age- and health-based laboratory studies, electrocardiogram, and a chest radiograph should be obtained, following the same criteria established for any other significant open surgical procedure that is undertaken with general anesthesia.

Especially in patients presenting with severe chronic obstructive pulmonary disease (COPD), further studies (i.e., arterial blood gases and pulmonary function tests) are required. In severe COPD, helium as an alternative insufflant should be considered. Severe cardiac arrhythmias have to be evaluated and treated accordingly because hypercarbia and the resulting acidosis may have adverse effects on the myocardium.

Absolute contraindications to laparoscopic surgery include uncorrectable coagulopathy, intestinal obstruction, abdominal wall infection, massive hemoperitoneum or hemoretroperitoneum, generalized peritonitis or retroperitoneal abscess, and suspected malignant ascites.

Relative contraindications to laparoscopic surgery necessitate careful risk-benefit analysis and extensive informed

consent. The following conditions should alert the surgeon to potential difficulties with a laparoscopic approach.

Morbid Obesity. Laparoscopic procedures in morbidly obese patients are technically challenging. Difficulties include inadequate length of instruments, decreased range of motion of instruments, need for higher pneumoperitoneum pressures to elevate the abdominal wall, and poor anatomic orientation owing to excessive amounts of adipose tissue. Traditionally, these difficulties translated into a higher rate of associated complications; in a multi-institutional review of laparoscopy in 125 morbidly obese individuals, one or more intraoperative or postoperative complications occurred in 30% (Mendoza et al, 1996). In comparison to open surgery, however, it has been found that the laparoscopic approach to renal and adrenal procedures actually has a lower complication rate than the open approach. **In a comparison of major laparoscopic renal and adrenal procedures** (N = 21) versus similar open procedures (N = 21) in obese patients (body mass index of 30 or greater), although operative time was longer in the former group (210 minutes vs. 185 minutes; $P = .16$), the laparoscopic group had significantly superior outcomes regarding blood loss (100 mL vs. 350 mL; $P = .001$), resumption of oral intake and ambulation (less than 1 day vs. 5 days; $P = .001$), narcotic analgesic requirements (12 mg vs. 279 mg; $P = .001$), median hospital stay (<1 day vs. 5 days; $P = .001$), and convalescence (3 weeks vs. 9 weeks; $P = .001$). The overall complication rate in the laparoscopic group was 29% (19% major, 10% minor) versus 67% in the open group (33% major, 33% minor) ($P = .16$) (Fazeli-Matin et al, 1999). These findings have been further confirmed at several other centers (Fugita et al, 2004; Kapoor et al, 2004).

With regard to laparoscopic radical prostatectomy in obese men, it has been found that while the operation can be performed without compromising pathologic outcomes, obese patients have a greater risk of perioperative complications (26% vs. 5%) (Ahlering et al, 2005).

Extensive Prior Abdominal or Pelvic Surgery. When extensive intra-abdominal or pelvic adhesions are suspected, close attention must be given to the possible site of Veress needle insertion as well as to the possibility of obtaining open access with a Hasson-style cannula. Alternatively, in these patients, a retroperitoneal approach may be preferable to a transperitoneal approach, or the procedure can be initiated retroperitoneally and the peritoneum then entered (Cadeddu et al, 1999).

A patient history of prior retroperitoneal surgery increases the difficulty of reentering the retroperitoneal space and therefore should be approached with caution. Subsequent attempts at extraperitoneoscopy or retroperitoneoscopy should only be considered by individuals with considerable experience and comfort with this approach. In our experience, prior percutaneous renal procedures do not necessarily constitute a contraindication to subsequent retroperitoneoscopy, provided that entry is away from the area of the prior nephrostomy tube placement (e.g., Petit's triangle).

Pelvic Fibrosis. Pelvic fibrosis owing to previous peritonitis and/or pelvic surgery may constitute a severe technical challenge to the laparoscopic surgeon when surgery of the lower urinary tract is indicated. Similar problems may be encountered when trying to perform pelvic lymph node dissection in patients who have a hip prosthesis; leakage of the polymethylmethacrylate cement can create a dense inflammatory reaction and fibrosis.

Organomegaly. Known or preoperatively diagnosed organomegaly necessitates a cautious approach when obtaining the pneumoperitoneum. The site of Veress needle insertion must be chosen at a safe distance from any enlarged organs. Alternatively, open access with the Hasson cannula may be considered. Open access should be considered in cases of marked hepatomegaly or splenomegaly.

Ascites: Benign Etiology. Patients with severe ascites are under increased risk of injury to the bowel owing to closer proximity of bowel loops to the anterior peritoneum. In addition, a watertight wound closure is required and firm wound dressing should be applied to prevent prolonged postoperative leakage. An open-cannula approach to achieving the pneumoperitoneum in these patients is recommended.

Pregnancy. Initial access to the abdomen must be obtained at a safe distance from the fundus of the gravid uterus. As such, trocar placement is usually performed more cephalad on the abdominal wall, depending on the fundus of the uterus. The left or right (i.e., Palmer's point) upper quadrant in the subcostal midclavicular line is often the preferred site of access. Prolonged intra-abdominal pressures of 15 mm Hg or greater may result in hypotension, owing to significantly reduced venous return because the vena cava is already mechanically compromised by the enlarged uterus. Prolonged CO_2 pneumoperitoneum, which may result in maternal hypercarbia and acidosis with subsequent adverse effects on the fetus, should be avoided. Accordingly, a working pneumoperitoneum of 10 mm Hg is recommended in the pregnant patient. As pregnancy progresses beyond the 20th week, the technical possibility of performing laparoscopic procedures decreases significantly, correlating with the increasing size of the gravid uterus. Both cholecystectomy and adrenalectomy have been successfully accomplished in the pregnant female (Nezhat et al, 1997).

Hernia. A *diaphragmatic hernia* may result in leakage of a significant amount of CO_2 into the mediastinum, which, although rarely seen, may eventually result in clinical problems (e.g., pneumopericardium) (Knos et al, 1991).

Any evidence of uncorrected or surgically corrected *umbilical hernia* should rule out the umbilicus as a site for obtaining a pneumoperitoneum.

Iliac or Aortic Aneurysm. This condition needs to be evaluated by the vascular surgeon. If the aneurysm does not warrant immediate surgical correction, insertion of the Veress needle should be performed in the left upper quadrant to stay well away from the area of the aneurysm. Of course, open access with the Hasson technique can be employed. Insertion of accessory trocars must be done under strict endoscopic control to avoid the area of the aneurysm. **Alternatively, the retroperitoneal laparoscopic approach can be employed** (Sung and Gill, 1999).

Informed Consent

Although laparoscopic surgery is generally associated with decreased pain and morbidity, it should be remembered that
there is considerable potential for serious complications, similar to that associated with standard open incisional surgery.** It is essential for the patient to understand the inherent risk with all laparoscopic procedures that the procedure may need to be converted from a traditional laparoscopic to a hand-assisted approach or to open surgery owing to hemorrhage, bowel injury, failure to progress, or other complications at any point during the intraoperative or postoperative course.

All alternative forms of surgical or nonsurgical treatment (if applicable), with their known advantages and disadvantages, must be discussed. The patient needs to be aware of both complications unique to laparoscopy (e.g., fatal gas embolism, problems owing to hypercarbia, postoperative crepitus, pneumothorax, or electrosurgical bowel injury due to capacitive coupling or insulation failure) and procedure-specific complications (e.g., damage of obturator nerve in pelvic lymphadenectomy).

Time spent obtaining informed consent is well invested. It is both the patient's right and the physician's protection. A good beginning augurs a good end.

Bowel Preparation

For extraperitoneoscopy and retroperitoneoscopy, no bowel preparation is needed. For transperitoneal laparoscopic procedures, a light mechanical bowel preparation can be given in an effort to decompress the bowel. Usually, a clear liquid diet and a Dulcolax suppository or half a bottle of magnesium citrate the day before the procedure are sufficient. The need for a full mechanical (e.g., GoLYTELY, 2 to 4 L, or 3 ounces of Fleet Phospho-Soda followed by a clear liquid diet and Fleet enema) and antibiotic (e.g., neomycin, 1 g by mouth, and metronidazole, 500 mg by mouth; three doses of each the day before surgery, plus 1 g of intravenous cefotetan on call to the operating room) bowel preparation becomes an issue only if one anticipates encountering dense intra-abdominal adhesions or if the surgery involves entering the bowel (e.g., enteric augmentation of the bladder or enteric conduit formation).

Preparation of Blood Products

Serum type and screen are sufficient for diagnostic laparoscopy or procedures associated with a low chance of major hemorrhage (e.g., varicocelectomy, pelvic operations). More extensive laparoscopic procedures (e.g., laparoscopic nephrectomy), especially early in one's experience, should be managed like any other major open surgical procedure, with two units of packed red blood cells available before surgery. The patient should also be provided with the option of donating two units of autologous blood. This is most important during one's initial major laparoscopic cases; with experience, a "type and hold" suffices because the need for transfusion among patients undergoing major laparoscopic procedures, such as radical nephrectomy or radical nephroureterectomy, is quite low (3% to 12%), with an estimated average blood loss in the range of 106 to 255 mL (Dunn et al, 2000; Jeschke et al, 2000; Ono Y, 1999; Shalhav et al, 2000). Similarly, the transfusion rate with laparoscopic radical prostatectomy is low (2.5% at experienced centers) such that a type and hold is sufficient (Guillonneau et al, 2000).

Optional Preoperative Endourologic and Radiologic Procedures

Preoperative computed tomography (CT), spiral angiographic three-dimensional CT, and magnetic resonance imaging (MRI) are helpful in depicting the anatomic relationship of the operative site to adjacent organs and/or blood vessels. The necessary studies required as part of a routine metastatic workup for cancer are still mandatory. For laparoscopic partial nephrectomy or in the patient with ureteropelvic junction obstruction, preoperative spiral CT angiography with three-dimensional reconstruction is essential. These studies depict the renal vasculature and, in the case of a renal mass, will clearly delineate the plane of dissection. For the latter situation, coronal and sagittal views should also be requested. When laparoscopic nephrectomy is performed for large malignant renal tumors (i.e., >10 cm), preoperative embolization of the renal artery may be considered; this procedure allows the surgeon to secure and divide the renal vein earlier in the transperitoneal laparoscopic procedure. In other disease states, preoperative placement of a ureteral catheter or a percutaneous drainage catheter can be quite helpful as intra-operative filling (e.g., with indigo carmine–stained saline), and drainage of the surgical site can aid greatly in its identification and subsequent treatment (e.g., pyeloplasty, lymphocele or intrarenal cyst, calyceal diverticulum).

A variety of catheters, both opaque and light bearing, can be placed in the ureter to facilitate ureteral identification and dissection in laparoscopic nephrectomy, pyeloplasty, nephroureterectomy, ureterolysis, ureterolithotomy, and retroperitoneal lymph node dissection. The need for preplacement of a ureteral stent is dependent on the pathology and the surgeon's prior laparoscopic experience.

IN THE OPERATING ROOM
Setup of the Operating Room

The operating room has to provide enough space to accommodate all necessary personnel and the technologic equipment required by both the laparoscopist and the anesthesiologist. Positioning of equipment, surgeon, assistants, nurses, anesthesiologist, and other support staff should be clearly defined and established for each standard laparoscopic case. All equipment must be fully functional and in operating condition before any laparoscopic procedure is started (Table 7–1). A separate tray with open laparotomy instruments must be ready for immediate use in the event of

complications or problems necessitating open incisional surgery.

Patient Positioning and Draping

Positioning of the patient depends primarily on the laparoscopic procedure to be performed. Most intra-abdominal laparoscopic procedures start with the patient in a supine position with the arms secured at the sides of the body. In the Trendelenburg or lateral position, tape and security belts applied across the chest and thighs provide safe and stable positioning of the patient; shoulder braces should not be used. In the lateral position, all bony prominences must be carefully padded; likewise, the point of contact between any of the positioning straps and the hip or shoulder should be padded. In the lateral position, the bottom leg is flexed approximately 45 degrees while the upper leg is kept straight; a pillow is placed between the legs as a cushion and also to elevate the upper leg so that it lies level with the flank, thereby obviating any undue stretch on the sciatic nerve. A shoulder support is placed under the downside shoulder. Application of active warming systems may prevent hypothermia, should a lengthy laparoscopic procedure be anticipated.

A host of new advances in padding and table mounted accessories are now available that when used appropriately can markedly decrease the incidence of iatrogenic neuromuscular injuries. Disposable foam padding has now been replaced by gel pads that are less bulky and appear to provide superior cushioning (AliMed Inc., Dedham, MA). Table-mounted accessories for all major commercial operating room tables now exist that aid in safely and effectively positioning patients in the lateral decubitus position and in the prone position. Specifically, for lateral decubitus positioning the buttock and upper back can be supported by gel pad–reinforced stabilizer bars that mount on the side rails of the table. The entire bed and especially the kidney rest can also be covered with gel pads, and the upper arm can be supported on a table-mounted adjustable armboard. Special head supports for the lateral decubitus position are also available.

The full extent of the abdominal wall should be prepared and draped from nipples to pubis. In some procedures it is of advantage to extend the preparation to the knees and to drape the external genitalia into the surgical field. For example, gently pulling on the testis may help identify the intrapelvic location of the vas deferens and spermatic vessels, transvaginal palpation facilitates laparoscopic bladder neck suspension, and free access to the urethral meatus enables the performance of auxiliary procedures such as flexible cystoscopy or manipulation of ureteral catheters during a laparoscopic nephroureterectomy or for stent placement at the end of a laparoscopic pyeloplasty.

Before major transperitoneal procedures, placement of a nasogastric/orogastric tube and a Foley catheter is usually performed to decompress the stomach and bladder, respectively, thereby decreasing the chance of injury of abdominal contents during insertion of the Veress needle and the initial trocar. In contrast, for an extraperitoneal or retroperitoneal approach, a nasogastric/orogastric tube is not needed. Pneumatic compression stockings are applied for antiembolic prophylaxis. The administration of 5000 units of subcutaneous heparin preoperatively is also an option.

Table 7–1. Instruments to be Checked before Making a Skin Incision for Obtaining the Pneumoperitoneum

Irrigation-aspiration unit is working.
Electrosurgical unit is working.
CO_2 tank is full, with extra CO_2 tank in the room.
Camera is white balanced, and light source is working.
Insufflation is checked for flow and response to kinking of the tubing.
Veress needle is checked for flow and proper tip retraction.

Strategic Placement of Operative Team and Equipment

Standard Laparoscopic Carts. Traditionally, the mandatory hardware for laparoscopic procedures (monitor, light source, insufflator) is located on carts or "towers" that can be rolled around the operating room and be adapted to various types of surgical procedures and approaches. If only one monitor is used (as in intrapelvic procedures), it is typically placed at the foot of the table or between the legs if the patient is in stirrups or on split-leg positioners. If two monitors are used, they are positioned on either side of the table opposite the primary surgeon and the assisting surgeon, respectively, to allow an unobstructed view.

The main laparoscopic cart should contain the monitor for the primary surgeon as well as the insufflator, placed at the surgeon's eye level to allow continuous monitoring of the CO_2 pressure. The light source, camera controls, and any recording device are also on this cart. Placement of a *sterile* plastic sheet over the front of this cart enables the surgical team to alter the intensity of the light as well as the pneumoperitoneum pressure with a blunt sterile forceps.

Integrated Endoscopy Systems. More recently, most major manufacturers of endoscopy equipment offer "integrated" systems that consist of flat panel displays and equipment towers that are mounted on adjustable ceiling booms. Thus, the display monitors can be suspended over the patient and placed directly in front of the surgeon. This feature greatly reduces eye and body strain. Furthermore, the tower containing the light source, camera system, and insufflator can be placed in any area around the patient depending on the operation at hand. The more sophisticated systems are frequently controlled by a touch screen display used by the surgeon or a nurse or by voice command, instead of manually adjusting instruments at the tower level. In addition to the laparoscopic equipment, other aspects of the operating room environment can be controlled such as the room lighting, input from digital radiology systems, and recording devices. Although they are not a necessity, these types of systems offer unique advantages with regard to operating room efficiency and greatly improve the ergonomics for the operating surgeon.

Placement of the Operative Team. The surgeon usually stands opposite the area of surgical interest and the assistant stands on the ipsilateral side of the table. The second assistant stands on the contralateral side of the table (Fig. 7–1). With two monitors in use, the instrument table and the scrub nurse are on the side of the surgeon toward the end of the table (see Fig. 7–1). Incoming lines from insufflator, suction/irrigation, and electrosurgical devices enter from the contralateral side of the table. Optional technology (e.g., harmonic scalpel, argon beam coagulator) must be arranged in an orderly fashion using either preexisting or improvised pockets of the surgical drape. Again, these lines ideally should enter the field from the contralateral side of the table or from the ipsilateral head of the table. Robotic devices for electronically controlled or voice-controlled camera manipulation should be brought into the operative area from the contralateral side of the table to prevent any limitation of the assistant's maneuverability during the procedure. Additional technology (e.g., laparoscopic ultrasound probe) may be moved to the operating table depending on the surgeon's needs as well as on the availability of space.

To provide more comfortable positioning of the surgeon's arms, a 6 × 4-foot, 6-inch lift can be used, because most

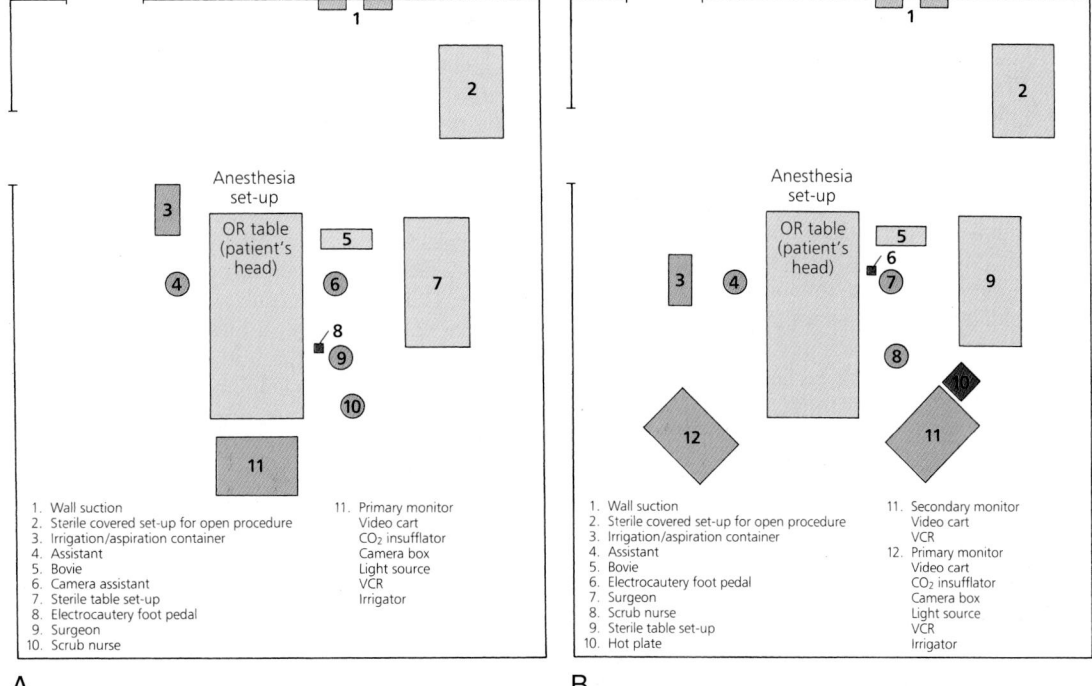

A

1. Wall suction
2. Sterile covered set-up for open procedure
3. Irrigation/aspiration container
4. Assistant
5. Bovie
6. Camera assistant
7. Sterile table set-up
8. Electrocautery foot pedal
9. Surgeon
10. Scrub nurse

11. Primary monitor
    Video cart
    CO_2 insufflator
    Camera box
    Light source
    VCR
    Irrigator

B

1. Wall suction
2. Sterile covered set-up for open procedure
3. Irrigation/aspiration container
4. Assistant
5. Bovie
6. Electrocautery foot pedal
7. Surgeon
8. Scrub nurse
9. Sterile table set-up
10. Hot plate

11. Secondary monitor
    Video cart
    VCR
12. Primary monitor
    Video cart
    CO_2 insufflator
    Camera box
    Light source
    VCR
    Irrigator

Figure 7–1. Setup of operative room with one monitor (**A**) and with two monitors (**B**). (From Clayman RV, McDougall EM [eds]: Laparoscopic Urology. St. Louis, Quality Medical Publishing, 1993.)

operating tables designed prior to widespread use of laparoscopy cannot be lowered sufficiently to allow the surgeon to hold the laparoscopic instruments with his or her elbows held comfortably at the side rather than extended laterally. This is most important during suturing. Several newer tables recently on the market, however, can be set at very low elevations (e.g., 60 cm for the Maquet Alphamaxx [Getinge USA Rochester, NY]) so that platforms are not needed.

Transperitoneal Procedures. The patient is positioned in a modified lateral decubitus position for transperitoneal laparoscopic renal surgery procedures. This is approximately a 30-degree angle to the table and allows for more effective lateral retraction of the kidney and exposure of the renal vessels during the hilar dissection. The kidney rest may be elevated at the outset and the table slightly flexed if necessary to provide adequate exposure for port placement; after port placement, the kidney rest should be completely lowered. The surgeon and camera assistant usually stand on the contralateral side of the table from the operative side. The second assistant stands on the contralateral side of the table to the surgeon (see Fig. 7–1). With two monitors in use, the instrument table and the scrub nurse are on the side of the surgeon toward the end of the table (see Fig. 7–1). Incoming lines from insufflator, suction/irrigation, and electrosurgical devices enter from the contralateral side of the table. Optional technology (e.g., harmonic scalpel, argon beam coagulator) must be arranged in an orderly fashion using either preexisting or improvised pockets of the surgical drape. Again, these lines ideally should enter the field from the contralateral side of the table or from the ipsilateral head of the table. Robotic devices for electronically controlled or voice-controlled camera manipulation should be brought into the operative area from the contralateral side of the table to prevent any limitation of the tableside assistant's maneuverability during the procedure. Additional technology (e.g., laparoscopic ultrasound probe) may be moved to the operating table depending on the surgeon's needs as well as on the availability of space.

Retroperitoneal Procedures. For retroperitoneal procedures the patient is placed in the true, 90-degree lateral decubitus position with the body at a right angle to the table. All of the proper steps for padding in this position should be followed (see earlier). The kidney rest is raised and the table is angled (broken) at the hip to accentuate and increase the distance between the 12th rib and the iliac crest. Maximizing this distance is paramount with regard to port placement. The operative field should include the space between the costal margin and the iliac crest and from the umbilicus to the spine. Both the primary surgeon and the camera assistant stand facing the patient's back. The scrub nurse/tech stands facing the patient's front, and instruments are handed across the patient accordingly.

Extraperitoneal Procedures. For extraperitoneal procedures the patient is positioned in the supine position with the legs level on split-leg positioners or elevated in stirrups that have knee and leg supports to avoid perineal nerve injury. The table is angled (broken) slightly at the hip to accentuate the pelvis. The patient's arms are tucked at the sides; plastic sleds can be used to support the arms. Adequate padding should be applied to the arms and legs. A slightly snug chest strap should be placed directly across the patient's chest. The table is placed in the 30-degree Trendelenburg position. Genitalia are draped into the operative field, which extends from the mid chest to thighs and from midaxillary line to midaxillary line. The surgeon stands on the side of the table where he or she is comfortable and the assistant stands on the opposite side. The scrub assistant also stands on the side of the table opposite the surgeon.

PERFORMING THE PROCEDURE
Before the Initial Incision

A checklist ensuring that all essential equipment is present and operational should be completed just before initiating the pneumoperitoneum (see Table 7–1). Specifically, this list should include (1) light cable on the table, connected to the light source and operational; (2) laparoscope connected to the light cable and to the camera, with an image that has been white balanced and focused using a white gauze sponge; (3) operational irrigator/aspirator; (4) insufflator tubing connected to the insufflator, which is turned on to allow the surgeon to see that there is proper flow of CO_2 through the tubing; kinking of the tubing should result in an immediate increase in the pressure recorded by the insufflator, with concomitant cessation of CO_2 flow; (5) an extra tank of CO_2 in the room; and (6) a Veress needle, checked to ensure that its tip retracts properly and that, when it is connected to the insufflator tubing, the pressure recorded with 2-L/min CO_2 flow through the needle is less than 2 mm Hg.

Achieving Transperitoneal Access
Pneumoperitoneum

The insufflant system (i.e., insufflator, tubing, and chosen gas) is essential for establishing a pneumoperitoneum. This is brought into use after either closed (i.e., Veress needle) or open (i.e., Hasson cannula or hand-assist device) access to the peritoneal cavity is established. If hand-assisted laparoscopy is to be performed, the pneumoperitoneum can be established directly after placement of the hand port.

Most commonly, CO_2 is used as the insufflant because it does not support combustion and is very soluble in blood (LD_{50} for CO_2 is 1750 mL (air = 357 mL) (Bordelon and Hunter, 1994). However, in patients with chronic respiratory disease, CO_2 may accumulate in the bloodstream to dangerous levels. Accordingly, in these patients, helium may be used for insufflation once the initial pneumoperitoneum has been established with CO_2 (Leighton et al, 1993). The drawback of helium is that it, like air, is much less soluble in blood than CO_2; however, its use precludes problems of hypercarbia. For this reason, even in patients with chronic respiratory disease, the procedure is initiated with CO_2 and then the change is made during the case to helium if necessary. Other gases that were once used for insufflation (room air, oxygen, nitrous oxide) are no longer routinely used because of their potential side effects (e.g., air embolus, intra-abdominal explosion, potential to support combustion). "Noble gases" such as xenon, argon, and krypton are inert and nonflammable but are not routinely used for insufflation because of their high cost and poor solubility in blood.

To begin, insufflator pressure is set at 15 mm Hg with a rate of gas flow of 1 L/min. Once safe entry into the peritoneal cavity has been achieved (i.e., 500 mL of insufflant has entered the abdominal cavity at < 15 mm Hg pressure), the pressure can be increased to 20 to 25 mm Hg and flow can be increased to 2 L/min for the Veress needle or to the maximal insufflator flow setting if an open access method (e.g., Hasson cannula) is used. The 14-gaugeVeress needle cannot deliver flow rates greater than 2 L/min.

KEY POINT: INSUFFLATION

■ The insufflated CO_2 is cold (21°C) and is not humidified (Ott, 1991a). Whereas this results in minimal cooling of the patient, it likely contributes to problems of fogging of the endoscope during the procedure. Accessory devices for insufflators that warm and humidify laparoscopic gas to physiologic conditions are available. However, the benefit of this technology is minimal. Indeed, warming the insufflant by itself may be of no benefit or even detrimental (Bessell et al, 1995); however, humidification appears to be of value and may decrease postoperative pain somewhat (Hamza et al, 2005).

Closed Technique: Veress Needle

Sites for Needle Passage. Disposable (70- or 120-mm, 14-gauge, and 2-mm outer diameter) as well as nondisposable (metal) Veress needles can be used. Proper needle function is ensured before the procedure. The blunt tip of the needle is tested to make sure it retracts easily; also, the needle is connected to the CO_2 line to ensure that there is no resistance to gas inflow. Lastly, saline is flushed through the needle with the tip manually occluded to make sure there is no leakage at the juncture between the shaft and hub of the needle.

With the patient in the supine position, the head of the bed is lowered 10 to 20 degrees; insertion of the Veress needle is commonly accomplished at the superior border of the umbilicus (Fig. 7–2). There are certain advantages to

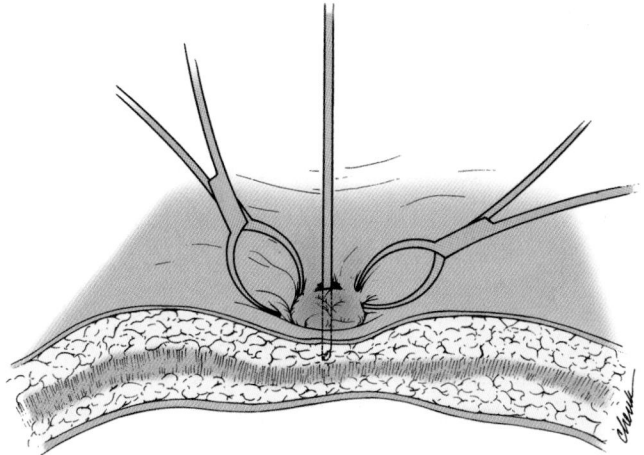

Figure 7–2. Insertion of Veress needle at umbilicus. The towel clips stabilize the abdominal wall as the needle is advanced. (From Clayman RV, McDougall EM [eds]: Laparoscopic Urology. St. Louis, Quality Medical Publishing, 1993.)

choosing the umbilical area as the site for initial trocar placement: the abdominal wall is thinnest, and postoperative cosmesis is excellent. However, this point of entry is fraught with the potential for injury to a major vessel, in particular the left common iliac, aorta, or vena cava.

Another important factor with regard to passing the Veress needle is body habitus, In obese patients, the umbilicus tends to migrate inferiorly. In nonobese patients the umbilicus lies in its commonly described position, directly above the bifurcation of the aorta and vena cava. Thus, for umbilical access in nonobese patients the Veress needle should be passed through the abdominal wall angled toward the pelvis to avoid injury to the bowel and great vessels that lie directly beneath. In more obese patients, because the umbilicus lies more caudad, less angulation is needed and the Veress needle should be passed perpendicular to the umbilical incision (Loffer and Pent, 1976). In addition, it has also been found that pneumoperitoneum pressure and volume as well as the ease of trocar or needle insertion is not significantly effected by body habitus. In a combined human and porcine study, McDougall and associates prospectively performed pressure-volume analysis on 41 individuals undergoing transperitoneal laparoscopic procedures and found that 94% of the maximal intraperitoneal volume is achieved with an insufflation pressure of 15 mm Hg. Additional pressure did not significantly increase volume. Furthermore, in the porcine component of the study, elevation of the pneumoperitoneum pressure above 15 mm Hg did not significantly ease bladed trocar insertion (McDougall et al, 1994). Hence, the pneumoperitoneum pressure need never be raised above 15 mm Hg unless it is done so in the setting of a vascular venous injury to control bleeding (a discussion of this technique is outlined below).

If the patient is in a lateral decubitus position, then the Veress needle is passed 2 fingerbreadths medial and 2 fingerbreadths superior to the anterior superior iliac spine. Just before insertion of the Veress needle, a 12-mm incision is made in the previously described area, in anticipation of placing a 10- to 12-mm trocar. The subcutaneous tissues are spread with a Kelly clamp, and the anterior fascia is secured with two Allis clamps. The abdominal wall is stabilized, but not lifted, with the two Allis clamps. The Veress needle is grasped at midshaft and is passed perpendicularly through the 12-mm incision using a gentle, steady pressure; two points of resistance are traversed: the abdominal wall fascia and the peritoneum. With this approach, the only organ at risk is the bowel; neither a vascular organ nor a major vessel can be injured using this insertion site.

Other potential insertion sites when the patient is either supine or in a lateral decubitus position are Palmer's point (i.e., subcostal in the midclavicular line on the right side) and the corresponding site on the left side. In this instance, stabilization or even a slight upward tension on the Allis clamps is essential; the needle if inserted too deeply will potentially hit the liver or the spleen, so care must be exercised. However, injury to the large bowel is distinctly remote with this approach. Chung and coworkers (2003) applied this method of laparoscopic access and trocar placement in 622 consecutive cases. Prior abdominal surgery had been performed in 192 patients (31%), and the body mass index was 30 or greater in 98 patients. Blind Veress needle placement was successful in 579 (93%) and was not associated with laterality, type of surgery, or prior surgery. In 34 cases (5%), a minor laceration to the liver was managed conservatively without sequelae; and in 21 cases (3%), the omentum or falciform ligament was traversed without significant injury. No major complications, such as vascular or hollow-organ perforation, were caused by either the Veress needle or trocar. No patient developed an incisional hernia at the upper quadrant trocar site (Chung et al, 2003).

Aspiration/Irrigation/Aspiration. With the use of a 10-mL syringe containing 5 mL of saline, the Veress needle is aspirated to check for blood or bowel contents. If this test result is negative, then the saline is injected into the abdominal cavity; this should occur without any resistance. Next, the plunger of the syringe is again withdrawn; no fluid should return into the barrel of the syringe. Lastly, the syringe is detached from the Veress needle, and any fluid left in the hub of the needle should fall swiftly into the peritoneal cavity.

Hanging Drop Test. If there is any question about the proper placement of the needle in the peritoneal cavity, a drop of saline can be placed on the hub of the Veress needle. The drop should fall swiftly into the spacious peritoneal cavity as the abdominal wall is lifted by the Allis clamps.

Advancement Test. If the needle has truly just entered the peritoneal cavity, then the surgeon ought to be able to advance the needle 1 cm deeper without the tip meeting any resistance. Resistance at this stage usually means the needle is still in the preperitoneal space and needs to be advanced (Fig. 7–3).

Once proper needle placement is verified, insufflation is started at 1 L/min. If free flow of CO_2 is noted (i.e., intra-abdominal pressure remains less than 15 mm Hg), then after 0.5 L has entered the abdomen the flow can be increased to maximal capacity (2 L/min through a 14-gauge needle). As soon as the preset limit of 15 mm Hg of intra-abdominal pressure is reached, free flow stops.

In a previously operated abdomen, Veress needle insertion should be performed in an unscarred quadrant of the abdomen (preferably the left upper quadrant). Alternatively, if there is no scar-free area, then an open technique should be used.

Closed Technique: Blind Trocar Insertion. Although controversial, this approach has been popular in the gynecologic literature. This method is performed via a subumbilical 12-mm transverse incision; the rectus sheath on either side of the incision is grasped with a towel clip, and a surgeon on either side lifts the abdominal wall upward. It is claimed that this creates a distance of 6 to 8 cm between the underside of the abdominal wall and the underlying viscera. A 5-mm incision is made in the elevated rectus sheath, and a 10- to 12-mm disposable shielded or optical view trocar is passed vertically. In a prospective randomized study, comprising 578 patients, the direct insertion technique was found to be associated with fewer complications (4.2.%) than a standard Veress insertion (complications in 14.6%); also of note, entry failure occurred in only 0.7% of the direct trocar insertion patients versus 4.6% of the Veress needle group (Gunenc et al, 2005). To date, use of this method has not been reported in the urologic literature.

Open Access Techniques. A pneumoperitoneum can be more easily, and in one's early experience, more safely established using an open technique; however, its use involves making a larger incision and increases the chances of port-site gas leakage during the procedure. The open technique is recommended specifically when extensive adhesions are

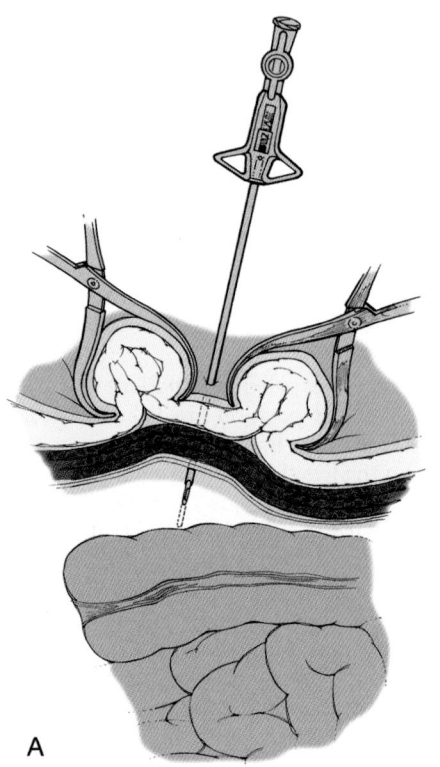

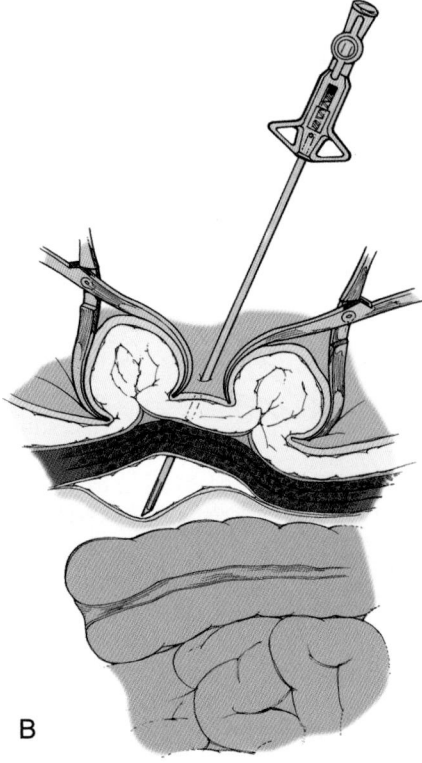

A   B

Figure 7–3. Advancement test. **A,** When the Veress needle is placed correctly inside the abdominal cavity, the tip can be advanced for 1 to 2 cm without encountering resistance; the red indicator in the hub of the needle does not move, indicating a lack of resistance to needle advancement. The atraumatic tip of the needle is extended. **B,** If the Veress needle is in the preperitoneal space, any attempt at further advancement is met with increasing resistance, indicating incorrect placement. Also, the indicator in the needle's hub moves up, indicating that the sharp surface of the Veress needle is exposed.

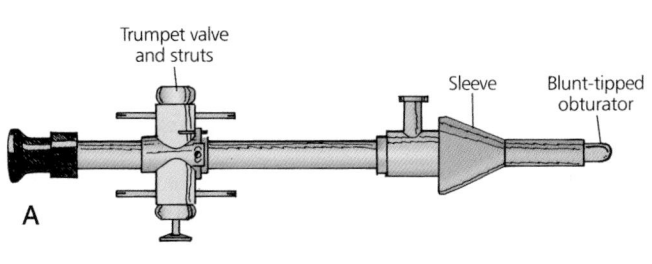

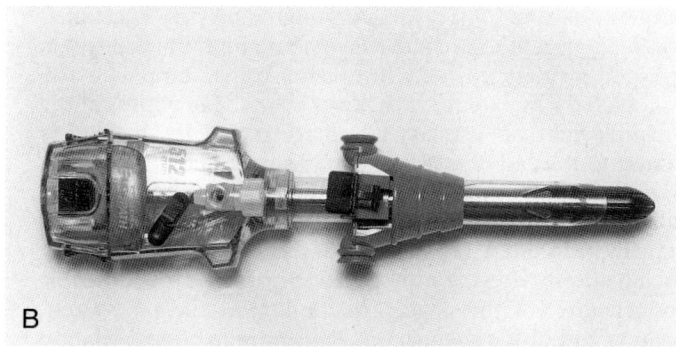

Figure 7–4. Hasson cannula: nondisposable (**A**) and disposable (**B**). (**A** from Clayman RV, McDougall EM [eds]: Laparoscopic Urology. St. Louis, Quality Medical Publishing, 1993.)

anticipated (Fig. 7–4). Studies in general surgery have shown the open technique to be as efficient as the closed approach and slightly more or equally as safe (Bonjer et al, 1997).

In the unscarred abdomen, a 2-cm semicircular incision is made at the lower edge or slightly below the umbilicus. The fascia and peritoneum are opened individually with a transverse incision, sufficient to accommodate the surgeon's index finger. After visual and digital confirmation of entry into the peritoneal cavity, two 0-0 silk traction sutures are placed on either edge of the fascia. Next, the Hasson cannula is advanced through the incision with the blunt tip protruding. The funnel-shaped adapter of the Hasson cannula is advanced until it rests firmly in the incision, and it is then tightened onto the cannula with the attached screw; fixation to the abdominal wall is provided with the fascial sutures that are wrapped around the struts on the funnel-shaped adapter of the Hasson cannula, thereby anchoring it in place. After removal of the obturator, free flow of CO_2 into the peritoneal cavity is achieved by attaching the CO_2 tubing to the cannula. The insufflator can be set at maximum inflow, thereby creating the pneumoperitoneum quickly.

A far simpler type of open cannula is to use a cannula equipped with a balloon retention device (e.g., Bluntport, U. S. Surgical Inc., Norwalk, CT). Once the cannula is positioned in the abdominal cavity, the balloon is inflated; the cannula is pulled upward until the balloon is snug on the underside of the abdominal wall. Next, the soft foam collar on the outside surface of the cannula is now slid downward until it is snug on the skin; at this point it is locked in place. This process creates an excellent seal, precluding gas leakage as well as subcutaneous emphysema.

Hand Port Access. If the hand port is going to be placed in the midline, then the midline should be marked before placing the patient in the 45-degree (modified) flank position. The pneumoperitoneum can be obtained before or after making the hand port incision, but if one wishes to ensure the minimum size of the skin incision then the incision should be made after obtaining the pneumoperitoneum because this places the skin on stretch. Therefore, this method will be discussed in detail. However, if the surgeon has little experience with achieving a pneumoperitoneum, the safest maneuver is to place the hand port via a 7-cm open incision and then create the pneumoperitoneum through the hand port.

After obtaining a pneumoperitoneum, the surgeon should carefully plan out the hand port entry site as well as the addi-

tional instrument and camera port sites. Every hand port device has a "footprint" that can be drawn on the abdominal wall; that footprint varies depending on the diameter of the external appliance. Care should be taken to plan out the additional trocar sites carefully to avoid interference between the hand port and the instrument ports. After the footprint is traced, the hand port incision site is marked; the length of the incision should correspond to the surgeon's glove size (i.e., 7 glove size = 7-cm incision). The skin is incised, and the fascia is divided. The peritoneum is entered, and the insufflation is temporarily stopped. The inner transabdominal coupling portion of the device is placed, and the external appliance is attached. Additional 5-mm or 10- to 12-mm ports can be placed rapidly under manual control with the surgeon's intra-abdominal hand being used to guide the additional trocars through the abdominal wall. Alternatively, a trocar can be placed through the hand port and the abdomen can be reinsufflated. A laparoscope can then be placed through the port and the rest of the trocars can be placed under direct vision. These two techniques minimize the risk of injury to intra-abdominal structures.

Gasless Technique. The gasless open technique avoids the use of insufflants entirely and allows the surgeon to use familiar and readily available open surgical instrumentation. After open entry into the peritoneal cavity, one of several different mechanical devices (retractors, wires, or rods) is used to lift the abdominal wall to create a suitable working space (Araki et al, 1993; Kitano et al, 1993).This technique has gained some popularity in Japan but is rarely used in the United States or Europe because the exposure is compromised owing to the cone-shaped working space created by the lifting modality (Igarashi et al, 2000; Watanabe et al, 2002).

Instrumentation for Developing the Extraperitoneal Space

Balloon Dilation

Gradual distention of a balloon dilator in an extraperitoneal space atraumatically displaces the mobile fat and moves the peritoneum forward relative to the immobile body musculature. This device thus creates a working space equivalent to the size of the balloon.

Commercially Available Balloons. A commercially available trocar-mounted preperitoneal balloon dissector (PDB) (U.S.

Surgical, Norwalk, CT) is commonly employed. The transparent, high-tensile strength silicone balloon is inflated with a sphygmomanometer bulb insufflator using room air. The balloon has a maximum capacity of 800 mL (40 pumps of the inflating bulb). A primary advantage is that the balloon is affixed to the end of a stiff, hollow, transparent, plastic shaft. The shaft allows precisely directed placement of the balloon dilator (see later). Furthermore, since the laparoscope can actually be inserted into the shaft of the balloon dilator during the inflation process, it provides the capability for endoscopic confirmation of the proper positioning of the transparent balloon and of the adequacy of the controlled radial dilation of the extraperitoneal area. Balloon dilators are commercially available in two different shapes: a round balloon for retroperitoneal dilation and a horizontally oriented, oblong-shaped balloon for dilation of the pelvic extraperitoneal space (Fig. 7–5).

Self-Styled Dilators. Gaur's original (1992) version of the balloon dilator was a size 7 surgeon's glove mounted on a No. 8 red rubber catheter. The external end of the catheter was connected to a sphygmomanometer bulb insufflator, and the balloon was insufflated to 110 mm Hg. After this initial description, several other self-styled dilators were described: the middle finger of a size 7 to 8 glove, two fingers of a 7 to 8 glove tied over each other for additional strength, a sterile condom, and the cot of an O'Connor-style drape mounted on a 16- or 18-French red rubber or whistle-tip catheter (Chiu et al, 1995; Webb et al, 1993). The device may be backloaded into an Amplatz sheath to facilitate introduction through a laparoscopic port. Although it is economically advantageous, drawbacks of the self-styled balloon include the lack of a stiff shaft to manually direct the balloon into a specific location for precise dilation as well as the inability to endoscopically monitor the dilation process from within the balloon.

An ex-vivo laboratory study demonstrated that increasing volumes of saline induced gradual pressure increments within the finger of a glove. At a volume of 1000 mL, the average pressure was 15 mm Hg. Pressures remained 15 mm Hg at 1500 mL and increased to 17 mm Hg at 2000 mL (McDougall et al, 1994). In practice, there is no need to exceed the 1000-mL limit. Also, latex balloons have less tensile

strength than silicone balloons, making them more likely to rupture. Regardless, with either balloon setup, on the few occasions that either type of balloon has ruptured there has been no obvious complication. However, the latex balloon has a tendency to rupture into multiple pieces whereas the Silastic balloon usually leaves only one large fragment, making retrieval an easier task.

Complications associated with balloon dilation stem from improper balloon placement or balloon rupture. Intramuscular dilation may result in hernia formation, or inadvertent peritoneal disruptions may occur (Gaur, 1992; Adams et al, 1996).

Manual Dilation. Creation of a working space within the retroperitoneum may be achieved exclusively with a combination of digital and laparoscopic instrument dissection (Rassweiler et al, 1998). After access to the extraperitoneal area is gained, to-and-fro movements of the laparoscope are performed to create a working space (McKernan, 1995). This technique has been employed to perform various simple and advanced procedures in the retroperitoneum (Abbou et al, 1999; Rassweiler et al, 1998). Although it is effective, potential disadvantages of this technique include frequent cleaning of the laparoscope and the lack of clear landmarks initially due to the smaller working space.

Gasless Preperitoneal Laparoscopy

Extraperitoneoscopy. The commercially available Laprofan-Laprolift system (U.S. Surgical, Norwalk, CT) has been used to retract the anterior abdominal wall after preliminary balloon dilation of the pelvic extraperitoneal space through an infraumbilical incision (Etwaru et al, 1994). The Laprofan consists of a specialized fan retractor with 10-cm blades. Inserted through the infraumbilical incision, the blades of the fan, articulated to 90 degrees, are spread open under the anterior abdominal wall. The Laprofan is then connected to the Laprolift, which consists of a motorized arm attached to the operating table to provide a vertical lift. Because CO_2 insufflation is not necessary to distend the extraperitoneal space, in contrast to conventional extraperitoneal laparoscopy, the risk of developing hypercarbia is eliminated by use of the gasless technique. As such, valveless trocars can be used, and the use of conventional open surgical instruments can be resorted to, if necessary. However, compared with conventional laparoscopy, this technique provides limited exposure, especially in obese patients (Goldberg and Maurer, 1997). Although procedures such as pelvic lymphadenectomy and bladder neck suspension have been performed, the gasless technique has not gained widespread acceptance (Etwaru et al, 1994; Davila, 1995; Goldberg and Maurer, 1997).

Gasless Assisted Retroperitoneoscopy. Gasless assisted retroperitoneoscopy has been employed to perform adrenalectomy, nephrectomy, nephroureterectomy, live-donor nephrectomy, partial nephrectomy, and pyeloplasty (Etwaru et al, 1994; Davila, 1995; Chung et al, 1996; Stackl et al, 1996; Suzuki et al, 1996; Yang et al, 1996; Goldberg and Maurer, 1997; Sakakibara et al, 2000). After balloon dilation, the Laprofan-Laprolift system is used. Visualization is afforded by a laparoscope introduced through a trocar, while the actual procedure is performed open, through a 4- to 6-cm incision, using either open surgical or laparoscopic instruments.

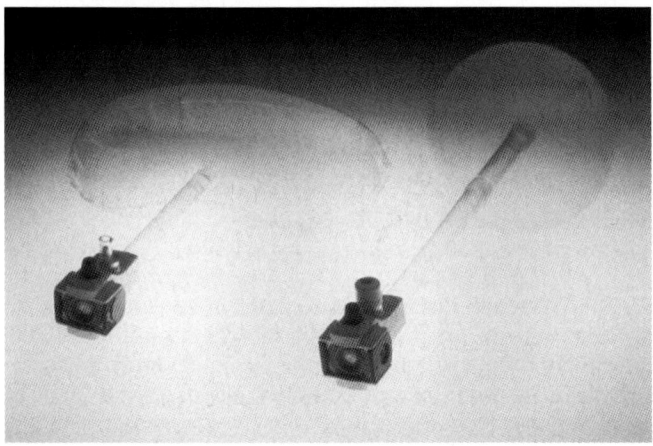

Figure 7–5. Commercially available balloon dilators are either round (for retroperitoneal dissection) or oblong (for pelvic extraperitoneal dissection).

Retroperitoneoscopy

Open (Hasson) Technique. This is the most commonly employed technique because it affords the greatest precision during development of the retroperitoneal space (Gill, 1998). Initial access is obtained through a 2- to 2.5-cm, transverse incision in the midaxillary line, just below the tip of 12th rib. The wound is opened with a pair of S-retractors. Under direct vision, the posterior layer of the lumbodorsal fascia is incised and muscle fibers are split or divided. The retroperitoneal space is entered, under direct vision, by making a small incision in the anterior thoracolumbar fascia with an electrocautery blade or by bluntly piercing the fascia digitally or with a hemostat. Care should be taken that this fascial opening is snug around the index finger and no larger, so that intraoperative air leak is minimized. Index finger palpation of the belly of the psoas muscle posteriorly and the Gerota's fascia–covered inferior pole of the kidney anteriorly confirms proper entry into the retroperitoneal space (Fig. 7–6). The index finger is employed to digitally create a space in this precise location for placement of the balloon dilator; this is usually aimed in a cephalad direction (Fig. 7–7). Thus, balloon dilation is performed anterior to psoas muscle and fascia and outside of and posterior to Gerota's fascia (Fig. 7–8). In cases involving definitive ureteric mobilization (retroperitoneoscopic donor nephrectomy, nephroureterectomy, ureterolitho-

tomy, pyeloplasty), a second balloon dilation is performed caudad to the primary site of dilation (Gill et al, 1995) (Fig. 7–9). Similarly, during a retroperitoneoscopic adrenalectomy, it is helpful after the initial balloon dilation to move the balloon up higher in the retroperitoneum and perform a second even more cephalad balloon dilation along the undersurface of the diaphragm (Sung and Gill, 2000) (Fig. 7–10).

Closed (Veress) Technique. Access to the retroperitoneum has been achieved by placement of a Veress needle in the inferior lumbar (Petit's) triangle (Capelouto et al, 1994; McDougall et al, 1994; Sung and Gill, 2000). CO_2 insufflation creates a small pneumoretroperitoneum; this is followed by blind insertion of the primary trocar. The laparoscope is then employed to bluntly create a space for placement of secondary ports. In contrast to transperitoneal laparoscopy, no actual, preexisting space is available in the retroperitoneal fat for accurate placement of the needle. Furthermore, standard tests to confirm appropriate position of the needle tip (as described in the preceding section on transperitoneal laparoscopy) may not apply. Occasionally, the needle tip may inadvertently be placed in the quadratus lumborum muscle. Pneumoinsufflation in this superficial location may result in trauma to and splaying of muscle fibers, precluding successful retroperitoneoscopic access and necessitating conversion to transperitoneal laparoscopy (Capelouto et al, 1994). Alternatively, the needle may be positioned too deeply, resulting in inadvertent creation of a pneumoperitoneum, thereby technically complicating the retroperitoneoscopic procedure from the outset. As mentioned, the open Hasson technique is safer, more precise, and quicker, and allows performance of balloon dilation, thus making it the preferred access technique for retroperitoneoscopy.

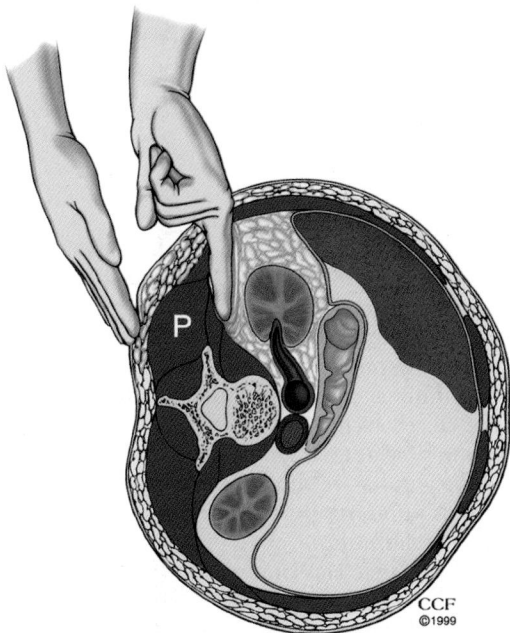

Figure 7–6. Access into the right retroperitoneum. Through the primary port incision at the tip of the lowest (12th) rib, open access is gained into the retroperitoneum after piercing the thoracolumbar fascia. Finger dissection is performed anterior to the psoas muscle and fascia to create a space for insertion of the balloon dilator. Confirmation that the finger dissection is indeed being performed in the proper plane is obtained by palpating the psoas and erector spinae muscles between the retroperitoneally located index finger and the fingertips of the opposite hand positioned on the patient's back. The fat-covered lower pole of the kidney can be palpated in a cephalad direction by turning the finger clockwise in the retroperitoneum on the right side. (Adapted from Hsu TH, Sung GT, Gill IS: Retroperitoneoscopic approach to nephrectomy. J Endourol 1999;13:713-718.)

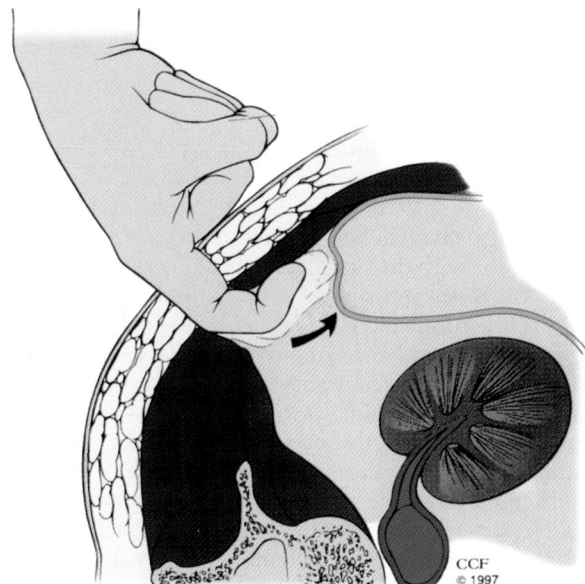

Figure 7–7. After retroperitoneal access by the open Hasson technique, blunt digital dissection may be performed to reflect the peritoneum medially, thus creating space for the safe insertion of the anterior port. (Adapted from Gill IS: Retroperitoneal laparoscopic nephrectomy. Urol Clin North Am 1998;25:343-360.)

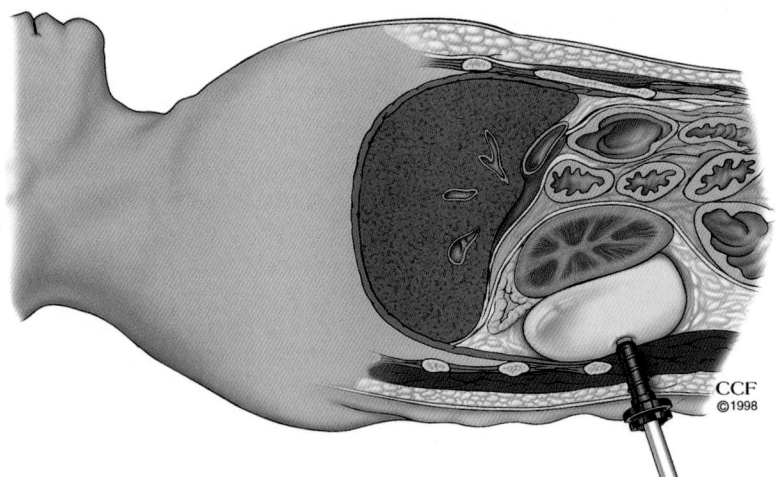

Figure 7–8. Balloon dilation in the posterior pararenal space facilitates the creation of a working space for retroperitoneal laparoscopic nephrectomy *(coronal view).*

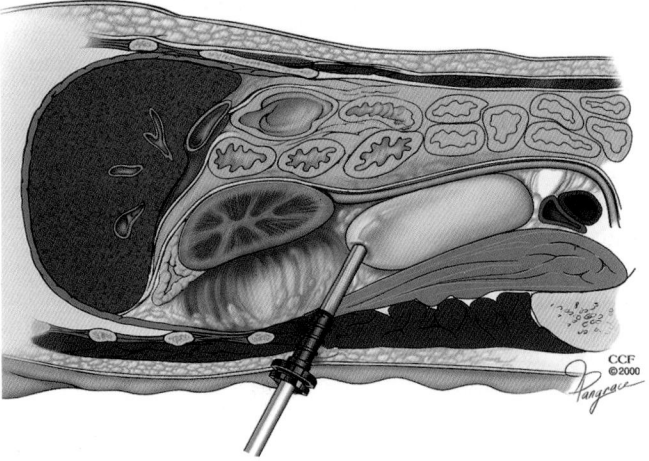

Figure 7–9. Secondary balloon dilation caudally is particularly useful for procedures requiring retroperitoneal ureteric dissection, such as radical nephroureterectomy and live-donor nephrectomy.

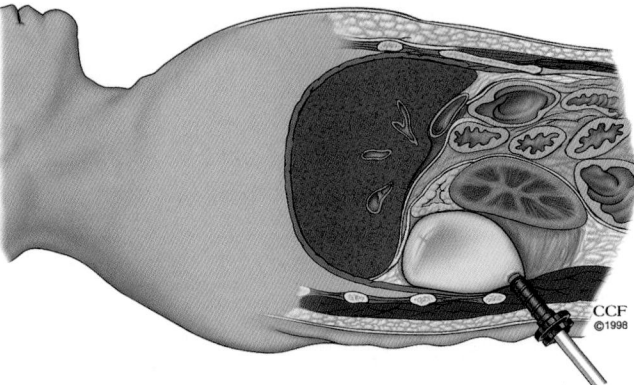

Figure 7–10. Secondary balloon dilation cranially is employed when performing retroperitoneoscopic adrenalectomy.

Extraperitoneoscopy

Open (Hasson) Technique. A 1.5- to 2-cm curvilinear incision is made along the inferior umbilical crease. The anterior rectus sheath is incised vertically for 1.5 cm, and the rectus muscle is separated in the midline to expose the posterior rectus sheath. With the surgeon's index finger positioned posterior to the rectus muscle and anterior to the posterior rectus sheath, gentle tunneling motions are made in a caudal direction until the area of the symphysis pubis is reached. At this distal location, the fascia transversalis is punctured with the fingertip, and gentle side-to-side digital dissection is performed in the prevesical space, posterior to the pubic bone. Into this predeveloped space, the balloon dilator is inserted and distended to create an adequate working space. Balloon dilation effectively displaces the prevesical fat and reflects the peritoneum cephalad. The balloon is initially inflated in the midline and then reinflated on either side to further expand the working area (Meraney and Gill, 2001).

Closed Technique. Similar to retroperitoneoscopy, closed access to the extraperitoneal space has been described (Lee et al, 1998). Apart from the inherent disadvantages associated with blind trocar insertion, such as iatrogenic injury to the bladder (Lee et al, 1998), a major drawback of this technique is that the primary port is located in relatively close proximity to the pubic symphysis. Unlike the open Hasson technique, in which the peritoneum is mechanically reflected cephalad, thereby creating a more voluminous craniocaudal space, during the closed technique the relatively undisplaced peritoneum may preclude wider separation between port sites. The secondary ports are thus positioned somewhat closer to the symphysis pubis, resulting in a steeper working angle and suboptimal visualization.

Caveat: The classic Hasson cannula requires the placement of two 0-0 silk sutures into the fascia, which are then affixed to the cone shaped portion of the cannula to effect a seal between the cannula and the fascia. This arrangement invariably results in a significant leakage of gas because the seal is never air tight. Indeed, in earlier studies of retroperitoneoscopy, excessive subcutaneous emphysema and higher CO_2 levels were the norm owing to use of the standard Hasson cannula (Wolf et al, 1995; Ng et al, 1999); this situation was completely reversed with the introduction of the open-access blunt port, which has a balloon to secure it on the underside of the abdominal wall and a soft foam cuff to secure it to the outer abdominal wall, thereby effecting an air-tight seal (Ng et al, 1999).

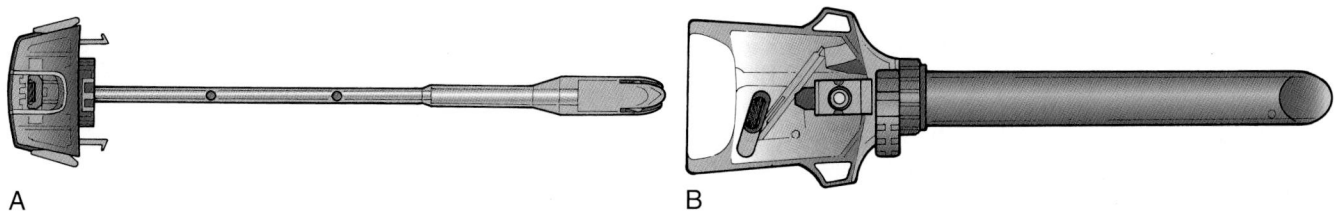

Figure 7–11. Laparoscopic trocar (disposable). Obturator with built-in safety shield (**A**) and cannula (**B**).

Trocar Technology and Placement

Types of Trocars. Trocars enable the laparoscopist to introduce working instruments into the gas-filled abdomen. They also maintain or reestablish a pneumoperitoneum by conveying the insufflant and may serve as pathways for delivering dissected tissue from the surgical area to the outside of the abdomen. Typically, a trocar consists of an **outer hollow sheath** (also called a cannula or port) and an inner sharp obturator, which is removed as soon as the outer sheath has entered the peritoneal cavity (Fig. 7–11).

A variety of nondisposable and disposable trocars are available. Standard models range from 3 to 20 mm in diameter and 5 to 15 cm in length. A variety of valves allow the surgeon to exchange instruments through the port without the escape of significant amounts of gas. Trapdoor or flap valves are found in disposable ports; thus, it is necessary to depress the valve lever to open the valve widely during retrieval of tissue or needles. More recently, a disposable multiseal valve has become available; the entire valve is removable as needed when retrieving tissue specimens. These valves are of greatest advantage when used in 10-mm or larger trocars because they allow passage of 5- and 10-mm instruments without the need for a separate reducer. In reusable trocars, a trumpet valve design is often used; the drawback to this valve is that it can be abrasive on the insulation of electrosurgical laparoscopic instruments.

Initially, only sharp-tipped/bladed trocars were available. These tips had a variety of shapes: conical, pyramidal, or eccentric; the obturator thus incised the various layers of tissue as it entered the peritoneal cavity. To protect the underlying viscera from the sharp tip of these trocars, a plastic safety shield was incorporated into the disposable trocars that would spring forward to shield the blade once the trocar entered the gas-filled abdomen (see Fig. 7–11). However, bladed and sharp-tipped trocars should be largely of historical interest because they have been superceded by noncutting dilating trocars. These trocars enter the abdomen by spreading the abdominal wall musculature rather than cutting it. As such, there is less chance of injuring an abdominal wall vessel and the resulting entry site is less prone to subsequent herniation; indeed, the risk of either of these complications appears to be 10-fold less with blunt versus sharp trocars. As with the older sharp trocars, there are both disposable and nondisposable blunt trocar units. The Step Needle/Sleeve (U.S. Surgical, Norwalk, CT) is a disposable system that uses a needle port with an outer diameter of 2.1 mm (6.5 French) that incorporates a Veress needle introducer. After correct and successful puncture of the abdomen and establishment of the pneumoperitoneum, the Veress needle introducer is removed and

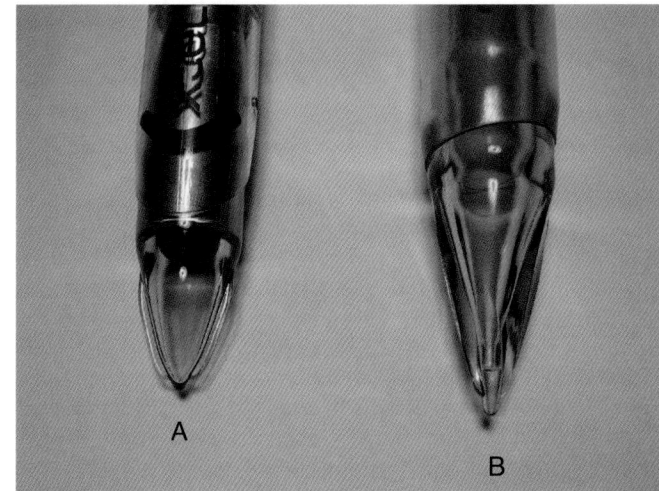

Figure 7–12. Examples of visual fascial dilating "bladeless" trocar systems. **A,** Endopath Xcel Bladeless Trocar (Ethicon, New Brunswick, NJ). **B,** Optical Separator System (Applied Medical Rescources, Rancho Santa Margarita, CA).

the needlescopic port serves either as a camera-bearing sheath of a 1.9-mm needlescope or as a working port for needlescopic scissors or graspers used to perform needlescopic surgery. Alternatively, the needle can carry the initial port into the abdomen; this is an expandable port that in its collapsed state is 2.1 mm at the distal tip and 3.8 mm along the body of the trocar. This trocar can then be expanded by passage of a blunt-tipped obturator to expand the collapsed sheath to 5 mm, 10 mm, or 12 mm, depending on the surgeon's needs. The port has an adjustable seal that allows introduction of laparoscopic instruments within a range of 4.4 to 12 mm in diameter. Thus, the tissues of the abdominal wall are stretched rather than incised, thereby precluding the need for placement of fascial sutures at the end of the procedure. Other blunt-tipped trocars are produced by all of the major trocar manufacturers. These devices have a variety of tips that enable their placement by spreading the tissues; they also have a clear plastic tip such that the surgeon can pass an endoscope into the trocar to endoscopically monitor its passage through the abdominal wall and its entry into the gas-filled abdomen (Fig. 7–12). One of the blunt-tipped disposable trocars incorporates a curved cutting blade that is trigger activated by the surgeon as the clear port is passed under endoscopic control (i.e., VISIPORT Plus RPF Single Use Optical Trocar with VERSAPORT Plus RPF Converterless Trocar Sleeve, U.S. Surgical, Norwalk, CT). This hybrid of a blunt and sharp trocar is used sparingly due to the cutting blade, which can injure vessels or viscera; also the port site created by passage of this trocar requires a sutured closure of the fascia. The reusable EndoTip system (Karl Storz, Culver City, CA) is a screwlike device that has no sharp points or cutting edges. It comes in a 5-, 10-, and 12-mm design; however, the 10- and 12-mm trocars require use of a cumbersome reducer system because they are not of a multiseal design (see later). It is introduced by rotating the cannula in a controlled manner, with the laparoscope monitoring the penetration of the various tissue layers. Unlike the action of trocars with a sharp tip, the tissue is not cut but is only displaced and bluntly dilated, thereby preserving the closing mechanism of the overlying muscle and fascia. Owing to its innovative design, this device reduces injury to the intra-abdominal organs, stays securely in place, and seals the point of entry against any inadvertent loss of gas. Also, on its removal, the fascia does not need to be sutured, when it is placed in a non-midline area; however, others do not place a suture even with midline placement provided that postoperative palpation of the entry site reveals a small defect (Siqueira et al, 2004).

All primary and some secondary trocars have side-arm insufflation line input valves and a small distal hole near the tip to prevent formation of a vacuum, which may suck viscera into the cannula when the cannula is removed (see Fig. 7–11). Some less-expensive, smaller trocars do not have side-arm stopcocks and can be used only as secondary trocars. Reducers allow downsizing of working channels in 10-mm or larger trocars to accommodate smaller, 5-mm working instruments without any leakage of CO_2; however, the development of multiport technology has resulted in valves that can accommodate 5- to 12-mm instruments without the need for a reducer. The aforementioned development saves significant time during a long procedure. In addition, different retention mechanisms prevent dislocation of cannulas: threaded sleeves, adjustable threaded sleeves, expandable arms, inflatable balloons, or simple fixation to the abdominal wall with No. 2 nonabsorbable stay sutures.

When reusable trocars are used, they must be checked frequently. The obturator needs to be sharp; if it is dull, it should be sent to the manufacturer to be resharpened; however, again at this time we recommend against the use of any sharp trocars throughout the laparoscopic procedure. Similarly, the trumpet valve found in some reusable trocars needs meticulous care, cleaning, and inspection after each procedure.

Hand-Assist Devices. The first generation of hand port devices consisted of the Handport, Intromit, and Pneumosleeve. As with most first-generation laparoscopic devices, they were adequate with regard to functionality but each one had several aspects that left much to be desired (Stifelman and Nieder, 2002). These products have now been replaced by a second generation of devices that have improved on the original designs: The Gelport (Applied Medical, Rancho Santa Margarita, CA), the Omniport (Advanced Surgical Concepts, Wicklow, Ireland), and the LapDisc (Ethicon Endosurgery, Cincinnati, OH) (Fig. 7–13).

The Gelport consists of a gel-like disc that easily admits the surgeon's hand and then molds around the wrist and arm. To set up the three-piece Gelport system the surgeon inserts the

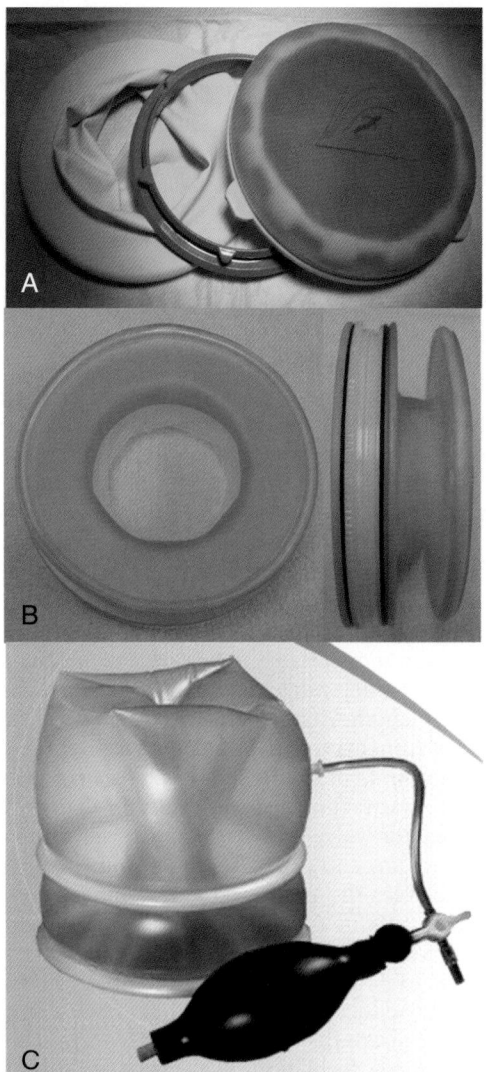

Figure 7–13. Components of currently available hand-assisted laparoscopy devices. **A,** The Gelport (Applied Medical, Rancho Santa Margarita, CA). **B,** LapDisc (Ethicon Endosurgery, Cincinnati, OH). **C,** Omniport (Advanced Surgical Concepts, Wicklow, Ireland).

lubricated wound protector and then stretches the portion protruding from the incision over a baseplate. A gel disc is then snapped on top of the baseplate. The Gelport offers the advantages of never losing a pneumoperitoneum upon hand exchange because it immediately seals after hand removal and it does not require adjustment to maintain a seal. It comes in 10- and 12-cm diameters.

The Omniport is a balloon-like device that anchors itself as one piece across the abdominal wall. The inflated device also creates a seal between itself and the surgeon's wrist. The device has a smaller footprint (12 cm), but it must be uninflated and reinflated each time a hand is exchanged, which loses the pneumoperitoneum.

The LapDisc is another one-piece unit that has an inner diaphragm that is used to anchor it across the abdominal wall and an outer appliance that dials down a thin plastic sheet, like a camera iris, that wraps around the surgeon's wrist.

Although this device has a low profile footprint (12 cm) it does result in loss of the pneumoperitoneum every time the hand is removed and reinserted.

In a recent study, 130 urologists participating in a series of hand-assist courses evaluated the different devices for a variety of features. The overall scores in this study were 8.6, 7.4, and 7.3 on a scale of 10 (10 being best) for the GelPort, LapDisc, and OmniPort, respectively (Patel and Stifelman, 2004). Advantages of the Gelport included sturdiness, ease of hand exchange, maintenance of the pneumoperitoneum, as well as the ability to pass both a hand and a laparoscopic instrument simultaneously.

Placement of Initial Trocar. For pelvic procedures, the patient is usually positioned with the head slightly down, and the intra-abdominal CO_2 pressure is kept at 15 mm Hg. However, some laparoscopists prefer to increase the intra-abdominal pressure to 20 to 25 mm Hg to further tense the peritoneum and add a bit more volume (i.e., 5%) to the pneumoperitoneum itself.

After establishment of a Veress needle pneumoperitoneum (i.e., closed technique), the edges of the wound and subcutaneous tissue are spread with a blunt forceps, following which the underlying anterior abdominal wall fascia may be secured and stabilized with an atraumatic Allis clamp. Next, the trocar is held in the dominant hand with the middle finger extending along the shaft and the trocar is inserted using a twisting downward motion. If the surgical site is in the mid to upper abdomen, then the trocar is passed perpendicular to the umbilical incision; however, for pelvic procedures, the trocar is directed 70 degrees caudally. Proof of entering the gas-filled intraperitoneal cavity is the sound of CO_2 escaping from the open side arm. After the side arm is closed, the obturator is removed, and the CO_2 insufflation line is connected to the side port of the trocar. If using a clear blunt port, a 0-degree laparoscopic lens is placed, so the entire entry of the trocar is endoscopically monitored.

For procedures such as nephrectomy or nephroureterectomy, the patient is placed in the flank (i.e., lateral decubitus) position and the pneumoperitoneum pressure is increased to 25 mm Hg. The edges of the initial incision, which is 2 fingerbreadths medial and 2 fingerbreadths superior to the anterior superior iliac spine or subcostal in the midclavicular line (e.g., Palmer's point on the right), are supported on either side by Allis clamps or towel clips. The trocar is passed perpendicular to the skin incision in the manner described for the transumbilical approach.

When an **open technique** is performed, the Hasson-style cannula used to obtain access to the abdomen also serves as the initial trocar.

Transperitoneal Approach: Abdominal Inspection. The sterile, handheld laparoscopic camera is connected to a 0- or 30-degree, 10-mm laparoscope. Next, the light cord is connected to the laparoscope, and the camera is white balanced by pointing the lens at a white gauze pad and pressing the designated button until the indicator on the television screen signals completion of this step; the camera image is also brought into focus on the gauze pad. Finally, the tip of the prewarmed endoscope is dipped into povidone-iodine solution or wiped with a commercial antifogging fluid, cleansed with a dry gauze pad, and passed into the initial trocar. Although

it is a minor extra expense, a dedicated fluid warmer to warm the shaft of the standard endoscope is a very useful adjunct. Newer endoscopes that have electronics embedded in the tip of the shaft should not be submerged in water.

The **entire abdomen** is inspected systematically. Initially, abdominal inspection is performed to rule out any injury to the underlying viscera that may have occurred during access or placement of the initial trocar. Then, if the patient is supine, the following pelvic anatomic landmarks are visualized: bladder, urachus, medial umbilical ligaments, and internal inguinal rings, followed by the appendix and the lower parts of the colon; in the male, the vasa deferentia can sometimes be seen, whereas in the female, the round ligaments, uterus, and ovaries are viewed. Next, turning toward the upper abdomen, the liver, gallbladder, spleen, stomach, omentum, and small bowel are visualized. However, abdominal inspection is usually limited to the superior ipsilateral half of the abdomen if the patient has undergone insufflation and port placement in the lateral decubitus position.

Hand-Assist Placement. The hand-assist device can be placed either as an initial "port" or as a secondary port depending on the surgeon's preference. To be sure, the former approach is easier because the procedure then begins with making a standard midline (for right or left renal surgery) or right lower quadrant (i.e., for right renal surgery) 6.5- to 7.5-cm incision at the planned hand-assist site. The peritoneal cavity is entered in the standard open surgical fashion, following which the hand-assist device is placed. Next, a blunt cannula is passed through the hand-assist device and a pneumoperitoneum is established. Alternatively, a Veress or Hasson pneumoperitoneum may be initially established, and the hand-assist device can then be placed under endoscopic monitoring. Before initiating a hand-assist procedure, the surgeon is advised to wrap the arm/glove seam on the hand that is to be used through the hand port either with a 1010 drape or an Ioban (3M, St. Paul, MN) "sticky drape" to waterproof his or her arm; if a 1010 drape is used, the surgeon will need to place a second glove on the hand-port hand.

Additional blunt ports can be rapidly and safely placed using the surgeon's one hand to place the port while the intra-abdominal hand is used to palpate the tip of the trocar and hence guide its entry into the abdomen. Lastly, the use of brown gloves is recommended because they do not reflect the light from the laparoscope and are thus easier to see (Wolf, 2005).

Secondary Trocar Placement

Transperitoneal: Standard. Number, size, and exact location of secondary trocars depend largely on the intended laparoscopic procedure. Their configuration should be planned so that neither the tips nor handles of the cannulas cross or come into close contact with one another, respectively (a problem termed *crossing swords* and *rollover*, respectively) such that adequate working space is provided for all instruments to be used during a particular procedure. In general, it is reasonable to place the ports in a four-point diamond pattern such that the site of the operation is encircled within the diamond. This is particularly of importance when considering reconstructive renal procedures, as the angle of the plane to the site of renal reconstruction should be less than 55 degrees while the angle between the surgeon's suturing instruments should be in the 25- to 45-degree range (Rassweiler and Frede, 2002).

Secondary trocars are placed under direct optical control. The 30-degree lens is ideal for this portion of the procedure because turning the lens 180 degrees away from the surgical site provides the surgeon with a panoramic view of the anterior abdominal wall. The operative lights are dimmed, and the tip of the laparoscope is moved upward toward the intended site of port placement, thereby, in the thin patient, transilluminating any superficial blood vessels that need to be avoided while passing the trocar. With a No. 12 hook or No. 15 small blade, a skin incision is made just wide enough to accept the selected cannula. When placing secondary ports it is of great importance to direct them toward the intended surgical field to provide tension-free maneuverability of the laparoscopic instruments. This is especially important in obese patients. Similar to placement of the initial port, all secondary ports are advanced through the abdominal wall using a slow, twisting motion and constant pressure. If necessary, the abdominal wall can be elevated by towel clips placed at the edges of the skin incision made for port entry, to facilitate safe advancement of trocars into the peritoneal cavity. Each secondary port is passed into the peritoneal cavity under meticulous endoscopic monitoring. After placement of the second port equal to or larger than 10 mm, the laparoscope is advanced through this port to inspect the entry site of the first trocar into the peritoneal cavity, to rule out any inadvertent injury to the bowel, underlying viscera, or to an abdominal wall vessel. To prevent dislocation, ports that do not possess self-retaining mechanisms may be anchored to the skin using No. 2 nonabsorbable sutures. In this regard, it is very important for the surgeon to never use a plastic retention sleeve with a metal cannula; this combination creates a situation in which stray electrosurgical current may injure the bowel or other structures adjacent to the cannula since the plastic sleeve insulates the abdominal wall, resulting in increased current density along the metal intra-abdominal portion of the cannula.

Transperitoneal: Hand-Assist. When the hand-assist device is in place, then secondary trocars can be placed via digital guidance. After inspection of the abdomen rules out any potentially interfering adhesions, the surgeon's index finger is placed on the underside of the abdominal wall at the planned site of trocar placement. A skin incision is made over the surgeon's index finger, and the nonbladed trocar is passed with the other hand and guided into the abdominal cavity. This is a very rapid and safe way to place all of the secondary nonbladed trocars.

Retroperitoneoscopy Approach. After controlled balloon dilation of the retroperitoneum, the balloon dilator is replaced with a 10-mm Bluntport (U.S. Surgical, Norwalk, CT). A feature unique to this port is the presence of an internal doughnut-shaped fascial retention balloon and an external adjustable foam cuff, a combination that effectively creates an airtight seal at the location of the primary port site (Fig. 7–14). Use of this device minimizes CO_2 leakage around the 1.5-cm primary port incision, thus reducing the incidence of subcutaneous emphysema and hypercarbia. In our experience, this is far superior to the reusable Hasson cannula; with this device efforts directed at minimizing gas leak, such as placing a deep mattress stay suture or placing petroleum jelly gauze around the cannula, were rarely effective. For retroperitoneoscopy, a

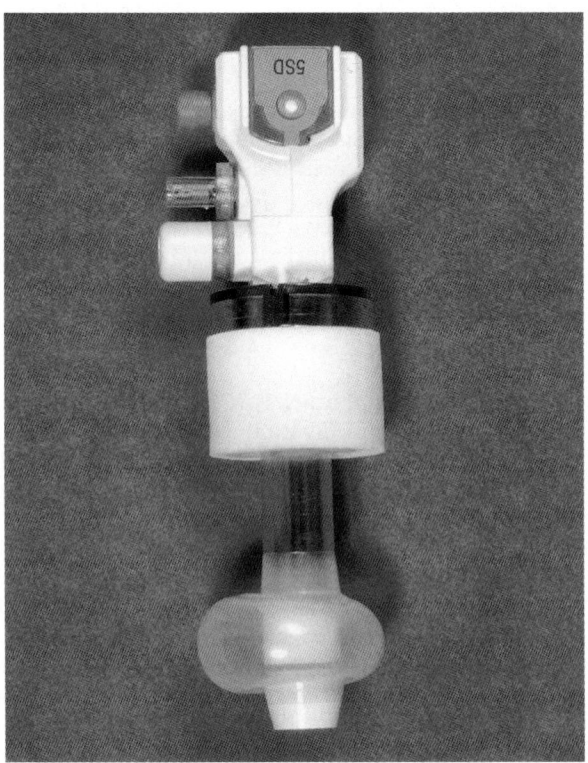

Figure 7–14. After open Hasson access into the retroperitoneum, placement of a Bluntport, which consists of a foam cuff and an internal, doughnut-shaped, fascial retention balloon, prevents carbon dioxide leakage around the port during retroperitoneal laparoscopy. The use of this device as the primary port is a critical factor in minimizing air leak and subcutaneous emphysema during retroperitoneoscopic surgery.

three-port ("I" distribution) approach is employed by Gill (Gill, 1998; Hsu et al, 1999) while others prefer a four- ("T" distribution) (i.e., the authors) or five- ("W" distribution) port placement (Abbou et al, 1999). A 30-degree laparoscope is used, and all secondary nonbladed ports are introduced under laparoscopic or digital control. The posterior secondary port is placed at the lateral border of the paraspinal muscles along the inferior border of the lowermost (12th) rib, and an anterior port is placed at the anterior axillary line, subcostal; thus the three ports are all in a line, hence an "I" configuration. A fourth port may be placed, in the middle axillary line, two to three fingerbreadths above the anterosuperior iliac spine (Fig. 7–15) near Petit's triangle; thereby creating a "T" configuration. Placement of this anterior port any closer to the iliac crest limits the amount of cephalad angulation of the cannula. A fifth port can be placed just lateral to the anterior axillary line and on the same level as the fourth port, thereby creating a "W" configuration. Depending on the anticipated technical difficulty of the procedure, patient obesity, and tumor size, for the "I" configuration, two 12-mm secondary ports or one 5-mm port and one 12-mm secondary port are used. In either situation, a 12-mm port is routinely placed for the surgeon's dominant hand to allow interchangeable use of various large-caliber instruments, including a 10-mm Endoclip applier, a 12-mm EndoGIA stapler, a 10-mm right-angle dissector, and a 10-mm reusable expandable retractor. The two secondary ports should be inserted as far apart as possible to minimize the possibility of instrument tips clashing

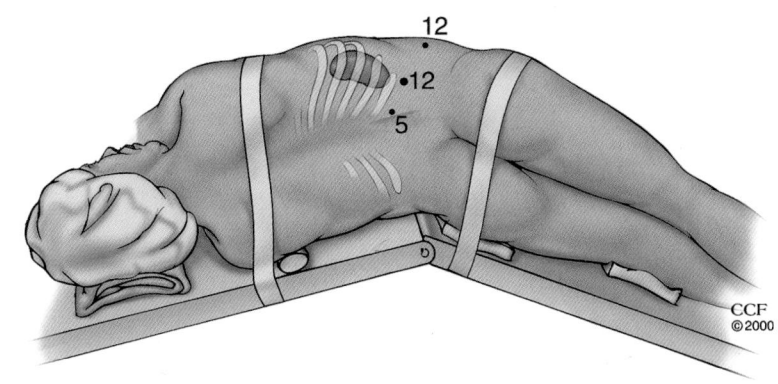

Figure 7-15. For retroperitoneal laparoscopy, the patient is positioned in the standard full-flank position. The kidney rest is elevated, and the operating table is flexed to maximize the space between the iliac crest and the lowest rib. A three-port approach is employed. **A,** The primary port is placed inferior to the tip of the 12th rib. **B,** An anterior port is placed near the anterior axillary line 3 cm cephalad to the iliac crest. **C,** A posterior port is placed at the junction of the lateral border of the paraspinal muscles and the 12th rib. (*Note:* After port placement, the kidney rest is lowered.)

within the retroperitoneum. The additional two ports can be 5, 10, or 12 mm, depending on the surgeon's preference. Contrary to common conception, the occurrence of an inadvertent peritoneotomy during retroperitoneoscopy does not usually interfere with the subsequent steps of the procedure, and conversion to a transperitoneal laparoscopic technique is not mandatory (Gill et al, 2000).

Extraperitoneal Access to the Pelvis. After balloon dilation, the Bluntport is inserted at the infraumbilical incision. The retention balloon is inflated, and the foam cuff is cinched down. The extraperitoneal space is insufflated with CO_2 at a pressure of 12 to 15 mm Hg, and secondary ports are introduced under visual control. Depending on the procedure to be performed, three to four secondary ports are inserted in a triangle-, diamond-, fan-, or W-shaped configuration. Pneumoextraperitoneum is reduced to 10 to 12 mm Hg for the remainder of the procedure. Unlike with retroperitoneoscopy, the occurrence of a peritoneotomy during extraperitoneoscopy may interfere with the performance of subsequent extraperitoneal dissection, and conversion to a transperitoneal technique may be required (Meraney and Gill, 2001).

Robotic Considerations. If a robotic procedure is planned, then the camera port is a 12-mm trocar site and the two auxiliary ports are both 8 mm. The ports need to be at least 8 to 10 cm apart to reduce the possibility of the robotic arms clashing with each other. In addition, if the patient is in a flank position, then the lowest port placement should not be inferior to the umbilicus or else the arm may be blocked from a full range of motion by the patient's upside leg. An assistant's port is placed either in between the arms of the robot or on a line below the robotic arms. The latter position seems preferable, as the assistant does not need to work in between the arms of the robot.

Laparoscopic Instrumentation

Instrumentation for Visualization

To create a laparoscopic image, four components are required: the laparoscope, light source, camera, and monitor. To record the image, video recorders and video printers are available. Laparoscopes that are most commonly used have 0- or 30-degree lenses (range, 0 to 70 degrees) and a size of 10 mm (range, 2.7 to 12 mm); however, newer deflectable laparoscopes now also exist that can deflect in four directions up to

90 degrees (Olympus, Melville, NY). Image transmission uses an objective lens, a rod-lens system with or without an eyepiece, and a fiberoptic cable. From the eyepiece, the optical image is magnified and transferred to the camera and onto the monitor. Light is transmitted from the light source through the fiberoptic cable onto the light post of the laparoscope. Some newer laparoscopes have a mini CCD camera mounted at the tip (EndoEYE, Olympus, Melville, NY) that improves image quality. Historically the advantage of the larger laparoscopes is that they are able to provide a wider view, better optical resolution, and a brighter image. However, today, some 5-mm laparoscopes can provide an image that rivals traditional 10-mm scopes.

A special variant is the offset "working laparoscope," which includes a working channel for passage of basic laparoscopic instrumentation; use of this type of laparoscope enables the surgeon to work in direct line with the image and may allow a reduction in the number of trocars needed to accomplish a particular procedure. However, the working channel occupies space that would otherwise be used for the optical system; hence, the resulting image is usually of lesser quality compared with that of laparoscopes without this feature.

The **camera system** consists of a camera and a video monitor. All currently made cameras can be gas or liquid sterilized, thereby facilitating their use and limiting possible intraoperative contamination. The camera is attached directly to the end of the laparoscope and transfers the view of the surgical field through a cable to the camera box unit. After reconstruction of the optical information, the image is displayed on one or two video monitors.

A wide variety of cameras are currently available: single-chip, single-chip/digitized, three-chip, three-chip/digitized, interchangeable fixed-focus lenses, zoom lenses, beam splitter, and direct coupler. Three-chip cameras are superior to single-chip cameras in that they provide a higher-quality image with superior color resolution. Again, some endoscopes have the added advantage of having the chip directly at the tip of the laparoscope such that the images are directly processed without interruption, thereby improving image quality (EndoEYE, Olympus, Melville, NY).

To obtain a "true" upright image of the surgical field on the monitor, the camera's orientation mark must be placed at the 12-o'clock position. With 0-degree laparoscopes, the camera is locked to the eyepiece in the "true" position. In contrast, with the 30-degree laparoscope, the camera is loosely attached to the eyepiece of the laparoscope so the laparoscope can be rotated. Accordingly, the assistant must hold the camera in the "true" upright position with one hand while rotating the laparoscope through a 360-degree arc to peer over and around vascular and other intra-abdominal structures; the 30-degree lens thus provides the surgeon with a more complete view of the surgical field than does a 0-degree lens. A more recent advancement in laparoscope technology is the four-way deflectable endoscope (EndoEYE Deflectable Tip Video Laparoscope, Olympus, Melville, NY), which offers many potential angles from which to view a structure, but this requires an adept assistant.

Three-Dimensional Laparoscopic Systems. Three-dimensional laparoscopic systems offer the surgeon the distinct advantage of depth perception. All 3-D laparoscopes are similar in that the laparoscope has two lenses (one for the left eye and one for the right eye) such that each eye sees a different image. In this way binocular vision is maintained. The most commonly used 3-D vision system currently in use is the InSite Vision System (Intuitive Surgical, Sunnyvale, CA), which provides vision for the da Vinci Surgical Robotic System. The laparoscope and camera are heavy but are controlled by a robotic arm that is under direct control of the surgeon from the ergonomic console. The surgeon maintains a steady, magnified 3-D view of the surgical field.

Hand-held 3-D laparoscopic systems are also available but currently require the surgeon to wear headgear with miniature video screens to display the 3-D image (EndoSite 3-D Digital Vision System, Viking Systems Inc., LaJolla, CA). With these systems it is often useful to employ the use of a robotic camera manipulator such as the AESOP system because the slight movements associated with hand-held camera manipulation can be distracting when displayed in 3-D.

The most vexing problem with the laparoscope is fogging of the lens. To prevent fogging of the laparoscope after insertion into the warm intraperitoneal cavity, it is advisable to initially warm the laparoscope in a container holding warm saline before it is passed into the abdomen. The most efficient way to warm the scope is to use a dedicated solution warming basin that is long enough to accommodate the laparoscope. In addition, wiping the tip with a commercial defogging fluid or with povidone-iodine solution is also recommended. Should moisture buildup occur between eyepiece and camera, both components must be disconnected and carefully cleansed with a dry gauze pad.

Video monitors are available in 13- or 19-inch standard sizes or 18-inch flat panel displays. A larger monitor does not produce a better picture; indeed, given the same number of lines on both monitors, a higher-resolution image is obtained with the smaller screen. To obtain a better image, more lines of resolution are needed. High-resolution monitors have 1125 lines of resolution but must be matched with a camera system of similar capability; to date, these monitors have not made their way into the operating room. Flat-panel video monitors are becoming more popular; one advantage is that these screens are usually mounted on a ceiling boom that allows the surgeon to obtain a clear view of both the monitor and the surgical field with the patient in any position. In addition, the flat screen can be lowered and angled close to the surgical site, thereby reducing the "disconnect" between the surgeon's line of sight and the actual operating field.

Light sources use high-intensity halogen, mercury, or xenon vapor bulbs with an output of 250 to 300 watts. In addition to manual control of brightness, some units have automatic adjustment capabilities to prevent too much illumination, which may result in a "washed-out" image. Any breakage of fibers in the fiberoptic cable, which may occur during sterilization and/or improper handling, results in decreased light transfer from the light source to the laparoscope. Newer light cables are transparent, allowing the surgeon to actually see when light-bearing cables have been damaged.

Videocassette recorders (VCR), digital video recorders (DVR), and video printers serve for documentation of laparoscopic procedures. VCRs are very reliable for taping procedures but are very cumbersome when it comes to storing, viewing, and editing for replay. Newer systems that use digital tapes, compact discs, or digital video discs are much more compact and easier to use when it comes to replaying and editing for video production. With regard to still images, the newer digital recorders have the advantage of storing thousands of images and maintain the ability to print paper copies of the desired images.

Instrumentation for Grasping and Blunt Dissection

Most graspers and dissectors are used in their 5-mm size but are available in a range from 3 to 12 mm, in predominantly reusable forms. Grasping instruments have either single-action (only one jaw moves during opening) or double-action (both jaws move) tip design.

Wide variations exist with regard to configuration of tip, surface characteristics of jaws, handle design, and possible electrosurgical properties. Tip designs include blunt-coarse, pointed (dolphin), straight (duck bill), curved (Maryland), and angled. The surface of the jaws may be atraumatic or traumatic. Serrated or smooth surfaces allow gentle tissue manipulation in atraumatic graspers (e.g., bowel forceps with a 3-cm long grasping jaw); other forceps have disposable soft inserts that are changed after each procedure (e.g., A-Trac Laparoscopic Grasping System, Applied Medical Resources, Rancho Santa Margarita, CA). Traumatic graspers have toothed or clawed surfaces on their jaws to allow them to grasp and hold tissues firmly. In addition, they may be equipped with tip-rotating and articulating features.

Depending on the design of the handle, grasping instruments may be locking or nonlocking. Most nonlocking forceps have a scissors-type handle. Different designs allow for locking capabilities; in particular, bar-type and spring-loaded locking handles are convenient when prolonged grasping of tissue is required (Fig. 7–16).

In addition to articulating instruments, both the laparoscopic suction apparatus as well as the "heel" of the hook electrode can be used for effective and rapid blunt dissection. Along these same lines, the development of laparoscopic "peanuts" (i.e., 5- and 10-mm gauze-tipped disposable dissectors) has been most helpful. These dissectors can be twirled or moved side to side or up and down in an area of adipose tissue to rapidly tease away the fat surrounding vital structures such as the renal hilum or the adrenal gland.

Water Jet Dissection. Water jet dissectors such as the Helix Hydro-Jet (ERBE, Tubingen, Germany) use an extremely thin,

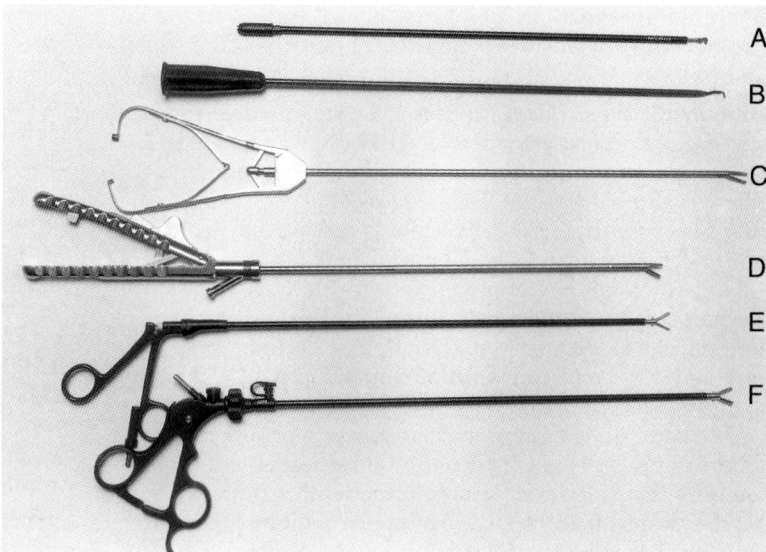

Figure 7–16. Laparoscopic ultrasonic knife (**A**), hook electrode (**B**), needle drivers (**C** and **D**), and graspers (**E**, nonlocking and **F**, locking).

high-pressure laminar liquid jet to develop a cleavage plane in tissues. Pressures of 250 to 350 psi are sufficient for dissecting soft tissue while leaving vascular and nervous structures intact (Shekarriz et al, 2004). The device is activated using a foot pedal, and the water jet is administered from a 5-mm wand. This device may have particular application in parenchymal transection as in partial nephrectomy or in nerve-sparing procedures such as during RPLND (Basting et al, 2000; Shekarriz et al, 2004).

Instrumentation for Incising and Hemostasis.

Laparoscopic scissors, scalpels, electrocautery, and lasers (CO_2, neodymium:yttrium-aluminum-garnet [Nd:YAG], or potassium titanyl phosphate [KTP]) are used to incise or cut tissue during laparoscopic surgery.

Laparoscopic scissors are available in disposable and nondisposable forms. The blades of laparoscopic scissors are shorter than their open surgical counterparts. The configuration of the tip may be useful for selected situations: serrated tips for cutting fascia, hooked tips for cutting sutures, microscissors for spatulating the ureter during a pyeloplasty, and curved tips for dissection. Incision of the tissue is achieved using either an electrosurgical ("hot") or a mechanical ("cold") approach. The scissors may come with either permanent blades or with replaceable tips; the latter ensures "sharp" scissors for each procedure. In addition, the shaft of the scissors may rotate and, in some disposable scissors, even articulate. The latter feature is particularly helpful when spatulating the ureter during a pyeloplasty.

A **laparoscopic scalpel** is also available. It is of particular use for incision of the ureter during laparoscopic ureterolithotomy.

For **electrosurgical incision** of tissue, a selection of different electrodes is available: needle electrodes (Corson type) produce fine cuts that are useful in making peritoneal incisions, spatula electrodes are used in blunt dissection and cutting, and hook electrodes (J and L configurations) are of particular value during dissection of vessels because tissue can be pulled away from delicate structures before the cutting

current is activated (see Fig. 7–16). The thinner the metal tip of the probe, the higher the density of the electrical current and the greater the cutting power.

As with all insulated instruments, certain precautions must be followed during monopolar electrosurgery to avoid local or distant transmitted thermal injury. Consequently, the electrosurgical probe should not be activated unless the metal part is in complete view. The insulation of the electrosurgical instrument should be carefully checked for any damage. The probe should not be activated unless it is in direct contact with the tissue to be incised. Also, use of the monopolar electrosurgical instrument through a metal rather than a plastic cannula decreases the chances of inadvertent electrosurgical injury owing to capacitive coupling. In this regard, one should never use a metal trocar in conjunction with an outer plastic retaining ring because stray current can no longer be harmlessly dissipated through the metal cannula directly to the surrounding peritrocar abdominal wall and, hence, any juxtaposed visceral structure may be damaged in an area remote to the laparoscopist's vision. The same precautions apply when using monopolar equipped grasping forceps, which might be used during a procedure to obtain hemostasis.

To avoid the potential dangers of stray current from use of monopolar electrosurgical equipment, the surgeon can use monopolar current in conjunction with active electrode monitoring (Encision Inc., Boulder, CO). This instrumentation is constructed such that there is ongoing feedback during activation of the electrosurgical current; as such, any break in the insulation of the shaft results in immediate deactivation of the instrument.

Floating Ball Electrode (Monopolar Device). The Endo FB3.0 floating ball electrode (TissueLink Medical Inc., Dover, NH) is a saline-cooled radiofrequency surface coagulator/sealer. Skimming an FB3.0 floating ball over a tissue surface in small circles seals the tissue, stopping the flow of blood and other fluids by effectively shrinking the natural collagen in the tissue. The wet energy from the FB3.0 cools tissue and keeps temperatures less than 100°C, preventing tissue charring and eschar formation. This device has been proven to be quite useful for coagulating the parenchymal bed after partial nephrectomy prior to application of a hemostatic agent and/or bolster (Stern et al, 2004; Urena et al, 2004).

Bipolar Electrosurgical Devices. The laparoscopic surgeon can also use bipolar electrosurgical devices, which require less energy for performance than their monopolar counterparts. There is also a decreased likelihood of injury to surrounding tissue because the electrical current is passing only from one jaw to the other, thereby precluding the potential problems of capacitive coupling commonplace with monopolar electrosurgical current. With bipolar current, the extent of coagulative damage is less than with monopolar electrosurgery: 1 to 6 mm versus 5 to 7 mm with monopolar current (Landman et al, 2003).

The latest development in laparoscopic bipolar electrosurgical equipment is the LigaSure vessel-sealing system (Valleylab, Boulder, CO). The system consists of a 5- or 10-mm grasper/dissector connected to a bipolar radiofrequency generator. When the vascular structure is grasped by the instrument, the tissue is evaluated by a feedback-response system that subsequently delivers the optimal energy required to seal the vessel effectively. Owing to the high-current and low-voltage output, the vascular structure enclosed by the jaws of the instrument degrades quickly and a protein-based seal is presumably created; this mechanism of electrical current delivery to the tissues results in less charring and less collateral thermal damage (1 to 3 mm) (Landman et al, 2003). An audible signal alerts the surgeon that the sealing of the vessel is complete; the instrument has a trigger-activated blade that the surgeon can then use to cut the sealed tissue. Vessels up to and including 7 mm appear to be effectively occluded with this device (Carbonell et al, 2003; Landman et al, 2003); however, in practice most surgeons limit use of the LigaSure to the occlusion of only veins in the 5 mm and less range (e.g., adrenal, ascending lumbar, or gonadal veins).

Laser Instrumentations. Lasers (CO_2, KTP, Nd:YAG, holmium) are most frequently used through the working channel of an operating laparoscope. The CO_2 laser provides excellent cutting and vaporization of surface lesions; it requires a rigid handpiece and probe. In contrast, the 400- and 600-μm KTP fibers are flexible and allow for noncontact cutting and fulguration. Nd:YAG laser fibers are also flexible and allow noncontact fulguration and contact cutting. Holmium laser fibers are also flexible and are used in a contact mode for cutting. Fibers with sculpted tips provide more precise cutting. Laser-specific goggles must be worn during all laser-related procedures by every individual in the operating room, including the patient. In urologic laparoscopy, lasers are not routinely used; likewise, in general surgery they have largely been supplanted by electrosurgical instruments. Only in gynecology is the CO_2 laser used extensively, generally in the treatment of endometriosis.

Ultrasound Instrumentation. Ultrasonic technology is another option for cutting and hemostasis in endoscopic surgery. It provides an especially attractive alternative to monopolar electrosurgery when one is working around particularly delicate tissues or operating on patients with an implanted pacemaker/cardioverter defibrillator (Gossot et al, 1999; Strate et al, 1999). In ultrasonic surgery, electrical energy is transformed into mechanical energy by the use of a piezo-

electric crystal system. Mechanical vibrations produced by this system in the tip of the instrument are capable of causing the following effects on tissue: cavitation, coaptation/coagulation, and cutting (Strate et al, 1999). Two different forms of ultrasonic technology are available for laparoscopic surgery: the ultrasonic cavitational aspirator and the ultrasonically activated scalpel ("harmonic knife") or shears ("harmonic shears"). The ultrasonic cavitational aspirator fragments and aspirates tissue with a high water content (e.g., fat cells) (Payne, 1994). Collagen-rich tissues, such as nerves or blood vessels, are largely preserved. Its tip oscillates at 23 kHz and has an excursion from side to side of 200 to 360 μm (Gossot et al, 1999). Although this technology is helpful in dissecting and identifying vessels, it is not widely used owing to its slowness, lack of hemostasis, and splashback during its use which may obscure the laparoscopist's vision. It has been most extensively used during adrenalectomy in patients with Cushing's disease to help clear away the abundant fat that surrounds the adrenal gland in these patients (Suzuki et al, 1995; Takeda et al, 1997; Gossot et al, 1999).

In the ultrasonically activated harmonic scalpel/shears, electrical energy is produced by a power-supply generator and transformed into mechanical vibration at the tip of the instrument via a piezoelectric crystal interface (see Fig. 7–16) (Suzuki et al, 1995; Takeda et al, 1997; Gossot et al, 1999). Mechanical vibration with a tip excursion of 80 to 200 μm (at a frequency of 55.5 kHz) is subsequently transferred to the tip of the instrument. Multifunctionality (grasping, cutting, dissecting, and coagulation) is provided with the shears. In addition to the absent risk of local thermal damage and tissue charring because of a working temperature of less than 80°C, the depth of penetration is limited to the targeted tissue within a diameter of 1 mm (Landman et al, 2003). Reduced tissue charring may result in a reduced rate of postoperative adhesions (Amaral and Chrotstek, 1997). In addition, the harmonic scalpel eliminates other problems associated with monopolar electrosurgery, specifically, problems of remote site tissue damage owing to capacitive coupling, insulation defects in the instrumentation, and direct coupling. Potential disadvantages of the harmonic technology include slowness to achieve the desired effect and the fact that the metal portion of the shears becomes quite hot during activation and must not come into direct contact with any bowel surrounding the area of dissection.

Other Instrumentation. The **argon beam coagulator** provides a noncontact form of electrocoagulation. Electrical current originating from a monopolar electrosurgical generator is conducted to the tissue via an ionized argon gas stream. The gas stream blows away blood from the tissue, resulting in better exposure of the bleeding site and, hence, more effective delivery of the fulguration current. Argon is a colorless, odorless, inert gas that clears the body within one respiratory cycle (Quinlan et al, 1992). Holding the handpiece at an oblique 60-degree angle within 1 cm of the surface of the target tissue provides optimal coagulation effects. During argon beam coagulation, the side arm on one of the laparoscopic ports must be opened to prevent buildup of excessive intra-abdominal pressures. Because argon beam coagulation has its major advantage when hemostasis must be achieved over a diffusely bleeding surface, its most practical indication in laparoscopic urologic surgery is during partial nephrectomy or wedge excision of a small renal tumor.

Surgical Pharmaceuticals. Recently, a vast array of topical hemostatics, sealants, and glues have entered the surgical realm. These agents, depending on their individual properties, can be used for a variety of surgical tasks and have become a valuable addition to the surgeon's tray.

Fibrin-Based Glue. Fibrin glue has been used for hemostasis in parenchymal beds (e.g., after partial nephrectomy or to seal a liver laceration), to bond tissue layers together (e.g., as after ureteropelvic junction or bladder repair), and to separate tissue layers (after vesicovaginal fistula repair). The two components of the fibrin glue, fibrinogen and thrombin, are delivered through separate channels and then combine at the tip of the delivery system during application to the tissue. Fibrin glue has an adhesive quality once dry where it essentially hardens into a rubbery coagulum. Tisseel VH Fibrin Sealant (Baxter, Glendale, CA) has the maximum concentration of human fibrinogen available. It can be delivered via a laparoscopic applicator in liquid form or in an aerosolized form. One disadvantage of Tisseel is that it requires a preparation time of 20 minutes before it can be applied by the surgeon. Thus, if the application at hand requires immediate application (bleeding), fibrin glue is not a viable option. Another fibrin-based sealant that can be delivered in a similar manner is Crosseal (Johnson & Johnson, New Brunswick, NJ). This agent comes frozen and thus requires no reconstitution. Thus, once thawed, it can be available in a minute. Another advantage is that it contains no bovine serum components and hence can be used in individuals with allergies to bovine-derived products.

Non–Fibrin-Based Surgical Hemostats. In contrast to the fibrin-based glues, other hemostatic agents such as thrombin-soaked oxidized cellulose particles (FloSeal, Baxter, Glendale, CA) have no adhesive capability at all but are excellent hemostatic agents in the presence of active bleeding from parenchymal surfaces such as a partial nephrectomy bed, liver/spleen laceration, or in an oozing adrenal bed. This agent is also prepared by the scrub assistant and takes 2 minutes to prepare. It is applied via a tube applicator with a syringe. It is most effective when pressure is applied after its delivery; this can be done either via an instrument (e.g., 10-mm gauze-tipped dissector) or with a bolster.

Avitene Microfibrillar Collagen Hemostat (Davol, Cranston, RI) is an active collagen hemostat that accelerates clot formation by enhancing platelet aggregation and the release of fibrin. Similar to FloSeal, it has no tissue-sealing capability but is useful for counteracting parenchymal bleeding. EndoAvitene is available in a preloaded endoscopic delivery system designed for use in endoscopic procedures. Developed to easily pass through standard trocars and cannulas, it is available in both 5- and 10-mm diameters.

Chemical-Based Sealants. BioGlue (CryoLife, Inc., Kennesaw, GA) is a two-component adhesive composed of purified bovine serum albumin (BSA) and glutaraldehyde. The solutions are mixed during application from a controlled delivery system. The glutaraldehyde then cross-links the BSA molecules to each other and then to the tissue protein at the site of use. Once applied, the agent polymerizes within 20 to 30 seconds and reaches its full bonding strength within 2 minutes. The delivery system comes ready for immediate use. BioGlue is a sealant and must be applied to a dry field and allowed to dry. Thus it cannot be used to counteract active bleeding but can be used to seal a raw, nonbleeding surface.

CoSeal (Baxter, Glendale, CA) is a completely synthetic product comprising two distinct polyethylene glycol polymers that chemically bond together to seal tissue surfaces, suture lines, and synthetic grafts. It does not require thawing, heating, or light activation and hence can be ready in 1 minute. It must be applied to a dry (nonbloody) surface because it does not interact with the clotting cascade and hence is not useful in the setting of active hemorrhage.

Now that the benefits of such substances have come into the spotlight in surgery, there are a myriad of agents available that all have different properties, advantages, and disadvantages. Further, newer agents are always coming onto the market. The most important factor is that the surgeon be familiar with the properties of these various agents and should choose one that is most appropriate for the job at hand. A comparison of popular hemostatic agents is outlined in (Table 7–2).

Instrumentation for Suturing and Tissue Anastomosis

Suturing and knot tying are among the most difficult tasks in laparoscopic surgery. A significant amount of practice is needed to achieve a sufficient level of proficiency. **Laparoscopic needle holders** have one fixed jaw and one jaw that opens by squeezing the spring-loaded handle of the instrument (see Fig. 7–16). Owing to the length and narrow shaft of the needle holders, they all have a locking mechanism to

Table 7–2.   Some Commonly Used Topical Tissue Sealants and Hemostatic Agents

Agent	Company/Producer	Active Ingredients0	Key Uses/ Properties	Time to Set Up
Tisseel	Baxter, Glendale, CA	Fibrinogen CaCl Aprotinin Thrombin	Topical hemostasis Tissue glue	20 min
CrossSeal	Johnson and Johnson, New Brunswick, NJ	Fibrinogen CaCl Aprotinin Thrombin	Topical hemostasis Tissue glue	Immediate
FloSeal	Baxter, Glendale, CA	Crosslinked gelatin granules Thrombin	Topical hemostasis	2 min
EndoAvetine	Davol, Cranston, RI	Avetine Microfibrillar collagen powder	Topical hemostasis	Immediate
BioGlue	CryoLife Inc., Kennesaw, GA	Bovine serum abumin and glutaraldehyde	Tissue sealant	Immediate
CoSeal	Baxter, Glendale, CA	Two polyethylene glycol polymers	Tissue sealant	Immediate

secure the needle in their jaws. This is done with a ratchet, spring-loaded, or Castroviejo-type mechanism. Some needle holders also possess a valuable feature that allows the jaws to rotate around the main axis relative to the handle. The handles may be straight or provide a pistol-type grip. Most needles can be introduced directly through a 10- or 12-mm port. Knot pushers, which work independent of the suture material, either slide (Clarke-Riech) or cinch (Gazayerli) the knot into place. Integral knot pushers are part of a system that contains a preformed ligature loop. As soon as the loop of the pre-knotted suture is passed over the tissue to be secured, the knot is delivered and secured around the target tissue with the integral pusher. The suture is then cut, and the plastic knot pusher is removed and discarded. Although these devices that aid in knot tying are helpful in certain situations, there is no substitute for practicing and mastering intracorporeal knot tying, which is the most reliable method for tying knots laparoscopically.

The Endo Stitch (U.S. Surgical, Norwalk, CT) device is an innovative, disposable, 10-mm instrument that facilitates laparoscopic suture placement and knot tying (Adams et al, 1995). The suture is secured to the center of a straight needle with pointed ends, thereby allowing tissue penetration in either direction. The needle is shuttled back and forth between the jaws of the instrument after each passage through the tissue, applying a long-known principle used in sewing machines. In this way, passing the needle through the tissue and regrasping the needle after it has traversed the tissue become simple tasks because they are done by a one-handed squeeze of the handle and a flip of the needle-securing lever, respectively. Use of this sewing apparatus has had a major impact on decreasing operative times, especially in laparoscopic pyeloplasty (Chen et al, 1998). However, with time, most reconstructive laparoscopists have become sufficiently facile with standard laparoscopic needle holders such that use of the Endo Stitch has become less common.

LapraTy clips (Ethicon, Somerville, NJ) are a very useful adjunct to suturing and knot tying. These small clips are made of absorbable polydioxanone and can be secured to the end of a single strand of 1-0, 2-0, 3-0, or 4-0 coated Vicryl. The clip acts as a knot, thereby precluding time-consuming intracorporeal laparoscopic knot tying. These clips provide secure anchoring of sutures for up to 14 days in low-tension to mid-tension environments. When they are used to secure a single suture, the suture must have a pre-tied loop on its end; the needle is passed through the tissues to be secured and is then passed through the pre-tied loop. Next, the suture is pulled taut, thereby tightening its hold on the encircled tissue; the LapraTy clip is then affixed to the suture material just as it exits the loop. For a running suture, the LapraTy clip can be used both to anchor the end of the suture and to secure the suture on completion of the run; this combination has worked very well during pyeloplasties with the Endo Stitch. It has also been found to be useful for anchoring bolsters during renorrhaphy for laparoscopic partial nephrectomy (Orvieto et al, 2004).

One major advance in laparoscopic suturing capability has been the advent of robotic surgical systems such as the da Vinci Surgical System (Sunnyvale, CA). This system offers a 3-D vision system, tremor reduction, motion scaling, and articulating needle drivers with 6 degrees of freedom that can mimic the motions of the surgeon's own hands and wrists.

The result is superb precision during laparoscopic suturing such as in radical prostatectomy or pyeloplasty; in addition, the handling of this equipment is identical to the movements one has learned using instrument suturing/knot tying during open surgery.

Instrumentation for Stapling and Clipping

Stapling Devices. Various stapling devices are available: manual linear cutting and noncutting and powered linear cutting and noncutting (Fig. 7–17). The Endo-GIA Universal 12-mm stapler/linear cutting device (U.S. Surgical, Norwalk, CT) requires a 12-mm port and delivers two triple-staggered rows of staples and simultaneously cuts between the rows. The universal stapler can be loaded with a variety of 30-, 45-, or 60-mm loads. Similarly, the ETS-Flex 45 stapler (Ethicon, Somerville, NJ) also requires a 12-mm port and delivers two triple rows of staples while cutting between row 3 and row 4. Articulating/roticulating staplers are available from both companies. These disposable devices can be reloaded multiple times during a procedure. Each staple load cartridge is color-coded depending on the size of the staples: 2.0-mm staples (gray) or 2.5-mm staples (white) are preferred for vascular (renal vein) stapling, whereas 3.8-mm (blue) and 4.8-mm (green) staples are used in thicker tissues (ureter, bowel, bladder). In addition, for laparoscopic live donor nephrectomy, a single Endo-TA (linear noncutting) stapler can be used to secure the patient-side of the renal vein, thereby providing a longer donor renal vein because there is no need to trim staples from the vessels before anastomosis (Meng et al, 2003). Linear noncutting staplers deliver either three or four staple rows, 30 or 60 mm long. In addition to renal vein ligation these staplers can also be used to close an enterotomy after a side-to-side bowel anastomosis. When using laparoscopic staplers, special attention must be paid to the markers on the cartridge to ensure that all the targeted tissue is properly situated within the markers before the cartridge is closed and fired. The stapler should not be fired across any previously

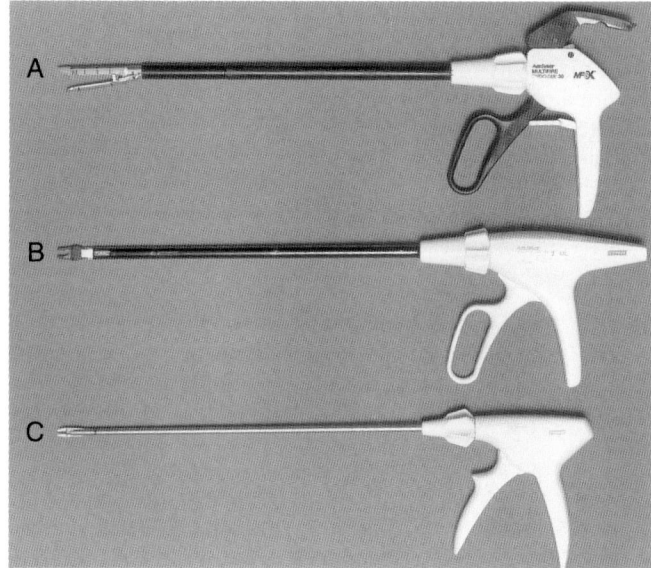

Figure 7–17. Laparoscopic stapler (**A**) and clip applier: 10 mm (**B**) and 5 mm (**C**).

placed clips because this may cause stapler malfunction. Indeed, in a 9-year review of stapler use (1992-2001), Brown and Woo (2004) noted FDA-recorded reports of 112 mortalities and 2,180 injuries attributed to use of the stapler; overall, malfunctions were reported 22,804 times.

Clipping Devices. Disposable and nondisposable clip appliers are available from different manufacturers (see Fig. 7–17). Generally, they contain occlusive clips ranging in size from 6 to 11 mm; they require either 10- or 12-mm laparoscopic ports. A 5-mm disposable clip applier is also available with 9-mm clips. Disposable clip appliers possess a rotating shaft and multifire, self-reloading features, whereas nondisposable instruments have to be reloaded for each clip to be deployed at the site of surgery and often do not have a rotating shaft. A right-angled clip applier that fits through a 10-mm trocar and deploys an 8-mm titanium clip is also available (U.S. Surgical, Norwalk, CT).

Electrocoagulation must be avoided in the vicinity of clips placed for occlusion of vessels to prevent conductive tissue necrosis and subsequent clip dislocation. To ensure reliable function, the closed ends of the occlusive clips must be seen extending slightly beyond the targeted vessel and should be placed perpendicular to the longitudinal axis of the vessel.

In addition to the metal "crush" type clips just described, polymer clips that completely encircle and lock down around vessels are available (Hem-O-Lok polymer ligation clip system Weck Closure Systems, Research Triangle Park, NC). These clips are more secure than the traditional metal clips (Joseph et al, 2004) and do not conduct electrical current. Removal of a clip is possible but difficult should a structure be clipped in error. They are available in four sizes (M, ML, L, and XL). Up to 10 mm of tissue can be ligated through a 5-mm trocar and up to 16-mm of tissue can be ligated through a 10-mm trocar.

Instrumentation for Specimen Entrapment

Various organ entrapment and retrieval systems are available. Depending on the size of the tissue and on whether in-situ morcellation or intact organ retrieval is planned, the laparoscopic surgeon is able to choose among different-sized sacks, materials, and designs. Studies have been conducted to test organ retrieval bags for permeability to tumor cells and bacteria before and after morcellation, as well as for stability during morcellation and resistance to tearing forces (Rassweiler et al, 1998; Urban et al, 1993). The originally designed (1990) LapSac (Cook Urological, Spencer, IN), which is made of nylon with a polyurethane inner coating and a polypropylene drawstring, is the least susceptible to tearing (Eichel et al, 2004) or leakage of cells. However, deployment of the LapSac and subsequent organ entrapment remain challenging endeavors. To aid in the opening of the LapSac, the neck of the sack can be modified using a double wrap (every other hole) of a nitinol guide wire, such that both ends of the guide wire exit the sack similar to the drawstring (Sundaram et al, 2002). The outward expansion of the nitinol guide wire serves to "open" the neck of the sack. The drawstring is then cut and removed. The sack is loaded onto a nondisposable two-tine LapSac introducer (i.e., Cook Urological, Spencer, IN). For a right kidney, the sack is rolled from top to bottom in a clockwise manner, whereas for a left kidney it is rolled from top to bottom in a counterclockwise manner; the handles of the two-

tine introducer and the ends of the nitinol guide wire should all be on the same side. This ensures that as the sack is unwound in the abdomen the bottom of the sack remains anterior to the body the sack, thereby facilitating its complete expansion in the abdomen. If this is not done, then the bottom of the sack lies posterior to the body of the sack and the surgeon needs to expend additional energy and time to move the bottom of the sack caudad. As a rule, it is easiest to deploy the LapSac via the uppermost 12-mm port site; if an 8 × 10-inch sack is being used (i.e., the largest available sack) the cannula is removed and the LapSac is passed under endoscopic guidance via the 12-mm incision site. Once the sack is completely in the abdomen, it is then unwound and the introducer is removed; the 12-mm port is replaced and the laparoscope is moved to this port. Atraumatic grasping forceps are then used to unfurl the sack. The sack is further expanded by passing the laparoscope into it and moving the endoscope in an ever-widening circle as it is being withdrawn; the nitinol guide wire at the neck of the sack further aids the opening of the sack. The tabs of the mouth of the sack can be secured with locking grasping forceps, and the specimen can then be moved into the sack. Up to a 2-kg specimen can be secured within the LapSac.

Other entrapment sacks offer marked advantages when the only goal is organ entrapment and intact removal, rather than morcellation. These sacks have spring wires that, when activated by the surgeon, deploy the bag after its introduction into the abdomen; this facilitates tissue entrapment because the broad wire supports stabilize the opened sack, thereby allowing the surgeon to literally scoop the specimen into the sack (Fig. 7–18). The entrapped specimen can easily be withdrawn through a hand-assist site or by enlarging a laparoscopic port site, usually to 5 to 7 cm for most specimens.

Instrumentation for Morcellation

Various techniques of tissue morcellation have been used in laparoscopic surgery. The simplest method for fragmentation of tissue within the entrapment sack is use of the index finger or ring forceps. The first mechanical morcellation devices worked by punching out pieces of tissue (i.e., serrated-edge macro-morcellators) (Semm, 1991). They were designed for removing relatively small amounts of tissue. The advent of laparoscopic nephrectomy resulted in the development of a foot-activated, aspirating, electrical morcellator for tissue fragmentation and evacuation (Cook Urological, Spencer, IN) (Clayman et al, 1992). However, this instrument is no longer available, having been removed from the market in 2001. Traditionally, ring forceps or a large Kelly clamp have been used. Recently, however, it has been shown that ring forceps are the preferred instrument for manual morcellation because they are less likely to puncture the entrapment sack (Eichel et al, 2004). If morcellation is performed intracorporeally, the entrapment sack should be a LapSac; however, a variation reported by Landman and colleagues for morcellation uses one of the plastic entrapment sacks. In this method, the morcellation is performed above the abdominal wall, by extending the extraction site incision to 3 cm in length. All tissue is fragmented and removed under direct vision above the abdominal surface; at no time is the morcellating instrument out of the direct vision of the surgeon. With this approach, specimens could be morcellated rapidly, with the

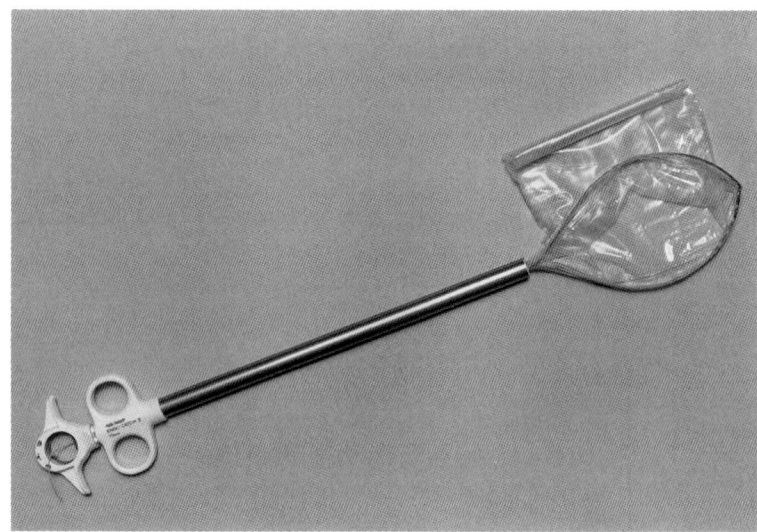

Figure 7–18. Organ retrieval bag.

entire entrapment and morcellation process taking only 13 minutes for clinical specimens as large as 700 g; also fragment size increased from 1.5 to 4.5 g, which might afford better tissue assessment with regard to capsular, vascular, or renal sinus fat invasion (Landman et al, 2003).

When morcellating a renal malignancy, the neck of the sack is triply draped to preclude any contamination: a towel drape, sticky drape (Ioban, 3M, St. Paul, MN), and nephrostomy drape are commonly used. At the end of the morcellation procedure, the morcellating surgeon and assistants re-gown and re-glove. The extraction site can be bathed in povidone-iodine in an effort to further reduce the chance of any wound seeding.

Instrumentation for Aspiration and Irrigation

Available as disposable and nondisposable devices, a combination of aspiration and irrigation abilities in one instrument is most practical. The aspirator, which is connected to a suction system, consists of a 5- or 10-mm metal tube, with suction controlled by either a one-way stopcock or a spring-controlled trumpet valve. The irrigation channel is also operated by either a one-way stopcock or a trumpet valve. The irrigation fluid is pressurized within a range from 250 to 700 mm Hg to allow for effective delivery of the irrigant and flushing of any bleeding site for accurate hemostasis. Usually, saline or lactated Ringer's solution is used as the irrigation fluid. Heparin (5000 units/L) may be added to prevent blood clots from forming should there be any intraoperative bleeding. Furthermore, a broad-spectrum antibiotic (e.g., cefazolin sodium, 1 g/L) may be added to the irrigant at the end of the procedure if one desires to further wash the surgical site just before exiting the abdomen.

Instrumentation for Retraction

Retractors greatly facilitate laparoscopic surgery. They help expose the area of surgical interest by holding away tissue and organs (e.g., liver, spleen, bowel). Sometimes, they also facilitate vascular dissection by putting tissue and/or organs closely associated with the vascular structures on stretch. Many varieties of retractors with different features are available. The simplest retractor is a metal bar with an atraumatic tip or a curved saddle shape; the latter is helpful for retracting a vessel during lymph node dissection. Similarly, the disposable laparoscopic "peanut" is very helpful as it can both dissect and atraumatically retract tissue.

However, the most useful retractors are the expanding types: fan retractors with three or four atraumatic finger-like extensions, fan retractors with V-hinge joints, balloon retractors, and kite-style instruments (e.g., PEER retractors (Jarit, Hawthorne, NY) (Brooks, 1993). The 5-mm kite-style retractor provides a 2 × 3-cm retracting area, whereas the 10-mm instrument doubles the area of direct retraction to 4 × 3 cm (Fig. 7–19); this type of retractor is very helpful for firm retraction such as on the kidney to put the renal hilum on stretch.

Another type of retractor is malleable and thus can be shaped to the needs of the surgeon. The Diamond-Flex angled 80-mm triangular retractor (Snowden Pencer, Tucker, GA) can be adapted to many different angles, curves, and shapes, and the surgeon can lock in its particular configuration. This feature is of particular value when retraction of the liver is required. This instrument forms a broad retracting surface 8 cm in length.

Retraction of tubelike structures (e.g., vessels, ureter) can also be achieved by placing a suture, a vessel loop, or an umbilical tape around the tissue and applying traction either with a grasper inside the abdomen or by pulling the ends of the retraction loop out of the abdomen through a small stab incision using a Carter-Thomason device (Carter, 1994) or a Keith needle on the end of the suture (see the later section "Exiting the Abdomen"). The retraction loop can then be secured under slight tension on the surface of the abdomen with a small hemostat clamp. **Alternatively, 2-mm needlescopic graspers can be employed to provide intraoperative retraction of tubular structures.**

External mechanical devices such as the Endoholder (Codman, Raynham, MA) can be used to keep grasping forceps or locking retractors in place. This device is usually mounted on the side of the table opposite the surgeon; the malleable free arm of it is then affixed to the shaft of a grasping forceps or laparoscopic retractor. When the surgeon has employed the retractor to its given purpose, the malleable arm of the external mechanical device is locked in place, thereby

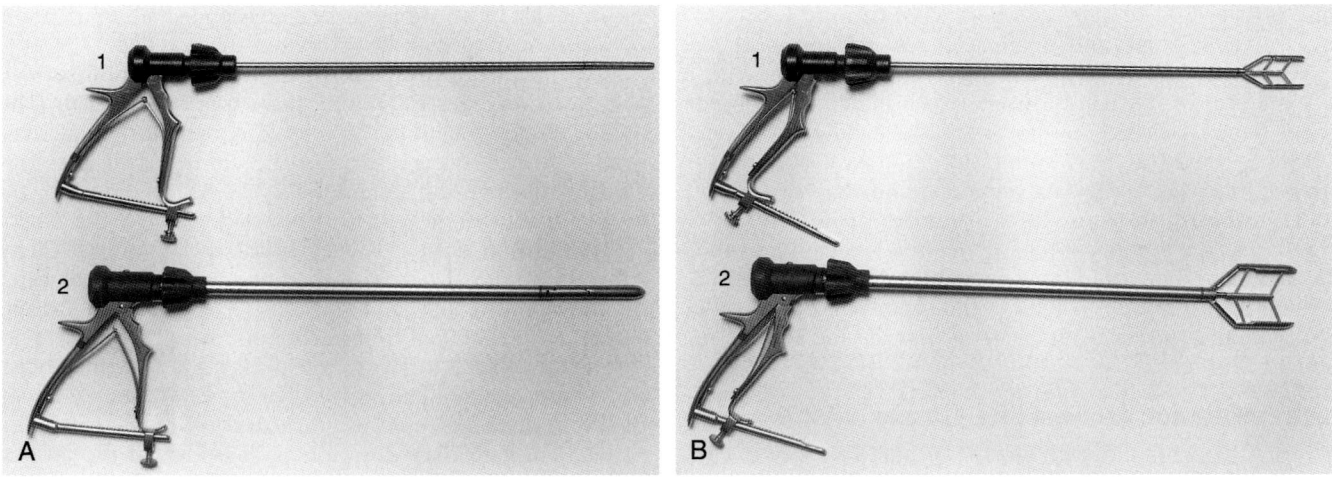

Figure 7–19. PEER retractor. **A,** Closed: 5 mm (1) and 10 mm (2). **B,** Open: 5 mm (1) and 10 mm (2).

providing reliable, continued traction. In most cases, this device can take the place of a second surgical assistant.

Also, for blunt retraction, the surgeon's hand, placed via a hand-assist device is most helpful. In this regard two key aspects for retraction are of note. First is the concept that the hand should be deployed such that the palm faces the laparoscope as much as possible. Hence, tissue is brought by the hand toward the laparoscope. In this regard, it is helpful to use a brown glove that will not reflect the light as much as the standard glove. A second helpful maneuver is the "C" configuration, as described by Strup, to dissect the renal hilum. In this maneuver, the forearm is passed through the hand-assist device parallel to the aorta/cava while the palm faces laterally. The wrist is flexed to 45 to 90 degrees to allow the fingers to lift the kidney while the thumb pushes inferomedially to retract the tissues overlying the renal hilum. Accordingly, excellent traction and countertraction is achieved that speeds hilar dissection (Wolf, 2005).

Exiting the Abdomen

Port Removal

Port removal and fascial closure are key elements of the procedure that, if not performed in a step-by-step, organized fashion, can result in major, possibly fatal, complications. Herniation, possible bowel incarceration, and postoperative hemorrhage are the results of a poorly performed or haphazard closure.

Before port removal is initiated, the operative site and the intra-abdominal entry sites of the cannulas must be carefully inspected with intra-abdominal pressure lowered to 5 mm Hg. After achieving perfect hemostasis, the surgical site is irrigated with the option of leaving behind 500 to 1000 mL of irrigation fluid, which contains cefazolin, 1 g/L, and heparin, 5000 U/L. Whether this maneuver truly results in a lower incidence of postoperative adhesions or in less infection is undetermined. To avoid any possible herniation of intra-abdominal contents into the previous port sites, removal of all laparoscopic ports must be undertaken strictly under visual control.

In the rare case in which bladed trocars are used, after inspection at 5 mm Hg, the first 10- or 12-mm port is removed and the fascia at the entry site is secured with 0-0 Vicryl. This is most efficiently accomplished using a commercially available suture passing device such a Carter-Thomason suture passer (see later) (Inlet Medical, Eden Prairie, MN) (Carter, 1994). This suture is not tied at the time of placement, but instead a 10-mm plastic introducer rod is passed back into the abdominal cavity through the port site incision. The 10-mm cannula is then slid over the 10-mm plastic introducer, and the plastic introducer is removed. In this manner, the ports can continue to be used for the passage of the 10-mm laparoscope and the passage of a grasping forceps to facilitate the closure of each 10-mm port site. Accordingly, all fascial sutures are placed under direct endoscopic control as the 10-mm laparoscope is moved from port to port to visualize the placement of each suture. After all fascial sutures have been placed, each 5-mm port is removed under endoscopic control at 5 mm Hg pressure; 5-mm ports are not closed in the adult but are closed in the pediatric patient. Then each of the non–endoscope-bearing 10-mm ports can be removed under endoscopic control, and the fascial suture can be tied and the closure inspected endoscopically. The final 10-mm port is removed with the endoscope in place to assess for any bleeding along the tract; however, the hemostasis of this port site should have been ensured at the time of placement of the fascial closure suture. In this manner, each port is visually assessed for any bleeding at 5 mm Hg, thereby precluding the possibility of removing a port and missing an injured vessel. After removal of all ports, the CO_2 is allowed to pass out passively through the 5-mm port sites.

However, currently with the swing from bladed to non-bladed trocars, the need for port closure for even 12-mm ports has come into question. Reports by Shalhav have shown that 12 mm ports regardless of site (i.e., midline vs. transmuscular) do not require fascial closure (Siqueira et al, 2004). To date, there has been one report of herniation through an unclosed adult 12-mm port (Lowry et al, 2003). In the literature, the switch from bladed to blunt trocars has resulted in a marked decrease in abdominal wall bleeding (from 0.83% to only 0.16%) and in port site hernia formation (1.83% to 0.19%) (Hashizume and Sugimachi, 1997; Thomas et al, 2003).

With regard to the hand-assist device, it should be removed before removal of the other port sites. The hand-assist device wound is closed as one would close a typical abdominal wound; however, recent data support an interrupted closure with nonabsorbable suture (Troxel and Das, 2005).

After closure, the pneumoperitoneum is reestablished and the other port sites are closed as previously described. Proceeding in this fashion precludes the chance of injuring the bowel or omentum beneath the hand-port site and ensures an airtight closure.

Instrumentation for Port Site Closure

A variety of possibilities for closure of port sites exists. The **simplest method** is retracting the skin with Sinn retractors, grasping the fascia with Kocher clamps, and suturing it with absorbable 0-0 suture. However, in any patient with a body mass index greater than 30, this is very difficult to accomplish.

Fortunately, several **devices for complete** en bloc closure of fascia, muscle, and peritoneum under direct vision have been developed (Carter, 1994; Monk et al, 1994; Garzotto et al, 1995; Elashry et al, 1996). These work well in patients of all sizes.

The **Carter-Thomason needlepoint suture passer** (Inlet Medical, Eden Prairie, MN) consists of a 5- or 10-mm cone that has two integrated, hollow, angled, cylindrical passages located 180 degrees opposite each other (Fig. 7–20). With the sharp-needlepoint, single-action grasper, the 0-0 Vicryl suture is inserted through one of the cylinders in the metal or plastic cone, thereby traversing muscle, fascia, and peritoneal layers in an ever-widening angle; the end of the suture is grasped with a 5-mm grasper via one of the other ports. The needlepoint grasper is reintroduced through the other cylinder of the cone; the intraperitoneal end of the suture is grasped by the needlepoint grasper and pulled out of the abdomen. The cone is slid off both ends of the suture. Subsequently, closure of the fascia, muscle layer, and peritoneum is accomplished by tying the suture. **The Carter-Thomason needlepoint device not only is helpful for wound closure but also can be used as a fifth port during nephrectomy to help hold the sack open or to encircle the ureter with a vessel loop through a small stab incision.**

The **disposable Endo Close** suture carrier (U.S. Surgical, Norwalk, CT) is a device with a spring-loaded suture carrier at its tip. Loaded with a suture, the device traverses fascia, muscle, and peritoneum alongside the port. After reinsertion on the opposite side of port entry, it is reloaded with the

suture, aided by a 5-mm grasper, and is pulled out again under optical control so that the suture can then be tied.

A far simpler, less-expensive, homemade solution is available to all surgeons for closing ports in a large patient. This **angiocatheter technique** applies the previously described principles. A 14-gauge, sheathed needle is passed alongside the port through the abdominal layers. After removal of the needle, a 0-0 Vicryl suture is inserted through the angiocatheter sheath until it is deep inside the peritoneal cavity. After the sheath is removed, the same maneuver is repeated on the opposite side, but this time a 30-inch 0-0 Prolene suture folded in half is passed into the peritoneal cavity through the sheath to act as a retrieving loop. A 5-mm grasper passed through another port is then passed through the loop of 0-0 Prolene and used to grasp the end of the 0-0 Vicryl suture. The 0-0 Vicryl suture is pulled through the Prolene loop and released. By pulling the Prolene loop upward through the angiocatheter sheath, the entrapped 0-0 Vicryl suture is then retrieved from the abdomen. After the angiocatheter sheath is removed, the two ends of the suture can be tied.

All 5-mm sheaths are removed under optical control at 5 mm Hg. In adults, the fascia of the 5-mm port entry sites is not sewn closed; however, in children, these port sites require closure with a single absorbable suture.

Closure of the Skin

The skin of all 10-mm port sites is closed with subcuticular 4-0 absorbable suture. Adhesive strips are applied to all port sites to close (for incisions smaller than 10 mm) or to further approximate (for incisions 10 mm or larger) the skin. As an alternative, the skin can be closed using octylcyanoacrylate glue. This has been found to speed up closure time and provide an equivalent cosmetic result compared with suturing (Sebesta and Bishoff, 2004).

POSTOPERATIVE PATIENT MANAGEMENT

Limited laparoscopic procedures (e.g., laparoscopic varicocelectomy, diagnostic laparoscopy) may allow discharge of patients the same day on an outpatient basis. More extensive procedures may require 1 to 3 days of hospital stay. The patient is usually given clear liquids on returning to the outpatient area or the hospital floor. A regular diet is provided either the evening of surgery or the morning thereafter.

Ambulation depends on the type of procedure performed as well as the overall health status and morbidity of the patient before surgery. The healthy patient after a minor or major laparoscopic procedure is encouraged to ambulate within 4 or 12 hours, respectively, after the procedure. Pneumatic compression stockings for prophylaxis against deep venous thrombosis are left on until the patient is fully ambulatory.

The Foley catheter is removed either while the patient is still in the operating room (pneumoperitoneum less than 2 hours) or later in the day or the next morning (pneumoperitoneum more than 2 hours). Indwelling Foley time will vary after laparoscopic radical prostatectomy or cystectomy with continent urinary diversion. Nasogastric tubes are removed in the operating room immediately on completion of the procedure

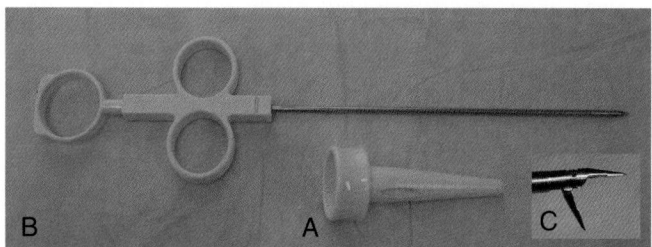

Figure 7–20. Carter-Thomason device. Cone (**A**); needle-point, single-action grasper (**B**); and tip of grasper in open condition (**C**).

for most procedures but may be left in longer if bowel is used for urinary diversion or augmentation depending on surgeon preference.

Antibiotics, with one dose having been administered before the procedure, are continued over 24 hours. Laboratory values are obtained in a standardized manner (hemoglobin, hematocrit, sodium, bicarbonate, chloride, potassium, creatinine) postoperatively and the next morning or as needed. In general, for a healthy patient undergoing an uneventful laparoscopic procedure, no laboratory studies are needed. However, after a major procedure or for high-risk patients, postoperative and 24-hour laboratory studies are warranted. This is especially important in the patient with pulmonary disease because the greatest risk of hypercarbia may occur 2 to 3 hours after the procedure. After an uncomplicated laparoscopic procedure, a postoperative chest radiograph is no longer recommended (Simon et al, 2005).

Parenteral analgesia (e.g., morphine, ketorolac tromethamine) is given as needed on the day of surgery and is usually replaced by oral pain medication on the first postoperative day. If irrigant is purposely left in the abdomen at the end of the procedure, the male patient should be advised that he may notice some scrotal swelling as he ambulates. This is due to the irrigation fluid and will resolve over several days as it is absorbed.

PHYSIOLOGIC CONSIDERATIONS IN THE ADULT

The rapidly expanding number of newly developed laparoscopic procedures in operative urology has resulted in an increasing need for urologists as well as anesthesiologists to familiarize themselves with both the physiology and the potential complications of the pneumoperitoneum. This is especially important now that laparoscopic urology has moved on to even more complicated ablative and reconstructive surgery, requiring patient exposure to the pneumoperitoneum for a prolonged period of time.

Choice of Insufflant

Carbon Dioxide

CO_2 is the insufflant most commonly used for laparoscopic surgery. Owing to its properties (colorless, noncombustible, and inexpensive), it is favored by most laparoscopists. Prolonged postoperative distention of the abdomen does not occur, because CO_2 is quickly absorbed (Wolf and Stoller, 1994). It is highly soluble in water and easily diffuses in body tissues. Because of its high diffusion coefficient relative to oxygen and other respiratory gases, it readily moves out of the peritoneal cavity, owing to a high diffusion gradient caused by the difference in concentration of CO_2 between the intraperitoneal space and the surrounding components (e.g., blood). However, the characteristic of rapid absorption, which lessens the chance of a CO_2 gas embolus, may also lead to potential problems (e.g., hypercapnia, hypercarbia, associated cardiac arrhythmias). In particular, patients with COPD may not be able to compensate for the absorbed CO_2 by increased ventilation; this may result in dangerously elevated levels of CO_2 in these patients. CO_2 also stimulates the sympathetic nervous system, which results in an increase in heart rate, cardiac contractility, and vascular resistance. Lastly, CO_2 is also stored in various body compartments (e.g., viscera, bones, muscles). After prolonged laparoscopic procedures, it may take hours before the patient has eliminated the extra CO_2 that has accumulated in these storage areas; again, this is more often the case in patients with pulmonary compromise (Lewis et al, 1972; Puri and Singh, 1992; Tolksdorf et al, 1992; Wolf and Stoller, 1994). Therefore, as previously noted, all patients, and in particular those with pulmonary disease, must be closely monitored for several hours after a lengthy laparoscopic procedure for possible signs or symptoms of hypercarbia.

Alternative Gases

Nitrous oxide is less irritating to the peritoneum and causes fewer acid-base changes and cardiovascular adverse effects (e.g., arrhythmias) compared with CO_2 (Scott and Julian, 1972; El-Minawi et al, 1981; Minoli et al, 1982; Sharp et al, 1982). However, some studies have shown that nitrous oxide insufflation reduces cardiac output and increases mean arterial pressure (MAP), heart rate, and central venous pressure (Marshall et al, 1972; Shulman and Aronson, 1984). Because nitrous oxide supports combustion, it can be used only during laparoscopic procedures that do not involve the use of electrosurgical instruments.

Helium is an inert and noncombustible insufflant. Initial studies performed in various animal models showed favorable effects on arterial partial pressure of CO_2 and pH with no evidence of hypercarbia (Fitzgerald et al, 1992; Leighton et al, 1993; Rademaker et al, 1995). These results were corroborated by clinical studies (Bongard et al, 1991; Fitzgerald et al, 1992; Leighton et al, 1993; Neuberger et al, 1994; Rademaker et al, 1995; Jacobi et al, 1997). As such, helium is particularly useful for the patient with pulmonary disease in whom hypercarbia would be poorly tolerated. Likewise, if hypercarbia develops during a laparoscopic procedure with CO_2, rather than aborting the procedure or converting to an open approach, the surgeon can change the insufflant to helium and usually salvage the case (Brackman et al, 2003). There is also evidence that the use of helium may cause a decrease in tumor cell growth and inflammatory reactions within the peritoneal cavity (Jacobi et al, 1997; Jacobi et al, 1999; Dahn et al, 2005). Most recently, it has been demonstrated that helium insufflation can be used for laparoscopic procedures (e.g., cholecystectomy, appendectomy, hernia repair) performed under local and regional anesthesia in high-risk patients, not only because of its favorable metabolic features but also owing to its lack of peritoneal irritation and its association with decreased postoperative pain (Crabtree and Fishman, 1999). However, laparoscopists have to bear in mind that helium may be associated with a higher risk of gas embolism because of its lower blood solubility. As such, it should likely not be used when extraperitoneal insufflation is needed, owing to an increased risk of pneumothorax. When helium is going to be used, it is advised to initially obtain the pneumoperitoneum with CO_2 and then change to helium, thereby lowering the chances of a helium gas embolus. Also, helium is significantly more expensive than CO_2. Lastly, when using helium a separate "yolk" (i.e., line from the gas tank to the insufflator) is needed; accordingly, one needs to make sure that a "helium yolk" is available in the operating room or make arrangements to have one provided when performing laparoscopy on patients with severe pulmonary compromise.

Other insufflants (e.g., room air, oxygen) have been used to establish a pneumoperitoneum in the past. However, possible serious side effects (e.g., air embolus, intra-abdominal explosion, combustion with oxygen and room air) have terminated their clinical use. Other options for insufflants include some of the other noble gases (e.g., xenon, argon, krypton), which are inert and nonflammable; however, their widespread clinical use has not been adopted.

Choice of Pneumoperitoneum Pressure

Overall, the most commonly selected pressure for performing laparoscopy is 15 mm Hg. However, McDougall and colleagues (1994) showed a marked reduction in oliguria when working at 10 mm Hg. In contrast, Kavoussi preferred a pressure of 20 mm Hg, noting increased insufflant filling volume of 22% and possibly less venous bleeding during the procedure (Adams et al, 1999). In contrast, McDougall and colleagues (1994) noted that, despite the increased volume, there was only a very small increase in abdominal girth at higher pressures. Indeed, recent studies support a pressure of 12 mm Hg, as this results in no perturbations in cardiac parameters (i.e., no change in stroke volume) versus a pressure of 15 mm Hg (Mertens zur Borg et al, 2004). Working at lower pneumoperitoneum pressures has also been found to reduce postoperative pain (Sarli et al, 2000).

Various cardiovascular, renal, and respiratory effects seen during different intra-abdominal pressures in the supine state are summarized in Table 7–3. It is of note that these physiologic parameters may be further altered (i.e., overridden or reversed), owing to the health of the individual patient and to changes in the patient's position.

Cardiovascular Effects of the Pneumoperitoneum

Venous Flow

Animal studies have shown that the effects of the pneumoperitoneum on venous return depend on atrial pressures,

which, in turn, are a reflection of the hydration state of the subject (Ivankovich et al, 1975; Diamant et al, 1978; Kashtan et al, 1981). If atrial pressures are low (normal or hypovolemic state), then, during a pneumoperitoneum of up to 20 mm Hg, venous return is reduced, owing to increased compression of the vena cava from the pneumoperitoneum. If atrial pressures are high (hypervolemic state), the vena cava resists elevated intra-abdominal pressure and venous return is actually enhanced. However, these principles apply only to an intra-abdominal pressure of up to 20 mm Hg. By further increasing pneumoperitoneum pressures, especially to 40 mm Hg and above, capacitance vessels are collapsed, vascular resistance increases, blood flow decreases markedly, and venous return is significantly reduced. Lower-extremity venous return is also reduced by elevated intra-abdominal pressures. Reduced venous blood flow in the lower extremities could facilitate deep vein thrombosis; however, this remains a rare complication of laparoscopy clinically (Jorgensen et al, 1993).

These pathophysiologic insights, gained through animal experiments, have been corroborated by clinical studies (Kelman et al, 1972; Motew et al, 1973; Lee, 1975; Jorgensen et al, 1993). As a result of these trials, intra-abdominal pressures during laparoscopy should not be allowed to exceed 20 mm Hg over extended periods (Arthur, 1970; Seed et al, 1970; Lee, 1975), and a working pressure of 10 to 12 mm Hg is recommended.

Cardiac Arrhythmias

Tachycardia and ventricular extrasystoles may be seen as results of hypercapnia (Scott and Julian, 1972). Peritoneal irritation may lead to vagal stimulation and subsequently to bradyarrhythmias (Doyle and Mark, 1989). Also, dysrhythmias can serve as clinical warning signs for the occurrence of pneumothorax, hypoxia, and gas embolism (Wolf and Stoller, 1994).

Unreliability of Central Venous Pressure Readings

As previously noted, intravenous pressures may actually rise with low intra-abdominal pressures. In addition, increasing intra-abdominal pressures may artificially elevate central venous pressure readings, owing to an increase in intrathoracic pressure. Therefore, it is important for the anesthetist *not* to rely on central venous pressure readings for any clinical decision-making. If information regarding vascular volume and central venous pressure is needed, a Swan-Ganz catheter should be placed.

Respiratory Effects of the Pneumoperitoneum

Pressure-Mediated Effects

Because of increased intra-abdominal pressure, diaphragmatic motion is limited. Pulmonary dead space remains unchanged, but functional reserve capacity decreases (Wolf and Stoller, 1994). The average peak airway pressure needed to keep up a constant tidal volume increases parallel to the increasing intra-abdominal pressure (Alexander et al, 1969; Motew et al, 1973; Wolf and Stoller, 1994).

Although usually not of great clinical importance in a healthy patient population, it is advisable to use positive end-

Table 7–3.	**Pressure Effects: 5, 10, 20, and 40 mm Hg**			
Effects	*5 mm Hg*	*10 mm Hg*	*20 mm Hg*	*40 mm Hg*
Cardiovascular				
Heart rate	↑	↑	↑	↓
Mean arterial pressure	↑	↑	↑	↑
Systemic vascular resistance	↑	↑	↑	↑
Venous return	→/↓	↓↑	↓↑	↓
Cardiac output	→/↓	→/↑	→/↓	↓
Renal				
Glomerular filtration rate	→	↓	↓↓	↓↓
Urine output	→	↓	↓↓	↓↓
Respiratory				
End-tidal CO_2	→	→/↑	→/↑	↑
P_{CO_2}	→	↑	↑	↑
Arterial pH	→	→/↓	↓	↓

CO_2, carbon dioxide; P_{CO_2}, partial pressure of carbon dioxide.

expiratory pressure techniques when patients with lung disease undergo general anesthesia for a laparoscopic procedure (Ekman et al, 1988; Wolf and Stoller, 1994; Hazebroek et al, 2002).

Non–Pressure-Related Respiratory Effects

The head-down position has an adverse effect on respiration. It elevates the diaphragm and decreases vital capacity. It can also lead to a dislocation of the endotracheal tube that, in turn, may cause right main-stem bronchus intubation. Although of little clinical significance in healthy patients, the head-down position may cause pulmonary edema in patients with increased left-sided heart pressures (Prentice and Martin, 1987). During lengthy procedures performed with the patient in the head-down position it is useful to limit fluid administration if possible because it will minimize facial swelling postoperatively.

Renal and Other Visceral Effects of the Pneumoperitoneum

Oliguria

Increased intra-abdominal pressure was found to be associated with a significant decrease in urinary output. A number of investigators, with the oldest study dating back to 1923, have observed oliguria and anuria associated with an ongoing increase in intra-abdominal pressure (Thorington and Schmidt, 1923; Harmann et al, 1982; Richards et al, 1983). Decreased renal vein blood flow and direct renal parenchymal compression, rather than marked hormonal changes or ureteral compression, have been shown to be the likely reasons for the oliguric state (Chiu et al, 1994; McDougall et al, 1996). Of interest, renal cortical blood flow decreased with increasing intra-abdominal pressures, whereas renal medullary blood flow increased up to pressures of 20 mm Hg; above this level, medullary blood flow also decreased (Chiu et al, 1994). In a porcine study, neither application of dopamine nor insertion of ureteral catheters was able to improve oliguria, owing to elevated intra-abdominal pressure (McDougall et al, 1996). These changes occurred regardless of intraperitoneal or extraperitoneal insufflation. Of note, oliguria was not a problem if a gasless, abdominal wall lift method was used to establish the working space in the abdomen.

These experimental findings in animals have been corroborated in the clinical setting (Iwase et al, 1992; Chang et al, 1994; McDougall et al, 1996); however, at least one recent study did show that low dose dopamine (2 μg/kg/min) can prevent the dip in urine output associated with pneumoperitoneum (Perez et al, 2002). Whether antidiuretic hormone and plasma arginine vasopressin, both of which have been measured at increased levels by some investigators, play a major role in oliguria during clinical laparoscopic procedures remains unclear (Melville et al, 1985; Solis Herruzo et al, 1989). In general, if one desires to avoid an oliguric state during a laparoscopic procedure, a pressure of 10 mm Hg or less is recommended. In addition, clinically the use of furosemide (Lasix) (mg dose = 20 times the patient's creatinine), mannitol (12.5 to 25 g dose), and dopamine at 2 μg/kg/min can help to overcome oliguria. With this regimen and judicious fluid administration, the patient can usually be maintained with a urine output in excess of 100 mL/hr. The key is to use these pharmaceutical modalities in lieu of excessive hydration and fluid boluses (Perez et al, 2002).

Effects on Mesenteric Blood Flow and Intestinal Motility

Decreased blood flow during laparoscopic procedures was found not only in the kidney but also in mesenteric vessels and other organs (e.g., liver, pancreas, stomach, spleen, small and large intestines (Caldwell and Ricotta, 1987; Ishizaki et al, 1993; Hashikura et al, 1994). This may rarely lead to mesenteric thrombosis with catastrophic results. This complication may take days to develop (Schorr, 1998).

Open, incisional abdominal surgery usually results in some postoperative impairment of gastric and intestinal emptying owing to intestinal paralysis (physiologic ileus) (Kemen et al, 1991). Interestingly, clinical observation and studies undertaken during laparoscopic and open surgical cholecystectomy have shown that laparoscopic surgery causes less significant disturbances of the gastrointestinal motility pattern, therefore resulting in no or less postoperative physiologic ileus than occurs with open surgery (Sezeur et al, 1993; Halevy et al, 1994). The exact mechanisms responsible for this difference have yet to be defined, but it is postulated that perhaps it is the hypercarbia (Aneman et al, 2000). In fact, intestinal perfusion does not change significantly during prolonged pneumoperitoneum at a pressure of 15 mm Hg with CO_2 or helium (Goitein et al, 2005).

Also, despite the increased intra-abdominal pressures associated with laparoscopy, there has been no increased incidence of gastroesophageal reflux and regurgitation in patients undergoing laparoscopic procedures (Schippers et al, 1992).

Acid-Base Metabolic Effects of Pneumoperitoneum

Animal and human studies have demonstrated that prolonged laparoscopic procedures may result in hypercarbia and respiratory acidosis (Motew et al, 1973). Because there is no increase in ventilatory dead space during laparoscopy, the resulting respiratory acidosis has been attributed to transperitoneal absorption of CO_2 during establishment and maintenance of the pneumoperitoneum (Motew et al, 1973; Leighton et al, 1993). Although the resulting mild respiratory acidosis does not adversely affect otherwise normal patients and can be corrected by increasing the minute ventilation, increased absorption of CO_2 can become dangerous in patients with COPD because of their impaired ability to release pulmonary CO_2. To ensure proper monitoring of acid-base status, intermittent arterial blood gas sampling should be performed in patients with COPD and during any laparoscopic procedure that requires more than 1 hour of CO_2 insufflation.

Pneumoinsufflation with CO_2 results in variable amounts of gas absorption, thereby raising the P_{CO_2} in the blood. CO_2 is absorbed from the peritoneal membrane during transperitoneal laparoscopy and from preperitoneal adipose and connective tissue during retroperitoneoscopy and extraperitoneoscopy (Collins, 1981). Others have also implicated the disrupted microvascular and lymphatic channels for CO_2 absorption during preperitoneal laparoscopy (Glascock et al, 1996). The potential for developing hypercarbia exists during both transperitoneal and preperitoneal laparoscopy.

Conceivably, this assumes greater importance in patients with preexisting airway and cardiovascular compromise. Although transperitoneal and retroperitoneoscopic approaches are routinely employed safely at numerous centers worldwide, vigilant perioperative anesthetic management is essential to prevent the development of potential complications related to CO_2 buildup.

End-tidal CO_2 and O_2 saturation are monitored intraoperatively using a capnometer. Furthermore, arterial blood gases are obtained during prolonged laparoscopic procedures and in patients with increased risk of developing hypercarbia (owing to airway disease, renal failure, congestive heart failure, or advanced age). A rise in end-tidal CO_2 should prompt the anesthesiologist to adjust the respiratory rate and tidal volume to enhance CO_2 elimination. Simultaneously, the surgeon should decrease the insufflation pressure of CO_2 or, if need be, desufflate the abdomen completely until the hypercarbia has been resolved. Several studies have demonstrated that CO_2 absorption during either laparoscopic approach (transperitoneal or retroperitoneal) increases significantly during the initial 30 to 60 minutes of the procedure and reaches a steady-state plateau thereafter (Wolf et al, 1995; Ng et al, 1999). Which one of the two approaches is associated with greater CO_2 absorption is debated. Although some studies have demonstrated greater absorption during transperitoneal laparoscopy (Giebler et al, 1997), others have demonstrated greater absorption during retroperitoneal laparoscopy using a standard Hasson cannula (Wolf et al, 1995). However, in the Cleveland Clinic experience, no significant clinical difference was seen (Ng et al, 1999), provided a blunt port type Hasson cannula was used that tightly sealed the site of entry between the balloon and soft cuff carried on the shaft of the cannula.

Hemodynamic Effects Related to Patient Position and Type of Approach

Several animal and human studies have examined hemodynamic changes owing to different surgical positions (Kelman et al, 1972; Joris et al, 1993; Williams and Murr, 1993). In the supine position, cardiac output remains unchanged or decreases when intra-abdominal pressures are less than 15 mm Hg, whereas MAP and systemic vascular resistance increase (Pearle, 1996). If pneumoperitoneum pressures are increased beyond 20 mm Hg, cardiac output is reduced because of decreasing venous return.

Changes in patient position have a marked impact on hemodynamic parameters. Specifically, in the head-up position, heart rate increases, MAP decreases, systemic vascular resistance increases, and cardiac output decreases; in contrast, in the head-down position, heart rate drops, MAP rises, systemic vascular resistance falls, and cardiac output increases (Pearle, 1996). These results show that the head-down position is favorable for the laparoscopy patient because of higher cardiac output caused by increased venous return. However, this beneficial effect is completely negated if pneumoperitoneum pressure is increased to 30 to 40 mm Hg; at pressures this high, the concomitant decrease in venous return results in a decrease in cardiac output.

There is some evidence that the extraperitoneal approach may be beneficial in this regard compared with transperitoneal laparoscopy. Giebler and coworkers demonstrated that transperitoneal laparoscopy was associated with more pronounced changes in cardiac output ($P = .001$), pulmonary artery pressure ($P = .007$), central venous pressure ($P = .001$), iliac venous pressure ($P = .001$), and inferior vena caval pressure gradient ($P = .00001$) as compared with retroperitoneal laparoscopy (Giebler et al, 1997). With regard to pelvic laparoscopy, Meininger and associates (2004) compared the effects of prolonged intraperitoneal and extraperitoneal CO_2 insufflation on hemodynamics and gas exchange. With both insufflation methods, arterial CO_2 pressure increased rapidly, reaching higher levels with extraperitoneal insufflation. Therefore, patients managed with extraperitoneal insufflation required a significantly higher minute ventilation. Heart rate and central venous pressure increased in both groups, whereas mean arterial blood pressure and pH decreased.

Hormonal and Metabolic Effects during Laparoscopic Surgery

As in other surgical procedures, several hormones (e.g., β-endorphin, cortisol, prolactin, epinephrine, norepinephrine, dopamine) have been noted to increase during laparoscopic surgery as a response to tissue manipulation, intraoperative trauma, and postoperative pain (Cooper et al, 1982; Lehtinen et al, 1987; Lefebvre et al, 1992). The clinical significance of increased serum arginine vasopressin levels seen in open surgery and in response to intraperitoneal insufflation during laparoscopy remains unexplained (Cochrane et al, 1981; Melville et al, 1985; Solis Herruzo et al, 1989).

Several adverse metabolic changes observed during open cholecystectomy are less pronounced with laparoscopic cholecystectomy: (1) reduced postoperative plasma glucose elevation, (2) less decrease in insulin sensitivity, and (3) reduced hepatic stress response (Thorell et al, 1993; Jakeways et al, 1994; Glerup et al, 1995). In addition, conventional open surgery results in a number of other, potentially adverse, reactions: muscle proteolysis, increased intestinal mucosal protein synthesis, and increased hepatic protein synthesis (Fischer, 1995).

One important feature of the catabolic response is a complex intraorgan shift of nitrogen; this reaction has been best characterized in the liver (Glerup et al, 1995). The conversion of amino acids to urea by the liver is much higher after open incisional cholecystectomy than it is after laparoscopic cholecystectomy; hence, the catabolic reaction of the body is decreased with a laparoscopic versus an open, incisional approach (Fischer, 1995). Indeed, in the laparoscopic patient, the reduced postoperative hepatic catabolic stress associated with reduced tissue loss of amino-nitrogen may, in some way, be responsible for the more rapid convalescence that is the hallmark of laparoscopy in general. Lastly, catabolic responses, in the form of released cytokines and opioids, owing to augmented neurohumoral stimuli resulting from incisional tissue trauma, may also be lessened with a laparoscopic approach (Fischer, 1995).

Immunologic Effects of Laparoscopic Surgery

A number of animal and clinical studies measuring a wide spectrum of inflammatory response mediators (e.g., C-reactive protein, interleukin-6) and other markers of cellular immune functions (e.g., pan-T cells [CD3], helper T cells [CD4], suppressor cells [CD8], and natural killer cells [CD16], delayed-type hypersensitivity skin tests, serial phytohemagglutinin-induced T cell proliferation) have suggested that laparoscopic procedures generally result in less immunosuppression than do their open surgical counterparts (Kloosterman et al, 1994; Trokel et al, 1994; Cristaldi et al, 1997; Karayiannakis et al, 1997; Nguyen et al, 1999; Bolla and Tuzzato, 2003). This may also play a role in hastening convalescence after laparoscopic procedures. Some data have also suggested that the CO_2 pneumoperitoneum in and of itself, as opposed to exposure of tissues to room air, results in a more favorable immunologic state (Watson et al, 1995). Also, experimental evidence shows that less tumor cell growth occurs after laparoscopic procedures than after open procedures (Bouvy et al, 1997). Although these data are intriguing, further well-designed, prospectively randomized clinical studies are needed to compare immunologic responses after laparoscopic versus open surgical procedures for urologic cancer. Whether decrease in inflammatory response mediators and improved post-laparoscopic immune status will translate into a better long-term prognosis for patients with urologic cancers remains to be determined. Indeed, in a recent study by Olweny and colleagues in patients undergoing open or transperitoneal laparoscopic radical/total nephrectomy for renal cancer, there was no discernible difference in immunologic parameters; part of the explanation for this observation could well be secondary to the immunosuppressive effects of the tumor itself (Landman et al, 2004).

TROUBLESHOOTING IN LAPAROSCOPIC SURGERY

Historically, in large series, the overall incidence of laparoscopic complications in urology was in the range of 4%. Mortality was distinctly unusual, with a rate of 0.03% to 0.08% (Mintz, 1977; Winfield et al, 1991; Chapron et al, 1998; Fahlenkamp et al, 1999; Harkki-Siren et al, 1999). However, due to the increasing complexity of laparoscopic urologic procedures (e.g., nephrectomy, prostatectomy) and the continued decrease in simpler laparoscopic procedures (e.g., varicocelectomy, bladder neck suspension, pelvic lymph node dissection), laparoscopic complications in urology appear to be on the rise. In a recent update from Johns Hopkins University regarding transperitoneal laparoscopic retroperitoneal procedures (e.g., renal surgery, RPLND), Kavoussi and coworkers (1993) report a 0.2% mortality rate and a 12% overall complication rate. Of concern, the most often cited injury was vascular, occurring in 2.8% of patients, followed by bowel injury at 1.1% (Table 7–4). The authors attribute this increase to the larger number of surgeons now doing laparoscopy and moving through the learning curve, the addition of several new procedures that are substantially more challenging than past procedures (e.g., partial nephrectomy, RPLND), and the aging and higher risk of our population in general (Parsons et al, 2004). Of interest, the complications for pelvic laparoscopy, although higher than for retroperitoneal laparoscopy, are of a more minor nature. Indeed, Vallancien and associates (2002) noted a 22.6% overall complication rate among 1311 proce-

Table 7–4. Major Complications of Transperitoneal Abdominal Surgery

Total Procedures	894* (100% Abdominal)	1311† (84% Pelvic)
Overall complications	13.2%	22.6%
Intraoperative/postoperative	5.7%/7.5%	3.6%/19%
Deaths	0.2%	0%
Vascular injury	2.8%	0.5%
Bowel injury	1.1%	1.2%
Adjacent organ injury	1.1%	0.8%
Conversion rate	1.7%	1.7%

*Data from Parsons JK, Varkarakis I, Rha KH, et al: Complications of abdominal urologic laparoscopy: Longitudinal five-year analysis. Urology 2004; 63:27-32.
†Data from Vallancien G, Cathelineau X, Baumert H, et al: Complications of transperitoneal laparoscopic surgery in urology: Review of 1,311 procedures at a single center. J Urol 2002;168:23-26.

dures of which 84% were pelvic. There were no deaths and the most often injured organ was bowel at 1.2%; vascular injuries were cited in only 0.5% of the procedures (see Table 7–4).

Minimizing the Incidence of Complications during the Laparoscopic Learning Curve

Early in one's experience with laparoscopic surgery, it is wise to apply this minimally invasive approach to low-risk surgical candidates of normal body habitus. In addition, it is advisable and recommended by many laparoscopic organizations, as well as by hospital credentialing boards, that the neophyte laparoscopic surgeon seek training in three arenas: (1) in-depth instructional courses, including didactic, "live-case" transmissions and "hands-on" laboratory sessions; (2) preceptor training in which the surgeon-in-training views more than five or more procedures being done by an already skillful laparoscopic surgeon; and (3) a mentoring experience, during which a trained laparoscopic surgeon oversees the initial procedures performed by the surgeon-in-training (Society of American Gastrointestinal Endoscopic Surgeons, 2001). Further training can be obtained through self-teaching using videotapes and a pelvic trainer. The latter is extremely helpful for developing one's sense of laparoscopic proprioception and for becoming facile with laparoscopic suturing and knot tying. Data have clearly shown benefits for individuals who have taken the time to practice their laparoscopic skills using a pelvic trainer in all areas of laparoscopy (cutting, clipping, and suturing) compared with individuals who had no such training (Derossis et al, 1998). The role of laparoscopic simulators and 1-week mini-fellowships is still being determined. The value of the former can only be determined by as yet to be completed scientifically correct validation studies; the latter appears to be of value, providing higher "take" rates (i.e., 76%) than the usual 2-day hands-on course (McDougall et al, 2005).

Procedural Complications

Aside from training in manual skills, the neophyte laparoscopic surgeon must be educated with regard to prevention, recognition, and appropriate treatment of complications. Accordingly, the following section covers the myriad complications that can occur with any laparoscopic procedure. Recognition, resolution, and prevention of these various problems are discussed.

Complications Related to Obtaining the Pneumoperitoneum

Malfunction of Equipment. A successful outcome of any laparoscopic procedure depends not only on the manual skills of the surgeon but also on a proper working knowledge of all the high-technology equipment involved in performing these procedures. To ensure undisturbed functioning of all technology, the laparoscopist must be supported by a well-trained staff who are capable not only of quickly recognizing any equipment malfunction but also of providing immediate, adequate response to correct problems. In this regard, the Society of American Gastrointestinal Endoscopic Surgeons has issued a troubleshooting guide for video and electronic failure. Newer laparoscopy systems have become more simplified in some ways offering automatic settings, touch screen control, and voice command; however, these new systems can be more taxing as well because they offer a host of optional settings and capabilities. For integrated operating room systems offered by most major equipment manufacturers the surgeon and operating room staff need to receive in-depth training on the systems operation, capabilities, and limitations. In this way equipment failure will be minimized.

Complications Associated with Closed Access (Veress Needle Placement)

Preperitoneal Placement. Preperitoneal placement of the Veress needle may preclude successful trocar placement (see Fig. 7–3). If not recognized early, 1 to 2 L of CO_2 may be inflated; indeed, once this much CO_2 has been insufflated into the preperitoneal space, many signs indicative of correct intraperitoneal insufflation may be present (e.g., distention, tympanic sound on percussion). The first trocar is usually placed, and all signs of proper placement are evident.

The first sign of preperitoneal insufflation is that there may be a steep rise in pressure with only 500 mL of CO_2 plus, if more CO_2 is instilled, unequal distention of the abdomen occurs. If this early sign is missed, then the laparoscope reveals only fat after trocar placement; the intraperitoneal viscera are not seen.

The next step is to evacuate the CO_2 through the side arm of the trocar and proceed with an open insertion technique. The initial incision can be widened, and the peritoneal surface can be grasped with a pair of Allis clamps and incised. A Hasson cannula is then secured in place, as previously described, and the peritoneal cavity is insufflated.

Several steps can be taken to avoid this complication. First, if the Veress needle is preperitoneal on initial insufflation, pressures are usually higher than the maximal initial allowable pressure of 10 mm. Second, if the Veress needle is preperitoneal, it cannot be easily advanced 1 cm deeper without resistance. If one has truly entered the peritoneal cavity properly, the Veress needle can be moved 1 cm deeper without meeting any resistance (the "advancement test").

Vascular Injuries. During initial placement of the Veress needle at the umbilicus, minor or major intra-abdominal

blood vessels may be punctured by the 14-gauge needle. The first sign of intravascular entry is blood appearing in the hub of the needle. Aspiration results in additional blood filling the syringe. As long as the needle has not been manipulated, it can usually be withdrawn without excessive bleeding. An alternative site for Veress needle placement or open cannula insertion should be used at this point.

To prevent this problem, it is important when using an umbilical approach to direct the Veress needle toward the hollow of the pelvis. Passing the Veress needle via a 12-mm incision, bluntly spreading the subcutaneous fat, and grasping and stabilizing the anterior fascia with a pair of Allis clamps may help prevent this problem. These maneuvers become especially important in children, who have less space between intra-abdominal structures and the abdominal wall. Lastly, for a case in which this problem occurs, it is important that the path of the initial Veress needle passage be traced on entry into the peritoneal cavity to assess the site of vascular injury. Upon proper entry into the abdomen, the prior site of Veress needle passage is carefully inspected at a pressure of 5 mm Hg; any site of bleeding can be expeditiously treated by the application of thrombin-impregnated gelatin matrix (i.e., Floseal) or fibrin glue. Gentle pressure can be applied to the bleeding vessel. Likewise, any hemodynamic instability associated with loss of "working space" within the abdomen during the procedure should alert the surgeon to the possibility of an expanding retroperitoneal bleeding.

Prevention of vascular complications can be further achieved in one of two manners. Using a nonumbilical site for Veress needle passage (i.e., just superior and medial to the iliac crest or subcostal in the midclavicular line) places no major vessels in danger. Also, the use of only blunt trocars decreases the chance of injury of the epigastric vessels by fivefold (reduced incidence from 0.83% to 0.16%) (Hashizume and Sugimachi, 1997; Thomas et al, 2003).

Visceral Injuries. During Veress needle placement, intra-abdominal organs may be punctured. The initial signs of this complication consist of aspiration of blood, urine, or bowel contents through the Veress needle or, in the case of a solid organ, high pressures on initial insufflation.

Management consists of simply removing the Veress needle. The Veress needle may then be reintroduced at a different site, or an open cannula placement can be pursued via a separate incision site. On entry into the abdomen, any bleeding site on the liver or spleen can be treated with an argon beam coagulator or the application of a surgical hemostatic (e.g., thrombin containing gelatin matrix or fibrin glue) (see earlier). Bowel or bladder entry of the Veress needle needs no further treatment other than needle withdrawal.

This problem can be readily prevented by placing a nasogastric tube and a transurethral indwelling bladder catheter to decompress the stomach and bladder, respectively, before Veress needle passage. Stabilization of the abdominal wall fascia with towel clips or Allis clamps at the time of Veress needle puncture may help provide more space for safe insertion of the Veress needle. Likewise, insufflation should never be initiated unless *all* of the signs for proper peritoneal entry (negative aspiration, easy irrigation of saline, negative aspiration of saline, positive drop test, and normal advancement test) have been observed.

Complications Related to Insufflation and Pneumoperitoneum

Bowel Insufflation. If entry into the bowel is not recognized at the time of irrigation and aspiration through the Veress needle, then the surgeon may well insufflate the small or large bowel. The first sign of this problem is asymmetrical abdominal distention. Associated signs may be passage of flatus and insufflation of only a small amount of CO_2 (less than 2 L) before high pressures are reached.

If this complication is suspected, then the insufflation line should be disconnected; the outflow of gas will immediately confirm bowel entry. The needle can be withdrawn, and open access cannula placement should be done at a different abdominal site.

Prevention of this problem is ensured if one properly performs the aspiration/irrigation/aspiration tests recommended for safe Veress needle placement and if one avoids sites of prior surgery. Similarly, initial open insertion may decrease the chances of this complication.

Gas Embolism. The CO_2 insufflant has favorable solubility in blood, as opposed to insufflants of air, helium, or nitrous oxide (LD_{50} = 1750 mL); however, use of CO_2 may still result in a gas embolus. The most common cause of CO_2 embolism is puncture of a blood vessel or organ with the Veress needle, followed by insufflation; this can occur only when the surgeon has ignored the previously described tests for proper entry into the peritoneal cavity. The first sign of intravascular insufflation is acute cardiovascular collapse. Other signs include dysrhythmias, tachycardia, cyanosis, and pulmonary edema. The diagnosis is usually made by the anesthesiologist based on an abrupt increase of end-tidal CO_2 accompanied by a sudden decline in oxygen saturation and then a marked decrease in end-tidal CO_2 (Loris, 1994). Sometimes, a "millwheel" precordial murmur can be auscultated (Keith et al, 1974). In addition, the anesthesiologist may notice foaming of any blood sample owing to the presence of insufflated CO_2.

The treatment is immediate cessation of insufflation and prompt desufflation of the peritoneal cavity. The patient, if at all possible, is turned into a left lateral decubitus position (i.e., right side up) to minimize right ventricular outflow problems. The patient is hyperventilated with 100% oxygen. Advancement of a central venous line into the right heart with subsequent attempts to aspirate gas may rarely be helpful. The use of hyperbaric oxygen and cardiopulmonary bypass have also been reported (McGrath et al, 1989; Diakun, 1991; Abdel-Meguid and Gomella, 1996).

This devastating complication can be precluded by meticulous attention to Veress needle and initial trocar placement and performance of each of the recommended tests for intraperitoneal entry. Insufflation should never be initiated if the surgeon has even the slightest doubt about correct positioning of the Veress needle; in this situation, the surgeon should withdraw the Veress needle and pass it at an alternative site or immediately proceed with open cannula access.

Barotrauma. Prolonged elevated pressures (higher than 15 mm Hg) may result in barotrauma (McGrath et al, 1989; Diakun, 1991; Abdel-Meguid and Gomelli, 1996). Prolonged high pressures may be caused by insufficient and infrequent monitoring of CO_2 pressure, malfunction of the insufflator, or additional pressures produced by auxiliary devices (e.g., argon beam coagulator, CO_2-cooled laser). Furthermore, barotrauma may be caused by ventilation techniques using positive end-expiratory pressure resulting in rupture of a pulmonary bleb or bulla.

The initial sign of barotrauma may be hypotension owing to decreased cardiac output secondary to an acute drop in venous return caused by compression of the vena cava. Also, a pneumothorax or pneumomediastinum may develop because of high ventilation pressures. Increased intra-abdominal pressures may induce a hiatal hernia as well.

The anesthesiologist usually alerts the surgeon to the problem of excessive intra-abdominal pressure; it usually presents as an increase in ventilation pressures. The surgeon should desufflate the abdomen and, once the hemodynamic changes have been reversed, reinitiate the pneumoperitoneum at 10 mm Hg. A malfunctioning insufflator should be replaced. Also, if one is using an argon beam coagulator or a CO_2-cooled laser device, the side arm on one port should be left open to allow high-pressure excess gas to readily escape.

These problems are avoided by the alert, meticulous surgeon. The insufflator should always be checked before initiating the procedure; at maximum inflow settings, gas should flow freely at less than 2 mm Hg pressure down the opened, unconnected insufflation line, and when the line is purposely kinked by the surgeon, the insufflator-recorded pressure should rise rapidly to its preset limit (usually 15 mm Hg), the inflow of CO_2 should cease, and the high pressure alarm should sound. Again, troubleshooting the insufflator should be part of the routine prelaparoscopy check in every case.

Subcutaneous Emphysema. This problem develops owing to improper placement of the Veress needle or, more commonly, to leakage of CO_2 around ports. The latter situation occurs when port site incisions are too large, when the procedure is particularly lengthy, or when high intra-abdominal pressures are used. The pathognomonic sign is crepitus over the abdomen and thorax; in male patients, a pneumoscrotum may also develop.

If the problem is due to improper placement of the Veress needle, then withdrawal of the Veress needle and open insertion are recommended. If the problem develops intraoperatively, the surgeon should check for gas leakage around a port site. If this is found, the surgeon can either place a purse-string suture around the port or, preferably, change the trocar to a larger size or switch to the balloon-based Hasson-type cannula that creates a tight seal between the intra-abdominal balloon and its outer soft foam cuff. Also, the surgeon should consider reducing the insufflation pressure.

This complication is eminently avoidable if the surgeon adheres to all the diagnostic tests for proper Veress needle placement and if the port site incisions are carefully tapered to the size of the port to be placed. In this regard, it is important to place each port so that it is pointing toward the surgical field, to avoid the continued forceful redirection of the port during the procedure that results in widening of the tissue tract around the port and subsequent escape of CO_2 into the surrounding subcutaneous tissues. In addition, the cannulas must be secured so they do not pull back into the abdominal wall tissues; to this end, the surgeon can use a screw-type cannula or may elect to simply use a suture to fix the side arm of the port to the skin, thereby precluding its retraction beyond a certain point. If the former solution is chosen, the surgeon must be careful to never use a plastic retaining collar with a metal trocar; this situation greatly increases the chance of inadvertent monopolar electrosurgical injury owing to stray current along the exposed shaft of the now partially insulated metal trocar. Also, the insufflator must be tested before each procedure to make sure it is functioning properly, so that when high pneumoperitoneum pressures develop, the inflow of CO_2 automatically ceases.

Two studies have demonstrated that the incidence of surgical emphysema is somewhat higher during retroperitoneal laparoscopy than during transperitoneal laparoscopy, albeit without any clinically significant sequelae: 45% versus 12.5%, $P = .09$ (Ng et al, 1999) and 94% versus 71%, $P = .07$ (Wolf et al, 1995). However, the risk of surgical emphysema and other CO_2-related sequelae during retroperitoneoscopic and extraperitoneoscopic surgery can be effectively minimized by adopting a variety of practical measures (Gill, 1998; Ng et al, 1999). Specifically working at a lower pressure is helpful (i.e., 12 mm Hg). In one study, in the initial 20 cases with an insufflation pressure of 15 mm Hg, subcutaneous emphysema was noted in three patients (15%); however, in the subsequent 180 cases, the insufflation pressure was maintained below 12 mm Hg and subcutaneous emphysema was noted in only two patients (1.1%) (Rassweiler et al, 1998). Also, use of the balloon-based Hasson cannula to seal the initial entry site is important. Invariably, the problem resolves itself during the initial 2 to 3 postoperative days.

Pneumomediastinum, Pneumothorax, and Pneumopericardium. Gas leaking along major blood vessels through congenital defects or secondary enlargement of openings in the diaphragm may lead to pneumomediastinum, pneumopericardium, or pneumothorax (Kalhan et al, 1990; Pascual et al, 1990; See et al, 1993; Abreu et al, 2004). Although a pneumomediastinum is usually not associated with specific clinical symptoms, a pneumopericardium may result in impaired cardiac function. The incidence of this complication is estimated to be 0.8% (Abreu et al, 2004). The diagnosis is rarely made during the procedure unless cardiac impairment occurs. Usually, the diagnosis is made on a chest radiograph taken in the recovery room. However, if there is sudden cardiac decompensation during a procedure, the same maneuvers are undertaken as described for treatment of a suspected gas embolism—interruption of the procedure and desufflation of the abdomen. If there is a strong suspicion of pericardial tamponade, pericardiocentesis is indicated.

A pneumothorax may be associated with pneumomediastinum, barotrauma, or direct puncture of the pleural space with a trocar (Doctor and Hussain, 1973; Kalhan et al, 1990; Pascual et al, 1990). The incidence of this complication in a recent series was 1.6% (Abreu et al, 2004). The earliest signs of this problem may be the development of subcutaneous emphysema, especially in the neck and chest area. More ominous signs, such as hypotension and decreased breath sounds with an increase in ventilatory pressure, are indicative of a *tension* pneumothorax. Although a chest radiograph will confirm the diagnosis, the development of pulmonary collapse with loss of breath sounds on one side mandates immediate decompression of the chest by passage of a 16-gauge needle via the second or third intercostal space in the midclavicular line followed by tube thoracostomy if a tension pneumothorax is suspected (See et al, 1993).

Of note, the occurrence of pulmonary complications appears to be greater with a retroperitoneal approach. Indeed, in one large series, 90% of these complications were associated with retroperitoneoscopy, whereas only 10% of these problems occurred in patients undergoing transperitoneal laparoscopy (Abreu et al, 2004).

Prevention of these problems is similar to the means to avoid subcutaneous emphysema: keep the intra-abdominal pressure at 15 mm Hg or less, make sure all port site incisions are tight around the laparoscopic cannulas, and make sure all cannulas are well seated in the peritoneal cavity. In addition, all trocars must remain below the 12th rib. While dissecting in the upper quadrants of the abdomen, especially during retroperitoneal laparoscopic surgery, the surgeon should be aware of the anatomic relationships of the kidneys, adrenal glands, and great vessels to the diaphragm to avoid direct injury.

Complications during Open Access (Hasson Technique). Potential problems associated with the open access are similar to, albeit less frequent than, problems associated with a closed Veress needle pneumoperitoneum. The biggest major risk in this regard is injury to underlying viscera while traversing the peritoneum. In a densely scarred abdomen, the bowel may be adherent to the underside of the abdominal wall and hence may still be injured. If a bowel injury is recognized early, it can often be repaired via the same incision that was made for insertion of the Hasson cannula. Although vascular injury with this approach is distinctly rare, the surgeon must realize that even with open access this devastating complication can occur (Hanney et al, 1999).

The only minor risk in using the open access technique is failure of the surgeon to obtain secure transfascial retaining sutures on either side of the cannula. If this is not done, the bulb of the Hasson cannula will not be seated tightly into the incision, thereby resulting in significant leakage of gas and subsequent subcutaneous emphysema. One way to prevent this problem is to also place a purse-string suture in the fascia to better secure it to the bulb of the Hasson cannula. In addition, one Hasson type cannula (Bluntport, U.S. Surgical, Norwalk, CT) has a retention balloon that can be inflated in the peritoneal cavity and then drawn up tightly against the underside of the abdominal wall; an outer foam sealing ring can then be advanced down the extra-abdominal shaft of the cannula, thereby sandwiching the abdominal wall between the inflated balloon and the foam seal, effectively precluding any leakage of gas during the case. This is especially effective when doing retroperitoneoscopic procedures.

Complications Related to Initial "Blind" Placement of the First Trocar after Obtaining a Veress Needle Pneumoperitoneum. This section should be prefaced with a comment about recent trocar technology. With the advent of nonbladed trocars (several of which also have clear tips for direct visualization of individual abdominal wall layers during port placement), the likelihood of catastrophic injuries to vital structures should be minimal (Thomas et al, 2003). If bladed trocars are used, then the surgeon must take extreme care not to allow the blade to cause injury.

Injury to Gastrointestinal Organs. Perforation of small or large intestine with passage of the primary port is the most common cause of trocar-induced injury of gastrointestinal

organs. Other organs (e.g., stomach) are affected much less frequently. Given the lateral positioning of the spleen and liver, injury of these organs with the passage of the primary trocar is distinctly unusual. The first sign that one has entered the bowel depends on whether the injury is through one wall or both walls ("through-and-through" injury) of the bowel. In the former instance, as soon as the laparoscope is introduced, the surgeon sees the mucosal folds of the interior of the bowel. However, with a through-and-through injury, the diagnosis is not made until the first secondary trocar is passed; at that time, the surgeon should routinely pass the laparoscope through the secondary port to inspect the puncture site of the initial port. The trocar will be seen passing completely through both walls of the bowel. If the surgeon fails to perform this maneuver routinely, this injury will not be noted until the end of the case when the trocars are being removed. A missed bowel injury of this nature leads to peritonitis and possible death.

In the case of a one-wall injury of the bowel, the surgeon can elect to leave the trocar in place and pass a second trocar in another location using an open access technique. On inspection of the abdomen, the site of injury to the bowel will be immediately apparent because the initial trocar will still be residing in the bowel. At this time, the surgeon may elect to open and repair the bowel or, if laparoscopically skilled, may place two more ports and proceed to close the bowel using laparoscopic suturing or stapling techniques.

When the injury to the bowel is a through-and-through injury, the safest path is to open and proceed with repair; alternatively, if particularly skilled, one may consider laparoscopic repair. In either case, the abdomen should be irrigated with 4 to 5 L of saline containing an antibiotic solution and the patient must be placed on broad-spectrum, triple-drug antibiotic coverage.

This complication is best prevented by use of an open access technique (Hasson). In addition, to decrease the risk of stomach perforation, patients should refrain from oral intake for 12 hours before surgery. To decompress the stomach, a nasogastric or orogastric tube should be placed before puncture of the abdomen with the Veress needle. Lastly, mechanical and antibiotic bowel preparation in patients with a history of extensive prior abdominal surgery is recommended.

Injury to Intra-abdominal Vessels. Major vascular injury is a rare but serious complication that occurs in 0.11% to 2% of cases (Hanney et al, 1995; Geers and Holden, 1996; Lin and Grow, 1999; Usal et al, 1998; Vallancien et al, 2002; Parsons et al, 2004) (Fig. 7–21). It is far more common in procedures related to retroperitoneal, as opposed to pelvic, laparoscopy. The aorta and common iliac arteries are most frequently involved. The inferior vena cava is less affected because of its lateral location in relation to the aorta; likewise, the common iliac vein is rarely involved given its posterior position in relation to the common iliac artery. Rarely, in a patient with adhesions or prior surgery, intestinal mesenteric vessels servicing a "fixed" loop of bowel may be injured.

The first sign of a major vascular complication is the onset of sudden hypotension and associated tachycardia. If the trocar has not been moved, then, as the obturator is withdrawn, the diagnosis is made immediately based on whether there is a pulsatile (arterial) or nonpulsatile (venous) profuse return of blood from the trocar sheath. If the trocar has been

displaced from the injured vessel, then, depending on the vessel injured, the surgeon will see blood rapidly accumulating in the abdominal cavity; a mesenteric hematoma; or, rarely, blood that preferentially accumulates retroperitoneally, in which case, the space within the peritoneal cavity will appear to be markedly reduced and actively decreasing because of the expanding retroperitoneal hematoma.

The response to this complication must be rapid. A vascular or trauma surgeon should be called to the room. If blood is coming through the trocar, then the trocar should be closed and left in place. An emergency laparotomy is done, and the trocar is followed to its point of entry into the vessel. Controlling sutures can be placed on either side of the trocar or a Satinsky clamp can be placed to isolate the area of injury, so that, as the trocar is withdrawn, the wound can be rapidly controlled.

If the injury is discovered at the time of passage of the laparoscope (i.e., the trocar is no longer residing in the vessel), then the sheath and laparoscope can be swung up to the underside of the abdominal wall and an immediate cutdown can be done on top of the laparoscope and sheath, thereby providing for a rapid and safe laparotomy. The site of injury must be rapidly located and controlled. Again, the aid of a vascular or trauma surgeon in this case is quite helpful.

The best way to handle this complication is to never have to experience it. In this regard, knowledge of the exact location and possible anatomic variations of major intra-abdominal blood vessels is mandatory. The CT scan should be reviewed before passage of any trocars to look for caval or other abnormalities of the great vessels. Owing to limited intraperitoneal space, special care must be given to trocar placement in children. Strict adherence to laparoscopic guidelines, such as ensuring that all the safety signs of passage of a Veress needle are present before proceeding with trocar passage, obtaining an adequate pneumoperitoneum before trocar passage (intra-abdominal pressure may be raised to 25 mm Hg temporarily for placement of the primary trocar), passing the initial trocar under direct endoscopic control (i.e., clear plastic port) and avoiding initial trocar passage through an abdominal scar, are important in helping to prevent this problem.

With regard to hemorrhage, when the situation is recognized but controlled, the surgeon has the ability to "prepare" for subsequent conversion. In that regard, a second suction unit should be obtained, the vascular or trauma surgeon should be in attendance, and the anesthesiologist has time to make sure the patient is well hydrated and that blood is in the room for transfusion. Furthermore, it is helpful to consider having a "hemorrhage" tray available in the operating room at all times (Table 7–5). This laparoscopic tray should contain a

Table 7–5. **Contents of Hemorrhage Tray for Laparoscopic Surgery**
Laparoscopic Satinsky clamp
Ten-millimeter suction/irrigation tip
Endostitch device with 4-0 absorbable suture
LapraTy clip applier and a packet of LapraTy clips
Six-inch length of 4-0 vascular suture on an SH needle with a LapraTy clip preplaced on the end
Two laparoscopic needle drivers
Topical hemostatic agent of choice

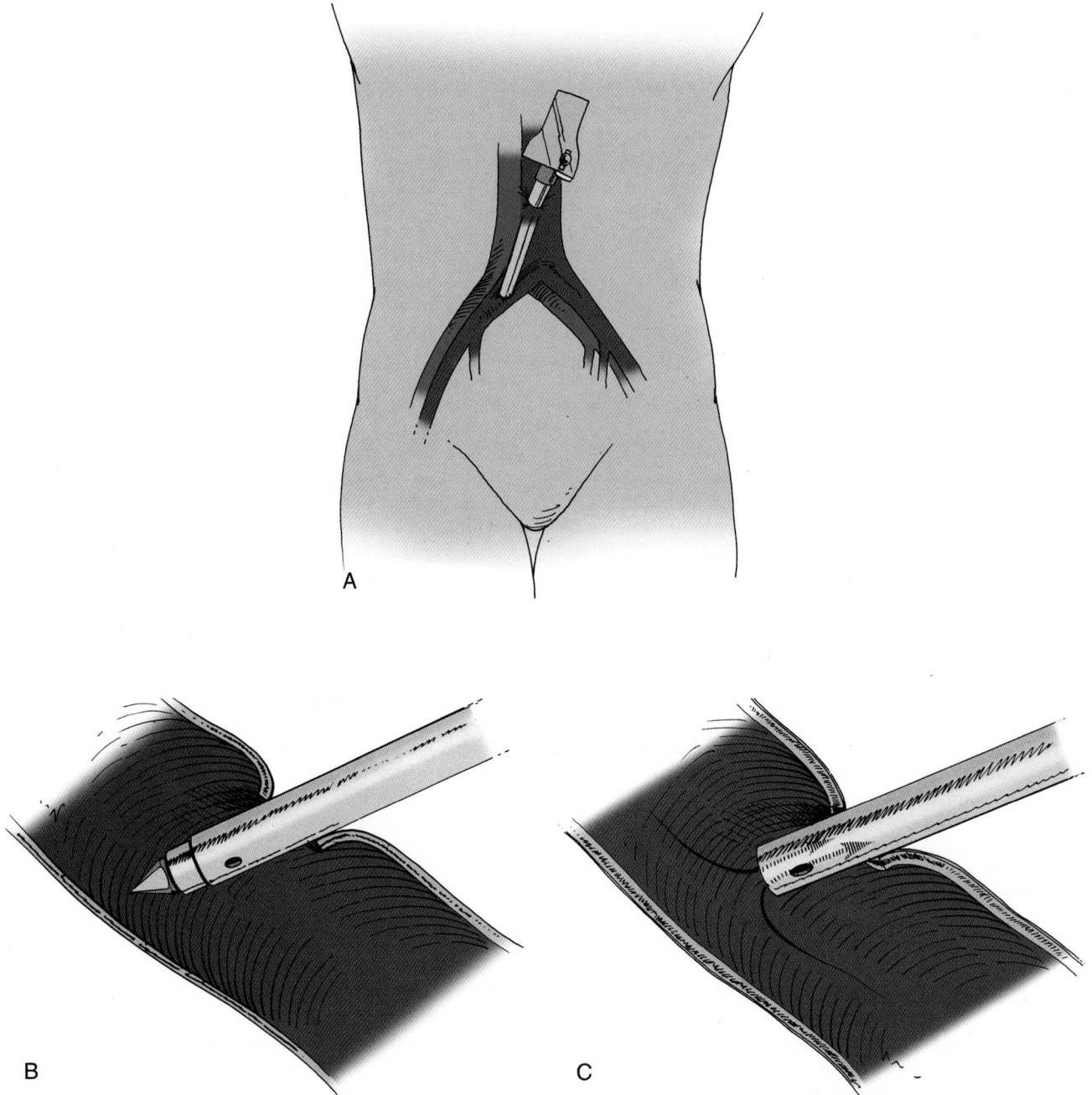

Figure 7–21. **A** and **B**, The right common iliac artery has been punctured by a trocar. **C**, As soon as the obturator is removed, blood fills the cannula. (From Clayman RV, McDougall EM [eds]: Laparoscopic Urology. St. Louis, Quality Medical Publishing, 1993.)

Satinsky clamp, a 10-mm suction tip for large clot evacuation, an Endo Stitch device with 4-0 Vicryl suture, a LapraTy clip applier, and a rack of LapraTy clips (6 clips per rack), two laparoscopic needle holders, and 4-0 vascular suture. With this tray available, some injuries to major venous structures (e.g., inferior vena cava) can be successfully resolved laparoscopically.

Injury to the Urinary Tract. Urinary tract injuries during laparoscopy are most commonly associated with trocar passage. The incidence of this problem varies widely as reported in the gynecologic literature: 0.02% to 8.3% range (Ostrzenski and Ostrzenski, 1998; Lin and Grow, 1999).

Usually, these injuries occur to the bladder at the time of initial trocar placement. Chances of this problem occurring have been greatly reduced by the introduction of blunt trocars.

Trocar injuries of the urinary tract have reportedly affected only the bladder. The initial sign of this problem is pneumaturia or macroscopic hematuria. The diagnosis is confirmed by retrograde intravesical instillation of indigo carmine diluted with saline; this allows the surgeon to rapidly identify the cystotomy site. The injury can be repaired laparoscopically, either with laparoscopic suturing techniques or by use of the laparoscopic tissue stapler; extensive defects may require open surgical repair (Ostrzenski and Ostrzenski,

1998). These injuries should always be closed and not left to heal "on their own" with prolonged Foley catheter drainage.

Prevention of this problem is simple. Preoperative placement of a urethral catheter to drain the bladder is recommended for all major laparoscopic urologic cases. Not only does it largely preclude bladder injury, but it also provides the necessary means for monitoring urine output during major laparoscopic urologic procedures.

Complications Related to Placement of Secondary Trocars

Bleeding at the Cannula Site. Blood dripping from the port entry site and onto the underlying abdominal viscera is the first sign of an injured abdominal wall vessel. The exact site of hemorrhage is determined by cantilevering the trocar into each of the four quadrants and noting which positioning of the trocar tamponades the bleeding.

Definitive therapy for this problem can be undertaken in one of three ways. The simplest method, albeit the most costly, is the insertion of curved electrosurgical scissors or forceps through another port; this instrument can be articulated up into the port site to electrocoagulate the bleeding site.

The least expensive method is to suture the area of hemorrhage. This can be accomplished by inserting a straight Keith needle with a 0-0 absorbable suture from the outside of the abdomen at one side of the affected quadrant and then grasping the needle with laparoscopic forceps and pushing it back out of the abdomen at the opposite side of the affected quadrant until it can be recovered on the surface of the abdomen (Fig. 7–22). This broad suture is then tied over a gauze 4 × 4-inch bolster on the abdominal surface; the port can be used throughout the procedure. Alternatively, various port closure devices, in particular the Carter-Thomasen device, may be used to similarly pass a suture to control the bleeding (Ortega, 1996).

This problem can often be avoided by routinely transilluminating the abdominal wall before trocar placement so large surface vessels can be avoided. In addition, the routine spreading of the subcutaneous tissues of the proposed port site with a blunt clamp (e.g., Kelly clamp) is also helpful. Also, the use of only blunt trocars reduces the chance of vascular wall injury nearly 10-fold. Finally, careful laparoscopic inspection of the peritoneal surface before each secondary port site placement is helpful to identify the area of the inferior epigastric vessels as well as any overlying peritoneal vessels, which can then be avoided; in this regard, no port site should be placed less than 6 cm off the midline (Hashizume and Sugimachi, 1997).

Position-Related Problems. Three potential problems may occur when the secondary trocars are not properly positioned: "crossing swords," "striking handles," and "rollover." The problem of "crossing swords" is due to the trocars being placed too close to one another; as a result, the intra-abdominal portions of two trocars cross each other so that the two cannot easily be used to deliver instruments to the same surgical site (Fig. 7–23). Similarly, the problem of "striking handles" is also due to trocars being placed too close to one another; as a result, the upper portions of the trocars strike one another on the abdominal surface, again precluding delivery of instruments to a specific surgical site. "Rollover" is a variant of the crossing swords problem, but it occurs between the

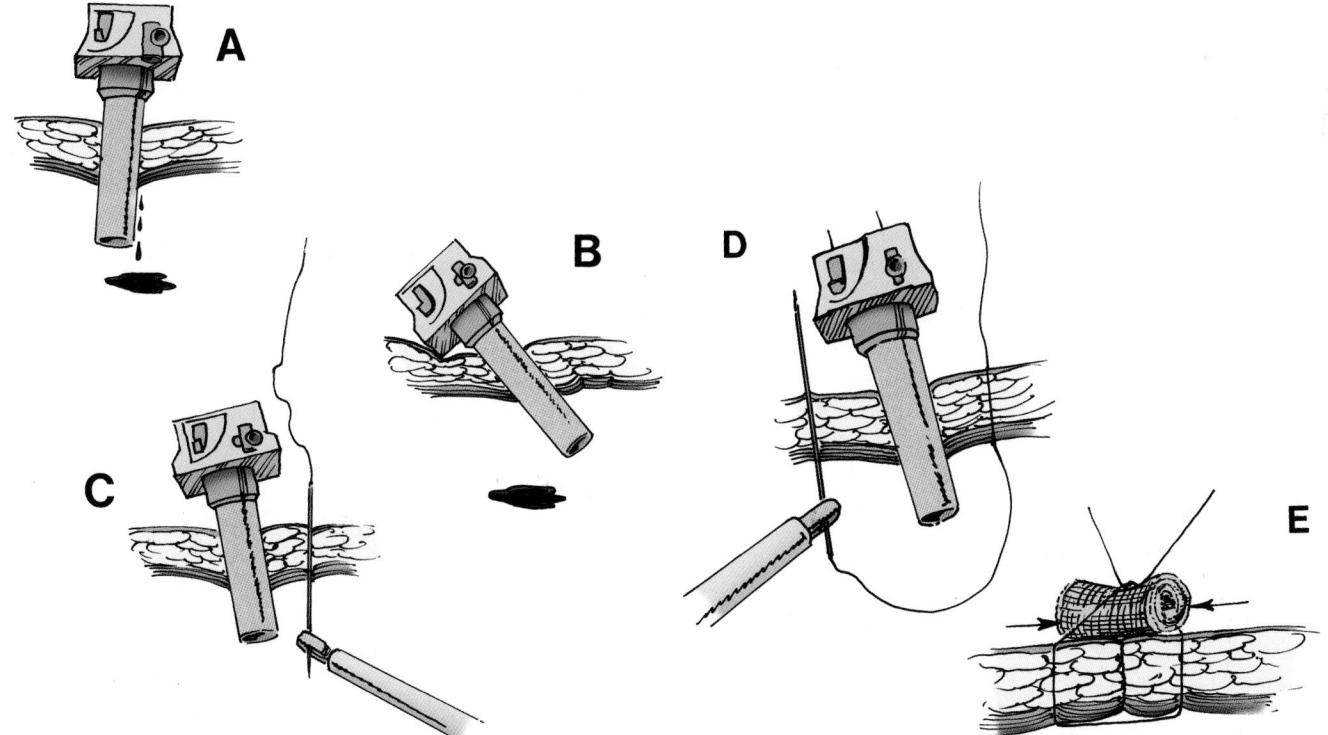

Figure 7–22. **A,** Bleeding at the cannula site. **B,** Cannula can be cantilevered into each of the four different quadrants to identify the source of bleeding. **C** and **D,** Straight Keith needle may be used to traverse the site of bleeding. **E,** Suture is tied down over a gauze bolster. (From Clayman RV, McDougall EM [eds]: Laparoscopic Urology. St. Louis, Quality Medical Publishing, 1993.)

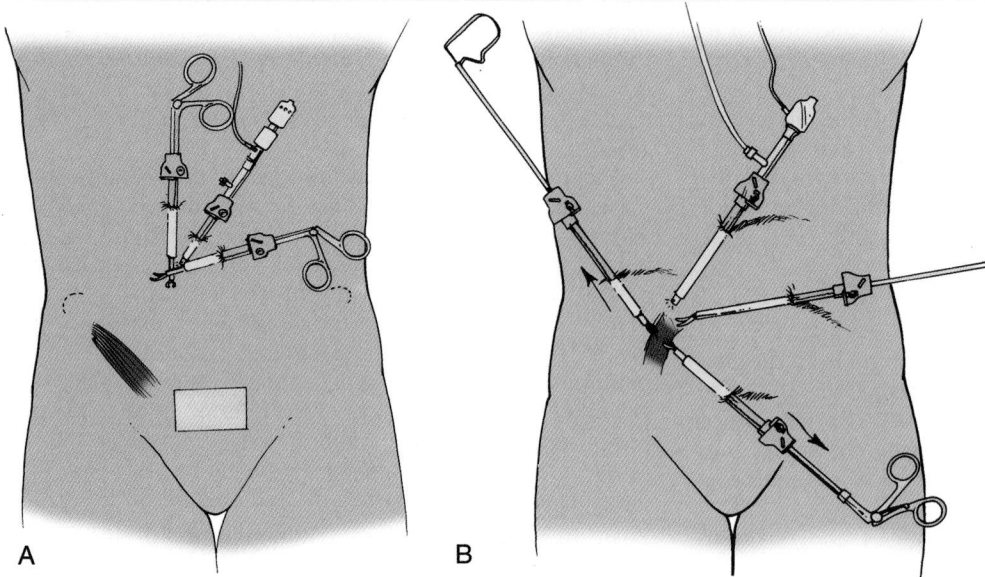

Figure 7–23. **A,** The cannulas have been placed too close to each other; hence, the intra-abdominal portions of the cannulas are also too close to each other, thereby impairing use of instruments passed through the ports. **B,** Correct spacing of the trocars eliminates this problem. (From Clayman RV, McDougall EM [eds]: Laparoscopic Urology. St. Louis, Quality Medical Publishing, 1993.)

laparoscope and an instrument. Instead of running parallel to the surgical site, the primary cannula holding the laparoscope and one of the instrument-holding secondary ports are pointed toward each other; as the instrument is advanced toward the surgical site, it strikes and is deflected by the larger laparoscope, thereby rolling over the laparoscope and hence suddenly moving out of the field of view.

Usually these problems are a minor annoyance, and the surgeon and assistant need to experience the problem only once to adjust for it. Specifically, to avoid the problem of "striking handles," the sheaths can be withdrawn a bit from the abdomen, thereby increasing the space between the handles of the trocars. The problems of "crossing swords" and "rollover" can be remedied by moving the handles of the crossing trocars closer to one another, thereby moving the tips of the trocars farther apart. When this is done to correct a "rollover," the surgical site may be displaced into one corner of the monitor; however, the desired delivery of the instrument to the surgical site can then be accomplished.

The best way to handle these situations is not to create them. Accordingly, proper placement and direction of each trocar are essential. For some procedures, such as pyeloplasty, they may be accomplished by placing all the trocars on the same line (i.e., midline) so they are all working parallel to each other, whereas, for procedures such as nephrectomy, the goal is to place the trocars so that they surround the surgical site, forming a diamond pattern within which the kidney lies. Also, the surgeon should avoid advancing sheaths too far into the abdomen. This can be accomplished by selecting the proper length of trocar for each patient. Lastly, if trocar interactions become particularly vexing during a procedure, the surgeon should not hesitate to place an additional 5-mm secondary trocar in a more conducive site to eliminate the problem.

Complications Related to General Anesthesia Unique to Laparoscopy

Cardiac Arrhythmias and Cardiac Arrest. Cardiac arrhythmias are frequently seen during anesthesia in laparoscopic procedures. The most common arrhythmia is sinus tachycar-

dia; bradyarrhythmias (e.g., atrioventricular dissociation, nodal rhythm, sinus bradycardia) may develop independently or in combination with tachycardia during the same procedure (Myles, 1991). Conditions leading to development of arrhythmias are CO_2 insufflation, hypercapnia, increased vagal tone owing to traction on pelvic or peritoneal structures, Trendelenburg position, anesthetic drugs (especially halothane in combination with spontaneous ventilation), preoperative patient anxiety, endobronchial intubation, and gas embolism (Harris et al, 1984; Myles, 1991). In rare cases, asystolic cardiac arrest and cardiovascular collapse may develop (Shifren et al, 1992).

The role of the anesthesiologist throughout the laparoscopic procedure is of paramount importance. Continuous monitoring of cardiovascular (electrocardiogram, arterial blood pressure) and pulmonary (capnometry, in-line oxygen, airway pressures and tidal volume, frequent arterial blood gas analyses) parameters is essential. Invasive cardiac monitoring should be instituted in patients with heart disease (using a Swan-Ganz catheter) or in high-risk (i.e., ASA 3 or 4) patients when prolonged and complicated laparoscopic procedures are expected, especially since a central venous pressure line cannot be relied on for accurate readings during laparoscopy.

Because hypercarbia is one of the most common underlying causes of cardiac arrhythmias, it is essential to monitor and control this problem. Overall, hypercapnia can be corrected rapidly by adjustment of ventilatory rate and tidal volume, use of positive end-expiratory pressure as needed, and reduction of intra-abdominal pressure to 10 mm Hg. The surgeon can also desufflate the abdomen for 5 to 10 minutes to allow the anesthesiologist to "catch up" and correct the hypercarbia; pneumoperitoneum can then be reinitiated at a lower pressure (5 to 10 mm Hg).

In rare cases, if the hypercarbia cannot be controlled by these maneuvers, helium should be substituted for CO_2 as the insufflant; however, this is a rare event and one that can usually be predicted before the procedure. For patients with severe pulmonary compromise, it is prudent to have a tank of helium and the proper helium yoke available in the operating room so the insufflant can be easily switched. Alternatively, argon gas can be used in the acute situation, as it is readily available in many operating rooms due to the argon beam coagulator.

In the event of cardiac arrest, the surgeon should immediately desufflate the abdomen and provide cardiac massage (compressions) while the anesthesiologist administers 100% oxygen and appropriate drug therapy. If a CO_2 embolus is suspected, additional maneuvers, such as turning the patient to a left lateral decubitus position and attempting to aspirate the embolus, can be attempted.

Preventive measures include avoidance of excessive intra-abdominal pressures (more than 25 mm Hg) over a prolonged period of time and avoidance of certain anesthetic agents and combinations (e.g., halothane and spontaneous ventilation). Premedication with atropine may prevent excessive vagal stimulation (Wolf and Monk, 1996).

Changes in Blood Pressure. Hypertension may be caused by inadequate general anesthesia, elevated intra-abdominal pressures, or hypercarbia. Hypotension may be the result of hypoxia, pneumothorax, pneumomediastinum, gas embolus, or hemorrhage (Abdel-Meguid and Gomella, 1996).

Intermittent or continuous noninvasive blood pressure measurements or invasive monitoring of intra-arterial (e.g., radial artery) pressure is part of all laparoscopic procedures. In the event of a marked change in blood pressure, one of the aforementioned conditions must be ruled out. The initial response of the surgeon, provided that there is neither active bleeding nor evidence of retroperitoneal hemorrhage, is to desufflate the abdomen. In addition to desufflation, therapy specific to an underlying laparoscopic cause may include CO_2 elimination by increased ventilation; increased oxygen saturation; treatment of an underlying pneumothorax, pneumomediastinum, or gas embolus; and pharmacologic (vasodilators or vasoconstrictors) therapy.

Aspiration of Gastric Contents. Aspiration of gastric contents may occur more frequently in patients with a hiatal hernia, significant obesity, diabetes with a history of gastroparesis, or any form of gastric outlet obstruction (Hanley, 1992). The combination of elevated intra-abdominal pressures from the pneumoperitoneum, morbid obesity, and use of the Trendelenburg position increases the likelihood of this complication (Abdel-Meguid and Gomella, 1996).

The diagnosis is easily made because the problem usually occurs during intubation, with associated coughing. The response to suspected aspiration depends on the intubation status of the patient. If the patient is not intubated, the head should be turned sideways and all gastric secretions should be vigorously suctioned. If the endotracheal tube is already in place, it should be left in situ and aggressive suctioning should be initiated. If aspiration of gastric contents occurs postoperatively, reintubation with mechanical ventilation and positive end-expiratory pressure may be indicated (Hagberg and Boin, 1999). Neither corticosteroid nor broad-coverage antibiotic administration is indicated (Tasch, 1999).

To prevent this problem in high-risk patients, oral or intravenous administration of 10 mg of metoclopramide is recommended. This medication may decrease the incidence of aspiration by increasing the tone of the lower esophageal sphincter. In addition, in patients with known gastro-esophageal reflux, histamine-2 blockers reduce gastric acidity and attendant morbidity if aspiration of gastric contents should occur (Hanley, 1992; Abdel-Meguid and Gomella, 1996). Also, in patients with known gastroesophageal reflux or other predisposing factors for gastric aspiration, a cuffed endotracheal tube should always be placed. Lastly, among these high-risk patients, administration of atropine should be avoided because it decreases the tone of the lower esophageal sphincter (Duffey, 1979).

Hypothermia. The patient's body core temperature may drop during prolonged laparoscopic procedures, especially if there is leakage of insufflant around the port sites. The CO_2 that is used is typically neither warm nor humidified. The resulting decrease in temperature may be 0.3°C for each 50 L of CO_2 insufflated (Ott, 1991a). The ambient operating room temperature may exacerbate this effect.

The clinical effects of hypothermia are well described. Core body temperatures around the 35°C level may result in (1) increased bleeding tendency owing to impaired platelet function, reduced activity of coagulation factors in the coagulation cascade, and enhanced fibrinolysis; (2) increased adrenergic response with vasoconstriction and increased arterial blood pressure; (3) prolonged recovery time owing to increased blood gas solubility; (4) twofold to threefold increase in the incidence of early postoperative myocardial ischemia in high-risk patients; and (5) impaired wound healing and increased susceptibility to wound infections (Rosenberg and Frank, 1999).

In general, there are no specific anesthetic symptoms that can be appreciated intraoperatively except for cardiac arrhythmias. In particular, atrial fibrillation may occur in extreme cases of hypothermia (body core temperature around 30°C). In such a case, if the patient undergoes arrest, cardiac resuscitative efforts should be prolonged because the patient must be warmed for resuscitative efforts to have their proper impact. The problem is combated by use of warm intravenous fluid and application of active warming systems.

In almost all cases, hypothermia can be avoided. Adjuncts to support the patient's body temperature include intravenous fluid warming, active warming by forced-air systems, circulating warm-water mattresses, and radiant heaters (Rosenberg and Frank, 1999). In addition, warming and humidifying CO_2 to physiologic levels, especially when a prolonged laparoscopic procedure is anticipated, is helpful (Ott, 1991b). However, warming the insufflant alone should be avoided, because this causes a drying of the intraperitoneal tissues and has been associated with increased postoperative patient discomfort (Slim et al, 1999).

Complications Related to the Surgical Procedure

Bowel Injury: Electrosurgical Etiology. Electrosurgically induced thermal injury may occur because of one of four mechanisms: inappropriate direct activation, coupling to another instrument, capacitive coupling, and insulation failure. Active electrode trauma by unintended activation causes direct bowel or other organ injury; it may occur when the instrument is left unobserved within the peritoneal cavity or when electrode activation is carried out by someone other than the primary surgeon. Furthermore, active electrode trauma may be seen when coagulation extends beyond the intended site and reaches other adjacent structures (e.g., bowel, blood vessels, nerves, ureter); this is more commonly seen when high electrocoagulation settings (i.e., >30 watts) are used instead of blended or pure cutting current. Direct coupling may occur when the active electrosurgical instrument touches another instrument that is in direct contact with other tissue (e.g., bowel). If this happens outside the field of view provided by the laparoscope, it may remain unnoticed by the surgical team. Injury owing to capacitive coupling occurs when the surrounding charge, which is intrinsic to all activated monopolar electrodes, is not allowed to conduct back to and disperse via the abdominal wall (Zucker et al, 1995; Munro, 1997). This condition may develop when a metal cannula is anchored to the skin with a nonconductive plastic grip, which, as previously noted, should never be done (Fig. 7–24). As a result, the electrical field, which builds up around the activated electrosurgical instrument, cannot be conducted to the abdominal wall because the plastic retainer acts as an insulator. This may lead to a high power density along the portion of the metal cannula that is inside the abdomen; the electrical charge built up on the cannula can then travel to other tissues in contact with the cannula. Similarly, capacitive coupling may constitute a risk when electrosurgical probes are used through operating laparoscopes, which are, in turn, inserted through plastic sheaths. The metal shaft of the laparoscope then becomes a repository for electrical current and may discharge this energy to any tissue in contact with the laparoscope. In general, the side-arm operating laparoscope is rarely used during urologic procedures. The risk of this complication is also increased when older generators with high voltage output and/or electrodes with thicker diameters are used, especially in coagulation rather than cutting mode (Munro, 1997). Lastly, insulation breakdown may allow current to escape along the shaft of the instrument, thereby harming tissues that are otherwise outside the field of view of the laparoscope. Insulation breakdown along the shaft of the instrument may be a result of repeated use, resterilization, or

mechanical damage to the instrument during repeated insertion through a trocar. Intraoperatively, thermal injuries of the bowel may present as whitish spots on the serosal lining. In severe cases, the muscularis mucosae or the intestinal lumen may be seen. However, in many patients, the event of thermal injury of the bowel is not realized at the time of the procedure. Postoperatively, the patient with unrecognized bowel trauma may not develop fever, nausea, or signs of peritonitis for many days; indeed, the full extent of the bowel necrosis may take up to 18 days to fully develop (Abdel-Meguid and Gomella, 1996). Therefore, the problem often does not become manifest until the patient has actually been discharged from the hospital.

Accordingly, bowel injury must be ruled out for any patient who develops a fever beyond postoperative day 1 or who complains of increasing abdominal discomfort. Abdominal radiographs are notoriously inaccurate because the CO_2 from the laparoscopy may remain as "free air" for upwards of 9 days after the procedure; however, an ileus pattern is usually present. The more sensitive test is an abdominal CT scan with oral contrast accompanied by delayed films, usually 6 or more hours after the initial oral contrast load. Laboratory values may be remarkable for leukocytosis with an associated left shift (i.e., increased percentage of neutrophils); in some patients, the latter occurs in the face of a normal or even low leukocyte count, making the "left shift" a more reliable sign than the absolute white cell count.

Minor postoperative thermal injuries of the bowel, discovered late in the postoperative period (i.e., >5 to 7 days postoperatively) may be managed conservatively, aided by administration of antibiotics and an elemental diet. Indeed, a closed fistula may develop that will heal with this approach. However, if the patient does not respond rapidly or develops worsening peritonitis, open surgical exploration is mandatory. Thermal injury caused by monopolar cautery often results in tissue damage that extends beyond the visible area of necrosis. With this in mind, the surgeon

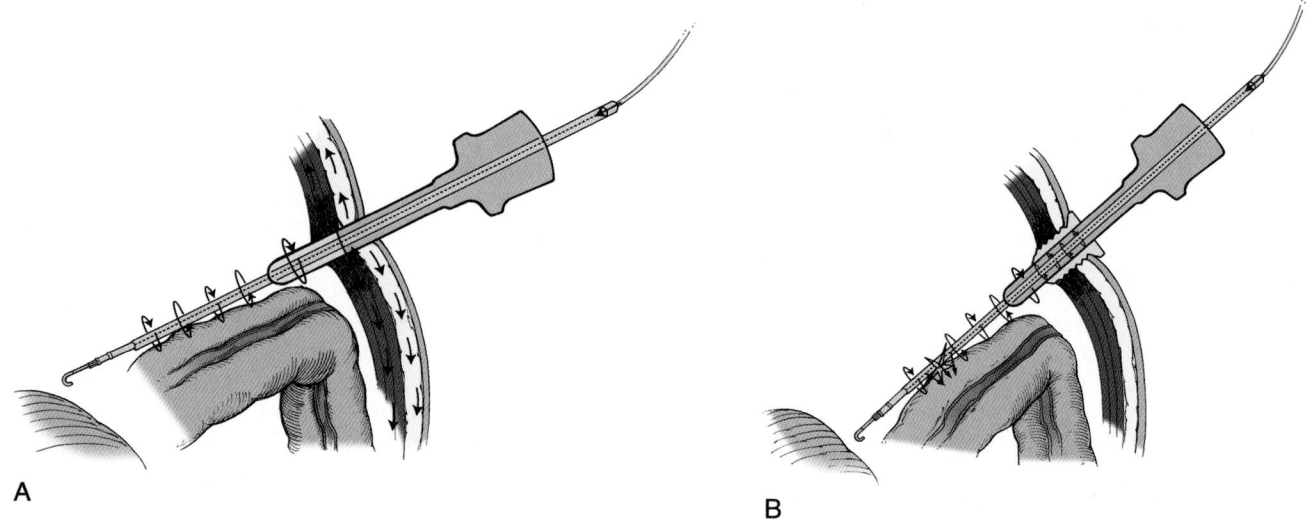

A **B**

Figure 7–24. Capacitive coupling. **A,** Charge surrounding the activated monopolar electrode is conducted back to the all-metal cannula and dispersed by the abdominal wall. **B,** The electrosurgical instrument is being used through a metal cannula that has been anchored to the skin with a nonconductive plastic grip; accordingly, the electrical field cannot be conducted to the abdominal wall because the plastic retainer acts as an insulator; a stronger electrical charge is thus conducted to any other tissue in contact with the cannula.

should perform a bowel resection with a safety margin of 6 cm on either side before completing an end-to-end anastomosis (Abdel-Meguid and Gomella, 1996).

Thermal injury caused by bipolar electrosurgery is more confined to the visible area of damage. These injuries only occur due to direct firing of the instrument on the bowel. If the injury is small, it can be managed by simple excision of the defect and closure of the bowel wall. Bipolar injuries that involve more than half of the circumference of the bowel should be treated by excision of the affected segment of the bowel followed by end-to-end anastomosis (Abdel-Meguid and Gomella, 1996).

The goal of every laparoscopic surgeon is to never experience a thermal complication. To this end there are several actions the surgeon can take to lessen the risks. First, electrosurgical instruments must be carefully inspected before use for any "breaks" in the insulation; if these are found, the instrument must be sent out to be recoated. Next, electrosurgical instruments should never be left untended within the abdomen; when not in use, they must be removed from the abdomen. Also, control of electrode activation should be performed *only* by the primary surgeon. The foot pedal should be placed so that only the surgeon can depress it. Furthermore, some newer laparoscopic instruments such as the 5-mm Ligasure (ValleyLab, Boulder, CO) are designed with ergonomic thumb-operated mechanisms that only the operative surgeon can activate. Also, isolation of the area to be cauterized from the surrounding tissues (vessels, nerves, ureter), as well as use of bipolar electrocautery, reduces the risk of thermal injury to other tissues. In addition, the electrosurgical device should never be activated unless the entire extent of the metal portion of the instrument is in view. In this manner, both inadvertent direct injury to adjacent tissue and direct coupling to another instrument can be avoided. Problems of capacitive coupling can be precluded by not creating a situation in which a mixture of conducting and nonconducting elements are used by the surgeon (e.g., metal trocars combined with plastic retainers, electrosurgical devices through operating laparoscopes passed through plastic trocars). In addition, use of modern generators and small-diameter electrodes significantly decreases the risk of capacitive coupling (Munro, 1997), as does greater use of blended or pure cutting current. The high voltages needed for pure coagulation current pose the greatest threat for electrosurgical injury, especially through the mechanism of capacitive coupling and insulation failure. Lastly, an active electrode monitoring system (Encision, Boulder, CO) is extremely helpful; with this device, any sudden break in the insulation of the electrosurgical instrument (e.g., with scissors or hook electrode) results in immediate shutdown of the electrosurgical current.

Bowel Injury: Mechanical. Inadvertent mechanical damage can be caused by a wide variety of sharp and blunt instruments (e.g., laparoscopic graspers, scissors, retractors). This type of injury is more visible to the surgeon and is usually discovered intraoperatively or at the end of the procedure when the surgical site is irrigated. Direct visual identification during the procedure allows the surgeon to repair the injury laparoscopically, even though the patient has not had a formal bowel preparation. Given its localized nature, bowel resection is rarely necessary. The abdomen should be irrigated copiously

at the end of the procedure with 4 to 5 L of an antibiotic-containing solution. If the situation is missed during the procedure, then postoperatively symptoms develop much earlier than with an electrosurgical injury. Fever, nausea, ileus, and peritonitis develop in the very early postoperative period. Diagnosis is confirmed by an abdominal CT scan with oral contrast material. This type of injury should be managed with immediate return to the operating room to correct the problem by local excision or resection of bowel with subsequent end-to-end anastomosis and copious irrigation of the abdomen (see earlier).

Delicate handling of tissue with laparoscopic instruments by the main surgeon and the assistants is essential to avoiding this complication. Likewise, it is important that introduction of laparoscopic instruments into the peritoneal cavity be done under strict visual control. Instruments should never be left untended; if they are not in use, they should be withdrawn from the abdominal cavity. Prudence, economy of motion, and deftness of touch are essential characteristics of both the successful open and laparoscopic surgeon.

Vascular Injury. Fortunately, direct vascular injury during laparoscopic dissection is a rare event. The use of only blunt trocars, the small nature of the instrumentation, the limitations on surgical speed, and the magnification of the surgical field by the laparoscope all combine to decrease this potential problem.

During right renal dissection, in particular, the chance of a vena caval or renal vein injury is very real. When this occurs, the surgeon can undertake several steps to resolve the bleeding. First, the pneumoperitoneum pressure can be raised to 25 mm Hg, thereby slowing or stopping any venous bleeding. Using the irrigator/aspirator, the blood can be cleared and the bleeding site identified; if need be a second insufflator can be brought into the room and connected to maintain pneumoperitoneum pressure even during use of suction at the site of injury. Next, via one of the 12-mm ports, a gauze sponge can be introduced into the abdomen and handled with a grasping forceps, thereby allowing the surgeon to identify and tamponade the area of bleeding. If the injury is small, it may respond to simple tamponade; alternatively, a hemostatic patch and/or fibrin glue or thrombin-impregnated granules (e.g., Floseal) may be applied. If the injury is larger, then the surgeon must decide whether to obtain a vascular consult and proceed to convert to an open procedure or to attempt securing the injury with a laparoscopic Satinsky clamp and proceed with intracorporeal suturing, either freehand or with an Endo Stitch and 6 inches of a 4-0 Vicryl suture with a LapraTy clip secured at its end. Care should be taken to use a laparoscopic grasper to introduce the LapraTy clip into the abdomen first, followed by the Endo Stitch device; the shaft of the Endo Stitch cannot be passed alongside the LapraTy clip because the two together are too broad to pass side by side through a 12-mm cannula. With the Endo Stitch device a running suture is done, with the initial LapraTy clip serving as the distal "knot"; after the defect is closed, the suture is again secured with a LapraTy clip. One caveat is important: specifically, the holes caused by the Endo Stitch needle and suture both passing through the tissue alongside one another may ooze slightly after the repair; this can be nicely controlled by the application of thrombin-impregnated granules (e.g., Floseal). Throughout this period, it is essential for the anesthesiologist to administer sufficient fluids or blood replacement to preclude a hypovolemic state because the patient has a higher risk of possible air embolism if this occurs (O'Sullivan et al, 1997).

If the surgeon is able to gain temporary control of the vessel with a grasper, then it is often helpful to place an extra 5-mm port that can be used by the assistant for suction/irrigation. This allows the surgeon to repair the bleeding site using two hands.

Alternatively, the surgeon can convert from standard laparoscopy to a hand-assisted approach. The hand in this case is valuable because it can rapidly tamponade the bleeding site. In this regard, it is recommended, if at all possible, to pinch the sidewalls of the vein (e.g., inferior vena cava) closed rather than just putting direct pressure on the top of the injury; the latter approach has a tendency to result in a gradual enlargement of the hole in the vein. Also, by pinching the hole closed, a Satinsky clamp can be more easily passed beneath the surgeon's fingers to more securely gain control in preparation for a sutured repair.

Minor arterial injuries usually respond to tamponade. Larger aortic or renal artery injuries are much more difficult to resolve laparoscopically. Although the latter, if they occur during a planned nephrectomy, can be handled by expeditiously dividing the renal artery with a vascular stapler, the former almost invariably leads to open repair. In this case, the area of injury should be tamponaded with a laparoscopic forceps. A vascular surgeon can be called into the room, and the surgeon can proceed to rapidly make a midline incision by swinging one of the midline ports up to the underside of the abdominal wall and cutting down on the shaft of the port. The tamponading laparoscopic forceps directs the surgeon immediately to the site of injury, which can then be properly repaired.

As mentioned previously in this chapter, because most bleeding episodes are unexpected, it is wise to have a hemorrhage tray equipped with all instruments necessary to control bleeding. In most cases, a successful outcome is heavily dependent on a rapid and effective response on the part of the surgeon, which is only possible if the equipment is immediately available and the operating room team is knowledgeable and efficient. A hemorrhage tray that can quickly be opened in case of a vascular injury containing all needed instruments is highly recommended (see Table 7–5).

Injury to the Urinary Tract

Bladder Injury. Electrocautery dissection, blunt and sharp dissection (with laparoscopic scissors), and laser dissection have been identified as intraoperative causes of bladder injury. Concomitant bladder or pelvic anomalies or pathologic conditions (acute or chronic inflammation, prior pelvic or bladder surgery, endometriosis, malignant infiltration, bladder diverticula, amyloidosis, or previous radiation) are predisposing factors that increase the chances of this complication (Ostrzenski and Ostrzenski, 1998).

When a bladder injury has occurred, the intraoperative signs may be subtle. One of the first signs is the presence of blood or gas in the Foley catheter bag. Also, the surgeon may notice clear fluid welling up in the pelvis, although this sign is often obscured if irrigation has been used during the procedure.

Postoperatively, if the bladder injury was missed, the patient may develop oliguria and urinary ascites; this may be accompanied by hyponatremia and, rarely, hyperkalemia with mild elevation of serum creatinine due to the peritoneal absorption of urine. Patients who have been discharged from the hospital owing to the minor nature of their laparoscopic procedure may contact their physician complaining of lower abdominal discomfort, abdominal swelling, fever, and, in the case of a gynecologic procedure, vaginal discharge.

The intraoperative suspicion of a bladder injury can be confirmed by the injection of saline mixed with indigo carmine through the Foley catheter. Postoperatively, the diagnosis can be made by radiologic examinations (pelvic ultrasound, pelvic CT scan, and/or voiding cystogram). Similarly, an endoscopic examination with the injection of 5 mL of indigo carmine intravenously is helpful if a vesical fistula is suspected; the surgeon can then look for blue-tinged vaginal or rectal discharge (Chapron et al, 1995; Ostrzenski and Ostrzenski, 1998).

The intraoperative diagnosis of a bladder injury can be followed by laparoscopic repair: suturing with absorbable suture, closing the defect with a laparoscopic stapler, or using preformed suture loops to encircle and secure the cystotomy (Poffenberger, 1996; Ostrzenski and Ostrzenski, 1998). More extensive defects may require open incisional repair.

When bladder injury is diagnosed postoperatively, the surgeon must first determine whether the drainage is extraperitoneal or intraperitoneal. Extraperitoneal injury without any complicating additional problems may be treated by simple placement of a transurethral indwelling Foley catheter. Intraperitoneal drainage is an indication for subsequent laparoscopic or open repair.

Prevention of bladder injury requires preoperative placement of a Foley catheter. Strict adherence to basic laparoscopic principles remains the hallmark of uncomplicated laparoscopic procedure; in this regard, avoidance of excessive coagulation near the bladder and dissection with exact knowledge of bladder anatomy (urachus, medial umbilical, and vesicocervical ligaments) are key.

Ureteral Injury. Ureteral injury is usually a result of thermal damage caused by dissection using monopolar electrocautery in the immediate vicinity of the ureter. Its incidence in laparoscopic hysterectomy is 1%; it may also occur during laparoscopic ablation of endometriosis and tubal ligation and has been reported during pelvic lymphadenectomy and laparoscopic radical prostatectomy (Baumann et al, 1988; Grainger et al, 1990; Poffenberger, 1996; Liu et al, 1997; Ostrzenski and Ostrzenski, 1998; Guillonneau et al, 2002).

The intraoperative diagnosis is made by the astute laparoscopist when urine is welling up in the wound. However, if irrigation has been used during the procedure, this sign is invariably obscured. As opposed to a bladder injury, macroscopic hematuria or pneumaturia is distinctly unusual with this injury.

Typically, ureteral injuries remain unnoticed throughout the laparoscopic procedure. Within 2 to 3 days after surgery, patients may present with abdominal and/or flank pain, fever, signs of peritonitis, and leukocytosis (Grainger et al, 1990; Liu and McFadden, 2000).

Most of these diagnoses are made during the postoperative period when an intravenous pyelogram or abdominal/pelvic CT scan is ordered owing to the patient's complaint of flank pain, abdominal swelling, and/or the physical signs of urinary ascites. Depending on the function of the contralateral kidney and the amount of urine leakage, serum chemistries may reveal hyponatremia and, rarely, hyperkalemia with a mild elevation in the serum creatinine level.

If identified intraoperatively, the injury can be repaired laparoscopically. If the injury is due to mechanical trauma, simple closure of the defect can be accomplished with laparoscopic suturing techniques followed by stent placement. If the injury is due to monopolar electrosurgical current, then a formal resection of the affected area and an end-to-end spatulated ureteroureterostomy and stent placement are indicated; ureteral reimplantation is indicated if the level of injury is at the ureterovesical junction. This can be done laparoscopically but usually will require conversion to an open procedure. An indwelling ureteral stent is placed.

If the problem is detected in the postoperative period, the first step is to place an indwelling ureteral stent and a bladder drainage catheter. Once a cystogram reveals reflux without extravasation, the bladder drainage catheter can be removed. The stent is left in place for 6 to 8 weeks. Careful follow-up is necessary to rule out the development of a ureteral stricture that may require endourologic or formal surgical repair.

Prevention of this injury again harkens back to the importance of the surgeon's knowledge of laparoscopic anatomy and the course of the ureter with regard to its topographic relation to other anatomic structures (medial umbilical ligament, round ligament or vas deferens, and common iliac artery). During dissection, the use of monopolar electrosurgical coagulation current should be used with great discretion around the ureter. In particular, a "cutting" rather than "coagulation" mode should be used whenever possible; when employing "coagulation" current the wattage should not exceed 30 watts. In addition, fine-tipped electrosurgical instruments should be employed, and the duration of discharge should be brief (i.e., multiple short bursts of current rather than a continuous 2- to 5-second discharge).

Pancreatic Injury. Injury to the pancreas during left sided laparoscopic adrenalectomy or radical nephrectomy is most commonly associated with mechanical retraction. The tail of the pancreas overlies the adrenal and may be injured during dissection of the medial aspect of the adrenal and the securing of the splenorenal ligament. The incidence of this complication is 2.1% for radical left nephrectomy and 8.6% for left adrenalectomy (Varkarakis et al, 2004). Of note, the diagnosis is rarely made intraoperatively; indeed, 75% of pancreatic injuries are diagnosed during the postoperative period. Among the few in whom this diagnosis is made intraoperatively, general surgery consultation can be obtained and the injury possibly repaired by freeing up the tail of the pancreas and excising the injured portion with an Endo-GIA stapler. However, more commonly the patient presents postoperatively with abdominal discomfort. Evaluation reveals an elevated serum lipase and amylase, as well as a leukocytosis. A CT scan reveals a fluid collection that can often be drained percutaneously. A nasogastric tube is placed and oral intake is stopped. When drainage drops below 50 mL/24 hr, the drain can be removed, followed by removal of the nasogastric tube and initiation of a low fat diet. Of note, the average hospital stay among patients with this complication was 18 days.

Prevention of this complication requires the surgeon to widely dissect the line of Toldt and the splenophrenic attachments. The latter are freed to the level of the diaphragm. The colon is broadly refelected from Gerota's fascia, and the splenocolic and splenorenal ligaments are divided. With these maneuvers, the spleen and colon rotate medially, carrying with them the tail of the pancreas, well away from the area of dissection.

Splenic Injury. The advent of laparoscopic surgery has been associated with a significant decrease in incidental splenectomy with a fall from 4.3% to only 1.5%. These injuries are invariably discovered intraoperatively and can effectively be treated with argon beam coagulation or with one of the newer hemostatic agents such as fibrin glue or thrombin-impregnated granules. Avoidance of this complication is best achieved by wide mobilization of the spleen during left radical/total nephrectomy. To this end the splenophrenic attachments as well as the splenocolic and splenorenal ligaments need to be divided. Retraction in the area of the spleen should never be on the spleen itself but beneath the area of the splenocolic ligament such that the retractor is placed on these thicker tissues (Cooper et al, 1996; Simon et al, 2004). Also, in this regard, the laparoscopic surgeon must be ever vigilant of the splenic vein. This often tortuous vein may run parallel and in close proximity to the upper pole of the left kidney.

Injury to Nerves. There is no problem more vexing to physician and patient alike than a postoperative nerve injury; a technically and surgically successful procedure is marred by an acute complication in a totally unrelated area. This problem is invariably due to patient positioning in combination with the duration of the procedure. The exact incidence of this problem is not known, but in a recent survey of neuromuscular injuries associated with laparoscopic urologic surgery completed by 18 urologists from 15 institutions in the United States, it was found that out of a total of 1651 procedures there were 46 neuromuscular injuries in 45 patients, or 2.7%. This included abdominal wall neuralgia (14), extremity sensory deficit (12), extremity motor deficit (8), clinical rhabdomyolysis (6), shoulder contusion (4), and back spasm (2) (Wolf et al, 2000). If the patient is inadequately positioned and/or padded, nerve damage may result owing to abnormal nerve stretching or compression. Among position-related nerve injuries, the brachial plexus appears to be most at risk. Injury may be inflicted in several ways: (1) abduction of the arm beyond 90 degrees, (2) extreme outward rotation of the head of the humerus, and (3) compression damage when shoulder braces are used in the Trendelenburg position, which pushes the clavicle into the retroclavicular space. Other nerves that can be affected by positioning include the femoral nerve, owing to extreme lateral rotation and abduction of the hip joint, and the sciatic nerve, owing to stretching along the superior leg when the patient is in the lateral decubitus position (Hershlag et al, 1990; Abdel-Meguid and Gomella, 1996). In addition, nerves may be injured during the surgery itself because of either direct mechanical injury or monopolar electrosurgical current. In this regard, the nerves most susceptible to damage in urologic laparoscopy are the obturator nerve during pelvic lymphadenectomy and the genitofemoral nerve during radical nephrectomy/nephroureterectomy.

The diagnosis is invariably made postoperatively. On awakening from anesthesia, the patient complains of weakness or inability to contract the affected musculature, paresthesias, and/or anesthesia of the innervated skin areas.

Mechanical or electrosurgical injury to a nerve during laparoscopy may be recognized intraoperatively. A common example is transection of the obturator nerve during pelvic lymphadenectomy. A neurosurgical consultation can be obtained, and the nerve can be repaired with 6-0 suture using an open or laparoscopic approach.

In contrast, nerve palsy owing to positioning is recognized only postoperatively, often in the postanesthesia recovery room or on the first postoperative day when the patient tries to ambulate. From both a medical and a legal standpoint, a neurology consultation should be obtained as soon as the patient calls the surgeon's attention to a possible nerve injury. Neurologic examination with possible nerve conduction studies to document acute damage is important. Physical therapy may facilitate recovery. However, recovery in these cases, if it does not occur within the first few postoperative days, is often slow, requiring months.

Prevention is paramount. A host of new advances in padding and table-mounted accessories are now available that when used appropriately can markedly decrease the incidence of iatrogenic neuromuscular injuries. Disposable foam padding has now been replaced by gel pads that are less bulky and provide superior cushioning (AliMed Inc., Dedham, MA). Indeed, in the supine position, pressures at the sacrum with a standard polyurethrane filled mattress are threefold higher than with a fluid-filled mattress. The former pressures are as high as 159 mm Hg, well in excess of the 20- to 60-mm Hg pressure found in the human capillaries (Keller et al, 2005). Table-mounted accessories for all major commercial operating room tables now exist that aid in safely and effectively positioning patients in the lateral decubitus position and in the prone position. Specifically, for lateral decubitus positioning the buttock and upper back can be supported by gel pad–reinforced stabilizer bars that mount on the side rails of the table. The entire bed and especially the kidney rest can also be covered with gel padding, and the upper arm can be supported on a table-mounted adjustable armboard. Special head supports are also available. If the arms are to be at the patient's side, they should be pronated to protect the brachial plexus. If the patient is to be in a lateral decubitus position, all bony prominences should be padded with additional gel pads (i.e., hip, knee, and ankle on the downside leg). Padding should also be placed beneath Velcro straps and tape, which may be used on the upside hip and shoulder. The kidney rest, if used, should be lowered after the pneumoperitoneum or retroperitoneum is obtained and trocars placed. Shoulder braces should not be used because of the risk of brachial plexus injury. Instead, a well-padded wide strap directly across the upper chest is an excellent way to secure the patient when in the extreme Trendelenburg position, which is often required during laparoscopic radical prostatectomy. Extreme abduction of the hip is also to be avoided. Padding must be checked each time the table position is changed. Lastly, as with all areas of laparoscopy, judicious use of coagulation current and knowledge of anatomy are key to avoiding direct nerve injury during the procedure.

Complications Related to Exiting the Abdomen

Bowel Entrapment. During removal of laparoscopic ports and release of the pneumoperitoneum, omentum or bowel may be entrapped at one of the port sites. If missed during the process of cannula removal, then in the early postoperative period, usually on the second or third postoperative day, the patient develops an ileus and point tenderness at the port site incision.

The treatment is laparoscopic. The pneumoperitoneum is reestablished via one of the unaffected port sites, and three ports are replaced: one for the camera and two for grasping forceps. The entrapped bowel is visualized, and an atraumatic bowel clamp is placed on the bowel on either side of the area of herniation. Once this is done, the skin sutures of the affected port site are carefully cut and the wound is opened; the surgeon manually reduces the bowel into the abdominal cavity. The bowel can then be carefully inspected; if it appears viable, which is usually the case, it can be left in place and the port site closed. Rarely is formal bowel resection and anastomosis required.

This particular problem is the result of a technical error. Indeed, most laparoscopic ports have a hole drilled into the side of the port, within a few millimeters of the end of the port's shaft. This hole equalizes the pressure in the port and the abdomen as the port is pulled out of the abdomen, thereby precluding any bowel being withdrawn with the port. Furthermore, if each port site is endoscopically inspected at the time of cannula removal, bowel or omentum that may have entered the port site can be readily identified and pulled back into the abdominal cavity. When the last endoscope-bearing port is removed, the assistant should pull up on the closure sutures or on a fascial clamp and the surgeon should back the cannula out of the wound and up onto the shaft of the endoscope so that the endoscope is the last thing to leave the abdomen. This maneuver, again, visually assures the surgeon that no bowel or omentum has entered the track of the final trocar.

Bleeding at the Sheath Site. This problem has been previously discussed under the heading of trocar placement. However, there are times when this problem does not become apparent until the end of the procedure due to tamponade from the trocar itself. Again, it is essential to inspect each trocar site at 5 mm Hg to rule out this problem. Its resolution and avoidance are as previously described.

Complications in the Early Postoperative Period

Acute Hydrocele. When significant amounts of irrigation fluid are used during a laparoscopic case in a male, it is not unusual for this fluid to accumulate in the scrotum if the patient has a patent processus vaginalis or a small hernia. The problem is usually not recognized until late in the first postoperative day when the patient is ambulating. The scrotum enlarges noticeably, and there may be dull, aching scrotal discomfort.

Direct visual inspection and transillumination suffice to make the diagnosis. If possible underlying testicular pathology is a concern, a scrotal ultrasound can be obtained.

Treatment of acute hydrocele is simply observation and scrotal support. Reabsorption of fluid occurs within a week.

Preventative effort with regard to this problem involves aspiration of irrigation fluid at the end of the procedure.

Scrotal and Abdominal Ecchymosis. This is another problem that may not become apparent until the second postoperative day. It is usually a result of delayed subcutaneous bleeding from one of the port sites. There are no specific symptoms, but the purplish discoloration of a large area of skin surrounding a port site is very disconcerting to the patient and family. Indeed, with pelvic ports, the discoloration in the male patient may involve the scrotum, too. There is no specific treatment other than observation and reassurance. The purplish discoloration of the skin eventually turns yellow and then disappears. The patient should be informed of these expected changes in color to preclude further alarm. The best method of prevention is to observe each port entry site after port removal to check for evidence of bleeding.

Pain. Pain may be localized or diffuse. If postoperative pain is limited to a port site, it may be secondary to herniation (immediate or late) or to infection (late). Localized pain combined with a subcutaneous bulge may indicate a rectus sheath hematoma, bleeding and hematoma formation at a port site, or a hernia. Pain at a port site without swelling may be due to a particularly broad fascial suture or palpation of the knot of a port site fascial suture in a thin patient. Early in the postoperative course, port site discomfort is to be expected; however, if it appears to be increasing on subsequent postoperative days, then herniation should be suspected.

Immediate, severe, diffuse abdominal pain may be related to the release of noxious material during the procedure (e.g., cyst fluid in patients with autosomal-dominant polycystic kidney disease) or to a bowel injury. Immediate postoperative scapular discomfort may be a result of the CO_2 pneumoperitoneum itself causing some irritation of the diaphragm; unfortunately, this discomfort may be sufficiently severe to mimic the symptoms of a pulmonary embolus. Of note is that this pain is invariably along the area of the right posterior shoulder region. Delayed diffuse abdominal discomfort and development of peritoneal signs or simply ongoing abdominal discomfort accompanied by low-grade fever may be due to an unsuspected bowel injury; usually, this is the result of a monopolar electrosurgical injury and may present as late as 18 days after the procedure. Of note, these patients may not have a leukocytosis; however, the differential usually shows a left shift.

The cause of localized pain can usually be discerned by the astute surgeon. A fascial knot or hematoma causing localized port site pain can be readily palpated; similarly, a port site hematoma is discernible by the firm mass it produces. When none of these signs is present in a patient complaining of localized pain over a port site, a hernia should be suspected; a CT scan readily reveals the diagnosis.

For diffuse pain, an associated low-grade fever and mild leukocytosis with a left shift are hallmarks of bowel injury. This is best diagnosed by a CT scan with oral contrast material and a repeat CT scan 6 to 8 hours later. If chest pain is present, an electrocardiogram plus cardiac enzymes as well as a spiral CT of the chest with intravenous contrast or ventilation/perfusion scan of the lungs plus arterial blood gas analy-

sis should be performed to rule out myocardial infarction and pulmonary embolism, respectively.

The treatment of localized pain is directed by the diagnosis. Thus, for localized pain owing to a hematoma or a fascial suture, time, reassurance, and a heating pad are all that is necessary. For a port site hernia, laparoscopic reduction, as previously described, is the next step. The treatment of diffuse pain is guided by the results of the CT scan. For suspected bowel injury, if it is early in the postoperative course (i.e., if the patient is still in the hospital), reexploration and surgical correction are indicated. If the bowel injury is detected late and the CT scan shows that it is already confined, then it can be managed as a closed fistula with observation and an elemental or parenteral diet; it often takes months for the problem to completely resolve when managed nonsurgically.

Prevention of most of these causes of postoperative pain requires a meticulous, careful inspection of the entire abdomen before ending the procedure. Various methods have been tried, with variable success, to decrease discomfort owing to the pneumoperitoneum; these have included placement of a drain to help expel all the CO_2, flushing of the abdomen with nitrous oxide at the end of the procedure to expel the CO_2 and replace it with a less irritating gas, and selective bathing of the surgical site with a solution of local anesthetic (e.g., bupivacaine).

Incisional Hernia. In adults, the occurrence of an incisional hernia is usually confined to port sites larger than 10 mm. However, in the pediatric population, this complication can occur even with 5-mm ports. The patient usually complains of localized discomfort accompanied by nausea and signs of an ileus. Rarely, diffuse abdominal pain and/or signs of a complete bowel obstruction may be present. On examination, there is tenderness and, at times, swelling overlying a port site. A plain film of the abdomen may show an ileus pattern; however, the definitive study is an abdominal CT scan, which can actually reveal the bowel protruding above the fascial level.

Laparoscopic repair with dissection of the hernia and subsequent intra-abdominal closure can be attempted. The method for performing this procedure has already been described. In complicated cases in which a strangulated hernia is suspected or confirmed laparoscopically, open surgical repair is indicated.

This problem is most easily avoided by performing a meticulous fascial suture closure of all bladed trocar entry sites equal to or larger than 10 mm in all adults. This should always be done under direct endoscopic monitoring. In children, it is advisable to perform fascial closure of any port site 5 mm or larger. The fascial layer is usually closed with an absorbable 0-0 suture as previously described. For patients in whom only nonbladed trocars have been used, fascial closure is indicated only of the midline ports or any port site that has been stretched (e.g., passage of a LapSac entrapment sack). Indeed, some authors recommend no closure even of midline nonbladed trocar sites. Although there has been one report of a hernia developing after use of a nonbladed trocar, this is distinctly rare (Lowry et al, 2003). Indeed, the incidence of postoperative hernia formation has been noted to fall from 1.8% to 0.19% for use of bladed and

nonbladed larger trocars, respectively (Boike et al, 1995; Hashizume and Sugimachi, 1997; Thomas et al, 2003). **Of note, with midline hand-assist approaches, a higher incidence of hernia formation has been identified than would otherwise be expected: 4% to 7.3%. As such, some authors have recommended closure of this midline incision with interrupted nonabsorbable suture rather than the more rapid, running, absorbable closure** (Troxel and Das, 2005).

Deep Venous Thrombosis. Although it seems reasonable to expect decreased venous return and, hence, increased stasis with concomitant higher risk of deep venous thrombosis in patients undergoing laparoscopy, this is not the case. Indeed, there is no evidence that this complication occurs more often during laparoscopic procedures versus open incisional surgery (Abdel-Meguid and Gomella, 1996).

Signs of deep venous thrombosis include localized calf tenderness with associated swelling. However, most patients with postoperative deep venous thrombosis have a subclinical course. Indeed, unfortunately, the most common clinical scenario is detection of a deep venous thrombosis only after a patient has developed a pulmonary embolus, after which impedance plethysmography and/or Doppler ultrasonography of the legs is obtained.

Treatment is immediate anticoagulation, initially with heparin and then with warfarin. In patients with a pulmonary embolus who are not candidates for anticoagulation, a caval filter is placed under radiographic control.

The problem can be avoided to some extent through the use of pneumatic sequential compression devices and/or mini-dose heparin and early postoperative ambulation. Currently the American College of Chest Physicians recommends either pneumatic compression stockings or heparin (i.e., mini-dose heparin or low-molecular-weight heparin) for all major urologic procedures (Goldhaber, 2004). Pneumatic compression stockings should be placed preoperatively and continued for 48 to 72 hours postoperatively. Additionally, in morbidly obese patients or in individuals at high risk for thrombosis, the addition of unfractionated perioperative heparin (5000 units 2 hours preoperatively and then every 12 hours postoperatively) has also been recommended (Clagett et al, 1995; Capan and Miller, 1999). However, **with specific respect to upper retroperitoneal (renal/adrenal/ureter) laparoscopic procedures at least one recent study by Montgomery and Wolf indicated that sequential pneumatic compressive stockings (SCD) provide equivalent DVT prophylaxis compared with subcutaneous fractionated heparin (FH) and that the use of FH may increase the incidence of hemorrhagic complications.** Three-hundred and forty-four patients (172 in each group) nonrandomly received FH or SCD as prophylaxis for deep venous thrombosis beginning on the day of surgery. In both groups the rate of thrombotic complication was 1.2%. The rate of hemorrhagic complication was 9.3% in the FH group, of which 7.0% were considered major. The hemorrhagic complication rate was only 3.5% in the SCD group, with 2.9% considered major ($P = .045$). **Thus, after urologic laparoscopy of the upper retroperitoneum, subcutaneous fractionated heparin is associated with increased hemorrhagic complications, without a reduction in thrombotic complications, compared with sequential compression devices** (Montgomery and Wolf, 2005); however, it must be stressed that this was a nonrandomized study obtained from a prospective database augmented by retrospective chat review.

Wound Infections. Superficial wound infections may occur at any of the port entry sites. This problem usually presents as local tenderness, redness, and swelling; rarely, it is accompanied by a low-grade fever. Incision and drainage of the port site are both diagnostic and therapeutic; antibiotic therapy is routinely administered.

Prevention of this complication is similar to open surgery and includes attention to antiseptic preparation and sterile draping of the abdominal wall, irrigation of each port site at the end of the procedure, and meticulous closure of the wound. Overall, this is a rare complication with standard laparoscopy. However, with the hand-assist approach a higher incidence of wound infections has been noted. In a recent report, the postoperative wound infection rate at the hand-assist site was 9% (Nelson and Wolf, 2002).

Rhabdomyolysis. Rhabdomyolysis is a devastating complication after laparoscopic surgery. The exact incidence of this problem is not known, but in a recent survey of neuromuscular injuries associated with laparoscopic urologic surgery completed by 18 urologists from 15 institutions in the United States it was found that out of a total of 1651 procedures there were 6 cases of clinical rhabdomyolysis (Wolf et al, 2000). In a more recent study, it was estimated that the occurrence of this problem among patients undergoing retroperitoneal laparoscopic procedures (e.g., renal, ureteral, adrenal) was 1% (Reisiger et al, 2005). Rhabdomyolysis is invariably associated with male patients undergoing laparoscopic renal procedures in excess of 5 hours. In most of these cases, egg crate foam has been used for padding and the kidney rest has been employed for the entire case.

The problem presents immediately in the postanesthesia recovery room with the patient complaining of severe pain in the downside hip area. Brown urine may also be noted. The serum creatine phosphokinase will invariably exceed 5000 units/dL. The treatment is hydration and alkalinization; these maneuvers are undertaken to try to prevent subsequent renal failure. The more difficult and ominous problem is that of long-term disability caused by the muscle necrosis. Extended physical therapy is often required.

Prevention of this problem is essential. This can to some extent be done by avoiding use of the kidney rest or employing it for only the earliest part of the case (i.e., less than an hour). Use of gel or fluid padding on the operative table (see section on "Patient Positioning and Draping") may also be helpful, along with avoiding any hypotension during the procedure (Cadeddu et al, 2001; Kuang et al, 2002; Parsons et al, 2004; Reisiger et al, 2005).

Late Postoperative Complications

Complications beyond the 3-week postoperative period are rare. These include primarily lymphatic complications and incisional hernia. The latter has been addressed in the prior discussion because it can also appear as an early postoperative complications.

Lymphocele Formation. Lymphocele formation is most commonly associated with pelvic procedures, such as pelvic lymph node dissection (1.3% incidence) (Kavoussi et al, 1993) or with renal transplantation. The lymphocele may take weeks to develop and may occur despite a transperitoneal approach. Presentation may be by a mass effect, but the astute clinician should realize that it may also present due to local compression causing lower extremity edema and, in rare cases, venous thrombosis and pulmonary embolism.

The lymphocele is diagnosed readily by CT. Treatment is immediate percutaneous drainage. Sclerosant therapy can be used to treat the lymphocele; however, if unsuccessful or if the lymphocele is not amenable to percutaneous drainage, then a transperitoneal laparoscopic marsupialization procedure is usually successful. At the time of the procedure, a tag of omentum can be placed into the opening made in the lymphocele to try to prevent closure of the opening and recurrence.

Prevention of lymphocele formation requires marked attention to clipping suspected lymphatic structures. Electrocoagulation does not work to seal lymphatics. Similarly, the impact of bipolar or harmonic devices on lymphatic patency is unreported to date.

Chylous Ascites. After left-sided retroperitoneal surgery (i.e., left radical nephrectomy, donor nephrectomy, left-sided retroperitoneal lymph node dissection), the patient may return complaining of a distended abdomen. Although this complaint is commonplace in the initial few days after a laparoscopic procedure, due to the pneumoperitoneum, irrigation fluid, and/or ileus, it is distinctly rare late in the patient's course. There is no associated fever; pain or bowel dysfunction and routine laboratory studies are within normal limits. If the suspicion is high for chylous ascites, one may opt to simply place the patient on a low-fat, medium-chain triglyceride diet and observe. Usually the condition is self-limited and resolves without any intervention.

If the presentation is not straightforward, then an abdominal CT will reveal the underlying problem and diagnose the presence of ascites. It tapped, the fluid should be sent for culture, complete blood cell count, triglycerides, cholesterol, and electrolytes. The chylous ascitic fluid may well have elevations in the level of lymphocytes, cholesterol, and triglycerides, the latter two being particularly more likely if following a fatty meal.

Treatment is usually dietary as previously noted. One may also consider giving somatostatin (Leibovitch et al, 2002). In the rare situation, where the fluid does not resolve with these conservative measures or if the patient is symptomatic, the fluid can be tapped once or twice. If it continues to accumulate, then an open or laparoscopic exploration is undertaken; before the procedure, the patient should be given a "fatty" meal or an intravenous load of hyperalimental lipids, which should create a whitish discoloration of the lymphatic fluid and make the injured lymphatic chain more visible. Once identified, the leaking lymphatic channel is dissected and secured with either suture or clips (Molina et al, 2003).

Prevention of this type of problem is extremely difficult because the lymphatics are not readily visible during the procedure. In addition, with the recent advent of avoiding clips around the renal hilum, the problem may become more prevalent. To date, instances of post-laparoscopic chylous ascites have been cited only sparingly in the literature (Leibovitch et al, 2002; Molina et al, 2003). However, we believe that because the condition is usually self-limited and responds well to dietary measures, it is likely underreported.

LIMITATIONS AND ADVANTAGES OF TRANSPERITONEAL VS. EXTRAPERITONEAL APPROACH TO THE FLANK AND PELVIS
Transperitoneal Laparoscopy vs. Retroperitoneoscopy

Limitations. Retroperitoneoscopy is associated with unique anatomic orientation and a relatively restricted initial working area compared with transperitoneal laparoscopy. This results in a steeper learning curve with the former technique. Moreover, the fact that a comparatively limited space is available necessitates precise accuracy regarding the strategic placement of ports. The degree of technical difficulty increases in the presence of large-sized specimens. Additionally, retroperitoneoscopic entrapment of these larger specimens may be difficult. The latter problem can be overcome by laparoscopically creating an intentional peritoneotomy at the end of the procedure to allow entrapment of the specimen within the larger peritoneal cavity. Laparoscopic reconstruction and intracorporeal suturing are technically demanding procedures; in the retroperitoneal space, reconstruction can be more challenging compared with transperitoneal laparoscopy.

If a patient has a history of prior open retroperitoneal surgery, subsequent attempts at retroperitoneoscopy should be approached with extreme caution. However, as mentioned earlier in this chapter, prior percutaneous renal procedures do not necessarily constitute a contraindication to subsequent retroperitoneoscopy. Lastly, of interest is an increase in pulmonary complications after retroperitoneoscopy versus transperitoneal laparoscopy (see earlier).

Advantages. With retroperitoneoscopy, morbidity that is usually associated with the transperitoneal approach is commonly avoided (Kavoussi et al, 1993). The risks of inadvertent bowel injury and postoperative ileus are minimized, although not eliminated. This results in a slightly more rapid postoperative recovery. During retroperitoneoscopy and extraperitoneoscopy, the bowel can be effectively and safely retracted within its peritoneal cover. Although out of sight, the bowel should never be out of mind, because bowel injuries can still occur. Transperitoneal laparoscopy may be associated with an increased incidence of postoperative shoulder-tip pain, a feature rarely associated with retroperitoneoscopy. In addition, extraperitoneoscopy and retroperitoneoscopy are associated with a significantly lower incidence of postoperative trocar site hernias.

A significant benefit of this technique is that a previous transperitoneal procedure does not preclude the performance of this form of laparoscopy. Also, rapid and direct access to the renal hilum is a hallmark of retroperitoneoscopy. Furthermore, if a partial nephrectomy is planned, it may be more effective to approach a posterior tumor from the retroperitoneal approach whereas anterior tumors are often more easily approached from the transperitoneal approach.

Transperitoneal vs. Extraperitoneal Pelvic Surgery

The transperitoneal approach to the pelvis offers easy access to all areas of the pelvic cavity after which the space of Retzius, iliac/obturator fossa, or the rectovesical space is entered directly through the peritoneum. Working space is maximized since the peritoneum does not limit camera or instrument motion once it is incised. The potential down sides associated with this approach, however, are that it is possible to cause mechanical or thermal injury to the bowel and it may be necessary to utilize more extreme Trendelenburg positioning or additional retraction of the bowel to prevent it from impinging on the operative field. The possibility of prolonged ileus has also been suggested; however, in the largest prospective study to date comparing 165 transperitoneal versus 165 extraperitoneal laparoscopic radical prostatectomy patients, Ruiz and colleagues (2004) did not find significant differences between the two groups in terms of hospital stay or medical and surgical complications. Operative time was half an hour shorter in the extraperitoneal group (220.0 min vs. 248.5 min; $P < .0001$), but there was also a trend toward higher positive margins in patients with pT2 (organ confined) cancers in the extraperitoneal group (17.0% vs. 13.0%; $P = 0.42$). In another study by Erdogru and associates (2004), patients were matched with regard to important preoperative attributes; the authors found no significant difference between the extraperitoneal and transperitoneal approaches regarding all important parameters. One undeniable advantage in favor of the extraperitoneal approach is that it avoids the necessity of lysis of adhesions in patients who have had prior abdominal surgery. In contrast, for patients who have had prior laparoscopic inguinal hernia repair, a transperitoneal approach is more advantageous.

In summary, for most cases there does not seem to be a clear advantage to using a transperitoneal versus extraperitoneal approach for laparoscopic pelvic surgery. In selected cases described earlier there may be advantages of one approach over the other. The usual guide is that of surgeon preference.

SUMMARY

Yesterday's humor is today's reality. Cartoons in the 1990s often depicted several surgeons standing around an operating table on which was a patient in whom numerous laparoscopic ports had been placed. The caption was "Can anyone open?" Although this concern has been a rallying cry for the maximally invasive surgeon, the less invasive surgeon sees this as a manifestation of the progress that has occurred in the past 15 years. Laparoscopic procedures unthinkable in early 1990 are now routine; open procedures unbearable are now passé. To be sure, the price will be less proficient open surgeons. The benefit will be more proficient laparoscopic surgeons who can handle any procedure and any complication without the massive incisions of yore. We would hope that in the near future a similar cartoon may show a group of urologists in an image-guidance suite or in an office gathered around a patient with the caption: "Can anyone do laparoscopy?" Such should be the final endpoint of our surgical and pharmacologic paths of discovery. At that point Osler's 20th century admonition, "Diseases that harm require treatments that harm less" will be truly fulfilled. We are as yet still on the bridge to the future.

Acknowledgment

The authors would like to acknowledge the contributions to this chapter of Drs. Inderbir S. Gill, MD, MCh; Kurt Kerbl, MD; and Anoop M. Meraney, MD. All were among the authors of this chapter when it first appeared in the eighth edition of Campbell's Urology. Many of their original thoughts and contributions are part of the current text.

SUGGESTED READINGS

Adams JB, Micali S, Moore RG, et al: Complications of extraperitoneal balloon dilation. J Endourol 1996;10:375-378.

Ahlering TE, Woo D, Eichel L, et al: Robot-assisted versus open radical prostatectomy: A comparison of one surgeon's outcomes. Urology 2004;63:819-822.

Cadeddu JA, Wolfe JS Jr, Nakada SY, et al: Complications of laparoscopic procedures after concentrated training in urological laparoscopy. J Urol 2001;166:2109-2111.

Dunn MD, Portis AJ, Shalhav AL, et al: Laparoscopic vs. open radical nephrectomy: A 9-year experience. J Urol 2000;164:1153-1159.

Elashry OM, Wolf JS, Nakada SY, et al: Comparative clinical study of port closure techniques following laparoscopic surgery. J Am Coll Surg 1996;183:335-344.

Erdogru T, Teber D, Frede T, et al: Comparison of transperitoneal and extraperitoneal laparoscopic radical prostatectomy using match-pair analysis. Eur Urol 2004;46:312-319; discussion 320.

Landman J, Kerbl K, Rehman J, et al: Evaluation of a vessel sealing system, bipolar electrosurgery, harmonic scalpel, titanium clips, endoscopic gastrointestinal anastomosis vascular staples and sutures for arterial and venous ligation in a porcine model. J Urol 2003;169:697-700.

Leighton T, Liu S, Bongard F: Comparative cardiopulmonary effects of carbon dioxide versus helium pneumoperitoneum. Surgery 1993;113:527-531.

Mertens zur Borg IR, Lim A, Verbrugge SJ, et al: Effect of intra-abdominal pressure elevation and positioning on hemodynamic responses during carbon dioxide pneumoperitoneum for laparoscopic donor nephrectomy: A prospective controlled clinical study. Surg Endosc 2004;18:919-923.

Reisiger K, Landman J, Kibel A, et al: Laparoscopic renal surgery and the risk of rhabdomyolysis: diagnosis and treatment. Urology 2005;66:29-35.

Wolf JS: Tips and tricks for hand-assisted laparoscopy. AUA Update Series 2005;24:10-15.

SECTION IV

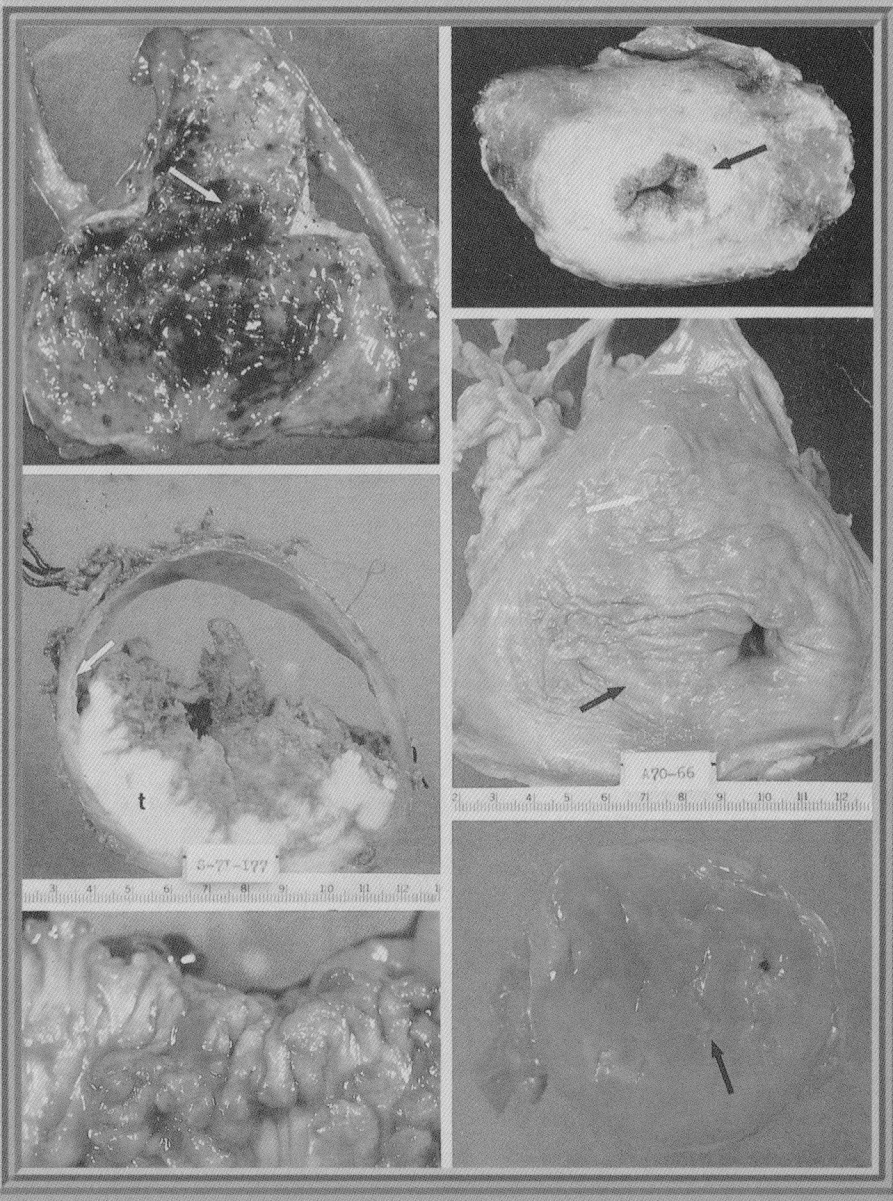

INFECTIONS AND INFLAMMATION

8 Infections of the Urinary Tract

ANTHONY J. SCHAEFFER, MD •
EDWARD M. SCHAEFFER, MD, PhD

Urinary tract infections (UTIs) are common, affect men and women of all ages, and vary dramatically in their presentation and sequelae. They are a common cause of morbidity and can lead to significant mortality. Although the urinary tract is normally free of bacterial growth, bacteria that generally ascend from the rectal reservoir may cause UTIs. When bacterial virulence increases or host defense mechanisms decrease, bacterial inoculation, colonization, and infection of the urinary tract occur. Careful diagnosis and treatment result in successful resolution of infections in most instances. A better understanding of the pathogenesis of UTI and the role of host and bacterial factors has improved the ability to identify patients at risk and prevent or minimize sequelae. Clinical manifestations can vary from asymptomatic bacterial colonization of the bladder to irritative symptoms such as frequency and urgency associated with bacterial infection; upper tract infections associated with fever, chills, and flank pain; and bacteremia associated with severe morbidity, including sepsis and death. New antimicrobial agents that achieve high urinary and tissue levels, that can be administered orally, and that are not nephrotoxic have significantly reduced the need for hospitalization for severe infection. Shorter-course therapy and prophylactic antimicrobial agents have reduced the morbidity and cost associated with recurrent cystitis in women. Although the vast majority of patients respond promptly and are cured by therapy, early identification and treatment of patients with complicated infections that place them at significant risk remains a clinical challenge to urologists.

DEFINITIONS

UTI is an inflammatory response of the urothelium to bacterial invasion that is usually associated with bacteriuria and pyuria.

***Bacteriuria* is the presence of bacteria in the urine, which is normally free of bacteria.** It has been assumed to be a valid indicator of either bacterial colonization or infection of the urinary tract. Although this is usually true, studies in animals (Hultgren et al, 1985; Mulvey et al, 1998) and humans (Elliott et al, 1985) have indicated that bacteria may be in the urothelium in the absence of bacteriuria. Alternatively, bacteriuria may represent bacterial contamination of an abacteriuric specimen during collection.

The possibility of contamination increases as the reliability of the collection technique decreases from suprapubic aspiration to catheterization to voided specimens. The term *significant bacteriuria* has a clinical connotation and is used to describe the number of bacteria in a suprapubically aspirated, catheterized, or voided specimen that exceeds the number usually caused by bacterial contamination of the skin, the

223

urethra, or the prepuce or introitus, respectively. Hence, it represents a UTI.

Bacteriuria can be *symptomatic* or *asymptomatic*. When it is detected by population studies (screening surveys), *screening* bacteriuria is a more precise and descriptive term than asymptomatic bacteriuria, especially because the latter term is clinically useful for describing the presence or absence of symptoms in an individual patient.

***Pyuria*, the presence of white blood cells (WBCs) in the urine, is generally indicative of infection and an inflammatory response of the urothelium to the bacterium.** Bacteriuria without pyuria is generally indicative of bacterial colonization without infection of the urinary tract. Pyuria without bacteriuria warrants evaluation for tuberculosis, stones, or cancer.

Infections are often defined clinically by their presumed site of origin.

Cystitis describes a clinical syndrome of dysuria, frequency, urgency, and occasionally suprapubic pain. These symptoms, although generally indicative of bacterial cystitis, may also be associated with infection of the urethra or vagina or noninfectious conditions such as interstitial cystitis, bladder carcinoma, or calculi. Conversely, patients may be asymptomatic and have infection of the bladder and possibly the upper urinary tract.

***Acute pyelonephritis* is a clinical syndrome of chills, fever, and flank pain that is accompanied by bacteriuria and pyuria, a combination that is reasonably specific for an acute bacterial infection of the kidney.** The term should not be used if flank pain is absent. It may have no morphologic or functional components detectable by routine clinical modalities. There may be serious difficulties in diagnosing spinal cord–injured and elderly patients who may be unable to localize the site of their discomfort.

Chronic pyelonephritis describes a shrunken, scarred kidney, diagnosed by morphologic, radiologic, or functional evidence of renal disease that may be postinfectious but is frequently not associated with UTI. Bacterial infection of the kidney may cause a *focal, coarse scar* in the renal cortex overlying a calyx, almost always accompanied by some calyceal distortion (Fig. 8–1), which can be detected radiographically or by gross examination of the kidney. Less commonly, renal scarring from infection can result in atrophic pyelonephritis or generalized thinning of the renal cortex, with a small kidney appearing radiographically similar to one with postobstructive atrophy (Fig. 8–2).

UTIs may also be described in terms of the anatomic or functional status of the urinary tract and the health of the host.

Uncomplicated describes an infection in a healthy patient with a structurally and functionally normal urinary tract. The majority of these patients are women with isolated or recurrent bacterial cystitis or acute pyelonephritis, and the infecting pathogens are usually susceptible to and eradicated by a short course of inexpensive oral antimicrobial therapy.

*A **complicated*** infection is associated with factors that increase the chance of acquiring bacteria and decrease the efficacy of therapy (Table 8–1). **The urinary tract is functionally or structurally abnormal, the host is compromised, and/or the bacteria have increased virulence or antimicrobial resistance. The majority of these patients are men.**

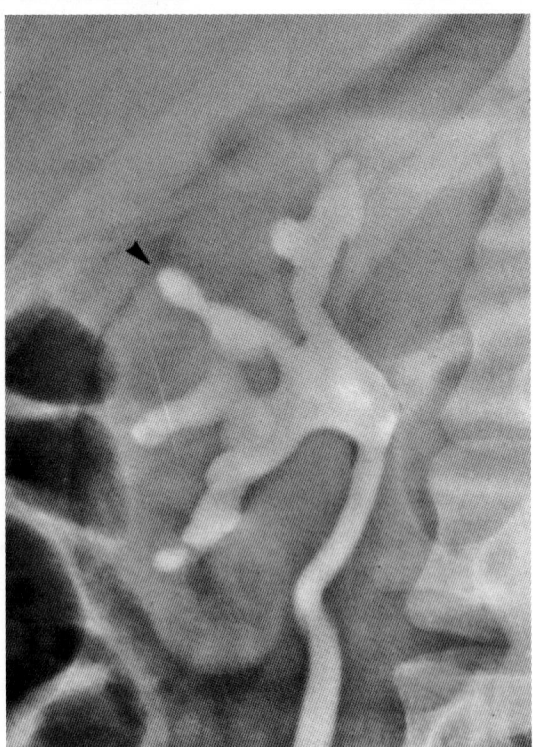

Figure 8–1. Excretory urogram (IVU) demonstrates focal, coarse scarring in the right kidney of an 18-year-old girl with a history of many recurrent fevers between 2 months and 2 years of age. A cystogram when the patient was 2 years old established an atrophic left kidney with marked reflux up to the left kidney and slight reflux up to the right kidney. IVU at the age of 6 years established severe atrophy of the left kidney. She had no infections between the ages of 6 and 15 years. Several reinfections occurred at the age of 15 years, and they ceased with prophylactic therapy. Her blood pressure has remained normal, and her serum creatinine level was 0.9 mg/dL at the age of 18 years. At 21 years of age she stopped antimicrobial prophylaxis for 18 months without infections or introital colonization with Enterobacteriaceae. Note that all calyces are blunted and that one extends to the capsule (*arrowhead*) because of atrophy of the overlying cortex.

Table 8–1. **Factors That Suggest Complicated UTI**
Functional or anatomic abnormality of urinary tract
Male gender
Pregnancy
Elderly
Diabetes
Immunosuppression
Childhood UTI
Recent antimicrobial agent use
Indwelling urinary catheter
Urinary tract instrumentation
Hospital-acquired infection
Symptoms for more than 7 days at presentation

Reprinted from Schaeffer AJ: Urinary tract infections. In Gillenwater JY, et al (eds): Adult and Pediatric Urology. Philadelphia, Lippincott Williams & Wilkins, 2002, p 212.

Renal diseases that reduce the concentrating ability of the kidney or neurologic conditions that alter bladder-emptying capabilities are commonly encountered functional abnormalities. Examples of anatomic abnormalities include obstruction associated with calculi or enlargement of the prostate or congenital or acquired sites of residual urine, such as calyceal or

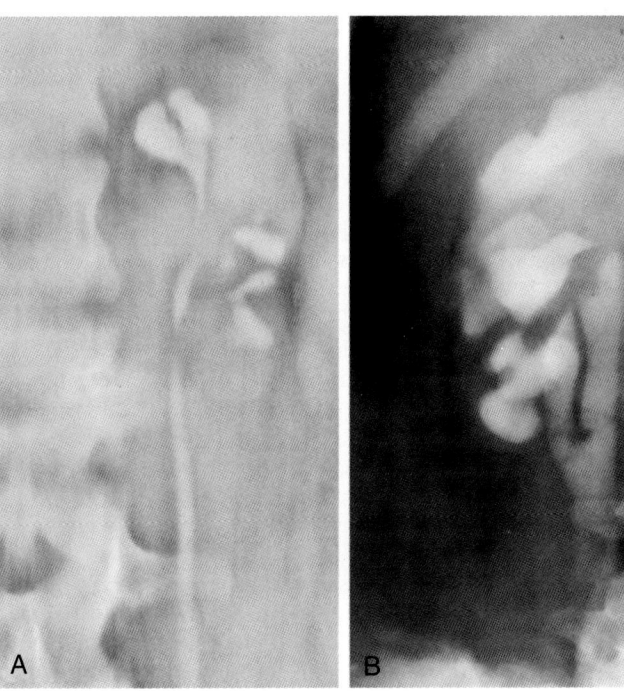

Figure 8–2. **A,** IVU of the contralateral left kidney from the same patient as in Figure 8–1. The severe pyelonephritic atrophy, undoubtedly caused by febrile urinary infections during early infancy with reflux into different segments of the kidney, produced irregular cortical scarring. Note how all the calyces extend to the capsule with irregular, intervening areas of cortex. **B,** Pyelonephritic atrophy, suggestive of postobstructive atrophy, in a 20-year-old woman with spina bifida, neurogenic bladder, and many episodes of fever and bacteriuria in early childhood. Observe the uniform, regular atrophy of the renal cortex that suggests reflux of bacteria simultaneously into virtually all nephrons. This type of pyelonephritic atrophy is uncommon compared with that shown in **A** and is characteristic of obstruction with superimposed infection.

bladder diverticula. A complicated infection is frequently caused by bacteria that have increased virulence and are resistant to many antimicrobial agents.

Chronic is a poor term that should be avoided in the context of UTIs, except for chronic bacterial prostatitis, because the duration of the infection is not defined.

UTIs may also be defined by their relationship to other UTIs.

A *first* or *isolated* infection is one that occurs in an individual who has never had a UTI or has one remote from a previous UTI.

An *unresolved* infection is one that has not responded to antimicrobial therapy.

A *recurrent* infection is one that occurs after documented, successful resolution of an antecedent infection.

The term *reinfection* describes a new event associated with reintroduction of bacteria into the urinary tract from outside.

Bacterial persistence **refers to a recurrent UTI caused by the same bacteria reemerging from a focus within the urinary tract, such as an infectious stone or the prostate.** *Relapse* is frequently used interchangeably. These definitions require careful clinical and bacteriologic assessment and are important because they influence the type and extent of the patient's evaluation and treatment.

Prophylactic antimicrobial therapy **is the prevention of reinfections of the urinary tract by the administration of antimicrobial drugs.** If the term is used correctly in reference to the urinary tract, it can be assumed that bacteria have been eliminated before prophylaxis is begun. **Surgical antimicrobial prophylaxis entails treatment with an antimicrobial agent before and for a** *limited* **time after a procedure to prevent local or systemic postprocedural infections.**

Suppressive antimicrobial therapy **is the suppression of a focus of bacterial persistence that cannot be eradicated.** A low, nightly dosage of an antimicrobial agent usually results in the urine showing no growth, as in the case of a small infection stone or in a bacterial prostatitis caused by *Escherichia coli.* Suppressive is also a useful term when recurrent acute symptoms are prevented in a poor-risk patient, such as one with a large staghorn infection calculus, in whom the antimicrobial agent reduces but does not eliminate the bacteria in the urine.

Domiciliary **or** *outpatient UTIs* occur in patients who are not hospitalized or institutionalized at the time they become infected. **The infections are generally caused by common bowel bacteria** (e.g., Enterobacteriaceae or *Enterococcus faecalis*) that are susceptible to most antimicrobial agents.

Nosocomial **or** *health care–associated UTIs* **occur in patients who are hospitalized or institutionalized,** and these are caused by *Pseudomonas* and other more antimicrobial-resistant strains.

KEY POINTS: DEFINITIONS

- Infection of the urinary tract occurs when bacterial virulence increases and/or host defense mechanisms decrease.

- The majority of patients respond promptly to short courses of antimicrobial therapy.

- Early identification and treatment of complicated UTIs is essential to prevent major sequelae or death.

INCIDENCE AND EPIDEMIOLOGY

UTIs are considered to be the most common bacterial infection. They account for more than 7 million visits to physicians' offices and necessitate or complicate over 1 million office visits and 1 million emergency department visits, resulting in 100,000 hospitalizations annually (Patton et al, 1991; Hooton and Stamm, 1997; Foxman et al, 2000). **They account for 1.2% of all office visits by women and 0.6% of all office visits by men** (Schappert, 1997).

The overall prevalence of bacteriuria in women has been estimated at 3.5%, with prevalence generally increasing with age in a linear trend (Evans et al, 1978). Surveys screening for bacteriuria have shown that about 1% of schoolgirls (aged 5 to 14 years) (Kunin et al, 1962) have bacteriuria and that this figure increases to about 4% by young adulthood and then by an additional 1% to 2% per decade of age (Fig. 8–3). **Nearly 30% of women will have had a symptomatic UTI requiring antimicrobial therapy by age 24, and almost half of all women will experience a UTI during their lifetime.** The prevalence of bacteriuria in young women is 30 times more than in men. However, **with increasing age, the ratio of women to men with bacteriuria progressively decreases. At least 20% of women and 10% of men older than 65 years have bacteriuria** (Boscia and Kaye, 1987).

The incidence of bacteriuria also increases with institutionalization or hospitalization and concurrent disease (Sourander, 1966). In a study of women and men older than 68 years, Boscia and colleagues (Boscia and Kaye, 1987) found that 24% of functionally impaired nursing home residents had bacteriuria compared with 12% of healthy domiciliary subjects (Boscia et al, 1986). UTIs account for approximately 38% of the 2 million nosocomial infections each year (Sedor and Mulholland, 1999). Greater than 80% of nosocomial UTIs are secondary to an indwelling urethral catheter (Sedor and Mulholland, 1999). The incidence of UTIs is also increased during pregnancy and in patients with spinal cord injuries, diabetes, multiple sclerosis, and human immunodeficiency virus (HIV) infection/acquired immunodeficiency syndrome (AIDS).

The financial impact of community-acquired UTIs is nearly $1.6 billion in the United States alone (Foxman, 2002); the annual cost of nosocomial UTIs has been estimated to range from between $515 million and $548 million (Jarvis, 1996).

Little is known about the natural history of untreated bacteriuria in women because most are treated when they are diagnosed, but a few studies in which treatment with antimicrobial agents is compared with placebo have been done. These show that 57% to 80% of bacteriuric women who are untreated or treated with placebo clear their infections spontaneously (Guttmann, 1973; Mabeck, 1972). Mabeck (1972) found that 8 of 53 bacteriuric women placed on placebo needed treatment with an antimicrobial agent because of symptoms, but 32 of the remaining 45 women cleared without treatment within a month, and 43 of the 45 had spontaneously cleared of bacteriuria within 5 months; only 2 women remained persistently bacteriuric.

Once a patient has an infection, he or she is likely to develop subsequent infections. Many adults had UTIs as children, underscoring the importance of genotypic factors in UTIs (Gillenwater et al, 1979). Of 45 women with untreated UTIs whose infection cleared, 20 (46%) had recurrences within a year (Mabeck, 1972).

When women with recurrent bacteriuria were followed after treatment, about one sixth (37 of 219) had a very high recurrence rate (2.6 infections per year), whereas the remaining women had a recurrence rate of only 0.32 per year (Mabeck, 1972). Similar separation was seen in a prospective study, in which only 28.6% of 60 women who experienced their first symptomatic UTI had recurrent infections over the first 18 months of observation, as opposed to recurrences in 82.5% of 106 women who had had previous UTIs (Harrison et al, 1974). **Other investigators also have found that the probability of recurrent UTIs increases with the number of previous infections and decreases in inverse proportion to the elapsed time between the first and the second infections** (Mabeck, 1972). Of these recurrent infections, 71% to 73% are caused by reinfection with different organisms, rather than recurrence with the same organism (Mabeck, 1972; Guttmann, 1973).

Women with frequent reinfections have a rate of 0.13 to 0.25 UTIs per month (1.6 to 3.1 infections per year) when the infections are treated with antimicrobial agents (Mabeck, 1972; Guttmann, 1973; Kraft and Stamey, 1977; Vosti, 2002).

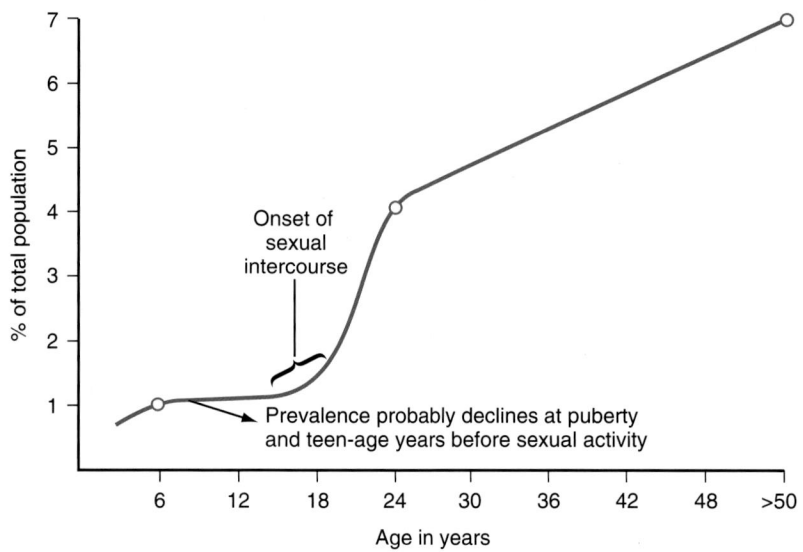

Figure 8–3. Prevalence of bacteriuria in females as a function of age. (From Stamey TA: The Prevention of Recurrent Urinary Infections. New York, Science and Medicine, 1973.)

In a prospective long-term study of 235 women with more than 1000 confirmed infections studied over a period ranging from 1 to nearly 20 years, about half of the patients had clusters of infections, which ranged in frequency from 2 to 12 infections per cluster.

Infections were followed by remission-free intervals that averaged approximately 1 year. **Most reinfections occurred after 2 weeks** (Harrison et al, 1974) and within 5 months (Mabeck, 1972), and most occurred early in this interval (Kraft and Stamey, 1977; Vosti, 2002) (Fig. 8–4). Rates of reinfection were independent of bladder dysfunction, radiologic changes of chronic pyelonephritis, and vesicoureteral reflux (Guttmann, 1973). The reinfections did not occur evenly over time. In the Stanford series, 23 women with frequent recurrent infections were studied with monthly urine cultures when asymptomatic and with immediate cultures when symptomatic for cystitis, for a mean of 3 years. Thirty-four percent of infections were followed by infection-free intervals of at least 6 months (average, 12.8 months), and 22 of the 23 women had such intervals. However, even these long intervals were followed by further infections (Kraft and Stamey, 1977), thus underscoring the importance of genotypic factors in the pathogenesis of UTIs in women (Schaeffer et al, 1981).

When the Stanford data (Kraft and Stamey, 1977) on recurrent UTIs in highly susceptible females are analyzed by examining sets of infections separated by remissions of at least 6 months, 69% of the sets contain only one infection. After this first set, the remaining sets show a 33% remission rate in infections, which means a patient who has two or more infections within 6 months has only a 33% probability of remaining free of infection for the next 6 months. Therefore, **if antimicrobial prophylaxis is started after the second or any succeeding infection within a set, about one third of the women will be treated unnecessarily. The remaining two thirds of the women still risk more infections.**

Whether a patient receives no treatment at all, or short-term, long-term, or prophylactic antimicrobial treatment, the risk of recurrent bacteriuria remains the same; prophylactic antimicrobial therapy reduces reinfections but does not alter the underlying predisposition to recurring infection. Asscher and associates (1973) found that reinfections occurred in 17 patients (34%) treated with a 7-day course of nitrofurantoin and in 13 patients (29%) receiving placebo during a 3- to 5-year follow-up. Mabeck (1972) found that 46% (20 of 43) of untreated patients had recurrent infections by 12 months compared with about 40% of treated patients who had recurrences. Both studies suggest that it makes little difference whether a UTI is cured with an antimicrobial agent or is allowed to clear spontaneously—the susceptibility to recurrent UTI remains the same. Moreover, patients with frequent UTI who take prophylactic antimicrobial agents for extended periods (≥6 months) may decrease their infections during the time of prophylaxis but the rate of infection returns to the pretreatment rate after prophylaxis is stopped (Vosti, 1975; Stamm et al, 1980a). Even long interruptions in the pattern of recurrence, therefore, do not appear to alter the patient's basic susceptibility to infections.

The sequelae of complicated UTIs are substantial. It is well established that in the presence of obstruction, infection stones, diabetes mellitus, and other risk factors, UTIs in adults can lead to progressive renal damage (Freedman, 1975). **The long-term effects of uncomplicated recurrent UTIs are not completely known, but, so far, no association between recurrent infections and renal scarring, hypertension, or progressive renal azotemia has been established** (Asscher et al, 1973; Freedman, 1975). Indeed, one investigator was unable to find a single case of unequivocal nonobstructive chronic pyelonephritis in 22 patients in whom chronic pyelonephritis was the cause of end-stage renal failure (Schechter et al, 1971). Similar data were reported by Huland and Busch (1982).

In pregnant women, the prevalence and rate of recurrent infection are the same but their bacteriuria progresses to acute clinical pyelonephritis more frequently than in nonpregnant women. This variation in the natural history of recurrent infections in females is discussed in a later section on UTIs in pregnancy.

KEY POINTS: INCIDENCE AND EPIDEMIOLOGY

- UTIs are the most common bacterial infection.
- They cause significant morbidity but do not cause renal damage unless comorbidities are present.
- Antimicrobial therapy reduces morbidity and the time to recurrent bacteriuria, but the risk of recurrence remains the same.

PATHOGENESIS

UTIs are a result of interactions between the uropathogen and the host. Successful infection of the urinary tract is determined in part by the virulence factors of the bacteria, the inoculum size, and the inadequacy of host defense mechanisms. These factors also play a role in determining the ultimate level of colonization and damage to the urinary tract. Whereas increased bacterial virulence appears to be necessary to overcome strong host resistance, bacteria with minimal virulence factors are able to infect patients who are significantly compromised.

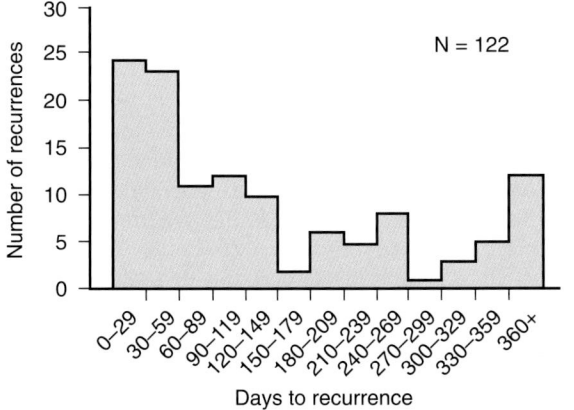

Figure 8–4. Days between recurrent UTIs grouped by 30-day intervals. (From Kraft JK, Stamey TA: The natural history of symptomatic recurrent bacteriuria in women. Medicine 1977;56:55.)

Routes of Infection

Ascending Route

Most bacteria enter the urinary tract from the bowel reservoir via ascent through the urethra into the bladder. Adherence of pathogens to the introital and urothelial mucosa plays a significant role in ascending infections. This route is further enhanced in individuals with significant soilage of the perineum with feces, women who use spermicidal agents (Hooton et al, 1996; Foxman, 2002; Handley et al, 2002), and patients with intermittent or indwelling catheters.

Although cystitis is often restricted to the bladder, approximately 50% of infections can extend into the upper urinary tract (Busch and Huland, 1984). The weight of clinical and experimental evidence strongly suggests that most episodes of pyelonephritis are caused by retrograde ascent of bacteria from the bladder through the ureter to the renal pelvis and parenchyma. Although reflux of urine is probably not required for ascending infections, edema associated with cystitis may cause sufficient changes in the ureterovesical junction to permit reflux. Once the bacteria are introduced into the ureter, they may ascend to the kidney unaided. However, this ascent would be greatly increased by any process that interferes with the normal ureteral peristaltic function. Gram-negative bacteria and their endotoxins, as well as pregnancy and ureteral obstruction, have a significant antiperistaltic effect.

Bacteria that reach the renal pelvis can enter the renal parenchyma by means of the collecting ducts at the papillary tips and then ascend upward within the collecting tubules. This process is hastened and exacerbated by increased intrapelvic pressure from ureteral obstruction or vesicoureteral reflux, particularly when it is associated with intrarenal reflux.

Hematogenous Route

Infection of the kidney by the hematogenous route is uncommon in normal individuals. However, the kidney is occasionally secondarily infected in patients with *Staphylococcus aureus* bacteremia originating from oral sites or with *Candida fungemia*. Experimental data indicate that infection is enhanced when the kidney is obstructed (Smellie et al, 1975).

Lymphatic Route

Direct extension of bacteria from the adjacent organs via lymphatics may occur in unusual circumstances, such as a severe bowel infection or retroperitoneal abscesses. There is little evidence that lymphatic routes play a significant role in the vast majority of UTIs.

Urinary Pathogens

Most UTIs are caused by facultative anaerobes usually originating from the bowel flora. Uropathogens such as *Staphylococcus epidermidis* and *Candida albicans* originate from the flora of the vagina or perineal skin.

***E. coli* is by far the most common cause of UTIs, accounting for 85% of community-acquired and 50% of hospital-acquired infections.** Other gram-negative Enterobacteriaceae, including *Proteus* and *Klebsiella*, and gram-positive *E. faecalis* and *S. saprophyticus* are responsible for the remainder of most community-acquired infections. Nosocomial infections are caused by *E. coli*, *Klebsiella*, *Enterobacter*, *Citrobacter*, *Serratia*, *Pseudomonas aeruginosa*, *Providencia*, *E. faecalis*, and *S. epidermidis* (Kennedy et al, 1965). Less common organisms such as *Gardnerella vaginalis*, *Mycoplasma* species, and *Ureaplasma urealyticum* may infect patients with intermittent or indwelling catheters (Josephson et al, 1988; Fairley and Birch, 1989).

The prevalence of infecting organisms is influenced by the patient's age. For example, *S. saprophyticus* is now recognized as causing approximately 10% of symptomatic lower UTIs in young, sexually active females (Latham et al, 1983) whereas it rarely causes infection in males and elderly individuals. A seasonal variation with a late summer to fall peak has been reported (Hovelius and Mardh, 1984).

Fastidious Organisms

Anaerobes in the Urinary Tract

Although symptomatic anaerobic infections of the urinary tract are documented, they are uncommon. However, the distal urethra, perineum, and vagina are normally colonized by anaerobes. Whereas 1% to 10% of voided urine specimens are positive for anaerobic organisms (Finegold, 1977), anaerobic organisms found in suprapubic aspirates are much more unusual (Gorbach and Bartlett, 1974). Clinically symptomatic UTIs in which only anaerobic organisms are cultured are rare, but these organisms must be suspected when a patient with bladder irritative symptoms has cocci or gram-negative rods seen on microscopic examination of the centrifuged urine (catheterized, suprapubic aspirated, or voided midstream urine) and routine quantitative aerobic cultures fail to grow organisms (Ribot et al, 1981).

Anaerobic organisms are frequently found in suppurative infections of the genitourinary tract. In one study of suppurative genitourinary infections in males, 88% of scrotal, prostatic, and perinephric abscesses included anaerobes among the infecting organisms (Bartlett and Gorbach, 1981). The organisms found are usually *Bacteroides* species, including *B. fragilis*, *Fusobacterium* species, anaerobic cocci, and *Clostridium perfringens* (Finegold, 1977). The growth of clostridia may be associated with cystitis emphysematosa (Bromberg et al, 1982).

Mycobacterium tuberculosis and Other Non-Tuberculous Mycobacteria

Mycobacterium tuberculosis and other non-tuberculous mycobacteria may be found when cultures for acid-fast bacteria are requested; they do not grow under routine aerobic conditions and may be found during evaluation for sterile pyuria. It has been emphasized that the mere presence of mycobacteria may not indicate tissue infection. Therefore, factors such as symptoms, endoscopic or radiologic evidence of infection, abnormal urine sediment, the absence of other pathogens, repeated demonstration of the organism, and the presence of granulomas should be considered before therapy is instituted (Brooker and Aufderheide, 1980; Thomas et al, 1980). (*M. tuberculosis* is discussed in Chapter 14, "Tuberculosis and Other Opportunistic Infections of the Genitourinary System.")

Chlamydia

Chlamydiae are not routinely grown in aerobic culture but have been implicated in genitourinary infections. (Their role in the urinary tract is discussed in Chapter 11, "Sexually Transmitted Diseases.")

Bacterial Virulence Factors

Virulence characteristics play a role in determining both if an organism will invade the urinary tract and the subsequent level of infection within the urinary tract. It is generally believed that uropathogenic strains resident in the bowel flora, such as uropathogenic *E. coli* (UPEC), can infect the urinary tract not by chance but rather by the expression of virulence factors that enable them to adhere to and colonize the perineum and urethra and migrate to the urinary tract where they establish an inflammatory response in the urothelium (Schaeffer et al, 1981; Yamamoto et al, 1997; Schlager et al, 2002). The same virulence factors can be found on bacterial strains that cause recurrent UTI in patients (Foxman et al, 1995). Some of these virulence determinants are located on one of approximately 20 UPEC specific pathogenicity-associated islands ranging in size from 30 to 170 kb (Hacker, 1999; Oelschlaeger et al, 2002). These pathogenicity islands collectively increase the size of the pathogen genome by about 20% over a commensal strain. A recent genomic analysis of a UPEC strain revealed the presence of genes for putative chaperone-usher systems as well as autotransporter proteins that may function as adhesins, toxins, proteases, invasins, serum resistance factors, or motility mediators (Henderson and Nataro, 2001). One UPEC-specific autotransporter, Sat, seems toxic to urinary tract cells in vitro (Guyer et al, 2000) and can cause cytoplasmic vacuolation and severe histologic damage in mouse kidneys (Guyer et al, 2002). Another toxin, hemolysin HlyA, forms pores in a variety of host cell membranes (Uhlen et al, 2000). In addition to proteases and toxins, UPEC produces several iron acquisition systems, including aerobactin (Johnson et al, 1988; Johnson, 2003) and the more recently described IroN system (Russo et al, 1999; Sorsa et al, 2003). Lastly, most UPEC strains produce an acid polysaccharide capsule that protects the bacteria from phagocytosis by human polymorphonuclear leukocytes and inhibits activation of complement (Johnson, 2003).

Early Events in UPEC Pathogenesis

Bacterial Adherence

It is well established that bacterial adherence to vaginal and urothelial epithelial cells is an essential step in the initiation of UTIs. This interaction is influenced by the adhesive characteristics of the bacteria, the receptive characteristics of the epithelial surface, and the fluid bathing both surfaces. Bacterial adherence is a specific interaction that plays a role in determining the organism, the host, and the site of infection. Portions of this section on bacterial adherence have been published (Schaeffer et al, 1981).

Bacterial Adhesins. UPEC expresses a number of adhesins that allow it to attach to urinary tract tissues (Mulvey, 2002). These adhesins are classified as either fimbrial or afimbrial, depending on whether the adhesin is displayed as part of a

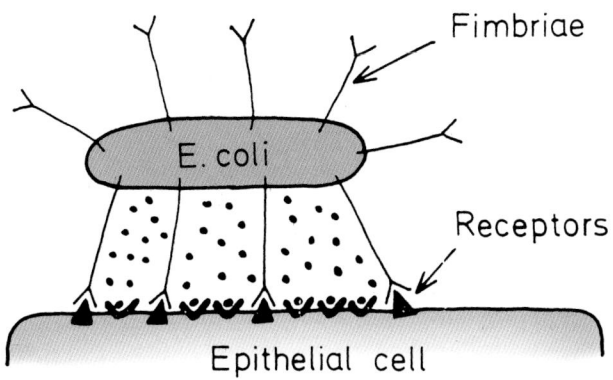

Figure 8–5. Bacterial adherence. Adhesins on pili (fimbriae) mediate attachment to specific epithelial cell receptors.

rigid fimbria or pilus (Fig. 8–5). Bacteria may produce a number of antigenically and functionally different pili on the same cell; others produce a single type; in some, no pili are seen (Klemm, 1985). A typical piliated cell may contain 100 to 400 pili. The pilus is usually 5 to 10 nm in diameter, is up to 2 μm long, and appears to be composed primarily of subunits known as pilin (Klemm, 1985). Pili are defined functionally by their ability to mediate hemagglutination of specific types of erythrocytes. The most well-described pili are types 1, P and S.

Type 1 (Mannose Sensitive) Pili. Type 1 pili are commonly expressed on both nonpathogenic and pathogenic *E. coli* and appear to facilitate bacterial colonization of the vaginal mucosa and bladder. These pili mediate hemagglutination of guinea pig erythrocytes (Duguid et al, 1979). The reaction is inhibited by the addition of mannose; thus type 1 pili are termed mannose-sensitive hemagglutination (MSHA) (Svenson et al, 1984; Reid and Sobel, 1987).

Type 1 pili consist of a helical rod composed of repeating FimA subunits joined to a 3-nm wide distal tip structure containing the adhesin FimH (Jones et al, 1995). Binding of the FimH adhesin to mannosylated host receptors present on the uroepithelium is critical to the ability of *E. coli* to colonize the vaginal introitus, urethra, and bladder and cause cystitis (Kunin, 1987; Connell et al, 1996; Thankavel et al, 1997).

The role of type 1 pili as a virulence factor in UTIs has been established. This evidence has been obtained (1) from the analysis of bacteria isolated from the urine of patients with UTIs, which were found to express mannose-sensitive (MS) adhesins (Ljungh and Wadstrom, 1983); (2) from studies with animal models (Fader and Davis, 1982; Hagberg et al, 1983a; Hagberg et al, 1983b; Hultgren et al, 1985; Iwahi et al, 1983) in which inoculation of type 1 piliated organisms into the bladder resulted in significantly more colonization of the urinary tract than inoculation of nonpiliated organisms; and (3) from the observation that anti-type 1 pili antibodies and competitive inhibitors such as methyl-α-d-mannopyranoside protected mice from contracting UTIs (Aronson et al, 1979; Hultgren et al, 1985). **Recent studies have demonstrated that interactions between FimH and receptors expressed on the luminal surface of the bladder epithelium are critical for the ability of many UPEC strains to colonize the bladder and cause disease** (Connell et al, 1996; Langermann et al, 1997; Thankavel et al, 1997; Mulvey et al, 1998).

The luminal surface of the bladder is lined by umbrella cells. The apical surfaces of umbrella cells appear as a quasi-crystalline array of hexagonal complexes composed of four integral membrane proteins known as uroplakins (Sun, 1996). In vitro binding assays have shown that two of the uroplakins, UPIa and UPIb, can specifically bind UPEC expressing type 1 pili (Wu et al, 1996).

The ability of type 1 pili to mediate attachment to the uroplakins in vivo has been investigated using a mouse cystitis model and microscopic techniques (Malaviya and Abraham, 1998). Shortly after inoculation, numerous bacteria can be found attached to the urothelial surface as detected by scanning electron microscopy (Mulvey et al, 1998) (Fig. 8–6). Bacteria adhered both singly and in large groups and can be inhibited by the soluble FimH receptor analog and d-mannose. Electron microscopy revealed that FimH containing type 1 pili could interact directly with uroplakins.

***P (Mannose Resistant) Pili.* P pili confer tropism to the kidney, the designation "P" standing for pyelonephritis** (Mulvey, 2002). P pili, which are found in most pyelonephritogenic strains of UPEC, mediate hemagglutination of human erythrocytes that is not altered by mannose and is thus termed mannose-resistant hemagglutination (MRHA) (Kallenius and Mollby, 1979). The adhesin PapG, at the tip of the pilus, recognizes the α-d-galactopyranosyl-(1-4)-β-d-galactopyranoside moiety present in the globoseries of glycolipids (Kallenius et al, 1980; Leffler and Svanborg-Eden, 1980), which are found on P-blood group antigens and on uroepithelium (Svenson et al, 1983).

The MRHA adhesins of UPEC that do not show the digalactoside-binding specificity have been provisionally named X adhesins (Vaisanen et al, 1981). In some strains of UPEC, hemagglutination is mediated by nonpiliated adhesins or hemagglutinins (Duguid et al, 1979).

Svanborg-Eden and coworkers (1976) were the first to report a correlation between bacterial adherence and severity of UTIs. They showed that UPEC strains from girls with acute pyelonephritis had high adhesive ability whereas strains causing asymptomatic bacteriuria or from the feces of healthy girls had low bacterial adherence. Between 70% and 80% of the pyelonephritic strains, but only 10% of the bowel isolates, had adhesive capacity. Furthermore, P pili were present in 91% of urinary strains causing pyelonephritis, 19% of strains causing cystitis, and 14% of strains causing asymptomatic bacteriuria but only 7% of bowel isolates from healthy children, highlighting the correlation between bacterial adherence and UTIs (Kallenius et al, 1981).

Whereas MRHA and P pili are strongly associated with pyelonephritis, these virulence factors are not associated with renal scarring and reflux due to bacterial infection (Vaisanen et al, 1981). Studies suggest minimal correlation between P-piliated *E. coli* strains and recurrent pyelonephritis with gross reflux in girls (Lomberg et al, 1983). Thus, it would appear that P pili in acute pyelonephritis are important mainly in nonrefluxing or minimally refluxing children.

***Other Adhesins.* S pili, which bind to sialic acid residues via the SfaS adhesin, have been associated with both bladder and kidney infection (Mulvey, 2002). F1C pili bind to glycosphingolipids in renal epithelial cells and induce an interleukin-8 inflammatory response (Backhed et al, 2002).

UPEC also expresses a group of afimbrial adhesins (AFA), which have been clustered with the Dr adhesin family for their recognition of decay-accelerating factor and for their similar genetic structure. Decay-accelerating factor is found on numerous different epithelial sites, and Dr adhesins are known to bind to many locations throughout the urinary tract (Anderson et al, 2004a).

Phase Variation of Bacterial Pili in Vivo

Early evidence for the role of type 1 and P pili in adherence in UTIs in humans was contradictory. Pili were visible by electron microscopy on *E. coli* in the urine of 31 of 37 patients (Ljungh and Wadstrom, 1983). Conversely, no MS adhesins were found in 22 of 24 urine isolates from patients with indwelling catheters (Ofek et al, 1981), and 19 of 20 samples from patients with acute UTIs were devoid of pili and nonadherent until subcultured in broth (Harber et al, 1982). Assessment of pili production by clinical *E. coli* isolates demonstrates that environmental growth conditions can produce rapid changes in pilus expression (Duguid et al, 1966; Goransson and Uhlin, 1984; Hultgren et al, 1986), wherein cells switch back and forth between piliated and nonpiliated phases (Eisenstein, 1981). For example, some bacteria grown in a broth medium express pili whereas the same strain grown on the same medium in a solid state will cease production of pili. **This process, called phase variation, can also occur in vivo and has obvious biologic and clinical implications.** For example, the presence of type 1 pili may be advantageous to the bacteria for adhering to and colonizing the bladder mucosa but disadvantageous because the pili enhance phagocytosis and killing by neutrophils (Silverblatt et al, 1979).

An animal model of ascending UTIs and studies of bacterial isolates from different sites in patients with UTI provide evidence that phase variation can occur during *E. coli* UTI in vivo. Type 1 piliated *E. coli* organisms that were capable of phase variation were introduced into the mouse bladder in the piliated phase, and the bacteria recovered from the bladder and urine 24 or more hours after inoculation were tested for

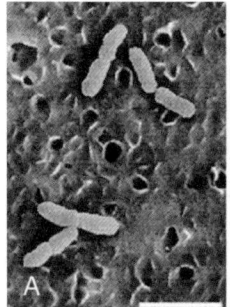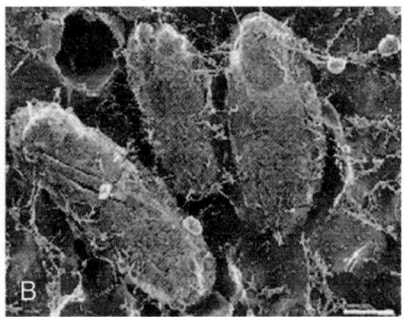

Figure 8–6. Type 1 pilus–mediated bacterial attachment to the bladder epithelium. After inoculation of C57BLy6 mice with type 1–piliated *Escherichia coli,* numerous bacteria *(yellow)* can be found attached to the luminal surface of the bladder *(blue)* as detected by scanning electron microscopy (EM) (**A**) and high-resolution freeze-dry deep-etch EM (**B**). Type 1 pili mediating bacterial attachment were resolved with the high-resolution technique. The scalloped appearance of the bladder surface is attributable to the presence of the uroplakin plaques (0.5 μm in diameter). *Bars* = 3 μm (**A**) and 0.5 μm (**B**). (From Mulvey MA, Schilling JD, Martinez JJ, Hultgren SJ: Bad bugs and beleaguered bladders: Interplay between uropathogenic *Escherichia coli* and innate host defenses. Proc Natl Acad Sci U S A 2000;97:8829-8835.)

piliation. All of the animals had bladder colonization, and 78% of the bacteria recovered showed type 1 piliation. The bacteriologic state of the urine often differed from that of the bladder. The urine was sterile in 59% of the animals with bladder colonization, and the organisms recovered from the urine were often nonpiliated.

When bladder and kidney cultures were examined 1, 3, and 5 days after intravesical inoculation of piliated bacteria, organisms recovered from the bladder remained piliated, whereas organisms recovered from the kidney showed significantly less piliation (Schaeffer et al, 1987) (Fig. 8–7).

Studies in humans using indirect immunofluorescence of fresh urine bacteria have confirmed in vivo expression and phase variation of pili. Analysis of the urine of adults with lower UTI detected type 1 pili in 31 of 41 specimens and P pili in 6 of 18 specimens (Kisielius et al, 1989). The piliation status of the bacterial population in the urine was heterogeneous, varying from predominantly piliated to a mixture of piliated and nonpiliated cells (Fig. 8–8). Strains isolated from different sites in the urogenital tract showed variation in the state of piliation. These results demonstrate that type 1 and P pili are expressed and subject to phase variation in vivo during acute UTIs.

This process of phase variation has obvious biologic and clinical implications. For example, the presence of type 1 pili may be advantageous to the bacteria for initially adhering to and colonizing the bladder mucosa. Subsequently, type 1 pili may be unnecessary for strains in suspension in urine and in fact detrimental because they enhance apoptosis, phagocytosis, and killing by neutrophils (Silverblatt et al, 1979; Mulvey et al, 1998). In the kidney, P pili may then take over as the primary mediator of bacterial attachment via their binding to the glycolipid receptors (Stapleton et al, 1995).

Epithelial Cell Receptivity

Vaginal Cells

The significance of epithelial cell receptivity in the pathogenesis of ascending UTI has been studied initially by examining adherence of E. coli to vaginal epithelial cells and uroepithelial cells collected from voided urine specimens. Fowler and Stamey (1977) established that certain indigenous micro-

organisms (e.g., lactobacilli, *S. epidermidis*) avidly attached themselves to washed epithelial cells in large numbers. When vaginal epithelial cells were collected from patients susceptible to reinfection and compared with such cells obtained from controls resistant to UTI, the *E. coli* strains that cause cystitis adhered much more avidly to the epithelial cells from the susceptible women. **These studies established increased adherence of pathogenic bacteria to vaginal epithelial cells as the first demonstrable biologic difference that could be shown in women susceptible to UTI.**

Subsequently, **Schaeffer and colleagues (1981) confirmed these vaginal differences in women, but in addition they observed that the increased bacterial adherence was also characteristic of buccal epithelial cells.** As can be seen in Figure 8-9, there is a striking similarity in the ability of both cell types to bind to the same *E. coli* strain. In addition, there was a significant relationship between vaginal cell and buccal cell receptivity. Seventy-seven different *E. coli* strains were tested for their ability to bind to vaginal and buccal epithelial cells. A direct nonlinear relationship between buccal and vaginal adherence in controls and patients was confirmed for urinary, vaginal, and anal isolates. Thus, high vaginal cell receptivity was associated with high buccal cell receptivity.

These observations emphasize that the increase in receptor sites for UPEC on epithelial cells from women with recurrent UTIs is not limited to the vagina and thus suggest that a genotypic trait for epithelial cell receptivity may be a major susceptibility factor in UTIs. This concept was extended by examining the human leukocyte antigens (HLAs), which are the major histocompatibility complex in humans and have been associated statistically with many diseases (Schaeffer et al, 1983). The A3 antigen was identified in 12 (34%) of the patients, which is significantly higher than the 8% frequency observed in healthy controls. Thus, HLA-A3 may be associated with increased risk of recurrent UTIs.

Variation in Receptivity. A small variation in both vaginal cell and buccal cell receptivity may be observed from day to day in healthy controls. Adherence ranges from 1 to 17 bacteria per cell and appears to be both cyclic and repetitive. When adherence was correlated with the days of a woman's menstrual cycle, higher values were noted in the early phase, diminishing shortly after the time of expected ovulation

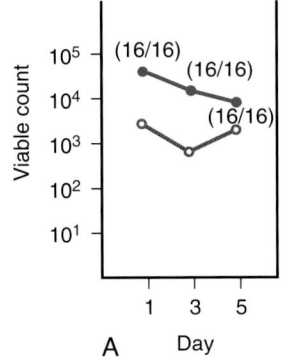
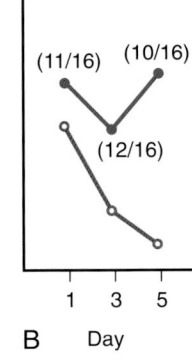
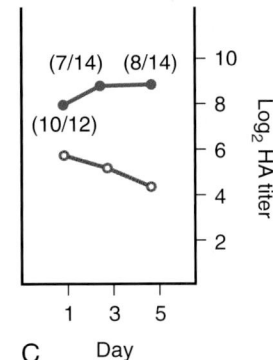

Figure 8–7. Time study after intravesical inoculation with *E. coli* strain I-I49 that compared the mean viable bacteria count (•) and hemagglutination (HA) titer (o) for bladders (**A**), kidneys (**B**), and urine specimens (**C**) from the same animals. Each point is the mean of all the animals tested. The numbers in parentheses show the proportion of animals inoculated that gave positive cultures. The HA titers were tested after 18 hours of growth on agar. The HA titer of bacteria recovered from the kidney decreased significantly by day 5 (*P* < 0.001). (**A** to **C**, from Schaeffer AJ, Schwan WR, Hultgren SJ, Duncan JL: Relationship of type 1 pilus expression in *Escherichia coli* to ascending urinary tract infections in mice. Infect Immun 1987;55:373-380.)

SECTION IV

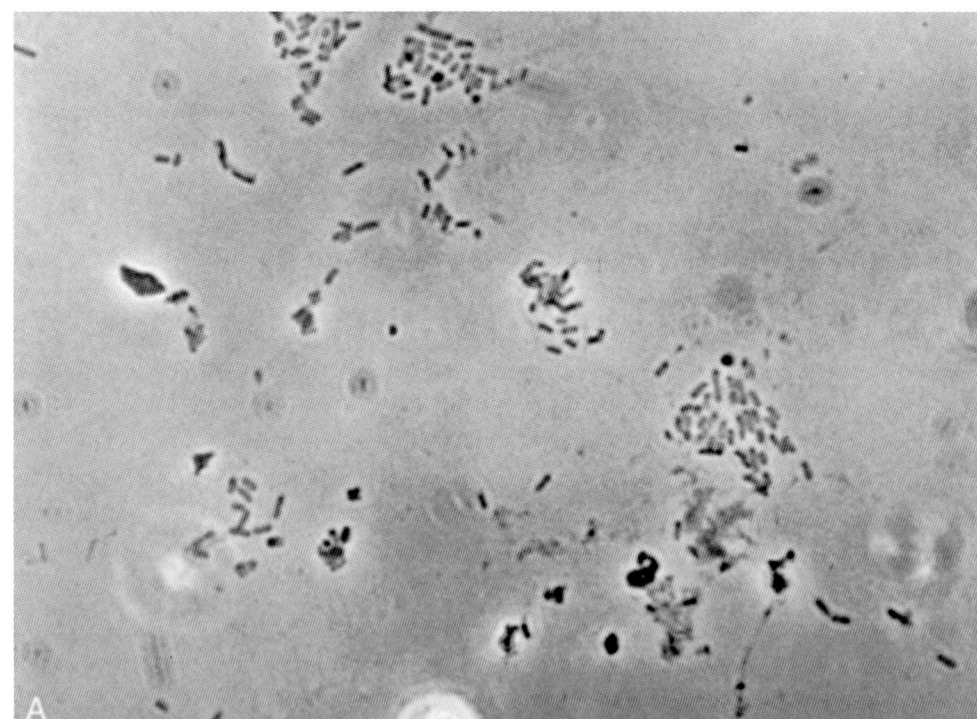

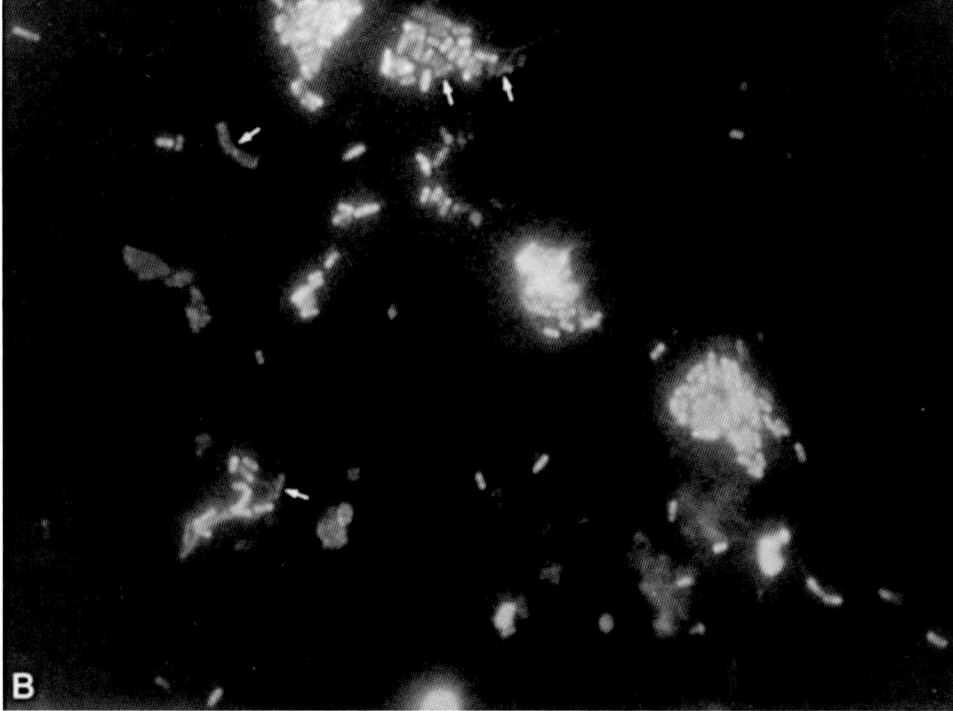

Figure 8–8. Phase-contrast micrograph (**A**) and immunofluorescence micrograph (**B**) of a sample stained with antiserum to type 1 pili of strain I-49 and with FITC-conjugated second antibody against nonadherent *E. coli* in the urine of a patient with acute UTI show a mixture of piliated and nonpiliated (*arrows* in **B**) cells. (**A** and **B**, from Kisielius PV, Schwan WR, Amundsen SK, et al: In vivo expression and variation of *Escherichia coli* type 1 and P pili in the urine of adults with acute urinary tract infections. Infect Immun 1989;57:1656.)

(day 14). The number of bacteria per epithelial cell often correlated with the value obtained on the same day of the menstrual cycle 1 or 2 months previously. Premenopausal women are particularly susceptible to attachment of uropathogenic *E. coli* and nonpathogenic lactobacilli at certain times during the menstrual cycle and to *E. coli* during the early stages of pregnancy. **The importance of such hormones as estrogens in the pathogenesis of UTI is therefore a matter of great interest,**

especially because the clinical urologist may see women who have recurrent cystitis at regular intervals, possibly in response to these hormonal changes.

Reid and Sobel (1987) found that uropathogens attached in larger numbers to uroepithelial cells from women older than 65 years of age than to cells from premenopausal women 18 to 40 years of age. Raz and Stamm (1993) noted that susceptibility to recurrent UTI was increased by the lowered

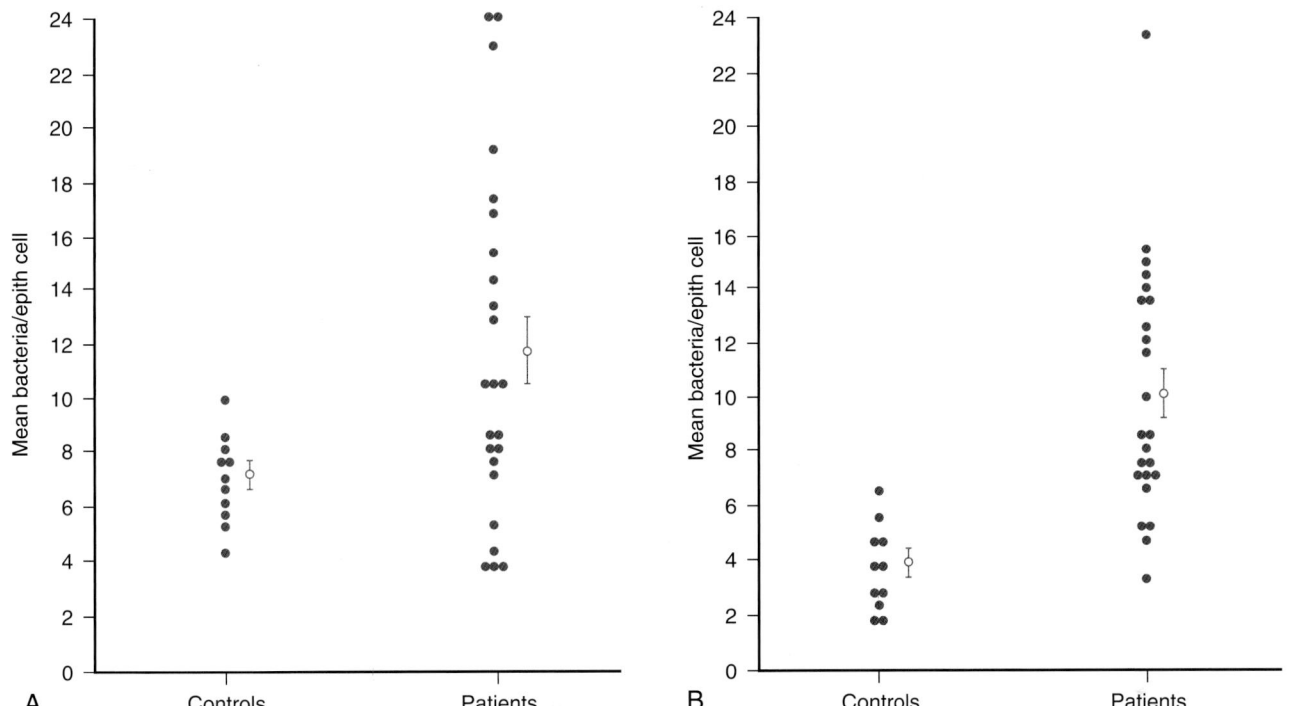

Figure 8–9.   In vitro adherence of *E. coli* to vaginal (**A**) and buccal (**B**) cells from healthy controls and patients with recurrent UTIs. Values represent an average of 14 (**A**) and 11 (**B**) determinations in each individual. The *open circles* and *bars* represent the means + SEM. (**A** and **B,** from Schaeffer AJ, Jones JM, Dunn JK: Association of in vitro *Escherichia coli* adherence to vaginal and buccal epithelial cells with susceptibility of women to recurrent urinary tract infections. N Engl J Med 1981;304:1062-1066.)

estrogen levels found in the postmenopausal women and that estrogen replacement decreased uropathogenic bacterial colonization and the incidence of UTI.

Blood group antigens and carbohydrate structures bound to membrane lipids or proteins also constitute an important part of the uroepithelial cell membrane. The presence or absence of blood group determinants on the surface of uroepithelial cells may influence an individual's susceptibility to a UTI. Sheinfeld and associates (1989) determined the blood group phenotypes in women with recurrent UTI and compared them with those of age-matched women controls. Women with Lewis Le(a−b−) and Le(a+b−) phenotypes had a significantly higher incidence of recurrent UTIs than women with Le(a−b+) phenotypes. There was no significant difference in the distribution of ABO or P blood group phenotypes. The Lewis antigen controls fucosylation. The protective effect in women with the Le(a−b+) phenotype may be due to fucosylated structures at the vaginal cell surface or in the overlying mucus, which decreases availability of putative receptors for *E. coli* (Navas et al, 1993). The nonsecretor status has also been associated with female acute uncomplicated pyelonephritis, especially in premenopausal women (Ishitoya et al, 2002). Stapleton and coworkers (1992) have shown that unique *E. coli*–binding glycerides are found in vaginal epithelial cells from nonsecretors but not from secretors. **These studies individually and collectively support the concept that there is an increased epithelial receptivity for *E. coli* on the introital, urethral, and buccal mucosa that is characteristic of women susceptible to recurrent UTIs and may be a genotypic trait.**

The possibility that vaginal mucus might influence bacterial receptivity was investigated by Schaeffer and colleagues (1994). Type 1 piliated *E. coli* bound to all of the vaginal fluid specimens (Venegas et al, 1995). The binding capacity of vaginal fluid from women colonized with *E. coli* in vivo was greater than that from noncolonized women (Schaeffer et al, 1999). The importance of vaginal fluid in bacteria/epithelial cell interactions was investigated in an in vitro model that measured the effect of vaginal fluid on the binding of bacteria to an epithelial cell line (Gaffney et al, 1995). Vaginal fluid from colonized women enhanced binding of bacteria to epithelial cells. Conversely, vaginal fluid from noncolonized women inhibited adherence. Thus, the vaginal fluid appears to influence adherence to cells and, presumably, vaginal mucosal colonization. Subsequent studies demonstrated that secretory IgA is the primary glycoprotein responsible for vaginal fluid receptivity (Rajan et al, 1999).

Bladder Cells

FimH binds mannosylated residues on the uroplakin molecules covering bladder superficial epithelial cells. Whereas UPEC can be seen randomly attached to the epithelium immediately after inoculation in an animal model, an isogenic *fimH*-mutant cannot colonize mouse bladders (Mulvey et al, 2000). High-resolution freeze-fracture electron microscopy has shown that the tips of these pili, including the adhesins, are buried in the central cavity of the uroplakin hexameric rings (Mulvey et al, 2000) (see Fig. 8–10A). Thus **fimH-mediated binding to the bladder epithelium is the initial step in the intricate cascade of events leading to UTIs.**

UPEC Persistence in the Bladder. Soon after attachment to the epithelium, UPEC is quickly internalized into the bladder superficial cells (Martinez and Hultgren, 2002; Anderson et al, 2004a) (Fig. 8–10). FimH is essential for UPEC invasion; isogenic fimH-mutants do not invade, and invasion of wild-type bacteria can be inhibited by the addition of mannose. In addition, polystyrene latex beads coated with fimH are quickly internalized in a process identical to bacteria expressing type 1 pili. This process is the result of localized actin rearrangement and engulfment of the bound bacterium by zippering of the membrane around the microorganism (Martinez and Hultgren, 2002). Invasion into the superficial epithelium of the bladder allows UPEC to establish a new niche in an effort to protect itself from the host innate immune response (Anderson et al, 2004a).

Once intracellular, the UPEC organisms rapidly grow and divide within the cell cytosol, forming small clusters of bacteria termed early intracellular bacterial communities (IBCs) (Anderson et al, 2004a; Justice et al, 2004). As they grow, the bacteria maintain their typical rod shape of approximately 3 μm and form a loosely organized cluster, with microorganisms randomly oriented in the cell cytoplasm. Between 6 to 8 hours after inoculation, early IBCs show a drop in bacterial growth rate resulting in doubling times greater than 60 minutes, a significant shortening of the bacterial morphology to an average of 0.7 μm, and a phenotypic switch into a biofilm-like community (Justice et al, 2004).

Biofilms shield bacteria from environmental challenges such as antimicrobial agents and the host immune response (Donlan and Costerton, 2002). Characteristics of the biofilm that increase protection include the slower growth rate of the bacteria with associated physiologic changes, expression of factors that inhibit antimicrobial activity, and the inability of the antimicrobial agent to penetrate the biofilm matrix (Anderson et al, 2004a). The biofilm also protects the bacteria from neutrophils because they are unable to effectively penetrate the IBC and engulf the bacteria. In animal models, bacteria on the edge of IBCs eventually detach, differentiate to typical rod morphology, become motile, and then escape the host cell into the bladder lumen in a process called fluxing (Mulvey et al, 2001) (see Fig. 8–10D). These bacteria may become highly filamentous, reaching up to 70 μm or greater in length. This process occurs by approximately 24 hours after inoculation (Justice et al, 2004). It is possible that the filaments may help the bacteria evade the immunologic response.

The escaped bacteria readhere and reinvade superficial cells to lead to second IBC formation. In subsequent rounds, further IBC formation occurs. After a few days, the invasive bacteria become more quiescent. In animal models, the bacteria can persist in this dormant reservoir state for some time before reemerging to cause recurrent UTIs (Anderson et al, 2004b).

Natural Defenses of the Urinary Tract

Periurethral and Urethral Region

The normal flora of the vaginal introitus, the periurethral area, and the urethra usually contain microorganisms such

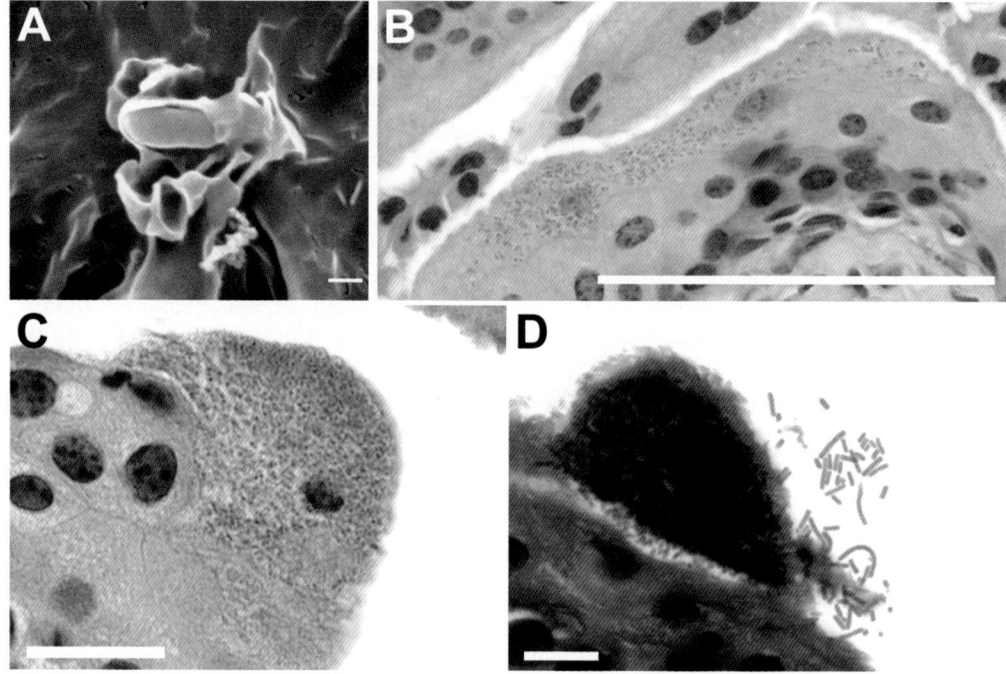

Figure 8–10. UPEC binds, invades, and multiplies inside the superficial cells of the bladder epithelium. **A,** Scanning electron microscopy shows a single UPEC bound to the surface of a bladder cell. Type 1 pilus–mediated contact between bacterium and host cell initiates signaling cascades in the bladder cell, leading to localized actin rearrangements and membrane protrusions around the bacterium. Scale bar, 0.5 μm. **B,** Once inside the bladder superficial cells, UPEC rapidly multiplies to form disordered bacterial clusters in the host cell cytoplasm, called an early IBC. Bacteria are visible as dark-staining rods inside the cell in this hematoxylin and eosin (H&E)-stained thin bladder section. Scale bar, 100 μm. **C,** H&E-stained thin bladder section reveals a middle IBC, wherein the constituent bacteria have organized themselves into a biofilm-like state within the bladder cell. Scale bar, 20 μm. **D,** A late IBC, visible by H&E staining, is typified by detachment of peripheral bacteria and fluxing of these organisms into the bladder lumen. Scale bar, 10 μm. (From Anderson GG, Martin SM, Hultgren SJ: Host subversion by formation of intracellular bacterial communities in the urinary tract. Microbes Infect 2004;6:1094-101.)

as lactobacilli, coagulase-negative staphylococci, corynebacteria, and streptococci that form a barrier against uropathogenic colonization (Fair et al, 1970; Pfau and Sacks, 1977; Marrie et al, 1978). Changes in the vaginal environment related to estrogen, cervical IgA (Stamey et al, 1978), and low vaginal pH (Stamey and Timothy, 1975) may alter the ability of these bacteria to colonize. More commonly, however, acute changes in colonization have been associated with use of antimicrobial agents and spermicidal agents that alter the normal flora and increase the receptivity of the epithelium for uropathogens.

Little is known about the factors that predispose patients to urethral colonization with uropathogens. The proximity of the urethral meatus to the vulvar and perianal areas suggests that contamination occurs frequently. The nature of urethral defense mechanisms other than flow of urine is largely unknown. Bacterial multiplication in the normal urethra may be inhibited by the indigenous flora (Chan et al, 1984). Although colonization of the periurethral and urethral regions is prerequisite to most infections, the ability of the organisms to overcome the normal defense mechanisms of the urine and the bladder is clearly pivotal.

Urine

In general, fastidious organisms that normally colonize the urethra will not multiply in urine and rarely cause UTIs (Cattell et al, 1974). In contrast, urine will usually support the growth of nonfastidious bacteria (Asscher et al, 1968). Urine from normal individuals may be inhibitory, especially when the inoculum is small (Kaye, 1968). The most inhibitory factors are the osmolality, urea concentration, organic acid concentration, and pH. Bacterial growth is inhibited by either very dilute urine or a high osmolality when associated with a low pH. Much of the antimicrobial activity of urine is related to a high urea and organic acid content (Solomon et al, 1983). From a clinical perspective, however, these conditions do not appear to significantly distinguish between patients who are susceptible or resistant to infection.

The presence of glucose in the urine may facilitate infections. This is consistent with the increased frequency and severity of infection in diabetes (Asscher et al, 1968). Urine obtained from pregnant women exhibits a more suitable pH for growth of *E. coli* in all stages of gestation (Asscher et al, 1973). Uromodulin (Tamm-Horsfall protein), a kidney-derived mannosylated protein that is present in an extraordinarily high concentration in the urine (greater than 100 mg/mL), may play a defensive role by saturating all the mannose-binding sites of the type 1 pili, thus potentially blocking bacterial binding to the uroplakin receptors of the urothelium (Duncan, 1988; Kumar and Muchmore, 1990).

Bladder

Bacteria presumably make their way into the bladder fairly often. Whether small inocula of bacteria persist, multiply, and infect the host depends in part on the ability of the bladder to empty (Cox and Hinman, 1961). Additional factors responsible for defense involve both innate and adaptive immunity and exfoliation of epithelial cells.

Immune Response

Pathogen Recognition. The host recognition of the pathogen is mediated by a series of pathogen-associated molecular pattern receptors (PAMPs), such as Toll-like receptors (TLRs) (Anderson et al, 2004a), which provide the link between recognition of invading organisms and development of the innate immune response. TLRs recognize molecular patterns that are conserved among many species of pathogens, such as lipopolysaccharide (LPS) and peptidoglycan (PG), and activate signaling pathways that initiate immune and inflammatory responses to kill pathogens. Superficial bladder epithelial cells express TLR4 on their membranes, which along with CD14 recognize LPS from the bacteria and activate the innate immune response (Anderson et al, 2004b). The newly identified TLR11, which recognizes UPEC and protects the kidneys from ascending infection, is also expressed on uroepithelial cells as well as renal cells (Zhang et al, 2004).

The innate system response to an infection in the bladder or kidneys is primarily local inflammation.

The innate immune response occurs more rapidly than the adaptive response and involves a variety of cell types, including polymorphonuclear leukocytes, neutrophils, macrophages, eosinophils, natural killer cells, mass cells, and dendritic cells. In addition, increased transcription of inducible nitric oxide synthase by polymorphonuclear leukocytes results in high levels of nitric oxide and related breakdown products that also have toxic effects on the bacteria (Poljakovic et al, 2001; Poljakovic and Persson, 2003). The innate response aids in establishing adaptive immunity due to interactions of macrophages, dendritic cells, and natural killer cells with T and B lymphocytes. Adaptive immunity involves the specific recognition of pathogens by T and B lymphocytes and production of high-affinity antibodies, a process that occurs 7 to 10 days after infection.

The urinary tract is part of the secretory immune system. Most of the human and experimental animal studies have focused on the immune response to bacterial infections of the upper tract and colonization of the vaginal introitus. Kidney infections are accompanied by both serum and local kidney immunoglobulin synthesis and the appearance of type-specific antibodies in the urine. Antibodies in serum against the O antigen and, to a lesser extent, the K antigen of the infecting *E. coli* strain have been found (Salit et al, 1988). Serum antibodies directed at type 1 and P pili have also been identified after acute pyelonephritis (Rene et al, 1982; de Ree and van den Bosch, 1987). In pyelonephritis, IgG and SIgA also appear in the urine and may become evident before antibodies are detected in the serum. These antibodies are synthesized locally within the kidney and may enhance bacterial opsonization and ingestion by local phagocytic cells. These antibodies may have further protective function. Svanborg-Eden and Svennerholm (1978) showed that IgG and SIgA derived from the urine of patients with acute pyelonephritis reduced in vitro adherence of the same strain of *E. coli* to uroepithelial cells. Similarly, immunization with *E. coli* P pili resulted in immunoglobulin production in experimental animals that prevented ascending pyelonephritis by reducing the adhesive capacity of the invading autologous uropathogenic *E. coli* (Roberts and Phillips, 1979; O'Hanley, 1983).

Neutrophils from the urinary tract appear to be essential for bacterial clearance, and their recruitment plays a pivotal role in resistance to UTIs (Haraoka et al, 1999). In mice, a UTI will spontaneously resolve in most cases; however, in mice with specific genetic backgrounds, a UTI can persist. This suggests that the presence or absence of specific host genes may determine how effectively a UTI will be resolved (Hopkins et al, 1998). Small deficiencies in human responses could lead to a variety of infection outcomes. For example, in mice, TLR11 appears to recognize uropathogenic *E. coli* and protect the kidneys from ascending infection. Humans have a truncated form of TLR11 that is probably inactive, thus increasing susceptibility to pyelonephritis. In addition, a recent study of inflammatory responses in women with recurrent UTIs revealed that neutrophils from these patients displayed reduced levels of CD16, decreased bacterial phagocytosis, and lower generation of reactive oxygen intermediates (Mysorekar et al, 2002).

The possibility that immunologic factors may be modified to reduce susceptibility to infection has been explored primarily through immunization in animal and human systems. For example, in a monkey model, vaccination with P fimbria has been shown to reduce adherence of P-fimbriated *E. coli* to uroepithelial cells and prevent acute pyelonephritis (Roberts and Phillips, 1979). Similarly, vaccination of mice with FimH adhesin prevents cystitis in mice (Langermann et al, 1997). Vaccination of women may reduce colonization of the vaginal introitus and subsequent ascending bacteria (Uehling et al, 1994).

Induced Exfoliation. Mulvey and colleagues (1998) **demonstrated that exfoliation and excretion of infected and damaged superficial cells is mediated by type 1 piliated bacteria that induce programmed cell death.** By utilizing an in vivo mouse model, it has been demonstrated that mice that exhibit a strong exfoliation response to UPEC infiltration are unlikely to form IBCs (Anderson et al, 2004a). However, mice with a much milder exfoliation response tend to form biofilms, which become sequestered in the bladder and presumably could lead to recurrent UTIs. **It has also been shown that many uropathogenic bacteria can suppress NFκB, increase apoptosis, and decrease the inflammatory responses** (Klumpp et al, 2001), **a process that could lead to subsequent bacterial invasion into deeper tissues. Thus, in some instances apoptosis may be a bacterial offense maneuver rather than a host defense.**

Alterations in Host Defense Mechanisms

Obstruction

Obstruction to urine flow at all anatomic levels is a key factor in increasing host susceptibility to UTI. Obstruction inhibits the normal flow of urine, and the resulting stasis compromises bladder and renal defense mechanisms. Stasis also contributes to the growth of bacteria in the urine and their ability to adhere to the urothelial cells. In the animal model of experimental hematogenous pyelonephritis, the kidney is relatively resistant to infection unless a ureter is ligated. Under these circumstances, only the obstructed kidney becomes infected (Beeson and Guze, 1956). Clinical observations support the role of obstruction in pathogenesis of UTI and in increasing severity of infection. **Mild episodes of cystitis or pyelonephritis can become life-threatening when obstruction to urine flow becomes present. Although obstruction clearly increases the severity of infection, it need not be a**

predisposing factor. For example, men with large residual urine may remain uninfected for years. However, if they are catheterized, even small inocula may lead to severe infections that are difficult to eradicate.

Vesicoureteral Reflux

Hodson and Edwards (1960) first described the association of vesicoureteral reflux, UTI, and renal clubbing and scarring. Children with gross reflux and UTIs usually develop progressive renal damage manifested by renal scarring, proteinuria, and renal failure. Those with a lesser degree of reflux usually improve or completely recover spontaneously or after treatment of the UTI. In adults, the presence of reflux does not appear to decrease renal function unless there is stasis and concurrent UTIs.

Underlying Disease

There is a high incidence of renal scarring in patients with underlying conditions that cause chronic interstitial nephritis, virtually all of which produce primary renal papillary damage. These conditions include diabetes mellitus, sickle cell disorders, adult nephrocalcinosis, hyperphosphatemia, hypokalemia, analgesic abuse, sulfonamide nephropathy, gout, heavy-metal poisoning, and aging (Freedman, 1979).

Diabetes Mellitus

An increased incidence of clinical asymptomatic and symptomatic UTIs appears to occur in women with diabetes mellitus, but there is no substantial increase among diabetic men (Vejlsgaard, 1973; Ooi et al, 1974; Forland et al, 1977; Meiland et al, 2002). Diabetes also results in three times more hospitalizations for acute pyelonephritis among women (10.86/10,000) than for men (3.32/10,000) (Nicolle et al, 1996). Autopsy studies have shown the incidence of pyelonephritis to be fourfold to fivefold higher in diabetic than in nondiabetic individuals (Robbins and Tucker, 1944). However, such studies may be misleading because it is difficult to distinguish renal parenchymal changes resulting from pyelonephritis from the interstitial inflammatory changes of diabetic nephropathy.

Although most UTIs in diabetic patients are asymptomatic, diabetes appears to predispose the patient to more severe infections. One study using antibody-coated bacteria techniques to localize the site of infection showed the upper urinary tract to be involved in nearly 80% of diabetic patients with UTIs (Forland et al, 1977). This evidence of increasing immunologic response in diabetic patients who acquire bacteriuria suggests renal parenchymal involvement and a potential increase in morbidity. There is no evidence that increased frequency of infection is due to glycosuria, but this condition may contribute to infection severity (Geerlings et al, 2000).

Infections are frequently caused by atypical organisms such as yeast and result in upper tract infections and significant sequelae such as emphysematous pyelonephritis, papillary necrosis, perinephric abscess, or metastatic infection (Wheat, 1980; Stapleton, 2002).

Renal Papillary Necrosis

The role of infection in the development and progression of renal papillary necrosis (RPN) is controversial. **Multiple**

Table 8–2. Conditions Associated with Renal Papillary Necrosis

Diabetes mellitus
Pyelonephritis
Urinary tract obstruction
Analgesic abuse
Sickle cell hemoglobinopathies
Renal transplant rejection
Cirrhosis of the liver
Dehydration, hypoxia, and jaundice of infants
Miscellaneous: renal vein thrombosis, cryoglobulinemia, renal
  candidiasis, contrast media injection, amyloidosis, calyceal arteritis,
  necrotizing angiitis, rapidly progressive glomerulonephritis,
  hypotensive shock, acute pancreatitis

From Eknoyan G, Qunibi WY, Grissom RT, et al: Renal papillary necrosis: An update. Medicine 1982;61:55.

predisposing conditions have been associated with the development of RPN, particularly diabetes, analgesic abuse, sickle cell hemoglobinopathy, and obstruction (Table 8–2). In the excellent review of RPN by Eknoyan and colleagues (1982), 67% of the patients (18 of 27) with RPN had an acute or chronic UTI. In only 4 patients (22%) was pyelonephritis alone associated with RPN. In the remaining 14 patients, several of the conditions that can be associated with RPN were present in addition to the UTI. All 4 patients with urinary tract obstruction had concomitant UTI. In 9 of the RPN patients, there was no evidence of infection at all. These figures emphasize that, although any of the recognized factors in Table 8–2 alone may cause RPN, the coexistence of multiple factors, such as diabetes or obstruction and infection, increases the risk of developing RPN.

Clinically, RPN is a spectrum of disease. Patients may have an acute fulminating illness with rapid progression or may have a chronic disease that is incidentally discovered on excretory urography. Some patients may chronically pass necrotic tissue in their urine (Hernandez et al, 1975), and some may never pass papillae (Lindvall, 1978). Although the diagnosis may be made from the passage of necrotic papillae in the urine, most often it is made from the excretory urogram. The radiographs show various degrees of renal involvement with either medullary or papillary changes causing irregular sinuses or medullary cavities or classic ring shadows (Eknoyan et al, 1982; Lindvall, 1978). Retained necrotic papillae may calcify, especially in association with infection. Furthermore, this necrotic tissue may form the nidus for chronic infection. Opportunistic fungal infections have been reported (Madge and Lombardias, 1973; Juhasz et al, 1980; Vordermark et al, 1980; Tomashefski and Abramowsky, 1981). Renal sonography may be useful to diagnose RPN (Buonocore et al, 1980; Hoffman et al, 1982).

The early diagnosis of RPN is important to improve prognosis and reduce morbidity. In addition to chronic infection, patients with analgesic abuse–associated papillary necrosis may have an increased incidence of urothelial tumors; routine urinary cytologic examinations may be helpful to diagnose these tumors early (Jackson et al, 1978). In patients who have analgesic abuse–induced RPN, the disease stabilizes if the analgesic intake is stopped (Gower, 1976). Furthermore, adequate antimicrobial therapy to control infection and early recognition and treatment of

ureteral obstruction caused by sloughed necrotic tissue can minimize a decline in renal function. A patient who suffers from an acute ureteral obstruction due to a sloughed papilla and who has a concomitant UTI has a urologic emergency. In this case, immediate removal of the obstructing papilla by stone basket (Jameson and Heal, 1973) or acute drainage of the kidney by ureteral catheter or percutaneous nephrostomy is necessary.

Other conditions that may increase the susceptibility of the kidney to infection include hypertension and vascular obstruction (Freedman, 1979). Association of renal infection with several other renal diseases, including glomerulonephritis, atherosclerosis, and tubular necrosis, which are not associated with papillary necrosis, does not lead to pyelonephritis and scarring.

Human Immunodeficiency Virus

UTIs are fivefold more prevalent in HIV-positive individuals than in control subjects (Schonwald et al, 1999). Furthermore, the pathologic flora are more reminiscent of complicated UTIs. It also appears that HIV-positive patients with UTIs have a tendency for recurrence and require longer treatment.

Pregnancy

The prevalence of bacteriuria in pregnant women varies from 4% to 7%, and the incidence of acute clinical pyelonephritis ranges from 25% to 35% in untreated bacteriuric women (Stamey, 1980). This is probably the result of dilation of the ureters and pelvis of the kidney secondary to pregnancy-related hormonal alterations. It is not surprising that untreated bacteriuria in the first trimester is accompanied by a substantial increase in the incidence of acute pyelonephritis, because half of these women have upper tract bacteriuria (Fairley et al, 1966). Untreated bacteriuria involving these dilated upper tracts would be expected to produce a significant number of abnormalities that should be radiologically apparent. Kincaid-Smith and Bullen (1965) performed a culture on 4000 women at their first antenatal visit. Of 240 bacteriuric women, 148 returned for excretory urography 6 weeks after delivery. Approximately 40% of these patients had radiologic abnormalities consistent with pyelonephritis or analgesic nephritis. Brumfitt and colleagues (1967) showed that the incidence of radiologic abnormalities in bacteriuria of pregnancy was proportional to the difficulty in clearing the infection. Patients who responded promptly to a single course of therapy had a 23% incidence of radiologic abnormalities, but those who remained bacteriuric despite repeated therapeutic efforts had a 65% incidence of radiologic changes. Thus, prolonged bacteriuria and pyelonephritis of pregnancy appear to be associated with significant radiologic abnormalities. However, there is little evidence to suggest that bacteriuria of pregnancy or acute pyelonephritis of pregnancy causes these renal radiologic abnormalities.

Spinal Cord Injury with High-Pressure Bladders

Of all patients with bacteriuria, no group compares in severity and morbidity with those who have spinal cord injury. Nearly all these patients require catheterization early after their injuries because of bladder overactivity or flaccidity, and significant numbers develop ureterectasis, hydronephrosis, reflux, and renal calculi. Bacteriologic and urodynamic advances in the management of these patients have vastly reduced their morbidity and mortality. Special problems associated with spinal cord injury are presented in a later section.

KEY POINTS: PATHOGENESIS

- Most UTIs are caused by bacteria, usually originating from the bowel flora.

- Bacterial virulence factors, including adhesin, play a role in determining which bacteria invade and the extent of infection.

- Increased epithelial cell receptivity predisposes patients to recurrent UTIs and is a genotypic trait.

- Obstruction to urine flow is a key factor in increasing host susceptibility to UTIs.

CLINICAL MANIFESTATIONS

Symptoms and Signs

Cystitis is usually associated with dysuria, frequency, urgency, suprapubic pain, and hematuria. Lower tract symptoms are commonly present and usually predate the appearance of upper tract symptoms by several days. Pyelonephritis is classically associated with fever, chills, and flank pain. Nausea and vomiting may be present. Renal or perirenal abscess may cause indolent fever and flank mass and tenderness. In the elderly, the symptoms may be much more subtle (e.g., epigastric or abdominal discomfort) or the patient may be asymptomatic (Romano and Kaye, 1981). Patients with indwelling catheters often have asymptomatic bacteriuria, but fever associated with bacteremia may occur rapidly and become life threatening.

Diagnosis

Presumptive diagnosis of UTI is made by direct or indirect analysis of the urine and is confirmed by urine culture. Assessment of the urine provides clinical information about the status of the urinary tract. The urine and the urinary tract are normally free of bacteria and inflammation. False-negative urinalysis and culture can occur in the presence of UTI, particularly early in an infection when the numbers of bacteria and WBCs are low or diluted by increased fluid intake and subsequent diuresis. Occasionally, the urine may be free of bacteria and WBCs despite bacterial colonization and inflammation of the uroepithelium (Elliott et al, 1985; Hultgren et al, 1985). False-positive urinalysis and culture are caused by contamination of the urine specimen with bacteria and WBCs during collection. This is most likely to occur in voided specimens but can also occur during urethral catheterization. Suprapubic aspiration of bladder urine is least likely to cause contamination of the specimen; therefore, it provides the most accurate assessment of the status of bladder urine.

Urine Collection

Voided and Catheterized Specimens. Diagnostic accuracy can be improved by reducing bacterial contamination when the urine is collected. In circumcised men, voided specimens require no preparation. For men who are not circumcised, the foreskin should be retracted and the glans penis washed with soap and then rinsed with water before specimen collection. The first 10 mL of urine (representative of the urethra) and a midstream specimen (representative of the bladder) should be obtained. Prostatic fluid is obtained by performing digital prostatic massage and collecting the expressed prostatic fluid on a glass slide. In addition, collection of the first 10 mL of voided urine after massage will reflect the prostatic fluid added to the urethral specimen. Catheterization of a male patient for urine culture is not indicated unless the patient cannot urinate.

In women, contamination of a midstream urine specimen with introital bacteria and WBCs is common, particularly when the woman has difficulty spreading and maintaining separation of the labia. Therefore the female should be instructed to spread the labia, wash and cleanse the peri-urethral area with a moist gauze, and then collect a midstream urine specimen. Cleansing with antiseptics is not recommended because they may contaminate the voided specimen and provide a false-negative urine culture. If the voided specimen shows evidence of contamination as indicated by vaginal epithelial cells and lactobacilli on urinalysis, catheterization should be performed and a midcatheterized specimen collected.

The incidence of catheter-induced UTI is determined primarily by the population at risk, varying from 1% in non-hospitalized, healthy women (Turck et al, 1962) **to 20% in women hospitalized on a medical ward** (Thiel and Spuhler, 1965). **The easiest way to prevent catheter-induced infections is to give a single dose of an oral antimicrobial agent, such as trimethoprim-sulfamethoxazole (TMP-SMX).** However, because antimicrobial usage encourages development of bacterial resistance, prophylaxis should be limited to high-risk patients.

Suprapubic Aspiration. Suprapubic aspiration is highly accurate, but because it carries some morbidity there is limited clinical usefulness except for a patient who cannot urinate on command, such as patients with spinal cord injuries. It is highly useful in newborns (Newman et al, 1967) and in patients with paraplegia. A single aspirated specimen reveals the bacteriologic status of the bladder urine without introducing urethral bacteria, which can start a new infection.

Before a suprapubic aspiration is performed, the patient should force fluids until the bladder is full. The site of the needle puncture is in the midline, between the symphysis pubis and the umbilicus and directly over the palpable bladder. The full bladder in the male is usually palpable because of its greater muscle tone; unfortunately, the full bladder in the female is frequently not palpable. In such patients, the physician performing the aspiration must rely on the observation that suprapubic pressure directly over the bladder produces an unmistakable desire to urinate. After determining the approximate site for needle puncture, the local area is shaved and the skin is cleansed with an alcohol sponge; a cutaneous wheal is raised with a 25-gauge needle and any local anesthetic. A 3.5-inch spinal, 22-gauge needle is introduced through the anesthetized skin. The progress of the needle is arrested just below the skin within the anesthetized area, and with a quick plunging action, similar to that of any intramuscular injection, the needle is advanced into the bladder. Most patients experience more discomfort from the initial anesthetization of the skin than they feel during the second stage when the needle is advanced into the bladder. After the needle has been introduced, a 20-mL syringe is used to aspirate 5 mL of urine for culture and 15 mL of urine for centrifugation and urinalysis. The obturator is reintroduced into the needle, and both needle and obturator are withdrawn. A small dressing is placed over the needle site in the skin. If urine is not obtained with complete introduction of the needle, the patient's bladder is not full and is usually deep within the retropubic area. When no urine is obtained on the first attempt, it is probably wise to wait until the bladder is full.

Urinalysis

For patients with urinary symptoms, microscopic urinalysis for bacteriuria, pyuria, and hematuria should be performed. Urinalysis provides rapid identification of bacteria and WBCs and presumptive diagnosis of UTI. Usually, the sediment from an approximately 5- to 10-mL specimen obtained by centrifugation for 5 minutes at 2000 rpm is analyzed. Microscopic bacteriuria is found in more than 90% of infections with counts of 10^5 colony-forming units (cfu) per milliliter of urine or greater and is a highly specific finding (Stamm, 1982; Jenkins et al, 1986). However, bacteria are usually not detectable microscopically with lower colony count infections (10^2 to 10^4/mL). **This important error (i.e., a false-negative result) occurs because of the limitation imposed by the microscope on the volume of urine that can be observed.** If the volume of urine that can easily rest beneath a standard 22-mm cover glass is carefully measured (0.01 mL) and the number of high dry fields (×570 magnification) present beneath the cover glass is estimated, it is disturbing to find that one high dry field represents a volume of approximately 1/30,000 mL. There are excellent studies showing that the bacterial count must be approximately 30,000/mL before bacteria can be found in the sediment, stained or unstained, spun or unspun (Sanford et al, 1956; Kunin, 1961). For these reasons, a negative urinalysis for bacteria never excludes the presence of bacteria in numbers of 30,000/mL and less.

The second error of urinalysis (i.e., a false-positive result) is the reverse of the first error: bacteria are seen in the microscopic sediment but the urine culture shows no growth. The voided urine from a female patient can contain many thousands of lactobacilli and corynebacteria. These bacteria are readily seen under the microscope; and although they are gram-positive, they often appear gram-negative (gram-variable) if stained. Strict anaerobes, usually gram-negative bacilli, also make up a significant mass of the normal vaginal flora (Marrie et al, 1978).

In practice, these problems can be minimized by using other information provided by urinalysis that can help the clinician to decide whether a patient has a UTI (Stamm et al, 1982b). **The validation of the midstream urine specimen can be questioned if numerous squamous epithelial cells (indicative of preputial, vaginal, or urethral contaminants) are present.**

Pyuria and hematuria are good indicators of an inflammatory response. Although the number of WBCs per high-power field in a centrifuged urine sample is useful, it is important to remember that other factors can influence the number of cells seen. These include the state of hydration; the intensity of tissue reaction; the method of urine collection; the volume, speed, and time of centrifugation; and the volume in which the sediment is resuspended.

Significant pyuria can be determined simply and reliably with a microscope by accurately examining the centrifuged sediment or by using a hemocytometer to count the number of WBCs in the unspun urine. One to 2 WBCs per high-power field (HPF) in sediment from a centrifuged specimen represents about 10 WBCs/mm^3 in an unspun specimen. More than 2 WBCs per HPF in a centrifuged specimen or 10 WBCs/mm^3 of urine correlates well with the presence of bacteriuria and is rarely seen in nonbacteriuric patients (Stamm et al, 1981). In clinical studies, determination of pyuria in voided urine specimens has a reported sensitivity of 80% to 95% and a specificity of 50% to 76% for UTI (depending on the definition of infection, the patient population, and the method used to evaluate for pyuria) (Stamm, 1982; Schultz et al, 1984; Wong et al, 1984; Wigton et al, 1985).

The absence of pyuria should cause the diagnosis of UTI to be questioned until urine culture data are available. Conversely, many diseases of the urinary tract produce significant pyuria in the absence of bacteriuria. Whereas tuberculosis is the well-recognized example of abacterial pyuria, staghorn calculi and stones of smaller size can produce intense pyuria with clumps of WBCs in the absence of UTI. Almost any injury to the urinary tract, from chlamydial urethritis to glomerulonephritis and interstitial cystitis, can elicit large numbers of fresh polymorphonuclear leukocytes (glitter cells). Depending on the stage of hydration, the intensity of the tissue reaction producing the cells, and the method of urine collection, any number of WBCs can be seen in the microscopic sediment in the presence of an uninfected urinary tract.

Microscopic hematuria is found in 40% to 60% of cases of cystitis and is uncommon in other dysuric syndromes (Stamm et al, 1980b; Wigton et al, 1985). **Thus, microscopic bacteriuria and hematuria lack sensitivity but are highly specific for UTIs.**

Rapid Screen Methods. Biochemical and enzymatic tests have been devised to detect bacteriuria and pyuria (Pezzlo, 1988). The Griess test detects the presence of nitrite in urine that is formed when bacteria reduce the nitrate normally present in urine. Tests for detecting pyuria by determining leukocyte esterase activity have also been developed (Chernow et al, 1984). In a study comparing traditional urine culture with these indirect tests, the combination of nitrite and leukocyte esterase tests (either test positive) had a sensitivity of 71% and a specificity of 83% when compared with 10^3 cfu/mL or greater of urine cultures (Pfaller and Koontz, 1985). However, several investigators (Pels et al, 1989; Hurlbut and Littenberg, 1991) noted substantial variability in the sensitivity and specificity results, which could be markedly influenced by the types of patients and infections chosen to evaluate the tests. This concept of spectrum bias was illustrated by a study that reported differences in the sensitivity of reagent strip testing, ranging from 56% to 92%, by changing only the groups of patients included in the analysis. Although false-positive results are relatively uncommon, the borderline sensitivity of these tests, especially among patients with less characteristic symptoms of UTIs, does not allow these inexpensive tests to replace careful microscopic urinalysis in symptomatic patients (Semeniuk and Church, 1999). Their main role is in screening asymptomatic patients (Pezzlo, 1988).

Urine Culture

Two techniques for urine culture are available. Direct surface plating of a known amount of urine on split-agar disposable plates is the traditional quantitative culture technique used by most microbiology laboratories. One half of the plate is blood agar, which grows both gram-positive and gram-negative bacteria, and the other is desoxycholate or eosin-methylene blue (EMB), which grows gram-negative bacteria (some of them, such as *E. coli*, in a very characteristic manner). Simple curved-tip eye droppers are sufficient to deliver about 0.1 mL of urine onto each half of the plate. After overnight incubation, the number of colonies is estimated, often identified (after some experience), and multiplied by 10 to report the number of cfu per milliliter of urine. The technique has been presented elsewhere in detail (Stamey, 1980).

A simpler but somewhat less accurate technique is the use of dip slides (Fig. 8–11). These inexpensive plastic slides are attached to screw-top caps; they have soy agar (a general nutrient agar to grow all bacteria) on one side and EMB or Mac-Conkey's agar for gram-negative bacteria on the opposite side. A slide is dipped into urine, the excess is allowed to drain off, and the slide is replaced in its plastic bottle and incubated. The volume of urine that attaches to the slide is between 1/100 mL and 1/200 mL. Hence, the colony count is 100 to 200 times the number of colonies that become visible with incubation. In actual practice, the growth is compared with a visual standard and reported as such. The species of bacteria is more difficult to recognize when this technique is used, but the technique is completely adequate.

It is emphasized that the urine must be refrigerated immediately on collection and should be cultured within 24 hours of refrigeration. One advantage to the dip slide is the ease with which the urine can be immediately cultured without the necessity of refrigeration. Patients can culture their own urine at home, keep the slide at room temperature, and bring it to the office within 48 hours.

Although most bacteria allowed to incubate for several hours in bladder urine reach cfu counts of 10^5/mL, this statistical number is fraught with two limitations. The first is that 20% to 40% of women with symptomatic UTIs present with bacteria counts of 10^2 to 10^4 cfu/mL of urine (Stamey et al, 1965; Mabeck, 1969; Kunz et al, 1975; Kraft and Stamey, 1977), probably because of the slow doubling time of bacteria in urine (every 30 to 45 minutes) combined with frequent bladder emptying (every 15 to 30 minutes) from irritation. **Thus, in dysuric patients, an appropriate threshold value for defining significant bacteriuria is 10^2 cfu/mL of a known pathogen** (Stamm and Hooton, 1993). Fortunately, most of these patients have symptoms of UTI and most have pyuria on urinalysis.

The second limitation of the 10^5 cutoff is overdiagnosis. Women susceptible to infection often carry large numbers of pathogenic bacteria on the perineum that contaminate otherwise sterile bladder urine. Uncircumcised men may harbor uropathogenic bacteria on their foreskins. In the original studies by Kass (1960), a single culture of 10^5 cfu/mL or more had a 20% chance of representing contamination. There is no statistical way to avoid these two major limitations on the interpretation of the midstream voided culture in women and in uncircumcised men without careful preparation.

Localization

Kidney

Fever and Flank Pain. Fever and flank pain are thought to indicate pyelonephritis, but few studies have tested the hypothesis. Aggressive localization studies in children and adults (Huland and Busch, 1982; Busch and Huland, 1984), as well as in patients with end-stage renal disease (Huland et al,

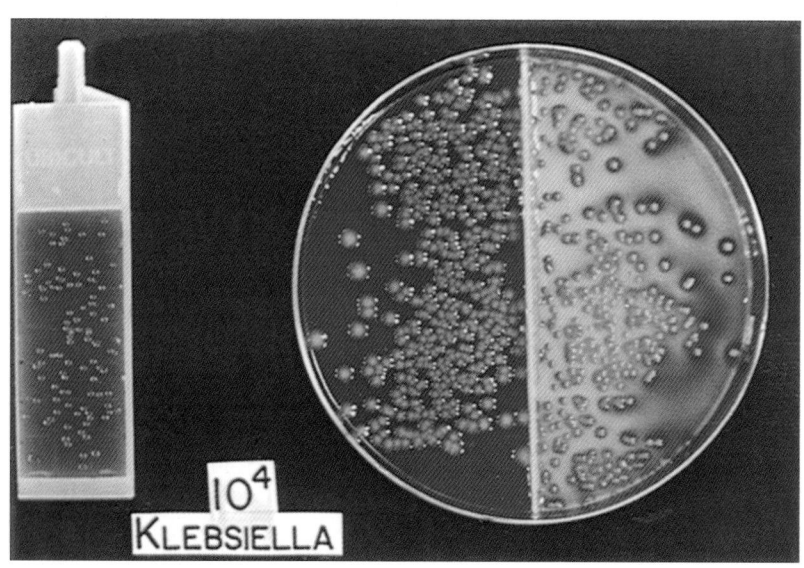

Figure 8–11. The dip slide on the left is compared with a split-agar surface plate on the right. The urine contained 10,000 colonies of *Klebsiella* per milliliter (about 200 times the number of colonies on the dip slide and 10 times the number on either side of the split-agar plate).

Table 8–3. Clinical Examples of Ureteral Catheterization Studies in Localizing the Site of Bacteriuria

Source	Bladder Infection (bacteria/mL)	Left Renal Infection (bacteria/mL)	Right Renal Infection (bacteria/mL)	Bilateral Renal Infection (bacteria/mL)
CB	>10^5	5,000	>10^5	4,000
WB	900	300	1,000	20
LK_1	20	2,000	20	400
LK_2	0	2,200	0	350
LK_3	0	2,500	0	500
LK_4	0	2,200	0	400
RK_1	10	0	10,000	260
RK_2	0	0	10,000	220
RK_3	0	0	8,000	300
RK_4	0	0	12,000	250

CB, catheterized patient, cystoscopic specimen; LK_1, LK_2, etc., serial cultures of urine from the left kidney; RK_1, RK_2, etc., serial cultures of urine from the right kidney; WB, controlled, "wash bladder" specimen collected after copious irrigation of the bladder.

1983), have shown substantial incidences of fever and even flank pain in bacteriuric patients in whom infection was localized to the bladder (see the later section on "Acute Pyelonephritis").

Ureteral Catheterization. **Ureteral catheterization allows not only separation of bacterial persistence into upper and lower urinary tracts but also separation of the infection between one kidney and the other, and even localization of infection to ectopic ureters or to nonrefluxing ureteral stumps (by using saline solution irrigation)** (Stamey, 1980).

Stamey began in 1959 to localize the site of bacteriuria by ureteral catheterization studies; the technique was published in 1963 (Stamey and Pfau, 1963) and the results in 1965 (Stamey et al, 1965). The technique is simple but exacting; the urologist should consult a more detailed description (Stamey, 1980) before actually performing this localization technique. The validity depends on controlling the number of bacteria from the bladder that contaminate the ureteral catheters as they pass through the bladder into the ureteral orifices. The bladder must be thoroughly irrigated before both ureteral catheters are passed into a small volume of residual irrigating fluid. A sample is obtained through both ureteral catheters simultaneously, and then each catheter is passed into the ureter or renal pelvis. Four serial cultures are obtained from each kidney. It is mandatory that the patient be started on the appropriate antimicrobial agent before leaving the cystoscopy room. In addition to quantitative bacterial counts on each specimen, determination of either specific gravity or urine creatinine levels on the renal samples can be very helpful in interpreting a change in diuresis in relation to bacterial counts. Examples of infections localized to the bladder, to one kidney, and to both kidneys have been published (Stamey, 1980). Clinical examples of results from each site are shown in Table 8–3.

When this technique was applied to large numbers of bacteriuric patients, 45% were found to have bladder infection only; 27%, unilateral renal bacteriuria; and 28%, bilateral renal bacteriuria (Table 8–4) (Stamey et al, 1965). These figures have been confirmed by at least five investigators in three countries (the United States, England, and Australia) and can be taken as a good approximation for any general bacteriuric adult population. **Although renal stones and other kidney abnormalities in the presence of bacteriuria can increase the proportion of renal infections, the urologist**

Table 8–4. Localization of UTIs in 95 Females and 26 Males with Bacteriuria

Number and Sex	Bladder Only	Unilateral Renal Bacteriuria	Bilateral Renal Bacteriuria
95 females	38 (40%)	27 (28%)	30 (32%)
26 males	16 (62%)	6 (26%)	4 (15%)
121 combined	54 (45%)	33 (27%)	34 (28%)

From Stamey TA, Govan DE, Palmer JM: The localization and treatment of urinary tract infections: The role of bactericidal urine levels as opposed to serum level. Medicine 1965;44:1.

should never assume the kidney is involved if an important decision is to be made.

Tissue and Stone Cultures. It is clinically useful to culture stones removed from the urinary tract to document that bacteria reside within their interstices. Tissue cultures are primarily useful for research information.

Using sterile technique at the operating table, the surgeon places the stone or fragment of tissue into a sterile culture tube containing 5 mL of saline solution; the culture is packed in ice and sent to the bacteriologic laboratory, where, after agitation of the stone or tissue in the 5 mL of saline solution, 0.1 mL is surface-streaked on both blood agar and EMB agar. The saline solution is then poured off the specimen; and, with sterile forceps, the stone or tissue is transferred to a second 5 mL of sterile saline solution. After agitation to ensure a reasonable washing action, the saline solution is again decanted and the specimen is transferred to a third 5 mL of saline solution and finally to a fourth 5 mL of saline solution. This last saline solution wash is cultured quantitatively in the same manner as the first. The remainder of this fourth 5 mL of saline solution is poured with the stone into a sterile mortar and pestle dish.

After the stone is crushed (or the tissue is ground in a tissue blender) in the fourth saline solution wash, 0.1 mL is again cultured on both blood agar and EMB agar. The difference in colony counts between the first and the fourth saline solution washes represents the washing effect of the saline solution transfers on the surface bacteria of the stone or tissue. The difference between the fourth saline wash before and after crushing (or grinding, for tissue) represents the difference between surface bacteria and bacteria within the specimen.

Prostate and Urethral Localization Studies. The technique for localizing infections to the urethra or prostate is covered in detail in Chapter 9, "Inflammatory Conditions of the Male Genitourinary Tract: Prostatitis and Related Conditions, Orchitis, and Epididymitis."

KEY POINTS: CLINICAL MANIFESTATIONS

■ The urine and the urinary tract are normally free of bacteria and inflammation.

■ Bacteriuria and WBCs provide a presumptive diagnosis of UTI.

■ In diagnosing patients, 10^2 cfu/mL confirms a symptomatic UTI.

IMAGING TECHNIQUES

Imaging studies are not required in most cases of UTI because clinical and laboratory findings alone are sufficient for correct diagnosis and adequate management of most patients. However, infection in most men or a compromised host, febrile infections, signs or symptoms of urinary tract obstruction, failure to respond to appropriate therapy, and a pattern of recurrent infections suggesting bacterial persistence within the urinary tract warrant imaging for identification of underlying abnormalities that require modification of medical management or percutaneous or surgical intervention.

Indications

Radiologic studies are unnecessary for evaluation of most women with genitourinary infections. Several reports of women patients with recurrent UTIs show that excretory urograms are unnecessary for routine evaluation if women who have special risk factors are excluded (Fair et al, 1979; Engel et al, 1980; Fowler and Pulaski, 1981; Fairchild et al, 1982). In none of these studies was information that was useful in the management of these patients obtained from excretory urograms. Furthermore, excluding excretory urograms in the routine evaluation of such patients represents a substantial financial saving.

However, in high-risk patients, including women with febrile infections and most men, radiologic studies may determine acute infectious processes that require further intervention or may find the cause of complicated infections.

First, radiologic procedures are needed in patients with risk factors that may require intervention in addition to antimicrobial treatment (Table 8–5).

A UTI associated with possible urinary tract obstruction must be evaluated. These are patients with calculi, especially infection (struvite) stones; ureteral tumors; ureteral strictures; congenital obstructions; or previous genitourinary surgery, such as ureteral reimplantation or urinary diversion procedures, that may have caused obstruction. Patients with diabetes mellitus can develop special complications from UTIs;

Table 8–5. Indications for Radiologic Investigation in Acute Clinical Pyelonephritis

Potential ureteral obstruction (e.g., due to stone, ureteral stricture, tumor)
History of calculi, especially infection (struvite) stones
Papillary necrosis (e.g., patients with sickle cell anemia, severe diabetes mellitus, analgesic abuse)
History of genitourinary surgery that predisposes to obstruction, such as ureteral reimplantation or ureteral diversion
Poor response to appropriate antimicrobial agents after 5 to 6 days of treatment
Diabetes mellitus
Polycystic kidneys in patients in dialysis or with severe renal insufficiency
Neuropathic bladder
Unusual infecting organisms, such as tuberculosis, fungus, or urea-splitting organisms (e.g., *Proteus*)

Table 8–6. Correctable Urologic Abnormalities That Cause Bacterial Persistence

Infection stones
Chronic bacterial prostatitis
Unilateral infected atrophic kidneys
Ureteral duplication and ectopic ureters
Foreign bodies
Urethral diverticula and infected periurethral glands
Unilateral medullary sponge kidneys
Nonrefluxing, normal-appearing, infected ureteral stumps after nephrectomy
Infected urachal cysts
Infected communicating cysts of the renal calyces
Papillary necrosis
Perivesical abscess with fistula to bladder

they may acquire emphysematous pyelonephritis or papillary necrosis. Impacted necrotic papillae may cause acute ureteral obstruction. Patients with polycystic kidney disease who are on dialysis are particularly prone to developing perinephric abscesses.

Urologic imaging is indicated in patients whose symptoms of acute clinical pyelonephritis persist after 5 to 6 days of appropriate antimicrobial therapy; they often have perinephric or renal abscesses. In addition, patients with unusual organisms, including urea-splitting organisms (e.g., *Proteus* species), should be examined for abnormalities within the urinary tract, such as obstructing stones, strictures, or fungus balls.

The second reason for radiologic evaluation is to diagnose a focus of bacterial persistence. **In patients whose bacteriuria fails to resolve after appropriate antimicrobial therapy or who have rapid recurrence of infection, abnormalities that cause bacterial persistence should be sought.** Although these patients are uncommon, it is important to identify them because they may have correctable urologic abnormalities that represent the only surgically curable causes of recurrent UTIs. Acquired or congenital urologic abnormalities that can cause unresolved or recurrent UTIs are listed in Table 8–6.

Plain Film of the Abdomen

The plain film of the abdomen (kidney, ureter, and bladder) is useful for the rapid detection of radiopaque calculi and unusual gas patterns in emphysematous pyelonephritis. It may show abnormalities, such as an absent psoas or abnormal renal contour, that suggest perirenal or renal abscess, but these findings are nonspecific.

Plain Film Renal Tomograms

Plain film renal tomograms show small or poorly calcified stones despite overlying gas and fecal shadows. Struvite and uric acid stones that contain small amounts of calcium may be seen on these films but not on routine plain films of the abdomen. Tomograms also localize findings (calcifications or gas) to the kidney.

Excretory Urogram

The excretory urogram has been a routine examination to evaluate patients with complicated infection problems but is not required in uncomplicated infections. The radiologic features of acute clinical pyelonephritis are discussed in a later section on that subject. The excretory urography study is useful to determine the exact site and extent of urinary tract obstruction; however, it is not the best screening test for hydronephrosis, pyonephrosis, or renal abscess.

Voiding Cystourethrogram

The voiding cystourethrogram is an important examination in assessing vesicoureteral reflux. It may be used to evaluate patients with neuropathic bladders and the rare female patient who has a urethral diverticulum causing her persistent infections.

Ultrasonography

The renal ultrasound study is an important renal imaging technique because it is noninvasive, easy to perform, and rapid, and offers no radiation or contrast agent risk to the patient. It is particularly useful in identifying calculi and hydronephrosis, pyonephrosis, and perirenal abscesses. A single radiograph for calculi should accompany ultrasonography. Ultrasonography is also useful for diagnosing postvoid residual urine. A disadvantage is that the study is dependent on the interpretative and performance skills of the examiner. Furthermore, the study may be technically poor in patients who are obese or who have dressings, drainage tubes, or open wounds overlying the area of interest.

Computed Tomography (CT) and Magnetic Resonance Imaging (MRI)

The radiologic modalities that offer the best anatomic detail are CT and MRI. They are more sensitive than excretory urography or ultrasonography in the diagnosis of acute focal bacterial nephritis, renal and perirenal abscesses, and radiolucent calculi (Kuhn and Berger, 1981; Mauro et al, 1982; Wadsworth et al, 1982; Soulen et al, 1989; Soler et al, 1997). When used to localize renal and perirenal abscesses, CT improves the approach to surgical drainage and permits percutaneous approaches. MRI has not superseded CT in the evaluation of renal inflammation, but it has provided some advantages in delineating extrarenal extension of inflammation.

Radionuclide Studies

Hippuran I-131 and technetium ^{99m}Tc glucoheptonate scans are used to detect focal parenchymal damage, renal function impairment, and decreased renal perfusion in acute renal infections (McAfee, 1979). Although gallium-67 scanning has been reported to be useful in the diagnosis of pyelonephritis and renal abscess, it is uncommonly required and may be positive in noninfectious entities. Indium-111–labeled WBC studies have limited efficacy in establishing the presence of an inflammatory focus, particularly when the patient's clinical presentation does not suggest an infectious process.

KEY POINTS: IMAGING TECHNIQUES

- Imaging studies are not required in most women with UTIs.

- Men and compromised patients or those who do not respond to therapy require imaging to identify abnormalities.

- CT and MRI provide the best anatomic data on the site, cause, and extent of infection.

PRINCIPLES OF ANTIMICROBIAL THERAPY

Therapy for UTIs must ultimately eliminate bacterial growth in the urinary tract. This can occur within hours if the proper antimicrobial agent is used (Stamey, 1980). **Efficacy of the antimicrobial therapy is critically dependent on the antimicrobial levels in the urine and the duration that this level remains above the minimal inhibitory concentration of the infecting organism** (Hooton and Stamm, 1991). **Hence, resolution of infection is closely associated with the susceptibility of the bacteria to the concentration of the antimicrobial agent achieved in the urine** (McCabe and Jackson, 1965; Stamey et al, 1965, 1974). The concentration of useful antimicrobial agents in the serum and urine of healthy adults is shown in Table 8–7, which demonstrates that the urinary levels are often several hundred times greater than the serum levels. Inhibitory concentrations in urine are achieved after oral administration of all commonly used antimicrobial agents, except for the macrolides (erythromycin). The question of serum levels versus urinary levels is a practical one because the policy of testing antimicrobial susceptibility agents at concentrations obtainable only in the serum discourages the physician from using drugs that are effective at the urinary level, for example, oral penicillin G for *E. coli* and *Proteus mirabilis* and tetracycline for *P. aeruginosa*.

The concentration of the antimicrobial agent achieved in blood is not important in treatment of uncomplicated UTIs. Blood levels are critical in patients with bacteremia and febrile urinary infections consistent with parenchymal involvement of the kidney and prostate.

Table 8-7. Serum and Urinary Antimicrobial Levels in Adults*

Antimicrobial Agent	Dose (mg)	Peak Serum Level (mg/L)	Percentage Bound to Protein	Half-Life Serum Peak (hr)	Mean (Active) Urine Levels* (g/mL)	Dose Excreted in Urine (%)	Dose Active in Urine (if Different) (%)
Ampicillin	250 PO QID	3 at 2 hr	15	1	350	42	–
Carbenicillin	764 PO QID	11-17 at 1.5 hr	60	1.2	1000	40	–
Cephalexin	250 PO QID	9 at 2 hr	12	0.9	800	98	–
Ciprofloxacin	500 PO BID	2.3 at 1.2 hr	35	3.9	200	30	–
Colistin	75 IM BID	1.8 at 4 hr	10	2	34	75	50
Gentamicin	1 mg/kg IM TID (200 mg/day)	4 at 1 hr	Negligible	2	125	80	–
Kanamycin	500 IM BID	18 at 1 hr	Negligible	2	750	94	–
Levofloxacin	500 mg PO QD	6.0 mg/L	30-50	6	N/A	95	95
Nalidixic acid	1000 PO QID	34 at 2-23 hr	85	1.5	75	79	5
Nitrofurantoin	100 PO QID	<2		0.3	150	42	–
Norfloxacin	400 PO BID	1.5 at 1.5 hr	15	3.3	170	27	–
Penicillin G	500 PO QID	1 at 1 hr	60	0.5	300	20	–
Sulfamethizole	250 PO QID		98	10	700	95	85
Tetracycline hydrochloride	250 PO QID	2-3 at 4 h	31	6	500	60	–
TMP-SMX	160/800 PO BID	1.7/32 at 2 hr	45/66	10/9	150/400	55/50	–/37
Trimethoprim	100 PO BID	1.0 at 2-4 hr	45	10	92	55	–

TMP-SMX, trimethoprim-sulfamethoxazole.
*These average urinary concentrations are based on the amount of biologically active drug excreted by normal kidneys at a urine flow rate of 1200 mL/24 hr.
From Stamey TA: The Pathogenesis and Treatment of Urinary Infections. Baltimore, Williams & Wilkins, 1980, p 59, with modifications.

In patients with renal insufficiency, dosage modifications are necessary for agents that are cleared primarily by the kidneys and cannot be cleared by another mechanism. In renal failure, the kidneys may not be able to concentrate an antimicrobial agent in the urine; hence, difficulty in eradicating bacteria may occur. Urinary tract obstruction may also reduce concentration of antimicrobial agents within the urine.

A decision regarding the antimicrobial selection and the duration of therapy must consider the spectrum of activity of the drug against the known pathogen or the most probable pathogens based on the presumed source of acquisition of infection, whether the infection is judged to be uncomplicated or complicated, potential adverse effects, and cost. An often underemphasized but important characteristic is the drug's impact on the bowel and vaginal flora and the hospital bacterial environment. Bacterial susceptibility will vary dramatically in patients exposed to antimicrobial agents and in individuals in inpatient and outpatient settings. It is imperative that each clinician keep abreast of changes that affect antimicrobial use and susceptibility patterns.

Bacterial Resistance

In the last several years, the frequency and spectrum of antimicrobial-resistant UTIs have increased in both the hospital and community. The increasing frequency of drug resistance has been attributed to combinations of microbial characteristics, bacterial selection pressure due to antimicrobial use, and societal and technologic changes that enhance the transmission of drug resistance (Cohen, 1992).

Bacterial resistance may occur because of inherited chromosomal-mediated resistance or by acquired chromosomal- or extrachromosomal (plasmid)-mediated resistance due to exposure of an organism to antimicrobial agents.

Inherited chromosomal resistance exists in a bacterial species because of the absence of the proper mechanism on which the antimicrobial agent can act. For example, Proteus and Pseudomonas species are always resistant to nitrofurantoin.

Acquired chromosomal resistance occurs during therapy for UTIs. Before antimicrobial therapy, relatively resistant bacteria called mutators may be present in the urine at very low concentrations. Frequencies in mutations for high-level antimicrobial resistance are 1000-fold higher in mutators than in normal strains, indicating the increased adaptability of these strains (Miller et al, 2004). The remainder of the bacteria, which are susceptible to the administered antimicrobial agent, will be eradicated by therapy, but within 24 to 48 hours a repeat urine culture will show high bacterial counts of the resistant mutant. In essence, the antimicrobial therapy has selected out the resistant mutant. This phenomenon is most likely to occur when the antimicrobial level in the urine is close to or below the minimal inhibitory concentration of the drug. Selection of resistant clones in the course of therapy for a previously sensitive bacteriuric population occurs between 5% and 10% of the time, clearly not an insignificant factor and one that must be considered in resolving bacteriuria. Underdosing and noncompliance, as well as diuresis induced by increased fluid intake, can contribute to this process. Therefore, the clinician should select an antimicrobial agent with a urinary concentration that exceeds the minimal inhibitory concentration by the widest margin possible, avoid underdosing, and emphasize patient compliance.

Extrachromosomal-mediated resistance may be acquired and transferable via plasmids, which contain the genetic material for the resistance. This so-called R-factor resistance occurs in the bowel flora and is much more common than selection of preexisting mutants in the urinary tract. All antimicrobial classes are capable of causing plasmid-mediated resistance. However, for the fluoroquinolones resistance is rarely transmitted by plasmids, and nitrofurantoin plasmid-mediated resistance has not been reported.

Hence, patients previously exposed to β-lactams, aminoglycosides, sulfonamides, TMP, and tetracycline will often have R-factor resistance to both the antimicrobial agent to which the bacteria were exposed and also to other antimicrobial agents. In addition, the plasmids carrying the resistant genetic material are transferable both within species and across genera. Thus, for example, a patient receiving tetracycline may harbor several bowel strains that are resistant to tetracycline, ampicillin, sulfonamides, and TMP. **Because the bowel flora is the major reservoir for bacteria that ultimately colonize the urinary tract, infections that occur after antimicrobial therapy and that can cause plasmid-mediated resistance are commonly caused by organisms with multidrug resistance. However, resistant _E. coli_ in the bowel flora that infect the urinary tract almost always show susceptibility to nitrofurantoin or to the quinolones.**

Antimicrobial resistance is also influenced by the duration and amount of antimicrobial agent used. For example, documented increased use of fluoroquinolones in the hospital setting has been directly associated with increased resistance of bacteria (particularly _Pseudomonas_) to the fluoroquinolones. Resistance tends to increase the longer the agent is used. Conversely, reduction in duration of therapy and in the amount of the drug used may lead to reemergence of more susceptible strains.

Most studies reporting antimicrobial resistance have been based on surveys of laboratory isolates, generally without correlation with clinical or epidemiologic factors (e.g., the presence and nature of symptoms, age, sex, and whether the infection was complicated). Gupta and colleagues (1999) determined the prevalence of and trends in antimicrobial resistance among uropathogens isolated from a large, well-defined population of women with acute uncomplicated cystitis. Over a 5-year period, the prevalence of resistance to TMP/SMX, ampicillin, and cephalothin increased significantly, whereas resistance to nitrofurantoin and ciprofloxacin remained uncommon. **However, fluoroquinolone resistance of _E. coli_ has increased from less than 1% to 10% in hospitalized patients** (Karlowsky et al, 2003). In a transplant unit, where fluoroquinolones are commonly administered prophylactically, _E. coli_ resistance can be 80%. **Previous use of fluoroquinolones and the presence of underlying urologic diseases were the strongest determinants for UTIs caused by resistant strains** (Ena et al, 1995). Fluoroquinolone resistance is an increasing problem in some European countries. A multiple-resistant phenotype involving fluoroquinolone

resistance is now present in most countries in Europe, and this phenotype is selected for not only by the use of quinolones but also by the use of ampicillin, sulfamethoxazole, and TMP/SMX (Kahlmeter and Menday, 2003). This is a concern because fluoroquinolones, which are associated with chromosomal-mediated but not plasmid-mediated resistance, are the current drug of choice for patients who have been exposed to agents causing plasmid-mediated resistance.

The clinical significance of these in vitro trends in resistance has been addressed in studies that correlated in vitro resistance to TMP/SMX with clinical outcome in uncomplicated cystitis and pyelonephritis (Gupta and Stamm, 2002). Clinical failures occurred in 40% to 50% of women if the bacteria were resistant and the bacteriologic failure approached 60%. (For further information on the role of TMP-SMX in prophylaxis, see the later section of this chapter on "Bladder Infections.")

Antimicrobial Formulary

The mechanism of action, reliable coverage, and common adverse reactions, precautions, and contraindications for antimicrobial agents used in the treatment of UTIs are indicated in Tables 8–8, 8–9, and 8–10, respectively.

Trimethoprim/Sulfamethoxazole

The combination of TMP-SMX has been the most widely used antimicrobial agent for the treatment of acute UTIs. TMP alone is as effective as the combination for most uncomplicated infections and may be associated with fewer side effects (Johnson and Stamm, 1989); however, the addition of SMX contributes to efficacy in the treatment of upper tract infection via a synergistic bactericidal effect and may diminish the emergence of resistance (Burman, 1986). TMP alone or in combination with SMX is effective against most common uropathogens, with the notable exception of _Enterococcus_ and _Pseudomonas_ species. **TMP and TMP-SMX are inexpensive and have minimal adverse effects on the bowel flora. Disadvantages are relatively common adverse effects, consisting primarily of rashes and gastrointestinal complaints** (Cockerill and Edson, 1991).

Nitrofurantoin

Nitrofurantoin is effective against common uropathogens, but it is not effective against _Pseudomonas_ and _Proteus_ species (Iravani, 1991). **It is rapidly excreted from the urine**

Table 8–8. Mechanism of Action of Common Antimicrobials Used in the Treatment of UTIs

Drug or Drug Class	Mechanism of Action	Mechanisms of Drug Resistance
β-Lactams (penicillins, cephalosporins, aztreonam)	Inhibition of bacterial cell wall synthesis	Production of β-lactamase Alteration in binding site of penicillin-binding protein Changes in cell wall porin size (decreased penetration)
Aminoglycosides	Inhibition of ribosomal protein synthesis	Downregulation of drug uptake into bacteria Bacterial production of aminoglycoside-modifying enzymes
Quinolones	Inhibition of bacterial DNA gyrase	Mutation in DNA gyrase-binding site Changes in cell wall porin size (decreased penetration) Active efflux
Nitrofurantoin	Inhibition of several bacterial enzyme systems	Not fully elucidated—develops slowly with prolonged exposure
Trimethoprim-sulfamethoxazole	Antagonism of bacterial folate metabolism	Draws folate from environment (enterococci)
Vancomycin	Inhibition of bacterial cell wall synthesis (at different point than β-lactams)	Enzymatic alteration of peptidoglycan target

Table 8–9. Reliable Coverage of Antimicrobials Used in the Treatment of UTIs of Commonly Encountered Pathogens*†

Antimicrobial Agent or Class	Gram-Positive Pathogens	Gram-Negative Pathogens
Amoxicillin or ampicillin	Streptococcus Enterococci	Escherichia coli Proteus mirabilis
Amoxicillin with clavulanate	Streptococcus Enterococci	E. coli P. mirabilis Klebsiella species
Ampicillin with sulbactam	Staphylococcus (not MRSA) Enterococci	P. mirabilis Haemophilus influenzae, Klebsiella species
Antistaphylococcal penicillins	Streptococcus Staphylococcus (not MRSA)	None
Antipseudomonal penicillins	Streptococcus Enterococci	Most, including Pseudomonas aeruginosa
First-generation cephalosporins	Streptococcus Staphylococcus (not MRSA)	E. coli P. mirabilis Klebsiella species
Second-generation cephalosporins (cefamandole, cefuroxime, cefaclor)	Streptococcus Staphylococcus (not MRSA)	E. coli, P. mirabilis H. influenzae, Klebsiella species
Second-generation cephalosporins (cefoxitin, cefotetan)	Streptococcus	E. coli, Proteus species (including indole-positive) H. influenzae, Klebsiella species
Third-generation cephalosporins (ceftriaxone)	Streptococcus Staphylococcus (not MRSA)	Most, excluding P. aeruginosa
Third-generation cephalosporins (ceftazidime)	Streptococcus	Most, including P. aeruginosa
Aztreonam	None	Most, including P. aeruginosa
Aminoglycosides	Staphylococcus (urine)	Most, including P. aeruginosa
Fluoroquinolones	Streptococcus*	Most, including P. aeruginosa
Nitrofurantoin	Staphylococcus (not MRSA) Enterococci	Many Enterobacteriaceae (not Providencia, Serratia, Acinetobacter) Klebsiella species
Trimethoprim-sulfamethoxazole	Streptococcus Staphylococcus	Most Enterobacteriaceae (not P. aeruginosa)
Vancomycin	All, including MRSA	None

*Depends on the antimicrobial agent.
†MRSA, methicillin-resistant Staphylococcus aureus.

Table 8–10. Common Adverse Reactions, Precautions, and Contraindications for Antimicrobial Agents Used in Treatment of UTI

Drug or Drug Class	Common Adverse Reactions	Precautions and Contraindications
Amoxicillin or ampicillin	Hypersensitivity (immediate or delayed) Diarrhea (esp. with ampicillin), GI upset AAPMC Maculopapular rash (not hypersensitivity) Decreased platelet aggregation	Increased risk of rash with concomitant viral disease, allopurinol therapy
Amoxicillin with clavulanic acid	Increased diarrhea, GI upset with amoxicillin/clavulanic acid	
Ampicillin with sulbactam	Same as amoxicillin with ampicillin	
Antistaphylococcal penicillins	Same as with amoxicillin/ampicillin GI upset (with oral agents) Acute interstitial nephritis (esp. with methicillin)	
Antipseudomonal penicillins	Same as with amoxicillin/ampicillin Hypernatremia (these drugs are given as sodium salt; esp. carbenicillin, ticarcillin) Local injection site reactions	Use with caution in patients very sensitive to sodium loading
Cephalosporins	Hypersensitivity (less than with penicillins) GI upset (with oral agents) Local injection site reactions AAPMC Positive Coombs' test Decreased platelet aggregation (esp. with cefotetan, cefamandole, cefoperazone)	Should not be used in patients with immediate hypersensitivity to penicillins; may use with caution in patients with delayed hypersensitivity reactions

(continued)

Table 8–10.   Common Adverse Reactions, Precautions, and Contraindications for Antimicrobial Agents Used in Treatment of UTI—Cont'd

Drug or Drug Class	Common Adverse Reactions	Precautions and Contraindications
Aztreonam	Hypersensitivity (less than with penicillins)	Less than 1% incidence of cross reactivity in penicillin- or cephalosporin-allergic patients; may be used with caution in these patients
Aminoglycosides	Ototoxicity: vestibular and auditory components Nephrotoxicity: nonoliguric azotemia Neuromuscular blockade with high levels	Avoid in pregnant patients Avoid if possible in patients with severely impaired renal function, diabetes, or hepatic failure Use with caution in myasthenia gravis patients (owing to potential for neuromuscular blockade) Use with caution with other potentially ototoxic and nephrotoxic drugs
Fluoroquinolones	Mild GI effects; dizziness, lightheadedness; photosensitivity CNS effects, including dizziness, tremors, confusion, mood disorder, hallucinations Tendon rupture	Avoid in children or pregnant patients due to arthropathic effects Concomitant antacid or iron or zinc or sucralfate use dramatically decreases oral absorption; use another antimicrobial agent or discontinue sucralfate use while on quinolones Space administration of quinolones from antacids or iron or zinc products by at least 2 hr to ensure adequate absorption Ensure adequate patient hydration These agents can significantly increase theophylline plasma levels (ciprofloxacin and enoxacin seem to have a greater effect than norfloxacin or ofloxacin); avoid quinolones or monitor theophylline levels closely These agents can lower seizure threshold; avoid in patients with epilepsy and in patients with other risk factors (medications or illness) that may lower the seizure threshold Monitor glucose levels in patients on antidiabetic agents because hypoglycemia and hyperglycemia have been reported in patients treated concurrently with fluoroquinolones and antidiabetic agents These agents can enhance warfarin effects; closely monitor coagulation tests
Nitrofurantoin	GI upset Peripheral polyneuropathy (esp. in patients with impaired renal function, anemia, diabetes, electrolyte imbalance, vitamin B deficiency, and debilitated) Hemolysis in patients with G6PD deficiency Pulmonary hypersensitivity reactions can range from acute to chronic and include cough, dyspnea, fever, and interstitial changes	Do not use in patients with low creatinine clearance (<50 mL/min) because adequate urine concentrations will not be achieved Use with caution in patients predisposed to peripheral polyneuropathy or with G6PD deficiency Monitor long-term patients closely Avoid concomitant probenecid use, which blocks renal excretion of nitrofurantoin Avoid concomitant magnesium or quinolones, which are antagonistic to nitrofurantoin
Trimethoprim-sulfamethoxazole	Hypersensitivity, rash GI upset Photosensitivity Hematologic toxicity (AIDS patients)	Higher incidence of all adverse reactions occurs in AIDS patients and the elderly Avoid in pregnant patients Avoid in patients receiving warfarin; concomitant use can significantly elevate prothrombin time Increased risk exists of hematologic effects in folate- or G6PD-deficient patients Ensure adequate hydration to avoid crystallization of drug in urinary tract
Vancomycin	"Red-man's syndrome": flushing, fever, chills, rash, hypotension (histaminic effect) Nephrotoxicity and/or ototoxicity when combined with other nephrotoxic and/or ototoxic drugs Local injection site reactions	Use with caution with other potentially ototoxic and nephrotoxic drugs

AAPMC, antimicrobial-associated pseudomembranous colitis; GI, gastrointestinal; G6PD, glucose-6-phosphate dehydrogenase.
From McEvoy GK (ed): American Hospital Formulary Service Drug Information. Bethesda, MD, American Society of Health-System Pharmacists, 1995.

but does not obtain therapeutic levels in most body tissues, including the gastrointestinal tract. Therefore, it is not useful for upper tract and complicated infections (Wilhelm and Edson, 1987). **It has minimal effects on the resident bowel and vaginal flora and has been used effectively in prophylactic regimens for more than 40 years.** Acquired bacterial resistance to this drug is exceedingly low.

Cephalosporins

All three generations of cephalosporins have been used for the treatment of acute UTIs (Wilhelm and Edson, 1987). In general, as a group, activity is high against Enterobacteriaceae and poor against enterococci. First-generation cephalosporins have greater activity against gram-positive organisms as well as common uropathogens such as *E. coli* and *Klebsiella pneumoniae* whereas second-generation cephalosporins have activity against anaerobes. Third-generation cephalosporins are more reliably active against community-acquired and nosocomial gram-negative organisms than other β-lactam antimicrobials. **Selective pressure engendered by these broad-spectrum agents should limit their use to complicated infections and situations in which parenteral therapy is required and resistance to standard antimicrobial agents is likely. They are also useful during pregnancy.**

Aminopenicillins

Ampicillin and amoxicillin have been used often in the past for the treatment of UTIs, but the emergence of resistance in 40% to 60% of common urinary isolates has lessened the usefulness of these drugs (Hooton and Stamm, 1991). The effects of these agents on the normal bowel and vaginal flora can predispose patients to reinfection with resistant strains and often lead to candidal vaginitis (Iravani, 1991). The addition of the β-lactamase inhibitor clavulanate to amoxicillin greatly improves activity against β-lactamase–producing bacteria resistant to amoxicillin alone. However, its high cost and frequent gastrointestinal side effects limit its usefulness. The extended-spectrum penicillin derivatives (e.g., piperacillin, mezlocillin, azlocillin) retain ampicillin's activity against enterococci and offer activity against many ampicillin-resistant gram-negative bacilli. **This makes them attractive agents for use in patients with nosocomially acquired UTIs and as the initial parenteral treatment of acute uncomplicated pyelonephritis acquired outside of the hospital, although less expensive agents are equally effective.**

Aminoglycosides

When combined with TMP-SMX or ampicillin, aminoglycosides are the first drugs of choice for febrile UTIs. Their nephrotoxicity and ototoxicity are well recognized; hence, careful monitoring of patients for renal and auditory impairment associated with infection is indicated. **Once-daily aminoglycoside regimens have been instituted to maximize bacterial killing by optimizing the peak concentration-to-minimal inhibitory concentration ratio and reduce potential for toxicity** (Fig. 8–12) (Nicolau et al, 1995). Administering an aminoglycoside as a single daily dose can take advantage not only of its concentration-dependent killing ability but also of two other important characteristics: time-dependent toxicity and a more prolonged post-antimicrobial effect (Gilbert, 1991; Zhanel et al, 1991). The regimen consists

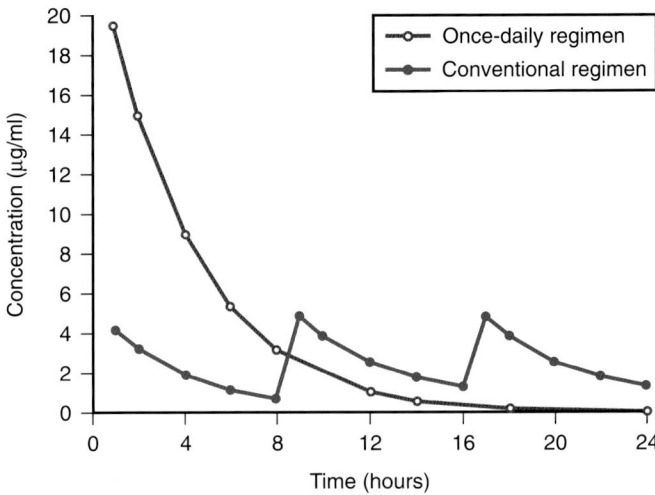

Figure 8–12. Simulated concentration-versus-time profile of once-daily (7 mg/kg every 24 hours) and conventional (1.5 mg/kg every 8 hours) regimens for patients with normal renal function. (From Nicolau DP, Freeman CD, Belliveau PP, et al: Experience with a once-daily aminoglycoside program administered to 2,184 adult patients. Antimicrob Agents Chemother 1995;39:650-655.)

of a fixed 7 mg/kg dose of gentamicin or 5-7 mg/kg tobramycin. Subsequent interval adjustments are made by using a single concentration in serum and a nomogram designed for monitoring of once-daily therapy (Fig. 8–13). Antimicrobial doses are given at the interval determined by the drug concentration of a sample obtained after the start of the initial infusion. For example, if the serum concentration was 7 mg/mL 10 hours after the start of the infusion, subsequent 7 mg/kg doses would be given every 36 hours. This regimen is clinically effective, reduces the incidence of nephrotoxicity, and provides a cost-effective method for administering aminoglycosides by reducing ancillary service times and serum aminoglycoside determinations.

Aztreonam

Aztreonam has a similar spectrum of activity as the aminoglycosides, and as with all β-lactams, it is not nephrotoxic. However, its spectrum of activity is less broad than the third-generation cephalosporins. **It should be used primarily in patients who have penicillin allergies.**

Fluoroquinolones

Fluoroquinolones share a common predecessor in nalidixic acid and inhibit DNA gyrase, a bacterial enzyme integral to replication. The fluoroquinolones have a broad spectrum of activity that makes them ideal for the empirical treatment of UTIs. **They are highly effective against Enterobacteriaceae, as well as *P. aeruginosa*. Activity is also high against *S. aureus* and *S. saprophyticus*, but, in general, antistreptococcal coverage is marginal.** Most anaerobic bacteria are resistant to these drugs; therefore, the normal vaginal and bowel flora are not altered (Wright et al, 1993). **Bacterial resistance initially appeared to be uncommon, but it is being reported at an increasing rate because of indiscriminate use of these agents** (Wright et al, 1993; Vromen et al, 1999).

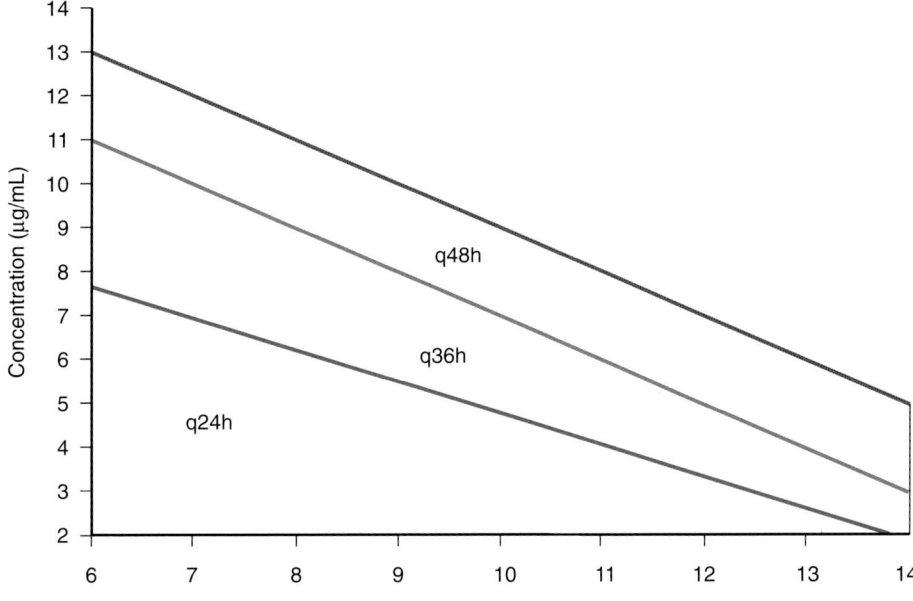

Figure 8–13. ODA nomogram for gentamicin and tobramycin at 7 mg/kg. (From Nicolau DP, Freeman CD, Belliveau PP, et al: Experience with a once-daily aminoglycoside program administered to 2,184 adult patients. Antimicrob Agents Chemother 1995;39:650-655.)

These drugs are not nephrotoxic, but renal insufficiency prolongs the serum half-life, requiring adjusted dosing in patients with creatinine clearances of less than 30 mL/min. Adverse reactions are uncommon; gastrointestinal disturbances are more common. Hypersensitivity, skin reactions, mild central and peripheral nervous system reactions, and even acute renal failure have been reported (Hootkins et al, 1989). Achilles tendon disorders, including rupture, have been estimated to occur in 20 cases per 100,000 and therefore fluoroquinolone use should be discontinued at the first sign of tendon pain (Greene, 2002). The mechanism of tendon rupture is unclear, but ciprofloxacin stimulates matrix-degrading protease activity from fibroblasts and exerts an inhibitory effect on fibroblast metabolism and synthesis of matrix ground substance, factors that may contribute to tendinopathy (Williams et al, 2000). Administration of the fluoroquinolones to immature animals has caused damage to the developing cartilage; therefore, they are currently contraindicated in children, adolescents, and pregnant or nursing women (Christ et al, 1988). **There are important drug interactions associated with the fluoroquinolones. Antacids containing magnesium or aluminum interfere with absorption of fluoroquinolones** (Davies and Maesen, 1989). Certain fluoroquinolones (enoxacin and ciprofloxacin) elevate plasma levels of theophylline and prolong its half-life (Wright et al, 1993). For most uncomplicated UTIs, the fluoroquinolones have been only slightly more effective than TMP-SMX. However, as resistance to TMP-SMX increases, the fluoroquinolones have distinct advantages in empirical treatment of patients recently exposed to antimicrobial agents and in the outpatient treatment of complicated UTIs (Dalkin and Schaeffer, 1988; Gupta et al, 1999). **They may be considered as first-line agents in areas where a significant level of resistance (greater than 20%) exists (in common bacteria) to agents such as ampicillin and TMP-SMX.**

Choice of Antimicrobial Agents

Many antimicrobial agents have been shown to be effective in the treatment of UTIs. **Factors important in aiding selection of empirical therapy include whether the infection is complicated or uncomplicated; the spectrum of activity of the drug against the probable pathogen; a history of hypersensitivity; potential side effects, including renal and hepatic toxicity; and cost.** In addition, favorable or unfavorable effects of the antimicrobial agent on the vaginal and bowel flora are important in women with recurrent UTIs. The bacterial susceptibility and cost of the drug vary dramatically among inpatient and outpatient settings throughout the country. It is imperative, therefore, that each clinician keep abreast of changes in bacterial susceptibility and cost and use current information when choosing antimicrobial agents.

Duration of Therapy

The duration of therapy needed to cure a UTI appears to be related to a number of variables, including the extent and duration of tissue invasion, the bacterial concentration in urine, the achievable urine concentration of the antimicrobial agent, and risk factors (see later) **that impair the host and natural defense mechanisms.**

KEY POINTS: PRINCIPLES OF ANTIMICROBIAL THERAPY

- Effective antimicrobial therapy must eliminate bacterial growth in the urinary tract.
- Antimicrobial resistance is increasing because of excessive utilization.
- Antimicrobial selection should be influenced by efficacy, safety, cost, and compliance.

ANTIMICROBIAL PROPHYLAXIS FOR COMMON UROLOGIC PROCEDURES
Principles

Surgical antimicrobial prophylaxis entails treatment with an antimicrobial agent before and for a *limited* time after a procedure to prevent local or systemic postprocedural infections. For most procedures, prophylaxis should be initiated between 30 minutes and 120 minutes before the procedure (Bratzler and Houck, 2004). **Efficacious levels should be maintained for the duration of the procedure and, in special circumstances, a limited time (24 hours, at most) after the procedure** (Bratzler and Houck, 2004). Although prospective studies addressing prophylaxis for urologic procedures exist, most focus on only a narrow spectrum of procedures. However, application of the principles of these studies with additional consideration of both the patient and the type of procedure provides a framework for determining when and what type of antimicrobial prophylaxis may be indicated. An additional, nontraditional type of prophylaxis in urology entails periprocedural treatment of the urinary tract with an antimicrobial agent to prevent local or systemic sequelae from the manipulation of colonized hardware such as a stent or urethral catheter.

A wide array of patients undergo invasive procedures in urology. The ability of a host to respond to bacteriuria or bacteremia and the sequelae of a possible infection are two important considerations when assessing the need for antimicrobial prophylaxis. Factors that affect the host's ability to respond to infection include advanced age, anatomic anomalies, poor nutritional status, smoking, chronic corticosteroid use, other concurrent medication use, and immunodeficiencies such as untreated HIV infection (Table 8–11). Additionally, chronic indwelling hardware, infected endogenous material such as stones, distant infectious sites, and prolonged hospitalizations also increase the risk of infectious complications by increasing the local bacterial concentration and/or altering the spectrum of bacterial flora. The potential seeding of artificial heart valves or prosthetic joints increases the sequelae of a systemic infection in hosts who otherwise may not be at an increased risk of infection. Thus, a thorough

Table 8–11. Host Factors That Increase the Risk of Infection

Advanced age
Anatomic anomalies
Poor nutritional status
Smoking
Chronic corticosteroid use
Immunodeficiency
Chronic indwelling hardware
Infected endogenous/exogenous material
Distant coexistent infection
Prolonged hospitalization

Data from Cruse PJ: Surgical wound infection. In Wonsiewicz MJ (ed): Infectious Disease. Philadelphia, WB Saunders, 1992, pp 758-764; and Mangram AJ, et al: Guideline for prevention of surgical site infection, 1999. Hospital Infection Control Practices Advisory Committee. Infect Control Hosp Epidemiol 1999;20:250-278; quiz 279-280.

history and examination of the patient is crucial in directing antimicrobial prophylaxis before a urologic procedure.

The type of procedure will also help direct the timing, duration, and spectrum of antimicrobial prophylaxis needed (see Table 8–12 for a summary of antimicrobial prophylaxis recommendations). Consideration should be given to the extent of the local tissue injury incurred and the anticipated type of flora at the site.

Antimicrobial prophylaxis is not without morbidity because allergic complications, although rare, may result in minor reactions such as rash or gastric disturbances or significant sequelae such as early withdrawal of therapy, allergic nephritis, or anaphylaxis.

Urethral Catheterization and Removal

The indications for the routine use of prophylactic antimicrobial agents before urethral catheterization vary and depend on the health, sex, and specific living circumstances of the individual patient as well as on the indication for catheterization (Schaeffer, 2006). **The risk of infection after one-time urethral catheterization is 1% to 2% in healthy domiciliary women; however, this risk rises significantly in hospitalized patients** (Turck et al, 1962; Thiel and Spuhler, 1965). Thus, for patients with risk factors for infection (see Table 8–11), antimicrobial prophylaxis with an oral agent such as TMP-SMX or a fluoroquinolone should decrease the risk of postprocedural infection (see Table 8–12).

Prolonged use of an indwelling urethral catheter is common in hospitalized patients and is associated with an increased risk of bacterial colonization, with a 3% to 10% incidence of bacteriuria per catheter day in one study and 100% incidence of bacteriuria with long-term catheterization (>30 days) (Kass, 1956; Nickel et al, 1985; Liedl, 2001). Prophylactic administration of antimicrobial agents during catheterization is not generally recommended because bacterial resistance can develop rapidly and complicate subsequent antimicrobial treatment (Clarke et al, 2005).

The natural history of bacteriuria after catheter removal has not been comprehensively studied. Harding and associates (1991) reported that in asymptomatic bacteriuric women who had been catheterized for 4 to 6 days, 25% developed a UTI within 14 days of catheter removal. In this study, 1-day treatment with TMP-SMX was as effective as a 10-day course at resolving infections. Similar studies on the natural history of postcatheterization bacteriuria have not been performed in male patients. Thus, potential benefits of antimicrobial treatment around catheter removal have not been fully investigated. Note that antimicrobial treatment before removal of an indwelling catheter in a patient suspected of having bacteriuria is not considered prophylaxis but rather is treatment for a presumptive UTI and duration of treatment generally should follow previously outlined guidelines for uncomplicated or complicated UTIs.

Data from Polastri and colleagues (1990) suggest that antimicrobial prophylaxis for chronic indwelling catheter changes is not indicated. In their study of 46 catheter changes, bacteremia occurred 4% of the time and when noted was associated with very low concentrations of bacteria in the cultures. Systemic sequelae were not noted.

Table 8–12. Guide For Antimicrobial Prophylaxis for Uncomplicated Urologic Procedures			
Procedure	*Ideal Host*	*Host with Risk Factors*	*Duration*
Urethral catheterization and removal	No absolute indication	Oral fluoroquinolone Bactrim DS	Single dose, <24 hr Single dose, <24 hr
Urodynamics	No absolute indication	Oral fluoroquinolone Bactrim DS	Single dose, <24 hr <24 hr
Transrectal prostate biopsy	Oral fluoroquinolone	Consider culture-directed treatment if infection suspected	1–4 days
Extracorporeal shockwave lithotripsy	Bactrim DS Oral fluoroquinolone	If infectious stone, treat preoperatively for UTI	Single dose, <24 hr Single dose, <24 hr
Endoscopic Procedures (Lower Urinary Tract)			
Diagnostic			
Urethroscopy, cystoscopy	No absolute indication	Cefazolin Oral fluoroquinolone Bactrim DS	Single dose, <24 hr Single dose, <24 hr Single dose, <24 hr
Therapeutic			
Prostate resection	Ampicillin + gentamicin or oral/IV fluoroquinolone (while catheter in place)	Ampicillin + gentamicin or oral/IV fluoroquinolone (consider culture-directed preoperative treatment if infection suspected)	While catheter in place
Bladder tumor resection	Ampicillin + gentamicin or oral/IV fluoroquinolone	Ampicillin + gentamicin or oral/IV fluoroquinolone	Single dose, <24 hr
Endoscopic Procedures (Upper Urinary Tract)			
Ureteroscopy	Ampicillin + gentamicin or oral/IV fluoroquinolone	Ampicillin + gentamicin or oral/IV fluoroquinolone	Single dose, <24 hr
Percutaneous renal surgery	Ampicillin + gentamicin Fluoroquinolone	Ampicillin + gentamicin Fluoroquinolone	Single dose, <24 hr Single dose, <24 hr
Open and Laparoscopic Procedures			
Radical nephrectomy	Cefazolin	Cefazolin	Length of procedure
Procedures with open urinary tract	Cefazolin Vancomycin or clindamycin for β-lactam allergic	Cefazolin Vancomycin or clindamycin for β-lactam allergic	Length of procedure Length of procedure
Reconstruction with colon or appendix	Cefotetan or cefoxitin Clindamycin + gentamicin, aztreonam, or ciprofloxacin for β-lactam allergic	Cefotetan or cefoxitin Clindamycin + gentamicin, aztreonam, or ciprofloxacin for β-lactam allergic	Length of procedure Length of procedure
Dirty wound including dependent trauma, abscess or nondirected genitourinary perforation	N/A	Treatment dose with broad coverage, narrowed coverage directed at culture-proven organisms	Variable; case

Drug doses: ampicillin, 25 mg/kg/dose; gentamicin, 1.5 mg/kg/dose; cefazolin, 25 mg/kg/dose.
From Bratzler DW, Houck PM: Antimicrobial prophylaxis for surgery: An advisory statement from the National Surgical Infection Prevention Project. Clin Infect Dis 2004;38:1706-1715.

Urodynamics

Urodynamics, like cystoscopy, is a minimally traumatic procedure with limited urothelial injury that poses a small risk of local infection in hosts with normal anatomy and immune response. Several recent studies support this notion. In a series of women with urinary incontinence randomized to receive 1 day of nitrofurantoin or placebo, Cundiff and coworkers (1999) noted no difference in postprocedural UTI (5% vs. 7%) 1 week after evaluation. Similarly, Peschers and associates (2001) reported infections 1 week after multichannel urodynamics in 5% and 6% in nondiabetic women treated with placebo or cotrimoxazole. Most series examining the use of antimicrobial prophylaxis exclude patients with altered anatomy such as large prostates or comorbidities, including neurogenic bladder, spinal cord injury, or diabetes, all factors that increase the risk of infection. This is illustrated in work performed by Payne and colleagues in which frequencies of

bacteriuria after urodynamics were much higher in men (36%) compared with the women studied (15%) (Payne et al, 1988). **In sum, contemporary studies suggest antimicrobial prophylaxis for urodynamic evaluation of uninfected females undergoing urodynamics for incontinence does not significantly lower rates of bacteriuria and infection; however, antimicrobial prophylaxis should be considered for patients with a more complex clinical history or anatomy such as men with large postvoid residuals or spinal cord–injured patients.**

Transrectal Ultrasound-Guided Prostate Biopsy

The use of prophylactic antimicrobials for transrectal ultrasound-guided prostate biopsy reduces postprocedural fever and UTI in most studies. The class and duration of antimicrobial treatment are more varied and controversial. One major population-based screening program reported fever (>38.5° C [101.3° F]) in 3.5% of cases utilizing 1 day of TMP-SMX for most cases and ciprofloxacin for patients with comorbid conditions. This series did not report the frequency of UTIs. Alternatively, Sieber and associates (1997) reported a 0.1% rate of UTI in a large community-based practice in men given 4 days of ciprofloxacin. More recent studies suggest a single-dose/day of fluoroquinolones is as effective as 3 days of treatment (Sabbagh et al, 2004). Together these data suggest that a minimum of 1 day of an antimicrobial agent is indicated for transrectal ultrasound-guided prostate biopsies and that in otherwise healthy men confounding factors including cost of drugs can help direct the class and duration of therapy (Griffith et al, 2002).

Shockwave Lithotripsy

The incidence of UTIs after shockwave lithotripsy is reported to range from 0% to 28% without antimicrobial prophylaxis. A recent meta-analysis of contemporary randomized controlled trials examined the utility and cost-effectiveness of antimicrobial prophylaxis for shockwave lithotripsy and demonstrated, in individuals with sterile preprocedure urine cultures, a reduction in the rate of UTIs after shockwave lithotripsy from 5.7% to 2.1% (Pearle and Roehrborn, 1997). This analysis also demonstrated cost-effectiveness of prophylaxis when consideration was given for the treatment of the rare but more morbid complications of urosepsis and pyelonephritis. A history of a recent UTI or of infectious stones should warrant a full treatment course of antimicrobial agents before shockwave lithotripsy.

Endoscopic Procedures: Lower Urinary Tract

Cystoscopy

Cystoscopy is a minimally traumatic procedure with limited urothelial injury performed on a diverse spectrum of patients including young healthy women and older men. Several prospective trials (Manson, 1988; Clark and Higgs, 1990; Burke et al, 2002) of patients with preprocedure sterile urine report culture-proven rates of UTI between 2.2% and 7.8% after cystoscopy without antimicrobial prophylaxis. In Clark's report the risk of infection was higher in patients with a previous history of UTI. In a similarly designed study, Rane and colleagues (2001) report a significantly higher postprocedure culture-proven infection rate of 21% without antimicrobial prophylaxis. The dramatic differences in culture-proven infections are unclear; however, in all the studies single doses of antimicrobial agents reduced infections to between 1% and 5%. In none of these studies were significant systemic infections reported after the cystoscopic procedures.

Together these studies illustrate two key concepts: (1) despite appropriate periprocedural preparation, a small inoculum of bacteria is likely introduced into the bladder during cystoscopy and (2) the significance of the bacteriuria is dependent on host factors, including the ability to mount an appropriate immune response to bacterial inoculation and the ability to clear the bacterial inoculation. For example,

in a man with urinary retention, a small inoculum of bacteria could persist and divide in the retained fraction of urine and result in a symptomatic infection. In a host with a reduced ability to respond to infection this bacteriuria could become significant. In contrast, a middle-aged woman undergoing cystoscopy for microscopic hematuria is more likely to efficiently empty her bladder and clear the inoculum but may be exposed to an increased inoculum of bacteria if inappropriately prepared for the examination. **Thus, although not absolutely indicated for simple cystoscopy, we recommend prophylaxis when aberrant host factors could increase the probability or significance of an infection** (see Table 8–12). A single dose of a fluoroquinolone is commonly used, but the best drug and number of doses has not been well studied.

Transurethral Resection of the Prostate and Bladder

Therapeutic transurethral lower urinary tract procedures increase the risk of localized infections compared with simple diagnostic cystoscopy. Although not delineated in any prospective studies, several risk factors likely increase infectious complications, including trauma to the mucosa, increased duration and/or degree of difficulty of the procedure, pressurized irrigants, and manipulation or resection of infected material. The most well-studied lower urinary tract procedure is transurethral resection of the prostate. In a meta-analysis of 32 studies (Berry and Barratt, 2002), a risk reduction was noted in bacteriuria from 26% to 9% on postoperative urine cultures obtained 2 to 5 days after the procedure for patients treated with prophylactic antimicrobial agents. Similarly, septicemia (defined as rigors, persistently elevated temperature [>38.5° C], and an elevated C-reactive protein level) decreased from 4.4% to 0.9% with antimicrobial prophylaxis. The most effective antimicrobial classes included fluoroquinolones, aminoglycosides, cephalosporins, and TMP/SMX (Bactrim, cotrimoxazole). Single doses of antimicrobial agents did lower the relative risk of bacteriuria but not as significantly as antimicrobial agents administered for short courses (2 to 5 days) while the urethral catheter remained in place. Although continuation of antimicrobial therapy while the catheter is in place is not truly prophylaxis, continuation of the initial prophylactic antimicrobial agent for an anticipated short period of time (with catheter in place) does not increase the risk of developing antimicrobial-resistant organisms. No recent trials have investigated prophylaxis for transurethral resection of bladder tumors; however, evidence from transurethral resection of the prostate procedures would suggest that prophylaxis would reduce bacteriuria in these procedures.

Patients who are known preoperatively to have UTIs should have the infections eradicated before the procedure is started; hence, in these patients, preoperative antimicrobial agents are therapeutic and not prophylactic. Failure to eradicate bacteriuria results in bacteremia in 50% of patients (Morris et al, 1976).

Diagnostic and therapeutic upper tract studies are performed with pressurized irrigants and may induce urothelial injury. Prophylaxis with antimicrobial agents that cover uropathogens is indicated.

Endoscopic Procedures: Upper Urinary Tract

Ureteroscopy

Diagnostic and therapeutic upper tract endoscopic procedures have an increased risk of localized infections compared with simple diagnostic cystoscopy due to several factors, including increased trauma to the mucosa, increased duration and/or degree of difficulty of most ureteroscopic procedures, increased pressure of irrigants, and (when applicable) manipulation or resection of infected material. The use of antimicrobial prophylaxis is supported by a randomized trial by Knopf and colleagues (2003) in which prophylactic fluoroquinolone administration significantly reduced postprocedure UTIs in a healthy population of individuals with ureteral stones and uninfected preoperative urine. If an infection or infectious material is suspected, culture and a full treatment course of an appropriate antimicrobial is recommended before the procedure.

Percutaneous Procedures

Percutaneous renal surgery is commonly performed for large renal stones, ureteropelvic junction obstruction, and transitional cell carcinoma surveillance. Pyrexia and bacteremia occur frequently and likely stem from a combination of renal parenchymal injury, pressurized irrigation, and, in some cases, manipulation of infectious stones. Several studies demonstrated a relationship between the risk of postoperative infectious complications (including bacteriuria and sepsis) and the duration of the procedure and amount of irrigant used (Dogan et al, 2002). If preoperative urine cultures are positive, treatment of the infection should occur before surgery. Conversely, if preoperative cultures are negative, antimicrobial prophylaxis covering common urinary pathogens should be instituted (see Table 8–12).

Open and Laparoscopic Surgery

Open surgical procedures can be classified as clean, clean contaminated, contaminated, and dirty (Table 8–13). **Antimicro-bial prophylaxis is indicated for clean contaminated and contaminated wounds, whereas antimicrobial treatment with an appropriate agent should be instituted for dirty-infected wounds.** To date, no large studies have evaluated the risk of surgical site infections for different laparoscopic urologic procedures. However, data in the general surgery literature suggest that the laparoscopic approach lowers the risk of surgical site infections (Kluytmans, 1997). Clean surgeries in urology include radical nephrectomy if the urinary tract is not entered. All urologic procedures where the urinary tract is opened electively are considered clean contaminated procedures, whereas entry into an infected urinary tract is considered a contaminated procedure and carries a higher rate of surgical site infection (Cruse, 1992). Antimicrobial agents should be active against the most likely infecting organism and should be administered within 1 hour of the procedure and discontinued 24 hours after because several studies have failed to demonstrate beneficial effects of long courses of prophylaxis (Conte et al, 1972; Goldmann et al, 1977). In the United States, first-generation cephalosporins are commonly used for prophylaxis of clean contaminated procedures because they have low incidences of allergic reactions, long half-lives, and low cost. For patients with a β-lactam allergy, the 2004 National Surgical Infection Prevention Project (NSIPP) guidelines recommend either vancomycin or clindamycin. Prophylaxis for urinary reconstruction with intestine requires increased anaerobic coverage, and thus use of second-generation cephalosporins is recommended (Bratzler and Houck, 2004). When use of the colon or appendix is anticipated for urologic reconstruction, the 2004 NSIPP recommendations include orally administered antimicrobial bowel preparation (neomycin plus erythromycin or neomycin plus metronidazole) 18 to 24 hours before surgery and parenteral cefotetan or cefoxitin 30 to 60 minutes before incision (Bratzler and Houck, 2004). Recommendations for patients with a β-lactam allergy include clindamycin plus gentamicin, aztreonam, or ciprofloxacin. Dirty wounds in urology include all abscesses and traumatic perforation of the genitourinary tract. Treatment of a dirty wound should begin with broad coverage of anticipated organisms and intraoperative wound cultures. Subsequent therapy and treatment duration depends on the sensitivities of the cultured organism.

Special Considerations

Patients with Risk of Endocarditis

The risk of endocarditis after urologic procedures is low; however, **the urinary tract is the second most common site of entry of organisms that cause endocarditis** (Dajani et al, 1997). In 1997 the American Heart Association updated their recommendations on the prevention of bacterial endocarditis. Recommendations are based on the patient's risk of developing endocarditis and the likelihood that a procedure will cause bacteremia with an organism that can cause endocarditis. Prophylaxis is recommended for both high- and moderate-risk patients. High-risk patients include individuals with prosthetic heart valves, previous bacterial endocarditis, cyanotic congenital heart disease, and systemic-pulmonary shunts or conduits. Moderate-risk patients include other congenital malformations (excluding isolated secundum atrial septal

Table 8–13.	**Surgical Wound Classification**
Clean	Uninfected wound without inflammation or entry into the genital, urinary, or alimentary tract
	Primary wound closure ± closed drainage
Clean Contaminated	Uninfected wound with controlled entry into the genital, urinary, or alimentary tract
	Primary wound closure ± closed drainage
Contaminated	Uninfected wound with major break in sterile technique (gross spillage from gastrointestinal tract or nonpurulent inflammation)
	Open fresh accidental wounds
Dirty Infected	Wound with preexisting clinical infection or perforated viscera
	Old traumatic wounds with devitalized tissue

Adapted from Mangram AJ, Horan TC, Pearson ML, et al: Guideline for prevention of surgical site infection, 1999. Hospital Infection Control Practices Advisory Committee. Infect Control Hosp Epidemiol 1999;20:250-278; quiz 279-280.

Table 8–14. Antimicrobial Regimens for Patients at Risk for Endocarditis

Patient Type	Antimicrobial Recommendation
High risk	Ampicillin, 2.0 g IM or IV, + gentamicin, 1.5 mg/kg (not to exceed 120 mg) 30 min preoperatively, and ampicillin, 25 mg/kg, or amoxicillin, 25 mg/kg 6 hr postoperatively
High risk with ampicillin or amoxicillin allergy	Vancomycin, 1.0 g over 1-2 hr, + gentamicin, 1.5 mg/kg (not to exceed 120 mg) 30 min preoperatively
Moderate risk	Amoxicillin, 2.0 g 1 hr preoperatively
Moderate risk with ampicillin or amoxicillin allergy	Vancomycin, 1.0 g IV over 1-2 hr, completed ≤ 30 min preoperatively

Adapted from Dajani AS, Taubert KA, Wilson W, et al: Prevention of bacterial endocarditis: Recommendations by the American Heart Association. JAMA 1997;277:1794-1801.

Table 8–15. Antimicrobial Regimens for Patients with Indwelling Orthopedic Hardware

Patient Type	Antimicrobial Recommendation
Total joint inserted > 2 years ago, pins, plates, screws + no host risk factors	Not recommended empirically
Total joint inserted < 2 years ago or aberrant host factor(s)	Oral quinolone or ampicillin, 2 g IV, + gentamicin, 1.5 mg/kg IV, 30-60 min before procedure Substitute vancomycin, 1 g IV, over 1-2 hr before procedure if ampicillin allergy

From American Urological Association, American Academy of Orthopaedic Surgeons: Antibiotic prophylaxis for urological patients with total joint replacements. J Urol 2003;169:1796-1797.

defects, surgically repaired atrial septal defects, ventricular septal defects, or patent ductus arteriosus, acquired valvular dysfunction, hypertrophic cardiomyopathy, and mitral valve prolapse with valvular regurgitation and/or thickened leaflets). Antimicrobial prophylaxis is not recommended for patients with congenital malformations, including isolated secundum atrial septal defects, surgically repaired atrial septal defects, ventricular septal defects or patent ductus arteriosus, previous coronary artery bypass graft surgery, benign heart murmurs, previous Kawasaki disease, or rheumatic fever without valvular dysfunction or implanted pacemakers or defibrillators. Prophylaxis should be initiated for urologic procedures, including those involving an obstructed urinary tract, prostatic surgery, urinary reconstruction with intestine, percutaneous renal surgery, cystoscopy, and urethral dilation; conversely, prophylaxis is not recommended for simple urethral catheterization.

Enterococcus faecalis (enterococci) is the most common organism causing endocarditis after urologic procedures (Dajani et al, 1997). The recommended antimicrobial regimens are described in Table 8–14.

Patients with Indwelling Orthopedic Hardware

Bacterial seeding of implanted orthopedic hardware is a rare but morbid event. A joint commission of the American Urological Association, the American Academy of Orthopaedic Surgeons, and infectious disease specialists convened in 2003 and released an advisory statement on antimicrobial prophylaxis for urologic patients with total joint replacement (American Urological Association and American Academy of Orthopaedic Surgeons, 2002) (Table 8–15). In general, antimicrobial prophylaxis for urologic patients with total joint replacements, pins, plates, or screws is not indicated. Prophylaxis is advised for individuals at higher risk of seeding a prosthetic joint, including those with recently inserted implants (within 2 years) and/or host risk factors as delineated earlier. Prophylaxis on the basis of potential seeding of a prosthetic joint should be instituted for procedures including stone manipulation, transmural incision of the urinary tract, upper tract endoscopic procedures, procedures involving bowel segments, and transrectal prostate biopsy. Additionally, patients with recent prosthetic joints or

compromised host factors and urinary diversions, indwelling stents or catheters, a recent history of urinary retention, or UTIs should receive antimicrobial prophylaxis before urinary tract procedures. The AUA Advisory Statement recommends for these patients either an oral quinolone or ampicillin, 2 g IV (vancomycin, 1 g IV over 1 to 2 hours for ampicillin-allergic patients), and gentamicin, 1.5 mg/kg IV, 30 to 60 minutes before the procedure.

KEY POINTS: ANTIMICROBIAL PROPHYLAXIS FOR COMMON UROLOGIC PROCEDURES

■ Antimicrobial prophylaxis entails treatment with an antimicrobial agent before and for a limited time after a procedure to prevent local or systemic postprocedural infections.

■ The type of procedure and competency of the host defenses determine the need for antimicrobial prophylaxis.

■ Special considerations for antimicrobial prophylaxis include patients with a risk of endocarditis and patients with indwelling orthopedic hardware.

BLADDER INFECTIONS
Uncomplicated Cystitis

Most cases of uncomplicated cystitis occur in women. Each year, approximately 10% of women report having had a UTI and more than 50% of all women have at least one such infection in their lifetime (Foxman et al, 2000). Uncomplicated cystitis occasionally occurs in prepubertal girls, but it increases greatly in incidence in late adolescence and during the second and fourth decades of life. Twenty-five to 30 percent of women 20 to 40 years of age have a history of UTIs (Kunin, 1987). **Although it is much less common, young men may also experience acute cystitis without underlying structural or functional abnormalities of the urinary tract**

Table 8–16.	**Risk Factors for UTIs**

Reduced Urine Flow

Outflow obstruction, prostatic hyperplasia, prostatic carcinoma,
    urethral stricture, foreign body (calculus)
Neurogenic bladder
Inadequate fluid uptake (dehydration)

Promote Colonization

Sexual activity—increased inoculation
Spermicide—increased binding
Estrogen depletion—increased binding
Antimicrobial agents—decreased indigenous flora

Facilitate Ascent

Catheterization
Urinary incontinence
Fecal incontinence
Residual urine with ischemia of bladder wall

(Krieger et al, 1993). Risk factors (Table 8–16) include sexual intercourse and use of spermicides (Hooton et al, 1996; Foxman, 2002; Handley et al, 2002). Sexual transmission of uropathogens has been suggested by demonstrating identical *E. coli* in the bowel and urinary flora of sex partners (Johnson and Stamm, 1989).

Clinical Presentation

The presenting symptoms of cystitis are variable but usually include dysuria, frequency or urgency, and suprapubic pain (Fig. 8–14). Hematuria or foul-smelling urine may develop. The probability of cystitis in a woman with these symptoms alone or in combination is 50% to 90%, respectively (Bent et al, 2002). When a woman who previously has had cystitis has symptoms suggesting a recurrence, the probability that an infection is present is about 90% (Gupta et al, 2001). Because acute cystitis, by definition, is a superficial infection of bladder mucosa, fever, chills, and other signs of dissemination are not present. Some patients may experience suprapubic tenderness, but most have no diagnostic physical findings. In women, physical examination should include the possibility of vaginitis, herpes, and urethral pathology, such as a diverticulum.

A remarkably narrow spectrum of etiologic agents with highly predictable profiles of antimicrobial susceptibility cause infections in young women with acute uncomplicated cystitis. *E. coli* **is the causative organism in 75% to 90% of cases of acute cystitis in young women** (Latham et al, 1983; Ronald, 2002). *S. saprophyticus,* **a commensal organism of the skin, is the second most common cause of acute cystitis in young women, accounting for 10% to 20% of these infections** (Jordan et al, 1980). **Other organisms less commonly involved include** *Klebsiella* **and** *Proteus* **species and** *Enterococcus.* **In men,** *E. coli* **and other Enterobacteriaceae are the most commonly identified organisms.**

Laboratory Diagnosis

The presumptive laboratory diagnosis of acute cystitis is based on microscopic urinalysis, which indicates microscopic pyuria, bacteriuria, and hematuria. The presence of pyuria has a sensitivity of 95% and a specificity of 70%. The presence of bacteria is less sensitive but more specific (40% to 70% and 85% to 95%, respectively, depending on the number

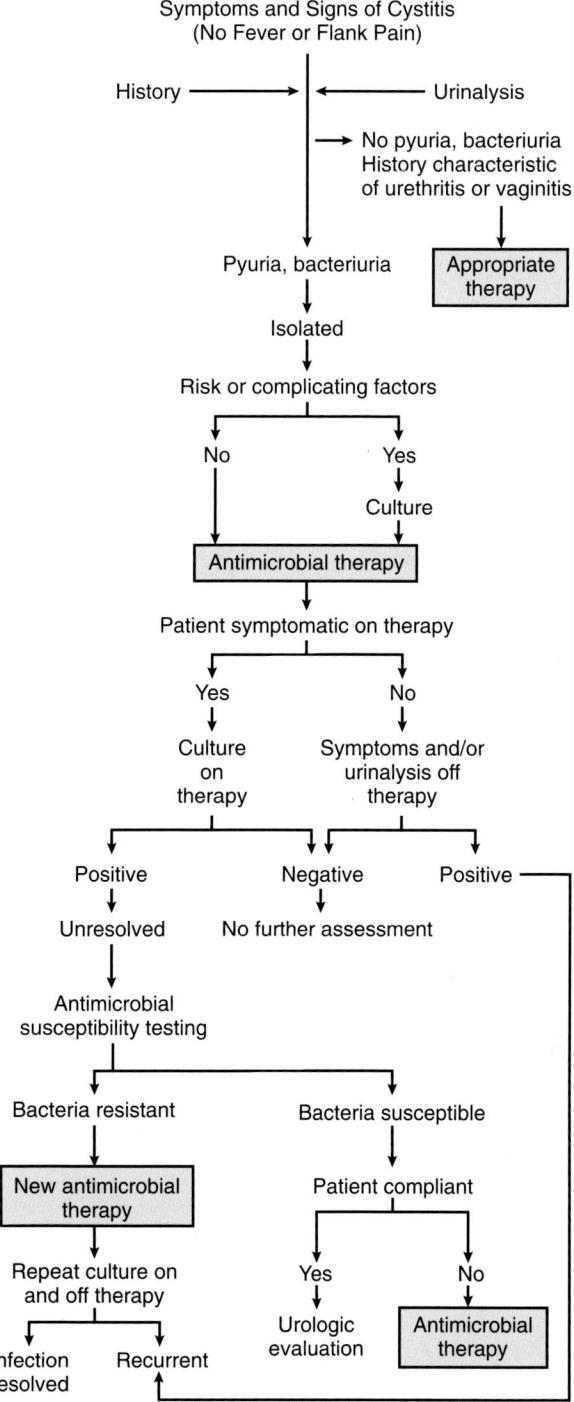

Figure 8–14. Management of acute cystitis.

of bacteria observed) (Fihn, 2003). Indirect dipstick tests for bacteria (nitrite) or pyuria (leukocyte esterase) may also be informative and more convenient but are less sensitive than microscopic examination of the urine. Dipsticks are most accurate when the presence of either nitrite or leukocyte esterase is considered a positive result (sensitivity of 75% and specificity of 82%, respectively) (Hurlbut and Littenberg, 1991). **Urine culture remains the definitive test; and in symptomatic patients, the presence of 10^2 cfu/mL or more of urine usually indicates infection** (Stamm et al, 1982b).

However, routine urine cultures are often not necessary. It is generally more cost-effective to manage many patients who have symptoms and urinalysis findings characteristic of uncomplicated cystitis without an initial urine culture because treatment decisions are usually made and therapy is often completed before culture results are known (Komaroff, 1986). This position was supported by a cost-effectiveness study (Carlson and Mulley, 1985) in which it was estimated that the routine use of pretherapeutic urine cultures for lower UTI increases costs by 40% but decreases the overall duration of symptoms by only 10%.

Thus, in women with recent onset of symptoms and signs suggesting acute cystitis and in whom factors associated with upper tract or complicated infection are absent, a urinalysis that is positive for pyuria, bacteriuria, or hematuria, or a combination should provide sufficient documentation of UTI and a urine culture may be omitted (McIsaac et al, 2002). A urine culture should be obtained for patients in whom symptoms and urine examination findings leave the diagnosis of cystitis in doubt. Pretherapeutic cultures and susceptibility tests are also essential in the management of patients with recent antimicrobial therapy or UTI. In these situations, various pathogens may be present and antimicrobial therapy is less predictable and must be tailored to the individual organism (Stamm, 1986).

Differential Diagnosis

Cystitis must be differentiated from other inflammatory infectious conditions in which dysuria may be the most prominent symptom, including vaginitis, urethral infections caused by sexually transmitted pathogens, and miscellaneous noninflammatory causes of urethral discomfort (Komaroff, 1984). Characteristic features of the history, physical examination, and voided urine or other specimens allow patients with dysuria to be assigned to one of these diagnostic categories. Vaginitis is characterized by irritative voiding associated with vaginal irritation and is subacute in onset. A history of vaginal discharge or odor and multiple or new sexual partners is common. Frequency, urgency, hematuria, and suprapubic pain are not present. Physical examination reveals a vaginal discharge, and examination of vaginal fluid demonstrates inflammatory cells. Differential diagnosis includes herpes simplex virus, gonorrhea, *Chlamydia,* trichomoniasis, yeast, and bacterial vaginosis. Urethritis causes dysuria that is usually subacute in onset and is associated with a history of discharge and new or multiple sexual partners. Frequency and urgency of urination may be present but are less pronounced than in patients with cystitis, and fever and chills are absent. Urethral discharge with inflammatory cells or initial pyuria in the male is characteristic. The common causes of urethritis include gonorrhea, *Chlamydia,* herpes simplex virus, and trichomoniasis. Appropriate cultures and immunologic tests are indicated. Urethral injury associated with sexual intercourse, chemical irritants, or allergy may also cause dysuria. A history of trauma or exposure to irritants and a lack of discharge or pyuria are characteristic.

Management

Antimicrobial Selection. Oral antimicrobial agents for treatment of acute uncomplicated cystitis are listed in Table 8–17. **TMP and TMP-SMX are effective and inexpensive agents for empirical therapy,** resulting in bacteriologic cure (i.e., eradication of the pathogen from the urine) within 7 days after the start of treatment in approximately 94% of women (Warren et al, 1999). **They are recommended in areas where the prevalence of resistance to these drugs among *E. coli* strains causing cystitis is less than 20%** (Warren et al, 1999). The probability of resistant strains can be predicted in part

Table 8–17. Treatment Regimens for Acute Cystitis

Circumstances	Route	Drug	Dosage (mg)	Frequency per dose	Duration (days)	Cost per day*
Women						
Healthy	Oral	Ciprofloxacin	500 mg	BID	3	$0.50
		Levofloxacin	500 mg	QD		$5.07
		TMP-SMX	1 double-strength tablet (160-800 mg)	BID		$0.26
		Trimethoprim	100 mg	BID		$1.32
		Nitrofurantoin macrocrystals	100 mg	BID		$3.24
		Norfloxacin	400 mg	BID		
Symptoms for >7 days, recent UTI, age >65 yr, diabetes, diaphragm use		TMP-SMX or Fluoroquinolone	As above	As above	7	As above
Pregnancy	Oral	Amoxicillin	250 mg	TID	7	$0.68
		Cephalexin	500 mg	QID		$1.76
		Nitrofurantoin macrocrystals	As above	As above		As above
		TMP-SMX*	As above	As above		As above
Men						
Healthy and age < 50 yr	Oral	TMP-SMX	As above	As above	7	As above
		Fluoroquinolone	As above	As above		As above

*Use of TMP-SMX during the first trimester of pregnancy is cautioned because there is early potential for teratogenicity and late potential for kernicterus post-delivery.

From Schaeffer AJ: Urinary tract infections. In Gillenwater JY, et al (eds): Adult and Pediatric Urology. Philadelphia, Lippincott Williams & Wilkins, 2002, pp 211-272.

from the history of recent antimicrobial usage. Women who have taken TMP-SMX recently are approximately 16 times as likely to be infected with an isolate resistant to this agent compared with women who have not taken the antimicrobial agent recently. In addition, those who have taken any other antimicrobial agent are more than twice as likely to be infected with a resistant isolate (Brown et al, 2002). With a 30% rate of resistance to TMP-SMX, the bacteriologic eradication rate is predicted to be 80% and the clinical cure rate is predicted to be 85% (Gupta et al, 2001). When used alone, TMP is as efficacious as TMP-SMX and is associated with fewer side effects, presumably because of the absence of the sulfa component (Harbord and Gruneberg, 1981). It can be prescribed to patients who are allergic to sulfa. However, TMP can cause hypersensitivity and rashes that may be erroneously attributed to sulfa (Alonso et al, 1992).

Nitrofurantoin has maintained an excellent level of activity over three decades and is well tolerated, but it is more expensive than TMP-SMX and it is considerably less active against aerobic gram-negative rods other than *E. coli*. Furthermore, it is usually prescribed for 7 days and causes gastrointestinal upset. It is not associated with plasmid-mediated resistance, however, so it is an excellent choice for patients with recent exposure to most other antimicrobial agents. The high in vitro resistance to ampicillin and sulfonamide and the high cost of amoxicillin/clavulanate and the cephalosporins limit their usefulness.

The fluoroquinolones offer excellent activity, and they are well tolerated. Resistance to the fluoroquinolones remains below 5% in most places (Fihn et al, 1988). Twice-daily and once-daily extended-release fluoroquinolones are equally effective (Henry et al, 2002). Their use for uncomplicated cystitis should be limited to patients with allergy to less costly drugs, to patients with previous exposure to antimicrobial agents causing bacterial resistance, and to areas where the prevalence of resistance to TMP or TMP-SMX is 20% or greater (Warren et al, 1999; Hooton et al, 2004).

The effects of an antimicrobial agent on the vaginal flora are also important in recurrence of bacteriuria (Fihn et al, 1988). The concentrations of TMP and the fluoroquinolones that have been studied in vaginal secretions are high, eradicating *E. coli* but minimally altering normal anaerobic and microaerophilic vaginal flora (Hooton and Stamm, 1991). Single-dose regimens using these drugs are less effective than multiple-day regimens in this regard (Fihn et al, 1988), which probably explains why there are more early recurrent infections after single-dose therapy with these drugs. Nitrofurantoin and β-lactam drugs are generally not effective in eliminating *E. coli* from the vagina.

Duration of Therapy. Three-day therapy is the preferred regimen for uncomplicated cystitis in women (Norrby, 1990; Warren et al, 1999). In an excellent review of more than 300 separate clinical trials of single-dose, 3-day, or 7-day treatment with TMP, TMP-SMX, fluoroquinolones, and β-lactam antimicrobial therapies, it was concluded that, irrespective of the antimicrobial used, 3-day therapy is more effective than single-dose therapy. Three-day therapy with TMP-SMX, TMP, amoxicillin, or cloxacillin has been associated with cure rates similar to longer courses of therapy and an incidence of adverse effects about as low as that seen with single-dose

therapy and lower than seen with longer courses of therapy (Charlton et al, 1976; Kunin, 1985; McCue, 1986; Warren et al, 1999). Because 7-day therapy often causes more adverse effects, it is recommended only for women with symptoms of 1 week or more, men, and individuals with possible complicating factors. Other options include nitrofurantoin, perhaps as 7-day therapy, and fosfomycin single-dose therapy; each of these requires further study. β-Lactams as a group are less effective in treatment of cystitis than TMP, TMP-SMX, and the fluoroquinolones.

Seven-day therapy is the preferred regimen in uncomplicated cystitis in men.

Cost of Therapy. The cost of treating a UTI involves not only the initial evaluation and cost of the drug but also what occurs subsequently. The most important prediction of high cost-effectiveness is high efficacy against the most common urinary pathogen, *E. coli*. The lower the effectiveness against this bacterium, the greater the number of revisits, cases of progression to pyelonephritis, and follow-up costs. Antimicrobial cost is a poor prediction of cost-effectiveness, as illustrated by the finding that the most expensive and least expensive drugs, the fluoroquinolones and TMP-SMX, are approximately equally cost-effective (Rosenberg, 1999). Both of these drugs are more cost-effective than nitrofurantoin and amoxicillin.

Follow-Up

Approximately 90% of women are asymptomatic within 72 hours after initiating antimicrobial therapy (Fihn et al, 1988). **Follow-up visit or culture is not required in young women who are asymptomatic after therapy. A follow-up visit, urinalysis, and urine culture are recommended in older women or those with potential risk factors and in men. Urologic evaluation is unnecessary in women and is usually unnecessary in young men who respond to therapy** (Lipsky, 1989; Abarbanel et al, 2003). **However, UTIs in most men should be considered complicated until proven otherwise.** Andrews and associates (2002) showed that approximately 50% of men with UTIs have a significant abnormality. Furthermore, if a patient does not respond to therapy, appropriate microbiologic urologic evaluations should be undertaken for the causes of unresolved and complicated UTIs.

Asymptomatic Bacteriuria

Asymptomatic bacteriuria is a microbiologic diagnosis based on the isolation of a specified quantitative count of bacteria in a properly collected specimen of urine from a patient who is without symptoms or signs referable to UTI. In healthy individuals, the absence of symptoms is clear cut, but in, for example, catheterized or neurologically comprised patients, it may be difficult to discern whether the UTI is truly asymptomatic. Kass (1962) originally proposed that for asymptomatic women two consecutive voided urine specimens with isolation of the same bacterial strain in quantitative counts of 10^5 cfu/mL is consistent with asymptomatic bacteriuria. In men, a single clean-catch voided specimen with similar counts is adequate. A single catheterized urine specimen with a solitary isolate with a quantitative count of 10^2 cfu/mL identifies bacteriuria in women or men (Nicolle et al, 2005). The prevalence of pyuria with asymptomatic bacteriuria ranges from approximately 30% in young women

(Hooton et al, 2000) to 100% in catheterized patients. In addition, many coexisting factors, such as stones, can incite inflammation in these patients and therefore the presence or absence of pyuria is not sufficient to diagnose bacteriuria, nor does it differentiate symptomatic from asymptomatic patients or provide indication for antimicrobial treatment (Nicolle et al, 2005).

The prevalence of asymptomatic bacteriuria varies widely and depends on the age, sex, and the presence of other genitourinary abnormalities (Table 8–18). *E. coli* is the most common isolate among patients with bacteriuria, and it contains fewer virulence characteristics than isolates from patients with symptomatic infections (Svanborg and Godaly, 1997). Other Enterobacteriaceae (e.g., *P. mirabilis*) and grampositive uropathogens, including group B streptococci and coagulase-negative staphylococci, become more prevalent in concert with increased underlying abnormalities. For patients who are institutionalized and/or with indwelling urologic devices, *P. aeruginosa*, *Proteus*, and other highly resistant organisms are more prevalent.

Management of asymptomatic bacteriuria is determined by the population and their risk for adverse outcome, which can be prevented with antimicrobial treatment of asymptomatic bacteriuria (Nicolle et al, 2005) (Table 8–19). **These recommendations are based on the observation that in adult populations asymptomatic bacteriuria has not been shown to be harmful.** Furthermore, although persons with bacteriuria are at increased risk of symptomatic urinary tractions, treatment of asymptomatic bacteriuria does not decrease the frequency of symptomatic infections or improve other outcomes. **Thus, in populations other than those for** whom treatment has been documented to be beneficial (e.g., pregnant women and patients undergoing urologic interventions), screening for or treatment of asymptomatic bacteriuria is not appropriate and should be discouraged (Nicolle et al, 2005).

Complicated Cystitis

Complicated UTIs are those that occur in a patient with a compromised urinary tract or that are caused by a very resistant pathogen (Table 8–20). **These complicating factors may be readily apparent from the severity of the presenting illness or the past medical history. However, they may not be obvious at first and may only become evident from subsequent failure of the patient to respond to appropriate therapy** (see discussion on unresolved or recurrent UTIs, later).

The clinical spectrum ranges from mild cystitis to life-threatening kidney infections and urosepsis (kidney infections and urosepsis are discussed subsequently). These infections can be caused by a broad range of bacteria with resistance to multiple antimicrobial agents. Therefore, urine cultures are mandatory to identify the bacteria and its antimicrobial susceptibility.

Because of the wide range of host conditions and pathogens and a lack of adequate controlled trials, guidelines for empirical therapy are limited. For patients with mild to moderate illness who can be treated as an outpatient

Table 8–18. Prevalence of Asymptomatic Bacteriuria in Selected Populations

Population	Prevalence, %	Reference
Healthy, premenopausal women	1.0-5.0	Nicolle, 2003
Pregnant women	1.9-9.5	Nicolle, 2003
Postmenopausal women aged 50-70 years	2.8-8.6	Nicolle, 2003
Diabetic patients		
Women	9.0-27	Zhanel, 1991
Men	0.7-11	Zhanel, 1991
Elderly persons in the community		
Women	10.8-16	Nicolle, 2003
Men	3.6-19	Nicolle, 2003
Elderly persons in a long-term care facility		
Women	25-50	Nicolle, 1997
Men	14-50	Nicolle, 1997
Patients with spinal cord injuries		
Intermittent catheter use	23-89	Bakke and Digranes, 1991
Sphincterotomy and condom catheter in place	57	Waites, 1993
Patients undergoing hemodialysis	28	Chaudhry, 1993
Patients with indwelling catheter use		
Short-term	9-23	Stamm, 1991
Long-term	100	Warren, 1982

From Nicolle LE, Bradley S, Colgan R, et al: Infectious Diseases Society of America guidelines for the diagnosis and treatment of asymptomatic bacteriuria in adults. Clin Infect Dis 2005;40:643-654.

Table 8–19. Screening for and Treatment of Asymptomatic Bacteriuria

Premenopausal nonpregnant women	Not recommended
Pregnant women	Recommended
Diabetic women	Not recommended
Older persons residing in the community	Not recommended
Elderly institutionalized subjects	Not recommended
Subjects with spinal cord injuries	Not recommended
Patients with indwelling urethral catheters	Not recommended
	Note: Antimicrobial treatment of asymptomatic women with catheter-associated bacteriuria that persists 48 hours after catheter removal may be considered.
Urologic interventions	Recommended
Immunocompromised patients and transplant patients	Not recommended

From Nicolle LE, Bradley S, Colgan R, et al: Infectious Diseases Society of America guidelines for the diagnosis and treatment of asymptomatic bacteriuria in adults. Clin Infect Dis 2005;40:643-54.

Table 8-20. Complicating Host Factors

Functional/structural abnormalities of urinary tract
Recent urinary tract instrumentation
Recent antimicrobial agent use
Diabetes mellitus
Immunosuppression
Pregnancy
Hospital-acquired infection

Table 8–21. Treatment of Complicated UTIs

Common Pathogens	Mitigating Circumstances	Recommended Empirical Treatment
E. coli, Proteus species, Klebsiella species, Pseudomonas species, Serratia species, enterococci, staphylococci	Mild-to-moderate illness, no nausea or vomiting—outpatient therapy Severe illness or possible urosepsis—hospitalization required	Oral* norfloxacin, ciprofloxacin, or ofloxacin for 10-14 days Parenteral† ampicillin and gentamicin, ciprofloxacin, levofloxacin, ceftriaxone, aztreonam, ticarcillin-clavulanate or imipenem-cilastin until fever gone; then oral* trimethoprim-sulfamethoxazole, norfloxacin, ciprofloxacin, or levofloxacin for 14-21 days

*Oral regimens for pyelonephritis and complicated UTI are as follows: trimethoprim-sulfamethoxazole, 160 to 800 mg q12h; norfloxacin, 400 mg q12h; ciprofloxacin, 500 mg q12h; levofloxacin, 500 mg/day.

†Parenteral regimens are as follows: ciprofloxacin, 400 mg q12h; levofloxacin, 500 mg/day; gentamicin, 1 mg/kg q8h; ceftriaxone, 1 to 2 g/day; ampicillin, 1 g q6h; imipenem-cilastin, 250 to 500 mg q6-8h; ticarcillin-clavulanate, 3.1 g q6h; and aztreonam, 1 g q8-12h.

Modified from Stamm WE, Hooton TM: Management of urinary tract infections in adults. N Engl J Med 1993;329:1328-1334. Copyright 1993 Massachusetts Medical Society. All rights reserved.

with oral therapy, the fluoroquinolones provide a broad spectrum of activity with excellent urine and tissue levels and safety. If the susceptibility pattern of the pathogen is known, TMP-SMX may be effective (Table 8–21).

For more ill, hospitalized patients, intravenous ampicillin plus gentamicin provides suitable coverage against most pathogens. Other parenteral agents can be used for special situations. Therapy can be modified when the susceptibility data are available.

Because therapy will be compromised without addressing the complicating factor(s), every effort should be made to correct any underlying urinary tract abnormalities and treat host factors that exacerbate the infection.

Therapy is usually continued for 10 to 14 days and switched from parenteral to oral therapy when possible. Urine cultures should be performed on and 7 to 14 days off therapy to validate efficacy.

Unresolved UTIs

Clinical Presentation

Unresolved infection indicates that initial therapy has been inadequate in eliminating symptoms and/or bacterial growth in the urinary tract. If the symptoms of UTI do not resolve by the end of treatment or if symptoms recur shortly after therapy, urinalysis and urine culture with susceptibility testing should be obtained. If the patient's symptoms are significant, empirical therapy with a fluoroquinolone is appropriate pending results of the culture and susceptibility testing.

The causes of unresolved bacteriuria during antimicrobial therapy are shown in Table 8–22. **Most commonly, the bacteria are resistant to the antimicrobial agent selected to treat the infection.** Typically, the patient has received the antimicrobial therapy in the recent past and developed bowel colonization with resistant bacteria. β-Lactams, tetracycline, and sulfonamides are notorious for causing plasmid-mediated R factors that simultaneously carry resistance to multiple antimicrobial agents. **The second most common cause is development of resistance in a previously susceptible population of bacteria during the course of treatment of UTIs. This problem occurs in approximately 5% of the patients receiving antimicrobial therapy. It is easy to recognize clinically because the culture on therapy shows that the previ-**

Table 8–22. Causes of Unresolved Bacteriuria, in Descending Order of Importance

Bacterial resistance to the drug selected for treatment
Development of resistance from initially susceptible bacteria
Bacteriuria caused by two different bacterial species with mutually exclusive susceptibilities
Rapid reinfection with a new, resistant species during initial therapy for the original susceptible organism
Azotemia
Papillary necrosis from analgesic abuse
Giant staghorn calculi in which the "critical mass" of susceptible bacteria is too great for antimicrobial inhibition
Self-inflicted infections or deception in taking antimicrobial drugs (a variant of Munchausen's syndrome)

ous susceptible population has been replaced by resistant bacteria of the same species. It can be shown that resistant organisms were actually present before contact with the initial antimicrobial agent, but they were present in such low numbers that it was impossible to detect by in vitro susceptibility studies before therapy. When the antimicrobial concentration in the urine is insufficient to kill all the bacteria present, the more resistant forms will emerge. This characteristically is seen in patients who are underdosed or who are poorly compliant and hence have inadequate dose regimens. **The third cause is the presence of an unsuspected, second pathogen that was present initially and is resistant to the antimicrobial therapy chosen.** Treatment of the dominant organism unmasks the presence of the second strain. **The fourth cause is rapid reintroduction of a new resistant species while the patient is undergoing initial therapy.** Rapid reinfection that mimics unresolved bacteriuria should alert the clinician to the possibility of an enterovesical fistula.

If the culture obtained on therapy shows that the initial species is still present and susceptible to the antimicrobial chosen to treat the infection, the unresolved infection must be caused by either inability to deliver an adequate concentration of antimicrobial agents into the urinary tract or an excessive number of bacteria that "override" the antimicrobial activity. In patients with azotemia, a determination of urinary antimicrobial concentrations usually shows that the level of the drug is below the minimal inhibitory concentration of the infecting organism.

In patients with papillary necrosis, severe defects in the medullary concentrating ability dilute the antimicrobial agent. A large mass of bacteria within the urinary tract is most commonly associated with a giant staghorn calculus. Even though adequate urinary levels of bactericidal drugs are present, the concentration is inadequate to sterilize the urine. This occurs because even susceptible bacteria cannot be inhibited once they reach a certain critical density, particularly if attached to a foreign body.

The last cause of unresolved bacteriuria occurs in those patients who have variants of Munchausen's syndrome. These patients secretly inoculate their bladders with uropathogens or omit their oral antimicrobial agents while steadfastly asserting that they never miss a dose. The patient with Munchausen's syndrome presents with a horrendous clinical history and invariably a normal collecting system on excretory urography. Careful bacteriologic observations usually indicate the implausibility of the clinical picture.

Laboratory Diagnosis

Urinalysis and urine culture are mandatory to determine the cause of unresolved bacteriuria. The first four causes that are associated with resistant bacteria require no further evaluation. However, if reculture shows that the bacteria is sensitive to the antimicrobial agent the patient is taking, renal function and radiologic evaluation should be performed to identify renal or urinary tract abnormalities.

Management

Initial empirical antimicrobial selection should be based on the assumption that the bacteria are resistant. Therefore, an antimicrobial agent different from the original agent should be selected. Fluoroquinolones offer excellent coverage in most cases and should be given for 7 days. When the bacterial susceptibilities are available, adjustments can be made if necessary. Urine cultures should be performed during and 7 days after therapy to ensure microbiologic efficacy.

Recurrent UTIs

Recurrent UTIs are caused by either reemergence of bacteria from a site within the urinary tract (bacterial persistence) or new infections from bacteria outside the urinary tract (reinfection). **Clinical identification of these two types of recurrence is based on the pattern of recurrent infections (Fig. 8–15). Bacterial persistence must be caused by the same organism in each instance, and infections that occur at close intervals are characteristic. Conversely, reinfections usually occur at varying and sometimes long intervals and often are caused by different species. The distinction between bacterial persistence and reinfection is important in management because patients with bacterial persistence can usually be cured of the recurrent infections by identification and surgical removal or correction of the focus of infection. Conversely, women with reinfection usually do not have an alterable urologic abnormality and require long-term medical management. Reinfections in men are uncommon and may be associated with an underlying abnormality, such as urethral stricture; therefore, at a minimum, endoscopic evaluation is indicated.**

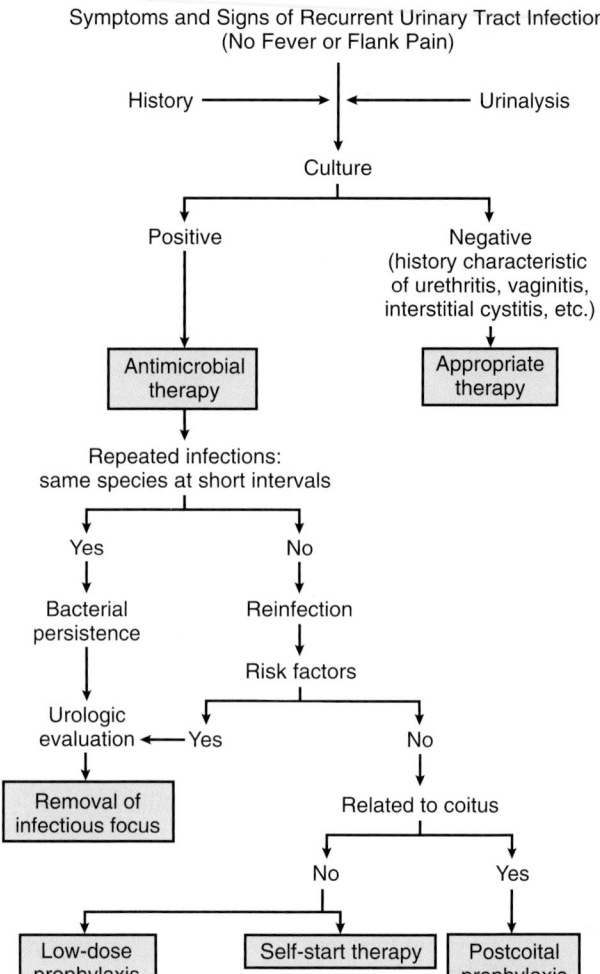

Figure 8–15. Management of recurrent UTI.

Bacterial Persistence

Once the bacteriuria has resolved (i.e., the urine shows no growth for several days after the antimicrobial agent has been stopped), recurrence with the same organism can arise from a site *within* the urinary tract that was excluded from the high urine concentrations of the antimicrobial agent. The 12 correctable urologic abnormalities that cause bacteria to persist within the urinary tract between episodes of recurrent bacteriuria are listed in Table 8–6. The relationship of these abnormalities to bacterial persistence, as well as the documentation that surgical excision removes the infection as a source of recurrent bacteriuria, is presented elsewhere in detail (Stamey, 1980). Once the urologist recognizes that the cause of the patient's recurrent bacteriuria is bacterial persistence, Table 8–6 should serve as a checklist for known, correctable causes. Some of the causes are subtle, and many require cystoscopic localization of the infection with ureteral catheters to accurately define the focus of bacterial persistence.

Although patients with bacterial persistence are relatively uncommon, their identification is important because they represent the only surgically curable cause of recurrent UTIs. A systematic radiologic and endoscopic evaluation of the urinary tract is mandatory. Excretory urography or CT and cystoscopy provide the initial screening. Retrograde urography may be required in selected patients to delineate abnormalities, such as diverticulum or nonrefluxing ureteral stump.

Urea-Splitting Bacteria That Cause Struvite Renal Stones. The infection that ultimately leads to an infection stone commonly begins inconspicuously as inadequately treated cystitis. Alternatively, bacteriuria in most of these patients with struvite stones recurs almost immediately on stopping antimicrobial therapy, usually within 5 to 7 days. It is true that *P. mirabilis* is a common cause of bacteriuria (about 25% of people carry this organism in their normal bowel flora), and most patients with *P. mirabilis* cystitis do not form struvite stones. But struvite stones form in those patients who have a protracted infection with *P. mirabilis*, an infection that is often asymptomatic or minimally symptomatic. *P. mirabilis* causes intense alkalinization of the urine with precipitation of calcium, magnesium, ammonium, and phosphate salts and the subsequent formation of branched struvite renal stones. The bacteriologic consequences are substantial because the bacteria persist inside these struvite stones even when the urine shows no growth. Indeed, struvite infection stones, together with the occasional oxalate or apatite stone that becomes secondarily colonized, constitute the major cause of bacterial persistence in women in the absence of azotemia.

Underlying urinary tract abnormalities are not a prerequisite for this type of infection. However, patients with indwelling catheters, urinary diversions, or other urinary tract abnormalities are particularly susceptible to these infections. Urea-splitting organisms, such as *P. mirabilis*, cause infection stones that are relatively radiolucent. If such a stone is suspected, plain film tomograms or CT scans without contrast medium enhancement should be obtained (Greenberg et al, 1982). Medical management with continued suppressive antimicrobial therapy and acidification temporarily relieves symptoms and retards deterioration of renal function in some patients. Complete removal of the calculus is generally required for bacteriologic cure and to prevent renal damage due to obstruction (Silverman and Stamey, 1983). Percutaneous nephrolithotomy and extracorporeal shockwave lithotripsy are now the preferred treatment for most renal and upper ureteral calculi.

When extracorporeal shockwave lithotripsy is used to fragment infection stones, the patient should be maintained on appropriate antimicrobial therapy until the fragments pass. Occasionally, long-term antimicrobial therapy can result in eradication of bacteriuria even if some fragments persist after lithotripsy, presumably because the shockwaves have rendered the entrapped bacteria more susceptible to antimicrobial therapy (Michaels et al, 1988). **If percutaneous or open surgery is used, all the residual particles of struvite stones must be removed at surgery to prevent recurrent bacteriuria from bacterial persistence in the calculus.** Rocha and Santos (1969) have shown that soaking these stones in iodine and alcohol for 6 hours will not kill the bacteria within the interior of the stone. The importance of recognizing this fact is twofold: **(1) The bacteria cannot be killed by antimicrobial therapy, even though the urine may show no growth for months or even years** (Shortliffe et al, 1984), **and (2) any**

fragments left behind at the time of surgical removal leave residual bacteria within the interstices of the stone; these bacteria ensure recurrence of the staghorn calculus with its attendant morbidity.

If fragments remain after surgery, a small, multiholed polyethylene catheter should be left for postoperative irrigation with Renacidin or Suby G solution (Silverman and Stamey, 1983). Follow-up radiographs are essential to ensure that all the stone fragments are removed, and cultures must demonstrate that the urease-splitting bacteria are eradicated.

Most of the other congenital or acquired abnormalities listed in Table 8–6 require surgical removal for eradication of the source of bacterial persistence. Chronic bacterial prostatitis is treated initially with long-term antimicrobial therapy and, in select cases, by radical transurethral resection (Meares, 1978).

In patients in whom the focus of infection cannot be eradicated, long-term, low-dose antimicrobial suppression is necessary to prevent symptoms of infection. The antimicrobial drugs used for low-dose prophylaxis will also be effective for bacterial suppression if the persistent strain is susceptible. These include nitrofurantoin, TMP-SMX, cephalexin, and the fluoroquinolones.

Reinfections

Patients with recurrent infections caused by different species or occurring at long intervals almost invariably have reinfections. These reinfections most often occur in women and girls and are associated with ascending colonization from the bowel flora. Reinfections in men are often associated with a urinary tract abnormality. The possibility of a vesicoenteric or vesicovaginal fistula should be considered when the patient has any history of pneumaturia, fecaluria, diverticulitis, obstipation, previous pelvic surgery, or radiation therapy. Evaluation of the patient with presumed reinfections must be individualized.

Failure to recognize and correct abnormalities that reduce formation, transmission, and elimination of urine by the urinary tract increases the incidence of reinfection in susceptible patients and reduces the effectiveness of antimicrobial therapy. Abnormalities should be corrected and urinary tract function restored by medical, pharmacologic, or surgical management. A thorough urologic evaluation is essential in all men and in women with evidence of upper tract infections (fevers, chills, flank pain, hemorrhagic cystitis, or other risk factors, such as history of unexplained hematuria, obstructive symptoms, neurogenic bladder dysfunction, renal calculi, fistula, analgesic abuse, or severe disease such as diabetes mellitus). In women, diaphragm-spermicide use has been associated with an increased risk of UTI and vaginal colonization with *E. coli* (Hooton et al, 1991b). Spermicides containing the active ingredient nonoxynol-9 may provide a selective advantage in colonizing the vagina, perhaps by a reduction in vaginal lactobacilli and through enhancement of adherence of *E. coli* to epithelial cells (Hooton et al, 1991a; Gupta et al, 2000). Thus, spermicides should be discontinued in women with recurrent UTI and other forms of contraception should be used. In postmenopausal women, the risk of infection is reduced by estrogen replacement (Raz and Stamm, 1993).

Postmenopausal women have frequent reinfections (Hooton et al, 1991c; Raz and Stamm, 1993). These infections are sometimes attributable to residual urine after voiding, which is often associated with bladder or uterine prolapse. In addition, the lack of estrogen causes marked changes in the vaginal microflora, including a loss of lactobacilli and increased colonization by *E. coli* (Raz and Stamm, 1993). Estrogen replacement frequently restores the normal vaginal environment, allows recolonization with lactobacilli, and thus eliminates bacterial uropathogenic colonization. A reduced incidence of UTIs has been documented with this approach (Raz and Stamm, 1993).

Urinary tract imaging will demonstrate the anatomy of the urinary tract and provide reasonable assessment of its functional status. In healthy women, upper tract abnormalities associated with reinfections are very rare; therefore, routine urologic imaging is not indicated. Cystoscopy should be performed in men or women who have frequent reinfections and symptoms suggestive of obstruction, bladder dysfunction, and fistula. If the patient has residual urine that is judged to be significant (e.g., 100 mL) and due to a narrowing of the urethra, a single dilation of the urethra to improve bladder emptying would appear appropriate. There is little evidence, however, that repeated urethral dilation is indicated in the routine management of most women.

Antimicrobial management in women who have had two or more symptomatic UTIs over a 6-month period or three or more episodes within a 12-month period involves one of three regimens: low-dose continuous prophylaxis, self-start intermittent therapy, or postintercourse prophylaxis.

Low-Dose Continuous Prophylaxis
Biologic Basis of Successful Prophylaxis: Antimicrobial Effect on Bowel and Vaginal Bacterial Flora. The success of prophylaxis depends, in large part, on the effect an antimicrobial agent has on the introital and bowel reservoirs of pathogenic bacteria. Antimicrobial agents that eliminate pathogenic bacteria from these sites and/or do not cause bacterial resistance at the sites can be effective for antimicrobial prophylaxis of UTIs (Table 8–23). Winberg and his colleagues were among the first to emphasize that oral antimicrobial therapy causes resistant strains in the bowel flora and subsequent resistant UTIs (Lincoln et al, 1970; Winberg et al, 1973).

With 7- to 10-day therapy, the disadvantage of a resistant bowel flora is not as great because rapid reinfections are relatively uncommon (Kraft and Stamey, 1977). Nevertheless, the increase in resistant strains of *E. coli*, as well as the proliferation of other Enterobacteriaceae species, *Candida albicans*, enterococci, and other pathogenic bacteria in the bowel and vaginal flora that accompanies even short-term, full-dose oral administration of tetracyclines, ampicillin, sulfonamides, amoxicillin, and cephalexin, is well documented (Sharp, 1954; Daikos et al, 1968; Hinton, 1970; Lincoln et al, 1970; Datta et al, 1971; Gruneberg et al, 1973; Winberg et al, 1973; Toivanen

Table 8–23. Low-Dose Prophylaxis for Recurrent UTIs In Women

Investigators	Regimen	Infections per Patient-Year
Bailey et al (1971)	Nitrofurantoin, 50 or 100 mg daily	0.09
	Nitrofurantoin, 50 mg daily	0.19
	Placebo	2.1
Harding and Ronald (1974)	Sulfamethoxazole, 500 mg daily	2.5
	TMP-SMX, 40 and 200 mg daily	0.1
	Methenamine mandelate, 2 g daily, plus ascorbic acid, 2 g	1.6
Kasanen et al (1974)	Nitrofurantoin, 50 mg daily	0.32
	Methenamine hippurate, 1 g daily	0.39
	Trimethoprim, 100 mg daily	0.13
	TMP-SMX, 80 and 400 mg daily	0.19
Gower (1975)	Cephalexin, 125 mg daily	0.10
Stamey et al (1977)	TMP-SMX, 40 and 200 mg daily	0.00
	Nitrofurantoin macrocrystals, 100 mg daily	0.74
Harding et al (1979)	TMP-SMX, 40 and 200 mg daily three times weekly	0.1
Stamm et al (1980)	TMP-SMX, 40 and 200 mg daily	0.15
	Trimethoprim, 100 mg daily	0.00
	Nitrofurantoin macrocrystals, 100 mg daily	0.14
	Placebo	2.8
Brumfitt et al (1981)	Nitrofurantoin, 50 mg twice daily	0.19
	Methenamine hippurate, 1 g twice daily	0.57
Harding et al (1982)	TMP-SMX, 40 and 200 mg three times weekly	0.14
Brumfitt et al (1983)	Trimethoprim, 100 mg daily	1.53
	Methenamine hippurate, 1 g daily	1.38
	Povidone-iodine wash, twice daily	1.79
Wong et al (1985)	TMP-SMX, 40 and 200 mg daily	0.2
	Self-administered cotrimoxazole, 4 × 80 and 400 mg	2.2
Martinez et al (1985)	Cephalexin, 250 mg daily	0.18
Brumfitt et al (1985)	Trimethoprim, 100 mg daily	1.00
	Nitrofurantoin macrocrystals, 100 mg daily	0.16
Nicolle et al (1989)	Nitrofurantoin, 200 mg daily	0.00
	Norfloxacin, 200 mg daily	0.00
Raz and Boger (1991)	Norfloxacin, 200 mg daily	0.04

TMP-SMX, trimethoprim-sulfamethoxazole.
From Nicolle LE, Ronald AR: Recurrent urinary tract infection in adult women: Diagnosis and treatment. Infect Dis Clin North Am 1987;1:793-806.

et al, 1976; Ronald et al, 1977; Preiksaitis et al, 1981). These ecologic changes may interfere with antimicrobial prophylaxis in the urinary tract and must be considered in the choice of prophylactic agents.

Effective Drugs. The oral antimicrobial agents with minimal adverse effects on the bowel and vaginal flora are TMP-SMX or TMP alone, nitrofurantoin, cephalexin (in minimal dosage), and the fluoroquinolones.

TMP-SMX eradicates gram-negative aerobic flora from the bowel and vaginal fluid. Because the bowel is a reservoir for organisms that may colonize the periurethral area and subsequently cause episodes of acute cystitis in young women, infection is prevented by eliminating the pathogens from this reservoir. In addition, vaginal fluid measurements of TMP and SMX in patients showed that TMP infused across the noninflamed vaginal wall and produced concentrations that exceeded serum levels (Stamey and Condy, 1975); SMX was undetectable in vaginal fluid. These observations on diffusion and concentration of TMP and vaginal fluid and on the effects of TMP-SMX in clearing Enterobacteriaceae from the rectal and vaginal flora clearly indicate why TMP-SMX is such a powerful prophylactic agent for the prevention of reinfections in the female. These important biologic effects occur in addition to the bactericidal levels of TMP-SMX that are present in the urine during nightly prophylaxis.

Kasanen and his colleagues in Finland (Kasanen et al, 1978) studied the bowel flora in volunteers and patients who took 100 mg of TMP per day for periods of 3 weeks to 36 months; 4 of 20 patients treated for long periods developed coliforms resistant to TMP ($>8 \mu g/mL$). Svensson and his associates (1982) gave 100 mg of TMP once daily for 6 months to 26 patients with recurrent UTIs. The infection recurrence rate before prophylaxis was 26 per 100 months compared with 3.3 recurrences per 100 months during prophylaxis ($P = .001$). The postprophylactic infection rate returned to 23 recurrences per 100 months. It is important to note that all *E. coli* UTIs after prophylaxis were sensitive to TMP, that the number of rectal Enterobacteriaceae was markedly reduced during prophylaxis, and that, although a 10% incidence of TMP-resistant organisms from rectal swabs was observed less than 1 month into prophylaxis, there was no significant further accumulation of resistant bacteria. This 10% incidence of TMP-resistant Enterobacteriaceae is virtually the same as was found in patients receiving 40 mg of TMP and 200 mg of SMX nightly in combination (Stamey and Condy, 1975).

These studies on TMP alone suggest that it should be as effective as TMP-SMX for prophylactic prevention of recurrent UTIs. Stamm and coworkers (1980a) noted only one resistant strain of *E. coli* in 316 rectal, urethral, and vaginal isolates from 15 patients receiving 100 mg of TMP and 15 others receiving 40 mg of TMP with 200 mg of SMX nightly for 6 months; their unbelievably low recovery of TMP-resistant *E. coli* was due to their method of sampling, which did not include streaking cultures from these colonization sites directly onto media containing TMP.

These studies on TMP-SMX and TMP prophylactic therapy usually have been limited to 6 months to test continuing susceptibility in patients with reinfections. Two studies (Pearson et al, 1979; Harding et al, 1982), however, continued TMP-SMX prophylaxis from 2 to 5 years without showing any increase in "breakthrough" infections or any increase in TMP-resistant recurrent infections. Indeed, in the 15 patients treated for 2 years with one-half tablet of TMP-SMX thrice weekly (Harding et al, 1982), 100 of 116 cultures from the periurethral area (91%) and 60 of 97 cultures from the anal canal (68%) showed no aerobic gram-negative bacilli at these colonization sites.

In view of all these studies that indicate minimal bowel flora in patients who take oral TMP-SMX or TMP alone, it is remarkable that Murray and colleagues (1982) reported TMP-resistant bowel gram-negative bacteria in 42 of 46 students who took TMP-SMX for 2 weeks in a diarrhea-preventive study in Mexico. This study would suggest that TMP-resistant strains are endemic in Mexico and should serve as a precaution to those who want to preserve the prophylactic efficacy of TMP-SMX in the United States.

Nitrofurantoin, which does not alter the bowel flora, is present for brief periods at high concentrations in the urine and leads to repeated elimination of bacteria from the urine, presumably interfering with bacterial initiation of infection. Because of either its complete absorption in the upper intestinal tract or its degradation and inactivation in the intestinal tract, it produces minimal effects on bowel flora (Stamey et al, 1977). Unlike the situation in prophylaxis with TMP-SMX, which eliminates colonization, in prophylaxis with nitrofurantoin, colonization of the vaginal introitus with Enterobacteriaceae continues throughout therapy. The bacteria colonizing the vagina nearly always remain susceptible because of the lack of bacterial resistance in the bowel flora.

The urologist should know the adverse reactions to nitrofurantoin; according to Holmberg and associates (1980), nitrofurantoin accounted for 10% to 12% of all adverse drug reactions reported in Sweden. The two largest groups consisted of acute pulmonary reactions (43%) and allergic reactions (42%). Neuropathy, blood dyscrasias, liver damage, and chronic pulmonary reactions constituted the remainder. These appeared to be acute hypersensitivity reactions, with 65% to 83% of the patients showing eosinophilia in the blood smears. **The risk of an adverse reaction increases with age, with the greatest number occurring in patients older than 50 years. Patients on long-term therapy should be monitored. If a patient develops a chronic cough, the drug should be discontinued and a chest radiograph obtained.**

Fairley and his associates (1974) first reported on the prophylactic efficacy of 500 mg of cephalexin per day in preventing recurrent infections during a 6-month period of observation. Of the 22 patients, 17 remained free of infection, an impressive record because several patients had papillary necrosis, chronic pyelonephritis, and even renal calculi. Gower (1975) treated 25 women with 125 mg of cephalexin nightly for 6 to 12 months and found only 1 infection, whereas 13 of 25 women receiving a placebo had infection. In a study of hospitalized patients with a mean age of 78 years, 125 mg/day of cephalexin was as effective as 250 mg/day in the 50% of patients whose urine remained sterile (Sourander and Saarimaa, 1975).

Martinez and coworkers (1985) studied the effect on the vaginal and rectal flora of 250 mg of cephalexin nightly for 6 months in 23 patients with reinfections of the urinary tract. Throughout prophylaxis, 22 of the 23 patients maintained a sterile urine; a single patient developed two enterococcal UTIs, both of which responded to nitrofurantoin. No change was detected in the rectal or vaginal carriage of Enterobacteriaceae. More importantly, not a single resistant strain of *E. coli* was detected in 154 cultures obtained at monthly intervals during cephalexin therapy. All rectal and vaginal cultures were streaked on Mueller-Hinton agar containing 32 μg of cephalexin per milliliter. These results are in contrast to those of Preiksaitis and colleagues (1981), who found rectal Enterobacteriaceae resistance in 38% of patients when cephalexin was administered at a dose of 500 mg four times daily for 14 days. **Cephalexin at 250 mg or less nightly is an excellent prophylactic agent because bowel flora resistance does not develop at this low dosage.**

With short-course fluoroquinolone therapy (Hooton et al, 1989), eradication of Enterobacteriaceae from the bowel and vaginal (Nord, 1988; Tartaglione et al, 1988) flora has been documented, observations that have been exploited in the use of these agents for prophylaxis. More recently, Nicolle and coworkers (1989) documented the prophylactic efficacy of norfloxacin for the prevention of recurrent UTIs in women. Of 11 women who completed 1 year of prophylaxis (200 mg orally), all remained free of infection. By comparison, the majority of individuals receiving placebos developed UTIs; the infection rate in the placebo group was similar to that previously reported in populations of women with recurrent UTIs. The drug was well tolerated. In addition to preventing symptomatic UTIs, norfloxacin virtually eradicated periurethral and bowel colonization with aerobic gram-negative organisms. A larger study by Raz and Boger (1991) confirmed these results.

Because the fluoroquinolones are expensive and can be used only in nonpregnant women, we favor their use only when antimicrobial resistance or patient intolerance to TMP-SMX, TMP, nitrofurantoin, or cephalexin occurs. Further studies are required to determine the minimal effective regimen and efficacy of the fluoroquinolones for prophylaxis of recurrent UTIs in women.

Efficacy of Prophylaxis. **Prophylactic therapy has been repeatedly documented as being effective in the management of women with recurrent UTIs, with recurrences decreased by 95% when compared with placebo or with the patients' prior experiences as controls.** These reported results of prophylaxis, together with agents and doses, have been summarized by Nicolle and Ronald (1987) (see Table 8–23). These studies consistently show a remarkable reduction in the reinfection rate from 2.0 to 3.0 per patient-year to 0.1 to 0.4 per patient-year with the use of prophylaxis. Urinary antiseptics, such as methenamine mandelate or hippurate, have resulted in some decrease in recurrences, but they are not as effective as antimicrobial agents.

Prophylactic therapy requires only a small dose of an antimicrobial agent, which is generally given at bedtime for 6 to 12 months. If a woman experiences symptomatic reinfection during prophylactic therapy, full therapeutic dosing may be used with the prophylactic agent or another antimicrobial agent used to treat the infection. Then, antimicrobial prophylaxis may be reinstituted. If a patient experiences symptomatic reinfection immediately after cessation of prophylactic therapy, reinstitution of nightly prophylaxis is an effective alternative and results in no increase in adverse effects (Harding et al, 1982).

Low-dose continuous prophylaxis is indicated when the urine culture shows no growth (usually when a patient has completed antimicrobial therapy). Nightly therapy is then begun with one of the following drugs: (1) nitrofurantoin, 50 to 100 mg half-strength (HS) (Stamey et al, 1977); (2) TMP-SMX, 40 to 200 mg (Stamm et al, 1982a); (3) TMP, 50 mg (Stamm et al, 1982a); or (4) Keflex, 250 mg (Martinez et al, 1985). Patients will have less than one UTI per year while taking these regimens. Every-other-night therapy is also effective and is probably practiced by most patients. When breakthrough infections occur, they are not necessarily accompanied by symptoms; therefore, we advocate monitoring for infections every 1 to 3 months, even in asymptomatic patients. Breakthrough infections usually respond to full-dose therapy with the drug used for prophylaxis. However, cultures and susceptibility tests may indicate that another drug is indicated. After the infection is cured, prophylaxis may be reinstituted. Low-dose prophylaxis is usually discontinued after about 6 months, and the patient is monitored for reinfection. Approximately 30% of women will have spontaneous remissions that last up to 6 months (Kraft and Stamey, 1977). Unfortunately, many of the remissions are followed by reinfections, and low-dose prophylaxis must be reinstituted. At this point, many patients prefer an alternative form of management.

Self-Start Intermittent Therapy. With self-start intermittent therapy, the patient is given a dip slide device to culture the urine and is instructed to perform a urine culture when symptoms of UTI occur (Schaeffer and Stuppy, 1999; Blom et al, 2002). The patient is also provided a 3-day course of empirical, full-dose antimicrobial therapy to be started immediately after performing the culture. It is important that the antimicrobial agent selected for self-start therapy have a broad spectrum of activity and achieve high urinary levels to minimize development of resistant mutants. In addition, there should be minimal or no side effects on the bowel flora. Fluoroquinolones are ideal for self-start therapy because they have a spectrum of activity broader than any of the other oral agents and are superior to many parenteral antimicrobials, including aminoglycosides. Nitrofurantoin and TMP-SMX are acceptable alternatives, although they are somewhat less effective. Antimicrobial agents such as tetracycline, ampicillin, SMX, and cephalexin in full doses should be avoided because they can give rise to resistant bacteria (Wong et al, 1985).

The culture is brought to the office as soon as possible. If the culture is positive and the patient is asymptomatic, a culture is performed 7 to 10 days after therapy to determine efficacy. In most cases, the therapy is limited to two inexpensive dip slide cultures and a short course of antimicrobial therapy. If the patient has symptoms that do not respond to initial antimicrobial therapy, a repeat culture and susceptibility testing of the initial culture specimen are performed and therapy adjusted accordingly. If symptoms of infection are not associated with positive cultures, urologic evaluation should be performed to rule out other causes of irritative bladder symptoms, including carcinoma in situ, interstitial cystitis, and neurogenic bladder dysfunction. Our experience with this technique has been very favorable, and we find that it is particularly attractive to patients who have less frequent infections and are willing to play an active role in their diagnosis and management.

Post-intercourse Prophylaxis. Antimicrobial management through post-intercourse prophylaxis is based on research establishing that sexual intercourse can be an important risk factor for acute cystitis in women (Nicolle et al, 1982). Diaphragm users have a significantly greater risk of UTI than do women who use other contraceptive methods (Fihn et al, 1985). Post-intercourse therapy with antimicrobial agents, such as nitrofurantoin, cephalexin, TMP-SMX, or a fluoroquinolone taken as a single dose, will effectively reduce the incidence of reinfection (Pfau et al, 1983; Melekos et al, 1997).

Other Strategies. Cranberry juice contains proanthocyanidins that block adherence of pathogens to uroepithelial cells in vitro (Foo et al, 2000). Randomized trials in low-risk patients show that 200 to 750 mL daily of cranberry or lingonberry juice or cranberry-concentrate tablets reduce the risk of symptomatic, recurrent infection by 12% to 20% (Avorn et al, 1994; Kontiokari et al, 2001; Stothers, 2002). However, the actual cranberry content of juices and tablets varies substantially; therefore their efficacy is not predictable (Consumer Reports, 2001; Klein, 2002). Furthermore, other trials of cranberry products show no benefit and there is no evidence that they are effective for treatment of UTIs (Jepson et al, 2001; Raz et al, 2004).

Other factors, such as hygiene, frequency and timing of voiding, wiping patterns, use of hot tubs, and type of undergarments, have not been shown to predispose women to recurrent infection and there is no rationale for giving women specific instructions regarding them.

KEY POINTS: BLADDER INFECTIONS

- Uncomplicated cystitis should be treated for 3 days.
- Asymptomatic bacteriuria should be treated only in pregnant women and prior to urologic intervention.
- Recurrent UTIs due to bacterial persistence require urologic management; reinfections can be managed medically.

KIDNEY INFECTIONS
Renal Infection (Bacterial Nephritis)

Although renal infection is less prevalent than bladder infection, it often is a more difficult problem for the patient and his or her physician because of its often varied and morbid presentation and course, the difficulty in establishing a firm microbiologic and pathologic diagnosis, and its potential for significantly impairing renal function. **Although the classic symptoms of acute onset of fever, chills, and flank pain are usually indicative of renal infection, some patients with these symptoms do not have renal infection. Conversely, significant renal infection may be associated with an insidious onset of nonspecific local or systemic symptoms, or it may be entirely asymptomatic.** Therefore, a high clinical index of suspicion and appropriate radiologic and laboratory studies are required to establish the diagnosis of renal infection.

Unfortunately, **the relationship between laboratory findings and the presence of renal infection often is poor. Bacteriuria and pyuria, the hallmarks of UTI, are not predictive of renal infection. Conversely, patients with significant renal infection may have sterile urine if the ureter draining the kidney is obstructed or the infection is outside of the collecting system.**

The pathologic and radiologic criteria for diagnosing renal infection may also be misleading. Interstitial renal inflammation, once thought to be caused predominantly by bacterial infection, is now recognized as a nonspecific histopathologic change associated with a variety of immunologic, congenital, or chemical lesions that usually develop in the absence of bacterial infection. Infectious granulomatous diseases of the kidney often have either radiologic or pathologic characteristics that mimic renal cystic disease, neoplasia, or other renal inflammatory disease.

The effect of renal infection on renal function is varied. Acute or chronic pyelonephritis may transiently or permanently alter renal function, but nonobstructive pyelonephritis is no longer recognized as a major cause of renal failure (Baldassarre and Kaye, 1991; Fraser et al, 1995). However, pyelonephritis, when associated with urinary tract obstruction or granulomatous renal infection, may lead rapidly to significant inflammatory complications, renal failure, or even death.

Interstitial renal inflammation is a nonspecific cellular response of the renal interstitium that may or may not be complicated by fibrosis and varying degrees of tubular or glomerular damage. It generally has been believed that bacterial infection of the kidney, such as pyelonephritis, was the most common cause of interstitial renal inflammation and subsequent development of serious renal disease. More recently, however, the nonspecific nature of the histopathologic changes of interstitial renal inflammation has been appreciated. As a result of urologic evaluations of patients with chronic preexisting interstitial renal inflammation, it is now recognized that interstitial renal inflammation is associated with immunologic reactions, congenital lesions, or papillary damage in the absence of bacterial infection and that bacterial infection is often a secondary event. Thus, histologic evidence alone is too often assumed indicative of bacterial nephritis and is not sufficient to establish whether interstitial changes in the kidney are either primary or secondary to bacterial infection or of noninfectious causes.

Pathology

The opportunity for pathologic confirmation of acute bacterial nephritis is rare. The kidney may be edematous. Focal acute suppurative bacterial nephritis caused by hematogenous dissemination of bacteria to the renal cortex is characterized by multiple focal areas of suppuration on the surface of the kidney (Fig. 8–16). Histologic examination of the renal cortex shows focal suppurative destruction of glomeruli and tubules. Adjacent cortical structures and the medulla are not involved in the inflammatory reaction. Acute ascending pyelonephritis is characterized by linear bands of inflammation extending from the medulla to the renal capsule (Fig. 8–17). Histologic examination usually reveals a focal wedge-shaped area of acute interstitial inflammation with the apex of the wedge in the renal medulla. Polymorphonuclear leukocytes or a

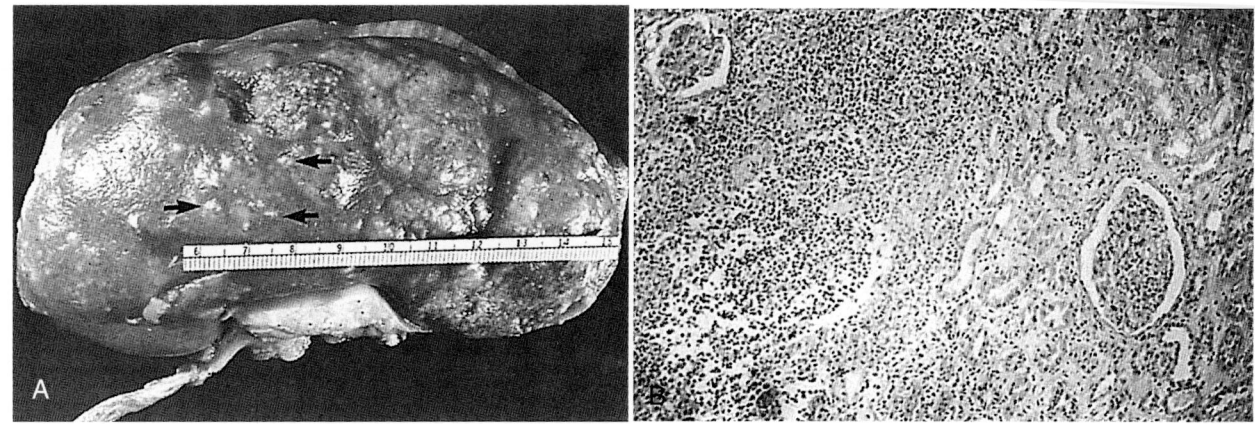

Figure 8–16. Acute focal suppurative bacterial nephritis. **A,** Surface of kidney. *Arrows* indicate focal areas of suppuration. **B,** Renal cortex showing focal suppuration destruction of glomeruli and tubules. (From Schaeffer AJ: Urinary tract infections. In Gillenwater JY, et al [eds]: Adult and Pediatric Urology. Philadelphia, Lippincott Williams & Wilkins, 2002, pp 211-272.)

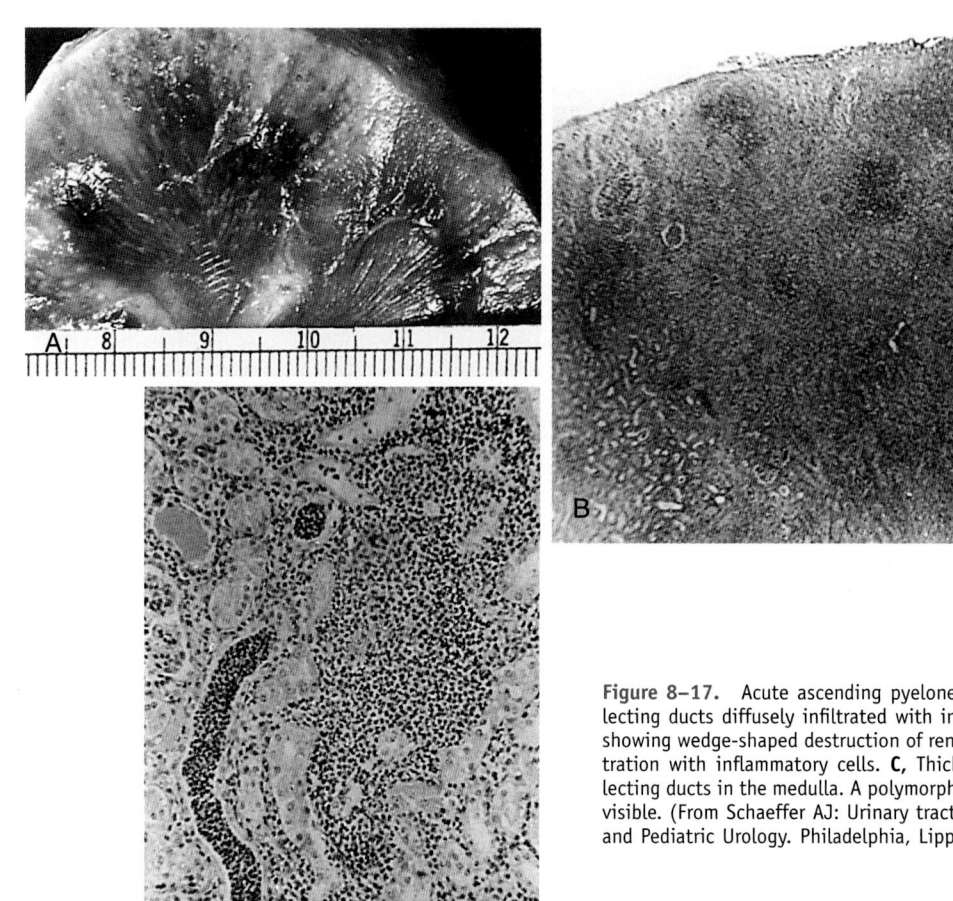

Figure 8–17. Acute ascending pyelonephritis. **A,** Cortical structures, tubules, and collecting ducts diffusely infiltrated with inflammatory cells. **B,** Section of the renal cortex showing wedge-shaped destruction of renocortical structures as a result of ascending infiltration with inflammatory cells. **C,** Thickened and inflamed tissue surrounding the collecting ducts in the medulla. A polymorphonuclear cast of segmented neutrophils is clearly visible. (From Schaeffer AJ: Urinary tract infections. In Gillenwater JY, et al [eds]: Adult and Pediatric Urology. Philadelphia, Lippincott Williams & Wilkins, 2002, pp 211-272.)

predominantly lymphocytic and plasma cell response are seen. Bacteria also may be present.

The changes that appear to be most specific for chronic pyelonephritis are evident on careful gross examination of the kidney and consist of a cortical scar associated with retraction of the corresponding renal papilla (Hodson, 1965a, 1965b; Heptinstall, 1974; Freedman, 1979). The kidney shows evidence of patchy involvement with numerous chronic inflammatory foci mainly confined to the cortex but also involving the medulla (Fig. 8–18).

The scars may be separated by intervening zones of normal parenchyma, causing a grossly irregular renal outline. The microscopic appearance, as with most chronic interstitial disease, includes the presence of lymphocytes and plasma cells. Although glomeruli within scars may be surrounded by a cuff of fibrosis or be partially or completely hyalinized, glomeruli outside these severely scarred zones are relatively normal. Vascular involvement is variable, but in patients with hypertension, nephrosclerosis may be found. Papillary abnormalities include deformity, sclerosis, and sometimes necrosis. Studies in animals have clearly indicated the critical role of the papilla in the initiation of pyelonephritis (Freedman and Beeson, 1958). However, these changes are not necessarily specific for bacterial infection and may occur in the absence of infection as a result of other disorders such as analgesic abuse, diabetes, and sickle cell disease.

The classic pathologic description of chronic pyelonephritis has traditionally been that of Weiss and Parker (1939); however, their autopsy studies included late stages of the disease, which are often complicated by hypertension and vascular changes and are best referred to as end-stage kidneys. They repeatedly emphasized that patients with this form of renal disease did not always have clinical evidence of bacterial infections of the urinary tract sufficient to explain the severe loss of renal tissue. Stamey and Pfau (1963) presented a case of pure symptomatic pyelonephritis, incurable with drug therapy and uncomplicated by vascular hypertension. The microscopic sections together with Heptinstall's comments

represent an unusual opportunity to study the pathologic characteristics of this disease in its purest form.

Acute Pyelonephritis

Although pyelonephritis is defined as inflammation of the kidney and renal pelvis, the diagnosis is clinical. True infection of the "upper urinary tract" can be proved by catheterization tests (ureteral catheterization or bladder washout) as described in this chapter, but these are impractical and unnecessary in most patients with acute pyelonephritis. None of the noninvasive tests that have been developed to determine infection in the kidney or bladder are totally reliable.

Clinical Presentation. The clinical spectrum ranges from gram-negative sepsis to cystitis with mild flank pain (Stamm and Hooton, 1993). **The classic presentation is an abrupt onset of chills, fever (100° F or greater), and unilateral or bilateral flank or costovertebral angle pain and/or tenderness. These so-called upper tract signs are often accompanied by dysuria, increased urinary frequency, and urgency.**

Although some authors regard loin pain and fever in combination with significant bacteriuria as diagnostic of acute pyelonephritis, it is clear from localization studies using ureteral catheterization (Stamey and Pfau, 1963) or the bladder washout technique (Fairley et al, 1967) that clinical symptoms correlate poorly with the site of infection (Stamey et al, 1965; Eykyn et al, 1972; Fairley, 1972; Smeets and Gower, 1973).

In a large study of 201 women and 12 men with recurrent UTIs, Busch and Huland (1984) showed that fever and flank pain are no more diagnostic of pyelonephritis than they are of cystitis. Of patients with flank pain and/or fever, over 50% had lower tract bacteriuria. Conversely, patients with bladder symptoms or no symptoms frequently had upper tract bacteriuria. Approximately 75% of patients give a history of previous lower UTIs.

On physical examination, there often is tenderness to deep palpation in the costovertebral angle. Variations of this clinical presentation have been recognized. Acute pyelonephritis may also simulate gastrointestinal tract abnormalities with abdominal pain, nausea, vomiting, and diarrhea. Asymptomatic progression of acute pyelonephritis to chronic pyelonephritis, particularly in compromised hosts, may occur in the absence of overt symptoms. Acute renal failure may be present in the rare case (Richet and Mayaud, 1978; Olsson et al, 1980).

Laboratory Diagnosis. The patient may have leukocytosis with predominance of neutrophils. **Urinalysis usually reveals numerous WBCs, often in clumps, and bacterial rods or chains of cocci.** Leukocytes exhibiting Brownian motion in the cytoplasm (glitter cells) may be present if the urine is hypotonic, but they are not in themselves diagnostic of pyelonephritis. **The presence of large amounts of granular or leukocyte casts in the urinary sediment is suggestive of acute pyelonephritis.** A specific type of urinary cast characterized by the presence of bacteria in its matrix has been demonstrated in the urine of patients who have had acute pyelonephritis (Fig. 8–19) (Lindner et al, 1980). Bacteria in the casts were not easily distinguished by simple brightfield

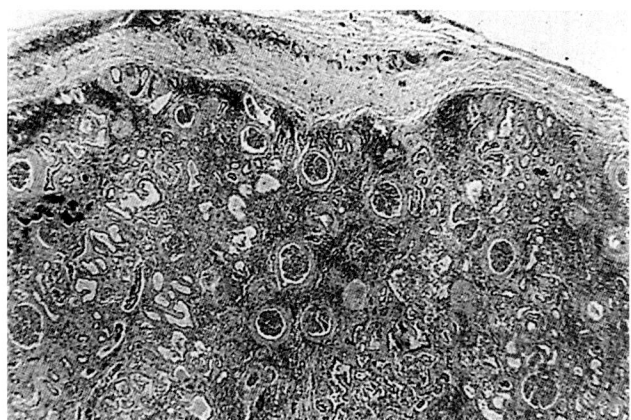

Figure 8–18. Chronic pyelonephritis. The renal cortex shows thickened fibrous capsule and focal retracted scar on surface of kidney. Focal destruction of tubules in center of picture is accompanied by periglomerular fibrosis and scarring. (From Schaeffer AJ: Urinary tract infections. In Gillenwater JY, et al [eds]: Adult and Pediatric Urology. Philadelphia, Lippincott Williams & Wilkins, 2002, pp 211-272.)

SECTION IV

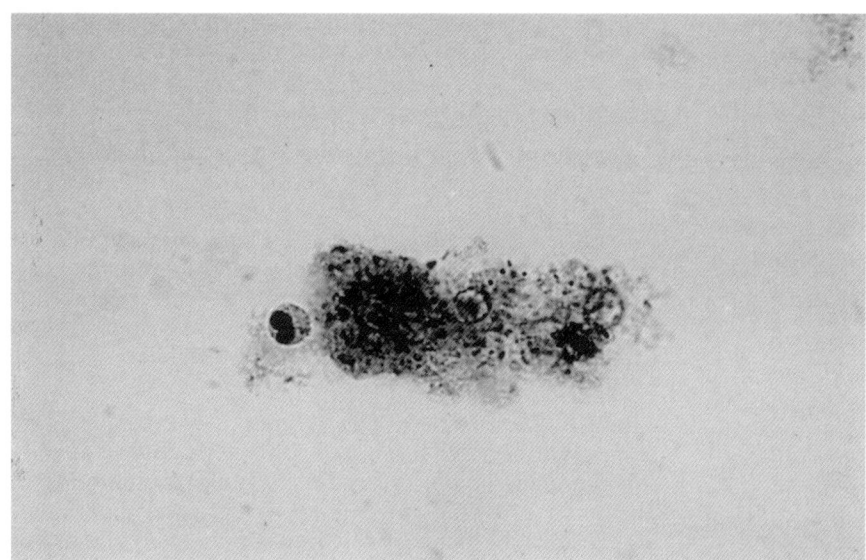

Figure 8–19. Brightfield micrograph of a mixed bacterial leukocyte cast from patient with acute pyelonephritis. Only the bacteria and the nucleus of a leukocyte stain strongly. Many bacteria are clearly demonstrated by through-focusing (toluidine blue O stain, magnification ×640). (From Lindner LE, Jones RN, Haber MH: A specific urinary cast in acute pyelonephritis. Am J Clin Pathol 1980;73:809-811.)

microscopy without special staining of the sediment. Staining of the sediment with a basic dye such as dilute toluidine blue or KOVA (I.C.L. Scientific, Fountain Valley, CA) stain demonstrated the bacteria in casts without difficulty. Blood tests may show leukocytosis with a predominance of neutrophils, increased erythrocyte sedimentation rate, elevated C-reactive protein levels, and elevated creatinine levels if renal failure is present. In addition, creatinine clearance may be decreased. Blood cultures may be positive.

Bacteriology. Urine cultures are positive, but about 20% of patients have urine cultures with fewer than 10^5 cfu/mL and, therefore, negative results on Gram staining of the urine (Rubin et al, 1992).

E. coli, which constitutes a unique subgroup that possesses special virulence factors, accounts for 80% of cases. If vesicoureteral reflux is absent, a patient bearing the P blood group phenotype may have special susceptibility to recurrent pyelonephritis caused by *E. coli* that have P pili and bind to the P blood group antigen receptors (Lomberg et al, 1983). Bacterial K antigens and endotoxins also may contribute to pathogenicity (Kaijser et al, 1977). Many cases of community-acquired pyelonephritis are caused by a limited number of multi-antimicrobial resistant clonal groups (Manges et al, 2004).

More resistant species, such as *Proteus, Klebsiella, Pseudomonas, Serratia, Enterobacter,* or *Citrobacter* should be suspected in patients who have recurrent UTIs, are hospitalized, or have indwelling catheters, as well as in those who required recent urinary tract instrumentation. Except for *E. faecalis, S. epidermidis* and *S. aureus,* gram-positive bacteria rarely cause pyelonephritis.

Blood cultures are positive in about 25% of cases of uncomplicated pyelonephritis in women, and the majority replicate the urine culture and do not influence decisions regarding therapy. Therefore, blood cultures should not be routinely obtained for the evaluation of uncomplicated pyelonephritis in women. However, they should be considered in men and women with severe toxicity or risk factors such as

pregnancy because bacteremia and sepsis are common (Velasco et al, 2003).

Radiologic Findings. *Excretory Urogram.* Excretory urography is usually performed after institution of adequate therapy and resolution of the patient's symptoms; therefore, it is not surprising that most patients with pyelonephritis have a normal excretory urogram (Silver et al, 1976; Wicks and Thornbury, 1979). If obtained during acute pyelonephritis, the most common radiologic abnormality is renal enlargement, which occurs from generalized renal edema as a consequence of the inflammatory process (Fig. 8–20A). An overall length of 15 cm or a length 1.5 cm greater than the unaffected side has been established as a criterion for the diagnosis of renal enlargement in acute pyelonephritis (Silver et al, 1976; Wicks and Thornbury, 1979; Corriere and Sandler, 1982). Focal renal enlargement, less common than generalized enlargement, may appear as a renal mass. Indeed, this finding, focal bacterial nephritis or acute lobar nephronia, has been emphasized only since 1978 as causing a renal mass (Rosenfield et al, 1979). This mass must be differentiated from a neoplasm or intrarenal abscess (Little et al, 1965; Barth et al, 1976; Teplick et al, 1979; McDonough et al, 1981; Funston et al, 1982; Konetschnik et al, 1982; Sotolongo et al, 1982). Although other radiologic modalities may be needed to differentiate the lesion from a neoplasm or intrarenal abscess, time and treatment cause the mass to disappear; however, scarring may occur.

The inflammatory response may also cause cortical vasoconstriction, which is presumably responsible for the diminished nephrogram and delayed appearance of the pyelogram, as well as compression of the collecting structures, so that the calyces have an attenuated or spidery appearance. In addition to these abnormalities, calyceal and ureteral dilation (without any obstructive cause) may be seen during acute pyelonephritis (Kass et al, 1976; Silver et al, 1976; Harrison and Shaffer, 1979; Teplick et al, 1979). This may be caused by the bacterial endotoxins that impair ureteral peristalsis. Although ureteral dilation may occur with infection, this diagnosis

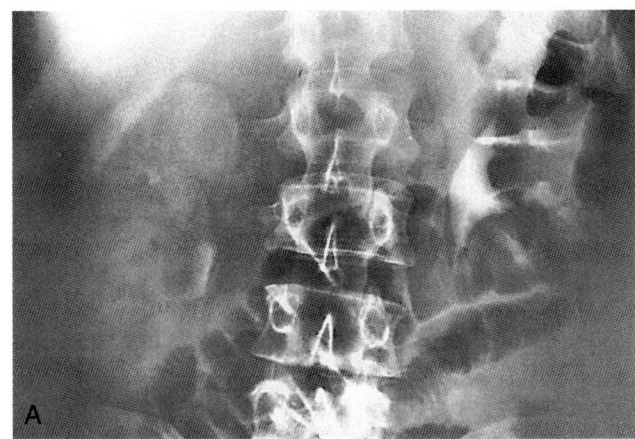

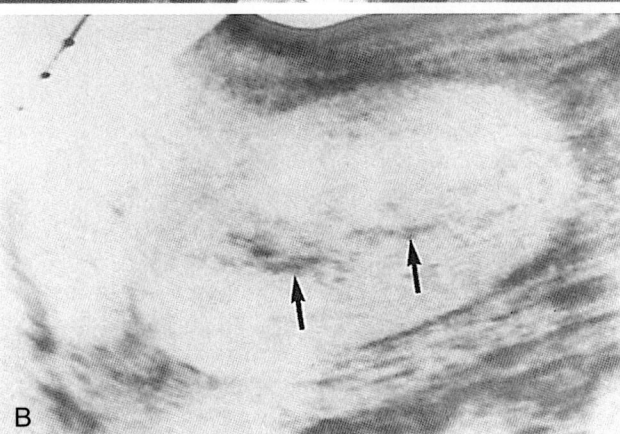

Figure 8–20. Acute pyelonephritis. **A,** Excretory urogram. Ten-minute film demonstrates enlarged right kidney with minimum function. Findings are consistent with edema. **B,** Ultrasound of the right kidney demonstrates renal enlargement, hypoechoic parenchyma, and compressed central collecting complex *(arrows)*. (From Schaeffer AJ: Urinary tract infections. In Gillenwater JY, et al [eds]: Adult and Pediatric Urology. Philadelphia, Lippincott William & Wilkins, 2002, pp 211-272.)

should not be made until obstruction, either past or present, has been excluded.

Parallel lucent renal pelvic and ureteral streaks have been seen in acute pyelonephritis (Harrison and Shaffer, 1979). These are probably caused by mucosal edema.

Renal Ultrasonography and Computed Tomography. **These studies are commonly used to evaluate patients initially for complicated UTIs or factors or to reevaluate patients who do not respond after 72 hours of therapy** (see later). Ultrasound (see Fig. 8–20B) and CT show renal enlargement, hypoechoic or attenuated parenchyma, and a compressed collecting system. They also may delineate focal bacterial nephritis and obstruction. When parenchymal destruction becomes pronounced, a more disorganized parenchyma and abscess formation associated with complicated renal and perirenal infections may be identified (Soulen et al, 1989).

Pathology. In acute pyelonephritis, the kidney may be grossly enlarged (Freedman, 1979). The capsule strips easily, and suppuration may soften areas of parenchyma. There are usually small, yellow-white cortical abscesses mixed with parenchymal hyperemia. Histologically, the parenchyma shows a focal,

patchy infiltrate of neutrophils. Bacteria are often in the infiltrate. Early in the inflammatory process, this infiltrate is limited to the interstitium, but, later, linear bands of inflammation extend from the papillae to the cortex in a wedge-shaped manner. Abscesses may cause tubular destruction; the glomeruli are usually spared.

Differential Diagnosis. Acute appendicitis, diverticulitis, and pancreatitis can cause a similar degree of pain, but the location of the pain often is different. Results of the urine examination are usually normal. Herpes zoster can cause superficial pain in the region of the kidney but is not associated with symptoms of UTI; the diagnosis will be apparent when shingles appear.

Management.

Initial Management. Infection in patients with acute pyelonephritis can be subdivided into (1) uncomplicated infection that does not warrant hospitalization, (2) uncomplicated infection in patients with normal urinary tracts who are ill enough to warrant hospitalization for parenteral therapy, and (3) complicated infection associated with hospitalization, catheterization, urologic surgery, or urinary tract abnormalities (Fig. 8–21).

It is critical to determine whether the patient has an uncomplicated or complicated UTI because significant abnormalities have been found in 16% of patients with acute pyelonephritis (Shen and Brown, 2004). In patients with presumed uncomplicated pyelonephritis who will be managed as outpatients, initial radiologic evaluation can usually be deferred. **However, if there is any reason to suspect a problem or if the patient will not have reasonable access to imaging if there should be no change in condition, we prefer renal ultrasound to rule out stones or obstruction.** In patients with known or suspected complicated pyelonephritis, CT provides excellent assessment of the status of the urinary tract and the severity and extent of the infection.

Hospitalization, initially with complete bed rest, intravenous fluids, and antipyretics, is required for patients with significant toxicity. Patients with less severe disease may be managed as outpatients. Upper tract obstruction, if suspected, should be ruled out by ultrasonography or CT.

An obstructed kidney has difficulty concentrating and excreting antimicrobial agents. In addition, obstruction in effect creates a potential abscess, pyonephrosis, which can rapidly destroy the renal parenchyma and endanger the patient's life. Any substantial obstruction must be relieved expediently by the safest and simplest means.

Until the results of the culture and susceptibilities are available, broad-spectrum antimicrobial therapy should be instituted (Table 8–24). A Gram stain of the urine sediment is helpful to guide the selection of the initial empirical antimicrobial therapy. In all cases, antimicrobial therapy should be active against potential uropathogens and achieve antimicrobial levels in renal tissue as well as urine.

For patients who will be managed as outpatients, single-drug oral therapy with a fluoroquinolone is more effective than TMP-SMX for patients with domiciliary infections (Talan et al, 2000). Many physicians administer a single parenteral dose of an antimicrobial agent (ceftriaxone, gentamicin, or a fluoroquinolone) before initiating oral therapy (Israel et al, 1991; Pinson et al, 1994). If a gram-positive

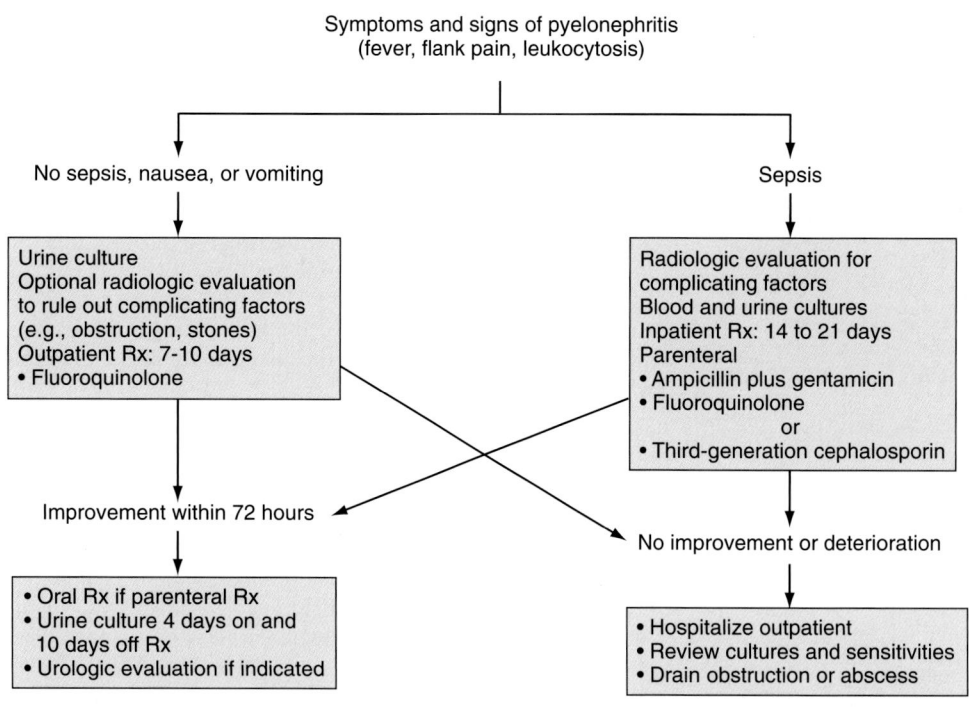

Figure 8–21. Management of acute pyelonephritis.

Table 8–24. **Treatment Regimens for Acute Complicated and Uncomplicated Pyelonephritis in Women**

Circumstances	Route	Drug	Dosage	Frequency per Dose	Duration (days)
Outpatient—moderately ill, no nausea or vomiting	Oral	TMP-SMX	160 to 800 mg	BID	10-14
		Ciprofloxacin	500 mg	BID	
		Levofloxacin	500 mg	QD	
		Norfloxacin	400 mg	BID	
Inpatient—severely ill, possible sepsis	Parenteral	TMP-SMX	160 to 800 mg	BID	14
		Ampicillin and gentamicin	1 g	QID	
			1.5 mg/kg	TID	
		Ciprofloxacin	400 mg	BID	
		Levofloxacin	500 mg	QD	
		Ceftriaxone	1 to 2 g	QD	
		Take until afebrile, then take oral TMP-SMX or fluoroquinolone			
Pregnant	Parenteral	Ceftriaxone	1 to 2 g	QD	14
		Ampicillin and gentamicin	1 g	QID	
			1 mg/kg	TID	
		Aztreonam	1 g	TID-QID	
		Take until afebrile, then take:			
	Oral	Cephalexin	500 mg	BID	

TMP-SMX, trimethoprim-sulfamethoxazole.
Modified from Stamm WE, Hooton TM: Management of urinary tract infections in adults. N Engl J Med 1993;329:1328-1334. Copyright 1993 Massachusetts Medical Society. All rights reserved.

organism is suspected, amoxicillin or amoxicillin/clavulanic acid is recommended (Warren et al, 1999).

If a patient has an uncomplicated infection but is sufficiently ill to require hospitalization (high fever, high WBC count, vomiting, dehydration, evidence of sepsis), has complicated pyelonephritis, or fails to improve during the initial outpatient treatment period, the patient should be admitted and treated with intravenous antimicrobial agents. A parenteral fluoroquinolone, an aminoglycoside with or without ampicillin, or an extended-spectrum cephalosporin with or without an aminoglycoside is recommended (Warren et al, 1999). If gram-positive cocci are causative,

ampicillin/sulbactam with or without an aminoglycoside is recommended.

Subsequent Management. Even though the urine usually becomes sterile within a few hours of starting antimicrobial therapy, patients with acute uncomplicated pyelonephritis may continue to have fever, chills, and flank pain for several more days after initiation of successful antimicrobial therapy (Behr et al, 1996). They should be observed.

Ambulatory patients should be treated with a fluoroquinolone for 7 days (Talan et al, 2000). Fluoroquinolone therapy is associated with greater bacteriologic and clinical cure rates than 14-day TMP-SMX therapy (Talan et al, 2000).

Alterations in antimicrobial therapy may be made depending on the patient's clinical response and the results of the culture and susceptibility tests. Susceptibility tests should also be used to replace potentially toxic drugs, such as aminoglycosides, with less toxic drugs, such as the fluoroquinolones, aztreonam, and cephalosporins.

Patients with complicated pyelonephritis and positive blood cultures should be treated for 7 days with parenteral therapy. If blood cultures are negative, 2- to 3-day parenteral therapy is sufficient. In either case, an appropriate oral antimicrobial drug (fluoroquinolone; TMP, TMP-SMX, or amoxicillin or amoxicillin/clavulanic acid for gram-positive organisms) should be continued in full dosage for an additional 10 to 14 days.

Unfavorable Response to Therapy. When the response to therapy is slow or the urine continues to show infection, an immediate reevaluation is mandatory. Urine and blood cultures must be repeated and appropriate alterations in antimicrobial therapy made on the basis of susceptibility testing. Radiologic investigation is indicated to attempt to identify unsuspected obstructive uropathy, urolithiasis, or underlying anatomic abnormalities that may have predisposed the patient to infection, prevented a rapid therapeutic response, or caused complications of the infectious process, such as renal or perinephric abscess. **In patients with fever lasting longer than 72 hours, these studies are most helpful for ruling out obstruction and identifying renal and perirenal infections** (Soulen et al, 1989). Radionuclide imaging may be useful to demonstrate functional changes associated with acute pyelonephritis (decrease in renal blood flow, delay in peak function, and delay in excretion of the radionuclide) (Fischman and Roberts, 1982) and cortical defects associated with vesicoureteral reflux.

Follow-Up. Repeat urine cultures should be performed on the fifth to the seventh day of therapy and 10 to 14 days and 4 to 6 weeks after discontinuing antimicrobial therapy to ensure that the urinary tract remains free of infections. Between 10% and 30% of individuals with acute pyelonephritis relapse after a 14-day course of therapy. Patients who relapse usually are cured by a second 14-day course of therapy, but occasionally a 6-week course is necessary (Tolkoff-Rubin et al, 1984; Johnson and Stamm, 1987).

Depending on the clinical presentation and response and initial urologic evaluation, some patients may require additional evaluation (e.g., voiding cystourethrogram, cystoscopy, bacterial localization studies) and correction of an underlying abnormality of the urinary tract. Raz and colleagues (2003) evaluated the long-term impact of acute pyelonephritis in women. Scanning with ^{99m}Tc-dimercaptosuccinic acid (^{99m}Tc-DMSA) 10 to 20 years after acute pyelonephritis revealed scars in approximately 50% of the patients but changes in renal function were minimal and not associated with renal scarring.

Acute Focal or Multifocal Bacterial Nephritis

Acute focal or multifocal bacterial nephritis is an uncommon, severe form of acute renal infection in which a heavy leukocyte infiltrate is confined to a single renal lobe (focal) or multiple lobes (multifocal).

Clinical Presentation. The clinical presentation of patients with acute bacterial nephritis is similar to that of patients with acute pyelonephritis but usually is more severe. About half of the patients are diabetic, and sepsis is common. Generally, leukocytosis and UTI resulting from gram-negative organisms are found; more than 50% of the patients are bacteremic (Wicks and Thornbury, 1979).

Radiologic Findings. The diagnosis must be made by radiologic examination. The urographic findings are those of a mass, most commonly poorly marginated and suggestive of renal abscess or tumor (Fig. 8–22A). The mass has slightly less nephrographic density than the surrounding normal renal parenchyma.

Ultrasonography and CT aid in establishing the diagnosis. On ultrasonography, the lesion is typically poorly marginated and relatively sonolucent with occasional low-amplitude echoes that disrupt the cortical medullary junction (Corriere and Sandler, 1982) (see Fig. 8–22B). **Enhancement with a contrast agent is necessary with CT studies because the lesion is difficult to visualize on the unenhanced study** (see Fig. 8–22C). **Wedge-shaped areas of decreased enhancement are seen.** No definite wall is evident, and frank liquefaction is absent. Conversely, abscesses tend to have liquid centers, are usually round, and are present both before and after contrast medium enhancement. More chronic abscesses may also show a ring-shaped area of increased enhancement surrounding the lesion (Corriere and Sandler, 1982). Gallium scanning reveals uptake that is in the region of and larger than the previously demonstrated mass (Rosenfield et al, 1979). In patients with multifocal disease, the findings are similar but multiple lobes are involved.

Management. Acute bacterial nephritis probably represents a relatively early phase of frank abscess formation. In a series of cases reported by Lee and coworkers (1980), a patient with acute focal bacterial nephritis progressed to abscess formation. **Treatment includes hydration and intravenous antimicrobial agents for at least 7 days, followed by 7 days of oral antimicrobial therapy.** Patients with bacterial nephritis typically respond to medical therapy, and follow-up studies will show resolution of the wedge-shaped zones of diminished attenuation. **Failure to respond to antimicrobial therapy is an indication for appropriate studies to rule out obstructive uropathy, renal or perirenal abscess, renal carcinoma, or acute renal vein thrombosis.** Long-term follow-up studies performed in a few patients with multifocal disease have demonstrated a decrease in renal size and focal calyceal deformities suggestive of papillary necrosis (Davidson and Talner, 1978).

Emphysematous Pyelonephritis

Emphysematous pyelonephritis is an acute necrotizing parenchymal and perirenal infection caused by gas-forming uropathogens. The pathogenesis is poorly understood. **Because the condition usually occurs in diabetic patients, it has been postulated that the high tissue glucose levels provide the substrate for microorganisms such as *E. coli*, which are able to produce carbon dioxide by the fermentation of sugar** (Schainuck et al, 1968). Although glucose fermentation may be a factor, the explanation does not account for the rarity of emphysematous pyelonephritis despite the high frequency of gram-negative UTI in diabetic patients, nor

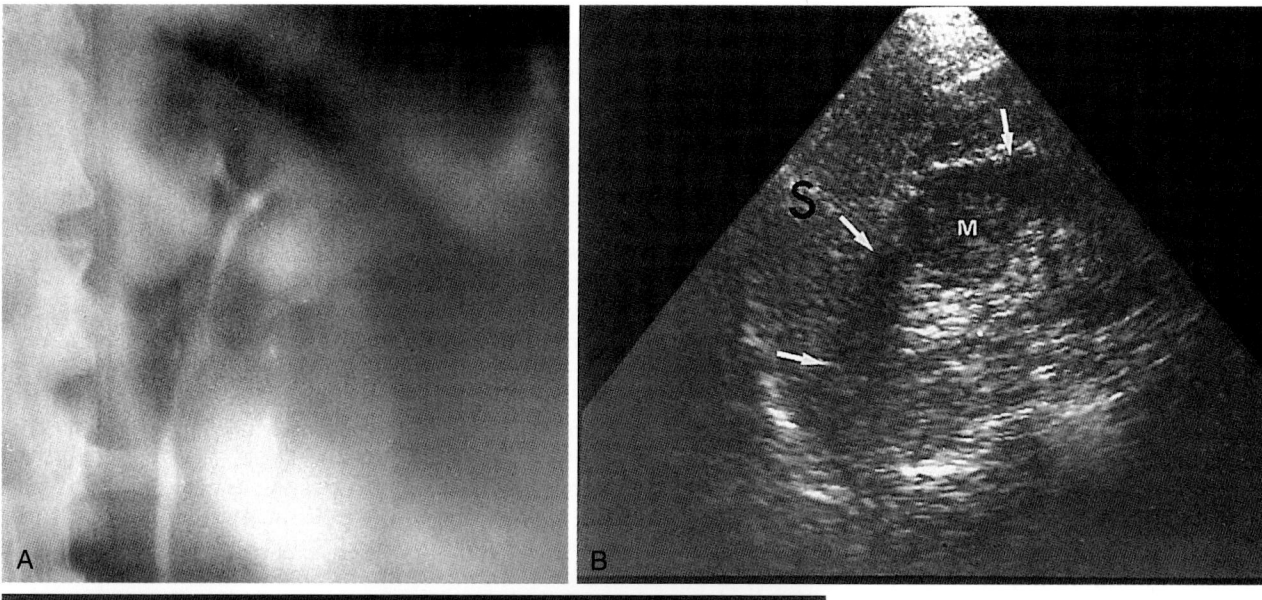

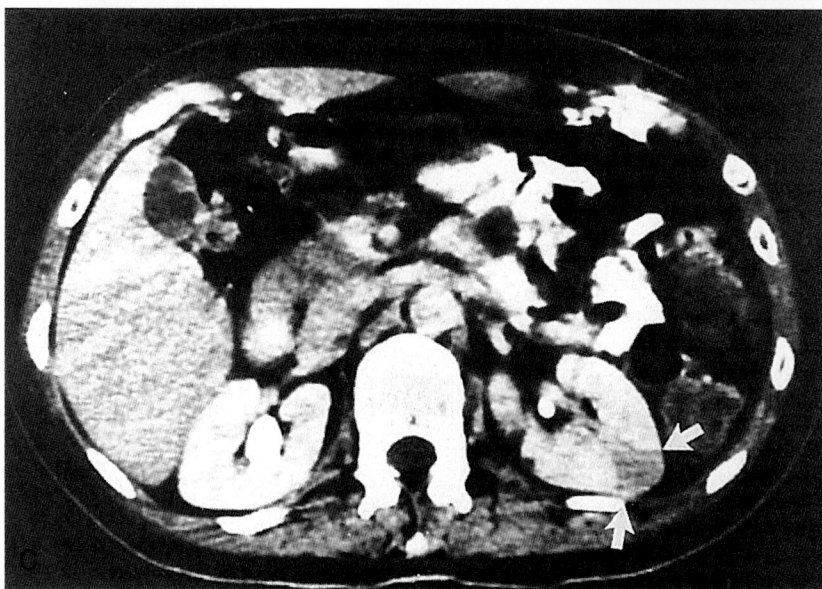

Figure 8–22. Acute focal bacterial nephritis. **A,** Excretory urogram. Five-minute tomogram demonstrates normally functioning upper and lower poles and a poorly marginated midrenal mass with poor function and absent collecting system visualization. **B,** Ultrasound; longitudinal view of the left kidney demonstrates spleen (S) and left kidney *(arrows)*. Note irregular midpole mass (M) of slightly higher echo texture than surrounding normal renal parenchyma. **C,** Contrast medium–enhanced CT scan demonstrates a wedge-shaped area of low density *(arrows)* in the middle portion of the left kidney. The findings resolved after antimicrobial therapy. (From Schaeffer AJ: Urinary tract infections. In Gillenwater JY, et al [eds]: Adult and Pediatric Urology. Philadelphia, Lippincott Williams & Wilkins, 2002, pp 211-272.)

does it explain the rare occurrence of the condition in nondiabetic patients.

In addition to diabetes, many patients have urinary tract obstruction associated with urinary calculi or papillary necrosis and significant renal functional impairment. It seems more reasonable to postulate that impaired host response caused by local factors, such as obstruction, or a systemic condition, such as diabetes, allows organisms with the capability of producing carbon dioxide to use necrotic tissue as a substrate to generate gas in vivo. Thus, emphysematous pyelonephritis should be considered a complication of severe pyelonephritis rather than a distinct entity. The overall mortality rate has been reported to be between 43% (Freiha et al, 1979) and 19% (Huang and Tseng, 2000).

Clinical Presentation. All of the documented cases of emphysematous pyelonephritis have occurred in adults (Hawes, 1983). Juvenile diabetic patients do not appear to be at risk. Women are affected more often than men.

The usual clinical presentation is severe, acute pyelonephritis, although in some instances a chronic infection precedes the acute attack. **Almost all patients display the classic triad of fever, vomiting, and flank pain** (Schainuck et al, 1968). Pneumaturia is absent unless the infection involves the collecting system. Results of urine cultures are invariably positive. *E. coli* is most commonly identified. *Klebsiella* and *Proteus* are less common.

Radiologic Findings. The diagnosis is established radiographically. Tissue gas that is distributed in the parenchyma may appear on abdominal radiographs as mottled gas shadows over the involved kidney (Fig. 8–23). This finding is often mistaken for bowel gas. A crescentic collection of gas over the upper pole of the kidney is more distinctive. As the infection progresses, gas extends to the perinephric space and retroperitoneum. This distribution of gas should not be confused with cases of emphysematous pyelitis in which air is in the collecting system of the kidney.

Emphysematous pyelitis is secondary to a gas-forming bacterial UTI, often occurs in nondiabetic patients, is less serious, and usually responds to antimicrobial therapy.

Excretory urography is rarely of value in emphysematous pyelonephritis because the affected kidney usually is nonfunctioning or poorly functioning. Because of the significant risk of contrast nephropathy in critically ill, dehydrated diabetic patients with abnormal renal function, retrograde pyelography rather than excretory urography is advisable to demonstrate obstruction. Obstruction is demonstrated in approximately 25% of the cases. Ultrasonography usually demonstrates strong focal echoes suggesting the presence of

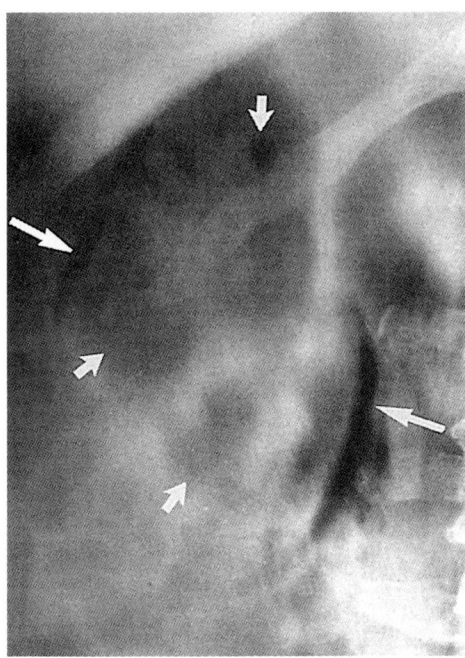

Figure 8–23. Emphysematous pyelonephritis; plain film. Extensive perinephric *(long arrows)* and intraparenchymal *(short arrows)* gas secondary to acute bacterial pyelonephritis. (From Schaeffer AJ: Urinary tract infections. In Gillenwater JY, et al [eds]: Adult and Pediatric Urology. Philadelphia, Lippincott William & Wilkins, 2002, pp 211-272.)

intraparenchymal gas (Brenbridge et al, 1979; Conrad et al, 1979). **CT is the imaging procedure of choice in defining the extent of the emphysematous process and guiding management** (Figs. 8–24 and 8–25). **An absence of fluid in CT images or the presence of streaky or mottled gas with or without bubbly and loculated gas appears to be associated with rapid destruction of renal parenchyma and a 50% to 60% mortality rate** (Wan et al, 1996; Best et al, 1999). The presence of renal or perirenal fluid, the presence of bubbly or loculated gas or gas in the collecting system, and the absence of streaky or mottled gas patterns is associated with a less than 20% mortality rate. A nuclear renal scan should be performed to assess the degree of renal function impairment in the involved kidney and the status of the contralateral kidney.

Management. Emphysematous pyelonephritis is a surgical emergency. Most patients are septic, and fluid resuscitation and broad-spectrum antimicrobial therapy are essential. If the kidney is functioning, medical therapy can be considered (Wan et al, 1996; Best et al, 1999). Nephrectomy is recommended for patients who do not improve after a few days of therapy (Malek and Elder, 1978). If the affected kidney is nonfunctioning and not obstructed, nephrectomy should be performed because medical treatment alone is usually lethal. If a kidney is obstructed, catheter drainage must be instituted. If the patient's condition improves, nephrectomy may be deferred pending a complete urologic evaluation. Although there are isolated case reports of retention of renal function after medical therapy combined with relief of obstruction, most patients require nephrectomy (Hudson et al, 1986).

Renal Abscess

Renal abscess or carbuncle is a collection of purulent material confined to the renal parenchyma. Before the antimicrobial era, 80% of renal abscesses were attributed to hematogenous seeding by staphylococci (Campbell, 1930). Although experimental and clinical data document the facility for abscess formation in normal kidneys after hematogenous inoculation with staphylococci, widespread use of antimicrobial agents since about 1950 appears to have diminished the propensity for gram-positive abscess formation (DeNavasquez, 1950; Cotran, 1969).

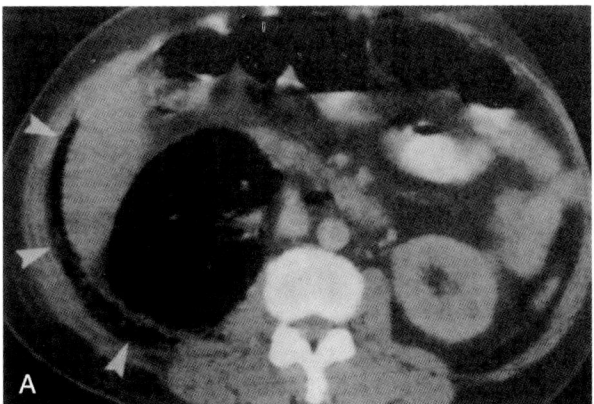
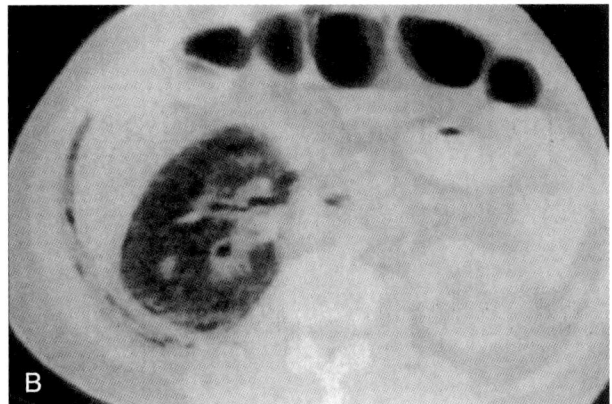

Figure 8–24. Type I emphysematous pyelonephritis with complete renal destruction in a 49-year-old woman. **A,** CT scan of the right kidney shows complete destruction with gas *(arrowheads)* extending beyond the renal fascia. **B,** CT scan with a modified lung window display shows the characteristic streaky gas in the completely destroyed kidney. The patient died on arrival in the emergency department. (**A** and **B,** from Wan YL, Lee TY, Bullard MJ, Tsai CC: Acute gas-producing bacterial renal infection: Correlation between imaging findings and clinical outcome. Radiology 1996;198:433-438.)

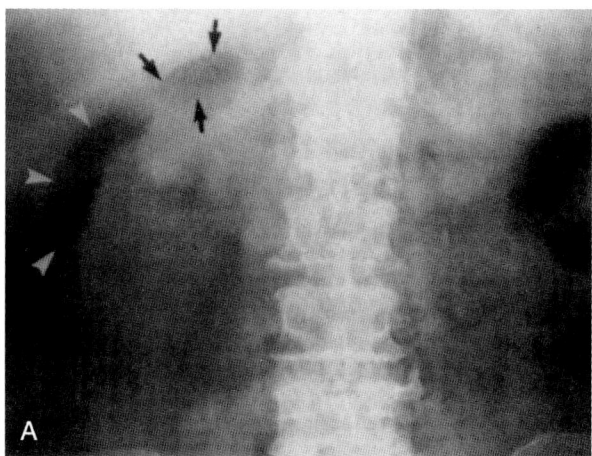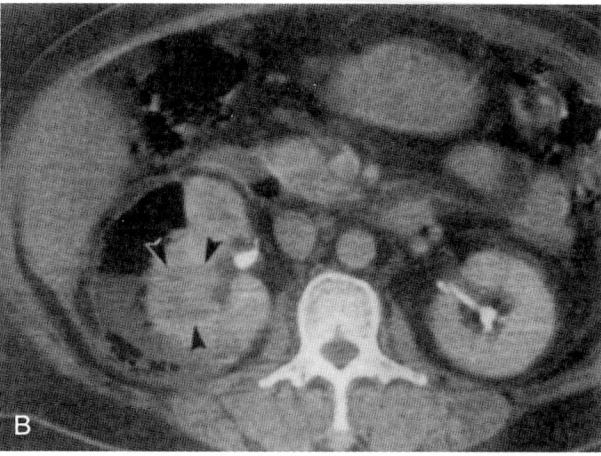

Figure 8–25. Type II emphysematous pyelonephritis in a 57-year-old woman. **A,** Radiograph shows crescent-shaped *(arrowheads)* and loculated *(arrows)* gas in the right renal area. **B,** CT scan obtained after administration of contrast material shows a low-attenuation area *(arrowheads)* in the right kidney due to acute pyelonephritis as well as a subcapsular abscess with fluid and bubbly and loculated gas. The patient survived after percutaneous drainage was performed. (**A** and **B,** from Wan YL, Lee TY, Bullard MJ, Tsai CC: Acute gas-producing bacterial renal infection: Correlation between imaging findings and clinical outcome. Radiology 1996;198:433-438.)

Since about 1970, gram-negative organisms have been implicated in the majority of adults with renal abscesses. Hematogenous renal seeding by gram-negative organisms may occur, but this is not likely to be the primary pathway for gram-negative abscess formation. Clinically, there is no evidence that gram-negative septicemia antedates most lesions. Further, gram-negative hematogenous pyelonephritis is virtually impossible to produce in animals unless the kidney is traumatized or completely obstructed (Cotran, 1969; Timmons and Perlmutter, 1976). The partially obstructed kidney rejects bloodborne gram-negative inocula as well as a normal kidney. Thus, ascending infection associated with tubular obstruction from prior infections or calculi appears to be the primary pathway for the establishment of gram-negative abscesses. Two-thirds of gram-negative abscesses in adults are associated with renal calculi or damaged kidneys (Salvatierra et al, 1967). Although the association of pyelonephritis with vesicoureteral reflux is well established, the association of renal abscess with vesicoureteral reflux has been infrequently noted (Segura and Kelalis, 1973). More recent observations, however, indicate that reflux is frequently associated with renal abscesses and persists long after sterilization of the urinary tract (Timmons and Perlmutter, 1976).

Clinical Presentation. The patient may present with fever, chills, abdominal or flank pain, and occasionally weight loss and malaise. Symptoms of cystitis may occur. Occasionally, these symptoms may be vague and delay diagnosis until surgical exploration or, in more severe cases, autopsy (Anderson and McAninch, 1980). **A thorough history may reveal a gram-positive source of infection 1 to 8 weeks before the onset of urinary tract symptoms. The infection may have occurred in any area of the body.** Multiple skin carbuncles and intravenous drug abuse introduce gram-positive organisms into the bloodstream. Other common sites are the mouth, lungs, and bladder (Lyons et al, 1972). Complicated UTIs associated with stasis, calculi, pregnancy, neurogenic bladder, and diabetes mellitus also appear to predispose the patient to abscess formation (Anderson and McAninch, 1980).

Laboratory Diagnosis. The patient typically has marked leukocytosis. The blood cultures are usually positive. Pyuria and bacteriuria may not be evident unless the abscess communicates with the collecting system. **Because gram-positive organisms are most commonly bloodborne, urine cultures in these cases typically show no growth or a microorganism different from that isolated from the abscess.** When the abscess contains gram-negative organisms, the urine culture usually demonstrates the same organism isolated from the abscess.

Radiologic Findings. The urographic findings depend on both the nature and the duration of the infection. Differentiation between early renal abscesses and acute pyelonephritis can be difficult because most of the former are small. In patients in whom abscess formation has progressed from an episode of acute bacterial nephritis or those in whom the kidney has been seeded by an outside infection, radiologic examination may demonstrate generalized renal enlargement with distortion of the renal contour on the affected side. Renal fixation on aspiratory and expiratory films and obliteration of the corresponding psoas shadow may also be evident. Scoliosis is often present, with a concavity of the curve facing the affected kidney. If renal involvement is diffuse, the nephrogram is delayed or even absent. When an abscess is more localized, the findings may be similar to those of acute focal bacterial nephritis.

In a more chronic abscess, the predominant urographic abnormalities are those of a renal mass lesion. The calyceal system may be poorly defined or show distortion or even amputation (Resnick and Older, 1982). Nephrotomography usually reveals a relative radiolucency in the involved area. Occasionally, the excretory urogram appears normal despite the presence of a renal abscess, particularly if the abscess involves the anterior or posterior portion of the kidney without impinging on the parenchyma or collecting system.

Ultrasonography and CT are helpful in distinguishing abscess from other inflammatory renal diseases. **Ultrasonography is the quickest and least expensive method to demonstrate a renal abscess. An echo-free or low-**

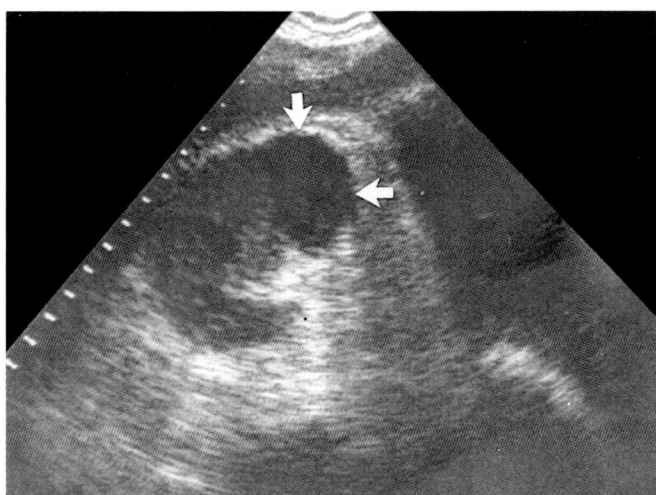

Figure 8–26. Acute renal abscess. Transverse ultrasonographic scan of the right kidney demonstrates a poorly marginated rounded focal hypoechoic mass *(arrows)* in the anterior portion of the kidney.

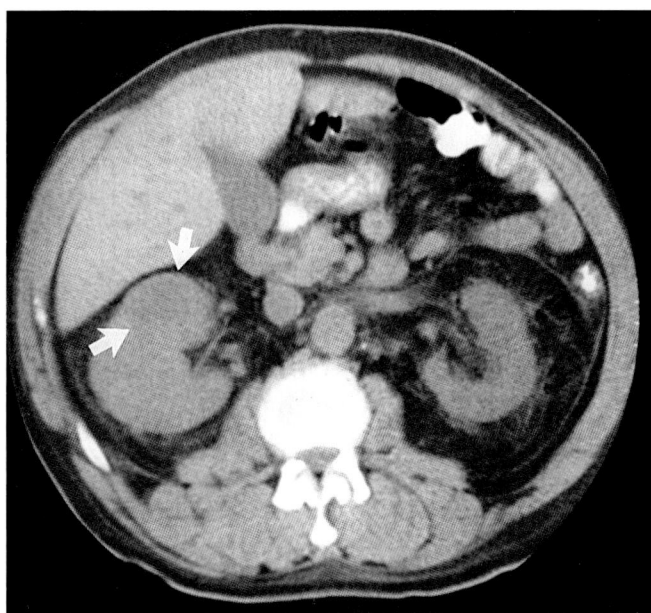

Figure 8–27. Acute renal abscess. Nonenhanced CT scan through the mid pole of the right kidney demonstrates right renal enlargement and an area of decreased attenuation *(arrows)*. After antimicrobial therapy, a follow-up scan showed complete regression of these findings.

echodensity space-occupying lesion with increased transmission is found on the sonogram (Fig. 8–26). The margins of an abscess are indistinguishable in the acute phase, but the structure contains a few echoes and the surrounding renal parenchyma is edematous (Fiegler, 1983). Subsequently, the appearance tends to be that of a well-defined mass. The internal appearance, however, may vary from a virtually solid lucent mass to one with large numbers of low-level internal echoes (Schneider et al, 1976). The number of echoes depends on the amount of cellular debris within the abscess. The presence of air results in a strong echo with a shadow. Differentiation between an abscess and a tumor is impossible in many cases. Arteriography is used infrequently to demonstrate abscesses. The center of the mass tends to be hypervascular or avascular, with increased vascularity at the cortical margins and lack of vascular displacement and neovascularity.

CT appears to be the diagnostic procedure of choice for renal abscesses, because it provides excellent delineation of the tissue. On CT, abscesses are characteristically well defined both before and after contrast agent enhancement. The findings depend in part on the age and severity of the abscess (Baumgarten and Baumgartner, 1997). Initially, CT shows renal enlargement and focal, rounded areas of decreased attenuation (Fig. 8–27). After several days of the onset of the infection, a thick fibrotic wall begins to form around the abscess. An echo-free or slightly echogenic mass due to the presence of necrotic debris is seen. CT of a chronic abscess shows obliteration of adjacent tissue planes, thickening of Gerota's fascia, a round or oval parenchymal mass of low attenuation, and a surrounding inflammatory wall of slightly higher attenuation that forms a ring when the scan is enhanced with contrast material (Fig. 8–28). The ring sign is caused by the increased vascularity of the abscess wall (Callen, 1979; Gerzof and Gale, 1982).

Radionuclide imaging with gallium or indium is sometimes useful in evaluating patients with renal abscesses (see prior sections in this chapter and Chapter 4, "Urinary Tract Imaging: Basic Principles").

Management.   Although the classic treatment for an abscess has been percutaneous or open incision and drainage, there

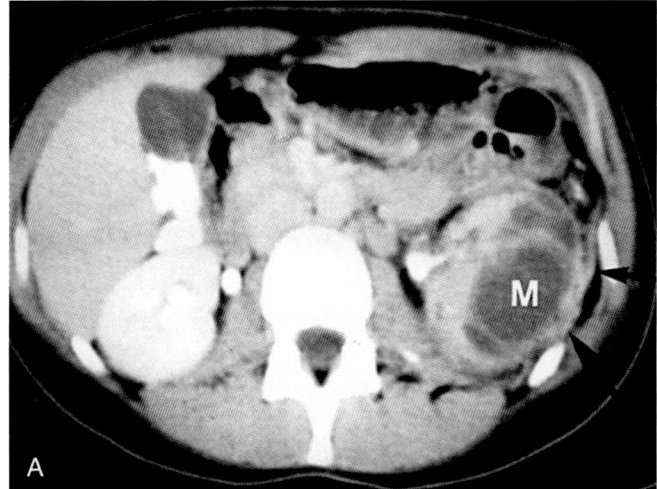
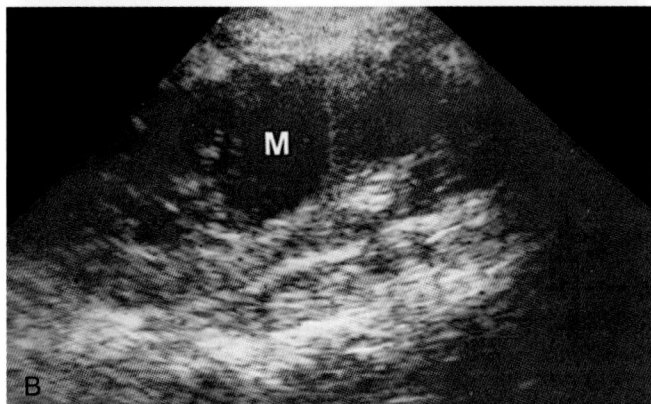

Figure 8–28. Chronic renal abscess. **A,** Enhanced CT scan shows an irregular septated low-density mass (M) extensively involving the left kidney. Note thickening of perinephric fascia *(arrowheads)* and extensive compression of the renal collecting system. Findings are typical of renal abscess. **B,** Ultrasound longitudinal scan demonstrates a septated hypoechoic mass (M) occupying much of the renal parenchymal volume.

is good evidence that the intravenous use of antimicrobial agents and careful observation of a small abscess less than 3 cm in diameter, if begun early enough in the course of the process, may obviate surgical procedures (Hoverman et al, 1980; Levin et al, 1984; Shu et al, 2004). **CT- or ultrasound-guided needle aspiration may be necessary to differentiate an abscess from a hypervascular tumor.** Aspirated material can be cultured and appropriate antimicrobial therapy instituted on the basis of the findings.

The selection of empirical antimicrobial therapy is dependent on the presumed source of the infection. When hematogenous dissemination is suspected, the pathogenic organism most frequently is penicillin-resistant *Staphylococcus,* and the antimicrobial of choice therefore is a penicillinase-resistant penicillin (Schiff et al, 1977). If a history of penicillin hypersensitivity is present, the recommended drugs are either cephalosporin or vancomycin. Cortical abscesses that occur in the abnormal urinary tract are associated with more typical gram-negative pathogens and should be treated empirically with intravenous third-generation cephalosporins, antipseudomonal penicillins, or aminoglycosides until specific therapy can be instituted. Patients should have serial examinations with ultrasonography or CT until the abscess resolves. A clinical course contrary to this should lead to the suspicion of misdiagnosis or an uncontrolled infection with the development of perinephric abscess or infection with an organism resistant to the antimicrobial agents used in therapy.

Abscesses 3 to 5 cm in diameter and smaller abscesses in immunocompromised hosts or those that do not respond to antimicrobial therapy should be drained percutaneously (Fernandez et al, 1985; Fowler and Perkins, 1994; Siegel et al, 1996). Surgical drainage, however, currently remains the procedure of choice for most renal abscesses greater than 5 cm in diameter.

Infected Hydronephrosis and Pyonephrosis

Infected hydronephrosis is bacterial infection in a hydronephrotic kidney. The term *pyonephrosis* refers to infected hydronephrosis associated with suppurative destruction of the parenchyma of the kidney, in which there is total or nearly total loss of renal function (Fig. 8–29). Where infected hydronephrosis ends and pyonephrosis begins is difficult to determine clinically. Rapid diagnosis and treatment of pyonephrosis are essential to avoid permanent loss of renal function and to prevent sepsis.

Clinical Presentation. The patient is usually very ill, with high fever, chills, flank pain, and tenderness. Occasionally, however, a patient may have only an elevated temperature and a complaint of vague gastrointestinal discomfort. A previous history of urinary tract calculi, infection, or surgery is common. **Bacteriuria may not be present if the ureter is completely obstructed.**

Radiologic Findings. The ultrasonographic diagnosis of infected hydronephrosis depends on demonstration of internal echoes within the dependent portion of a dilated pyelocalyceal system. CT is nonspecific but may show thickening of the renal pelvis, stranding of the perirenal fat, and a striated nephrogram. The urographic findings are those of urinary tract obstruction and depend on the degree and duration of

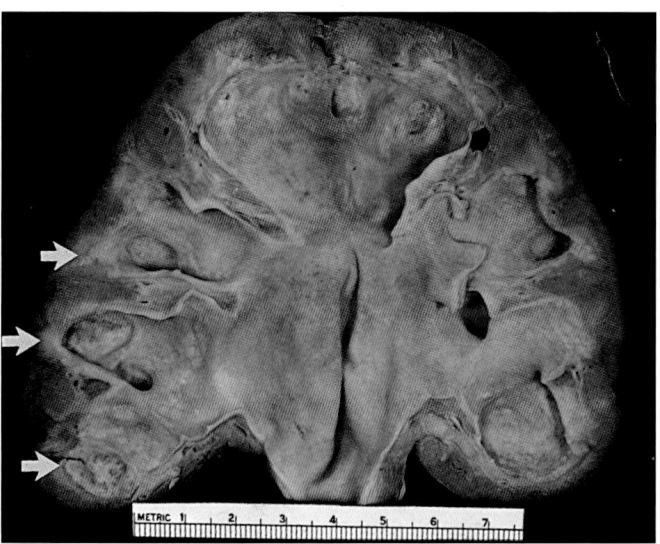

Figure 8–29. Pyonephrosis-gross specimen. The kidney shows marked thinning of the renal cortex and medulla, suppurative destruction of the parenchyma *(arrows),* and distention of the pelvis and calyces. Previous incision released a large quantity of purulent material. The ureter showed obstruction distal to the point of section.

obstruction. Typically, the obstruction is of long standing, and excretory urography shows a poorly functioning or nonfunctioning hydronephrotic kidney. Ultrasound demonstrates hydronephrosis and fluid debris levels within the dilated collecting system (Corriere and Sandler, 1982) (Fig. 8–30A). The diagnosis of pyonephrosis is suggested if focal areas of decreased echogenicity are seen within the hydronephrotic parenchyma.

Management. Once the diagnosis of pyonephrosis is made, the treatment is initiated with appropriate antimicrobial drugs and drainage of the infected pelvis. A ureteral catheter can be passed to drain the kidney, but if the obstruction prevents this, a percutaneous nephrostomy tube should be placed (Camunez et al, 1989) (see Fig. 8–30B). When the patient becomes hemodynamically stable, other procedures are usually needed to identify and treat the source of the obstruction.

Perinephric Abscess

Perinephric abscess usually results from rupture of an acute cortical abscess into the perinephric space or from hematogenous seeding from sites of infection. Patients with pyonephrosis, particularly when a calculus is present in the kidney, are susceptible to perinephric abscess formation. Diabetes mellitus is present in approximately one third of patients with perinephric abscess (Thorley et al, 1974; Edelstein and McCabe, 1988). In about one third of the cases, perinephric abscess is caused by hematogenous spread, usually from sites of skin infection. A perirenal hematoma can become secondarily infected by the hematogenous route or by direct extension of a primary renal infection. When a perinephric infection ruptures through Gerota's fascia into the pararenal space, the abscess becomes paranephric. Paranephric abscesses may also result from infectious disorders of the bowel, pancreas, or pleural cavity. Conversely, perinephric or psoas abscess may

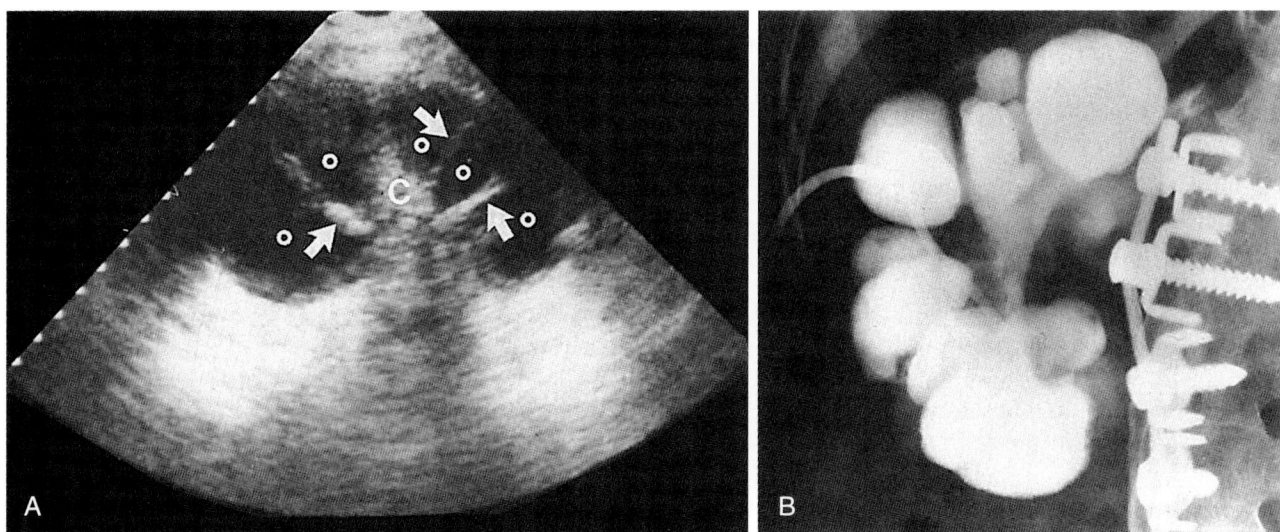

Figure 8–30. Pyonephrosis. **A,** Longitudinal ultrasound scan of the right kidney demonstrates echogenic central collecting complex (C) with radiating echogenic septa *(arrows)* and thinned hypoechoic parenchyma. Multiple dilated calyces (o) with diffuse low-level echoes are seen. **B,** Antegrade pyelogram performed through a percutaneous nephrostomy catheter correlates well with the ultrasound image. Dilated pus-filled calyces are demonstrated. The renal pelvis is obliterated by chronic scarring and stone disease. The kidney did not regain function. (From Schaeffer AJ: Urinary tract infections. In Gillenwater JY, et al [eds]: Adult and Pediatric Urology. Philadelphia, Lippincott Williams & Wilkins, 2002, pp 211-272.)

be the result of bowel perforation, Crohn's disease, or spread of osteomyelitis from the thoracolumbar spine. *E. coli, Proteus,* and *S. aureus* account for most infections.

Clinical Presentation. The onset of symptoms is typically insidious. Symptoms are present for more than 5 days in most patients with perinephric abscess compared with only about 10% of patients with pyelonephritis. The clinical presentation may be similar to that of pyelonephritis; however, more than one third of patients may be afebrile. An abdominal or flank mass can be felt in about half of the cases. Psoas abscess should be suspected if the patient has a limp and flexion and external rotation of the ipsilateral hip. Laboratory features include leukocytosis, elevated levels of serum creatinine, and pyuria in more than 75% of cases. Edelstein and McCabe (1988) showed that results of urine cultures predicted perinephric abscess isolates in only 37% of cases; a blood culture, particularly with multiple organisms, was often indicative of perinephric abscess but identified all organisms in only 42% of cases. **Therefore, therapy based on the results of urine and blood cultures often may be inadequate. Pyelonephritis usually responds within 4 to 5 days of appropriate antimicrobial therapy; perinephric abscess does not. Thus, perinephric abscess should be suspected in a patient with UTI and abdominal or flank mass or persistent fever after 4 days of antimicrobial therapy.**

Radiologic Findings. Excretory urography is abnormal in 80% of cases. However, the abnormalities are not specific. Classically, the radiographic features of perinephric abscess have been the absence of psoas shadow, a mass in the perirenal area often associated with indistinct renal outlines, and an elevated or immobile diaphragm. With large abscesses, the soft tissue density may extend to the pelvis following the renal fascia. In patients with perinephric abscess secondary to gas-forming organisms, bubbled collections of extraluminal gas are seen surrounding the kidney (Love et al, 1973).

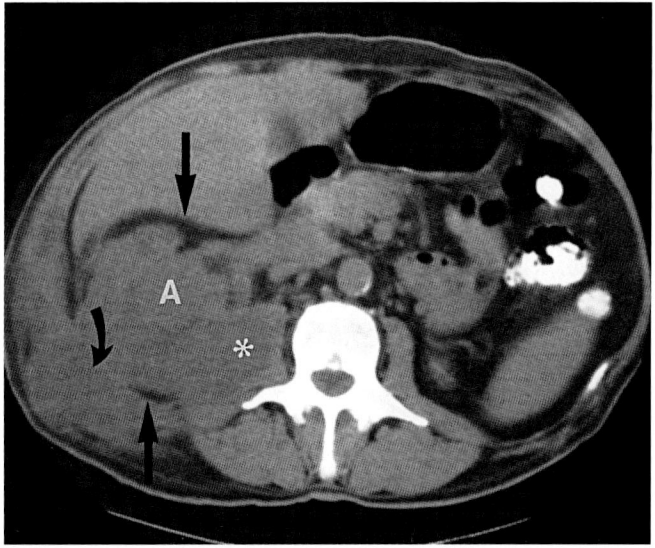

Figure 8–31. Nonenhanced CT scan through the lower pole of the right kidney (previous left nephrectomy) shows extensive perinephric abscess. Extensive abscess (A) distorts and enlarges the renal contour, infiltrates perinephric fat *(straight arrows)*, and also extends into the psoas muscle *(asterisk)* and the soft tissues of the flank *(curved arrow)*. Also note that normal renal collecting system fat has been obliterated by the process.

CT is particularly valuable for demonstrating the primary abscess. In some cases, the abscess is confined to the perinephric space; however, extension to the flank or psoas muscle may occur (Fig. 8–31). CT is able to show with exquisite anatomic detail the route of spread of infection into the surrounding tissues (Fig. 8–32). This information may be helpful in planning the approach for surgical drainage. Ultrasound demonstrates a diverse sonographic appearance ranging from a nearly anechoic mass displacing the kidney to

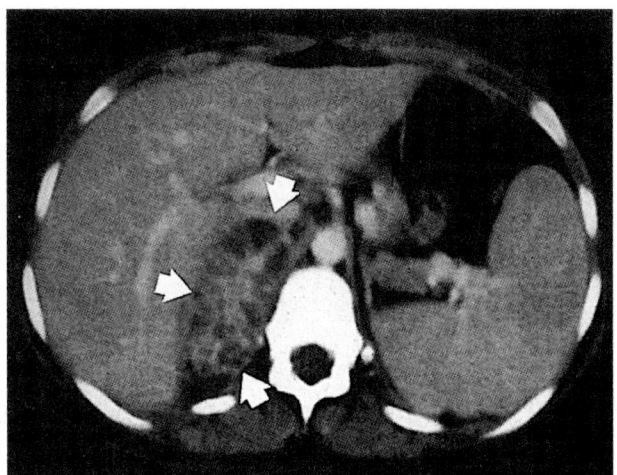

Figure 8–32. Perinephric abscess involving the right adrenal gland. CT scan shows large right pararenal mass *(arrows)* with multiple low-density areas within. At surgery, a large pararenal abscess with extensive involvement of the right adrenal was found. (From Schaeffer AJ: Urinary tract infections. In Gillenwater JY, et al [eds]: Adult and Pediatric Urology. Philadelphia, Lippincott Williams & Wilkins, 2002, pp 211-272.)

an echogenic collection that tends to blend with normally echogenic fat within Gerota's fascia (Corriere and Sandler, 1982). Occasionally, a retroperitoneal or subdiaphragmatic infection may spread to the paranephric fat that is outside Gerota's fascia. The clinical symptoms of insidious onset of fever, flank mass, and tenderness are indistinguishable from those associated with perinephric abscess. UTI, however, is absent. Ultrasonography and CT can usually delineate the abscess outside Gerota's fascia.

Management. Although antimicrobial agents are useful to control sepsis and to prevent spread of infection, the primary treatment for perinephric abscess is drainage; reports of successful treatment by antimicrobial agents alone are unusual (Herlitz et al, 1981). A detailed analysis of 52 perinephric abscess patients by Thorley and colleagues (1974) supports this tenet. In this study, half the patients were admitted to medical services and the other half to surgical services; 65% of those admitted to medical services died, whereas 23% of those admitted to surgical services died. These mortality rates reflect differences in the population of patients. Those admitted to the medical services were usually sicker and had higher temperatures, more underlying diseases, and vaguer symptoms. More importantly, none of those admitted to medical wards had an admission diagnosis of perinephric abscess, whereas 73% of those admitted to surgical wards did. Although 71% of all the patients had eventual surgical treatment of their perinephric abscesses, the diagnostic delay of those patients admitted to medical services postponed definitive treatment and consequently caused higher mortality.

Although surgical drainage, or nephrectomy if the kidney is nonfunctioning or severely infected, is the classic treatment for perinephric abscesses, renal ultrasonography and CT make percutaneous aspiration and drainage of small perirenal collections possible (Haaga and Weinstein, 1980; Elyaderani et al, 1981; Edelstein and McCabe, 1988). Haaga and Weinstein (1980), however, consider percutaneous

drainage to be contraindicated in large abscess cavities filled with thick, purulent fluid.

Gram stain identifies the pathogenesis and guides antimicrobial therapy. An aminoglycoside together with an anti-staphylococcal agent, such as methicillin or oxacillin, should be started immediately. If the patient has a penicillin hypersensitivity, cephalothin or vancomycin may be used.

Once the perinephric abscess has been drained, the underlying problem must be dealt with. Some conditions such as renal cortical abscess or enteric communication require prompt attention. Nephrectomy for pyonephrosis may be performed concurrent with drainage of the perinephric abscess if the patient's condition is good. In other instances, it is best to drain the perinephric abscess first and correct the underlying problem or perform a nephrectomy when the patient's condition has improved.

Perinephric Abscess versus Acute Pyelonephritis. It has already been emphasized that the greatest obstacle to the treatment of perinephric abscess is the delay in diagnosis. **In the series of Thorley and colleagues (1974), a common misdiagnosis was acute pyelonephritis. In their review, they found that two factors differentiated perinephric abscess and acute pyelonephritis: (1) most patients with uncomplicated pyelonephritis were symptomatic for less than 5 days before hospitalization, whereas most with perinephric abscesses were symptomatic for longer than 5 days; and (2) no patient with acute pyelonephritis remained febrile for longer than 4 days once appropriate antimicrobial agents were started. All patients with perinephric abscesses had a fever for at least 5 days, with a median of 7 days. Similar results were noted by Fowler and Perkins** (1994).

Patients with polycystic renal disease who undergo hemodialysis may be particularly susceptible to the progression from acute UTIs to perinephric abscess. Of 445 patients undergoing chronic hemodialysis at the Regional Kidney Disease Program in Minneapolis, 5.4% had polycystic kidney disease and 33.3% of these patients developed symptomatic UTIs (Sweet and Keane, 1979). Eight (62.5%) developed perinephric abscesses, and 3 of these patients died. According to the investigators, all UTIs, even those that progressed to perinephric abscesses, were promptly treated with appropriate antimicrobial agents, and all patients in this group became afebrile and asymptomatic when the agents were stopped. Yet later, after various times, symptoms attributable to perinephric abscess developed in 8 of the patients.

Chronic Pyelonephritis

In patients without underlying renal or urinary tract disease, chronic pyelonephritis secondary to UTI is a rare disease and an even more rare cause of chronic renal failure. In patients with underlying functional or structural urinary tract abnormalities, however, chronic renal infection can cause significant renal impairment. Hence, it is essential that appropriate studies be used to diagnose, localize, and treat chronic renal infection.

The prevalence of chronic pyelonephritis has also been assessed in patients undergoing dialysis for end-stage renal disease. Despite a 2% to 5% prevalence of bacteriuria in women, pyelonephritis uncomplicated by obstruction or urinary tract malformation does not cause end-stage renal disease. Schechter and colleagues (1971) analyzed the cause for renal failure in 170 patients referred to them for dialysis. Chronic pyelonephritis was the primary cause of end-stage renal disease in 22 (13%) but was usually associated with an underlying structural defect. Unequivocal nonobstructive chronic pyelonephritis was not found. The authors also observed that symptomatic infections tended to occur before the onset of azotemia in most patients with chronic pyelonephritis. Similarly, Huland and Busch (1982) evaluated 161 patients with end-stage renal disease and found that 42 had chronic pyelonephritis. However, in addition to a history of UTIs, these 42 patients had complicating defects, such as vesicoureteral reflux, analgesic abuse, nephrolithiasis, or obstruction. Nonobstructive uncomplicated UTI alone was never found to be the cause of renal insufficiency. Thus, using end-stage renal disease seen at autopsy or at the dialysis clinic as an indicator, the prevalence of uncomplicated chronic bacterial pyelonephritis is rare.

In addition, the role of bacterial infection in development of chronic renal disease can be assessed in patients with renal interstitial and tubular damage similar to that which has classically been called chronic pyelonephritis. The frequency with which various potential causes of interstitial damage are operative in patients with interstitial nephritis was assessed by Murray and Goldberg (1975). These investigators not only concluded that UTI is rarely the sole cause of chronic renal disease in the adult but also observed that 89% of their azotemic patients had a readily identifiable primary cause of their interstitial nephritis. Thus, when patients with a clinical diagnosis of chronic interstitial nephritis are selected as the starting point, it is easy to associate many factors with this disease, but UTI does not seem to be one of them.

Clinical Presentation. There are no symptoms of chronic pyelonephritis until it produces renal insufficiency, and then the symptoms are similar to those of any other form of chronic renal failure. If a patient's chronic pyelonephritis is thought to be an end result of many episodes of acute pyelonephritis, a history of intermittent symptoms of fever, flank pain, and dysuria may be elicited. Similarly, urinary findings and the presence of renal infection correlate poorly. Bacteriuria and pyuria, the hallmarks of UTI, are not predictive of renal infection. Conversely, patients with significant renal infection may have sterile urine if the ureter draining the kidney is obstructed or the infection is outside of the collecting system.

The pathologic and radiologic criteria for diagnosing renal infection may also be misleading. Asscher (1980) has tabulated eight long-term follow-up studies from the literature on kidneys of adults with UTIs. The data from these reports on 901 patients show that bacteriuria present in otherwise healthy adults for long periods may be associated with nonexistent or extremely minimal evidence of kidney damage. Conversely, patients who have chronic pyelonephritis may have negative urine cultures.

Radiologic Findings. The diagnosis of chronic pyelonephritis can be made with the greatest confidence on the basis of pyelographic findings. The essential features are asymmetry and irregularity of the kidney outlines, blunting and dilation of one or more calyces, and cortical scars at the corresponding site (Fig. 8–33). In the absence of stones, obstruction, and

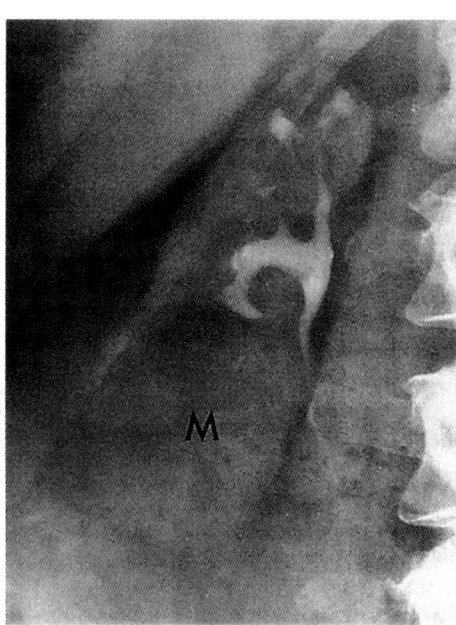

Figure 8–33. Chronic pyelonephritis. Ten-minute excretory urogram demonstrates irregular renal outline with upper pole parenchymal atrophy. Note significant loss of renal cortical thickness over blunted and dilated calyces. Lower pole mass (M) is a simple cyst. (From Schaeffer AJ: Urinary tract infections. In Gillenwater JY, et al [eds]: Adult and Pediatric Urology. Philadelphia, Lippincott Williams & Wilkins, 2002, pp 211-272.)

tuberculosis, and with the single exception of analgesic nephritis with papillary necrosis (which can be readily excluded by history), chronic pyelonephritis is virtually the only disease that produces a localized scar over a deformed calyx (Stamey, 1980). In advanced pyelonephritis, calyceal distortion and irregularity together with cortical scars complete the picture. Hodson (1965a) pointed out that renal infarction, an extremely rare condition, may closely resemble pyelonephritic scars but that the renal pyramid remains with renal infarction in contradistinction to pyelonephritis.

Pathology. In chronic pyelonephritis, the gross kidney is often diffusely contracted, scarred, and pitted. The scars are Y-shaped, flat, broad-based depressions with red-brown granular bases. The scarring is often polar with underlying calyceal blunting. The parenchyma is thin, and the corticomedullary demarcation is lost. **Histologic changes are patchy.** There is usually an interstitial infiltrate of lymphocytes, plasma cells, and occasional polymorphonuclear cells. Portions of the parenchyma may be replaced by fibrosis, and, although glomeruli may be preserved, periglomerular fibrosis is often seen. In some affected areas, glomeruli may be completely fibrosed and tubules atrophied. Leukocyte and hyaline casts are sometimes present in the tubules; the latter may cause resemblance to the thyroid colloid, hence the description *renal thyroidization* (Braude, 1973). In general, the changes are nonspecific; they also may be seen in toxic exposures, postobstructive atrophy, hematologic disorders, postirradiation nephritis, ischemic renal disease, and nephrosclerosis.

Management. Management of radiographic evidence of pyelonephritis should be directed at treating infection, if present; preventing future infections; and monitoring and preserving renal function. The treatment of existing infection must be based on careful antimicrobial susceptibility tests and selection of drugs that can achieve bactericidal concentrations in the urine and yet are not nephrotoxic. Achievement of acceptable bactericidal levels of a drug in the urine of a patient with chronic pyelonephritis may be difficult because the diminished concentrating ability of pyelonephritis may impair excretion and concentration of the antimicrobial agent. The duration of antimicrobial therapy is often prolonged to maximize the chance of cure. With patients in whom renal damage develops or progresses in the presence of UTI, the working hypothesis should be that there is an underlying renal, usually papillary, lesion or underlying urologic condition, such as obstruction or calculus, that has increased susceptibility to renal damage. Appropriate nephrologic and urologic evaluation should be undertaken to identify and, if possible, correct these abnormalities.

Bacterial "Relapse" from a Normal Kidney

The concept that bacteria persist in the renal parenchyma between bacteriuric episodes and cause "relapsing" UTIs was based on a study by Turck and colleagues (1968) that suggested that bacterial persistence could be recognized by simply identifying two consecutive recurrent infections with the same organism. Unfortunately, this study did not indicate whether the urine was cultured during therapy to ensure that the original infection had actually been eradicated. It is possible that some of these so-called relapses were in fact unresolved initial infections and that ureteral edema associated with catheterization may have impeded clearance of the initial infecting strain.

Subsequent studies summarized by Stamey (1980) and Forland and associates (1977) have shown that in a **normal urinary tract recurrent infections are not caused by relapse from bacterial persistence in the kidney.** With ureteral catheterization techniques, Cattell (1973) localized the site of bacteriuria in 42 patients who had follow-up for 6 months after therapy. He analyzed the response to antimicrobial therapy of 2 weeks' duration. Of the 26 patients who were cured of their initial infection, 16 had recurrence with the same organism, 8 had upper tract infections, and 8 had bladder bacteriuria.

If bacterial persistence in the kidney is a major problem after therapy, we would expect patients who have more recurrent infections to also have more relapses than those who have less frequent recurrences. Mabeck (1972) analyzed this, however, and found that with an increasing number of recurrences, the relationship among treatment failure, relapse, and reinfection remained unchanged. Thus, bacteria do not persist in normal kidneys between recurrent UTIs (Stamey, 1980) and recurrences with the same strain are not caused by "relapse" from the kidney.

Although it is known that certain adults have increased risk of renal damage from bacteriuria (this subject is discussed in detail in the pathogenesis section on alterations in host defense mechanisms), acute clinical pyelonephritis does not cause scarring in most adults with normal urinary tracts. **Most of the changes of chronic pyelonephritis seem to occur in infancy, probably because the growing kidney is most susceptible to scarring. In a review that examined the long-term effect of UTIs in adults, it was concluded that renal damage is rare in nonobstructive UTIs** (Stamey, 1980) but

that it does occur (Bailey et al, 1969; Davies et al, 1972; Davidson and Talner, 1973; Feldberg, 1982). In most reports of renal change after acute nonobstructive bacterial pyelonephritis, calyceal and papillary distortion similar to that occurring in papillary necrosis is seen but focal cortical scars characteristic of chronic pyelonephritic changes are absent. Instead, the urograms show generalized shrinkage of the kidneys after the acute infection. Two of the four patients reported by Davidson and Talner (1978) had diabetes in addition to pyelonephritis.

The natural history of patients with chronic pyelonephritis is discussed in Chapter 112, "Infection and Inflammation of the Pediatric Genitourinary Tract" (see the sections on course and prognosis), because these changes are usually discovered in childhood. A few studies have examined the prognosis in cases that were discovered in adults. In a longitudinal study of patients with the radiologic changes of bilateral chronic pyelonephritis defined by focal parenchymal scarring and calyceal clubbing, the calculated 5-year survival rate was 95% and the 10-year survival rate was 86% (Gower, 1976). The survival rate for patients with changes of unilateral chronic pyelonephritis was 100% at both 5 and 10 years. During the study period of 5 to 135 months, this investigator also observed that bacteriuria that was found in patients more than 20% of the time could not be correlated with deteriorating renal function; however, infection was often associated with the appearance or growth of renal calculi.

The relationships of the pyelonephritic kidney with end-stage renal disease and hypertension have been examined. In one report of 161 patients with end-stage renal disease requiring dialysis, 42 patients (26%) had "chronic pyelonephritis" with bacteriuria in the past or at the time they were studied (Huland and Busch, 1982). However, a complicating factor was involved in all of the 42 patients with chronic pyelonephritis and end-stage renal disease: 66.7% had vesicoureteral reflux; 14.3%, analgesic abuse; 11.9%, nephrolithiasis; 4.8%, pyelonephritis during pregnancy; and 2.4%, hydronephrosis. The association between hypertension and the pyelonephritic kidney has been addressed by Pfau and Rosenmann (1978), who concluded that the association of chronic pyelonephritis and hypertension is usually coincidental. Their conclusion agrees with that of a study by Parker and Kunin (1973) that examined 74 women who had been admitted to the hospital 10 to 20 years previously for pyelonephritis. Only 14.5% of these women had hypertension, a rate similar to that found in a random female population of the same age.

Infectious Granulomatous Nephritis

Xanthogranulomatous Pyelonephritis

Xanthogranulomatous pyelonephritis is a rare, severe, chronic renal infection typically resulting in diffuse renal destruction. Most cases are unilateral and result in a nonfunctioning, enlarged kidney associated with obstructive uropathy secondary to nephrolithiasis. Xanthogranulomatous pyelonephritis is characterized by accumulation of lipid-laden foamy macrophages. It begins within the pelvis and calyces and subsequently extends into and destroys renal parenchymal and adjacent tissues. It has been known to imitate virtually every other inflammatory disease of the kidney, as well as renal cell carcinoma, on radiographic examination (Malek and Elder, 1978; Tolia et al, 1980). In addition, the microscopic appearance of xanthogranulomatous pyelonephritis has been confused with clear cell adenocarcinoma of the kidney on frozen section and has led to radical nephrectomy (Anhalt et al, 1971; Malek and Elder, 1978; Flynn et al, 1979; Lorentzen and Nielsen, 1980; Tolia et al, 1980). The entity is uncommon and is found in only about 0.6% (Malek et al, 1972) to 1.4% (Ghosh, 1955) of patients with renal inflammation who are evaluated pathologically.

Pathogenesis. The primary factors involved in the pathogenesis of xanthogranulomatous pyelonephritis are nephrolithiasis, obstruction, and infection (Gregg et al, 1999). Nephrolithiasis has been noted in as many as 83% of the patients in various series; approximately half of the renal stones have been of the staghorn type (Parsons et al, 1983; Chuang et al, 1992; Nataluk et al, 1995). It has been proposed clinically and demonstrated experimentally that primary obstruction followed by infection with *E. coli* can lead to tissue destruction and collections of lipid material by macrophages (Povysil and Konickova, 1972). These macrophages (xanthoma cells) are distributed in sheets around parenchymal abscesses and calyces and are intermixed with lymphocytes, giant cells, and plasma cells. The bacteria appear to be of low virulence because spontaneous bacteremia has rarely been described. Other possible interrelated factors include venous occlusion and hemorrhage, abnormal lipid metabolism, lymphatic blockage, failure of antimicrobial therapy in UTI, altered immunologic competence, and renal ischemia (Friedenberg and Spjut, 1963; Mering et al, 1973; Goodman et al, 1979; McDonald, 1981; Tolia et al, 1981). The concept that xanthogranulomatous pyelonephritis is related to incomplete bacterial degradation and altered host response has received mixed support (Nielsen and Lorentzen, 1981; Khalyl-Mawad et al, 1982). Thus it appears that there is probably no single factor that is instrumental in the pathogenesis of this disease. Rather, there is an inadequate host acute inflammatory response within an obstructed, ischemic, or necrotic kidney.

Pathology. The kidney is usually massively enlarged and has a normal contour. Xanthogranulomatous pyelonephritis may be diffuse, as in approximately 80% of the patients, or segmental. In the diffuse form of the disease, the entire kidney is involved, whereas in segmental xanthogranulomatous pyelonephritis, only the parenchyma surrounding one or more calyces or one pole of a duplicated collecting system is involved. On sectioning, the kidney usually demonstrates nephrolithiasis and peripelvic fibrosis. The calyces are dilated and filled with purulent material, but fibrosis surrounding the pelvis usually prevents dilation. The papillae are often destroyed by papillary necrosis (Goodman et al, 1979). In advanced stages of the disease, multiple parenchymal abscesses are filled with viscous pus and lined by yellowish tissue (Fig. 8–34A). The cortex is often thin and is often replaced by xanthogranulomatous tissue. The capsule is often thickened, and extension of the inflammatory process into the perinephric or paranephric space is common (Goodman et al, 1979; McDonald, 1981; Gregg et al, 1999).

On microscopic examination, the yellowish nodules that line the calyces and surround the parenchymal abscesses contain dark sheets of lipid-laden macrophages (foamy histiocytes with small, dark nuclei and clear cytoplasm) intermixed with lymphocytes, giant cells, and plasma cells (see Fig. 8–34B). Xanthogranulomatous cells are not specific to xanthogranulomatous pyelonephritis but may be present anywhere inflammation or obstruction coexists. The origin of the fatty substance is disputed. Cholesterol esters that make up a part of the lipid might be derived from lysis of erythrocytes after hemorrhage (Saedd and Fine, 1963).

Clinical Presentation. Xanthogranulomatous pyelonephritis should be suspected in patients with UTIs and a unilateral enlarged nonfunctioning or poorly functioning kidney with a stone or a mass lesion indistinguishable from malignant tumor. **Most patients present with flank pain (69%), fever and chills (69%), and persistent bacteriuria (46%)** (Malek and Elder, 1978). **Additional vague symptoms, such as malaise, may be present. On physical examination, 62% of the patients had a flank mass and 35% had previous calculi** (Malek and Elder, 1978). Less commonly, hypertension, hematuria, or hepatomegaly is the presenting complaint. The medical history is often positive for UTIs and urologic instrumentation (Malek and Elder, 1978; Flynn et al, 1979; Goodman et al, 1979; Grainger et al, 1982; Yazaki et al, 1982; Petronic et al, 1989; Eastham et al, 1994; Nataluk et al, 1995). Diabetics also appear to be at greater risk of developing the disease (Eastham et al, 1994). Although it may occur at any age, the peak incidence of xanthogranulomatous pyelonephritis is in the fifth to the seventh decade. Women are more commonly affected than men. There is no predilection for either kidney.

Bacteriology and Laboratory Diagnosis. Although review of the literature shows *Proteus* to be the most common organism involved with xanthogranulomatous pyelonephritis (Anhalt et al, 1971; Tolia et al, 1981), *E. coli* is also common. The prevalence of *Proteus* organisms may reflect their association with stone formation and subsequent chronic obstruction and irritation. Malek and Elder (1978), in their analysis of 26 cases, found that renal tissue cultures grew bacteria in 22 of 23 cases. Anaerobes also have been cultured (Malek and Elder, 1978).

Approximately 10% of patients have mixed cultures. About one third of patients have no growth in their urine, probably because many patients have recently taken or are taking antimicrobial agents when cultures are obtained. The infecting organism may be revealed only by tissue cultures obtained during surgery. Urinalysis usually shows pus and protein. In addition, blood tests often reveal anemia and may show hepatic dysfunction in up to 50% of the patients (Malek and Elder, 1978).

Xanthogranulomatous pyelonephritis is almost always unilateral; therefore, azotemia or frank renal failure is uncommon (Goodman et al, 1979; Gregg et al, 1999).

Radiologic Findings. Fifty to 80 percent of patients show the classic triad of unilateral renal enlargement with little or no function and a large calculus in the renal pelvis (Elder, 1984). At times, the enlargement may be localized and resemble a renal mass. Less commonly, excretory urography demonstrates delayed function and hydronephrosis, which may be

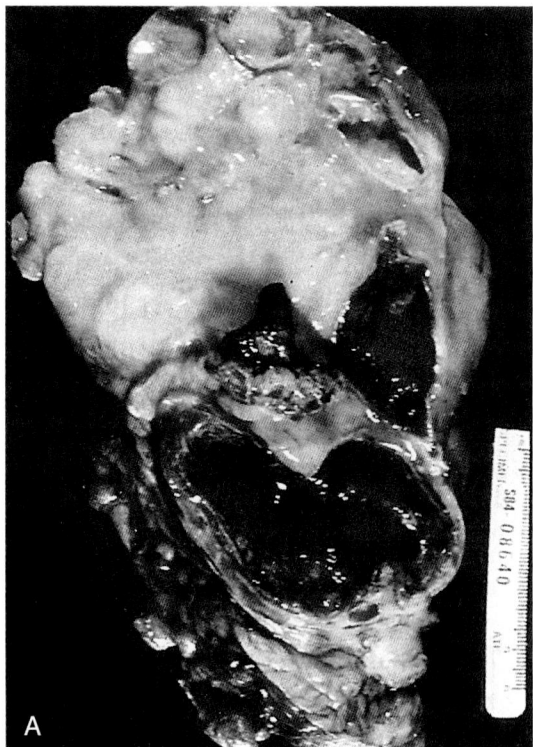

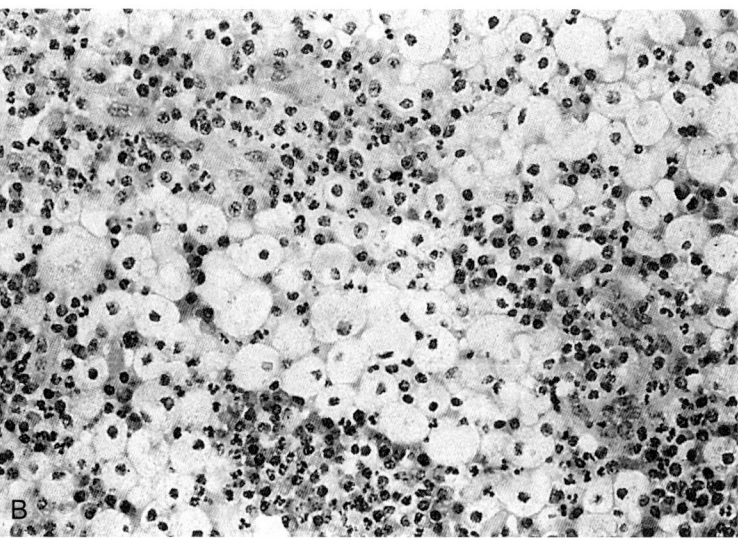

Figure 8–34. Xanthogranulomatous pyelonephritis. **A,** Gross specimen. Kidney is massively enlarged, measuring 23 × 12 cm; the normal architecture is replaced by a shaggy yellow upper pole mass corresponding to xanthogranulomatous inflammation and numerous distorted and dilated calyces. **B,** Microscopically, the shaggy yellow tissue is composed primarily of lipid-laden histiocytes mixed with other inflammatory cells. (From Schaeffer AJ: Urinary tract infections. In Gillenwater JY, et al [eds]: Adult and Pediatric Urology. Philadelphia, Lippincott Williams & Wilkins, 2002, pp 211-272.)

massive. Smaller calcifications within the mass are not uncommon but are much less specific (Fig. 8–35). Although there is abundant intracellular fat, the plane almost never demonstrates significant lucency (Hartman, 1985). Retrograde pyelography may show the point of obstruction and dilation of the renal pelvis and calyces. If there is extensive parenchymal damage, contrast studies may demonstrate an ulcerated pyelocalyceal system with multiple irregular filling defects.

CT is probably the most useful radiologic technique in evaluating patients with xanthogranulomatous pyelonephritis (Fig. 8–36). **CT usually demonstrates a large, reniform mass with the renal pelvis tightly surrounding a central calcification but without pelvic dilatation** (Solomon et al, 1983; Goldman et al, 1984; Hartman, 1985). Renal parenchyma is replaced by multiple water-density masses representing dilated calyces and abscess cavities filled with varied amounts of pus and debris. On enhanced scans, the walls of these cavities demonstrate a prominent blush owing to the abundant vascularity within the granulation tissue. The cavities themselves, however, fail to enhance, whereas tumors and other inflammatory lesions usually do. The CT scan is particularly helpful in demonstrating the extent of renal involvement and may indicate whether adjacent organs or the abdominal wall are involved by xanthogranulomatous pyelonephritis (Eastham et al, 1994; Kaplan et al, 1997).

Sonography usually demonstrates global enlargement of the kidney (Merenich and Popky, 1991). The normal renal architecture is replaced by multiple hypoechoic fluid-filled masses that correspond to debris-filled, dilated calyces or foci of parenchymal destruction (Fagerholm, 1983; Hartman et al, 1984). With focal involvement, a solid mass involving a

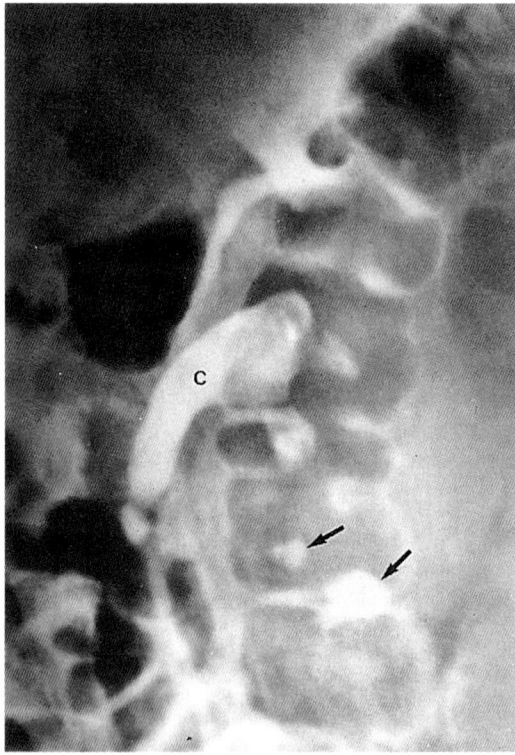

Figure 8–35. Xanthogranulomatous pyelonephritis. Ten-minute excretory urogram shows lower-pole enlargement and nonfunction. Note a large pelvic calculus (C) and several smaller parenchymal calculi *(arrows)*. The upper pole of the bifid collecting system functions normally. (From Schaeffer AJ: Urinary tract infections. In Gillenwater JY, et al [eds]: Adult and Pediatric Urology. Philadelphia, Lippincott Williams & Wilkins, 2002, pp 211-272.)

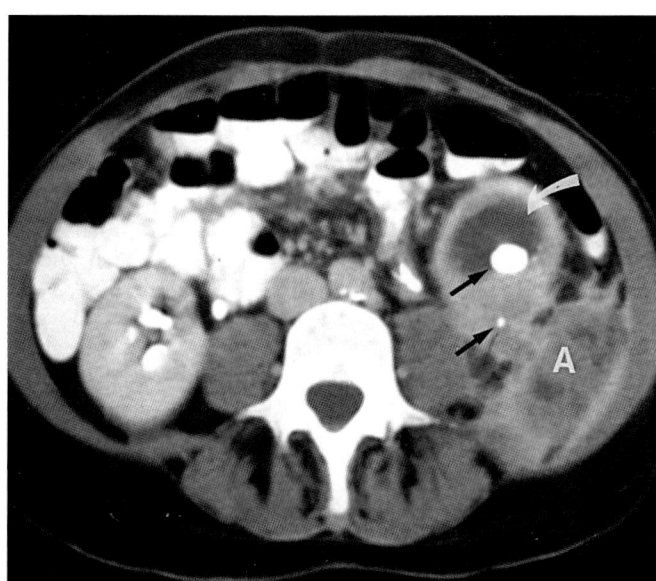

Figure 8–36. Xanthogranulomatous pyelonephritis. Enhanced CT scan shows collecting system and parenchymal calculi *(straight arrows)* with lower pole pyonephrosis *(curved arrow)* and an irregular, predominantly low-density perinephric abscess (A) extending into the soft tissues of the flank.

segment of the kidney is demonstrated with an associated calculus in the collecting system or ureter. Renal cell carcinoma and other solid renal lesions must be considered in the differential diagnosis (Elder, 1984).

Radionuclide renal scanning using ^{99m}Tc-DMSA is used to confirm and quantify the differential lack of function in the involved kidney (Gregg et al, 1999). MRI has not yet superseded CT in the evaluation of renal inflammation, but it provides some advantages in delineating extrarenal extension of inflammation (Soler et al, 1997). Lesions of xanthogranulomatous pyelonephritis may appear as cystic foci of intermediate intensity signal on T1-weighted images and hyperintensity on T2-weighted images. Arteriography shows hypervascular areas, but there may be some hypovascular areas (Malek and Elder, 1978; Van Kirk et al, 1980; Tolia et al, 1981). Therefore, radiologic studies, although distinctive, often cannot differentiate between xanthogranulomatous pyelonephritis and renal cell carcinoma.

Differential Diagnosis. Diagnosis of segmental xanthogranulomatous pyelonephritis without calculi may be difficult. Xanthogranulomatous pyelonephritis in association with massive pelvic dilation cannot be distinguished from pyonephrosis. When xanthogranulomatous pyelonephritis occurs within a small contracted kidney, the radiographic findings are nonspecific and nondiagnostic. Renal parenchymal malacoplakia may show renal enlargement and multiple inflammatory masses replacing the normal renal parenchyma, but calculi are usually not present. Renal lymphoma may be associated with multiple hypoechoic masses surrounding the contracted, nondilated pelvis, but lymphoma is usually clinically obvious, and renal involvement is usually bilateral and not associated with calculi (Hartman, 1985).

Management. The primary obstacle to the correct treatment of xanthogranulomatous pyelonephritis is incorrect diagnosis. In the past, the diagnosis was made postoperatively

as in Malek and Elder's series of 26 patients (1978) in which only 1 of the patients was correctly diagnosed preoperatively. Today with CT technology, the diagnosis of xanthogranulomatous pyelonephritis is made preoperatively nearly 90% of the time (Eastham et al, 1994; Nataluk et al, 1995). Antimicrobial therapy may be necessary to stabilize the patient preoperatively, and, occasionally, long-term antimicrobial therapy will eradicate the infection and restore renal function (Mollier et al, 1995). Because the renal abnormality may be diagnosed preoperatively as a renal tumor and/or is diffuse, nephrectomy is usually performed. If localized xanthogranulomatous pyelonephritis is diagnosed preoperatively or at exploration, it is amenable to partial nephrectomy (Malek and Elder, 1978; Tolia et al, 1980; Osca et al, 1997).

The lipid-laden macrophages associated with xanthogranulomatous pyelonephritis, however, closely resemble clear cell adenocarcinoma and may be difficult to distinguish solely on the basis of frozen section. Furthermore, xanthogranulomatous pyelonephritis has been associated with renal cell carcinoma, papillary transitional cell carcinoma of the pelvis or bladder, and infiltrating squamous cell carcinoma of the pelvis (Schoborg et al, 1980; Pitts et al, 1981; Tolia et al, 1981). Therefore, if malignant renal tumor cannot be excluded, nephrectomy should be performed. When diffuse and extensive disease into the retroperitoneum exists, removal of the kidney and perinephric fat may be needed. Under these circumstances, the surgery may be difficult and may involve dissection of granulomatous tissue from the diaphragm, great vessels, and bowel (Malek and Elder, 1978; Flynn et al, 1979). It is important to remove the entire inflammatory mass because in nearly three fourths of patients, xanthogranulomatous tissue is infected. If incision and drainage alone are performed rather than nephrectomy, the patient may continue to suffer from protracted debilitating illness and may develop a renal cutaneous fistula; an even more difficult nephrectomy will then be necessary. An early case matched series of laparoscopic nephrectomies performed for xanthogranulomatous pyelonephritis concluded that the benefits of laparoscopic surgery do not extend to the treatment of this disease (Bercowsky et al, 1999); however, a larger review of a modern xanthogranulomatous pyelonephritis experience suggests that laparoscopic nephrectomy is a reasonable approach to the treatment of this disease.

Malacoplakia

Malacoplakia, from the Greek word meaning "soft plaque," is an unusual inflammatory disease that was originally described to affect the bladder but has been found to affect the genitourinary and gastrointestinal tracts, skin, lungs, bones, and mesenteric lymph nodes. It is an inflammatory lesion described originally by Michaelis and Gutmann (1902). It was characterized by von Hansemann (1903) as soft, yellow-brown plaques with granulomatous lesions in which the histiocytes contain distinct basophilic inclusions or Michaelis-Gutmann bodies. Although its exact pathogenesis is unknown, malacoplakia probably results from abnormal macrophage function in response to a bacterial infection, which is most often *E. coli.*

Pathogenesis. The pathogenesis is unknown, but several theories are popular. In 93 patients who had cultures of urine, diseased tissue, or blood, 89.4% had coliform infections (Stanton and Maxted, 1981). Moreover, 40% of the patients in this review had an immunodeficiency syndrome, autoimmune disease, carcinoma, or another systemic disorder. This association of coliform infections and compromised health status in patients with malacoplakia is well recognized.

It is hypothesized that bacteria or bacterial fragments form the nidus for the calcium phosphate crystals that laminate the Michaelis-Gutmann bodies. Most investigations into the pathogenesis of this disease support theories that a defect in intraphagosomal bacterial digestion accounts for the unusual immunologic response that causes malacoplakia.

Pathology. The diagnosis is made by biopsy. The lesion is characterized by large histiocytes, known as *von Hansemann cells,* and small basophilic, extracytoplasmic, or intracytoplasmic calculospherules called Michaelis-Gutmann bodies, which are pathognomonic (Fig. 8–37). Electron microscopy has revealed intact coliform bacteria and bacterial fragments within phagolysosomes of the foamy-appearing malacoplakic histiocytes (Lewin et al, 1976; Stanton and Maxted, 1981). In their review of the subject, Stanton and

Maxted (1981) and Esparza and associates (1989) emphasized that, although pathognomonic for the disease, Michaelis-Gutmann bodies may be absent in early malacoplakia and are not necessary for the diagnosis.

It has been shown that macrophages in malacoplakia involving the kidney and bladder contain large amounts of immunoreactive α_1-antitrypsin (Callea et al, 1982). The amount of α_1-antitrypsin remains unchanged during the morphogenetic stages of the pathologic process. Macrophages from other pathologic processes, closely resembling malacoplakia but without Michaelis-Gutmann bodies, do not contain α_1-antitrypsin except for a few macrophages in tuberculosis and xanthogranulomatous pyelonephritis. Therefore, **immunohistochemical staining for α_1-antitrypsin may be a useful test for an early and accurate differential diagnosis of malacoplakia.**

Clinical Presentation. Most patients are older than 50 years. The ratio of females to males with malacoplakia within the urinary tract is 4:1, but this disparity does not occur in other body tissues (Stanton and Maxted, 1981). The patients often are debilitated, are immunosuppressed, and have other chronic diseases. The symptoms of bladder malacoplakia

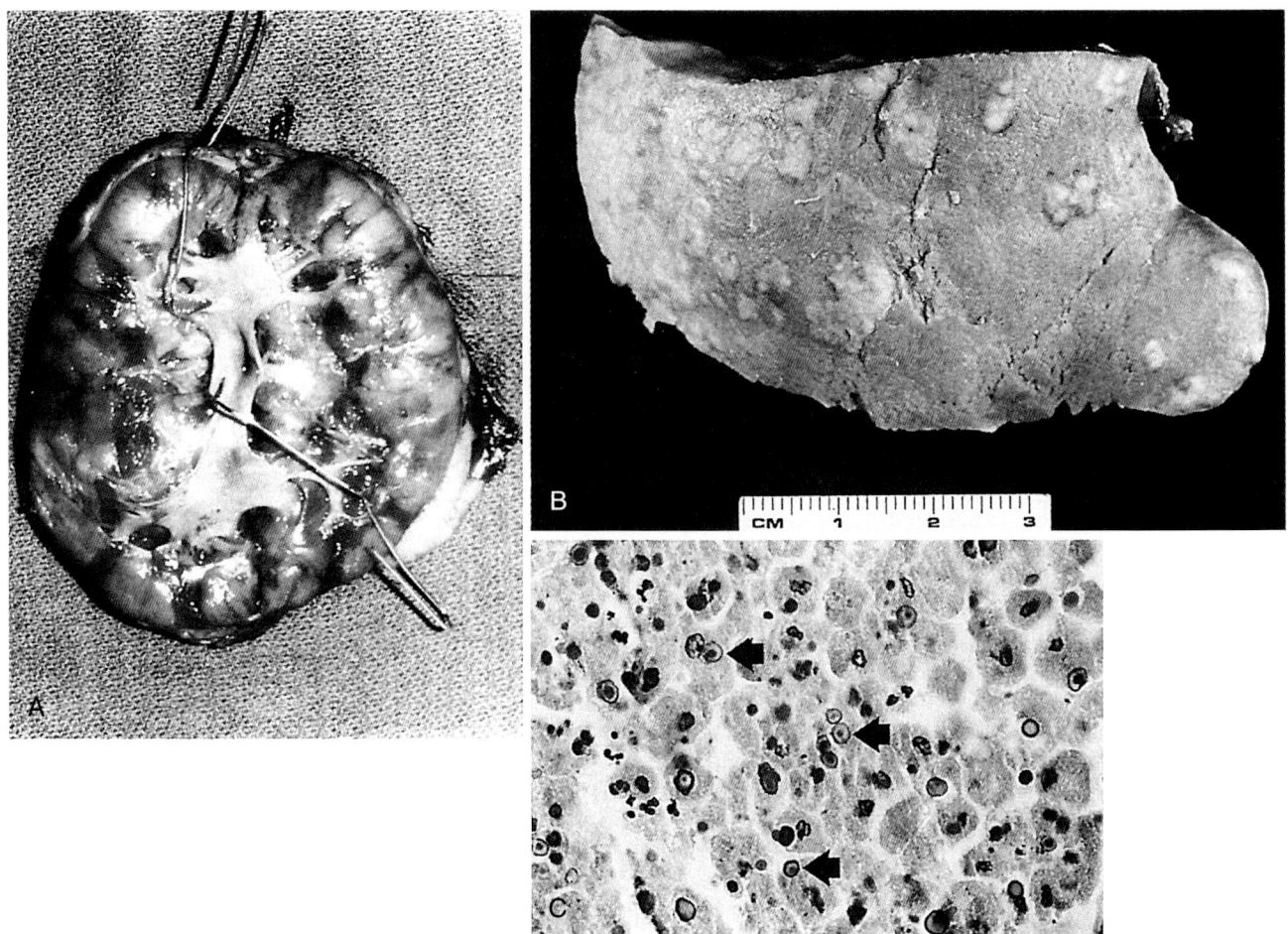

Figure 8–37. Renal parenchymal malacoplakia. **A,** Cut surface demonstrates extensive cortical and upper medullary replacement by multifocal, confluent, tumor-like masses. **B,** Cortical surface exhibits multiple, firm, plaquelike lesions. **C,** Hallmark of malacoplakia is demonstration of the Michaelis-Gutmann body *(arrows),* which represents incompletely destroyed bacteria surrounded by lipoprotein membrane (hematoxylin-eosin stain). (From Hartman DS: Radiologic pathologic correlation of the infectious granulomatous diseases of the kidney: I and II. Monogr Urol 1985;6:3.)

are bladder irritability and hematuria. Cystoscopy reveals mucosal plaques or nodules. As these lesions progress, they may become fungating, firm, sessile masses that cause filling defects of the bladder, ureter, or pelvis on excretory urograms. The distal ureter may become strictured or stenotic and cause subsequent renal obstruction or nonfunction (Sexton et al, 1982). A typical patient with renal parenchymal disease may have one or more radiographic masses and chronic *E. coli* infections. Renal parenchymal malacoplakia may be complicated by renal vein thrombosis and inferior vena cava thrombosis (McClure, 1983). When malacoplakia involves the testis, epididymo-orchitis is present. Malacoplakia of the prostate is rare, but, when it occurs, it may be confused with carcinoma clinically (Shimizu et al, 1981). Mortality can exceed 50%, and the morbidity can be substantial (Stanton and Maxted, 1981).

Radiologic Findings. **Multifocal malacoplakia on excretory urography typically presents as enlarged kidneys with multiple filling defects.** Renal calcification, lithiasis, and hydronephrosis are absent. The multifocal nature is best appreciated by using ultrasonography, CT, or arteriography. Sonographic examination may demonstrate renal enlargement and distortion of the central echo complex. The masses are often confluent, resulting in an overall increase in the echogenicity of the renal parenchyma (Hartman et al, 1980). On CT, the foci of malacoplakia are less dense than the surrounding enhanced parenchyma (Hartman, 1985). Arteriography typically reveals a hypovascular mass without peripheral neovascularity (Cavins and Goldstein, 1977; Trillo et al, 1977).

Unifocal malacoplakia on excretory urography appears as a noncalcified mass that is indistinguishable from other inflammatory or neoplastic lesions. Ultrasonography and CT may demonstrate a solid or cystic structure, depending on the degree of internal necrosis. Angiography may demonstrate neovascularity (Trillo et al, 1977). Extension beyond the kidney, which can occur with either multifocal or uniform malacoplakia, is best demonstrated by CT.

Differential Diagnosis. The differential diagnosis includes renal cystic disease, neoplasia, and renal inflammatory disease (Hartman, 1985). Malacoplakia should be considered when one or more renal masses are observed, particularly in female patients with recurrent UTIs with *E. coli*, altered immune response syndromes, or cystoscopic evidence of malacoplakia or filling defects in the collecting system (Charboneau et al., 1980). Malacoplakia should also be suspected when these radiographic findings occur in a renal transplant patient who has persistent UTI despite appropriate antimicrobial therapy. Cystic disease generally can be excluded by careful sonographic and CT evaluations. Renal involvement with metastatic disease or lymphomas usually occurs late in the course of the disease, which is well established. Multifocal renal cell carcinoma is most often seen in the context of von Hippel-Lindau disease with its other clinical manifestations. Patients with xanthogranulomatous pyelonephritis usually have signs and symptoms of UTI. As with malacoplakia, the involved kidney is enlarged but renal calculi and obstruction are common. Multiple renal abscesses are often associated with hematogenous dissemination resulting from cardiac disease.

Management. Management of malacoplakia should be directed at control of the UTIs, which should stabilize the disease process. This subject is well reviewed by Stanton and Maxted (1981). Although multiple long-term antimicrobial agents, including many antituberculosis agents, have been used, the sulfonamides, rifampin, doxycycline, and TMP are thought to be especially useful because of their intracellular bactericidal activity (Maderazo et al, 1979). Fluoroquinolones are taken up by macrophages directly and have also proven effective in the management of malacoplakia (Vallorosi et al, 1999). Other investigators have used ascorbic acid and cholinergic agents such as bethanechol in conjunction with antimicrobial therapy and have reported good results (Abdou et al, 1977; Zornow et al, 1979; Stanton et al, 1983). Both agents are thought to increase intracellular cyclic guanosine monophosphate levels, which have been postulated as the biologic defect causing macrophage dysfunction. Surgical intervention, however, may be necessary if the disease progresses in spite of antimicrobial treatment. Nephrectomy is usually performed for the treatment of symptomatic unilateral renal lesions.

The long-term prognosis appears to be related to the extent of the disease. When parenchymal renal malacoplakia is bilateral or occurs in the transplanted kidney, death usually occurs within 6 months (Bowers and Cathey, 1971; Deridder et al, 1977). Patients with unilateral disease usually have a long-term survival after nephrectomy.

Renal Echinococcosis

Echinococcosis is a parasitic infection caused by the larval stage of the tapeworm *Echinococcus granulosus*. The disease is prevalent in dogs, sheep, cattle, and humans in South Africa, Australia, New Zealand, Mediterranean countries (especially Greece), and some parts of the former Soviet Union. In the United States, the disease is rare, but it is found in immigrants from Eastern Europe or other foreign endemic areas or as an indigenous infection among American Indians in the Southwest and in Eskimos (Plorde, 1977).

Pathogenesis and Pathology. **Echinococcosis is produced by the larval form of the tapeworm, which in its adult form resides in the intestine of the dog, the definitive host.** The adult worm is 3 to 9 mm long. The ova in the feces of the dog contaminate grass and farmlands and are ingested by sheep, pigs, or humans, the intermediate hosts. Larvae hatch, penetrate venules in the wall of the duodenum, and are carried by the bloodstream to the liver. Those larvae that escape the liver are next filtered by the lungs. Approximately 3% of the organisms that escape entrapment in the liver and lungs may then enter the systemic circulation and infect the kidneys. The larvae undergo vesiculation, and the resultant hydatid cyst gradually develops at a rate of about 1 cm/yr. Thus, the cyst may take 5 to 10 years to reach pathologic size.

Echinococcosis cysts of the kidney are usually single and located in the cortex (Nabizadeh et al, 1983). The wall of the hydatid cyst has three zones: a peripheral zone of fibroblasts derived from tissues of the host becomes the adventitia and may calcify; an intermediate laminated layer becomes hyalinized; and a single inner layer is composed of nucleated epithelium and is called the *germinal layer*. The germinal layer gives rise to brood capsules that increase in number, become vacuolated, and remain attached to the germinal membrane by a pedicle. New larvae (scoleces) develop in large numbers from

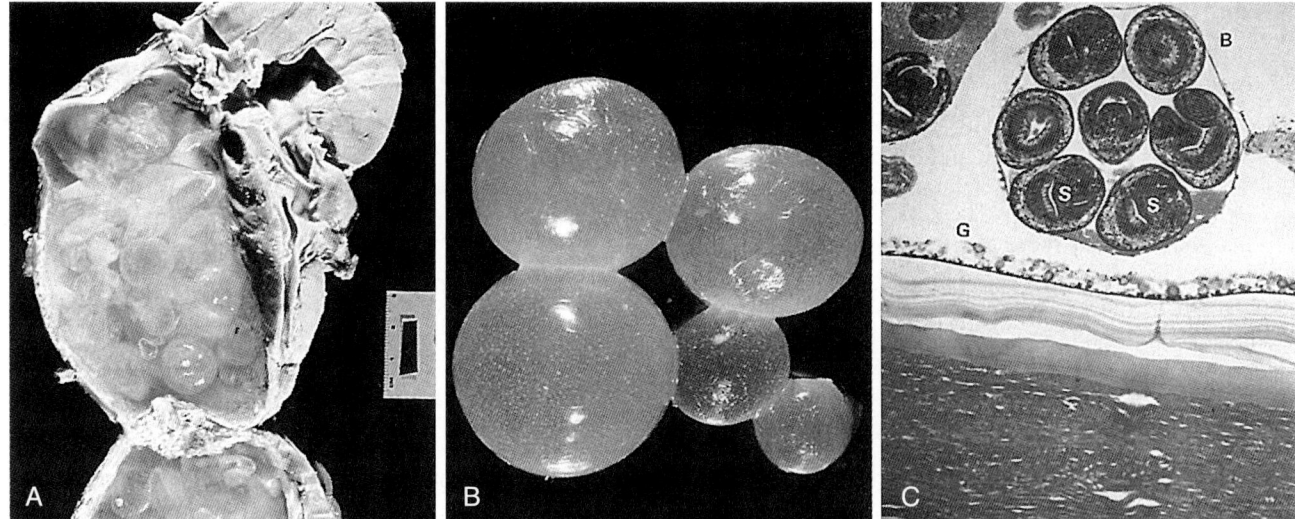

Figure 8–38. Echinococcosis. **A,** Gross specimen. A cystic mass measuring 7 × 11 cm in lower pole. Smaller daughter cysts are identified within the larger cystic mass. **B,** Gross specimen. Daughter cysts represent brood capsules that have detached and move freely. **C,** Photomicrograph. Brood capsules (B) arising from the germinal layer (G) contain viable and degenerating scoleces (S). (From Hartman DS: Radiologic pathologic correlation of the infectious granulomatous diseases of the kidney: III and IV. Monogr Urol 1985;6:26.)

the germinal layer within the brood capsule (Fig. 8–38). The hydatid cyst is also filled with fluid. When brood capsules detach, they enlarge and move freely in the fluid and are then called daughter cysts. Hydatid sand is composed of free larvae and daughter cysts.

Clinical Presentation. The symptoms of echinococcosis are those of a slowly growing tumor. Most patients are asymptomatic or have a flank mass, dull pain, or hematuria (Gilsanz et al, 1980; Nabizadeh et al, 1983). Because the cyst is focal, it rarely affects renal function. Rarely, the cyst ruptures into the collecting system, and the patient may experience severe colic and passage of debris resembling grape skins in the urine (hydatiduria). The cyst may also rupture into an adjacent viscus or the peritoneal cavity. The fluid is extremely antigenic (Hartman, 1985).

Laboratory Diagnosis. If cyst rupture occurs, the definitive diagnosis can be established by identifying daughter cysts in the urine or by identifying the laminated wall of the cyst (Sparks et al, 1976). Fewer than half of the patients have eosinophilia. The most reliable diagnostic test uses partially purified hydatid arc 5 antigens in a double-diffusion test (Coltorti and Varela-Diaz, 1978). Complement fixation, HA, and the Casoni intradermal skin tests are less reliable but, when combined, are positive in about 90% of patients (Sparks et al, 1976).

Radiologic Findings. Excretory urography typically shows a thick-walled cystic mass, occasionally calcified (Buckley et al, 1985). If the cyst ruptures into the collecting system, daughter cysts may be outlined in the pelvis as an irregular mass or as multiple solitary lesions (Gilsanz et al, 1980). Occasionally, direct filling of the cyst with contrast medium occurs.

Ultrasonography and CT are useful in characterizing the mass. Ultrasonography usually demonstrates a multicystic or multiloculated mass. A sudden change in position may demonstrate bright falling echoes corresponding to hydatid sand, which can be observed during real-time evaluation of hydatid cysts (Saint Martin and Chiesa, 1984).

On CT, several patterns of renal echinococcosis may be recognized. The most specific is a cystic mass with discrete, round daughter cysts and a well-defined enhancing membrane (Martorana et al, 1981). The less specific pattern is that of a thick-walled multiloculated cystic mass (Gilsanz et al, 1980). The presence of daughter cysts within the mother cyst differentiates the lesion from a simple renal cyst and from renal abscesses, infected cysts, and necrotic neoplasm.

Both CT and ultrasonography are useful in evaluating the liver. Angiography is seldom required. **Diagnostic aspiration should not be performed because of the danger of rupture and spillage of the highly antigenic cyst contents and risk of fatal anaphylaxis.** Nevertheless, Baijal and coworkers (1995) described a percutaneous management of renal hydatidosis as a minimally invasive diagnostic and therapeutic option.

Management. The prognosis of echinococcosis is good but depends on the site and size of the cysts. Medical treatment with benzimidazole compounds such as mebendazole has shown limited success with significant side effects (Nabizadeh et al, 1983).

Surgery remains the mainstay of treatment of renal echinococcosis (Poulios, 1991). The cyst should be removed without rupture to reduce the chance of seeding and recurrence. If the cyst wall is calcified, the larvae are probably dead and the risk of seeding is low, although a daughter cyst may be viable. If the cyst ruptures or cannot be removed and marsupialization is required, the contents of the cyst initially should be aspirated and filled with a scolicidal agent such as 30% sodium chloride, 0.5% silver nitrate, 2% formalin, or 1% iodine for approximately 5 minutes to kill the germinal portion (Sparks et al, 1976; Nabizadeh et al, 1983; Shetty et al, 1992).

KEY POINTS: KIDNEY INFECTIONS

■ Acute pyelonephritis classically presents as the abrupt onset of chills, fever, and flank or costovertebral angle tenderness but can present as symptoms as mild as cystitis or as severe as sepsis.

■ Emphysematous pyelonephritis is a life-threatening infection diagnosed radiographically by the presence of gas in the parenchyma or collecting system and managed surgically.

■ Renal abscesses are well delineated by CT and are classically managed with intravenous antimicrobial agents and drainage.

■ Pyonephrosis is a bacterial infection in a hydronephrotic kidney. Prompt diagnosis is critical; treatment entails intravenous antimicrobial agents and drainage of the obstructed renal unit.

■ Xanthogranulomatous pyelonephritis is a chronic renal infection that is often found in poorly functioning renal units obstructed secondary to nephrolithiasis. Xanthogranulomatous pyelonephritis can be mistaken for renal tumors.

■ Malacoplakia is an unusual inflammatory disease thought to result from abnormal macrophage function. Michaelis-Gutmann bodies are lysosomal inclusion bodies that characterize this disease microscopically.

Table 8–25. Characteristics of Sepsis

General	Fever (core temperature > 38.3° C)
	Hypothermia (core temperature < 36° C)
	Heart rate > 90 min, 1 or 2 SD above the normal value for age
	Tachypnea
	Altered mental status
	Significant edema or positive fluid balance (20 mL/kg over 24 hr)
	Hyperglycemia (plasma glucose >120 mg/dL or 7.7 mol/L) in the absence of diabetes
Inflammatory	Leukocytosis (WBC count > 12,000/μL)
	Leukopenia (WBC count < 4000/μL)
	Normal WBC count with > 10% immature forms
Organ Dysfunction	Arterial hypoxemia (PaO2/FIO2 >300)
	Acute oliguria (urine output 0.5 ml/kg 1 hr for at least 2 hrs)
	Creatinine increase of 0.5 mg/dL
	Coagulation abnormalities (INR 1.5 or aPTT > 60 sec)
	Ileus (absent bowel sounds)
	Thrombocytopenia (platelet count <100,000/μL)
	Hyperbilirubinemia (plasma total bilirubin > 4 mg/dL or 70 mmol/L)
Tissue Perfusion	Hyperlactatemia (>1 mmol/L)
	Decreased capillary refill or mottling

INR, International normalized ration; aPTT, activated partial thromboplastin time.
From Levy MM, Fink MP, Marshall JC, et al: 2001 SCCM/ESICM/ACCP/ATS/SIS International Sepsis Definitions Conference. Crit Care Med 2003;31:1250-1256.

BACTEREMIA, SEPSIS, AND SEPTIC SHOCK

Sepsis is a clinical syndrome characterized by extremes of body temperature, heart rate, respiratory rate, and WBC count that occurs in response to an infection. A typical host response to infection involves localized containment and elimination of bacteria and repair of damaged tissue. This process is facilitated by macrophages and dendritic cells and orchestrated by CD4+ T helper cells via the release of both proinflammatory and anti-inflammatory molecules (cytokines, chemokines, interferons). Sepsis occurs when a local infectious process becomes an uncontrolled systemic bloodborne inflammatory response resulting in damage to tissues or organs remote from the initial site of infection or injury.

Definitions

Bacteremia: the presence of viable bacteria in the blood.
Systemic inflammatory response syndrome (SIRS): a clinical syndrome characterized by the 2001 International Sepsis Definitions Conference (Levy et al, 2003) as extremes of body temperature, heart rate, ventilation, and immune response. A detailed list of diagnostic criteria is presented in Table 8–25. **SIRS can occur in response to multiple insults including systemic infection, trauma, thermal injury or a sterile inflammation.**

Sepsis: SIRS and infection either documented or strongly suspected.
Septic shock: an extreme form of sepsis complicated by organ dysfunction and persistent circulatory failure despite fluid and pharmacologic resuscitation.

Pathophysiology

Initial studies of pathophysiologic features of septic shock concentrated on the interactions of LPS from the gram-negative bacterial cell wall with various innate immune system pathways. More recent investigations now focus on understanding the activation and regulation of both the innate and acquired immune systems and the array of cytokines that are released during localized and systemic inflammatory responses.

Bacterial Cell Wall Components in Septic Shock

The exotoxins produced by some bacteria (e.g., exotoxin A produced by *P. aeruginosa*) can initiate septic shock. **However, the bacteria themselves, and in particular their cell wall components, are primarily responsible for the development of septic shock. These components activate numerous innate immunologic pathways including macrophages, neutrophils, and dendritic cells and the complement system. The prime initiator of gram-negative bacterial septic shock is endotoxin, an LPS component of the bacterial outer membrane.** Endotoxin can directly activate the coagulation, complement, and fibrinolytic systems, leading to the release of small molecules that cause vasodilation and increased endothelial permeability (Tapper and Herwald, 2000).

Cytokine Network

Monocytic cells appear to have a pivotal role in mediation of the biologic effects of SIRS and septic shock. Monocytes can remove and detoxify LPS and be beneficial to the host. However, LPS-stimulated monocytes produce cytokines such as tumor necrosis factor (TNF) and interleukin (IL)-1. The intravascular activation of inflammatory systems involved in septic shock is mainly the consequence of an overproduction of these and other cytokines. Production of these cytokines is modulated by CD4+ T helper cells. Type 1 CD4+ T helper cells release proinflammatory cytokines including TNF-α, interferon-γ, and IL-2. These cytokines are also produced by macrophages, endothelial cells, and other cells stimulated by microbial products. The systemic release of large amounts of the cytokine TNF is associated with death from septic shock in humans (Waage et al, 1987; Calandra et al, 1988; Girardin et al, 1988). However, despite the fact that TNF is classically regarded as a central mediator of pathophysiologic changes associated with sepsis, the role of attenuation of this and other proinflammatory cytokines remains unclear. For example, in one animal model of peritonitis, survival was worsened by the administration of antibodies blocking TNF (Eskandari et al, 1992). Also, patients suffering from rheumatoid arthritis treated with TNF-α agents remain susceptible to the development of septic shock. Lastly, a meta-analysis of clinical trials utilizing anti-inflammatory agents in sepsis suggested these agents were generally harmful in all but a small subset of patients (Hotchkiss and Karl, 2003). More recently, anti-inflammatory cytokines, including IL-4 and IL-10, released by type II CD4+ T helper cells, have also been noted to be elevated in sepsis, further illustrating the complex regulation of the both proinflammatory and anti-inflammatory cytokines in a septic patient. In summary, the release of both proinflammatory and anti-inflammatory cytokines are elements of early sepsis; however, the role of cytokine modulation in the treatment of sepsis remains unclear.

Clinical Presentation and Diagnosis

Early signs of the systemic inflammatory response syndrome include temperature extremes (>38° C [100.4° F] or <36° C [96.8° F]), tachycardia (heart rate > 90 beats per minute), tachypnea, and altered mental status. The classic bedside findings differentiating septic shock from other types of shock include a warm patient, brisk capillary refill and a bounding pulse reflecting pyrexia, peripheral vasodilation, and decreased systemic vascular resistance. Other diagnostic criteria include evidence of organ dysfunction such as hypotension, oliguria, or ileus and laboratory abnormalities including leukocytosis or leukopenia, hyperbilirubinemia, hyperlactatemia, hyperglycemia, coagulation abnormalities, and elevated C reactive protein and procalcitonin (see Table 8–25 for complete list of Consensus Conference criteria). The classic clinical presentation of fever and chills followed by hypotension is manifest only in about 30% of patients with

gram-negative bacteremia (McClure, 1983). **Even before temperature extremes and the onset of chills, bacteremic patients often begin to hyperventilate. Thus, the earliest metabolic change in septicemia is a resultant respiratory alkalosis.** In critically ill patients, **the sudden onset of hyperventilation should lead to blood drawing for culture and careful evaluation of the patient. Changes in mental status can also be important clinical clues.** Although the most common pattern is lethargy or obtundation, an occasional patient may become excited, agitated, or combative. Cutaneous manifestations such as the bull's-eye lesion associated with *P. aeruginosa* may be identified.

Metastatic infections secondary to genitourinary tract bacteremia have been described (Siroky et al, 1976). In this review of 137 patients who developed metastatic infections from bacteremia with a genitourinary source, 79% had undergone prior urologic instrumentation, 59% developed skeletal infections, mainly of the spine; and 29% developed endocarditis, most commonly caused by *E. faecalis*.

Bacteriology

In classic studies of sepsis syndrome and septic shock, gram-negative bacteria were predominant organisms isolated in 30% to 80% of cases and gram-positive bacteria in 5% to 24% (Ispahani et al, 1987; Calandra et al, 1988; Bone, 1991). Although *E. coli* is the most common organism causing gramnegative bacteremia, many nosocomial catheter-associated infections are caused by highly resistant gram-negative organisms: *P. aeruginosa*, *Proteus*, *Providencia*, and *Serratia*. *Acinetobacter* and *Enterobacter* are also emerging as important nosocomial pathogens. In a large series, *E. coli* caused about one third of the cases; the *Klebsiella-Enterobacter-Serratia* family, approximately 20%; and *Pseudomonas*, *Proteus*, *Providencia*, and anaerobic species, approximately 10% each (Kreger et al, 1980). Anaerobic organisms may cause bacteremia when the source is a postsurgical intra-abdominal abscess or transrectal prostatic biopsy. **More recent studies suggest the incidence of sepsis caused by both gram-positive bacterial and fungal organisms are increasing** (Martin et al, 2003) **and reinforce the need for initial broad-spectrum antimicrobial coverage.**

Management

The principles of management of sepsis include resuscitation, supportive care, monitoring, administration of broadspectrum antimicrobial agents, and drainage or elimination of infection (Dellinger et al, 2004; Sessler et al, 2004). Although the identification and early intervention of sepsis by the urologist is important, the use of expert consultants is also recommended because management of sepsis and the critically ill patient is complex and always evolving.

Principles of resuscitation include support of the airway and breathing and optimization of perfusion. Intubation and mechanical ventilation may be required in patients who are obtunded and are unable to protect their airway. Supplemental oxygen may be instituted, but supranormal oxygen delivery is no longer considered a goal of therapy (Dellinger et al, 2004). Tissue perfusion should first be optimized with fluid resuscitation to restore mean circulating filling pressures. If additional blood pressure support is needed, vasoactive agents including phenylephrine, norepinephrine, and dopamine can be instituted; however, low-dose dopamine administration for renal protection is no longer recommended by critical care experts. Other principles of resuscitation and supportive care include optimization of oxygen delivery, the use of stress-dose corticosteroid therapy, correction of coagulopathies if clinically significant, maintenance of blood glucose levels below 150 mg/dL, and implementation of hemofiltration as needed.

Identification of the presumptive source of infection and cultures from corresponding fluids and blood should be obtained before the initiation of antimicrobial therapy. Multiple blood cultures for aerobic and anaerobic organisms should be obtained. In addition, all potential sources of bacteremia must be cultured (i.e., urine, sputum, and wounds). Careful attempts to identify the source of infection should be made, because the choice of appropriate antimicrobial coverage depends on the organisms that are thought most likely to cause the infection. The severity of the underlying disease and the possibility of synergistic interactions are also important considerations. If the urinary tract is the most likely portal of entry, an aminoglycoside (gentamicin, tobramycin, or amikacin), alone or in combination, is usually the drug of choice. **Three clinical factors have been predictive of the subsequent isolation of a resistant pathogen: (1) the use of an antimicrobial drug in the last month, (2) advanced age, and (3) male sex** (Leibovici et al, 1992). If the infection is hospital acquired, or if the patient has had multiple infections or is immunocompromised or severely ill, an aminoglycoside and anti-*Pseudomonas* penicillin (carbenicillin, ticarcillin, or piperacillin) or a third-generation cephalosporin should be used. When identification and drug susceptibilities of the offending organism are known, antimicrobial therapy should be changed to use the lowest cost, least toxic antimicrobial with the narrowest antimicrobial coverage. Antimicrobial treatment should be continued until the patient has been afebrile for 3 to 4 days and is clinically stable. Local infections that may have provided the focus for the bacteremia should be treated individually as appropriate.

Recent clinical trials have supported the use of recombinant human activated protein C (drotrecogin alfa), an inhibitor of multiple inflammatory and coagulation pathway components, in the treatment of septic shock. The randomly controlled trial noted significantly lower mortality rates (24.7% vs. 30.8%) in the group treated with activated protein C (Bernard et al, 2001). Shock involves the activation of multiple inflammatory pathways, and it is thought that activated protein C acts to attenuate some of these inflammatory cascades in sepsis. Specific targets of activated protein C include the inhibition of the coagulation factors Va and VIIIa, inhibition of macrophage production of TNF, limitation of thrombin-induced inflammation, and inhibition of plasminogen activator inhibitor. However, the exact pathways through which it acts to reduce mortality in sepsis is poorly understood. Exclusion criteria for the use of drotrecogin alfa exist because potentially significant side effects can occur, including an increased risk of serious bleeding. Thus its use at our institutions is initiated only under the direction of a critical care specialist and pharmacist.

KEY POINTS: BACTEREMIA, SEPSIS, AND SEPTIC SHOCK

- Sepsis is a clinical syndrome characterized by extremes of body temperature, heart rate, respiratory rate, and WBC count that occurs in response to an infection.

- The principles of management of sepsis include resuscitation, supportive care, monitoring, administration of broad-spectrum antimicrobial agents, and drainage or elimination of infection.

BACTERIURIA IN PREGNANCY

Asymptomatic bacteriuria is one of the most common infectious complications of pregnancy. The prevalence of bacteriuria does not change with the occurrence of pregnancy and ranges from 2% to 7% (Hooton et al, 2000). The risk of acquiring bacteriuria during pregnancy increases with duration of pregnancy (Norden and Kass, 1968; Campbell-Brown et al, 1987; Stenqvist et al, 1989), lower socioeconomic class, multiparity, and sickle cell traits (Patterson and Andriole, 1987; Stenqvist et al, 1989).

The site of bacteriuria in the pregnant female patients probably also reflects the situation before conception. In two studies that localized the origin of the bacteriuria, one using the Stamey ureteral catheterization technique and the other the Fairley bladder washout, upper tract infections were found in 44% and 24.5% of pregnant female patients, respectively (Fairley et al, 1966; Heineman and Lee, 1973). In nonpregnant females with recurrent bacteriuria, Stamey (1980) has reported about a 50% probability that the origin is in the upper tract. With other techniques, which may reflect the severity of tissue infection rather than the location of infection, the results are similar; approximately 50% of women with screening bacteriuria of pregnancy are fluorescent antibody-positive (Fa+) and thus have evidence of upper tract infection (Harris et al, 1976). Fairley and his group (1973) found that the site of infection is unrelated to the likelihood that pyelonephritis will develop during pregnancy.

Spontaneous resolution of bacteriuria in pregnant women is unlikely unless treated. Nonpregnant patients often clear their asymptomatic bacteriuria (Hooton et al, 2000), **but pregnant women become symptomatic more frequently and tend to remain bacteriuric** (Elder et al, 1971).

Pyelonephritis develops in 1% to 4% of all pregnant women (Sweet, 1977) **and in 20% to 40% of pregnant women with untreated bacteriuria** (Pedler and Bint, 1987; Wright et al, 1993). **Of the women who develop pyelonephritis during pregnancy, 60% to 75% acquire it during the third trimester** (Cunningham et al, 1973), **when hydronephrosis and stasis in the urinary tract are most pronounced.** From 10% to 20% of pregnant women who get pyelonephritis develop it again before or just after the delivery (Cunningham et al, 1973; Gilstrap et al, 1981). Moreover, a third of pregnant women who develop pyelonephritis have a documented prior history of pyelonephritis (Gilstrap et al, 1981). Treatment of screening bacteriuria of pregnancy decreases the incidence of acute pyelonephritis during pregnancy from a range of 13.5% to 65% to a range of 0% to 5.3% (Sweet, 1977).

In Sweet's excellent review (1977) of bacteriuria and pyelonephritis during pregnancy, he suggests that patients with a renal source of bacteriuria are more likely to have persistent postpartum bacteriuria than those with cystitis alone. In addition, those women with persistent bacteriuria may have an increased incidence of impaired creatinine clearance and urinary concentrating ability and an increased incidence of radiographic changes compatible with chronic pyelonephritis. His review of 12 studies revealed that follow-up excretory urograms in pregnant women with bacteriuria showed an 8% to 33% incidence of radiologic changes compatible with chronic pyelonephritis; the incidence of all urinary tract abnormalities in this group was 18% to 80%.

Zinner and Kass (1971) estimated that approximately 10% of bacteriuric pregnant females have pyelographic evidence of pyelonephritis, and, in their study, these abnormalities were most common in women who had bacteriuria 10 to 14 years after pregnancy. The highest incidence of radiographic changes of pyelonephritis was found in women who had their infections localized to the upper urinary tract (Fairley et al, 1966). In this study, abbreviated excretory urograms were performed within a few days of localization of the infection by ureteral catheterization. Six women (30%) with upper UTIs revealed radiographic renal abnormalities compatible with chronic pyelonephritis on the side to which the infection was localized, and two (10%) had nonexcretion of one kidney with infection in the contralateral one. No patient with an infection localized to the bladder showed radiographic evidence of pyelonephritis.

In their evaluation of renal function, Zinner and Kass (1971) found that women who had had bacteriuria during pregnancy and had it again 10 to 14 years later on follow-up showed significantly lower mean maximal urine osmolalities than those who were not bacteriuric on follow-up. Others have found evidence of decreased creatinine clearance and concentrating ability in bacteriuric women post partum (Sweet, 1977). It is unlikely, however, that uncomplicated bacteriuria in pregnant women produces changes in kidney appearance or function different from those found in nonpregnant bacteriuric women. After following 40 bacteriuric women during pregnancy, Kincaid-Smith (1978) stated that there was no difference in renal size or function between 6 months and 4 years after delivery. Pregnancy, therefore, may provide the opportunity for bacteriuria to be discovered, but this bacteriuria probably reflects only a susceptibility to UTI that was present at conception. **The increased likelihood that bacteriuria may progress to acute pyelonephritis during pregnancy alters the morbidity of bacteriuria for this group.** Treatment of asymptomatic bacteriuria found early in pregnancy has been shown to decrease the prevalence of subsequent acute pyelonephritis from 28% to less than 3% (Sweet, 1977).

Pathogenesis

The anatomic and physiologic changes induced by the gravid state significantly alter the natural history of bacteriuria (Patterson and Andriole, 1987). **These changes may cause pregnant women to be more susceptible to pyelonephritis and may require alteration of therapy.** These changes have been well summarized in several reviews (Davison and Lindheimer, 1978; Waltzer, 1981).

Anatomic and Physiologic Changes during Pregnancy

Increase in Renal Size

Renal length increases approximately 1 cm during normal pregnancy. It is thought that this does not represent true hypertrophy but is the result of increased renal vascular and interstitial volume. No histologic changes have been identified in renal biopsies (Waltzer, 1981).

Smooth Muscle Atony of the Collecting System and Bladder

The collecting system, especially the ureters, undergoes decreased peristalsis during pregnancy, and most women in their third trimester show significant ureteral dilatation (Davison and Lindheimer, 1978; Kincaid-Smith, 1978; Waltzer, 1981) (Fig. 8–39). This hydroureter has been attributed both to the muscle-relaxing effects of increased progesterone during pregnancy and to mechanical obstruction of the ureters by the enlarging uterus at the pelvic brim. Progesterone-induced smooth muscle relaxation also may cause an increased bladder capacity (Waltzer, 1981).

Bladder Changes

The enlarging uterus displaces the bladder superiorly and anteriorly. The bladder becomes hyperemic and may appear congested endoscopically (Waltzer, 1981). Estrogen stimulation probably causes bladder hypertrophy as well as squamous changes of the urethra (Waltzer, 1981).

Augmented Renal Function

The transient increases in glomerular filtration rate and renal plasma flow during pregnancy have been well summarized by several authors and are probably secondary to the increase in cardiac output (Zacur and Mitch, 1977; Davison and Lindheimer, 1978; Kincaid-Smith, 1978; Waltzer, 1981). Glomerular filtration increases by 30% to 50%, and urinary protein excretion increases. The significance of these physiologic changes is apparent when the normal serum creatinine and urea nitrogen values for pregnant women are surveyed (Table 8–26). Values considered normal in nonpregnant women may represent renal insufficiency during pregnancy.

Davison and Lindheimer (1978) recommend that pregnant patients with serum creatinine levels greater than 0.8 mg/dL or urea nitrogen levels greater than 13 mg/dL undergo further

Table 8–26. Average Values for Serum Creatinine and Urea Nitrogen		
	Nonpregnant Females (mg/dL)	Pregnant Females (mg/dL)
Serum creatinine	0.7	0.5
Urea nitrogen	13.0	9.0

Data from Davison JM, Lindheimer MD: Renal disease in pregnant women. Clin Obstet Gynecol 1978;21:411.

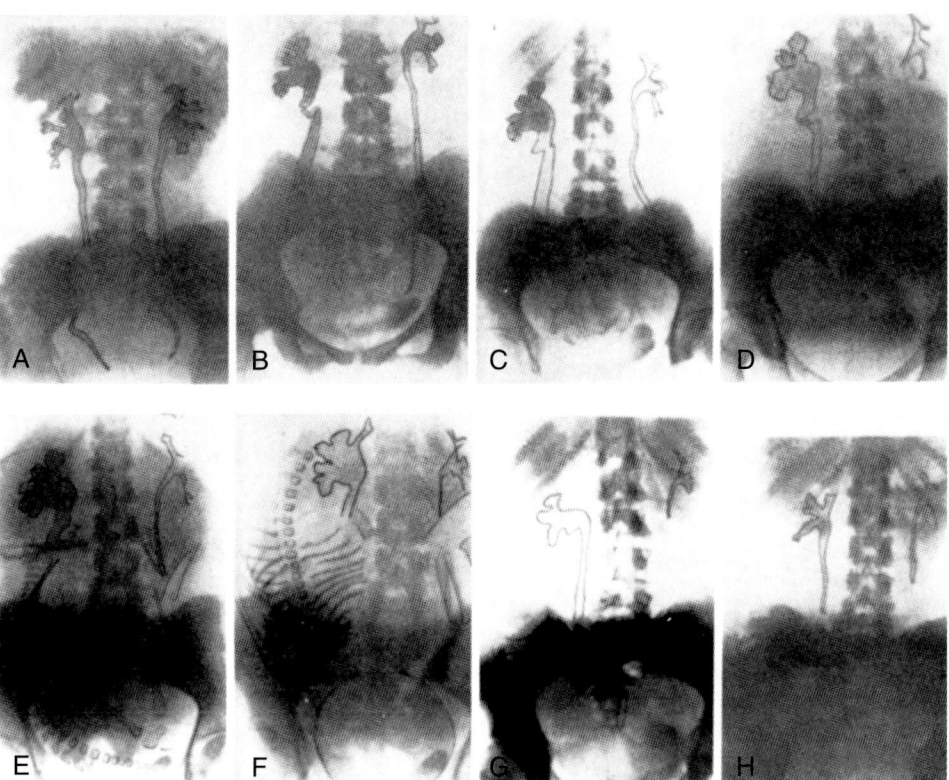

Figure 8-39. Progressive hydroureter and hydronephrosis observed on IVGs during a normal pregnancy. **A,** At 15 weeks; **B,** 18 weeks; **C,** 22 weeks; **D,** 26 weeks; **E,** 34 weeks; **F,** 39 weeks; **G,** 1 week post partum; **H,** 6 weeks post partum. Bilateral hydroureter and hydronephrosis are shown as early as 15 weeks (**A**). **B** to **H,** Successive urograms are from one patient during a normal pregnancy. Dilation occurs mainly on the right side, and both urinary tracts are normal by 6 weeks after delivery. (**A** to **H,** from Hundley JM, Walton HJ, Hibbits JT, et al: Physiologic changes occurring in the urinary tract during pregnancy. Am J Obstet Gynecol 1935;30:625-649.)

evaluation of renal function. Similarly, urinary protein in pregnancy is not considered abnormal until greater than 300 mg of protein in 24 hours is excreted.

These significant physiologic changes in pregnancy, which may develop as early as the first trimester, lead to urinary stasis and mild hydroureteronephrosis, and contribute to development of pyelonephritis.

Recent studies of *E. coli* adhesins and their respective specific tissue receptors have established an adhesin-based mechanism of pyelonephritis-induced preterm births and low birth weights in mice (Kaul et al, 1999). There is a higher incidence of *E. coli*–bearing Dr adhesins during the third trimester of pregnancy in women with gestational pyelonephritis (Nowicki et al, 1994) and an upregulation of Dr adhesin in the kidney, endometrium, and placenta during the third trimester of pregnancy (Martens et al, 1993). When infected intravesically with *E. coli*–bearing Dr adhesin, nearly 90% of mice that were hyporesponsive to bacterial lipopolysaccharide and had a deficient immune response delivered preterm, compared with 10% of mice infected with *E. coli* without Dr adhesin. Also, there was a significant reduction in fetal birth weight in the Dr adhesin–infected group. Bacterial tissue culture showed systemic spread of the *E. coli*–bearing Dr adhesins to the placentae and fetuses.

Complications Associated with Bacteriuria during Pregnancy

Prematurity and Prenatal Mortality

In the preantimicrobial era, pregnant women with symptomatic UTIs and bacterial pyelonephritis were reported to have a high incidence of prematurity, low birth weight, and death (Gilstrap et al, 1981). The relationship between asymptomatic bacteriuria and prematurity is less clear. Gilstrap and colleagues (1981) found no difference in pregnancy among patients treated for asymptomatic bacteriuria as compared with nonbacteriuric controls. **However, because women with asymptomatic bacteriuria are at higher risk for developing a symptomatic UTI that results in adverse fetal sequelae, complications associated with bacteriuria during pregnancy, and pyelonephritis and its possible sequelae, such as sepsis in the mother, all women with asymptomatic bacteriuria should be treated** (Smaill, 2001).

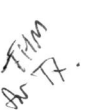

Maternal Anemia

Although several studies suggest that bacteriuria untreated during pregnancy is associated with maternal anemia, not all studies support this. Some difficulties in interpreting the results of these surveys have been caused by inadequate documentation of bacteriuria. In one survey in which urine cultures were obtained by suprapubic aspiration, the data suggest that pregnant patients requiring three or more treatments for bacteriuria have lower levels of serum hemoglobin and folate than controls (McFadyen et al, 1973). In another study from England, investigators showed a statistically significant difference in the incidence of anemia between 410 bacteriuric pregnant women and 409 control pregnant women (Williams et al, 1973). In this survey, 14.6% of bacteriuric women and 10% of control women were anemic at the first prenatal visit. This separation increased during the third trimester (32 weeks), when 25% of women treated with placebo alone had anemia, but only 16.8% of those women treated with antimicrobial agents had anemia. Furthermore, in the 31 untreated (placebo-treated) bacteriuric women who subsequently developed pyelonephritis, the incidence of anemia was 45.2%. These investigators concluded that "untreated bacteriuria increases the likelihood of developing anemia during pregnancy and that this risk is enhanced by the development of acute pyelonephritis, even if it is treated promptly."

Laboratory Diagnosis

Significant false-negative rates occur if screening is conducted by urinalysis or reagent strip testing (Preston et al, 1999; McNair et al, 2000). **Therefore, an initial screening culture should be performed in all pregnant women during the first trimester** (Stenqvist et al, 1989). If the culture shows no growth, repeat cultures are generally unnecessary because patients who have no growth in their urine early in their pregnancy are unlikely to develop bacteriuria later (Norden and Kass, 1968; McFadyen et al, 1973). Pregnant women with a history of recurrent UTI or vesicoureteral reflux may benefit from antimicrobial prophylaxis (Bukowski et al, 1998).

Management

Selection of an antimicrobial agent to treat the bacteriuria must be made, however, with special considerations given to maternal and fetal toxicity. The physiologic changes of pregnancy may decrease tissue and serum drug concentrations. Maternal expanded fluid volume, the distribution of the drug in the fetus, increased renal blood flow, and increased glomerular filtration decrease the serum drug concentration. If the culture is positive, special consideration must be given to the selection of antimicrobial agents chosen to treat infection to prevent fetal toxicity. The pathogens are similar to those seen in nonpregnant women (MacDonald et al, 1983). Table 8–27 lists the antimicrobial agents and dosing for use in pregnancy. The aminopenicillins and cephalosporins are considered safe and generally effective throughout pregnancy. In

patients with penicillin allergy, nitrofurantoin is a reasonable alternative. It may be used safely during the first two trimesters in patients without glucose-6-phosphate dehydrogenase deficiency. Given the low efficacy of short-course β-lactam therapy in nonpregnant women, it is prudent to describe a full 3- to 7-day course of therapy in pregnant women. Follow-up cultures should be obtained to document absence of infection. If the culture is positive, the cause of bacteriuria must be determined to be lack of resolution, bacterial persistence, or reinfection. If the infection is unresolved, proper selection and administration of another drug probably will solve the problem. If the problem is bacterial persistence or rapid reinfection, antimicrobial suppression of infection or prophylaxis (Pfau and Sacks, 1992) throughout the remainder of the pregnancy should be considered.

Pregnant women with acute pyelonephritis should be hospitalized and treated initially with parenteral antimicrobial agents. More than 95% of these patients respond within 24 hours using ampicillin and an aminoglycoside (Cunningham et al, 1973) or cephalosporins (Sanchez-Ramos et al, 1995). Appropriate oral agents should then be given for at least 14 days (Faro et al, 1984). After the treatment course is completed, low-dose prophylaxis with nitrofurantoin, amoxicillin, or cephalexin has been shown to be effective in preventing reinfection (Van Dorsten et al, 1987; Sandberg and Brorson, 1991). The efficacy of postcoital prophylaxis with either cephalexin (250 mg) or nitrofurantoin (50 mg) has been reported (Pfau and Sacks, 1992).

Drugs that are relatively contraindicated during pregnancy include the fluoroquinolones, TMP, chloramphenicol, erythromycin, tetracycline, sulfonamides, and nitrofurantoin. Fluoroquinolones are contraindicated because of their effects on immature cartilage. TMP may have teratogenic effects and should be avoided, especially in the first trimester. The "gray baby" syndrome is a toxic effect of chloramphenicol on neonates resulting from the inability of the infant to metabolize or excrete the drug. Erythromycin may cause cholestatic

Table 8–27. Oral Antimicrobial Agents Used in Pregnancy

Drug	Dosage	Comments
Agents Considered Safe		
Penicillins		
Ampicillin	500 mg QID	Extensively used
Amoxicillin	250 mg TID	Safe and effective
Penicillin V	500 mg QID	Used less frequently but achieves excellent urinary levels
Cephalosporins		
Cephalexin	500 mg QID	Extensively used
Cefaclor	500 mg QID	Somewhat more effective against gram-negatives
Nitrofurantoin	100 mg QID	May result in hemolytic anemia in patients with G6PD deficiency
Sulfisoxazole	1 g, followed by 500 mg QID	May cause kernicterus in the newborn; also may cause hemolytic anemia when G6PD deficiency is present; especially avoid in last few weeks of gestation
Agents That Should Be Avoided		
Fluoroquinolones		Possible damage to immature cartilage
Chloramphenicol		Associated with "gray baby" syndrome
Trimethoprim		May cause megaloblastic anemia because of anti–folic acid action
Erythromycin		Associated with maternal cholestatic jaundice
Tetracyclines		May cause acute liver decompensation in the mother and inhibition of new bone growth in the fetus

G6PD, glucose-6-phosphate dehydrogenase.
Adapted from Schaeffer AJ: Urinary tract infections. In Gillenwater JY, Grayhack JT, Howards SS, Mitchell ME (eds): Adult and pediatric urology. Philadelphia, Lippincott Williams & Wilkins, 2002, pp 211–272.

jaundice in the mother. Tetracycline may cause fetal malformations and maternal liver decompensation. Sulfonamides may cause kernicterus and neonatal hyperbilirubinemia and should be avoided in the third trimester. Nitrofurantoin can cause hemolytic anemia in both mother and child when glucose-6-phosphate dehydrogenase deficiency is present.

Pregnancy in Women with Renal Insufficiency

With current management of recurrent UTIs, infections alone are no contraindication to pregnancy. In patients who have renal insufficiency with or without UTIs, Davison and Lindheimer (1978) emphasize that renal function should be carefully evaluated by both serum creatinine levels and creatinine clearance before a woman is counseled about conceiving or continuing a pregnancy. Although little is known about the outcome of pregnancies with differing degrees of renal insufficiency, it is known that normal pregnancy is rare if the preconception serum creatinine level exceeds 3 mg/dL (about 30 mL/min clearance).

One retrospective analysis of 44 pregnancies in women with preexisting renal disease provides some helpful guidelines about the degree of renal impairment beyond which pregnancy is inadvisable (Bear, 1976). In this study, patients were divided into those with mild renal disease and serum creatinine levels less than 1.5 mg/dL and those with renal disease and serum creatinine levels greater than 1.6 mg/dL. In those with mild renal disease, 34 of 35 pregnancies resulted in normal live births; and although the serum creatinine level remained fixed during the pregnancy (it did not decrease as expected during a normal pregnancy), the pregnancy appeared to have no remote effect on renal function. Conversely, pregnancy in 8 patients with serum creatinine levels greater than 1.6 mg/dL was complicated in all cases, and the incidences of prematurity, delivery by cesarean section, hypertension, and worsening proteinuria and renal insufficiency during pregnancy were increased; 4 of the 8 patients progressed to severe renal failure or death within 18 months. These data have caused Bear (1976) to recommend that conception is ill advised in patients with less than 50% of normal renal function (serum creatinine levels > 1.7 mg/dL or about 50 mL/min clearance).

BACTERIURIA IN THE ELDERLY

UTIs in the elderly are a common and expanding health problem (Kaye, 1980). In 2003, there were almost 34 million Americans older than 65 years (U.S. Census Bureau, 2003). As the life expectancy increases, the diagnosis, treatment, morbidity, and mortality of UTIs in the elderly will assume increasing importance.

Epidemiology

At least 20% of women and 10% of men older than 65 years have bacteriuria (Boscia and Kaye, 1987). In contrast to young adults, in whom bacteriuria is 30 times more prevalent in women than in men, the ratio in women to men with bacteriuria progressively decreases to 2:1. Most elderly patients

> ### KEY POINTS: BACTERIURIA IN PREGNANCY
>
> - Screening for bacteriuria with a culture should be performed in all pregnant women during the first trimester.
> - The prevalence of bacteriuria does not change with the occurrence of pregnancy; however, unlike in nonpregnant women, spontaneous resolution of bacteriuria in pregnant women is unlikely.
> - All pregnant women with bacteriuria should be treated.
> - Bacteriuria more commonly progresses to acute pyelonephritis during pregnancy.
> - Pyelonephritis develops in 1% to 4% of all pregnant women (Sweet, 1977) and in 20% to 40% of pregnant women with untreated bacteriuria.
> - Pregnant women with acute pyelonephritis should be hospitalized and treated initially with parenteral antimicrobial agents.

with bacteriuria are asymptomatic; estimates among women living in nursing homes range from 17% to 55%, as compared with 15% to 31% for their male cohorts (Nicolle, 1994). The prevalence of bacteriuria in the elderly increases with age (Table 8–28) (Sourander, 1966; Brocklehurst et al, 1968) and concurrent disease (Fig. 8–40) and may exceed 50% in selective groups (Boscia and Kaye, 1987; Schaeffer, 1991). Risk factors can be compounded. In a study of 373 women and 150 men older than 68 years, 24% of functionally impaired nursing home residents had bacteriuria compared with 12% of healthy domiciliary subjects (Boscia et al, 1986). Longitudinal studies have clarified the dynamic aspect of bacteriuria in the elderly with frequent, spontaneous alteration between positive and negative urine cultures (Monane et al, 1995) (Fig. 8–41). There is only a small pool of elderly patients with persistent bacteriuria (Kaye, 1980). The incidence of asymptomatic bacteriuria is much more common than is apparent from a single survey, implying that most elderly will eventually have episodes of bacteriuria (Boscia et al, 1986).

Pathogenesis

The pathophysiology of increased susceptibility is multifactorial and poorly understood. **Age-related changes include decline in cell-mediated immunity, neurogenic bladder**

Table 8–28.	Bacteriuria in Two Population Surveys	
Age (yr)	**Men (%)**	**Women (%)**
65-70	2-3	20-21
>80	21-22	23-50

Data from Brocklehurst JC, Dillane JB, Griffiths L, et al: Prevalence and symptomatology of urinary infection in an aged population. Gerontol Clin 1968;10:242-253; and Sourander LB: Urinary tract infections in the aged: An epidemiological study. Ann Med Intern Fenn 1966;55(Suppl 45):7-55.

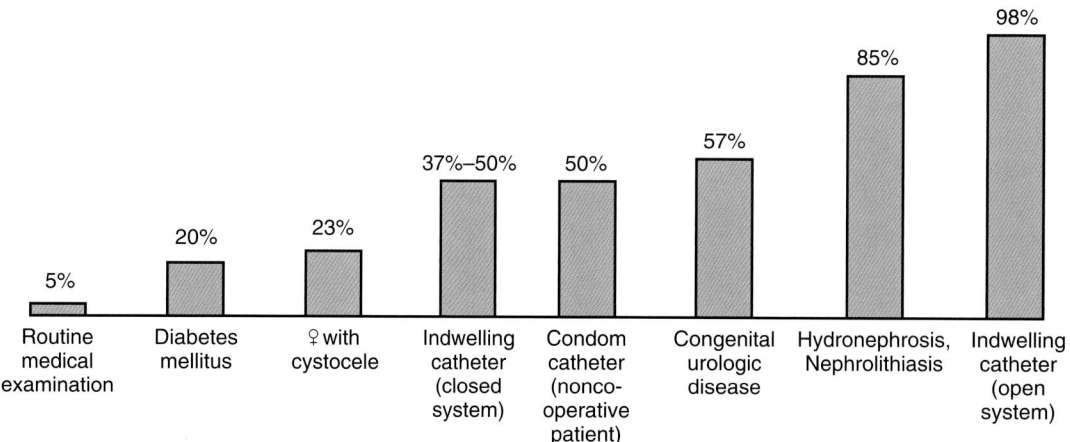

Figure 8–40. Frequency of significant bacteriuria related to underlying disease. (Adapted from Jackson GG, Arana-Sialer JA, Andersen BR: Profiles of pyelonephritis. Arch Intern Med 1962;110: 663-675.)

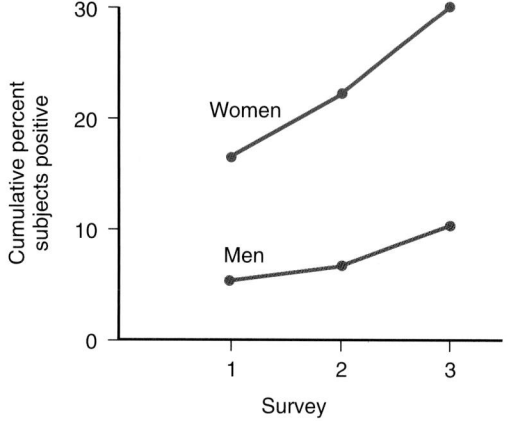

Figure 8–41. Cumulative percentage of subjects (age = 65 years) with at least one positive urine culture survey result over three surveys performed at 6-month intervals. (From Boscia JA, Kobasa WD, Knight RA, et al: Epidemiology of bacteriuria in an elderly ambulatory population. Am J Med 1986;80:208.)

dysfunction, increased perineal soiling as a result of fecal and urinary incontinence, increased incidence of urethral catheter placement, and, in women, changes in the vaginal environment associated with estrogen depletion (Schaeffer, 1991; Raz and Stamm, 1993). Increased receptivity of uroepithelial cells (Reid et al, 1984) and a decrease in prostatic and vaginal antimicrobial factors associated with changes in pH and levels of zinc and hormones have been observed (Boscia et al, 1986). Bacteriologic characteristics of infection in the elderly differ from those in younger patients (Baldassarre and Kaye, 1991). *E. coli* remains the most common uropathogen, causing 75% of these infections. There is a significant increase in the incidence of *Proteus, Klebsiella, Enterobacter, Serratia,* and *Pseudomonas* species, as well as enterococci. Bacteriuria due to gram-positive bacteria is much more common in elderly men than in elderly women (Jackson et al, 1962). *S. saprophyticus* is not seen in this population. Polymicrobial bacteriuria is more common among the elderly (Nicolle et al, 1987). **The shift in the pattern of uropathogens, the high frequency of polymicrobial infections, and antimicrobial resistance in UTIs in the elderly are due in large part to the high frequency of institutionalization and hospitalization,**

catheterization, and antimicrobial usage in this population (Fig. 8–42).

Laboratory Diagnosis

Diagnosis of bacteriuria and UTIs in the elderly can be difficult. **Urinary tract symptoms are often absent, and concomitant disease can mask or mimic UTI. Even severe upper tract infections may not be associated with fever or leukocytosis** (Baldassarre and Kaye, 1991). Therefore a high index of suspicion is warranted, and diagnosis should rely on the results of a carefully obtained urinalysis and culture. The presence of greater than 10^5 cfu/mL of urine remains the standard for diagnosis in these patients. However, counts of 10^2 or more bacteria are clinically significant in catheterized specimens (Kunin, 1987; Nicolle et al, 2005).

Pyuria alone is not a good predictor nor an indication for antimicrobial treatment of bacteriuria in this population (Ouslander et al, 1996; Nicolle et al, 2005). Boscia and associates (1989) reported that more than 60% of women with pyuria of 10 WBCs/mm^3 or greater (noted in midstream specimens) did not have a concurrent bacteriuria. However, the absence of pyuria was a good predictor of the absence of bacteriuria.

Because urinary tract abnormalities can often predispose and complicate bacteriuria in the elderly, a thorough urologic evaluation is warranted. Renal dysfunction, calculi, hydronephrosis, urinary retention, neurogenic bladder dysfunction, and other abnormalities should be identified by serum creatinine measurement, excretory urography, CT, ultrasonography, urodynamics, and/or cystoscopy. The timing and sequence of these tests should be dictated by the clinical setting.

Significance of Screening Bacteriuria

Screening for asymptomatic bacteriuria in elderly residents in the community or long-term care facilities is not recommended (Nicolle et al, 1983; Nordenstam et al, 1986; Boscia et al, 1987; Abrutyn et al, 1994). There is no documented relationship between asymptomatic bacteriuria and uncomplicated UTIs and worsening renal function in this population. The treatment of asymptomatic bacteriuria to improve incontinence has not been justified (Baldassarre and Kaye, 1991;

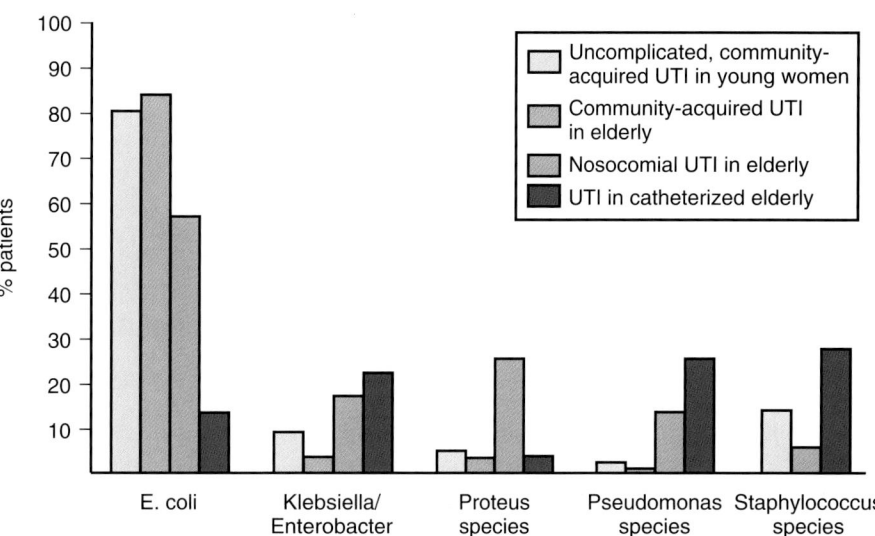

Figure 8-42. Microbiology of urinary tract infections. (Data compiled from Stark RP, Maki DG: Bacteriuria in the catheterized patient: What quantitative level of bacteriuria is relevant? N Engl J Med 1984;311:560-564; Kunin CM: Detection, Prevention, and Management of Urinary Tract Infections, 4th ed. Philadelphia, Lea & Febiger, p xiii; Nicolle LE, Bjornson J, Harding GKM: Bacteriuria in elderly institutionalized men. N Engl J Med 1983;309:1420-1425; Krieger JN, Kaiser DL, Wenzel RP: Urinary tract etiology of bloodstream infections in hospitalized patients. J Infect Dis 1983;148:57-62.)

Ouslander et al, 1995). Although studies have demonstrated decreased survival in bacteriuric patients compared with nonbacteriuric control subjects, it is unclear whether increased mortality rates and bacteriuria are causally related (Baldassarre and Kaye, 1991; Abrutyn et al, 1994).

Studies that have found a significantly increased mortality among persons with bacteriuria have looked at populations that were heterogeneous in terms of age and underlying disease (Dontas et al, 1981; Latham et al, 1985). An age difference of only 2 years increases mortality by 20% (Dontas et al, 1968). Therefore, in the studies mentioned previously (Dontas et al, 1968) and others (Abrutyn et al, 1994), it is not clear how much of the observed association between bacteriuria and mortality was due to differences in age between the bacteriuric and the abacteriuric groups. In a study of bacteriuria and mortality in a homogeneous 70-year-old population, the association between bacteriuria and mortality was weaker and linked to fatal diseases not attributable to bacteriuria (Dontas et al, 1968). Nicolle and associates (1987) randomized institutionalized women with bacteriuria to treatment or observation and followed these patients for more than 1 year. Treatment did not result in improved survival and was associated with a number of adverse effects.

Bacteriuria that leads to UTIs in elderly subjects in the presence of underlying structural urinary tract abnormalities (e.g., obstruction with hydronephrosis) or systemic conditions (e.g., severe diabetes mellitus) are clinically significant, can lead to renal failure, and require prompt therapy. In addition, UTIs caused by urea-splitting bacteria, such as *Proteus* or *Klebsiella* species that cause formation of infection stones, may also lead to severe renal damage.

Sepsis and its sequelae (sepsis syndrome and septic shock) are increasingly common in the elderly. This is in part due to the aggressive use of catheters (Kunin et al, 1992) and other invasive equipment, implantation of prosthetic devices, and the administration of chemotherapy to cancer patients or corticosteroids in other immunosuppressed patients with organ transplants or inflammatory diseases. In addition, modern medical care has given longer life spans to the elderly and patients with metabolic, neoplastic, or immunodeficiency disorders, who remain at increased risk for infection.

Management

Prospective randomized comparative trials of antimicrobial or no therapy in elderly male and female nursing home residents with asymptomatic bacteriuria consistently document no benefit of antimicrobial therapy. There was no decrease in symptomatic episodes and no improvement in survival. In fact, treatment with antimicrobial therapy increases the occurrence of adverse drug effects and reinfection with resistant organisms and increases the cost of treatment. **Therefore, asymptomatic bacteriuria in elderly residents of long-term care facilities should not be treated with antimicrobial agents.**

If patients present with lower tract symptoms, 7 days of therapy is recommended. For individuals presenting with fever or more severe systemic infection 10 to 14 days of therapy is recommended. The goal in this population is to eliminate symptoms but not sterilize the urine (McMurdo and Gillespie, 2000).

The 10% to 15% decrease in susceptibility of uropathogens to β-lactams, TMP-SMX, and fluoroquinolones in isolates from nursing home residents is disturbing and most likely due to a pattern of empirical prescribing in the nursing homes. In contrast, the susceptibility of isolates from patients with acute uncomplicated UTI in an outpatient setting has not changed appreciably in 10 years. The difference in susceptibility between the isolates from the outpatient and nursing home settings can be attributed to the presence of additional risk factors for antimicrobial resistance in the latter group. These risk factors include frequent antimicrobial usage, overcrowding, underlying pathology, and the presence of catheters and other invasive devices. Antimicrobial use needs to be guided by current surveillance studies of targeted uropathogenic bacteria and implemented (Vromen et al, 1999).

The elderly population is more susceptible than young patients to the toxic and adverse effects of antimicrobial agents (Grieco, 1980; Carty et al, 1981; Boscia et al, 1986) because the metabolism and excretion of antimicrobial agents may be impaired, and resulting increased serum levels can further damage renal function. Interactions with other medications can occur (Stahlmann and Lode, 2003). The safety margin between therapeutic and toxic doses is significantly narrowed. Therefore, antimicrobial agents must be used judiciously, and dosing and drug levels should be carefully monitored.

The fluoroquinolones are effective in this population, and the side effects are not more apparent than in a younger population. However, fluoroquinolones can cause QT interval prolongation, and therefore, they should be avoided in patients with known prolongation of the QT interval, patients with uncorrected hypokalemia or hypomagnesemia, and patients receiving some antiarrhythmic agents (Stahlmann and Lode, 2003).

Chondrotoxicity of fluoroquinolones has led to restricted use in pediatric patients, but there is no indication that similar effects could occur in joint cartilage of adults. Tendinitis and tendon ruptures have occurred in rare cases. Chronic renal diseases, concomitant use of corticosteroids, and age older than 60 years have been recognized as risk factors for fluoroquinolone-induced tendon disorders (Stahlmann and Lode, 2003).

KEY POINTS: BACTERIURIA IN THE ELDERLY

- Bacteriuria is very common in both elderly women and men.

- Screening for bacteriuria is not recommended in elderly patients because there is no relationship between asymptomatic bacteriuria and uncomplicated UTIs or deteriorating renal function; asymptomatic bacteriuria should not be treated.

- Infections of the urinary tract may present as subtle signs, and a high index of suspicion is often required for diagnosis.

- Treatment of symptomatic UTI requires modifications for physiologic and pathophysiologic conditions of the elderly.

CATHETER-ASSOCIATED BACTERIURIA

Catheter-associated bacteriuria is the most common hospital-acquired infection, accounting for up to 40% of such infections and more than 1 million per year (Haley et al, 1985; Stamm, 1991). **The development of bacteriuria in the presence of an indwelling catheter is inevitable and occurs at an incidence of approximately 10% per day of catheterization.** Intermittent catheterization has been associated with rates of bacteriuria of less than 1% in healthy individuals and 15% in elderly hospitalized patients (Turck et al, 1968). The most important risk factors associated with increased likelihood of developing catheter-associated bacteriuria are duration of catheterization, female gender, absence of systemic antimicrobial agents, and catheter-care violations (Stamm, 1991). Most catheter-associated UTIs are asymptomatic. In patients with short-term catheter placement, only 10% to 30% of bacteriuric episodes produce typical symptoms of acute infection (Haley et al, 1981; Hartstein et al, 1981). Similarly,

although patients with long-term catheters are bacteriuric, the incidence of febrile episodes occurs at a rate of only 1 per 100 days of catheterization (Warren, 1991). **The extra direct cost associated with catheter-associated UTIs is about $600 per year per patient.** The nosocomial costs for *E. coli* infections with relatively susceptible strains are considerably lower than for those caused by resistant gram-negative bacteria, which often require expensive parenteral antimicrobial therapy (Tambyah et al, 2002).

Pathogenesis

Bacteria enter the urinary tract of a catheterized patient by several routes. Bacteria can be introduced at the time of initial catheter placement by either mechanical inoculation of urethral bacteria or contamination from poor technique. Subsequently, the bacteria most commonly gain access via a periurethral or intraluminal route (Stamm, 1991). In women, periurethral entry is the most prevalent. Daifuku and Stamm (1984) found that among 18 women who developed catheter-associated bacteriuria, 12 had antecedent urethral colonization with the infecting strain. Bacteria may also enter the drainage bag and follow the intraluminal route to the bladder. This route is particularly common in patients who are clustered among other patients with indwelling catheters (Maizels and Schaeffer, 1980; Tambyah et al, 1999).

The urinary catheter system provides a unique environment that allows for two distinct populations of bacteria: those that grow within the urine and another population that grows on the catheter surface. A biofilm represents a microbial environment of bacteria embedded in an extracellular matrix of bacterial products and host proteins that often lead to catheter encrustation (Stamm, 1991). Certain bacteria, particularly of the *Pseudomonas* and *Proteus* species, are adept at biofilm growth, which may explain their higher incidence in this clinical setting (Mobley and Warren, 1987). The uropathogens isolated from the catheterized urinary tract often differ from those found in noncatheterized ambulatory patients. *E. coli* is still the most common organism isolated, but *Pseudomonas, Proteus,* and *Enterococcus* species are very prevalent (Warren, 1991). In patients with long-term catheterization of more than 30 days, the bacteriuria is usually polymicrobial and the presence of four or five pathogens is not uncommon (Warren et al, 1982). Although certain species may persist for long periods, the bacterial populations in these patients tend to be dynamic.

Clinical Presentation

Most patients are asymptomatic. Suprapubic discomfort and development of fever, chills, or flank pain may indicate a symptomatic UTI.

Laboratory Diagnosis

Significant bacteriuria in patients with catheters is present when greater than 100 cfu/mL is present because even this low level progresses to greater than 10^5 cfu/mL in almost all patients (Maizels and Schaeffer, 1980; Stark and Maki, 1984). Pyuria is not a discriminate indicator of infection in this population.

Management

Careful aseptic insertion of the catheter and maintenance of a closed dependent drainage system are essential to minimize development of bacteriuria. The catheter-meatal junction should be cleaned daily with water, but antimicrobial agents should be avoided because they lead to colonization with resistant pathogens, such as *Pseudomonas.*

Incorporation of silver oxide (Schaeffer et al, 1988) or silver alloy (Saint et al, 1998) into the catheter and hydrogen peroxide into the drainage bag has been reported to decrease the incidence of bacteriuria in some studies (Schaeffer et al, 1988) but not in other populations (Stamm, 1991). The major benefit of silver alloy is in decreasing the likelihood of bacteriuria in hospitalized adults catheterized short term (Newton et al, 2002; Saint et al, 2000; Brosnahan et al, 2004). If an asymptomatic catheterized patient has had an indwelling catheter for 3 or more days, and will have the catheter removed, a dipstick test can be used to rule out bacteriuria (Tissot et al, 2001). **Concurrent administration of systemic antimicrobial agents transiently decreases the incidence of bacteriuria associated with short-term catheterization, but after 3 to 4 days the incidence of bacteriuria is similar to the rate in catheterized patients not taking systemic antimicrobials agents, and the prevalence of resistant bacteria and side effects is substantial.** The concept of instilling nonvirulent bacteria into the bladder to completely block colonization and infection by pathogens has been tested in patients with spinal cord injuries (Hull et al, 2000). Patients successfully colonized with the nonvirulent strain had reduced symptomatic UTI and a subjective improvement in quality of life.

Patients with indwelling catheters should only be treated if they become symptomatic (e.g., febrile). Urine cultures should be performed before initiating antimicrobial therapy. The antimicrobial agent should be discontinued within 48 hours of resolution of the infection. If the catheter has been indwelling for several weeks, encrustation may shelter bacteria from the antimicrobial agent; therefore, the catheter should be changed.

When a catheter is to be removed and there is a high probability of bacteriuria or the dipstick test is positive, a culture should be obtained 24 hours before removal (Tissot et al, 2001). **If the probability is low or the dipstick is negative, a culture may not be necessary. The patient should be started on empirical antimicrobial therapy such as TMP-SMX or a fluoroquinolone just before de-catheterization and maintained on therapy for 2 days. A post-therapy culture should be obtained 7 to 10 days later to confirm the eradication of the bacteriuria.**

MANAGEMENT OF UTI IN PATIENTS WITH SPINAL CORD INJURY

Patients with spinal cord injury have unique concerns that affect the risk, diagnosis, and management of UTIs, which are all considered complicated.

Epidemiology

UTIs are among the most common urologic complications of spinal cord injury. It has been estimated that approximately

---

KEY POINTS: CATHETER-ASSOCIATED BACTERIURIA

- Careful aseptic insertion of the catheter and maintenance of a closed dependent drainage system are essential to minimize development of bacteriuria.

- The development of catheter associated bacteriuria is inevitable.

- If an infection is suspected in a catheterized patient, a culture should be obtained and antimicrobial therapy initiated before de-catheterization.

- Only symptomatic catheter-associated UTIs require treatment.

- Antimicrobial therapy should be continued for 2 to 3 days and a post-therapy culture obtained 7 to 10 days later.

33% of spinal cord–injured patients have bacteriuria at any time (Stover et al, 1989) and that eventually almost all of spinal cord–injured patients will become bacteriuric and many will suffer significant morbidity and mortality. One prospective study of patients on intermittent catheterization or condom catheterization reported an incidence of significant bacteriuria of 18 episodes per person per year and an annual incidence of febrile UTIs of 1.8 per person per year (Waites et al, 1993). In addition, UTI is the most common cause of fever in the spinal cord–injured patient (Beraldo et al, 1993). **The 1992 National Institute on Disability and Rehabilitation Research Consensus Conference (1993) examined the problems associated with UTIs in spinal cord–injured patients. Among the risk factors identified were impaired voiding, overdistention of the bladder, elevated intravesical pressure, increased risk of urinary obstruction, vesicoureteral reflux, instrumentation, and increased incidence of stones. Other factors that have been implicated are decreased fluid intake, poor hygiene, perineal colonization, decubiti and other evidence of local tissue trauma, and reduced host defense associated with chronic illness** (Gilmore et al, 1992; Waites et al, 1993).

Pathogenesis

The method of bladder management has profound impact on UTI. The National Institute on Disability and Rehabilitation Research Consensus Conference (1993) noted that indwelling catheters were most likely to lead to UTI and that the vast majority of patients with an indwelling catheter for 30 days are bacteriuric. Suprapubic catheters and indwelling urethral catheters eventually have an equivalent infection rate (Kunin et al, 1987; Tambyah and Maki, 2000; Biering-Sorensen, 2002). However, the onset of bacteriuria may be delayed using a suprapubic catheter compared with a urethral catheter. During a 2-year period, 170 patients with spinal cord injury were evaluated regarding type of urinary drainage and infection (Warren et al, 1982). In patients using indwelling urethral catheters, all urine cultures were positive. The corresponding values for the suprapubic catheter group were 44%. Condom drainage systems are also associated with an incidence of bacteriuria from 63% (Dukes, 1928) to almost 100% (Pyrah et al, 1955).

Since its introduction by Lapides and colleagues (1972), clean (but not sterile) intermittent catheterization (CIC) has earned general recognition in the management of spinal cord injury patients (National Institute on Disability and Rehabilitation Research, 1993). **Although never rigorously compared with indwelling urethral catheterization, CIC has been shown to decrease lower tract complications by maintaining low intravesical pressure and reducing the incidence of stones** (Stover et al, 1989). CIC also appears to reduce complications associated with an indwelling catheter, such as UTI, fever, bacteremia, and local infections such as epididymitis and prostatitis. Weld and Dmochowski (2000) followed 316 patients with spinal cord injury with different bladder management for a mean of 18.3 years and recorded all complications. The CIC group had statistically significantly lower complication rates compared with the urethral catheterization group and no significantly higher complication rates relative to all other management methods for each type of complication studied. Thus, it is generally agreed that CIC places patients with spinal cord injury at the lowest risk for significant long-term urinary tract complications (Stamm, 1975).

There is conflicting evidence over the value of sterile versus nonsterile or "no touch" methods of CIC. Some studies have reported a lower incidence of infection in patients treated with sterile techniques (Foley, 1929), whereas others have not (Pyrah et al, 1955; Nyren et al, 1981). Bennett and coworkers (1997) reported on a sterile method of CIC that uses an introducer tip to bypass the distal 1.5 cm of the urethra and showed a significant decrease in UTI with the use of the urethral introducer tip. Different types of catheters have been used for CIC. The low-friction catheters might be less traumatic for the urethra (Casewell and Phillips, 1977; Garibaldi et al, 1980), but their impact on bacteriuria and UTI has to be studied.

Clinical Presentation

The majority of patients with spinal cord injury with bacteriuria are asymptomatic. Because of a loss of sensation, patients usually do not experience frequency, urgency, or dysuria. More often, they complain of flank, back, or abdominal discomfort, leakage between catheterizations, increased spasticity, malaise, lethargy, and/or cloudy, malodorous urine. UTI is the most common cause of fever in spinal cord–injured patients (Beraldo et al, 1993).

Bacteriology and Laboratory Diagnosis

Urinalysis will show bacteriuria and pyuria. Pyuria is not diagnostic of infections, because it may occur from the irritative effects of the catheter. The National Institute on Disability and Rehabilitation Research Consensus Statement (1993) recommended the following criteria for the diagnosis of significant bacteriuria in spinal cord–injured patients. Any detectable bacteria from indwelling or suprapubic catheter aspirates was considered significant because the vast majority of patients with an indwelling catheter and low-level bacteri-

uria showed an increase to greater than 10^5 cfu/mL within a short period of time (Cardenas and Hooton, 1995). For patients on CIC, greater than or equal to 10^2 cfu/mL was considered significant. For catheter-free males, a clean voided specimen showing greater than or equal to 10^4 cfu/mL was considered significant.

Bacteriuria in patients with spinal cord injury differs from that in patients with intact spinal cords in its etiology, complexity, and antimicrobial susceptibility and is influenced by the type and duration of catheterization. E. coli is isolated in approximately 20% of patients. Enterococci, *P. mirabilis*, and *Pseudomonas* are more common among spinal cord–injured patients than patients with intact spinal cords. Other common organisms are *Klebsiella* species, *Serratia* species, *Staphylococcus*, and *Candida* species. Most bacteriuria in short-term catheterization is of a single organism, whereas patients catheterized for longer than a month will usually demonstrate a polymicrobial flora caused by a wide range of gram-negative and gram-positive bacterial species (Edwards et al, 1983). Such specimens commonly have two to four bacterial species, each at concentrations of 10^5 cfu/mL or more (Monson and Kunin, 1974; Nickel et al, 1987). Some may have up to six to eight species at that concentration (Monson and Kunin, 1974). This phenomenon is due to an incidence of new episodes of bacteriuria approximately every 2 weeks and the ability of these strains to persist for weeks and months in the catheterized urinary tract (Edwards et al, 1983; Gabriel et al, 1996). Two of the most persistent species are *E. coli* and *Providencia stuartii*. *P. stuartii* is rarely found outside the long-term catheterized urinary tract and may use the catheter itself as a niche (Lindberg et al, 1975; Hockstra, 1999).

Management

Because of the diverse flora and high probability of bacterial resistance, a urine culture must be obtained before initiating empirical therapy. For afebrile patients, an oral fluoroquinolone is the agent of choice (Cardenas and Hooton, 1995). β-Lactams, TMP-SMX, and nitrofurantoin are not recommended because of the high prevalence of bacterial resistance to these drugs. An indwelling catheter should be changed to ensure maximal drainage and eliminate bacterial foci in catheter encrustations. **Spinal cord–injured patients with fever or chills are usually admitted and treated with a parenteral aminoglycoside and a penicillin or a third-generation cephalosporin** (Cardenas and Hooton, 1995).

If clinical improvement does not occur within 24 to 48 hours, reculture and adjustment of antimicrobial therapy based on the initial culture and susceptibility should be performed. Imaging studies should be obtained to rule out obstruction, stones, and abscess. The duration of therapy is not established, but 4 to 5 days is recommended for the mildly symptomatic patient and 10 to 14 days for sicker patients (Cardenas and Hooton, 1995). Post-therapy cultures are usually not necessary because asymptomatic recolonization is common and not clinically significant. However, if a ureasplitting bacterium is identified, a follow-up culture should be obtained to ensure its eradication. Spinal cord–injured patients with recurrent symptomatic UTIs should undergo urinary tract imaging and urodynamic testing and a review of their bladder management program with particular attention to catheter drainage, intermittent catheterization techniques, and frequency of intermittent catheterization or voiding schedule (Cardenas and Hooton, 1995).

Antimicrobial prophylaxis is not supported for most patients who have neurogenic bladder caused by spinal cord injury (Morton et al, 2002). Antimicrobial prophylaxis did not significantly decrease symptomatic UTIs and resulted in an approximately twofold increase in antimicrobial-resistant bacteria.

Recurrent UTIs may be associated with high storage pressures, and intervention to decrease storage pressure may decrease the incidence of symptomatic UTI. Evidence from studies in spinal cord–injured patients suggests that bladder catheterization for longer than 10 years is associated with an increased risk of carcinoma of the bladder. West and colleagues (1999) examined two databases with more than 33,000 spinal cord–injured patients and identified 130 patients with bladder cancer (0.4%) during a 5-year period. Several risk factors for bladder cancer have been proposed. Vereczky and associates (Weyrauch and Bassett, 1951) tested different risk factors based on the outcome of 153 spinal cord–injured patients in which 7 were diagnosed with bladder cancer. Of a total of 31 possible predictors, only duration of catheterization was significant. **Chronic infection and inflammation of the bladder mucosa could be the carcinogenic stimulus in these patients (Pyrah et al, 1955). Nitrosamines produced in infected urine have also been implicated** (Najenson et al, 1969).

For further discussion of spinal cord injury and urinary infection, see Chapter 59, "Lower Urinary Tract Dysfunction in Neurologic Injury and Disease."

KEY POINTS: MANAGEMENT OF UTI IN PATIENTS WITH SPINAL CORD INJURY

- UTI in patients with spinal cord injury commonly presents as fever, flank, back, or abdominal discomfort, leakage between catheterizations, increased spasticity, malaise, lethargy, and/or cloudy, malodorous urine.
- The majority of spinal cord–injured patients with bacteriuria are asymptomatic.
- Only symptomatic patients require therapy.
- Urine culture before the initiation of empirical therapy is essential because spinal cord–injured patients often culture diverse flora with a high probability of bacterial resistance.
- Clean intermittent catheterization places patients with spinal cord injury at the lowest risk for significant long-term urinary tract complications.
- Chronic infection can be carcinogenic.

FUNGURIA

Funguria is usually associated with predisposing factors, including indwelling catheters, antimicrobial therapy, diabetes mellitus, hospitalization, and immunosuppressed states (Krcmery et al, 1999).

Clinical Presentation

Fungi may invade the kidneys as the result of hematogenous spread from other sources of infection or the gastrointestinal tract. *C. albicans* accounts for approximately 50% of positive fungal cultures (Michigan, 1976). *Candida glabrata* is the second most common fungus, representing 10% to 15% of positive fungal cultures. *C. glabrata* is a normal commensal organism of the gastrointestinal tract and vagina and probably colonizes the urinary tract by ascending infection.

Asymptomatic funguria, implying urinary colonization rather than infection, is common. Invasive infection is suggested by the presence of irritative voiding symptoms and pyuria. Renal or perinephric abscesses and fungus balls (also known as bezoars) may result from funguria. These patients may demonstrate symptoms suggestive of pyelonephritis with flank pain and fever. However, fungal balls may develop in the collecting system of asymptomatic patients.

Laboratory Diagnosis

The criteria for diagnosis are unclear. Particularly in women, vaginal or perineal colonization may contaminate urine specimens. Microscopic examination can reveal fungi budding forms or pseudohyphae. The presence of pyuria does not correlate well with the presence of symptoms or the degree of funguria. Cultures of 10,000 to 15,000 cfu/mL have been suggested as cutoff points for infection (Kozinin et al, 1978). Regardless of the count, a positive culture requires evaluation.

Management

A treatment algorithm for genitourinary fungal infection has been presented by Wise (1990) (Fig. 8–43). **Before antifungal therapy, predisposing factors to funguria should be eliminated.** Unnecessary indwelling catheters should be removed and the nutritional status should be optimized. Discontinuation of broad-spectrum antimicrobial agents reduces fungal colonization. The majority of patients with asymptomatic funguria do not require treatment. Up to 75% of patients will clear spontaneously (Kauffman et al, 2000). However, if a patient is symptomatic or requires eradication of funguria before urologic surgery, topical, oral, or parenteral therapy is indicated.

If, after removal of the catheter, fungal infection persists, amphotericin B may be instilled intravesically for up to 1 week. Fifty milligrams of amphotericin B dissolved in 1 L of sterile water is introduced into the bladder via a three-way catheter over a 24-hour period (Wise et al, 1982). Alternatively, 200 to 300 mL of irrigant may be instilled for 1 to 2 hours with clamping of the catheter. Fluconazole is commonly used as a bladder irrigant, while amphotericin B is used more rarely (e.g., in cases of resistant fungal infections) (Wise, 2005). Amphotericin B may also be instilled via nephrostomy tube for upper tract fungal infection.

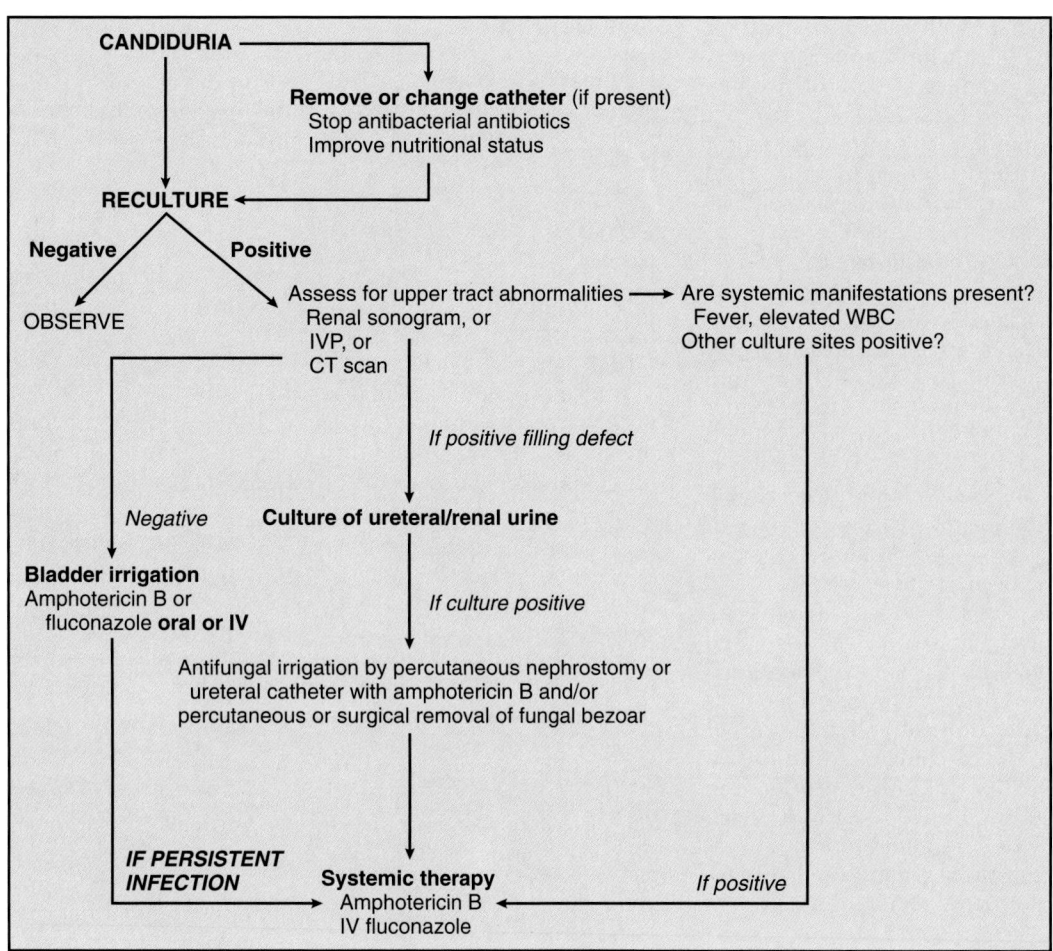

Figure 8–43. Treatment algorithm for management of suspected candiduria. IVP, excretory pyelogram (Wise, 1990).

Funguria also may be treated effectively with oral agents. Flucytosine is readily absorbed from the gastrointestinal tract and is primarily excreted renally. A dosage of 100 to 200 mg/kg per day in four divided doses for 2 to 3 weeks is recommended. Dosing adjustments should be made for patients with renal insufficiency. Wise and associates (Wise et al, 1980) reported success (as defined by a decrease in colony counts or clinical improvement) in 212 of 225 patients treated for 21 to 28 days. Fungal resistance was reported in 14 of the patients. Flucytosine may be used in combination with amphotericin B bladder irrigation. Side effects include an elevation in liver function test results, diarrhea, and agranulocytosis.

Fluconazole is a triazole antifungal agent that is readily absorbed from the gastrointestinal tract and is excreted predominantly in unchanged form in the urine. Dosing is typically 200 mg for the first day followed by 100 mg daily for 10 to 14 days. Success rates of greater than 75% to 80% have been reported in studies treating *Candida* species with limited numbers of patients (Nito, 1989; Bamberger et al, 1992; McGuire and Wise, 1992). Oral fluconazole has been shown to be as effective and safe as amphotericin B bladder irrigation for treatment of older adults with funguria (Jacobs et al, 1996). The most common side effects present in 60% of patients include nausea, headache, rash, abdominal pain, vomiting, and diarrhea (Grant and Clissold, 1990).

Patients with renal candidiasis and disseminated infection are usually treated with intravenous amphotericin B.

Amphotericin B acts in a fungicidal fashion by binding to the fungal cell membranes, eventually resulting in disruption of the internal cellular components. Fungal resistance is uncommon. Because excretion is primarily biliary, amphotericin B may be administered to patients with renal insufficiency with caution because of its nephrotoxic effects, but without need for dosing adjustment. Side effects of significance with amphotericin B include chills, rigor, fevers, phlebitis, bone marrow toxicity, and potassium and magnesium depletion. After an initial dose of 1 mg, the dose may be increased gradually in daily increments of 5 mg to a maintenance dose of 0.3 to 1.2 mg/kg. Daily dosing should not exceed 50 mg. Although strict guidelines for duration of total amount of therapy do not exist, most renal infections require between 500 mg and 1.5 g to 2 g over a 6- to 12-week period (Medoff and Kobayashi, 1980). Liposomal amphotericin is an effective alternative in patients who are at risk for nephrotoxic side effects. Fluconazole has not been used extensively for upper tract infections, but when given intravenously, it has been shown to be effective in treating systemic candidiasis in critically ill patients (Kujath and Lerch, 1989; Anaissie et al, 1991; Corbella et al, 1992; Graninger et al, 1993).

The presence of fungal balls and accompanying obstruction should be assessed in patients with suspected upper tract funguria. Fungal balls typically involve *Candida* species because of their propensity to develop pseudohyphae. Patients with upper tract obstruction are especially prone to fungemia.

The patients often require the placement of percutaneous nephrostomy tubes to relieve the obstruction. This tube may then be used to instill antifungal irrigant or to provide a tract for access for percutaneous endourologic removal of the fungal ball. (For more information, see Chapter 14, "Tuberculosis and Other Opportunistic Infections of the Genitourinary System.")

KEY POINTS: FUNGURIA

■ Funguria is commonly associated with predisposing factors including indwelling catheters, antimicrobial therapy, diabetes mellitus, hospitalization, and immunosuppressed states.

■ Symptomatic funguria may be treated with topical, oral, or parenteral antifungal therapy.

OTHER INFECTIONS

Fournier's Gangrene

Fournier's gangrene is a form of necrotizing fasciitis occurring about the male genitalia. It is also known as idiopathic gangrene of the scrotum, streptococcal scrotal gangrene, perineal phlegmon, and spontaneous fulminant gangrene of the scrotum (Fournier, 1883, 1884). As originally reported by Baurienne in 1764, and by Fournier in 1883, it was characterized by an abrupt onset of a rapidly fulminating genital gangrene of idiopathic origin in previously healthy young patients that resulted in gangrenous destruction of the genitalia. The disease now differs from these descriptions in that it involves a broader age range, including older patients (Bejanga, 1979; Wolach et al, 1989), follows a more indolent course, and has a less abrupt onset; and, in approximately 95% of the cases, a source can now be identified (Macrea, 1945; Burpee and Edwards, 1972; Kearney and Carling, 1983; Jamieson et al, 1984; Spirnak et al, 1984).

Infection most commonly arises from the skin, urethra, or rectal regions. An association between urethral obstruction associated with strictures and extravasation and instrumentation has been well documented. **Predisposing factors include diabetes mellitus, local trauma, paraphimosis, periurethral extravasation or urine, perirectal or perianal infections, and surgery such as circumcision or herniorrhaphy.** In cases originating in the genitalia, the infecting bacteria probably pass through Buck's fascia of the penis and spread along the dartos fascia of the scrotum and penis, Colles' fascia of the perineum, and Scarpa's fascia of the anterior abdominal wall. In view of the typical foul odor associated with this condition, a major role for anaerobic bacteria is likely. Wound cultures generally yield multiple organisms, implicating anaerobic-aerobic synergy (Meleney, 1933; Miller, 1983; Cohen, 1986). Mixed cultures containing facultative organisms (*E. coli, Klebsiella,* enterococci) along with anaerobes (*Bacteroides, Fusobacterium, Clostridium,* microaerophilic streptococci) have been obtained from the lesions.

Clinical Presentation

Patients frequently have a history of recent perineal trauma, instrumentation, urethral stricture associated with sexually transmitted disease, or urethral cutaneous fistula. Pain, rectal bleeding, and a history of anal fissures suggest a rectal source of infection. Dermal sources are suggested by history of acute and chronic infections of the scrotum and spreading recurrent hidradenitis suppurativa or balanitis.

The infection commonly starts as cellulitis adjacent to the portal of entry. Early on, the involved area is swollen, erythematous, and tender as the infection begins to involve the deep fascia. Pain is prominent, and fever and systemic toxicity are marked (Paty and Smith, 1992). The swelling and crepitus of the scrotum quickly increase, and dark purple areas develop and progress to extensive gangrene. If the abdominal wall becomes involved in an obese patient with diabetes, the process can spread very rapidly. Specific genitourinary symptoms associated with the condition include dysuria, urethral discharge, and obstructed voiding. Alterations in mental status, tachypnea, tachycardia, and temperature greater than 38.3° C (101° F) or less than 35.6° C (96° F) suggest gram-negative sepsis.

Laboratory Diagnosis and Radiologic Findings

Anemia occurs secondary to a decreased functioning erythrocyte mass caused by thrombosis and ecchymosis coupled with decreased production secondary to sepsis (Miller, 1983). Elevated serum creatinine levels, hyponatremia, and hypocalcemia are common. Hypocalcemia is believed to be secondary to bacterial lipases that destroy triglycerides and release free fatty acids that chelate calcium in its ionized form.

Because crepitus is often an early finding, a plain film of the abdomen may be helpful in identifying air. Scrotal ultrasonography is also useful in this regard. Biopsy of the base of an ulcer is characterized by superficially intact epidermis, dermal necrosis, and vascular thrombosis and polymorphonuclear leukocyte invasion with subcutaneous tissue necrosis. Stamenkovic and Lew (1984) noted that the use of frozen sections within 21 hours after the onset of symptoms could confirm a diagnosis earlier and lead to early institution of appropriate treatment.

Management

Prompt diagnosis is critical because of the rapidity with which the process can progress. The clinical differentiation of necrotizing fasciitis from cellulitis may be difficult because the initial signs including pain, edema, and erythema are not distinctive. However, the presence of marked systemic toxicity out of proportion to the local finding should alert the clinician. Intravenous hydration and antimicrobial therapy are indicated in preparation for surgical débridement. Antimicrobial regimens include combinations of ampicillin plus sulbactam or a parenteral third-generation cephalosporin such as ceftriaxone, gentamicin, and clindamycin. If there is no response to clindamycin, chloramphenicol may be used.

Immediate débridement is essential. In the patient in whom diagnosis is clearly suspected on clinical grounds (deep pain with patchy areas of surface hypoesthesia or crepitation, or bullae and skin necrosis), direct operative intervention is indicated. Extensive incision should be made through the skin and subcutaneous tissues, going beyond the areas of involvement until normal fascia is found. Necrotic fat and fascia should be excised, and the wound should be left open. A second procedure 24 to 48 hours later is indicated if there is any question about the adequacy of initial débridement. Orchiectomy is almost never required, because the testes have their own blood supply independent of the compromised fascial and cutaneous circulation to the scrotum. Suprapubic diversion should be performed in cases in which urethral trauma or extravasation is suspected. Colostomy should be performed if there is colonic or rectal perforation. Hyperbaric oxygen therapy has shown some promise in shortening hospital stays, increasing wound healing, and decreasing the gangrenous spread when used in conjunction with débridement and antimicrobials (Paty and Smith, 1992). Once wound healing is complete, reconstruction, for example, using myocutaneous flaps, improves cosmetic results.

Outcome

The mortality rate averages approximately 20% (Cohen, 1986; Baskin et al, 1990; Clayton et al, 1990) but ranges from 7% to 75%. Higher mortality rates are found in diabetics, alcoholics, and those with colorectal sources of infection who often have a less typical presentation, greater delay in diagnosis, and more widespread extension. Regardless of the presentation, Fournier's gangrene is a true urologic emergency that demands early recognition, aggressive treatment with antimicrobial agents, and surgical débridement to reduce morbidity and mortality.

Periurethral Abscess

Periurethral abscess is a life-threatening infection of the male urethra and periurethral tissues. Initially, the area of involvement can be small and localized by Buck's fascia. However, when Buck's fascia is penetrated, there can be extensive necrosis of the subcutaneous tissue and fascia. Fasciitis can spread as far as the buttocks posteriorly and the clavicle superiorly. Rapid diagnosis and treatment are essential to reduce the morbidity and high mortality historically associated with this disease.

Pathogenesis

Periurethral abscess is frequently a sequela of gonorrhea, urethral stricture disease, or urethral catheterization. Frequent instrumentation is also associated with periurethral abscess formation. The source of the infecting organism is the urine. Gram-negative rods, enterococci, and anaerobes are most frequently identified. The presence of multiple organisms is common. Anaerobes, normal residents of the male urethra, are also frequently found in wound cultures.

Clinical Presentation

Presenting signs and symptoms include scrotal swelling in 94% of patients, fever (70%), acute urinary retention (19%), spontaneously drained abscess (11%), and dysuria or urethral discharge (5% to 8%). The average interval between initial symptoms and presentation is 21 days. Urinalysis of the first glass specimen reveals pyuria and bacteriuria.

Management

Treatment consists of immediate suprapubic urinary drainage and wide débridement. Antimicrobial therapy with an aminoglycoside and a cephalosporin is usually adequate for empirical coverage. More selective antimicrobial therapy can

be instituted when the antimicrobial susceptibility of the organisms is available. Perineal urethrostomy or chronic suprapubic diversion occasionally has been helpful to prevent recurrences, and it should be considered in patients with diffuse stricture disease. The presence of a malignancy is unusual, but biopsy is important.

KEY POINTS: OTHER INFECTIONS

■ Fournier's gangrene is necrotizing fasciitis arising from the perineal skin, scrotum, urethra, or rectum.

■ Emergent surgical débridement and broad-spectrum antimicrobial agents are the essentials of treatment of Fournier's gangrene.

■ Periurethral abscess can occur secondarily to urethral stricture or catheterization; treatment entails surgical débridement, suprapubic urinary drainage, and antimicrobial agents.

SELECTED READINGS

Anderson GG, Dodson KW, Hooton TM, et al: Intracellular bacterial communities of uropathogenic *Escherichia coli* in urinary tract pathogenesis. Trends Microbiol 2004;12:424-430.

Asscher AW, Chick S, Radford N, et al: Natural history of asymptomatic bacteriuria in nonpregnant women. In Brumfitt W, Asscher AW (eds): Urinary Tract Infection. London, University Press, 1973, p 51.

Dajani AS, Taubert KA, Wilson W, et al: Prevention of bacterial endocarditis: Recommendations by the American Heart Association. JAMA 1997;277: 1794-1801.

Eknoyan G, Qunibi WY, Grissom RT, et al: Renal papillary necrosis: An update. Medicine (Baltimore) 1982;61:55-73.

Elliott TS, Reed L, Slack RC, et al: Bacteriology and ultrastructure of the bladder in patients with urinary tract infections. J Infect 1985;11:191-199.

Foxman B: Epidemiology of urinary tract infections: Incidence, morbidity, and economic costs. Am J Med 2002;113(Suppl 1A):5S-13S.

Gupta K, Scholes D, Stamm WE: Increasing prevalence of antimicrobial resistance among uropathogens causing acute uncomplicated cystitis in women. JAMA 1999;281:736-738.

Hooton TM, Stamm WE: Management of acute uncomplicated urinary tract infection in adults. Med Clin North Am 1991;75:339-357.

Hultgren SJ, Porter TN, Schaeffer AJ, et al: Role of type 1 pili and effects of phase variation on lower urinary tract infections produced by *Escherichia coli.* Infect Immun 1985;50:370-377.

Hultgren SJ, Schwan WR, Schaeffer AJ, et al: Regulation of production of type 1 pili among urinary tract isolates of *Escherichia coli.* Infect Immun 1986;54:613-620.

Mabeck CE: Treatment of uncomplicated urinary tract infection in nonpregnant women. Postgrad Med J 1972;48:69-75.

Martinez JJ, Hultgren SJ: Requirement of Rho-family GTPases in the invasion of type 1–piliated uropathogenic *Escherichia coli.* Cell Microbiol 2002;4:19-28.

Mulvey MA: Adhesion and entry of uropathogenic *Escherichia coli.* Cell Microbiol 2002;4:257-271.

Mulvey MA, Schilling JD, Martinez JJ, et al: Bad bugs and beleaguered bladders: Interplay between uropathogenic *Escherichia coli* and innate host defenses. Proc Natl Acad Sci U S A 2000;97:8829-8835.

Mulvey MA, Lopez-Boado YS, Wilson CL, et al: Induction and evasion of host defenses by type 1–piliated uropathogenic *Escherichia coli.* Science 1998; 282:1494-1497.

National Institute on Disability and Rehabilitation Research: The prevention and management of urinary tract infections among people with spinal cord injuries. National Institute on Disability and Rehabilitation Research consensus statement. January 27-29, 1992. SCI Nurs 1993;10:49-61.

Nicolle LE, Bradley S, Colgan R, et al: Infectious Diseases Society of America guidelines for the diagnosis and treatment of asymptomatic bacteriuria in adults. Clin Infect Dis 2005;40:643-654.

Schaeffer AJ, Jones JM, Dunn JK: Association of in vitro *Escherichia coli* adherence to vaginal and buccal epithelial cells with susceptibility of women to recurrent urinary-tract infections. N Engl J Med 1981;304:1062-1066.

Stamey TA: Pathogenesis and Treatment of Urinary Tract Infections. Baltimore, Williams & Wilkins, 1980.

Stamey TA, Govan DE, Palmer JM: The localization and treatment of urinary tract infections: The role of bactericidal urine levels as opposed to serum levels. Medicine (Baltimore) 1965;44:1-36.

Stamm WE: Recent developments in the diagnosis and treatment of urinary tract infections. West J Med 1982;137:213-220.

Stamm WE: Catheter-associated urinary tract infections: Epidemiology, pathogenesis, and prevention. Am J Med 1991;91:65S-71S.

Turck M, Goffe B, Petersdorf RG: The urethral catheter and urinary tract infection. J Urol 1962;88:834-837.

Vromen M, van der Ven AJ, Knols A, et al: Antimicrobial resistance patterns in urinary isolates from nursing home residents: Fifteen years of data reviewed. J Antimicrob Chemother 1999;44:113-116.

Warren JW, Abrutyn E, Hebel JR, et al: Guidelines for antimicrobial treatment of uncomplicated acute bacterial cystitis and acute pyelonephritis in women. Infectious Diseases Society of America (IDSA). Clin Infect Dis 1999;29:745-758.

Inflammatory Conditions of the Male Genitourinary Tract: Prostatitis and Related Conditions, Orchitis, and Epididymitis

J. CURTIS NICKEL, MD

PROSTATITIS

RELATED CONDITIONS

PROSTATITIS
Historical Aspects

Legneau may have been the first to describe inflammation of the prostate gland in 1815, but it was Verdes, in 1838, who presented the first accurate description of the pathology of prostatitis (Von Lackum, 1928). The modern era describing the clinical presentation, pathology, and microscopic evaluation of prostate-specific specimens was firmly established by Young, Gereghty, and Stevens (1906) by the turn of the 20th century. Bacterial and cytologic localization studies of the lower urinary tract were described shortly thereafter (Hitchens and Brown, 1913) and standardized by 1930 (Von Lackum, 1927, 1928; AC Nickel, 1930; JC Nickel 1999a).

The primary form of therapy during most of the 20th century was repetitive prostate massage (Farman, 1930; O'Conor, 1936; Henline, 1943; Campbell, 1957). With the introduction of sulfanilamide in the 1930s, antimicrobial therapy became the main therapeutic approach (Ritter and Lippow, 1938). However, even in the 1950s and 1960s, the significance of inflammatory cells and bacteria in the expressed prostatic secretion (EPS) was questioned (O'Shaughnessy et al, 1956; Bowers and Thomas, 1958; Bourne and Frishette, 1967), and it was even recognized that, in many cases, antibiotics may be little better than placebo in the treatment of prostatitis (Gonder, 1963).

The next era of prostatitis management began in the 1960s with Meares and Stamey's (1968) description of the four-glass lower urinary tract segmented localization study.

With this insight, prostatic massage as the mainstay of prostatitis therapy was abandoned and antimicrobial therapy was rationalized for the very small percentage of patients with bacteria localized to prostate-specific specimens. Unfortunately, the vast majority of patients who were diagnosed with a nonbacterial cause continued to suffer the indignities of dismal urologic management (Nickel, 1998a). Over the past decade **the establishment of new definitions and a classification system, evolving understanding of the etiopathogenesis, and randomized placebo-controlled trials with validated outcome indices have made evidence-based management a real possibility.**

Epidemiology

Utilizing data from the National Ambulatory Medical Care Surveys (NAMCS), McNaughton-Collins and colleagues (1998) noted from 1990 to 1994 that there were almost 2 million U.S. physician visits annually with prostatitis listed as the diagnosis. Approximately 5% of visits to U.S. urologists were reported to be for inflammatory diseases of the prostate (Schappert, 1994). In the mid 1990s, the average Wisconsin urologist saw a mean of 173 (median, 100) prostatitis patients per year (Moon, 1997). A similar Canadian survey showed that Canadian urologists saw a mean of 22 (median, 11) prostatitis patients per month, 38% newly diagnosed (Nickel et al, 1998a). **Prostatitis is the most common urologic diagnosis in men younger than 50 years and the third most common urologic diagnosis in men older than 50 years (after benign prostatic hyperplasia [BPH] and prostate cancer), representing 8% of male urology office visits** (McNaughton-Collins et al, 1998). Based on both a physician survey study in Dane County, Wisconsin (Moon, 1997), and a survey of younger men from a Wisconsin National Guard unit (Moon et al, 1997), it was estimated that 5% of young men (aged 20 to 50 years) have a history of prostatitis. In the

Netherlands, de la Rosette and colleagues (1992a) noted that 4% of respondents reported a history of prostatitis whereas researchers in Finland reported a 14% overall lifetime prevalence in that country (Mehik et al, 2000). McNaughton-Collins and colleagues (2002) noted that 16% of health care professionals in the United States report either a previous or current diagnosis of prostatitis. Roberts and associates (1998) reviewed the medical records of 2113 men from July 1992 through February 1996 (a median of 50 months' follow-up) in the Olmsted County community-based cohort in Minnesota and found the overall prevalence of a physician's diagnosis of prostatitis was 9%.

Many of these epidemiologic studies are limited by physicians' or patients' long-term recollection and the unreliability of a physician's coding or diagnosis of prostatitis. **Population-based studies employing the validated National Institutes of Health Chronic Prostatitis Symptom Index (NIH-CPSI)** (Litwin et al, 1999) **to determine the prevalence of prostatitis-like symptoms in the general population of men showed widely variant results (8.0% in Malaysia** [Cheah et al, 2003], **6.6% in Canada** [Nickel et al, 2001b], **2.7% in Singapore** [Tan et al, 2002], **and approximately 2.2% in older men in Olmsted County** [Roberts et al, 2002]). Prospective practice audit studies have shown that as many as 12% of men presenting to Italian urologists are diagnosed with prostatitis (Rizzo et al, 2003), whereas only 2.8% of men had a clinical diagnosis of prostatitis in a similar study carried out in Canada (Nickel et al, 2005c). Symptoms of prostatitis wax and wane, with approximately one third to one half of patients experiencing relief of symptoms over a 1-year period (O'Leary et al, 2001; Nickel et al, 2002; Turner et al, 2004).

It has traditionally been believed that prostatitis is a disease of young men. Epidemiologic studies described in this section confirm that prostatitis affects men of all ages, unlike BPH and prostate cancer, which are predominantly diseases of older men. Compared with men aged 66 years and older, the odds of a prostatitis diagnosis are 1.6-, 2.6-, and 2.1-fold greater in men aged 18 to 35, 36 to 50, and 51 to 65 years, respectively, in the Olmsted County study (Roberts et al, 1998). The age-specific prevalence of a physician-assigned diagnosis of prostatitis was highest in patients between the ages of 20 and 49 years and increased again in those older than 70 years. The accumulative probability of having a diagnosis of prostatitis (acute or chronic) by 85 years of age was 26%. In the Canadian prevalence study (Nickel et al, 2001b), there was no significant difference in the prevalence of prostatitis-like symptoms in men younger than 50 years (11.5% reported at least mild symptoms over the past week) compared with men older than 50 years (8.5% reported at least mild symptoms over the past week). As many as 20% of men diagnosed with BPH also have prostatitis-like symptoms (Nickel, 2005a).

Chronic prostatitis (CP) is associated with substantial costs and significant predicted resource consumption (Calhoun et al, 2004; Turner et al, 2004), a factor that needs increased attention when evaluating the incidence and treatment of this prevalent condition.

Histopathology

For the pathologist, *prostatitis* is defined as an increased number of inflammatory cells within the prostatic

KEY POINTS: EPIDEMIOLOGY

- Two to 10 percent of men currently experience prostatitis-like symptoms.
- Nine to 16 percent of men have had a diagnosis of prostatitis.
- Prostatitis represents 3% to 12% of male outpatient visits to urologists.

parenchyma (Cotran et al, 1999). Prostatic inflammation may (or may not) be noted in patients with a diagnosis of prostatitis (True et al, 1999), BPH (Nickel et al, 1999c), or prostate cancer (Zhang et al, 2000) and is noted in autopsy series in as many as 44% of prostate tissue samples from men without any definitive prostate disease (McNeal, 1968).

A consistent description of fairly distinct, although often coexisting, patterns of chronic inflammation can be found in the prostate gland of patients with or without prostate disease. **The most common pattern of inflammation is a lymphocytic infiltrate in the stroma immediately adjacent to the prostatic acini** (Kohnen and Drach, 1979; Nickel et al, 1999b). The intensity of the inflammatory process varies considerably from only scattered lymphocytes to dense lymphoid nodules. Stromal lymphocytic infiltrates frequently coexist with periglandular inflammation. Sheets, clusters, and occasional nodules of lymphocytes and scattered plasma cells are seen within the fibromuscular stroma with no apparent relationship to the ducts and acini. Infiltrates of inflammatory cells restricted to the glandular epithelium and lumen are found in association with prostatitis and BPH and are a rare isolated finding in asymptomatic patients. The intraepithelial inflammatory cells may be neutrophils, lymphocytes, or macrophages, or all of these, whereas neutrophils and macrophages are typically found in the lumen. Figure 9–1 illustrates the various inflammatory patterns seen in a prostate specimen of a patient with CP.

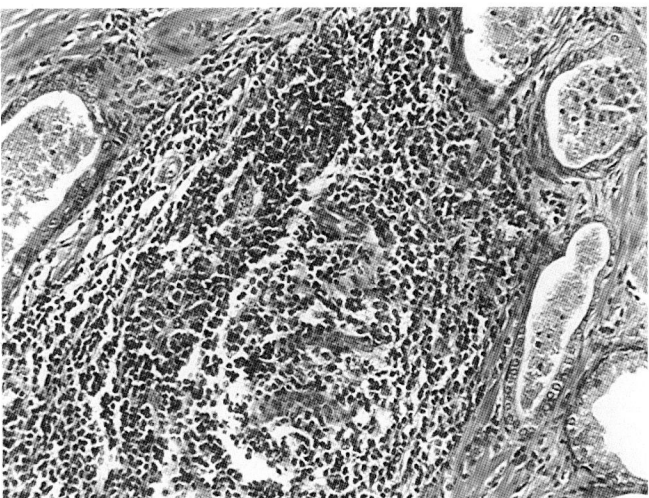

Figure 9–1. Histologic preparation of a prostate specimen demonstrating areas of glandular, periglandular, and stromal inflammation (×400). (Courtesy of Dr. Alexander Boag.)

Corpora amylacea, which may develop from the deposition of prostatic secretions around a sloughed epithelial cell or other irritant, are not usually associated with inflammation unless they become large enough to distend or obstruct the prostatic gland (Attah, 1975). Prostatic calculi may contribute to prostatic inflammation by obstructing central prostate ducts and thus preventing drainage or providing a nidus in which bacteria can survive host defenses and antibiotics (Meares, 1974; Roberts et al, 1997).

Granulomatous prostatitis presents a nonspecific and variable histologic pattern typified by heavy lobular, mixed, inflammatory infiltrates that include abundant histiocytes, lymphocytes, and plasma cells. Small, discrete granulomas may be present, or the pattern may be typified by well-defined granulomas. Granulomatous prostatic inflammation is a common consequence of surgery (Eyre et al, 1986) or bacillus Calmette-Guérin (BCG) therapy (Lafontaine et al, 1997) and a rare event in patients with systemic tuberculosis (Saw et al, 1993).

A consensus group of urologists and pathologists have developed a classification system to describe histologic inflammatory patterns in the prostate (Nickel et al, 2001d), but it is only useful for comparative research purposes.

Etiology

Microbiologic Causes

Gram-Negative Uropathogens. **Acute bacterial prostatitis is a generalized infection of the prostate gland and is associated with both lower urinary tract infection (UTI) and generalized sepsis. Chronic bacterial prostatitis is associated with recurrent lower UTIs (i.e., cystitis) secondary to areas of focal uropathogenic bacteria residing in the prostate gland. The most common cause of bacterial prostatitis is the Enterobacteriaceae family of gram-negative bacteria, which originate in the gastrointestinal flora.** The most common organisms are strains of *Escherichia coli*, which are identified in 65% to 80% of infections (Stamey, 1980; Lopez-Plaza and Bostwick, 1990; Weidner et al, 1991b; Schneider et al, 2003). *Pseudomonas aeruginosa, Serratia* species, *Klebsiella* species, and *Enterobacter aerogenes* are identified in a further 10% to 15% (Meares, 1987; Weidner et al, 1991b).

Urovirulence factors play a significant role in the pathogenesis of bacterial prostatitis (Ruiz et al, 2002; Johnson et al, 2005). For instance, bacterial P-fimbria (or pili) binds to the urothelial receptors, and this subsequently facilitates ascent into the urinary tract as well as establishing deep infections in the prostate gland itself (Dilworth et al, 1990; Neal et al, 1990; Andreu et al, 1997). Colonization of the lower urinary tract by *E. coli* is also facilitated by the presence of the type 1 fimbria, also known as mannose-sensitive fimbria. The receptor is a common moiety of the uroepithelial uromucoid; this association has been shown to be important in the development of cystitis in humans, and its presence in prostatitis has also been documented (Correll et al, 1996). Phase variation of type 1 pili during the establishment of acute bacterial prostatitis may occur in the setting of prostatitis (Schaeffer, 1991). Multiple virulence factors appear to be necessary to produce prostatitis (Mitsumori et al, 1999; Ruiz et al, 2002). Bacteria

reside deep in the ducts of the prostate gland and when threatened with host defense and antimicrobial therapy, tend to form aggregates (also called biofilms); this appears to be a protective mechanism that allows bacteria to persist in the prostate gland even when the cystitis is treated with antibiotics (Nickel and Costerton, 1993; Nickel et al, 1994).

Gram-Positive Bacteria. Enterococci are believed to account for 5% to 10% of documented prostate infections (Drach, 1974a; Meares, 1987; Bergman, 1994). The role of other gram-positive organisms, which are also commensal organisms in the anterior urethra, is controversial (Jimenez-Cruz et al, 1984; Fowler and Mariano, 1984b; Krieger et al, 2002). An etiologic role for gram-positive organisms such as *Staphylococcus saprophyticus*, hemolytic streptococci, *Staphylococcus aureus*, and other coagulase-negative staphylococci has been suggested by a number of authors (Drach, 1974a, 1986; Bergman, 1994). Nickel and Costerton (1992) have shown coagulase-negative *Staphylococcus* to be present in the EPS as well as transperineal prostate biopsy tissue of men with CP (microscopy and culture). Although this and other studies (Carson et al, 1982; Pfau, 1983; Bergman et al, 1989; Wedren, 1989) suggested that coagulase-negative staphylococci are involved in the pathogenesis of CP, these studies did not conclusively demonstrate that these bacteria were actually causing the inflammation and symptom-complex rather than simply colonizing the prostate (Krieger et al, 2002). However, eradication of gram-positive bacteria in the prostate of men experiencing recent onset of prostatitis symptoms resulted in similar clinical results compared with men with gram-negative uropathogens localizing to the prostate (Nickel et al, 2005e). In both cases, eradication of the bacteria localized to the prostate was strongly correlated with a good clinical outcome (Nickel et al, 2005e).

Anaerobic Bacteria. In studies in which the prostate-specific specimens were cultured anaerobically, anaerobic bacteria could be identified in a small number of patients (Nielsen and Justesen, 1974; Mardh and Colleen, 1975; Szoke et al, 1998). This has not been a consistent finding, and the role of anaerobic bacteria is essentially unknown.

***Corynebacterium* Infection.** *Corynebacterium* species have usually been acknowledged as prostate nonpathogens but have been suggested as potential etiologic agents in this disease (Riegel et al, 1995; Domingue, 1998). Domingue and colleagues (1997) suggested that these difficult-to-culture coryneforms could be missed by routine culturing of EPS. Direct Gram staining of the EPS showed gram-variable pleomorphic coccobacillary rods that do not usually grow on routine media. The presence of these pleomorphic swollen rods was also shown by fluorescent acridine orange staining. Tanner and associates (1999), using polymerase chain reaction techniques, were able to identify a bacterial signal (phylogenetically gram-positive organisms with predominance of *Corynebacterium* species) in 65% of 17 patients with CP. Approximately half these patients tended to respond to antimicrobial therapy, whereas patients in whom molecular signals for these bacteria could not be identified did not.

***Chlamydia* Infection.** **The evidence supporting the role of *Chlamydia trachomatis* as an etiologic agent in chronic prostatic inflammation is both confusing and conflicting.** Mardh and Colleen (1972) found that one third of men with

CP had antibodies to *C. trachomatis* compared with 3% of controls. Shortliffe and coworkers (1992) found that 20% of patients with nonbacterial prostatitis had antichlamydial antibody titers in the prostatic fluid. Koroku and associates (1995) detected *C. trachomatis*–specific immunoglobulin A (IgA) in 29% of men with chronic nonbacterial prostatitis. Bruce and colleagues (1981) found that 56% of patients with "subacute or chronic prostatitis" were infected with *C. trachomatis* (examining early morning urine, prostatic fluid, or semen). In a follow-up study, Bruce and Reid (1989) found that 6 of 55 men with abacterial prostatitis, including 31 believed to have chlamydial prostatitis, met strict criteria for positive diagnosis for chlamydial prostatitis based on identification of the organisms by culturing or immunofluorescence. Kuroda and colleagues (1989) identified *C. trachomatis* in the urethras of 20% of men with prostatitis. Other investigators have come to similar conclusions (Nilsson et al, 1981; Weidner et al, 1983). Chlamydia has also been isolated in prostate tissue specimens. Poletti and coworkers (1985) isolated *C. trachomatis* from prostate samples obtained by transrectal aspiration biopsy of men with "nonacute abacterial prostatitis." Abdelatif and colleagues (1991) identified intracellular *Chlamydia* employing "in-situ hybridization techniques" in transurethral prostate chips from 30% of men with histologic evidence of "chronic abacterial prostatitis." Shurbaji and associates (1998) identified *C. trachomatis* in paraffin-embedded secretions in 31% of men with histologic evidence of prostatitis compared with none in patients with BPH without inflammation.

Although Mardh and Colleen (1972) suggested that *C. trachomatis* may be implicated in as many as one third of men with CP, their follow-up studies employing culturing and serologic tests could not confirm *C. trachomatis* as an etiologic agent in idiopathic prostatitis (Mardh and Colleen, 1975; Mardh et al, 1978). Shortliffe and Wehner (1986) came to a similar conclusion when they evaluated antichlamydial antibody titers in prostatic fluid. Twelve percent of controls (compared with 20% of patients with nonbacterial prostatitis) had detectable antibodies. Berger and coworkers (1989) could not culture *C. trachomatis* from the urethras in men with CP nor did they find a serologic or local immune response to *C. trachomatis* in such patients. Doble and associates (1989b) were not able to culture or detect by immunofluorescence *Chlamydia* in transperineal biopsies of abnormal areas of the prostate in men with chronic abacterial prostatitis. Krieger and colleagues (1996b) were only able to find *Chlamydia* in 1% of prostate tissue biopsies in men with CP. A further localization and culture series by Krieger and associates (2000) also failed to culture *Chlamydia* from either urethral or prostate specimens. Further elucidation of the role of chlamydial etiology of prostate infection is required to make any definitive statement on the association between isolation of this organism and its prostatic origin and effect (Weidner et al, 2002).

***Ureaplasma* Infection.** *Ureaplasma urealyticum* is a common organism isolated from the urethra of both asymptomatic men and men with nonspecific urethritis. Weidner and colleagues (1980) found high *U. urealyticum* concentrations in prostate-specific specimens in patients with signs and symptoms of abacterial prostatitis. Isaacs and associates

(1993) cultured *U. urealyticum* from prostate secretion in 8% of patients with chronic nonbacterial prostatitis. Fish and Danziger (1993) found significant *U. urealyticum* concentrations in 13% of patients with prostatitis. Treatment with specific antimicrobial therapy cleared the organisms in all cases. Ohkawa and associates (1993a) isolated *U. urealyticum* cells from the prostates of 18 of 143 patients with CP. Antibiotics eradicated the organism in all, improved the symptoms in 10, and cleared the leukocytes in the EPS in 4 (Ohkawa et al, 1993b).

Other investigators (Mardh and Colleen, 1975), employing similar techniques, were unable to implicate *U. urealyticum* in patients with nonbacterial prostatitis. The problems encountered in all these studies include the absence of controls and the fact that it was difficult to account for possible urethral contamination in collecting specific prostate specimens.

Other Microorganisms. *Candida* (Golz and Mendling, 1991; Indudhara et al, 1992) and other mycotic infections such as aspergillosis and coccidioidomycosis (Schwarz, 1982; Chen and Schijf, 1985; Campbell et al, 1992; Truett and Crum, 2004) have been implicated in prostatic inflammation. In most cases, however, it was usually an isolated finding in immunosuppressed patients or those with systemic fungal infection. Viruses (Doble et al, 1991; Benson and Smith, 1992) have also been implicated in prostatic inflammation, but no systematic evaluation of the role of these agents in prostatitis has been undertaken. *Trichomonas* has been described in the prostate glands of patients complaining of prostatitis-like symptoms (Kuberski, 1980; Gardner et al, 1996; Skerk et al, 2002a).

Nonculturable Microorganisms. There are significant limitations to the culture techniques employed to attempt to identify etiologic microorganisms associated with prostatitis (Lowentritt et al, 1995; Domingue et al, 1997; Domingue, 1998). Bacteria may exist in aggregated biofilms adherent to the prostatic ductal walls or within the obstructed ducts in the prostate (Nickel and MacLean, 1998). Nickel and Costerton (1993) observed that 60% of patients with previously diagnosed chronic bacterial prostatitis who progressed to sterile EPS cultures but continued to have symptoms despite antimicrobial therapy had positive cultures (with an organism similar to the initial organism) in prostate biopsy specimens. These organisms appeared to persist in small aggregates or biofilms in the ducts and acini of the prostate gland.

Berger and associates (1997) cultured urine specimens and transperineal prostate biopsies specifically for commensal and fastidious organisms. These investigators demonstrated that, in prostate biopsy cultures, men with evidence of inflammation in EPS are more likely to have bacteria isolated, positive cultures for anaerobic bacteria, higher total bacterial counts, and more bacterial species isolated than men without EPS inflammation. Krieger and colleagues (1996b), Riley and coworkers (1998), and Tanner and associates (1999) used a combination of clinical, culture, and molecular biologic methods (polymerase chain reaction [PCR]) and found a strong correlation between inflammation and EPS and the detection of bacteria-specific 16S rRNA (gram-negative and gram-positive organisms) in the prostate tissue. But other researchers did not show any association between culture and

PCR findings in men with nonbacterial prostatitis compared with men with prostatitis symptoms (Lee et al, 2003; Keay et al, 1999; Leskinen et al, 2003). Shoskes and associates (2005) demonstrated the possibility that nanobacteria associated with prostatic calculi may be implicated in some cases of CP.

It has been estimated that less than 10% of all environmental bacteria have been identified (Domingue, 1998), so it is possible that fastidious and nonculturable microorganisms might be present in the prostate gland and that such organisms might be involved in the inflammatory process and subsequent development of symptoms.

Altered Prostatic Host Defense

Risk factors that allow bacterial colonization or infection of the prostate with potentially pathogenic bacteria include intraprostatic ductal reflux (Kirby et al, 1982); **phimosis** (VanHowe, 1998); **specific blood groups** (Lomberg et al, 1986); **unprotected penetrative anal rectal intercourse; UTIs; acute epididymitis** (Berger et al, 1987); **indwelling urethral catheters and condom catheter drainage** (Meares, 1998); **and transurethral surgery, especially in men who have untreated, infected urine** (Meares, 1989). Secretory dysfunction of the prostate characterized by an alteration in the composition of prostatic secretions can be diagnostic of patients with prostatitis, that is, a decrease in the levels of fructose; citric acid; acid phosphatase; the cations zinc, magnesium, and calcium; and the zinc-containing prostatic antibacterial factor, whereas pH, the ratio of isoenzymes lactate dehydrogenase-5 to lactate dehydrogenase-1, inflammatory proteins such as ceruloplasmin, and complement C3 are increased (Meares, 1989). These defined alterations in the prostate secretory function have also been blamed for adversely affecting the normal antibacterial nature of prostatic secretions. A decrease in prostatic antibacterial factor may reduce the intrinsic antibacterial activity of the prostatic fluid (Fair et al, 1976), whereas the alkaline pH may hamper diffusion of certain basic antimicrobial drugs into the prostatic tissue and fluid (Fair and Cordonnier, 1978). However, it is not known whether these compositional changes are a cause or a consequence of inflammation.

Dysfunctional Voiding

Anatomic or neurophysiologic obstruction resulting in high-pressure dysfunctional flow patterns has been implicated in the pathogenesis of the prostatitis syndrome. Blacklock (1974, 1991) demonstrated that bladder neck, prostatic, and urethral anatomic abnormalities predisposed some men to developing prostatitis. Urodynamic studies confirm that many patients, particularly those with prostatodynia, have decreased maximal urinary flow rates and obstructive-appearing flow patterns (Barbalias et al, 1983; Ghobish, 2002). On videourodynamic studies, many patients with prostatitis syndromes show incomplete funneling of the bladder neck as well as vesicourethral dyssynergic patterns (Kaplan et al, 1994, 1997; Hruz et al, 2003). In a study of 48 treatment-refractory CP patients with no associated infection, Hruz and colleagues (2003) determined that 29 (60%) had bladder neck hypertrophy diagnosed by endoscopic and urodynamic criteria. This dyssynergic voiding may lead to an autonomic overstimulation of the perineal-pelvic neural system, with subsequent development of a chronic neuropathic pain state. Alterna-

tively, this high-pressure dysfunctional voiding may result in intraprostatic ductal reflux in susceptible individuals (see the next section).

Intraprostatic Ductal Reflux

Reflux of urine and possibly bacteria into the prostatic ducts has been postulated as one of the most important etiologic mechanisms involved in the pathogenesis of chronic bacterial and nonbacterial prostatic inflammation. Anatomically, the ductal drainage of the peripheral zone is more susceptible than other prostatic zones to intraprostatic ductal reflux (Blacklock, 1974, 1991). Kirby and associates (1982) instilled a carbon particle solution into the bladders of men diagnosed with nonbacterial prostatitis. Carbon particles were found in the EPS macrophages and prostatic acini and ductal system after surgery in men with nonbacterial prostatitis. Persson and Ronquist (1996) noted high levels of urate and creatinine in EPS, which they postulated was caused by urine reflux into the prostatic ducts. Terai and coworkers (2000) provided molecular epidemiologic evidence for ascending infection in acute bacterial prostatitis.

Prostatic calculi are composed of substances found only in urine, not in prostatic secretions (Sutor and Wooley, 1974; Ramiraz et al, 1980), further evidence that urinary intraprostatic reflux occurs and likely contributes to the formation of prostatic calculi. If pathogenic bacteria reflux into the prostate gland, they may exist in protected aggregates within prostatic calculi themselves. High culture counts of pathogens encrusted in prostatic calculi have been demonstrated by Eykyn and colleagues (1974). This type of bacterial colonization in protective bacterial aggre-gates or biofilms associated with prostatic calculi may lead to recalcitrant CP and subsequent recurrent UTIs despite what seems to be adequate antibiotic therapy. Ludwig and coworkers (1994), employing transrectal ultrasonography, showed that men with chronic inflammatory prostatitis had a significantly increased frequency of prostatic calculi compared with men without prostate inflammation (prostatodynia). The inflammation resulting from chemical, bacterial, or immunologic stimulation has been shown to possibly cause an increase in intraprostatic pressures, measurable with transperineally inserted pressure transducers (Mehik et al, 2002).

Immunologic Alterations

The local prostatic immune system is activated by infection in bacterial prostatitis. In acute bacterial prostatitis, serum and prostatic fluid antigen-specific (i.e., bacterial antigen) IgG and IgA can be detected immediately after the onset of infection, and, after successful antibiotic therapy, they decline to normal levels over the next 6 to 12 months (Fowler and Mariano, 1984a; Meares, 1977, 1998; Kumon, 1992). Prostate-specific antigen levels can be markedly elevated during an acute episode of bacterial prostatitis (Dalton, 1989; Moon et al, 1992; Neal et al, 1992) and slowly resolve to normal levels over the course of 6 weeks, provided there is no recrudescence of the infection. In chronic bacterial prostatitis, no serum immunoglobulin elevation is detected whereas prostatic fluid IgA and IgG levels are both increased (Shortliffe and Wehner, 1986; Kumon, 1992). After successful antibiotic therapy, IgG levels return to normal after several months but the IgA (particularly secretory IgA) levels remain elevated for almost 2 years (Shortliffe et al, 1981a,b; Fowler and Mariano, 1984a). Antibody-coated bacteria detected in urine, EPS, and semen are another prominent feature of chronic bacterial prostatitis (Riedasch et al, 1984, 1991).

Noninfectious inflammation (nonbacterial prostatitis) might also be secondary to immunologically mediated inflammation due to some unknown antigen or perhaps even related to an autoimmune process. IgA and IgM antibody levels (not microorganism-specific) are elevated (Shortliffe and Wehner, 1986; Shortliffe et al, 1989, 1992), and similar antibodies as well as fibrinogen and complement C3 (Vinje et al, 1983; Doble et al, 1990) have been identified in prostatic biopsies from patients with CP. Both animal model studies (Donadio et al, 1998; Ceri et al, 1999; Lang et al, 2000) and human studies (Alexander et al, 1997; Batstone et al, 2002; John et al, 2003) have suggested that prostatitis may be an autoimmune process. A number of candidates have been suggested for the self-antigen, including PSA (Ponniah et al, 2000). Other specific immunologic and neuroendocrine alterations such as cytokine production (Alexander et al, 1998; Jang et al, 2003) and nerve growth factor (Miller et al, 2002) have a subsequent role to play in the process of inflammation. Specifically, interleukin (IL)-10 has been implicated in the etiology and clinical manifestations in CP (Miller et al, 2002; Shoskes et al, 2002), but other cytokines such as IL-1β and tumor necrosis factor-α (TNF-α) have also been implicated (Nadler 2000). There may be a genetic phenotype that promotes specific immunologic parameters that predispose to immunologically induced prostatic inflammation (Shoskes et al, 2002; Riley et al, 2002). These immunophenotypic patterns have even been observed in noninflammatory category IIIB CP/chronic pelvic pain syndrome (CPPS) (Barghorn et al, 2001). **Whatever the initiating event, the immunologic cascade appears to have an important role in the development of prostatitis in those patients who develop prostatic inflammation** (Moon, 1998; Kumon, 1999).

Chemically Induced Inflammation

Investigators have demonstrated that urine and its metabolites (e.g., urate) are present in the prostatic secretion of patients with CP (Persson and Ronquist, 1996). These investigators have hypothesized that the prostatic inflammation and subsequent symptoms may be simply due to a chemically induced inflammation secondary to the noxious substances in the urine that have refluxed into the prostatic duct.

Neural Dysregulation/Pelvic Floor Musculature Abnormalities

Some investigators (Zermann et al, 1999) **propose that the sensory or motor disturbances or both consistent with neural dysregulation of the lower urinary tract may be a consequence of acquired abnormalities in the central nervous system.** Zermann and Schmidt (1999) describe 103 patients with chronic pelvic pain whom they evaluated at a specialized neurourologic unit. They showed that a majority of the men had insufficient conscious control of their somatically innervated striated pelvic floor muscles. The patients showed various levels of identity with their pelvic floor muscles, but none was able to demonstrate the full range of pelvic floor contraction and relaxation repetitively and effort-

lessly. This was true whether or not there was evidence of inflammation. They conclude that their findings reflect a functional disassociation between the central nervous system and the peripheral target, the pelvic floor muscles.

Other clinicians (Anderson, 1999; Potts, 2003) believe that the source of the pain is specifically at the pelvic musculature attachment area at the sacrum, coccyx, ischial tuberosity, pubic rami, and endopelvic fascia. These areas are immediately adjacent to the prostate and bladder and can be recognized by the demonstration of a hyperirritable spot or myofascial trigger point that is painful on compression. It is hypothesized that the formation of myofascial trigger points in this area results from mechanical abnormalities in the hip and lower extremities, chronic holding patterns such as those that occur during toilet training, sexual abuse, repetitive minor trauma and constipation, sports that create chronic pelvic stimulation, trauma or unusual sexual activity, recurrent infections, and surgery (Anderson, 1999). More recently, it has been hypothesized that the pain experienced in some men with CPPS may be explained by pudendal nerve entrapment, which causes subsequent neuropathic pain (Antolak et al, 2002).

Interstitial Cystitis–like Cause

Interstitial cystitis is an ill-defined CPPS occurring primarily in females, and a number of investigators have hypothesized that chronic nonbacterial prostatitis may have a similar cause. Unfortunately, the cause of interstitial cystitis remains unknown, but the pathogenic mechanisms are theorized to be very similar to those that cause CP/CPPS in men (Sant and Nickel, 1999; Eisenberg et al, 2003; Parsons 2003). Some researchers have proposed in some patients diagnosed with prostatitis that a bladder-orientated interstitial cystitis mechanism actually accounts for the symptoms and the prostate is only indirectly involved (Sant and Kominski, 1997). Certainly, the pain and voiding symptoms of interstitial cystitis and CP overlap to some extent (Miller et al, 1995; Novicki et al, 1998; Sant and Nickel, 1999; Forrest and Schmidt, 2004), and men with CP have cystoscopic (Berger et al, 1998), urodynamic (Siroky et al, 1981), and potassium sensitivity testing (Parsons et al, 2002, 2005) findings very similar to those of patients with interstitial cystitis. However, Yilmaz and coworkers (2004) did not confirm positive potassium sensitivity testing in prostatitis patients and Keay and colleagues (2004) have shown that men diagnosed with CP (pain only) have normal antiproliferative factor activity while men diagnosed with interstitial cystitis (pain and irritative voiding symptoms) have detectable levels of urine antiproliferative factor.

Psychological Cause

Psychological factors have always been considered to play an important role in the development or exacerbation of both of the CP syndromes. Some researchers who have investigated the psychopathology of CP concluded that this syndrome should be viewed as a psychosomatic disorder (Mendlewich et al, 1971; Mellan et al, 1973; Keltikangas-Jarvinen et al, 1982). De la Rosette and associates (1993b) compared a group of 50 CP patients with a group of 50 patients seen for vasectomy and showed that, although there were significant statistical differences between the groups (with CP patients scoring consistently higher personality disorder scores), these differences in scores were quite small compared with those between prostatitis and psychiatric patients. Berghuis and coworkers (1996) compared 51 CP patients with a group of 34 men without any chronic pain condition and concluded that depression and psychological disturbances are common among CP patients. Egan and Krieger (1994) compared CP patients with those seeking treatment for chronic low back pain. Major depression was more common in prostatitis patients, but back pain caused more somatically focused depression and anxiety. Ku and coworkers (2002) suggested that depression and weak masculine identity may be associated with an early stage of CP. These more recent studies demonstrate that psychological factors are involved in the disease, but it seems unjustified to label this group of patients as neurotic or as having a psychopathologic condition. A recent analysis of the large NIH Chronic Prostatitis Cohort showed that psychological variables could predict pain experience (Tripp et al, 2004).

An Interrelated, Pluricausal, Multifactorial Etiology

It is likely that the CP syndrome has a multifactorial etiology, either a spectrum of etiologic mechanisms or, more likely, a progression or cascade of events after some initiating factor. In an important review on mechanisms involved in the pathogenesis of CP, Pontari and Ruggieri (2004) concluded that "the symptoms of chronic prostatitis/chronic pelvic pain syndrome appear to result from an interplay between psychological factors and dysfunction in the immune, neurological and endocrine systems." Figure 9–2 describes a hypothetical scenario that could potentially involve most of the proposed and interrelated causes described in this section.

KEY POINTS: ETIOLOGY

- Gram-negative Enterobacteriaceae and enterococci are responsible for most cases of bacterial prostatitis.

- CPPS is caused by an interrelated cascade of inflammatory, immunologic, neuroendocrine, and neuropathic mechanisms that begin with an initiator in a genetically or anatomically susceptible man.

Definition and Classification

Traditional Classification

The traditional classification system is based on the landmark paper by Meares and Stamey (1968) describing the differential diagnosis of the prostatitis syndromes. This classic paper described in great detail the serial cultures (and treatment) in four patients with CP and introduced the so-called Meares-Stamey four-glass test. This localization test, which segmentally assesses inflammation and cultures of the male lower urinary tract, is described in detail in the section "Lower Urinary Tract Evaluation." **Based on 10 years of clinical experience with this test, a classification system describing four categories of prostatitis was described by Drach and colleagues in 1978. Differentiation of the four categories depended on an analysis of prostatic fluid, which included microscopy (examination for white blood cells [WBCs], inflammatory cell clumps, mucus debris, oval fat bodies, and macrophages) and culturing (identifying traditional uropathogens).**

Acute bacterial prostatitis was diagnosed when prostatic fluid was clinically purulent, systemic signs of infectious disease were present, and bacteria were cultured from prostatic fluid. Chronic bacterial prostatitis was diagnosed when pathogenic bacteria were recovered in significant numbers from a purulent prostatic fluid in the absence of a concomitant UTI or significant systemic signs. Nonbacterial prostatitis was diagnosed when significant numbers of bacteria could not be cultured from prostatic fluid, but the fluid consistently revealed microscopic purulence. Prostatodynia was diagnosed in the remaining patients who had persistent pain and voiding complaints as in the previous two categories but who had no significant bacteria or purulence in the prostatic fluid. This clinical differentiation of the prostatitis syndromes is now referred to as the *traditional* classification system (Table 9–1).

The significant limitations of this classification system included the abandonment by most physicians of the rigorous Meares-Stamey four-glass test (Moon, 1997; Nickel et al, 1998a; McNaughton-Collins et al, 1999, 2000), the realization that only the very rare patient would be subsequently diagnosed with chronic bacterial prostatitis, the perception that patients responded to specific therapy (e.g., antibiotics) independent of this classification system, and the dawning

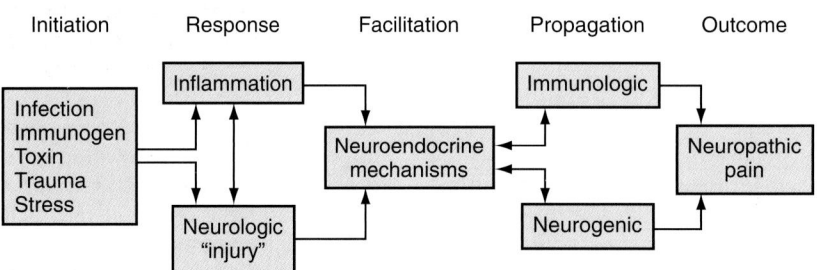

Figure 9–2. It is very likely that the etiology and pathogenesis of chronic prostatitis/chronic pelvic pain syndrome (category III CPPS) involves a pluricausal, multifactorial mechanism. An initiating stimulus such as infection, reflux of some "toxic" or "immunogenic" urine substance, perineal/pelvic "trauma," and/or psychological stress starts a cascade of events in an anatomically or genetically susceptible man, resulting in a local response of either inflammation or neurogenic injury (or both). Further immunologic or neuropathic (possibly interrelated) mechanisms mediated by neuroendocrine pathways propagate or sustain the chronicity of the initial (or ongoing) event. The final outcome is the clinical manifestation of chronic perineal/pelvic pain symptoms associated with local and central neuropathic mechanisms.

Table 9-1. Classification System for the Prostatitis Syndromes

Traditional	National Institutes of Health	Description
Acute bacterial prostatitis	Category I	Acute infection of the prostate gland
Chronic bacterial prostatitis	Category II	Chronic infection of the prostate gland
	Category III Chronic Pelvic Pain Syndrome (CPPS)	Chronic genitourinary pain in the absence of uropathogenic bacteria localized to the prostate gland employing standard methodology
Nonbacterial prostatitis	Category IIIA (Inflammatory CPPS)	Significant number of white blood cells in expressed prostatic secretions, post–prostatic massage urine sediment (VB3), or semen
Prostatodynia	Category IIIB (Noninflammatory CPPS)	Insignificant number of white blood cells in expressed prostatic secretions, post–prostatic massage urine sediment (VB3), or semen
	Asymptomatic Inflammatory Prostatitis (AIP)	White blood cells (and/or bacteria) in expressed prostatic secretions, post–prostatic massage urine sediment (VB3), semen, or histologic specimens of prostate gland

realization that, in many cases, patients presenting with prostatitis syndromes were not easily classified into one of these categories (e.g., patients in whom specific cultures were negative because of previous antibiotic therapy or those with CP thought to have a cause other than the prostate gland) (Nickel, 1998a).

National Institutes of Health Classification

The limitations of the traditional diagnostic algorithm and traditional classification system led to the development of the NIH classification system (see Table 9–1) (Krieger et al, 1999). The new definition recognized that pain is the main symptom in "abacterial chronic prostatitis" (with variable voiding and sexual dysfunction), and it was the optimal criterion to differentiate CP patients from control patients or patients experiencing other genitourinary problems (e.g., BPH). **This classification differed from the traditional system in two main areas, the descriptions of category III CPPS, and category IV asymptomatic inflammatory prostatitis.**

Category I is identical to the acute bacterial prostatitis category of the traditional classification system. Category II is identical to the traditional chronic bacterial prostatitis classification. Category III is defined as the "presence of genitourinary pain in the absence of uropathogenic bacteria detected by standard microbiological methodology." This syndrome is further categorized into category IIIA, or inflammatory CPPS (based on the presence of excessive leukocytes in EPSs or post–prostatic massage urine or semen), and category IIIB—noninflammatory CPPS (no significant leukocytes in similar specimens). Category IV, or asymptomatic inflammatory prostatitis, addressed one of the major problems and omissions of the traditional classification system. Patients are classified as having category IV prostatitis by the presence of significant leukocytes (or bacteria or both) in prostate-specific specimens (EPS, semen, and tissue biopsies) in the absence of typical chronic pelvic pain.

The NIH International Prostatitis Collaborative Network met in Washington in 1998 and confirmed the value of this classification system, not only in clinical research studies but also in clinical practice (Nickel et al, 1999c).

KEY POINT: CLASSIFICATION

■ The NIH classification of the prostatitis syndromes has now become recognized as the best system for research and clinical practice.

Clinical Presentation

Category I: Acute Bacterial Prostatitis

Acute bacterial prostatitis, category I, is a rare but important lower urinary tract infectious disease. It is characterized by an acute onset of pain combined with irritative and obstructive voiding symptoms in a patient with manifestations of a systemic febrile illness. The patient typically complains of urinary frequency, urgency, and dysuria. Obstructive voiding complaints including hesitancy, poor interrupted stream, strangury, and even acute urinary retention are common. The patient complains of perineal and suprapubic pain and may have associated pain or discomfort of the external genitalia. In addition, there are usually significant systemic symptoms including fever, chills, malaise, nausea and vomiting, and even frank septicemia with hypotension. The combination and severity of symptoms in category I, acute bacterial prostatitis, are variable from patient to patient. Approximately 5% of patients with acute bacterial prostatitis may progress to chronic bacterial prostatitis (Cho et al, 2005).

Category II: Chronic Bacterial Prostatitis

The most important clue in the diagnosis of category II, chronic bacterial prostatitis, is a history of documented recurrent UTIs. From 25% to 43% of patients diagnosed with chronic bacterial prostatitis employing a four-glass test had a history of recurrent UTIs (Weidner and Ludwig, 1994; Wright et al, 1994). Patients may be relatively asymptomatic between acute episodes, or they may present with a long history of a CPPS, which is described extensively in the next section. The prevalence of bacterial prostatitis ranges from 5% to 15% of prostatitis cases (Schaeffer et al, 1981; Krieger and Egan, 1991; Weidner and Ludwig, 1994). In one of the largest and most comprehensive clinical series, Weidner and associates (1991b) found significant bacteriuria (with uropathogenic organisms) in 4.4% of patients with symptoms of CP.

Category III: Chronic Pelvic Pain Syndrome

The presenting symptoms of inflammatory category IIIA CPPS (chronic nonbacterial prostatitis) are indistinguishable from those of patients with noninflammatory category IIIB disease (prostatodynia). The symptoms experienced by patients with CP/CPPS have been studied extensively by Krieger and colleagues (1996a). They evaluated 50 patients with CP seen in a prostatitis clinic (compared with 75 control patients). Alexander and Trissel (1996) surveyed a cohort of 163 prostatitis patients on the Internet. The symptoms were best defined in the development of prostatitis symptom scores by Neal and Moon (1994), Brahler and coworkers (1997), Krieger and colleagues (1996a), and Nickel and Sorensen (1996b). **The predominant symptom in all these studies was pain, which was most commonly localized to the perineum, suprapubic area, and penis but can also occur in the testes, groin, or low back. Pain during or after ejaculation is one of the most prominent, important, and bothersome feature in many patients** (Shoskes et al, 2004). Irritative and obstructive voiding symptoms including urgency, frequency, hesitancy, and poor interrupted flow are associated with this syndrome in many patients. Erectile dysfunction and sexual disturbances have been reported in patients with CPPS (Mehik et al, 2001; Liang et al, 2004; Zaslau et al, 2005) but are not pathognomonic features of this syndrome. The best description of the CP/CPPS patient was provided by the NIH Chronic Prostatitis Cohort Study (Schaeffer et al, 2002). A detailed description of 488 men with CP/CPPS noted that the most frequently reported pain/discomfort was in the perineum, followed by pain/discomfort in the suprapubic area. Over half of the men had pain/discomfort during or after sexual climax.

By definition, the syndrome becomes chronic after 3 months' duration. The symptoms tend to wax and wane over time; approximately one third of patients improve over 1 year (usually patients with shorter duration and fewer symptoms) (Nickel et al, 2002; Turner et al, 2004).

The impact of this condition on health status is significant. The quality of life of many patients diagnosed with CP/CPPS is impaired. Wenninger and associates (1996), employing a generic health status measure, the Sickness Impact Profile, showed that the mean scores were within the range of scores reported in the literature for patients with a history of myocardial infarction, angina, or Crohn's disease. McNaughton-Collins and coworkers (2001b) employed similar quality of life assessment instruments in the NIH Chronic Prostatitis Cohort of almost 300 patients and confirmed this finding. These investigators noted that the mental health component was affected more than the physical component of the quality of life assessment. CP/CPPS patients' quality of life was lower than those observed in the most severe subgroups of men with congestive heart failure and diabetes mellitus. This significant impact on quality of life has also been reported in a cohort of CP/CPPS men evaluated in a primary care setting (Turner et al, 2002).

Category IV: Asymptomatic Inflammatory Prostatitis

Category IV, asymptomatic inflammatory prostatitis, by definition, does not cause symptoms. The patients present with BPH, an elevated prostate-specific antigen (PSA) level, prostate cancer, or infertility. Subsequent microscopy of EPS or semen, and histologic examination of BPH chips, prostate cancer specimens, or prostate biopsies disclose evidence of prostatic inflammation.

Symptom Assessment

In a syndrome such as CP/CPPS, in which the objective parameters of the disease are unknown, controversial, or not validated, evaluation outcomes become of critical importance. In a syndrome defined primarily by its symptom complex, analysis of specific prostatitis-like symptoms, the quality of

life, the patient's functional status, and the patient's satisfaction with medical care will result in not only better evaluation of the prostatitis patient but also improved therapeutic follow-up. Scientifically validated symptom indices not only improve the care of patients but also optimize clinical decision making in terms of comparing clinical trial outcomes. Since the early 1990s, several different symptom indices have been described in clinical research (Neal and Moon, 1994; Krieger et al, 1996a; Nickel and Sorensen, 1996b; Brahler et al, 1997; Chiang et al 1997) and have been sporadically employed in clinical practice (McNaughton-Collins and O'Leary, 1999). Although each of these symptom indices was successful at the time it was developed for the specific purpose or study, none was believed to be ideal for use in general research or clinical practice, because they were not validated according to the rigorous standards that now must be met for an accepted urologic disease-specific index (O'Leary et al, 1992).

The NIH Chronic Prostatitis Collaborative Research Network (CPCRN) developed a reproducible and valid instrument to measure the symptoms and quality of life of CP for use in research protocols as well as clinical practice (Litwin et al, 1999). The steps followed in the development of the NIH-CPSI included a systematic literature review, focus groups, cognitive testing, an expert panel review, a validation test, and psychometric analyses. The final index consists of nine questions that address the three most important domains of the CP experience. Pain (which is the primary symptom of CP/CPPS) was captured in four questions that focused on its location, severity, and frequency. Urinary function, the second most important component of patients' symptoms, was captured in two questions, one concerning irritative and the other obstructive function. The quality of life, or impact, was captured in three additional questions that asked about the effect of symptoms on daily activities. The NIH-CPSI (Fig. 9–3) has now been accepted by the international prostatitis research community as an accepted outcome measure (Nickel et al, 1999c), has shown validity and responsiveness in primary care samples (Turner et al, 2003), and is at present being translated and validated in many languages other than English (Collins et al, 2001; Kunishima et al, 2002; Leskinen et al, 2003; Schneider et al, 2004). The symptom index has also proved its usefulness in the evaluation and follow-up of patients in general clinical urologic practice (Nickel, 1999b).

KEY POINT: SYMPTOM ASSESSMENT

- The validated NIH-CPSI is a useful research and clinical tool for evaluating CPPS patients.

Lower Urinary Tract Evaluation

Physical Examination

Physical examination is an important part of the evaluation of a prostatitis patient, but it is usually not helpful in making a definitive diagnosis or further classifying a prostatitis patient. It assists in ruling out other perineal, anal, neurologic, pelvic, or prostate abnormalities and is an integral part of the lower urinary tract evaluation by providing prostate-specific specimens.

In category I, acute bacterial prostatitis, the patient may be systemically toxic, that is, flushed, febrile, tachycardic,

NIH-Chronic Prostatitis Symptom Index (NIH-CPSI)

Pain or Discomfort

1. In the last week, have you experienced any pain or discomfort in the following areas?

	Yes	No
a. Area between rectum and testicles (perineum)	❑ 1	❑ 0
b. Testicles	❑ 1	❑ 0
c. Tip of the penis (not related to urination)	❑ 1	❑ 0
d. Below your waist, in your pubic or bladder area	❑ 1	❑ 0

2. In the last week, have you experienced:

	Yes	No
a. Pain or burning during urination?	❑ 1	❑ 0
b. Pain or discomfort during or after sexual climax (ejaculation)?	❑ 1	❑ 0

3. How often have you had pain or discomfort in any of these areas over the last week?

❑ 0 Never
❑ 1 Rarely
❑ 2 Sometimes
❑ 3 Often
❑ 4 Usually
❑ 5 Always

4. Which number best describes your AVERAGE pain or discomfort on the days that you had it, over the last week?

❑	❑	❑	❑	❑	❑	❑	❑	❑	❑	❑
0	1	2	3	4	5	6	7	8	9	10

NO PAIN — PAIN AS BAD AS YOU CAN IMAGINE

Urination

5. How often have you had a sensation of not emptying your bladder completely after you finished urinating, over the last week?

❑ 0 Not at all
❑ 1 Less than 1 time in 5
❑ 2 Less than half the time
❑ 3 About half the time
❑ 4 More than half the time
❑ 5 Almost always

6. How often have you had to urinate again less than two hours after you finished urinating, over the last week?

❑ 0 Not at all
❑ 1 Less than 1 time in 5
❑ 2 Less than half the time
❑ 3 About half the time
❑ 4 More than half the time
❑ 5 Almost always

Impact of Symptoms

7. How much have your symptoms kept you from doing the kinds of things you would usually do, over the last week?

❑ 0 None
❑ 1 Only a little
❑ 2 Some
❑ 3 A lot

8. How much did you think about your symptoms, over the last week?

❑ 0 None
❑ 1 Only a little
❑ 2 Some
❑ 3 A lot

Quality of Life

9. If you were to spend the rest of your life with your symptoms just the way they have been during the last week, how would you feel about that?

❑ 0 Delighted
❑ 1 Pleased
❑ 2 Mostly satisfied
❑ 3 Mixed (about equally satisfied and dissatisfied)
❑ 4 Mostly dissatisfied
❑ 5 Unhappy
❑ 6 Terrible

Scoring the NIH-Chronic Prostatitis Symptom Index Domains

Pain: Total of items 1a, 1b, 1c, 1d, 2a, 2b, 3, and 4 = ____

Urinary Symptoms: Total of items 5 and 6 = ____

Quality of Life Impact: Total of items 7, 8, and 9 = ____

Figure 9–3. The National Institutes of Health Chronic Prostatitis Symptom Index (NIH-CPSI) captures the three most important domains of the prostatitis experience: pain (location, frequency, and severity), voiding (irritative and obstructive symptoms), and quality of life (including impact). This index is useful in research studies and clinical practice. (From Litwin MS, McNaughton-Collins M, Fowler FJ, et al: The NIH Chronic Prostatitis Symptom Index [NIH-CPSI]: Development and validation of a new outcome measure. J Urol 1999:162;369-375. Reprinted with permission.)

tachypneic, and even hypotensive. The patient usually has suprapubic discomfort and perhaps has clinically detectable acute urinary retention. Perineal pain and anal sphincter spasm may complicate the digital rectal examination. The prostate itself is usually described as hot, boggy, and exquisitely tender. The expression of prostatic fluid is believed to be totally unnecessary and perhaps even harmful.

The physical examination of a patient with category II, chronic bacterial prostatitis, and category III CPPS is usually unremarkable (except for pain). Careful examination and palpation of external genitalia, groin, perineum, coccyx, external anal sphincter (tone), and internal pelvic floor and side walls may pinpoint prominent areas of pain or discomfort. **The digital rectal examination should be performed after the patient has produced pre–prostatic massage urine specimens (see later). The prostate may be normal in size and consistency, and it has also been described as enlarged and boggy (loosely defined by the author as softer than normal).**

The degree of elicited pain during prostatic palpation is variable and is unhelpful in differentiating a prostatitis syndrome. The prostate should be carefully checked for prostatic nodules before a vigorous prostatic massage is performed to produce prostate-specific specimens (EPS and post–prostatic massage urine sample).

Lower Urinary Tract Cytologic Examination and Culture Techniques

In patients presenting with category I, acute bacterial prostatitis, a urine culture is the only laboratory evaluation of the lower urinary tract required. It has been suggested that the vigorous prostatic massage necessary to produce EPS can exacerbate the clinical situation, although such fears have never been substantiated in the literature. A midstream urine specimen will show significant leukocytosis and bacteriuria microscopically, and culturing usually discloses typical uropathogens. Blood cultures may show the same organism.

In 1968, Meares and Stamey described the classic four-glass urine collection technique to distinguish urethral, bladder, and prostate infections in men with CP, and for 3 decades this has remained the "gold standard" for the evaluation of this lower urinary tract syndrome. The voided bladder-1 (VB1) specimen includes the first 10 mL of urine and represents the urethral specimen. The voided bladder-2 (VB2) specimen is similar to a midstream urine collection and represents the bladder urine. EPS should be collected directly into a sterile container during prostatic massage. The voided bladder-3 (VB3) specimen, the first 10 mL of urine voided after prostatic massage, includes any EPS trapped in the prostatic urethra. The three urine specimens are centrifuged for 5 minutes and the sediment examined under high power for leukocytes (including aggregates of leukocytes), macrophages, oval fat bodies, erythrocytes, bacteria, and fungal hyphae. A wet mount of a drop of EPS can be examined under a coverslip in a similar manner. Some researchers (Muller et al, 2001; Krieger et al, 2003) point out that quantitative determination of the EPS WBC concentration by a counting chamber method is superior to the standard wet mount method but probably only indicated in research studies. In fact, the NIH

Chronic Prostatitis Cohort Study (Schaeffer et al, 2002; Nickel et al, 2003a) suggested that leukocyte determination did not appear to add significant clinical information to the assessment of a patient with CP/CPPS. All four specimens are sent to the laboratory for quantitative culturing. Figure 9–4 illustrates the technique and interpretation of the four-glass test.

Category II, chronic bacterial prostatitis, is diagnosed if there is a 10-fold increase in bacteria in the EPS or VB3 specimen compared with the VB1 and VB2. In a patient who has acute cystitis, this localization is impossible; and in this case, patients can be treated with a short course (1 to 3 days) of therapy with antibiotics such as nitrofurantoin, which penetrates the prostate poorly but eradicates the bladder bacteriuria. Subsequent localization of bacteria in the post–prostatic massage urine or EPS is then diagnostic of category II prostatitis. Category IIIA CPPS (chronic nonbacterial prostatitis) is diagnosed when no uropathogenic bacteria are cultured, but excessive leukocytosis (usually defined as more than 5 to 10 WBCs per high-power field [HPF]) is noted in the prostate-specific specimens (EPS or VB3 or both). Category IIIB CPPS (prostatodynia) is diagnosed when no uropathogenic bacteria are cultured and there is no significant leukocytosis noted on microscopic examination of EPS or the sediment of VB3.

Although the four-glass test remains the gold standard diagnostic evaluation of prostatitis patients, numerous surveys (Moon, 1997; Nickel et al, 1998a; McNaughton-Collins et al, 1999b; McNaughton-Collins et al, 2000) have confirmed that clinicians have more or less abandoned this time-consuming and expensive rigorous evaluation. **The pre–prostatic massage and post–prostatic massage test (or two-glass test), originally suggested by Weidner and Ebner** (1985) **and popularized by Nickel** (1995, 1996, 1997a), **is a simple, cost-effective screen to categorize CP patients.** The patient provides a midstream pre–prostatic massage urine specimen and a urine specimen (initial 10 mL) after prostatic massage. Microscopy (sediment) and culturing of these two screening urine specimens allows categorization of the majority of patients presenting with CP. Figure 9–5 illustrates the technique and interpretation of the two-glass pre-massage and post–prostatic massage test.

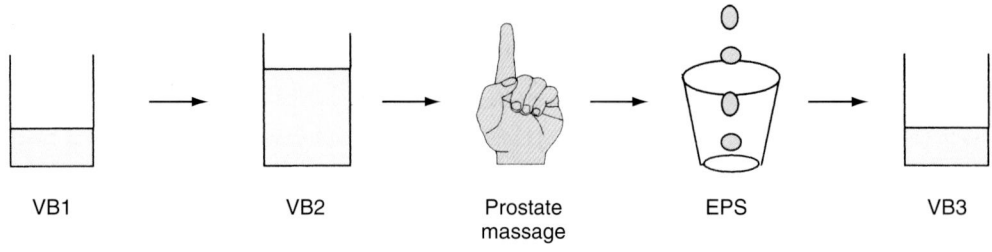

VB1 → VB2 → Prostate massage → EPS → VB3

Figure 9–4. Technique and interpretation of the Meares-Stamey four-glass lower urinary tract localization test for chronic prostatitis/chronic pelvic pain syndrome.

4-Glass test (Meares-Stamey test)

Classification	Specimen	VB$_1$	VB$_2$	EPS	VB$_3$
CAT II	WBC	−	+/−*	+	+
	Culture	−	+/−*	+	+
CAT IIIA	WBC	−	−	+	+
	Culture	−	−	−	−
CAT IIIB	WBC	−	−	−	−
	Culture	−	−	−	−

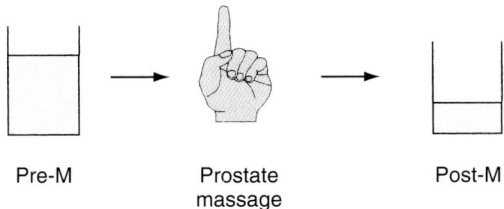

Pre-M | Prostate massage | Post-M

2-Glass test (PPMT)

Classification	Specimen	Pre-M	Post-M
CAT II	WBC	+/–*	+
	Culture	+/–*	+
CAT IIIA	WBC	–	+
	Culture	–	–
CAT IIIB	WBC	–	–
	Culture	–	–

Figure 9–5. Technique and interpretation of the pre- and post-massage two-glass lower urinary tract localization test for chronic prostatitis/chronic pelvic pain syndrome.

In a retrospective personal series and a review of series in the literature, Nickel (1997a) noted that this test had 91% sensitivity and specificity compared with the gold standard Meares-Stamey test. Its limitations were thought to be due to the exclusion of the urethral and EPS specimen. However, in patients without clinical urethritis, Krieger and associates (2000) demonstrated that urethral swabs are more efficient in picking up urethral inflammation than VB1. But in this series of 235 patients, only 3% had more than 1 WBC/HPF. Therefore, urethral specimens rarely detected significant urethral inflammation, and in this series rarely did cultured organisms change the direction of clinical therapy in prostatitis patients (without clinical urethritis). In the same study (Krieger et al, 2000) comparing EPS with post–prostatic massage urine, the investigators demonstrated that EPS examination detected 76%, whereas post–prostatic massage urine examination detected 82% of the patients who had inflammation on one or both tests. Ludwig and associates (2000), in a series of 328 patients in whom both EPS and VB3 were obtained, demonstrated that VB3 is almost as accurate as EPS (92% sensitivity; 99% specificity) in detecting prostate-specific inflammation. Seiler and coworkers (2003) came to the same conclusion in their study of 143 CP patients. Nickel and colleagues from the NIH CPCRN (2005d) examined a cohort of 353 CP/CPPS men with complete four-glass data and noted that the two-glass test predicted a positive four-glass result with clinically acceptable accuracy (high specificity; lower sensitivity) This test, however, is only a screening test, and in patients in whom it is important to localize bacteria to the prostate versus the urethra (e.g., patients with recurrent UTIs, suspicion of urethral abnormality), a follow-up VB1 or urethral swab may be very helpful. If typical urethral organisms are localized to the prostate when the pre–prostatic massage and post–prostatic massage test is used and the clinician is inclined to consider them pathogenic and subsequently treat the patients, urethral and EPS specimens to definitively localize the specific bacteria to the prostate are appropriate. As a general rule, it is always best to examine the EPS (if it can be obtained) microscopically.

Microbiologic Considerations. Both the traditional and the NIH classification systems depend on culturing for standard uropathogens. The Enterobacteriaceae (e.g., *E. coli, Serratia, Klebsiella, Proteus, Pseudomonas*) represent the most common uropathogens, followed by gram-positive enterococci. However, as discussed in the section "Etiology," other gram-positive organisms that typically colonize the urethra (*Staphylococcus epidermidis, Staphylococcus saprophyticus, Streptococcus* species, *Corynebacterium,* and *Bacteroides*) can be localized to the prostate specimens, including semen (>10-fold colony-forming unit count in prostate-specific specimens compared with pre–prostatic massage specimens), and their association with the prostatic inflammation symptom complex remains unclear. At this time, these patients are still considered category III CPPS, but as more research results become available, this may change as our understanding of bacterial pathogenicity in the prostate gland evolves (Nickel and Moon, 2005; Nickel et al, 2005e).

Cytologic Considerations.

The differentiation of the two subtypes of category III CPPS depend on cytologic examination of the urine or EPS or both. The urine specimens are centrifuged for 5 minutes, and the sediment is resuspended under a coverslip and examined at high power (300× to 400×) while the wet mount of a drop of EPS is examined under a coverslip at the same power. WBCs have traditionally been reported as numbers of leukocytes per high-power field (Fig. 9–6). There is no validated cut-off point for the level of WBCs per high-power field that is required to differentiate an inflammatory from a noninflammatory CPPS. Although the suggested limits have ranged from as low as 2 (Anderson and Weller, 1979) to as high as 20 (Blacklock and Beavis, 1974), the consensus appears to favor 5 to 10 WBCs/HPF in EPS as the upper level of normal (Meares and Stamey, 1968; Pfau et al, 1978; Schaeffer et al, 1981). But inflammatory cells in the EPS fluctuate over time (Anderson and Weller, 1979; Schaeffer et al, 1981) and with the frequency of ejaculation (Jameson, 1967; Yavascaoglu et al, 1999). A disadvantage of looking at a drop of prostatic fluid or urine sediment is that the cells may clump or aggregate, which renders quantifying them virtually impossible. Also, an unstained specimen does not allow differentiation of the type of WBC present (e.g., polymorphonuclear leukocytes, lymphocytes, monocytes, macrophages). If accuracy is required (i.e., research), then the white blood cells can be counted in a glass hemacytometer (so they may be quantified as cells per square millimeter) and subsequently stained to differentiate the inflammatory cell subtype (Anderson and Weller, 1979).

The clinical relevance of adding cytologic examination of semen specimens (which is difficult without special staining

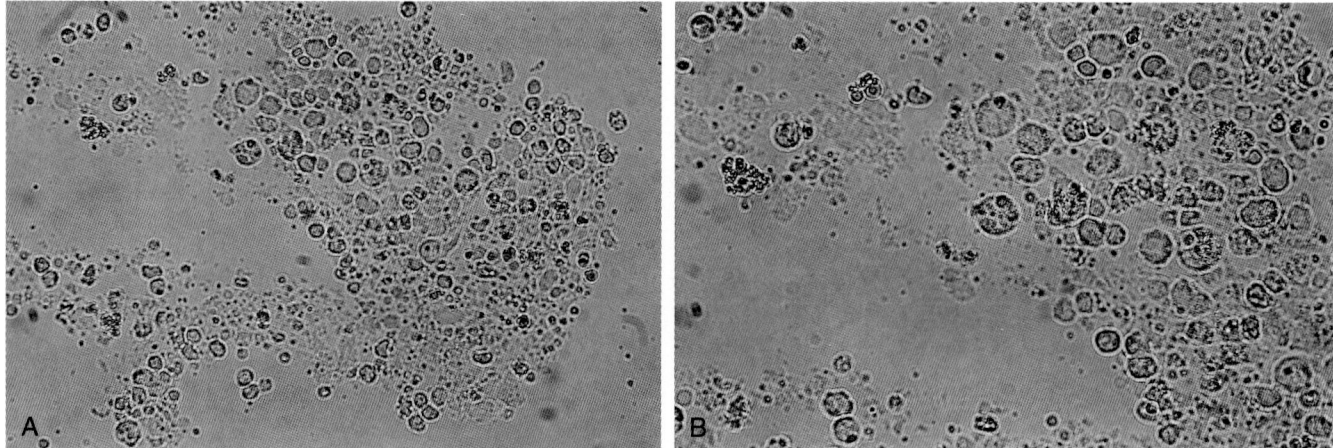

Figure 9–6. **A** and **B**, Unstained photomicrographs showing individual white blood cells, clumps of white blood cells, and lipid-laden macrophages in the expressed prostatic secretion (EPS) of a patient with category IIIA CPPS (**A**, ×250; **B**, ×400).

techniques) is unknown. Certainly, semen examination increases the percentage of patients identified as inflammatory category IIIA CPPS (Krieger et al, 2000).

Nickel and colleagues (2003a) compared the number of WBCs in the EPS in patients with CP/CPPS to EPS specimens from normal asymptomatic control men and noted that although there was a statistically significant difference in WBC counts in the CP/CPPS men, the clinical significance was not apparent (e.g., 50% of CPPS men had >5 WBCs/HPF compared with 40% of control men). The relevance of examining urine and EPS for WBCs in routine clinical practice has been challenged (Nickel et al, 2003a). However, some investigators (Nickel, 2002d) have recommended that urine cytology (for malignant cells) become a standard diagnostic test for men presenting with prostatitis-like symptoms, particularly if the symptom-complex includes irritative voiding symptoms, dysuria, and/or suprapubic/bladder pain.

Urodynamics

Pain is the dominant symptom in patients presenting with CP/CPPS, but a wide constellation of irritative and obstructive voiding symptoms are associated with this syndrome. Proposed causes to account for the persistent irritative and obstructive voiding symptoms include detrusor vesical neck or external sphincter dyssynergia, proximal or distal urethral obstruction, and fibrosis or hypertrophy of the vesical neck (Orland et al, 1985; Blacklock, 1974, 1986; Bates et al, 1975; Theodorou et al, 1999). These abnormalities can be clarified and diagnosed by urodynamics, particularly video-urodynamics. Others have suggested that men with defined primary voiding dysfunction have been misdiagnosed with CP (Webster et al, 1980; Siroky et al, 1981; Murnaghan and Millard, 1984). Siroky and associates (1981) noted that urodynamics revealed that 50% of 47 men with recurrent voiding symptoms, perigenital pain, or both, previously diagnosed as CP had bladder areflexia with non-relaxing perineal floor (striated muscle spasm), and another 36% had bladder hyperreflexia with appropriate striated sphincter relaxation. Barbaralis (1990) and Barbaralis and colleagues (1983) noted decreased peak and mean urinary flow rates, a significantly elevated maximal urethral closing pres-

sure, and incomplete funneling of the bladder neck accompanied by urethral narrowing at the level of the external urinary sphincter during voiding with urodynamic evaluation of men diagnosed with CP. Hellstrom and colleagues (1987) also noted elevated urethral pressures, "hyperreflexia" of the external urethral sphincter, and intraprostatic reflux in three patients with unremitting symptoms of chronic nonbacterial prostatitis.

Kaplan and associates (1994, 1996, 1997) postulated that chronic lower urinary tract symptoms in young men are often misdiagnosed as chronic nonbacterial prostatitis when in fact they indicate a cohort of men with undiagnosed chronic voiding dysfunction. This conclusion is based on the video-urodynamic studies of 137 consecutive men 50 years of age or younger diagnosed with CP (Kaplan et al, 1996). They demonstrated a variety of urodynamic abnormalities, including 54% of patients with primary vesical neck obstruction, 24% with functional obstruction localized to the membranous urethra (pseudodyssynergia), 17% with impaired bladder contractility, and 5% with an acontractile bladder. They noted detrusor instability in 49% of the men. Simple documentation of uroflowmetry and residual urine bladder scan abnormalities may suggest proceeding to more sophisticated urodynamics (Ghobish, 2000). Other groups dispute the benefits of urodynamics and have noted very few urodynamic abnormalities in patients presenting with classic CP symptoms (Mayo et al, 1998).

Endoscopy

Clinical experience (rather than controlled clinical studies) suggests that lower urinary tract endoscopy (i.e., cystoscopy) is not indicated in the majority of men presenting with CP/CPPS. However, cystoscopy is indicated in patients in whom the history (e.g., hematuria), lower urinary tract evaluation (e.g., VB1 urinalysis), or ancillary studies (e.g., urodynamics) indicate the possibility of a diagnosis other than CP/CPPS. In these patients, occasionally lower urinary tract malignancy, stones, urethral strictures, bladder neck abnormalities and so forth that can be surgically corrected are discovered. Cystoscopy can probably be justified in men refractory to standard therapy.

Transrectal Ultrasonography

Transrectal ultrasonography has become one of the best radiologic methods to evaluate prostate disease and has become an especially helpful clinical tool for the assessment of prostate volume and ultrasound guidance of biopsy needles. The diagnostic value of ultrasonography in differentiating benign from malignant prostate disease is controversial, and the further differentiation of the various benign conditions of the prostate is even more so. Di Trapani and colleagues (1988) described inhomogeneous echo structures, constant dilatation of periprostatic venous plexus, elongated seminal vesicles, and thickening of the inner septa in patients with prostatitis. Doble and Carter (1989) described seven ultrasound signs associated with the presence of symptoms of CP compared with controls; and although the sensitivity increased with higher leukocyte counts, the signs were not sufficiently specific to differentiate clinical groups.

Peeling and Griffiths (1984) describe the heterogeneity of the echo pattern and prostatic calculi as ultrasound features related to prostatitis. Ludwig and coworkers (1994) described the ultrasound features such as prostatic calcifications and seminal vesicle abnormalities that appear to be indicative of signs of inflammation but not proof of the presence of CP. Harada and associates (1980) concluded that the presence of stones is not related to a specific prostate disease process. De la Rosette and colleagues (1992b) performed ultrasonography in 22 patients with nonbacterial prostatitis and compared the results with those of a control group of 22 patients without lower urinary tract symptoms. This study indicated that there were no significant differences in ultrasound patterns of patients with nonbacterial prostatitis and the control group. Others have employed color Doppler ultrasonography (Veneziano et al, 1995) and automated computer analysis (de la Rosette et al, 1995) in an attempt to improve the value of transrectal ultrasonography in the evaluation of prostatitis patients; however, the results are not conclusive enough to indicate that this is a clinically useful tool.

Transrectal ultrasonography can be valuable in diagnosing medial prostatic cysts in patients with prostatitis-like symptoms (Dik et al, 1996), **diagnosing and draining prostatic abscesses** (Granados et al, 1992), **or diagnosing and draining obstructed seminal vesicles** (Littrup et al, 1988). It is not required in all cases of acute bacterial prostatitis but rather only in those patients who are failing appropriate antimicrobial therapy (Horcajada et al, 2003).

Prostate Biopsy

Occasionally, because of an elevated PSA level or abnormal digital rectal examination, prostate biopsy is indicated (Kawakami et al, 2004). Some clinicians will consider starting patients with elevated screening PSA levels and a history of prostatitis or symptoms of CPPS on antibiotics, but this practice is really only rational in patients with acute or chronic bacterial prostatitis (Nickel, 2002c), conditions that invariably lead to elevated PSA levels. The diagnosis of CP/CPPS should only be used as a reason against a prostate biopsy if the clinician is looking for an excuse not to biopsy (Nickel, 2002c). A comprehensive review on PSA and prostatitis is available (Kawakami et al, 2004).

Out of desperation, urologists sometimes resort to prostate biopsy in an attempt either to demonstrate histologic evidence of prostatic inflammation or to culture an organism that cannot be cultured employing the standard approach. The importance and interpretation of prostate biopsies in CP performed for reasons other than prostate cancer screening is unclear. Doble and associates (1990) demonstrated immune complexes in the prostate of patients with prostatitis but found culture of the prostatic tissue unhelpful (Doble et al, 1989a). Nickel and Costerton (1993) were able to confirm the presence of potentially uropathogenic bacteria in patients with a documented history of chronic bacterial prostatitis in whom EPS cultures became sterile after antibiotic therapy. Berger and associates (1997) also confirmed the presence of potential uropathogenic bacteria in prostate biopsies (which correlated to some extent with prostatic inflammation in EPS) in patients in whom the same bacteria did not grow standard prostatic specimens (such as EPS). Krieger and colleagues (1996b) demonstrated the possible presence of microorganisms in the prostate gland of a majority of men with CP syndrome using the molecular biologic technique of polymerase chain reaction. **At this time, histologic, culture, and molecular biologic evaluations of prostate biopsies in patients with CP/CPPS remain research tools only.**

Other

Wishnow and associates (1982) found that control patients (10 patients) and men with chronic abacterial prostatitis (4 patients) had no antibodies to gram-negative bacterial antigens, in contrast to men with bacterial prostatitis (6 patients). They hypothesized that immunologic analysis may provide a better diagnostic tool than culturing and microscopy. Shortliffe and coworkers (1981a, 1981b, 1986, 1989, 1992) found that the total IgA and IgG levels in the prostatic fluid in men with chronic abacterial prostatitis were higher than those of controls. They also discovered that prostatic fluid from control or abacterial prostatitis patients did not contain specific antibodies to gram-negative urinary pathogens (in contrast to men with bacterial prostatitis). Nickel and colleagues (2001a) used a similar antibody screening procedure in evaluation of 102 men with CP/CPPS who were subsequently treated with quinolone antibiotics. However, "antibody-positive" patients did not have a better response to antibiotic therapy than "antibody-negative" patients after 12 weeks of therapy. Li and associates (2001) demonstrated increased endotoxin concentrations in EPS and VB3 of men with bacterial prostatitis and inflammatory category IIIA CPPS and suggested that endotoxin levels might be used to identify these categories of CP patients.

Alexander and colleagues (1998) discovered that men with chronic abacterial prostatitis had higher mean levels of the proinflammatory cytokines (IL-1α and TNF-α) in seminal plasma compared with controls. Ruggieri and coworkers (2000) noted that levels of both IL-1α and IL-8 were significantly higher in semen in category IIIA patients (leukocytes) than in category IIIB patients, but there was no statistically significant difference in levels of TNF-α, IL-1α, or IL-6. This group found no correlation between cytokine levels and the number of leukocytes in EPS. Nadler and colleagues (2000) found that mean levels of IL-1α in EPS were higher in men with inflammatory chronic abacterial prostatitis and noninflammatory chronic bacterial prostatitis compared with controls. Hochreiter and associates (2000a) did find a direct significant correlation between the number of leukocytes in EPS and IL-1α levels in EPS. The sensitivity or specificity of these immunologic tests are really unknown and are not yet indicated in clinical practice.

Marmar and associates (1980) hypothesized that zinc levels in EPS would be a useful marker for prostatitis and found that, indeed, zinc levels in men with chronic abacterial prostatitis and bacterial prostatitis were significantly lower than zinc levels in control patients and men with prostatodynia. However, Zaichick and colleagues (1996) found no differences in zinc levels between patients with chronic abacterial prostatitis, BPH, and controls. At this time, the measurement of zinc levels in prostatic or semen specimens is clinically unhelpful.

Tanner and associates (1999) detected positive signals (rRNA-based molecular technique with prostatic fluid) in 65% of patients with CP. Seven of 11 patients with bacterial signals but none of 6 patients without bacterial signals were improved on antibiotic therapy. The same group (Shoskes and Shahed, 2000) subsequently confirmed this finding with a larger cohort of patients. These results are intriguing, and controlled studies evaluating the potential clinical significance of differentiating patients based on molecular biologic techniques are required.

A diagnostic algorithm that provides a practical approach to the workup of the majority of men presenting with CP/CPPS is shown in Figure 9–7. Table 9–2 shows the tests recommended by the NIH Third International Prostatitis Collaborative Network (Nickel, 2003).

KEY POINTS: LOWER URINARY TRACT EVALUATION

■ Mandatory evaluation includes history, physical examination, urinalysis, and urine culture.

■ Recommended evaluation includes lower urinary tract localization test, NIH-CPSI, flow rate, residual urine determination, and urine cytology.

Treatment

In this section the rationale for each of the various treatments advocated for the prostatitis syndromes is presented, followed by a review of the clinical trial data that support (or not) the use of those specific therapeutic modalities in clinical practice. Recent rigorous prospective studies in chronic bacterial

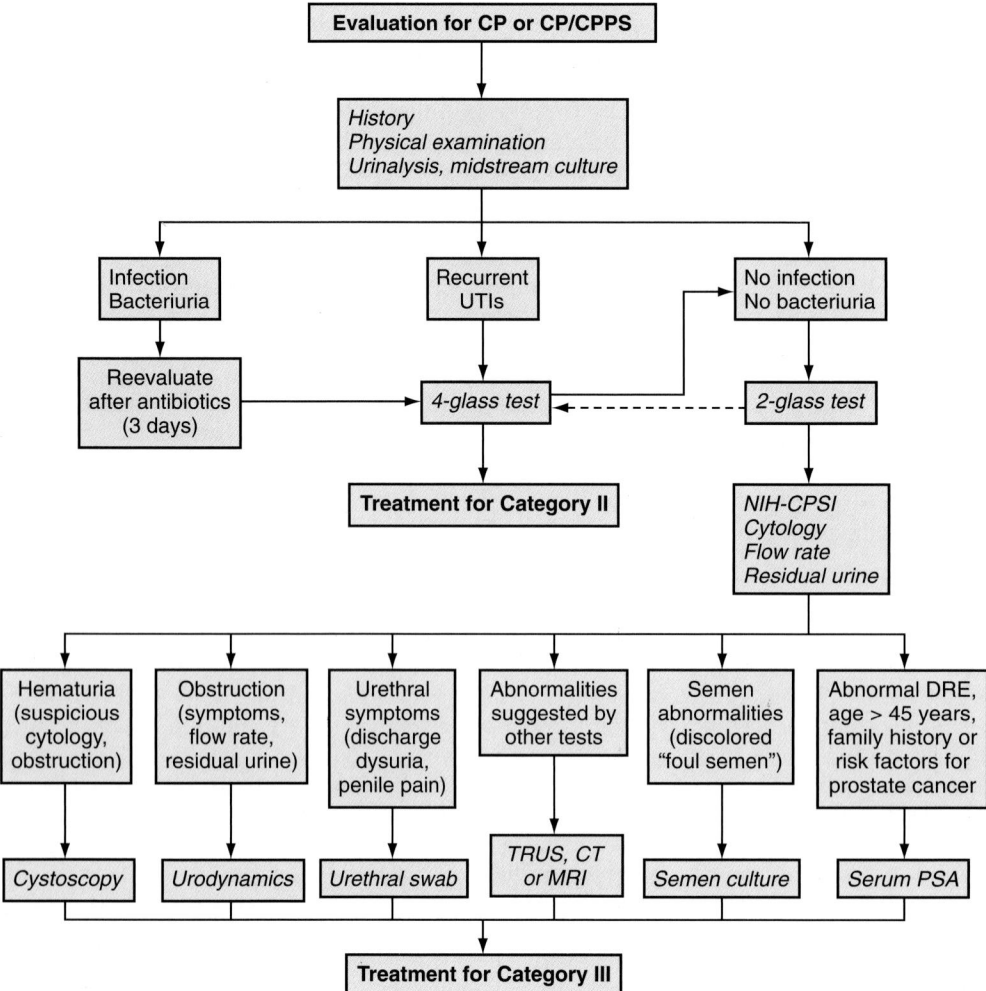

Figure 9–7. A suggested diagnostic algorithm for the evaluation of patients presenting with chronic prostatitis and chronic pelvic pain syndrome. UTIs, urinary tract infections; TRUS, transrectal ultrasound; CT, computed tomography; MRI, magnetic resonance imaging, DRE; digital rectal examination; PSA, prostate-specific antigen.

Table 9-2. **Suggested Evaluation of a Man with CPPS***
Mandatory
History
Physical examination, including digital rectal examination
Urinalysis and urine culture
Recommended
Lower urinary tract localization test
Symptom inventory or index (NIH-CPSI)
Flow rate
Residual urine determination
Urine cytology
Optional
Semen analysis and culture
Urethral swab for culture
Pressure flow studies
Video urodynamics (including flow electromyography)
Cystoscopy
Transrectal ultrasound
Pelvic imaging (ultrasound, CT, MRI)
Prostate-specific antigen

*See text for explanation, rationale, and description of each test (Nickel, 2002).

prostatitis and randomized placebo-controlled trials employing standardized definitions and validated outcomes in CP/CPPS has allowed us to develop evidence-based treatment strategies in a therapeutic field that used to be based on poor clinical data, dogma, and anecdotal experience (McNaughton-Collins et al, 2001b, 2001a; Nickel, 2002a, 2002b, 2004).

Medical Therapy

Antimicrobial Agents

Rationale. It is generally accepted that acute and chronic bacterial prostatitis are etiologically secondary to bacterial infection of the prostate gland. Many urologists further believe that, although bacteria are only cultured in 5% to 10% of cases of prostatitis, bacteria may be the cause of prostatitis in a significant percentage of patients presenting with this syndrome. **Antimicrobial therapy is most commonly prescribed for the CP syndromes** (Moon, 1997; Nickel et al, 1998a; McNaughton-Collins et al, 2000a, 2001), independent of culture status.

Pharmacology and Pharmacokinetics. Most antimicrobial pharmacokinetic studies were performed in animal models (dogs and rats) (Madsen et al, 1978; Nickel, 1997b). Stamey (1980) and Stamey and associates (1970) found that acid antibiotic drugs can be detected in prostatic secretions only in very low concentrations, even when plasma concentrations of the drug are very high. Alkaline antibiotic drugs are found in concentrations greater than the simultaneous plasma levels. In dogs, this was explained by the presence of a pH gradient across the prostate epithelium. This phenomenon of ion trapping, and the fact that drug penetration was believed to be a passive transport mechanism based on diffusion and concentration, suggested that drug penetration is dependent on the lipid solubility, degree of ionization, degree of protein binding, and size and shape of the antimicrobial molecule. In dogs, the pH of plasma was found to be 7.4 whereas that of prostatic secretion is 6.4. Therefore, in this model, weak acids (low pKa) concentrate on the plasma side

whereas antibiotics with higher pKas (weak bases) concentrate in the prostatic secretion.

Because infection may alter the local prostatic environment, thus changing the pharmacokinetic parameters, animal models were developed that introduced infection into the process (Baumueller and Madsen, 1977; Madsen et al, 1994; Nickel et al, 1995). All these animal studies (with and without infection) showed that trimethoprim concentrates in prostatic secretion and prostatic interstitial fluid (exceeding plasma levels) whereas sulfamethoxazole and ampicillin do not. The fluoroquinolones, which are neither pure acids nor bases but have characteristics of both, being zwitterionic drugs (e.g., those that have two pKa values) (Gasser et al, 1986), should allow drug concentration in the prostate at various pH ranges. In the dog model, ciprofloxacin and norfloxacin did not concentrate in prostatic secretion as predicted, and this may be accounted for by their lipid solubility and protein-binding characteristics. Carbenicillin, which for years was the only antibiotic approved by the U.S. Food and Drug Administration for the treatment of bacterial prostatitis, could not be detected in prostatic secretion at all. Aminoglycosides did not concentrate in prostatic secretion and for unknown reasons may not follow the rules of nonionic diffusion of drugs across biologic membranes.

It is difficult to extrapolate the animal pharmacokinetic studies to humans (Sharer and Fair, 1982). Fair and Cordonnier (1978) found that the prostatic secretion of normal men is slightly alkaline (pH approximately 7.3) but also that the pH of prostatic secretion in men with prostatic infection is markedly increased (pH approximately 8.3). This has been confirmed in other studies (Anderson and Fair, 1976; Blacklock and Beavis, 1978; Pfau et al, 1978), and because the pH gradation is crucial to ion trapping, we should not apply the results from animal studies directly to humans. Unfortunately, drug diffusion studies are difficult to carry out in humans, and most studies determine antibiotic concentrations in transurethrally resected BPH adenomas. These studies are further complicated because the high drug concentrations in urine can substantially alter the results. Employing a method to reduce urine contamination, Naber and coworkers (1999) demonstrated that for most fluoroquinolones, the ratio of concentrations in prostatic fluid to concentrations in plasma is less than 1 (norfloxacin ratio 0.12, ciprofloxacin ratio 0.18 to 0.26, lomefloxacin ratio 0.48). Concentrations in seminal fluid usually exceed corresponding plasma concentrations of ciprofloxacin and ofloxacin, with ciprofloxacin demonstrating the highest seminal fluid-to-plasma ratio (Naber, 1999). The numerous studies evaluating fluoroquinolone concentrations in prostatic tissue demonstrated that the fluoroquinolone concentration in the adenoma tissue is usually higher than that in plasma.

Clinical Trial Data. Unless the patient has a significant anatomic abnormality of the lower urinary tract or develops a prostate abscess, antimicrobial therapy is universally successful in eradicating the bacteria and curing the patient presenting with acute bacterial prostatitis. In the acutely inflamed prostate gland, the pharmacokinetic considerations described in the previous section probably do not play a significant role in antibiotic penetration, and it is believed that most antibiotics achieve reasonable intraprostatic concentrations in the acute phase of the disease. Although prospective clinical trial data are unavailable, most experts suggest therapy initially with parenteral antibiotics (depending on the seriousness of the infection), followed by oral antibiotics with wide-spectrum antimicrobial activity (Becopoulos et al, 1990). The most common drugs suggested for initial therapy (Neal, 1999) are a combination of penicillin (i.e., ampicillin) and an aminoglycoside (i.e., gentamicin), second- or third-generation cephalosporins, or one of the fluoroquinolones. Once the acute infection has settled down, therapy should be continued with one of the oral antimicrobial agents appropriate for the treatment of chronic bacterial prostatitis (e.g., trimethoprim or fluoroquinolones). The duration of optimal therapy is unknown; between 2 and 4 weeks has been suggested (Nickel, 1998b; Bjerklund-Johansen et al, 1998).

In the 1970s to 1990s, the most commonly used antimicrobial agent in CP was trimethoprim-sulfamethoxazole (co-trimoxazole) (Moon, 1997; Nickel et al, 1998a) and, to a lesser extent, trimethoprim alone. In patients with chronic bacterial prostatitis, eradication of pathogens (the only objective measurement in most CP studies) with trimethoprim-sulfamethoxazole or trimethoprim alone ranged from a low of 0% (Smith et al, 1979) to a high of 67% (Paulson and White, 1978), with most studies demonstrating an efficacy rate of between 30% and 50% (Meares, 1973, 1975, 1978; Drach, 1974b; McGuire and Lytton, 1976). It appears that longer-duration therapy (90 days) provides the best clinical results. Trimethoprim-sulfamethoxazole is less effective, both in bacterial eradication and cost-effectiveness, when compared with the newer fluoroquinolones (Kurzer and Kaplan, 2002).

Except for the well-studied fluoroquinolones, most antibiotics (including minocycline, cephalexin, and carbenicillin) do not demonstrate significant clinical efficacy in clinical studies in which patients were followed for sufficient time (Paulson and White, 1978; Oliveri et al, 1979; Mobley, 1981). One notable exception has been the macrolides, erythromycin (Mobley, 1974), azithromycin (Skerk et al, 2003), and clarithromycin (Skerk et al, 2002b), particularly when *C. trachomatis* is implicated.

The fluoroquinolones have demonstrated improved therapeutic results, especially in CP caused by *E. coli* and other members of the Enterobacteriaceae but not necessarily in prostatitis due to *P. aeruginosa* or enterococci. Naber (1999) analyzed the many studies available in the literature evaluating fluoroquinolones in CP and found eight comparable studies in which the diagnosis was obtained by localization studies and in which the patients were observed for a sufficient time after completion of therapy (Weidner et al, 1987; Pust et al, 1989; Heidler, 1990; Schaeffer and Darras, 1990; Pfau, 1991; Weidner et al, 1991a; Ramirez et al, 1994; Koff, 1996) evaluating norfloxacin, ciprofloxacin, ofloxacin, and lomefloxacin. In 2005 Naber (reported at the 6th International Consultation on New Developments in Prostate Cancer and Prostate Disease, Paris, June 2005) added three more studies that met these strict criteria (Naber et al, 2000; Naber et al, 2002; Bundrick et al, 2003). These studies are described in Table 9–3. For CP caused by *E. coli*, a treatment duration of 1 month for the fluoroquinolones seems to be superior to the usual 3-month treatment with trimethoprim-sulfamethoxazole. In microbiologically diagnosed chronic bacterial prostatitis, eradication of bacteria is associated with both short-term and long-term clinical success (Nickel et al, 2005e). This appears to be true in men with recent onset of prostatitis associated with bacterial localization with the traditional uropathogens (gram-negative uropathogens and enterococci species) as well as nontraditional bacteria (gram-positive such as coagulase-negative *Staphylococcus* and *Streptococcus* species) (Nickel et al, 2005e). A number of investigators (Baert and Leonard, 1988; Jimenez-Cruz et al, 1988; Yamamoto et al, 1996) have advocated direct injection of antibiotics into the prostate gland, but this method has never been rigorously evaluated or become popular among urologists.

Table 9–3. Clinical Trials of Fluoroquinolone Treatment of Chronic Bacterial Prostatitis*

Antibiotic	Dose (mg)	Duration of Therapy (days)	No. of Patients	Bacteriologic Cure (%)	Follow-Up (mo)	Reference
Norfloxacin	400[†]	28	14	64	6	Schaeffer and Darras (1990)
Norfloxacin	400[†]	174	42	60	8	Petrikkos et al (1991)
Ciprofloxacin	500[†]	14	15	60	12	Weidner et al (1987)
Ciprofloxacin	500[†]	28	16	63	21-36	Weidner et al (1991)
Ciprofloxacin	500[†]	60-150	7	86	12	Pfau (1991)
Ciprofloxacin	250[†]	21-42	34	62	6	Heidler (1990)
Ciprofloxacin	500[†]	28	34	76	6	Naber et al (2001)
Ciprofloxacin	500[†]	28	78	72	6	Naber et al (2002)
Lomefloxacin	400[‡]	28	75	63	6	
Ofloxacin	200[†]	14	21	67	12	Pust et al (1989)
Ofloxacin	300[†]	42	30	57	6	Ramirez et al (1999)
Lomefloxacin	400[‡]	42				
Ofloxacin	200[†]	42	33	60	6	
Lomefloxacin	400[‡]	42		67		Koff (1996)
Ciprofloxacin	500[‡]	28	125	56 (clinical[§])	6	Bundrick et al (2003)
Levofloxacin	500[‡]	28	136	53 (clinical[§])	6	

*Naber (1999) reviewed the world literature in respect to clinical trials of fluoroquinolone treatment of chronic bacterial prostatitis and noted only eight studies in which the diagnosis of prostatitis was obtained by localization studies and in which the patients were observed for at least 6 months. Naber has subsequently expanded his list of suitable available trials in 2005 (reported at the 6th International Consultation on New Developments in Prostate Cancer and Prostate Disease, Paris, June 2005).
[†]Twice a day.
[‡]Once a day.
[§]Clinical success at 6 months: bacterial eradication post therapy was 75% for levofloxacin and 77% for ciprofloxacin.

Many studies evaluating physicians' practice patterns in CP syndromes (de la Rosette et al, 1992a; Moon, 1997; Nickel et al, 1998a; McNaughton-Collins et al, 1998, 2000) have confirmed that most patients diagnosed with CP, irrespective of culture results, are treated with antimicrobial therapy. Older studies have generally indicated that approximately 40% of patients with nonbacterial CP have some symptomatic improvement with antimicrobial therapy (Berger et al, 1989; Weidner, 1992; de la Rosette et al, 1993a; Ohkawa et al, 1993b; Bergman, 1994; Bjerklund-Johansen et al, 1998; Tanner et al, 1999; Nickel et al, 2001a). Antibiotic therapy may benefit CPPS patients by three different mechanisms: a strong placebo effect, the eradication or suppression of noncultured microorganisms (Nickel et al, 2001a), or the independent anti-inflammatory effect of some antibiotics (Yoshimura et al, 1996; Galley et al, 1997). It has been suggested by a European consensus group evaluating the role of antibiotics in the treatment of CP (Bjerklund-Johansen et al, 1998) that antibiotics should be considered empirical treatment for category IIIA CPPS but the benefits should be appraised after a minimum of 2 to 4 weeks of therapy. However, recent research may lead to a review of those recommendations. Two multicenter randomized placebo-controlled studies have assessed the efficacy of 6 weeks of levofloxacin (Nickel et al, 2003b) and ciprofloxacin (Alexander et al, 2004) in men with CP/CPPS. In these trials the participants had chronic symptoms for a long duration (many years) and had been heavily treated (including treatment with antibiotics). In the study by Nickel and associates (2003b), 80 patients were randomized to levofloxacin or placebo, while in the NIH-sponsored study reported by Alexander and colleagues (2004), 196 men with CP/CPPS were randomized in a two-by-two factorial design to ciprofloxacin, tamsulosin, the combination of ciprofloxacin and tamsulosin, or placebo. In both of these prospective designed controlled multicenter trials, no significant difference was reported between the fluoroquinolone and placebo in terms of symptom amelioration. **Antibiotics should not be prescribed for previously treated men with CP/CPPS of long duration.**

α-Adrenergic Blocker Therapy

Rationale. Patients with CP/CPPS have significant lower urinary tract symptoms, which appear to be related to poor relaxation of the bladder neck during voiding (Barbalias et al, 1983; Murnaghan and Millard, 1984; Blacklock, 1986; Hellstrom et al, 1987; Barbalias, 1990; Kaplan et al, 1997). The subsequent turbulent "dysfunctional" voiding may predispose the patient to reflux of urine into the prostatic ducts, causing intraprostatic inflammation and subsequently pain (Kirby et al, 1982). **The bladder neck and prostate are rich in α-adrenergic receptors, and it is hypothesized that α-adrenergic blockade may improve outflow obstruction, improving urinary flow and perhaps diminishing intraprostatic ductal reflux.**

Clinical Trial Data. A number of older clinical trials suggested that the α-adrenergic blockers diphenoxybenzamine (Dunzendorfer et al, 1983), phenoxybenzamine (Osborn et al, 1981), alfuzosin (de la Rosette et al, 1992c; Barbalias et al, 1998), terazosin (Neal and Moon, 1994; Barbalias et al, 1998; Lacquaniti et al, 1999; Gul et al, 2001), doxazosin (Evliyaoglu and Burgut, 2002), and tamsulosin (Lacquaniti et al, 1999)

resulted in significant symptomatic improvement of prostatitis-related symptoms. However, these trials were small, most were uncontrolled, and outcome measures were not validated. The study by Barbalias and associates (1998) further seemed to indicate that the combination of antibiotics and α-adrenergic blockers improved the clinical result in patients with chronic bacterial prostatitis.

Four randomized placebo-controlled trials with clearly defined CP/CPPS patients (NIH classification) and employing the NIH-CPSI as the outcome parameter have confirmed the efficacy of α-adrenergic blockers but only in men who have recent-onset disease, who are not heavily pretreated, and who are on therapy for longer than 6 weeks. Cheah and coworkers (2003) randomized 86 patients with CP to either terazosin or placebo for 14 weeks. Patients on terazosin had a 50% reduction in mean symptom score compared with 37% in the placebo-treated group. Terazosin resulted in modest but significant improvement in all domains of the NIH-CPSI. Mehik and colleagues (2003) followed 19 patients randomized to 6 months of alfuzosin treatment and 20 patients to 6 months of placebo therapy, and both groups were followed for a further 6 months after discontinuing the active or placebo medication. Patients in the alfuzosin group had a significant amelioration of symptoms compared with the placebo therapy group that was evident at 4 months and became even more clinically significant by 6 months. At 6 months 65% of alfuzosin patients were rated as responders compared with 24% of placebo group. The beneficial effect appeared to wear off over the next 6 months after the alfuzosin was discontinued. Nickel and colleagues (2004b) randomized 57 men with CP/CPPS to tamsulosin 0.4 mg or placebo after a 2-week placebo run-in and followed the two groups for 6 weeks. Patients treated with tamsulosin had a statistically significant (but only modest clinically significant) treatment effect compared with placebo patients. A significant treatment effect was not observed in patients who had mild symptoms, but patients with severe symptoms (75th percentile) had a statistically and clinically significant response compared with placebo. It appears that the response to α-adrenergic blockers is durable, for a least up to 24 to 38 weeks (Mehik et al, 2003; Cheah et al, 2004). In contrast, the results from the NIH Chronic Prostatitis Collaborative Research Network Randomized Controlled Trial (Alexander et al, 2004) comparing 6 weeks of ciprofloxacin, tamsulosin, and the combination of ciprofloxacin and tamsulosin to placebo in very chronic and heavily pretreated patients failed to show any improvement in patients treated with tamsulosin (± ciprofloxacin) compared with patients treated with placebo. **The lessons learned from these very well designed and implemented studies were that α-adrenergic blockers provided significant symptom amelioration only after more than 6 weeks of therapy in less heavily treated patients with recent onset of moderate to severe symptoms.**

Anti-inflammatory Agents and Immune Modulators

Rationale. Prostatic inflammation is associated with category IIIA CPPS, and elevated cytokine levels are noted in the semen (Alexander et al, 1998; Ruggieri et al, 2000) and EPS (Nadler et al, 2000; Hochreiter et al, 2000b) of patients with inflammatory CPPS. **Nonsteroidal anti-inflammatory drugs, corticosteroids, and immunosuppressive drugs theoreti-**

cally should improve the inflammatory parameters within the prostate and possibly result in a reduction of symptoms (Pontari, 2002).

Clinical Trial Data. Canale and associates (1993a) found that nimesulide (a nonsteroidal anti-inflammatory drug) quickly reduced inflammatory-type symptoms such as dysuria, strangury, and painful ejaculation. A second study by Canale's group (1993b) found that by the rectal route, keto-profen was inferior to nimesulide (both drugs were used as suppositories). Prednisolone has been suggested as a potent anti-inflammatory for CP (Bates and Talbot, 2000), and a randomized study presented by Dimitrakov and associates (2004) indicates that high-dose methylprednisolone (followed by rapid tapering of dose) may have more efficacy than placebo, even after 12 months, but the side-effect profile makes this type of therapy less attractive. The new class of cyclooxygenase-2 inhibitors has proved successful for long-term treatment of other chronic inflammatory conditions such as rheumatoid arthritis and chronic osteoarthritis, and many urologists employed these medications for prostatitis patients with some anecdotal successes reported. The results of a North American randomized control trial comparing the cyclooxygenase-2 inhibitor rofecoxib to placebo indicated that many men with CPPS benefited (in terms of pain and quality of life) from rofecoxib therapy compared with placebo. In this study in which 161 patients were randomized to rofecoxib 25 mg, rofecoxib 50 mg, or placebo, only patients on the high dose showed any clinical improvement compared with the placebo. Very few patients, however, had complete resolution of their symptoms (Nickel et al, 2003c). Another study from China (Zeng et al, 2004) assessing the effectiveness of two doses of the cyclooxygenase-2 inhibitor celecoxib also demonstrated a dose-dependent response (200 mg twice a day for 6 weeks was more effective than 200 mg once a day). At this time, high-dose, long-duration therapy with cyclooxygenase-2 inhibitors is not recommended.

Because the clinical and pathologic characteristics are similar to those of interstitial cystitis, Wedren (1987) compared the efficacy of pentosan polysulfate, a glycosaminoglycan drug that has been used in the treatment of interstitial cystitis, with placebo. In this small study, the treated group was noted to have a statistically significant improvement in symptoms but the major symptom that improved was nonspecific myalgia and arthralgia. An uncontrolled pilot study evaluating oral pentosan polysulfate in 32 men with CPPS demonstrated amelioration of symptoms and improvement in the quality of life in over 40% after treatment for 6 months (Nickel et al, 2000). The results of a multicenter, randomized, placebo-controlled trial that randomized 100 men to pentosan polysulfate, 900 mg/day (three times the usual dose), or placebo indicated this medication provided modest benefit for some men with CPPS (Nickel et al, 2005b).

Thalidomide, a cytokine-modulating drug, was assessed in 30 men with chronic abacterial prostatitis and abnormal semen cytokine levels (IL-2, -6, -8, and -10 and TNF-α) in a randomized placebo-controlled trial (Guercini et al, 2005). Despite a significant reduction in cytokine levels in semen, no difference in symptom relief was noted.

The potential of various anti-inflammatories, immune modulators, and cytokine inhibitors makes these classes of drugs potentially useful in the CP syndromes, but clinical

efficacy will have to be determined in future prospective clinical trials.

Muscle Relaxants

Rationale. Many investigators believe that CPPS is the ultimate reflection of a smooth and skeletal neuromuscular dysregulatory phenomenon in the perineum or pelvic floor (Osborn et al, 1981; Egan and Krieger, 1997; Anderson, 1999; Zermann and Schmidt, 1999). **The use of α-adrenergic blockers to relax smooth muscle** (see the previous section "α-Adrenergic Blocker Therapy") **and skeletal muscle relaxants combined with adjuvant medical and physical therapies has been advocated and promoted** (Anderson, 1999; Zermann and Schmidt, 1999).

Clinical Trial Data. In one of the few studies to compare muscle relaxants to placebo, Osborn and associates (1981) conducted a prospective double-blind study comparing phenoxybenzamine, baclofen (a striated muscle relaxant), and placebo in 27 patients with prostatodynia (category IIIB). Patients were treated with each agent for 1 month in a crossover trial. Symptomatic improvement was seen in 37% of the patients treated with baclofen compared with 8% treated with placebo. Simmons and Thin (1985) compared diazepam with an antibiotic in patients with chronic abacterial prostatitis and found no difference in symptom improvement between the diazepam group (8 of 11 men improved) and the antibiotic group (7 of 12 men improved). Unfortunately, **these studies were hindered by a lack of controlled and defined entry criteria and no quantified measurement of patients' responses.**

Hormone Therapy

Rationale. Prostate growth and function are influenced by the local hormonal milieu, especially by androgens. Theoretically, anti-androgens (including 5α-reductase inhibitors) could result in regression of prostatic glandular tissue (inflammation is believed to begin at the level of the ductal epithelium), improved voiding parameters (especially in older patients with BPH and prostatitis), and reduced intraprostatic ductal reflux (Nickel, 1999c).

Clinical Trial Data. Holm and Meyhoff (1996) were the first to note that the 5α-reductase inhibitor finasteride had potential in alleviating symptoms by observing the effect of finasteride therapy in four patients with CP or prostatodynia. Leskinen and colleagues (1999) randomized 41 patients with chronic idiopathic prostatitis (i.e., nonbacterial prostatitis and prostatodynia) to treatment with placebo (25%, or 10 patients) or finasteride (75%, or 31 patients) for 1 year. Compared with placebo, finasteride reduced prostatitis and BPH symptom scores; however, there was no statistically significant difference in pain between the two groups. The baseline characteristics of the two groups were not comparable, and the enrolled patients consisted of an unknown mixed population with inflammatory and noninflammatory prostatitis syndromes. A randomized open-label comparative trial in 64 CP/CPPS men showed significantly more improvement in men treated for a year with finasteride compared with saw palmetto, an herbal therapy (Kaplan et al, 2004). A randomized controlled trial compared the reduction of NIH-CPSI in 64 men with CP/CPPS randomized to finasteride or placebo (Nickel et al, 2004c). Six months of finasteride resulted in a numerical but not statistically significant reduction in symptoms compared with the symptom reduction noted in the placebo group. **Finasteride cannot be recommended as a monotherapy except perhaps in men with associated BPH.**

Testosterone and dihydrotestosterone are not the only hormones with a possible effect on prostate inflammation; estrogens may also play a role. A number of small, poorly controlled studies (Cavallini, 2001; Saitta et al, 2001) suggested that mepartricin (a drug that lowers estrogen levels in the prostate) may be useful in the treatment of CP/CPPS. A small prospectively designed randomized controlled trial assigned 26 men with CP/CPPS to 60 days therapy with mepartricin or placebo (De Rose et al, 2004). The study showed a statistical and perhaps clinically significant benefit (60% vs. 20% improvement, respectively) that should stimulate further research in the role of hormonal manipulation (in this case estrogens) in the treatment of CP/CPPS.

Phytotherapeutic Agents

Rationale. A number of plant extracts have been shown in many in-vitro experiments to have 5α-reductase activity, α-adrenergic blockade activity, effects on bladder contractility, and anti-inflammatory properties (Lowe and Fagelman, 1999; Shoskes, 2002).

Clinical Trial Data. Three specific phytotherapeutic agents have been tested in clinical trials, Cernilton, a bee pollen extract (Buck et al, 1989; Rugendorff et al, 1993), Quercetin, a natural bioflavonoid (Shoskes et al, 1999), and *Serenoa repens,* an extract of the saw palmetto berry (Kaplan et al, 2004, Reissigl et al, 2004). Rugendorff and coworkers (1993) noted that over half of 72 CP patients without other lower urinary tract abnormalities had favorable improvements in pain and irritative voiding symptoms when treated with Cernilton. No control group was included in this study. Shoskes and associates (1999) randomized 15 patients to the bioflavonoid Quercetin and 13 patients to placebo for 1 month. Sixty-seven percent of the patients in the treatment group were considered responders compared with only 20% of the patients in the placebo arm. Kaplan and associates (2004) did not note any appreciable long-term improvement in any CP/CPPS parameters when compared with 12 months of finasteride in a randomized open-label comparative study. However, Reissigl and colleagues (2004) reported that there was a moderate/marked improvement in over 60% of 72 CP/CPPS patients after 12 months of therapy with *Serenoa repens* compared with less than 25% in the 70 men in the placebo-treated group. However, further follow-up did not support the durability of this therapy (Reissigl et al, 2005). Phytotherapy for CP/CPPS may look promising, but further multicenter randomized controlled trials with well-characterized, standardized, and stable herbal components should be considered to assess their role in therapy.

Allopurinol

Rationale. Persson and Ronquist (1996) theorized that the intraprostatic ductal reflux of urine increases the concentration of metabolites containing purine and pyrimidine bases in the prostatic ducts, causing inflammation.

Clinical Trial Data. Persson and associates (1996) compared allopurinol therapy with placebo in a double-blind controlled study in 54 men. The allopurinol groups had lower levels of serum urate, urine urate, and EPS urate and xanthine. With variations in accepted statistical methodology, the inves-

tigators were able to show a difference in the mean patient-reported discomfort score between the study and the control groups at certain times in this trial with 330 days of follow-up. However, a reexamination of the data employing more standardized statistical analyses did not convince other groups that changes in the urine and prostatic secretion of purine and pyrimidine bases resulted in significant amelioration of symptoms in this particular trial (Nickel et al, 1996a).

KEY POINTS: MEDICAL THERAPY

The following medical therapies have been evaluated in standardized randomized placebo controlled trials in CPPS:

- Antibiotics, α-adrenergic blockers, anti-inflammatory agents, hormonal therapies, phytotherapies

The following medical therapies have shown benefits in placebo or sham-controlled studies in CPPS:

- Marked benefit—none

- Moderate benefit—α-adrenergic blockers

- Modest benefit—anti-inflammatory agents, phytotherapies

Physical Therapy

Prostatic Massage. Prostatic massage has been the principal therapy for prostatitis since the turn of the 20th century (O'Conor, 1936; Campbell, 1957). With the introduction of the scientific approach advocated by Meares and Stamey in 1968, prostatic massage became important only as a diagnostic tool, but as a therapy, it was abandoned by urologists. Currently, it is regaining some popularity, primarily because of the failure of standard medical therapy in patients with refractory symptoms of CP. Its benefits are believed to arise from draining theoretically occluded prostatic ducts and improving circulation and antibiotic penetration (Hennenfent and Feliciano, 1998). Independent but uncontrolled studies (Nickel et al, 1999a; Shoskes and Zeitlin, 1999) describe clinical benefits in one third to two thirds of patients treated with repetitive prostatic massage (two to three times per week) for 4 to 6 weeks along with antibiotic therapy. **Some patients do appear to improve with prostatic massage, but a panel of North American "prostatitis experts" (Nickel et al, 1999) could not come to a consensus on the potential overall benefit or even the mechanism of achieving that benefit if it does occur.** Frequent ejaculation may achieve the same function as prostatic massage (Yavascaogalu et al, 1999).

Perineal or Pelvic Floor Massage and Myofascial Trigger Point Release. Most clinicians recognize that men with CP syndromes, especially the noninflammatory category or prostatodynia, have specific anatomic areas that cause discomfort. Anderson (1999) believes that prolonged or chronic tension, distention, or distortion in the muscle bands (e.g., in the perineum) leads to a painful trigger point that is responsible for the pain. Predisposing factors leading to the formation of myofascial trigger points in the perineum or pelvis may include mechanical abnormalities in the hip and lower extremities, chronic urinary holding patterns (dysfunctional toilet training), sexual abuse, repetitive minor trauma, constipation, trauma, unusual sexual activity, recurrent infections or surgery, and perhaps stress and anxiety. Treatment of these trigger points includes heat therapy, physiotherapy massage, ischemic compression, stretching, anesthetic injections, acupuncture, electroneural modulation, and mind-body interactions such as progressive relaxation exercises, yoga, and hypnosis (Potts, 2000). Anderson and associates (2005) report that employing these techniques with a team consisting of a urologist, physiotherapist, and psychologist results in more than half of patients having or demonstrating a clinically detectable improvement. These methods have yet to be tested in a prospective rigorous fashion, and there certainly is the potential for significant placebo effect in these alternate forms of therapy.

Pudendal Nerve Entrapment Therapy. It has been hypothesized that the symptoms of CPPS could be caused by entrapment of the pudendal nerve, perhaps between the sacrotuberous and sacrospinous ligaments, in the canal of Alcock or by the falciform process of the sacrotuberous ligament (Robert et al, 1998). Pudendal nerve blocks (Thoumas et al, 1999; McDonald et al, 2000) and neurolysis surgery (Robert et al, 1993; Mauillon et al, 1999) have been suggested for treatment. The role of the pudendal nerve in chronic perineal pain deserves more scientific scrutiny.

Biofeedback. It is possible that the voiding and pain symptoms associated with CPPS may be secondary to some form of pseudodyssynergia during voiding or repetitive perineal muscle spasm; biofeedback has the potential to improve this process. Kaplan and associates (1997), Nadler (2002), and Ye and colleagues (2003) have demonstrated in small uncontrolled studies that biofeedback does ameliorate specific prostatitis-like symptoms in some men. Controlled clinical trials will be necessary to evaluate this mode of therapy.

Acupuncture. Acupuncture is an accepted traditional Chinese therapy for chronic pain, including prostatitis (Ge et al, 1988; Katai, 1992; Ikeuchi and Iguchi, 1994). Chen and Nickel (2003) determined in a pilot study of 12 treatment refractory men that acupuncture was safe and provided effective and durable symptom improvement. A larger sham-controlled study is required to confirm these encouraging initial results.

Psychological Support. Data from the NIH Prostatitis Cohort (Tripp et al, 2005) support a biopsychosocial model that associates the chronic pain of CPPS with depression and suggests that physicians may be able to advise patients to avoid certain pain coping strategies that can be associated with greater depression.

Minimally Invasive Therapies

Balloon Dilatation. Lapatin and coworkers (1990) employed balloon dilatation in an uncontrolled trial of seven patients with nonbacterial prostatitis and prostatodynia and showed improvement in voiding symptoms during a 1- to 5-month follow-up. Pain and discomfort were not assessed. This treatment effect has never been substantiated, and balloon dilatation has not been routinely employed in clinical practice.

Suzuki and coworkers (1995) combined the potential beneficial effects of balloon dilatation with prostatic hyperthermia in five men with CP and demonstrated significant improvement in symptoms in one patient and partial improvement in three. Nickel and associates (1998b) were not able to duplicate this beneficial effect in a small pilot trial evaluating the "hot balloon" (heating by radiofrequency energy rather than laser energy).

Minimally Invasive Surgery. Chiang and associates (1997) employed transurethral needle ablation (TUNA) of the prostate in seven patients with chronic nonbacterial prostatitis, assessed the patients before and after therapy (6 months of follow-up) employing a modification of the Symptom Severity Index (Nickel and Sorensen, 1996b), and reported favorable results in four. A follow-up study by Chiang and Chiang (2004) showed significant improvement in symptoms in the majority of 32 patients treated with TUNA. But Leskinen and colleagues (2002) investigated the effectiveness and durability of TUNA in 25 patients randomized to TUNA and 8 patients randomized to sham treatment. They reported that the efficacy of TUNA in CPPS is comparable to sham treatment and so could not recommend TUNA as therapy for CPPS. Serel and colleagues (1997) also reported significantly meaningful beneficial effects in 30 patients with chronic abacterial prostatitis and prostatodynia employing the neodymium:yttrium-aluminum-garnet laser. Ruedi and colleagues (2003) suggested that high-frequency electrostimulation may be harnessed to treat CP. Sham control trials will be required before this or any other minimally invasive therapy can be recommended.

Microwave Hyperthermia and Thermotherapy. It is believed that the heat applied to the prostate gland by the microwave process could shorten the natural resolution of the inflammatory process, perhaps by accelerating the process of fibrosis or scar formation in the area of chronic inflammation. In addition, heat therapy, particularly with the higher temperatures achieved with transurethral microwave thermotherapy, could alter the afferent nerve fibers that convey the objective symptom of pain from the inflamed prostate gland (intraprostatic sympathectomy) (Perachino et al, 1993). It may even be possible that the microwave energy kills nonculturable or cryptic bacteria within the prostate gland (Sahin et al, 1998).

Although many uncontrolled trials employing heat therapy have shown benefit (Nickel, 1999d; Zeitlin, 2002), only three published studies have used sham controls. Vassily and associates (1999) noted symptom improvement in 75% of men in a transrectal microwave hyperthermia-treated group compared with 52% of men in the sham-treated group. Shaw and colleagues (1993) documented treatment success (defined as a greater than 50% improvement in symptoms) in 55% of the men in a transrectal microwave hyperthermia group (15 patients) compared with 10% of patients treated with sham therapy (13 patients) at 3 months. Nickel and Sorensen (1996b) examined the safety and efficacy of transurethral microwave thermotherapy (TUMT) in 20 men randomized to therapy or sham. At 3 months' follow-up, the patients treated by TUMT had significantly improved symptom scores compared with sham-treated patients (7 of 10 men treated with TUMT had a favorable result compared with 1 of 10 men treated with a sham therapy). A recently reported study in men with CPPS treated with cooled TUMT using the NIH-CPSI as an outcome (Kastner et al, 2004) again suggested that thermotherapy remains a promising treatment for intractable CP, particularly when it is associated with concomitant BPH. Whereas this prospective study showed a significant reduction in NIH-CPSI score compared with baseline in 35 men followed for 12 months, it was not a randomized sham-controlled trial. **Heat therapy appears to be a promising therapeutic approach but, until larger-scale studies are performed, should be restricted to patients with refractory or end-stage symptoms.**

Surgery

In acute bacterial prostatitis (category I), urinary obstruction is a very common symptom. Traditionally, it has been suggested that the insertion of a suprapubic cystotomy tube is the optimal therapy because an indwelling Foley catheter may further obstruct urethral ducts, resulting in the potential to develop prostate abscesses (Dajani and O'Flynn, 1968; Pai and Baht, 1972; Weinberger et al, 1988). In most patients, however, an in-and-out catheterization to relieve the initial obstruction or short-term (12 hours) indwelling catheterization with a small-caliber Foley catheter is appropriate. **A developing prostate abscess, best detected with transrectal ultrasonography or computed tomography (CT)** (Rovik and Doehlin, 1989), **in patients who fail to respond quickly to antibiotics is optimally drained by the transurethral incision route** (Pai and Baht, 1972). However, transperineal incision and drainage (Granados et al, 1992) must be considered when the abscess has penetrated beyond the prostatic capsule or penetrated through the levator ani muscle. More recently it has been suggested that percutaneous drainage of the abscess is the most effective and less morbid procedure (Varkarakis et al, 2004).

Surgery does not have an important role in the treatment of most CP syndromes unless a specific indication is discovered during the evaluation of the patient (Kirby, 1999). These indications are usually noted during specific and ancillary investigations such as cystoscopy, transrectal ultrasonography, urodynamics, or CT or magnetic resonance imaging (MRI). Certainly, patients with urethral strictures benefit from surgical correction. Kaplan and associates (1994) have suggested that men with chronic nonbacterial prostatitis-like symptoms and urodynamic evidence of vesical neck obstruction benefit from endoscopic incision of the bladder neck.

Radical transurethral resection of the prostate (Barnes et al, 1982; Sant et al, 1984) has been advocated in patients who have either relapsing or refractory chronic bacterial prostatitis (category II) secondary to bacterial persistence within the prostate gland. Although prostatic calculi are not pathognomonic of prostatitis (Harada et al, 1980), it has been clearly shown that bacteria can persist in protective biofilms or aggregates within the interstices or on the surface of the calculus material (Meares, 1974; Nickel et al, 1994). Theoretically, removal of all the infected material, including potentially infected calculi, can be achieved (with appropriate intraoperative radiographs or ultrasound studies), but except for small anecdotal case series (Barnes et al, 1982; Sant et al, 1984) there is no substantial proof in the literature as to the efficacy of major prostate surgery in category II CP. Radical transurethral resection of the prostate has not been advocated for category III CPPS, but open radical prostatectomy has been shown anecdotally to benefit a few patients with symptoms of nonbacterial prostatitis or prostatodynia, or both (Davis and Weigel, 1990; Frazier et al, 1992). **No definitive clinical series or long-term follow-up has ever been presented, and this type of surgery should not be encouraged or recommended at this time.**

Table 9-4. Medical Therapy for Chronic Prostatitis and Chronic Pelvic Pain Syndrome

Class of Treatment	Specific Therapy	Dose	Duration of Therapy (wk)	Evidence
Antibiotics	Trimethoprim-sulfamethoxazole	160/800 mg BID	12	Naber (1999) and Meares (1998) for review
	Norfloxacin	400 mg BID	4-12	
	Ciprofloxacin	500 mg BID	4-12	
	Ofloxacin	300 mg BID	4-12	See Table 9-2 for summary of clinical trial data
	Lomefloxacin	400 mg QD	4-12	
	Levofloxacin	500 mg QD	4-12	
α-Adrenergic blockers	Terazosin	5 mg QD	>14	Cheah et al (2003)
	Alfuzosin	2.5 mg TID (10 mg QD)	>12	Mehik et al (2003)
	Tamsulosin	0.4 mg QD	>6	Nickel et al (2004), Alexander et al (2004)
Phytotherapy	Pollen extract	1 tab TID	24	Buck et al (1989), Rugendorff et al (1993)
	Quercetin	500 mg BID	4	Shoskes et al (1999)
	Saw palmetto	150 mg QD	24	Reissigl et al (2004)
Anti-inflammatory agents	Nimesulide	100 mb BID	2-4	Canale et al (1993)
	Rofecoxib	25-50 mg QD	>6	Nickel et al (2003)
	Other NSAIDs Indomethacin Diclofenac Ibuprofen	Various	2-4	Evans (1999)
	Pentosan polysulfate	100 mg TID	24	Wedren (1987), Nickel et al (1999, 2005)
Hormonal agents	Finasteride	5 mg QD	24	Leskinen et al (1999), Nickel et al (2004)
	Mepartricin	40 mg QD	8	De Rose et al (2004)

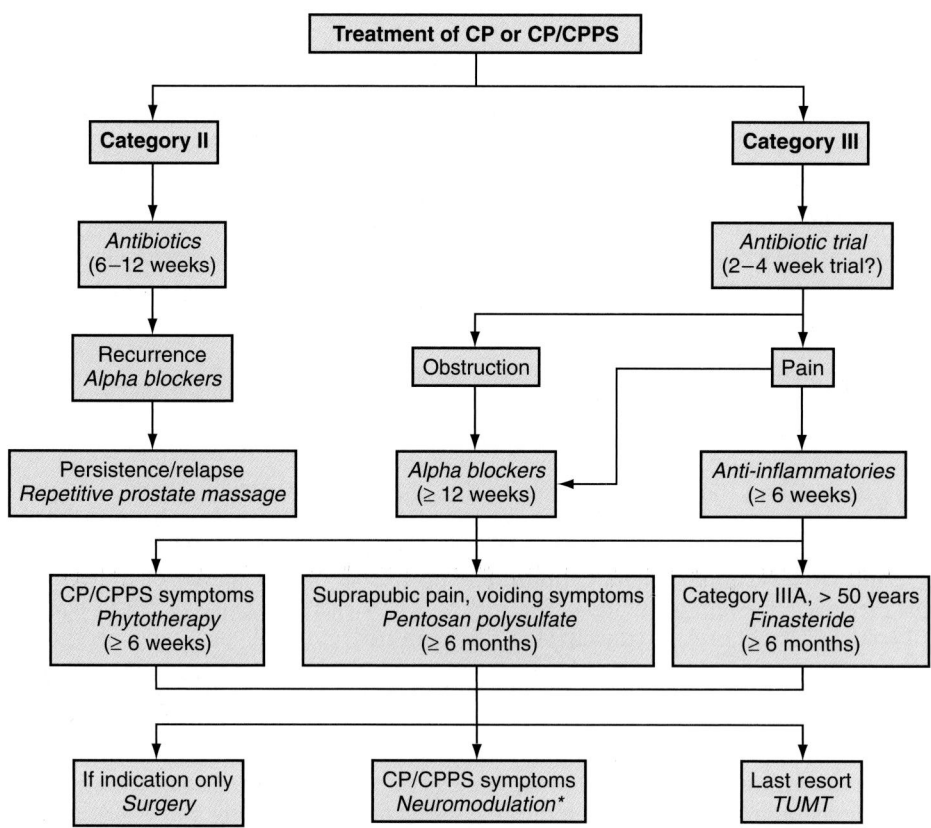

Figure 9–8. A suggested therapeutic algorithm for the treatment of patients presenting with chronic prostatitis/chronic pelvic pain syndrome. TUMT, transurethral microwave thermotherapy.

*amitriptyline, gabapentin, biofeedback, massage therapy, acupuncture, neurostimulation

Treatment Summary

Acute bacterial prostatitis is relatively simple to treat; eradicate the bacteria with appropriate antibiotic therapy. Chronic bacterial prostatitis can be assessed objectively by short- and long-term eradication of bacteria, but long-term symptom amelioration sometimes eludes us. Our standard therapies for CP/CPPS, when used as monotherapy, offer only modest improvement in symptoms (Nickel, 2004a). Multimodal therapy employing multiple concurrent treatment strategies may offer the best results at this time (Shoskes et al, 2003). However, a number of well-controlled prospective studies did not demonstrate increased efficacy by combining α-adrenergic blockers and antibiotics (Alexander et al, 2004) or α-adrenergic blockers and anti-inflammatory agents (Batstone et al, 2005). The explanation for this difficulty in treating CP may be that the patients become peripherally and centrally sensitized and treatment targeted to the initiators of the process may not work as well when the condition becomes chronic (Yang et al, 2003). Table 9–4 describes the various standard medical therapies that are currently recommended, whereas Figure 9–8 shows a suggested treatment algorithm. Further investigations should focus not only on the mechanisms inducing the symptoms, including the pain, but also on the mechanisms maintaining the pain.

To evaluate and compare the many clinical trials assessing the various therapies advocated for CP/CPPS, it is important to clearly define and classify the patient population (NIH classification system), determine results by employing a standardized outcome index (NIH-CPSI), prospectively compare a treated group to a similar group randomized to placebo, and fulfill the requirements of peer review for publication in a reputable journal (Nickel et al, 1999c; Propert et al, 2002). In the past several years, a significant number of such trials have been published (Nickel, 2004), allowing the reader to assess and compare the efficacy of antibiotics, α-adrenergic blockers, anti-inflammatory agents, phytotherapies, and hormonal agents in CP/CPPS (Table 9–5).

RELATED CONDITIONS
Seminal Vesiculitis

Seminal vesiculitis can occur as a consequence of local bacterial infection in acute and chronic bacterial prostatitis (Zeitlin, 1999) or acute epididymitis (Furuya et al, 2004) and patients can present with seminal vesicle abscesses (Stearns, 1963; Kennelly and Oesterling, 1989). Seminal vesicle abscesses, diagnosed clinically by a positive ejaculate culture and imaged traditionally by seminal vesiculography (Dunnick et al, 1982; Baert et al, 1986) but now with CT (Patel and Wilbur, 1987), transrectal ultrasonography (Littrup et al, 1988), MRI (Sue et al, 1989), or recently with ^{99m}Tc-ciprofloxacin radioisotope scan (Choe et al, 2003), can be managed with antibiotic therapy, transrectal aspiration, and, if necessary, an operation to remove the seminal vesicles. Traditionally, seminal vesiculectomy was performed as a difficult open procedure,

Table 9–5. Clinical Trials Evaluating Treatments for CP/CPPS*

Active Agent	Reference	Duration	Patients (n) Active	Patients (n) Placebo	Responders (%) Active	Responders (%) Placebo	Change in NIH-CPSI Active	Change in NIH-CPSI Placebo	Effect Treatment
Levofloxacin	Nickel et al (2003)	6 wk	35	45	42	37	−5.4	−2.9	2.5
Terazosin	Cheah et al (2003)	14 wk	43	43	NK	NK	−14.3†	−10.2	4.1
Alfuzosin	Mehik et al (2003)	24 wk	17	20	65	24	−9.9†	−3.8	6.1
Tamsulosin	Nickel et al (2004)	6 wk	27	30	52	33	−9.1†	−5.5	3.6
Ciprofloxacin	Alexander et al (2004)	6 wk	49	49	22	22	−6.2	−3.4	2.8
Tamsulosin			49		24		−4.4		1.0
Tamsulosin + ciprofloxacin			49		10		−4.1		0.7
Rofecoxib 25 mg	Nickel et al (2003)	6 wk	53	59	46	40	−4.9	−4.2	0.7
Rofecoxib 50 mg			49		63		−6.2		2.0
Pentosan polysulfate	Nickel et al (2005)	16 wk	51	49	37	18	−5.9	−3.2	2.7
Finasteride	Nickel et al (2004)	24 wk	33	31	33	16	−3.0	−0.8	2.2
Mepartricin	De Rose et al (2004)	8 wk	13	13	NK	NK	−15.0	−5.0	10.0
Quercetin	Shoskes et al (1999)	4 wk	15	13	67	20	−7.9†	−1.4	6.5

*These trials met the evidence-based criteria established by Nickel (see text).
†Significant difference between active and placebo (P < 0.05).
NK, not known.

but recently laparoscopic excision of the seminal vesicles was reported to be the least morbid procedure (Nadler and Rubenstein, 2001).

KEY POINT: SEMINAL VESICULITIS

■ Seminal vesiculitis is rare; is diagnosed by ultrasound, CT, or MRI; and is treated with antimicrobial therapy, aspiration, or excision of seminal vesicles.

Orchitis

Definition and Classification

By definition, *orchitis* is inflammation of the testis, but the term has been used to describe testicular pain localized to the testis without objective evidence of inflammation. Acute orchitis represents sudden occurrence of pain and swelling of the testis associated with acute inflammation of that testis. Chronic orchitis involves inflammation and pain in the testis, usually without swelling, persisting for more than 6 weeks. A classification (Nickel and Beiko, 2001) based on etiology is presented in Table 9–6.

Pathogenesis and Etiology

Isolated orchitis is a relatively rare condition and is usually viral in origin. It spreads to the testis by a hematogenous route. Most cases of orchitis, particularly bacterial, occur secondary to local spread of an ipsilateral epididymitis and are termed *epididymo-orchitis*. UTIs are usually the underlying

Table 9–6. Classification of Orchitis

Acute bacterial orchitis
  Secondary to UTI
  Secondary to STD
Nonbacterial infectious orchitis
  Viral
  Fungal
  Parasitic
  Rickettsial
Noninfectious orchitis
  Idiopathic
  Traumatic
  Autoimmune
Chronic orchitis
Chronic orchialgia

UTI, urinary tract infection; STD, sexually transmitted disease.

source in boys and elderly men. In young sexually active men, sexually transmitted diseases (STDs) are often responsible (Berger, 1998). Truly noninfectious orchitis is often idiopathic or related to trauma, although autoimmune disease has rarely been implicated (Pannek and Haupt, 1997). It may be impossible to clinically distinguish chronic orchitis from chronic orchialgia.

Bacterial orchitis is usually associated with epididymitis and is therefore often caused by urinary pathogens, including *E. coli* and *Pseudomonas*. Less commonly, *Staphylococcus* species or *Streptococcus* species are responsible. The most common sexually transmitted microorganisms responsible are *Neisseria gonorrhoeae*, *C. trachomatis*, and *Treponema pallidum*.

Mycobacterial infections can also cause orchitis, with tuberculosis (Chen et al, 2004) being much more common than leprosy. The most common cause of viral orchitis is mumps

(Jalal et al, 2004), but infectious mononucleosis has also been implicated (Weiner, 1997). Fungal infections occasionally involve the testis, with candidiasis, aspergillosis, histoplasmosis, coccidioidomycosis, blastomycosis, and actinomycosis all having been reported as causes of orchitis (Wise, 1998). Parasitic infections rarely cause orchitis in the Western Hemisphere, but filariasis has been described in some endemic areas of Africa, Asia, and South America and can be associated with elephantiasis (Hazen and Lichtenberg, 1998).

Diagnosis

In patients presenting with acute infectious orchitis, history discloses a recent onset of testicular pain, often associated with abdominal discomfort, nausea, and vomiting. These symptoms may be preceded by symptoms of parotitis in boys or young men, UTIs in boys or elderly men, or alternatively by symptoms of an STD in sexually active men. Although the process is usually unilateral, it is sometimes bilateral, especially if viral. Physical examination may reveal a toxic and febrile patient. The skin of the involved hemiscrotum is erythematous and edematous, and the testis is quite tender to palpation or can be associated with a transilluminating hydrocele. The patient should be clinically assessed for prostatitis and urethritis. For acute noninfectious orchitis, the clinical picture resembles the above description, except that these patients lack the toxic appearance and fever.

For chronic orchitis and orchialgia, there may have been a history of previous episodes of testicular pain, usually secondary to acute bacterial orchitis, trauma, or other causes. The patient has chronic testicular (and possibly epididymal) pain to a degree that could seriously affect his day-to-day functioning and quality of life. Patients with this diagnosis usually become very frustrated with this problem. On examination, the patient does not appear toxic and does not have a fever. The scrotum is not usually erythematous, but the testis may be somewhat indurated and is almost always tender to palpation.

Laboratory tests employed to assist in the diagnosis include urinalysis, urine microscopy, and urine culture. For a patient in whom an STD is suspected, a urethral swab should also be taken for culture. If the diagnosis is not evident from the history, physical examination, and these simple tests, scrotal ultrasonography should be performed (to rule out malignancy in patients with chronic orchitis/orchialgia). The most important differential diagnosis in young men and boys is testicular torsion. Testicular torsion is often difficult to differentiate from an acute inflammatory condition. Scrotal ultrasound (with use of Doppler imaging to determine testicular blood flow) is especially helpful in differential diagnosis (Mernagh et al, 2004), but occasionally it will miss the diagnosis (particularly with intermittent or partial torsion) and the clinician should err in favor of the surgically correctable diagnosis of torsion.

Treatment

General principles of therapy include bed rest, scrotal support, hydration, antipyretics, anti-inflammatory agents, and analgesics. Antibiotic therapy (specific for UTI, prostatitis, or STD) should be employed for infectious orchitis and is ideally based on culture and sensitivity testing but may be based on microscopic or Gram stain results. There are no specific antiviral agents available to treat orchitis caused by mumps, and the previously mentioned supportive measures are important. If early testing is negative or results are unavailable, empirical treatment should be initiated, directed at the most likely pathogens based on the available clinical information: a fluoroquinolone would be the best agent in this scenario. Most patients can be readily managed on an outpatient basis. Surgical intervention is rarely indicated, unless testicular torsion is suspected (as discussed previously). Spermatic cord blocks with injection of a local anesthetic may sometimes be needed to relieve the patient of severe pain. Abscess formation is rare, but if it does occur, percutaneous or open drainage is necessary.

Treatment of chronic orchitis/orchialgia is supportive. Anti-inflammatory agents, analgesics, support, heat therapies, and nerve blocks all have a role in ameliorating symptoms. It is generally believed that the condition is self-limited but could take years (and sometimes decades) to resolve. Orchidectomy is indicated only in cases where pain control is refractory to all other measures (and even this might not be successful in alleviating the chronic pain).

Epididymitis

Definitions and Classification

Epididymitis by definition is inflammation of the epididymis. Acute epididymitis represents sudden occurrence of pain and swelling of the epididymis associated with acute inflammation of the epididymis (Nickel et al, 2002). Chronic epididymitis refers to inflammation and pain in the epididymis, usually without swelling (but with induration in long-standing cases), persisting for over 6 weeks (Nickel et al, 2002). Inflammation is not always clinically evident in many cases of localized epididymal pain. A classification for epididymitis is presented in Table 9–7 (Nickel et al, 2002).

Pathogenesis and Etiology

Epididymitis usually results from the spread of infection from the bladder, urethra, or prostate via the ejaculatory ducts and vas deferens into the epididymis. The process starts in the tail of the epididymis then spreads through the body to the head of the epididymis. In infants and boys, epididymitis is often related to a UTI and/or an underlying genitourinary congenital anomaly (Merlini et al, 1998) or even the presence of a foreskin (Bennett, 1998). In elderly men, BPH and associated stasis, UTI, and catheterization is the most common cause of epididymitis. Bacterial prostatitis and/or seminal vesiculitis are associated with epididymal infection in postpubertal males of all ages (Furuya et al, 2004). In sexually active men younger than 35 years of age, epididymitis is commonly the result of an STD (Berger, 1998). In most cases of acute epididymitis, the testis is also involved in the process and referred to as epididymo-orchitis.

Chronic epididymitis may result from inadequately treated acute epididymitis, recurrent epididymitis, or some other cause including associations with other disease processes such as Behçet's disease (Cho et al, 2003). The etiology of chronic epididymalgia is usually unclear.

The most common causative microorganisms in the pediatric and elderly age groups are the coliform organisms that

Table 9-7. **Classification of Epididymitis**
Acute bacterial epididymitis
Secondary to UTI
Secondary to STD
Nonbacterial infectious epididymitis
Viral
Fungal
Parasitic
Noninfectious epididymitis
Idiopathic
Traumatic
Autoimmune
Amiodarone-induced
Associated with a known syndrome (e.g., Behçet's disease)
Chronic epididymitis
Chronic epididymalgia

UTI, urinary tract infection; STD, sexually transmitted disease.

cause bacteriuria (Berger et al, 1979). In men younger than the age of 35 who are sexually active with women, the most common offending organisms causing epididymitis are the usual bacteria that cause urethritis, namely *N. gonorrhoeae* and *C. trachomatis*. In homosexual men practicing anal intercourse, *E. coli* and *Haemophilus influenzae* are most commonly responsible. As with orchitis, viral, fungal, and parasitic microorganisms have all been implicated in epididymitis (Berger, 1998; Hazen and von Lichtenberg, 1998; Wise, 1998).

Diagnosis

Both acute infectious and acute noninfectious epididymitis present in much the same way as do acute infectious and acute noninfectious orchitis, respectively. Physical examination localizes the tenderness to the epididymis (although in many cases the testis is also involved in the inflammatory process and subsequent pain—referred to as epididymo-orchitis). The spermatic cord is usually tender and swollen. Early on in the process, only the tail of the epididymis is tender, but the inflammation quickly spreads to the rest of the epididymis and if it continues to the testis, the swollen epididymis becomes indistinguishable from the testis.

There may be no clinical or etiologic differentiation between chronic epididymitis and epididymalgia, and the patient usually presents with a long-standing history of pain (waxing and waning or constant) localized to the epididymis; and like chronic orchitis/orchialgia, these symptoms may have a significant impact on the patient's quality of life (Nickel et al, 2002).

Laboratory tests should include Gram stains of a urethral smear and a midstream urine specimen. Gram-negative bacilli can usually be identified in patients with underlying cystitis. If the urethral smear reveals the presence of intracellular gram-negative diplococci, a diagnosis of *N. gonorrhoeae* is established. If only WBCs are seen on the urethral smear, a diagnosis of *C. trachomatis* will be established two thirds of the time. A urethral swab and midstream urine specimen should be sent for culture and sensitivity testing. When an infant or young boy is diagnosed with epididymitis, he should be further evaluated with abdominopelvic ultrasound, voiding cystourethrography, and possibly cystoscopy (Shortliffe, 1998). If the diagnosis is uncertain, duplex Doppler scrotal ultrasonography to look for increased blood flow to the affected epididymis may be performed (also to rule out torsion, as described under "Orchitis") (Mernagh et al, 2004).

Treatment

A 4- to 6-week trial of antibiotics that would potentially be effective against possible bacterial pathogens and particularly *C. trachomatis* is appropriate for chronic epididymitis (Nickel, 2005). Anti-inflammatory agents, analgesics, scrotal support, and nerve blocks have all been recommended as empirical treatment (Nickel, 2005). It is generally believed that chronic epididymitis is a self-limited condition that will eventually "burn out," but this could take years (or even decades). Surgical removal of the epididymis (epididymectomy) should only be considered when all conservative measures have been exhausted and the patient accepts that the operation will have at best a 50% chance of curing his pain (Padmore et al, 1996).

KEY POINTS: ORCHITIS AND EPIDIDYMITIS

- Orchitis usually occurs with epididymitis (except for viral).

- Etiology of epididymitis and orchitis is usually related to age of patient.

- Acute presentation is usually related to infection or ischemia.

- In young patients, the most important differential diagnosis is torsion of the testis.

SUGGESTED READINGS

Alexander RB, Propert KJ, Schaeffer AJ, et al: Chronic Prostatitis Collaborative Research Network: Ciprofloxacin or tamsulosin in men with chronic prostatitis/chronic pelvic pain syndrome: A randomized, double-blind trial. Ann Intern Med 2004;141:581-589.

Drach GW, Fair WR, Meares EM, Stamey TA: Classification of benign diseases associated with prostatic pain: Prostatitis or prostatodynia? J Urol 1978;120:266.

Krieger JN, Nyberg LJ, Nickel JC: NIH consensus definition and classification of prostatitis. JAMA 1999;282:236-237.

Litwin MS, McNaughton-Collins M, Fowler FJ, et al: The National Institutes of Health chronic prostatitis symptom index: Development and validation of a new outcome measure. J Urol 1999;162:369-375.

McNaughton-Collins M, MacDonald R, Wilt JJ: Diagnosis and treatment of chronic abacterial prostatitis: A systematic review. Ann Intern Med 2000a;133:367-381.

Nickel JC: The three As of chronic prostatitis therapy: Antibiotics, alpha-blockers and anti-inflammatories: What is the evidence? BJU Int 2004;94:1230-1233.

Nickel JC: Clinical evaluation of the man with chronic prostatitis/chronic pelvic pain syndrome. Urology 2003;60(Suppl 6A):20-23.

Nickel JC, Alexander RB, Schaeffer AJ, et al: Leukocytes and bacteria in men with chronic prostatitis/chronic pelvic pain syndrome compared to asymptomatic controls. J Urol 2003;170:818-822.

Pontari MA, Ruggieri MR: Mechanisms in prostatitis/chronic pelvic pain syndrome. J Urol 2004;172:839-845.

Schaeffer AJ, Landis JR, Knauss JS, et al: Chronic Prostatitis Collaborative Research Network Group. Demographic and clinical characteristics of men with chronic prostatitis: The National Institutes of Health chronic prostatitis cohort study. J Urol 2002;168:593-598.

Weidner W, Schiefer HG, Krauss H, et al: Chronic prostatitis: A thorough search for etiologically involved microorganisms in 1461 patients. Infection 1991;19:119-125.

10 Painful Bladder Syndrome/ Interstitial Cystitis and Related Disorders

PHILIP M. HANNO, MD, MPH

Painful bladder syndrome/interstitial cystitis (PBS/IC) is a condition diagnosed on a clinical basis and requiring a high index of suspicion by the clinician. Simply put, it should be considered in the differential diagnosis of the patient who presents with chronic pelvic pain that is often exacerbated by bladder filling and associated with urinary frequency. The perception that the original term, *interstitial cystitis,* was not at all descriptive of the clinical syndrome or even the pathologic findings in many cases has led to the current effort to reconsider the name of the disorder and even the way it is positioned in the medical spectrum (Hanno, 2005). What was originally considered a bladder disease is now considered a chronic pain syndrome (Janicki, 2003) that may begin as a pathologic process in the bladder in most but not all patients and eventually can develop into a disease in a small subset of those affected that even cystectomy may not benefit (Hanno et al, 2005). Its relationship to other chronic pelvic pain syndromes including the chronic pelvic pain syndrome in men (previously referred to as nonbacterial prostatitis) is unclear (Chai, 2002; Hakenberg and Wirth, 2002).

PBS/IC encompasses a major portion of the "painful bladder" disease complex, which includes a large group of patients with bladder and/or urethral and/or pelvic pain, irritative voiding symptoms (urgency, frequency, nocturia, dysuria), and sterile urine cultures. Painful bladder conditions with well-established causes include radiation cystitis, cystitis caused by microorganisms that are not detected by routine culture methodologies, and systemic disorders that affect the bladder. In addition, many gynecologic disorders can mimic PBS/IC (Kohli et al, 1997; Howard 2003a, 2003b).

The symptoms are mostly allodynic, an exaggeration of normal sensations. Urinary frequency patterns can be related to fluid intake and age, and the signal or urge to void is considered an unpleasant or painful sensation by most persons (Burgio et al, 1991). There are no pathognomonic findings on pathologic examination, and even the finding of petechial hemorrhages on the bladder mucosa during cystoscopy after bladder hydrodistention under anesthesia is no longer considered the sine qua non of PBS/IC that it had been until a decade ago (Waxman et al, 1998). PBS/IC is truly a diagnosis of exclusion. It may have multiple causes and represent a final common reaction of the bladder to different types of insult.

HISTORICAL PERSPECTIVE

Recent historical reviews confirm that IC was recognized as a pathologic entity during the 19th century (Christmas, 1997; Parsons and Parsons, 2004). Joseph Parrish, a Philadelphia surgeon, described three cases of severe lower urinary tract symptoms in the absence of a bladder stone in an 1836 text and termed the disorder "tic douloureux of the bladder." Teichman and colleagues (2000) argue that this may represent the first description of IC. Fifty years later Skene (1887) used the term *interstitial cystitis* to describe an inflammation that has "destroyed the mucous membrane partly or wholly and extended to the muscular parietes."

Early in the 20th century, at a New England Section meeting of the American Urological Association, Guy Hunner reported on eight women with a history of suprapubic pain, frequency, nocturia, and urgency lasting an average of 17 years (Hunner 1915, 1918). He drew attention to the disease, and the red, bleeding areas he described on the bladder wall came to have the pseudonym "Hunner's ulcer." As Walsh (1978) observed, this has proven to be unfortunate. In the early part of the 20th century, the very best cystoscopes available gave a poorly defined and ill-lit view of the fundus of the bladder. It is not surprising that when Hunner saw red and bleeding areas high on the bladder wall he thought they were ulcers. For the next 60 years, urologists would look for ulcers and fail to make the diagnosis in their absence. The disease was thought to be a focal cystitis rather than a pancystitis.

Hand (1949) authored the first comprehensive review about the disease, reporting 223 cases. In looking back, his paper was truly a seminal one, years ahead of its time. Many of his epidemiologic findings have held up to this day. His description of the clinical findings bears repeating. "I have frequently observed that what appeared to be a normal mucosa before and during the first bladder distention showed typical interstitial cystitis on subsequent distention." He notes, "small, discrete, submucosal hemorrhages, showing variations in form…dot-like bleeding points…little or no restriction to bladder capacity." He portrays three grades of disease, with grade 3 matching the small-capacity, scarred bladder described by Hunner. Sixty-nine percent of patients had grade 1 disease, and only 13% had grade 3 disease.

Walsh (1978) coined the term *glomerulations* to describe the petechial hemorrhages that Hand had described. But it was not until Messing and Stamey (1978) discussed the "early diagnosis" of IC that attention turned from looking for an ulcer to make the diagnosis to the concepts that (1) symptoms and glomerulations at the time of bladder distention under anesthesia were the disease hallmarks and (2) the diagnosis was primarily one of exclusion.

KEY POINT: HISTORICAL PERSPECTIVE

■ Bourque's *Aunt Minnie (she is hard to define, but you know her when you see her)* description of IC is over 50 years old and is worth recalling. "We have all met, at one time or another, patients who suffer chronically from their bladder; and we mean the ones who are distressed, not only periodically but constantly, having to urinate often, at all moments of the day and of the night, and suffering pains every time they void. We all know how these miserable patients are unhappy, and how those distressing bladder symptoms get finally to influence their general state of health physically at first, and mentally after a while." (Bourque, 1951)

Although memorable and right on the mark, Bourque's description under "Key Point: Historical Perspectives" and others like it were not suitable for defining this disease in a manner that would help physicians make the diagnosis and design research studies to learn more about the problem. Physician interest and government participation in research were sparked through the efforts of a group of frustrated patients led by Dr. Vicki Ratner, an orthopedic surgery resident in New York City, who founded the first patient advocacy group, the Interstitial Cystitis Association, in the living room of her New York City apartment in 1984 (Ratner et al, 1992; Ratner and Slade, 1997). The first step was to develop a working definition of the disease. The modern history of PBS/IC is best viewed through the perspective of definition.

DEFINITION

Interstitial cystitis (IC) is a clinical diagnosis primarily based on symptoms of urgency/frequency and pain in the bladder and/or pelvis. The International Continence Society (ICS) prefers the term *painful bladder syndrome* (PBS), defined as "the complaint of suprapubic pain related to bladder filling, accompanied by other symptoms such as increased daytime and night-time frequency, in the absence of proven urinary infection or other obvious pathology" (Abrams et al., 2002). **The ICS reserves the diagnosis of IC for patients with "typical cystoscopic and histological features," without further specifying these.** In the absence of clear criteria for "IC," this chapter will refer to PBS/IC and IC interchangeably, because all but recent literature terms the syndrome "IC." Perhaps more than for most diseases, how we arrived at this point is instructive and critical to an overall understanding of PBS/IC.

"It resembles a constellation of stars; its components are real enough but the pattern is in the eye of the beholder" (Makela and Heliovaara, 1991). This evocative description of fibromyalgia could equally apply to PBS/IC. Indeed, it has been argued, not necessarily convincingly, that each medical specialty has at least one somatic syndrome (irritable bowel syndrome, chronic pelvic pain, fibromyalgia, tension headache, noncardiac chest pain, hyperventilation syndrome) that might be better conceptualized as a part of a general functional somatic syndrome than with the symptom-based classification that we have now that may be more a reflection of professional specialization and access to care (Wessely and White, 2004).

There are data to suggest that true urinary frequency in women can be defined as regularly having to void at intervals of less than 3 hours, and that of women older than age 40 years, 25% have nocturia at least once (Glenning, 1985; Fitzgerald and Brubaker, 2003). Whereas bladder capacity tends to fall in women by the eighth and ninth decades of life, bladder volume at first desire to void tends to rise as women age (Collas and Malone-Lee, 1996). Based on a 90th percentile cutoff to determine the ranges of normality, the highest normal frequency varies in the fourth decade range from 6 voids for men to 9 voids for women (Burgio et al, 1991). Large variation in the degree of bother with varying rates of frequency (Fitzgerald et al, 2002) makes a symptomatic diagnosis of PBS/IC based on an absolute number of voids subject to question, and frequency per volume of intake or even the concept of "perception of frequency" as a problem may be more accurate than an absolute number.

In an effort to define IC so that patients in different geographic areas, under the care of different physicians, could be compared, the National Institute of Diabetes and Digestive and Kidney Diseases (NIDDK) held a workshop in August 1987 at which consensus criteria were established for the diagnosis of IC (Gillenwater and Wein, 1988). These criteria were not meant to define the disease but rather to ensure that groups of patients included in basic and clinical research studies would be relatively comparable. After pilot studies testing the criteria were carried out, the criteria were revised at another NIDDK workshop a year later (Wein et al, 1990). These criteria are presented in Table 10–1.

Although meant initially to serve only as a research tool, the NIDDK "research definition" became a de facto definition of this disease, diagnosed by exclusion and colorfully termed a "hole in the air" by Hald (George, 1986). Certain of the exclusion criteria serve mainly to make one wary of a diagnosis of IC but should by no means be used for categorical exclusion

Table 10–1. National Institute of Diabetes and Digestive and Kidney Diseases (NIDDK) Diagnostic Criteria for Interstitial Cystitis

To be diagnosed with interstitial cystitis, patients must have either glomerulations on cystoscopic examination or a classic Hunner ulcer, and they must have either pain associated with the bladder or urinary urgency. An examination for glomerulations should be undertaken after distention of the bladder under anesthesia to 80 to 100 cm H_2O for 1 to 2 minutes. The bladder may be distended up to two times before evaluation. The glomerulations must be diffuse—present in at least three quadrants of the bladder—and there must be at least 10 glomerulations per quadrant. The glomerulations must not be along the path of the cystoscope (to eliminate artifact from contact instrumentation). The presence of any one of the following excludes a diagnosis of interstitial cystitis:

1. Bladder capacity of greater than 350 mL on awake cystometry using either a gas or liquid filling medium
2. Absence of an intense urge to void with the bladder filled to 100 mL of gas or 150 mL of liquid filling medium
3. The demonstration of phasic involuntary bladder contractions on cystometry using the fill rate just described
4. Duration of symptoms less than 9 months
5. Absence of nocturia
6. Symptoms relieved by antimicrobial agents, urinary antiseptic agents, anticholinergic agents, or antispasmodic agents
7. A frequency of urination while awake of less than 8 times per day
8. A diagnosis of bacterial cystitis or prostatitis within a 3-month period
9. Bladder or ureteral calculi
10. Active genital herpes
11. Uterine, cervical, vaginal, or urethral cancer
12. Urethral diverticulum
13. Cyclophosphamide or any type of chemical cystitis
14. Tuberculous cystitis
15. Radiation cystitis
16. Benign or malignant bladder tumors
17. Vaginitis
18. Age younger than 18 years

From Wein AJ, Hanno PM, Gillenwater JY: Interstitial cystitis: An introduction to the problem. In Hanno PM, Staskin DR, Krane RJ, Wein AJ (eds): Interstitial Cystitis. London, Springer-Verlag, 1990, pp 13-15.

of such a diagnosis. However, because of the ambiguity involved, these patients should probably be eliminated from research studies or categorized separately. In particular, exclusion criteria 4, 5, 6, 8, 9, 11, 12, 17, and 18 are only relative. What percentage of patients with idiopathic "sensory urgency" have IC is unclear (Frazer et al, 1990). The specificity of the finding of bladder glomerulations has come into question (Erickson, 1995; Waxman, et al, 1998; Tomaszewski et al, 2001). Similarly, the sensitivity of glomerulations is also unknown, but clearly patients with IC symptoms can demonstrate an absence of glomerulations under anesthesia (Awad et al, 1992; Al Hadithi et al, 2002). Bladder ulceration is extremely rare and accounts for less than 5% of patients in my experience and in the experience of others (Sant, 1991). A California series found 20% of patients to have ulceration (Koziol, 1994). Specific pathologic findings represent a glaring omission from the criteria, because there is a lack of consensus as to which pathologic findings, if any, are required for, or even suggestive of, a tissue diagnosis (Hanno et al, 1990, 2005; Tomaszewski et al, 1999, 2001).

The unexpected use of the NIDDK research criteria by the medical community as a definition of IC led to concerns that many patients suffering from this syndrome might be misdiagnosed. The multicenter Interstitial Cystitis Database (ICDB) study through NIDDK accumulated data on 424 patients with IC, enrolling patients from May 1993 through December 1995. Entry criteria were much more symptom driven than those promulgated for research studies (Simon et al, 1997) and are noted in Table 10–2. In an analysis of the defining criteria (Hanno et al, 1999a, 1999b), it appeared the NIDDK research criteria fulfilled their mission. Fully 90% of expert clinicians agreed that patients diagnosed with IC by those criteria in the ICDB indeed had the disorder. However, 60% of patients deemed to have IC by these experienced clinicians would not have met NIDDK research criteria. Thus, IC remains a clinical syndrome defined by some combination of chronic symptoms of urgency, frequency, and/or pain in the absence of other reasonable causation. **Whereas IC symptom and problem indices have been developed and validated** (O'Leary et al, 1997; Goin et al, 1998), **these are not intended to diagnose or define IC but rather to measure the severity of symptomatology and monitor disease progression or regression** (Moldwin and Kushner, 2004).

Recent international consultations have essentially agreed that the nomenclature of "interstitial cystitis" be revised to "painful bladder syndrome/interstitial cystitis." This recognizes that **it is the symptoms that drive treatment, and the question as to whether IC refers to a distinct subgroup of the painful bladder syndrome is, as yet, unclear.** The International Continence Society (ICS) definition of painful bladder syndrome (Abrams et al, 2002) of "suprapubic pain related to bladder filling, accompanied by other symptoms such as increased daytime and nighttime frequency in the absence of infection or other pathology" appears to be a useful one, highlighting, as it does, that pain is the primary component of PBS/IC. For purposes of PBS/IC, the symptom of pain should be broadened to include "pressure" and "discomfort." IC may be a subgroup that encompasses those patients with typical histologic and cystoscopic features (Peeker and Fall, 2002), but what these features are is still controversial and somewhat vague.

Table 10-2. Interstitial Cystitis Database (ICDB) Study Eligibility Criteria

1. Providing informed consent to participate in the study.
2. Willing to undergo a cystoscopy under general or regional anesthesia when indicated, during the course of the study.
3. At least 18 years of age.
4. Having symptoms of urinary urgency, frequency, or pain for more than 6 months.
5. Urinating at least 7 times per day, or having some urgency or pain (measured on linear analog scales).
6. No history of current genitorurinary tuberculosis.
7. No history of urethral cancer.
8. No history of bladder malignancy, high-grade dysplasia, or carcinoma in situ.
9. Males: no history of prostate cancer.
10. Females: no occurrence of ovarian, vaginal, or cervical cancer in the previous 3 years.
11. Females: no current vaginitis, clue cell, trichomonas, or yeast infections.
12. No bacterial cystitis in the previous 3 months.
13. No active herpes in the previous 3 months.
14. No antimicrobials for urinary tract infections in previous 3 months.
15. Never having been treated with cyclophosphamide.
16. No radiation cystitis.
17. No neurogenic bladder dysfunction (e.g., due to a spinal cord injury, stroke, Parkinson's disease, multiple sclerosis, spina bifida, or diabetic cystopathy).
18. No bladder outlet obstruction (determined by urodynamic investigation).
19. Males: no bacterial prostatitis for previous 6 months.
20. Absence of bladder, ureteral, or urethral calculi for previous 3 months.
21. No urethritis for previous 3 months.
22. Not having had a urethral dilation, cystometrogram, bladder cystoscopy under full anesthesia, or a bladder biopsy in previous 3 months.
23. Never having had an augmentation cystoplasty, cystectomy, cystolysis, or neuroectomy.
24. Not having a urethral stricture of less than 12 French.

From Simon LJ, Landis JR, Erickson DR, Nyberg LM: The Interstitial Cystitis Data Base Study: Concepts and preliminary baseline descriptive statistics. Urology 1997;49:64-75.

Urgency is a common complaint of this group of patients. The ICS definition of urgency (Abrams et al, 2002), "the complaint of a sudden compelling desire to pass urine, which is difficult to defer," could be interpreted as compatible with either detrusor overactivity or PBS/IC. Pain and pressure are more involved in the frequency of PBS/IC, and fear of incontinence seems the reason for the urgency of overactive bladder (Abrams et al, 2005). Thus, urgency is left out of the definition of PBS/IC because it would tend to obfuscate the borders of overactive bladder and PBS/IC and is unnecessary for definition purposes. Figure 10–1 is a graphic depiction of one view of the relationship between these two, sometimes confused, conditions. The 14% incidence of urodynamic detrusor overactivity in the PBS/IC patients (Nigro et al, 1997) is probably close to what one might expect in the general population if studied urodynamically (Salavatore et al, 2003).

EPIDEMIOLOGY

Epidemiology studies of PBS/IC are hampered by many problems (Bernardini et al, 1999). **The lack of an accepted definition, the absence of a validated diagnostic marker, and questions regarding etiology and pathophysiology make much of the literature difficult to interpret. This is most apparent when one looks at the variation in prevalence reports in the United States and around the world. These range from 1.2 per 100,000 population and 4.5 per 100,00 females in Japan** (Ito et al, 2000) **to a questionnaire-based study that suggests a figure in American women of 20,000 per 100,000** (Parsons and Tatsis, 2004)!

It has been estimated that the prevalence of chronic pain due to benign causes in the population is at least 10% (Verhaak et al, 1998). Numerous case series have, until recently, formed the basis of epidemiologic information regarding PBS/IC. Farkas and associates (1977) discussed

OVERACTIVE BLADDER (OAB) AND ITS RELATIONSHIP TO
PAINFUL BLADDER SYNDROME (PBS)

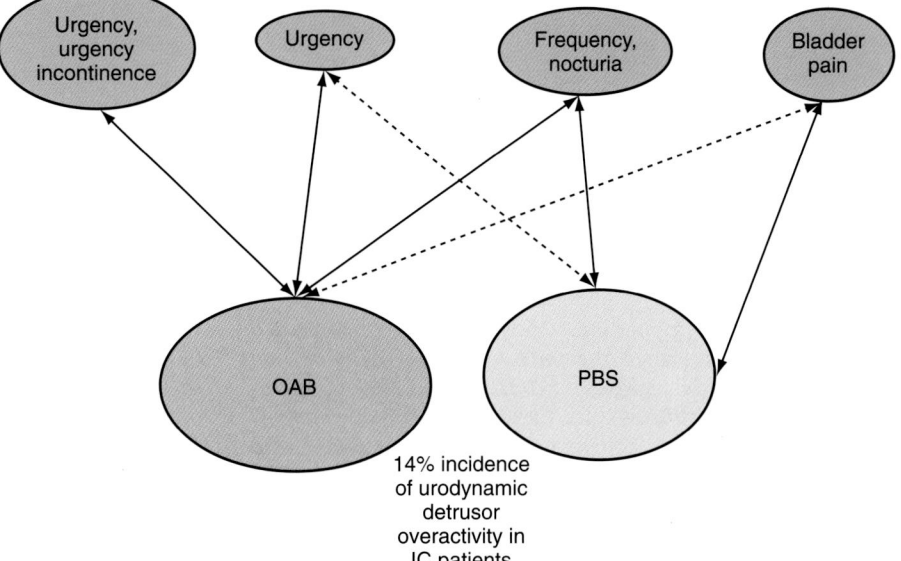

Figure 10–1. Relationship of overactive bladder (OAB) to painful bladder syndrome (PBS). (From Abrams PH, Hanno PM, Wein AJ: Overactive bladder and painful bladder syndrome: There need not be confusion. Neurourol Urodyn 2005;24:149-150.)

IC in adolescent girls. Hanash and Pool (1969) reviewed their experience with IC in men. Geist and Antolak (1970) reviewed and added to reports of disease occurring in child-hood. A childhood presentation is extremely rare and must be differentiated from the much more common and benign-behaving *extraordinary urinary frequency syndrome of childhood*, a self-limited condition of unknown etiology (Koff and Byard, 1988; Robson and Leung, 1993). Neverthe-less, there is a small cohort of children with chronic symptoms of bladder pain, urinary frequency, and sensory urgency in the absence of infection who have been evaluated with urodynamics, cystoscopy, and bladder distention and have findings consistent with the diagnosis of PBS/IC. In Close and colleague's review (1996) of 20 such children, the median age at onset was younger than 5 years and the vast majority of patients had long-term remissions with bladder distention.

A study conducted at the Scripps Research Institute (Koziol et al, 1993) included 374 patients at Scripps as well as some members of the Interstitial Cystitis Association, the large patient support organization. A more recent, but similar study in England (Tincello and Walker, 2005) concurred with the Scripps findings of urgency, frequency, and pain in the vast majority of these patients, devastating effects on quality of life, and often unsuccessful attempts at therapy with a variety of treatments. Although such reviews provide some information, they would seem to be necessarily biased by virtue of their design.

Several population-based studies have been reported in the literature, and these studies tend to support the reviews of selected patients or from individual clinics and the com-prehensive follow-up case-control study by Koziol (1994). The first population-based study (Oravisto, 1975) included "almost all the patients with interstitial cystitis in the city of Helsinki." This superb, brief report from Finland sur-veyed all diagnosed cases in a population approaching 1 million. The prevalence of the disease in women was 18.1 per 100,000. The joint prevalence in both sexes was 10.6 cases per 100,000. The annual incidence of new female cases was 1.2 per 100,000. Severe cases accounted for about 10% of the total. Ten percent of cases were in men. The disease onset was generally subacute rather than insidious, and full development of the classic symptom complex occurred over a relatively short time. IC does not progress continuously but usually reaches its final stage rapidly (within 5 years in the study by Koziol and colleagues (1993) and then continues without significant change in symptomatology. Subsequent major deterioration was found by Oravisto to be unusual. The duration of symptoms before diagnosis was 3 to 5 years in the Finnish study. Analogous figures in a classic American paper a quarter of a century earlier were 7 to 12 years (Hand, 1949).

Another early population study, this in the United States, first demonstrated the potential extent of what had been considered a very rare disease (Held et al, 1990). The fol-lowing population groups were surveyed: (1) random survey of 127 board-certified urologists, (2) 64 IC patients selected by the surveyed urologists and divided between the last patient with IC seen and the last patient with IC diagnosed, (3) 904 female patients belonging to the Interstitial Cystitis Associa-tion, and (4) a random phone survey of 119 persons from the U.S. population. This 1987 study reached the following conclusions:

1. There were 43,500 to 90,000 diagnosed cases of IC in the United States (twice the Finnish prevalence).
2. Up to a fivefold increase in IC prevalence occurred if all patients with painful bladder and sterile urine had been given the diagnosis, yielding up to a half million possible cases in the United States.
3. Median age at onset is 40 years.
4. Late deterioration in symptoms is unusual.
5. There is a 50% temporary spontaneous remission rate, with a mean duration of 8 months.
6. The incidence of childhood bladder problems is 10 times higher in IC patients versus controls.
7. The incidence of a history of urinary tract infection is twice that of controls.
8. Fourteen percent of IC patients were Jewish (15% in the sample of Koziol [1994]) versus 3% who were Jewish in a general population sample.
9. IC patients have a lower quality of life than dialysis patients.
10. Costs including lost economic production, in 1987, were $427 million.

Other population studies followed. Jones and Nyberg (1997) obtained their data from a self-report of a previous diagnosis of IC in the 1989 National Household Interview Survey. The survey estimated that 0.5% of the population, or more than 1 million people in the United States, reported having a diagnosis of IC. There was no verification of this self-report by medical records. Bade and associates (1995) did a physician questionnaire–based survey in the Netherlands yielding an overall prevalence of 8 to 16 per 100,000 females, with the diagnosis heavily dependent on pathology and pres-ence of mast cells. This prevalence in females compares to 4.5 per 100,00 in Japan (Ito et al, 2000). The Nurses Health Study I and II (Curhan et al, 1999) showed a prevalence of IC between 52 and 67 per 100,000 in the United States, twice the prevalence in the study of Held and associates (1990) and threefold greater than the study of Bade and coworkers (1995). It improved on previous studies by using a large sample derived from a general population and careful ascertainment of the diagnosis. If the 6.4% confirmation rate of their study were applied to the Jones and associates' National Health Interview Survey data, the prevalence estimates of the two studies would be nearly identical.

Leppilahti and colleagues (2002) and Miller and associates (1997) used the O'Leary-Sant IC Symptom and Problem Index (never validated for making a diagnosis per se) to select persons with IC symptoms from the Finnish population reg-ister. They calculated an incidence, based on an index score of 12 or greater, of 450/100,000. Roberts (2003), using a physi-cian diagnosis as the arbiter of IC, found annual incidence in Olmsted County, Minnesota, of 1.6 per 100,000 in women and 0.6 per 100,000 in men, a figure remarkably similar to the find-ings of Oravisto in Helsinki. The cumulative prevalence by age older than 80 years in the Minnesota study was 114 per 100,000, a figure comparable to that in the Nurses Health Study if one takes into account the younger age group in the Curhan data. Clemens and associates (2005) calculated a prevalence of diagnosed disease in a managed care population of 197 per 100,000 women and 41 per 100,000 men, but when the diagnosis was tested by eliminating those who had not been evaluated with endoscopy or in whom exclusionary conditions existed, the numbers dropped considerably.

Whether the considerable variability in prevalence in studies within the United States and around the world is related to methodology or true differences in incidence is an important question yet to be answered. Familial occurrence of PBS/IC has been reported (Dimitrakov, 2001). A hereditary aspect to incidence has been suggested by Warren and associates (2001, 2004) in a pioneering study. They found that adult female first-degree relatives of patients with IC may have a prevalence of IC 17 times that found in the general population. This, together with previously reported evidence showing a greater concordance of IC among monozygotic than dizygotic twins suggests but does not prove a genetic susceptibility to IC that could partially explain the discord in prevalence rates in different populations.

The ICDB cohort of patients has been carefully studied, and the findings seem to bear out those of other epidemiologic surveys (Propert et al, 2000). Patterns of change in symptoms with time suggest regression to the mean and an intervention effect associated with the increased follow-up and care of cohort participants. Although all symptoms fluctuated, there was no evidence of significant long-term change in overall disease severity. The data suggest that PBS/IC is a chronic disease and no current treatments have a significant impact on symptoms over time in the majority of patients. Quality of life studies suggest that PBS/IC patients are six times more likely than individuals in the general population to cut down on work time owing to health problems but only half as likely to do so as patients with arthritis (Shea-O'Malley and Sant, 1999). There is an associated high incidence of comorbidity, including depression, chronic pain, and anxiety and overall mental health (Michael et al, 2000; Rothrock et al, 2002; Hanno et al, 2005). There seems to be no effect on pregnancy outcomes (Onwude and Selo-Ojeme, 2003).

Most studies show a female-to-male preponderance of 5:1 or greater (Clemens et al, 2005; Hanno et al, 2005). In the absence of a validated marker, it is often difficult to distinguish PBS/IC from the chronic pelvic pain syndrome (nonbacterial prostatitis, prostatodynia) that affects males (Forrest and Schmidt, 2004), and the percentage of men with PBS/IC may actually be higher (Miller et al, 1995, 1997; Novicki et al, 1998). Men tend to be diagnosed at an older age and have a higher percentage of Hunner's ulcer in the case series reported (Novicki et al, 1998; Roberts et al, 2003).

Associated Diseases

Knowledge of associated diseases is relevant for the clues it engenders with regard to etiology and possible treatment of this enigmatic pain syndrome. In a case-control study, Erickson and associates (2001) found that patients with IC had higher scores than control subjects for pelvic discomfort, backache, dizziness, chest pain, aches in joints, abdominal cramps, nausea, palpitations, and headache. Buffington (2004) theorizes that a common stress response pattern of increased sympathetic nervous system function in the absence of comparable activation of the hypothalamic-pituitary-adrenal axis may account for some of these related symptoms. It has recently been hypothesized that panic disorder may some-

KEY POINTS: EPIDEMIOLOGY

Prevalence estimates per 100,000 persons (see text for details):

- United States: 35-24,000
- Netherlands: 7
- Finland: 10.6-450
- Japan: 1.2
- Female to male ratio = 5:1

An accurate country-by-country determination of PBS/IC prevalence and incidence is difficult to perform at the present time. Until specific diagnostic markers are verified and/or a set of agreed-upon diagnostic criteria based on well-designed published data are established, it seems most appropriate to use a more inclusive symptom specific definition of PBS/IC to permit an assessment of the population burden. Specifically, a validated questionnaire that can be administered in person or by telephone and that has been compared with a gold standard (disease marker in the future; expert opinion and diagnosis at present) is required to estimate within a given range the true extent of disease in populations around the world.

times be a part of a familial syndrome that includes IC, thyroid disorders, and other disorders of possible autonomic or neuromuscular control (Weissman et al, 2004).

Newly diagnosed patients are most concerned with the possibility that PBS/IC could be a forerunner of bladder carcinoma. **No reports have ever documented a relationship to suggest that IC is a premalignant lesion.** Utz and Zincke (1973) discovered bladder cancer in 12 of 53 men treated for IC at the Mayo Clinic. Three of 224 women were eventually diagnosed with bladder cancer. Four years later additional cases were reported (Lamm and Gittes, 1977). Tissot and associates (2004) reported 1% of 600 patients previously diagnosed as having IC were found to have transitional cell carcinoma as the cause of symptoms. Somewhat ominously, 2 of these patients had no hematuria. In all patients, irritative symptoms resolved after treatment of the malignancy. From these experiences has come the dictum that all patients with presumed IC should undergo cystoscopy, urine cytology, and bladder biopsy of any suspicious lesion to be sure that a bladder carcinoma is not masquerading as PBS/IC. It would seem that in the absence of microhematuria, and with a negative cytology, the risk of missing a cancer is negligible, but not zero. There is no evidence that PBS/IC itself is associated with a higher risk of bladder cancer or of transitions to cancer over time (Murphy et al, 1982).

A large-scale survey of 6783 individuals diagnosed by their physicians as having IC studied the incidence of associated disease in this population (Alagiri et al, 1997) (Fig. 10-2). Data from the 2405 responders were validated by comparison with 277 nonresponders. **Allergies were the most common association, with over 40% affected.** Allergy was also the

Prevalence rates ICA study group vs general population

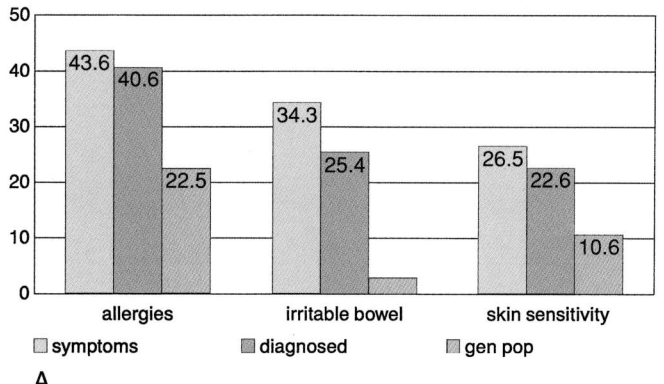

A

Prevalence rates ICA study group vs general population

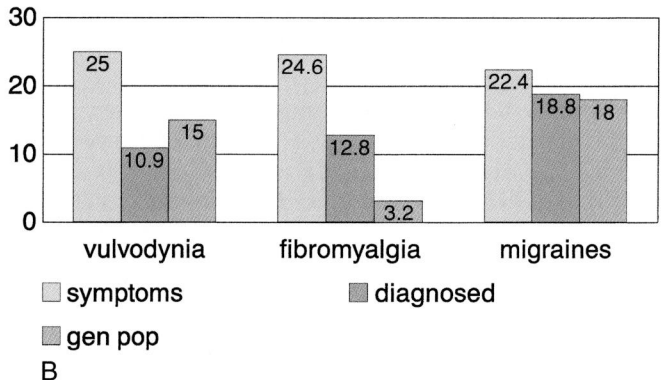

B

Prevalence rates ICA study group vs general population

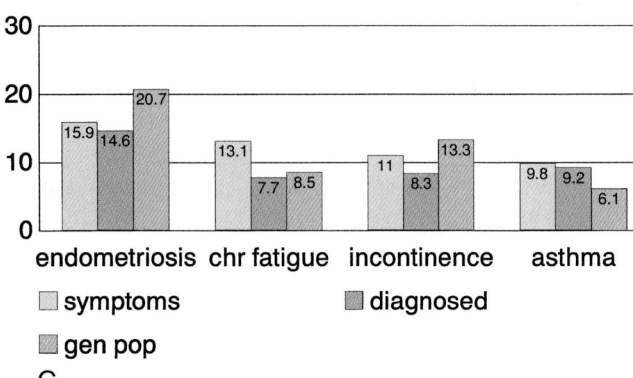

C

Prevalence rates ICA study group vs general population

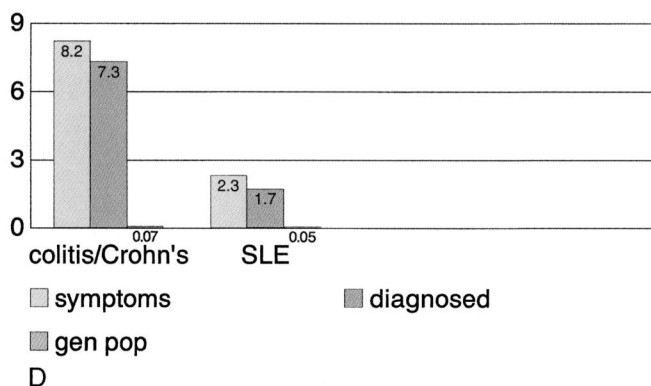

D

Figure 10–2. **A** to **D**, Comparison of disease prevalence rates between the Interstitial Cystitis Association (ICA) study group patients who report symptoms of a disorder, who have been diagnosed with a disorder, and the general population. SLE, systemic lupus erythematosus. (From Alagiri M, Chottiner S, Ratner V, et al: Interstitial cystitis: Unexplained associations with other chronic pain syndromes. Urology 1997;49[Suppl 5A]:52-57.)

primary association in Hand's study (Hand, 1949). Thirty percent of patients had a diagnosis of irritable bowel syndrome, a finding confirming that of Koziol (1994). Altered visceral sensation has been implicated in irritable bowel syndrome in that these patients experience intestinal pain at intestinal-gas volumes that are lower than those that cause pain in healthy persons (Lynn and Friedman, 1993), strikingly similar to the pain on bladder distention in IC.

Fibromyalgia, another disorder frequently considered functional because no specific structural or biochemical cause has been found, is also overrepresented in the IC population. This is a painful, nonarticular condition predominantly involving muscles; it is the most common cause of chronic, widespread musculoskeletal pain. It is typically associated with persistent fatigue, nonrefreshing sleep, and generalized stiffness. As in IC, women are affected at least 10 times more often than men (Consensus document, 1993). The association is intriguing because both conditions have nearly identical demographic features, modulating factors, associated symptoms, and response to tricyclic compounds (Clauw et al, 1997).

Vulvodynia, migraine headaches, endometriosis, chronic fatigue syndrome, incontinence, and asthma had similar prevalence as in the general population. Several publications have noted an association between IC and systemic lupus ery-

thematosus (SLE) (Fister, 1938; Boye et al, 1979; de la Serna and Alarcon-Segovia, 1981; Weisman et al, 1981; Meulders et al, 1992). The question has always been as to whether the bladder symptoms represent an association of these two disease processes or rather are a manifestation of lupus involvement of the bladder or even a myelopathy with involvement of the sacral cord in a small group of these patients (Sakakibara et al, 2003). The beneficial response of the cystitis of SLE to corticosteroids (Meulders et al, 1992) tends to support the latter view. No association with discoid lupus has been demonstrated (Jokinen et al, 1972). Although the actual numbers are small, the Alagiri study demonstrated a 30 to 50 times greater incidence of SLE in the IC group compared with the general population. Overall, the incidence of collagen vascular disease in the IC population is low. Parsons (1990) found only 2 of 225 consecutive IC patients to have a history of autoimmune disorder.

Inflammatory bowel disease was found in over 7% of the IC population Alagiri studied, a figure 100 times higher than in the general population. While unexplained at this time, abnormal leukocyte activity has been implicated in both conditions (Bhone et al, 1962; Kontras et al, 1971).

Another mysterious disorder that has been associated with IC is focal vulvitis. Vulvar vestibulitis syndrome is a constellation of symptoms and findings involving and limited to the vulvar vestibule consisting of (1) severe pain on vestibular touch to attempted vaginal entry, (2) tenderness to pressure localized within the vulvar vestibule, and (3) physical findings confined to vulvar erythema of various degrees (Marinoff and Turner, 1991). McCormack (1990) reported on 36 patients with focal vulvitis, 11 of whom also had IC. Fitzpatrick and associates (1993) have added three more cases. The concordance of these noninfectious inflammatory syndromes involving the tissues derived from the embryonic urogenital sinus and the similarity of the demographics argue for a common etiology.

An association has been reported between IC and Sjögren's syndrome, an autoimmune exocrinopathy with a female preponderance manifested by dry eyes, dry mouth, and arthritis but that can also include fever, dryness, and gastrointestinal and lung problems. Van De Merwe and coworkers (1993) investigated 10 IC patients for the presence of Sjögren's syndrome. Two patients had both the keratoconjunctivitis sicca and focal lymphocytic sialoadenitis, allowing a primary diagnosis of Sjögren's syndrome. Only 2 patients had neither finding. They later reported an incidence of 28% of Sjögren's syndrome in patients with IC (van de Merwe et al, 2003). The incidence of symptoms of PBS/IC in patients with Sjögren's syndrome has been estimated to be up to 5% (Leppilahti et al, 2003).

A negative correlation with diabetes has been noted (Parsons, 1990; Koziol, 1994).

Further epidemiologic studies are warranted, because the epidemiology of this disorder may ultimately yield as many clues into etiology and treatment as other avenues of research.

KEY POINTS: ASSOCIATED DISORDERS

- Allergies
- Irritable bowel syndrome
- Fibromyalgia
- Systemic lupus erythematosus
- Inflammatory bowel disease
- Focal vulvitis/vulvar vestibulitis
- Sjögren's syndrome

ETIOLOGY

It is likely that PBS/IC has a multifactorial etiology that may act predominantly through one or more pathways resulting in the typical symptom-complex (Holm-Bentzen et al, 1990; Levander, 2003; Mulholland and Byrne, 1994; Erickson, 1999; Keay et al, 2004b) (Fig. 10–3). There are an abundance of theories regarding its pathogenesis, but confirmatory evidence gleaned from clinical practice has proven sparse. Among numerous proposals that shall be further explored in this section are "leaky epithelium," mast cell activation, and

neurogenic inflammation, or some combination of these and other factors leading to a self-perpetuating process resulting in chronic bladder pain and voiding dysfunction (Elbadawi, 1997).

Animal Models

Until recently, lacking an easily available animal model of the naturally occurring disease, researchers have had to devise animal models to study isolated symptoms of PBS/IC, hoping to uncover the root causes of the symptomatology (Ruggieri et al, 1990). Bullock and associates (1992) reported a mouse model in which bladder inflammation could be induced by the injection of syngeneic bladder antigen. While demonstrating that a component in the Balb/cAN mouse is capable of inducing a bladder-specific, adoptively transferable, cell-mediated autoimmune response that exhibits many characteristics of clinical IC, the model became difficult to reproduce (Klutke et al, 1997).

A guinea pig model was used in which a solution was instilled containing a protein to which the animal had been previously immunized and which resulted in bladder inflammation (Christensen et al, 1990; Kim et al, 1992), and a rat model was used of allergic cystitis using a local challenge of ovalbumin in previously sensitized rats (Ahluwalia et al, 1998). Changes in the rat model were dependent on mast cell degranulation and activation of sensory C fibers.

Ghoniem and coworkers (1995) studied four female African green monkeys challenged with intravesical acetone. Not surprisingly, they exhibited symptoms of painful bladder syndrome. Rivas and associates (1997) performed similar experiments using dilute hydrochloric acid in a rat model. A rat model for neurogenic cystitis using pseudorabies virus demonstrated that inflammatory changes in the spinal cord can result in dramatic, neurogenically mediated changes in the bladder (Doggweiler et al, 1998).

The problem with all of these animal models relates to whether they mirror the human disease to any great extent. **Buffington (1994) has described what appears to be a naturally occurring animal model of PBS/IC.** Two thirds of cats with lower urinary tract disease have sterile urine and no evidence of other urinary tract disorders (Kruger et al, 1991). A portion of these cats experience frequency and urgency of urination, pain, and bladder inflammation (Houpt, 1991) (Fig. 10–4). Glomerulations have been observed in the bladders of these animals. GP-51, a glycosaminoglycan (GAG) commonly found in the surface mucin covering the mucosa of the normal human bladder and decreased in IC, shows a decreased expression in cats with this symptom-complex (Press et al, 1995), originally termed *feline urologic syndrome*. Bladder Aδ afferents in these cats are more sensitive to pressure changes than are afferents in normal cats (Roppolo et al, 2005). These cats also demonstrate an increase in baseline nitric oxide production in smooth muscle and mucosal strips when compared with healthy cats with evidence of altered mucosal barrier function (Birder et al, 2005).

Buffington and associates (1999) now refer to this disorder as *feline interstitial cystitis*. It is associated with urinary urgency, frequency, and pain with sterile urine, bladder mastocytosis, increased histamine excretion, increased bladder permeability, decreased urinary GAG excretion (Buffington et

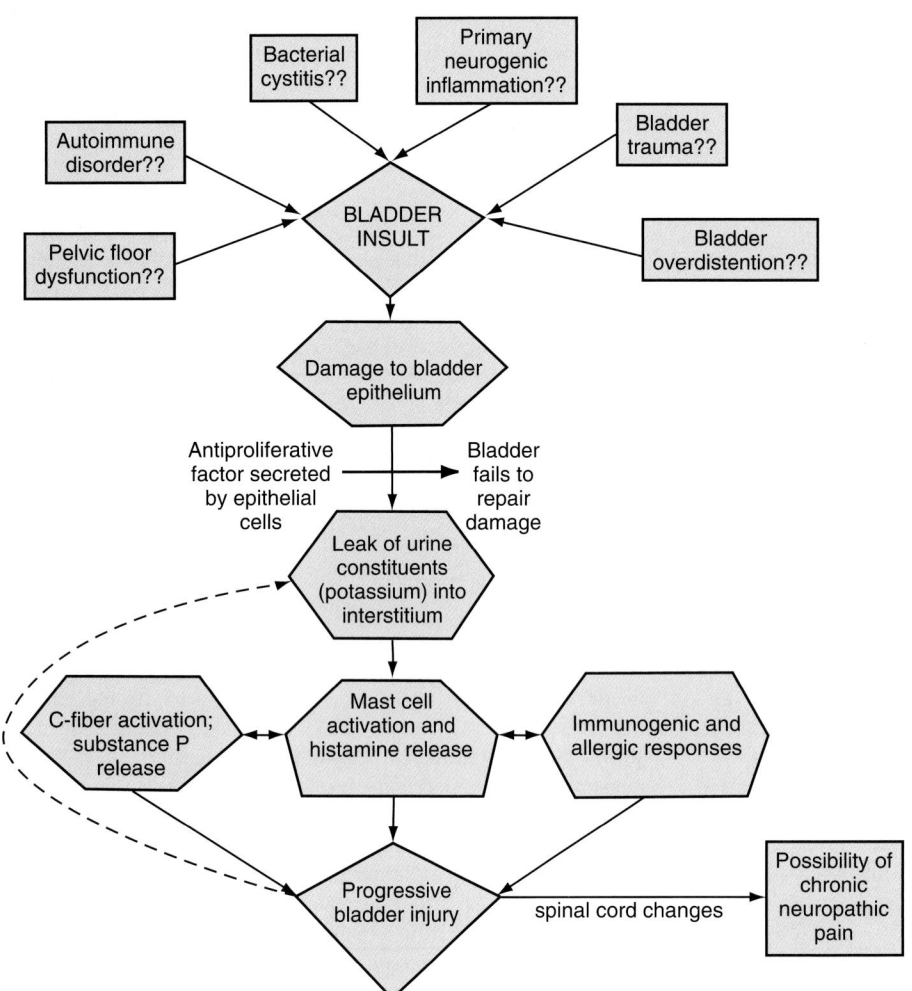

Figure 10–3. Hypothesis for etiologic cascade of painful bladder syndrome/interstitial cystitis.

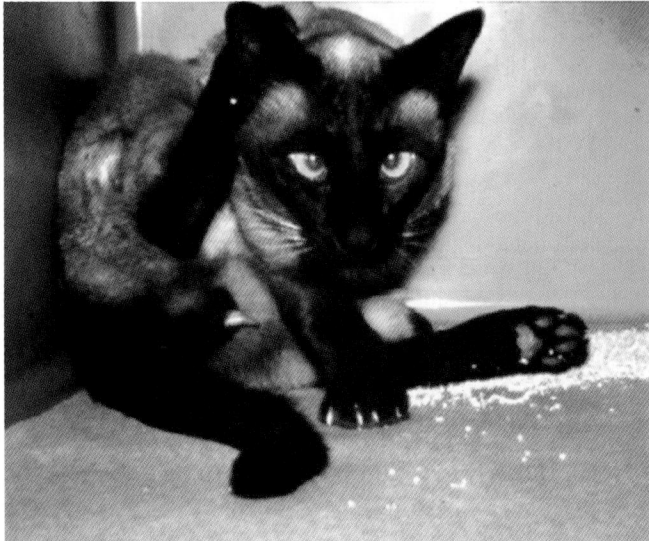

Figure 10–4. Photograph of cat suffering from feline interstitial cystitis. (Courtesy of Tony Buffington.)

al, 1996), and increased plasma norepinephrine concentrations (Buffington and Pacak, 2001b).

Although animal models can yield clues to etiology, all theories must ultimately be tested in humans with the disease.

Infection

Often, a diagnosis of PBS/IC is made only after a patient has been seen by a number of physicians and treated with antibiotics for presumed urinary tract infection without resolution of symptoms (Held et al, 1990). The symptom-complex looks to the patient and physician like an infectious process (Porru et al, 2004). The epidemiology of urinary tract infection and its predominance in women mirror the IC data (Warren, 1994). The acute to subacute onset in many patients has fascinated clinicians, who often associate an insidious onset with a chronic condition such as PBS/IC.

Reverse logic led some to suspect that antibiotics may be instrumental in causing IC (Holm-Bentzen et al, 1990). Most patients have been treated with antibiotics once or several times before the diagnosis is made. Numerous antibiotics, primarily in the penicillin family, can induce a cystitis (Bracis et al, 1977; Marx and Alpert, 1984; Moller, 1978; Chudwin et al, 1979; Cook et al, 1979), but no evidence has ever been documented that these antibiotics or the supposedly "surface active" nitrofurantoins or tetracyclines have any involvement in pathogenesis (Ruggieri et al, 1987; Levin et al, 1988).

To determine whether there is an infectious cause of IC certain procedures are necessary (Warren, 1994). Not just urine but bladder epithelium as well must be cultured for appropriate microorganisms, including bacteria, viruses, and fungi. Because some organisms might be culturable yet fastidious, special culture techniques should be used. Because some organisms in urine or tissue might be viable but nonculturable, specific nonculture techniques for discovery and identification should be employed. Most important, the same procedures must be carried out in a control population.

Attempts to show an infectious etiology go back to the dawn of the disease, but the case has never been a strong one (Duncan and Schaeffer, 1997). Hunner (1915) originally proposed that IC resulted from chronic bacterial infection of the bladder wall secondary to hematogenous dissemination. Harn and associates (1973) proposed a relationship between IC and streptococcal and post-streptococcal inflammation. They produced a progressive chronic inflammation in rabbit bladders by injecting small numbers of *Streptococcus pyogenes* in the bladder wall. The discovery that *Helicobacter pylori* is related to the pathogenesis of chronic atrophic gastritis and peptic ulcer disease and that antibiotic treatment can heal ulceration (Parsonnet et al, 1991; NIH Consensus Development Panel, 1994; Sung et al, 1995) has continued to focus attention by researchers in IC on the possibility that an infectious etiology is not only reasonable but will ultimately be found. Studies of *H. pylori* itself have failed to demonstrate an association with IC (Agarwal and Dixon, 2003; Atug et al, 2004; English et al, 1998; Haq et al, 2004). Wilkins and coworkers (1989) found bacteria in catheterized urine specimens and/or bladder biopsies in 12 of 20 patients with IC. However, eight of the isolates were fastidious bacteria, *Gardnerella vaginalis*, and *Lactobacillus* species and no control subjects were included in the study.

Negative studies far outnumber the positive ones. Hanash and Pool (1970) performed viral, bacterial, and fungal studies on 30 IC patients and failed to substantiate an infectious etiology. Hedelin and colleagues (1983) found only 3 of 19 IC patients to have urine cultures positive for *Ureaplasma urealyticum* and indirect hemagglutination antibodies to *Mycoplasma hominis* to be no greater than in controls. Potts and associates (2000) cultured *U. urealyticum* in 22 of 48 patients with "chronic urinary symptoms" and had great success in these patients (none of whom had established IC) with short courses of commonly prescribed antibiotics. Given the history of empirical use of antibiotics in the vast majority of IC patients, it is doubtful if this group represents even a small percentage of the IC-diagnosed population. Nevertheless, it illustrates that IC is a diagnosis of exclusion, and urine culture is critical while an empirical short course of antibiotics is certainly reasonable if the patient has not already been treated for presumed infection. Empirical use of doxycycline at a dose of 100 mg twice daily for 2 weeks followed by 100 mg daily for 2 weeks has been successfully used in this manner (Burkhard et al, 2004).

The development of highly sensitive, rapid, and specific molecular methods of identifying infectious agents by the direct detection of DNA or RNA sequences unique to a particular organism (Naber, 1994) resulted in a flurry of activity into the search for a responsible virus or microorganism. Hampson and coworkers (1993) could find no evidence of mycobacterial involvement in eight cases of IC using DNA probes. Haarala and coworkers (1996) confirmed an absence of bacterial DNA in the bladder of 11 IC patients with no documented history of urinary tract infection. Hukkanen and colleagues (1996) reported an absence of adenovirus and BK virus genomes in urinary bladder biopsies of IC patients. Domingue and associates' (1995) provocative finding of the presence of bacterial 16S rRNA genes in bladder biopsies from 29% of IC patients but not from control bladders, and their discovery of 0.22-μm filterable forms in culture of biopsy tissue from 14 of 14 IC patients and none of 15 control subjects has never been confirmed or repeated.

A preliminary study found a statistically significant increase in urine PCR to *Chlamydia pneumoniae* major outer membrane protein gene in patients with IC as compared with controls (Franke et al, 1999). Other studies have shown that similar percentages of both IC and control patient populations have nonculturable bacteria in their bladder on the basis of polymerase chain reaction studies of bladder biopsy specimens (Heritz et al, 1997; Keay et al, 1998a). The spirochete *Borrelia burgdorferi* has been found in the bladder biopsies and urine of patients with Lyme disease and can cause frequency, urgency, and nocturia. DNA studies have failed to show a role for *Borrelia* in IC (Haarala et al, 2000).

The role of infection in the pathogenesis of IC remains a mystery (Elbadawi, 1997; Elgavish et al, 1995). At this time there are little data to support the role of an infectious etiology but investigators keep returning to an infectious theory. New insights into the mechanisms by which bacteria adhere, grow, and persist in association with host tissue and form intracellular pods capable of subverting host defense mechanisms and allowing replication within epithelial cells lay the foundation for a possible role of infection in initiating the PBS/IC pathologic cascade (Kau et al, 2005). The University of Maryland group proposed a model of IC in which bladder epithelial damage such as that caused by bacterial cystitis may be the first step leading to a low-level inflammatory response we call IC (Keay and Warren, 1998). **Domingue and Ghoniem (1997) write that "It is logical to suggest that even if organisms are not causative agents, their presence may lead to immune and host-cell responses that could initiate or exacerbate an inflammatory state."**

If infection does play a role, it would be predicted that appropriate treatments to minimize microbial presence in the tissue would significantly improve the morbidity associated with IC. Durier's incredible series (1992) purporting to cure 27 of 27 IC patients with the use of up to five sequential antibiotics covering the anaerobic spectrum has never been duplicated. Warren and colleagues' (2000) prospective, double-blind, placebo-controlled, randomized trial of 50 patients may well prove the end of long-term empirical antibiotic treatment in established IC. Eighteen weeks of placebo or antibiotics (sequential doxycycline, erythromycin, metronidazole, clindamycin, amoxicillin, and ciprofloxacin for 3 weeks each) were administered. Most patients guessed the arm to which they were assigned. Of the 25 patients in the active arm, 80% had new non-urinary symptoms perceived as side effects. There was minimal improvement in some patients associated with the active arm of the study, but the conclusion that intensive antibiotics do not represent a major advance in therapy for IC seems well justified.

KEY POINT: ETIOLOGY (INFECTION)

■ Although the concept that a urinary tract infection may trigger IC in some patients is appealing, it is unlikely that active infection is involved in the ongoing pathologic process or that antibiotics have a role to play in treatment.

Autoimmunity/Inflammation

Immune/neuroimmune mechanisms may have an important role in the pathogenesis of PBS/IC. Excessive release of sensory nerve neurotransmitters and mast cell inflammatory mediators is thought to be responsible for the development and propagation of symptoms (Luo, 2005). Inflammation results in altered nerve growth factor content of the bladder and in morphologic changes in sensory and motor neurons innervating the bladder. Such neuroplasticity may be a possible explanation for the association of bladder inflammation with long-term symptoms and pain after inflammation subsides (Dupont et al, 2001).

For many years the possibility that IC may represent some type of autoimmune disorder has been considered. Narrowly defined, autoimmune diseases are clinical syndromes caused by the activation of T cells or B cells, or both, in the absence of an ongoing infection or other discernible cause (Davidson and Diamond, 2001). To establish a disease as autoimmune, three types of evidence can be marshaled: (1) direct evidence from transfer of pathogenic antibody or pathogenic T cells, (2) indirect evidence based on reproduction of the autoimmune disease in experimental animals, and (3) circumstantial evidence from clinical clues (Rose and Bona, 1993). Circumstantial evidence would include (1) association with other autoimmune diseases in the same individual or same family; (2) lymphocytic infiltration of target organ; (3) statistical association with a particular major histocompatibility complex haplotype; and (4) favorable response to immunosuppression.

Circumstantial evidence by itself cannot define an autoimmune disease, and at this point the case for autoimmunity in IC is far from clear. **Three different possibilities exist: (1) IC is caused by a direct autoimmune attack on the bladder, (2) some of the autoimmune symptoms and pathology of IC arise indirectly as a result of tissue destruction and inflammation from other causes, and (3) autoimmune phenomena in IC patients are coincident and unrelated to the disease** (Ochs and Tan, 1997).

Silk (1970) found bladder antibodies in 9 of 20 IC patients and none in 35 pathologic or normal control patients. Gordon and associates (1973) found anti-bladder antibodies present in biopsy specimens from 6 of 8 IC patients and in 3 of 5 control patients. No control patient demonstrated antibodies in the muscle, whereas 3 of 5 IC patients with muscle in the biopsy did so. Jokinen and associates (1972) looked at sera from 33 IC patients and found 28 with an antinuclear anti-

body (ANA) titer of 1:10 or greater, but no bladder-specific antibodies were detected with immunofluorescence. There was poor correlation between ANA titers and symptom severity. Jokinen and associates (1973) noted that elevated antibody titers against cell nuclei and crude kidney homogenate decreased within 12 months after cystectomy in 3 IC patients. All of this provided hints that IC could fall into the autoimmune group of diseases.

Oravisto summarized the world literature on this idea in 1980, concluding that the chronic course of disease, the absence of infection, the pathologic findings, the occurrence of antinuclear antibodies, and the reported responses to corticosteroids at that time provided strong circumstantial evidence of autoimmunity. He discounted the paucity of activated lymphocytes which speak against an autoimmune process. Studies on autoantibodies in PBS/IC have shown that these mainly consist of antinuclear antibodies (Jokinen et al, 1972) similar to the autoantibody profiles in some systemic diseases such as Sjögren's syndrome, well known to be of autoimmune origin (Tan, 1989; Leppilahti et al, 2003). Mattila (1982) presented evidence of immune deposits in the bladder vascular walls in 33 of 47 IC patients. Studying sera from 41 patients with IC, he concluded that the classical pathway activation of the complement system was involved, supporting the possibility that a chronic local immunologic process was indeed occurring (Mattila et al, 1983). The autoantibodies tested were found to be directed against cytoskeletal intermediate filaments. Because the autoantibodies have to gain access to intracellular structures to cause in vivo deposits, primary tissue injury of unknown etiology has to be postulated (Mattila and Linder, 1984).

Anderson and colleagues (1989) studied 26 patients with IC and compared them with a control group of similar age and sex with other urologic complaints. They performed a standard autoimmune profile and looked for specific antibodies to normal human bladder in the serum. Sixty-five percent of IC patients and 36% of controls demonstrated non–organ-specific antibodies; 40% of IC patients had ANAs; 75% of IC patients and 40% of controls had anti-bladder antibodies present in the serum. There was no increase in immunoglobulin deposition in the bladder epithelium in IC patients versus controls. Although IC patients demonstrated a nonspecific increase in antibody formation, this was not significantly different from a similar group of other urologic patients. The lack of specificity indicates the immunologic findings are likely secondary to inflammation rather than a primary etiology.

In a study looking for active immune cellular deposition in IC patients, no statistically significant difference between controls and nonulcerative IC patients was identified (Harrington et al, 1990). In contrast, the ulcerative IC group had focal sheets of plasma cells, aggregates of T cells, B cell nodules, a decreased or normal helper-to-suppressor cell ratio, and suppressor cytotoxic cells in germinal centers. Flow cytometry analysis of peripheral blood lymphocyte subsets showed increased numbers of secretory Ig–positive B cells and activated lymphocytes in the nonulcerative group and increased numbers of secretory Ig–positive cells and activated lymphocytes in the ulcerative group. These results may suggest a partial role for an immune mechanism in IC. Erickson and coworkers (1997) have also noted a major difference in inflammatory cell types as well as clinical features in IC patients with severe inflammation, suggesting two different patient groups with two different underlying pathophysiologies.

Hanno and colleagues (1990) found CD4 cell predominance in all layers of the bladder in IC patients. Christmas (1994) reported increased numbers of CD4+ and CD8+ T cells in bladder biopsies from patients with IC and bacterial cystitis as compared with controls. These T cells were present in the urothelium and submucosa but not in the detrusor. Control bladder tissue demonstrated only CD8 cells in the urothelium and both CD4+ and CD8+ cells in the submucosa. The number of plasma cells was significantly greater in IC patients than in normal controls and controls with bacterial cystitis.

MacDermott and colleagues (1991b) found a normal distribution of peripheral blood lymphocytes in IC patients, a finding not supportive of an autoimmune mechanism in the disease. The lamina propria showed a predominance of CD4 (helper T cells) lymphocytes over CD8 cells in both IC and other cystitis patients. The same pattern was seen in the epithelium of patients with bacterial or mechanical cystitis, but patients with IC had a predominance of CD8 lymphocytes in the urothelium—identical to control subjects. The findings suggest that the urothelium is not involved in the inflammatory reaction, as is the lamina propria, making the urothelium an unlikely source for the initiating factor.

Miller and coworkers (1992) investigated the function of peripheral blood lymphocytes from nonulcerative IC patients, testing the proliferative response and cytokine production of T cells to nonspecific mitogenic stimulation and the proliferative response of T cells to urine components. Proliferation and cytokine production after mitogen stimulation were the same for control subjects and IC patients. Moreover, no immunologic response to IC urine by autologous peripheral blood lymphocytes in in-vitro assays was observed. Their findings cast doubt on theories suggesting that IC is an autoimmune disease.

Numerous inflammatory mediators have been studied with regard to their relation to IC (Elgebaly et al, 1992; Felsen et al, 1994; Lotz et al, 1994; Steinert et al, 1994; Zuraw et al, 1994). Patients with PBS/IC exhibit varying degrees of inflammation that can separate them into clusters (Tomaszewski et al, 2001; Green et al, 2004). Bladder inflammation in IC is categorized by elevated urinary interleukin-6 (Erickson et al, 1997) and activation of the kallikrein-kinin system (Rosamilia et al, 1999b). The absence of urinary interleukin-1β in IC argues against an immunologic or autoimmune etiology of the disorder (Martins et al, 1994). Neurogenic inflammation may play a role in the etiology, because long-term exposure of afferent nerve terminals to inflammatory mediators can alter ion channels and result in bladder hyperalgesia (Buffington and Wolfe, 1998; Yoshimura and de Groat, 1999). Substance P itself does not seem to be the single initiator of inflammation in the bladder, and its blockade does not protect the bladder in animal models from inflammatory responses (Luber-Narod et al, 1997). Urinary nitric oxide synthase (NOS) activity is known to be elevated in patients with urinary infection and thought to play a role in the bladder's response to infection and in the inflammatory process that follows infection. The finding that urinary NOS activity is decreased in IC patients

has puzzled researchers but could explain the reduction in functional bladder capacity associated with the disorder (Smith et al, 1996; Foster et al, 1997).

Urothelial cell activation in IC may result in aberrant immune responses and immune activation within the bladder wall (Liebert et al, 1993) that could relate to pathogenesis of the disease but might not reflect initiating etiology (Ochs et al, 1994). It has been proposed that inflammatory and/or immune responses in IC could be exacerbated by persistent activation of the nuclear factor (NF)-kB (Abdel-Mageed and Ghoniem, 1998; Abdel-Mageed, 2003). Angiogenic factors such as platelet-derived endothelial cell growth factor/thymidine phosphorylase and transforming growth factor-β may be involved in the inflammatory process to induce painful symptoms in patients with IC or bladder carcinoma (Ueda et al, 2002).

The exact role of autoimmunity in IC remains controversial (Ochs and Tan, 1997). Suplatast tosilate, a new immunoregulator, has shown efficacy in a small, uncontrolled IC study in which improvements in symptoms and bladder capacity were correlated with changes in autoimmune parameters (Ueda et al, 2000). **Although the immune system remains a target for therapy, no clear indication of a primary role for autoimmunity as the cause of IC has been observed** (Liebert, 1997).

Mast Cell Involvement

Although mast cells are thought of primarily in the context of allergic disorders, and certain acute inflammatory responses, these cells have also been implicated in biologic responses as diverse as angiogenesis and wound healing, bone remodeling, peptic ulcer disease, atherosclerosis, and reactions to neoplasms (Galli, 1993). Mast cells remain one of the most enigmatic cells in the body. They secrete significant amounts of numerous proinflammatory mediators that contribute to a number of chronic inflammatory conditions, including stress-induced intestinal ulceration, rheumatoid arthritis, scleroderma, and Crohn's disease. They have been described even among the lowest order of animals, having been discovered in the frog mesentery over 100 years ago. Their raison d'etre may be for initiating and coordinating the host's inflammatory and immune responses against microbial pathogens (Abraham and Malaviya, 1997). Recently they have been implicated in a range of neuroinflammatory diseases, especially those worsened by stress (Theoharides, 2004; Theoharides and Cochrane, 2004). These include multiple sclerosis, migraines, inflammatory arthritis, atopic dermatitis, coronary inflammation, irritable bowel syndrome, and PBS/IC. They may be activated through their Fc receptors by immunoglobulins other than IgE, as well as by anaphylatoxins, neuropeptides, and cytokines to secrete mediators selectively without overt degranulation.

Mast cells have frequently been reported to be associated with IC, both as a pathogenetic mechanism and as a pathognomonic marker (Simmons, 1961; Bhone et al, 1962; Smith and Dehner, 1972; Larsen et al, 1982; Hofmeister et al, 1997). The association of bladder mastocytosis, IC, and irritable bowel syndrome (Pang et al, 1996) and chronic urticaria (Sant et al, 1997) is intriguing. Evidence of their importance is mounting, suggesting that they may serve as the final common pathway through which the symptomatic condition is expressed. Mast cells produce, among other compounds, histamine. Histamine release in tissue causes pain, hyperemia, and fibrosis, all notable features of IC.

Simmons (1961) was the first to suggest mast cells as a cause of IC. Contribution of mast cells to the cellular infiltrate in IC (Fig. 10–5) has been shown to vary from about 20% in nonulcer IC patients to 65% in patients with ulceration (Sant et al, 1988; Enerback et al, 1989). Mast cells participate in allergic reactions (hypersensitivity type I) during which IgE antibody is synthesized in response to specific antigens. IgE binds to mast cell receptors, and antigen binds to the IgE, leading to degranulation (Lagunoff et al, 1983). Other triggers of mast cell secretion include acetylcholine, anaphylatoxins, cationic peptides such as substance P, chemicals, contrast agents, cytokines, opioids, antihistamines, exercise, hormones, viruses, and bacterial toxins (Sant and Theoharides, 1994). Mast cells promote infiltration of neutrophils, T and B lymphocytes, monocytes, and eosinophils. T lymphocytes secrete substances capable of activating mast cells, thus perpetuating the cycle of inflammation (Kaplan et al, 1985).

Since the presence of mast cells within the bladder wall was first recognized (Simmons and Bunce, 1958), numerous investigators have tried to determine whether there is an increase in the number of mast cells in the bladder of patients with IC, or differences in their location or functional state (Larsen et al, 1982; Kastrup et al, 1983; Fall et al, 1987; Feltis et al, 1987; Lynes et al, 1987; Christmas and Rode, 1991). An increase in urothelial mast cells appears to be part of the generalized inflammatory cell reaction regardless of etiology and not a specific feature of IC, whereas the presence of increased numbers of mast cells in the detrusor is more specific for IC. However, one study did report detrusor mastocytosis in 64% of IC patients and 80% of a control group with other urologic disease, with no statistically significant difference between the mean number of detrusor mast cells in the two groups (Hanno et al, 1990).

Aldenborg and associates (1986) reported that mast cells are found predominantly in the detrusor muscle in patients with classic IC, but there is also a secondary population of

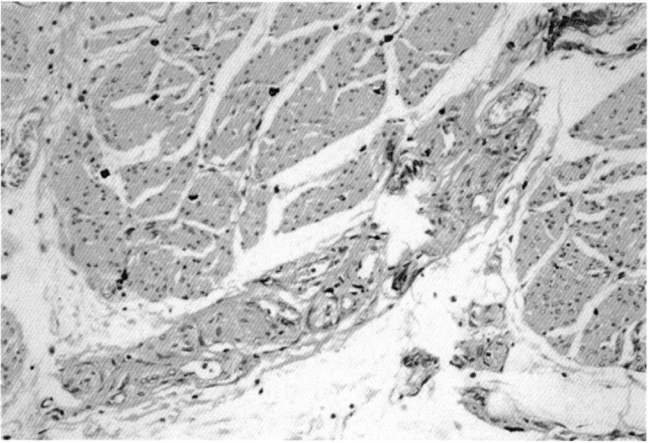

Figure 10–5. Giemsa stain shows detrusor mastocytosis and nerve hypertrophy in interstitial cystitis. (Original magnification, ×400.) (Courtesy of John Tomaszewski, Hospital of the University of Pennsylvania, Department of Pathology.)

mast cells in the lamina propria and the bladder epithelium, with staining characteristics distinct from those in the detrusor. None of these epithelial mast cells were found in controls. These findings were interpreted to indicate a transepithelial migration of mast cells in patients with IC. This second population of mast cells does not appear to be involved in the nonulcer type of IC (Aldenborg et al, 1989). This mucosal population of mast cells can also differ from the mast cells found in deeper tissues in physiologic responses and release of secretory products (Sant, 1991). The "mucosal mast cells" are susceptible to aldehyde fixation and require special fixation and staining techniques for proper demonstration. Detrusor mast cells are not susceptible to fixation techniques. Recent studies have shown that although all human mast cells contain the proteinase tryptase, there is a population of mast cells that also contain the proteinase chymase. The mast cell expansion in IC involves both types (Yamada et al, 2000). Mast cell activation is far more pronounced in the ulcerative form, which in addition displays prominent inflammation, in contrast to nonulcer IC, where it is sparse. Thus, the basic pathologic processes may differ (Peeker et al, 2000b). Because activated mast cells lose their histologically identifiable granules once degranulation occurs, estimates of mast cell density using standard histologic techniques may underestimate mast cell numbers (Sant and Theoharides, 1994).

Electron microscopy has confirmed that mast cells in IC are more likely to be degranulated or activated than those found in other conditions (Larsen et al, 1982; Theoharides and Sant, 1991; Theoharides et al, 1995). In at least a subpopulation of IC patients, this may be explained by increased stimulation of mast cells by stem cell factor (Pang et al, 1998). A chronic exposure of detrusor muscle to histamine in IC patients is suggested by the finding that there is an impairment of the direct contractile response to histamine in detrusor muscle affected by IC in comparison to control detrusor, suggesting a receptor desensitization (Palea et al, 1993). The clinical relationship between an increased number of mast cells and symptoms of IC has not been definitively established. Some studies have found no correlation (Lynes et al, 1987; Holm-Bentzen et al, 1987b; Dondore et al, 1996). Although mast cell infiltration in intestinal segments used for augmentation has been associated with pain and failure of the procedure (Kisman et al, 1991), others have shown that mast cell infiltration in intestine used in the urinary tract is the norm and not pathologic (MacDermott et al, 1990).

Many of the substances that have been shown to induce mast cell secretion are released from neurons that innervate the organ containing the mast cells (Christmas et al, 1990). The capsaicin-sensitive sensory neurons that innervate the bladder are thought to have a dual "sensory-efferent" function, in which an axon reflex–induced release of neuropeptides results in local inflammation (Barbanti et al, 1993; Foreman, 1987). Hand (1949) reported an increase in the submucosal nerve density in IC, a phenomenon confirmed by Christmas and colleagues (1990), who showed an increase in nerve fiber proliferation in IC but not in patients with bacterial or lupus cystitis. Increased innervation by nerves releasing substances affecting mast cells could lead to increased mast cell secretion. Among these substances is acetylcholine. Mast cells can be stimulated by cholinergic agonists to secrete serotonin (Theoharides and Sant, 1991). Substance P–containing fibers have been found to be increased in bladders from IC patients and are found adjacent to mast cells (Pang et al, 1995b). In mice, mast cells modulate the inflammatory response of the bladder to substance P and to *E. coli* lipopolysaccharide (Bjorling et al, 1999).

An increase in adrenergic but not cholinergic nerves in IC patients as compared with controls has been reported (Hohenfellner et al, 1992). These researchers also found increased numbers of neurons staining for vasoactive intestinal polypeptide and neuropeptide Y (NPY), both of which are associated with sympathetic nerves. Studies in rats have revealed that psychological stress can activate bladder mast cells via the action of sensory neuropeptides (Spanos et al, 1997; Alexacos et al, 1999). Diurnal cortical variations have been associated with symptom levels in PBS/IC (Lutgendorf et al, 2002), and the mast cell may represent a pathway for stress to be reflected in bladder symptomatology.

Mast cells can alter their environment by regulating tissue gene expression (Saban et al, 2001). The finding of increased synthesis of urinary leukotriene E4 in patients with IC and detrusor mastocytosis when compared with healthy control subjects suggests that cysteinyl-containing leukotrienes are involved in the inflammatory reaction observed in the urinary bladder of patients with IC and may be produced from tissue mast cells in the bladder wall or from macrophages (Bouchelouche et al, 2001a).

Could mast cell products be useful in diagnosing IC? They are not specific for PBS/IC and are increased in bladder carcinoma (Serel et al, 2004). Elevated histamine levels have been found in bladder biopsies of IC patients (Kastrup et al, 1983; Lynes et al, 1987; Enerback et al, 1989) as well as from bladder washings (Lundeberg et al, 1993). Holm-Bentzen and coworkers (1987) reported a significantly elevated urinary excretion of 1,4-methylimidazole acetic acid, the major metabolite of histamine. Others have found no differences between IC and controls in random spot tests of urinary histamine (Yun et al, 1992). Levels were elevated after hydrodistention in IC patients but not in control subjects, a possible consequence of hydrodistention and resultant mast cell degranulation. El Mansoury and associates (1994) found increased methylhistamine, a histamine metabolite, in spot and 24-hour urine samples from IC patients as compared with control subjects. While such an increase could still be interpreted as indicating a systemic rather than a bladder syndrome, subsequent findings of elevated mast cell tryptase in the urine of IC patients could only come from the bladder (Boucher et al, 1995). Erickson and colleagues (2004) reported that urine methylhistamine is not useful as an objective marker of response to bladder distention or as a predictor of response to distention or as a substitute for bladder biopsy to determine mast cell counts.

The realization that mast cells are associated with the syndrome of IC by no means diminishes the other multiple theories of causation. Their very presence could be related to injury from any of the proposed theories of etiology, and degranulation could likewise reflect a final common pathway resulting in pain and frequency from multiple causes. Rickard and Lagunoff (1995) proposed, based on results with mast cell granules and epithelial cells in tissue culture, that mast cells could contribute to failure of epithelialization of the bladder surface following injury by two potential mechanisms: (1)

inhibition of epithelial cell replication and (2) interference with epithelial cell spreading, thus resulting in the "leaky epithelium" found in some patients. Mast cells may actually be the mediator through which female hormones play a role, accounting for the 10:1 female to male preponderance of the disease (Vliagoftis et al, 1992; Pang et al, 1995a; Patra et al, 1995; Bjorling and Wang, 2001). Estradiol augments the secretion of mast cell histamine in response to substance P. It has been proposed that the symptoms of IC may depend on an imbalance of the relative number of estrogen receptors to progesterone receptors on bladder mast cells (Letourneau et al, 1996).

KEY POINT: ETIOLOGY (MAST CELL INVOLVEMENT)

- Mast cells are strategically localized in the urinary bladder close to blood vessels, lymphatics, nerves and detrusor smooth muscle (Saban et al, 1997). Studies strongly suggest that IC is a syndrome with neural, immune, and endocrine components in which activated mast cells play a central, although not primary, pathogenetic role in many patients (Elbadawi and Light 1996; Filippou et al, 1999).

Bladder Glycosaminoglycan Layer and Epithelial Permeability

Until the early 1970s, most investigators thought that the major barrier to free flow of urinary constituents was at the level of the epithelial cells. Tight junctions between urothelial cells, specialized "umbrella cells" lining the surface, and direct bactericidal activity of the vesical mucosa were thought capable of defense of the internal milieu from bacteria, molecules, and ions in the urine (Ratliff et al, 1994). Staehelin and colleagues (1972) proposed that lipid and other hydrophobically bonded materials were important in any barrier to permeability in the luminal membrane because permeants leaked through the interplaque regions if the particles alone limited transport. It has been shown that inflammation of the underlying muscle and lamina propria can disrupt the bladder permeability barrier by damaging tight junctions and apical membranes and causing sloughing of epithelial cells. Leakage of urinary constituents through the damaged epithelium may then exacerbate the inflammation in the deeper layers (Lavelle et al, 1998, 2000).

It was Parsons who hypothesized and popularized the concept that IC in a subset of patients is the result of some defect in the epithelial permeability barrier of the bladder surface glycosaminoglycans (Parsons and Hurst, 1990). The major classes of glycosaminoglycans (GAGs) include hyaluronic acid, heparin sulfate, heparin, chondroitin 4-sulfate and chondroitin 6-sulfate, dermatan sulfate, and keratan sulfate. These carbohydrate chains, coupled to protein cores, produce a diverse class of macromolecules, the proteoglycans (Trelstad, 1985). GAGs exist as a continuous layer on the bladder urothelium (Dixon et al, 1986; Cornish et al, 1990). Except heparin, all the other types of GAGs have been found on the bladder surface (Ruoslahti, 1988). The GAG layer functions as a permeability and antiadherence barrier. When impaired, its functions can be duplicated by exogenous GAG (Hanno et al, 1978). In the absence of this protective layer in the urinary bladder, its susceptibility to infection would increase and the production of nitric oxide in the urothelial cells, and of substance P in the intraepithelial afferent C-fiber terminals, increases. Consequently, the permeability of both the urothelium and the blood vessels in the mucous membrane increases and the blood flow slows due to vasodilatation (Hohlbrugger, 1999).

Parsons and Hurst reported a lower excretion of urinary uronic acid and glycosaminoglycans in IC patients than in normal volunteers and hypothesized that a leaky transitional epithelium might be absorbing these substances to its surface (Parsons and Hurst, 1990). The data are interesting in that one might expect urinary GAG to increase with injury to the bladder and decrease with resolution (Uehling et al, 1988). The San Diego group (Lilly and Parsons, 1990; Parsons et al, 1990) went on to show experimentally that one can damage the GAG layer with protamine sulfate with resultant back-diffusion of urea through the bladder lumen and that this urea loss can be prevented with a bladder instillation of exogenous GAG (heparin). By placing a solution of concentrated urea into the bladder of IC patients and measuring absorption versus controls, Parsons and colleagues (1991) found support for their theory in patients with IC. The rationale of the epithelial permeability school is nicely summarized in four publications (Parsons, 1993, 1994; Hurst et al, 1997; Hohlbrugger and Riedl, 2000) and provides a comprehensive, if somewhat imperfect, theory of the disorder.

Support for an epithelial abnormality from a different perspective has come from Bushman and associates (1994), who found aneuploid DNA profiles on barbotage specimens from IC patients that may signal an underlying abnormality of the epithelial cell population in some patients with IC. Wilson and colleagues (1995) identified a loss of type IV collagen in the urothelial basement membrane in 5 of 11 IC patients. Hurst's group studied bladder biopsies of IC patients and controls and concluded that there is a deficit of bladder luminal and basal proteoglycans associated with the disorder. The basal abnormality may reflect an altered urothelial differentiation program (Hurst et al, 1996). In a later study, IC bladder biopsies showed abnormalities in 24 of 27 patients when examined by immunohistochemical assessment of E-cadherin, ZO-1, uroplakin, and chondroitin sulfate (Slobodov et al, 2004). Erickson and coworkers (1996) measured a glycoprotein (epitectin) in the urine of IC patients and found a decrease compared with a control population, although a significant overlap was detected. Buffington and Woodworth (1997) gave 6 IC patients and 6 controls oral fluorescein dye. The IC patients had higher levels of fluorescein in their plasma and lower urinary excretion of the dye, suggesting altered membrane permeability and increased fluorescein reabsorption in the bladder wall of IC patients. Erickson and colleagues (1998) compared urinary levels of hyaluronic acid in IC patients and control subjects, reporting higher urinary hyaluronic acid in the patient group, possibly accounted for by leakage of this GAG across the epithelium.

Further data for an abnormal surface mucin came from Moskowitz and colleagues (1994), who studied biopsies from 23 IC patients with regard to the presence of a glycoprotein component of the surface mucin referred to as GP1 and compared the results to 11 normal controls. Qualitative GP1 changes in a majority of IC patients were identified. GP1 reactivity was noted in all control subjects but was absent in 35% of IC patients and diminished in 61%. This study may provide evidence of an abnormal bladder urothelium, but the effects of bladder distention in the IC group are unknown and may have contributed to the results. No pathologic controls were used, and no attempt was made to correlate GP1 reactivity with IC symptoms (Messing, 1994). Castration in female rabbits is associated with bladder mucosal changes resulting in increased mucosal permeability (Parekh et al, 2004). Birder and colleagues (2005) have shown that feline IC results in increased baseline production of nitric oxide due to inducible nitric oxide synthase. These changes in transmitter release may have a role in altering mucosal barrier properties.

Purportedly strong evidence for a population with mucosal leak has been reported (Parsons et al, 1994b). Parsons placed water or 0.4 M potassium chloride (KCl) intravesically into normal volunteers and IC patients. Water did not provoke pain in either group, but KCl provoked the symptom in 4.5% of normal individuals and 70% of IC patients. Symptomatic responses were reduced in patients on heparinoid therapy. Similar findings occur in patients with radiation cystitis (100%) (Parsons et al, 1994c), urinary infection (100%) (Parsons et al, 1998), detrusor instability (25%) (Parsons et al, 1998), "urethral syndrome" (55%) (Parsons et al, 2001), and greater than 80% of women with endometriosis, vulvodynia, and pelvic pain (Parsons et al, 2001, 2002b). Eighty-four percent of men with prostatitis also have a positive test (Parsons and Albo, 2002). The poor specificity of the KCl test does not suggest that it is providing unequivocal evidence of a permeability dysfunction. Because it is known that the normal bladder epithelium can never be absolutely tight, and there is always some leak, however small (Hohlbrugger, 1997), it is conceivable that the findings of pain with KCl are related to a hypersensitivity of the sensory nerves in this condition, rather than to pathologic epithelial permeability, at least in some patients. In fact, KCl administered intravesically to cats with feline IC seems to *inhibit* afferent firing of peripheral A fibers. Heightened sensitivity of afferent nerve fibers can explain KCl results without necessarily evoking increased permeability (Lutgendorf and Kreder, 2005; Roppolo et al, 2005). Intravesical administration of KCl has since been proposed as a diagnostic test for IC (Parsons et al, 1998) (see later).

How central abnormal epithelial permeability is to IC is, however, by no means clear. Tamm-Horsfall protein (THP), a high-molecular-weight glycoprotein synthesized exclusively by the ascending loop of Henle and the distal tubule of the kidney, has been studied as a potential marker of urothelial permeability. Fowler provided graphic data that the urothelium might be leaky in IC. With immunohistochemical techniques his group assayed the bladder biopsies of 14 IC patients and 10 normal controls for intraurothelial THP to assess indirectly the in-vivo permeability of the urothelium. Eight pathologic control subjects were also assessed. Ten of 14 IC patients versus 1 of 18 control subjects demonstrated intraurothelial THP (Fowler et al, 1988). Serum THP autoantibody is higher in PBS/IC patients versus controls (Neal et al, 1991). It is known that excretion rates of THP vary widely, even in repeat samples taken from the same individual (Reinhart et al, 1990). Subsequent studies in IC have failed to show differences in the presence of intraurothelial THP in the IC population versus controls and in antibody reactivity to THP (Stone et al, 1992; Stein et al, 1993). Bade and coworkers (1996) failed to find THP in the bladder tissue from 10 IC patients. Others have suggested that when THP is seen in bladder tissue, it is an incidental finding of no clinical significance. The finding of intraurothelial THP has not been shown to be a harbinger of IC or any other bladder disorder (Truong et al, 1994).

Finally, we must look at a body of literature that has failed to find GAG abnormality or hyperpermeability. Ultrastructural, biochemical, and functional studies of bladder GAG have not supported this theory (Collan et al, 1976; Dixon et al, 1986; Johansson and Fall, 1990; Ruggieri et al, 1991). Nickel's group (Nickel et al, 1993) reported sophisticated electron micrography using a specific anti-mucus, antisera stabilization technique to study the ultrastructural morphologic appearance of the GAG. No significant difference in the morphologic appearance of the mucus or GAG layer was noted in IC versus control subjects. Urinary chondroitin sulfates, heparan sulfate, and total sulfated glycosaminoglycans normalized to creatinine are not altered in IC (Erickson et al, 1997). Although an increased ratio of total GAGs to sulfated GAGs in IC may indicate an altered GAG layer, whether it reflects a cause or is a result of the primary pathologic process(es) is unknown (Wei et al, 2000). That leaves one to postulate an as yet unknown functional abnormality, rather than GAG deficiency, to account for any increase in permeability.

Chelsky and coworkers (1994) measured bladder permeability in IC using direct measurement by transvesical absorption of ^{99m}Tc-diethylenetriaminepentaacetic acid (DTPA). Whereas some IC patients had a more permeable bladder than others, the same was true for normal volunteers. Increased permeability in the IC group could not be demonstrated. However, three IC patients had marked absorption of DTPA and may represent a subpopulation of patients with increased epithelial permeability. Intravesical instillation of 10% and 20% ethanol in rabbits was reported to be a reliable quantitative measure of bladder hyperpermeability by the San Diego group (Monga et al, 2001) and subsequently failed to demonstrate bladder permeability in humans with IC (Gordon et al, 2003).

Neurobiology

Neuropeptides present in primary afferents and the dorsal horn of the spinal cord have an important role in the mediation of nociceptive input under normal conditions. Under pathologic conditions, such as chronic inflammation or after peripheral nerve injury, the production of peptides and peptide receptors is dramatically altered, leading to a number of functional consequences (Wiesenfeld-Hallin and Xu, 2001). **Inflammatory painful stimuli, especially if repeated, can chronically alter innervation, central pain-processing mechanisms, and tissue responses** (Steers and Tuttle, 1997). It has been known for some time that the sensory nervous system can generate some of the manifestations of inflammation (Foreman, 1987; Dimitriadou et al, 1991, 1992). Activation of

KEY POINT: ETIOLOGY (BLADDER GLYCOSAMINOGLYCAN LAYER AND EPITHELIAL PERMEABILITY)

■ Overall, it does seem that there is a population of IC patients with increased epithelial permeability. Increased mucosal permeability is nonspecific and a consequence of bladder inflammation and also occurs with cyclophosphamide-induced bladder injury, bacterial infection, and cystitis after intravesical challenge with antigen after sensitization (Engelmann et al, 1982; Kim et al, 1992). It may also be a consequence of aging itself (Jacob et al, 1978). Whether this represents a primary cause of IC or merely reflects the result of an as-yet-unidentified source of inflammation is unclear. Treatments that tend to damage GAG, including transurethral resection and laser of ulcerated areas, bladder distention, silver nitrate administration, and oxychlorosene (Clorpactin) administration and use of the organic solvent dimethyl sulfoxide (DMSO) have all been used with varying results to treat IC. Increased permeability and epithelial dysfunction must be only a part of the story.

capsaicin-sensitive afferent neurons locally and centrally may be involved in stress-related pathologic changes in the rat bladder (Ercan et al, 2001). Activation of sensory nerves, specifically pain fibers, is known to trigger neurogenic inflammation through release of neuropeptides such as substance P, neurokinin A, and calcitonin gene–related protein, and subsequent increase in vascular permeability, with leukocyte adhesion and tissue edema. The neuropeptide mediators have been shown to also cause degranulation of mast cells with release of additional potent mediators of inflammation and to lead to injury and increased permeability of epithelial surfaces (Elbadawi and Light, 1996). An increase in nerve fibers within the suburothelium and detrusor muscle in ulcerative IC has been noted (Lundeberg et al, 1993). A correlation was found between the number of nerve fibers and numbers of mast cells as well as between the number of nerve fibers and the amount of histamine. Consolidating the leaky urothelium theory and mast cell activation, neurogenic inflammation is an attractive proposal for etiology and can readily accommodate infectious, immunologic, and autoimmunologic mechanisms as factors (Elbadawi and Light, 1996).

Harrison and associates (1990) proposed that small-diameter sensory nerves in the bladder wall may have a role in the transmission of the sensation of pain and in the triggering of inflammatory reactions rather than forming the afferent limb of the micturition reflex. Abelli and colleagues (1991) demonstrated in the rat urethra that mechanical irritation alone can cause neuropeptide release from peripheral capsaicin-sensitive primary afferent neurons resulting in neurogenic inflammation. Extracellular adenosine triphosphate (ATP) can act through the purinergic receptor subtype $P2X_3$ to transmit a pain signal to the central nervous system. These subunits expressed by cultured IC bladder urothelial cells are upregulated during in-vitro stretch and may phenotypically mimic sensory neurons (Sun and Chai, 2004).

Several pieces of additional information support a theory of neurogenic inflammation. Levels of nerve growth factor are elevated in bladder biopsy specimens of IC patients (Lowe et al, 1997). Studies in rats using pseudorabies virus clearly show that bladder inflammation can be induced from a somatic structure through a neural mechanism and that central nervous system dysfunction can bring about a peripheral inflammation (Doggweiler et al, 1998; Jasmin et al, 1998). Pelvic nerve stimulation in the rat increases urothelial permeability that is antagonized by capsaicin, indicating both an efferent effect of afferent nerves and afferent mediated neuroepithelial interaction (Lavelle et al, 1999).

Numerous studies indicate increased sympathetic activity in IC. Hohenfellner and colleagues (1992) suggested that IC is associated with increased sympathetic outflow into the bladder and altered metabolism of vasoactive intestinal polypeptide and neuropeptide Y. Neuropeptide Y inhibits bladder afferents and therefore may be involved in autonomic disturbances affecting the bladder. Elevation of urinary catecholamines in IC patients and of plasma catecholamines in cats with feline IC has been observed (Buffington and Pacak, 2001a; Stein et al, 1999), as has an increased density and number of nerve fibers immunoreactive for tyrosine hydroxylase in IC patients (Peeker et al, 2000a). Whether these changes reflect a cause of IC or are merely the result of long-standing intense pain and a severely pathologic voiding pattern is unknown.

Galloway and colleagues (1991) proposed that the changes in IC may be explained by an increase in sympathetic discharge, analogous to that seen in reflex sympathetic dystrophy (RSD) of limbs. The pathology in RSD is the development of abnormal synaptic activity between sensory afferent and sympathetic efferent neurons. Nerve cells in the spinal cord become hypersensitive to sensory input, and this sustains abnormal sympathetic outflow and corresponding vasomotor dysregulation. The excess sympathetic outflow leads to constriction of blood vessels and tissue ischemia, setting up further sensory changes and perpetuating the cycle. In RSD, there is usually a trigger event leading to these changes. With the acute phase of RSD, regional signs of inflammation are evident in the affected extremity. One school of thought believes an inflammatory response to an injury initiates RSD. Increased capillary permeability is a direct result (Goris and Jan, 1998). Perhaps a urinary infection could trigger such a pathologic cycle in some IC patients?

Herbst and colleagues (1937) produced bladder lesions in a dog resembling the ulceration of IC by ligating the blood vessels to the posterior bladder wall and infecting the area with *Streptococcus viridans*. Studies using laser Doppler flowmetry have shown that when the bladder is distended under anesthesia, blood flow increases in control patients to a statistically significant degree as compared with IC patients (Irwin and Galloway, 1993; Pontari et al, 1999). Another study has purported to show that topical heparin therapy can normalize urothelial permeability and vesical blood flow in IC (Hohlbrugger et al, 1998). Decreased microvascular density has been described in the suburothelium but not in the deeper mucosa in bladder biopsies of women with IC (Rosamilia et al, 1999a). Hyperbaric oxygen has been suggested to be effec-

tive in the treatment of PBS/IC (van Ophoven et al, 2004b) as well as radiation-induced cystitis (Weiss and Neville, 1989).

If lumbar sympathetic blocks can decrease the pain of IC, a role of the sympathetic nervous system in IC pathogenesis is a reasonable supposition (Irwin et al, 1993; Doi et al, 2001). An increase in sympathetic activity has been demonstrated in cats with feline IC (Buffington and Pacak, 2001b; Buffington et al, 2002). Similar findings have been reported in a small study of IC patients (Dimitrakov et al, 2001) and sympathetic activity may be an underlying common denominator in many disorders associated with PBS/IC (Buffington, 2004).

Nevertheless, no studies performed to date can say any case of IC is related to the syndrome of RSD (Ratliff et al, 1994). No single test can be used to exclude sympathetically maintained pain, and there are no clear symptoms that predict sympathetically mediated pain (Baron, 2000). In the animal model, bladder ischemia is associated with detrusor overactivity or impaired detrusor contraction, not sensory urgency (Azadzoi et al, 1999). Those patients with RSD who have voiding symptoms rarely have a picture that would be confused with IC (Chancellor et al, 1996).

Before leaving the neurogenic theory of etiology, **it is important to note that the nervous system itself almost surely contributes to the chronic nature of this pain syndrome, regardless of initiating etiology** (Vrinten et al, 2001). Repetitious stimulation of a peripheral nerve, at sufficient intensity to activate C fibers, results in a progressive buildup of the magnitude of the electrical response recorded in the second-order dorsal horn neurons. This "wind-up" phenomenon is central to the concept of chronic pain. Biochemically it is dependent on activation of N-methyl-D-aspartate (NMDA) receptors in the spinal cord (Bennett, 1999). With persistent NMDA receptor activation, spinal cord cells undergo trophic changes, and the pain resulting from subsequent stimulation becomes exaggerated and prolonged. This "pain memory" in the spinal cord may be what causes IC patients to become refractory to different therapies (Brookoff, 1997). NMDA-receptor-driven formation of new connections in the spinal cord may account for the expansion of the pain field.

Upregulation of the CNS and augmented sensory processing has been referred to as non-nociceptive pain (Bennett, 1999). The four characteristic features of non-nociceptive pain would seem to apply very well to the clinical syndrome of IC (Table 10–3). Chronic neuropathic pain may continue

---

Table 10–3. Non-nociceptive Pain: Characteristic Clinical Features

1. The description of the pain seems inappropriate in comparison with the degree of tissue pathology, or no tissue pathology may be discernible.
2. Noxious stimuli result in a pain experience that is greater and more unpleasant than would normally be expected (hyperalgesia).
3. Normally non-noxious stimuli may result in pain (allodynia).
4. The extent of the pain boundary is greater than would be expected on the basis of the site of the original tissue pathology.

From Bennett RM: Emerging concepts in the neurobiology of chronic pain: Evidence of abnormal sensory processing in fibromyalgia. Mayo Clin Proc 1999;74:385-398.

after the resolution of tissue damage and persist on the basis of a maladaptive mechanism (Urban et al, 2002).

Burnstock's observation (1999) that ATP has a role in mechanosensory transduction by the epithelial lining of hollow viscus organs such as bladder has been followed up by Sun and colleagues (2001). Stretched epithelial cells lining hollow organs release ATP, which acts on purinergic nociceptive receptors on subepithelial sensory nerve terminals. ATP was significantly elevated in the urine of PBS/IC patients, and the stretch- activated release of ATP was augmented in IC urothelium.

KEY POINT: ETIOLOGY (NEUROBIOLOGY)

- Neurogenic inflammation may be the cause of some cases of IC or may be the result of other initiating etiologic events. It is not incompatible with the central role of the mast cell, or with the leaky epithelium theory. It conceivably could result in the appearance of autoimmune phenomena or result from an episode of infection. The central nervous system may also be implicated in dysregulation of the pelvic floor, resulting in chronic pelvic pain and contributing to IC (Zermann et al, 1999), and perhaps in the rare cases of IC that chronologically seem to relate to trauma or pelvic surgery (Zermann et al, 1998). It is an etiologic theory that provides fertile ground for new treatment possibilities.

Urine Abnormalities

Current theories of pathogenesis generally involve access of a component of urine to the interstices of the bladder wall, resulting in an inflammatory response induced by toxic, allergic, or immunologic means. The substance in the urine may be a naturally occurring one—a substance that acts as an initiator only in particularly susceptible individuals—or may act like a true toxin, gaining access to the urine by a variety of mechanisms or metabolic pathways (Wein and Broderick, 1994). Clemmensen and coworkers (1988) noted that 8 of 11 IC patients had positive skin reactions to patch tests with their own urine. Immediate reactions were not observed, and the histology suggested a toxic rather than an allergic reaction. Lynes and associates (1990) were unable to find a urinary myotropic substance unique to IC patients. The San Diego group found IC urine to result in higher cell death of cultured transitional cells than normal urine, suggesting a toxic compound in the urine of some IC patients (Parsons and Stein, 1990). They identified heat-labile, cationic components of low molecular weight that bind to heparin and that when separated from the bulk of urinary wastes are cytotoxic to urothelial cells as well as underlying smooth muscle cells (Parsons et al, 2000). They reported a 12% increase in 72-kD stress protein in cells treated with urine from IC patients compared with controls (Ito et al, 1998).

Others have not been able to demonstrate in-vitro cytotoxicity (Beier-Holgersen et al, 1994) or immunohistochemical

changes in the nociceptive centers in the spinal cord or bladder wall when IC urine was compared with control urine (Baykara et al, 2003). Efforts to induce an IC-like picture in the rabbit bladder from exposure to urine of IC patients have failed to demonstrate conclusive changes (Perzin et al, 1991; Ruggieri et al, 1993; Kohn et al, 1998). Increased levels of soluble mediators associated with activation of sensory neurons and/or mast cells have been found in the urine of both IC and bladder cancer patients (Okragly et al, 1999).

Circumstantial evidence for the toxicity of IC urine is suggested by the failure of substitution cystoplasty and continent diversions in some of these patients because of the development of pain or contraction of the bowel segment over time (Nielsen et al, 1990; Baskin and Tanagho, 1992; Trinka et al, 1993; Lotenfoe et al, 1995) and the histologic findings similar to IC found to occur in bowel used to augment the small-capacity IC bladder (McGuire et al, 1973; Singh and Thomas, 1996). Intestinal mucosa in contact with urine undergoes progressive changes as long as 3 years after surgery and the significance of the histologic IC-like changes has been questioned (MacDermott et al, 1990; Davidsson et al, 1996).

Antiproliferative Factor (APF)

The finding that cells from the bladder lining of normal controls grow significantly more rapidly in culture than cells from IC patients led Keay and associates (1996) at the University of Maryland to the discovery of an antiproliferative factor (APF) produced by the urothelium of IC patients. Normal bladder cells were cultured in the presence of urine from patients with IC, asymptomatic controls, bacterial cystitis, and vulvovaginitis. Only urine from IC patients inhibited bladder cell proliferation (Keay et al, 1998b). The presence of APF was found to be a sensitive and specific biomarker for IC (Keay et al, 2001) (Table 10-4). It was found in bladder urine but not in renal pelvic urine of IC patients, indicating production by the bladder urothelial cells (Keay et al, 1999).

Table 10-4. Prevalence of Urine Antiproliferative Factor Activity in Interstitial Cystitis Patients and Control Groups

Groups	No. of Patients (Positive/Total)	% Positive
Patients		
Interstitial cystitis	206/219	94
Controls		
Asymptomatic	10/113	9
Overactive bladder	2/32	6
Bacterial cystitis	7/58	12
Microscopic hematuria	2/19	10
Stress incontinence	1/10	10
Neurogenic bladder	0/11	0
Benign prostatic hypertrophy	1/14	7
Nonbacterial prostatitis	1/16	6
Vulvovaginitis	0/12	0
Miscellaneous	1/16	6

From Keay SK, Zhang CO, Shoenfelt J, et al: Sensitivity and specificity of antiproliferative factor, heparin-binding epidermal growth factor-like growth factor, and epidermal growth factor as urine markers for interstitial cystitis. Urology 2001;57:9.

Subsequent studies indicated that APF is associated with decreased production of heparin-binding epidermal growth factor–like growth factor (HB-EGF) (Keay et al, 2000, 2003b). APF activity was related to increased production of epidermal growth factor (EGF), insulin-like growth factor-1, and insulin-like growth factor–binding protein-3 by the bladder cells from IC patients but not by the cells from healthy bladders. Studies of IC patients and asymptomatic controls showed urine levels of APF, HB-EGF, and EGF to reliably separate out IC from controls (Keay et al, 2001; Erickson et al, 2002).

APF levels in the urine were found to discriminate between men with IC versus those with chronic pelvic pain syndrome (CPPS) or nonbacterial prostatitis (Keay et al, 2004a). APF activity dropped significantly in IC patients within 2 hours after hydrodistention (Chai et al, 2000b) and after 5 days of sacral neuromodulation (Chai et al, 2000a). Cell culture studies showed that APF actually caused decrease in HB-EGF and increase in EGF, mirroring the differences in urine levels of these growth factors between IC patients and controls and suggesting that APF is the primary abnormality (Keay et al, 2003b).

Whereas APF may prove to be a useful marker for PBS/IC, it may also unlock the etiology of the syndrome. It has been hypothesized by Keay and colleagues (2003a) that PBS/IC may result from an inhibition of bladder epithelial cell proliferation caused by the APF, which is mediated by its regulation of growth factor production from bladder cells. Conceivably, any of a variety of injuries to the bladder (infection, trauma, and overdistention) in a susceptible individual may result in PBS/IC if APF is present and suppresses production of HB-EGF (Keay and Warren, 1998). Theoretically, if production of APF could be "turned off" by genetic techniques, or its effects were nullified by exogenous HB-EGF growth factor, the clinical syndrome might be prevented.

APF has been purified (Fig. 10–6) and proved to be a frizzled 8 protein that belongs to a newly discovered family of proteins that seem to be important in the development of nerve tissues, skin, and the lining of organs (Keay et al, 2004b).

Studies are ongoing to confirm the research by Dr. Keay and colleagues and expand on its significance in diagnosis and development of a rational treatment approach (Rashid et al, 2004).

KEY POINT: ETIOLOGY (ANTIPROLIFERATIVE FACTOR)

■ Antiproliferative factor is a frizzled 8 protein produced by bladder uroepithelial cells of PBS/IC patients. It inhibits bladder cell proliferation and appears to be a sensitive and specific biomarker for IC. Initial studies suggest it can differentiate chronic pelvic pain syndrome in men/chronic nonbacterial prostatitis from PBS/IC. It causes a decrease in heparin binding epidermal growth factor-like growth factor and an increase in epidermal growth factor. It may ultimately unlock the etiology of the syndrome and could provide avenues for development of future therapies.

Other Potential Causes

Various other etiologic theories have been proposed (Ratliff et al, 1994), but none has received much scientific support. Voiding almost hourly, always having to be aware of how far the nearest restroom facilities are, and suffering constant pain would be expected to lead to psychological stress. However, could there be individual differences in the propensity to develop IC that result from a dysregulation of anxiety and mood (Nesse, 1999; Bodden-Heidrich, 2004)? **There are no data currently to suggest that stress *initiates* the chronic syndrome of IC, although it certainly can increase symptom severity** (Lutgendorf et al, 2000). Cats restricted to indoor living are five times more likely to have urinary problems as cats allowed outdoors (Buffington, 2002). Female patients with PBS/IC have been shown to have increased heart rate at

MEWGYLLEVT SLLAALALLQ RSSGAAAASA KELACQEITV PLCKGIGYNY TYMPNQFHD
TQDEAGLEVH QFWPLVEIQC SPDLKFFLCS MYTPICLEDY KKPLPPCRSV CERAKAGCAP
LMRQYGFAWP DRMRCDRLPE QGNPDTLCMD YNRTDLTTAA PSPPRRLPPP PPGEQPPSGS
GHGRPPGARP PHRGGGRGGG GGDAAAPPAR GGGGGGGKARP PGGGAAPCEP
GCQCRAPMVS VSSERHPLYN RVKTGQIANC ALPCHNPFFS QDERAFTVFW IGLWSVLCFV
STFATVSTFL IDMERFKYPE RPIIFLSACY LFVSVGYLVR LVAGHEKVAC SGGAPGAGGA
GGAGGAAAGA GAAGAGGP GGRGEYEELG AVEQHVRYET TGPALCTVVF LLLVYFFGMAS
SIWWVILSLT WFLAAGMKWG NEAIAGYSQY FHLAAWLVPS VKSIAVLALS SVDGDPVAGI
CYVGNQSLDN LRGFVLAPLV IYLFIGTMFL LAGFVSLFRI RSVIKQQDGP TKTHKLEKLM
IRLGLFTVLY TVPAAVVVAC LFYEQHNRPR WEATHNCPCL RDLQPDQARR PDYAVFMLKY
FMCLVVGITS GVWVWSGKTL ESWRSLCTRC CWASKGAAVG GGAGATAAGG
GGGPGGGGGG GPGGGGGPGG GGGSLYSDVS TGLTWRSGTA SSVSYPKQMP LSQV

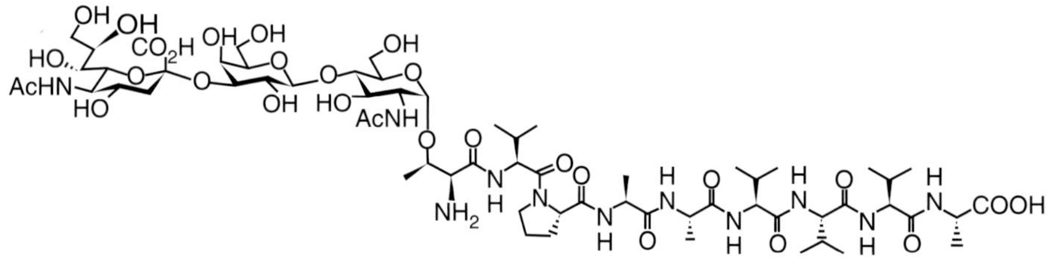

Figure 10–6. Composition and structure of antiproliferative factor (APF). (From Keay SK, Szekely Z, Conrads TP, et al: An antiproliferative factor from interstitial cystitis patients is a frizzled 8 protein-related sialoglycopeptide. Proc Natl Acad Sci U S A 2004;101:11803-11808.)

baseline and throughout a laboratory mental stress challenge but did not demonstrate greater autonomic reactivity to stress (Lutgendorf et al, 2004). Until stress can be shown to produce PBS/IC de novo in humans, it is just as reasonable to speculate that the stress is a result of the syndrome as a primary cause for it.

Speculation that abnormalities in or obstruction of lymphatics or vascular structures is causative has never been borne out. The fact that some of these patients have had hysterectomy probably relates more to the attempt of the physician to treat chronic pelvic pain than postsurgical change causing the IC syndrome (Chung, 2004).

The knowledge that there is at least a 5:1 female to male preponderance immediately makes the role of the hormonal milieu potentially important (Bjorling and Wang, 2001). Paradoxically, it is known that estrogens can control hematuria in hemorrhagic cystitis, perhaps by decreasing the fragility of the mucosal microvasculature of the bladder (Liu et al, 1990). Estradiol augments while the estrogen receptor blocker tamoxifen inhibits mast cell secretion (Vliagoftis et al, 1992). Bladder mast cells express high-affinity estrogen receptors, and there is a higher number of such cells present in patients with IC compared with controls. Although this may help explain why IC is so common in women, the hormonal role can only account for the propensity of IC to occur in females, not the ultimate etiology.

Pelvic floor dysfunction has been associated with PBS/IC for many years (Schmidt and Vapnek, 1991), **and uncontrolled trials suggest that treatment of the pelvic floor can be effective in ameliorating symptoms** (Lilius et al, 1973; Doggweiler-Wiygul et al, 2001; Holzberg et al, 2001; Weiss, 2001; Doggweiler-Wiygul and Wiygul, 2002; Oyama et al, 2004). Speculation that abnormalities of the pelvic floor muscular function may contribute to the etiology of some cases of the chronic pelvic pain syndrome in men are well accepted (Segura et al, 1979; Schmidt and Vapnek, 1991; Zermann et al, 1999), and a similar case might be made for patients with PBS/IC, although scientific support for a direct etiologic relationship is lacking.

PATHOLOGY

One can have pathology consistent with the diagnosis of IC, but there is no microscopic picture pathognomonic of this syndrome (Figs. 10–7 and 10–8). **The role of histopathology in the diagnosis of IC is primarily one of excluding other possible diagnoses.** One must rule out carcinoma and carcinoma in-situ, eosinophilic cystitis, tuberculous cystitis, as well as any other entities with a specific tissue diagnosis (Hellstrom et al, 1979; Johansson and Fall, 1990).

Although earlier reports described a chronic, edematous pancystitis with mast cell infiltration, submucosal ulcerations and involvement of the bladder wall, and chronic lymphocytic infiltrate (Smith and Dehner, 1972; Jacobo et al, 1974), these were cases culled from patients with severe disease and not representative of the majority of cases currently diagnosed. The pathologic findings in IC are not consistent. There has been a great variation in the reported histologic appearance of biopsy specimens from IC patients, and even variation among specimens taken from the same patients over time (Gillenwater and Wein, 1988).

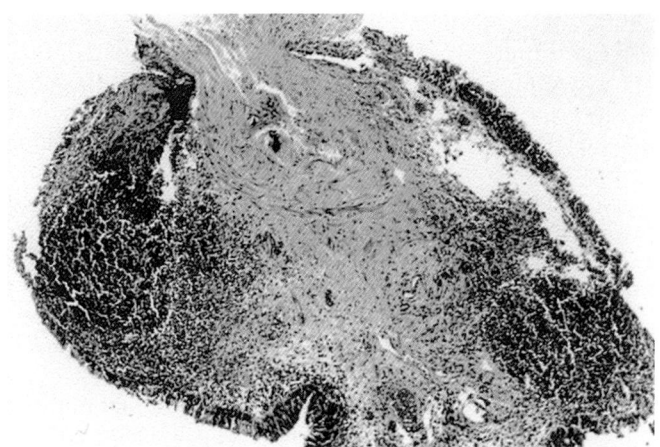

Figure 10–7. Nonulcerative form of interstitial cystitis with dense lymphoid infiltrate in the lamina propria. (H&E, original magnification, ×20.) (Courtesy of John Tomaszewski, Hospital of the University of Pennsylvania, Department of Pathology.)

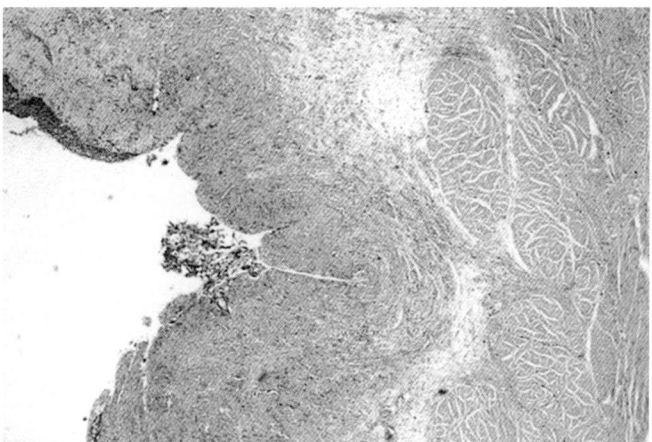

Figure 10–8. Knifelike Hunner's ulcer in interstitial cystitis. (H&E, original magnification, ×40.) (Courtesy of John Tomaszewski, Hospital of the University of Pennsylvania, Department of Pathology.)

Lepinard and colleagues (1984) reported a pancystitis affecting the three layers of the bladder wall. In nonulcerative disease the vesical wall was never normal, with epithelium being thinned and muscle being affected. Johansson and Fall (1990) looked at 64 patients with ulcerative disease and 44 with nonulcerative IC. The former group had mucosal ulceration and hemorrhage, granulation tissue, intense inflammatory infiltrate, elevated mast cell counts, and perineural infiltrates. The nonulcer group, despite the same severe symptoms, had a relatively unaltered mucosa with a sparse inflammatory response, the main feature being multiple, small, mucosal ruptures and suburothelial hemorrhages that were noted in a high proportion of patients. Because these specimens were almost all taken immediately after hydrodistention, how much of the admittedly minimal findings in the nonulcer group were purely iatrogenic is a matter of speculation. One can see completely normal biopsies in the nonulcerative IC group (Johansson and Fall, 1994). Transition from nonulcerative to ulcerative IC is a rare event (Fall et al, 1987), and pathologically the two types of IC may be completely separate entities. Whereas mast cells are more commonly seen in the detrusor in ulcerative IC (Holm-Bentzen et al, 1987b), they are also common in patients with idiopathic bladder instability (Moore et al, 1992). Mastocytosis in PBS/IC is best documented by tryptase immunocytochemical staining (Theoharides et al, 2001). Despite attempts to develop a diagnostic algorithm based on the detrusor to mucosa mast cell ratio and nerve fiber proliferation (Hofmeister et al, 1997), mast cell counts per se have no place in the differential diagnosis of this clinical syndrome.

Lynes and coworkers (1990) concluded that biopsy specimens are often not helpful in confirming the diagnosis. Although IC patients in his study had a higher incidence and degree of denuded epithelium, ulceration, and submucosal inflammation, none of these findings was pathognomonic. In addition, these "typical" findings occurred only in IC patients with pyuria or small bladder capacity. Epithelial and basement membrane thickness, submucosal edema, vascular ectasia, fibrosis, and detrusor muscle inflammation and fibrosis were not significantly different in the IC and control patients.

Attempts to definitively diagnose IC by electron microscopy have also been very unsuccessful. Collan's group (1976), in the first such study, wrote that the similarity of the ultrastructure of epithelial cells in controls and IC patients makes it improbable that the disease process originates in the epithelium. Other investigators found no differences in the morphologic appearances of the glycocalyx and of urothelial cells in patients with IC when compared with controls (Dixon et al, 1986). Anderstrom and colleagues (1989) saw no surface characteristics specific for IC but believed that the mucin layer covering the urothelial cells seemed reduced in IC compared with controls, a fact disputed in a very elegant paper (Nickel et al, 1993). Elbadawi and Light (1996) observed ultrastructural changes sufficiently distinctive to be diagnostic in specimens submitted for pathologic confirmation of nonulcerative IC. Marked edema of various tissue elements and cells appeared to be a common denominator of many observed changes. The wide-ranging discussion of the etiology of IC in Elbadawi's papers is fascinating, but the pathologic findings are potentially marred by the methodology, in that specimens were obtained after diagnostic hydrodistention (Elbadawi, 1997).

So what is the place of pathologic examination of tissue in IC? Attempts to classify the painful bladder by the pathoanatomic criteria described by Holm-Bentzen (1989) are of questionable value. There is a group of patients with what she and her colleagues describe as "nonobstructive detrusor myopathy" (Holm-Bentzen et al, 1985). In this series these patients with degenerative changes in the detrusor muscle often had residual urine, a history of urinary retention, and an absence of sensory urgency on cystometry with bladder capacities over 400 mL. Most would not be clinically confused with IC. A similar English series (Christmas et al, 1996), however, included patients who met NIDDK research criteria and associated detrusor myopathy with diminished detrusor compliance and ultimate bladder contracture.

The ICDB study worked backward from symptoms to pathology and concluded that certain symptoms are predictive of specific pathologic findings (Tomaszewski et al, 1999, 2001) (Table 10–5). Denson and coworkers (2000) analyzed forceps biopsies from 65 females and 4 males with PBS/IC. Ten

Table 10–5. Associations among Pathologic Features and Patient Symptoms

Night-Time Frequency
Mast cell count in lamina propria on tryptase stain
Complete loss of urothelium
Granulation tissue in lamina propria
Vascular density in lamina propria

Urinary Urgency
Percentage of submucosal granulation tissue

Urinary Pain
Percentage of mucosa denuded of urothelium
Percentage of submucosal hemorrhage

From Tomaszewski JE, Landi JR: Baseline associations among pathologic features and patient symptoms in the National Interstitial Cystitis Data Base. J Urol 1999;161S:28.

percent of specimens showed vasodilatation or submucosal edema. Inflammation was absent in 30% of patients and mild in another 41%. Cystoscopic changes did not correlate with degree of inflammation. Hanus and colleagues (2001) studied 84 biopsy specimens from 112 PBS/IC patients and reported a linear relationship between the mean bladder capacity under anesthesia and severity of glomerulations. They did not find a correlation between severity of symptoms and histopathologic changes observed by light or electron microscopy.

Rosamilia and colleagues reviewed the pathology literature pertaining to PBS/IC in two recent publications and presented their own data (Rosamilia et al, 2003; Hanno et al, 2005). They compared forceps biopsies from 35 control and 34 PBS/IC patients, 6 with bladder capacities less than 400 mL under anesthesia. Epithelial denudation, submucosal edema, congestion and ectasia, and inflammatory infiltrate were increased in the PBS/IC group. Submucosal hemorrhage did not differentiate the groups, but denuded epithelium was unique to the IC group and more common in those with severe disease. The most remarkable finding in this study was that histologic parameters were normal and indistinguishable from control subjects in 55% of IC subjects. Method of biopsy can be important in interpreting findings, because transurethral resection biopsies tend to show mucosal ruptures, submucosal hemorrhage, and mild inflammation (Johansson and Fall, 1990) while histology is normal approximately half the time with cold-cup forceps biopsies (Mattila, 1982; Lynes et al, 1990; Rosamilia et al, 2003).

KEY POINT: PATHOLOGY

■ Histopathology plays a supportive diagnostic role at most (Johansson et al, 1997). While recent studies suggest that a severely abnormal pathology may be associated with poor prognosis (McDougald, 2003; Nordling et al, 2003), this is not necessarily the case (MacDermott et al, 1991a). IC is a diagnosis of exclusion, and, at this point in time, excluding other diseases that are pathologically identifiable is the primary utility of bladder biopsy in this group of patients.

DIAGNOSIS

PBS/IC can be considered one of the chronic visceral pain syndromes, affecting the urogenital and rectal area, many of which are well described but poorly understood (Wesselmann et al, 1997; Wesselmann, 2001). **These include vulvodynia, orchialgia, penile pain, perineal pain, and rectal pain.** In men, many of the entities have now been folded into the rubric of the chronic pelvic pain syndrome and can be difficult to distinguish from PBS/IC (Hakenberg and Wirth, 2002; Forrest and Schmidt, 2004). The diagnosis of PBS/IC is by its very nature based on the definition. In the past this was by default, the symptom criteria enumerated by the NIDDK (Hanno et al, 1999a, 1999b) (see Table 10–1). It has now morphed largely into a diagnosis of chronic pain, pressure, or discomfort associated with the bladder, usually accompanied by urinary frequency in the absence of any identifiable cause (Hanno, 2005; Hanno et al, 2005). Diagnostic approaches vary widely, and general agreement on a diagnostic algorithm remains a future goal (Chai, 2002; Nordling, 2004; Nordling et al, 2004). The disorder can be very difficult to diagnose until symptoms become well established, unless one has a high level of suspicion (Porru et al, 2004). Frequency and pelvic pain of long duration related to the bladder unrelated to other known causes establishes a working diagnosis. It is often difficult for patients to distinguish between sensations of pain, pressure, discomfort, and urgency. Ask a patient why he or she voids hourly, and it is usually because of discomfort rather than convenience. Heavy reliance on other aspects of the NIDDK research criteria will result in underdiagnosing more than half of patients (Hanno et al, 1999b). IC symptom scales (O'Leary et al, 1997; Goin et al, 1998; Moldwin and Kushner, 2004), like the AUA symptom score for benign prostatic hyperplasia, are designed to evaluate the severity of symptomatology and monitor disease progression or regression with or without treatment. They have not been validated as diagnostic criteria.

One must rule out infection and less common conditions, including but not limited to carcinoma (Utz and Zincke, 1974; Tissot et al, 2004), eosinophilic cystitis (Hellstrom et al, 1979; Sidh et al, 1980; Littleton et al, 1982; Aubert et al, 1983; Abramov et al, 2004), malacoplakia, schistosomiasis, scleroderma (Batra and Hanno, 1997), and detrusor endometriosis (Sircus et al, 1988; Price et al, 1996). In men younger than the age of 50, video-urodynamics are useful to rule out voiding dysfunction resulting from vesical neck obstruction, "pseudo" dyssynergia, or impaired contractility (Kaplan et al, 1996). Musculoskeletal dysfunction may also play a role in causation or increasing symptom severity and should be looked for in the diagnostic phase of evaluation (Prendergast and Weiss, 2003). Reports of successful treatment of IC symptoms by laparoscopic adhesiolysis (Chen et al, 1997) or urethral diverticulum excision (Daneshgari et al, 1999) give credence to the fact that IC is a diagnosis of exclusion. Many drugs including cyclophosphamides, aspirin, nonsteroidal anti-inflammatory agents, and allopurinol have caused a nonbacterial cystitis that resolves with drug withdrawal (Bramble and Morley, 1997; Gheyi et al, 1999). **Various gynecologic problems can mimic the pain of IC** (Kohli et al, 1997). The pelvic congestion syndrome, a condition of the reproductive years and equally prevalent among parous and nulliparous women, is manifest by shifting location of pain, deep dyspareunia and postcoital pain, and exacerbation of pain after prolonged standing (Stones, 2003). Similar symptoms can be seen in PBS/IC. Other gynecologic disorders can include pelvic tumors, vaginal atrophy, vulvodynia, vestibulitis, pelvic relaxation, pelvic adhesive disease, levator ani myalgia, and undiagnosed chronic pelvic pain (Myers and Aguilar, 2002). Endometriosis probably causes pain, but that conclusion has to be regarded carefully, because it is based largely on one study (Sutton et al, 1997). Whiteside and Falcone (2003) point out that any claim linking endometriosis with pain fails to account for the common experience that identical lesions can be found in symptomatic and asymptomatic women (Vercellini, 1997). Between 2% and 43% of asymptomatic women are found to have endometriosis (Moen and Stokstad, 2002). Furthermore, there does not appear to be any risk for patients with asymptomatic mild endometriosis to develop symptoms even after greater than 10 years (Moen and Stokstad, 2002). While 70% to 90% of women with chronic pelvic pain have endometriosis, this does not definitively establish causation (Gambone et al, 2002). **Laparoscopy, which is not considered essential before initiating hormonal treatment of endometriosis** (Howard, 2003b), **should not be considered a part of any routine evaluation of PBS/IC unless a gynecologist believes it is likely to benefit the patient.**

A presumptive diagnosis can be made merely by ruling out known causes of frequency and pain/urgency in a patient with compatible chronic symptoms. Often this will involve a complete history, physical examination, appropriate cultures, and local cystoscopy. In the absence of microhematuria, the value of cytology is questionable (Duldulao et al, 1997) but something we still consider important, especially if bladder carcinoma in situ is a serious possibility, as in patients older than 40 and those with a smoking history. The recent report of a large series of PBS/IC patients indicating that 1% actually had transitional/cell carcinoma and that 4 of the 6 cancer patients did not have microhematuria provides evidence for the justification of local cystoscopic examination (Tissot et al, 2004).

It must be recognized that one may sacrifice a certain level of confidence in the diagnosis without the supporting evidence that can be furnished by additional studies. In a long-term illness such as IC, many patients and physicians ultimately want to base a diagnosis and treatment plan on the most complete data set possible (Rovner and Wein, 1999). A more thorough evaluation for IC would also include a urodynamic evaluation and cystoscopy under anesthesia with hydrodistention of the bladder (Hanno et al, 1990; Hanno, 1994a). Bladder biopsy is indicated only if necessary to rule out other disorders that might be suggested by the cystoscopic appearance. Cystoscopy under anesthesia with bladder distention has been important in the identification of Hunner's ulcer. Experimental data suggest that measurement of increased nitric oxide levels in the bladder can also accurately identify those with ulcerative disease (Logadottir et al, 2004). **The diagnosis is generally subject to more rigorous testing in Europe than in North America, where symptoms in the absence of other obvious causes seems to be the gold standard** (Nordling, 2004; Nordling et al, 2004; Hanno, 2005; Hanno et al, 2005).

Although sensations reported during cystometric bladder filling are subjective, they have a normal pattern and may be helpful in distinguishing bladder pathology (Wyndaele, 1998). Many dispute the need for urodynamic study, but we agree with Siroky (1994) that not only can it help to assess bladder compliance and sensation and reproduce the patient's symptoms during bladder filling, but it can also help to rule out detrusor overactivity. Women with pain on bladder filling can be indistinguishable from those with detrusor overactivity in their perception of bladder fullness (Creighton et al, 1991). One should be wary of diagnosing IC in patients with discrete, involuntary bladder contractions whose symptoms respond to anticholinergic therapy. The two problems coexist in 15% to 19% of patients (Gajewski and Awad, 1997; Kirkemo et al, 1997), but the pathophysiology is likely to be very different. Patients who respond to anticholinergic medication tend not to respond to standard therapy for IC (Perez-Marrero et al, 1987). If involuntary contractions are noted and the patient's symptoms of frequency and pain continue despite successful treatment, one is on firmer ground in considering a diagnosis of IC. Complex cases may benefit from full video-urodynamics studies (Carlson et al, 2001).

Cystometry in conscious IC patients generally demonstrates normal function, the exception being decreased bladder capacity and hypersensitivity. Pain on bladder filling that reproduces the patient's symptoms is very suggestive of IC. Bladder compliance in patients with IC is normal, because hypersensitivity would prevent the bladder from filling to the point of noncompliance (Siroky, 1994; Rovner and Wein, 1999). The possible addition of including a second cystometrogram after instillation of intravesical lidocaine to help to determine if pain is bladder related

is a provocative one worth further study (Teichman et al, 1997).

Long before it was considered a diagnostic tool, cystoscopy with hydrodistention of the bladder was used as a therapeutic modality for IC (Bumpus, 1930). Performing this procedure with the patient under anesthesia allows for sufficient distention of the bladder to afford visualization of either glomerulations or Hunner's ulcers (Figs. 10–9 and 10–10). After filling to 80 cm H_2O for 1 to 2 minutes, the bladder is drained and refilled. The terminal portion of the effluent is often blood tinged. Reinspection will reveal the pinpoint petechial hemorrhages that develop throughout the bladder after distention and are not usually seen after examination without anesthesia (Nigro and Wein, 1997).

Glomerulations are not specific for IC (Erickson, 1995; Waxman et al, 1998), **and only when seen in conjunction with the clinical criteria of pain and frequency can the finding of glomerulations be viewed as significant.** Glomerulations can be seen after radiation therapy, in patients with carcinoma, after exposure to toxic chemicals or chemotherapeutic agents, and often in patients on dialysis or after urinary diversion when the bladder has not filled for prolonged periods. They have been reported in the majority of men with prostate pain syndromes, begging the question as to whether the chronic pelvic pain syndrome in men is closely linked with IC (Berger et al, 1998). We have speculated that they may simply reflect the response of the bladder to distention after a prolonged period of chronic underfilling because of sensory urgency, rather than result from a primary pathologic process. While the presence of a Hunner's ulcer has been associated with pain and urinary urgency, neither the findings of bloody irrigating fluid nor glomerulations are strongly

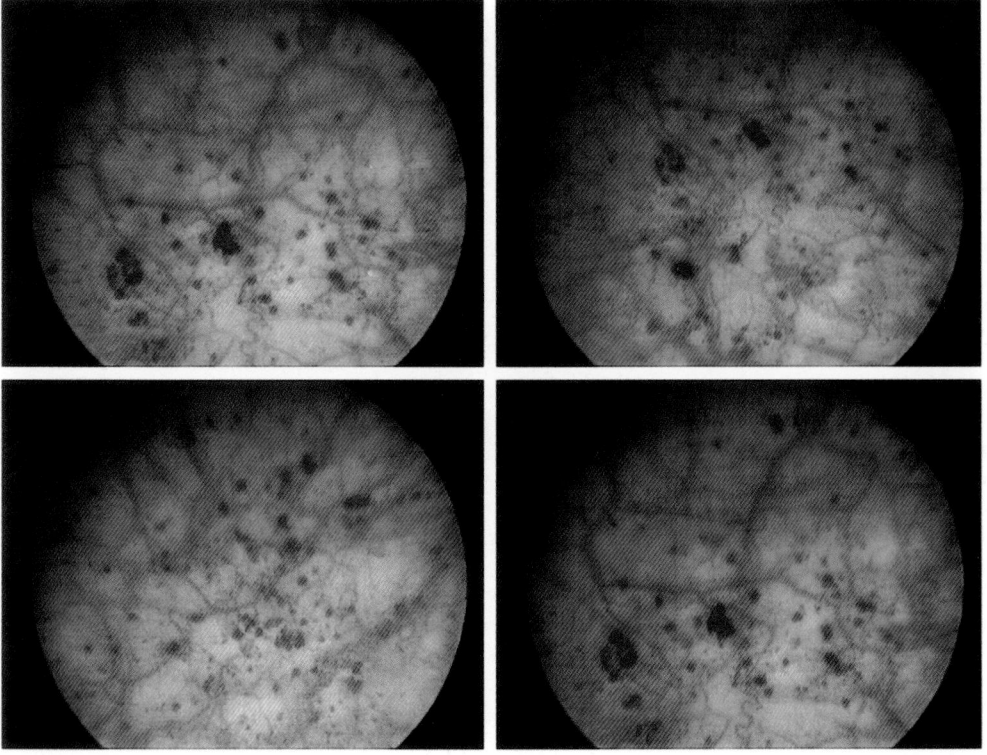

Figure 10–9. Typical appearance of glomerulations after bladder distention in a patient with nonulcerative interstitial cystitis.

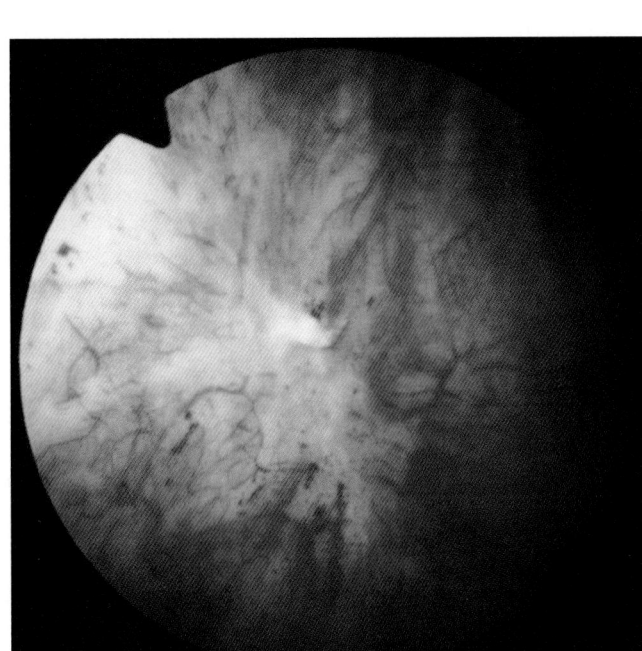

Figure 10–10. Typical appearance of Hunner's ulcer in a patient with interstitial cystitis before bladder distention.

associated with any particular symptom in patients in the ICDB (Messing et al, 1997).

Further confusion arises when the patient demonstrates the symptoms of IC but the cystoscopic findings under anesthesia are completely normal. This occurred in 8.7% of patients undergoing cystoscopy with hydrodistention entered into the ICDB (Messing et al, 1997). Awad and colleagues recognized this entity soon after the NIDDK research criteria had been described. They reported on a series of patients in whom the symptomatology, urodynamic evaluation, histology, and response to therapy was identical to IC, in whom findings on cystoscopy with hydrodistention were normal. It was referred to as "idiopathic reduced bladder storage" (Awad et al, 1992). **Clinical, urodynamic, and cystoscopic data strongly suggest that the presence of glomerulations is not selecting out a meaningful difference in patients with symptoms of PBS/IC** (Al Hadithi et al, 2002). The presence of glomerulations on cystoscopy under anesthesia meeting the NIDDK criteria may identify a group of patients with worse daytime frequency and nocturia and lower bladder capacity under anesthesia but does not have any relationship to biopsy findings, bladder pain, or urgency (Erickson et al, 2005). Ultimately, disease definitions are helpful only relative to the utility they provide in terms of treatment and prognosis, and it is likely that the definition of IC and therefore proper methods of diagnosis will continue to evolve.

Markers

What is the value of a "diagnostic test" in what is essentially a clinical syndrome defined by a symptom-complex? If a patient has chronic pain associated with the bladder usually accompanied by urinary frequency with no discernible cause, we diagnose PBS/IC. In essence, once we have ruled

out well-characterized pathologic entities, the patient makes the diagnosis by relating symptoms; much like a patient with impotence makes that diagnosis. Testing for impotence may give clues as to etiology, but we cannot rule out impotence in a patient who cannot function sexually by doing a test!

This is not to say that establishment of a valid diagnostic marker would not be a major advance in our understanding of IC. It will be important largely to the extent that it can predict prognosis in a given group of patients, predict response to therapy in a given group of patients, and/or distinguish between IC and another possible cause of the symptom-complex that has been diagnosed. Ultimately, marker identification may enable us to stratify patients with the symptom-complex in such a way that treatments will be specific to the specific etiology (disease) the patient has. Because various causes are identifiable, the diagnosis of IC may itself become a rarity, much as what has happened to "acute urethral syndrome" (Stamm et al, 1980).

In just such an effort, numerous investigators have looked at the mast cell as a possible diagnostic marker for IC. The results have been very contradictory, and at this time, in terms of the use of mast cell criteria in diagnosis, the issue remains moot (Kastrup et al, 1983; Lynes et al, 1987; Feltis et al, 1987; Holm-Bentzen et al, 1987; Hanno et al, 1990; Christmas and Rode 1991; Moore et al, 1992; Dundore et al, 1996; Hofmeister et al, 1997). Methylhistamine, a histamine metabolite found in the urine and thought to reflect mast cell activation, was not associated with symptom scores, response to bladder distention, cystoscopic findings, or bladder biopsy features including mast cell determination by tryptase staining (Erickson et al, 2004).

Attempts have been made to look at other markers (Erickson, 2001), including eosinophil cationic protein (Lose et al, 1987), glycosaminoglycan excretion (Hurst et al, 1993), and urinary histamine and methylhistamine (El Mansoury et al, 1994). Proposals for measuring smooth muscle isoactin expression (Rivas et al, 1997) and urinary levels of neurotrophin-3, nerve growth factor, glial cell line–derived neurotrophic factor, and tryptase (Okragly et al, 1999) have been suggested. Low levels of GP51, a urinary glycoprotein with a molecular weight of 5 kD have been documented in IC patients compared with normal controls and patients with other urinary tract diseases (Byrne et al, 1999). Even cell cultures (Elgavish et al, 1997) and the measurement of elevated nitric oxide levels in air instilled and incubated in the bladder have been proposed for office screening (Ehren et al, 1999; Lundberg et al, 1996).

The urine antiproliferative factor (APF) identified by Keay (see earlier) **may prove to be the most accurate marker of PBS/IC when confirmed by other centers. It appears to have the highest sensitivity and specificity of the variety of possible markers tested and fits nicely into an etiologic schema** (Keay et al, 2001; Erickson et al, 2002). It has also been shown to differentiate men with PBS/IC symptoms from controls and differentiate men with bladder-associated pain and irritative voiding symptoms from those with pelvic/perineal pain alone and other nonspecific findings compatible with the chronic pelvic pain syndrome in men, previously referred to as "nonbacterial prostatitis" (Keay et al, 2004a). This evidence that chronic pelvic pain syndrome and PBS/IC are very likely two different disorders will doubtless be the subject of future research.

Potassium Chloride Test

Parsons has championed an intravesical KCl challenge, comparing the sensory nerve provocative ability of sodium versus potassium using a 0.4 M KCl solution. Pain and provocation of symptoms constitutes a positive test. Whether the results indicate abnormal epithelial permeability in the subgroup of positive patients or hypersensitivity of the sensory nerves is unclear. Normal bladder epithelium can never be absolutely tight, and there is always some leak, however small (Hohlbrugger, 1997). The concentration of potassium used is 400 mEq/L, far exceeding the physiologic urinary concentrations of 20 to 80 mEq/L, depending on dietary intake (Vander, 1995). Healthy control subjects can distinguish KCl from sodium chloride, although they do not experience severe pain (Roberto et al, 1997). The hope is that this test may stratify patients into those who will respond to certain treatments (perhaps those designed to fortify the glycosaminoglycan layer), but to date this information is lacking (Teichman and Nielsen-Omeis, 1999).

Used as a diagnostic test for IC, the KCl test is not valid (Chambers et al, 1999). The gold standard in defining PBS/IC for research purposes has been the NIDDK criteria. These criteria are recognized to constitute a set of patients that virtually all researchers can agree have PBS/IC, although they are far too restrictive to be used in clinical practice (Hanno et al, 1999b). Thus, this group of patients should virtually all be positive if the KCl test is to have the sensitivity needed to aid in diagnosis. Up to 25% of patients meeting the NIDDK criteria will have a negative KCl test (Parsons et al, 1998). In the group it should perform the best in, it is lacking in sensitivity. When we look at the specificity side of the equation, in the universe of asymptomatic persons, it performs relatively well and is rarely positive, although a recent study reported a 36% false-positive rate in asymptomatic men (Yilmaz et al, 2004). It is in the patient population with confounding conditions for which we would want help in sorting out PBS/IC from other disorders. Twenty-five percent of patients with overactive bladder test positive, and virtually all patients with irritative symptoms from radiation cystitis and urinary tract infection test positive (Parsons et al, 1994b, 1998). The results with chronic prostatitis/chronic pelvic pain syndrome in men are variable, but 50% to 84% of men have been reported to test positive (Parsons and Albo, 2002; Yilmaz et al, 2004; Parsons et al, 2005). In women with pelvic pain, results are similar (Parsons et al, 2002b); and based on these findings, Parsons and colleagues (2000a) have expressed the view that PBS/IC may affect over 20% of the female population of the United States. Another way to interpret the findings would be that the KCl test is very nonspecific, missing a significant number of PBS/IC patients and overdiagnosing much of the population.

Cystometry employing KCl (0.3 M) has been compared with saline cystometry in patients with PBS/IC and those with detrusor overactivity (Philip and Irwin, 2004). Both groups show lowered volumes at first desire to void and lower cystometric capacity with KCl, raising the question as to whether potassium may act not on the urothelial sensory mechanism but rather on the detrusor muscle.

Prospective and retrospective studies looking at the KCl test for diagnosis in patients presenting with symptoms of PBS/IC have found no benefit of the test in comparison with standard techniques of diagnosis (Chambers et al, 1999; Gregoire et al, 2002; Kuo, 2003). The development of a painless modification of the KCl test (Daha et al, 2003) using cystometric capacity and a 0.2 M solution may improve acceptability among patients, but further research is needed to determine what place, if any, this test will have in the diagnostic or treatment algorithm for PBS/IC.

CLINICAL SYMPTOM SCALES

There are three published PBS/IC symptom questionnaires: the University of Wisconsin IC Scale, the O'Leary-Sant IC Symptom Index and IC Problem Index, and the Pelvic Pain and Urgency/Frequency (PUF) Scale.

The University of Wisconsin IC Scale (Table 10–6) includes 7 PBS/IC symptom items (1, 2, 10, 18, 21, 23, and 25) but has not been validated for identification or diagnosis of PBS/IC. It captures severity of symptom expression (Keller et al, 1994; Goin et al, 1998). PBS/IC patients do not appear to indiscriminately report higher scores than controls for different somatic and general complaints (Porru et al, 2005). Unlike the other two instruments, it addresses some quality-of-life issues, and this is an advantage when such issues are subjects of inves-

Table 10–6. **University of Wisconsin Symptom Instrument**	
Symptom	Score 1 to 6 (0 = Not at all; 6 = A lot)
1. Bladder discomfort	
2. Bladder pain	
3. Other pelvic discomfort	
4. Headache	
5. Backache	
6. Dizziness	
7. Feelings of suffocation	
8. Chest pain	
9. Ringing in ears	
10. Getting up at night to go to the bathroom	
11. Aches in joints	
12. Swollen ankles	
13. Nasal congestion	
14. Flu	
15. Abdominal cramps	
16. Numbness or tingling in fingers or toes	
17. Nausea	
18. Going to the bathroom frequently during the day	
19. Blind spots or blurred vision	
20. Heart pounding	
21. Difficulty sleeping because of bladder symptoms	
22. Sore throat	
23. Urgency to urinate	
24. Coughing	
25. Burning sensation in bladder	

From Sirinian E, Azevedo K, Payne CK: Correlation between 2 interstitial cystitis symptom instruments. J Urol 2005;173:835-840.

tigation. Its most attractive aspects are its clinically apparent face validity and its ease of implementation.

The O'Leary-Sant indices (Table 10–7) **form a validated questionnaire that was originally developed by focus groups, subjected to test-retest reliability analysis, and validated by administration to IC patients and asymptomatic controls** (O'Leary et al, 1997; Lubeck et al, 2001). The questionnaires center on three questions related to urgency/frequency and one on bladder-associated pain. They do not address generalized pelvic pain or symptomatology associated with sexual activity. This is not because these questions were not considered in the formulation of the questionnaire. Of 73 questions in the preliminary instrument covering domains of urinary symptoms, pain, sexual function, menstrual variability, and general health, only the four questions now in the instrument were needed to reliably and validly describe the illness experience of those with IC and distinguish these patients from those without the disorder (O'Leary and Sant, 1997).

The most recently published instrument is the PUF questionnaire (Parsons et al, 2002a) (Table 10–8). It was specifi-

cally designed to include questions that directly reflect a wide variety of the symptoms experienced by patients who are affected by this disorder. One third of the questions address pelvic pain, including pain anywhere in the pelvis: the vagina, labia, lower abdomen, urethra, perineum, testes, penis, or scrotum. A large study utilizing the PUF questionnaire has concluded that up to 23% of American females have PBS/IC (Parsons et al, 2002a). This makes one very wary as to the utility and face-validity of the PUF (Ito et al, 2003). A total score of 10 to 14 = 74% likelihood of positive potassium test (PST); 15 to 19, 76%; 20+, 91%. To the extent that the PST is suspect, the reliability of PUF data comes into question.

The O'Leary-Sant and University of Wisconsin instrument correlates strongly in a large population of patients with PBS/IC (Sirinian and Payne, 2001). **Treatment outcome studies have also used the Global Response Assessment, a balanced patient self-report on overall response to therapy developed for NIDDK-sponsored multicenter therapeutic trials** (Sant et al, 2003) (Table 10–9).

Table 10–7. O'Leary-Sant Indices

IC Symptom Index	IC Problem Index
During the past month...	During the past month how much has each of the following been a problem for you:
Q1. . . . how often have you felt the strong need to urinate with little or no warning? 0. Not at all 1. Less than 1 time in 5 2. Less than half the time 3. About half the time 4. More than half the time 5. Almost always	Q1. Frequent urination during the day 0. No problem 1. Very small problem 2. Small problem 3. Medium problem 4. Big problem
Q2. . . . how often have you had to urinate less than 2 hours after you finished urinating? 1. Less than 1 time in 5 2. Less than half the time 3. About half the time 4. More than half the time 5. Almost always	Q2. Getting up at night to urinate? 0. No problem 1. Very small problem 2. Small problem 3. Medium problem 4. Big problem
Q3. . . . how often did you most typically get up at night to urinate? 0. Not at all 2. A few times 3. Almost always 4. Fairly often 5. Usually	Q3. Need to urinate with little warning? 0. No problem 1. Very small problem 2. Small problem 3. Medium problem 4. Big problem
Q4. . . . have you experienced pain or burning in your bladder? 0. Not at all 2. A few times 3. Almost always 4. Fairly often 5. Usually	Q4. Burning, pain, discomfort, or pressure in your bladder? 0. No problem 1. Very small problem 2. Small problem 3. Medium problem 4. Big problem
Add the numerical values of the checked entries. Total score: _____	Add the numerical values of the checked entries. Total score: _____

From O'Leary MP, Sant GR, Fowler FJ Jr, et al: The interstitial cystitis symptom index and problem index. Urology 1997;49:58-63.

KEY POINT: CLINICAL SYMPTOM SCALES

■ Symptom scales have potential utility in PBS/IC. Their future development may enable reliable diagnosis of the syndrome on the basis of a questionnaire alone. A brief survey that reliably segregates PBS/IC from other urologic disorders would make the ability to diagnose the syndrome reliable, inexpensive, and available to all health care providers. It would aid in epidemiologic studies as well. Currently, such work sponsored by NIDDK is ongoing (http://kidney.niddk.nih.gov/about/Research_Updates/spr04/6.htm). Questionnaires and symptom scales can also be utilized to measure treatment outcome and are especially valuable in clinical research studies as well as for guiding therapy for individual patients. None of the questionnaires has been shown to be of value in diagnosis (Moldwin and Kushner, 2004).

ASSESSING TREATMENT RESULTS

The diversity of PBS/IC therapies underscores the lack of understanding about the treatment of this syndrome (Rovner et al, 2000). It has been not only a difficult condition to diagnose but also a difficult condition for which to assess therapeutic impact. There is a 50% incidence of temporary remission unrelated to therapy, with a mean duration of 8 months (Held et al, 1990). A somewhat surprising finding from the ICDB was that although there was initial improvement in symptoms partially due to regression to the mean (Sech et al, 1998) and the intervention effect, there was no evidence of a long-term change in average symptom severity over the 4-year course of follow-up (Propert et al, 2000). **In a chronic, devastating condition with primarily subjective symptomatology, no known cause, and no cure, patients are desperate and often seem to respond to any new therapy**

Table 10-8. Pelvic Pain and Urgency/Frequency Patient Symptom Scale (PUF)

PATIENT SYMPTOM SCALE
Patient's Name: _____ Today's Date: _____
Please circle the answer that best describes how you feel for each question.

	0	1	2	3	4	Symptom Score	Bother Score
1. How many times do you go to the bathroom during the day?	3-6	7-10	11-14	15-19	20+		
2. a. How many times do you go to the bathroom at night?	0	1	2	3	4+		
b. If you get up at night to go to the bathroom, does it bother you?	Never bothers	Occasionally	Usually	Always			
3. Are you currently sexually active. YES ____ NO ____							
4. a. If you are sexually active, do you now or have you ever had pain or symptoms during or after sexual activity?	Never	Occasionally	Usually	Always			
b. If you have pain, does it make you avoid sexual activity?	Never	Occasionally	Usually	Always			
5. Do you have pain associated with your bladder or in your pelvis (vagina, labia, lower abdomen, urethra, perineum, penis, testes or scrotum)?	Never	Occasionally	Usually	Always			
6. a. If you have pain, is it usually		Mild	Moderate	Severe			
b. Does your pain bother you?	Never	Occasionally	Usually	Always			
7. Do you still have urgency after you go to the bathroom?	Never	Occasionally	Usually	Always			
8. a. If you have urgency, is it usually		Mild	Moderate	Severe			
b. Does your urgency bother you?	Never	Occasionally	Usually	Always			

Symptom Score (1, 2a, 4a, 5, 6a, 7, 8a)

Bother Score (2b, 4b, 6b, 8b)

Total Score (Symptom Score + Bother Score)
Total score ranges are from 1 to 35.

From Parsons CL, Dell J, Stanford EJ, et al: Increased prevalence of interstitial cystitis: Previously unrecognized urologic and gynecologic cases identified using a new symptom questionnaire and intravesical potassium sensitivity. Urology 2000;60:573-578.

Table 10-9. Global Response Assessment (GRA)

−3: Markedly Worse
−2: Moderately Worse
−1: Slightly Worse
0: No Change
+1: Slightly Improved
+2: Moderately Improved
+3: Markedly Improved

From Sant GR, Propert KJ, Hanno PM, et al: A pilot clinical trial of oral pentosan polysulfate and oral hydroxyzine in patients with interstitial cystitis. J Urol 2003;170:810-815.

(Fig. 10–11). They are often victims of unorthodox health care providers with untested forms of therapy, some medical, some homeopathic, and some even surgical.

Placebo effects influence patient outcomes after any treatment, including surgery, in which clinician and patient beliefs are effective. **Placebo effects plus disease natural history and regression to the mean can result in high rates of good outcomes, which may be misattributed to specific treatment effects** (Gillespie et al, 1991; Gillespie, 1994; Turner et al, 1994; Propert et al, 2000). Unfortunately, few IC treatments have been subjected to a placebo-controlled trial. This is not to say that what seems effective is not but rather that a high index of skepticism is healthy, even in treatments tested by controlled trials (Schulz et al, 1995). While in many diseases an argument can be made against using a true placebo control as opposed to an orthodox treatment of approved or accepted value (Rothman and Michels, 1994), a good case for true placebo can readily be made for IC. The vagaries of the natural history, the general lack of progression of symptom severity over time, and the fact that it is not life threatening mean that there is little to lose and much to gain by subjecting new treatments to the vigorous scrutiny of placebo control. Many patients who volunteer for such trials have already run the gamut of accepted (though generally unproved) therapies. It has long been recognized in protocols that use subjective criteria for assessment that "improvement" may be expected in up to 35% of placebo-treated patients (Benson and Epstein, 1976). Because the spontaneous remission rate (though temporary) for IC is 11% (Oravisto and Alfthan, 1976) to 50% (Held et al, 1990), combined with the placebo improvement it can be difficult to prove efficacy. Even in placebo-controlled trials, it is reasonable to surmise that some degree of unblinding may occur as a result of somatic or psychological side effects of the active arm, impairing the validity of the trial results and giving the active arm a slight

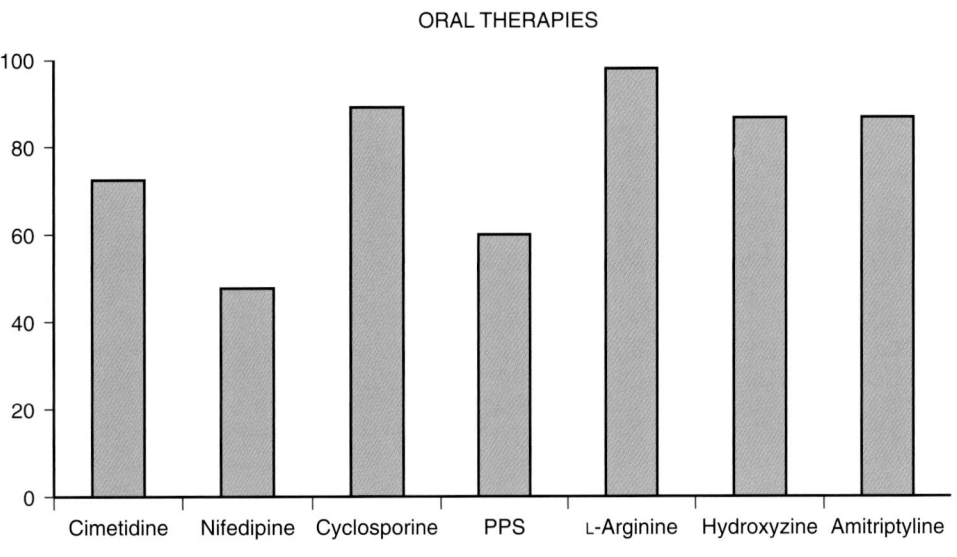

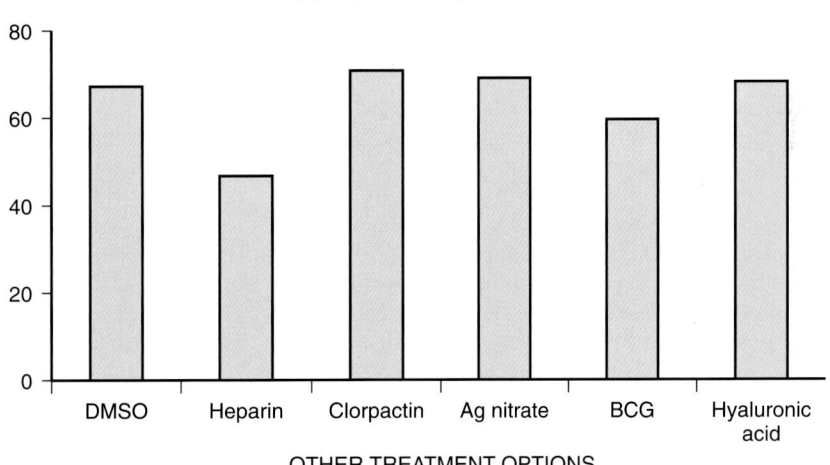

Figure 10–11. Selected reported treatment outcomes in uncontrolled studies in the interstitial cystitis literature: Percentage of patients initially improved. Ag nitrate, silver nitrate; BCG, bacillus Calmette-Guérin; DMSO, dimethyl sulfoxide; PPS, sodium pentosan polysulfate; TENS, transcutaneous electrical nerve stimulation.

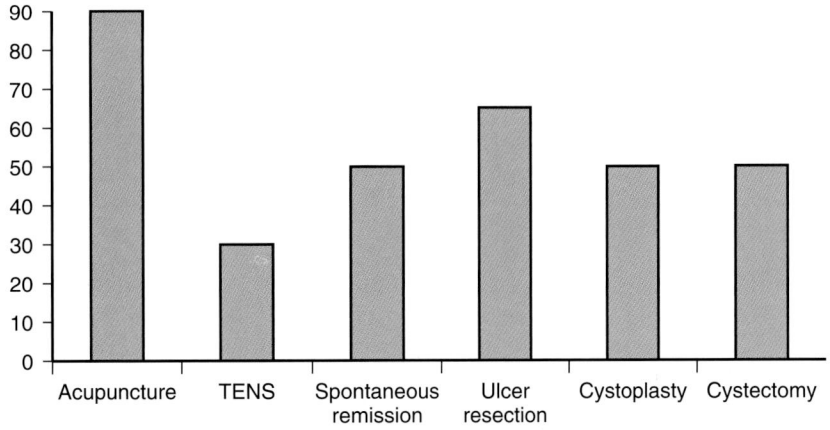

edge over placebo (DuBeau et al, 2005; Rees et al, 2005). This is of specific concern in PBS/IC and in any disorder in which primary outcomes may be subject to patient-specific psychological and physiologic factors.

The value of placebo-controlled trials is aptly illustrated by the recent decisions by pharmaceutical manufacturers not to pursue U.S. Food and Drug Administration approval for seemingly promising intravesical therapies for PBS/IC

(Morales et al, 1996; Chancellor and de Groat, 1999) after placebo-controlled trials failed to establish efficacy. These include low-concentration hyaluronic acid (Bioniche, Canada), high-concentration hyaluronic acid (SKK, Tokyo), and resiniferatoxin (ICOS, Bothell, WA). Nalmefene, an initially promising oral therapy in the 1990s (Stone, 1994), also failed phase 3 trials (IVAX, Miami, FL). Placebo trials are impractical in surgery, and it can be difficult to evaluate surgical reports. The many older medications currently used off-label might not meet success if tested in the stringent manner in which new molecular entities are tested. The expense of testing therapies currently used off-label often requires dependence on the largesse of government agencies such as the National Institutes of Health (Propert et al, 2002; Sant et al, 2003; Mayer and Interstitial Cystitis Clinical Trials Group, 2005).

Finally, when considering objective changes, the concept of statistical versus clinical significance is paramount. Investigators should, but rarely do, point out differences between statistical improvement and what they consider to be clinically significant improvement (Wein and Broderick, 1994). As Gertrude Stein reportedly stated, "A difference, to be a difference, must make a difference." An increase in bladder capacity of 30 mL may be statistically significant but clinically irrelevant. Number needed to treat and number needed to harm data (McQuay, 2003) may be particularly important in PBS/IC and have not typically been included in efficacy analysis.

CONSERVATIVE THERAPY

Once the diagnosis has been made one must decide whether to institute therapy or employ a policy of conservative "watchful waiting." If the patient has not had an empirical course of antibiotics for their symptoms by the time the PBS/IC diagnosis is made, such a trial is reasonable. Doxycycline has been reported efficacious in a recent Swiss study (Burkhard et al, 2004). Further attempts to alleviate symptoms with antibiotics are unlikely to be worthwhile and are not recommended in the absence of positive cultures (Warren et al, 2000). If the patient's symptoms are "livable," the withholding of immediate treatment is reasonable. While the concept of "livable" is certainly patient dependent, someone who gets up once or twice a night and voids every 2 to 3 hours during the day with minimal pain would certainly fall into this category. An educated patient is likely to realize that no treatment will make him or her perfect, and any therapy is a tradeoff among the inconvenience, chronicity of treatment, side effects, and the benefits. As with any decision in medicine, "perfect is the enemy of good." **Data that "early" treatment affects the natural history or course of the disease is lacking at this time, and an argument for the early institution of therapy cannot be supported on the basis of epidemiologic data or clinical trials.**

Patient education and empowerment **is an important initial step in therapy.** Taking advantage of on-line databases, interactive computer programs, electronic mail lists for disabled persons, telephone hotlines, educational videos, health magazines, and public libraries enables patients to make health choices that they can feel comfortable with (McCormick, 1997; Breau et al, 2003). It is important to reassure the patient (who often has already seen multiple doctors and had many tests) that the symptoms, although very bothersome, are not signs of a life-threatening disease. Patients are usually reassured after learning that they are not the only persons with these symptoms and that what they have is a part of a well-described syndrome. One must not forget the placebo effect, euphemistically termed "remembered wellness," as one of the physician's most therapeutic assets (Benson

and Epstein, 1976; Benson and Friedman, 1996; O'Reilly et al, 2004). The Interstitial Cystitis Association (Ratner et al, 1992) is an important resource for information and support for patients as well as a clearing house for ideas and funding for researchers and clinicians.

There are data that timed voiding and *behavioral modification therapy* **can be helpful in the short-term, especially in patients in whom frequency rather than pain predominates** (Chaiken et al, 1993; Barbalias et al, 2000). This can consist of diary keeping, controlled fluid intake, pelvic floor muscle training, and active attempts to increase voiding intervals. Parson's group reported success in 15 of 21 patients who had primarily frequency rather than pain, by gradually encouraging longer voiding intervals over time through voiding diary techniques (Parsons and Koprowski, 1991). A similar study with 15 patients concluded that although average voided volume increased by 65 mL after a month, the persistent sense of bladder fullness did not change from preintervention volumes (Mendelowitz and Moldwin, 1997).

While there are no randomized, controlled trials to prove it, many clinicians believe that stress reduction, exercise, warm tub baths, and efforts by the patient to maintain a normal lifestyle all contribute to overall quality of life (Whitmore, 1994). In a controlled study of 45 PBS/IC patients and 31 healthy control subjects, higher levels of stress were related to greater pain and urgency in patients with IC but not in the control group (Rothrock et al, 2001). Maladaptive strategies for coping with stress may impact adversely on symptoms (Rothrock et al, 2003). Biofeedback, soft tissue massage, and other physical therapies may aid in muscle relaxation of the pelvic floor (Mendelowitz and Moldwin, 1997; Meadows, 1999; Holzberg et al, 2001; Lukban et al, 2001; Markwell, 2001). Mendelowitz and Moldwin (1997) had a 69% success rate in 16 patients treated with electromyographic biofeedback, but treatment response did not correlate to changes in muscle identification, and the placebo effect may have been considerable. Acupuncture has been used for PBS/IC and many other chronic pain syndromes. There is limited evidence that it is more effective than no treatment for chronic pain, and there is inconclusive evidence that acupuncture is more effective than placebo, sham acupuncture, or standard care (Ezzo et al, 2000). PBS/IC results with acupuncture have been disappointing (Geirsson et al, 1993).

Elaborate dietary restrictions are unsupported by any literature, but many patients do find their symptoms are adversely affected by specific foods and would do well to avoid them (Koziol et al, 1993; Koziol, 1994). Often this includes caffeine, alcohol, and beverages that might acidify the urine such as cranberry juice. Anecdotal association of IC with many foods has spawned the recommendation of various "IC diets" with little in the way of objective, scientific basis (Table 10–10). The only placebo-controlled dietary study, while small, failed to demonstrate a relationship between diet and symptoms (Fisher et al, 1993). Bade and colleagues (1997) found that IC patients tend to have a healthier diet than the general population but could discern no rationale for dietary or fluid intake change other than decreasing caffeine intake. Nguan and coworkers (2005) performed a prospective, double-blind, crossover study consisting of crossover instillations of urine at physiologic pH (5.0) and neutral buffered pH (7.5). There was no statistically significant difference in sub-

Table 10–10. **Interstitial Cystitis Association Recommendations of Foods to Avoid**	
Milk/Dairy Products	*Nuts*
Aged cheeses	*Beverages*
Sour cream	Alcoholic beverages including beer and wine
Yogurt	Carbonated drinks
Chocolate	Coffee
Vegetables	Tea
Fava beans	Fruit juices
Lima beans	*Seasonings*
Onions	Mayonnaise
Tofu	Ketchup
Soybeans	Mustard
Tomatoes	Salsa
Fruits	Spicy foods: (Chinese, Mexican, Indian, Thai)
Apples	Soy sauce
Apricots	Miso
Avocados	Salad dressing
Bananas	Vinegar
Cantaloupes	*Preservatives and Additives*
Citrus fruits	Benzyl alcohol
Cranberries	Citric acid
Grapes	Monosodium glutamate
Nectarines	Artificial sweeteners
Peaches	Preservatives
Pineapples	Artificial ingredients
Plums	Food coloring
Pomegranates	*Miscellaneous*
Rhubarb	Tobacco
Strawberries	Caffeine
Juices from above fruits	Diet pills
Carbohydrates and Grains	Junk foods
Rye bread	Recreational drugs
Sourdough bread	Allergy medications with ephedrine or pseudoephedrine
Meats and Fish	Certain vitamins
Aged, canned, cured, processed, smoked meats and fish	

From www.ichelp.org

jective pain scores, suggesting that adjusting urine pH with diet or dietary supplements may have little influence on symptomatology. Orange and grapefruit juices, rich in potassium and citrate, tend to increase urinary pH (Wabner and Pak, 1993) but surprisingly are avoided by many IC patients based on "IC diet" recommendations. Urinary alkalinization may be worth trying, but supporting studies are lacking.

Unfortunately, education and self-help are often not sufficient, and most patients will require one or more of a variety of therapies.

ORAL THERAPY (Table 10–11)
Tricyclic Antidepressants

Amitriptyline has become a staple of oral treatment for IC. The tricyclic agents possess varying degrees of at least three major pharmacologic actions: (1) they have central and peripheral anticholinergic actions at some but not all sites, (2) they block the active transport system in the presynaptic nerve ending that is responsible for the reuptake of the released amine neurotransmitters serotonin and noradrenaline, and (3) they are sedatives, an action that occurs presumably on a central basis but perhaps is related to their antihistaminic properties. Amitriptyline, in fact, is one of the most potent tri-

cyclic antidepressants in terms of blocking H1-histaminergic receptors (Baldessarini, 1985). There is also evidence that they desensitize α_2- adrenergic receptors on central noradrenergic neurons. Paradoxically, they also have been shown to block α-adrenergic receptors and serotonin receptors. Theoretically, tricyclic agents have actions that might tend to stimulate predominantly β-adrenergic receptors in bladder body smooth musculature, an action that would further facilitate urine storage by decreasing the excitability of smooth muscle in that area (Barrett and Wein, 1987).

Hanno and Wein (1987) first reported a therapeutic response in IC after noting a "serendipitous" response to amitriptyline in one of their patients concurrently being treated for depression. The following year a similar report appeared relating a response to desipramine hydrochloride (Renshaw, 1988). By reasoning that a drug used successfully at relatively low dosages for many types of chronic pain syndromes, which would also have anticholinergic properties, β-adrenergic bladder effects, sedative characteristics, and strong H1 antihistaminic activity would seem to be ideal for IC, the first clinical trial was carried out with promising results (Hanno et al, 1989). A subsequent follow-up study (Hanno, 1994b) reported that in 28 of 43 patients who could tolerate therapy for at least a 3-week trial at a dosage of 25 mg at bedtime gradually increasing to 75 mg at bedtime over 2

Table 10–11. Some Oral Medications That Have Been Used for Treatment of PBS/IC

Drug	Randomized Control Trial	% Success
Amitriptyline	Yes	42%
Antibiotic regimens	Yes	48%
Anticholinergics and antispasmodics	No	Anecdotal
Azathioprine	No	50%
Benzydamine	Yes	0%
Chloroquine derivatives	No	50%
Cimetidine	Yes	65%
Cortisone and other steroids	No	80%
Cyclosporine	No	90%
Doxycycline	No	71%
Gabapentin	No	Anecdotal
Hormones	No	Anecdotal
Hydroxyzine	Yes	31%
L-Arginine	Yes	Not effective
Methotrexate	No	50%
Misoprostol	No	48%
Montelukast	No	90%
Nalmefene	Yes	Not effective
Narcotic analgesics	No	Anecdotal
Nifedipine	No	87%
Phenazopyridine	No	Anecdotal
Quercetin	No	92%
Sodium pentosan polysulfate	Yes	33%
Suplatast tosylate	Yes	Pending publication
Vitamin E	No	Anecdotal

Adapted from 3rd International Consultation on Incontinence.

weeks, there were 18 who had total remission of symptoms with a mean follow-up of 14.4 months, 5 dropped out because of side effects, and 5 derived no clinical benefit. Benefits were apparent within 4 weeks. All patients had failed hydrodistention and intravesical DMSO therapy. Sedation was the main side effect. Kirkemo and colleagues (1990) treated 30 patients and had a 90% subjective improvement rate at 8 weeks. Both studies noted that patients with bladder capacities over 450 to 600 mL under anesthesia seemed to have the best results. Another uncontrolled study of 11 patients with urinary frequency and pelvic pain (Pranikoff and Constantino, 1998) related success in 9 of the patients, with 5 reporting complete resolution of symptoms and 4 significant relief. Two patients could not tolerate the medication. In a 4-month intent-to-treat, placebo-controlled, double-blind trial of 50 patients, 63% on amitriptyline at doses of 25 to 75 mg (dose as tolerated) before bed reported good or excellent satisfaction versus 4% on placebo (van Ophoven et al, 2004a). At 19-month follow-up there was little tachyphylaxis and good response rates were observed in the entire spectrum of PBS/IC symptoms (van Ophoven and Hertle, 2005).

Amitriptyline has proven analgesic efficacy, with a median preferred dose of 75 mg in a range of 25 to 150 mg daily. This range is lower than traditional doses for depression of 150 to 300 mg. The speed of onset of effect is much faster (1 to 7 days) than reported in depression, and the analgesic effect is distinct from any effect on mood (McQuay and Moore, 1997). Tricyclic antidepressants are contraindicated in patients with long QT syndrome or significant conduction system disease

(bifascicular or trifascicular block) after recent myocardial infarction (within 6 months), unstable angina, congestive heart failure, frequent premature ventricular contractions, or a history of sustained ventricular arrhythmias. They should be used with caution in patients with orthostatic hypotension (Low and Dotson, 1998). Doses greater than 100 mg are associated with increased relative risk of sudden cardiac death (Ray et al, 2004).

Antihistamines

The use of antihistamines goes back to the late 1950s and stems from work by Simmons (1961) who postulated that the local release of histamine may be responsible for, or accompany the development of, IC. He reported on six patients treated with pyribenzamine. The results were far from dramatic, with only half of the patients showing some response. The therapy is notable for this disease in that it was very logically conceived. It has been Theoharides (1994) who has spearheaded mast cell research in this field and been a major modern proponent of antihistamine therapy. He has used the unique piperazine H1-receptor antagonist hydroxyzine, a first-generation antihistamine (Simons, 2004), which can block neuronal activation of mast cells (Minogiannis et al, 1998). In 40 patients treated with 25 mg before bed increasing over 2 weeks (if sedation was not a problem) to 50 mg at night and 25 mg in the morning, virtually every symptom evaluated improved by 30%. Only 3 patients had absolutely no response. As with many IC drug reports, these responses were evaluated subjectively and without being blinded or placebo controlled. A subsequent study suggested improved efficacy in patients with documented allergies and/or evidence of bladder mast cell activation (Theoharides and Sant, 1997a, 1997b). No significant response to hydroxyzine was found in an NIDDK placebo-controlled trial (Sant et al, 2003). Why an H2 antagonist would be effective is unclear, but uncontrolled studies show improvement of symptoms in two thirds of patients taking cimetidine in divided doses totaling 600 mg (Seshadri et al, 1994; Lewi, 1996). It proved effective in a double-blind, placebo-controlled trial (Thilagarajah et al, 2001), but histologic studies show the bladder mucosa to be unchanged before and after treatment, and the mechanism of any efficacy remains unexplained (Dasgupta et al, 2001).

Sodium Pentosan Polysulfate

Parson's suggestion that a defect in the epithelial permeability barrier, the glycosaminoglycan (GAG) layer, contributes to the pathogenesis of IC has led to an attempt to correct such a defect with the synthetic sulfated polysaccharide sodium pentosan polysulfate (PPS), a heparin analog available in an oral formulation, 3% to 6% of which is excreted into the urine (Barrington and Stephenson, 1997). It is sold under the trade name Elmiron. Studies have been contradictory.

Fritjofsson and associates (1987) treated 87 patients in an open multicenter trial in Sweden and Finland. Bladder volume with and without anesthesia was unchanged. Relief of pain was complete in 35% and partial in 23% of patients. Daytime frequency decreased from 16.5 to 13, and nocturia decreased from 4.5 to 3.5. Mean voided volumes increased by almost a tablespoon in the nonulcer group. Holm-Bentzen and colleagues (1987a) studied 115 patients in a double-blind, placebo-controlled trial. Symptoms, urodynamic parameters, cystoscopic appearance, and mast cell counts were unchanged after 4 months. Bladder capacity under anesthesia increased significantly in the group with mastocytosis, but this had no bearing on symptoms or awake capacity.

Parsons and coworkers (1983) had a more encouraging initial experience, and subsequently the results of two placebo-controlled multicenter trials in the United States were published (Mulholland et al, 1990; Parsons et al, 1993). In the initial study, overall improvement of greater than 25% was reported by 28% of the PPS-treated group versus 13% in the placebo group. In the latter study the respective figures were 32% on drug versus 16% on placebo. Average voided volume on PPS increased by 20 mL. No other objective improvements were documented. An NIDDK 2 × 2 factorial study to evaluate PPS and hydroxyzine looked at each drug used alone and in combination and compared results with a placebo group (Sant et al, 2003). Patients were treated for 6 months. No statistically significant response to either medication was documented. No significant trend was seen in the PPS treatment groups (34%) compared with non-PPS groups (18%). Of the 29 patients on PPS alone, 28% had global response (the primary endpoint) of moderately or markedly improved versus 13% on placebo, a number remarkably similar to the results in the 3-month pivotal trials, although not reaching statistical significance in the 6-month study. A subsequent industry sponsored trial showed no dose-related efficacy response in the range of 300 to 900 mg daily, but adverse events *were* dose related (Nickel et al, 2005).

Long-term experience with PPS is consistent with efficacy in a subset of patients that may drop below 30% of those initially treated (Jepsen et al, 1998). Tachyphylaxis seems to be uncommon in responders. Adverse events with PPS occurred in less than 4% of patients at the dose of 100 mg three times daily (Hanno, 1997) and include reversible alopecia, diarrhea, nausea, and rash. Rare bleeding problems have been reported (Rice et al, 1998). It promotes cellular proliferation in vitro in the MCF-7 breast cancer cell line, and caution has been suggested in prescribing it in groups at high risk for breast cancer and premenopausal females (Zaslau et al, 2004). A 3- to 6-month treatment trial is generally required to see symptom improvement. In a small trial, PPS has shown efficacy when administered intravesically (Bade et al, 1997). It may be of value in the management of radiation cystitis (Hampson and Woodhouse, 1994; Parsons, 1986) and cyclophosphamide cystitis (Toren and Norman, 2005), but its value in the treatment of PBS/IC seems marginal.

Miscellaneous Agents

Several oral therapies for IC have been tried and essentially been discarded, although some are being reinvestigated. Dees reported temporary improvement with **systemic corticosteroids** (Dees, 1953), but these drugs have not been found to be useful (Pool, 1967), and the risks of chronic administration are considerable. Prednisone at a dose of 25 mg daily for 1 to 2 months and then tapered as tolerated may be effective in patients with otherwise unresponsive ulcerative disease (Soucy and Gregoire, 2005). **Hormones** have been used

without success (Burford and Burford, 1958; Badenoch, 1971). **Vitamin E, anticholinergics,** and **antispasmodics** are not generally efficacious (Burford and Burford, 1958; Pool, 1967). **Immunosuppression and chloroquine derivatives** have been administered (Oravisto and Alfthan, 1976); about 50% of patients responded to some extent, but potential complications are significant and neither therapy has found general usage. Cyclosporine seemed to have some beneficial effect in a small, uncontrolled study (Forsell et al, 1996). A follow-up trial showed benefit in 20 of 23 patients treated for a minimum of 1 year (Sairanen et al, 2004). Low-dose oral methotrexate improved bladder pain in 4 of 9 patients and had no effect on voiding pattern (Moran et al, 1999). Benzydamine, a potent anti-inflammatory drug with strong analgesic effects, was initially reported to have a superb response rate in IC (Walsh, 1976), but a controlled follow-up trial demonstrated no responses in the first 12 patients, and the trial was discontinued (Walsh, 1977).

The **opiate antagonist nalmefene** was tried in an uncontrolled trial with promising results (Stone, 1994). It is known that mast cells degranulate and release histamines and other mediators when their endogenous opioid receptors are stimulated. In PBS/IC this theoretically could occur because of chronic endorphin release stimulated by the pain. By blocking the patient's own endogenous stimulation of mast cell degranulation, a "vicious cycle" could possibly be broken. Unfortunately, an unpublished, placebo-controlled trial failed to demonstrate the hoped-for efficacy.

The **calcium channel antagonist nifedipine** has been tried in an uncontrolled study for IC and urethral syndrome (Fleischmann, 1994). Nifedipine has been reported to inhibit detrusor contractions and depress cell-mediated immune functions. Of 9 IC patients treated for at least 4 months, 5 showed a 50% decrease in symptom scores and 33% were asymptomatic. Similar results were noted in patients treated for urethral syndrome. Misoprostol, an oral prostaglandin analog, demonstrated a 48% response in a 9-month open-label trial, although 64% of patients experience adverse drug effects (Kelly et al, 1998). A cytoprotective action was postulated as the mode of action. The **cysteinyl leukotriene D4 receptor antagonist montelukast,** a commonly used allergy medication, has shown potential benefits in a small, uncontrolled Danish study (Bouchelouche et al, 2001b).

Oral L-arginine, an over-the-counter amino acid preparation, was purported to increase nitric oxide–related enzymes and metabolites in the urine of IC patients and decrease symptoms (Smith et al, 1996; Smith et al, 1997), perhaps through relaxation of urinary tract smooth muscle. Later studies showed no change in bladder nitric oxide concentrations after treatment with L-arginine or any significant symptom improvement (Ehren et al, 1998; Korting et al, 1999). An open-label trial of the over-the-counter oral eucalyptus bioflavonoid Quercetin has suggested some efficacy (Katske et al, 2001).

Analgesics

The long-term, appropriate use of pain medications forms an integral part of the treatment of a chronic pain condition such as IC. Most patients can be helped markedly with medical pain management using pain medications commonly used for chronic neuropathic pain syndromes including antidepressants, anticonvulsants, and opioids (Wesselmann et al, 1997). Many nonopioid analgesics including acetaminophen and the nonsteroidal anti-inflammatory drugs (NSAIDs) and even antispasmodic agents (Rummans, 1994) have a place in therapy along with agents designed to specifically treat the disorder itself. Unlike opioids, with increasing doses acetaminophen, aspirin, and the other NSAIDs all reach a ceiling for their maximum analgesic effect ("Drugs for Pain," 1998). Gabapentin, introduced in 1994 as an anticonvulsant, has found efficacy in neuropathic pain disorders, including diabetic neuropathy (Backonja et al, 1998) and postherpetic neuralgia (Rowbotham et al, 1998). It demonstrates synergism with morphine in neuropathic pain (Gilron et al, 2005). It may give some benefit in chronic pelvic pain syndromes and PBS/IC (Sasaki et al, 2001).

With the results of major surgery anything but certain, the use of long-term opioid therapy in the rare patient who has failed all forms of conservative therapy over many years may also be considered. Opiates are seldom the first choice of analgesics in chronic pain states, but they should not be withheld if less powerful analgesics have failed (Portenoy et al, 1997; Bennett, 1999). This is a difficult decision that requires much thought and discussion between patient and urologist, and involvement of a pain specialist is indicated. A single practitioner has to take responsibility for pain treatment and write all prescriptions for pain medications (Brookoff, 1997). Opioids are effective for most forms of moderate and severe pain and have no ceiling effect other than that imposed by adverse effects. The common side effects include sedation, nausea, mild confusion, and pruritus. These are generally transient and easily managed. Respiratory depression is extremely rare if they are used as prescribed. Constipation is common, and a mild laxative is generally necessary. The major impediment to the proper use of these drugs when they are prescribed for long-term nonmalignant pain is the fear of addiction. Studies suggest the risk is low (Gourlay, 1994). The long-acting narcotic formulations that result in steady levels of drug over many hours are preferable.

Chronic pain patients often receive inadequate doses of short-acting pain medications, which put them on cycles of short-term relief, anxiety, and pain. It leads to doctor-shopping and drug-seeking behavior confused by physicians with drug addiction. Whereas physical dependence to opioids will be unavoidable, physical addiction, a chronic disorder characterized by the compulsive use of a substance resulting in physical, psychological, or social harm to the user and the continued use despite that harm, is rare. Chronic opioid therapy can be considered as a last resort in selected patients. It is best administered in a pain clinic setting, requiring frequent reassessment by both patient and physician (Portenoy and Foley, 1986).

INTRAVESICAL AND INTRADETRUSOR THERAPY (Table 10–12)

Intravesical lavage with one of a variety of preparations has remained a mainstay of treatment in the therapeutic armamentarium of IC. Perhaps the oldest of the intravesical therapies is *silver nitrate*. The use of silver nitrate has been

Table 10–12. Some Intravesical Medications That Have Been Used for Treatment of PBS/IC

Drug	Randomized Controlled Trial	% Success
Silver nitrate	No	60%
Clorpactin WCS-90	No	60%
Dimethylsulfoxide	Yes	70%
Bacillus Calmette-Guérin	Yes	No proven efficacy
Resiniferatoxin	Yes	No proven efficacy
Hyaluronic acid	Yes	No proven efficacy
Heparin	No	60%
Chondroitin sulfate	No	33%
Lidocaine	No	65%
Capsaicin	No	No demonstrated efficacy
Oxybutynin	No	Efficacy suggested
Doxorubicin	No	Anecdotal efficacy
Pentosan polysulfate	Yes	40%

Adapted from 3rd International Consultation on Incontinence.

attributed to Mercier (Pool and Rives, 1944), who reported in 1855 that excellent results with bladder instillations had been obtained in patients suffering from symptoms compatible with IC. Dodson (1926) advocated the use of solutions of silver nitrate in increasing strengths as the treatment of choice for this condition. Pool and Rives (1944) reported on 74 patients with IC treated with intravesical silver nitrate. The treatment was carried out as follows:

A urethral catheter is inserted and the contents of the bladder are evacuated. The bladder is then irrigated with a saturated solution of boric acid. Then 30 to 60 mL of a 1:5000 solution of silver nitrate is instilled into the bladder and permitted to remain there for 3 or 4 minutes if it does not cause intolerable irritation. At the end of this period the solution is permitted to run out through the catheter, which is then withdrawn. The patient usually experiences some dysuria and vesical irritability for 2 or 3 hours. Treatments are repeated every other day. At subsequent treatments, the concentration of silver nitrate in the solution is increased to 1:2500, 1:1000, 1:750, 1:500, 1:400, 1:200, and finally 1:100. If at any time the reaction is too severe, the concentration is increased more slowly.

The initial treatments are performed under general anesthesia, but later treatments are given on an outpatient basis. Ureteral reflux would be a contraindication, and it goes without saying that bladder biopsy would be contraindicated just before instillation for fear of extravasation. Twenty-three years later, Pool (1967) wrote that he still considered this treatment regimen the most efficacious form of treatment. He reported excellent results in 70% of patients with a mean response of 7.6 months. Burford and Burford (1958) reported a 14% cure rate and 79% improved figure. DeJuana and Everett (1977) had a 50% response rate in 102 patients.

O'Connor (1955) reported the use of intravesical *Clorpactin WCS 90*. Clorpactin is a generic term for closely related, highly reactive chemical compositions having a modified derivative of hypochlorous acid in a buffered base. Its activity is dependent on the liberation of hypochlorous acid and its resulting oxidizing effects, wetting and penetrating properties, and detergency. Wishard and associates (1957) treated 20 patients with 0.2% Clorpactin gently lavaged in the bladder for 3 to 5 minutes without anesthesia, of whom 14 reported subjective improvement. Murnaghan and coworkers (1970) noted improvement in 14 of 17 patients, although 10 required further treatment during the average 2-year follow-up. Most commonly, the treatments are given as described by Messing and Stamey (1978), using 0.4% solution administered at 10 cm H$_2$O under anesthesia. Multiple instillations can be given, with a 1-month pause after the first 2 instillations to await a therapeutic response. Their success rate was 72%, with average 6-month duration of response. La Rock and Sant (1995) noted a 50% to 55% meaningful improvement rate occurring within 4 to 6 weeks of treatment. A case of ureteral fibrosis complicating the treatment prompted the recommendation that vesicoureteral reflux be considered a contraindication to the procedure (Messing and Freiha, 1979). Our method of Clorpactin delivery is as follows:

Reflux is excluded with a cystogram. Under anesthesia the bladder is distended for 2 minutes at 60 to 80 cm H$_2$O and emptied. The perineum is shielded with a moistened towel. A solution of 0.4% freshly prepared Clorpactin (4 g in 1000 mL of sterile water) is instilled by gravity drainage (the Foley catheter held 10 cm above the level of the bladder) in 150- to 200-mL aliquots for a dwell time of 2 to 3 minutes and drained by gravity. This continues until the entire 1000-mL solution has been used. The bladder and introitus are then irrigated with normal saline, and the catheter is removed.

A mainstay of the treatment of IC is the intravesical instillation of *dimethyl sulfoxide (DMSO)* (Sant, 1987). DMSO is a product of the wood pulp industry and a derivative of lignin. It has exceptional solvent properties and is freely miscible with water, lipids, and organic agents. Pharmacologic properties include membrane penetration, enhanced drug absorption, anti-inflammatory action, analgesic action, collagen dissolution, muscle relaxation, and mast cell histamine release. In-vitro effects on bladder function belie its positive effects in vivo (Freedman et al, 1989), where histamine release has not been demonstrated after treatment (Stout et al, 1995). It has been suggested that DMSO actually desensitizes nociceptive pathways in the lower urinary tract (Birder et al, 1997). Tests for DMSO for treatment of human illness began in the 1960s in the areas of musculoskeletal inflammation and the cutaneous manifestations of scleroderma.

Stewart and colleagues (1968) are responsible for popularizing intravesical DMSO for IC. In the mid 1960s they applied it to the skin over the suprapubic area in a group of patients refractory to conventional forms of therapy. Results were poor, but intravesical delivery of 50 mL of a 50% solution instilled for 15 minutes by catheter and repeated at intervals of 2 to 4 weeks showed positive effects in 6 of 8 patients lasting 2 to 12 months. The lack of side effects, other than a garlic-like odor on the breath, or need for inpatient administration were significant breakthroughs over previous treatments. Further reports by this group confirmed safety and efficacy (Stewart et al, 1971, 1972; Stewart and Shirley, 1976; Shirley et al, 1978) with symptom-free intervals of 1 to 3 months in 73% of patients. Ek and colleagues (1978) reported a 70% success rate, but found most patients ultimately required re-treatment or further therapy with other modalities. Prospective series of Fowler (1981) and Barker and associates (1987) revealed symptomatic success rates of greater than 80%, although relapse was not uncommon. Fowler noted only

minimal improvements in functional bladder capacity and attributed the beneficial effects of DMSO to a direct effect on the sensory nerves of the bladder. Perez-Marrero and coworkers (1988) compared DMSO to saline and showed a 93% objective improvement and 53% subjective improvement compared with 35% and 18%, respectively, for saline. Patients with bladder instability do not respond (Emerson and Feltis, 1986).

With its ease of administration (Biggers, 1986), **lack of side effects, and dependable symptomatic results, DMSO certainly merits its place as a useful treatment for PBS/IC.** I generally administer 50 mL of 50% DMSO as a bladder "cocktail" with 10 mg of triamcinolone, 40,000 units of heparin, and 44 mEq of sodium bicarbonate. In-vivo studies on rat bladder strips exposed to various concentrations of DMSO for 7 minutes showed absence of electrical field stimulation contraction at a 40% concentration and diminished compliance at 30% concentration (Melchior et al, 2003). Concentrations of 25% or less had negligible effects in this model. How it relates to use of DMSO in humans is unknown. A rare case of eosinophilic cystitis has been reported after DMSO instillation (Abramov et al, 2004).

Exogenous glycosaminoglycans have been shown to be effective in providing an epithelial permeability barrier in bladders in which the epithelium has been injured with protamine (Nickel et al, 1998). *Heparin*, which can mimic the activity of the bladder's own mucopolysaccharide lining (Hanno et al, 1978), has anti-inflammatory effects as well as actions that inhibit fibroblast proliferation, angiogenesis, and smooth muscle cell proliferation. Because of its numerous effects, the possibility that heparin could be used for therapeutic reasons other than the control of coagulation has been the subject of much inquiry and speculation (Lane and Adams, 1993). Weaver and coworkers (1963) first reported intravesical heparin for IC treatment. Given intravesically, there is virtually no systemic absorption, even in an inflamed bladder (Caulfield et al, 1995). While uncontrolled studies suggested some beneficial effect for subcutaneous administration (Lose et al, 1983, 1985), the obvious risks of anticoagulation and osteoporosis have prevented this form of administration from undergoing further trials and general usage. Ten thousand units can be administered intravesically in sterile water either alone or with DMSO at varying intervals with good results reported (Perez-Marrero et al, 1993; 1994a). Kuo reported 50% or more improvement in the International Prostate Symptom Score in 29 of 40 women with IC treated with 25,000 units intravesically twice weekly for 3 months (Kuo, 2001). Parsons has used daily intravesical doses of 40,000 units of heparin in 20-mL sterile water administered by the patient daily and held for 30 to 60 minutes. "Reasonable improvement of symptoms" can be expected between 6 months and 2 years after starting therapy (Parsons, 2000). Adding alkalinized lidocaine to the heparin instillation provides better pain relief (Parsons, 2005). These encouraging outcomes must be kept in perspective, given that they are unproven by any placebo-controlled trial.

Another GAG analog, pentosan polysulfate, administered intravesically 300 mg twice weekly in 50 mL of normal saline, showed some modest benefit in a small trial (Bade et al, 1997). The nonsulfated GAG, hyaluronic acid, has also been used intravesically. Trials using 40 mg dissolved in 40-mL normal saline weekly for 4 to 6 weeks and then monthly treatments thereafter have had response rates varying from 71% (Morales et al, 1996) to 30% (Porru et al, 1997). In the summer of 2003, Bioniche Life Science and, in the spring of 2004, Seikagaku Corporation reported double-blind, placebo-controlled, multicenter clinical studies of their hyaluronic acid preparations (40 mg/mL or 200 mg/mL, respectively), and neither showed significant efficacy of sodium hyaluronate compared with placebo. These negative studies have not been published in peer-reviewed literature. Neither preparation has been approved for use for PBS/IC in the United States.

Hurst (2003) has shown by immunohistochemistry a deficit of chondroitin sulfate from the luminal bladder surface in IC patients. Small uncontrolled studies using intravesical chondroitin sulfate have shown success rates of 33% (Steinhoff et al, 2002) to 50% (Sorensen, 2003).

Doxorubicin (Khanna and Loose, 1990) and the mast cell stabilizer cromolyn sodium (Edwards et al, 1986; Kennelly and Konnak, 1995) have been tried in pilot trials with the promising results we come to expect in such studies. Follow-up studies are lacking, and these drugs have not become a part of the intravesical pharmacopoeia.

The use of intravesical bacillus Calmette-Guérin (BCG) for IC was first reported by Zeidman and colleagues in 1994. A subsequent randomized, prospective, double-blind, placebo-controlled trial of 30 patients treated weekly for 6 weeks and followed for a mean of 8 months noted a 60% response rate compared with a 27% placebo response (Peters et al, 1997). Surprisingly, BCG was tolerated as well as placebo. Even more surprisingly, 8 of 9 BCG responders continued to have an excellent response in all parameters measured at 27 months of follow-up (Peters et al, 1998). It is unclear how BCG achieved this result, but immunologic and/or anti-inflammatory mechanisms have been postulated (Peters et al, 1999). A double-blind crossover Swedish study comparing DMSO to BCG failed to substantiate BCG efficacy (Peeker et al, 2000c). A large multicenter randomized controlled trial by NIDDK comparing BCG to placebo found a 12% response rate for placebo compared with a 21% response for BCG. The small response rate failed to reach statistical significance at the $P = .05$ level, and this large study of 265 patients indicates that BCG has no place in the treatment of moderate to severe PBS/IC (Mayer and Interstitial Cystitis Clinical Trials Group, 2005). Although the BCG safety profile was considered acceptable in the NIDDK trial, adverse events were not uncommon, and rare hypersensitivity reactions to intravesical BCG can occur (Parker et al, 2004).

Efforts to bring new therapies directly to the bladder continue to be the focus of investigators. Oxybutynin has shown efficacy in preliminary studies when administered intravesically at doses of 10 mg dissolved in saline (Bade et al, 2000; Barbalias et al, 2000). Electromotive drug administration, the active transport of ionized drugs by the application of an electric current, using lidocaine and dexamethasone, has shown a 25% success rate up to 6 months after instillation (Rosamilia et al, 1997). A similar trial using repeated instillations noted success rates of 60% with a mean duration of 6.6 months (Riedl et al, 1997). Capsaicin, the main pungent ingredient in hot peppers of the genus *Capsicum,* is a specific neurotoxin that desensitizes C fiber afferent neurons. Resiniferatoxin, an ultrapotent analog of capsaicin, appears to have similar effects

with less of the acute pain and irritation associated with capsaicin application. Both compounds have been tested intravesically for the relief of detrusor overactivity (Chancellor and de Groat, 1999). Clinical trials for the use of these compounds in bladder pain and urgency/frequency could show this to be a new and viable treatment modality in the future, but current data on efficacy in IC are lacking (Lazzeri et al, 1996, 2000; Cruz et al, 1997). An unpublished phase 2 safety and proof of concept multicenter, placebo-controlled trial conducted by ICOS Corporation of Bothell, Washington, found no significant efficacy of resiniferatoxin compared with placebo, although no safety issues were identified (Interstitial Cystitis Association, 2004).

The therapeutic value of botulinum toxin type A (BTX-A) stems partially from its ability to temporarily inhibit acetylcholine release and cause flaccid paralysis in a dose-related manner. It can correct focal dystonia when injected into a muscle. In recent years there has been increasing evidence that BTX-A might also have analgesic properties (Rajkumar and Conn, 2004). Initially, this was thought to be due to relief of muscle spasm. However, botulinum has been shown to reduce peripheral sensitization by inhibiting the release of several neuronal signaling markers, including glutamate and substance P, and reducing c-*fos* gene expression. It may affect the sensory feedback loop to the central nervous system by decreased input from the muscle tissue, possibly by inhibiting acetylcholine release from gamma motor neurons innervating intrafusal fibers of the muscle spindle (Rosales et al, 1996). BTX-A has been used effectively for years in different conditions with muscular hypercontractions. Intradetrusor BTX administration blocks the acetic acid–induced calcitonin gene-related peptide (CGRP) release from afferent nerve terminals in the bladder mucosal layer in rats (Chuang et al, 2004). In an animal model of bladder permeability barrier disruption, intradetrusor BTX-A minimized bladder irritability and restored afferent neural responses to baseline levels (Vemulakonda et al, 2005). These results support clinical trials of BTX-A for the treatment of PBS/IC and other types of visceral pain (Chancellor and Yoshimura, 2004).

A multi-institutional case series using Botox or Dysport intradetrusor injections in 13 patients with refractory PBS/IC reported improvement in 9 patients. Improvements in symptoms lasted a mean of 3.72 months (range, 1 to 8 months). No systemic complications were observed, although 2 patients had a diminished flow with some need to strain to void (Smith et al, 2004). Rackley and colleagues at the Cleveland Clinic reported no change in objective or subjective outcome measures in a series of 10 PBS/IC patients in whom the trigone was spared in the injection technique (Rackley et al, 2005). At this time, Botox can be recommended for PBS/IC use only in the context of carefully controlled clinical trials.

NEUROMODULATION

As a chronic pain syndrome, it is reasonable to consider therapeutic options that directly interface with the nervous system in the treatment of PBS/IC. This approach is further supported by the association of pelvic floor dysfunction with pelvic pain syndromes (Zermann et al, 1999).

Pain diversion by *transcutaneous electrical nerve stimulation (TENS)* is routine in a variety of painful conditions. Fall and colleagues (1987) were the first to use electrical stimulation in IC, reporting on 14 patients treated successfully with long-term intravaginal stimulation and TENS (Fall et al, 1980). Subsequently, McGuire and associates (1983) noted improvement in 5 of 6 patients treated with electrical stimulation.

The primary intention in applying peripheral electrical nerve stimulation in IC is to relieve pain by stimulating myelinated afferents to activate segmental inhibitory circuits. As a secondary effect, urinary frequency may also be reduced. In the most complete review of the subject to date (Fall and Lindstrom, 1994), 33 patients with ulcerative IC and 27 patients with nonulcerative IC were treated by means of suprapubic TENS. Electrodes were positioned 10 to 15 cm apart immediately above the pubic symphysis. High- or low-frequency (2 to 50 Hz) TENS was employed. If there was no effect with high-frequency TENS after 1 month, low-frequency TENS was used. Thirty to 120 minutes of TENS was prescribed daily. Pain improved more than frequency. Good results or remission were described in 26% of nonulcer patients and in a surprising 54% of patients with ulcerative disease. The authors caution that the experience is based on open studies, relatively few patients, and the knowledge of a significant placebo effect with peripheral pain stimulation.

Acupuncture has been used to treat frequency, urgency, and dysuria (Chang, 1988). Twenty-two of 26 patients treated at the Sp. 6 point had clinically symptomatic improvement. A study looking at both acupuncture and TENS in IC showed limited effects of both modalities (Geirsson et al, 1993). *Lumbar epidural blockade* is the subject of a positive recent case report (Pelaez et al, 2004), but in an earlier series resulted in only short-term (mean 15 days) pain relief in IC (Irwin et al, 1993). An Australian double-blind placebo-controlled study of transdermal posterior tibial nerve laser therapy for IC showed no benefit in 56 patients when comparing active to placebo arms, but the placebo effect was remarkably strong, indicating the importance of such trials when evaluating invasive therapies (O'Reilly et al, 2004).

Direct sacral nerve stimulation has been explored in the treatment of IC and urgency/frequency and is referred to as neuromodulation, a technique whose urologic potential was developed through the basic and clinical research of Schmidt (1993). He and others have observed that patients who do best with this treatment modality are those who have identifiable pain *and* dysfunction in the pelvic muscles (Everaert et al, 2001; Siegel et al, 2001; Aboseif et al, 2002). Those patients reporting pelvic pain in the absence of demonstrable pelvic floor dysfunction and levator tenderness did poorly (Schmidt, 2001). As initially practiced, trial stimulation was performed with a percutaneous temporary electrode for a 3- to 4-day temporary stimulation period to access efficacy. The S3 nerve is most frequently used. A wire electrode is inserted into the foramen and connected to an external pulse generator (Medtronic Inc., Minneapolis, MN). If the trial is successful, the patient would be considered for implantation of a permanent neural prosthesis. More recently, a staged procedure has supplanted the traditional percutaneous approach, because the response to stimulation can be better assessed with more accurate lead placement and stability than through the more hit or miss percutaneous lead placement (Peters et al, 2003). Peters' test to implant rate increased from 52% to 94%. Other reports have noted a test to implant rate in the

percutaneous technique from 76% in 33 PBS/IC patients (Whitmore et al, 2003) to 40% in 211 patients with refractory urge incontinence, urgency-frequency syndrome, and urinary retention (Scheepens et al, 2002).

Neuromodulation has been shown to be effective in treating refractory urinary urge incontinence (Schmidt et al, 1999; Spinelli et al, 2001). Studies on therapeutic potential in PBS/IC followed (Van Kerrebroeck, 1999). The University of Maryland group described decrease in antiproliferative factor activity and normalization of HB-EGF levels in patients with successful test stimulation (Chai et al, 2000a). Peters and coworkers (2003) reported success in two thirds of PBS/IC patients with sacral nerve stimulation. Comiter (2003) found 17 of 25 patients were successful with test stimulation and went on to permanent implantation of the Interstim device (Medtronics, St. Paul, MN). Thirteen of 15 who underwent staged implantation were permanently implanted versus 4 of 10 undergoing percutaneous test stimulation. With a mean follow-up of 14 months, 16 of 17 patients were judged successful, giving intent to treat success rate of 64%. Although sacral neuromodulation can decrease narcotic requirements significantly in refractory PBS/IC, the majority of patients taking chronic narcotics for pain will likely continue to use them for pain relief even after implantation (Peters and Konstandt, 2004).

HYDRODISTENTION

Hydrodistention of the bladder under anesthesia, while technically a surgical treatment, is often the first therapeutic modality employed, often as a part of the diagnostic evaluation. Since there have been no standard methods of distention, results vary markedly. Frontz first suggested hydraulic overdistention of the bladder for IC in 1922, and Bumpus reported the first series 8 years later. Simple bladder filling at cystoscopy will give relief to some patients (Hald et al, 1986), whereas Dunn and colleagues (1977) reported on 25 patients who underwent distention under anesthesia to the level of the systolic blood pressure for up to 3 hours. Sixteen of the patients were symptom free with a mean follow-up of 14 months; 2 patients suffered bladder rupture. The bladder in IC patients can be very thin, and the possibility of perforation or rupture must always be kept in mind and discussed with the patient (Badenoch, 1971; Hamer et al, 1992). Prolonged distention probably has little or no benefit over a short-term distention measured in minutes (Taub and Stein 1994; McCahy and Styles, 1995). Using epidural anesthesia and a balloon distention technique to the mean arterial pressure for 3 hours continuously, Glemain and colleagues (2002) reported good but transient efficacy in patients with a bladder capacity of greater than 150 mL on predistention cystometry. In their prospective series of 30 patients, 18 had maintained a therapeutic response at 6 months and 13 at 1 year of follow-up. Moderate hematuria was almost universal, worsening of symptoms occurred in 5% of patients, and low back and hypogastric pain were common sequelae. There was one bladder rupture, one episode of sepsis, and one episode of prolonged retention.

Our method is to perform an initial cystoscopic examination (which is generally unremarkable), obtain urine for cytology, and distend the bladder for 1 to 2 minutes at a pressure of 80 cm H_2O. The bladder is emptied and then refilled to look for glomerulations or ulceration. A therapeutic hydraulic distention follows for another 8 minutes. Biopsy, if indicated, is performed after the second distention. Therapeutic responses in patients with a bladder capacity under anesthesia of less than 600 mL showed 26% with an excellent and 29% with a fair result compared with 12% excellent and 43% fair in patients with larger bladder capacities (Hanno and Wein, 1991). Most favorable responses were extremely brief, however, with the exceptional patient noting improvement for 6 months, thus being a candidate for repeat therapeutic distention.

Acute hydrodistention does not seem to result in any long-term bladder dysfunction (Kang et al, 1992; Lasanen et al, 1992). Any efficacy is probably related to damage to mucosal afferent nerve endings (Dunn et al, 1977). It has no benefits in patients with detrusor hyperreflexia or instability (Taub and Stein, 1994; McCahy and Styles, 1995). Over half of men with prostate pain and without bacteriuria may have glomerulations. Symptoms in this group have been reported to improve with hydrodistention (Berger et al, 1998). While many patients with IC have sensory urgency at awake capacities of less than 100 mL, hydrodistention under anesthesia seems to allow for "staging" of the disease, giving the clinician some idea of the capacity he or she has to work with conservative therapies. A capacity under anesthesia of under 200 mL would not bode well for the likelihood of success of medical therapy. Fortunately, these cases are relatively rare.

SURGICAL THERAPY

The surgical therapy of IC is an option after all trials of conservative treatment have failed, a point that cannot be overemphasized. IC, although a cause of significant morbidity, is a nonmalignant process with a temporary spontaneous remission rate of up to 50% (Held et al, 1990) **and does not directly result in mortality.** Deaths are either self-inflicted or the complications of therapy. Nowhere does the caveat "primum non nocere" bear more relevance; the treatment must be no worse than the disease process (Siegel et al, 1990). Surgery should be reserved for the motivated and well-informed patient who falls into the category of extremely severe, unresponsive disease, a group that comprises less than 10% of patients (Irwin and Galloway, 1994; Parsons, 2000).

Many surgical approaches have been employed for IC, and it is worth mentioning a few for historical perspective alone. Sympathectomy and intraspinal alcohol injections have been used to treat pelvic pain (Greenhill, 1947). Differential sacral neurotomy was reported in 3 patients with good results (Meirowsky, 1969) but, like most denervation procedures, never gained popularity because of subsequent poor results. Transvesical infiltration of the pelvic plexuses with phenol failed in 5 of 5 patients with IC (Blackford et al, 1984). With a significant complication rate of 17% (McInerney et al, 1991) it is rarely used. There are several reports on cystolysis going back to Richer in 1929 (Bourque, 1951). Worth and Turner-Warwick reported some short-term benefit, but unpredictable long-term results (Worth and Turner-Warwick, 1973; Worth, 1980). Freiha and Stamey (1979) used it in 6 IC patients with good results in 4. Albers and Geyer (1988) reported long-term follow-up in 11 IC patients and had only one success. Dener-

vation procedures have a notoriously high late-failure rate, and the procedure is not justified for IC (Walsh, 1985; Stone, 1991). In fact, Rogers (2003) has concluded that there exist no convincing clinical studies to recommend surgical procedures to interrupt visceral nerve pathways in women suffering with any type of chronic pelvic pain.

Transurethral resection of a Hunner's ulcer, as initially reported by Kerr (1971), can provide symptomatic relief. Fall (1985) resected ulcerated lesions in 30 patients resulting in initial disappearance of pain in all and a decrease in urinary frequency in 21. Similar results have been attained with the neodymium:yttrium-aluminum-garnet laser (Shanberg et al, 1985; Shanberg, 1989; Rofeim et al, 2001). Extreme caution is critical if using a laser in an IC bladder, because forward scatter through these thin bladders with resulting bowel injury is an ever-present danger. There would seem to be no justification in the literature for using the laser to treat areas of glomerulation or in the nonulcerative form of the disease (Shanberg and Malloy, 1997).

Supratrigonal cystectomy and the formation of an enterovesical anastomosis with bowel segments has been a popular surgical procedure for intractable IC. The diseased bladder is resected in its entirety, sparing only a 1-cm cuff around the trigone to which the bowel segment is anastomosed (Worth and Turner-Warwick, 1972; Irwin and Galloway, 1994). While it is not always clear in the literature how much bladder has been resected, the results reported using these procedures for IC have been mixed at best. Badenoch (1971) operated on 9 patients, with 4 becoming much worse and 3 ultimately undergoing urinary diversion. Flood and colleagues (1995) reviewed 122 augmentation procedures, 21 of which were done for IC. Patients with IC had the poorest results of any group, with only 10 having an "excellent" outcome. Wallack and colleagues (1975) reported two successes; Seddon and associates (1977) had success in 7 of 9 patients; and Freiha and coworkers (1980) ended up performing formal urinary diversion in 2 of 6 patients treated with augmentation cecocystoplasty. Weiss and associates (1984) had success in 3 of 7 patient treated with sigmoidocystoplasty, and Lunghi and colleagues (1984) had no excellent results in 2 patients with IC. Webster and Maggio (1989) reviewed their data in 19 patients and concluded that only patients with bladder capacities under anesthesia less than 350 mL should undergo substitution cystoplasty. Hughes and associates (1995) lowered the threshold to less than 250 mL.

More recent series on subtotal cystectomy plus augmentation have been somewhat more positive (Costello et al, 2000; Chesa et al, 2001). Peeker and associates (1998) had good results in all 10 patients with ulcerative IC but poor results in the 3 patients operated on with nonulcerative disease. They no longer perform the procedure in the latter group. Linn and colleagues (1998) had success in 20 of 23 patients (only 2 with ulcerative IC) treated with subtotal cystectomy and orthotopic bladder substitution with an ileocecal pouch. They recommend a supratrigonal cystectomy. A Spanish series reported success in 13 of 17 procedures with a mean follow-up of 94 months (Rodriguez Villamil et al, 1999). The University of Alabama group reported long-term success in 1 of 4 patients with orthotopic neobladders and 1 of 3 with augmentation cystoplasty (Lloyd, 1999). A German report on substitution cystoplasty sparing the trigone was quite enthusiastic, detailing a 78% pain-free rate in 18 patients treated with ileocecal augmentation (10) or ileal substitution (8) at a mean follow-up of 57 months (van Ophoven et al, 2002). Two patients failed to get any pain relief, and 4 required either long-term intermittent catheterization or suprapubic drainage to empty the neobladder.

Not all patients empty the bladder spontaneously after substitution cystoplasty. Although the need for clean intermittent catheterization would not obviate a successful outcome in the patient treated for bladder contraction from tuberculous cystitis, it can be a painful disaster in the IC patient. Nurse and colleagues (1991) have gone one step farther, recommending trigone biopsy before substitution cystoplasty. Diversion and/or total cystourethrectomy is recommended if the trigone is "affected" by IC. It is not clear how this is determined histologically, because IC has no pathognomonic findings by histology and generally is not a localized process. Nielsen and coworkers (1990) described 8 women treated with substitution cystoplasty. In 6 patients the procedure failed, and the results of postoperative biopsies from the trigone showed no difference in the amount of fibrosis, degree of degenerative changes in the muscle, and mast cell density between the 2 cured patients and the others.

There has been a controversy over whether the IC process can occur in a transposed bowel patch (McGuire et al, 1973; Kisman et al, 1991; Singh and Thomas, 1996), or even in the ureter (Smith and Christmas, 1996). If so, not only would this be a relative contraindication to the procedure, but it would also provide support for the view that a substance in the urine might be involved in pathogenesis. There is, however, evidence that inflammation and fibrosis are the usual reactions of bowel to exposure to urine and, therefore, pathologic findings alone would not be conclusive of spread of IC in those patients (MacDermott et al, 1990).

Augmentation cystoplasty has many potential complications from the rare incidence of bladder neoplasm (Golomb et al, 1989) to the more common complication of upper tract obstruction (Cheng and Whitfield, 1990). In the best of hands complications can involve almost 50% of patients, requiring surgical intervention in 25% (Khoury et al, 1992; Bunyaratavej et al, 1993). Whereas problems are more common in patients operated on for disorders other than IC, the risk-benefit ratio of substitution cystoplasty seems to have discouraged its use in the last several years.

Urinary diversion with or without cystourethrectomy is the ultimate surgical answer to the dilemma of IC, akin to cutting the "Gordian knot." If diversion alone is chosen, one must keep in mind potential problems that can befall the remaining bladder, including pyocystis, hemorrhage, severe pain, and unremitting feelings of incomplete emptying and spasm (Eigner and Freiha, 1990; Adeyoju et al, 1996). Bladder carcinoma has also been reported after urinary diversion but is not specifically associated with IC (Hanno and Tomaszewski, 1982). Cystourethrectomy is certainly indicated in patients who are miserable and have not only failed all other therapies but have demonstrated chronicity such that remission is considered extremely unlikely. Fortunately few patients fall into this category. Theoretically, conduit diversion seems to be reasonable if one is concerned about disease occurring in any continent storage type of reconstruction. The extended simple cystectomy performed for intractable IC may lend itself

to anterior enterocele formation from weakening of the anterior vaginal wall, and prevention of this entity is warranted at the time of cystectomy (Anderson et al, 1998).

Bejany and Politano (1995) reported excellent results in 5 patients treated with total bladder replacement and recommend neobladder reconstruction. Keselman and associates (1995) had 2 failures in 11 patients treated with continent diversion and attributed this to surgical complications. A Finnish group noted failure in 2 of 4 patients treated with cystectomy and conduit diversion because of persistent pain (Lilius et al, 1973). Baskin and Tanagho (1992) also cautioned about persistence of pelvic pain after cystectomy and continent diversion, discussing 3 such patients. A similar report followed (Irwin and Galloway, 1992). Webster and coworkers (1992) had 10 failures in 14 patients treated with urinary diversion and cystectourethrectomy. Ten patients had persistent pelvic pain, and 4 of them also complained of pouch pain. Only two patients had symptom resolution. An English study of 27 patients who underwent cystectomy and bladder replacement with a Kock pouch noted successful treatment of pain in all patients, but follow-up was limited (Christmas et al, 1996). Parsons (2000) suggests that pouch pain will occur in 40% to 50% of patients within 6 to 36 months of surgery.

Attempts have been made to improve results by limiting the operation to those without detrusor mastocytosis (Trinka et al, 1993) and those without "neuropathic pelvic pain" (Lotenfoe et al, 1995). Based on the experience of the past decades, it is unclear if these efforts will prove any more successful. It would seem that risks of failure peculiar to IC include both the development of pain over time in any continent storage mechanism that is constructed and the risk of phantom pain in the pelvis that persists despite the fact that the stimulus that initially activated the nociceptive neurons (diseased bladder) has been removed (Cross, 1994). Brookhoff (1997) has proposed trying a differential spinal anesthetic block before considering cystectomy. If the patient continues to perceive bladder pain after a spinal anesthetic at the T10 level, it can be taken as an indicator that the pain signal is being generated at a higher level in the spinal cord and that surgery on the bladder will not result in pain relief. Some patients with intractable urinary frequency will opt for simple conduit urinary diversion alone, feeling that their quality of life will be improved independent of the pain piece of the puzzle. Despite all of the problems, many patients will do well after major surgery and quality of life can measurably improve (Rupp et al, 2000). In the event of neobladder pain after subtotal cystectomy and enterocystoplasty or continent diversion, it appears safe to retubularize a previously used bowel segment to form a urinary conduit for a straightforward urinary diversion without significant risk of conduit pain (Elzawahri et al, 2004).

Forty years ago Pool (1967) recognized that "surgical treatment has not been the boon many had hoped it would be." "Diversion of the urine is not the entire answer to the situation. Removal of the lesion in the bladder has been of no benefit. Likewise, removal of almost the entire mobile portion of the bladder proved to be a failure." Blaivas and colleagues (2005) described results of augmentation enterocystoplasty and continent diversion in 76 consecutive patients with benign disease with a mean 9-year follow-up. All 7 patients with the diagnosis of IC were classified as failures whereas 67 of the remaining 69 patients were cured or improved. When one of the deans of major urologic reconstruction writes, "I find it very difficult to justify such extensive surgery (continent diversion, cystourethrectomy) with such limited results and for these reasons have not been involved in surgery for IC over the past 3 years" (Webster, 1993), it is obvious that one should think carefully and proceed with surgery only after a complete discussion with a very motivated and well-informed patient.

PRINCIPLES OF MANAGEMENT

The information currently available in the literature does not lend itself to easily formulating a diagnostic or treatment guideline. Different groups of "experts" would undoubtedly create different "best practices." The compromise approach devised by an experienced cross section of urologists and gynecologists from around the world at the International Consultation on Continence 2004 meeting in Monaco (Hanno et al, 2005) seems reasonable and allows for significant latitude in individual practice and to account for patient preference (Fig. 10–12).

KEY POINTS: PRINCIPLES OF MANAGEMENT

▪ History/Initial Assessment

Men or women with bladder pain, with or without a sensation of urgency, often with urinary frequency and nocturia (especially if drinking a normal amount of fluids) and no abnormal gynecologic findings to explain the symptoms should be evaluated for PBS/IC. The initial assessment consists of a frequency/volume chart, focused physical examination, urinalysis, and urine culture. Cytology and cystoscopy are recommended if clinically indicated.

Patients with infection should be treated and reassessed. Those with recurrent urinary infection, abnormal urinary cytology, and hematuria are evaluated with appropriate imaging and endoscopic procedures, and only if findings are unable to explain the symptoms are they diagnosed with PBS/IC.

▪ Initial Treatment

Patient education, dietary manipulation, nonprescription analgesics, and pelvic floor relaxation techniques comprise the initial management of PBS/IC. When these fail, or symptoms are severe and conservative management unlikely to succeed, oral medication or intravesical treatment can be prescribed.

▪ Secondary Assessment

If initial oral or intravesical therapy fails, or before beginning such therapy, it is reasonable to consider further evaluation that can include urodynamics, pelvic imaging, and cystoscopy with bladder distention and possible bladder biopsy under anesthesia. Findings of bladder overactivity suggest a trial of antimuscarinic therapy. Findings of Hunner's ulcer suggest therapy with transurethral fulguration or resection of the ulcer. Distention itself can have therapeutic benefit in up to one third of patients, although benefits rarely persist for longer than a few months.

▪ Refractory PBS/IC

Those patients with persistent, unacceptable symptoms despite oral and/or intravesical therapy are candidates for more aggressive modalities. These might include neuromodulation, pain clinic consultation, narcotic analgesia, and/or experimental protocols. The last step in treatment is usually some type of surgical intervention aimed at increasing the functional capacity of the bladder or diverting the urine stream. Augmentation (substitution) cystoplasty and urinary diversion with or without cystectomy have been used as a last resort with good results in selected patients.

▪ A Philosophy of Management

I believe that, because of the natural history of the disorder, it is best to cautiously progress through a variety of treatments. Whereas the shotgun approach, starting newly diagnosed patients on a variety of simultaneous medications, seems to have many adherents, employing (or adding) one treatment at a time makes the natural history of the disease itself an ally in the treatment process. One should encourage patients to maximize their activity and live as normal a life as possible, not becoming a prisoner of the condition. Although some activities or foods may aggravate symptoms, nothing has been shown to negatively affect the disease process itself. Therefore, patients should feel free to experiment and judge for themselves how to modify their lifestyle without the guilt that comes from feeling they have harmed themselves if symptoms flare. Dogmatic restriction and diet are to be avoided unless they are shown to improve symptoms in a particular patient.

URETHRAL SYNDROME

In 1945, the distinguished American physician Richard Cabot was quoted as having stated that "any pain within two feet of the female urethra for which one cannot find an adequate explanation should be suspected of coming from the female urethra" (Charlton, 1986). The term *urethral syndrome* was first mentioned in a clinicopathologic study of the female urethra in 1949 (Powell and Powell, 1949). It appeared in the British literature in 1965 when a group of New Zealand physicians used it to describe the 50% of their female patients with urinary symptoms without demonstrable infection (Gallagher et al, 1965). The urethral syndrome is a very nonspecific con-

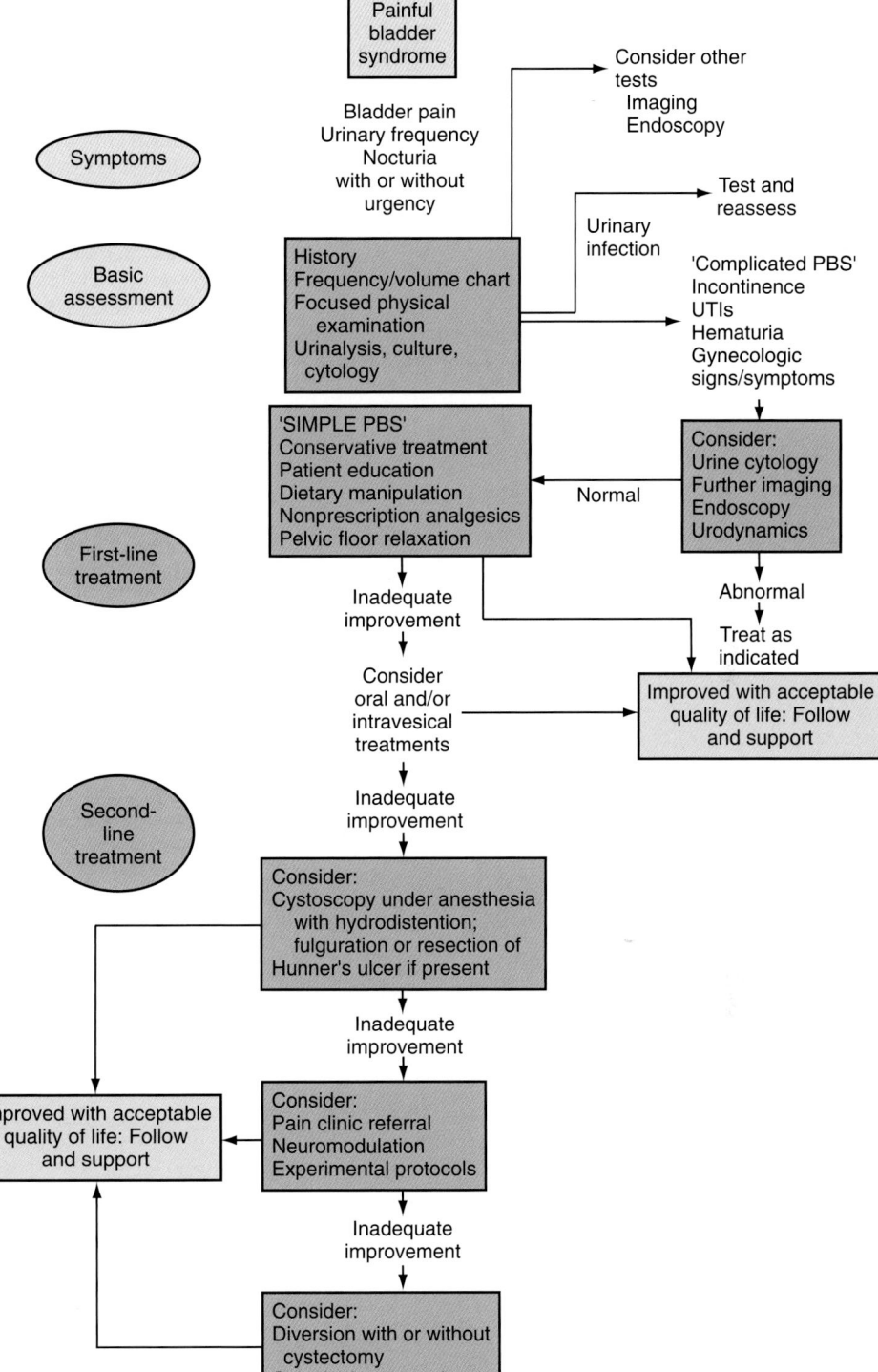

Figure 10–12. Suggested diagnosis and treatment algorithm for painful bladder syndrome. (From Hanno PM, Baranowski A, Fall M, et al: Painful bladder syndrome [including interstitial cystitis]. In Abrams P, Cardozo L, Khoury S, Wein A [eds]: Incontinence, 3rd ed. Paris, Health Publications, 2005, vol 2, pp 1456-1520.)

stellation of symptoms including urinary frequency, urgency, dysuria, and suprapubic discomfort without any objective findings of urologic abnormality to account for the symptoms. Although the symptoms are typically thought to occur in women, there is no reason to assume that a similar entity does not occur in men (Bodner, 1988; Hanno, 1995; Gittes and Nakamura, 1996). The frequency, urgency, and suprapubic, perineal, and low back pain of the chronic pelvic pain syn-

drome in men are certainly reminiscent of the urethral syndrome (Fowler, 1989; Gittes, 2002).

The urethral syndrome has been subdivided into an acute and a chronic condition. In the past, dysuric women with midstream urine cultures containing 10^5 bacteria/mL or greater were usually considered to have cystitis and those with lower-count bacterial cultures were said to have the urethral syndrome. Since about 1980, it has become apparent that infections of the urethra, urinary bladder, and vagina account for a large proportion of patients who develop the symptom-complex acutely. Therefore, the term *acute urethral syndrome,* implying as it does a mysterious cause and a urethral origin of the malady, has largely been abandoned in favor of identifiable etiologic diagnoses (Latham and Stamm, 1984; Hooton, 1988), many of which are found in the chapters on urinary tract infection and sexually transmitted diseases. Only a relatively small percentage of patients with acute urethral syndrome are found on investigation to have no cause for the

symptoms (Stamm et al, 1980; Stamm, 1987). It would be more accurate to categorize this group of patients by their symptoms than to give them a diagnosis of "acute urethral syndrome," which ultimately communicates little about the disorder.

Those patients with chronic symptoms and with no apparent cause constitute the *chronic urethral syndrome* category. This phantom diagnosis is one of exclusion and is rarely used in modern urologic texts. The symptomatic manifestations of IC and the chronic urethral syndrome are indistinguishable (Fowler, 1989; Hanno, 1995).

The concept of the urethral syndrome, chronic or acute, is now essentially a historical one and no longer alluded to in the modern medical literature. Some of the many causes of urinary frequency and urgency are listed in Table 10–13.

Table 10–13. Causes of Frequency and Urgency

Interstitial cystitis
Upper motor neuron lesion
Habit
Large fluid intake
Pregnancy
Bladder calculus
Urethral caruncle
Radiation cystitis
Large postvoid residual
Genital condylomata
Diabetes mellitus
Cervicitis
Periurethral gland infection
Atrophic urethral changes
Urinary tract infection
Chemical irritants: contraceptive foams, douches, diaphragm, obsessive washing
Overactive bladder
Vulvar carcinoma
Diuretic therapy
Bladder cancer
Urethral diverticulum
Pelvic mass
Chemotherapy
Bacterial urethritis
Renal impairment
Diabetes insipidus

SUGGESTED READINGS

Buffington CA, Chew DJ, DiBartola SP: On the definition of feline interstitial cystitis. J Am Vet Med Assoc 1999;215:186-188.
Elbadawi A: Interstitial cystitis: A critique of current concepts with a new proposal for pathologic diagnosis and pathogenesis. Urology 1997;49(Suppl):14-40.
Fall M, Johansson SL, Aldenborg F: Chronic interstitial cystitis: A heterogeneous syndrome. J Urol 1987;137:35-38.
Hand JR: Interstitial cystitis: Report of 223 cases (204 women and 19 men). J Urol 1949;61:291-310.
Hanno P, Baranowski A, Fall M, et al: Painful bladder syndrome (including interstitial cystitis). In Abrams PH, Wein AJ, Cardozo L (eds): Incontinence, 3rd ed. Paris, Health Publication, 2005, pp 1455-1520.
Keay S, Warren JW: A hypothesis for the etiology of interstitial cystitis based upon inhibition of bladder epithelial repair. Med Hypoth 1998;51:79-83.
Messing EM, Stamey TA: Interstitial cystitis: Early diagnosis, pathology, and treatment. Urology 1978;12:381-392.
Nordling J, Anjum FH, Bade JJ, et al: Primary evaluation of patients suspected of having interstitial cystitis (IC). Eur Urol 2004;45:662-669.
Oravisto KJ: Epidemiology of interstitial cystitis. Ann Chir Gynaecol Fenn 1975;64:75-77.
Parsons JK, Parsons CL: The historical origins of interstitial cystitis. J Urol 2004;171:20-22.
Pool TL: Interstitial cystitis: Clinical considerations and treatment. Clin Obstet Gynecol 1967;185-191.

11 Sexually Transmitted Diseases

TARA FRENKL, MD, MPH • JEANNETTE POTTS, MD

Screening and detecting sexually transmitted diseases (STDs) is a form of secondary prevention, which interrupts further transmission as well as progression of the infection and its sequelae. Unfortunately, primary prevention, by means of education and safe sex practices, has not been enough to significantly curb the prevalence and high cost of STDs.

People at high risk of contracting STDs are young adults between the ages of 18 and 28. It is also important to bear in mind that STDs rank among the top five risks of international travelers, along with diarrhea, hepatitis, and motor vehicle accidents (Mawhorter, 1997).

The brunt of the STD burden, both in risk and consequence, falls on women. When exposed to STDs, women are more likely to become infected and are much more likely to be asymptomatic. STDs can cause pelvic inflammatory disease, with subsequent risks of chronic pain syndromes, ectopic pregnancy, and infertility. Unfortunately, there is very little evidence that treatment will reverse the sequelae.

A urologist should have a high index of suspicion for underlying STD in women who present with recurrent urinary tract infections (UTIs) and in those who are symptomatic with sterile urine cultures. Up to 50% of women with signs of UTI during emergency department examination had subsequent positive cultures for STD (Berg et al, 1996). Physicians should maintain the same level of vigilance when treating women who have sex with women. Genital human papillomavirus (HPV) has been identified along with squamous intraepithelial lesions among lesbians and occurs among those who have not had sexual relations with men (Marrazzo et al, 1998).

Proctitis may occur in women and men who have anal sex. Causative organisms include *Neisseria gonorrhoeae, Chlamydia trachomatis, Treponema pallidum,* and herpes simplex virus (HSV). A discussion of human immunodeficiency virus (HIV) is beyond the scope of this chapter; however, it is important to remember that STDs—especially the ulcerative types—facilitate the transmission and infection of HIV. HSV type 2, in particular, may play a role in the transmission of HIV, because it has been identified more frequently than other STDs among HIV-concordant couples. Increased risk of HIV concordance has also been observed among couples who both have *Mycoplasma genitalium* antibodies (Perez et al, 1998).

New evidence is available that has shown that the spermicide nonoxynol-9 is not preventive against sexually transmitted infections and that frequent use may be actually detrimental by increasing the rate of genital ulceration and HIV transmission (Richardson, 2002).

It is imperative that the physician treating STDs make special efforts to be sure that his or her methods of diagnosis and treatment reflect the latest knowledge. To that end, the Centers for Disease Control and Prevention (CDC) periodically updates recommendations for STD treatment, which can be retrieved easily by checking the CDC website. Changes that occur in the interim will need to come from a review of current literature. The accurate diagnosis and treatment of a patient with an STD will allow the physician to treat not only the patient but also the sexual partner and possibly the couple's unborn children.

The most common STDs are discussed in the following pages. They include HSV, *Chlamydia* urethritis/cervicitis, lymphogranuloma venereum, syphilis, gonorrhea, chancroid, trichomoniasis, HPV, and scabies. Other sexually associated pathogens, which cause urethritis and vaginitides, are also discussed briefly.

EPIDEMIOLOGY AND TRENDS

It is estimated that over 15 million new cases of STDs are reported each year and over 65 million people are infected with incurable viral STDs (American Social Health Association, 1998). Approximately two thirds occur in adolescents and young adults. The most common STDs are HPV and HSV. **Of the top ten nationally notifiable infectious diseases in the United States in 2002, five were STDs** (CDC, 2003). This does not include HPV and HSV, because they are not reportable diseases.

The prevalence of HPV in the United States is approximately 20 million, and the incidence is 6.2 million. At least 50% of sexually active men and women acquire genital HPV infection at some point in their lives. By age 50, at least 80% of women will have acquired genital HPV infection (STD Facts, 2005).

In 2002, only 67 cases of chancroid were reported (CDC, 2003). Interesting, 76% were reported from the South Atlantic states, primarily from South Carolina. Overall, the rate of reported cases has declined 99% since 1987. *Haemophilus ducreyi* is difficult to culture, and therefore the infection could be underdiagnosed. Improved diagnostic testing by means of polymerase chain reaction (PCR) testing is now commercially available and may increase diagnostic capability.

The incidence of infection with *Chlamydia* has continued to rise since it became a notifiable disease in 1995. In 2003, 877,478 cases were reported to the CDC (CDC, 2004a). The reported number of cases of chlamydial infection was more than two times greater than the reported cases of gonorrhea. It is probable that this incidence is at least in part secondary to improved diagnostic ability and growth and implementation of screening programs in women.

Rates of gonorrhea have decreased slightly since 1998. Rates are particularly higher for non-Hispanic blacks (which is 24 times the rate for non-Hispanic whites) and for men who have sex with men (Fox et al, 2001; CDC, 2003). There has also been a significant increase in quinolone-resistant *N. gonorrhoeae*, especially in Hawaii and California. **Fluoroquinolones are not recommended for treatment of gonorrhea in these states or for individuals who may have acquired the infection in those states.**

The rates of primary and secondary syphilis have remained steady since 2000, with an incidence of 2.5/100,000 people in 2003, representing an increase from 2002 (CDC, 2004b). The rate has increased by 27% men and decreased by 21% among women. It has been proposed that this is secondary to outbreaks among males having sex with males in urban areas with high rates of coinfection with HIV and high-risk sexual behavior (CDC, 2002b). Rates continue to be particularly high in southern states and among African-Americans. During 2002-2003, primary and secondary syphilis cases declined 23.6% among women and 17.8% among African-Americans (CDC, 2004b). There is no evidence that screening high-risk individuals, including those with HIV or other STDs, or the general population reduces morbidity or mortality from syphilis. However, it has been shown that screening pregnant women reduces the prevalence of congenital syphilis (Coles et al, 1998).

Partner Notification

In the past, once an STD was reported to the health department, the health department notified past and present sexual partners of the patient. However, the increased incidence of HIV and threats of bioterrorism are competing for health department resources and many departments now only notify partners of patients with HIV or syphilis (Erbelding and Zenilman, 2005). Patients are now requested to notify their own partners, who are then expected to go for evaluation and treatment themselves. Problems with this proposal are evident, and already this concept has been shown to be ineffective (Macke and Maher, 1999). Golden and colleagues (2003) reported their success implementing an expedited treatment plan for partners that did not require medical evaluation. This was a randomized controlled trial in which patients in the expedited treatment group were given a "partner packet" of therapy to deliver to the partner themselves or, if they were unwilling to do so, the partner was notified by the physician staff and the packet was delivered by mail or could be picked up at a participating pharmacy. Both the patients and partners in the expedited treatment group had better outcomes than the control group. Although this approach is sensible, effective, and progressive, legal and clinical barriers may unfortunately prevent the widespread acceptance of this approach.

GENITAL ULCERS

Several sexually transmitted infections are clinically characterized by genital ulcers, most commonly HSV, syphilis, and chancroid. In 2002, it was estimated that over 45 million people had HSV whereas only 6862 cases of syphilis and 67 cases of chancroid were reported (CDC, 2003).

Although specificity for clinical diagnosis of genital ulcer disease is good (94% to 98%), sensitivity is quite low (31% to 35%) (DiCarlo and Martin, 1997). Inguinal lymph node findings did not contribute to diagnostic accuracy. Confirmatory cultures and serologic testing for syphilis, chancroid, and HSV should be performed whenever possible. Specifically, the CDC recommends (1) serology and either darkfield examination or direct immunofluorescence for *Treponema pallidum*, (2) culture or antigen test for HSV, and (3) culture for *H. ducreyi*. **One should bear in mind that patients may be coinfected with more than one STD. Approximately 10% of patients with chancroid are coinfected with HSV or syphilis.** HIV testing should also be considered in the management of patients with confirmed STD. Clinical characteristics of sexually transmitted genital ulcers are summarized in Table 11–1. Other causes that are not sexually transmitted, such as Behçet's syndrome, drug reaction, erythema multiforme, Crohn's disease, lichen planus, amebiasis, trauma, and carcinoma, must also be considered. **Empirical treatment for the most likely cause based on history and physical examination should be initiated as laboratory test results are pending.** If ulcers do not respond to therapy or appear unusual, a biopsy should be performed.

Table 11-1. Genital Ulcer Disease

Disease	Lesions	Lymphadenopathy	Systemic Symptoms
Primary syphilis	Painless, indurated, with a clean base, usually singular	Nontender, rubbery, nonsuppurative bilateral lymphadenopathy	None
Genital herpes	Painful vesicles, shallow, usually multiple	Tender, bilateral inguinal adenopathy	Present during primary infection
Chancroid	Tender papule, then painful, undermined purulent ulcer, single or multiple	Tender, regional, painful, suppurative nodes	None
Lymphogranuloma	Small, painless vesicle or papule progresses to an ulcer	Painful, matted, large nodes develop, with fistula tracts	Present after genital lesion heals

HERPES SIMPLEX VIRUS INFECTION

Diagnosis. Genital herpes infection is common, afflicting more than 50 million people in the United States. It is caused by HSV type 2 (HSV-2) in 85% to 90% of cases and HSV type 1 (HSV-1) in 10% to 15% of cases. HSV-1 is responsible for common cold sores but can be transmitted via oral secretions during oral-genital sex. Silent infection is common and may account for more than 75% of viral transmission (Langenberg et al, 1999). Up to 80% of women with HSV-2 antibodies have no history of clinical infection (White and Wardropper, 1997). The incubation period ranges from 1 to 26 days but is usually short, approximately 4 days. Nongenital infection of HSV-1 during childhood may be protective to some extent against subsequent genital HSV-2 infection in adults. When exposed to HSV-2, women with negative HSV-1 antibodies had a 32% risk of infection per year whereas women with positive antibodies had a 10% risk of infection per year (Baker, 1997).

Primary infection manifests as painful ulcers of the genitalia or anus and bilateral painful inguinal adenopathy. The initial presentations for HSV-1 and HSV-2 are the same. A group of vesicles on an erythematous base that does not follow a neural distribution is pathognomonic (Figs. 11–1 to 11–3). The differential diagnosis includes other STDs, such as primary syphilis and chancroid, as well as noninfectious disorders such as Crohn's disease, trauma, contact dermatitis, erythema multiforme, Reiter's syndrome, psoriasis, and lichen planus.

The initial infection is often associated with constitutional flulike symptoms. Sacral radiculomyelopathy is a rare manifestation of primary infection that has a greater association with primary anal HSV. Genital lesions, especially urethral lesions, may cause transient urinary retention in women. Recurrent episodes are usually less severe, involving only ulceration of the genital or anal area. Severe disease and complications of herpes include pneumonitis, disseminated infection, hepatitis, meningitis, and encephalitis. **Asymptomatic viral shedding can take place for up to 3 months after clinical presentation, thereby perpetuating risk of transmission** (Baker, 1997).

The diagnosis of genital herpes should not be made on clinical suspicion alone because the classic presentation of the ulcer occurs in only a small percentage of patients. **Women especially may present with atypical lesions such as abrasions, fissures, or itching** (Wald, 2004). Viral culture with subtyping has been the gold standard of diagnosis of herpes infection. Viral subtype should be determined in every patient because it important for prognosis and counseling. Women with HSV-2 have an average of four recurrences within the

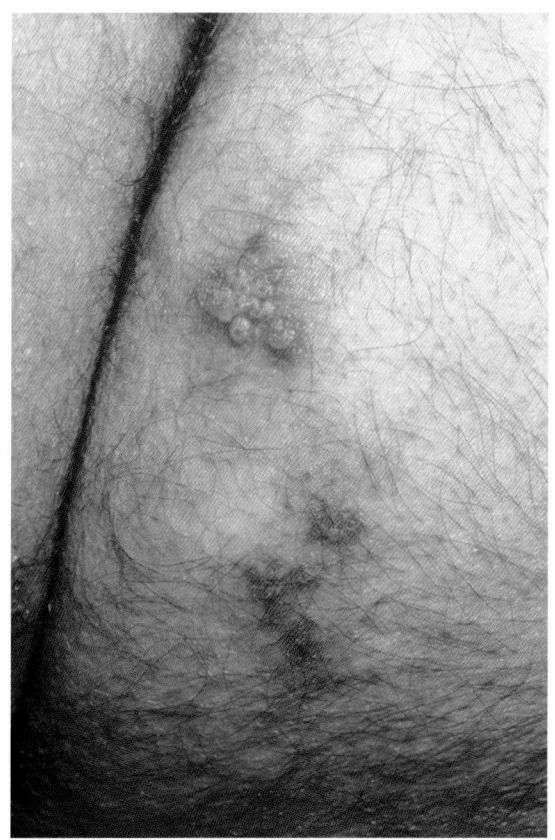

Figure 11–1. Typical vesicular eruption of herpes simplex virus.

first year, and women with HSV-1 have one recurrence in the first year. After the first year, HSV-1 rarely recurs while the rate of HSV-2 decreases but slowly (Bendedetti et al, 1994). Viral culture can generally isolate the virus in 5 days, is relatively inexpensive, and is highly specific. However, the sensitivity of viral culture ranges from 30% to 95% depending on the stage of the lesion and whether it is the primary infection or a recurrence. Viral load is highest when the lesion is vesicular and during primary infection. Therefore, viral culture has the highest sensitivity at these times and declines sharply as the lesion heals.

There are currently three U.S. Food and Drug Administration (FDA)-approved type-specific antibody assays (HerpeSelect HSV-1 and HSV-2 ELISA, HerpeSelect HSV-1 and HSV-2 Immunoblot, and Captia ELISA). These tests identify antibodies to HSV glycoproteins G-1 and G-2, which evoke a

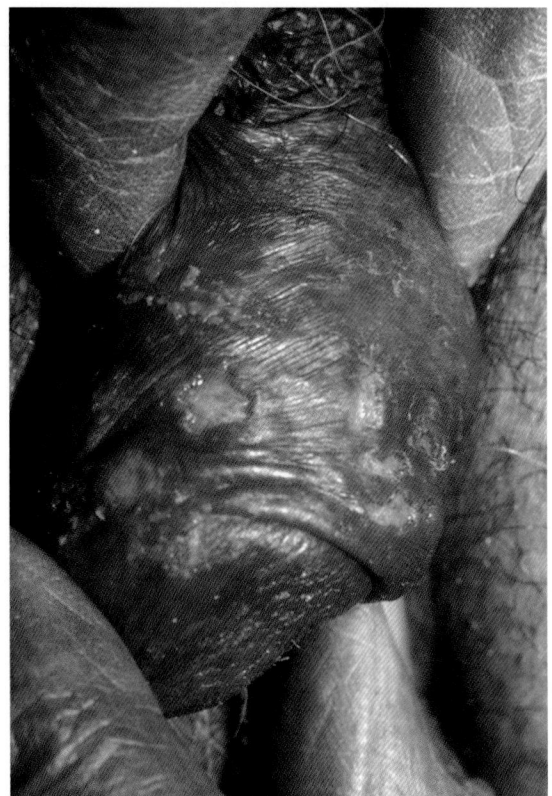

Figure 11–2. Herpes simplex virus infection on the penis.

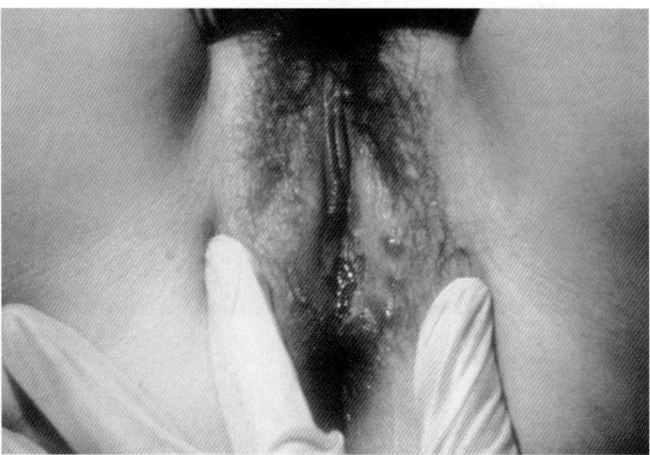

Figure 11–3. Vulvovaginal herpes simplex virus infection.

type-specific antibody response (Wald et al, 2002). These tests may also be able to identify recently acquired versus established HSV infection based on antibody avidity (Morrow et al, 2004).

Antigen detection kits are available but cannot distinguish reliably between HSV-1 and HSV-2. PCR testing has been shown to be 1.5 to 4 times as sensitive as viral culture, although no test is currently FDA approved. Samples are easy to attain and more stable than samples for viral culture. PCR testing will most likely replace viral culture as its availability increases and cost decreases.

Treatment. Antiviral therapies approved for treatment include oral acyclovir, valacyclovir, and famciclovir. Recommended antiviral regimens are listed in Table 11–2. **Topical antiviral medications are not effective.** Recurrences can be treated with an episodic or suppressive approach. When used for episodic treatment, medication must be initiated during the prodrome or within 1 day of the onset of lesions. Daily suppressive therapy has been shown to prevent 80% of recurrences and is an option for patients who suffer from frequent recurrences. It has been shown to decrease the frequency and duration of recurrences as well as viral shedding and therefore reduction in the rate of transmission. The safety and efficacy of daily suppressive therapy has been well documented.

CHANCROID

Diagnosis. Chancroid, caused by *Haemophilus ducreyi*, is the most common STD worldwide. It affects men three times more often than women. The incubation period ranges from 1 to 21 days. It causes a painful, nonindurated ulcer on the penis or vulvovaginal area. The ulcer has a friable base covered with a gray or yellow purulent exudate and a shaggy border. It can spread laterally by apposition to inner thighs and buttocks, especially in women. **It is associated with inguinal adenopathy that is typically unilateral and tender with tendency to become suppurative and fistulize** (Figs. 1–4 and 11–5). *H. ducreyi* is fastidious and difficult to culture. The special culture media is not widely available, and sensitivity of culture remains less than 80%. Gram stain of a specimen obtained from the undermined edge of the ulcer may be more helpful in identifying the short, fine, gram-negative streptobacilli, which are usually arranged in short, parallel chains. Recently, PCR assays have been shown to be a sensitive and specific means of detecting *H. ducreyi*. Although no PCR test is currently FDA approved, testing can be performed by com-

Table 11–2.	**Recommended Oral Treatment for Genital HSV Infection**		
Agent	*First Clinical Episode*	*Episodic Therapy*	*Suppressive Therapy*
Acyclovir	400 mg tid for 7-10 days *or* 200 mg five times a day for 7-10 days	400 mg tid for 5 days *or* 200 mg five times a day for 5 days *or* 800 mg bid for 5 days	400 mg bid
Famciclovir	250 mg bid for 7-10 days	125 mg bid for 5 days	250 mg bid
Valacyclovir	1 g bid for 7-10 days	500 mg bid for 3-5 days *or* 1 g/day for 5 days	500 mg/day *or* 1 g/day

Adapted from Centers for Disease Control and Prevention: Sexually transmitted diseases treatment guidelines 2002. MMWR Morbid Mortal Weekly Rep 2002;51(RR-6):14.

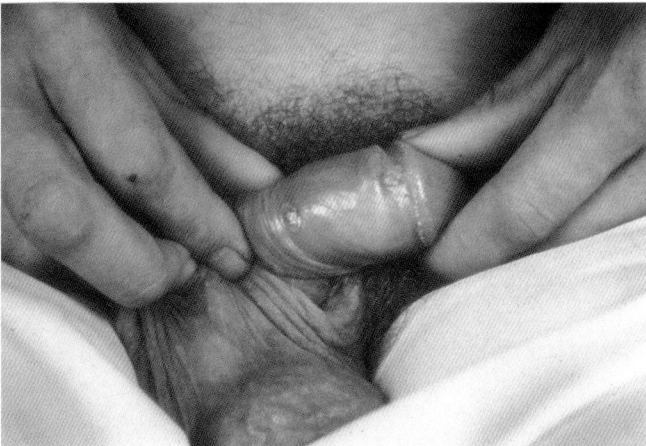

Figure 11–5. Chancroid lesion.

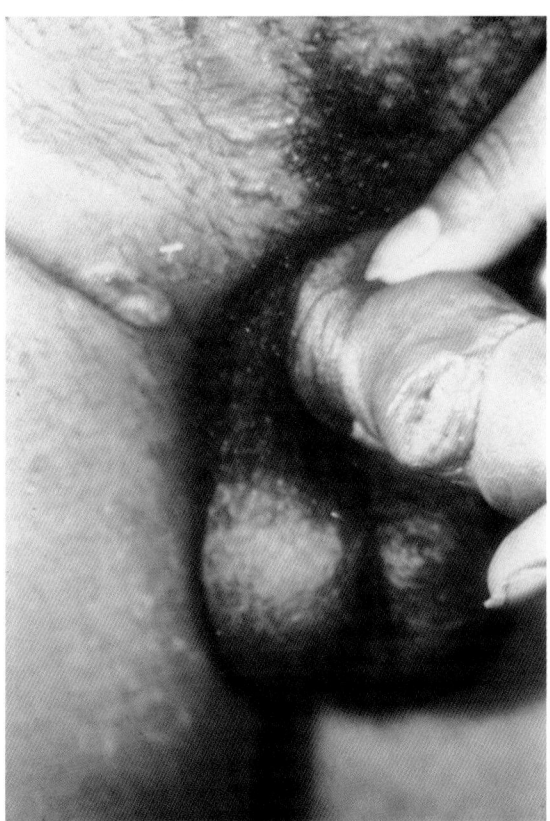

Figure 11–4. Chancroid with regional adenopathy.

mercial agencies. HIV and syphilis screening should be performed at the time of diagnosis and 3 months after treatment if initially negative.

Treatment. Single-dose treatments consist of azithromycin, 1 g orally, or ceftriaxone, 250 mg intramuscularly. Alternative regimens include ciprofloxacin, 500 mg twice daily for 3 days, or erythromycin base, 500 mg by mouth four times daily for 7 days. However, antibiotic susceptibility varies geographically. Resistance has been reported to ciprofloxacin and erythromycin in some regions. Ciprofloxacin is contraindicated during pregnancy and lactation. Subjective improvement should be noted within 3 days, and ulcers generally heal completely in 7 to 14 days. Healing may be slower in uncircumcised men with ulcers below the foreskin and in patients with HIV (Schmid, 1999). Patients should be reexamined in 5 to 7 days. Sexual partners should be examined and treated if sexual relations were held within 2 weeks before or during the eruption of the ulcer. Symptomatic relief of inguinal tenderness can be provided by needle aspiration or incision and drainage of the buboes.

SYPHILIS

Diagnosis. Syphilis is caused by the spirochete *Treponema pallidum.* Incubation periods range between 10 and 90 days. It is spread through contact with infectious lesions or body fluids. It can also be acquired in utero and through blood transfusion. Primary syphilis is characterized by a single painless, indurated ulcer occurring at the site of inoculation that

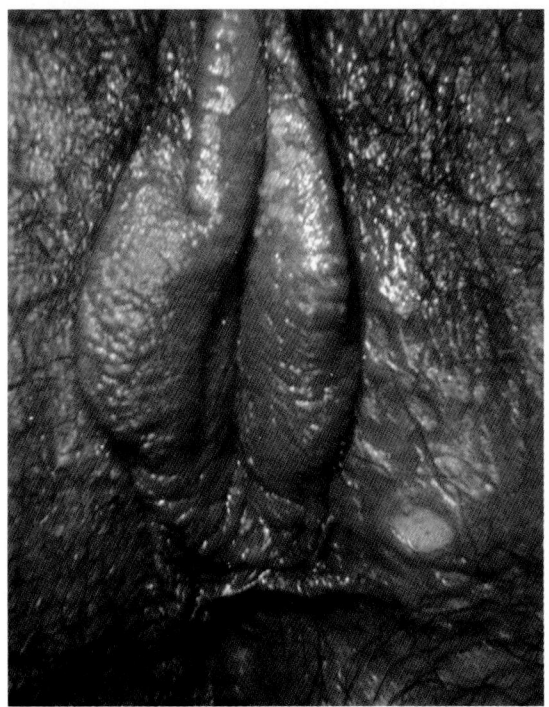

Figure 11–6. Syphilis with vulvar chancre.

appears about 3 weeks after inoculation and persists for 4 to 6 weeks (Figs. 11–6 and 11–7). The ulcer is typically found on the glans, corona, or perianal area on men and on the labial or anal area on women. It is often associated with bilateral, nontender inguinal or regional lymphadenopathy. Because the ulcer and adenopathy are painless and heal without treatment, primary syphilis often goes unnoticed.

Latent syphilis is defined as seroreactivity with no clinical evidence of disease. Early latent syphilis is latent syphilis acquired within the past year. All other latent syphilis is either referred to as late latent syphilis or latent syphilis of unknown duration.

Secondary syphilis usually begins 4 to 10 weeks after the appearance of the ulcer but may present as long as 24 months

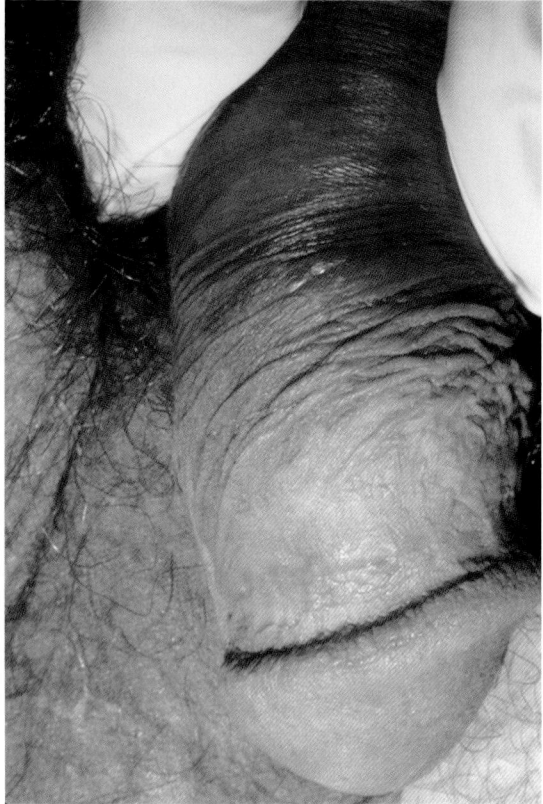

Figure 11–7. Syphilis with penile chancre.

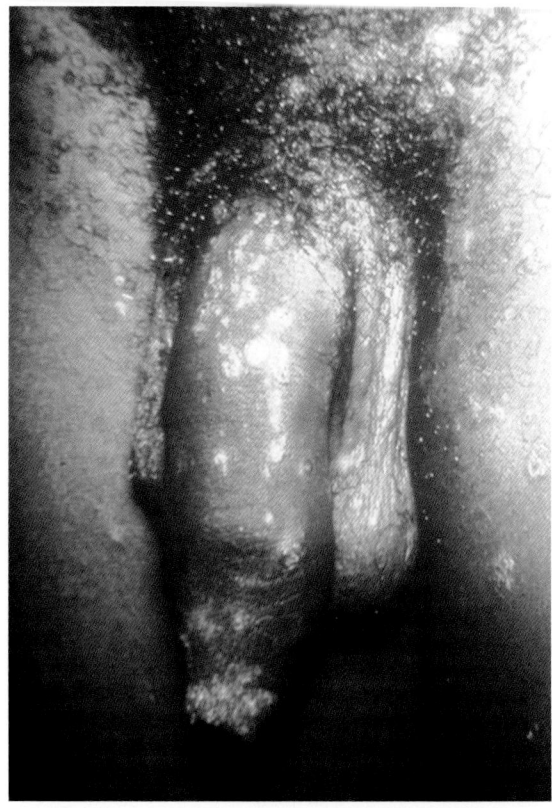

Figure 11–8. Secondary syphilis affecting the genitalia.

after the initial infection. Secondary syphilis manifests as mucocutaneous, constitutional, and parenchymal signs and symptoms (Figs. 11–8 and 11–9). Frequent early manifestations consist of maculopapular rash, which is commonly seen on the trunk and arms, and generalized nontender lymphadenopathy. After several days or weeks, a papular rash may accompany the primary rash. These papular lesions are associated with endarteritis and may therefore become necrotic and pustular. The distribution widens and commonly affects the palms and soles. **In the intertriginous areas, these papules may enlarge and erode to produce condyloma lata, which are particularly infectious.** Less common manifestations of secondary syphilis include hepatitis and immune complex–induced glomerulonephritis (Goldmeier and Guallar, 2003).

Approximately one third of untreated patients will develop tertiary syphilis. It is very rare in industrialized countries, except for occasional cases reported in HIV patients. **Syphilis is a systemic disease that can affect almost any organ or system, especially the cardiovascular, skeletal, and central nervous systems, and skin. Aortitis, meningitis, uveitis, optic neuritis, general paresis, tabes dorsalis, and gummas of the skin and skeleton are just some of the sequelae associated with tertiary syphilis.**

Darkfield microscopy and direct fluorescent antibody (DFA) tests specimens obtained from primary or secondary lesions. Darkfield microscopy is not widely available, but DFA testing of a fixed smear from a lesion can be performed at

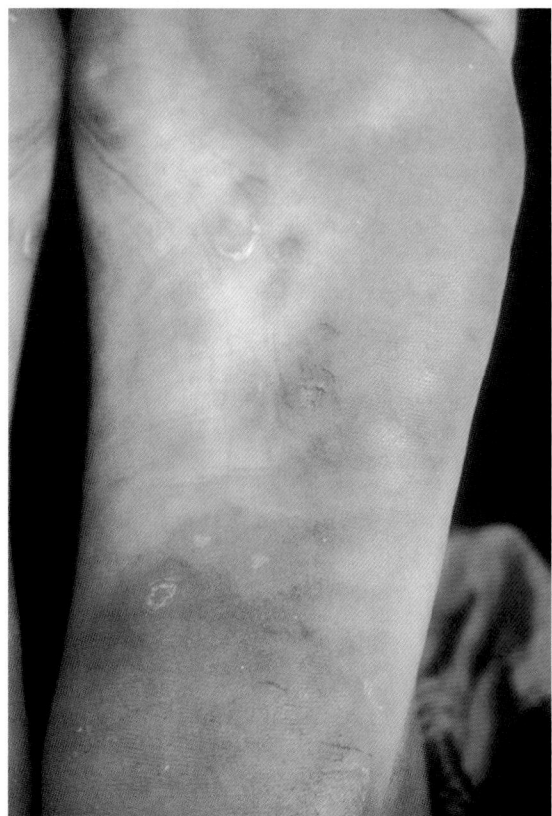

Figure 11–9. Secondary syphilis affecting the soles of the feet.

many commercial laboratories. Nontreponemal serologic testing with rapid plasma reagin (RPR) or Venereal Disease Research Laboratory (VDRL) are the most common methods of screening suspected individuals. Sensitivity is 78% and 86% for RPR and VDRL, respectively, in primary syphilis, 100% for both in secondary syphilis, and over 95% in tertiary syphilis (Hart, 1986). The false-positive rate is 1% to 2% and may be secondary to a large variety of causes (Golden et al, 2003). **Therefore, all positive tests should be confirmed with treponemal testing using *T. pallidum* particle agglutination (TP-PA) or fluorescent treponemal antibody absorbed (FTA-ABS) testing.** HIV can cause false-negative results by both treponemal and nontreponemal methods (Hicks et al, 1987; Erbelding et al, 1997). Positive treponemal antibody tests usually remain positive for life and do not correlate with disease activity. Nontreponemal antibody titers, RPR and VDRL, correlate with disease activity. These tests usually become negative 1 year after treatment. A low percentage of patients remain "serofast," never regaining a negative titer. A fourfold difference in titer is reflective of a clinically significant difference. A fourfold increase after therapy is indicative of ineffective therapy or reinfection (Johnson and Farnie, 1994). A fourfold decrease represents successful treatment. Following disease activity, the same test, either RPR or VDRL, should be performed at the same laboratory because the results are not interchangeable and may vary from laboratory to laboratory.

The U.S. Preventive Services Task Force recommends that pregnant women and people who are at higher risk for syphilis infection receive screening tests for the disease (Calonge, 2004). People at higher risk for syphilis include men who have sex with men and engage in high-risk sexual behavior, commercial sex workers, persons who exchange sex for drugs, and those in adult correctional facilities. The CDC recommends that HIV testing should be considered in the initial evaluation of all patients with syphilitic infection and that screening for hepatitis B and C, gonorrhea, and chlamydial infection also should be considered. The presence of chancres increases the risk of HIV acquisition twofold to fivefold (Greenblatt et al, 1988; Stamm et al, 1988).

Treatment. Benzthiazide penicillin G (2.4 million units intramuscularly as a single dose) remains the treatment of choice. Other parenteral preparations or oral penicillin are not acceptable substitutes. The **Jarisch-Herxheimer reaction** is a reaction consisting of headache, myalgia, fever, tachycardia, and increased respiratory rate that occurs within the first 24 hours after treatment with penicillin. Patients should be warned about the reaction, and it is usually managed with bedrest and nonsteroidal anti-inflammatory agents. It may cause fetal distress and preterm labor in pregnant women.

If the patient has penicillin allergy, doxycycline, 100 mg by mouth twice daily for 14 days, is an alternative. For late latent syphilis, latent syphilis of unknown duration, or tertiary syphilis, benzthiazide penicillin injection should be repeated weekly for a total of three doses or doxycycline therapy extended for a total of 4 weeks. In pregnancy, doxycycline should not be used and desensitization to penicillin is recommended if the patient has a penicillin allergy. Small

studies have shown that azithromycin or ceftriaxone may be potential alternatives for early syphilis, but insufficient data are available to make definitive recommendations (Augenbraun and Workowski, 1999; Gruber et al, 2000; Hook et al, 2002).

Tertiary syphilis is treated with aqueous crystalline penicillin G, 3 to 4 million units intravenously every 4 hours for 10 to 14 days, or with penicillin G procaine, 2.4 million units IM once daily, plus probenecid, 500 mg orally four times daily, with both drugs given for 10 to 14 days. Probenecid cannot be used in patients with an allergy to sulfa.

Patients should be followed with nontreponemal antibody titers at 6 and 12 month. Patients with HIV should be followed at 3, 6, 9, 12, and 24 months. A fourfold decrease in antibody titer is usually reflective of cure. The rate of treatment failure ranges from 4% to 21% (Parkes et al, 2004). Patients with treatment failure should be re-treated, and cerebrospinal fluid should be examined to exclude neurosyphilis. Patients with neurosyphilis require repeat examination of cerebrospinal fluid 3 to 6 months after therapy and every 6 months afterward until normal results are achieved.

LYMPHOGRANULOMA VENEREUM

Diagnosis. Lymphogranuloma venereum is caused by *Chlamydia trachomatis* types L1, L2, and L3 and is extremely rare in the United States. It still persists in parts of Africa, Asia, South America, and the Caribbean (Mabey and Peeling, 2002). The incubation period ranges from 3 to 30 days. The initial manifestation of infection is usually a single, painless ulcer on the penis, anus, or vulvovaginal area that goes unnoticed. **Patients usually present with painful unilateral suppurative inguinal adenopathy and constitutional symptoms that occur 2 to 6 weeks after resolution of the ulcer** (Figs. 11–10 and 11–11). Women and homosexual men may present with proctocolitis and perirectal or deep iliac lymph node enlargement if the primary lesion arises from the rectum or cervix. Significant tissue injury and scarring may occur, leading to labial fenestration, urethral destruction, anorectal fistulas, and elephantiasis of the penis, scrotum, or labia.

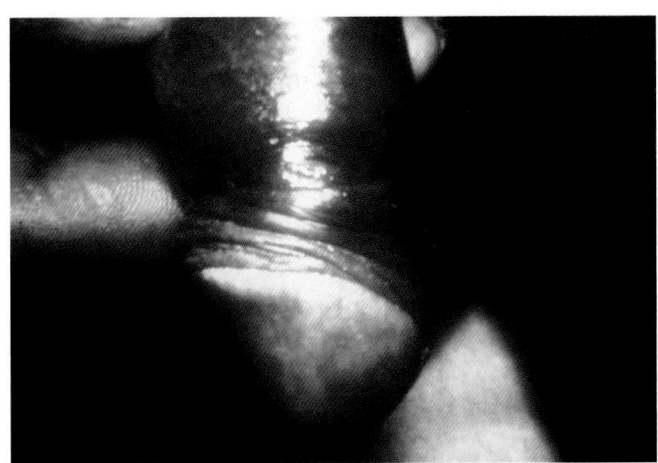

Figure 11–10. Lymphogranuloma venereum.

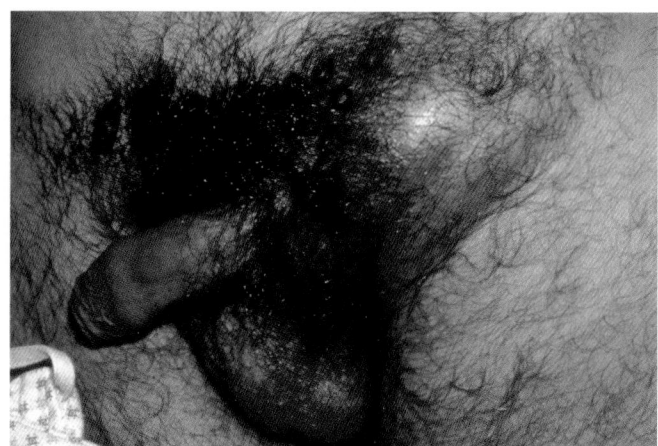

Figure 11–11. Lymphogranuloma venereum with inguinal adenopathy.

The diagnosis is mainly clinical, and cultures are positive in only 30% to 50% of cases. Complement fixation or indirect fluorescence antibody titers can confirm diagnosis. A complement fixation titer greater than 64 is diagnostic of infection. Other causes of inguinal adenopathy should be excluded.

Treatment. Antibiotic therapy for 3 weeks is necessary, using either doxycycline, 100 mg twice daily, or erythromycin, 500 mg four times daily. Doxycycline is contraindicated in pregnant and lactating women. Patients should be followed clinically until symptoms resolve. Sexual partners should be examined, tested for urethral or cervical infection, and treated if sexual relations were held within 30 days of the onset of symptoms.

CHLAMYDIA TRACHOMATIS INFECTION

Diagnosis. This is the most common bacterial STD in the United States and the most common worldwide. In the United States, it is most prevalent in sexually active adolescents and young adults. Virulent serotypes include D, E, F, G, H, I, J, and K. The incubation period ranges from 3 to 14 days.

The majority of both of men and women are asymptomatic. Approximately 50% of men experience lower urinary tract symptoms attributed to urethritis, epididymitis, or prostatitis and may notice clear or white urethral discharge. *C. trachomatis* is the most common cause of epididymitis in young men. Approximately 75% of women are asymptomatic and 40% with untreated infection will develop pelvic inflammatory disease (Rees, 1980). **The squamous cells of vaginal epithelium are relatively resistant to infection with *C. trachomatis*, but the columnar cells of the cervix are not. A mucopurulent endocervical discharge may be present.** Scarring of the fallopian tubes from chlamydial infection puts patients at risk for recurrent pelvic inflammatory disease with vaginal flora, ectopic pregnancy, pelvic pain, and infertility (Simms and Stephenson, 2000).

Chlamydia may also be transmitted to newborns during vaginal birth through exposure of the mother's infected cervix. Neonates may contract ocular, oropharyngeal, respiratory, urogenital, or rectal infection.

Selective screening has been shown to reduce the incidence of pelvic inflammatory disease (Scholes et al, 1996). Women should be screened annually until age 25 or if risk factors such as a new sexual partner are present. In women, screening may be accomplished by (1) a nucleic acid amplification test (NAAT) performed on an endocervical swab specimen, if a pelvic examination is acceptable; otherwise, an NAAT performed on urine; (2) an unamplified nucleic acid hybridization test, an enzyme immunoassay, or direct fluorescent antibody test performed on an endocervical swab specimen; or (3) culture performed on an endocervical swab specimen. In men, the options remain the same but intraurethral samples must be used.

NAATs utilizing PCR assays for urine are a highly sensitive and noninvasive means of screening men and women for chlamydial infection. NAATs have doubled the detection rate for asymptomatic infections compared with culture and antigen tests (Black et al, 2002; Watson et al, 2002). **This method should not replace pelvic examination or endocervical culture in symptomatic women because antibiotic sensitivity cannot be determined.** Specimens for culture can be obtained from urethral or cervical swabs, urine, or prostatic fluid. However, NAAT remains an alternative in patients when culture is not possible due to logistics or noncompliance. Urine NAAT is only slightly less sensitive than endocervical swab and because of its noninvasive nature can be used in venues where pelvic examinations are not performed, such as schools and prisons (Black et al, 2002). They may be used with urine or vaginal specimens but not oral or rectal samples. NAAT to test for cure should not be performed less than 3 weeks after treatment has been completed because dead organisms that may still be present will yield a false-positive test. NAATs are available that test for both infection with *Chlamydia* and *N. gonorrhoeae* from one sample. However, a positive result is nondiscriminatory between the two diseases and therefore further testing would be needed to determine which disease is present.

Treatment. Azithromycin, 1 g by mouth as a single dose, or doxycycline, 100 mg twice daily for 7 days, are primary treatments and equally effective. Alternative therapies include erythromycin base, 500 mg four times daily, erythromycin ethylsuccinate, 800 mg four times daily, ofloxacin, 300 mg twice daily, or levofloxacin, 500 mg daily for 7 days. Doxycycline, erythromycin estolate, and ofloxacin are contraindicated during pregnancy. Erythromycin base, erythromycin ethylsuccinate, and azithromycin are safe during pregnancy. Another alternative in pregnant women includes amoxicillin, 500 mg three times per day for 7 days. Partners should be examined, tested, and treated. Patients should refrain from sexual intercourse until both their and their partner's treatment is completed or 7 days after single-dose therapy. Reculture for cure is not needed for patients treated with doxycycline or a quinolone antibiotic. It is recommended 3 weeks after treatment with erythromycin because cure rates are lower with this regimen, in pregnant women, or if the patient has persistent symptoms. However, patients with *Chlamydia* are at high risk for reinfection and should be rescreened 3 to 4 months after treatment.

All sexual partners who came in contact with the patient within 60 days of diagnosis or symptom onset should be evaluated, tested, and treated for both *N. gonorrhoeae* and *C. trachomatis*. If more than 60 days has passed, the most recent sexual partner should be evaluated and treated. Sexual activity should be avoided until both partners complete treatment and are symptom free.

GONORRHEA

Diagnosis. Gonorrhea is caused by the gram-negative diplococcus *Neisseria gonorrhoeae*. The incubation period ranges from 3 to 14 days. Risk of infection after one exposure is 10% in men and 40% in women. Men will usually experience lower urinary tract symptoms attributed to urethritis, epididymitis, proctitis, or prostatitis, with associated mucopurulent urethral discharge. Women may have symptoms of vaginal and pelvic discomfort or dysuria. **As with *C. trachomatis*, the vaginal epithelium is resistant to infection with *N. gonorrhoeae* but the cervix is not. A mucopurulent endocervical discharge may be present. Many women are asymptomatic** (Table 11–3). Both symptomatic and asymptomatic infections can lead to pelvic inflammatory disease and its subsequent complications. Therefore, screening in all sexually active adolescents and women up to the age of 25 should be performed yearly. In addition, any women with risk factors such as a new sexual partner or multiple sexual partners should be screened. Manifestations of gonococcal dissemination are rare today and include arthritis, dermatitis, meningitis, and endocarditis.

The CDC recommends screening by culture on an endocervical swab specimen in women or an intraurethral swab in men (CDC, 2002c). Culture and sensitivity are important to monitor antibiotic susceptibility and resistance. Culture may be performed on urethra exudates if present. If transport and storage conditions are not conducive to maintaining the viability of *N. gonorrhoeae*, an NAAT or nucleic acid hybridization test can be performed. If it is not possible to obtain an intraurethral or endocervical specimen, NAAT may be performed on urine. Urine NAATs for *N. gonorrhoeae* have been shown to be less sensitive than endocervical and intraurethral swabs in asymptomatic men (Martin et al, 2000; Van der Pol et al, 2001).

Treatment. The most highly recommended treatment for gonorrhea is ceftriaxone, 125 mg intramuscularly as a single dose. It produces high, sustained blood levels that result in cure in over 99% of uncomplicated cases at all anatomic sites. Single oral-dose regimens including cefixime, 400 mg, ciprofloxacin, 500 mg, levofloxacin, 250 mg, or ofloxacin, 400 mg, have been shown to provide high cure rates of uncomplicated urogenital and anorectal infections. Cefixime, however, is no longer available in the United States. Other cephalosporins and quinolones have been shown to be effective but offer no advantage over the recommended regimens.

There has been growing concern regarding quinolone-resistant *N. gonorrhoeae*. **Areas where this organism is prevalent include parts of Asia, the Pacific, Hawaii, and California** (CDC, 2002). Quinolones are not advised as primary therapy in these regions or in patients who have had recent sexual encounters with people from these areas.

Quinolones are contraindicated during pregnancy. Spectinomycin, 2 g intramuscularly, can be used during pregnancy or in patients allergic to quinolones and cephalosporins. It is not as effective for pharyngeal infection.

Patients infected with gonorrhea are often coinfected with *C. trachomatis*. It has been recommended that patients undergo simultaneous dual treatment because the cost of treatment is less than that of chlamydial testing. Single-dose regimens given in the office also ensure compliance in patients who may otherwise not be able to afford the medication, comply with treatment, or return for follow-up. Patients undergoing dual therapy for chlamydial infection should receive azithromycin, 1.0 g as a single dose, or doxycycline, 100 mg twice a day for 7 days, in addition to one of the previously mentioned regimens for infection with *N. gonorrhoeae*.

All sexual partners who came in contact with the patient within 60 days of diagnosis or symptom onset should be evaluated, tested, and treated for both *N. gonorrhoeae* and *C. trachomatis*. If more than 60 days has passed, the most recent sexual partner should be evaluated and treated. Sexual activity should be avoided until both partners complete treatment and are symptom free.

Table 11–3. Differential Diagnosis of STDs in Women

	Vaginal Discharge	pH	WBC	Microscopy	Symptoms
Normal	White, thick, smooth	≤4.5	Absent	Lactobacilli	None
Candidiasis	White, thick, curdy	≤4.5	Absent	Mycelia	Vulvar pruritus, external or superificial dysuria
Trichomoniasis	Frothy or purulent	≥4.5	Present	Mobile trichomonads present, Amine odor	Vulvar erythema and edema, punctate strawberry lesions on cervix
Neisseria gonorrhoeae	None or mucopurulent discharge from cervicitis	≥4.5	Present	Gram-negative diplococci within or adjacent to polymorphonuclear leukocytes on Gram stain	Vaginal and pelvic discomfort, dysuria, most often asymptomatic
Chlamydia trachomatis	None or mucopurulent discharge from cervicitis	≥4.5	Present	Organisms not visualized	Vaginal and pelvic discomfort, dysuria, most often asymptomatic
Bacterial Vaginosis	Thin, white homogeneous	≥4.5	Absent	Paucity of lactobacilli (75% of patients), Amine odor, Clue cells	Fishy odor and increased vaginal discharge

TRICHOMONIASIS

Diagnosis. Trichomoniasis is one of the most common STDs, with approximately 174 million new cases reported worldwide each year and more than 8 million new cases reported yearly in North America (WHO, 1999). There is an increased incidence in developing countries and in women who have had multiple sexual partners. It is caused by the flagellated protozoan *Trichomonas vaginalis*, which can inhabit the vagina, urethra, Bartholin glands, Skene's glands, and prostate. It cannot infect the rectum or mouth. The human is its only known host. The incubation period ranges from 4 to 28 days.

It is typically asymptomatic in men but may produce short-lived symptoms of urethral discharge, dysuria, and urinary urgency. **Fifty percent of women are asymptomatic.** Clinical manifestations in women include the sudden onset of a frothy white or green, foul-smelling vaginal discharge, pruritus, and erythema. Other symptoms include dyspareunia, suprapubic discomfort, and urinary urgency. It has been associated with premature labor in pregnant women and with increased risk of HIV transmission (Cotch et al, 1997; Sorvillo et al, 1998).

Clinical examination may reveal a frothy discharge and the characteristic "strawberry vulva" or "strawberry cervix." However, clinical assessment alone is not specific enough for diagnosis. Typically, the vaginal discharge has an elevated pH. The motile protozoa, which are one to four times the size of polymorphonuclear cells, can also be seen on vaginal wet-mount smear or microscopic examination of urine. In men, the diagnosis is made with urethral culture or microscopic examination of the urine (preferably voiding bottle No. 1). Standard culture, transport culture kits, enzyme immunoassay, nucleic acid amplification, and immunofluorescence techniques are also available for confirmatory testing.

Treatment. Infected individuals and their sexual partners should be treated to prevent recurrence of infection. A single 2.0-g dose of metronidazole is effective in most cases and can be used in the second trimester of pregnancy. For nonpregnant treatment failures a longer course of metronidazole, 500 mg twice daily for 7 days, is recommended. The dosing regimens appear equally effective, but side effects, especially gastrointestinal side effects, are more common with the high-dose single therapy. Patients must abstain from alcohol consumption during therapy. Repeat testing at 5 to 7 days and 30 days should be performed if symptoms fail to resolve and treatment failure is suspected, and a course of metronidazole, 500 mg twice a day for 7 days, should be repeated, or 2 g once day for 3 to 5 days may be tried. Metronidazole gel for intravaginal application is available but is less than 50% effective as oral treatment. Patients allergic to metronidazole should be desensitized. **Clotrimazole and other agents have been tried as local intravaginal applications but have not been found to be effective** (duBouchet et al, 1997).

GENITAL WARTS

Diagnosis. Genital warts (condylomata acuminata) are caused by HPV. HPV is a DNA-containing virus that is spread by direct skin-to-skin contact. Over 100 types of HPV exist, and over 30 types can infect the genital area. Risk factors for acquiring HPV include multiple sexual partners, early age at onset of sexual intercourse, and having a sexual partner with HPV. Most infections are subclinical and asymptomatic. It has been shown that 60% of a group of female college students followed by Papanicolaou smear every 6 months for 3 years were infected with HPV at some point. The median duration of HPV infection was 8 months, with only 9% remaining infected after 2 years (Ho et al, 1998).

External visible warts are typically caused by HPV types 6 and 11. Patients may be infected with more than one type of HPV. Genital warts may appear anywhere on the external genitalia (Figs. 11–12 to 11–14). It has been suggested that inoculation occurs at the site of genital micro-trauma (Frydenberg and Malek, 1993). HPV has also been found on the cervix, vagina, urethra, anus, and on mucous membranes such as the conjunctiva, mouth, and nasal passages. Intra-anal warts are contracted via receptive anal sex. However, perianal warts are contracted by skin-to-skin contact and not exclusively through receptive anal intercourse.

Types 6 and 11 HPV are low risk for conversion to invasive carcinoma of the external genitalia. Some other types present in the anogenital region. Types 16, 18, 31, 33, 35, 39, 45, and 51 have been associated with cervical dysplasia and neoplasm in women and squamous intraepithelial neoplasia in men (Syrjanen 1981; Adam et al, 2000; Kulasingam et al, 2002). Over 99% of cervical cancers and 84% of anal cancers are

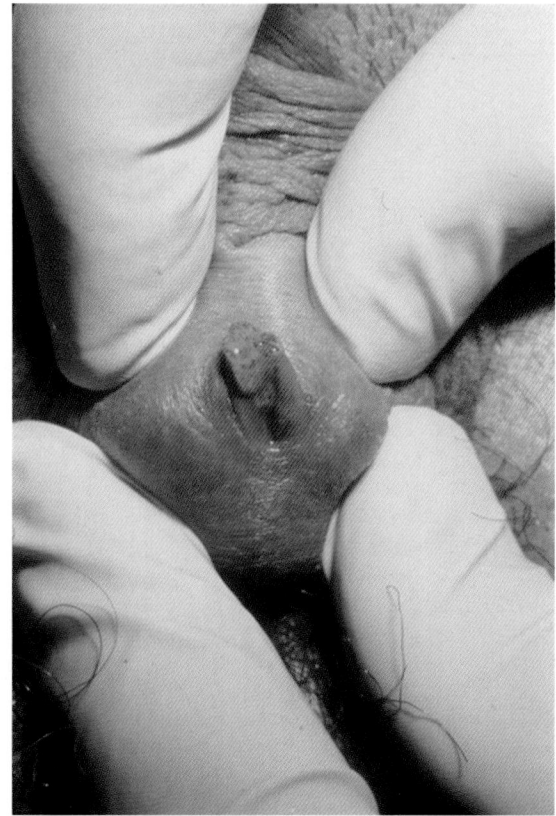

Figure 11–12. Meatal wart caused by human papillomavirus.

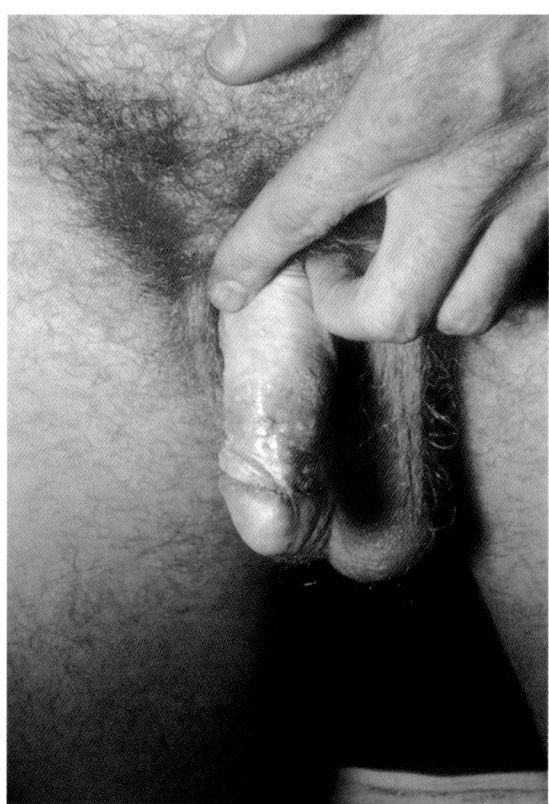

Figure 11–13.   Penile warts.

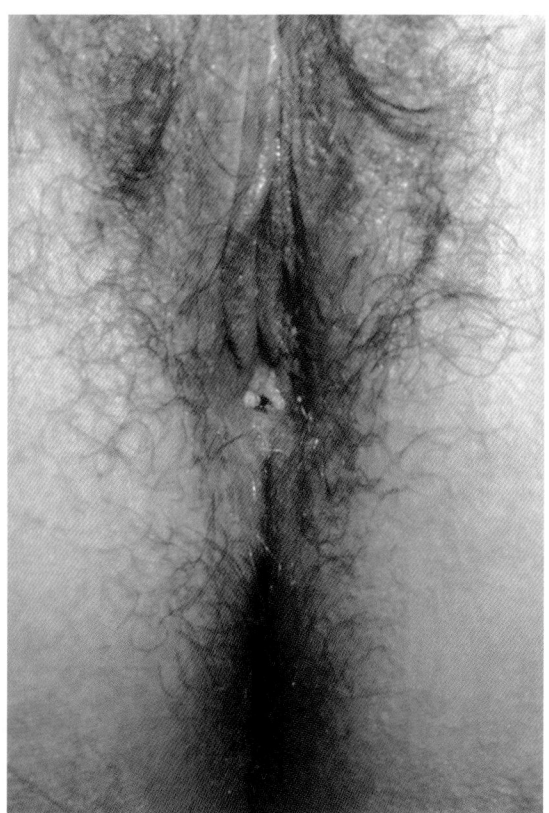

Figure 11–14.   Vaginal condylomata caused by human papillomavirus.

associated with HPV, most commonly HPV 16 and 18 (Frisch et al, 1997; Walboomers et al, 1999; Kulasingam et al, 2002). **Because HPV progresses rapidly in HIV-infected women, cervical cancer is considered one of the illnesses that defines the acquired immunodeficiency syndrome (AIDS).** Smoking may increase the risk of dysplastic progression and malignancy in both men and women.

In women, HPV may be associated with nonspecific symptoms, such as vulvodynia or pruritus. Malodorous vaginal discharge may also be a presenting sign, and the high rate of coinfection with other STDs observed in this setting may be a contributing factor.

The diagnosis is usually made through the visualization or palpation of nontender papillomatous genital lesions. Aceto-whitening with 3% to 5% acetic acid placed on a towel and wrapped around the genitalia may show subclinical, flat condylomata appearing as whitish areas. Using this method, it was shown that 50% to 77% of steady male partners of women with HPV infection and/or cervical neoplasia had subclinical HPV infection (Schneider et al, 1988). Conversely, female partners of men with genital warts have a high incidence of HPV infection (Campion et al, 1985). The benefit of evaluating and treating asymptomatic sexual partners of women with genital warts or abnormal Papanicolaou smears remains unclear. **Therefore, routine androscopy is not recommended.** Biopsies of genital warts are not routinely needed but should be undertaken in all instances of atypical, pigmented, indurated, fixed, or ulcerated warts. In addition, biopsy should be performed if the lesions persist or worsen after treatment and in immunocompromised patients.

Treatment. The CDC currently recommends that patients with genital warts be informed that HPV and recurrence is common among sexually active persons, the incubation period can be long and variable, and duration of infection and methods of prevention are not definitively known. The choice of therapy for genital warts depends on several factors, including wart size, number, and location, and patient and physician preference. Because genital warts spontaneously resolve with time, observation remains an option. Therapy can be patient applied or provider applied. Patient-applied therapies are less expensive and may be more effective than provider-applied therapy (Langley et al, 1999; Arican et al, 2004). Patients must be able to identify and access the lesion and be capable of carefully following the product instructions.

Recommended treatment choices for patient-applied therapy include podofilox 0.5% solution or gel and imiquimod 5% cream. Podofilox solution should be applied every 12 hours for 3 days, then off for 4 days with the option to repeat the treatment cycle four times. The total volume of solution used should not exceed 0.5 mL/day, and the total wart area should not be greater than 10 cm^2. It may be helpful to demonstrate the first application in the office. Imiquimod cream should be applied three times per week at bedtime for up to 16 weeks. The area should be thoroughly washed 6 to 10 hours after application. Imiquimod should not be used on vaginal lesions because it has been reported to cause chronic ulceration. Neither medication should be used in pregnancy.

Options for provider-applied therapy include cryotherapy with liquid nitrogen, electrosurgery, laser therapy, podophyllin resin 20% to 25%, trichloroacetic acid (TCA), or bichloroacetic acid (BCA) 80% to 90%, or surgical excision. Surgical excision may be accomplished by electrocautery or sharply with a tangential incision. Bleeding can generally be controlled with electrocautery or silver nitrate application. Surgical therapies appear to be equally effective with regard to clearance rates (Wiley et al, 2002). The advantages of surgical excision are that large warts or large areas can be addressed at one time. Carbon dioxide laser therapy is an alternative option for treatment.

Podophyllin 10% to 25% in compound tincture of benzoin is applied once and washed thoroughly 1 to 4 hours after treatment. Treatment may be repeated weekly as needed. Podophyllin is contraindicated during pregnancy. TCA and BCA should be carefully applied with a cotton-tipped applicator only to the warts at 1- to 2-week intervals. Patients will complain of a burning sensation, which should resolve in 2 to 5 minutes. Un-reacted acid should be removed with baking soda or talc. TCA and BCA are not recommended for keratinized or large warts. TCA is not absorbed and may be used during pregnancy.

Women with genital warts or a history of exposure should seek prompt gynecologic evaluation of the vagina and cervix. In the past, extensive vulvar lesions were treated with 5-fluorouracil cream but it was reported to cause ulceration and acquired adenosis and its use is no longer recommended.

Large or extensive lesions surrounding the meatus may herald the presence of urethral or bladder condylomata, warranting cystourethroscopy. Urethral or bladder lesions should be cystoscopically excised. Intraurethral 5% 5-fluorouracil cream used twice weekly may be useful. However, its use is limited by the great amount of inflammation produced. Cystoscopic evaluation should be considered with caution, because of the risk of transmitting the infection beyond the urethra and into the bladder. Considerations might include many and proximal urethral condylomata or other factors that would heighten suspicion for intravesical papillomas. We try to avoid traversing the external sphincter when performing limited urethroscopic examinations for the diagnosis of urethral condyloma or for the treatment of more distal lesions. Frequent serial ultrasounds of the distended bladder have been used for long-term surveillance of patients followed for recurrence of urethral condylomata.

Preliminary studies of prophylactic HPV-like particle vaccine have been performed with encouraging results (Evans et al, 2001; Ault et al, 2004). A vaccine containing eight of the most common HPV types associated with cancer could potentially prevent 95% of cervical cancer (Ault et al, 2004). Topical application of viable bacille Calmette-Guérin have also shown promising preliminary results, but larger studies are needed to fully evaluate its safety and efficacy (Metawea et al, 2005).

MOLLUSCUM CONTAGIOSUM

Diagnosis. Molluscum contagiosum virus (MCV) is a double-stranded DNA virus that belongs to the Poxviridae family and has worldwide geographic distribution. There are four known subtypes of MCV, but the subtype does not appear to influence disease presentation or course (Nakamura et al, 1995). MCV-1 is the most prevalent in the United States, whereas types 2 and 3 are more prevalent in Europe, Australia,

and in HIV-infected patients (Thompson et al, 1990, 1992; Porter and Archard, 1992). The incubation period ranges from 14 to 50 days (Fenner et al, 2001). MCV may be transmitted by skin-to-skin contact, fomites, or self-inoculation. It was once believed to cause only a benign, self-limiting childhood syndrome but is now also considered an STD in adolescents and adults. In children, lesions usually occur in clusters on the face and neck, chest, back, and extremities. In adults and adolescents, it is most commonly transmitted by sexual contact and lesions most frequently appear in the genital and inguinal regions, the inner thighs, and perineum. It less commonly affects mucosal areas such as the conjunctiva and oral mucosa. It should be remembered that in children it may spread by self-inoculation to the genital area.

MCV primarily infects the squamous epithelium and manifests as smooth, round, pearly papules, 2 to 5 mm in diameter, with a subtle central umbilication (Figs. 11–15 and 11–16). The lesions may have an erythematous or hypopigmented halo at the base. The papules are typically asymptomatic but may be associated with an eczematous, pruritic reaction. Giant lesions, more than 5 mm, can occur and seem to be more

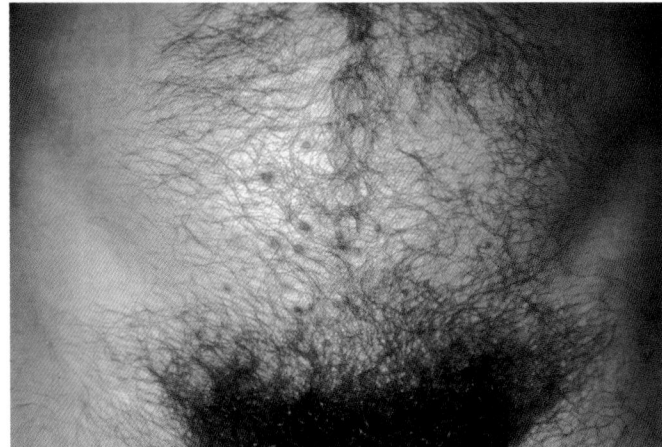

Figure 11–15. Molluscum contagiosum on abdomen.

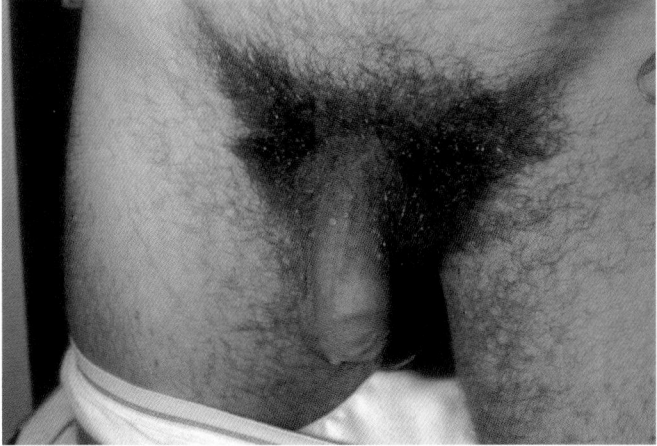

Figure 11–16. Molluscum contagiosum affecting penis.

common in immunocompromised patients. In immunocompetent persons the lesions usually spontaneously resolve within a few months and usually by 1 year but may take up to 5 years (Gottlieb and Myskowski, 1994; Smith et al, 1999).

Diagnosis is usually made on clinical suspicion and may be incidental. If confirmation is necessary, hematoxylin and eosin staining of a biopsy specimen may be performed. The presence of acidophilic, hyaline-filled Henderson-Patterson bodies, also known as molluscum contagiosum bodies, are pathognomonic. A squash preparation with methylene blue will also reveal the molluscum contagiosum bodies. It is recommended that the patients be tested for other STDs such as gonorrhea, chlamydia, and syphilis and carefully examined for coexistent condyloma acuminata and pediculosis pubis (Waugh, 1998). Careful consideration should also be given to HIV testing in patients with extensive multisite lesions, especially those involving the head and neck, and in lesions with a poor response to treatment.

Treatment. In most cases, MCV is benign and self-limiting and therefore requires no treatment. If the patient desires or if spread is of particular concern, destructive therapy with cautery, curettage, or cryotherapy with liquid nitrogen are sound options. All of these methods cause discomfort and may result in scarring. Lidocaine/prilocaine cream applied in an occlusive manner before the procedure should assist with discomfort. A topical antibiotic preparation should be applied afterward to prevent secondary infection.

Other topical therapies such as TCA, cantharidin, tretinoin, and podophyllotoxin have been reported for the treatment of MCV (Smith and Skelton, 2002). None is approved by the U.S. FDA for this indication, and all may result in pain and inflammation, especially in the genital area. Immunotherapy with imiquimod cream, either 1% or 5%, applied to lesions three times daily has been shown to be effective and appears especially useful in patients infected with HIV (Syed et al, 1998; Liota et al, 2000). Small studies in HIV-infected patients with recalcitrant lesions have also reported success with 1% cidofovir cream (Calista, 2000; Torro et al, 2000). Currently, cidofovir is commercially available only in an intravenous preparation.

SCABIES

Diagnosis. This infection is caused by the mite *Sarcoptes scabiei*. In adults, scabies is usually sexually transmitted, but this is not the case in children. The incubation period ranges from 2 to 6 weeks. Wavy, elongated papules are characteristic of the mite burrow. Eruption with pruritus is caused by an immune reaction to the mites, their eggs, and their feces. Susceptible areas include the penile shaft and glands, areolae, finger webs, and auxiliary folds (Fig. 11–17). Confirming the diagnosis may require microscopic evidence of the mite or eggs, which is retrieved by scraping the burrow with a scalpel blade coated with mineral oil. It can also usually be demonstrated if a thin shaving of skin from a papule is removed and placed on a glass slide and digested with heat and 10% potassium hydroxide.

Norwegian scabies, also known as crusted scabies, is caused by the same mite but occurs in immunocompromised or

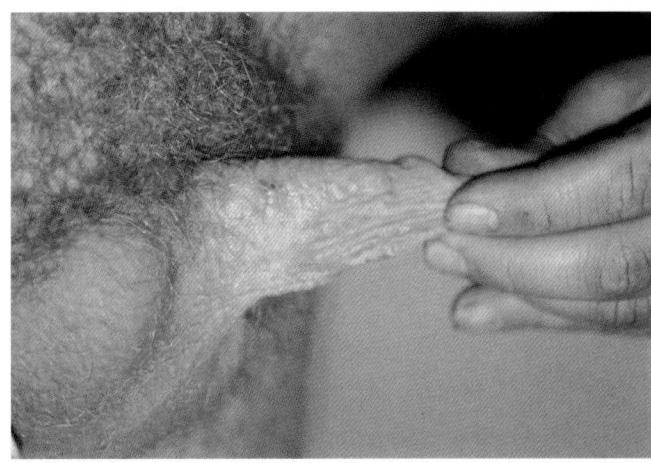

Figure 11–17. Scabies affecting shaft of penis.

debilitated persons. The parasite burden is much greater, resulting in many severe, deep, hyperkeratotic crusts that are characteristically less pruritic, most likely secondary to the host's immune compromise. The incubation period is shorter in patients with Norwegian scabies—usually less than 2 weeks (Kolar and Rapini, 1991).

Treatment. Permethrin cream (5%) should be applied to all areas of the body from the neck down and washed off 8 to 14 hours later. Alternative regimens include lindane (1%) lotion or cream applied in a similar fashion and removed after 8 hours. If necessary, treatment may be repeated in 1 week. **Lindane should not be used after a bath and is contraindicated in children younger than 2 years of age, pregnant and lactating women, and patients with extensive dermatitis.** Serious adverse side effects from lindane include seizures and aplastic anemia. An alternative to lotion or cream is oral ivermectin, 200 μg in a single dose, repeated 2 weeks later. Ivermectin therapy has been shown to be equally effective as permethrin cream and lindane lotion (Wendel and Rompalo, 2002). For young children or pregnant/lactating women, sulfur (3% to 6%) applied on 3 consecutive nights is an option. Sexual partners and close contacts should also be treated. Treatment of Norwegian scabies may require combined oral and topical therapy or repeated treatments. Lindane should be avoided in these patients because of their excessive dermatitis, which may lead to increased absorption.

Clothing or bed linen that may have been contaminated should be washed and dried by machine on a hot cycle or dry cleaned and removed from body contact for at least 72 hours. It should be noted that itching may persist for 2 to 3 weeks after adequate therapy.

PEDICULOSIS PUBIS

Diagnosis. Pediculosis pubis infection (phthiriasis, pubic lice) is caused by infection with the human louse *Phthirus pubis*. This species of lice has a proclivity for the pubic area, but the nits and lice can be seen in other areas with hair, such as the axilla, eyelashes, or scalp hair. The saliva of the lice causes a maculopapular or urticarial reaction in sensitized people and results in intense itching of the affected area. The presence of eggs (nits) attached to the hair shaft near the skin surface or the actual presence of an imbedded louse in the hair follicle is diagnostic. These lice can often be seen with the naked eye or with low-power magnification.

Treatment. Permethrin cream (5%) should be applied to all affected areas of the body and washed off 10 minutes later. Alternative regimens include lindane (1%) shampoo applied for 4 minutes and then thoroughly washed off. If necessary, treatment may be repeated in 1 week if symptoms persist. **Lindane should not be used after a bath and is contraindicated in children younger than 2 years of age and in pregnant or lactating women.** Although topical insecticidal preparations are the preferred treatment, trimethoprim-sulfamethoxazole can eliminate infections (Hutchinson and Farquhar, 1982). Pediculosis of the eyelashes is treated by applying an occlusive ophthalmic ointment, such as sterile petrolatum, to the eyelid margins two to three times a day for 10 days. Sexual partners within the past 30 days should also be treated. Clothing or bed linen that may have been contaminated should be washed and dried by machine on a hot cycle or dry cleaned and removed from body contact for at least 72 hours.

OVERVIEW OF OTHER SEXUALLY ASSOCIATED INFECTIONS
Mollicutes

Ureaplasma urealyticum, Mycoplasma hominis, and *Mycoplasma genitalium* are considered commensal organisms of the genital tract in both men and women. At least 60% of asymptomatic women have been shown to harbor *Ureaplasma* in their genital tract. **However, these organisms have also been implicated in cases of chronic prostatitis in men, urgency/frequency syndromes in women, and up to 40% of nongonococcal urethritis cases.** They have been isolated as the sole pathogen in symptomatic patients, who respond to antimicrobial therapy targeting these mollicutes. Women, especially young sexually active women, with urgency frequency syndrome with or without dysuria who have repeatedly negative urine cultures may benefit from culture and subsequent treatment for *Mycoplasma* and *Ureaplasma*. Culturing for this organism should also be considered in men with symptoms previously attributed to prostatitis or in men with prior history of STD exposure or infection.

Mollicutes have complex nutritional requirements and will not grow on routine culture medium. They cannot be visualized well with Gram stain. Confirming the presence of the organism from cervical, urethral, or urine specimens requires the visualization of characteristic colonies on specialized agar and color changes of urea broth. The organisms are highly sensitive to drying and must be promptly placed in the proper medium and delivered to the laboratory. If cultures are positive, treatment is recommended with subsequent surveillance for improvement in symptoms. Sexual partners should be evaluated and treated as well as refrain from sexual activity for 2 weeks during treatment.

Historically, this group of organisms was highly sensitive to tetracycline. Today, however, up to 30% of strains may be resistant, which may explain persistent symptoms in those patients treated empirically for nongonococcal urethritis or presumed *Chlamydia* infection. Most tetracycline-resistant strains remain sensitive to erythromycin. Currently, the initial recommended therapy is doxycycline, 100 mg twice daily for 2 weeks, or a single 1-g dose of azithromycin, which can be repeated after 10 to 14 days. Other alternatives include erythromycin, 500 mg four times daily, or ofloxacin, 300 mg twice daily for 10 to 14 days. Sexual partners should be evaluated and treated as well as refrain from sexual activity for 2 weeks during treatment.

Bacterial Vaginosis

Diagnosis. Bacterial vaginosis is caused by the overgrowth of *Gardnerella vaginalis,* anaerobic organisms, and *Mycoplasma hominis* and inhibition of normal vaginal flora, particularly *Lactobacillus.* The cause of disruption in the microflora has not been elucidated. Bacterial vaginosis increases a woman's risk of contracting infection with HIV, is associated with increased complications in pregnancy, and may be involved in the pathogenesis of pelvic inflammatory disease.

Patients may complain of a malodorous vaginal discharge, particularly after sexual intercourse, and nonspecific low-grade genital discomfort. Risk factors for bacterial vaginosis include an increased number of sexual partners, douching, abnormal uterine bleeding, and contraceptive use.

To examine vaginal discharge, a wet mount is performed by adding 2 drops of normal saline to the vaginal discharge on one microscope slide and 2 drops of 10% potassium hydroxide to another sample on a second slide. The whiff test is performed immediately after adding the potassium hydroxide. A fishy odor secondary to the release of amines is suggestive of bacterial vaginosis. The slide is then examined under the microscope using low and high power. Clue cells are white blood cells with bacteria attached to the cell membrane. Three of four of the following factors must be met to confirm the diagnosis: (1) thin, white vaginal discharge that covers the vagina, (2) vaginal pH greater than 4.5, (3) clue cells, and (4) positive whiff test. Vaginal cultures are not helpful in this setting; however, a Gram stain of the vaginal discharge can identify the relative change in concentrations of normal bacterial flora. There are commercially available DNA probes and card tests that can be useful for office diagnosis. Routine operative prophylaxis with metronidazole before hysterectomy has been shown to reduce postoperative infectious complications.

Treatment. Recommended primary therapy includes metronidazole, 500 mg twice daily for 7 days, clindamycin cream, 2% intravaginally at bedtime for 7 days, or metronidazole gel, 0.75% intravaginally at bedtime for 5 days. Alternative regimens include clindamycin, 300 mg by mouth twice daily for 1 week, metronidazole, 2 g in a single dose, and clindamycin ovules, 100 g intravaginally at bedtime for 3 days. Clindamycin cream and ovules may weaken latex condoms and diaphragms. Factors that disrupt the normal vaginal flora, such as douching, should be avoided. Treatment of the sexual partner has not been shown to prevent recurrence in two randomized trials and is therefore not recommended (Vejtorp et al, 1988; Colli et al, 1997).

Vulvovaginal Candidiasis

Vaginitis caused by *Candida albicans* is the most common type seen in the clinical setting but other species of *Candida* may also cause infection. The organism is present in the normal vagina and can also be found in the coronal sulcus of the penis. Sexual transmission with subsequent colonization and infection is possible. Predisposing factors for active infection include hormonal changes resulting from pregnancy or contraception, antibiotic use, systemic corticosteroids, or antimetabolites. Complicated vulvovaginal candidiasis is defined as recurrent, severe, non–*C. albicans* infections occurring in patients with altered immunity or pregnancy. Characteristically, thick, cheesy vaginal discharge is usually associated with vulvar irritation and itching. Patients may also experience vaginal discomfort, burning, dyspareunia, and external dysuria (CDC, 2002).

Diagnosis can be confirmed in a woman with signs and symptoms by findings of yeast or pseudohyphae on a wet preparation slide or Gram stain of the vaginal discharge. Often the yeast and pseudohyphae are seen better when 10% KOH is used. The pH of the vaginal discharge should be normal (<4.5). A vaginal culture may also be performed and is advised in patients with recurrent infections. Recurrent vulvovaginal candidiasis is defined as four or more episodes per year, and in 10% to 20% of patients *C. glabrata* and other candidal species are found.

Treatment. Over-the-counter antifungal vaginal creams, tablets, or suppositories of the topical azole class are generally effective, requiring 1- to 7-day regimens depending on the agent and dosage form. Treatment agents include butoconazole, clotrimazole, miconazole, and terconazole. The vaginal preparations may weaken latex condoms. An alternative to vaginal creams that is both effective and economical is fluconazole, 150 mg, as a single oral dose (Miller, 1997).

Recurring infections or complicated vulvovaginal candidiasis may require extended treatment of 14 days with vaginal preparations. Oral fluconazole therapy repeated 3 days after the initial dose also increases efficacy. Patients suffering from recurrent candidal vulvovaginitis require further evaluation to exclude HIV infection, diabetes, or other immune-compromised states, although in most women no cause is found. These patients often do well with maintenance therapy, but 30% to 40% will have recurrence once maintenance therapy is stopped. Treatment of sexual partners is not suggested in general but may be considered in patients with recurrent infections.

KEY POINTS: SEXUALLY TRANSMITTED DISEASES

- Bacterial STDs are decreasing in prevalence whereas the prevalence of viral STDs has increased significantly in recent years.

- The differential diagnosis for genital ulcers includes the following STDs: syphilis, chancroid, lymphogranuloma venereum, herpes simplex virus. Other causes also include diseases not transmittable through sexual activity: Behçet's syndrome, drug reaction, erythema multiforme, Crohn's disease, lichen planus, amebiasis, trauma, and carcinoma.

- Sensitivity of diagnosis made solely on the appearance of genitourinary ulcers is 35% at best.

- Confirmatory testing made by cultures, PCR, or serologic studies are important for appropriate treatment and eradication of the disease in both patients and their partner(s).

- Empirical treatments for vaginitides should be done with caution because the differential diagnosis is quite extensive. Women with chronic lower urinary tract symptoms should be thoroughly examined to exclude the possibility of vaginal pathology and/or STDs.

- The physician treating STDs should make special efforts to be sure that his or her methods of diagnosis and treatment reflect the latest knowledge. The CDC periodically updates its website with recommendations for STD treatment, since this topic has rapidly changing epidemiologic characteristics and treatment trends based on newly resistant strains.

SUGGESTED READINGS

Retiano M: Counseling patients with genital warts. Am J Med 1997;102:38-43.

STD Facts—Human Papilloma Virus. Available at CDC.gov/std/hpv/stdfact-hpv 2005.

Sulak PJ: Sexually transmitted diseases. Semin Reprod Med 2003;21:399-413.

White C, Wardropper AG: Genital herpes simplex infection in women. Clin Dermatol 1997;15:81-91.

12

Urologic Implications of AIDS and HIV Infection

JOHN N. KRIEGER, MD

HIV/AIDS EPIDEMIOLOGY

HIV VIROLOGY AND TARGETS FOR ANTIVIRAL THERAPY

PATHOGENESIS OF HIV INFECTION

TESTS TO DIAGNOSE AND MONITOR HIV INFECTION: WHAT THE UROLOGIST SHOULD KNOW

UROLOGIC MANIFESTATIONS OF HIV INFECTION

OCCUPATIONAL RISKS FOR HIV INFECTION IN UROLOGY

ANTIRETROVIRAL THERAPY

The acquired immunodeficiency syndrome (AIDS) is the most severe manifestation of infection with human immuno-deficiency virus (HIV). AIDS is defined by development of serious opportunistic infections, neoplasms, or other life-threatening conditions resulting from progressive immuno-suppression caused by HIV infection.

The first AIDS cases were described in 1981, and the number increased rapidly (Steinbrook, 2004; WHO, 2004). An estimated 34.6 to 42.3 million people worldwide are living with HIV infection. More than 20 million have died of AIDS (Joint United Nations Program on HIV/AIDS, 2004). In 2003 alone, 4.8 million people were infected and 2.9 million died of AIDS. Of all people 15 to 49 years of age worldwide, 1.1% are now infected with HIV (Steinbrook, 2004).

HIV/AIDS EPIDEMIOLOGY

In less than 15 years HIV reached pandemic proportions, with AIDS reported in over 190 countries (UNAIDS/WHO, 2001). It is also increasingly clear that the HIV pandemic consists of multiple separate epidemics, each with distinct characteristics. On a world scale, the epidemic has evolved predominantly into a heterosexually transmitted disease in the developing world and, increasingly, of underprivileged and marginalized populations in the industrialized world.

The impact of HIV infection is much different in the developing world than in the industrialized world. **At one time, AIDS was the leading cause of death among 25- to 44-year old men in Western European and North American cities and was the third most common cause of death for young women** (Carael et al 2004;Steinbrook, 2004). **With effective antiretroviral therapy, deaths attributed to AIDS are declining rapidly.**

By contrast, in many African cities AIDS represents the leading cause of death and of years of potential lost in men and the second most important cause of death in women. Life expectancy in the most affected sub-Saharan countries was reduced as much as 15 years by the year 2000, compared with projections without HIV infection.

Worldwide Perspective

The three main modes of HIV transmission have changed little: unprotected intercourse, contact with blood, and transmission from mother to child. Direct blood contact, such as sharing drug-injection equipment, results in the most efficient transmission. Globally, unprotected sexual intercourse between men and women is the predominant mode of HIV transmission (WHO, 2004).

The burden of HIV infection is greatest in the developing world (Steinbrook, 2004). Two thirds of HIV-infected persons are in Africa, where the epidemic exploded during the 1990s, and one fifth are in Asia, where the epidemic has been growing steadily (Steinbrook, 2004). Eight of nine countries with the most HIV-infected people are in sub-Saharan Africa. Estimates for India range from 2.2 to 7.6 million and for China from 430,000 to 1.5 million. For comparison, an estimated 950,000 people are living with HIV in the United States, 860,000 in the Russian Federation, and 680,000 in Brazil. Statistics highlight global disparities in availability of therapy. Overall, 2.2 million people died of AIDS in sub-Saharan Africa in 2003 (accounting for 76% of the global total). By comparison, in Western Europe, only 6000 people died of AIDS in 2003 (Table 12–1) (Joint United Nations Program on HIV/AIDS, 2004).

Developed World Perspective

The cumulative total of AIDS cases in the United States is more than 849,000 and more than 940,000 adults and

Table 12-1.   The Global HIV-AIDS Epidemic at the End of 2003

Region	No. of People Living with HIV-AIDS	Prevalence of HIV-AIDS among Adults (%)	No. of New HIV Infections in 2003	No. of Deaths due to AIDS in 2003
Total	37.8 million	1.1	4.8 million	2.9 million
Sub-Saharan Africa	25 million	7.5	3 million	2.2 million
South and Southeast Asia	6.5 million	0.6	850,000	460,000
Latin America	1.6 million	0.6	200,000	84,000
Eastern Europe and Central Asia	1.3 million	0.6	360,000	49,000
North America	1 million	0.6	44,000	16,000
East Asia	900,000	0.1	200,000	44,000
Western Europe	580,000	0.3	20,000	6,000
North Africa and Middle East	480,000	0.2	75,000	24,000
Caribbean	430,000	2.3	52,000	35,000
Oceania	32,000	0.2	5,000	700

From Joint United Nations Program on HIV/AIDS: 2004 Report on the Global AIDS Epidemic. Geneva, United Nations, July 2004.

children, respectively, living with HIV/AIDS (Carael et al, 2004; CDC, 2004; Steinbrook, 2004). Early in the epidemic, most infections occurred in men who have sex with men, but the incidence in this group leveled off by 1985 to 1987. However, HIV prevalence levels of 7% to 9% are still found among young homosexual and bisexual men in cities such as San Francisco and New York. The largest decline in the proportion of AIDS cases in the United States has occurred among homosexual and bisexual men, whereas cases acquired by heterosexual transmission have increased. Despite anti-retroviral therapy, blood screening, and treatment of sexually transmitted infections, the number of infections has remained at a plateau of 40,000 new HIV infections per year in the United States over the past decade (Mayer and Safren, 2004).

The HIV prevalence among injecting drug users has been increasing steadily, but with large regional differences (Carael et al, 2004). Since the late 1980s in the U.S. West Coast states, about 90% of people with AIDS are men who have sex with men, whereas in the Northeast, most new HIV infections occurred among injecting drug users. Young adults belonging to ethnic minorities (including men who have sex with men) are at considerably greater risk of infection than they were 5 years ago. For example, African Americans, who make up only 12% of the U.S. population, constituted 47% of AIDS cases reported in 2000.

Dynamics of the HIV Epidemic: Importance of Urologic Risk Factors

HIV epidemics may occur suddenly, reflecting circumstances that are not fully understood (Carael et al, 2004). For example, HIV seroprevalence among injecting drug users in Bangkok increased from zero in 1985-1986 to 16% in 1988 and to 40% to 60% in 1992. A number of the major risk factors are urologic (Table 12-2) (Carael et al, 2004). Early epidemiologic studies identified major risk factors, especially unprotected sexual intercourse with multiple partners or an infected partner, presence of sexually transmitted infections (STIs), or a history of STIs (Van de Perre et al, 1985; Kreiss et al, 1986; Cameron et al, 1989; Laga et al, 1994). More recent studies have highlighted sex differences in HIV transmission. For many monogamous women the main risk factor may be the sexual behavior of their steady partner.

Table 12-2.   HIV Infection Risk Associated with Sexual Behaviors Compared with Blood Exposure

Route/Type of Exposure	Risk of Infection Mean/Range (%)
Transfusion of contaminated blood	84-100
Intravenous drug use (needle sharing)	0.8
Receptive anal intercourse	0.3-0.8
Insertive anal intercourse	0.04-0.1
Occupational needlestick exposure	0.28-0.33
Insertive vaginal intercourse	0.03-0.09
Receptive vaginal intercourse	0.005-0.02
Insertive oral intercourse	0.003-0.008
Receptive oral intercourse	0.006-0.02

Data from Royce et al, 1997; Varghese et al, 2002; Henderson et al, 1986; Kaplan and Heimer, 1994; and Henderson, 2004.

Variable Rates of Sexual Transmission. Multiple cofactors affect HIV transmission, which is why estimates vary on the relative risk for specific exposures (see Table 12-2) (Royce et al, 1997; Vernazza and Eron, 1997). **The probability of HIV transmission associated with unprotected vaginal sexual intercourse is not constant from one contact to another; estimates range from 0.0005 to 0.002 per episode, in the absence of cofactors** (Carael et al, 2004).

Sexually Transmitted Infections. The presence of STIs suggests a marked risk of concurrent HIV. First, the modes of transmission of HIV and other STIs are similar. Second, genital ulcers as well as nonulcerative STIs facilitate HIV transmission (Cameron et al, 1989). Ulcerative STIs, including herpes, syphilis, and chancroid, enhance susceptibility to HIV per sexual act. Nonulcerative STIs, including gonorrhea, chlamydial infections, and trichomoniasis, are independent risk factors for HIV, with relative risks of 2.7 to 3.5 (Laga et al, 1994). Because syphilis infection facilitates acquisition and transmission of HIV, recent outbreaks of syphilis among men who have sex with men in major U.S. cities and reported increases in sexual behavior have raised concerns about potential increases in HIV transmission (CDC, 2004).

Several studies investigated aggressive diagnosis and treatment of STIs to limit HIV infection in high-risk populations, with apparently conflicting results. One study from Uganda employed syndromic management of STIs in an area where the epidemic was still in its early stages (i.e., 1% of the adult population were infected at the start). HIV incidence decreased in communities where the intervention was undertaken compared with control communities (Grosskurth et al, 1995). Different findings were reported in a study from Tanzania that employed periodic mass STI treatment of at-risk adults. This study found no decrease in HIV incidence (Wawer et al, 1999). In the latter study, the epidemic was more advanced (i.e., 16% of the adult population were infected at the start). In addition, there was a high rate of concomitant genital herpes that was not treated. Taken together, these findings suggest that efforts to decrease HIV spread through treating STIs should focus on specific treatment for individual patients, with aggressive diagnosis and treatment of STIs that are common in the community. The potential benefit of STI control programs may also prove greatest in areas of lower HIV prevalence. In communities where the epidemic is widespread, the likelihood of encountering a new partner who is HIV infected may be substantial, so the benefit of modifying a cofactor may be more limited (Mayer and Safren, 2004).

Antiretroviral Therapy and Genital Secretions. Only a small proportion of sexual exposures result in HIV transmission (Anderson and May, 1988). Transmission may occur by exposure to cell-free or cell-associated virus, and different factors may affect expression of virus concentrations in different body fluids (i.e., blood, semen, or cervicovaginal secretions) (Krieger et al, 1998; Chakraborty et al, 2001; Mayer and Safren, 2004). Although lower blood HIV levels are associated with lower transmission rates (Quinn et al, 2000), antiretroviral therapy may not make HIV-infected people noninfectious. In fact, sexual transmission of multidrug-resistant HIV has been well documented (Boden et al, 1999; Little et al, 1999). These observations underscore the need for HIV-infected patients to practice safer sex even if they are on therapy.

Circumcision Status. **Lack of male circumcision has been associated with an increased risk of acquiring STIs and HIV** (Auvert et al, 2001; Bailey et al, 2001; Mayer and Safren, 2004). The prepuce contains abundant cells that are susceptible to HIV infection (Patterson et al, 2002). These cells include T helper lymphocytes, monocyte/macrophage cells, Langerhans cells, and follicular dendritic cells. Follicular dendritic cells may be particularly important because of their mobility; they can bind HIV on their surface membrane and/or internalize it and migrate via draining lymphatics to distal sites, where propagation in submucosal lymphoid tissue can occur, with subsequent viral dissemination through the bloodstream. Thus, uncircumcised status appears to increase the risk for HIV infection (Moses et al, 1994; Lavreys et al, 1999). Prospective clinical trials are in progress to determine the effectiveness of male circumcision as an HIV prevention strategy (Bailey et al, 2002).

Gynecologic Factors. Female genital tract tissues vary in susceptibility to HIV infection. The stratified vaginal epithelium contains fewer cells with co-receptors than can bind HIV (Patterson et al, 1998). Thus, vaginal mucosa is less susceptible to HIV infection than the endocervix, which has a thinner, highly vascular layer, containing a much higher concentration of HIV-binding cells. Physiologic events that result in ectropion (i.e., increased exposure of the endocervix), such as the use of hormonal contraceptives or occult *Chlamydia tra-*

chomatis infection, increase susceptibility to HIV (Mostad et al, 2000; Moscicki et al, 2001).

Specific Sexual Behaviors. Calculation of precise risk for infection for each type of exposure is imprecise because many cofactors alter the amount of HIV in the genital tract (Mayer and Safren, 2004). Factors, such as a source with a high plasma viral load (Quinn et al, 2000) or concomitant STI, can greatly increase the average per-contact risk (Cohen et al, 1997; Wawer et al, 1999). Data used to generate per-contact risks are often based on cohort studies in which individuals recollect their risk during previous time intervals (often every 3 to 6 months). Recollections are often obtained about behaviors under the influence of drugs or alcohol.

Data from the developed world suggest that men are more likely to transmit HIV to their female partners (see Table 12–2) (Mayer and Safren, 2004). However, studies from Africa suggest that rates of male-to-female and female-to-male transmission were similar (Quinn et al, 2000). Reasons for this apparent difference in the efficiency of female-to-male transmission may include different rates of male circumcision or the prevalence of other STIs. For anal intercourse, the insertive partner is less likely to acquire HIV from an infected receptive partner than vice versa; but there appear to be sufficient susceptible cells in the distal male urethra and foreskin such that an insertive partner is still at substantial risk. One study suggested that, on average, receptive anal intercourse was more than seven times as efficient at transmitting HIV as insertive anal intercourse (DeGruttola et al, 1989).

Oral intercourse, either fellatio or cunnilingus, is a much less efficient way to acquire HIV. However, case reports show that oral exposure to ejaculate may transmit HIV (Mayer and Safren, 2004). The efficiency of oral transmission is less than that of unprotected vaginal intercourse, in the realm of less than 1/1000 contacts. However, animal studies demonstrate that HIV can be transmitted orally via lymphoid tissue in the oropharynx. Although HIV has been identified in preejaculatory secretions, there are no reliable case reports of HIV transmission through exposure to preejaculate without exposure to semen.

HIV VIROLOGY AND TARGETS FOR ANTIVIRAL THERAPY
The Virion

Although there are two HIV viruses, the focus in this chapter is on HIV-1 because there have been very few cases of HIV-2 in the developed world. HIV-2 is transmitted less readily than HIV-1, and the virus is less virulent. Both viruses have similar modes of transmission, and HIV-2 also causes an immunodeficiency syndrome. In this review, HIV refers to the clinical manifestations of infection caused by HIV-1.

HIV has a spherical shape with an outer envelope, variable surface projections, and an icosahedral capsid containing ribonucleoprotein complexed with a core shell (Fig. 12–1) (Liang and Wainberg, 2004). The HIV projections consist of envelope glycoproteins loosely associated with a lipid bilayer. Beneath the lipid layer, the matrix protein covers the internal surface of the viral coat. The capsid protein constitutes the shell of the cone-shaped core, and the nucleocapsid protein forms part of a nucleoid structure that also consists of reverse

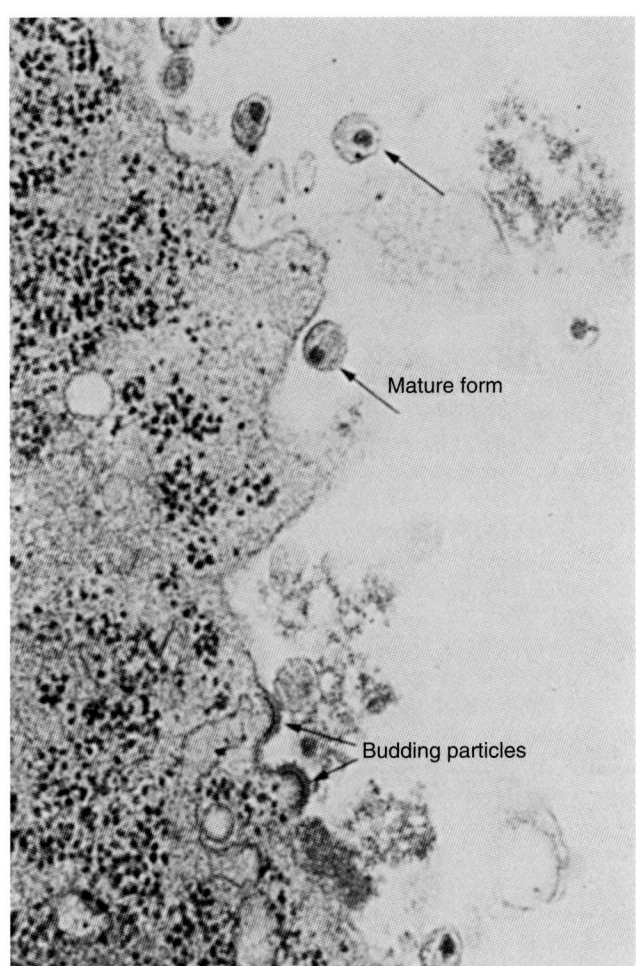

Figure 12–1. HIV virion. HIV has a spherical shape, an outer envelope, variable surface projections, and an icosahedral capsid containing ribonucleoprotein complexed with a core shell. (Electron micrograph courtesy of the Centers for Disease Control and Prevention.)

transcriptase, integrase, and two copies of the single-stranded viral genomic RNA (Liang and Wainberg, 2004).

HIV Replication Cycle (Fig. 12–2)

Viral Attachment, Fusion, and Uncoating. HIV initially attaches to the CD4 receptor on susceptible host cells. High-affinity interactions occur between the viral envelope glycoprotein and a specific region of the CD4 molecule (Pollard and Malim, 1998) on the surface of immature T cells and mature CD4+ T helper cells. In addition to CD4, a variety of co-receptors on lymphocytes and monocytes promote HIV entry into target cells after the initial binding (Cocchi et al, 1996). Two major co-receptors are CCR5 and CXCR4. Whereas cells of monocyte/macrophage origin generally express only the former, many lymphocyte populations express both co-receptor types. Differences in co-receptor expression help explain why HIV variants may be lymphocyte tropic, macrophage tropic, or both, and why some viruses are able to cause lymphocytes to fuse into giant cells. Other host cell membrane proteins also promote virus entry. One example is a C-type lectin (DC-Sign) that is highly expressed on dendritic

cells and binds to the HIV envelope glycoprotein (Liang and Wainberg, 2004).

Efforts are underway to develop compounds that antagonize HIV entry into susceptible cells by interfering with either the CD4 receptor or the co-receptors. Cell entry probably occurs by fusion of viral and cell membranes mediated by the viral transmembrane protein. **After fusion, the virion is uncoated by a proteolytic event mediated by the virion-encoded protease. A number of protease inhibitors that inhibit this step have proven to be very effective antiretroviral agents.**

Reverse Transcription. After entry, viral RNA is converted into DNA, which is then integrated into host cell chromosomal DNA. This process of reverse transcription occurs within 4 to 6 hours of infection and takes place mainly in the cytoplasm catalyzed by virion-encoded reverse transcriptase. The final products of reverse transcription are double-stranded viral DNA molecules. **This distinctive viral reverse transcription step has been the target of a number of effective antiretroviral agents.**

Integration. The products of reverse transcription are generated primarily in the cytoplasm of infected cells. The double-stranded DNAs are then transported into the nucleus where viral DNA is integrated into host cell chromosomal DNA.

Integration of viral DNA into the host chromosomal DNA is catalyzed by a virion-encoded integrase found in the viral particle. After reverse transcription of genomic viral RNA, viral integrase remains associated with viral DNA as a high-molecular-weight nucleoprotein preintegration complex. The integrase first removes two nucleotides from the 3′ end of viral DNA and then cleaves to target host DNA. This is followed by insertion of viral DNA into host cell DNA. After integration, HIV proviral DNA remains permanently associated with the host genetic material for as long as the cell lives. The viral integrase is currently under active investigation as a potential target for antiretroviral therapy.

Viral Gene Expression, Packaging, and Assembly. HIV exploits the host cell transcription and translation machineries to generate its own gene products. The primary RNA transcripts of the provirus are made by host cell RNA polymerase II. Cellular activation and proliferation signals result in the binding of transcription factors to the long terminal repeat and lead to increased rates of initiation of transcription. Tat and Rev are two key virion-encoded proteins that upregulate viral gene expression and replication, whereas HIV accessory proteins, including Nef, Vif, Vpu and Vpr, are crucial determinants of HIV virulence (Emerman and Malim, 1998). Host cellular ribosomes translate proviral mRNA into viral proteins (Liang and Wainberg, 2004). The HIV Gag proteins are the driving force for virus assembly.

Therapeutic Considerations. To date, the viral reverse transcriptase and protease enzymes have been the main targets of anti-HIV therapy. Reverse transcriptase is responsible for copying HIV RNA into DNA. However, this enzyme has an exceedingly high error rate (i.e., about one mutation per virus replication event) (Liang and Wainberg, 2004). This means that **mutants are constantly generated that have the potential for drug resistance.** Drug resistance to HIV occurs when these mutations result in altered forms of HIV reverse trans-

THE HIV-1 LIFE CYLCE

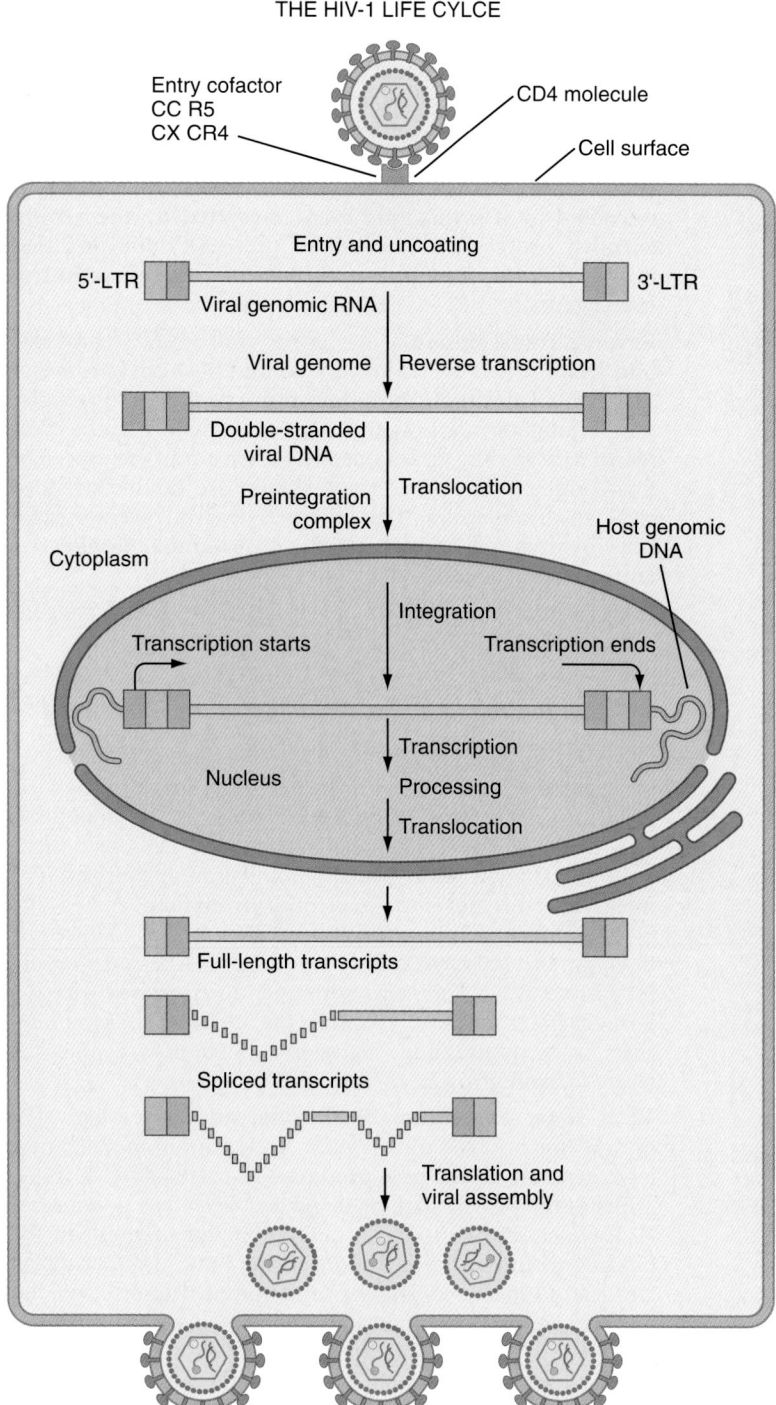

Entry cofactor
CC R5
CX CR4

CD4 molecule

Cell surface

Entry and uncoating

5'-LTR

Viral genomic RNA

3'-LTR

Viral genome   Reverse transcription

Double-stranded
viral DNA

Translocation

Preintegration
complex

Host genomic
DNA

Cytoplasm

Integration

Transcription starts   Transcription ends

Transcription

Nucleus

Processing

Translocation

Full-length transcripts

Spliced transcripts

Translation and
viral assembly

Figure 12–2. HIV replication cycle. The diagram illustrates the stages of HIV replication, including viral entry, uncoating, reverse transcription, integration, expression of proviral genome, viral assembly, and particle release. (From Liang C, Wainberg MA: Virology of HIV. In Cohen J, Powderly WG, Berkley SF, et al [eds]: Infectious Diseases, 2nd ed. Edinburgh, Mosby, 2004, vol 2, pp 1251-1255.)

criptase and protease that function, yet are not inhibited by antiviral agents. Because HIV uses cellular machineries to complete its life cycle, it is possible that cellular components might also be potential targets of anti-HIV compounds.

PATHOGENESIS OF HIV INFECTION

The prognosis and outcome of HIV infection changed dramatically with availability of highly active antiretroviral combination therapy (HAART). HAART has delayed the natural history and rate of progression, prolonging survival. However, initial optimism for immune reconstitution has been thwarted by information about HIV's pathogenic mechanisms and the limitations of HAART. **It is now clear that eradication of the virus is not possible with available antiviral drugs.**

Natural History of HIV Infection

The course of HIV infection is highly variable. In the absence of treatment, the typical course occurs over 8 to 12

years. **Three distinct phases have been defined: primary infection, chronic asymptomatic infection, and overt AIDS** (Pierre-Alexandre and Pantaleo, 2004).

Primary HIV Infection. Primary HIV infection is a transient symptomatic illness of variable severity. This acute syndrome occurs in 40% to 90% of patients. Clinical signs and symptoms generally appear 2 to 4 weeks after infection. The clinical presentation may mimic acute mononucleosis or other acute febrile illnesses, emphasizing the nonspecific nature of these symptoms and the difficulty of early diagnosis. **The self-limited syndrome generally lasts less than 14 days.**

Diagnosis of primary HIV infection depends on diagnostic testing. There are three laboratory characteristics: high plasma viremia often greater than 1 million HIV RNA copies/mL, a decrease in the blood CD4+ T cell count, and a large increase in the blood CD8+ T cell count. Subsequently, a marked decline in plasma viremia coincides with resolution of the clinical syndrome (Kahn and Walker, 1998). This decrease in viral load also correlates with the appearance of the virus-specific immune responses, particularly HIV-specific cytotoxic T lymphocytes, indicating that immune responses downregulate virus replication (Pantaleo et al, 1994; Musey et al, 1997). Standard laboratory assays used to diagnose HIV infection are usually negative during acute infection.

Chronic Asymptomatic HIV Infection. Primary HIV infection is followed by a long phase of clinical latency, usually lasting around 10 years. During this phase patients have neither signs nor symptoms. Relatively stable HIV replication levels and CD4+ T cell counts characterize this chronic phase.

This apparent clinical "stability" is deceptive. Although viral levels and the blood CD4+ T cell count are stable, this stability is only apparent in the blood. Virus replication and the accumulation of extracellular virus trapped in the follicular dendritic cell network are active in the lymphoid tissue, where progressive anatomic and functional deterioration occurs, leading to impaired specific immune responses (Pantaleo et al, 1993, 1998). Eventually, immunologic deterioration is reflected by a rapid increase in viremia levels and a drop in CD4+ T cell counts, resulting in transition to overt AIDS.

Overt AIDS. AIDS represents the end stage of HIV infection. This advanced stage of HIV disease is marked by low CD4+ T cell counts (<200 to 300 cells/μL) and appearance of constitutional symptoms. This phase may be complicated by the development of AIDS-defining opportunistic infections or malignancies. **Without antiretroviral therapy, AIDS usually leads to death in 2 to 3 years.** The risk for death and opportunistic infections increases significantly with CD4+ T cell counts less than 50 cells/μL.

Highly Variable Clinical Course. The clinical course of HIV infection is variable (Pierre-Alexandre and Pantaleo, 2004). Conceptually, patients may be classified in four categories: typical progressors, rapid progressors, slow progressors, or nonprogressors. **In 60% to 70% of HIV-infected patients, the median time between infection and the development of AIDS is 10 to 11 years, in the absence of therapy. These infected persons are "typical progressors."**

Ten to 20 percent of HIV infections progress rapidly. These "rapid progressors" develop AIDS less than 5 years after infection. After primary infection these patients' plasma virus levels are often greater than 10^5 HIV-1 RNA copies/mL and their CD4+ T cell counts start to decrease much earlier and more rapidly. HIV-specific immune responses are either never detected or are lost rapidly after the transition from the acute to the chronic phase of infection.

At the other extreme, 5% to 15% of HIV-infected people are "slow progressors," remaining free of AIDS for more than 15 years in the absence of therapy. Their CD4+ T cell counts remain stable, frequently greater than 500 cells/μL, and plasma HIV RNA levels are usually less than 10,000 copies/mL.

The slow progressors group includes a subgroup of long-term "nonprogressors." About 1% of HIV-infected people appear to fall into this category. Long-term nonprogressors have documented HIV infections for at least 8 to 10 years without antiretroviral therapy and have no signs of disease progression (e.g., constant high CD4+ T cells counts and either low [500 to 1000 HIV RNA copies/mL] or very low [<50 copies/mL] plasma virus levels).

Early Pathogenic Events Determine the Natural History

The most common route of HIV infection is sexual transmission at the genital mucosa (Royce et al, 1997). Animal models have provided important insights into the early pathogenic events. After intravaginal infection of rhesus monkeys, tissue dendritic cells (i.e., Langerhans cells that reside in the lamina propria adjacent to the vaginal epithelium) are the first potential target cells of HIV (Spira et al, 1996). These dendritic cells constitute a complex and highly developed system of antigen-presenting cells that are able to prime naive T cells. The ability of dendritic cells to attract and prime naive T cells can be explained by expression of a type II membrane protein with an external mannose binding, C-type lectin domain named DC-Sign (Steinman, 2000). It has been suggested that interaction between DC-Sign and the intracellular adhesion molecule (ICAM)-3 represents the initial contact between dendritic cells and resting T cells, a critical step for initiation of T cell immune responses. Dendritic cells express high levels of specific chemokines that target naive rather than memory T cells (Cameron et al, 1996).

After encountering HIV below the vaginal epithelium, Langerhans cells can either be infected or can pick up HIV virions (Steinman, 2000). Thus, DC-Sign–positive dendritic cells play the major role in the delivery of HIV to T cells, greatly amplifying the viral infection (Zhu et al, 1996). Subsequently, dendritic cells migrate to the internal iliac lymph nodes, where they target the T cell areas; they then present the viral antigens to activated virus-specific T cells. Therefore, dendritic cells play a key role, both in priming the initial HIV-specific immune response and in transporting HIV to the draining lymphoid tissue. Rapid recruitment and spreading of target cells (i.e., activated CD4+ T cells) confers a major advantage to HIV because these events occur before the appearance of virus-specific immune responses.

Within 2 days after infection, HIV can be detected in the draining lymphoid tissue. The virus then disseminates rapidly throughout the lymphoid system. Afterward, HIV enters the bloodstream, where viral replication can be detected in plasma 5 days after infection in the animal model. In humans, the time from mucosal infection and initial plasma viremia varies, ranging from 4 to 11 days (Pierre-Alexandre and Pantaleo, 2004). The clinical importance of these observations is that the risk of infection is increased by conditions that decrease genital mucosal barriers, especially lesions caused by inflammatory or infectious diseases, such as cervicitis, urethritis, and genital ulcers.

Critical Role of Lymphoid Tissue in Primary HIV Infection. Events in the lymphoid tissue play a central role in HIV infection. During primary infection the peak number of virus-expressing cells in the lymph node occurs at the same time as the peak of plasma viremia or shortly precedes it (Brodie et al, 1999; Musey et al, 1999; Pierre-Alexandre and Pantaleo, 2004). With the transition from primary to chronic infection, there is a switch from individual virus-expressing cells to virus trapped by the follicular dendritic cell network of lymph node germinal centers. This trapped virus becomes the dominant form of virus in lymph nodes, and this event is associated with a dramatic decrease in the number of individual cells expressing viral RNA, reflecting the role of the host immune system in partially containing HIV infection (Pantaleo et al, 1998).

Virus Escape and Establishment of Chronic HIV Infection. Early in primary HIV infection, vigorous virus-specific immune responses may contribute to both control of the initial peak of virus replication and reduction in plasma viremia (Musey et al, 1997; Kahn and Walker, 1998; Pantaleo et al, 1993, 1998). **However, HIV-specific immune responses cannot control HIV or block the eventual progression to symptomatic disease.** HIV differs from other viruses by targeting a broad spectrum of effector components of the antiviral immune response very early after infection (during the primary phase) and by rendering these mechanisms ineffective or reshaping them (Soudeyns and Pantaleo, 1999).

HIV escapes the host immune response by both virologic and immunologic mechanisms. Virologic mechanisms include formation of stable pool of latently infected CD4+ T cells containing HIV that is capable of replicating (Finzi et al, 1997; Wong et al, 1997), the genetic variability of HIV (Coffin, 1995), and trapping of infectious virions on the surface of follicular dendritic cells (Pantaleo et al, 1994). Rapid formation of a pool of latently HIV-infected CD4+ T cells is especially important. This event occurs before appearance of virus-specific immune responses. The pool of latently infected CD4+ T cells contains replication-competent HIV proviral DNA that represents a potential reservoir of wild-type virus with respect to known drug-induced mutations. This stable reservoir of HIV remains sheltered from the host immune responses and HAART (Chun et al, 1997; Wong et al, 1997). Initiation of HAART very early during primary HIV infection does have a significant impact on the size of this pool of CD4+ T cells. Decay of this pool of infected CD4+ lymphocytes is very slow and not much influenced by the effective suppression of virus replication. This reservoir of replication-competent virus represents a major obstacle to HIV eradication and long-term control of virus replication (Chun et al, 1997; Finzi et al, 1997; Wong et al, 1997).

Genetic variability is another efficient mechanism by which HIV escapes the host immune response. The virus possesses the intrinsic ability to mutate very rapidly. Both during primary and established chronic infection, rapid mutations ensure that the virus is able to escape both the humoral and cell-mediated virus–specific immune responses.

HIV also reshapes antiviral mechanisms by trapping of the virus on the surface of follicular dendritic cells in lymphoid germinal centers, as described earlier. For most infections, formation of immune complexes and their attachment to the follicular dendritic cell network represent mechanisms leading to clearance of the pathogen and to maintenance of effective immune responses. In HIV infection, however, these mechanisms lead to the formation of a stable reservoir of infectious virions, representing a continuous source for infection of CD4+ T cells that ultimately results in the destruction of the lymphoid tissue (Musey et al, 1997).

HIV escapes from the immune response through multiple immunologic mechanisms. These immunologic mechanisms for HIV escape include deletion of HIV-specific CD4+ T cell clones (Rosenberg et al, 1997); deletion of HIV-specific cytotoxic CD8+ T clones; generation of virus escape mutants (Soudeyns and Pantaleo, 1999); egress of cytotoxic T lymphocytes from lymph nodes; impaired function of antigen-presenting cells (Soudeyns and Pantaleo, 1999); and interference with the humoral neutralizing response.

In summary, virus escape and establishment of chronic HIV infection reflect the ability of HIV to target the host's antiviral immune response and reshape it into a self-defense mechanism. Primary infection is critical in the pathogenesis of HIV infection because events that occur during this stage determine both the pattern and the rate of disease progression.

Virologic Set Point. During the transition from primary to chronic infection, HIV plasma RNA levels reach a virologic set point that predicts the rate of disease progression (Mellors et al, 1996). The virologic set point varies among HIV-infected individuals and tends to remain stable in the same person during the chronic phase. The virologic set point that a person attains is determined by both the mechanisms involved in the establishment of chronic infection and by host factors that can modulate the course of HIV disease. **The plasma RNA load is the most accurate predictor of disease progression** (Mellors et al, 1996). The higher the plasma viral RNA load, the greater the risk of rapid progression to AIDS and death.

Prospects for HIV Eradication

Free HIV virions are eliminated with a half-life of 6 hours. In contrast, productively infected cells have a half-life of 1.6 days. It was hoped that HIV eradication was achievable within 2 to 3 years (Perelson et al, 1997). This goal could only be realized with complete and sustained suppression of HIV replication and if there were no pool of long-lived, latently infected cells to serve as a virus reservoir (Chun et al, 1997; Finzi et al, 1997; Wong et al, 1997).

Data from HIV-infected patients on long-term HAART significantly challenged these theories. There appears to be a pool of latently HIV-infected resting CD4+ T cells in HIV-infected patients who adhered to HAART for up to 3 years (Chun et al, 1997; Finzi et al, 1997; Wong et al, 1997). This pool is composed of quiescent memory CD4+ T cells with a longer half-life than the original estimate of 1 to 4 weeks. More importantly, these cells contain replication-competent HIV proviral DNA. After activation these cells are able to support efficient viral replication.

The extent of this HIV reservoir is quantitatively limited, estimated between 50,000 and 5 million resting memory CD4+ T cells for the whole body. However, this pool of cells has a half-life of 3 to 6 months, dramatically increasing estimates of the potential time required for HIV eradication.

The reservoir of HIV-infected cells originates from productively infected cells during primary infection (Pierre-Alexandre and Pantaleo, 2004). Initiation of HAART as early as 10 days after the onset of symptoms of primary HIV infection rapidly controls plasma viremia but does not preclude generation of this viral reservoir. These observations emphasize the rapidity with which HIV viral reservoirs are established and the limited ability of HAART to interfere with this pathogenic process. This pool of HIV-infected cells represents a major obstacle to HIV eradication.

In addition to their role as a viral reservoir, HIV-infected long-lived resting memory CD4+ T cells possess the ability to support virus production, albeit at low levels. Patients on HAART with a viral load below detectable levels with usual clinical assays may still have viral replication detectable with more sensitive tests (Pierre-Alexandre and Pantaleo, 2004). In these studies, 40% to 60% of patients still had low levels of viremia after 36 to 48 weeks of HAART.

Viral sanctuaries represent another potential source of residual HIV replication. **Sanctuaries are defined as cells and organs where the HIV can be sheltered or where HAART does not achieve therapeutic concentrations. Tissue sanctuaries include the lymphoid tissue, mucosa-associated lymphoid tissue, the genital organs, and the central nervous system, where the achievable concentration of antiviral drugs (especially protease inhibitors) may be suboptimal.** These sites may serve both as a potential source of low-level virus replication and as a reservoir of latently infected cells (Pierre-Alexandre and Pantaleo, 2004). Presence of viral sanctuaries, including the reproductive tract, with limited bioavailability of antiviral drugs further complicates the issue of HIV eradication. Current estimates are that it may take 5 to 10 years or more to eliminate HIV, considering a half-life of 4 months for the long-lived infected CD4+ cells and provided that effective and durable suppression of viral replication is achieved by HAART.

TESTS TO DIAGNOSE AND MONITOR HIV INFECTION: WHAT THE UROLOGIST SHOULD KNOW

HIV was first isolated in 1983, and the first diagnostic tests were marketed in 1985. Tests for diagnosis and monitoring of HIV infection have improved constantly (Kuritzkes, 2004; Reiss et al, 2004). Few areas in medicine have witnessed such rapid and widespread adaptation of molecular tools to everyday practice. Fortunately, the many tests for diagnosis and monitoring of HIV infection can be considered in three categories: diagnostic tests, viral load, and resistance assays.

Diagnostic Tests and Testing Algorithms

Assays have been developed to detect HIV antibodies in serum, whole blood, saliva, and urine (Kuritzkes, 2004). Most laboratories screen for anti–HIV-1 and anti–HIV-2 antibodies using an enzyme-linked immunosorbent assay (ELISA) based on antigens from viral lysates, recombinant or synthetic. Current third-generation HIV ELISAs have sensitivity and specificity approaching 100%. In contrast to earlier tests, which only detected IgG antibodies, these tests detect all classes of anti-HIV antibodies, substantially shortening the time to diagnosis after acute infection. A variety of rapid tests and "home tests" have also been developed.

Despite sensitivity of greater than 99%, a reactive HIV ELISA has relatively low positive predictive value in low-risk populations. Thus, the current testing algorithm includes a confirmatory test to exclude false-positive results. The Western blot is most widely used for confirmation. Some laboratories prefer immunoblotting for confirmation because immunoblots are simpler to standardize and are more sensitive in cases of recent seroconversion (Kuritzkes, 2004).

Clinical Application. After acute infection, HIV RNA can be detected from day 12. HIV RNA assays (see later) **have a sensitivity of 100% in diagnosing acute infection, but at the cost of lowered specificity (97%)** (Kuritzkes, 2004). **The first antibodies can generally be detected on day 21. However, development of a positive HIV antibody test can vary according to the patient and infecting strain. Beyond week 6 after infection, antibodies are detectable in almost all patients** (Kuritzkes, 2004). Since reactivity by the Western blot test lags seroconversion by ELISA, a positive ELISA in a patient with a negative or evolving Western blot can provide evidence of recent infection.

Testing is a two-stage process. Samples positive by an initial screening assay are retested to exclude clerical or laboratory error, and then a confirmatory assay is performed on repeatedly reactive sera to verify that the antibodies are directed against HIV. Confirmation of a reactive ELISA by a positive Western blot establishes the diagnosis of HIV infection. A negative Western blot suggests a false-positive ELISA or an acute infection.

Viral Load Monitoring

Assays to quantify HIV RNA, termed the "viral load," led to our current understanding of HIV pathogenesis and helped establish complete suppression of HIV replication as the ultimate goal for antiretroviral therapy (Kuritzkes, 2004). These assays are now standard. Performance characteristics of the commercially available assays are similar. Current commercial assays have a lower limit of quantitation of 50 to 80 HIV RNA copies/mL.

Clinical Application. Plasma HIV RNA levels correlate with clinical stage (Kuritzkes, 2004). Patients with symptomatic HIV infection or AIDS have significantly higher virus loads than patients with asymptomatic infection. The plasma HIV RNA load is also a powerful predictor of the risk of disease progression and death at all stages of disease. Current guidelines recommend obtaining two plasma HIV RNA measurements to determine the baseline or "set point" virus load before initiating antiretroviral therapy.

After antiretroviral therapy, the change in plasma HIV RNA provides important clinical information. Several large clinical trials showed significant correlations between the plasma HIV RNA reduction from baseline and the clinical benefit (De Gruttola et al, 2001). **The nadir in plasma HIV RNA levels is a marker for the duration of virus suppression** (Hirsch et al, 2000). **The early response to treatment predicts long-term outcome. Conversely, increasing plasma HIV RNA level suggests treatment failure.**

Increasing plasma HIV RNA level is the harbinger of potential development of retroviral drug-resistance (Reiss et al, 2004). This is not necessarily accompanied by an immediate decline in blood CD4+ lymphocyte numbers or by the development of clinical symptoms. Regular monitoring with plasma HIV RNA levels facilitates timely detection of drug-resistant HIV in patients on HAART.

HIV Drug-Resistance Assays

Various assays are available for assessing drug-resistance (Kuritzkes, 2004; Reiss et al, 2004). These assays can be considered as either genotypic or phenotypic assays. Genotypic assays evaluate HIV nucleotide sequences to detect critical drug-resistance mutations. Phenotypic assays estimate the concentration of antiviral drugs necessary to inhibit virus replication in vitro. Each approach has potential advantages and disadvantages. An important limitation is that both approaches measure characteristics of the predominant viral species but do not indicate the presence of minor species that may emerge as resistant variants during subsequent treatment.

Clinical Application. Clinical trials demonstrate the value of drug-resistance testing (Kuritzkes, 2004; Reiss et al, 2004). The risk of virologic failure during salvage therapy was reduced by 30% to 50% for each drug in the new regimen that was predicted to have activity (Kuritzkes, 2004; De Gruttola et al, 2001). Drug resistance remained an independent predictor of the likelihood of treatment failure even after controlling for treatment history.

Most experts recommend testing for drug resistance to guide the selection of salvage therapy for patients whose therapy is failing and in pregnant women (Hirsch et al, 2000). Resistance testing is also recommended for patients with acute HIV infection. Some experts also recommend that evidence for increasing transmission of drug-resistant HIV (Little et al, 2002) provides a rationale for testing of all patients before initiation of antiretroviral therapy, where affordable (Kuritzkes, 2004).

UROLOGIC MANIFESTATIONS OF HIV INFECTION
Nonmalignant Conditions

The genitalia may be involved in either early or late stages of HIV infection (Kho et al, 2004).

Primary HIV Infection

Primary HIV infection may be characterized by an acute exanthem, beginning 1 to 5 weeks after infection. Characteristic symptoms include fatigue, fever, and night sweats, accompanied by lymphadenopathy. The skin eruption consists of erythematous, round-to-oval macules and papules. The syndrome resolves with complete recovery.

Sexually Transmitted Infections

In many populations, the pattern of HIV acquisition parallels that of STIs (Quinn et al, 1988). **Thus, testing for HIV is recommended in anyone with a diagnosed STI, or at risk for STI** (CDC, 2002). **Accurate diagnosis of STIs is of exceptional importance in individuals at high risk for HIV infection because presence of an STI increases the risk of both transmitting and acquiring HIV infection. These infections may have more atypical and prolonged clinical manifestations in people with HIV infection.**

Genital Herpes Simplex Virus (HSV). HSV infection is common in HIV-infected persons (CDC, 2002). In these populations, HSV types 1 and 2 cause recurrent, severe, painful vesicles with an erythematous base. Untreated lesions may enlarge, becoming confluent ulcerations that persist with secondary bacterial infection. Sometimes ulceration occurs without well-defined vesicles ever being noted (Kho et al, 2004). Specific diagnosis is established by viral culture, other diagnostic tests, or biopsy.

In patients with intact immune function, the course of HSV is similar to other HSV-infected patients. Immunocompromised patients may have more prolonged and severe infections (CDC, 2002). Episodic or suppressive therapy with oral antiviral agents is often beneficial (Table 12–3) (CDC, 2002). Severe cases merit parenteral therapy with intravenous acyclovir (5 mg/kg every 8 hours) (CDC, 2002).

HSV resistance should be suspected if lesions persist or recur despite antiviral therapy. Viral culture and resistance testing should be obtained, if possible (CDC, 2002). Patients with acyclovir-resistant HSV strains require alternative agents, such as foscarnet (40 mg/kg intravenously every 8 hours until clinical resolution) or topical cidofovir gel (1% applied to

Table 12–3. Recommended Regimens for Treating Genital Herpesvirus Infections in HIV-Infected Patients

Episodic Treatment Regimens		
Drug	*Dosage*	*Duration*
Acyclovir	400 mg orally three times a day	5-10 days
Acyclovir	200 mg orally five times a day	5-10 days
Famciclovir	500 mg orally twice a day	5-10 days
Valacyclovir	1 g orally twice a day	5-10 days

Daily Suppressive Therapy	
Drug	*Dosage*
Acyclovir	400-800 mg orally twice or three times a day
Famciclovir	500 mg orally twice a day
Valacyclovir	500 mg orally twice a day

From Centers for Disease Control and Prevention: Sexually transmitted diseases treatment guidelines 2002. MMWR Morb Mortal Wkly Rep 2002;51:1.

lesions daily for 5 days, a preparation that is not commercially available but that must be compounded by a pharmacy).

Human Papillomavirus (HPV). Warts can develop in unusual locations, such as on the lips, tongue, and oral mucosa, in addition to the genitalia. Such lesions are treated using standard regimens (cryotherapy, podofilox, imiquimod, podophyllin resin, laser or excisional surgery) (CDC, 2002). However, in immunosuppressed patients genital lesions are resistant to treatment and patients may be at higher risk for recurrence (CDC, 2002).

In men, HPV affects the penis, urethra, scrotum, perineum, and rectal mucosa as condylomata acuminata, which are usually recognized as soft sessile lesions with finger-like projections (Fig. 12–3). In women, the spectrum of clinical disease is broad, with vulvar, vaginal, and cervical condylomata. Other clinical presentations of HPV infection include bowenoid papulosis and epidermodysplasia verruciformis. Bowenoid papulosis presents as small, brown, flat papules affecting the perianal and genital areas. Epidermodysplasia verruciformis consists of a widespread eruption of pink-red, flat, wartlike lesions distributed mostly on sun-exposed skin (Berger et al, 1991).

HPV infection increases the risk for carcinoma, especially in HIV-infected hosts. These lesions include cervical intraepithelial neoplasia in women and squamous cell carcinoma in men. Whenever extensive warts develop, the patient should be screened for HIV infection. Because there is an increased risk of anal cancer in HIV-infected homosexual men, screening for anal squamous intraepithelial neoplasia by cytology is recommended by some authorities. Until more data on the natural history of anal squamous intraepithelial neoplasia and the efficacy of treatment are available, routine screening is not recommended (CDC, 2002). Differential diagnosis of atypical and/or extensive genital warts includes squamous cell carcinoma in situ and squamous cell carcinoma. These cases are best diagnosed by biopsy. Treatment by various excisional procedures is often effective, but recurrence occurs frequently.

Syphilis. A high prevalence of syphilis is found in certain HIV-infected populations, particularly men who have sex with men (Quinn et al, 1988; CDC, 2002). In HIV-infected patients, primary infection with *Treponema pallidum* presents as the typical chancre. Secondary syphilis may present in classic papulosquamous form with involvement of palms, soles, and mucous membranes, but unusual presentations are common, such as verrucous plaques, extensive oral ulcerations, keratoderma, deep cutaneous nodules, and widespread gummas (Kho et al, 2004). The disease may progress faster from secondary to tertiary syphilis in HIV-infected patients. Early central nervous system relapse can also be more common.

Unusual serologic responses have been observed among HIV-infected persons with syphilis, usually higher than expected titers. False-negative tests have also been reported (CDC, 2002). Patients with clinical findings suggesting possible syphilis but with nonreactive or atypical serologic tests should have alternative diagnostic tests, such as biopsy of lesions, darkfield examination, or direct fluorescent antibody staining for diagnosis.

HIV-infected persons with early syphilis appear to be at increased risk for neurologic complications and higher risk for treatment failure with standard regimens. For primary and secondary syphilis in HIV-infected patients the current recommendation is benzathine penicillin G (2.4 million units IM). At least one dose is recommended, and some authorities recommend three doses at weekly doses, as recommended for late syphilis. Careful follow-up is recommended with repeated serologic studies for at least 24 months after treatment.

Chancroid. In the United States, chancroid usually occurs in discrete outbreaks. Chancroid is a cofactor for HIV transmission. Definitive diagnosis requires culture of *Haemophilus ducreyi* on special culture. Although polymerase chain reaction (PCR)-based tests are described, none is approved by the U.S. Food and Drug Administration. Probable diagnosis can be made if the patient has painful genital ulcers, no evidence of *T. pallidum* infection, and a negative test for HSV. The combination of a painful ulcer and tender inguinal adenopathy, symptoms occurring in one third of patients, suggests a diagnosis of chancroid. When accompanied by suppurative inguinal adenopathy, these signs are almost pathognomonic.

Recommended regimens for chancroid in HIV-infected patients are either ciprofloxacin, 500 mg orally twice daily for

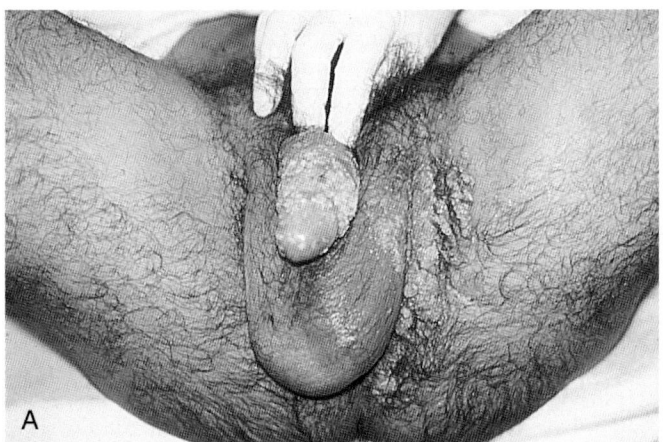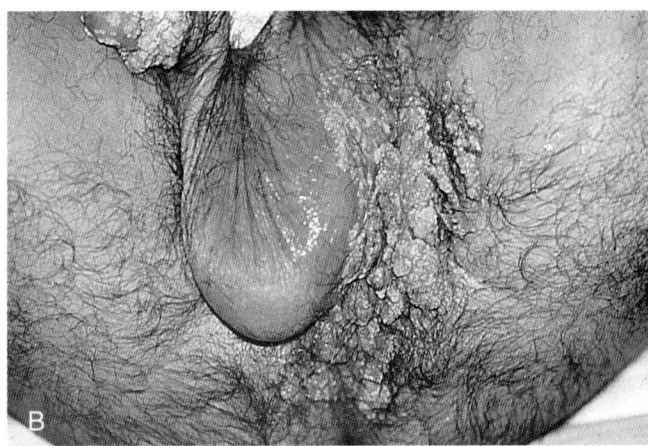

Figure 12–3.   A and **B,** AIDS patient with five active urogenital viral infections. Extensive genital condylomata were associated with areas of dysplasia and squamous intraepithelial neoplasia related to coinfection with human papillomavirus. Shedding of HIV, cytomegalovirus, and hepatitis B virus was documented in the patient's semen. Herpes simplex virus type 2 was cultured from active ulcers in the patient's inguinal crease.

3 days, or erythromycin base, 500 mg orally three times daily for 7 days (CDC, 2002). Alternative regimens are either azithromycin, 1 g as a single oral dose, or ceftriaxone, 250 mg as a single intramuscular dose; only limited data are available on the efficiency of these regimens so close follow-up is essential. HIV-infected patients with chancroid should be monitored closely because as a group these patients are more likely to experience treatment failure and to have ulcers that heal more slowly. HIV-infected patients may require longer courses of therapy, and treatment failures can occur with any regimen.

Urethritis. Patients with HIV infection are at risk for urethritis caused by the pathogens considered in Chapter 8, "Infections of the Urinary Tract." As the first rheumatic disease reported in HIV-infected patients, Reiter's syndrome, consisting of uveitis, urethritis, and arthritis, often presents in incomplete form (Solomon et al, 1991). The link between Reiter's syndrome and AIDS is poorly understood. The syndrome, particularly the urethral discharge, is usually refractory to antibiotic therapy.

Molluscum Contagiosum. Molluscum contagiosum is caused by a sexually transmitted poxvirus. This condition reportedly develops in 10% to 20% of AIDS patients (Kho et al, 2004). Characteristic lesions are umbilicated, dome-shaped, translucent 2- to 4-mm papules. Lesions can develop in any part of the body, especially the face and genital areas. In AIDS patients these lesions are widespread and may attain immense size (Izu et al, 1994). Most HIV-infected patients with extensive molluscum contagiosum have CD4+ counts of less than 250 cells/mL. In such immunosuppressed patients, diagnosis of molluscum contagiosum should be confirmed by histologic examination because the clinical appearance may simulate more serious infections such as cutaneous pneumocystosis, histoplasmosis and *Penicillium marneffei* infection, and cryptococcosis or cutaneous mycobacterial infection. Molluscum contagiosum is treated with cryotherapy, electrodesiccation, curettage, or topical application of keratolytic preparations (Kho et al, 2004).

HIV-Related Genitourinary Tract Infections

The genitourinary tract may be involved as the site or sequelae of HIV-related opportunistic infections (Randazzo et al, 1986; Stamm et al, 1988; Miles et al, 1989; Shevchuk et al, 1989; Pudney and Anderson, 1991; Wilson et al, 1992; Buzelin et al, 1994; Leibovitch and Goldwasser, 1994; Swartz et al, 1994; Trauzzi et al, 1994; Cespedes et al, 1995; Timmerman et al, 1995; Shevchuk et al, 1999; Appel et al, 2004; Kuritzkes, 2004).

Renal Infections. There has been a rise in drug-resistant tuberculosis in the United States. Persons with or at risk for HIV infection appear to be at increased risk for active infection with drug-resistant strains of *Mycobacterium tuberculosis*. Persons coinfected with HIV and *M. tuberculosis* have a greater likelihood of developing clinical tuberculosis, including renal and other extrapulmonary disease, that may be more difficult to diagnose and treat (Weiss et al, 1998).

Other renal infectious manifestations of AIDS include cytomegalovirus infection, aspergillosis, and toxoplasmosis. Cytomegalovirus infection is a common opportunistic infection in immunocompromised patients. Renal infection is most commonly noted in widespread disease in association with acute tubular necrosis (Kwan and Lowe, 1995). Although

it has been suggested that renal cytomegalovirus infection might facilitate the development of HIV-associated nephropathy (HIVAN), an autopsy study of 75 kidneys suggested that the two findings are unrelated (Nadasdy et al, 1992). Aspergillosis and toxoplasmosis are common opportunistic infections of the kidney. Both infections are treated with systemic therapy. Serious infections such as abscesses require percutaneous drainage, open drainage, or nephrectomy.

Prostatitis. The prostate is the site for varied opportunistic infections in HIV-infected patients. In one study, bacterial prostatitis was diagnosed in 17 (8%) of 209 men hospitalized for HIV (Leport et al, 1989). The clinical presentation varies based on the severity of the infection but includes fever, obstructive and irritative voiding symptoms, and a tender prostate on digital rectal examination with possible fluctuance. Superimposed urinary tract infections occurred in 22% of AIDS patients in one study (Kaplan et al, 1987). Diagnosis requires broad cultures, including aerobes, anaerobes, fungi, and mycobacteria. Prostatic abscesses require open, transrectal, or endoscopic drainage. Bacterial prostatitis requires prolonged courses of antibiotics with high levels of prostatic penetration. Fungal prostatitis is initially treated with two-agent therapy (often amphotericin and flucytosine) or one of the newer antifungal drugs, with long-term suppression for persistent or recurrent infections.

Epididymitis and Orchitis. The most common pathology in AIDS is testicular atrophy secondary to endocrine imbalances, febrile episodes, malnutrition, toxic effects of therapeutic agents, and testicular infections (Leibovitch and Goldwasser, 1994). Autopsy studies have demonstrated opportunistic testicular infection in up to 39% of AIDS patients (De Paepe et al, 1990). One study (Shevchuk et al, 1989) of 80 autopsies in AIDS patients demonstrated that 2 of 11 cases with systemic toxoplasmosis involved the testes, 4 of 48 cases of systemic cytomegalovirus infection involved the prostate while one involved the testes, and 1 of 27 cases of systemic candidiasis involved the prostate. Most patients' testes exhibited marked spermatogenic arrest, germ cell degeneration, peritubular fibrosis, and Leydig cell depletion, nonspecific findings that likely reflect severe systemic disease (Shevchuk et al, 1999). Other immunocompromised patients develop symptomatic genitourinary tract infections with both common and unusual organisms, for example, epididymitis caused by *Candida* (Swartz et al, 1994) or cytomegalovirus (Randazzo et al, 1986). Patients may be less likely to respond to medical therapy and to require surgery (Coburn, 1998).

Clinically, scrotal infections usually present as epididymo-orchitis. Relapse is common and may result in persistent symptoms or fulminant infection with abscess formation. Treatment requires initial antibiotic treatment followed by long-term maintenance suppression. The differential diagnosis of epididymitis or orchitis that does not respond to conventional therapy includes fungal, mycobacterial, and other opportunistic infections, in addition to testicular tumors (see later).

Impetigo, Abscesses, Cellulitis, Lymphadenitis, and Necrotizing Fasciitis. Impetigo, usually caused by *Staphylococcus aureus*, occurs in the inguinal area as in other common sites (the face, shoulders, and axilla). Typically the infection begins with painful red macules, progressing to pustules that rupture and produce a characteristic honey-colored crust (Kho et al, 2004). Soft tissue and deep-seated infections, including cellulitis, abscesses, and necrotizing fasciitis, may develop in HIV-infected patients.

Necrotizing fasciitis of the genitalia, also known as Fournier's gangrene, has a propensity to occur in immunocompromised hosts (Corman et al, 1999). This aggressive, progressive, necrotizing fasciitis has been documented as the presenting finding in previously undiagnosed AIDS patients (McKay and Waters, 1994). Treatment depends on rapid diagnosis, wide surgical débridement, hemodynamic support, and prolonged antibiotic therapy. Diverting colostomy and partial or complete scrotectomy are commonly necessary during operative débridement.

Voiding Dysfunction

Because HIV infection affects both the central and peripheral nervous systems, voiding dysfunction is common in patients with advanced infection (Hermieu et al, 1996). Urinary retention is the most common voiding dysfunction (54%) seen by urologists, although detrusor hyperreflexia (27%) and outflow obstruction (18%) have been documented during urodynamic evaluation of AIDS patients with voiding symptoms (Travers and Huybers, 1987; Kane et al, 1996). **Standard pharmacologic measures are preferred for patients with mild dysfunction, and routine urodynamic investigation has proven to be of low yield** (Gyrtrup et al, 1995). In our experience, voiding complaints often reflect the degree of systemic impairment; such symptoms often improve substantially after effective antiretroviral therapy. For patients with urinary retention, intermittent catheterization is the treatment of choice. When the patient lacks sufficient manual dexterity, indwelling urethral or suprapubic catheterization is employed.

Urolithiasis

Urinary calculi have been associated with several treatments for HIV infection. **The strongest association is with protease inhibitors, especially indinavir** (Daudon and Jungers, 2004). Kidney and ureteral stones are the most serious adverse effect observed so far in patients taking indinavir, appearing in 2% to 3% (Lerner et al, 1998; Katner et al, 2002), but rates as high as 12% to 24% have been reported (Hermieu et al, 1999; Reiter et al, 1999; Meraviglia et al, 2002). Renal secretion appears to increase urinary supersaturation with formation of indinavir urinary crystals, especially with indinavir dosages above 600 mg (Vella and Floridia, 2004). **The stones are nonopaque and may be associated with minimal findings on noncontrast computed tomographic examination** (Gentle et al, 1997; Blake et al, 1998; Schwartz et al, 1999).

Our experience is consistent with recommendations for conservative treatment in most cases, consisting of hydration, analgesics, and temporary cessation of indinavir (Hermieu et al, 1999; Kohan et al, 1999). Indications for intervention include persistent fever, intractable pain, inability to tolerate oral hydration, or obstruction of a solitary kidney. Indinavir crystals develop at pH 7.0 and can be dissolved when the pH is lowered to 4.0. This suggests that short-term urinary acidification may be valuable for stone dissolution (Kalaitzis et al, 2002). After resolution of the acute symptoms and passage of the stone, indinavir therapy can be restarted with aggressive

oral hydration (Clayman, 1998). Urinary calculi have also been associated with use of other protease inhibitors, such as nelfinavir (Engeler et al, 2002) and saquinavir (Green et al, 1998).

HIV-infected patients on protease inhibitors also form stones that do not contain protease inhibitors. One study of 24 HIV-infected patients with urinary calculi found that only 3 (29%) of 14 on indinavir had indinavir-containing stones (Nadler et al, 2003). Of 10 patients evaluated, 8 had metabolic abnormalities. Thus, metabolic evaluation may help prevent future stone episodes while avoiding the need to alter antiretroviral regimens in most patients.

Sulfadiazine therapy for toxoplasmosis has also been associated with obstructive nephropathy (Farina et al, 1995; Colebunders et al, 1999; Crespo et al, 2000). The obstructing calculi often appear radiolucent. Initial therapy should include hydration, discontinuation of the sulfadiazine, and urinary alkalinization (Crespo et al, 2000). Invasive interventions should be reserved for patients who fail such medical management (Colebunders et al, 1999).

HIV-Associated Nephropathy (HIVAN)

Glomerular diseases, particularly a unique "HIV-associated nephropathy" (HIVAN) have emerged as significant medical renal diseases in HIV-infected patients (Appel et al, 2004).

Epidemiology. HIVAN has been reported more often on the U.S. East Coast than the West Coast. In urban East Coast populations, the prevalence of HIVAN approached 90% in nephrotic HIV-infected patients compared with 2% in San Francisco, where most patients were white homosexuals (Appel et al, 2004; Ross and Klotman, 2004).

HIVAN occurs more frequently among HIV-infected black patients, with a black-to-white ratio of 12:1. HIVAN is the third leading cause of end-stage renal disease among 20- to 64-year-old blacks (following only diabetes and hypertension). Blacks also appear to have more severe renal disease, with heavier proteinuria, higher rate of the nephrotic syndrome, and greater renal insufficiency. Intravenous drug use has been the most common risk factor associated with HIVAN, but the disease has been seen in all HIV risk groups (Appel et al, 2004). There is no relationship between HIVAN and patient age, duration of HIV infection, types of opportunistic infections, or malignancies (Appel et al, 2004). The prevalence of HIVAN is reported to be 3.5% in HIV-infected clinic patients and 6.9% in autopsy series of HIV-infected patients (Shahinian et al, 2000).

Clinical Presentation. HIVAN usually occurs in patients with low CD4 counts, but overt AIDS is not a prerequisite (Appel et al, 2004). HIVAN typically presents as proteinuria in the nephrotic range (and often massive) and renal insufficiency (Appel et al, 2004). Other characteristics typical of the nephrotic syndrome are common in some series, including edema, hypoalbuminemia, hypercholesterolemia, and hypertension. Patients may also present with sub–nephrotic-range proteinuria and urinary sediment findings of microhematuria and sterile pyuria. Renal ultrasound shows echogenic kidneys with preserved or enlarged size despite severe renal insufficiency (Appel et al, 2004).

Pathology and Pathogenesis. Diagnosis of HIVAN is based on a renal biopsy showing characteristic focal segmental glomerulosclerosis with collapsing features and related mesangiopathies (Appel et al, 2004). Patients with HIVAN have a higher percentage of glomerular collapse, less hyalinosis, and greater visceral cell swelling than patients with classic, idiopathic focal segmental glomerulosclerosis or heroin nephropathy.

There are conflicting data on the potential for direct HIV infection of renal glomerular cells in vivo, but HIV appears to be able to infect glomerular endothelial cells and, to a lesser degree, mesangial cells in vitro (Marras et al, 2002; Appel et al, 2004). HIV replication may not be necessary for the development of HIVAN, and it is likely that a viral gene product or indirect effects on host cytokine production are involved in the pathogenesis.

Course and Treatment. During the early years of the epidemic HIVAN was characterized by rapid progression to end-stage renal disease (Appel et al, 2004). There was an almost universal requirement of dialysis within 1 year of diagnosis (Appel et al, 2004).

With the introduction of HAART, the rise in new cases of end-stage renal disease due to HIVAN slowed markedly (Kirchner, 2002; Appel et al, 2004). There are reports of patients with biopsy-documented or presumed HIVAN who experienced dramatic resolution of nephrotic syndrome and improved glomerular filtration rate on therapy (Appel, 2004). Antiretroviral therapy also appears to delay progression of HIVAN to end-stage renal disease. Thus, antiretroviral therapy is recommended for patients with early histologic lesions and milder proteinuria without renal deterioration. Other therapies that have been recommended include angiotensin-converting enzyme inhibitors, angiotensin II receptor blockers, and immunosuppressive therapy in selected patients (Appel, 2004).

Abnormal Urinalysis

Abnormalities on urinalysis are relatively common in HIV-infected persons. These findings include hematuria, pyuria, bacteriuria, and proteinuria. One study suggests that hematuria occurs in 25% of HIV-infected persons (Cespedes et al, 1995). Although hematuria may be related to many causes, genitourinary tumors appear to be uncommon, particularly in young men. Thus, complete urologic evaluation may safely be omitted in young men with asymptomatic microscopic hematuria (Cespedes et al, 1995). In contrast, we have seen a number of HIV-infected patients with urologic malignancies, including bladder, renal, and other tumors presenting with hematuria. These observations suggest that complete investigation is indicated in older patients and those with significant hematuria. Proteinuria is also common in certain populations of HIV-infected patients, as considered earlier.

Neoplasms

Many neoplasms occur in HIV-infected patients (Kho et al, 2004; Tirelli and Vaccher, 2004). Vascular and lymphoreticular neoplasms have been associated most strongly with HIV infection, particularly Kaposi's sarcoma (KS) and non-Hodgkin's lymphoma (NHL). **The risk of KS and NHL are increased 1000- and 100-fold, respectively, among HIV-infected patients compared with the general population**

(Tirelli and Vaccher, 2004). KS, primary central nervous system lymphoma, systemic intermediate/high-grade B-cell NHL, and invasive cervical cancer have been designated as AIDS-defining illnesses. Other malignancies reported to be associated with HIV infection include Hodgkin's disease, high-grade anal epithelial lesions, nonmelanomatous skin cancer, myeloma, and lung and testicular carcinoma (International Collaboration of HIV and Cancer, 2000; Tirelli and Vaccher, 2004). HAART radically changed the clinical spectrum of HIV infection in industrialized countries. During the mid 1990s, rates of opportunistic infections, KS, primary central nervous system lymphoma, and NHL decreased significantly (International Collaboration of HIV and Cancer, 2000; Grulich et al, 2001).

Kaposi's Sarcoma

KS is the most common vascular neoplasm and a significant causes of morbidity and mortality in certain HIV-infected populations (Cockerell, 1996).

Classification and Clinical Presentation. KS is classified into classic and epidemic forms. The classic form was first described in 1827 (Kho et al, 2004), occurring mainly in elderly Mediterranean men, black equatorial Africans, and patients with lymphoma or immune deficiencies. In contrast, epidemic KS is associated with AIDS.

KS ranges from an indolent to an aggressive disease with substantial morbidity and mortality. **Typical patients present with disseminated skin lesions,** often with lymph node and visceral involvement (Tirelli and Vaccher, 2004). Any skin area may be involved, including the genitalia. Three types of skin lesions are described: macule or patch, plaque, and nodule (Kho et al, 2004). Typical macules are oriented along skin cleavage lines and may be mistaken for blushes, purpura, or nevi. With time, the lesions darken and develop into raised, firm indurated purplish plaques, reflecting presence of abundant blood vessels, extravasated erythrocytes, and siderophages. Some lesions may ulcerate. Nodular lesions are dome-shaped, elevated, and usually purple. On palpation they are firm and may be ulcerated.

Epidemiology. KS incidence rates started to decline in the late 1980s, then dramatically so with the introduction of HAART in the mid 1990s (International Collaboration of HIV and Cancer, 2000; Grulich et al, 2001; Tirelli and Vaccher, 2004). Meta-analysis of 47,936 HIV-infected individuals from North America, Europe, and Australia found that the KS rate ratio for 1997-1999 versus 1992-1996 was 0.3 (International Collaboration of HIV and Cancer, 2000). The risk of KS among male homosexuals is greater than 100,000-fold higher than for other HIV-infected populations (Tirelli and Vaccher, 2004).

A new herpesvirus, called KS-associated herpesvirus or human herpesvirus 8 (Chang et al, 1994) **is essential for all forms of KS.** KS-associated herpesvirus transmission correlates with a history of STDs and number of male sexual partners. Co-infection with HIV and KS-associated herpesvirus increases the risk of developing KS 10,000-fold compared with KS-associated herpesvirus infection alone. The probability of developing KS after co-infection with both KS-associated herpesvirus and HIV approaches 50% over 10 years (Chang et al, 1994).

Pathology and Pathogenesis. KS is a proliferative disease characterized by angiogenesis, endothelial spindle cell growth (KS cells), inflammatory cell infiltration, and edema (Tirelli and Vaccher, 2004). These lesions reflect immune dysregulation characterized by CD8+ T-cell activation, production of Th1 cytokines, and angiogenic factors. This process induces generalized activation of endothelial cells.

Diagnosis and Management. An experienced observer can often make a presumptive diagnosis, but skin biopsy is usually necessary to confirm the diagnosis of KS.

No specific therapy is curative (Tirelli and Vaccher, 2004). Treatment needs to be individualized, based on the patient's clinical and immunologic status. HAART results in clinical improvement of KS lesions and prolongation of time to treatment failure (Lebbe et al, 1998; Levine and Tulpule, 2001). Numerous anecdotal reports document KS regression on HAART alone. Anti-KS activity of HAART appears to reflect immune system reconstitution and, to a lesser extent, suppression of HIV replication. HIV protease inhibitors are also potent anti-angiogenic molecules that may affect KS pathogenesis (Sgadari et al, 2002).

Localized, cutaneous KS lesions can be treated using radiation, laser, cryotherapy, or intralesional injections of antineoplastic drugs (Levine and Tulpule, 2001). Cytotoxic chemotherapy is indicated for patients who do not respond to HAART and patients with life-threatening or visceral disease. A wide variety of drugs, including *Vinca* alkaloids (vincristine, vinblastine), bleomycin, and doxorubicin individually and in combination, have produced tumor regression in 21% to 59% of patients, with lower rates for monotherapy. Paclitaxel is the newest systemic agent approved for the relapsed KS patient (Levine and Tulpule, 2001). Corticosteroid therapy should be avoided because it induces development of KS and may worsen preexisting KS lesions.

Prognosis for HIV-infected patients with KS depends primarily on their immune status and secondarily on the clinical stage of the KS lesions. Median survival of patients with CD4+ T-cell counts greater than 150/μL and early stage disease is 35 months. Patients with CD4+ T-cell counts less than 150/μL have poor median survival (13 months for early and 12 months for advanced stage disease, respectively) (Levine and Tulpule, 2001).

Non-Hodgkin's Lymphoma

A number of lymphoreticular malignancies of both B and T cells develop in HIV-infected patients. Most are based in the lymph notes and reticuloendothelial system, although the genital skin and genitourinary organs may be involved primarily or secondarily (Mearini et al, 2002; Kho et al, 2004; Tirelli and Vaccher, 2004). Patients usually present with advanced disease associated with a short median survival time. NHL is the most common lymphoreticular neoplasm.

Epidemiology and Clinical Presentation. NHL incidence decreased significantly after the introduction of HAART (Tirelli and Vaccher, 2004). Systemic NHL incidence decreased less than KS and later than the other AIDS-defining illnesses. Consequently, lymphoma has become the most common AIDS-associated cancer among patients receiving HAART (International Collaboration of HIV and Cancer, 2000; Grulich et al, 2001; Tirelli and Vaccher, 2004).

HIV-infected patients characteristically have widespread disease at presentation (Tirelli and Vaccher, 2004). They frequently have systemic symptoms, including fever, night sweats, and weight loss of more than 10%. At diagnosis of NHL, approximately 75% of HIV-infected patients have advanced disease, with frequent involvement of extranodal sites. Any body site may be affected, including the genitourinary tract.

Diagnosis and Treatment. NHL should be diagnosed by histologic examination of an incisional or excisional biopsy. Treatment consists of the usual therapy for systemic lymphoma. Optimal therapy has not been defined, and whether intensive or conservative chemotherapy regimens are indicated remains controversial. Prognosis for HIV-infected patients with lymphoma is poor, with a median survival of 5 to 10 months after diagnosis (Tirelli and Vaccher, 2004).

Squamous Genital Cancers: Role of HPV

HIV infection is associated with HPV-related anogenital neoplasms (Tirelli and Vaccher, 2004). **These lesions include cancers and precancerous lesions of the cervix, vulva, anus, and penis.** The risk of all HPV-associated cancers and their in-situ precursor lesions in both women and men is elevated across all HIV exposure categories (Tirelli and Vaccher, 2004). Risk factors include multiple sexual partners, cigarette smoking, and STDs, particularly HPV infection.

HPV sequences are found in more than 99% of cervical squamous cell carcinomas and in most anal cancers, with HPV type 16 present in 50% and types 18, 31, and 45 present in another 30%. High-grade intraepithelial precursor lesions have comparable rates of similar HPV types. HPV-associated oncogenesis results from upregulated expression of viral-encoded transforming proteins, particularly E6 and E7. These proteins interact with and inactivate the host cell tumor suppressor gene products, including RB and TP53. This results in upregulated cell cycle progression, deficient DNA repair, and, eventually, malignant transformation (Tirelli and Vaccher, 2004). The degree of HIV-related immunosuppression corresponds with the occurrence and severity of these anogenital tumors.

Testicular Cancer

There may be an increased incidence of germ cell and non–germ cell testicular tumors associated with HIV infection (Wilson et al, 1992; Kwan et al, 1995). **Retrospective review of 3000 patients enrolled in an HIV clinic found a 50 times greater rate of testicular neoplasms than in the general population** (Wilson et al, 1992). **Compared with HIV-noninfected patients, there is a greater risk of tumor bilaterality and a greater risk of high-grade testicular lymphoma** (Armenakas et al, 1992).

The therapeutic dilemma is that all accepted treatments for testicular neoplasms, except surveillance, result in additional immune suppression. Furthermore, patients with advanced HIV/AIDS often tolerate radiation and chemotherapy poorly. This may require major modifications of standard treatment protocols, resulting in decreased effectiveness. Despite these limitations, most experts recommend that HIV-infected patients with testicular neoplasms should receive standard treatment as indicated by the tumor histology and stage (Wilkinson and Carroll, 1990).

OCCUPATIONAL RISKS FOR HIV INFECTION IN UROLOGY

For reasons that are not completely understood occupational HIV infection remains relatively uncommon (Henderson, 2004).

Epidemiology

The CDC has recorded only 57 instances of documented occupational HIV infection. For each case, the worker sustained an occupational exposure, had a negative baseline serum sample, and then developed serologic evidence of HIV infection. In addition there have been 138 instances of probable or possible occupational HIV infection among U.S. health care workers (CDC, 2004). Of adults with AIDS, 5.1% have occurred in health care workers, including 122 surgeons. Approximately 60 cases of "possible or probable" occupational infection have been reported from outside the United States (Henderson, 2004). There were no documented cases of occupationally acquired AIDS/HIV infection among surgeons and 6 possible cases of occupational transmission among surgeons.

Risks Associated with Specific Exposures

Of the 57 health care workers who seroconverted after occupational exposures: 48 (84%) had percutaneous (puncture/cut injury) exposures; 5 (9%) had mucocutaneous (mucous membrane and/or skin) exposures); 2 (4%) had both percutaneous and mucocutaneous exposure; and 2 (4%) had an unknown route of exposure. Forty-nine health care personnel were exposed to HIV-infected blood; 3 to concentrated virus in a laboratory; 1 to visibly bloody fluid, and 4 to an unspecified fluid (CDC, 2004).

Many occupational cases of HIV transmission share common features. Most are percutaneous exposures, especially injection needlestick injuries. All clinical cases occurred after exposure to blood or grossly blood-stained fluids from HIV-infected patients. As yet, no case has been documented after a needlestick injury with a solid surgical needle (Henderson, 2004).

A retrospective, case-control study from the United States, France, and the United Kingdom identified five **risk factors for occupational infection: deep as compared with superficial exposure** ($P < .0001$), **blood visible on the device causing the exposure** ($P = .0014$), **the device had been placed in a source-patient's vein or artery** ($P = .0028$), **the source-patient died within 60 days of the exposure** ($P = .0011$, **and the exposed health care worker did not take zidovudine postexposure chemoprophylaxis** ($P = .0026$) (Cardo et al, 1997). **The first four factors are likely related to an increased inoculum.**

The importance of an inoculum effect is supported by other data. Transfusion of a unit of blood from an HIV-infected donor is associated with virtually 100% risk for

Table 12–4. Risk for HIV Infection Associated with Occupational Exposure

Type of Exposure	Percutaneous	Mucous Membrane
No. of longitudinal studies	27	21
No. of exposures	6807	2761
No. of documented infections	21	0/1
Infection rate per exposure	0.031%	0–0.11%

From Henderson DK: Preventing occupational infection with HIV in the health care environment. In Cohen J, Powderly WG, Berkley SF, et al (eds): Infectious Diseases, 2nd ed. Edinburgh, Mosby, 2004, vol 2, pp 1217-1222.

infection (Ward et al, 1987). The depth of a percutaneous exposure was an independent risk factor for occupational HIV infection (Cardo et al, 1997). In addition, all needlestick exposures associated with occupational transmission have been caused by hollow-bore needles (i.e., injection as compared with suturing needles), which contain more blood than solid needles.

Combining available data, health care workers have sustained more than 6800 percutaneous exposures to sharp devices contaminated with blood or other blood-stained body fluids from HIV-infected patients (Ippolito et al, 1999; Henderson, 2004). Twenty-one occupational HIV infections were documented, resulting in a risk of transmission per injury of 0.31% (Table 12–4). Thus, 1 in 324 parenteral exposures resulted in occupational HIV infection.

Other exposures represent a lower risk for infection. In rare circumstances, mucous membrane or cutaneous exposures may produce occupational infection (Chamberland et al, 1995). To date, more than 2700 exposures have been followed prospectively, with only one seroconversion (Ippolito et al, 1993). Thus, a maximum risk estimate for HIV infection is 0.11% per mucous membrane exposure. Occupational exposures other than percutaneous and mucous membrane exposures are even less likely to result in infection. Prospective studies (Friedland et al, 1990; Gershon et al, 1990), which include hundreds of person-years of follow-up, have not identified a single instance of transmission of HIV. Whereas exposures to other fluids are likely to be associated with some occupational risk, this risk is below measurable limits.

Interventions to Decrease Occupational Risk

Adherence to current guidelines might prevent one third of parenteral occupational exposures (Marcus, 1988). "Universal precautions" are based on the principle that health care workers should treat blood and blood-stained body fluids from all patients as potentially infectious (CDC, 1988). The CDC also recommends "standard precautions," focusing on the bidirectional spread of organisms to and from patients and health care providers. The recommendations emphasize that blood and blood-containing body fluids represent risk to health care workers and that health care workers should use barriers and take precautions to prevent occupational exposures. These recommendations are effective. For example, the act of piercing a latex glove with a needle covered with blood may reduce the blood inoculum by as much as 50% (Henderson, 2004).

Once exposure to HIV has occurred, the exposed site should be allowed to bleed freely and first aid should be administered. The wound should be cleansed and decontaminated as soon as patient safety permits. Wounds should be washed with soap and water and then irrigated with sterile saline, a disinfectant, or other suitable solution.

Postexposure Prophylaxis

Data have been accumulated that support postexposure chemoprophylaxis to reduce the risk of occupational HIV transmission. Postexposure prophylaxis has proven effective in animal models (Henderson and Gerberding, 1989; Henderson, 2004). The case-control study described earlier found that zidovudine chemoprophylaxis was associated with an 80% reduction in the risk for occupational infection (Cardo et al, 1997).

Current recommendations include a three-drug regimen for the most severe occupational exposures (i.e., zidovudine, lamivudine, and one of four additional agents) and a two-drug regimen for lesser exposures (i.e., zidovudine plus lamivudine or one of two other alternative two-drug regimens) (CDC, 2001). If the source patient is (or recently has been) receiving antiretroviral therapy, some authorities recommended use of alternative regimens (Henderson, 2004).

There are two major problems with antiretroviral prophylaxis after occupational exposure to HIV. First, these drugs have substantial toxicity. Data on healthy individuals, especially for the newer agents, are extremely limited (Henderson, 2004). Studies of antiretroviral prophylaxis after occupational HIV exposures in health care workers have demonstrated substantial side effects, often limiting completion of the regimen. Recently, use of nevirapine has been contraindicated because of the risk of severe liver toxicity, including hepatic failure. Virtually all marketed antiretroviral agents have potential for carcinogenicity, teratogenicity, and mutagenicity. Second, there have been documented failures of antiretroviral prophylaxis. Cases of zidovudine chemoprophylaxis failure (eight of which have clinical relevance) have appeared in the literature (Henderson, 2004). Thus, the potential risks and benefits of postexposure prophylaxis must be considered on a case-by-case basis.

ANTIRETROVIRAL THERAPY (Fig. 12–4)

Suppression of HIV replication is associated with a significant delay in the progression to AIDS and increased survival. Thus, the goal of antiretroviral treatment should be to obtain maximal and sustained suppression of HIV replication (Vella and Floridia, 2004).

The main tools for monitoring antiretroviral treatment are the plasma HIV RNA level and CD4+ lymphocyte count (O'Brien et al, 1996). **Previously untreated patients should reach undetectable plasma HIV RNA levels within 4 to 6 months accompanied by a concomitant rise in CD4+ counts. In this context "undetectable plasma HIV RNA level" does not mean eradication of the virus at other sites (lymphoid tissues, central nervous system, or genital tract)** (Perelson et al, 1997). Eradication of HIV from these viral reservoirs and sanctuaries is not yet a realistic goal.

From Monotherapy to HAART

In 1987, zidovudine, the first effective antiretroviral drug and prototype of the nucleoside reverse transcriptase inhibitors (NRTIs), was introduced. Zidovudine monotherapy remained the mainstay of treatment until it became evident that benefit was limited (Concorde Coordinating Committee, 1994). Clinical trials demonstrated that two-drug regimens induced a more profound and prolonged effect on viral load and CD4+ counts, delayed clinical progression, and increased patient survival (Hammer et al, 1996; Deeks et al, 1997). In 1995, protease inhibitors (PIs) became available. Combined with NRTIs, PIs produced a further reduction of HIV replication, often to undetectable levels (Deeks et al, 1997). Nonnucleoside reverse transcriptase inhibitors (NNRTIs), introduced after 1996, also proved highly effective. Availability of a rapidly increasing number of drugs and the evolving information has made HIV treatment extremely complex.

The objective of antiretroviral therapy is to prevent disease progression and prolong survival while maintaining quality of life. Long-term nonprogression will be achieved by reducing plasma viral load below 50 copies/mL on a long-term basis. Combinations of antiretroviral agents with minimal or no overlapping toxicity and demonstrated antiviral additive to synergistic effect is recommended to maximize the antiviral response (Montaner et al, 2004).

Available Drugs

The optimal treatment of HIV infection is a potent combination of drugs, termed highly active anti-retroviral therapy. Most HAART regimens are based on a dual nucleoside "backbone" plus an NNRTI or a PI (with the option of adding low-dose ritonavir to another PI for pharmacologic enhancement). Three-nucleoside regimens including abacavir are increasingly used because these regimens are easy to administer and are dual-class sparing (i.e., allow deferred use of PIs and NNRTIs).

Currently, antiretroviral drugs include six nucleoside reverse transcriptase inhibitors (RTIs) (zidovudine, didanosine, zalcitabine, stavudine, lamivudine, and abacavir), one nucleotide RTI (tenofovir disoproxil fumarate), three NNRTIs (nevirapine, delavirdine, and efavirenz), and six HIV PIs (saquinavir, ritonavir, indinavir, nelfinavir, amprenavir, and lopinavir (Table 12–5).

Reverse Transcriptase Inhibitors. RTIs act through at least two mechanisms. First, as "chain terminators," they block viral DNA elongation, stopping addition of further nucleosides. This mechanism depends on intracellular phosphorylation of RTIs to the corresponding triphosphates. Second, they act by competition/binding of the reverse transcriptase; NNRTIs act only through this mechanism and not as "chain terminators."

Protease Inhibitors. PIs act by binding to the catalytic site of HIV aspartic protease. This enzyme is critical for the post-translational processing of the polyprotein products into the functional core proteins and viral enzymes. By inhibiting this step, PIs release immature, noninfectious viral particles. However, unlike the RTIs, which provide no protection in established HIV infection, PIs are also active in chronically infected cells. PIs are combined with RTIs or with other PIs,

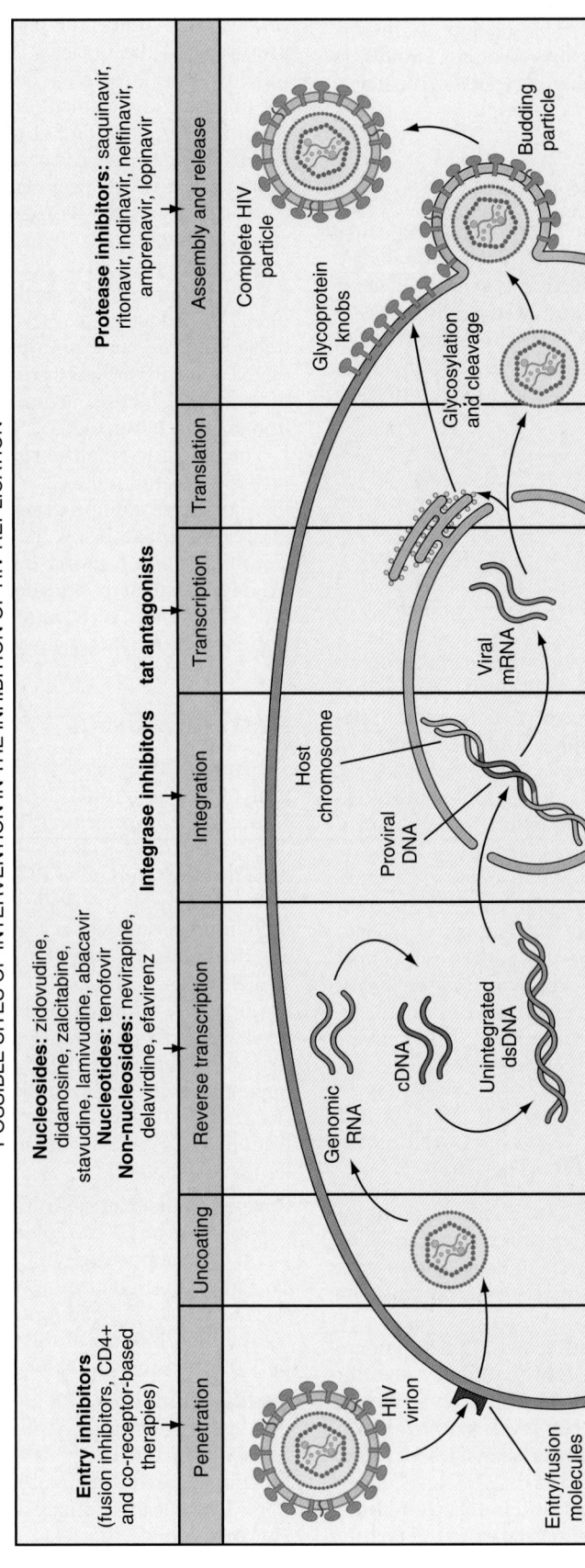

Figure 12–4. Antiretroviral therapy for HIV infection. Diagram illustrates potential sites of action for drug therapy. (From Vella S, Floridia M: HIV therapy: Antiviral therapy. In Cohen J, Powderly WG, Berkley SF, et al [eds]: Infectious Diseases, 2nd ed. Edinburgh, Mosby, 2004, vol 2, pp 1387-1398.)

Table 12–5. Antiviral Drugs Available for HAART Combination Regimens

Class	Drug	Trade Name
Nucleoside reverse transcriptase inhibitors (NRTIs)	Zidovudine (AZT)	Retrovir*†
	Didanosine (ddI)	Videx
	Zalcitabine (ddC)	Hivid
	Lamivudine (3TC)	Epivir*†
	Stavudine (d4T)	Zerit
	Abacavir (ABC)	Ziagen†
Nucleotide reverse transcriptase inhibitors	Tenofovir	Virend
Non-nucleoside reverse transcriptase inhibitors (NNRTIs)	Delaviridine (DLV)	Rescriptor
	Nevirapine (NVP)	Viramune
	Efavirenz (EFV)	Sustiva
Protease inhibitors (PIs)	Saquinavir (SAQ)	Invirase
	Rinonavir (RTV)	Norvir
	Nelfinavir (NFV)	Viracept
	Amprenavir (APV)	Agenerase
	Lopinavir (LPV)	Kaletra‡

*Also available as Combivir (300 mg AZT + 150 mg 3TC).
†Also available as Trizivir (300 mg AZT + 150 mg 3TC + 300 mg ABV).
‡Only available as Kaletra (133.3 mg lopinavir + 33.3 mg ritonavir).
From Vella S, Floridia M: HIV therapy: Antiviral therapy. In Cohen J, Powderly WG, Berkley SF, et al (eds): Infectious Diseases, 2nd ed. Edinburgh, Mosby, 2004, vol 2, pp 1387-1398.

taking advantage of a boosting effect on drug concentrations that occurs when PIs are co-administered.

Significant Urologic Side Effects. Of the RTIs, zalcitabine is associated with peripheral neuropathy and painful penile ulcers. Of the PIs, ritonavir should be used with caution among patients at high risk of bleeding. Indinavir is a potent PI that has been associated with urolithiasis (discussed earlier). In addition to drug-specific adverse events, long-term use HAART has highlighted a number of previously unrecognized adverse events. Some appear to be associated with a specific class of drugs, such as mitochondrial toxicity and lactic acidosis with NRTIs or hypoglycemia with PIs. Fat distribution changes (commonly described as lipodystrophy) represent a major clinical event. This syndrome presents as atrophic changes (peripheral fat loss involving face and limbs resembling Cushing's disease), hypertrophic changes (visceral or dorsocervical fat accumulation, breast enlargement), or both.

New Investigational Agents. Even with potent, multidrug regimens, virologic failure is frequent. This may depend on various factors, including low adherence, drug-resistant HIV strains, low drug levels in the plasma or tissues, and other undetermined factors. Targeted strategies are being developed to improve treatment efficacy, including development of new drugs with improved formulation and administration schedules, increased potency, and reduced toxicity. A number of agents in each of the available drug classes as well as drugs with novel mechanisms of action are in development. Desirable characteristics of this new generation of drugs include easier administration schedule, perfected pharmacokinetics, potency, tolerability, and the ability to inhibit HIV viruses that are resistant to the existing agents.

Evolving HIV Treatment Strategies

Growing appreciation of the difficulties of taking antiretroviral therapy on a long-term basis, the adverse effects of many regimens, and of their negative impact on quality of life has led to reevaluation of this early intervention strategy. Because "eradication" of HIV is not on the horizon, the goal of therapy must now be redirected toward the long-term management of a chronic infection (Vella and Floridia, 2004).

The decision to start treatment is now based first on the patient's disease stage, because it is clear that a symptomatic patient should be treated. For an asymptomatic patient, the decision is often driven by the CD4+ lymphocyte count and the plasma HIV RNA level (Montaner et al, 2004). **The CD4+ T lymphocyte count can be regarded as an immediate predictor of prognosis, whereas the plasma HIV RNA level indicates the level of actual HIV replication.** Other elements include the patient's commitment to therapy and knowledge of the limitations of current regimens.

In addition to a plethora of new antiretroviral agents targeting the HIV replication cycle, there are a number of strategies under active investigation to prevent HIV infection or to improve therapy. Two promising approaches are development of immune-based strategies and vaccines.

Immune-Based Strategies That May Be Combined with HAART

Because eradication of HIV with HAART probably cannot be achieved in less than 50 to 60 years (Montaner et al, 2004), the possibility of adding additional treatment to ensure immune restoration holds considerable appeal (Pollard and Onorato, 2004). Various strategies are under investigation to both enhance HIV-specific immune responses and to stimulate the general immune responses, such as therapeutic vaccination, structured treatment interruption, transfer of HIV-specific cell populations to enhance cell-mediated immunity, and transfer of pooled immune sera from donors who have HIV infection or of monoclonal antibodies directed against HIV. Such strategies may be of particular value for treating later-stage disease, whose high levels of viremia and previous exposure to therapy place them at greatest risk of developing resistance to therapeutic agents (Pollard and Onorato, 2004).

Vaccines to Prevent HIV Infection. Considerable efforts are being expended to develop an effective vaccine to prevent HIV infection (Rosenberg et al 1997; Amara et al, 2001; Shiver et al, 2002; Fast et al, 2004). HIV represents a formidable challenge. Its immune evasion mechanisms include molecular tricks to avoid neutralization by antibody, downregulation of immune functions, direct destruction of the CD4+ T cells that support both antibody and effector T-cell responses, and a very rapid mutation rate that gives rise to virus strains lacking the antigenic sites to which effective immune responses are directed.

Nevertheless, several lines of evidence suggest that vaccines may prove effective in preventing HIV infection or in preventing progression to AIDS (Fast et al, 2004). First, HIV infection occurs after only a small fraction of all exposures, suggesting that a modest immune defense might be effective. Second, the natural history of HIV infection is that, after an initial phase of rapid viral replication, immune responses may control HIV replication and slow its pathogenic effects for many years. Third, in primate models some vaccines can prevent infection or slow viral replication and disease progression. Immunization that induces mucosal responses is particularly effective against mucosal challenges, as would occur with sexual exposure (Amara et al, 2001; Shiver et al, 2002). A number of vaccines have been tested and, lacking credible immunogenicity data, abandoned. Several more promising vaccines have recently entered trials or are expected to do so soon.

SUGGESTED READINGS

Bailey RC, Plummer FA, Moses S: Male circumcision and HIV prevention: Current knowledge and future research directions. Lancet Infect Dis 2001;1:223.

Centers for Disease Control and Prevention: Updated U.S. Public Health Service guidelines for the management of occupational exposures to HBV, HCV, and HIV and recommendations for postexposure prophylaxis. MMWR Morb Mortal Wkly Rep 2001;50:1.

Daudon M, Jungers P: Drug-induced renal calculi: Epidemiology, prevention and management. Drugs 2004;64:245.

Krieger JN, Nirapathpongporn A, Chaiyaporn M, et al: Vasectomy and human immunodeficiency virus type 1 in semen. J Urol 1998;159:820.

Patterson BK, Landay A, Siegel JN, et al: Susceptibility to human immunodeficiency virus-1 infection of human foreskin and cervical tissue grown in explant culture. Am J Pathol 2002;161:867.

Pierre-Alexandre B, Pantaleo G: Pathogenesis: Immunopathogenesis of HIV-1 infection. In Cohen J, Powderly WG, Berkley SF, et al (eds): Infectious Diseases. Edinburgh, Mosby, 2004, vol 2, pp 1235-1249.

Quinn TC, Wawer MJ, Sewankambo N, et al: Viral load and heterosexual transmission of human immunodeficiency virus type 1. Rakai Project Study Group. N Engl J Med 2000;342:921.

Ross MJ, Klotman PE: HIV-associated nephropathy. AIDS 2004;18:1089.

Vella S, Floridia M: HIV therapy: Antiviral therapy. In Cohen J, Powderly WG, Berkley SF, et al (eds): Infectious Diseases. Edinburgh, Mosby, 2004, vol 2, pp 1387-1398.

World Health Organization: The world health report 2004—changing history. Accessed May 2004 at http://www.who.int/whr.

KEY POINTS: UROLOGIC IMPLICATIONS OF AIDS AND HIV INFECTION

- With effective antiretroviral therapy, deaths attributed to AIDS are declining rapidly in Western European and North American cities.

- In many African cities AIDS represents the leading cause of death and of years of potential lost in men and the second most important cause of death in women. Life expectancy in the most affected sub-Saharan countries was reduced as much as 15 years by the year 2000, compared with projections without HIV.

- The three main modes of HIV transmission have changed little: unprotected intercourse, contact with blood, and transmission from mother to child.

- Eradication of HIV is not possible with available antiviral drugs.

- In the absence of treatment, the typical course of HIV occurs over 8 to 12 years.

- Without antiretroviral therapy, AIDS usually leads to death in 2 to 3 years.

- In 60% to 70% of HIV-infected patients, the median time between infection and the development of AIDS is 10 to 11 years, in the absence of therapy.

- Ten to 20 percent of HIV infections progress rapidly, and these patients develop AIDS less than 5 years after infection.

- Five to 15 percent of HIV-infected people are "slow progressors," remaining free of AIDS for more than 15 years in the absence of therapy.

13 Cutaneous Diseases of the External Genitalia

RICHARD E. LINK, MD, PhD

Diagnosis and treatment of cutaneous diseases of the external genitalia remains an important element of urologic practice. Often overlooked during formal urologic residency training, this topic lies at the interface of three specialties: urology, infectious disease, and dermatology.

INTRODUCTION TO BASIC DERMATOLOGY

Dermatology is the clinical discipline focused on the biology and pathology of the skin. The diagnosis of skin disease depends critically on the history and physical examination, with laboratory testing often relegated to a peripheral and confirmatory role. In many cases, visual inspection alone suffices to narrow the diagnosis significantly.

The skin is divided into three layers: the epidermis, dermis, and subcutaneous tissue. The epidermis, composed of stratified squamous epithelium, can vary in thickness from 0.05 to 1.5 mm depending on location. The dermis, composed of collagen, elastin, and reticular fibers, can be divided into two layers: the thin superficial layer (papillary dermis) and the thicker deeper layer (reticular dermis).

Literally hundreds of cutaneous diseases exist that may involve the external genitalia. In addition, within each disease there may be significant variation in appearance and symptoms as the process evolves. For this reason, a methodical and systematic approach is essential to reach a rational diagnosis. The dermatologic history should focus on the duration, rate of onset, location, symptoms, family history, allergies, occupation, and previous treatment of the condition (Habif, 2004). Common symptoms include pruritus (itching), burning, and pain.

The physical examination should address the distribution of primary and secondary skin lesions. **It is important to perform a thorough skin survey and not focus solely on the area of affected genital skin.** Most skin conditions begin with a characteristic primary lesion that is an important key to diagnosis. Precise description of this lesion includes documenting its color (red, brown, black, yellow, blue, or green) and morphology (macule, papule, plaque, nodule, pustule, vesicle, bulla, or wheal; Table 13–1) (Habif, 2004). Because of the mucosal nature of genital skin, papular and macular lesions may present as erosions in this area (Margolis, 2002). Secondary skin lesions develop as the skin condition evolves or are caused by scratching or superinfection. A secondary lesion should also be classified morphologically as a scale, crust, erosion, ulcer, atrophy, or scar (Table 13–2).

Once gross morphology is determined, laboratory testing may serve to confirm the diagnosis. To identify cutaneous fungi such as dermatophytes and *Candida* species, potassium hydroxide (KOH) or periodic acid–Schiff (PAS) staining may be applied to scraped or touched skin specimens. KOH dissolves keratin, leaving fungal hyphal walls prominently visible under the microscope. Likewise, Tzanck preparations may aid in identifying viral agents such as herpes simplex, varicella-zoster, and molluscum contagiosum.

For difficult cases or those in which malignancy is suspected, skin biopsy may be indicated. A variety of techniques exist for this purpose, including curettage and punch, shave, incisional, and complete excisional biopsies. For small scrotal or phallic shaft lesions, these techniques can often be performed in the office setting under local anesthesia. For larger lesions or those involving the glans penis or urethral meatus, biopsy in the operating room is recommended.

Table 13-1. Primary Cutaneous Lesions

Primary Lesion	Description
Flat	
Macule	A circumscribed, **flat** discoloration that may be brown, blue, red, or hypopigmented
Elevated, solid	
Papule	An **elevated, solid** lesion up to 0.5 cm in diameter of variable color. Papules may become confluent to become plaques.
Nodule	A circumscribed, **elevated solid** lesion > 0.5 cm in diameter
Plaque	A circumscribed, **elevated**, superficial, **solid** lesion > 0.5 cm in diameter
Fluid-Filled	
Vesicle	A circumscribed **collection of free fluid** up to 0.5 cm in diameter
Bulla	A circumscribed **collection of free fluid** > 0.5 cm in diameter
Pustule	A circumscribed collection of leukocytes and free fluid (**pus**)
Wheal (hive)	A firm **erythematous plaque** resulting from **infiltration** of the dermis with fluid (may be transient)

From Habif TP: Clinical Dermatology: A Color Guide to Diagnosis and Therapy. Edinburgh, Mosby, 2004.

Table 13-2. Secondary Cutaneous Lesions

Secondary Lesion	Description
Scale	Excess dead epidermal cells that are produced by abnormal keratinization and shedding
Crust	A collection of dried serum and cellular debris (a scab)
Erosion	A focal loss of epidermis. Erosions do not penetrate below the dermoepidermal junction and heal without scarring.
Ulcer	A focal loss of epidermis and dermis that heals with scarring
Fissure	A linear loss of epidermis and dermis with sharply defined, vertical walls
Atrophy	A depression in the skin resulting from thinning of the epidermis or dermis
Scar	An abnormal formation of connective tissue implying dermal damage

From Habif TP: Clinical Dermatology: A Color Guide to Diagnosis and Therapy. Edinburgh, Mosby, 2004.

DERMATOLOGIC THERAPY

Medical therapy for dermatologic conditions consists of a broad range of topical and systemic compounds.

For systemic therapy, useful drug classes include antibiotics and antifungal, antiviral, anti-inflammatory, and antipruritic agents. Less commonly used agents, including chemotherapeutic drugs (e.g., methotrexate, cyclophosphamide), immunosuppressants (e.g., azathioprine, cyclosporine, tacrolimus), and hydroxyurea, are covered in the discussions of specific disease entities.

A lack of familiarity with cutaneous diseases affecting the genitalia may lower the threshold of urologists to prescribe systemic antibiotics for these conditions. Unfortunately, these agents carry significantly greater risks than topical preparations, including promotion of resistant organisms, interaction with other medications, and disruption of the normal bowel and vaginal flora. Similar caveats apply to systemic antifungal agents such as ketoconazole and fluconazole. Superficial dermatophytes, such as those causing tinea cruris, generally respond well to topical antifungal preparations. **Systemic antifungal agents are indicated for local infection with an extensive area of skin involved, disseminated mycoses with skin involvement, infection involving the hair follicles, or fungal infections in immunocompromised individuals** (Lesher and McConnell, 2003). In some cases, even in immunocompetent individuals, systemic antifungal agents are necessary to treat infections resistant to local therapy (Lesher, 1999).

Systemic anti-inflammatory agents, in particular the glucocorticosteroids (GCS), deserve additional attention. Oral GCS are absorbed in the jejunum, with peak plasma concentrations occurring in 30 to 90 minutes (Lester, 1989). Despite short plasma half-lives of 1 to 5 hours, the duration of effect of GCS lasts between 8 and 48 hours, depending on the agent (Nesbitt, 2003). These drugs have widespread anti-inflammatory effects. They release neutrophils from bone marrow but inhibit their movement to sites of inflammation in tissue. They also impair both T-cell activation and antigen presentation by dendritic cells (Nesbitt, 2003). **For short-term (= 3 weeks) treatment of dermatologic conditions such as allergic contact dermatitis** (Feldman, 1992), **a single morning dose of GCS is given to minimize suppression of the hypothalamic-pituitary-adrenal axis** (Myles, 1971). Prednisone is generally the GCS of choice owing to its low cost, intermediate duration of action, and variety of dosage forms, although methylprednisolone may be substituted to reduce mineralocorticoid effects (Wolverton, 2001). **Longer-term treatment with systemic GCS may lead to a wide variety of adverse effects, including osteoporosis, cataract formation, hypertension, obesity, immunosuppression, and psychiatric changes** (Nesbitt, 2003).

Topical preparations are the mainstay of therapy for a wide range of cutaneous diseases affecting the genitalia. Urologists tend to be less familiar with the use of these medications than dermatologists. **Topical medications can be broken down into five general classes: emollients, anti-inflammatory agents, antibiotics, antifungal agents, and chemotherapeutic agents.**

Topical preparations have both active ingredients and a vehicle that determines the rate at which the active ingredients are absorbed by the skin. Emollients restore water and lipids to the epidermis and are useful for dry skin diseases. Emollients should be applied to moist skin for maximal effect, such as after bathing. Preparations containing urea (e.g., Carmol, vanodine) or lactic acid (Lac-Hydrin, AmLactin) may be particularly potent hydrating agents (Habif, 2004).

Topical corticosteroids are potent anti-inflammatory agents available in a myriad of preparations and strengths. A detailed review of the use and dosing of topical corticosteroids is beyond the scope of this chapter, and the reader is directed to several excellent dermatology textbooks for more detail (Habif, 2004). **It is important to recognize that even topical corticosteroids can have significant adverse effects, both from systemic absorption and locally. Local effects include epidermal atrophy, dermal changes (telangiectasia,** hypopigmentation), allergic reactions, and alteration in the usual course of skin infections and infestations (Burry, 1973). In most cases, atrophy is a reversible process that can be expected to resolve over the course of several months (Sneddon, 1976). Atrophy is particularly troublesome if corticosteroids are applied under the foreskin, which can serve as an occlusive "dressing" and enhance penetration of the drug (Fig. 13–1) (Goldman and Kitzmiller, 1973).

A variety of physical modalities have also been applied to treat dermatologic problems, including ultraviolet light therapy, photodynamic therapy, laser therapy, and cryosurgery. Ultraviolet light therapy with UVB has been used to treat psoriasis, atopic dermatitis, and seborrheic dermatitis (Honigsmann and Schwarz, 2003). Psoralens, when combined with long-wave UVA radiation (PUVA therapy), can generate a phototoxic effect beneficial for treating psoriasis (Honigsmann, 2001), vitiligo (Honigsmann and Schwarz, 2003), atopic dermatitis (Morison, 1992), and lichen planus (Honigsmann and Schwarz, 2003). Photodynamic therapy (PDT) involves the use of cytotoxic oxygen radicals generated from photo-activated molecules to achieve a therapeutic response (Tope and Shaffer, 2003). PDT is a new arena of dermatologic therapy and holds promise for treating a variety of inflammatory and malignant skin conditions. Laser surgery and cryosurgery play a relatively small role in the management of genital lesions, although the CO_2 laser has been used effectively to manage genital condyloma accuminata.

ALLERGIC DERMATITIS

Allergic or "eczematous" dermatitis consists of a group of allergy-mediated processes leading to pruritic skin lesions (Table 13–3).

Atopic Dermatitis (Eczema)

Atopic dermatitis (AD) is a chronic relapsing dermatitis associated with intense pruritus and damage to the epidermis. **The characteristic lesions are erythematous papules and thin plaques with secondary excoriations** (Fig. 13–2) (Kang et al, 2003). In general, the lesions do not have a precise border, as is common for papulosquamous disorders (Margolis, 2002). Although any age can be affected, 90% of patients with AD

Table 13–3. **Differential Diagnosis of Allergic Dermatitis**
Eczema
Allergic dermatitis
Seborrheic dermatitis
Intertrigo
Contact dermatitis
Irritant dermatitis
Balanoposthitis
Zoon's balanitis
Candidal-related illness
Impetigo
Herpes simplex
Herpes zoster
Drug reaction

From Margolis DJ: Cutaneous diseases of the male external genitalia. In Walsh PC (ed): Campbell's Urology. Philadelphia, WB Saunders, 2002.

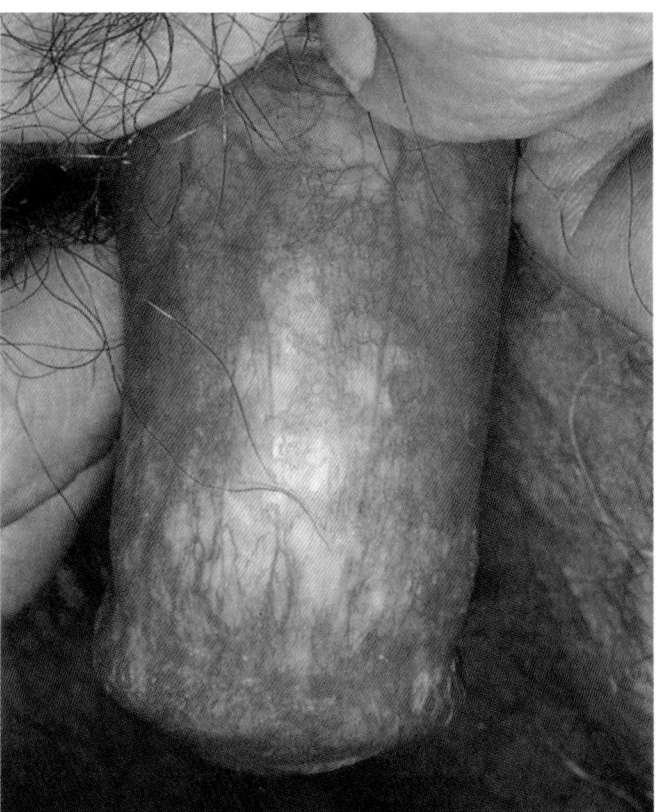

Figure 13–1. Steroid atrophy of penile shaft skin after application of corticosteroid under the foreskin for 8 weeks. (From Habif TP: Clinical Dermatology. Edinburgh, Mosby, 2004, p 36.)

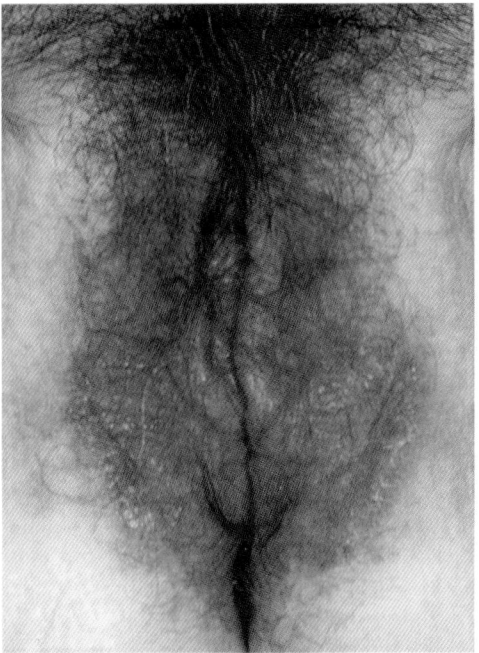

Figure 13–2. Eczema involving the vulva. (From du Vivier A: Atlas of Clinical Dermatology. London, Churchill Livingstone, 2002, p 687.)

manifest their condition before the age of 5 years (Rajka, 1989). AD is associated with susceptibility to irritants and proteins as well as the tendency to develop asthma and allergic rhinitis.

The genetic susceptibility to AD has been extensively explored. In a study of 372 patients with this disorder, 73% had a positive family history for atopy. Likewise, twin concordance studies have demonstrated a risk for having AD of 0.86 for monozygotic twins as compared with only 0.21 for dizygotic twins. These findings have spurred an intense search for genes involved in atopy and AD (Wollenberg and Bieber, 2000), although no single gene has been found to be a unique marker for the disease (Kang et al, 2003).

Intense pruritus is the hallmark of AD, and controlling the patient's urge to scratch is critical for successful treatment (Przybilla et al, 1994). Itching is often worse during evening hours and can be exacerbated by sweating or wool clothing (Kang et al, 2003). Scratching of lesions may contribute to the clinical complications of AD, including superinfection with *Staphylococcus aureus* (Ogawa et al, 1994). There is growing evidence that bacterial toxins may serve as superantigens that drive an inflammatory cascade sustaining atopic dermatitis (Skov and Baadsgaard, 2000; Skov et al, 2000).

Clinically, there is no pathognomonic laboratory test, biopsy result, or single clinical feature that allows the definitive diagnosis of AD. The association with a personal or family history of atopy is a critical clue to the diagnosis (Kang et al, 2003). For patients presenting with genital findings, extragenital involvement is common.

A variety of "trigger factors" have been implicated in the exacerbation of AD, including chemicals, detergents, and household dust mites. Removal of these factors from the environment may be beneficial on an individualized basis. Dust mite exposure, in particular, has received significant attention in the literature. Although several studies have demonstrated modest improvement in AD with mite reduction (Kubota et al, 1992; Tan et al, 1996), others report that reduction is associated with no significant clinical benefit (Colloff et al, 1989; Gutgesell et al, 2001).

Treatment of AD includes gentle cleaning with nonalkali soaps and the frequent use of emollients. Evaporation of liquid from the skin may trigger AD (Kang et al, 2003), thus very frequent bathing is not encouraged. Soaking may be helpful during episodes of bacterial superinfection but should be discontinued once the infection has resolved (Margolis, 2002). Topical corticosteroids may be needed to control pruritus but should only be used for short courses, with a rapid taper to avoid local complications of skin atrophy and pigment changes. Topical macrolide immunomodulatory agents such as tacrolimus and pimecrolimus have shown efficacy in the treatment of AD (Meagher et al, 2002; Nghiem et al, 2002), although experience with genital application is lacking. Antihistamines such as diphenhydramine may be helpful in breaking the "itch-scratch cycle," particularly when given before bedtime (Kang et al, 2003). Oral antistaphylococcal drugs have not been shown to significantly improve AD in one randomized, double-blind trial (Ewing et al, 1998). Systemic treatment with corticosteroids, cyclosporine, methotrexate, or azathioprine may be indicated rarely for severe, widely disseminated cases (Cooper, 1993; Salek et al, 1993).

Contact Dermatitis

Contact dermatitis can be broken down into two distinct entities: irritant contact dermatitis (ICD) and allergic contact dermatitis (ACD). Although the mechanisms differ significantly, the clinical presentation of ICD and ACD may be similar. Most notably, the affected area is usually sharply limited to an area of skin exposure to an allergen or irritating chemical. The primary mode of treatment is to identify and reduce exposure to the offending agent.

ICD results from a direct cytotoxic effect of an irritant chemical touching the skin and is responsible for approximately 80% of cases of contact dermatitis (Marks et al, 2002). Examples of offending agents include soaps, solvents, metal salts, and acid or alkali-containing compounds. Occupational ICD is a serious public health problem and contributes to costs on the scale of $1 billion annually in the United States (Cohen, 2000). The clinical manifestations of ICD depend on the identity of the irritating substance as well as the duration of contact, concentration, temperature, pH, and location of exposure. Acute ICD, such as might result from an occupational accident, generally peaks within minutes to hours after exposure and then begins to heal. Symptoms of burning, stinging, and soreness may be accompanied by erythema, edema, bullae, or frank necrosis in a sharply defined area corresponding to the exposed skin (Cohen and Bassiri-Tehrani, 2003). There are also a variety of subacute forms of ICD that result from repeated subthreshold skin insults. Pruritus is much more common in these more chronic conditions, and the skin lesions are less well demarcated. The mainstay of treatment for ICD lies in avoiding skin contact with the causative irritants through the use of protective clothing, safe occupational practices, and the use of skin barriers such as ointments or emollients (Berndt et al, 2000).

In contrast, allergic contact dermatitis (ACD) represents a local type IV hypersensitivity reaction to a skin allergen to which an individual has been previously sensitized. The typical appearance is a well-demarcated pruritic eruption, which may manifest as blistering or weeping in the acute phase or the development of scaly plaques more chronically (Mowad and Marks, 2003). In 2003, the North American Contact Dermatitis Group (NACDG) reported a long list of common allergens implicated in ACD based on patch testing results (Marks et al, 2003). Patch testing is a simple technique of exposing an area of skin to a variety of potential allergens in a grid template (Fig. 13–3). Generally performed by dermatologists, patch testing can help to confirm the diagnosis of ACD and the allergen involved. The most common sensitizing allergen identified by the NACDG was nickel sulfate, which is a common component of costume jewelry and belt buckles (Fig. 13–4). Although traditionally a cause of earlobe dermatitis from pierced earrings, nickel sensitivity may be a potential cause of genital ACD due to the increasing prevalence of genital piercing. Other important allergens include textile dyes, topical antibiotics, perfumes, and topical corticosteroids. Oral antihistamines may be helpful for the symp-

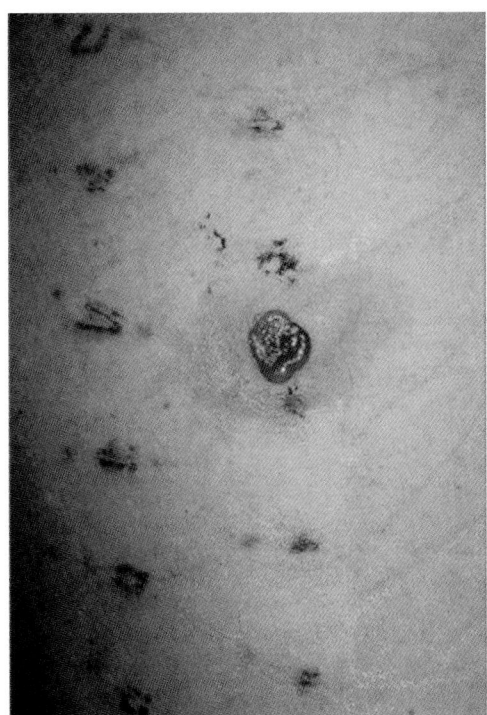

Figure 13–3. An example of patch testing with a positive response to nickel. (From Bolognia JL, Jorizzo JL, Rapini RP: Dermatology. Edinburgh, Mosby, 2003, p 233.)

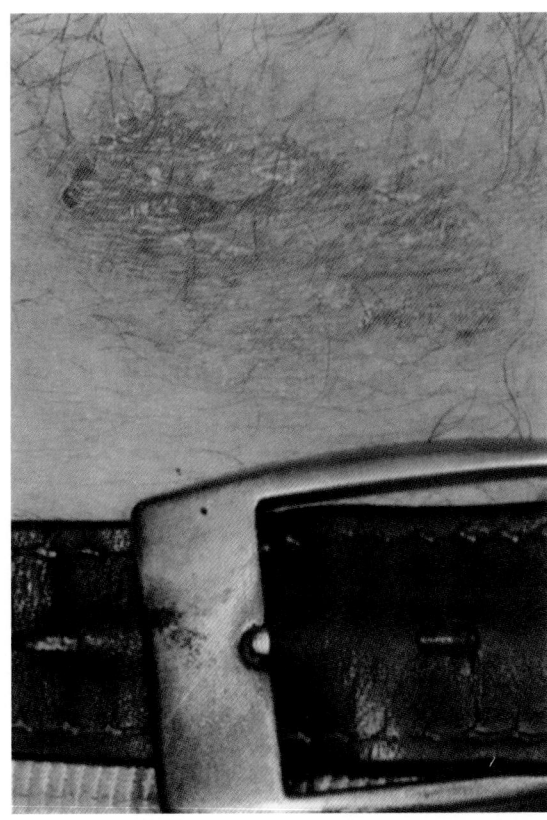

Figure 13–4. Contact dermatitis from belt buckle due to nickel allergy. (From Habif TP: Clinical Dermatology. Edinburgh, Mosby, 2004, p 94.)

tomatic control of ACD in combination with removal of the inciting allergen.

Erythema Multiforme and Stevens-Johnson Syndrome

Erythema multiforme (EM) is a generalized skin disease that may involve the genitalia. **EM can be subdivided into minor and major forms.**

EM minor was first described in 1860 by an Austrian dermatologist, Ferdinand von Hebra. **It is an acute, self-limited skin disease characterized by the abrupt onset of symmetrical fixed red papules that may evolve into target lesions** (Weston, 1996). EM is a clinical rather than a histologic diagnosis. Papules and target lesions are usually grouped and can be present anywhere on the body, including the genitalia (Fig. 13–5). There is also a predilection for involvement of the oral mucous membranes.

The majority of cases of EM minor are precipitated by herpesvirus types 1 and 2 (Schofield et al, 1993; Nikkels and Pierard, 2002), **with herpetic lesions usually preceding the development of target lesions by 10 to 14 days** (Lemak et al, 1986). Although continuous suppressive acyclovir may prevent EM episodes in patients with herpesvirus infection (Tatnall et al, 1995), administration of the drug after development of target lesions is of no benefit (Huff, 1988). The natural history of EM minor is spontaneous resolution after several weeks without sequelae (Schofield et al, 1993), although recurrences are common (Huff and Weston, 1989). Oral antihistamines may provide symptomatic relief. For immunosuppressed patients, the time course of EM minor

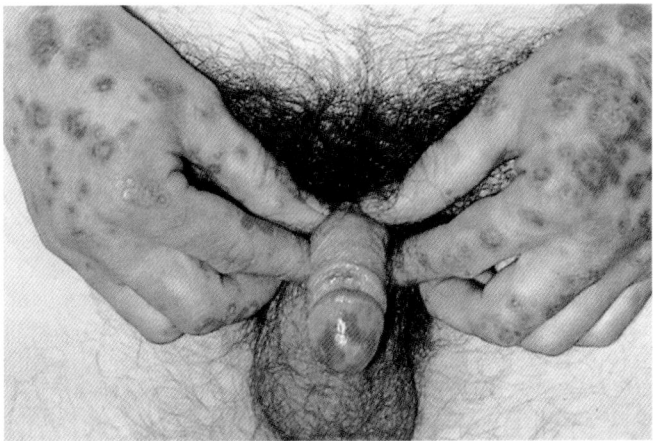

Figure 13–5. Erythema multiforme. Targetoid lesions of the hands and penis. (From Korting GW: Practical Dermatology of the Genital Region. Philadelphia, WB Saunders, 1981, p 16.)

outbreaks may be longer and the frequency of recurrence may be greater (Schofield et al, 1993).

The major form of EM has been called Stevens-Johnson syndrome (SJS) in the past, although there remains some controversy as to whether EM major and SJS are distinct entities (Bachot and Roujeau, 2003; Williams and Conklin, 2005). SJS is a much more serious illness than EM minor, with features similar to extensive skin burns. In its more severe forms, SJS may mimic life-threatening toxic epidermal necrolysis.

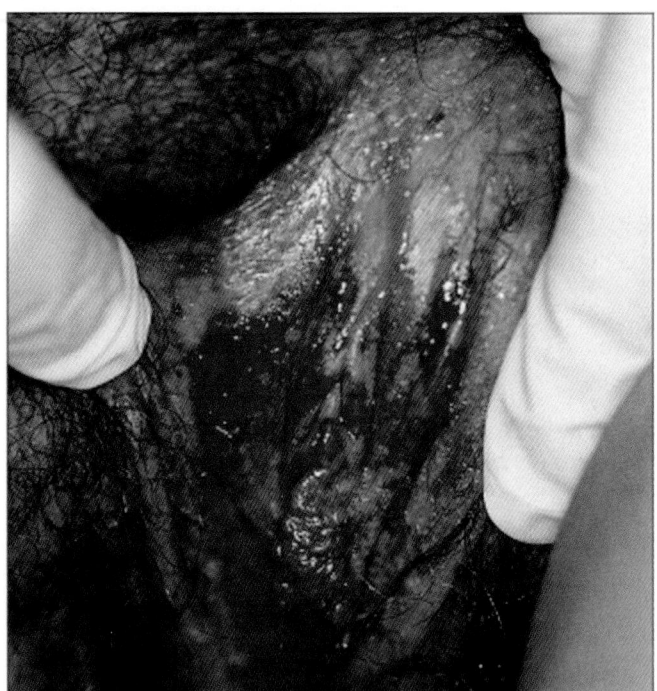

Figure 13–6. Labial erosions in a case of Stevens-Johnson syndrome. (From Bolognia JL, Jorizzo JL, Rapini RP: Dermatology. Edinburgh, Mosby, 2003, p 319.)

Table 13–4. **Differential Diagnosis of Papulosquamous Lesions**
Psoriasis
Seborrheic dermatitis
Dermatophyte infection
Erythrasma
Secondary syphilis
Pityriasis rosea
Discoid lupus
Mycosis fungoides
Lichen planus
Fixed drug eruption
Reiter's syndrome
Pityriasis versicolor
Bowen's disease
Extramammary Paget's disease

From Margolis DJ: Cutaneous diseases of the male external genitalia. In Walsh PC (ed): Campbell's Urology. Philadelphia, WB Saunders, 2002.

Psoriasis

Psoriasis is a common disease affecting up to 2% of the population (Christophers, 2001). For patients with a predisposition, which is likely polygenic in nature, triggering factors such as trauma, infection, psychological stress, or new medications can elicit a flare-up in the psoriatic phenotype. One third of affected patients have a family history of psoriasis (Melski and Stern, 1981; Hensler and Christophers, 1985; Margolis, 2002).

The characteristic lesion is a sharply demarcated erythematous plaque with silvery-white scales (van de Kerkhof, 2003). Its pattern can be limited to the elbows or knees or distributed over the entire surface of the skin. Although psoriasis can appear at any age, two peaks of onset have been identified: 20 to 30 and 50 to 60 years of age. Patients' complain of a significant impairment in their quality of life due to pruritus and the cosmetic impact of these visible plaques.

Psoriatic involvement of the genitalia is relatively common, although usually within the context of a generalized cutaneous disorder. **Patients may present with concerns for malignancy or sexually transmitted disease when psoriatic lesions are present on the genitalia.** The presence of characteristic lesions on the elbows, knees, buttocks, nails, scalp, and umbilicus may help direct the diagnosis (Fig. 13–7) (Margolis, 2002). When lesions are present in the inguinal folds and intergluteal cleft, scaling may be absent (so-called inverse psoriasis) (Goldman, 2000). When evaluating nonscaling erythematous plaques in the inguinal folds, the diagnosis of fungal involvement (i.e., tinea or *Candida* infection) should be considered. In circumcised men, psoriatic plaques are often present on the glans and corona, whereas in uncircumcised men lesions are commonly hidden under the preputial skin (Buechner, 2002). In some cases, however, psoriasis involves the entire penis and scrotum (Fig. 13–8).

Psoriasis is a chronic disease with a relapsing and remitting course. A variety of topical and systemic therapies have been developed and applied to this difficult problem. Despite the variety of therapy, however, as many as 40% of psoriasis sufferers express frustration at the ineffectiveness of current treatments (Krueger et al, 2001). **For genital psoriasis, the mainstay of therapy is the use of low-potency topical corticosteroid creams for short courses.** Examples include a

Admission to the intensive care unit or burn unit may significantly reduce morbidity and mortality in this condition (Wolf et al, 2005). **Most patients with SJS have a prodromal upper respiratory illness (fever, cough, rhinitis, sore throat, and headache) that progresses after 1 to 14 days to the abrupt development of red macules with blister formation and areas of epidermal necrosis. Genital involvement includes erythema and erosions of the labia (Fig. 13–6), penis, and perianal region.**

A vast array of inciting factors has been implicated in the development of SJS, with drug exposures being the most commonly identified. Nonsteroidal anti-inflammatory agents are the most frequent offending agents, followed by sulfonamides, tetracycline, penicillin, doxycycline, and anticonvulsants (Chan et al, 1990). In contrast to EM minor, there is rarely an association with an infectious agent (Weston, 2003). **SJS generally has a protracted course of 4 to 6 weeks and may have a mortality rate approaching 30%. Severe scarring of denuded skin may result in a range of complications, including joint contractures, vaginal stenosis, urethral meatal stenosis, and anal strictures** (Brice et al, 1990; Weston, 2003). Treatment involves immediate removal of the offending drug and supportive care similar to the management of severe burns. There is currently no strong evidence for any specific therapy for SJS (Weston, 2003), and the role of systemic corticosteroids in treating SJS remains controversial (Rasmussen, 1976; Tripathi et al, 2000; Weston, 2003).

PAPULOSQUAMOUS DISORDERS

Papulosquamous disorders are a disparate group of diseases that share a common primary lesion: scaly papules and plaques (Table 13–4).

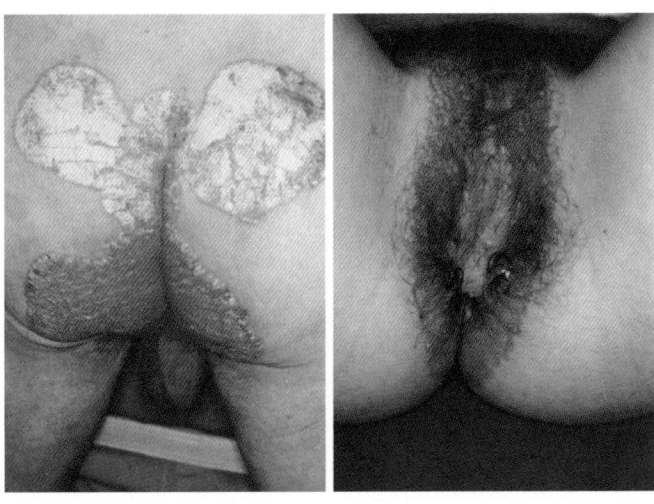

Figure 13–7. Psoriasis. Silver scales on an erythematous base. (From Callen JP, Greer DE, Hood AF, Paller AS: Color Atlas of Dermatology. Philadelphia, WB Saunders, 1993, p 320.)

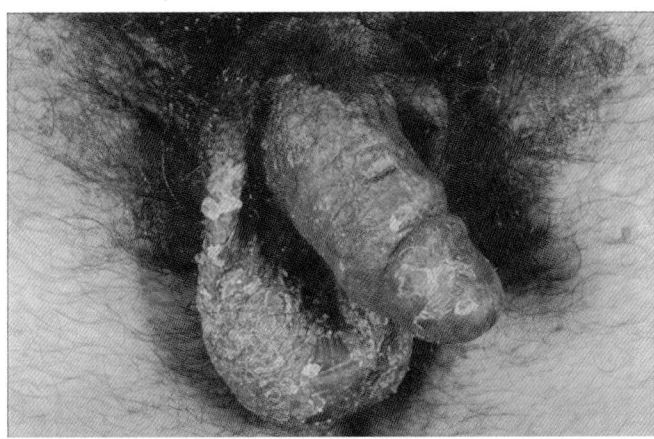

Figure 13–8. Psoriasis involving the entire penis and scrotum. (From Bolognia JL, Jorizzo JL, Rapini RP: Dermatology. Edinburgh, Mosby, 2003, p 130.)

Figure 13–9. Comparison of psoriasis (**A**) and Reiter's syndrome (**B**, balanitis circinata) involving the glans penis. Note the highly characteristic coalescence of lesions in this case of Reiter's syndrome forming a wavy pattern (arrow). (From Habif TP: Clinical Dermatology, Edinburgh, Mosby, 2004, p 217.)

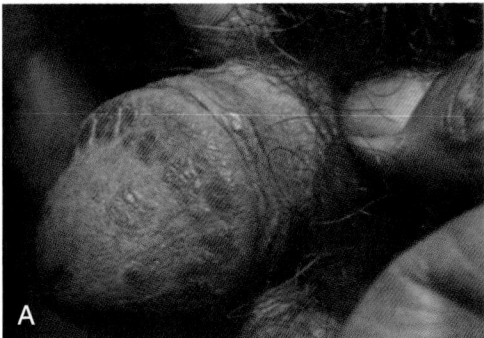

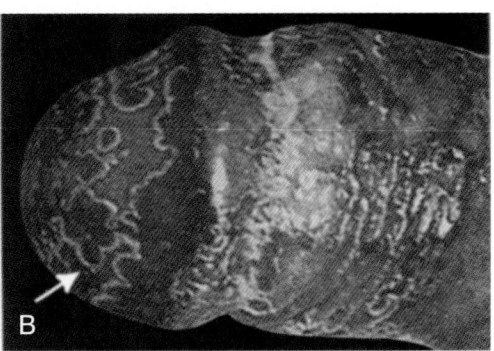

preparation of 3% liquor carbonis detergens in 1% hydrocortisone cream (Fisher and Margesson, 1998). These preparations should not be used for more than 2 weeks continuously on thin genital skin or in areas occluded by skin folds (Margolis, 2002). Other topical therapies for psoriasis include vitamin D₃ analogs, dithranol, and retinoids, although these agents may be too irritating for genital skin application. PUVA therapy has been used extensively to treat psoriasis. However, a dose-dependent increase in the risk of genital squamous cell carcinoma has been associated with high-dose PUVA therapy for psoriasis elsewhere on the body (Stern, 1990; Stern et al, 2002). Genital shielding during PUVA therapy is strongly recommended; therefore, this modality is contraindicated for treating psoriatic lesions localized to genital skin. For patients with extensive psoriasis, systemic therapy with methotrexate, cyclosporine, or retinoids may be appropriate. Experimental therapies that have shown promise in treating psoriasis include the 308-nm excimer laser (Gerber et al, 2003) and antibodies against T-cell surface molecules (Gottlieb et al, 2000), tumor necrosis factor (Chaudhari et al, 2001), or intracellular adhesion molecules (Gottlieb et al, 2000).

Reiter's Syndrome

Reiter's syndrome comprises urethritis, arthritis, ocular findings, oral ulcers, and skin lesions. The skin findings, particu-

larly when present on the genitalia, may be mistaken for psoriatic lesions (Fig. 13–9). Reiter's syndrome is more common in men than in women and is rarely diagnosed in children. **It is generally preceded by an episode of either urethritis (from *Chlamydia, Neisseria gonorrhoeae*) or gastrointestinal infection (*Yersinia, Salmonella, Shigella, Campylobacter, Neisseria,* or *Ureaplasma* species) and is more common in patients infected with human immunodeficiency virus (HIV)** (Rahman et al, 1992; Margolis, 2002). **There is a strong genetic association with the human leukocyte antigen (HLA)-B27 haplotype.** Whether cross-reactivity between bacterial antigens and HLA-B27 leads to autoimmunity in Reiter's syndrome remains controversial (Ringrose, 1999; Yu and Kuipers, 2003).

Conjunctivitis is the most common ocular manifestation, although iritis, uveitis, glaucoma, and keratitis may occur. Polyarthritis and sacroiliitis are the most common orthopedic complaints and may lead to chronic disability in a small minority of cases (van de Kerkhof, 2003). Psoriasiform skin lesions present on the penis are referred to as *balanitis circinata* (Fig. 13–10). **These lesions may be difficult to differentiate from psoriasis, and histologic analysis of biopsy specimens cannot consistently differentiate the two conditions** (Margolis, 2002). The course of Reiter's syndrome involving the genitalia is usually self-limited, lasting a few weeks to months. Lesions may respond to topical corticosteroids, and systemic therapy is rarely required.

Lichen Planus

Lichen planus (LP), the prototype of the lichenoid dermatoses, is an idiopathic inflammatory disease of the skin and mucous

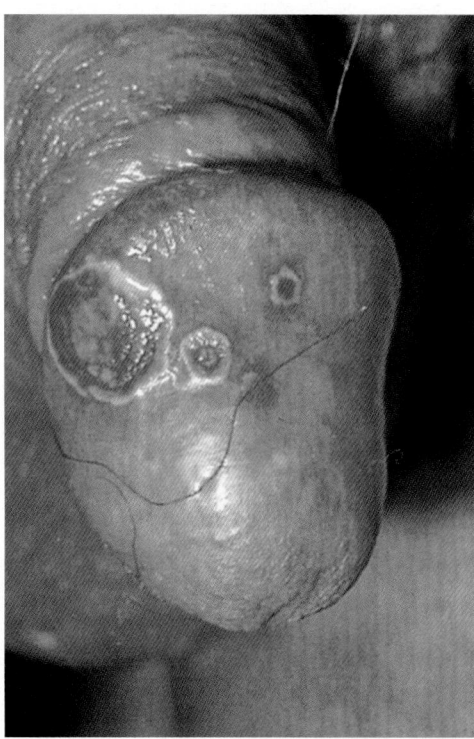

Figure 13–10. Erosive psoriasiform lesions of the glans penis (Reiter's syndrome; balanitis circinata) may also lack the wavy pattern, making them difficult to differentiate from genital psoriasis. (From Callen JP, Greer DE, Hood AF, Paller AS: Color Atlas of Dermatology. Philadelphia, WB Saunders, 1993, p 160.)

membranes. The characteristic "lichenoid tissue reaction" is demonstrated by epidermal basal cell damage that is associated with a massive infiltration of mononuclear cells in the papillary dermis (Shiohara and Kano, 2003). Cutaneous LP may affect up to 1% of the adult population (Boyd and Neldner, 1991), and oral lesions may be present in as many as 4% (Scully et al, 1998). The pathogenesis of LP appears to be related to an autoimmune reaction against basal keratinocytes that express altered self-antigens on their surfaces. (Morhenn, 1986).

The primary lesion of LP is a small, polygonal, violaceous, flat-topped papule. These lesions may be widely separated or coalesce into larger plaques, which may ulcerate, particularly on mucosal surfaces. LP commonly involves the flexor surfaces of the extremities, the trunk, the lumbosacral area, the oral mucosa, and the glans penis (Margolis, 2002). **On the genitalia, the clinical presentation of LP can be quite variable and includes isolated or grouped papules, a white reticular pattern, or an annular (ringlike) arrangement with or without ulceration** (Fig. 13–11). In some cases, the lesions appear to form linear patterns related to skin trauma (the so-called Koebner phenomenon; also seen with psoriasis). The differential diagnosis of LP includes squamous cell carcinoma, Bowen's disease, Zoon's balanitis, psoriasis, secondary syphilis, and lupus erythematosus; and biopsy may be necessary to establish the diagnosis, particularly when the lesions are ulcerated (Shiohara and Kano, 2003). Lichenoid reactions can also occur in response to ingested drugs and contact allergens, and a careful search for potential offending agents is appropriate.

The natural history of LP is benign, and the spontaneous resolution of cutaneous lesions has been observed in up to two thirds of cases after 1 year (Shiohara and Kano, 2003), **although the oral form may persist significantly longer** (Mignogna et al, 2000). Although bothersome pruritus is common with LP, asymptomatic lesions on the genitalia do not require treatment. The primary modality of treatment for symptomatic cutaneous LP is topical corticosteroids, with the caveats mentioned previously about their use on genital skin. For severe cases, systemic corticosteroids (15 to 20 mg/day; 2-

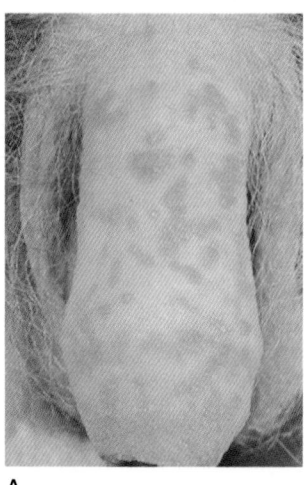
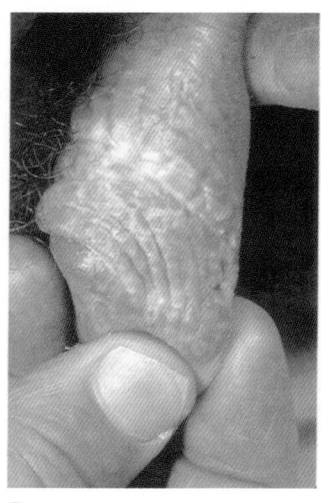
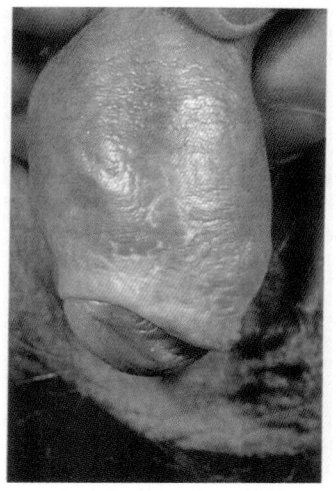
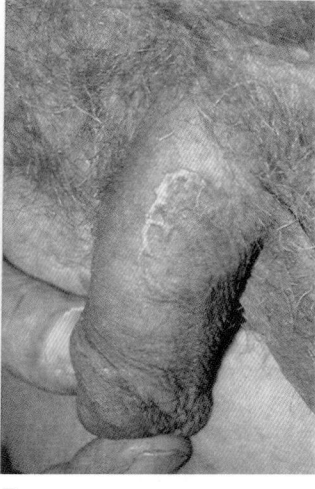

A   B   C   D

Figure 13–11. Various presentations of lichen planus on the male genitalia. **A** and **B,** Individual and grouped purple papules on the penile shaft; some oriented in a linear pattern. **C,** White reticular pattern sometimes seen in lichen planus. **D,** Annular (ringlike) arrangement with a shiny surface. (**A** from Korting GW: Practical Dermatology of the Genital Region. Philadelphia, WB Saunders, 1981, p 29; **B** to **D** from du Vivier A: Atlas of Clinical Dermatology. London, Churchill Livingstone, 2002, p 100.)

to 6-week course [Boyd and Neldner, 1991]) have been shown to shorten the time course to clearance of LP lesions from 29 weeks to 18 weeks (Cribier et al, 1998). Other systemic therapies for severe LP include cyclosporine, griseofulvin, metronidazole, and acitretin (Ho et al, 1990; Boyd and Neldner, 1991; Cribier et al, 1998; Buyuk and Kavala, 2000), although randomized trials demonstrating efficacy are generally lacking.

Lichen Nitidus

Lichen nitidus (LN) is an unusual inflammatory eruption characterized by tiny, discrete, flesh-colored papules arranged in large clusters. Although there is some debate as to whether LN may represent a variant of LP (Aram, 1988), the two entities are histologically distinct. LN has a dense, well-circumscribed, lymphohistiocytic infiltrate closely apposed to the epidermis (Shiohara and Kano, 2003). Commonly involved sites include the flexor aspects of the upper extremities, genitalia, trunk, and dorsal aspects of the hands. Nail involvement is common. Similar to LP, the natural history of LN is one of spontaneous resolution, with the majority of patients (69%) manifesting disease for less than 1 year (Lapins et al, 1978). Patients should be reassured that these genital lesions are not infectious and should resolve with time. For symptomatic pruritus, genital lesions usually respond to topical corticosteroids and oral antihistamines (Shiohara and Kano, 2003).

Lichen Sclerosus

Lichen sclerosus et atrophicus (LS) is a chronic inflammatory disease with a predilection for the external genitalia. LS is 6 to 10 times more prevalent in women than in men, generally presenting around the time of menopause (Wojnarowska and Cooper, 2003). For patients with genital LS, 15% to 20% have extragenital disease (Powell and Wojnarowska, 1999). LS is a scarring disorder characterized by tissue pallor, loss of architecture, and hyperkeratosis (Fig. 13–12). It tends to affect older men (>60 years of age) (Ledwig and Weigand, 1989) and can be associated with pain during voiding or erection (Margolis, 2002). The glans penis and foreskin are usually affected, and the perianal involvement common in women is usually absent. Preputial scarring from LS can lead to phimosis, and circumcision is usually curative, although recurrence in the circumcision scar may occur. The late stage of this disease is called *balanitis xerotica obliterans*, which can involve the penile urethra and result in troublesome urethral stricture disease.

Despite the similarities in name, LS shares little in common with LP and LN other than pruritus and a predilection for the genital region. **Another critical distinction is that LS has**

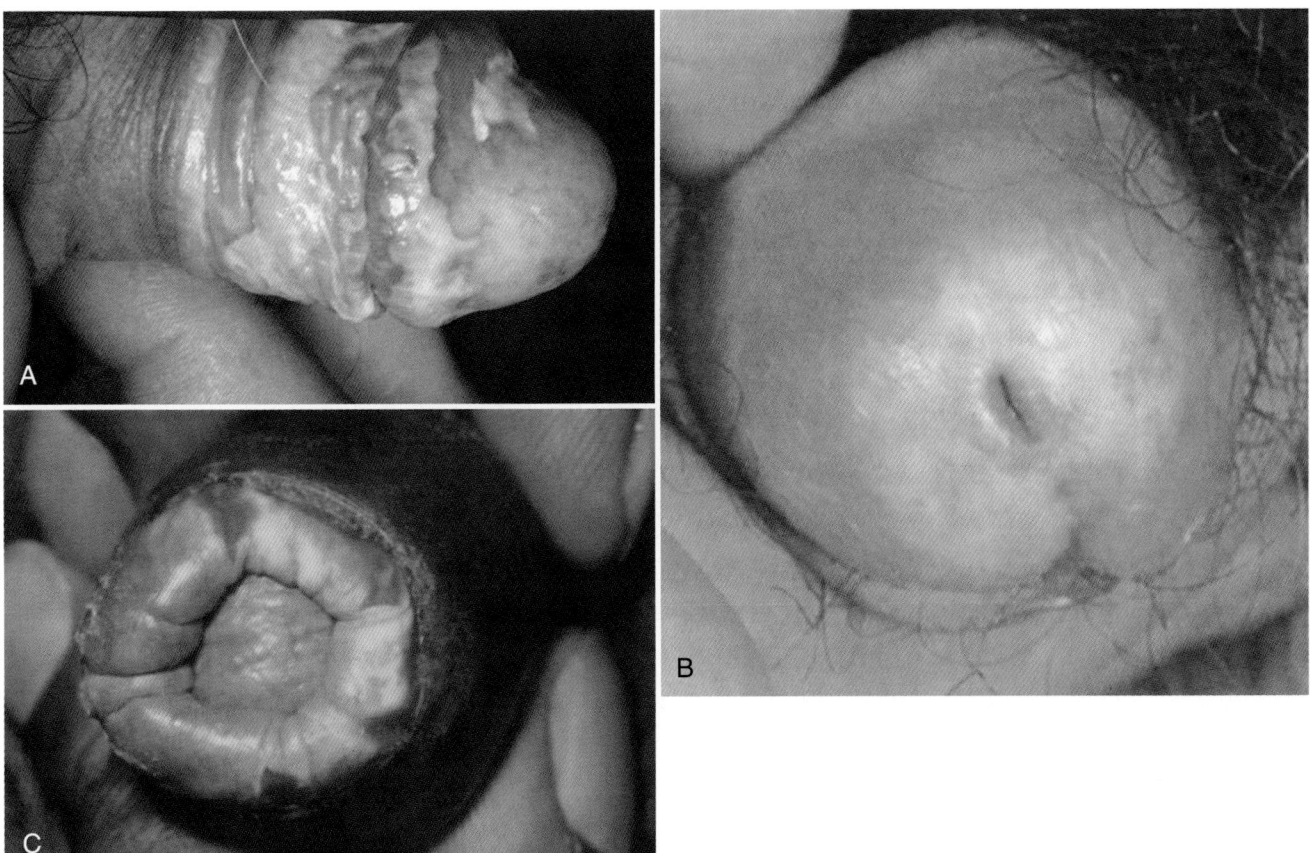

Figure 13–12. **A** to **C**, Lichen sclerosis et atrophicus (balanitis xerotica obliterans) of the penis. Note the erythematous and white plaques involving the penile shaft, preputial skin, and glans. (**A** from Callen JP, Greer DE, Hood AF, Paller AS: Color Atlas of Dermatology. Philadelphia, WB Saunders, 1993, p 327; **B** from du Vivier A: Atlas of Clinical Dermatology. London, Churchill Livingstone, 2002, p 716; **C** from Bolognia JL, Jorizzo JL, Rapini RP: Dermatology. Edinburgh, Mosby, 2003, p 1101.)

been associated with squamous cell carcinoma of the penis, particularly those variants not associated with human papillomavirus, and may represent a premalignant condition (Velazquez and Cubilla, 2003). LS has specific histologic features, including basal cell vacuolation, epidermal atrophy, dermal edema, collagen homogenization and focal perivascular infiltrate of the papillary dermis, and plugging of the ostia of follicular and eccrine structures (Margolis, 2002). Biopsy is worthwhile both to confirm the diagnosis and exclude malignant change (Powell and Wojnarowska, 1999).

From a management standpoint, long-term follow-up of patients with LS is important owing to the association with squamous cell carcinoma. The application of potent topical corticosteroids (e.g., clobetasol propionate 0.05%) for long courses (3 months) is well established as a treatment for LS in women and may both improve symptoms and reverse the disease process (Dalziel et al, 1991). This regimen is contrary to the usual policy of avoiding long courses of corticosteroid application to genital skin. The efficacy of similar approaches has not been confirmed in adult men, although benefits have been demonstrated in the pediatric age group (Kiss et al, 2001).

Fixed Drug Eruption

A fixed drug eruption occurs in response to oral medications, usually 1 to 2 weeks after the first exposure, and commonly involves the lips, face, hands, feet, and genitalia (Fig. 13–13). After subsequent reexposure to the drug, the reaction presents in the same location, usually within 24 hours (hence the term *fixed*). The most common medications causing this reaction are sulfonamides, nonsteroidal anti-inflammatory agents, barbiturates, tetracyclines, carbamazepine, phenolphthalein, salicylates, oral contraceptives, and salicylates (Kauppinen and Stubb, 1985; Stubb et al, 1989; Thankappan and Zachariah, 1991).

When present on the penile shaft or glans, these lesions are usually solitary inflammatory plaques that may be erosive and painful (Margolis, 2002). On the genitalia, the differential diagnosis includes herpes simplex infection or an insect bite. Removing the offending agent usually results in resolution of the lesion, although a postinflammatory brown pigmentation may remain.

Seborrheic Dermatitis

This common skin disease is characterized by the presence of sharply demarcated pink-yellow to red-brown plaques with a flaky scale. It shares a variety of features in common with eczematous dermatitis and could easily be grouped in that category. Common dandruff is a mild form of seborrheic dermatitis (SD) localized to the scalp. It has a predilection for areas rich in sebaceous glands and is generally present only during the first few months of life or after puberty, when seba-

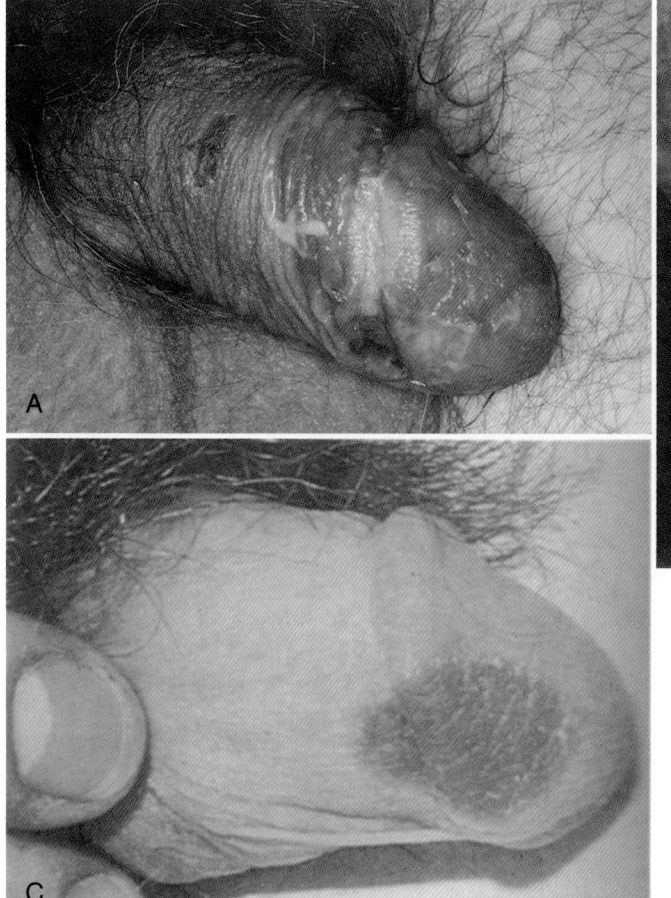
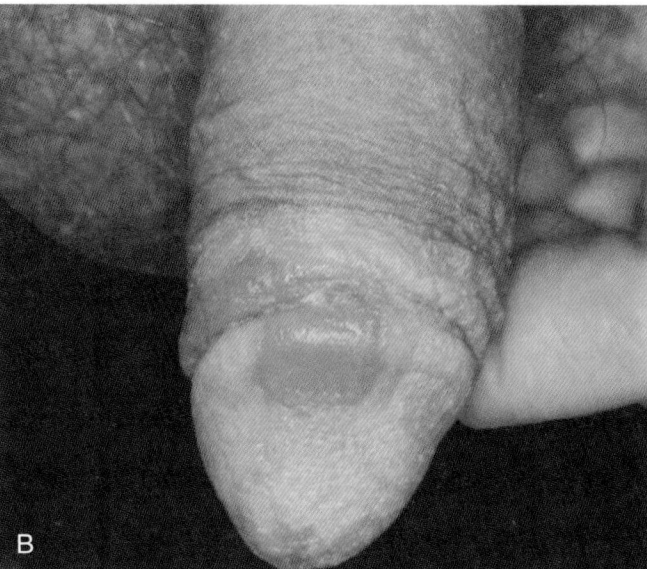

Figure 13–13. **A** to **C,** Fixed drug eruptions involving the penis. (**A** from Callen JP, Greer DE, Hood AF, Paller AS: Color Atlas of Dermatology. Philadelphia, WB Saunders, 1993, p 160; **B** from Bolognia JL, Jorizzo JL, Rapini RP: Dermatology. Edinburgh, Mosby, 2003, p 345; **C** from Habif TP: Clinical Dermatology. Edinburgh, Mosby, 2004, p 492.)

ceous glands are active. Common areas affected include the scalp, eyebrows, nasolabial folds, ears, and chest, although the anus, penis, and pubic areas may also be involved (Margolis, 2002). Circumcision may be somewhat protective against the development of SD. In one study of 357 patients, the risk of developing penile SD was 2.5 times greater in the uncircumcised state (Mallon et al, 2000).

Adult SD has a chronic relapsing course (Webster, 1991). **This condition is particularly common in patients with Parkinson's disease, and up to 83% of patients with the acquired immunodeficiency syndrome (AIDS) may manifest SD** (Froschl et al, 1990; Gupta and Bluhm, 2004). Particularly in immunosuppressed individuals, SD may involve a significant proportion of the body surface area. **Extensive and/or severe SD should raise concerns for possible underlying infection with HIV** (Fritsch and Reider, 2003). SD may be pruritic, and differentiation from psoriasis may occasionally be problematic. Unlike psoriasis, however, SD rarely involves the nails and tends to have a thinner associated scale.

Controversy concerning the etiology of SD revolves around a possible autoimmune response to a component of normal skin flora, the yeast *Malassezia furfur (Pityrosporum ovale)*. Although *M. furfur* can be isolated from the lesions of SD, the number of organisms is only about twice that observed in normal control skin (Nenoff et al, 2001). Likewise, severely SD affected HIV patients do not harbor more organisms than HIV patients without manifestations of SD (Pechere et al, 1999). Another factor potentially linked to SD is an elevated level of triglycerides and cholesterol at the skin surface (Fritsch and Reider, 2003).

Creams containing topical antifungal agents (e.g., ketoconazole) are the mainstay of SD treatment on the body and have a 75% to 90% response rate (Faergemann, 2000; Fritsch and Reider, 2003). For hair-bearing areas, "antidandruff" shampoos containing zinc, salicylic acid, selenium sulfide, tar, or ketoconazole are effective (Margolis, 2002). Because of the relapsing nature of SD, treatment often must be repetitive. Low-potency topical corticosteroids may play a role during the initial treatment of severe cases but should not be the primary mode of treatment for this chronic condition owing to local corticosteroid side effects.

VESICOBULLOUS DISORDERS

Vesicobullous disorders are uncommon conditions often characterized by autoimmune damage to the epidermis or basement membrane (Table 13–5). On the genitalia, the rupture of blisters and bullae may leave behind erosions (Margolis, 2002).

Pemphigus Vulgaris

Pemphigus is a family of autoimmune blistering diseases characterized by intraepidermal blisters due to the loss of keratinocyte cell-cell adhesion (Martel and Joly, 2001). These blisters are located in the deep epidermis close to the basal cell layer. The proposed immunopathology includes the development of autoantibodies directed against keratinocyte cell

Table 13–5. Differential Diagnosis of Vesicobullous Disorders

Bullous pemphigoid
Pemphigus vulgaris
Pemphigus foliaceus
Zoon's balanitis
Behçet's syndrome
Contact dermatitis
Dermatitis herpetiformis
Porphyria cutanea tarda
Herpes zoster
Herpes simplex
Lymphangioma circumscriptum
Impetigo
Fixed drug eruption
Factitial
Innocent trauma
Benign familial pemphigoid (Hailey-Hailey disease)

From Margolis DJ: Cutaneous diseases of the male external genitalia. In Walsh PC (ed): Campbell's Urology. Philadelphia, WB Saunders, 2002.

surface markers and desmosomes (Amagai et al, 1996; Zhou et al, 1997; Joly et al, 2000). **Almost all pemphigus patients will have painful oral mucosal erosions, and over half will have cutaneous blisters, which may involve the genitalia. Characteristic oral lesions are, therefore, an important clue to the diagnosis** (Fig. 13–14). The cutaneous blisters are thin walled and easily broken to leave behind a painful erosion. The loss of epidermal cohesion seen in pemphigus leads to the characteristic Asboe-Hansen sign: spreading of fluid under the adjacent normal-appearing skin away from the direction of pressure on the blister (Amagai, 2003). **In severe cases without appropriate treatment, pemphigus may be fatal due to the loss of the epidermal barrier function of large areas of affected skin.** Treatment of pemphigus usually depends on systemic corticosteroids, although minimization of corticosteroid dose is an important goal to limit side effects. The addition of immunosuppressive agents such as azathioprine and cyclophosphamide may be beneficial, owing to their corticosteroid-sparing effect (Amagai, 2003).

Bullous Pemphigoid

Bullous pemphigoid (BP) is a subepidermal blistering disease that is more common in men and generally afflicts patients older than 60 years of age (Rzany and Weller, 2001). There is enrichment for specific HLA class II alleles in BP patients as compared with normal controls (Delgado et al, 1996), supporting an autoimmune mechanism of pathogenesis. In BP, autoantibodies against specific proteins involved in cell-cell adhesion (BP180, BP230) are present. These proteins are components of hemidesmosomes, structures that mediate epidermal-stromal adhesion. Binding of autoantibodies to these structures leads to complement activation and a cascade of events resulting in tissue damage, epidermal-dermal separation, and blister formation (Kitajima et al, 1994; Lin et al, 1997).

Clinically, the presentation of BP can be highly variable. It generally begins with a nonbullous phase characterized by

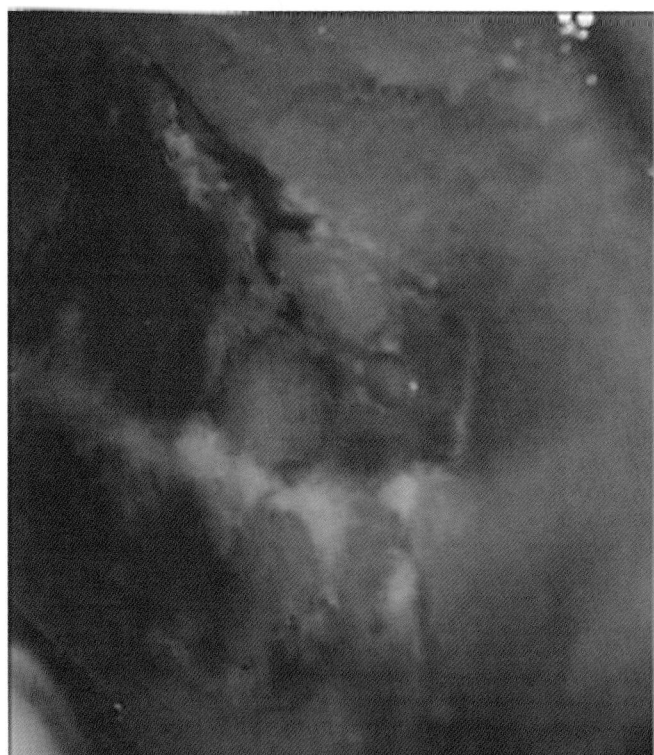

Figure 13–14. Characteristic painful oral mucosal erosions in pemphigus vulgaris. (From Bolognia JL, Jorizzo JL, Rapini RP: Dermatology. Edinburgh, Mosby, 2003, p 455.)

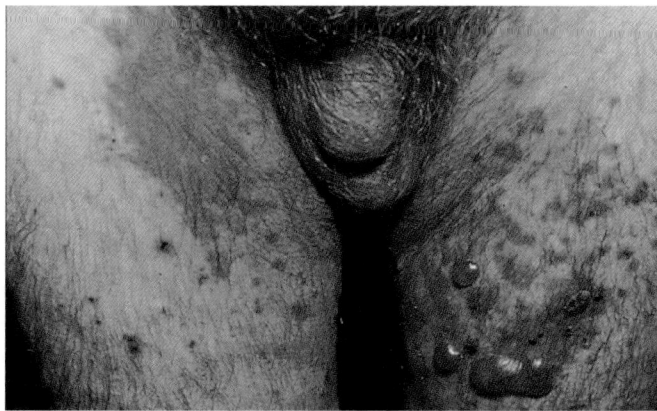

Figure 13–15. Bullous pemphigoid involving the inner thighs. Note the confluent plaques and tense blisters in the inguinal area. (From Bolognia JL, Jorizzo JL, Rapini RP: Dermatology. Edinburgh, Mosby, 2003, p 465.)

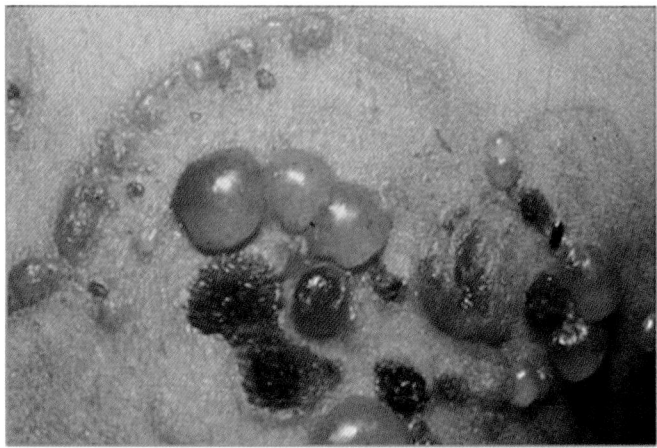

Figure 13–16. The circumferential and linear vesicle patterns typical of linear IgA bullous dermatosis. (From: Bolognia JL, Jorizzo JL, Rapini RP: Dermatology. Edinburgh, Mosby, 2003, p 485.)

severe itching and nonspecific skin findings. As the disease moves into the bullous phase, vesicles and blisters appear on normal skin or areas containing confluent erythematous plaques. The blisters are tense, tend to form on flexor surfaces, and may involve the inner thighs and genitalia (Fig. 13–15). Mucous membranes may also be involved, although less commonly than in pemphigus. **The diagnosis is made by a combination of clinical, histologic, and, often most importantly, immunohistochemical features such as the deposition of IgG antibodies along the basement membrane** (De Jong et al, 1996). Treatment of BP is similar to that described for pemphigus, with systemic corticosteroids and immunosuppressants playing primary roles (Kirtschig and Khumalo, 2004). For treatment-resistant cases, intravenous immunoglobulin or plasmapheresis may be beneficial (Hatano et al, 2003; Lee, et al, 2003; Ruetter and Luger, 2004; Wetter et al, 2005).

Dermatitis Herpetiformis and Linear IgA Bullous Dermatosis

Both of these entities are blistering autoimmune skin diseases associated with the deposition of IgA antibodies at the basement membrane.

Dermatitis herpetiformis (DH) is a cutaneous manifestation of celiac disease and is generally associated with gluten sensitivity (Karpati, 2004). It is most common in people of northern European origin. There is a close association of DH

with certain HLA class II DQ2 alleles (DQA1*0501, DQB1*02) (Reunala, 1998). Pruritic plaques, papules, and vesicles in a symmetrical distribution characterize DH. These vesicles may form "herpetiform" groups on an erythematous base. Patients may also complain of pain and burning over the lesions. Diagnosis can be confirmed by biopsy and direct immunofluorescence, which shows a granular pattern of IgA deposition at the basement membrane. Treatment includes the use of dapsone and a strict gluten-restricted diet (Frodin et al, 1981; Andersson and Mobacken, 1992).

Linear IgA bullous dermatosis (LABD), in contrast, is not associated with celiac disease. As the name implies, a linear pattern of antibody deposition at the basement membrane is found on immunohistochemistry. Characteristic clinical features include vesicles and bullae arranged in a combination of circumferential and linear orientations (Fig. 13–16). Treatment with either sulfapyridine or dapsone is usually effective in controlling LABD, and long-term spontaneous remission rates of 30% to 60% have been described (Wojnarowska et al, 1988).

Hailey-Hailey Disease

Hailey-Hailey disease (HH) is an autosomal dominant blistering dermatosis that usually develops within the second or third decade of life (Burge, 1992). **It has a predilection for the intertriginous areas, including the groin and perianal region** (Fig. 13–17). In women, disease in the inframammary folds is common although vulvar disease is unusual (Wieselthier and Pincus, 1993). Symptoms include an unfortunate combination of pruritus, pain, and a foul odor. Because heat and sweating exacerbate the condition, HH tends to worsen during the summer (Burge, 1992). Skin findings include confluent areas of vesicles and fragile blisters, which form due to aberrant keratinocyte cell adhesion. Lesions may be confined to the axilla or groin, and superinfection with yeast or bacteria may compound the problem. Histologic examination may be helpful in differentiating HH from impetigo, pemphigus, intertrigo, and Darier's disease (Margolis, 2002). **Treatment includes wearing lightweight, breathable clothing to avoid friction and sweating. Lesions may respond to topical or intralesional corticosteroids, with the caveats mentioned previously about the use of these agents on intertriginous skin. For disease resistant to medical therapy, wide excision and skin grafting have been effective, as have local ablative techniques such as dermabrasion and laser vaporization** (Hamm et al, 1994; Christian and Moy, 1999; Hohl et al, 2003).

NONINFECTIOUS ULCERS

Genital ulcers can be a result of both infectious and noninfectious causes (Table 13–6).

Aphthous Ulcers and Behçet's Disease

Aphthous ulcers are small, painful erosions that commonly involve the oral cavity but can occasionally be present on the genitalia. **When oral and genital aphthous ulcers coexist, the clinician should consider the diagnosis of Behçet's disease (BD).** BD is a generalized relapsing and remitting ulcerative mucocutaneous disease that likely involves a genetic predisposition and an autoimmune mode of pathogenesis (Sakane, 1997). Oxidative stress related to overproduction of superoxide radicals by neutrophils has also been implicated in the development of this condition (Freitas et al, 1998). BD has a

Table 13–6. Differential Diagnosis of Ulcers

Syphilis
Chancroid
Herpes simplex
Crohn's disease
Aphthous ulcer
Behçet's disease
Granuloma inguinale
Lymphogranuloma venereum
Factitial dermatitis
Wegener's granulomatosis
Leukocytoclastic vasculitis
Pyoderma gangrenosum

From Margolis DJ: Cutaneous diseases of the male external genitalia. In Walsh PC (ed): Campbell's Urology. Philadelphia, WB Saunders, 2002.

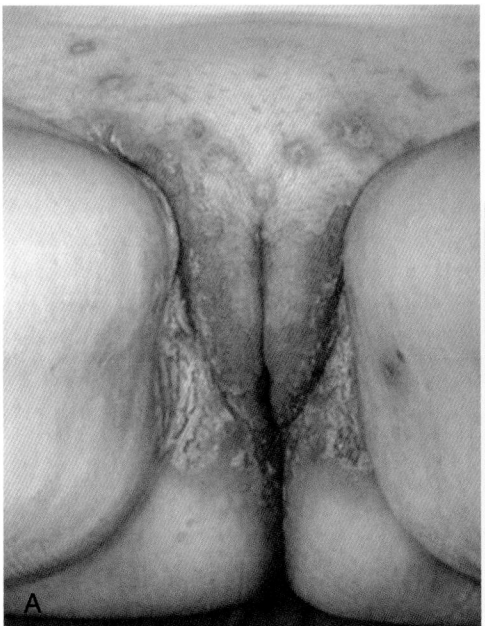 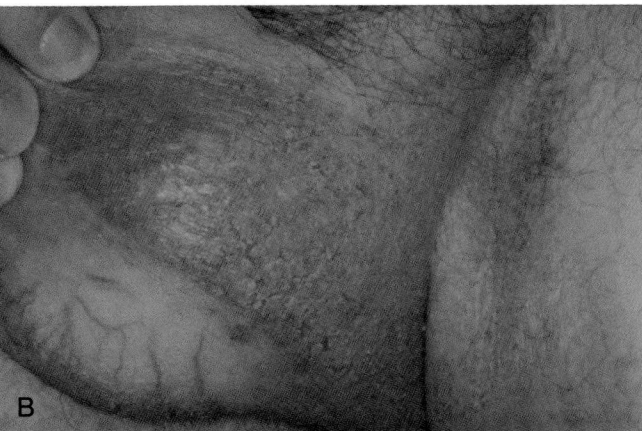

Figure 13–17. Genital presentations of Hailey-Hailey disease. **A,** The vulva and groin are covered in a vesicular eruption that has become confluent and macerated. **B,** Erythematous plaque with maceration of the inguinal canal and scrotum. (**A** from du Vivier A: Atlas of Clinical Dermatology. London, Churchill Livingstone, 2002, p 688; **B** from Bolognia JL, Jorizzo JL, Rapini RP: Dermatology. Edinburgh, Mosby, 2003, p 830.)

high prevalence in Turkey (80 per 100,000) and Japan (10 per 100,000) but is rare in the United States (0.12 per 100,000) (Arbesfeld and Kurban, 1988). Affected individuals may also suffer from epididymitis, thrombophlebitis, aneurysms, and gastrointestinal, neurologic, and arthritic problems (Koc et al, 1992; Tuzun et al, 1997; Cetinel et al, 1998; Krause et al, 1999; Aykutlu et al, 2002; Margolis, 2002).

Mucocutaneous lesions of the oral cavity and genitalia (Fig. 13–18) and ocular involvement (uveitis) form a triad of clinical features in BD. The genital lesions are larger and generally more painful than the oral lesions. Optic involvement occurs in 90% of cases and may lead to blindness (Moschella, 2003). The Behçet's International Study Group (1990) has defined the diagnosis as recurrent oral ulceration plus any two of the following: recurrent genital ulceration, eye lesions, cutaneous lesions, and skin sensitivity to needle puncture (pathergy test). Other causes for genital ulceration, however, including aphthous ulcers, syphilis, herpes simplex, and chancroid must be considered before a diagnosis of BD is made (Margolis, 2002). The clinical course of BD is protean, and randomized controlled trials in support of specific therapy are currently limited (Kaklamani and Kaklamanis, 2001). A wide range of topical and systemic agents has been applied to treat BD with variable success, including corticosteroids, dapsone, colchicine, and immunosuppressants (Moschella, 2003).

Pyoderma Gangrenosum

Pyoderma gangrenosum (PG) is a ulcerative skin disease associated with systemic illnesses, including inflammatory bowel disease, arthritis, collagen vascular disease, and myeloproliferative disorders (Moschella, 2003). **It most commonly affects women between the second and fifth decades of life and likely has an autoimmune pathogenesis given its association with other autoimmune diseases. Twenty to 50 percent of cases, however, are idiopathic.**

The classic morphologic presentation of PG is painful cutaneous and mucous membrane ulceration, often with extensive loss of tissue and a purulent base (Fig. 13–19). Although unusual, PG can involve the penis, scrotum, vulva, and peristomal sites (Cairns et al, 1994). As was the case in BD, no specific diagnostic laboratory test or histopathologic feature is pathognomonic for PG, although a history of underlying systemic disease may raise suspicion. Treatment includes a combination of local and systemic corticosteroid therapy with or without adjunctive immunosuppressants (i.e., cyclosporine) (Chow and Ho, 1996).

Traumatic Causes

Cutaneous lesions of the genitalia, including ulceration, can be caused by local trauma, which should be included in the

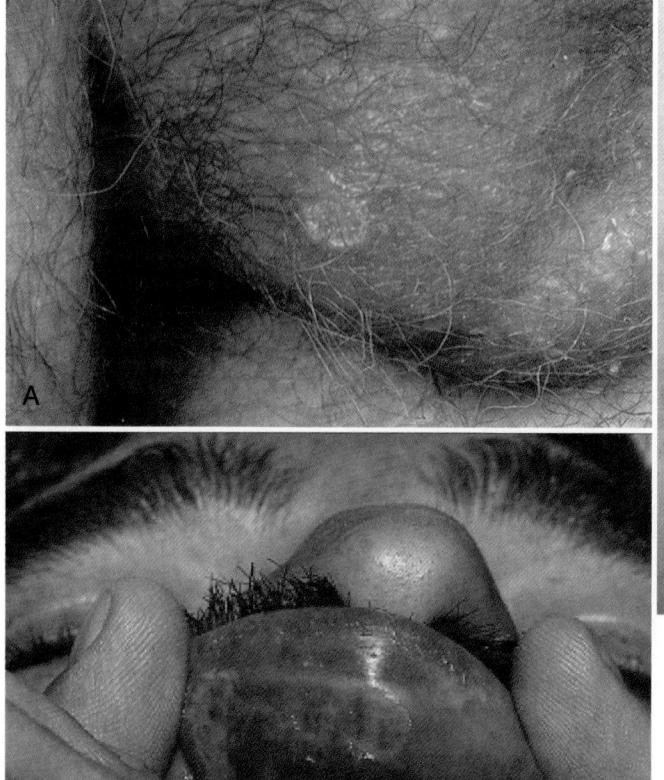

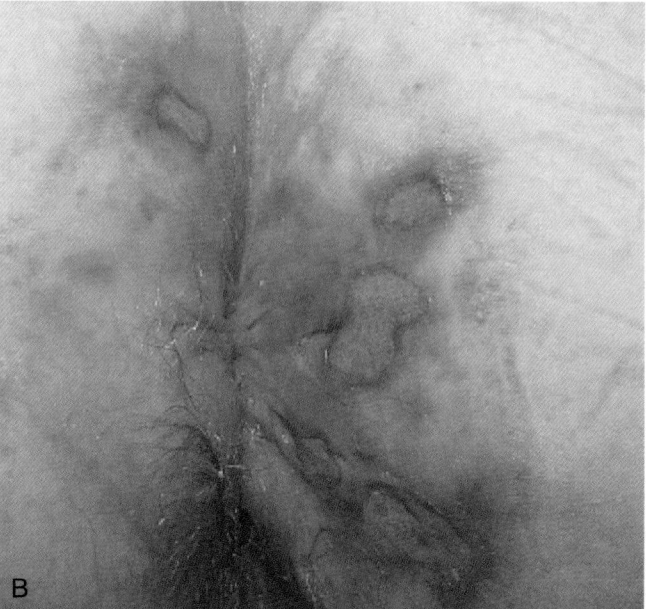

Figure 13–18. Scrotal (**A**), perianal (**B**), and oral (**C**) ulcers seen in Behçet's disease. (**A** from du Vivier A: Atlas of Clinical Dermatology. London, Churchill Livingstone, 2002, p 713; **B** and **C** from Bolognia JL, Jorizzo JL, Rapini RP: Dermatology. Edinburgh, Mosby, 2003, p 419.)

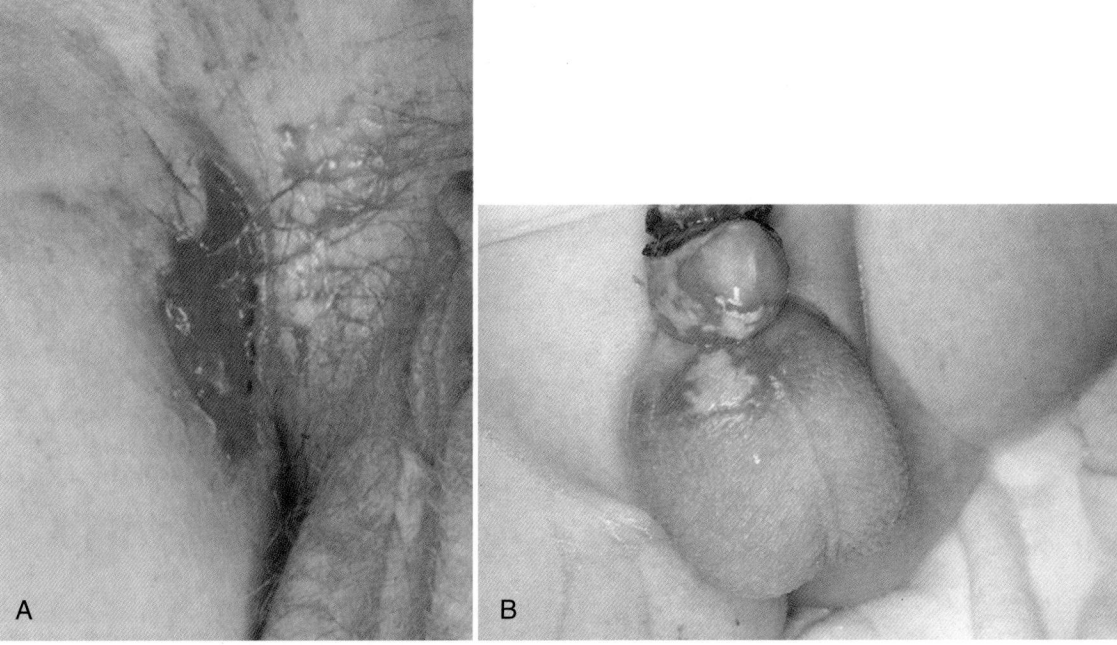

Figure 13–19. Pyoderma gangrenosum involving the inner thigh of a woman with rheumatoid arthritis (**A**) and the penis and scrotum (**B**) of another patient. (**A** from du Vivier A: Atlas of Clinical Dermatology, London, Churchill Livingstone, 2002, p 387; **B** from Callen JP, Greer DE, Hood AF, Paller AS: Color Atlas of Dermatology. Philadelphia, WB Saunders, 1993, p 330.)

differential diagnosis. **This can be either accidental ("innocent trauma") or self-inflicted ("factitial dermatitis").** Accidental injuries may be a result of trauma during sexual practices, ornamentation (i.e., piercing), or unusual hygiene practices (i.e., excessive cleaning) (Margolis, 2002). **Factitial dermatitis is a psychocutaneous disorder in which the individual self-inflicts cutaneous lesions usually for an unconscious motive.** An association between factitial dermatitis and borderline personality disorder appears to exist (Koblenzer, 2000). Other disorders to be considered include Münchausen syndrome by proxy and malingering if secondary gain issues exist.

INFECTIONS AND INFESTATIONS
Sexually Transmitted Diseases

Sexually transmitted diseases with genital cutaneous manifestations include lymphogranuloma venereum, granuloma inguinale, herpes simplex, chancroid, molluscum contagiosum, human papillomavirus, and syphilis (Fig. 13–20). These conditions are covered in detail in Chapter 11, "Sexually Transmitted Diseases."

Balanitis and Balanoposthitis

Balanitis is an inflammatory disorder of the glans penis. When the process involves the preputial skin in uncircumcised men it is termed *balanoposthitis.* In children, bacterial infections are the predominant cause. In adult men, the cause may be intertrigo, irritant contact dermatitis, local trauma, or can-

didal and bacterial infections (Fig. 13–21). Treatment includes removal of irritating agents, improved hygiene, topical antibiotics and antifungal agents, and occasionally short courses of low-potency topical corticosteroids (Margolis, 2002). When treatment fails, the differential diagnosis should include neoplastic diseases, Zoon's balanitis, psoriasis, and alternative infectious agents such as papillomavirus (Wikstrom, et al, 1994). Balanoposthitis tends to occur in patients with phimosis, and circumcision may be curative in select recurrent cases.

Cellulitis and Erysipelas

Cellulitis is an infection of the deep dermis and subcutaneous tissues most commonly caused by gram-positive organisms (*S. pyogenes* and *S. aureus*) (Lewis, 1998). In immunocompetent individuals, organisms usually gain entry to the site of infection through a break in the skin barrier. In immunocompromised patients, a bloodborne route of infection is more common. Systemic signs of illness include fever, chills, and general malaise. Local signs include erythema (rubor), warmth (calor), pain (dolor), and swelling (tumor) at the site with indistinct borders (Fig. 13–22). Treatment includes systemic antibiotics with activity against *S. pyogenes* and *S. aureus* species. In cases associated with diabetes, mixed flora may be present and antibiotic coverage should be broadened. Marking the zone of cellulitis at the onset of therapy is an important step to allow progression and resolution of cellulitis to be monitored during therapy.

Erysipelas is a superficial bacterial skin infection limited to the dermis with lymphatic involvement. It is commonly a disease at the extremes of age and often involves the face. In

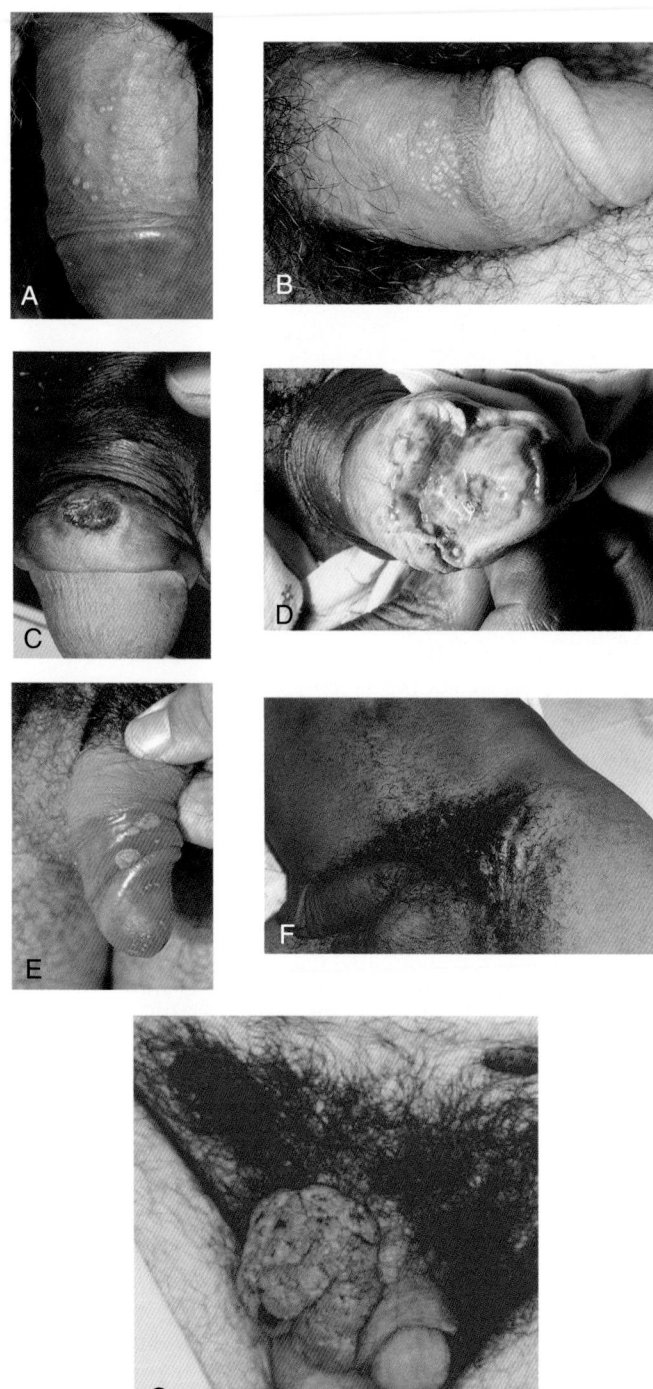

Figure 13–20. Genital lesions associated with sexually transmitted diseases. **A,** Herpes simplex virus. **B,** Molluscum contagiosum. **C,** Syphilitic chancre. **D,** Granuloma inguinale. **E,** Chancroid. **F,** Lymphogranuloma venereum. **G,** Condylomata acuminata. (From Callen JP, Greer DE, Hood AF, Paller AS: Color Atlas of Dermatology, Philadelphia, WB Saunders, 1993, pp 48, 177, 233, and 328-331.)

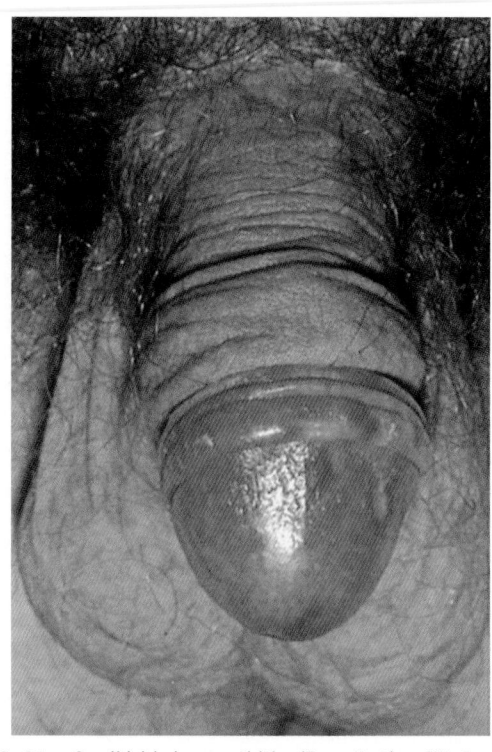

Figure 13–21. Candidal balanoposthitis. (From Korting GW: Practical Dermatology of the Genital Region. Philadelphia, WB Saunders, 1981, p 159.)

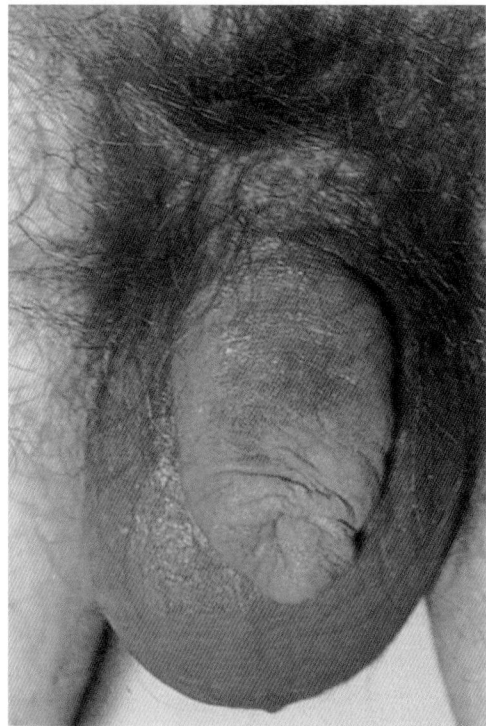

Figure 13–22. Penoscrotal cellulitis. (From Korting GW: Practical Dermatology of the Genital Region. Philadelphia, WB Saunders, 1981, p 37.)

contrast to the cutaneous lesion of cellulitis, erysipelas generally has a raised and distinct border at the interface with normal skin. The causative organism is usually *S. pyogenes*.

Fournier's Gangrene (Necrotizing Fasciitis of the Perineum)

Fournier's gangrene (FG) is a potentially life-threatening progressive infection of the perineum and genitalia (Morpurgo and Galandiuk, 2002). In the genital region, most cases of FG are caused by mixed bacterial flora, which include gram-positive, gram-negative, and anaerobic bacteria. Risk factors for developing FG include alcoholism, diabetes, malnutrition, advanced age, and peripheral vascular disease. However, group A streptococcal necrotizing fasciitis can occur in healthy immunocompetent individuals.

The hallmark of FG is a rapid progression from the signs and symptoms of cellulitis to blister formation and foul-smelling necrotic lesions (Fig. 13–23). **Infection may spread along fascial planes, and hence the exterior skin findings may represent only a small proportion of the underlying infected and necrotic tissue. The diagnosis of FG is a surgical emergency because progression from genitalia to perineum to abdominal wall may occur extremely rapidly (often within hours). The exclusion of FG, therefore, should be a priority during every consultation for soft tissue infection of the genitalia.** Pain out of proportion to the visible extent of infection should raise suspicion for FG. The skin may also have a grayish cast or fetid odor uncharacteristic of uncomplicated genital cellulitis. Imaging of the genitalia with plain radiographs or computed tomography (Amendola et al, 1994) may demonstrate gas bubbles within the tissue, although the delay associated with imaging should not delay surgical intervention in obvious cases.

Treatment involves a combination of broad-spectrum antibiotics and extensive surgical débridement to margins of healthy bleeding tissue. These patients will often require a second-look operation after 24 to 48 hours to exclude further disease progression (Gurdal et al, 2003). During surgical débridement for scrotal FG, the testes and other structures within the tunica vaginalis can almost always be spared, although loss of tissue in the abdominal wall may be extensive due to bacterial spread along fascial planes. The indications for adjunctive hyperbaric oxygen therapy in FG remain controversial, although several groups have reported favorable results (Dahm et al, 2000; Eke, 2000; Jallali et al, 2005). Despite aggressive modern management, the mortality of FG may be as high as 16% to 40% (Dahm et al, 2000; Eke, 2000; Blume et al, 2003; Yeniyol et al, 2004).

Folliculitis

Folliculitis is a common disorder characterized by perifollicular pustules on an erythematous base (Kelly, 2003). It occurs most frequently in heavily hair-bearing areas such as the scalp, beard, axilla, groin, and buttocks and can be exacerbated by local trauma from shaving, rubbing, or clothing irritation (Margolis, 2002). Patients may complain of pruritus or pain over the area or symptoms may be absent. Cultures are generally negative, although a variety of infectious organisms have been associated with folliculitis, including *S. aureus*, *Pseudomonas* species, fungi, and herpes simplex virus. Folliculitis has also been associated with the use of contaminated hot tubs and swimming pools, with the offending organism usually *Pseudomonas aeruginosa* (Fig. 13–24) (Gregory and Schaffner, 1987; Rolston and Bodey, 1992). Treatment of folliculitis includes good hygiene, removal of offending irritants, and appropriate topical or systemic antiviral, antibiotic, or antifungal agents.

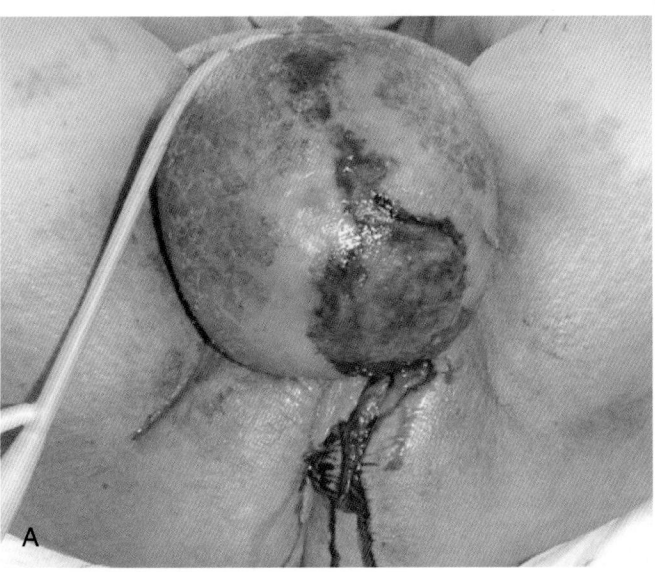
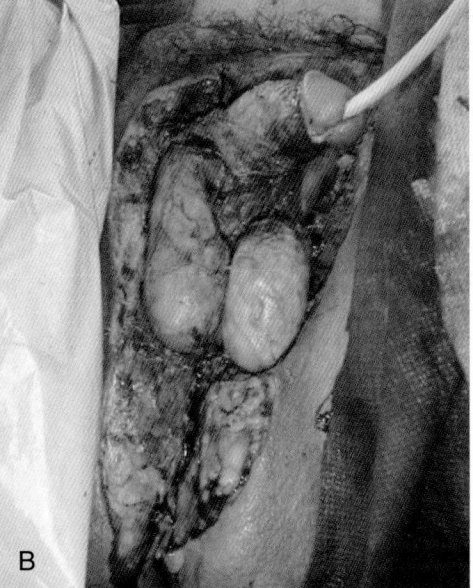

Figure 13–23. Fournier's gangrene of the scrotum. **A,** Surface appearance of scrotum and perineum showing area of frank necrosis. **B,** Extent of soft tissue débridement required to achieve margins of viable tissue. Note that the testes within their tunica vaginalis compartment are spared.

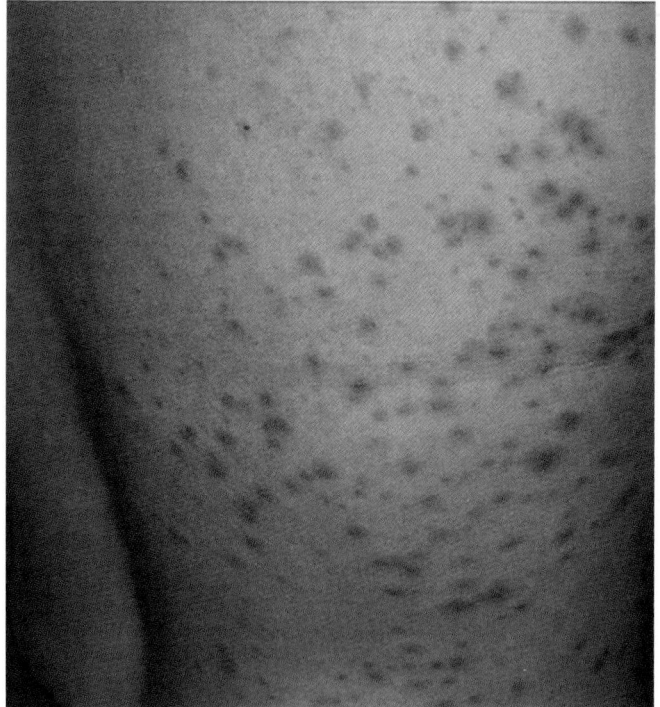

Figure 13–24. Pseudomonal folliculitis caused by the use of a hot tub. (From Bolognia JL, Jorizzo JL, Rapini RP: Dermatology. Edinburgh, Mosby, 2003, p 554.)

Furunculosis

Both furuncles and abscesses are walled-off collections of pus. **Although abscesses can occur anywhere on the body, a furuncle is by definition associated with a hair follicle.** Furuncles tend to occur in areas prone to minor trauma, including the groin and buttocks (Fig. 13–25). *S. aureus* is the most common causative organism, although anaerobes may be present. Risk factors include diabetes mellitus, obesity, poor hygiene, and immunosuppression (Brook and Finegold, 1981). Warm compresses may be beneficial, and larger lesions may require incision and drainage as for any abscess. When there is associated cellulitis, a systemic antibiotic with activity against staphylococci should be given.

Hidradenitis Suppurativa (Acne Inversa)

Hidradenitis suppurativa (HS) is a chronic disease of apocrine gland-bearing skin with a predilection for the axillae and anogenital regions (Kelly, 2003). **It generally begins after puberty, and a familial form with an autosomal dominant pattern of inheritance has been described** (Von Der Werth et al, 2000). Originally believed to be a disease of apocrine glands, HS is now thought to be an epithelial disorder of hair follicles (Jansen et al, 2001). Although superinfection of HS lesions may occur, bacterial infection does not appear to be the primary initiator. During the pathogenesis of HS, hair follicles become plugged and swollen. Rupture of follicular contents (including bacteria and keratin) into the surrounding dermis initiates a marked inflammatory response with the formation of abscesses and sinus tracts (Slade et al, 2003).

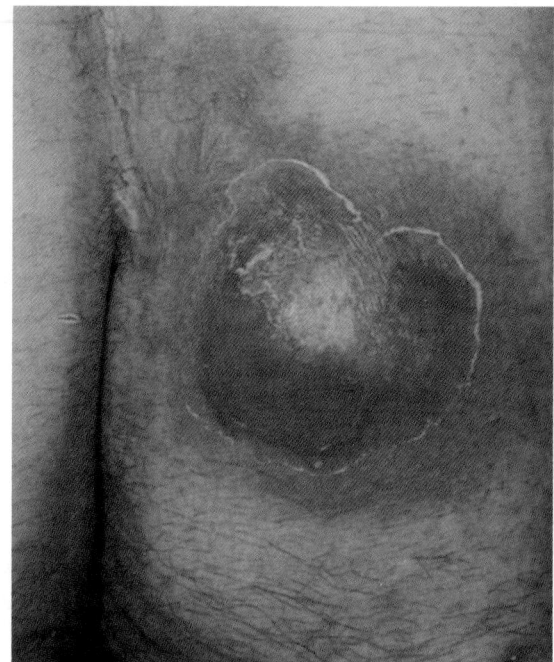

Figure 13–25. A large furuncle located on the buttocks. (From Habif TP: Clinical Dermatology. Edinburgh, Mosby, 2004, p 284.)

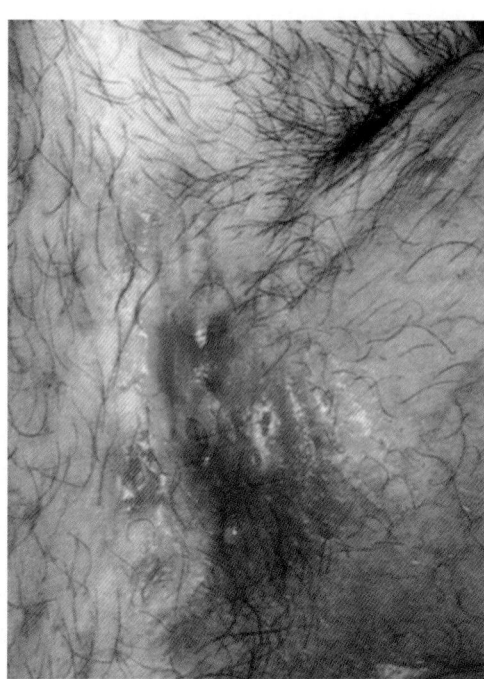

Figure 13–26. Hidradenitis suppurativa showing painful papules and draining sinus tracts. (From du Vivier A: Atlas of Clinical Dermatology. London, Churchill Livingstone, 2002, p 712.)

The clinical features of HS include painful inflammatory nodules and sterile abscesses developing in the axillae, groin, perianal, and inframammary areas (Fig. 13–26) (Kelly, 2003). Over time, draining sinus tracts and hypertrophic scars develop. Serious complications of HS can occur, including hypoproteinemia, secondary amyloidosis, the development of fistulas to the urethra (Gronau and Pannek, 2002), bladder, peritoneum, and rectum (Nadgir et al, 2001), and squamous cell carcinoma in areas of heavy scarring (Altunay et al, 2002; Rosenzweig et al, 2005).

Treatment of HS includes improvement in hygiene, weight reduction, and efforts to minimize friction and moisture in affected areas (i.e., loose undergarments, absorbent powder) (Kelly, 2003). Topical clindamycin may be beneficial in some patients. In a double-blind randomized trial, systemic therapy with tetracycline was no more effective than topical clindamycin in HS (Jemec and Wendelboe, 1998). Systemic corticosteroids may improve HS, but relapse is the rule after cessation of therapy (Slade et al, 2003). Lithium may exacerbate HS or limit its response to conventional medical therapy (Gupta et al, 1995). Although recurrent incision and drainage of HS lesions is discouraged, wide excision and skin grafting has been effective (Rompel and Petres, 2000; Bocchini et al, 2003). A variety of new approaches, including the use of the CO$_2$ laser to treat HS, are under investigation (Lapins et al, 1994).

Corynebacterium Infection (Trichomycosis Axillaris and Erythrasma)

Trichomycosis axillaris (TA) is a superficial bacterial infection of axillary and pubic hair caused by *Corynebacterium*. Yellow, red, or black nodules are visible on the hair shafts (Fig. 13–27), and there is frequently a characteristic odor (Blume et al, 2003). There is an association with hyperhidrosis (Margolis, 2002). The differential diagnosis includes infestation with pediculosis pubis or fungal infection (piedra) (Avram et al, 1987), although examination with magnification can generally distinguish TA from these conditions. Shaving can provide

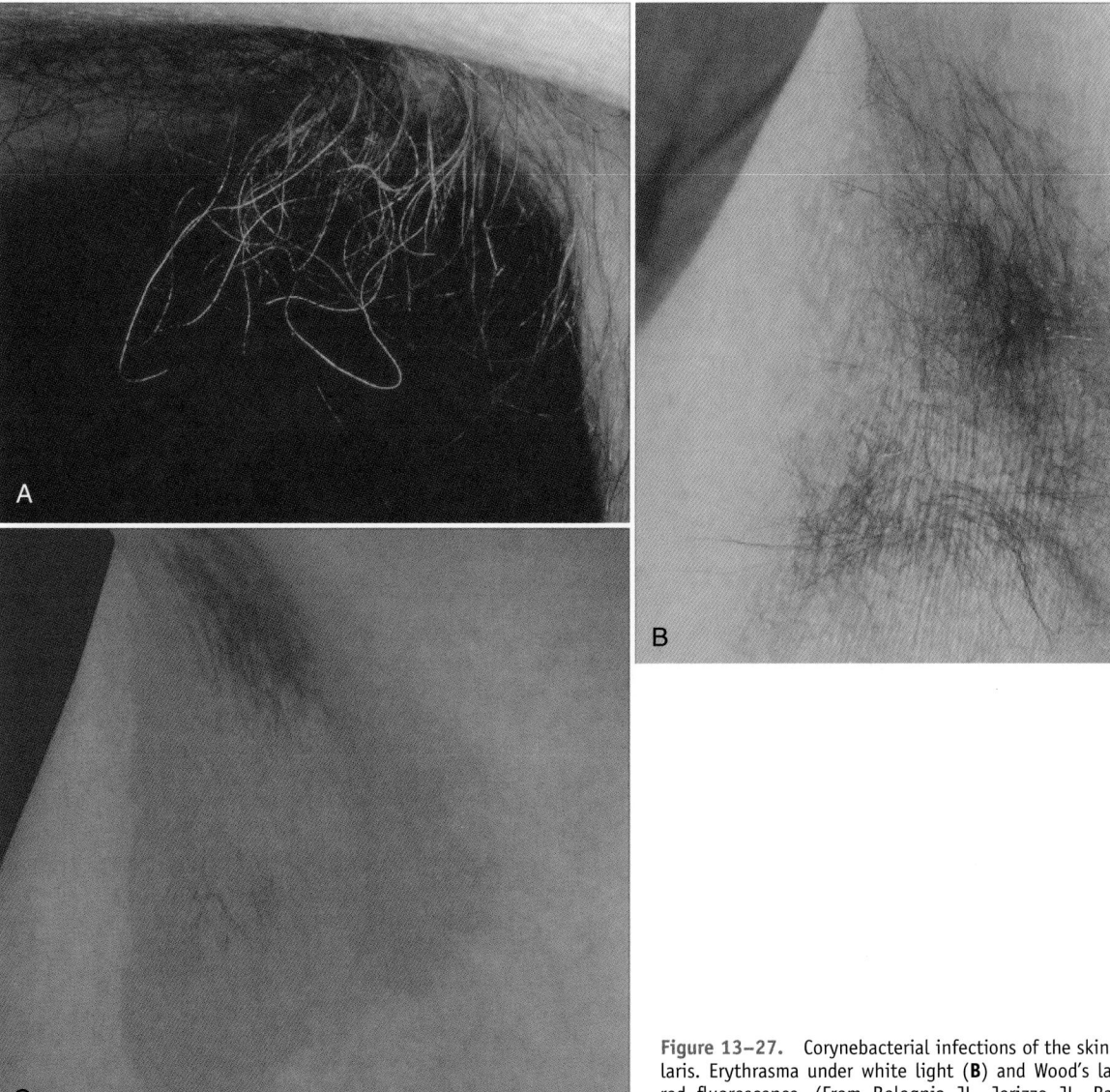

Figure 13–27. Corynebacterial infections of the skin. **A,** Trichomycosis axillaris. Erythrasma under white light (**B**) and Wood's lamp (**C**) showing coral-red fluorescence. (From Bolognia JL, Jorizzo JL, Rapini RP: Dermatology. Edinburgh, Mosby, 2003, pp 1128-1129.)

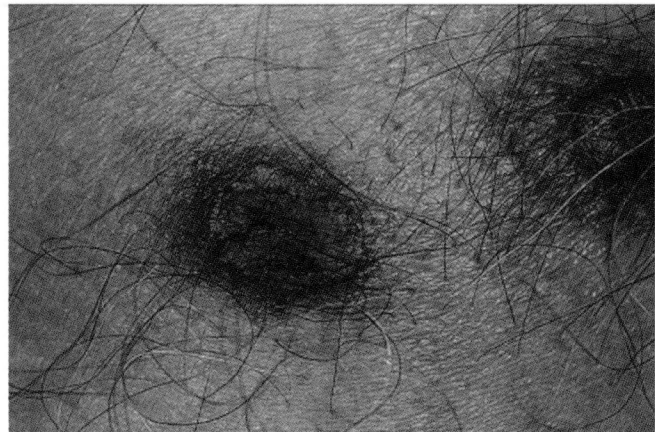

Figure 13–28. Ecthyma gangrenosum on the chest wall. Note the necrotic center and erythematous border around the lesion. (From Bolognia JL, Jorizzo JL, Rapini RP: Dermatology. Edinburgh, Mosby, 2003, p 1132.)

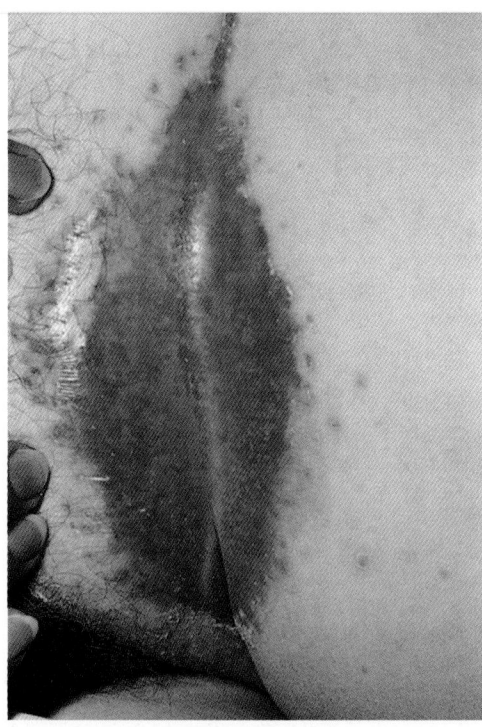

Figure 13–29. Candidal intertrigo with erythema, areas of tissue maceration, and satellite lesions. (From Callen JP, Greer DE, Hood AF, Paller AS: Color Atlas of Dermatology. Philadelphia, WB Saunders, 1993, p 318.)

immediate improvement, and antibacterial soaps may prevent further infection (Blume et al, 2003). For pubic TA, clindamycin gel, bacitracin, and oral erythromycin have also proven effective (Bargman 1984; Blume et al, 2003).

Erythrasma is a *Corynebacterium minutissimum* infection of the skin that results in sharply bordered, red-brown, scaling eruptions in moist areas, including the groin and axilla. These lesions may be pruritic or asymptomatic and may be confused with dermatophyte infection (tinea cruris) (Sindhuphak et al, 1985). Under a Wood light the lesions show a characteristic bright coral-red fluorescence (see Fig. 13–27) (Halprin, 1967). Effective treatments include antibacterial soaps, topical aluminum chloride, topical clindamycin, miconazole cream, and oral erythromycin (Holdiness, 2002).

Ecthyma Gangrenosum

Ecthyma gangrenosum (EG) is a rare cutaneous manifestation of pseudomonal septicemia that presents most commonly on the anogenital area in debilitated or immunosuppressed patients. The lesions of EG are tender grouped erythematous macules that may progress to form bullae or rupture to produce a gangrenous ulcer (Fig. 13–28) (Blume et al, 2003). On histologic examination, necrotizing vasculitis and gram-negative organisms are present. The differential diagnosis includes pyoderma gangrenosum, necrotizing vasculitis, cryoglobulinemia, and septic emboli containing other organisms including *Candida, Aspergillus, Citrobacter, Escherichia coli, Aeromonas hydrophila,* and *Fusarium* (Altwegg and Geiss, 1989; Martino et al, 1994; Gucluer et al, 1999; Reich et al, 2004). Consistent with the underlying sepsis, EG carries a poor prognosis, and immediate treatment with intravenous antipseudomonal antibiotics is indicated. Wound débridement may also be necessary (Collini et al, 1986).

Candidal Intertrigo

Fungal infection of macerated skin folds can occur with *Candida* species and involve the finger webs and intertriginous areas. Affected pruritic skin is reddened, and characteristic satellite lesions may be present (Fig. 13–29). The differential

diagnosis includes dermatophyte infection (tinea cruris), pemphigoid, psoriasis, seborrheic dermatitis, and contact dermatitis (Margolis, 2002). Fungal forms can be seen in scraped skin preparations after treatment with KOH, and culture is usually unnecessary. Topical treatment with imidazoles for at least 2 weeks is usually necessary for intertrigo, and occasionally oral antifungal agents are required (Cullin, 1977). Maneuvers to decrease moisture and skin maceration, such as the use of drying powders and loose clothing, may also help prevent relapse.

Dermatophyte Infection

Dermatophytes are fungi of three genera *(Trichophyton, Microsporum, Epidermophyton)* that have the propensity to invade and grow within keratinized tissues such as the skin, hair, and nails. These fungi produce keratinases, which break down keratin and facilitate invasion (Viani et al, 2001). In addition, mannans in the cell wall of some dermatophytes have immunoinhibitory effects (Dahl, 1994).

Tinea cruris is the term given to dermatophyte infection of the groin and genital area and is commonly known as "jock itch." More common in males than females, this condition is favored by hot, humid environments and concomitant dermatophyte infection of the feet *(tinea pedis)*. Obesity may also be a significant risk factor (Scheinfeld, 2004). The inner thighs and inguinal region are the most commonly affected areas, and the scrotum and penis are usually spared. **Significant scrotal involvement should raise suspicion for cutaneous candidiasis as an alternative diagnosis** (Sobera and Elewski, 2003). Characteristic lesions in tinea cruris are sharply demar-

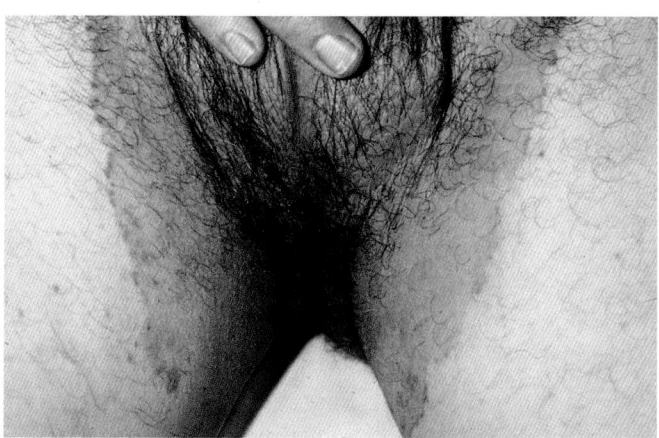

Figure 13–30. Dermatophyte infection of the groin (tinea cruris) showing areas of postinflammatory hyperpigmentation and active infection at the border of the lesions. (From Callen JP, Greer DE, Hood AF, Paller AS: Color Atlas of Dermatology. Philadelphia, WB Saunders, 1993, p 318.)

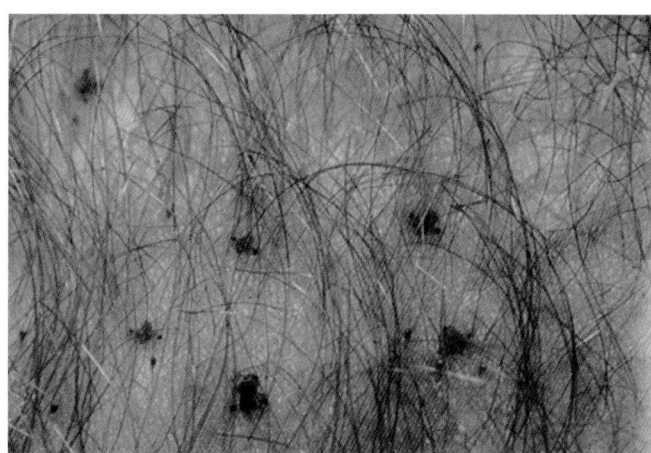

Figure 13–31. Pediculosis pubis. Several crab lice are visible. (From du Vivier A: Atlas of Clinical Dermatology. London, Churchill Livingstone, 2002, p 338.)

cated with a raised erythematous border (Fig. 13–30) and may be intensely pruritic. A variety of disorders can mimic dermatophyte infection, including seborrheic dermatitis, psoriasis, contact dermatitis, and erythrasma. The diagnosis of fungal infection can be confirmed with skin scrapings and a KOH preparation.

Good hygienic practices can be beneficial in preventing recurrent disease, including wearing loose clothing, cleaning of contaminated garments, weight reduction, and the use of topical powders to keep the intertriginous areas dry (Sobera and Elewski, 2003). Topical antifungal preparations are the primary agents for treatment, with the powdered forms having the added benefit of drying moist areas. **Care should be taken to treat only active disease and not the postinflammatory hyperpigmentation that can occur with recurrent chronic dermatophyte infection** (Margolis, 2002). Systemic antifungal agents are rarely necessary to treat groin infection with dermatophytes.

Infestation

Pediculosis pubis and scabies *(Sarcoptes scabiei)* are the most common infestations involving the genital region.

Infestation with the crab louse *(Phthirus pubis)* causes pediculosis pubis, a pruritic disorder of the genitalia, which may coexist with other sexually transmitted diseases (Opaneye et al, 1993; Varela et al, 2003). In one study of adolescent males, patients with pediculosis pubis had a more than twofold higher risk of concomitant gonorrhea or chlamydial infection than normal controls (Pierzchalski et al, 2002). Louse infestation is not limited to the genitalia and may involve other hair-bearing areas such as the eyelashes, beard, and axillae (Meinking, 1999). The diagnosis is confirmed by identification of crab lice attached to hairs (Fig. 13–31), often with associated perifollicular erythema. **Transmission of pediculosis pubis is usually though sexual contact, although contaminated clothing, bedding, and towels have also been implicated in some cases** (Meinking, 1999). **The standard treatment is application of 5% permethrin cream overnight to all affected hair-bearing areas with a repeat application 1**

week later (Meinking et al, 2003). Note that the second application of permethrin is important, because the rate of treatment success with a single application may be as low as 57% (Kalter et al, 1987). For rare cases refractory to topical therapy or those involving the eyelashes (tinea palpebrum), the addition of oral ivermectin may be curative (Burkhart and Burkhart, 2000).

Another important infestation involving the genitalia is scabies, caused by the female itch mite *Sarcoptes scabiei*. **Scabies is a worldwide problem, and factors such as overcrowding, delayed treatment of primary cases, and poor public awareness encourage spread** (Meinking et al, 2003). Transmission is common between close contacts and family members (Burkhart et al, 2000). The number of mites living on an immunocompetent host is usually small (<100) (Arlian et al, 1988), although far greater numbers may be recovered in cases of immunosuppression (so-called crusted scabies). The incubation period before symptoms develop after infestation can vary from days to months.

Severe pruritus is the hallmark of scabies and is often accentuated at night or after bathing (Meinking et al, 2003). In both sexes, the genital areas are commonly affected. Small erythematous papules are present and excoriations with secondary bacterial infection may occur (Fig. 13–32). **Thin, gray or white burrows may be visible and are pathognomonic for scabies infestation.** In the absence of visible burrows, a broad differential diagnosis must be considered, including atopic dermatitis, pyoderma, psoriasis, and other insect bites. As in the case of pediculosis pubis, the treatment of choice for scabies is 5% permethrin cream applied to the entire body overnight with a second application 1 week later. An alternative scabicide, lindane, is not favored owing to both central nervous system toxicity in children and a rising rate of resistance among mites (Purvis and Tyring, 1991; Elgart, 1996). Oral ivermectin is an alternate regimen that has been successfully used to treat scabies (Chouela et al, 2002; Heukelbach et al, 2004; Karthikeyan, 2005). **Note that pruritus may persist for several weeks despite successful treatment and that intimate contacts should also be treated to prevent reinfestation.**

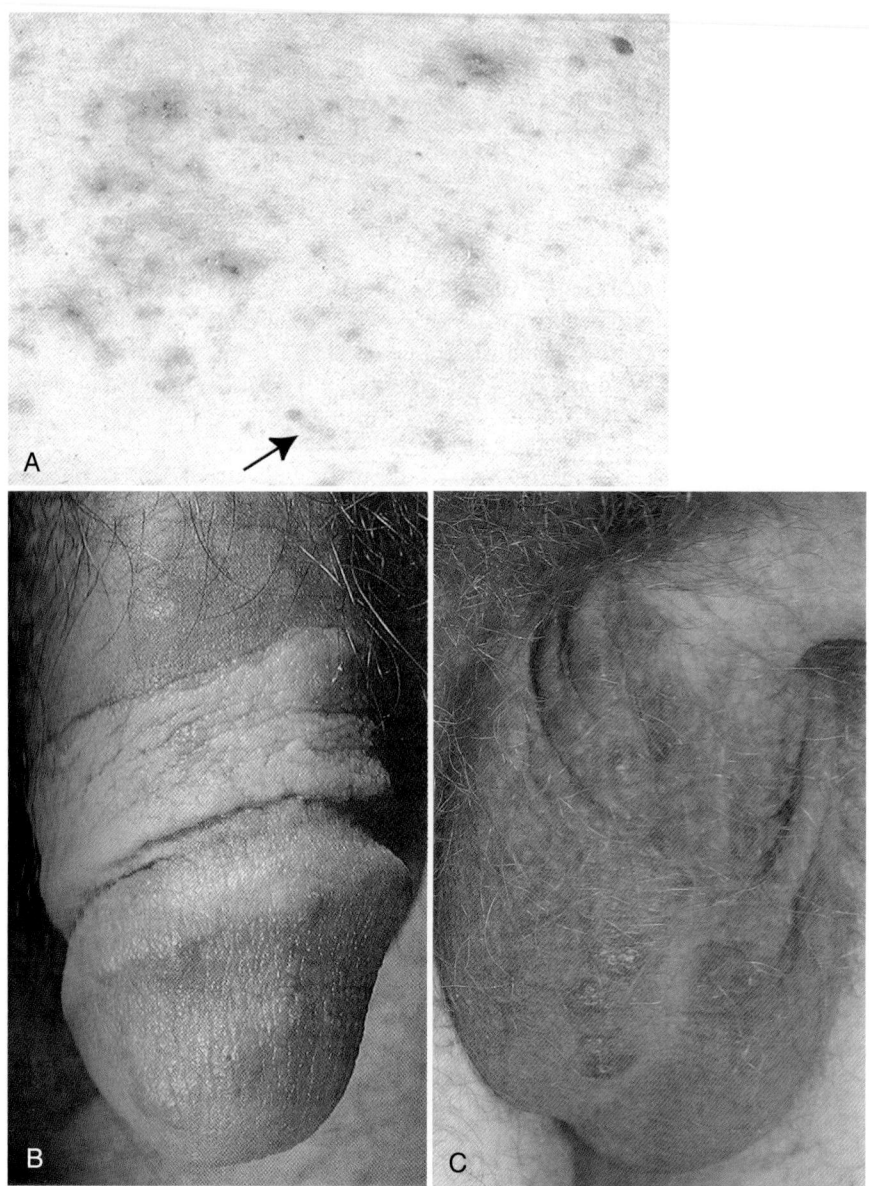

Figure 13–32. Scabies. **A,** Papular eruption with characteristic burrows visible *(arrow)*; **B** and **C,** Classic established genital scabies with eroded papules on the glans penis and scrotum. (**A** from du Vivier A: Atlas of Clinical Dermatology. London, Churchill Livingstone, 2002, p 332; **B** and **C,** Habif TP: Clinical Dermatology. Edinburgh, Mosby, 2004, p 501.)

NEOPLASTIC CONDITIONS
Squamous Cell Carcinoma in Situ

Squamous cell carcinoma in situ (SCCis) is a full-thickness intraepidermal carcinoma (Miller and Moresi, 2003). Bowen originally described this condition in 1912, hence the term *Bowen's disease.* On extragenital sites there is a strong association between SCCis and UV light exposure (Reizner et al, 1994). **Commonly presenting in the seventh decade of life with a slight female predominance** (Arlette, 2003; Hemminki and Dong, 2000), **SCCis usually has an indolent clinical course and rarely progresses to invasive disease. When it occurs on mucosal surfaces of the male genitalia, most notably the glans penis of uncircumcised men, this entity is referred to as erythroplasia of Queyrat** (Fig. 13–33). In that location, coinfection with human papillomavirus types 8, 16,

39, and 51 has been identified (Wieland et al, 2000). Other risk factors for SCCis include ionizing radiation, immunosuppression, thermal injury, arsenic exposure, chronic dermatoses, and lichen sclerosis of the glans penis (Euvrard et al, 1995; Nasca et al, 1999; Powell et al, 2001; Centeno et al, 2002; Arlette, 2003).

SCCis lesions are sharply demarcated, solitary, pink to red scaly plaques and may be confused with basal cell carcinoma, eczema, or psoriasis. When localized to the penile shaft, SCCis may have a more thickened, verrucoid appearance. Although usually asymptomatic, these lesions may also be pruritic or painful. The diagnosis is confirmed by histologic evaluation, and several areas should be sampled to exclude the presence of dermal invasion (Margolis, 2002).

Primary treatment of SCCis involves either surgical excision or tissue ablation. For accessible areas, such as the scrotum, simple excision with a 5-mm margin is favored (Bissada, 1992;

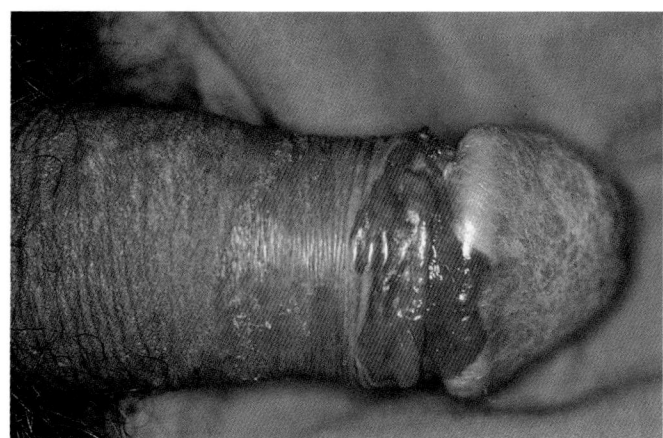

Figure 13–33. Erythroplasia of Queyrat. Squamous cell carcinoma involving the glans penis. (From Callen JP, Greer DE, Hood AF, Paller AS: Color Atlas of Dermatology. Philadelphia, WB Saunders, 1993, p 330.)

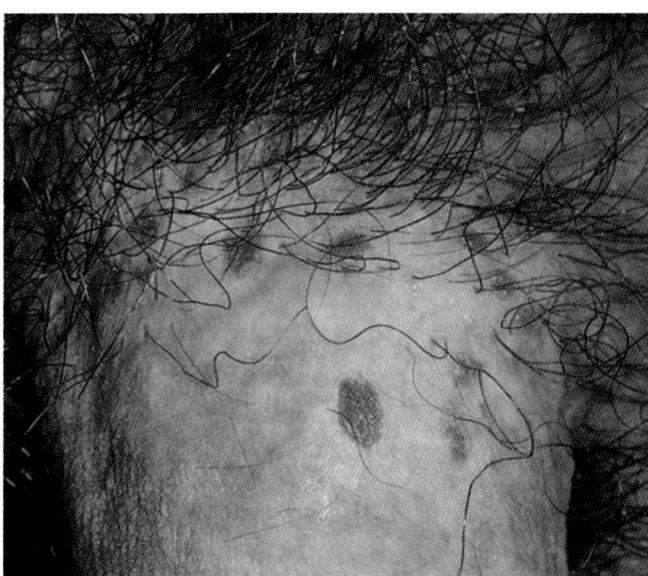

Figure 13–34. Bowenoid papulosis of the penile shaft. Note multiple brown verrucous papules on the penile shaft. (From Habif TP: Clinical Dermatology. Edinburgh, Mosby, 2004, p 343.)

Margolis, 2002). For areas where tissue preservation is more critical, Mohs' microsurgery, laser therapy, and cryoablation may have a role (Sonnex et al, 1982b; van Bezooijen et al, 2001; Leibovitch et al, 2005). Topical treatment with either 5-fluorouracil or imiquimod has also proven effective for management of selected cases of SCCis involving the genitalia (Gerber, 1994; Arlette, 2003; Micali et al, 2003).

Bowenoid Papulosis

Bowenoid papulosis (BP) is an uncommon condition found on the penis and vulva of sexually active adults, with a peak incidence in the third decade (Schwartz and Janniger, 1991). **It histologically resembles Bowen's disease except that the abnormal keratinocytes are spread discontinuously throughout the epidermis** (Margolis, 2002). Typical lesions are multiple, small, erythematous papules that may coalesce to form plaques with a verrucous surface similar to a genital wart (Fig. 13–34). There is a clear association with HPV type 16. **Female partners of men with BP have an increased risk of cervical neoplasia and should have close cervical follow-up** (Rosemberg et al, 1991). In men, however, BP generally has a benign course and spontaneous regression may occur (Eisen et al, 1983; Giam and Ong, 1986). Therefore, conservative local therapy with observation, topical agents (5-fluorouracil or imiquimod), or ablative measures (electrodissection, cryotherapy, laser therapy) is usually appropriate (Margolis, 2002).

Squamous Cell Carcinoma

Invasive squamous cell carcinoma involving the genitalia (Fig. 13–35) is covered in detail in Chapter 31.

Verrucous Carcinoma (Buschke-Löwenstein Tumor)

Verrucous carcinoma (VC) is a locally aggressive, exophytic, low-grade variant of squamous cell carcinoma that has little metastatic potential (Habif, 2004). **The Bushke-Löwenstein tumor is a VC of the anogenital mucosal surface and may

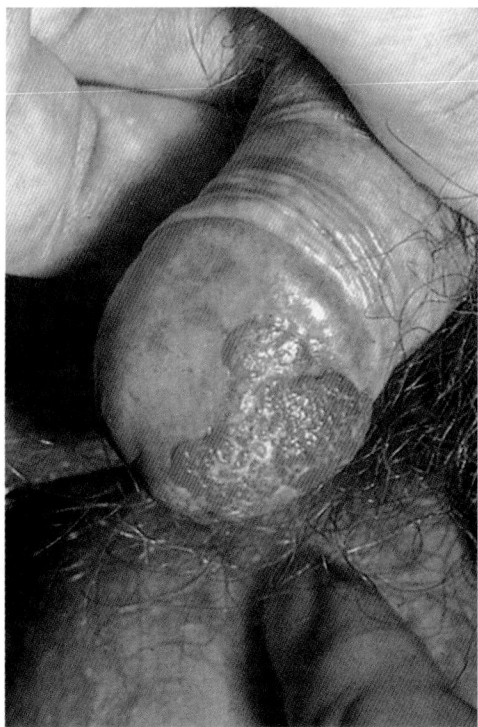

Figure 13–35. Squamous cell carcinoma. Exophytic erosive lesion with evident keratinization. (From Callen JP, Greer DE, Hood AF, Paller AS: Color Atlas of Dermatology. Philadelphia, WB Saunders, 1993, p 129.)

represent up to 24% of all penile tumors** (Schwartz, 1995). It most commonly occurs in uncircumcised men on the glans or prepuce, although similar lesions can be found on the vulva, vagina, cervix, or anus. VC has been associated with human papillomavirus types 6 and 11 infection but not with the more classically oncogenic types 16 and 18 (Yasunaga et al, 1993; Chan et al, 1994; Margolis, 2002).

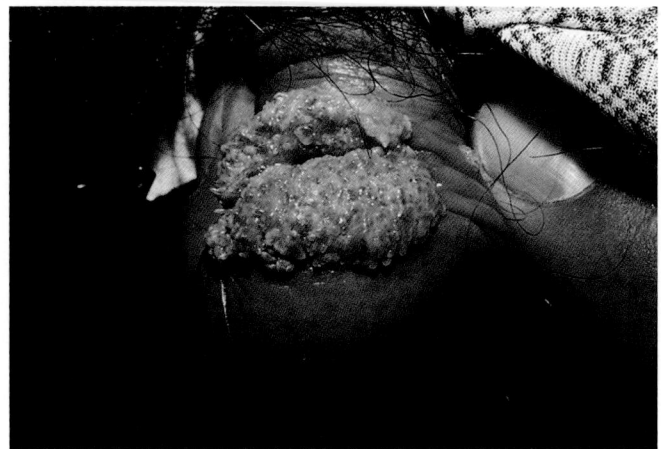

Figure 13–36. Verrucous carcinoma of the penis (Buschke-Löwenstein tumor). Note the exophytic and wartlike appearance. (From Callen JP, Greer DE, Hood AF, Paller AS: Color Atlas of Dermatology. Philadelphia, WB Saunders, 1993, p 330.)

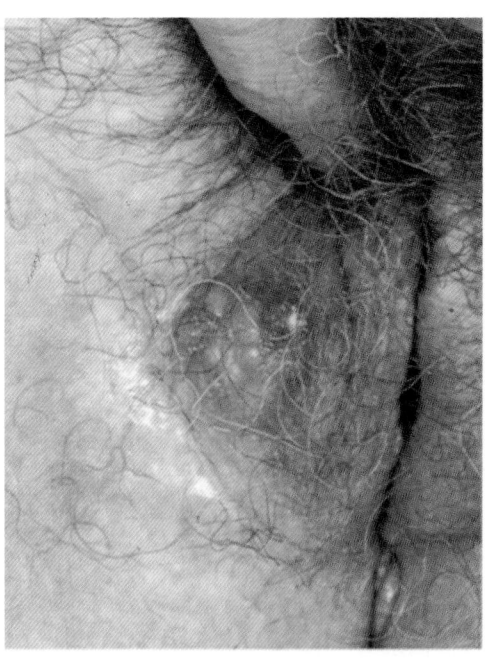

Figure 13–37. Basal cell carcinoma involving the vulva. (From du Vivier A: Atlas of Clinical Dermatology. London, Churchill Livingstone, 2002, p 688.)

VC lesions have a warty appearance and are often large and fungating when presenting on the genitalia (Fig. 13–36). Aside from genital sites, these lesions can also present within the oral and nasal cavities and plantar surfaces of the feet. They are slow growing and locally destructive, often extending deeply into underlying tissue. Treatment is preferably by local excision. **Primary radiation therapy is relatively contraindicated owing to the potential for anaplastic transformation with a subsequent increase in metastatic potential** (Stehman et al, 1980; Andersen and Sorensen, 1988; Fukunaga et al, 1994; Vandeweyer et al, 2001).

Basal Cell Carcinoma

Basal cell carcinoma (BCC) is the most common cutaneous neoplasm, arising most often on areas of chronically sun-exposed skin such as the head and neck. Genital BCC has also been described as a rare entity, most commonly involving the scrotal skin in the male and vulva in the female (Nahass et al, 1992; Benedet et al, 1997; Esquivias Gomez et al, 1999; Kinoshita et al, 2005). Several subtypes of BCC have been defined, including nodular, superficial, micronodular, and infiltrating. The nodular variant accounts for 60% of all BCCs and presents as a pearly, skin-toned papule or plaque often with telangiectases overlying the tumor (Fig. 13–37) (Miller and Moresi, 2003). These lesions may ulcerate and have a very low metastatic potential. Treatment is by local excision.

Kaposi's Sarcoma

Kaposi's sarcoma (KS) is a disease of endothelial cell origin. Whether KS is a neoplastic or hyperplastic process remains controversial, and evidence exists both for and against clonal expansion (Rabkin et al, 1997; Gill et al, 1998). Prior to the onset of the AIDS epidemic, KS was considered a chronic disease afflicting elderly men of Jewish, Mediterranean, or Eastern European decent ("classic KS") (Safai, 1987). However, infection with HIV-1 has increased the incidence of KS by more than 7000-fold (Miles, 1994; Margolis, 2002). KS generally affects HIV-infected patients with advanced immune impairment (CD4+ T-cell counts of < 500 cells/mm) (Tappero et al, 1993). Approximately 40% of homosexual men with AIDS have developed KS as compared with less than 5% in other risk groups (Rogers et al, 1987; North et al, 2003). There is also a clear association between infection with human herpesvirus 8 and the development of KS (Boshoff and Weiss, 1997; Weiss et al, 1998).

Classic KS in immunocompetent individuals presents as slowly growing blue-red pigmented macules on the lower extremities. Although oral and gastrointestinal lesions may occur, the genitalia are seldom involved. This is in contrast to the case with AIDS ("epidemic KS") in which a solitary genital lesion may be the first manifestation of KS (Lowe et al, 1989). **The clinical features of KS in AIDS patients are diverse, ranging from a single lesion to disseminated cutaneous and visceral disease** (Fig. 13–38). Lesions may coalesce to cover large areas of skin and may result in lymphatic or venous blockage leading to local edema (Margolis, 2002). When these lesions involve the glans penis, they can cause obstruction at the urethral meatus or fossa navicularis (Swierzewski et al, 1993).

Treatment must be tailored to the individual clinical case, and complete cure may be an unrealistic goal. For solitary lesions, local therapy such as surgical excision, laser treatment, cryotherapy, or intralesional injection of chemotherapeutic agents (i.e., vinblastine) may be beneficial (Chun et al, 1999; Schwartz, 2004; Heyns and Fisher, 2005). For extensive loco-regional disease, radiation therapy (15 to 30 Gy) has an objective response rate of more than 90% (Kirova et al, 1998; Cattelan et al, 2002). For widely disseminated KS, systemic chemotherapy with vincristine, doxorubicin, and bleomycin is preferred (Aversa et al, 1999).

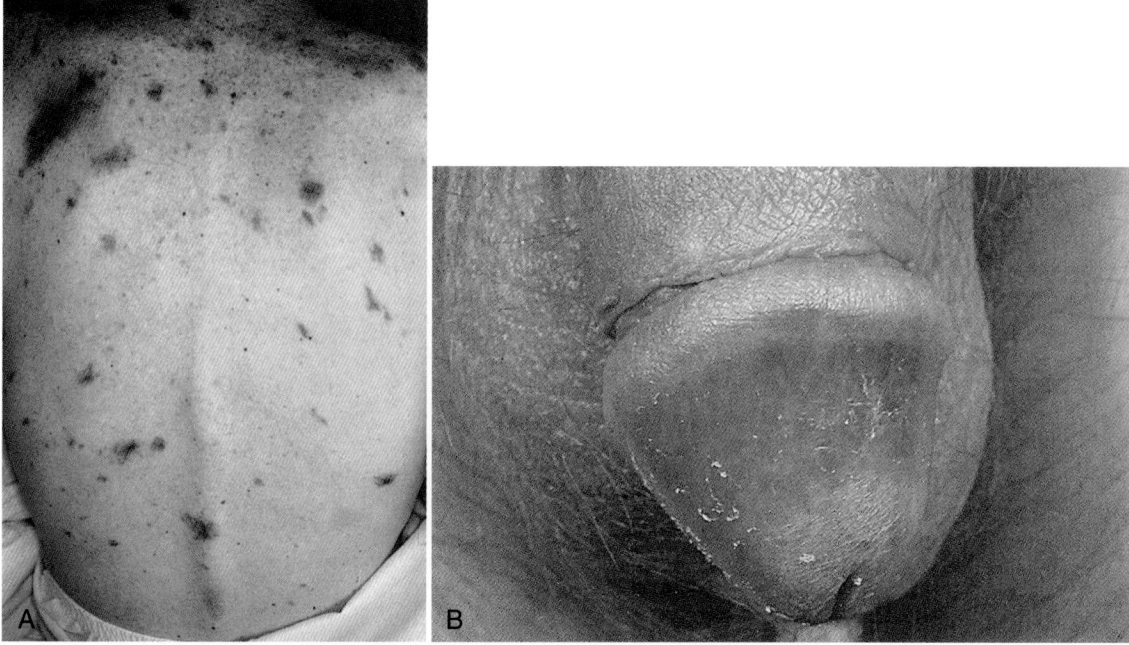

Figure 13–38. Kaposi's sarcoma. Classic macular lesions seen on the back (**A**) and glans penis (**B**). (**A** from Callen JP, Greer DE, Hood AF, Paller AS: Color Atlas of Dermatology. Philadelphia, WB Saunders, 1993, p 220; **B** from du Vivier A: Atlas of Clinical Dermatology. London, Churchill Livingstone, 2002, p 716.)

Pseudoepitheliomatous, Keratotic, and Micaceous Balanitis

Pseudoepitheliomatous, keratotic, and micaceous balanitis (PEKMB) is a rare entity characterized by the development of a thick, hyperkeratotic plaque on the glans penis of older men (Fig. 13–39). The term *micaceous* refers to the white, scaly appearance of the lesions (Child et al, 2000). PEKMB was originally thought to be a purely benign process, although several case reports have documented the presence of concurrent verrucous carcinoma associated with this lesion (Child et al, 2000). There remains controversy as to whether PEKMB is a premalignant condition (Read and Abell, 1981; Beljaards et al, 1987; Jenkins and Jakubovic, 1988). Histologic examination is essential to exclude the presence of squamous cell carcinoma and verrucous carcinoma (Margolis, 2002). PEKMB is characterized on histology by a hyperplastic epidermis, with ridges extending deeply into the dermis (Jenkins and Jakubovic, 1988). These lesions should be treated locally either by surgical excision or ablative techniques, and close follow-up is essential (Read and Abell, 1981; Bargman, 1985). There are also anecdotal reports of successful treatment using topical 5-fluorouracil cream (Bargman, 1985; Krunic et al, 1996).

Melanoma

Malignant melanoma is a neoplasm arising from melanocytes. The incidence of melanoma has risen 3% to 7% over the past several decades (Nestle and Kerl, 2003). Risk factors for development of the disease include family history, certain genetic markers, fair skin, and ultraviolet radiation exposure. Primary melanoma of the male genitalia is an uncommon entity, with only approximately 100 cases reported in the literature

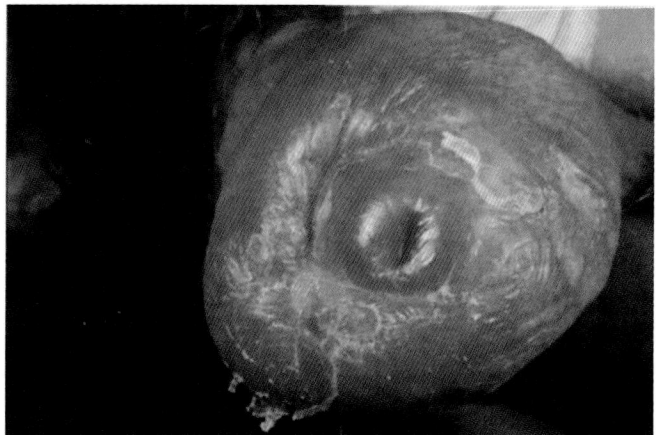

Figure 13–39. Pseudoepitheliomatous, keratotic, and micaceous balanitis. The glans becomes covered with mica (asbestos-like) scales and horny crusts. (From du Vivier A: Atlas of Clinical Dermatology. London, Churchill Livingstone, 2002, p 717.)

(Sanchez-Ortiz et al, 2005); and melanoma of the male urethra is even more rare (Oliva et al, 2000).

Genital melanoma usually presents as a pigmented macule or papule with an irregular border, although unpigmented lesions and ulceration may also be present (Margolis, 2002). **Early diagnosis is critical because local treatment of superficial lesions with wide local excision or partial penectomy can provide excellent disease control (Stillwell et al, 1988; Sanchez-Ortiz et al, 2005). In contrast, patients with biopsy-proven metastatic disease have a universally poor prognosis despite aggressive surgical management and multiagent cytotoxic chemotherapy.**

Extramammary Paget's Disease

Extramammary Paget's disease (EPD) is an uncommon intraepithelial adenocarcinoma of sites bearing apocrine glands (Zollo and Zeitouni, 2000). The majority of patients with EPD are elderly white females, and involvement of the male penis and scrotum is exceedingly rare (Park et al, 2001; van Randenborgh et al, 2002; Yang et al, 2005). The vulva is the most commonly involved genital site in women, followed by the perianal region in men (Wojnarowska and Cooper, 2003). **There is an important association between EPD and another underlying malignancy in 10% to 30% of cases** (Payne and Wells, 1994; Ng et al, 2001; Margolis, 2002). **In the male, associations between urethral, bladder, rectal, and apocrine malignancies with EPD have been described** (Hayes et al, 1997; Salamanca et al, 2004). It is critical, therefore, to perform a systematic evaluation for underlying carcinoma in cases of EPD.

The lesion in EPD is usually an erythematous plaque with a sharp border between normal and involved skin (Fig. 13–40). It may be asymptomatic, pruritic, or associated with burning pain. The diagnosis is confirmed histologically by the presence of vacuolated Paget's cells in the epidermis that stain for glandular cytokeratins, epithelial membrane antigen, and carcinoembryonic antigen (Wojnarowska and Cooper, 2003). Treatment generally involves surgical excision, although radiotherapy and topical imiquimod or 5-fluorouracil have also been used successfully (Sillman et al, 1985; Bewley et al, 1994; Brown et al, 2000, 2002; Guerrieri and Back, 2002; Moreno-Arias et al, 2003).

Cutaneous T-Cell Lymphoma

Cutaneous T-cell lymphoma (CTCL) represents a group of related neoplasms derived from T cells that home to the skin. It includes a variety of conditions, including mycosis fun-goides, Sezary's syndrome, lymphoid papulosis, and pagetoid reticulosis (Willemze, 2003). There is an increased risk of CTCL associated with HIV infection (Biggar et al, 2001). Although these disorders may involve the genitalia of both sexes, extragenital disease is usually also present. CTCL accounts for the majority of primary cutaneous lymphomas, with B-cell–derived lymphomas accounting for only 20% to 25% (Willemze et al, 1997, 2005). Definitive diagnosis depends on biopsy histopathology.

CTCL generally presents as pruritus, which must be differentiated from a variety of benign dermatoses, including psoriasis, eczema, superficial fungal infections, and drug reactions. Patients may subsequently develop hematologic involvement (Sézary's syndrome) and cutaneous plaques, erosions, ulcers, or frank skin tumors (Fig. 13–41) (Margolis, 2002). CTCL is a chronic condition that may progress over many years. Topical treatments include corticosteroids, nitrogen mustard, and carmustine, with complete remission rates of approximately 60% (Vonderheid et al, 1989; Zackheim et al, 1998). Other treatments include radiation therapy, phytotherapy (PUVA), and systemic treatment with chemotherapy, interferons, or retinoids (Hoppe et al, 1990; Olsen and Bunn, 1995; Diederen et al, 2003; Querfeld et al, 2005).

BENIGN CUTANEOUS DISORDERS SPECIFIC TO THE MALE GENITALIA
Angiokeratoma of Fordyce

Angiokeratomas of Fordyce (AF) are vascular ectasias of dermal blood vessels that may be visible on the penis and scrotum of adult men (Bechara et al, 2002). These lesions appear as 1- to 2-mm red or purple papules (Fig. 13–42A), and there may be associated generalized scrotal redness (Miller and James, 2002). This is usually a benign condition without systemic manifestations, although it may rarely be a

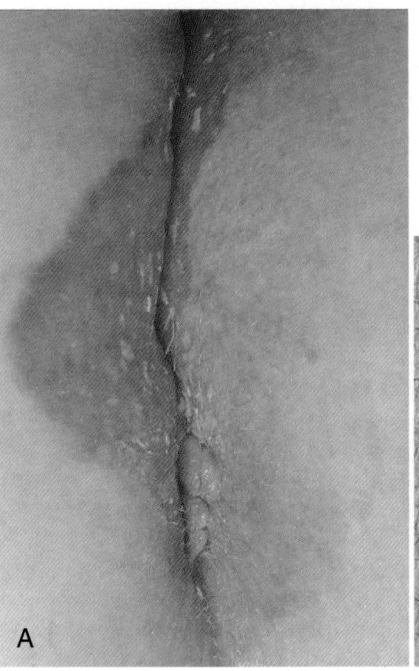
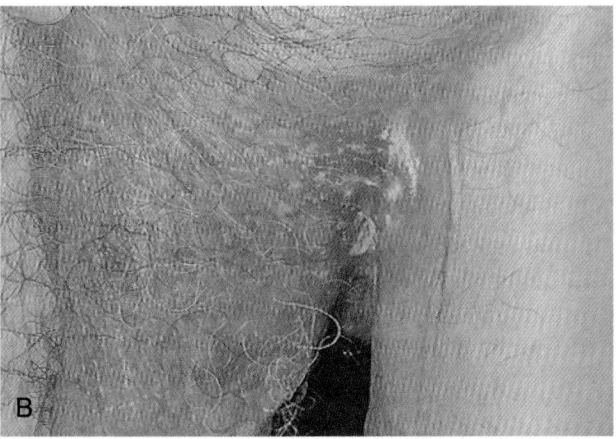

Figure 13–40. Extramammary Paget's disease involving the vulva (**A**) and base of scrotum (**B**). Note the well-demarcated border between the lesion and normal adjacent skin. (**A** from Habif TP: Clinical Dermatology. Edinburgh, Mosby, 2004, p 764; **B** from Bolognia JL, Jorizzo JL, Rapini RP: Dermatology. Edinburgh, Mosby, 2003, p 1108.)

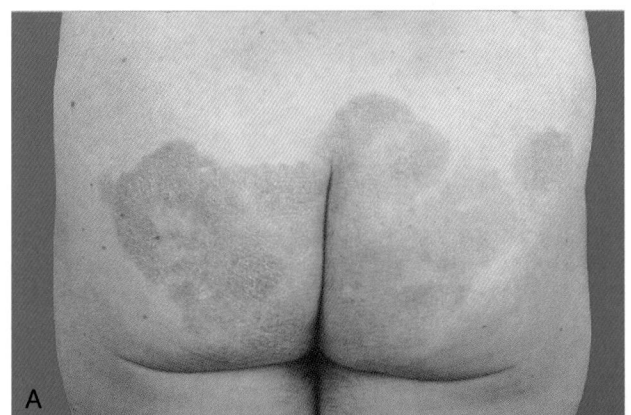

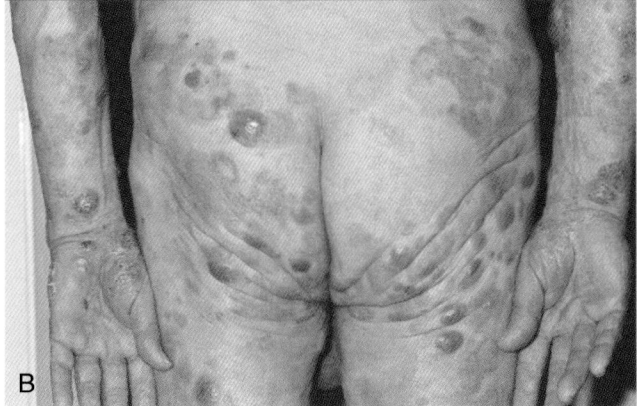

Figure 13–41. Mycosis fungoides (a cutaneous T-cell lymphoma) involving the buttocks. **A,** Limited plaque stage. **B,** A more advanced case with plaques, patches, and tumors. (From Bolognia JL, Jorizzo JL, Rapini RP: Dermatology. Edinburgh, Mosby, 2003, pp 1926-1927.)

source of troublesome scrotal bleeding (Taniguchi et al, 1994; Hoekx and Wyndaele, 1998). Similar lesions can be observed in Fabry's disease (see Fig. 13–42B), which is a rare glycogen storage deficiency. Although treatment is usually unnecessary for AF, several authors have reported success using erbium:YAG, KTP, and argon laser photocoagulation in select cases (Occella et al, 1995; Bechara et al, 2004).

Pearly Penile Papules

Pearly penile papules (PPP) are white, dome-shaped, closely spaced small papules located on the glans penis (see Fig. 13–42C). They are often arranged circumferentially at the corona. PPP are very common lesions found in up to 14% to 48% of young postpubertal adults, particularly if the penis is not circumcised (Rehbein, 1977; Khoo and Cheong, 1995; Sonnex and Dockerty, 1999). **Although PPP may occasionally be misdiagnosed as condylomata, the available evidence does not support a role for human papillomavirus in causing PPP and no association with cervical intraepithelial neoplasia in female partners has been demonstrated** (Hogewoning et al, 2003). Patients should be reassured that this is a benign condition that does not usually require treatment. If treatment is desired due to cosmetic concerns, local destruction with either the CO_2 laser or cryotherapy has been applied successfully (Ocampo-Candiani and Cueva-Rodriguez, 1996; Lane et al, 2002). **Histologically, these**

lesions are angiofibromas similar to the lesions seen on the face in tuberous sclerosis.

Zoon's Balanitis

Zoon's balanitis, also called plasma cell balanitis, occurs in uncircumcised men from the third decade onward (Pastar et al, 2004). Smooth, moist, erythematous, well-circumscribed plaques on the glans penis characterize the disease (see Fig. 13–42D). Shallow erosions may also be present (Yoganathan et al, 1994), and the lesions can be quite large (up to 2 cm in diameter) (Margolis, 2002). Squamous cell carcinoma and extramammary Paget's disease should be excluded, often by biopsy. Circumcision appears to be proof against development of the disease and can be performed to cure the majority of cases (Sonnex et al, 1982a; Ferrandiz and Ribera, 1984). For patients averse to circumcision, topical corticosteroids may provide symptomatic relief and laser therapy may also have a role (Baldwin and Geronemus, 1989; Tang et al, 2001; Albertini et al, 2002; Retamar et al, 2003; Wojnarowska and Cooper, 2003).

Sclerosing Lymphangitis

Nonvenereal sclerosing lymphangitis is a rare penile lesion consisting of an indurated, slightly tender cord involving the coronal sulcus and adjacent penile skin (Gharpuray and Tolat, 1991; Rosen and Hwong, 2003). It is usually flesh colored but may occasionally be red. A mechanism related to thrombosis of lymphatic vessels has been proposed. There is an association with vigorous sexual activity, and resolution usually occurs within several weeks (Sieunarine, 1987; Margolis, 2002).

Median Raphe Cyst

Median raphe cysts occur in young men on the ventral aspect of the penis, most commonly near the glans (Stone, 2003). Although these cysts are believed to develop from aberrant urethral epithelium, they do not communicate with the urethra (Asarch et al, 1979). Treatment is by surgical removal.

Ectopic Sebaceous Glands

Ectopic sebaceous glands on the penile shaft may be visible as pin-sized papular lesions, which may be mistaken for verruca (see Fig. 13–42E) (Margolis and Wein, 2002).

COMMON MISCELLANEOUS CUTANEOUS DISORDERS
Skin Tag

Skin tags (acrochordons, fibroepithelial polyps) are soft, skin-colored, pedunculated lesions that can be present anywhere on the body. Although usually asymptomatic, these lesions may be painful secondary to local trauma or torsion and infarction in rare cases. These are common lesions, and up to 50% of all individuals may have at least one skin tag (Banik and Lubach, 1987). **It is important to distinguish these lesions from the hamartomatous skin lesions (multiple fibrofolliculomas)**

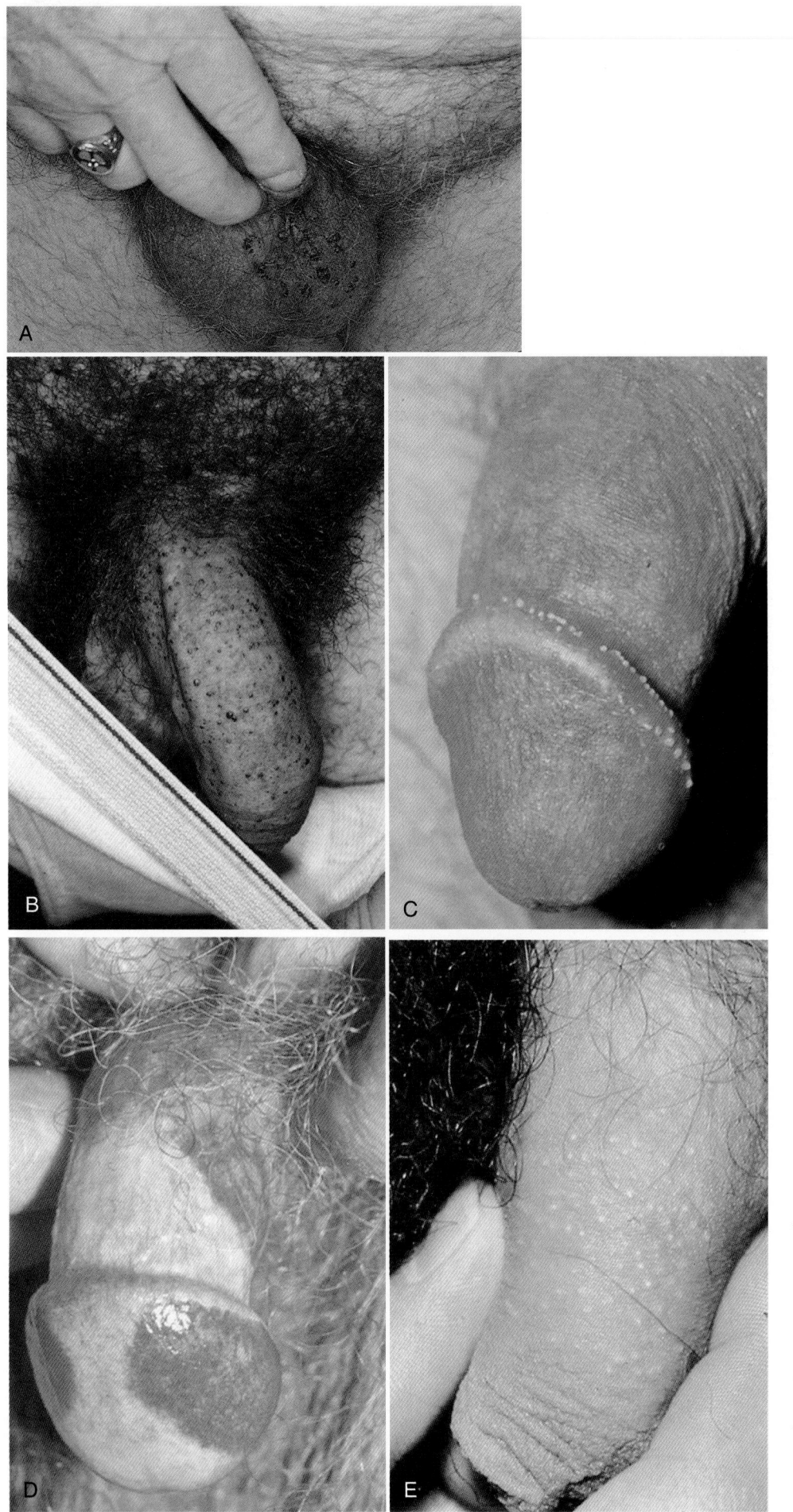

Figure 13–42. Benign cutaneous disorders specific to the male genitalia. **A,** Angiokeratoma of Fordyce showing purple scrotal vascular malformations. **B,** Fabry's disease, a glycogen storage deficiency with associated purple vascular malformations on the penile shaft. **C,** Pearly penile papules located on the corona of the glans penis. **D,** Zoon's balanitis of the glans penis. **E,** Ectopic sebaceous glands on the penile shaft. (**A, B,** and **E** from Callen JP, Greer DE, Hood AF, Paller AS: Color Atlas of Dermatology. Philadelphia, WB Saunders, 1993, pp 3, 327, and 328; **C** and **D** from Korting GW: Practical Dermatology of the Genital Region. Philadelphia, WB Saunders, 1981, pp 5 and 159.)

associated with Birt-Hogg-Dubé syndrome, which are histologically distinct from common skin tags (De la Torre et al, 1999).

Epidermoid Cysts

Epidermoid or epidermal-inclusion cysts (EC) are the most common cutaneous cysts and can be found anywhere on the body, including the genitalia. They are particularly common on the scrotum (Fig. 13–43E). **The term *sebaceous cyst* should be avoided because the contents of these cysts is not of sebaceous origin** (Stone, 2003). Although not painful at baseline, rupture of the cyst wall can lead to a severe inflammatory reaction that is extremely painful. Definitive treatment requires surgical excision of the entire cyst wall to prevent cyst recurrence. Inflamed or superinfected epidermoid cysts may require incision and drainage and antibiotic therapy if there is adjacent cellulitis. Dystrophic calcification of scrotal epidermoid cysts may be a cause of scrotal calcinosis (Dare and Axelsen, 1988; Michl et al, 1994).

Seborrheic Keratosis

Seborrheic keratoses are very common brown macules, plaques, and papules affecting individuals older than 30 years of age and increasing in frequency with advancing age. They are most common on the face, neck, and trunk, although any body site except the palms, soles, and mucous membranes may be affected. The degree of pigmentation can vary significantly, and darker lesions may be confused with melanoma or warts (Pierson et al, 2003). **These lesions have a waxy, "stuck-on" appearance** (see Fig. 13–43D), **and patients may note that they drop off spontaneously and regrow** (Margolis, 2002). Treatment by shave excision or destruction with liquid nitrogen is usually performed for cosmetic reasons. **An abrupt increase in the size and number of multiple seborrheic keratoses has been termed *Leser-Trélat syndrome* and has been implicated as a cutaneous marker of internal malignancy** (Chiba et al, 1996; Heaphy et al, 2000; Vielhauer et al, 2000; Ginarte et al, 2001).

Lentigo Simplex

Lentigo simplex is a condition characterized by the presence of brown-pigmented macules unrelated to sunlight exposure (see Fig. 13–43A). These lesions can be found anywhere on the body, including the mucous membranes and nail beds. In the genital area (genital lentiginosis), these lesions present commonly on the labia, vaginal introitus, perineum, and glans penis (penile melanosis). The lesions of lentigo simplex are usually smaller than those seen in melanocytic nevi. Although usually benign, the lesions of lentigo simplex may deserve biopsy evaluation in cases with atypical shape or coloration. **Finally, the combination of multiple pigmented lesions associated with intestinal polyposis should raise suspicion for Peutz-Jeghers syndrome.**

Mole (Nevus)

A mole or nevus of the skin is composed of slightly altered melanocytes called "nevus cells" arranged in a cluster. The location of the cluster determines the type of nevus. Junctional nevi are located between the epidermis and dermis and are usually flat, tan to black, small (<5 mm), and sharply bordered (Margolis, 2002). Intradermal nevi have clusters within the dermis and are usually small (<5 mm) and lighter in color with sharp borders. Compound nevi have clusters in both locations and are usually darker and raised as a papule (see Fig. 13–43B). As for any pigmented lesion, irregularity in coloration or border and rapid change over time are indications for excisional biopsy.

Dermatofibroma

Dermatofibromas are small hyperpigmented nodules that occur most commonly on the lower extremities and occasionally on the genitalia. Pinching of these lesions causes a downward movement of the tumor (the so-called dimple sign) (Kamino and Pui, 2003). These are benign lesions with a characteristic histologic pattern of spindle-shaped fibroblasts and myofibroblasts arranged in fascicles. Treatment by surgical excision is usually unnecessary and may leave a scar that is cosmetically inferior to the original lesion (Kamino and Pui, 2003).

Neurofibroma

Neurofibromas are common tumors composed of neuromesenchymal tissue with residual nerve axons. They can be present anywhere on the body, including the labia and scrotum (Yoshimura et al, 1990; Singh et al, 1992; Mishra et al, 2002; Kantarci et al, 2005). They are usually skin colored, soft, or rubbery nodular lesions and may be pedunculated. **Digital pressure on the lesion causes invagination or so-called button-holing** (Habif, 2004). These can be solitary lesions or multiple, which should raise suspicion for neurofibromatosis or von Recklinghausen's disease.

Capillary Hemangioma

Capillary hemangiomas are proliferations of blood vessels that are either present at birth or develop rapidly during the neonatal period. These lesions can involve the anogenital region and lead to bleeding or cause obstruction of the urethra, vagina, or anus (Sharma et al, 1981; Roberts and Devine, 1983). The majority will involute during childhood or early adolescence (Margolis, 2002).

Vitiligo

Vitiligo is an acquired disorder of skin depigmentation that affects 0.5% to 2% of the population (Ortonne, 2003). It may present at any age, and the pathogenesis remains a topic of intense research effort. Large patches of skin become completely amelanotic, appearing white although the tissue is otherwise normal. The borders with unaffected skin are usually sharp and well defined. This condition is particularly noticeable in darker-skinned individuals and on body sites that are normally hyperpigmented. Vitiligo limited to the genitalia has been observed in less than 0.3% of the male population (Moss and Stevenson, 1981). Lesions have a tendency to enlarge circumferentially over time and may develop at sites of local

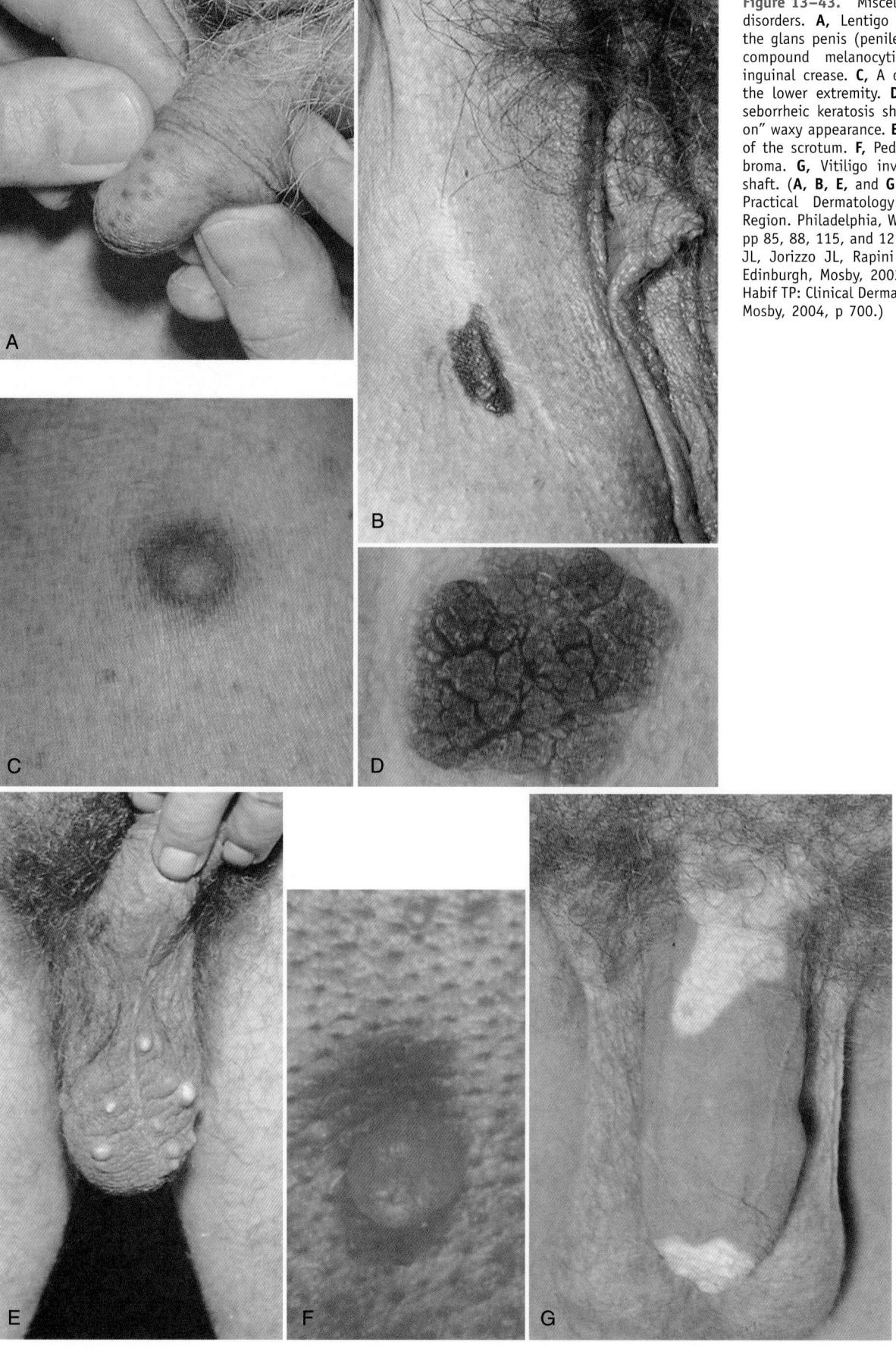

Figure 13–43. Miscellaneous cutaneous disorders. **A,** Lentigo simplex involving the glans penis (penile melanosis). **B,** A compound melanocytic nevus in the inguinal crease. **C,** A dermatofibroma on the lower extremity. **D,** A characteristic seborrheic keratosis showing the "stuck-on" waxy appearance. **E,** Epidermoid cysts of the scrotum. **F,** Pedunculated neurofibroma. **G,** Vitiligo involving the penile shaft. (**A, B, E,** and **G** from Korting GW: Practical Dermatology of the Genital Region. Philadelphia, WB Saunders, 1981, pp 85, 88, 115, and 121; **C** from Bolognia JL, Jorizzo JL, Rapini RP: Dermatology. Edinburgh, Mosby, 2003, p 1865; **D** from Habif TP: Clinical Dermatology. Edinburgh, Mosby, 2004, p 700.)

trauma (Koebner phenomenon). Genital vitiligo must be differentiated from lichen sclerosis and postinflammatory hypopigmentation (Margolis, 2002). Treatments include repigmentation with topical cosmetics, UV exposure, PUVA therapy, and skin grafting.

SUGGESTED READINGS

Bhattacharya M, Kaur I, Kumar B Lichen planus: A clinical and epidemiological study. J Dermatol 2000;27:576-582.

Bolognia JL, Jorizzo JL, Rapini RP: Dermatology. Edinburgh, Mosby, 2003.

Criteria for diagnosis of Behçet's disease. International Study Group for Behçet's Disease. Lancet 1990;335:1078-1080.

Eke N: Fournier's gangrene: A review of 1726 cases. Br J Surg 2000;87:718-728.

Karpati S: Dermatitis herpetiformis: Close to unravelling a disease. J Dermatol Sci 2004;34:83-90.

Krueger G, Koo J, Lebwohl M, et al: The impact of psoriasis on quality of life: Results of a 1998 National Psoriasis Foundation patient-membership survey. Arch Dermatol 2001;137:280-284.

Leibovitch I, Huilgol SC, Selva D, et al: Cutaneous squamous carcinoma in situ (Bowen's disease): Treatment with Mohs micrographic surgery. J Am Acad Dermatol 2005;52:997-1002.

Mallon E, Hawkins D, Dinneen M, et al: Circumcision and genital dermatoses. Arch Dermatol 2000;136:350-354.

Morpurgo E, Galandiuk S: Fournier's gangrene. Surg Clin North Am 2002;82:1213-1224.

Reunala T: Dermatitis herpetiformis: Coeliac disease of the skin. Ann Med 1998;30:416-418.

Rompel R, Petres J: Long-term results of wide surgical excision in 106 patients with hidradenitis suppurativa. Dermatol Surg 2000;26:638-643.

Sanchez-Ortiz R, Huang SF, Tamboli P, et al: Melanoma of the penis, scrotum and male urethra: A 40-year single institution experience. J Urol 2005;173:1958-1965.

Stern RS, Bagheri S, Nichols K: The persistent risk of genital tumors among men treated with psoralen plus ultraviolet A (PUVA) for psoriasis. J Am Acad Dermatol 2002;47:33-39.

Wolf R, Orion E, Marcos B, Matz H: Life-threatening acute adverse cutaneous drug reactions. Clin Dermatol 2005;23:171-181.

Wollenberg A, Bieber T: Atopic dermatitis: From the genes to skin lesions. Allergy 2000;55:205-213.

KEY POINTS: CUTANEOUS DISEASES OF THE EXTERNAL GENITALIA

- The diagnosis of cutaneous diseases of the external genitalia depends critically on a thorough history and physical examination. Extragenital findings may provide the key to diagnosis. The urologist should perform a thorough skin survey and not focus solely on the area of affected genital skin.

- The side effects of topical corticosteroids are significant, both from systemic absorption and locally. Adverse effects may be worsened if these agents are applied under the foreskin, which may serve as an occlusive dressing. In general, when applied to genital skin, only low-potency topical corticosteroids should be used for short treatment courses.

- Cutaneous disorders of the external genitalia can be broken down into the general categories of allergic, papulosquamous, vesicobullous, ulcerative, infectious, neoplastic, and miscellaneous diseases.

- Histopathologic analysis of biopsy specimens plays an important role in differentiating cutaneous diseases with similar clinical features and in excluding malignancy.

- Local treatment modalities including the use of laser energy, photodynamic therapy, ultraviolet radiation, and cryotherapy are being applied successfully to a variety of genital cutaneous disorders and offer an alternative to surgical excision in some cases.

14 Tuberculosis and Parasitic and Fungal Infections of the Genitourinary System

SARAH J. McALEER, MD • CHRISTOPHER W. JOHNSON, MD • WARREN D. JOHNSON, JR., MD

GENITOURINARY TUBERCULOSIS

PARASITIC DISEASES OF THE GENITOURINARY SYSTEM

FUNGAL DISEASES OF THE GENITOURINARY SYSTEM

GENITOURINARY TUBERCULOSIS
History

The disease known as "consumption" has been observed in humans for over 7000 years (Myers, 1952). The remains of skeletons from about 4000 BC show the characteristic changes of tuberculosis (TB). It was a common disease in Egypt around 1000 BC (Morse et al, 1964), and during the 1700s in Europe infections reached epidemic proportions. Almost one fourth of the deaths in England during that period were caused by "consumption" (Colby, 1954). Finally in 1882, Koch (1882) discovered the cause of TB. He observed the organism in patients, grew it outside the body, and reproduced the disease in a susceptible host. The Koch postulates have since become the basis for the study of all infectious diseases. Ehrlich then discovered the acid-fast nature of the bacillus in 1882.

The pathogenesis of renal TB remained obscure until Medlar (1926) published his classic studies on patients who had died from pulmonary TB, none of whom had any clinical evidence of genitourinary disease. He reviewed 100,000 serial sections from the kidneys of 30 patients. Microscopic lesions were found in the renal cortex, and almost all were bilateral. It was Medlar and associates (1949) who suggested that these pathologic changes should be termed "metastatic" rather than "secondary," because it was clear that the kidneys had become infected through the bloodstream at the time of the primary infection.

Surgical intervention for genitourinary TB was introduced in 1870, when the first nephrectomy was performed for pyonephrosis by Bryant (Wise and Marella, 2003). The prognosis for these patients was poor, and 85% of them died before the introduction of antituberculous medications. The greatest milestone in the treatment of TB was the discovery of the antituberculous drugs, starting with streptomycin in 1944, followed by *para*-aminosalicylic acid in 1946, isoniazid (INH) in 1952, and rifampicin in 1966. These discoveries were followed by the introduction of shorter courses of chemotherapy for all forms of tuberculosis.

Epidemiology
Incidence

The World Health Organization (WHO) estimates that one third of the world's population is infected with *Mycobacterium tuberculosis* and there are 8 to 10 million new active cases of TB each year (WHO, 1997). **In the United States, the number of reported cases declined annually until 1985, when the trend was dramatically reversed.** The factors responsible for this increase included the emergence of the acquired immunodeficiency syndrome (AIDS), immigration, and the neglect and deterioration of the public health infrastructure. However, since 1992, the number of cases of TB in the United States has decreased annually and is now at the lowest rate in our history (Centers for Disease Control and Prevention [CDC], 2005). The worldwide trends, as reported by the WHO, have not shown the same improvement (Dolin et al, 1993). Furthermore, in 2004, foreign-born persons accounted for 54% of TB cases in the United States (CDC, 2005).

The interaction between human immunodeficiency virus (HIV) infection and TB has been a major obstacle to the control of TB. **Globally, TB is the most common opportunistic infection in AIDS patients** (Pape et al, 1983; WHO, 1997; Perlman et al, 1999). The probability that an HIV-infected person who was previously infected with *M. tuberculosis* will develop active TB is 10% per year. In contrast, a normal host without HIV infection and a similar *M. tuberculosis* experience will have a 5% to 10% lifetime probability of developing active TB. Studies in New York City showed that among patients with both TB and AIDS, almost two thirds had

436

developed TB within 6 months of their diagnosis of AIDS (CDC, 1987). Block and Snider (1990) reported that 2.6% of patients with AIDS had extrapulmonary TB. It is recommended that all people with HIV infection undergo tuberculin testing so that those who react to tuberculin can be offered treatment for latent infection. It is also recommended that all people who contract TB be offered testing for HIV.

Genitourinary TB remains an important, but uncommon form of TB. **In 1999, 1.2% of patients in New York City had the genitourinary tract as the primary site of disease** (New York City Department of Health, 2000) (Table 14–1). The prevalence of genitourinary TB nationally is comparable with the New York experience. The percentage of patients in the United States with extrapulmonary TB who had genitourinary involvement was 17.9% in 1977, 11.9% in 1986, and 5% in 2003 (CDC, 2003; Goldfarb and Salman, 2004). In Great Britain, the prevalence of genitourinary TB has decreased from 4.5% to 2.6% in the period 1983 to 1993 (Gow, 1998).

Transmission and Development of Disease

Almost all *M. tuberculosis* infections are acquired by the inhalation of aerosolized droplet nuclei, which reach the pulmonary alveoli. Rarely, TB has been acquired by aerosolization from a patient's skin ulcer or during an autopsy (Frampton, 1992; Templeton et al, 1995). The greatest risk of transmission is exposure to a patient with either laryngeal or cavitary pulmonary TB. In the latter instance, sputum contains up to 10^8 bacilli/mL. It has been estimated that the efficiency of a single cough in aerosolizing organisms is equivalent to talking with a patient for 5 minutes (Bates and Stead, 1993).

The probability that a person will become infected depends on the duration of exposure to the source case, the size of the bacillary inoculum inhaled, and the infectivity of the mycobacterial strain. Up to 50% of the active disease

occurs within 2 years of infection, which is why antituberculous prophylaxis is recommended if there is evidence of new infection (purified protein derivative [PPD] of tuberculin test conversion to positive) or exceptionally heavy exposure (Styblo, 1980; CDC, 2000). In contrast, virtually all AIDS patients with a PPD test develop active TB during their lifetime unless antituberculous prophylaxis is offered or another opportunistic infection develops and is fatal (Pape et al, 1993; CDC, 1998b; Bloom and Small, 1998).

Genitourinary TB is caused by metastatic spread of the organism through the bloodstream during the initial infection. The kidney is usually the primary organ infected in urinary disease, and other parts of the urinary tract become involved by direct extension. The initial infection occurs in the renal cortex, where the bacilli can remain dormant within granulomas for decades. This dormant infection then becomes activated due to failure of the local immune response. **The primary site for infection of the genital tract is often the epididymis in men and the fallopian tubes in women, also by hematogenous spread. Similar to urinary disease, the infection then spreads to adjacent organs by direct extension.** The transmission of genital TB from male to female is very rare despite the fact that men with genital TB can have *M. tuberculosis* in the semen (Sutherland et al, 1982).

Immunology and Pathogenesis

The development of disease depends on the interaction between the pathogen and the host immune response. *M. tuberculosis* is the paradigm of the successful intracellular pathogen (Ellner, 1997). Although the organism evokes both a humoral and a cellular immune response, it is the latter that determines the outcome of an infection. T lymphocytes interact with mycobacterial antigens to proliferate and to generate cytokines that, in turn, activate macrophages to become more mycobactericidal (Orme et al, 1993). These mononuclear phagocytes also release a number of factors (tumor necrosis factor-α, transforming growth factor-β) that, together with the lymphocyte secretory products, determine the character of the pathologic lesion and the outcome of the infection.

During the initial primary pulmonary infection, the *M. tuberculosis* organisms multiply and evoke an inflammatory reaction. In spite of this reaction, there is still little resistance to the multiplication of the bacteria, and rapid spread occurs, first by way of the lymphatics and then through the bloodstream. After several weeks, the rate of multiplication decreases as the aforementioned host response develops and the dissemination ceases. At this stage, the individual shows evidence of delayed hypersensitivity, coincident with the macrophages acquiring the ability to inhibit the multiplication of *M. tuberculosis*. **Most persons control the initial infection and develop no clinical illness. They have dormant bacilli, which may begin to produce disease years later after debilitating disease, trauma, corticosteroids, immunosuppressive therapy, diabetes, or AIDS.**

Pathology and Clinical Features

Urologists should always consider the diagnosis of genitourinary TB in a patient presenting with vague, longstanding urinary symptoms for which there is no obvious

Table 14–1. New York City Department of Health: 1999 Tuberculosis Control Program Information Summary		
	No. Cases	**%**
Tuberculosis Cases by Primary Site of Disease		
Pulmonary	1073	73.5
Lymphatic	152	10.4
Pleural	69	4.7
Miliary	38	2.6
Bone or joint	36	2.5
Meningeal	22	1.5
Genitourinary	17	1.2
Peritoneal	12	0.8
Other	41	2.8
Total	1460	100.0
Tuberculosis Cases by All Sites of Disease		
Only pulmonary disease	998	68.4
Only extrapulmonary disease	287	19.7
Both pulmonary and extrapulmonary	175	12.0
Total	1460	100.0

From New York City Department of Health: Tuberculosis in New York City, 1999 Information Summary. New York, New York City Department of Health, 2000.

cause (Garcia-Rodriguez et al, 1994). The symptoms and signs of genitourinary TB vary in both intensity and duration. **Most patients affected are aged 20 to 40 years, and the male to female ratio is 2:1.** This has remained unchanged over many years. **Genitourinary TB is very uncommon in children** because the symptoms of renal TB do not appear for 3 to 10 or more years after the primary infection (Ustvedt, 1947). It is therefore unlikely that the disease will be seen in a child younger than 5 years (Chattopadhyay et al, 1997).

Tuberculosis of the Kidney, Ureter, and Bladder

The patient usually complains of **frequent painless micturition.** Urgency is uncommon. The urine is classically characterized by a sterile pyuria; however, up to 20% of patients do not have any leukocytes in the urine (Gow, 1976). Commonly, **the symptoms are intermittent.** Overt hematuria is present in only 10% of patients, but **microscopic hematuria is present in up to 50%.** Renal or suprapubic pain is a rare presenting symptom and usually means extensive involvement of the kidney and bladder. Ureteral colic is uncommon and occurs only if a small flake of calcification or a clot passes down the ureter. Recurrent cystitis is also a warning sign of urinary TB. If the cause is not confirmed and the symptoms persist or recur, investigation should be conducted repeatedly, because *M. tuberculosis* may be difficult to isolate from the urine.

Kidney. Renal TB is caused by the activation of a prior bloodborne renal infection. The organisms in the kidney settle in the blood vessels, usually those close to the glomeruli. Caseating granulomas develop and consist of Langhans giant cells surrounded by lymphocytes and fibroblasts. The course of the infection depends on the virulence of the organism and the resistance of the host.

The healing process results in fibrous tissue and calcium salts being deposited, producing the classic calcified lesion. One may also develop papillary necrosis and strictures in the calyceal stem or at the pelviureteral junction. There can be extensive calcification (Fig. 14–1), which can lead to parenchymal destruction and eventual "autonephrectomy." The mycobacterium can remain dormant within these calcifications for years. In one study, 28% of all large areas of calcification that were excised had viable *M. tuberculosis* in the calcified matrix (Wong and Lan, 1980).

Hypertension may rarely occur as a complication of severe unilateral TB and reduced renal blood flow, but it is unusual in a patient with a contralateral functional kidney. The role of the individual kidney in causing the hypertension can be predicted by the selective measurement of renal vein renin in a unilateral tuberculous kidney. This is critical because many patients with genitourinary TB have essential hypertension, which is unrelated to tuberculosis. These patients should have standard medical treatment for hypertension combined with antituberculous chemotherapy.

Ureter. Tuberculous ureteritis is always an extension of the disease from the kidney and leads to fibrosis and stricture formation. The site most commonly affected is the ureterovesical junction (UVJ). The disease rarely involves the ureteropelvic junction (UPJ) and is even less common in the middle third of the ureter. Very occasionally, the whole of the ureter is involved. In such patients, the kidney shows

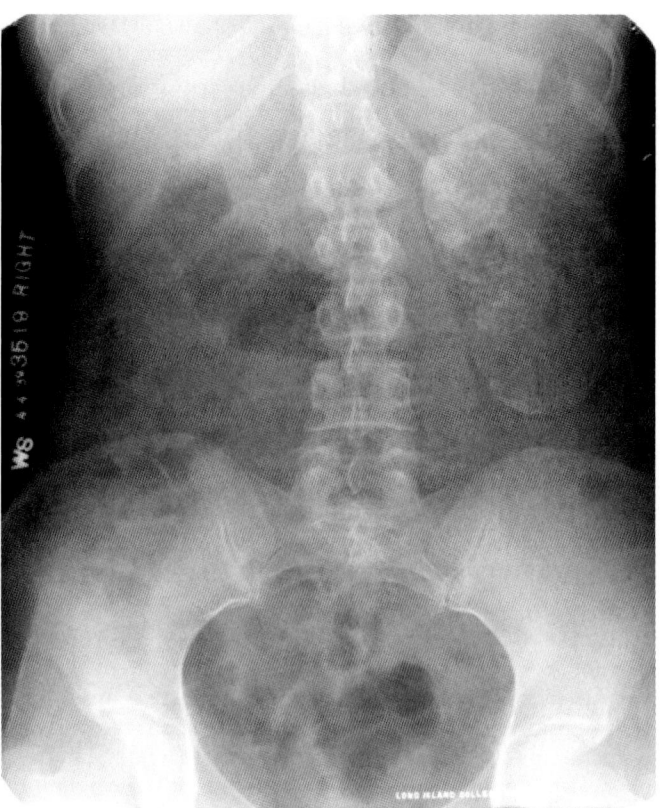

Figure 14–1. KUB radiographic view in a patient with left renal tuberculosis with associated calcifications.

extensive disease, is often nonfunctioning, and is calcified (Fig. 14–2A). UVJ strictures are typically less than 5 cm in length (Fig. 14–3), and the area of fibrosis is localized. Unless a large part of the ureter is involved, the stricture is confined to the intermural part of the ureter or an area just proximal to it.

Bladder. Bladder lesions are without exception secondary to renal TB. The earliest forms of infection start around one or another ureteral orifice, which becomes inflamed and edematous (see Fig. 14–2B). As the area of mild inflammation progresses, granulations appear and may completely obscure the ureteral orifice (see Fig. 14–2C). Tuberculous ulcers are rare but can appear in any part of the bladder (see Fig. 14–2D). Occasionally, the whole of the bladder is covered by inflamed, velvety granulations with ulceration (see Fig. 14–2H). If the disease continues to progress, bladder wall fibrosis and contraction can occur and the ureteral orifice may assume the classic golf-hole appearance (see Fig. 14–2E and F). With modern chemotherapy, this advanced disease is now a rare occurrence. Healed mucosal lesions have a stellate appearance (see Fig. 14–2G).

Tuberculosis of the Epididymis and Testis

Hematospermia is a rare presenting symptom of genital TB. However, Yu and coworkers (1977) reported an 11% incidence in 65 TB patients during a period of 10 years. All these patients had other clinical evidence of genitourinary TB. TB should be considered in patients who are seen with repeated attacks of hematospermia as the only presenting symptom, even if there is no other evidence of genitourinary TB.

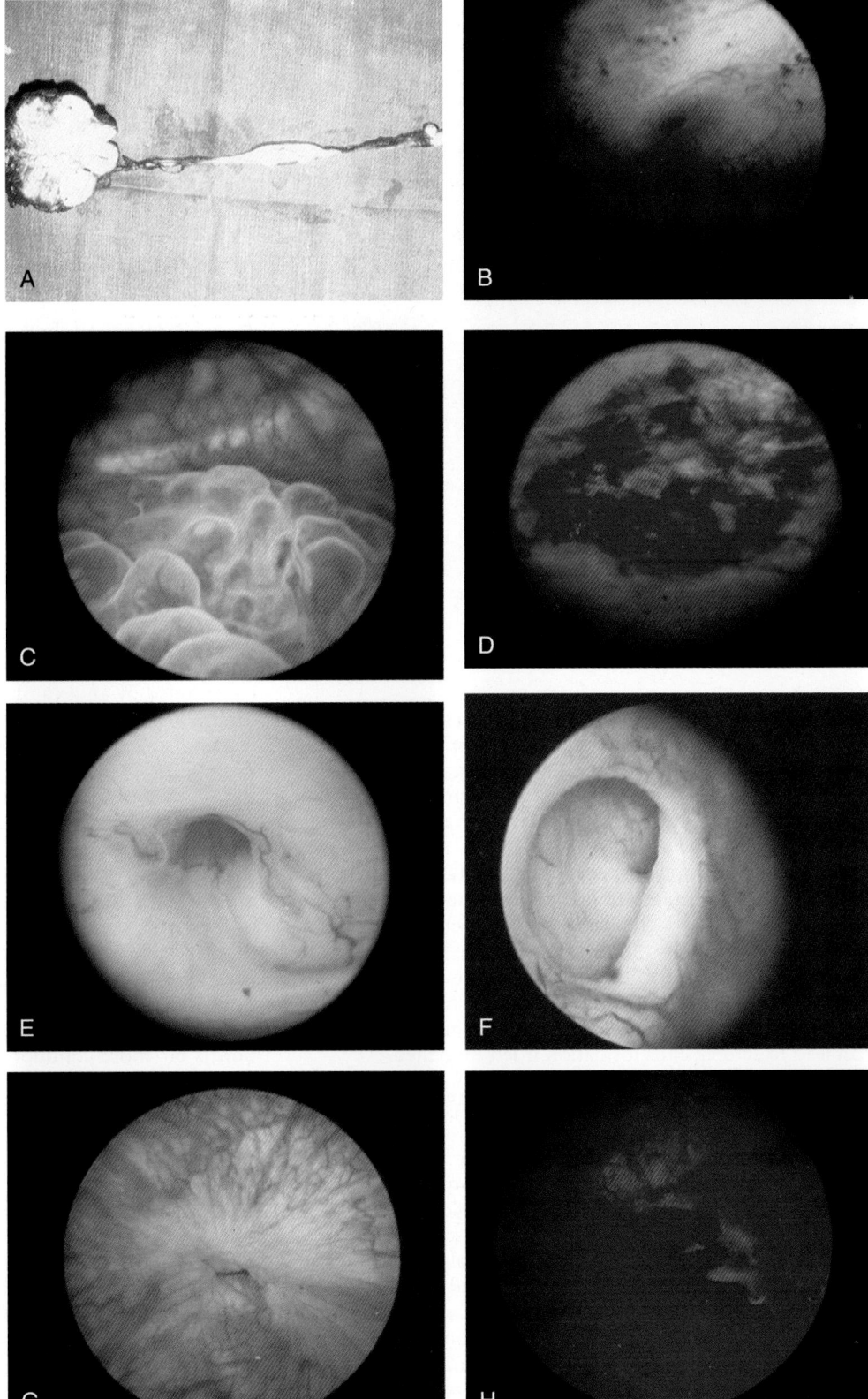

Figure 14–2. A, Extensive tuberculosis of the kidney and ureter with calcification and stricture formation. **B,** Acutely inflamed ureteric orifice. **C,** Tuberculous bullous granulations. **D,** Acute tuberculous ulcer. **E,** Tuberculous golf-hole ureter. **F,** Tuberculous golf-hole ureter, severely withdrawn. **G,** Healed tuberculous lesion. **H,** Acute tuberculous cystitis with ulceration.

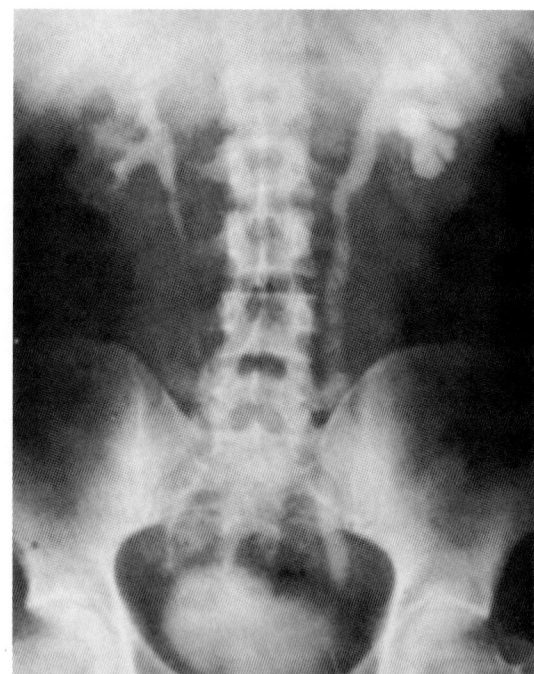

Figure 14–3. Stricture at the distal left ureter.

Tuberculous epididymitis may be the first and only presenting symptom of genitourinary TB. The usual presentation is a painful, inflamed scrotal swelling that is difficult to differentiate from acute epididymo-orchitis. The globus minor alone is affected in 40% of cases. The disease usually develops in young, sexually active males, and in 70% of patients there is a previous history of TB. **TB of the testis is almost always secondary to infection of the epididymis via direct extension** (Macmillan, 1954). Tuberculous orchitis with no epididymal involvement is very rare.

Tuberculous epididymitis can also present as infertility due to scarring of the epididymis or multiple vasal obstructions (Paick et al, 2000; Fraietta et al, 2003). Very rarely the disease can lead to scrotal sinus formation if left untreated.

Tuberculosis of the Prostate, Penis, and Urethra

TB of the prostate is uncommon, and in many cases the pathologist diagnoses it incidentally after a transurethral resection. Very rarely, in acute fulminating cases, the disease spreads rapidly, and cavitation may lead to a perineal sinus (Sporer and Auerback, 1978).

TB of the penis and of the urethra are also very unusual manifestations (Lal et al, 1971; Symes and Blandy, 1973). Many years ago, however, TB of the penis was not uncommonly seen as a complication of ritual circumcision, when it was the usual practice for the operators, many of who had open pulmonary TB, to suck the circumcised penis (Lewis, 1946).

Primary TB of the penis appears as a superficial ulcer of the glans. Clinically, it is indistinguishable from malignant disease, although it can also progress to cause a tubercular cavernositis with involvement of the urethra (Venkataramaiah et al, 1982). Rarely, the lesion occurs as a solid nodule (Baskin

and Mee, 1989) or as a cavernositis with ulceration (Ramesh and Vasanthi, 1989).

Finally, TB of the urethra is caused by spread from another focus in the genital tract. Its rarity is difficult to understand in view of the almost constant exposure of the urethra to infected urine. In the acute phase, there is a urethral discharge with involvement of the epididymis, prostate, and other parts of the renal tract. Urethral strictures can also develop, leading to a slowing of the urinary stream or retention.

Microbiology and Diagnosis

The *M. tuberculosis* complex is composed of *M. tuberculosis*, *M. bovis*, *M. microti*, and *M. africanum*. **M. tuberculosis is the cause of most human disease, and humans are the only reservoir for this organism.** In practical terms, genitourinary TB is synonymous with disease due to *M. tuberculosis*. *M. bovis* infection, acquired from the ingestion of contaminated cow's milk, has been virtually eradicated in the United States but remains a problem in some developing countries (Yaqoob et al, 1990).

Tuberculin Test

The tuberculin test is accomplished by intradermal injection of a PPD of tuberculin. An inflammatory reaction develops at the site and reaches a maximum between 48 and 72 hours after injection. This reaction consists of a central indurated zone surrounded by an area of erythema; it is assessed by measuring the diameter of the indurated area. A person's ability to respond to the local concentration of the injection may be decreased by malignancy, nutritional deficiencies, corticosteroid therapy, irradiation, and AIDS.

The CDC has recommended three cut points for defining a positive tuberculin reaction: induration of 5 mm to less than 10 mm, 10 mm to less than 15 mm, and 15 mm or greater (CDC, 2000). The individuals who correspond to each of these cut points are identified in Table 14–2.

A positive reaction is considered an indication that the person has been infected, but it cannot be regarded as an indication of active tuberculous disease or that the patient's symptoms are caused by TB. However, *M. tuberculosis* infection is far more common than nontuberculous disease in a patient with a positive tuberculin test. The CDC (2000) has detailed the indications and regimens for the treatment of latent TB.

Urine Examination

The urine is examined for red blood cells and leukocytes, and the pH and concentration are noted. The urine is also cultured for organisms such as *Escherichia coli*. Secondary bacterial infection is found in about 20% of cases; however, **"sterile pyuria" is the classic urinary finding on routine urinalysis and culture. Up to 50% of patients will also have microhematuria.**

Urine culture is traditionally used for diagnosis because acid-fast bacilli (AFB) smears are often negative. Cultures, however, take 6 to 8 weeks because *M. tuberculosis* is slow growing, with a doubling time of 15 to 20 hours. Furthermore, the organism is intermittently excreted; therefore, at least three, but preferably five, consecutive early morning specimens of urine should be cultured. Each specimen

Table 14–2. **Criteria for Tuberculin Positivity, by Risk Group**

Reaction ≥ 5 mm of Induration

HIV-positive persons
Recent contacts of tuberculosis (TB) case patients
Fibrotic changes on chest radiograph consistent with prior TB
Patients with organ transplants and other immunosuppressed patients (receiving the equivalent of ≥ 15 mg/day of prednisone for 1 mo or more)*

Reaction ≥10 mm of Induration

Recent immigrants (i.e., within the last 5 yr) from high-prevalence countries
Injection drug abusers
Residents and employees† of the following high-risk congregate settings: prisons and jails, nursing homes and other long-term facilities for the elderly, hospitals and other health care facilities, residential facilities for patients with AIDS, and homeless shelters
Mycobacterial laboratory personnel
Persons with the following clinical conditions that place them at high risk: silicosis, diabetes mellitus, chronic renal failure, some hematologic disorders (e.g., leukemias and lymphomas), other specific malignancies (e.g., carcinoma of the head or neck and lung), weight loss of ≥ 10% of ideal body weight, gastrectomy, and jejunoileal bypass
Children younger than 4 yr or infants, children, and adolescents exposed to adults at high risk

Reaction ≥15 mm of Induration

Persons with no risk factors for TB

*Risk of TB in patients treated with corticosteroids increases with higher doses and longer duration.
†For persons who are otherwise at low risk and are tested at the start of employment, a reaction of ≥ 15 mm induration is considered positive.
From Centers for Disease Control and Prevention: Targeted tuberculin testing and treatment of latent tuberculosis infection. MMWR Morb Mortal Wkly Rep 2000;49:24.

should be inoculated on Löwenstein-Jensen culture medium to isolate *M. tuberculosis,* bacille Calmette-Guérin (BCG), and the occasional nontuberculous mycobacteria. It is particularly important to collect all specimens into sterile containers, because unsterilized containers may be contaminated with environmental bacteria. Mycobacterial drug sensitivity testing should be performed on all isolates. The sensitivity of urine culture is as high as 80% to 90%. Cultures from the female genital tract or male seminal fluid on the other hand are usually negative and are therefore unreliable.

Each specimen of urine should be inoculated as soon as possible after collection, because the longer the urine remains in contact with organisms, the less likely it is that the mycobacterium will grow. Newer diagnostic methods are available that utilize fluorescence microscopy. An additional technique is the radiometric culture method, based on the release of radioactive carbon dioxide, which is detected by a special instrument. It is also used for drug susceptibility testing (Salfinger and Pfyffer, 1994).

M. tuberculosis can be distinguished from nontuberculous mycobacteria between the second and the fifth days after the culture is started. Culture confirmation tests using DNA probes are now widely available for different mycobacteria and allow species specification within a few hours. This can help to distinguish *M. tuberculosis* from nontuberculous mycobacteria, which are usually not pathologic but result from

skin contamination or urethral colonization (Goldfarb and Salman, 2004).

Molecular methods, including nucleic acid hybridization and polymerase chain reaction (PCR) of either DNA or rRNA, have been developed to more rapidly identify TB. Typically, sensitivity for these techniques falls in between that of urine culture and urine AFB staining. Moussa and colleagues (2000), however, found that when analyzing pooled urine samples for an *M. tuberculosis* species–specific DNA insertion sequence, the sensitivity and specificity were 96% and 98%, respectively. Pooled urine samples are recommended because urinary excretion of the organism is intermittent and may be missed with a single specimen. Although these molecular methods may ultimately supplant traditional techniques for mycobacterial isolation and identification, they are only complementary at present.

Radiography

There are a number of reviews covering the different procedures for the diagnostic imaging of genitourinary TB (Chung et al, 1997; Wang et al, 1997; Valentini et al, 1998; Engin et al, 2000).

Plain Radiographs

Plain radiographs of the urinary tract are important because they show calcification in the kidneys and in the lower genitourinary tract (see Fig. 14–1). Tuberculous ureteral calcification is very uncommon unless there is extensive renal calcification, but it must be distinguished from that seen in schistosomiasis. In the former, all calcification is intraluminal and appears as a cast of the ureter, which is thickened and not dilated (Hartman et al, 1977). In schistosomiasis, the calcification is mural and the ureter is generally dilated and tortuous. Calcification rarely occurs in the bladder wall and seminal vesicles except in advanced disease. A calcified psoas abscess can simulate renal calcification, and an intravenous urogram or preferably a computed tomography (CT) scan should be obtained to confirm the diagnosis. Plain radiographs of the chest and spine are also obtained to exclude any evidence of old or active pulmonary or spinal disease.

Intravenous Urography

High-dose intravenous urography (IVU) has traditionally been the gold standard tool to diagnose and evaluate genitourinary TB. It is still used in common practice but in many institutions has been replaced by CT. The IVU provides functional information relating to ureteral peristalsis, which gives an indication of the extent of the disease, the amount of fibrosis that is present, and the length of a stricture, particularly at the UVJ.

Renal lesions can also be visualized on IVU. They may appear as a distortion of a calyx, as a calyx that is fibrosed and completely occluded (lost calyx from infundibular stenosis) (Fig. 14–4) (Sherwood, 1980), as multiple small calyceal deformities, or as severe calyceal and parenchymal destruction (Fig. 14–5). Other manifestations of genitourinary TB that can be visualized on IVU include ureteral dilatation above a UVJ stricture or a rigid fibrotic ureter with multiple strictures. The cystographic phase of the IVU can give valuable information about the condition of the bladder, which may be small and

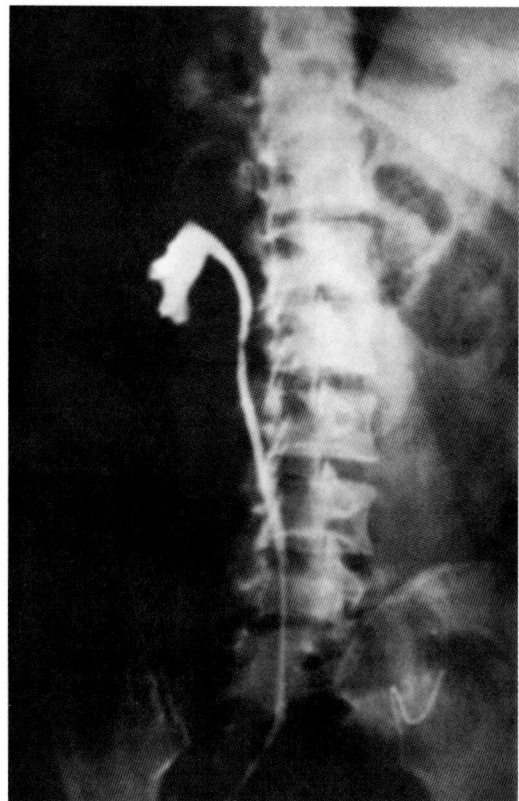

Figure 14–4. Occluded calyx.

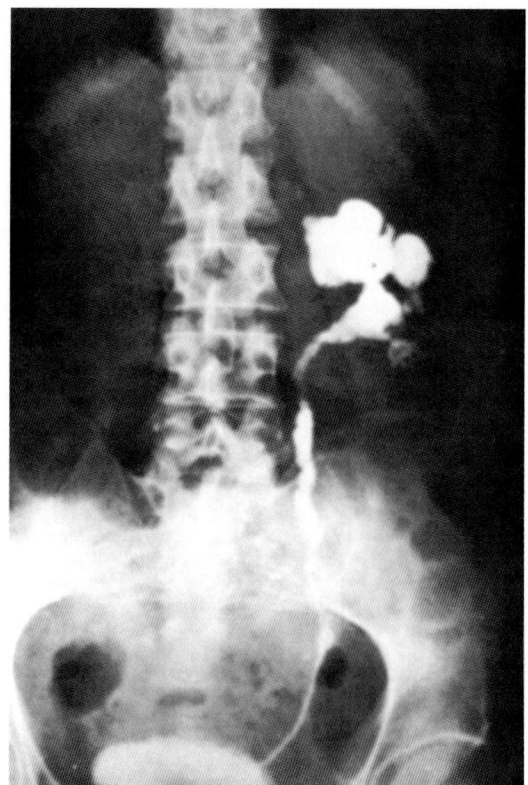

Figure 14–5. Severe calyceal and parenchymal destruction.

contracted (thimble bladder) (Fig. 14–6) or irregular, with filling defects and bladder asymmetry.

Computed Tomography

CT has become more widely available and has arguably replaced IVU as the imaging modality of choice for the diagnosis and evaluation of genitourinary TB. The latest CT software allows for the creation of three-dimensional reconstructed images, adding another dimension to the images that a CT scan can produce. It is at least the equal of IVU in identifying calyceal abnormalities, hydronephrosis or hydroureter, autonephrectomy, amputated infundibulum, urinary tract calcifications, and renal parenchymal cavities (Wang et al, 2003) (Fig. 14–7). In a retrospective study of 53 patients with the diagnosis of genitourinary TB, the most common findings on CT were parenchymal scarring (79%), hydrocalycosis, hydronephrosis or hydroureter (67%), and thickening of the walls of the renal pelvis, ureters, or bladder (61%) (Wang et al, 2003). **These findings are not specific and therefore, as with IVU, one must look for multiple abnormalities and consider them in conjunction with the patient's history and presentation.**

Unlike IVU, however, CT can identify extrapulmonary manifestations of TB in addition to other genitourinary findings such as adrenal, prostatic, or seminal vesicle necrosis or caseation (Premkumar and Newhouse, 1988; Harisinghani et al, 2000).

Ultrasonography

Ultrasonography is of limited value. It can, however, be used to monitor the size of kidney lesions during chemotherapy or

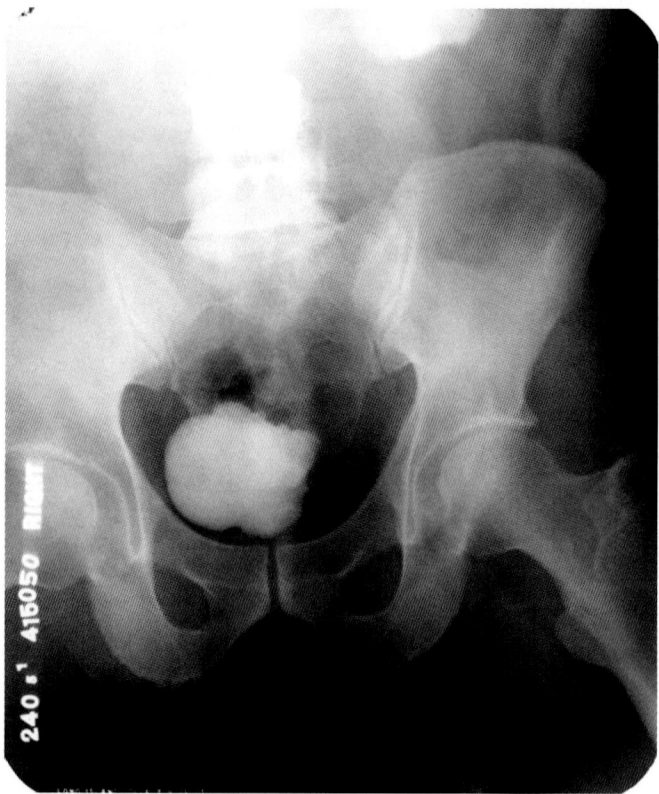

Figure 14–6. The cystogram portion of an intravenous pyelogram in a patient with left renal tuberculosis. Note the contracted left side of the bladder that is secondary to fibrosis from the tuberculosis.

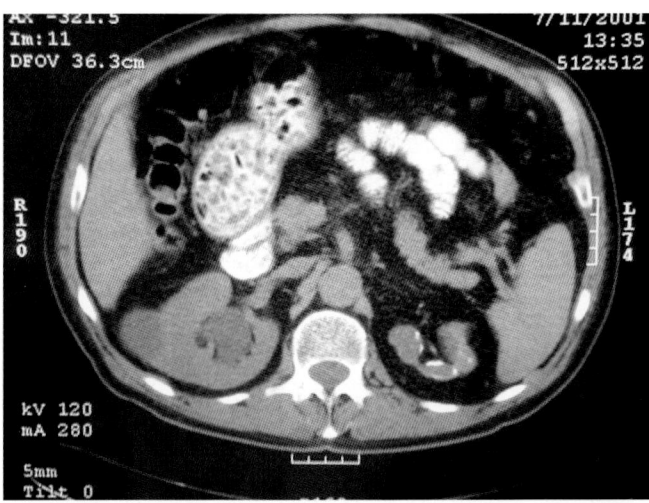

Figure 14–7. CT after oral contrast medium in a patient with bilateral tuberculosis. The right kidney is hydronephrotic secondary to infundibular stenosis but has retained good function. The left kidney is an end-stage nonfunctioning atrophic kidney with calcification.

to monitor the volume of a contracted bladder during treatment. This is of value to assess the need for future intervention.

Cystoscopy and Biopsy

Cystoscopy is rarely indicated in the diagnosis of genitourinary TB. It has some place, however, in assessing the extent of the disease or the response to chemotherapy. Occasionally, the appearance of the bladder suggests extensive TB, but *M. tuberculosis* cannot be cultured from the urine and the upper urinary tract appears normal. In this situation, the most likely diagnosis is an acute interstitial cystitis.

Cystoscopy must always be performed with the patient under general anesthesia with a muscle relaxant to reduce the risk of hemorrhage. The phase of bladder filling should be performed under direct vision. Biopsy is usually only necessary to rule out malignancy and is not advised before the initiation of medical therapy.

Retrograde Pyelography

Retrograde pyelography is now rarely necessary, but there are two indications for its use. The first is a stricture at the lower end of the ureter, when it is necessary to try to delineate its length and the amount of obstruction and dilatation above the stricture. The examination is performed under direct vision and a bulb-tipped catheter used to introduce contrast agent into the ureteral orifice. A stent can also be placed in this setting if a stricture is causing significant obstruction.

The second indication for retrograde pyelography is ureteral catheterization, which may be required to obtain urine samples for culture from each kidney if it is not certain from which side the organisms are coming. In such cases, a No. 5 French catheter is passed into the renal pelvis. To increase the output of urine a diuretic may be infused intravenously during the examination.

Percutaneous Antegrade Pyelography

Percutaneous antegrade pyelography is an alternative to retrograde pyelography for visualizing a nonfunctioning kidney

or for determining the condition of a renal unit when access cannot be obtained in a retrograde manner. It can also be used to aspirate the contents of the renal pelvis so that they can be sent for diagnostic examination or to aspirate the contents of tuberculous cavities to estimate the quantity of drugs that has penetrated the walls. Finally, percutaneous access allows for percutaneous nephrostomy tube placement for maximal drainage of a kidney if access cannot be achieved or is insufficient, in a retrograde manner.

Arteriography, Radioisotope Investigation, and Magnetic Resonance Imaging

Arteriography, radioisotope investigation, and magnetic resonance imaging are rarely indicated. They have very little application in the management of genitourinary TB because they do not provide additional information over the other imaging modalities.

Antituberculous Drugs

Isoniazid

Isoniazid (INH) was introduced in 1952. It is highly active against *M. tuberculosis* and is bactericidal at higher concentrations. It inhibits the synthesis of mycolic acids in *M. tuberculosis* by affecting the enzyme mycolase synthetase, which is unique to mycobacteria. Seventy percent of all administered INH is excreted by the kidneys, most in an inactive form (Mitchell et al, 1976). It is widely distributed in the body, and tissue levels are similar to serum levels. Dose modification in renal failure is usually not necessary but is recommended in hepatic failure, especially in persons who are slow hepatic acetylators.

INH is associated with hepatic "toxicity" in 10% to 20% of patients, usually in the form of asymptomatic elevations in transaminase levels. This occurs after 6 to 8 weeks of therapy and may normalize with continued INH treatment. Patients are advised to discontinue INH therapy if they develop symptoms suggestive of hepatitis (fatigue, nausea, anorexia), because severe hepatic necrosis has been reported (Kopanoff et al, 1978). Peripheral neuropathy in patients taking higher-than-standard INH doses is due to enhanced pyridoxine excretion and is prevented by daily supplemental oral pyridoxine (vitamin B_6) therapy.

Rifampicin

Rifampicin is one of a group of antibiotics that is isolated from *Streptomyces mediterranei*. Rifampicin acts to inhibit bacterial RNA synthesis by interfering with DNA-directed RNA polymerase of sensitive bacteria (Hartmann et al, 1967). The drug is lipid soluble, enters macrophages, and is excreted in the urine (Kunin et al, 1969).

Hepatotoxicity is the major adverse reaction to rifampicin (Wallace, 2000). Liver failure requires a moderate reduction in dosage, but full doses can be given with renal insufficiency. There are significant drug interactions between rifampicin and more than 100 drugs, including oral contraceptives, corticosteroids, and a number of antiretroviral drugs (Strayhorn et al, 1997). Drug-drug interactions occur primarily between rifampicin and other drugs that are metabolized by the hepatic cytochrome P450 system.

Streptomycin

Streptomycin was isolated from *Streptomyces griseus* in 1944. It belongs to a group of antibiotics known as the aminoglycosides and must be given intramuscularly. It interferes with bacterial protein synthesis by its ability to bind to a particular protein or proteins of the 30S unit of bacterial ribosomes so that faulty proteins are produced (Luzzatto et al, 1968). It penetrates the walls of tuberculous abscesses in lethal concentrations even in caseous material. Streptomycin is not active against intracellular mycobacteria. High concentrations are obtained in the urine. Isolates resistant to streptomycin are not resistant to other aminoglycosides. **Streptomycin is ototoxic, but this is reversible if the drug is discontinued immediately after the appearance of symptoms.**

Pyrazinamide

Pyrazinamide, a derivative of nicotinamide, was synthesized in 1952. The mechanism of action appears to be through the inhibition of fatty acid synthetase I of *M. tuberculosis* (Zimhony et al, 2000). After doses higher than currently recommended, hepatotoxicity was reported in up to 15% of patients (McLeod et al, 1959). Nausea and vomiting are common.

Ethambutol

Ethambutol was discovered in 1961. It is active against *M. tuberculosis* strains resistant to INH and other commonly used antituberculous drugs. It is well absorbed after oral administration. About 80% is excreted in the urine as active unchanged drug; dosage should be adjusted in renal failure. It enters cells and inhibits mycobacterial cell wall synthesis. Ethambutol rarely causes retrobulbar neuritis and should be discontinued if ocular changes occur. Changes in visual acuity and red-green color perception are early findings, and these parameters should be tested at baseline and every 4 to 6 weeks.

Medical Treatment

It is very sobering to reflect that before the advent of chemotherapy 50% of persons with active pulmonary TB died within 2 years and that TB accounted for approximately 25% of all adult deaths in Europe during the early Industrial Revolution (Styblo, 1980). Today, despite the confounding variables of deteriorating health care systems in areas of civil unrest, drug resistance, and AIDS, the mortality should be negligible if treatment is prompt and appropriate and if medications are taken as prescribed.

The cornerstone of antituberculous therapy is multidrug treatment to decrease the duration of therapy and diminish the likelihood that drug-resistant organisms will develop. Directly observed therapy is indicated for many patients. Therapy has become increasingly complex, with Treatment Guidelines from *The Medical Letter* 2004 listing 18 first- and second-line drugs (Table 14–3). It is therefore prudent that even "experts" consult the most reliable and current sources for up-to-date information on dosage, toxicity, drug interactions, and use in special situations (e.g., pregnancy, renal failure, lactation) (Bartlett, 2000; Gilbert et al, 2000; Wallace, 2000; The Medical Letter, 2004).

The current recommendation of the CDC and American Thoracic Society is to treat compliant patients with drug-sensitive genitourinary TB for 6 to 9 months (Iseman, 2000). There is now, however, abundant evidence that the 6-month regimens are effective for most forms of TB, including genitourinary TB (Cek et al, 2005), with the exception of disseminated TB, TB osteomyelitis, and TB meningitis. **The common factor in these 6-month regimens is the initial use of rifampicin, INH, pyrazinamide, and ethambutol** (American Thoracic Society, 2003; The Medical Letter, 2004). Patients should be seen 3, 6, and 12 months after the course of chemotherapy has finished. At each visit, three consecutive early morning specimens of urine should be cultured.

All the drugs should be administered in one dose, and they may be taken together at night just before bedtime, with or without milk. This has been found to be the best way of achieving maximal patient tolerance (Israili et al, 1987). Corticosteroids may also be useful in cases of acute tuberculous disease to decrease inflammation and stricture formation (Horne and Tulloch, 1975); however, this is largely based on anecdotal experience and is not universally advocated (Gow, 1970).

The rate at which patients can be rendered noninfectious is dramatic. In patients with renal TB, it is almost impossible to isolate *M. tuberculosis* from the urine after 2 weeks of chemotherapy. There are several aspects of genitourinary TB that make it very responsive to short-course chemotherapy. First, fewer organisms are involved in the renal form of the disease than in the pulmonary form. Second, there are high concentrations of INH, rifampicin, pyrazinamide, and streptomycin in the urine. Third, INH and rifampicin pass freely into renal cavities in high concentration. Finally, all these drugs reach adequate concentrations in the kidney, ureters, bladder, and prostate.

Multidrug-resistant tuberculosis (MDR) TB emerged as a major public health problem in the past decade. Risk factors for MDR TB include prior treatment and residence in countries with known high MDR TB rates (e.g., India, Russia, Dominican Republic). Treatment regimens for MDR TB patients must be designed according to the organism's sensitivity and continued for 18 to 24 months or 12 to 18 months after cultures become negative (The Medical Letter, 2004).

Surgery

Surgical treatment has undergone many changes since the 1970s, but in general **it has become an adjuvant to medical therapy in the treatment of genitourinary TB. Previously it was believed that all diseased tissue must be excised. This is now debated, and the current focus is on organ preservation and reconstruction as opposed to excision** (Mochalova and Starikov, 1997). **Furthermore, when surgical intervention is mandated it should be delayed until medical therapy has been administered for at least 4 to 6 weeks.**

Excision of Diseased Tissue

Nephrectomy. Classically the indications for nephrectomy were (1) a nonfunctioning kidney with or without calcification; (2) extensive disease involving the whole kidney, together with hypertension and UPJ obstruction; and (3) coexisting renal carcinoma. Although the second and third indications remain, it is not mandated that nonfunctioning

Table 14–3. Antituberculosis Drugs

Drug/Formulation	Adult Dosage (Daily)	Main Adverse Effects
First-Line Drugs		
Isoniazid (INH)* 100, 300 mg tabs 50 mg/5 mL syrup 100 mg/mL injection	5 mg/kg (max 300 mg) PO, IM, IV	Hepatic toxicity, peripheral neuropathy
Rifampin (Rifadin, Rimactane) 150, 300 mg caps 600 mg injection powder	10 mg/kg (max 600 mg) PO, IV	Hepatic toxicity, flulike syndrome, pruritus
Rifabutin[†] (Mycobutin) 150 mg caps	5 mg/kg (max 300 mg) PO	Hepatic toxicity, flulike syndrome, uveitis, neutropenia
Pyrazinamide 500 mg tabs	20-25 mg/kg PO	Arthralgias, hepatic toxicity, hyperuricemia, gastrointestinal upset
Ethambutol[‡] (Myambutol) 100, 400 mg tabs	15-25 mg/kg PO	Decreased red-green color discrimination, decreased visual acuity
Second-Line Drugs		
Streptomycin[§]	15 mg/kg IM (max 1 g)	Vestibular and auditory toxicity, renal damage
Capreomycin (Capastat)	15 mg/kg IM (max 1 g)	Auditory and vestibular toxicity, renal damage
Kanamycin (Kantrex and others)	15 mg/kg IM, IV (max 1 g)	Auditory toxicity, renal damage
Amikacin (Amikin)	15 mg/kg IM, IV (max 1 g)	Auditory toxicity, renal damage
Cycloserine[¶] (Seromycin and others)	10-15 mg/kg in two doses (max 500 mg bid) PO	Psychiatric symptoms, seizures
Ethionamide (Trecator-SC)	15-20 mg/kg in two doses (max 500 mg bid) PO	Gastrointestinal and hepatic toxicity, hypothyroidism
Ciprofloxacin (Cipro and others)	750-1500 mg PO, IV	Nausea, abdominal pain, restlessness, confusion
Ofloxacin (Floxin)	600-800 mg PO, IV	Nausea, abdominal pain, restlessness, confusion
Levofloxacin (Levaquin)	500-1000 mg PO, IV	Nausea, abdominal pain, restlessness, confusion
Gatifloxacin[¶] (Tequin)	400 mg PO, IV	Nausea, abdominal pain, restlessness, confusion
Moxifloxacin[¶¶] (Avelox)	400 mg PO, IV	Nausea, abdominal pain, restlessness, confusion
Aminosalicylic acid (PAS; Paser)	8-12 g in 2-3 doses PO	Gastrointestinal disturbance

*Pyridoxine, 10 to 25 mg, should be given to prevent neuropathy in malnourished or pregnant patients and those with HIV infection, alcoholism, or diabetes.

[†]For use with amprenavir, fosamprenavir, nelfinavir, or indinavir, the rifabutin dose is 150 mg/day or 300 mg two to three times a week. For use with atazanavir, ritonavir alone or combined with other protease inhibitors, and lopinavir/ritonavir, the rifabutin dose is further decreased to 150 mg every other day or three times weekly. For use with efavirenz, the rifabutin dose is increased to 450-600 mg/day or 600 mg two to three times weekly. No dose adjustment is needed for use with nevirapine.

[‡]Some clinicians use 25 mg/kg/day during the first one or two months or longer if organism is isoniazid resistant. Decrease dosage if renal function diminished.

[§]When oral drugs are given daily, streptomycin is generally given five times per week (15 mg/kg, or a maximum of 1 g per dose) for an initial 2- to 12-week period and then (if needed) two to three times per week (20 to 30 mg/kg, or a maximum of 1.5 g per dose). For patients >59 years old, dosage is reduced to 10 mg/kg/d (max 750 mg/d). Dosage should be decreased if renal function is diminished.

[¶]Some authorities recommend pyridoxine, 50 mg, for every 250 mg of cycloserine to decrease the incidence of adverse neurologic effects.

[¶¶]No published clinical data on dosage for tuberculosis.

From The Medical Letter: Drugs for Tuberculosis. Treatment Guidelines from The Medical Letter, 2004;28:83-88.

kidneys must be excised if the patients are otherwise asymptomatic (Bloom et al, 1970; Wechsler and Lattimer, 1975). This is in contrast to previous recommendations, such as that made by Kerr and coworkers (1969, 1970), which called for the removal of diseased or nonfunctional organs. The success of medical management has shifted this paradigm. However, if a patient is symptomatic with pain, sinus formation, hematuria, or hypertension, then nephrectomy may alleviate these symptoms. Skutil and Obsitnik (1987) have advocated nephrectomy for some patients with persistent tuberculous cystitis or those with secondary development of nephrolithiasis.

Nephrectomy, when indicated, is most commonly performed through an open approach given the difficult dissection due to inflammation and scarring. However, in experienced hands it can be performed laparoscopically (Hemal et al, 2000; Lee et al, 2002).

Partial Nephrectomy. Partial nephrectomy is now rarely performed because, with modern chemotherapy, the response of a local lesion in the kidney is rapid and effective. There are only two indications for such intervention: (1) the localized polar lesion containing calcification that has failed to respond after 6 weeks of intensive chemotherapy and (2) an area of calcification that is slowly increasing in size and is threatening to gradually destroy the whole kidney. Partial nephrectomy is difficult to justify in the absence of calcification.

Abscess Drainage. Open surgical drainage of an abscess is unnecessary in the current management of genitourinary TB, because, with modern radiographic techniques, the contents of an abscess can be aspirated in a minimally invasive manner. This is a satisfactory method of treatment and largely obviates surgery. It also allows the contents to be cultured for viable organisms.

Epididymectomy. The incidence of tuberculous epididymitis is declining, but exploration of the scrotum with a view to epididymectomy is still occasionally required. **The main indication is a caseating abscess that is not responding to**

chemotherapy. Another indication is a firm swelling that has remained unchanged or has slowly increased in size despite the use of antibiotics and antituberculous chemotherapy. One serious complication after epididymectomy is testicular atrophy, which occurs in 6% of patients. It is seen in severe disease where because of the inflammation surrounding the cord, dissecting the globus major from the vascular pedicle is extremely difficult. Involvement of the testis is uncommon; therefore, orchiectomy is required in only 5% of cases.

Epididymectomy should be performed through a scrotal incision. The globus minor is dissected first, followed by the body of the epididymis, and finally the globus major. The vas is then isolated and brought out in the groin through a separate stab incision to prevent the formation of a subcutaneous abscess.

Reconstructive Surgery

Ureteral Strictures. As previously noted, the most common site for tuberculous stricture is at the UVJ; stricture may also occur at the UPJ and, rarely, in the middle third of the ureter. Very occasionally, the disease may involve the entire ureter and cause complete stenosis, fibrosis, and even calcification.

In the acute phase of the illness the patient may benefit from placement of a double J stent or a percutaneous nephrostomy tube to allow for adequate drainage of the renal unit. Additionally for severe UPJ obstructions where a double J stent cannot be passed from below, a percutaneous nephrostomy tube can be placed and the pelvis irrigated with antituberculous drugs. Again this is rarely necessary because typically by the time the patient develops a UPJ obstruction the greater part of the kidney has already been destroyed.

Strictures of the lower end of the ureter, however, occur in approximately 9% of patients. A number of these strictures result from edema and respond to chemotherapy alone. Therefore, after the initiation of chemotherapy, the stricture should be monitored by IVU or CT. If there is deterioration or no improvement after 3 weeks, some have advocated adding corticosteroids. If there is deterioration or no improvement after a 6-week period, then surgical reimplantation or dilatation may be necessary.

The specific method of surgical repair for ureteral strictures is dependent on the location of the stricture and the degree of stenosis. Endoscopic dilatation and endopyelotomy, for example, have been utilized in select instances. They are less invasive but are only appropriate for relatively short strictures and may have lower success rates compared with open techniques. Open surgical management is dependent on the location of the structure.

When surgery is indicated for a UVJ stricture, **the entire stricture should be excised and the healthy ureter reimplanted into the bladder. Unless the stricture has been present for a considerable period, the muscle improves after the obstruction has been relieved and normal peristalsis recommences.** A reflux-preventing technique should be employed whenever possible, and, for success to be guaranteed, a submucosal tunnel of at least 2 cm is necessary. When choosing the location for the neocystotomy, one must be careful to avoid any diseased areas of the bladder; however, because the tuberculous infection is almost always localized to the area around the infected ureteral orifice, this is usually not difficult.

If the stricture is longer than 5 cm, a direct reimplantation often cannot be achieved. In these cases, either a psoas hitch (Turner-Warwick, 1965) or a Boari flap procedure (Gow, 1968) may be necessary. However, in patients with concomitant tuberculous cystitis this may be difficult secondary to a small, noncontractile bladder.

UPJ and midureteral strictures are rare and can be managed, when necessary, as one would manage other benign strictures at the same location. It is important, however, to note that **stricture recurrence is a common complication and therefore all patients should be followed carefully with periodic imaging.**

Augmentation Cystoplasty. The urinary bladder, besides being a contractile organ for expelling urine, is also a reservoir. In determining the appropriate treatment, both of these aspects must be considered. The main symptoms that warrant consideration of an augmentation cystoplasty are intolerable frequency of micturition, both day and night, together with pain, urgency, and hematuria. With severe disease **the bladder can lose elasticity and compliance, leaving a capacity of less than 100 mL.** The goal of augmentation is to increase the bladder capacity while retaining as much of the bladder as possible. Inflammation of the bladder is not a contraindication to surgery, but a two-layer closure and the routine use of omentum wrapped around the anastomosis reduces complications.

Like augmentation cystoplasties for other disease entities, ileum, stomach, or colon can be utilized depending on the individual patient and surgeon preference. **Furthermore, renal failure is not a contraindication to surgery.** Kuss and coworkers (1970) believe that **patients with a creatinine clearance of more than 15 mL/min should be accepted for augmentation cystoplasty.** Renal function can also improve in some patients after this procedure (Ramanathan et al, 1998).

Lower urinary tract infection is seen as a postoperative complication of urinary diversion or bladder augmentation. It is often symptomless and difficult to eradicate, so low-dose antibiotics taken continuously for 6 months or longer may be required.

Urinary Conduit Diversion. Urinary diversion, as opposed to augmentation, may be necessary in a select group of patients. There are three indications for permanent urinary diversion: (1) a history of psychiatric disturbance or obvious subnormal intelligence, (2) enuresis not related to small bladder capacity, and (3) intolerable diurnal symptoms with incontinence that has not responded to chemotherapy or bladder dilatation. Ileal or colonic segments are both satisfactory conduits.

Occasionally, patients desire takedown of their urinary diversion. Normal anatomy can frequently be restored, but a careful study of the dysfunctional bladder is necessary to ensure that the disease is quiescent, that there is no bladder outlet obstruction, and that there is adequate detrusor activity and bladder compliance. For this purpose, a full urodynamic study is necessary.

Orthotopic Neobladder. Finally, as orthotopic neobladders are being used with increased frequency for urinary reconstruction after cystectomy for malignant disease, it is also being applied to patients with TB. Hemal and Aron (1999) presented their early data in four patients who have undergone orthotopic neobladder construction for end-stage tuberculosis of the bladder. Their data are encouraging but will require longer follow-up and additional investigation to see if there is any advantage over augmentation.

Vasal or Epididymal Obstruction

Patients with infertility secondary to genital tuberculous disease causing vasal or epididymal obstruction often require in-vitro fertilization to achieve pregnancy. Surgical intervention has been generally unsuccessful (Paick et al, 2000).

Vaccine Prospects

A major international research effort is underway to develop safe and effective new TB vaccines. This research has been facilitated by the sequencing of the complete genome of *M. tuberculosis*. Candidate vaccines, including DNA and recombinant vaccines and attenuated mycobacteria, should soon be available for clinical trials (CDC, 1998a, 1999; Doherty and Andersen, 2000). In the meanwhile, **BCG is still used in many developing countries.**

It was in 1925 that Calmette and Guérin (1925) developed a method of attenuating the virulence of *M. bovis* by repeated subculture, eventually obtaining a permanently avirulent strain they called bacille Calmette-Guérin. The degree of protection is variable, from 80% among urban schoolchildren in the United Kingdom and North American Indians to nil among schoolchildren in Georgia (United States) and in the southern Indian general population (Ten Dam et al, 1976). The reason for this variation is unknown. It has been suggested that BCG acts not by preventing infection but by limiting the multiplication and spread of *M. tuberculosis*. Despite the variation of the response, the procedure is relatively safe and inexpensive.

However, **the use of BCG remains controversial.** In the first place, protection appears to last for only about 15 years. Second, a proportion of subjects in any age group will have been previously infected, and BCG cannot affect these individuals. Third, there is a chance of complications, including lymphadenitis, lupus vulgaris, and "BCG-itis." Fourth, the vaccine does not decrease the incidence of infection. Because of these inconsistencies, most developed countries have stopped mass BCG vaccination and have taken the view that the complications outweigh any possible benefits. In developing countries, the vaccine is given as soon as possible after birth (Ten Dam and Hitze, 1980). Furthermore, if the subsequent level of tuberculin positivity is low, many workers recommend revaccination a few years later. However, there is worldwide variation, and each region should perform studies to identify the optimal time for vaccination.

Intravesical BCG Therapy

Morales and associates (1976) **first introduced intravesical BCG for the treatment of superficial bladder cancer in 1976.** It is generally well tolerated and provides excellent long-term results, making it the most commonly used intravesical therapy. **The precise mechanism of action has not been clearly delineated, but the attenuated bacillus, from the *M. bovis* strain, is thought to induce a cellular immune reaction, which is effective in reducing the recurrence rate of carcinoma in situ and superficial urothelial carcinoma.** Both Alexandroff and colleagues (1999) and Bevers and coworkers (2004) include concise descriptions of the immune response in their reviews of BCG immunotherapy.

There is no uniformly accepted regiment for administering BCG. Typically, patients are given one vial intravesically on a weekly basis for 6 weeks. Many maintenance regimens have been established to help delay cancer recurrence; however, with increased frequency of administration side effects are more common. **To avoid systemic absorption and therefore reduce the risk of major adverse reactions, one should wait 1 to 3 weeks after transurethral resection before starting BCG treatment. Similarly, patients with immunosuppression, traumatic catheterizations, or hematuria should not be given BCG.**

BCG is generally well tolerated, but **60% to 80% of patients will experience cystitis and 5% will develop serious infection** (O'Donnell, 2005). Common minor reactions to BCG include dysuria, frequency, hematuria, and low-grade fevers (<38.3°C [101°F]). These symptoms typically occur after the third treatment and can usually be managed with supportive medications such as acetaminophen, phenazopyridine, oxybutynin, or diphenhydramine (Lamm, 1992). The next intravesical treatment, however, should be delayed until after these symptoms abate. Granulomatous prostatitis is also seen but is usually asymptomatic. It can, however, cause an elevation in the prostate-specific antigen level.

Major reactions to BCG include systemic infection and even sepsis. These infections are uncommon but need to be recognized and treated expeditiously. Gonzalez and coworkers (2003) characterized these reactions as either early or late complications of intravesical BCG. Early presentation, usually developing weeks after administration, is characterized by high fever (39.4°C [103°F]), generalized symptoms such as sweats and malaise, or systemic infection (most commonly pneumonitis and hepatitis). Symptoms in these patients are due to systemic infection in an immunocompetent host who is sensitized by the ongoing therapy. Late presentation on the other hand represents reactivation of the BCG infection. It is characterized by more organ-specific, localized disease involving one or multiple areas of the body (e.g., genitourinary tract, vascular tree, vertebrae). In either instance **antituberculous therapy is indicated and intravesical BCG should no longer be administered.**

BCG sepsis is the most serious complication of intravesical administration, and, although rare, it can be fatal. It is characterized by high fevers, rigors, and hypotension. It can mimic gram-negative sepsis with patients developing mental status changes, disseminated intravascular coagulation, and respiratory failure (Lamm, 1992). Treatment is **antituberculous chemotherapy.** Depending on the severity of the disease, treatments range from INH alone for 3 months to triple therapy for 6 months. In these instances, it is important to involve an infectious disease specialist for specific treatment regiments. Even though these complications are not common, the urologist must know how to recognize them so that treatment is not delayed.

PARASITIC DISEASES OF THE GENITOURINARY SYSTEM

Parasitic diseases are a major health problem today, especially in developing countries, but the human urogenital tract is regularly affected by only a few species of parasites (Richens, 2004). Two are discussed in detail: *Schistosoma haematobium,* a digenetic blood fluke that causes severe urinary tract disease, and filarial roundworms of the genera *Wuchereria, Brugia,* and *Onchocerca,* which can give rise to funiculoepididymitis, hydrocele, genital elephantiasis, and chyluria. Genitourinary involvement due to other parasites (except sexually transmitted protozoa) is either subordinate to systemic manifestations or rare.

Millions of people harbor parasites, but symptomatic infections are substantially less common. Therefore, parasitic infection must be clearly differentiated from parasitic disease, which constitutes a small fraction of total prevalence, depending on the intensity of infection and other factors.

Modern human mobility and jet travel bring "tropical diseases" into the offices of physicians far from endemic areas. The most important requirement for recognition of parasitic infections is awareness, based on knowledge of common clinical presentations, pathogenesis, and geographic distribution of parasitic diseases. Therefore, evaluation must include careful history taking, including the question, "Where have you been?" Finally, current knowledge of the prevalence and the best available drugs for different parasites can be obtained from the Division of Parasitic Diseases, Center for Infectious Diseases, Centers for Disease Control and Prevention, Atlanta, GA 30333.

Urinary Schistosomiasis

History

Schistosomiasis is a chronic disease caused by schistosomes, a genus of digenetic parasitic trematodes. The paired adult male and female worms cohabit the venous plexuses of the abdominal viscera. *S. mansoni* and *S. japonicum* reside in the mesenteric veins, leading to gastrointestinal or hepatic disease, whereas **S. haematobium worm pairs dwell principally in the perivesical venous plexus and cause urinary schistosomiasis.** Schistosomiasis caused by *S. haematobium* is discussed in this chapter.

Urinary schistosomiasis has been a scourge of the Middle East and Africa for millennia and is still a major cause of disease and death in these areas. Egyptian physicians of the XIIth dynasty (1900 BC) recognized hematuria as the cardinal sign and symptom of the disease. Theodore Bilharz, a German pathologist working in Cairo in the late 1800s, first described worm pairs in mesenteric veins at autopsy and linked these to eggs found in human excreta.

Biology and Life Cycle

The life cycle of *S. haematobium* is outlined in Figure 14–8. Briefly, the adult *S. haematobium* worms, which measure 1.5 cm in length, reside in vesical and pelvic venules and lay eggs within the venules of the human host. Male and female worms pair and attach to the blood vessel endothelia, remaining in intimate contact with the blood and producing and depositing 200 to 500 eggs per day. During its estimated mean life span of 3 to 6 years (Butterworth et al, 1988), a single worm pair spawns 250,000 to 600,000 eggs; moreover,

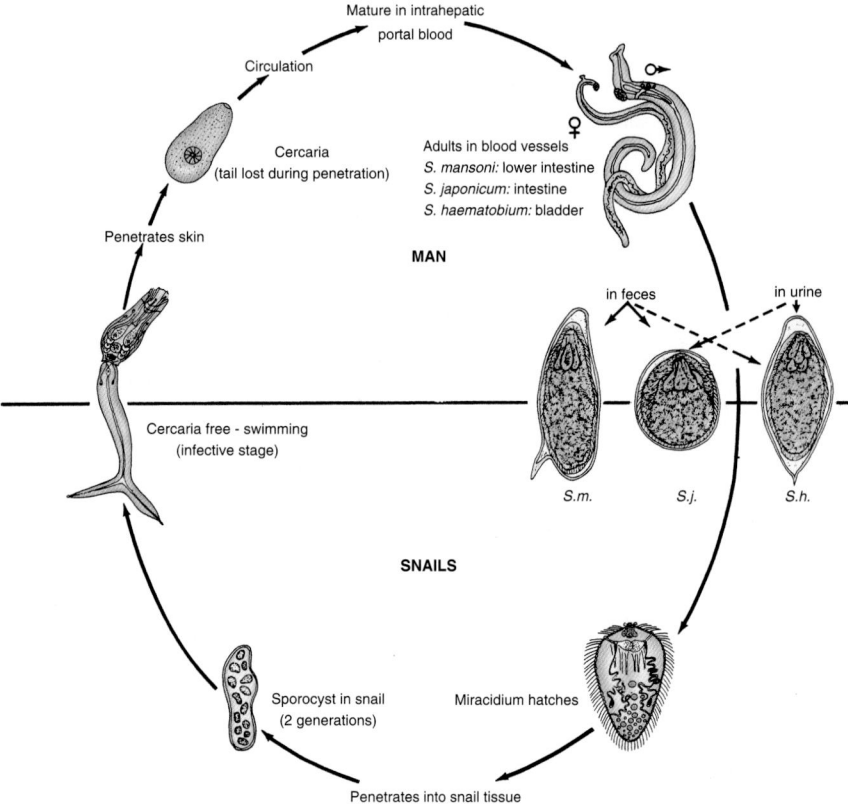

Figure 14–8. Life cycle of a schistosome. (From U.S. Department of Health and Human Services, Public Health Service Publications. Washington, DC, U.S. Government Printing Office, 1964.)

occasional worm pairs may persist as long as 30 years (De Gentile et al, 1988).

According to experimental data, **20% of the eggs cross into the lumina of the hollow viscera in which they are laid and are excreted in the urine** or feces whereas some of the eggs are swept into the bloodstream to microembolize to the microvasculature of lungs, liver, and other sites (Cheever and Anderson, 1971). A portion of the eggs trapped in tissues is destroyed by the host's granulomatous response. Finally, the remaining entrapped eggs become calcified and accumulate in the viscera at the rate of 90 to 100 eggs per worm pair per day (Cheever et al, 1977).

S. haematobium eggs measure 80 to 150 μm, are ovoid, and are terminally spined, which differentiates them from laterally spined *S. mansoni* eggs. The only other schistosome that is pathogenic for humans and has terminally spined eggs, *S. intercalatum*, is rarely seen outside limited foci in the Republic of Zaire, Gabon, and Cameroon (WHO, 1993); thus, terminally spined eggs in the urine, feces, or human tissue are always diagnostic of *S. haematobium* infection.

Egg maturation begins in utero from a single oocyte, and it continues for several days until the miracidium forms. Mature miracidia remain viable within eggs for less than 3 weeks. If not extruded into water within that period, they die and the eggs degenerate. **In active infection, all egg stages are seen, whereas in cured or inactive infection only degenerated (dark) or calcific eggs appear in the tissues or excreta.**

On deposition into fresh water (not salt), the miracidia emerge as short-lived, ciliated larvae that swim and seek hosts. Guided by phototropism and by snail trace minerals, **they find and enter snails** of *Bulinus* species (Ross et al, 2002), migrate through their tissues, and transform into successive generations of sporocysts. Each miracidium develops into a sporocyst, which produces 20 to 40 daughter sporocysts, each of which, in turn, produces 200 to 400 cercariae. The cercariae escape the daughter sporocyst, migrate to the snail's surface, and emerge into surrounding fresh water. This enormous asexual multiplication from a single miracidium to 10^5 cercariae compensates for the attrition during aquatic parts of the life cycle. The cercariae move through water by vibratory movements to find the human host. They then penetrate unbroken skin; if they fail to penetrate skin within a few hours, they die.

At penetration, the cercarial body becomes a schistosomulum. After a short rest in the dermis, the schistosomulum begins its migratory, growth, pairing, and maturation processes, which in *S. haematobium* may require 80 to 110 days. Schistosomula initially congregate in the lung and in the liver as growth of the worms accelerates. Finally, adults pair off and move to the pelvis (in the case of *S. haematobium*) where egg laying begins and is maintained until the death of the worm.

The immune response to the different stages of *S. haematobium* is very complex. **Some acquired resistance has been demonstrated in humans** (Chan et al, 1996). This resistance may depend on the age of the host or perhaps the duration and intensity of infection. Significant cellular and humoral host responses develop (Phillips and Colley, 1978; Butterworth, 1993; Mwatha et al, 1998; De Jesus et al, 2002: Pearce and MacDonald, 2002; Leutscher et al, 2005) as schistosomula become adults. These responses partially abrogate (but do not

eliminate) subsequent reinfection in experimental animals (Cheever et al, 1988a, 1988b) and human adults (but not children) (Hagan et al, 1985, 1987; Woolhouse et al, 1991), via eosinophil-mediated killing (Hagan et al, 1991). **These responses are ineffective against the adult worms, which by themselves do not produce significant disease in the host.**

An interesting observation has been made regarding the integrity of the immune system, AIDS, and egg excretion (Karanja et al, 1997). Patients who were infected with *S. mansoni* and were seropositive for HIV had similar levels of circulating schistosomal antigen but excreted fewer eggs than individuals who were HIV negative. Egg excretion in the HIV-seronegative group was significantly higher than that of the seropositive group. These observations are compatible with the hypothesis that the transit of schistosome eggs through tissue in the human host is facilitated by a competent immune system and that the efficiency of this process decreases in schistosomiasis patients co-infected with HIV.

Epidemiology

Of the 200 million persons afflicted with schistosomiasis, 80 to 90 million are infected by *S. haematobium* (Mahmoud and Abdel Wahab, 1990; WHO, 1998, 2002; Engels et al, 2002) and as many as 10 to 40 million persons have obstructive uropathy and other complications secondary to their disease. Transmission of *S. haematobium* occurs in 53 countries in the Middle East and in most of the African continent. In Southwest Asia, the disease is found in Southern Yemen, Yemen, Saudi Arabia, Lebanon, Syria, Turkey, Iraq, and Iran (WHO, 1998).

Furthermore, in both clinical and autopsy studies, the prevalence of infection and its intensity, as measured by egg excretion or tissue egg burden, are related (Smith et al, 1974b). The tissue egg burden, in turn, is related to the severity of the disease and to the frequency of complications. Autopsies indicate that severe uropathy is uncommon when the frequency of infection in a population is below 30% but increases linearly after this threshold is exceeded (Cheever et al, 1978).

Pathogenesis and Pathology

Schistosomal disease results directly from the granulomatous host response to schistosome eggs (Phillips and Colley, 1978; Cheever et al, 1985; Waine and McManus, 1997). The host responds to egg antigens by forming granulomas around the egg, which is T cell–dependent (Cheever et al, 1985). In patent human infections, all stages of granulomas are simultaneously present. Furthermore, the spectrum of serious disease ascribed to *S. haematobium* results from the interaction of four factors: intensity, duration, activity, and focality. These variables determine the morbidity, mortality, and treatment of urinary schistosomiasis.

Even though *S. haematobium* adult worm pairs are widely distributed throughout the pelvic venous plexuses, egg laying occurs chiefly in the pelvic lower urinary tract, thus leading to its pathologic manifestations (Cheever et al, 1977). Furthermore, *S. haematobium* deposits eggs in groups, rather than singly, and thus produces composite granulomas rather than unioval granulomas. Of note, *S. mansoni* also lays eggs in the lower urinary tract, especially in heavy infections, but no lower urinary tract lesions have been ascribed solely to *S. mansoni* (Cheever et al, 1978).

Viable adult worm pairs, sustained egg laying, and a vigorous granulomatous host response characterize active urinary schistosomiasis. Microscopic examination shows that the polypoid patch consists of scattered or massed composite granulomas separated by edematous granulation tissue diffusely infiltrated by eosinophils, lymphocytes, and plasma cells. Grossly, these areas of granulomatous inflammation result in large, bulky, hyperemic, and polypoid masses projecting into the lumen (Fig. 14–9). Schistosomal polyposis of the urinary bladder consists of multiple large inflammatory polyps and is related to heavy localized egg burdens during the active stage of the disease (Smith et al, 1977c). In endemic areas, polypoid patches occur mainly in children through their early teens. However, 60% of polypoid lesions of the urinary bladder in patients with schistosomiasis result from conditions other than schistosomiasis, such as polypoid cystitis (Smith et al, 1974a). As egg laying then ceases, entrapped eggs are destroyed or calcified and the inflammation wanes, being supplanted by fibrous tissue to produce the sandy patches characteristic of chronic urinary schistosomiasis.

Inactive urinary schistosomiasis, which occurs after adult worms have died, is characterized by the absence of viable eggs in tissues or urine and the presence of "sandy patches"—relatively flat, tan mucosal lesions of various depth, often not sharply defined (Fig. 14–10). Urinary excretion of dead or calcified eggs during this later stage is rare; however, the bladder wall may contain sufficient numbers of calcified eggs to outline the circumference of the bladder on radiographs. Patients also develop schistosomal obstructive uropathy as a result of chronic disease. There are two components to schistosomal obstructive uropathy: obstruction and

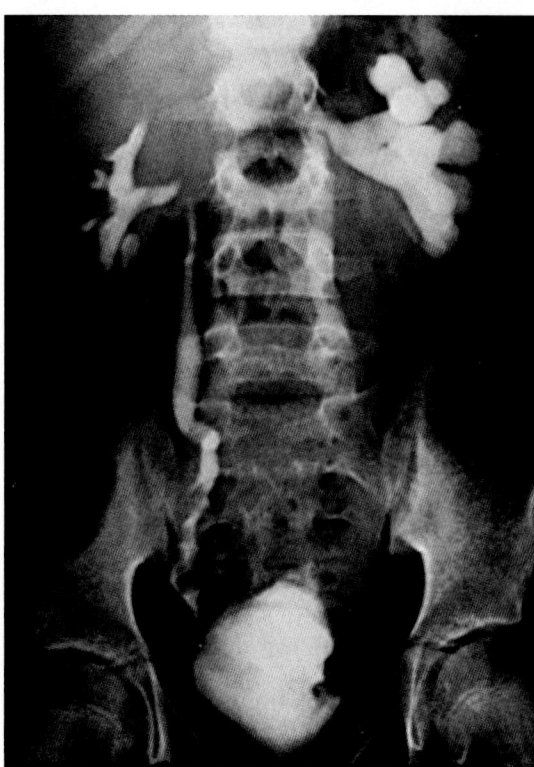

Figure 14–9. Intravenous urogram in an Egyptian boy shows scalloping of the bladder and right lower ureter by schistosomal polypoid lesions.

its effect on the proximal ureter. Schistosomal obstructive uropathy is usually bilaterally asymmetrical (Smith et al, 1974a). It may occur at the ureteral meatus (1%), interstitial ureter (10% to 30%), juxtavesical ureter (20% to 60%), lower third (pelvic) of the ureter (15% to 50%), or a contiguous combination of these areas (30% to 60%) (Gelfand, 1948; Smith et al, 1977b; Al-Shukri and Alwan, 1983). The results of these obstructions are hydroureter and hydronephrosis (Fig. 14–11). Three types of hydroureter are associated with schistosomal obstruction: segmental (i.e., cylindrical or fusiform), tonic, and atonic (Smith et al, 1977b). Segmental ureteral dilatations constitute 25% of schistosomal obstructive uropathy; nearly 80% of these are in the lower ureter and are accompanied by concentric ureteral muscular obliteration by fibrosis and sandy patches. Segmental lesions are rarely associated with important hydronephrosis. Tonic hydroureter, found in 25% to 30% of patients with schistosomal obstructive uropathy, is a dilated, tortuous, thick-walled, and trabeculated ureter with marked ureteral muscle hypertrophy and retarded peristaltic action. It involves the entire ureter proximal to an obstructive lesion, often a functional stenosis, and is often accompanied by significant hydronephrosis, which usually resolves after relief of obstruction (Smith et al, 1977b). Atonic hydroureter, seen in 35% of patients with schistosomal obstructive uropathy, is a markedly dilated, very tortuous, thin-walled ureter, without peristalsis and with atrophic fibrotic ureteral muscle.

Hydroureter usually precedes hydronephrosis (Lehman et al, 1973; Smith et al, 1974a, 1977b; Cheever et al, 1978). Schistosomal hydronephrosis passes from progressive renal pelvic dilatation, then medullary atrophy, to nearly total medullary effacement, before cortical atrophy ensues (Smith et al, 1974a, 1977b). This progression explains abrogation of tubular function (especially maximal urine concentration) before compromise of glomerular function (Lehman et al, 1971, 1973).

Finally, another pathologic sequelae of schistosomiasis is bladder cancer. Urinary schistosomiasis has been linked to the development of bladder cancer since the turn of the century. **Bladder cancer in the setting of _S. hematobium_ has an early onset (40 to 50 years) and a high frequency of squamous cell carcinomas (60% to 90%),** with 5% to 15% adenocarcinomas (Cheever, 1978; Lucas, 1982; Al-Shukri et al, 1987; Thomas et al, 1990; Bedwani et al, 1998). **More than 40% of squamous call carcinomas associated with schistosomiasis are well-differentiated or verrucous carcinomas that are exophytic and carry a good prognosis.** Most occur on the posterior (40% to 50%) and lateral walls (30%) of the bladder. Exophytic tumors constitute about 70% of schistosomal bladder cancers, and 25% are ulcerative endophytic tumors. It should be noted, however, that some unselected autopsy series from the same regions have shown similar frequencies of bladder cancer in patients without schistosomiasis (Smith et al, 1974a; Cheever et al, 1978).

Clinical Manifestations

Acute Schistosomiasis. Acute schistosomiasis, also called **Katayama fever,** is rarely found among endemic populations, but the first and presumably heavy exposure of a noninfected traveler may result in **fever, lymphadenopathy, splenomegaly, eosinophilia, urticaria, and other manifestations of a serum**

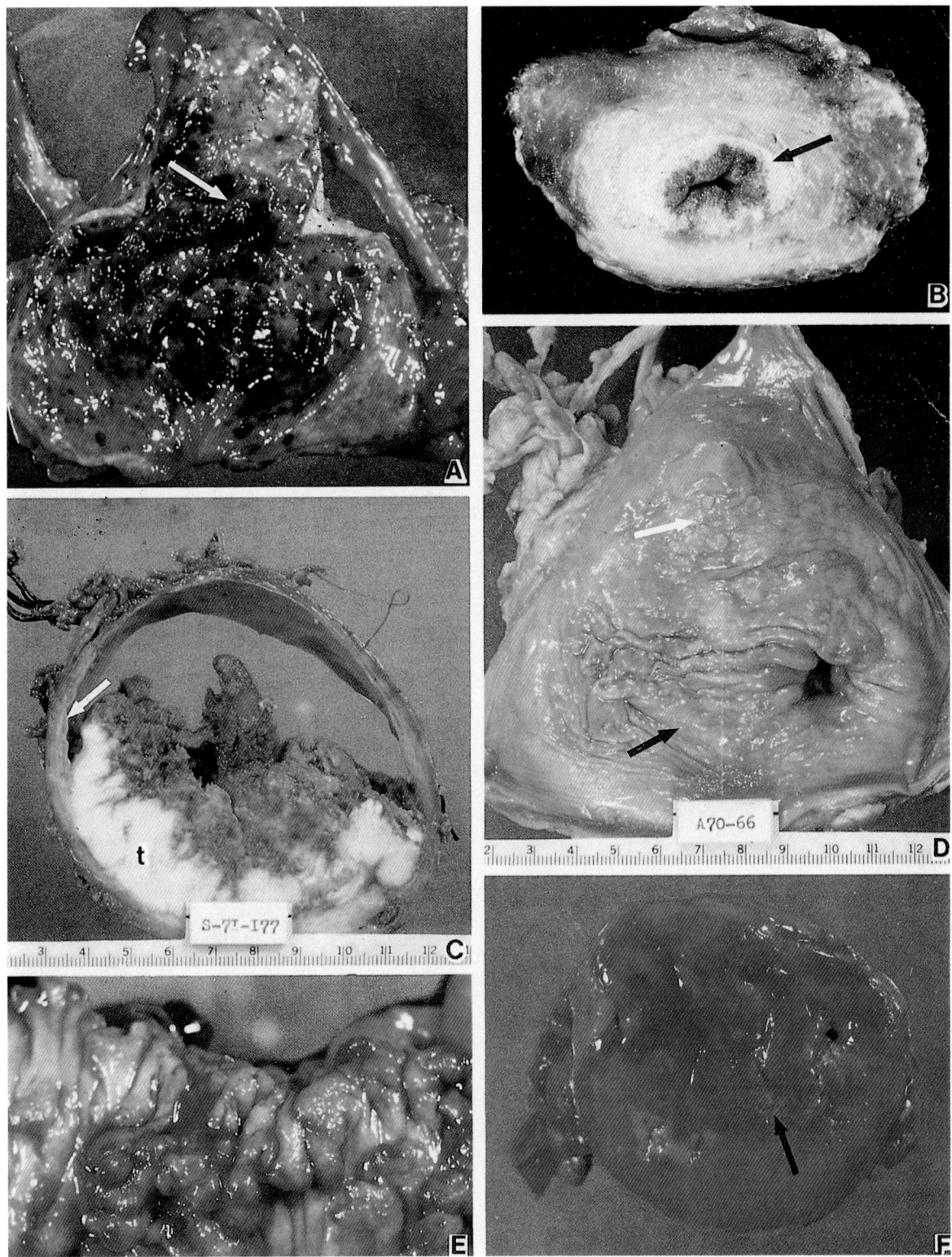

Figure 14–10. Macroscopic appearance of human urinary schistosomiasis. **A,** Urinary bladder opened with an anterior Y incision. The posterior and apical walls have many erythematous, granular, sessile, and pedunculated polyps *(arrow)*, characteristic of the early active stage of urinary schistosomiasis. **B,** Coronal section through the apex of a formalin-fixed urinary bladder. The lamina propria has been expanded and is replaced by a yellow-tan, finely granular sandy patch *(arrow)*, which is characteristic of chronic inactive foci. Small sandy patches are sprinkled through the fibrotic, atrophic detrusor muscle, even in perivesical fat. The more superficial erythematous portion of the lamina propria contains some viable eggs with granulomatous response (chronic active stage of urinary schistosomiasis). **C,** Coronal section through the middle of a urinary bladder after formalin inflation and fixation. The lamina propria *(arrow)* has been replaced by a concentric sandy patch, most prominent at the margin of the exophytic, moderately differentiated squamous cell carcinoma. The bladder wall is attenuated except for the tumor (t). No evidence of recent oviposition was found in the lower urinary tract (chronic inactive stage of urinary schistosomiasis, usually found with the bilharzial bladder cancer syndrome). **D,** Urinary bladder opened with anterior Y incision shows several features of severe chronic inactive urinary schistosomiasis. The entire lamina propria has been replaced by a sandy patch. Foci of epidermization are seen at or near the *white arrow*. The left ureteral orifice *(right)* is markedly dilated (the so-called golf-hole ureter of schistosomal uropathy). The right ureteral orifice *(point of black arrow)* is markedly stenotic. **E,** Rectosigmoid colon with polyposis. Numerous sessile and pedunculated polyps are seen. Many are erythematous, indicative of active oviposition with granuloma formation. Some have necrotic hemorrhagic tips. **F,** Mucosal surface of partial cystectomy specimen (4- to 5-cm ellipse) from a patient with the chronic inactive stage of the disease. There is a stellate chronic schistosomal ulcer. Despite the inactivity of the disease, these ulcers may bleed profusely. Pale mucoid flecks at the margin of the ulcer *(arrow)* are areas of adenoid (goblet cell) metaplasia.

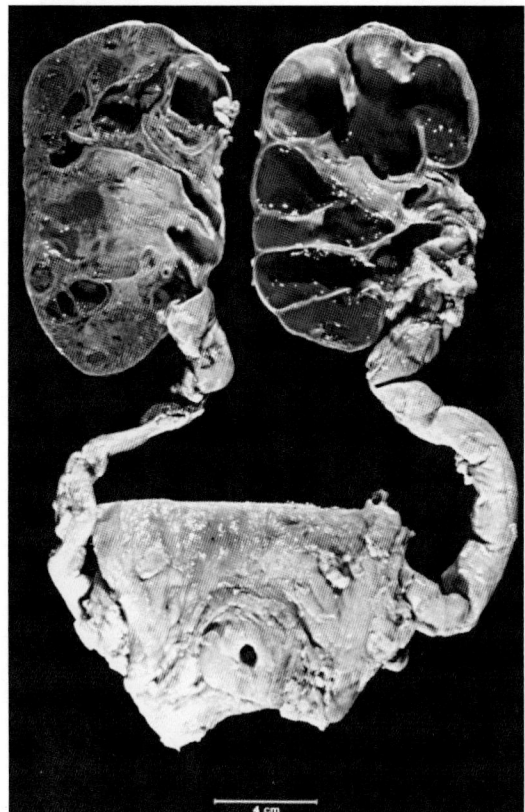

Figure 14–11. Schistosomal obstructive uropathy. The urinary bladder and ureters were fixed by inflation with formalin, and the bladder was sectioned coronally. The left hydroureter *(right)* is dilated (external diameter, 2 cm) and thin walled throughout its extravesicular course (interstitial ureteral stenosis is behind the bladder) and appears to be an atonic ureter; it is tortuous and kinked. The left kidney exhibits stage IV (end-stage) hydronephrosis with complete medullary and nearly complete cortical atrophy, and its pelvis is filled with sterile gelatinous rusty material; this is simple, uncomplicated hydronephrosis. The right ureter exhibits a moderately thick walled hydroureter (probably tonic), with stages II to III hydronephrosis and complicating acute and chronic pyelonephritis. The patient died of septicemia secondary to the right renal pyelonephritis, and the urinary schistosomiasis is therefore classified as an underlying cause of death.

sickness–like disease (Doherty et al, 1996; De Jesus et al, 2002). This syndrome may be fulminant in *S. japonicum* infection, probably as a result of the prodigious fecundity of *S. japonicum,* but it is rare in infection with *S. haematobium.* Acute schistosomiasis generally occurs 3 to 9 weeks after infection, coinciding with the onset of egg laying and often preceding the occurrence of eggs in the urine, but it may be delayed for more than 4 months (Young et al, 1986).

Acute schistosomiasis may be associated with ectopic egg laying as worms meander toward the pelvic venous plexuses and become delayed or lost. Ectopic eggs incite granulomas in such aberrant sites as the skin (Edington et al, 1975), epididymis (Elem et al, 1989), or spinal cord or nerve roots or both (Pitella, 1997).

Chronic Schistosomiasis. Chronic schistosomiasis is far more common than acute disease and has several different clinical manifestations. When the infection enters an "active" stage, eggs are deposited in tissues, traverse the bladder or rectosigmoid mucosa, and are excreted in the urine (and less

regularly in the feces). This prepatent period is usually 2 to 3 months but may last over 7 months (Young et al, 1986). **The classic clinical presentation of active schistosomiasis is hematuria with terminal dysuria.** Hematuria may be sufficient to cause anemia (Wilkins et al, 1985). Patients may also develop polypoid lesions of the bladder during this phase that can present clinically as a urethral or ureteral obstruction or bleed enough to produce clot retention. In endemic foci, active disease usually begins in childhood and nearly all children eventually suffer dysuria and hematuria; indeed, hematuria in males may be seen as a sign of puberty.

S. haematobium egg burdens of seminal vesicles and the ejaculatory ducts are high, and schistosome eggs, blood, or both may appear in the ejaculate before they appear in the urine. These patients may present with scrotal pain or a testicular mass. Egg burdens of the uterus, vagina, and testes are lower than those of the epididymis, ovaries, and fallopian tubes (Cheever et al, 1977, 1978; Helling-Giese et al, 1996).

S. haematobium causes genital disease in 30% of infected women (Poggensee and Feldmeier, 2001; Kjetland et al, 2005). Schistosomal cervicitis and vaginitis are often asymptomatic but may manifest similarly to cervicitis and vaginitis of other causes (Williams, 1967). A routine Papanicolaou smear may reveal terminally spined eggs. Schistosomal lesions of the vagina and cervix may predispose patients to the acquisition of HIV infection and AIDS, just as ulcerating sexually transmitted diseases (Feldmeier et al, 1994). At term in pregnancy, schistosome eggs have been found in the placenta and amniotic fluid, but there are no documented reports of fetal schistosomiasis.

The schistosomal "contracted bladder" syndrome occurs most frequently during the late chronic active stage, when egg burdens in tissue are highest. It manifests as constant, deep lower abdominal and pelvic pain, urgency, frequency, and incontinence (Duvie, 1986). Whereas the trigone appears normal or minimally hyperemic and edematous, the detrusor muscle is indurated and thickened, as is the entire bladder wall, and the bladder lumen is reduced to as little as 50 mL of functional capacity.

After some years, active infection enters a more quiescent period, in which egg deposition and excretion continues at a lower rate and symptoms are diminished. Over 30% of light infections "resolve" spontaneously in some endemic areas (Rutasitara and Chimbe, 1985). However, although symptoms are absent, silent obstructive uropathy may develop throughout this phase, as fibrosis replaces polypoid lesions and the bladder and ureters undergo irreversible damage. A slow, insidious evolution may result in enormous hydroureters and hydronephrosis with few symptoms.

Patients finally enter a **chronic inactive phase,** in which viable eggs are no longer detected in urine or tissues. Signs and symptoms at this stage are caused by sequelae and complications rather than by the schistosomal infection itself. Of patients with schistosomal obstructive uropathy, 40% to 60% present to urologists during this stage of their disease (Smith and Christie, 1986). In heavily endemic areas, nonfunctioning kidneys are commonly found in apparently well patients.

In up to 50% of patients, chronic or acute bacterial urinary tract infection is superimposed on their schistosomal obstructive uropathy. Bacterial urinary tract infections associated with schistosomal obstructive uropathy are usually ascending infections caused by the same organisms that cause infections in patients without schistosomiasis. **Chronic or recurrent urinary tract infections caused by *Salmonella* species,** often associated with intermittent bacteremia, are another finding in many patients with urinary schistosomiasis (King, 2001). *Salmonella* organisms reside in the apical invaginations of the schistosome tegument, where they are protected from host defenses and antibiotics. Both conditions usually respond to antischistosomal drug treatment alone or in combination with antibiotics but not to antibiotic therapy alone.

Another manifestation of schistosomal disease is the development of **bladder ulcers,** which occur in two types (Smith et al, 1977a). Acute schistosomal ulcers will rarely present in the active stage, when a necrotic polyp sloughs into the urine. The more common chronic schistosomal ulcer is a late sequelae of heavy infection. This lesion is associated with a constant "burning" micturition and intense pelvic and suprapubic pain. Over 90% of these patients have a history of previous urinary schistosomiasis, 20% have histories of previous sequelae and complications, and 10% have had previous surgical intervention for urinary schistosomiasis. Gross hematuria and gross pyuria are found in over half of these patients.

Diagnosis

The presence of **terminally spined eggs in urinary sediment is diagnostic** of active *S. haematobium* infection. In moderate to heavy infections, eggs are almost always present in a routine examination of urinary sediment. In lighter infections, routine urinalysis does not always reveal eggs, so the sedimentation or filtration of a 10-mL volume of urine may be necessary (Mott, 1983). *S. haematobium* egg excretion peaks between 10 AM and 2 PM. This circadian phenomenon reverses in night-shift workers without any variation induced by athletic activity or water loading (McMahon, 1976).

Ova are excreted in the urine in proportion to the viable worm burden in lower urinary tract tissues (Smith et al, 1974b; Smith and Christie, 1986). **The intensity of the current infection in its early stages can be estimated by examination of urine and quantitation of urinary egg excretion. This also correlates with prognosis.**

Eggs may also be seen in rectal or bladder mucosal biopsy specimens. If eggs are not found in several urine specimens, rectal biopsy should be attempted before bladder biopsy, because eggs are nearly as common in the rectum and the hazard of urinary tract infection is avoided. **A squash preparation of the biopsy specimen between glass slides is preferable to histopathologic analysis** because its sensitivity is greater and it may permit a determination of egg viability.

Serologic tests (Western blot) that are sensitive and specific for *S. haematobium* are available at the CDC (Tsang and Wilkins, 1997; Al-Sherbiny et al, 1999). The tests are highly sensitive and about 95% specific. They may be useful in diagnosing infection when eggs are not present but do not distinguish between acute infection and chronic disease. **Although serologic testing is a valuable diagnostic and epidemiologic tool, finding eggs is the gold standard for diagnosis of active infection.** In chronic inactive urinary schistosomiasis, in which egg excretion is uncommon, patients with severe sequelae can have negative urine examinations even when there are 10^6 eggs/g of tissue (Smith et al, 1974b). In these instances,

radiographic (Lehman et al, 1973) and serologic diagnoses are superior.

Radiography is an important diagnostic tool in the evaluation of the sequelae and complications of urinary schistosomiasis. A plain radiograph of the abdomen may reveal calcification within the urinary tract. **The classic presentation of a calcified bladder, which looks like a fetal head in the pelvis, is pathognomonic of chronic urinary schistosomiasis** (Fig. 14–12). The seminal vesicles, prostate, posterior urethra, distal ureters, and, in rare instances, the colon may also be calcified. **The earliest radiographic changes appear to be striations in the ureters and renal pelvis** (Hugosson, 1987). Ureteral calcification is typically mural, and the ureter is dilated. This differs from the calcification seen in tuberculous disease, which forms a cast of a nondilated ureter.

Hydroureter, hydronephrosis, nonfunctioning kidney, ureteral stenosis, and bladder and ureteral filling defects such as polypoid lesions are readily observed in a standard intravenous urogram. In the presence of severe obstructive uropathy, delayed films are often needed to discern distended ureters and kidneys. Postvoid films may indicate bladder neck obstruction with retention. Fluoroscopy can differentiate

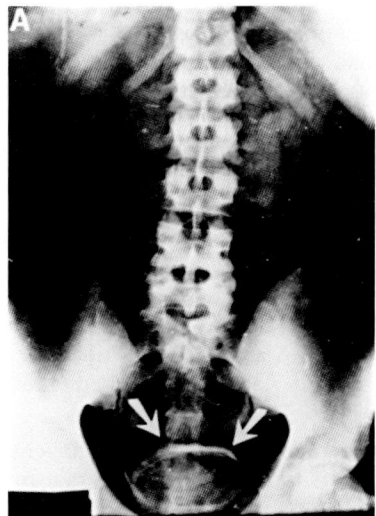

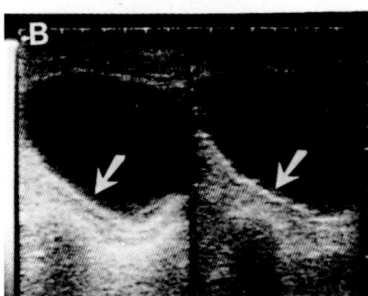

Figure 14–12. Bladder calcification in a 30-year-old Egyptian farmer. **A,** Plain x-ray film of the abdomen shows a rim of calcification surrounding the urinary bladder *(arrows).* **B,** Abdominal ultrasound study shows a bright line surrounding the bladder with a definite dark rim behind it *(arrows).* (**A** and **B,** Courtesy of G. Thomas Strickland, MD. From Abdel-Wahab MF, Ramzy I, Esmat G, et al: Ultrasound for detecting *Schistosoma haematobium* urinary tract complications: Comparison with radiographic procedures. J Urol 1992;148:346.)

tonic and atonic ureters (Abdel-Halim et al, 1985) and identify nonstenotic, immotile ureters. CT, however, can detect both obstructive uropathy and calcified lesions in the urinary tract and the colon (Jorulf and Linstedt, 1985) and thus complements or substitutes for IVU.

Another useful imaging modality is vesicocystourethrography. It indicates the presence of vesicoureteral reflux, which occurs in 25% of infected ureters. Abdominal ultrasonography is also a useful method to detect focal thickening of the bladder wall and polypoid lesions of the urinary tract, hydroureter, and hydronephrosis in endemic areas, and it detects heavily calcified patches (Medhat et al, 1997). Reeder and Palmer (1981) provide additional details on the radiography of urinary schistosomiasis.

Treatment

Medical Management. The development of safe and effective antischistosomal drugs has dramatically changed the management of schistosome infection (WHO, 1993; Richter, 2003). All patients with schistosomiasis should be treated regardless of the intensity or apparent activity of their infection. **Praziquantel is the drug of choice for all *Schistosoma* species** (The Medical Letter, 2004). It is active against all clinical forms and stages of the disease after the first 3 to 4 weeks of infection. Praziquantel interferes with ion transport in the schistosome tegument, resulting in calcium and sodium fluxes, metabolic alterations, and sudden contraction of the parasite's musculature. **Cure rates with praziquantel for *S. haematobium* infection are 83% to 100%** (Mott et al, 1985). The drug also has activity against most other flukes and tapeworms, which is a great advantage in the developing world. The current recommendation is two oral doses of 40 mg/kg in 1 day for *S. haematobium* (The Medical Letter, 2004). Praziquantel is extremely well tolerated, with gastrointestinal complaints (nausea, vomiting, diarrhea, and anorexia) being the major side effects. Headache, dizziness, and fever are occasionally reported. The lack of serious side effects has made it the agent of choice in national mass chemotherapy programs (King et al, 1990).

Surgical Management. The efficacy of current drug therapy for schistosomiasis is sufficiently good that one should not electively operate for schistosomal disease without first treating medically and then reevaluating the need for surgery (Cioli et al, 1995). **In general, surgery is reserved for complications that have not responded to adequate medical treatment within a reasonable follow-up time (e.g., obstructive uropathy) or for those mandating immediate intervention, such as intractable bladder hemorrhage.**

Significant prostatitis and hypertrophy are uncommon in schistosomiasis, and no evidence of bladder outlet obstruction was associated with *S. haematobium* infections in autopsy studies (Smith et al, 1974a; Cheever et al, 1977, 1978). However, clinical studies consistently report cystoscopic (Fam, 1964), urodynamic (Sabha and Nilsson, 1988), and postvoid residual urine, which are evidence of functional bladder outlet obstruction and may require intervention in patients with severe inactive urinary schistosomiasis (Abdel-Halim, 1984). Schistosomal epididymitis commonly manifests as induration and enlargement with variable scrotal pain; surgery is often performed for suspicion of testicular tumor.

As previously discussed, schistosomal disease of the urinary bladder leads to a spectrum of outcomes, including schistosomal polyposis, sandy patches, "contracted bladder," schistosomal ulceration, urothelial hyperplasia, metaplasia, dysplasia, and bladder cancer. In particular instances, such as the chronically contracted bladder, surgical intervention is indicated and takes the form of vesical denervation, urinary diversion, ileocystoplasty, or hydrodistention. Any treatment, however, must be done in conjunction with medical chemotherapy. Chronic deep bladder ulcers may necessitate a partial cystectomy, because fulguration rarely produces either symptomatic relief or healing of the ulcer. Urothelial hyperplasia is strongly associated with severe urinary schistosomiasis whereas **urothelial metaplasia and dysplasia commonly accompany schistosomal bladder cancer** (Khafagy et al, 1972). Treatment of bladder cancer secondary to schistosomiasis is usually surgical and discussed elsewhere in this textbook.

The most common sequelae of urinary schistosomiasis result from ureteral involvement causing obstructive uropathy (Lehman et al, 1973; Smith et al, 1974a; Cheever et al, 1978; Smith and Christie, 1986). Hydroureter and hydronephrosis are related to the intensity of *S. haematobium* infection. **Because ureteral obstruction seen during active schistosomiasis is most often caused by concentric or hemiconcentric polypoid lesions that "girdle" the ureteral muscle in the intramural and adjacent extravesical ureter, it responds well to medical management alone.** Complete resolution of deteriorated renal function occurs within 1 to 2 months of antischistosomal chemotherapy when obstruction is caused by active disease (Lehman et al, 1973). In one study it was reported that chemotherapy not only reverses schistosomal obstructive uropathy but also prevents it, even in people who continue to get reinfected (Subramanian et al, 1999). In late chronic active and inactive urinary schistosomiasis, on the other hand, anatomic obstruction is more prominent.

Anatomic ureteral stenosis, with or without calculi, has been identified in up to 80% of obstructions (Lehman et al, 1973; Smith et al, 1977b; Al-Shukri and Alwan, 1983; El-Nahas et al, 2003). **Therefore, when there is residual ureteral stenosis after successful chemotherapy it is usually amenable to surgical intervention. Depending on the extent and location of the stricture, procedures involving excision or dilatation have been used.** Balloon dilatation has reportedly proved effective with anatomic stenosis (Jacobsson et al, 1987), but mechanical dilatation is frequently followed by repeat stenosis (Wishahi, 1987). When the ureteral meatus, intermural ureter, ureterovesical junction, or lower ureter is involved, a variety of plastic operations to reconstruct a functional valve are available. Most of these procedures are variants of the Leadbetter-Politano operation (Politano and Leadbetter, 1958; Leadbetter and Leadbetter, 1961). Although highly effective for some patients (Smith et al, 1977b; Al-Shukri and Alwan, 1983), other authors have noted restenosis (Umerah, 1981).

In long or multisegmental lesions, excision of the affected portion leaves inadequate residual ureter for reimplantation; in these cases, surgeons have successfully employed the Boari-Ockerblad bladder flap, Boari-Küss flap, ileal conduit, suprapubic intravesical ureterostomy, and ureteroileocystostomy with care to have an isoperistaltic direction of the ileal segment (Abdel-Halim, 1980, 1984; Al-Shukri and Alwan,

1983; Abu-Aisha et al, 1985). Isolated meatal stenosis may be amenable to simple meatoplasty (Al-Shukri and Alwan, 1983). When a ureter is hopelessly obstructed, long-term nephrostomy drainage or creation of an ileal ureter can provide relief.

Prognosis

Tens of millions of people are infected with *S. haematobium*, but **most have mild infections, and the prognosis is good. However, the morbidity and mortality of schistosomiasis are determined by the overall intensity of infection.** No mortality was observed in areas in which the prevalence of schistosomiasis and frequency and severity of schistosomal obstructive uropathy were low (Nigeria), but when Egypt had a prevalence of 50%, mortality approached 10% (Smith et al, 1974a; Cheever et al, 1978). **Among patients with severe disease, mortality reached 50% in 2 to 5 years** (Lehman et al, 1970).

Patients who die of schistosomal obstructive uropathy (bilateral end-stage hydronephrosis) are usually in their 20s, have early-stage disease, and have heavy total egg burdens. Patients who develop the complications of pyelonephritis and urothelial cancer are usually older than age 40 (Christie et al, 1986; Smith and Christie, 1986).

The prognosis for persons with demonstrable urinary tract lesions has dramatically improved with therapy with praziquantel. In children with obstructive polyps the uropathy usually completely resolves within 2 to 6 weeks of treatment. For patients with chronic obstructive uropathy due to sandy patches and fibrosis, the prognosis is less clear. Some individuals tolerate advanced obstructive uropathy with little, if any, deterioration in renal function. **Schistosomal obstructive uropathy, urolithiasis, bladder outlet obstruction, and bacterial cystitis all predispose to pyelonephritis.** Bacterial superinfection is a serious prognostic event and should be treated as vigorously and as soon as possible. Furthermore, for those who develop a bladder malignancy, their prognosis is dependent on the aggressiveness of their tumor.

Prevention and Control

Travelers in endemic areas should be advised of the hazard of infected fresh water streams, rivers, ponds, and lakes and should avoid contact with such water. Boiling of the water kills the cercariae. Measures of control in endemic areas have utilized several approaches: destruction of the snail host, elimination of urine and fecal contamination of water, and reduction of contact with infected water (WHO, 1993). In many endemic areas, such measures are expensive, unfeasible, or poorly tolerated by the local population. Therefore, mass therapy by drugs has been emphasized, and all major control campaigns today include drug treatment as a major component, often age-directed or annual or both (King et al, 1991; Engels et al, 2002; WHO, 2002). Vaccines to prevent disease or to reduce infection are not currently available (Pearce, 2003).

Genital Filariasis

Filarial diseases are classified as either lymphatic or nonlymphatic. **Wuchereria bancrofti accounts for 90% of cases of human lymphatic filariasis** and is widespread throughout the tropics. It is an exclusively human parasite without animal reservoirs. *Brugia malayi* and *B. timori*, which cause the remainder of human lymphatic filariasis, have been found in primates and felines and are confined to the Far East. **Nonlymphatic filariasis is caused by *Onchocerca volvulus*,** the agent of African river blindness, which is known to cause massive inguinal lymphadenopathy, "hanging groin," and scrotal elephantiasis.

Lymphatic Filariasis

The symptoms of bancroftian and brugian filariasis range from acute lymphatic inflammation characterized by fever, localized lymphangitis, and transitory lymphadenopathy to chronic lymphatic dilatation with hydrocele, elephantiasis of the limbs, and chyluria (Ottesen, 1989; Dreyer et el, 2000). Lymphatic filariasis affects 120 million persons living in 73 countries, with India accounting for 40% of the global infections (Ramaiah et al, 2000).

Biology and Life Cycle. The lymphatic filariae are elongated (100×0.3 mm for female and 40×0.1 mm for male *W. bancrofti*) nematodes. **Their cycle proceeds from human to mosquito and back.** The most common urban vectors of *W. bancrofti* are the ubiquitous *Culex pipiens* complex, but filariae have adapted to a wide variety of mosquitoes in different areas. Only small portions of mosquito bites (1%) are infective, even in hyperendemic areas, and obstructive lymphatic disease occurs in persons who have been repeatedly infected over many years.

Female mosquitoes ingest microfilariae with their blood meals. These rapidly become infective larvae and go to the mosquitoes' salivary glands. The infective larvae are then deposited on the skin during the next mosquito feeding. Although unable to traverse unbroken skin, the infective larvae can enter the bite site or can cross the normal conjunctiva or buccal mucosa (Ah et al, 1974; Sullivan and Chernin, 1976). **The adult filaria then migrates to and lives in the larger lymphatic vessels. *W. bancrofti* adults have a predilection for periaortic, iliac, inguinal, and intrascrotal lymph vessels, whereas *B. malayi* prefers inguinal and more distal lymphangioles.**

Most of the mature *Wuchereria* female is composed of the uterus, which contains all stages, from eggs to mature microfilariae. Microfilarial discharge into the blood is regulated by a feedback system that maintains a constant level of microfilaremia. There is, however, no constant relationship between the number of worms and the level of microfilaremia. Indeed, microfilaremia is found in only 30% to 40% of all infections. The timing of peak microfilaremia in each endemic focus corresponds to the peak feeding period of local mosquito vectors.

Pathology and Pathogenesis. Epidemiologic findings and animal experiments clearly indicate that host reactions to microfilariae differ from those to adult worms. Although pathologic and clinical features differ between patients from endemic and from nonendemic areas, significant humoral and cellular immune responses develop in both groups (Steel et al, 1996). Filaria-specific IgE titers rise, and IgE-eosinophil–mediated killing of microfilariae has been noted in vitro. However, patients from endemic regions manifest IgG_4 blocking antibodies and antigen-specific suppressor T cells. The extent of immune downregulation correlates with an absence of pathologic sequelae and the presence of microfilaremia (Piessens, 1982; Davis, 1989; Ottesen, 1989).

Early Infection. Lesions of established infection do not remit but either persist actively or result in significant scarring and lymphatic obstruction. Lesions may appear at the worms' nesting areas (funiculoepididymitis, orchitis, filarial lymphangitis, filarial abscess), in their lymphatic distribution (e.g., hydrocele, lymphadenitis, genital edema), or both. Dying or dead adult filariae are often detected in surgically excised tissue, which suggests that worm death provokes the inflammatory response.

The lesions vary from nodular inflammation, simulating neoplasm, to suppuration, simulating acute bacterial disease. Histologically, nodular lesions show massive granulomas around cuticular fragments or necrotic filaria. **Tissue eosinophilia is a useful diagnostic hint but may be absent.** The most acute subcutaneous filarial lesions simulate fluctuant abscesses with bacteriologically sterile but purulent exudate that surrounds a dying worm (O'Connor and Hulse, 1935).

Episodic filarial inflammation eventually abates, leaving obliterated lymphatics surrounded by poorly organized scar tissue. A palpable mass or indurated cord may develop. The consequences of lymphatic obstruction vary with the location of the obstruction, but the common feature is the accumulation of lymphedema or hydrocele fluid associated with lymphoid infiltrates.

Late Infection. The complications of late infection include huge hydroceles and scrotal and penile elephantiasis (Fig. 14–13). **Lymphangiographic studies reveal that the initial obliteration of lymphatic vessels is bypassed by collateral formation. As these collaterals become progressively obstructed, lymph dilatation follows.** Lymphangiograms in late filariasis show poorly draining networks of communicating lymph vessels extending through lymphedematous tissues into superficial dermal layers (Kanetkar et al, 1966).

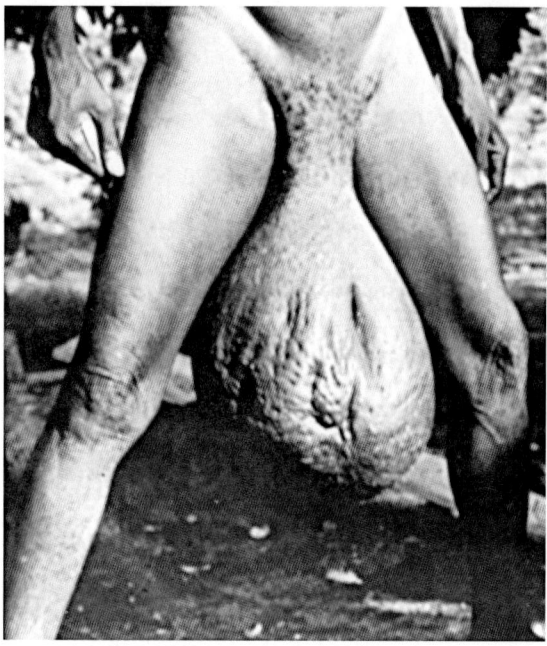

Figure 14–13. Huge hydrocele and scrotal elephantiasis. (Courtesy of Dr. B. H. Kean. From Zaiman H: A Pictorial Presentation of Parasites, Valley City, ND.)

Although bacteria play no role in chyluria, and filarial hydrocele is rarely superinfected, elephantiasis and lymph scrotum are often superinfected (Olszewski et al, 1997). To further confirm the role of infection, it has been noted that classic elephantiasis can be prevented when patients with lymphedema are instructed to use antiseptic soap and are treated with antibiotics (Maher and Ottesen, 2000). Thus, bacterial infection is an important contributing factor to the development of sequelae (Dreyer et al, 2000).

Serial autopsy studies of men show that the tail of the epididymis and the lower spermatic cord are the most constant locations of worms (Galindo et al, 1962). Correspondingly, funiculoepididymitis and hydrocele are the most common consequences of bancroftian filariasis. Assuming that heavy infections saturate the preferred habitat and compel adult filariae to spread centrifugally to increasingly distant sites, saturation of inguinal lymphatic trunks (yielding scrotal edema) initiates encroachment into femoral lymphatics (causing elephantiasis of lower extremities) and proximally to renal lymphangioles (producing lymph varices whose intrapelvic rupture causes chyluria).

Clinical Manifestations. Clinical lymphatic filariasis manifests as one of four forms: (1) asymptomatic, (2) filarial fevers, (3) chronic lesions, and (4) tropical eosinophilia.

Asymptomatic Infection. Persons in endemic areas may have positive serologic or skin test reactivity to filarial antigens but no microfilaremia and no clinical evidence of filariasis. Asymptomatic microfilaremia may occur in patients with downregulated effector immune responses. They develop both antigen-specific T-cell–effector mechanisms and IgE antibodies, but these are made ineffective by filarial antigen-specific suppressor T-cell subsets and blocking IgG_4 antibodies (Ottesen, 1989). Such individuals probably developed tolerance to filarial antigens in utero (Weil et al, 1983). In addition, generation of elevated levels of interleukin-12 has been noted in individuals with chronic microfilaremia (King et al, 1995).

Filarial Fevers. Patients with "filarial fever" sustain episodic fevers, lymphangitis-lymphadenitis, funiculoepididymitis, transient edema, and small acute hydroceles. **They are typically amicrofilaremic.** Expatriates residing in endemic areas long enough to sustain repeated filarial infections constitute one moiety of the filarial fever group; unlike patients with endemic filarial fever who inexorably progress to chronic abnormalities, their disease abates, presumably because repatriation averts further infection.

Chronic Filariasis. Early established filariasis progresses to the late chronic stage with a series of **progressive lesions: funiculoepididymitis, hydrocele, orchitis, scrotal and penile elephantiasis, lymph scrotum, and chyluria. These do not resolve with treatment** (Fan et al, 1995).

Funiculoepididymitis. Most symptomatic cases of filarial funiculoepididymitis appear before the patients' fourth decade. The attack may be isolated, with remission, or may be repetitive and progressive. Pain radiating to the testis and simulating ureteral colic may accompany the systemic symptoms.

Palpable cordlike swelling may mimic an intrascrotal tumor or torsion of the cord and be accompanied by hydrocele or soft tissue edema. Eosinophilia is common. Varicocele or thrombosis of the pampiniform plexus may complicate inflammation, augmenting pain and discomfort. Bacterial superinfection of acute filarial corditis, a rare but often lethal complication, brings exquisite pain, high fever, and septic thrombophlebitis.

Mild cases may involute spontaneously, but, in an endemic setting, they more often augur future recurrences or the development of chronic lymphedema or both (Kazura et al, 1995). The disease frequently simulates malignancy and many patients ultimately undergo operations, including orchiectomy. Even in severe filarial funiculitis, the spermatic cord is usually intact and patent. Sterility due to filariasis is rare, as is orchitis.

Hydrocele. In endemic areas, differentiation of filarial from idiopathic hydrocele is difficult on either clinical or laboratory grounds. Microfilariae or adult worms are rarely detected in the hydrocele fluid, but a milky or sediment-rich hydrocele fluid suggests a filarial origin. Hydrocele accompanied by nodules in the cord or epididymis and a history of travel to or residence in an endemic area suggests filariasis. Discovery of a thick, fibrous tunica, especially with cholesterol or calcium deposits, should also suggest a diagnosis of filariasis. Tunical calcification is very rare in idiopathic hydrocele.

Scrotal and Penile Elephantiasis. Mild scrotal edema is not unusual during early infection or with established hydrocele. Penile edema on the other hand is unusual, and the monstrous elephantine enlargements of the scrotum or penis depicted in textbooks occur largely in populations without access to medical care. Elephantiasis of the limbs poses the differential diagnosis between filarial and other causes, but genital elephantiasis is rarely due to other causes, such as malignancy.

Chyluria. Chyluria occurs with or without microfilaremia, usually in young adults. It occurs earlier in the natural history of filariasis than genital elephantiasis. Dying worms provoke lymphatic obstruction with proximal lymphangiolar dilatation. Rupture of a lymphatic varix into the urinary collecting system has been demonstrated by lymphangiography. Chyluria may initially alarm patients but often is disregarded and may result in severe protein loss, leading to hypoalbuminemia and anasarca. Chyluria is usually intermittent and may spontaneously remit with bed rest.

Tropical Pulmonary Eosinophilia. Tropical pulmonary eosinophilia occurs in patients with an allergic response to microfilarial antigens; such patients are amicrofilaremic (Ong and Doyle, 1998). This syndrome is characterized by marked, sustained peripheral eosinophilia only temporarily affected by corticosteroids but responsive to antifilarial drugs. There is an absence of classic filarial lesions such as lymphedema or funiculoepididymitis. However, the presence of lymphadenopathy that can be marked enough to mimic lymphoma and symptomatic pulmonary infiltrates suggest asthma (Danaraj et al, 1966). Patients develop very high levels of filaria-specific IgE and pulmonary reticulonodular densities on chest radiographs that reveal an eosinophilic interstitial pneumonitis on biopsy. The frequency of this syndrome varies markedly between endemic foci and is most common in southern India and Singapore.

Diagnosis. Careful history taking and physical examination are paramount in suggesting a filarial lymphedema. TB, schistosomiasis haematobia, and gonorrhea may also produce funiculoepididymitis. Idiopathic hydrocele with or without varicocele or hernia is common in tropical and non-tropical areas, but hydrocele occurs at an earlier age and in greater frequency in areas of endemic filariasis (Jachowski et al, 1962).

The histologic finding of adult worms is a diagnostically definitive but an insensitive technique. The presence of microfilariae in peripheral blood, chylous urine, or hydrocele fluid is also diagnostic. Blood samples must be taken when peak microfilaremia occurs (e.g., midnight in the case of nocturnal periodic *W. bancrofti*). Peripheral blood is best examined by thick-drop technique with Giemsa stain. It is important to remember that filaremia may be absent in both early and late filariasis, after treatment with a microfilaricide, and in tropical pulmonary eosinophilia. Immunoassays for measuring antibody and circulating antigens, as well as molecular biologic assays for detecting parasite DNA, have been developed (Harnett et al, 1998).

Direct ultrasonographic observation of adult filariae has been reported in lymph vessels of microfilaremic and otherwise asymptomatic patients made possible by energetic movements of the worms ("filarial dance sign") (Amaral et al, 1994; Chaubal et al, 2003). Lymphangiography may distinguish filariasis from other causes of lymphatic obstruction, especially in conditions with reduced numbers and competence of lymph vessels. Plain radiographs may reveal calcified worms, which are diagnostic.

Treatment and Prevention. There has been dramatic progress in the development of new control strategies and treatment programs for filariasis in the past decade. **The new methodology seeks to control transmission through mass treatment programs and to control disease through treatment of individual patients** (Ottesen et al, 1997). **Three drugs, used singly or in various combinations and doses, are currently employed: diethylcarbamazine (DEC), ivermectin, and albendazole** (Shenoy et al, 1999). DEC has been used for over 50 years and remains the standard against which all new drugs must be compared. DEC is approved by the U.S. Food and Drug Administration but is currently available only through the CDC.

All patients with filarial infection, whether symptomatic or not, should be treated with DEC, 6 mg/kg/day in three divided dose for 2 weeks (Noroes et al, 1997; The Medical Letter, 2004). The objective of this therapy is to kill the adult worms and to abolish microfilaremia. **Side effects, including fever, headache, nausea, vomiting, and arthralgias, may occur within 1 to 2 days of initiating treatment.** The symptoms are due to dying filariae, and the severity is directly proportional to the magnitude of the microfilaremia. Patients with high microfilarial counts should start with lower doses of DEC for the first several days to minimize these side effects. Premedication with corticosteroids or antihistamines may also decrease these symptoms.

Ivermectin in a single oral dose of 200 to 400 μg/kg has a microfilaricidal effect comparable to that of DEC. However, it has no effect on adult filariae. In contrast, **albendazole** kills both adults and microfilariae in lymphatic disease (Ottesen et al, 1999; Bookaire et al, 2002; Gardon et al, 2002). These medications are the cornerstone of the mass treatment programs, which are successfully interrupting transmission by reducing the microfilariae available to the mosquito vectors in endemic areas.

Use of elastic stockings and elevation of extremities are important adjunctive measures in reducing lymphedema. Meticulous skin care and aggressive treatment of secondary infections may halt or even reverse the lymphedema and prevent the development of elephantiasis (Ottesen et al, 1997). Abdominal binders have been used to increase intra-abdominal pressure in an effort to stop chyluria but are controversial because they may increase chyluria in some patients (Ahrens, 1970). Finally, diagnostic retrograde lymphangiography curatively scleroses lymphatic fistulas in 48% of patients (Gandhi, 1976). Thus, **surgical correction is unnecessary in many of these cases and operative intervention is challenging because the varices are hard to identify and eliminate.**

Genital elephantiasis is rarely amenable to surgery. Additionally, procedures such as lymphadenectomy may further compromise lymph drainage and exacerbate complications. There are, however, a few instances when surgical intervention is necessary to treat the complication of filariasis. For example, patients with filarial funiculoepididymitis should first undergo a thorough workup for malignant, filarial, and bacterial causes of their symptoms. Then, appropriate antibiotics should be prescribed for bacterial disease, and treatment of the filariasis may require surgical decompression or excision of filarial nodules, preserving the testis and cord. When funiculoepididymitis is recurrent, painful, and deforming or complicated by blood vessel involvement, more radical surgery is warranted. Next, for the treatment of large or symptomatic hydroceles, hydrocelectomy is indicated. Excision of the intact hydrocele sac is the treatment of choice; an alternative method is inversion with partial excision (Jachowski et al, 1962). Small hydroceles that do not enlarge can be ignored. Finally, a variety of procedures have been devised to remove redundant tissue and to reconstruct the scrotum or vulva.

With regard to prevention of disease, DEC has been used as a prophylactic drug, given as an annual dose of 6 mg/kg. Trials with prophylactic ivermectin have had similar salutary effects. Major control methods however depend on the use of residual insecticides, the use of domestic mosquito netting, and the reduction of mosquito-breeding sites.

Onchocerciasis

Onchocerca volvulus is the agent of African river blindness and of severe, debilitating, chronic dermatitis. Onchocerciasis is **common throughout tropical Africa, and endemic foci also exist in Central and South America.** This filaria differs sharply from *Brugia* and *Wuchereria*: (1) it is transmitted by black flies of the *Simulium* species, (2) adult worms inhabit subcutaneous tissue and cause palpable fibrous nodules in which they are encapsulated, and (3) microfilariae travel through the dermis (and the eye) but are not in the peripheral blood. Diagnosis and estimation of infection intensity are made by microscopic examination of skin snips immersed in normal saline solution for 20 to 30 minutes under a coverslip on a slide or with Giemsa stain. Serologic and antigen detection tests have also been developed (Vincent et al, 2000; Pischke et al, 2002).

In the late stages, when blindness and atrophic dermatitis are the principal infirmities, onchocercal infection may produce "hanging groin" or scrotal elephantiasis. Excised surgical specimens show atrophy and fibrosis in the inguinal lymph nodes with subcutaneous edema and fibrosis superimposed on the usual onchocercal dermatitis (Connor et al, 1970). Onchocerciasis is occasionally accompanied by giant inguinal lymphadenopathy, which may be an antecedent to hanging groin.

A single oral dose of ivermectin (150 µg/kg) repeated every 2 to 6 months until the patient is asymptomatic has proved to be a successful onchocercal microfilaricide with few side reactions (Greene et al, 1985; The Medical Letter, 2004). **DEC should not be used for treatment of this disease** because of the severe allergic immune responses to microfilariae dying in the skin and other sites (the Mazzotti reaction). Ivermectin distribution has been successfully used for curbing *O. volvulus* transmission in an international campaign against African river blindness under the auspices of the WHO (Dull and Meredith, 1998). A recent advance with potential therapeutic implications is the demonstration that a 6-week course of doxycycline renders the female worm sterile by reducing the symbiotic *Wolbachia* endobacteria in the females (Hoerauf, 2003).

Other Parasitic Diseases of the Genitourinary Tract

This section describes parasitic infections that are rare or in which urogenital manifestations are overshadowed by the disease in other organs. These include the intestinal helminth *Enterobius*; the larval tapeworm of hydatid disease; and *Entamoeba histolytica*.

Enterobiasis

The common **intestinal pinworm *Enterobius vermicularis*, which is ubiquitous worldwide,** occasionally migrates from its nocturnal swarming site, the anus, into the vagina upward, reaching the peritoneal cavity by way of the uterus and fallopian tubes. In that unnatural habitat, worm movement and egg laying may continue, producing inflammation of the pelvic peritoneum with pain, fever, simulated acute appendicitis, or other lesions. Dead worms and eggs incite granulomas and adhesions. **Treatment of pelvic enterobiasis is simply effected with pyrantel pamoate, mebendazole, or albendazole** (The Medical Letter, 2004).

Hydatid Disease

No part of the human anatomy is invulnerable to hydatid cysts, but renal hydatids occur in only about 2% of cases (Musacchio and Mitchell, 1966). **The hydatid is the larval form of *Echinococcus granulosus*, whose definitive host is the dog and whose principal intermediate host is the sheep.** The major endemic loci of hydatid disease are sheep-herding areas, such as Australia, Argentina, Greece, Spain, and the Middle East. In addition, feral life cycles lead to sporadic human cases in sites without sheep. Echinococcal cysts of other species are found in Alaska, Siberia, parts of Europe (*Echinococcus multilocularis*) (Rausch, 1967), and Central America (*Echinococcus vogeli*) (D'Alessandro, 1979). In each instance, humans acquire the cysts by accidentally eating eggs excreted in the feces of dogs or alternative feral hosts.

In the kidney and other sites, hydatid cysts evolve by slow, asymptomatic, concentric growth over years and may invoke pressure symptoms or flank pain, depending on their location and size. Cysts can reach over 20 cm in diameter (Fig. 14–14). A host fibrous shell with scant inflammatory reaction envelops the cyst.

The most common urologic presentation is of **chronic dull flank or lower back discomfort from cystic pressure** (Gogus et al, 2003). The cysts seldom affect renal function. Diagnosis can be made by plain film radiography, ultrasonography, or CT, which show a thick-walled, fluid-filled spherical cyst, often with a calcific cyst wall (Horchani et al, 2001). Serologic testing (available through state laboratories or the CDC) has proved useful but has a sensitivity of only 60% to 90%. **Albendazole, 400 mg twice daily for 1 to 6 months, is the recommended medical therapy. Some patients may require surgical excision of their cysts owing to the size or location of the lesions** (Handa and Harjai, 2005). **Praziquantel and albendazole have been recommended preoperatively or in the case of operative spillage of cyst contents** (The Medical Letter, 2004). Rupture of cysts may result in systemic anaphylaxis. Spillage of cystic products into the peritoneum or the bloodstream may result in metastatic cysts.

Amebiasis

E. histolytica **is a rare cause of renal abscess** (Brandt and Perez Tamayo, 1970). Liver abscesses invariably accompany the abscess. The right kidney is more frequently involved.

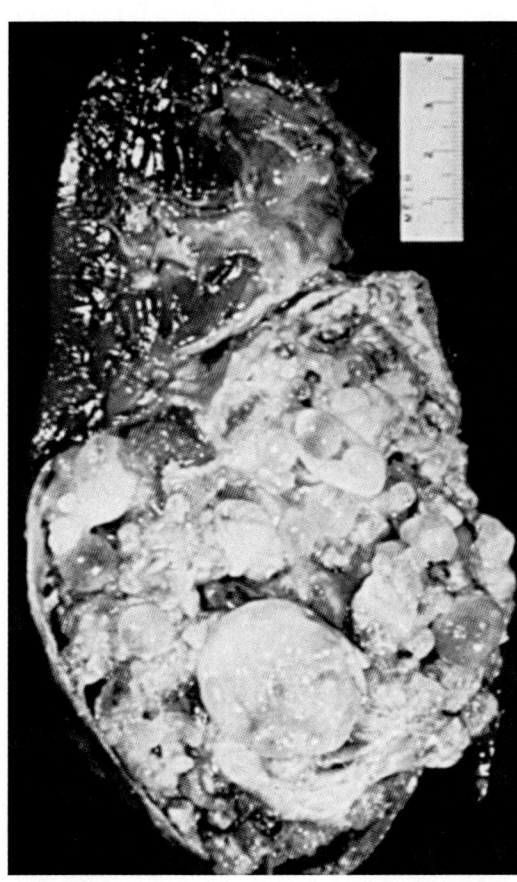

Figure 14–14. Echinococcosis of the human kidney.

Hematuria may be a prominent manifestation, especially if the abscess induces renal vein thrombosis. Medical therapy (metronidazole or tinidazole) must be promptly instituted (The Medical Letter, 2004). Surgery, if necessary, should be delayed until drug therapy has been initiated; otherwise, disastrous spread of amebic infection is likely (Grigsby, 1969). Good reviews on the pathology (Brandt and Perez Tamayo, 1970), surgery (Grigsby, 1969), and medical management of amebiasis (Ravdin, 2000) are available.

FUNGAL DISEASES OF THE GENITOURINARY SYSTEM

The genitourinary tract is rarely the site of primary fungal infection, with the exception of *Candida* species; however, it may be involved as part of a systemic infection. Aspergillosis, cryptococcosis, and phycomycosis are usually encountered in the genitourinary tract as part of the disseminated disease in the immunocompromised host. Blastomycosis, histoplasmosis, and coccidioidomycosis may involve the genitourinary tract as either part of a primary infection or as the result of "reactivation" disease in the immunocompromised patient (AIDS, corticosteroids, malignancy, neutropenia). The treatment of these infections is directed at the multisystem disease, including the genitourinary tract. There are excellent reviews and texts, which describe these diseases and their therapy (Pappas et al, 2004; The Medical Letter, 2005; Mandell et al, 2005).

Candidiasis

The terms *thrush, moniliasis,* and *yeast* have been used interchangeably to describe a clinical entity caused by fungal species of *Candida,* particularly *C. albicans.* Thrush has been known since the days of Hippocrates (Rippon, 1988). In 1890, Schmorl reported renal involvement in a patient with disseminated candidiasis. Lundquist reported primary renal mycosis in 1931 (Odds, 1988); and in 1948, Moulder described cystoscopic findings of "thrush of the urinary bladder." In the subsequent decades there has been a marked increase in candidal infections related to the use of broad-spectrum antibiotics, indwelling central venous catheters, Foley catheters, and immunosuppressive therapy (Edwards, 1991).

Epidemiology and Predisposing Factors

During the decade 1980 to 1990, approximately 350,000 infections were reported to the National Nosocomial Infections Surveillance System (NNISS) (Edwards, 1991). **Fungi were responsible for 7.9% of the infections, and *Candida* accounted for 6.2% of the total number of infections.** Recent studies revealed that *Candida* species accounted for 10.1% of intensive care unit infections, which ranked them fourth after *Pseudomonas aeruginosa* (12.4%), *Staphylococcus aureus* (12.3%), and coagulase-negative staphylococci (10.2%) (Jarvis and Martone, 1992; Zaoutis et al, 2005). Fungi, primarily *Candida,* caused 5% of infections in renal transplant patients.

The NNISS data from 1989 to 1999 indicated a significant decrease in the incidence of *C. albicans* and an increase in other *Candida* species. In this report, *C. albicans* represented

59% of candidemias followed by *C. glabrata* (12%), *C. parapsilosis* (11%), *C. tropicalis* (10%), and *C. krusei* (1.2%) (Trick et al, 2002). **Predisposing factors for candidemia and primary sites of infection included intravascular catheters (65%), total parenteral nutrition (42%), urinary tract (11%), gastrointestinal tract (8%), and respiratory tract (7%)** (Taylor et al, 1994). In a study of hospital-acquired fungemia, Klein and Watanakunakorn (1979) noted that a positive urine culture for *Candida* species occurred in 18 of 31 patients (58%) before the development of positive blood cultures, whereas urine cultures became positive in 20 of 25 patients (80%) after fungemia. **These numbers are significantly lower in asymptomatic or minimally symptomatic patients** (Kauffman, 2005).

In an extensive review of *C. albicans* urinary tract infections, Fisher and associates (1982) **cited diabetes, antibiotic administration, corticosteroid therapy, urine flow turbulence, congenital anomalies, neurogenic bladder, indwelling catheters, and ileal conduits as factors that enhance the patient's vulnerability to these infections.** Hamory and Wenzel (1978) evaluated 98 hospital patients with candiduria (>10,000 to 15,000 colonies/mL). Patients who developed candiduria had a longer period of urethral catheter drainage (12 vs. 6 days) and antibiotic therapy (16 vs. 7 days) than non-candiduria patients.

In a multicenter study of 861 patients with a documented single episode of candiduria, the major associated illnesses included diabetes mellitus (39%), urinary tract disease (37.7%), malignancy (22.2%), and malnutrition (17%). Surgical procedures were associated with candiduria in 52.3% of patients. Indwelling urethral catheters were present in 77.6% of patients. Microbiologic and clinical outcomes were documented in 61.1% of patients. There were 105 deaths (19.8%) in this series, of which 2 (0.4%) were directly attributable to candidiasis, whereas the majority of deaths were related to comorbid conditions (Kauffman et al, 2000).

Clinical Manifestations

Cutaneous Infection. Candidal infection can occur in the skin around ileostomies and cutaneous pyelostomies (Schonebeck, 1986). Postoperative wound infections cause erythema and pustules at the incision site (Wise, 1989). Identification of the fungus by smear or culture of the wound exudate confirms the diagnosis; and if it is an isolated finding the infection can be treated with topical antifungal agents. However, cutaneous infection may be a sign of disseminated disease and other potential sites of infection such as the oral cavity, respiratory system, gastrointestinal tract, and genitourinary system should be evaluated.

Infection of the Female Genitalia. Vulvovaginitis is commonly caused by *C. albicans*. In addition to the previously mentioned risk factors, oral contraceptives and pregnancy put women at increased risk for vulvovaginitis. AIDS also increases the vulnerability to vaginal colonization and persistent infection (Schuman et al, 1998). Clinical signs include yellowish white vaginal discharge and gray-white pseudomembranous exudate in the vagina and vulva. Pruritic symptoms are proportional to the number of organisms found in the vaginal discharge (Odds, 1988). Diagnosis can be established by microscopic detection of *Candida* species

in vaginal exudate or by culture. **Treatment with oral fluconazole (a single 150-mg dose)** (The Medical Letter, 2005) **is as effective as topical intravaginal therapy in the treatment of vulvovaginal candidiasis** (Table 14–4) (Andersen et al, 1989). Recurrent infections are more difficult to eradicate and may require weekly therapy (Sobel et al, 2004).

Infection of the Male Genitalia. In a study of 135 unselected men, *C. albicans* was the most frequent "yeast" found in the coronal sulcus and meatus. The incidence was similar in both circumcised (14%) and uncircumcised (17%) men; however, clinical manifestations of infection were greater in uncircumcised men (Davidson, 1977). These patients can be treated with topical therapy in most cases. Epididymitis and orchitis are unusual manifestations of candidal infection that are managed with systemic therapy and possibly surgery.

Infection of the Bladder and Prostate. The patient with candiduria is usually asymptomatic. Only 4% of patients in a multicenter study of 861 patients with candiduria had frequency, dysuria, urgency, hematuria, or renal colic (Kauffman et al, 2000). Cystoscopy may demonstrate white patches on the bladder wall and areas of mucosal edema and erythema (Hopfer, 1985; Rippon, 1988). A gray-white "snow effect" may obscure visualization. Microscopic examination of the exudate demonstrates inflammatory cells, among which yeast forms and pseudohyphae can be seen (Zincke et al, 1973). Accretions of the candidal pseudohyphae can develop with formation of fungus balls that may require surgical removal (Fig. 14–15) (Chisholm and Hutch, 1961; Harold et al, 1977). Emphysematous cystitis has been observed in diabetic patients (Comiter et al, 1996; Singh and Lytle, 1983). Therapy is discussed in the treatment section (see Table 14–4).

Prostatic emphysematosa secondary to *C. albicans* has been reported in diabetic patients. Emphysematous prostatitis or prostatic abscesses require 4 to 6 weeks of systemic therapy with surgical drainage, preferably performed in a transurethral manner (Yu and Provet, 1992; Lentino et al, 1984) (Fig. 14–16).

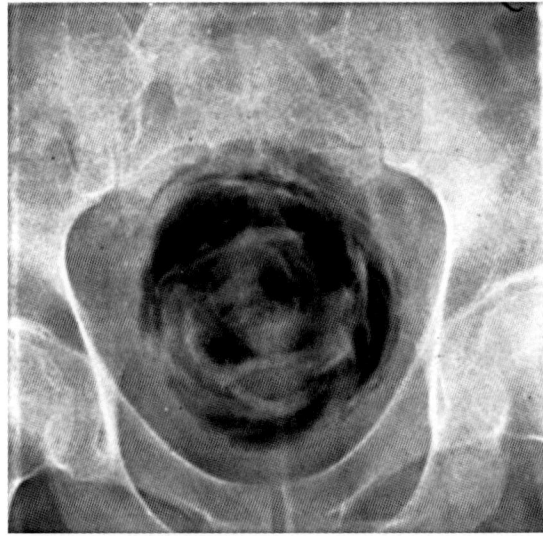

Figure 14–15. Radiographic appearance of a large fungal bezoar in the bladder of 48-year-old diabetic man.

Table 14-4. Treatment of Fungal Infections

Infection/Drug of Choice	Dosage*	Duration†	Alternatives
Aspergillosis			
Amphotericin B	1-1.5 mg/kg/day IV‡	> 10 wk	Itraconazole, 200 mg
Voriconazole§	6 mg/kg IV q12h × 1 day, then 4 mg/kg IV q12h, then 200 mg PO bid		IV bid × 2 days, then 200 mg IV qd × 12 days or 200 mg PO tid × 3 days; either followed by 200 mg PO bid Caspofungin 70 mg IV × 1day, then 50 mg IV once daily
Blastomycosis¶			
Itraconazole	200 mg PO bid	6-12 mo	Fluconazole 400-800 mg PO once daily
Amphotericin B	0.5-1.0 mg/kg/day IV3	6-12 wk	
Candidiasis¶			
*Vulvovaginal Topical Therapy***			
Butoconazole, clotrimazole, miconazole, tioconazole, or terconazole	Once daily (available as intravaginal creams, ointments, tablets, ovules or suppositories)	1-7 days	
Systemic Therapy			
Fluconazole	150 mg PO once††	1 day	Itraconazole 200 mg PO bid × 1 day Ketoconazole 200 mg PO bid × 5 days
Candidemia¶			
Fluconazole	400-800 mg IV once daily, followed by PO	2 wk after afebrile and blood cultures negative	
Caspofungin	70 mg IV × 1 day, then 50 mg IV once daily		
Amphotericin B	0.5-1 mg/kg/day IV‡		
Urinary‡‡			
Fluconazole	200 mg IV or PO once daily	7-14 days	Flucytosine 25 mg/kg PO qid¶¶¶
Amphotericin B§§	0.3-0.5 mg/kg/day IV‡	7-14 days	
Coccidioidomycosis¶¶			
Itraconazole	200 mg PO bid	>1 yr	
Fluconazole	400-800 mg PO once daily	>1 yr	
Amphotericin B	0.5-0.7 mg/kg/day IV‡	>1 yr	
Cryptococcosis			
Amphotericin B + Flucytosine followed by	0.5-1 mg/kg/day IV‡ 100 mg/kg/d PO	2 wk	
Fluconazole	400 mg PO once daily	8 wk	Itraconazole 200 mg PO bid
Maintenance***	200 mg PO once daily		Amphotericin B 0.5-1 mg/kg IV weekly‡
Histoplasmosis¶			
Itraconazole	200 mg PO bid	6-18 mo	Fluconazole 400-800 mg PO once daily
Amphotericin B	0.5-1.0 mg/kg/day IV‡	10-12 wk	
Chronic Suppression*			
Itraconazole	200 mg PO once daily or bid		Amphotericin B 0.5-1 mg/kg IV weekly‡
Mucormycosis			
Amphotericin B	1-1.5 mg/kg/day IV‡	6-10 wk	

*Usual dosage. Some patients may need dosage adjustment for renal or hepatic dysfunction or when used with interacting drugs.

†The optimal duration of treatment with these drugs is often unclear. Depending on the disease and its severity, they may be continued for weeks or months or, particularly in immunocompromised patients, indefinitely.

‡Dosage of amphotericin B deoxycholate. Usual doses of lipid-based formulations for treatment of invasive fungal infection are amphotericin B lipid complex (Abelcet), 5 mg/kg/day; liposomal amphotericin B (AmBisome), 3-5 mg/kg/day; amphotericin B cholesteryl sulfate (Amphotec), 3-4 mg/kg/day. For treatment of aspergillosis and mucormycosis, the dosage of AmBisome is 5 mg/kg/day and doses up to 15 mg/kg/d have been used. For treatment of cryptococcal meningitis in HIV-infected patients, the dosage of AmBisome is 6 mg/kg/day.

§In one large controlled trial, voriconazole was more effective than amphotericin B for treatment of invasive aspergillosis (Herbrecht R, et al: N Engl J Med 2002;347:408).

¶Patients with severe illness or central nervous system involvement should receive amphotericin B.

¶¶*Candida albicans* is generally highly susceptible to fluconazole. *C. krusei* infections are resistant to fluconazole. *C. glabrata* infections are often resistant to low doses but may be susceptible to high doses of fluconazole. *C. lusitaniae* may be resistant to amphotericin B.

**Non–*C. albicans* species, such as *C. glabrata* and *C. krusei*, respond to boric acid, 600 mg intravaginally daily × 14 days, or to topical flucytosine cream (Sobel JD, et al: Am J Obstet Gynecol 2003;189:1297).

††May be repeated in 72 hours if patient remains symptomatic.

‡‡Asymptomatic candiduria usually does not require treatment.

§§Bladder irrigation with amphotericin B has been used to treat candidal cystitis but does not treat disease beyond the bladder.

¶¶¶Divided into four doses every 6 hours. Dosage must be decreased in patients with diminished renal function. When given with amphotericin B, some physicians recommend beginning flucytosine at 75 mg/kg/day divided q6h, until the degree of amphotericin nephrotoxicity becomes clear or flucytosine blood levels can be determined.

"Itraconazole is the drug of choice for nonmeningeal coccidioidomycosis.

***Suppressive for patients with HIV infection.

Adapted from The Medical Letter: Antifungal Drugs. Treatment Guidelines from The Medical Letter 2005;30:7-14.

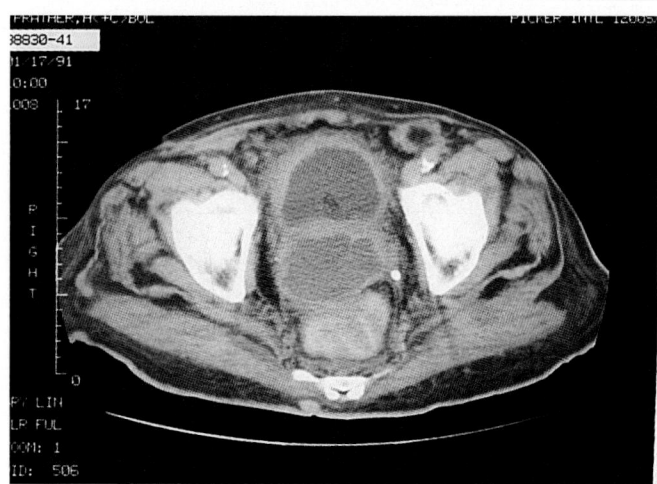

Figure 14–16. CT demonstrates a prostatic abscess cavity caused by *Candida*. (From Yu S, Provet J: Prostatic abscess due to *Candida tropicalis* in a non-acquired immunodeficiency syndrome patient. J Urol 1992;148: 1536-1538.)

Infection of the Ureter and Kidney. Candidal renal infection may present as a classic pyelonephritis with flank pain and fever. The upper tract of the urinary system is subject to the same risks for infection as the lower urinary tract and may have additional vulnerability in the presence of an obstructive uropathy (Blum, 1966; Shelp et al, 1966). Renal colic may be caused by the passage of fungal balls that obstruct the collecting system. **The kidney is a major target organ associated with candidemia** (Luno and Tortoledo, 1985). Genitourinary candidal infection may be either the result or the cause of systemic infection. Experimental and clinical studies indicate that hematogenous candidal infection can cause pyelonephritis, abscess formation, papillary necrosis, and obstruction (Hurley and Winner, 1963; Lehner, 1964). Microscopic study demonstrates yeast forms or pseudohyphae in the glomeruli, interstitium, and tubules. The proliferation of tubular pseudohyphae causes intrarenal obstructive uropathy. In later stages of hematogenous infection, larger fungal accretions develop that can cause obstruction of the renal collecting system (Louria et al, 1962; Hurley and Winner, 1963; Luno and Tortoledo, 1985).

In a retrospective study of 50 patients with genitourinary fungal infections, 25 (50%) had "complex" infections as defined by upper tract involvement and/or a positive culture requiring systemic antifungal therapy. The other 25 patients (50%) had "simple" infections that were confined to the bladder. Obstructive uropathy was associated with 88% of patients with complex infections and 20% of patients with simple infections. Fourteen patients (56%) required surgical intervention (Weinstein et al, 1995).

Fungal accretions are known to cause ureteral (Keane at al, 1993) or UPJ obstruction (Stein et al, 1993; Scerpella and Alhalel, 1994). Diagnosis is established by the identification of fungi in the urine and imaging studies (ultrasound, intravenous urography, CT) that document obstructive uropathy and/or soft tissue densities within the renal collecting system, pelvis, or ureter (Stein et al, 1993).

Predisposing conditions for **pyelonephritis** include candidal cystitis, ileal conduits (Schonebeck, 1986), and chronic neurogenic bladder disease (Sandin et al, 1991). Histologic findings in the renal pelvis may be similar to those found in the bladder, namely, edema, erythema, and pseudoexudate (Hopfer, 1985). Candidal organisms have also been found in association with renal pelvic lithiasis (Sales and Mundy, 1973; Bhattacharya et al, 1982). For the treatment of these infections, nephrostomy tubes and systemic antifungal agents have been utilized with success (Bell et al, 1993; Scerpella and Alhalel, 1994).

Perinephric abscesses secondary to *Candida* have been reported primarily in diabetic patients. Predisposing factors were noted to be surgery (including renal transplantation) and prolonged antibiotic therapy. Fever and flank pain were the most common clinical findings. Treatment with systemic therapy and surgical drainage or nephrectomy may be required (High and Quagliarello, 1992).

Systemic Candidal Infection and Co-infection. Disseminated candidal infection is documented by culture of *Candida* species from other sites, such as blood, wound, oropharynx, or gastrointestinal tract. Funduscopic examination may demonstrate retinal exudate caused by candidal endophthalmitis (Kozinn et al, 1978). Candidemia may also occur synchronously or metachronously with staphylococcal or enterococcal infections (Meunier-Carpentier et al, 1981) or bacteremia secondary to *Klebsiella, Serratia, Bacteroides, Enterobacter,* and *Proteus* species or *Escherichia coli* (Dyess et al, 1985). In a study of 83 patients with fungemia, Dyess and colleagues (1985) noted that 17% of blood cultures were positive for bacteria before fungemia whereas 28 blood cultures (20%) had synchronous bacterial and fungal positivity.

Candidal Infection in Pediatric Patients. Indwelling intravascular catheters, broad-spectrum antibiotics, prematurity, and low birth weight have been associated with the development of renal candidal infection in infants (Robinson et al, 1987), with *C. albicans* being the most prevalent organism. A 1993 survey indicated that candidemia accounted for 21% of the nosocomial bloodstream infections in children, and intravenous lines, prolonged hyperalimentation, and candiduria were cited as significant risk factors (MacDonald et al, 1998). The manifestation, diagnosis, and evaluation is similar to that of adults; however, a delay in the diagnosis for pediatric patients resulted in a 50% mortality rate (Noe and Tonkin, 1982; Bartone et al, 1988). Percutaneous nephrostomy tubes or pyelotomies and systemic antifungal therapy are utilized for treatment (Gokhale et al, 1993; Keizer et al, 1993).

Diagnosis

Microscopic examination of the urine reveals *Candida* with budding forms or pseudohyphae. Pyuria and hematuria may be present but are not specific findings. Urinary casts containing fungal material are diagnostic of renal infection and are demonstrated by Papanicolaou stain (Gregory et al, 1984). *Candida* species can also be cultured from the urine using a variety of laboratory media. Species differentiation is dependent on germ tube growth and carbohydrate fermentation (Hopfer, 1985).

Urinary candidal colony counts are usually not helpful in differentiating colonization from infection, particularly in the presence of indwelling urinary catheters (Navarro et al, 1997).

Furthermore, there are no laboratory studies that reliably indicate an upper tract or invasive infection (Fisher et al, 1995). Blood cultures, for example, were positive in fewer than half of patients with histologically proven renal candidiasis (Kozinn et al, 1978). Whole-cell agglutination, agar cell diffusion, latex agglutination, counterimmunoelectrophoresis, antibody-coated latex particles, and radioimmunoassays have been utilized to help improve diagnosis but with unreliable results (de Repentigny and Reiss, 1984; Suits et al, 1989; de Repentigny, 1992). PCR, on the other hand, can identify candidal cellular components (Buchman et al, 1990; Kan, 1993). PCR amplification of the candidal actin gene provided a 100% sensitivity and specificity for the detection of candiduria (Muncan and Wise, 1996), **making the use of PCR efficacious for the detection of occult candidemia in critically ill patients** (Talluri et al, 1998).

Radiography

Candida species can form accretions, known as fungal balls or bezoars, which cause obstruction of the urinary collecting system, pelvis, ureter, or bladder. Cystography and intravenous, retrograde, or percutaneous pyelography may delineate filling defects caused by these bezoars (Fig. 14–17)

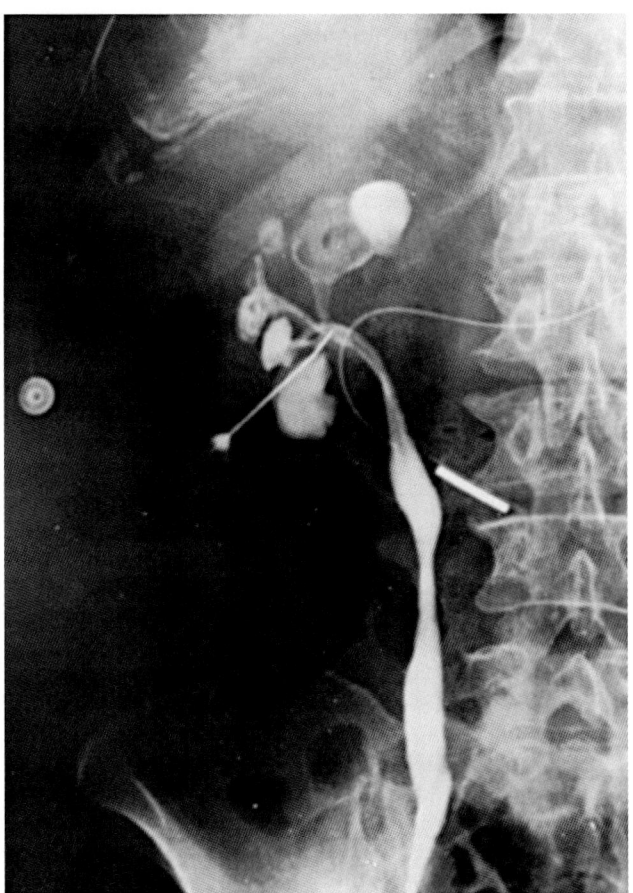

Figure 14–17. Antegrade nephrostogram demonstrates a filling defect caused by fungal accretion. (From Wise GJ: Genitourinary candidal infection. AUA Update Series 1989;8:197.)

(Chisholm and Hutch, 1961; Blum, 1966; Shelp et al, 1966; Bhattacharya et al, 1982; Beilke and Kirmani, 1988). Nephrostomy tubes also provide access for the collection of material for microscopic study or culture, drainage, and access for percutaneous removal of a fungal bezoar (Bartone et al, 1988; Doemeny et al, 1988). Other radiographic modalities are ultrasonography and CT, which can demonstrate fungal material within the collecting system (Dembner and Pfister, 1977; Aragona et al, 1985) and evaluate for urinary obstruction. In CT studies of the renal collecting system, the fungal accretion appears as a mass lesion with less attenuation than a calculus (Doemeny et al, 1988). Magnetic resonance imaging has little clinical relevance for the evaluation of fungal infections.

Treatment

The treatment of candiduria is controversial because there are no strict criteria for distinguishing colonization from infection and there have been few controlled treatment trials. **It should be emphasized that *Candida* species in the urine may represent contamination of the specimen during collection or colonization, without true infection. However, the persistence of candiduria requires evaluation and consideration of treatment.** The Infectious Diseases Society of America has developed guidelines for the treatment of candidal infections (Pappas et al, 2004). **It has recommended systemic antifungal therapy in very low birth weight infants, in patients undergoing renal transplantation or urinary tract instrumentation, and in symptomatic patients.** Table 14–4 lists the recommended drugs, dosages, and duration of therapy for the different types of *Candida* infections (The Medical Letter, 2005).

Removal of an indwelling urinary catheter or intravenous line, cessation of antibiotic therapy, and improvement of nutritional status may eliminate candidal colonization or infection (Urinary tract candidosis, 1988). Elimination of hyperalimentation catheters has decreased the number of episodes of fungemia (Klein and Watanakunakorn, 1979). These authors have noted similar findings after the removal or change of indwelling urethral catheters or ureteral stents. In a multicenter study of 861 patients with a single episode of candiduria, 14% resolved spontaneously. Forty-one (35%) of 116 patients cleared their funguria with catheter removal alone (Kauffman et al, 2000).

The persistence of candiduria in some patients is not uncommon in clinical practice. Furthermore, asymptomatic candiduria does not lead to candidemia or pyelonephritis in most patients. It is also an uncommon cause of chronic renal failure in the absence of obstruction. If candiduria does not resolve after removal of the indwelling urinary catheter or stopping the antibiotic therapy, then the initiation of treatment can be considered.

Systemic Treatment for Urinary Tract Infection. Fluconazole administered by mouth or by intravenous route achieves high urine levels (Urinary tract candidosis, 1988). Orally administered fluconazole (100 mg twice daily for 10 days) eradicated candiduria in 19 of 20 critically ill patients (Nassoura et al, 1993) and achieved eradication rates similar to that for amphotericin bladder irrigations (Fan-Harvard et al, 1995). An elevated serum creatinine value was associated with a reduced rate of fungal eradication from the urine related to lower urinary levels of fluconazole (Sobel et al, 2000). **Fluconazole is active against most *Candida* species, except *C. krusei* and many strains of *C. glabrata*.**

Miconazole and ketoconazole are poorly excreted by the kidney, have low urinary concentrations, and are inferior to fluconazole. Flucytosine is not recommended for candidal urinary tract infection because of its potentially lethal bone marrow toxicity, colitis, and the rapid development of drug resistance when used alone.

Intravenous amphotericin B has been used to control recalcitrant urinary candidal infection (Fisher et al, 1995). Intravenous liposomal amphotericin B has been used, but there is concern over whether it achieves adequate urinary levels in those with compromised renal function (Ralph et al, 1991; Agustin et al, 1999).

Local Treatment of Urinary Tract Infections. Irrigation of the bladder with amphotericin B via a Foley catheter can be considered but does not appear to offer any advantage over oral or intravenous therapy. Bladder irrigation with amphotericin may clear the candiduria more rapidly than intravenous amphotericin or oral fluconazole, but eradication rates 1 to 4 weeks after treatment were similar for all regimens (Leu and Huang, 1995). **Most studies utilized a dose of 50 mg of amphotericin B/1000 mL of water or 5% dextrose/water administered at 40 mL/hr (1 L/day).**

Localized renal pelvic and collecting system candidal infections have also been treated successfully with amphotericin B irrigants with dose schedules similar to those of bladder irrigations (Wise et al, 1982). Low-dose amphotericin B (10 to 24 mg/day for up to 15 days) has been advocated as a renal irrigation in infants with localized upper tract candidiasis (Bartone et al, 1988).

Systemic Therapy for Treatment of Invasive or Disseminated Infection. Patients with candidemia and invasive disease may be treated with either fluconazole, caspofungin, or amphotericin B (see Table 14–4) (The Medical Letter, 2005). The choice of drugs will be influenced by cost (Table 14–5), intravenous access, drug toxicity, and the patient's comorbidities. Consultation with an infectious diseases expert is recommended for these patients with multisystem invasive disease. Amphotericin B has been the "gold standard" for treatment of patients with invasive or disseminated infection; however, caspofungin also has been shown to be effective. Fluconazole, given intravenously and then orally for at least 2 weeks, is also efficacious (see Table 14–4).

Percutaneous, Endoscopic, and Surgical Treatment. Foley catheter placement, ureteral stenting, or placement of a percutaneous nephrostomy tube may be necessary in the case of an obstructive uropathy caused by a candidal infection. If these drainage tubes are chronic, they may need to be changed to facilitate the eradication of the infection. These interventions should be used in conjunction with antifungal treatment by irrigant and/or systemic therapy. **Definitive correction of a urogenital anomaly (i.e., by pyeloplasty) or acquired disease (i.e., bladder outlet obstruction) should only be undertaken after eradication of the infection** (Ang et al, 1993).

Table 14–5. Cost of Antifungal Agents

Drug	Daily Dosage	Cost($)*
Amphotericin B Formulations		
Amphotericin B deoxycholate generic (Abbott)	1-1.5 mg/kg IV	23.28
Fungizone (Sandoz)		40.90
Amphotericin B lipid complex (ABLC)	5 mg/kg IV	920.00
Abelcet (Enzon)		
Liposomal amphotericin B (L-AmB)	3-5 mg/kg IV	1318.80
AmBisome (Fujisawa)		
Amphotericin B colloidal dispersion (ABCD)	3-4 mg/kg IV	480.00
Amphotec (InterMune)		
Azoles (Parenteral)		
Fluconazole Diflucan (Pfizer)	200-400 mg IV once	162.19
Itraconazole Sporanox (Ortho Biotech)	200 mg IV once	203.44
Voriconazole Vfend (Pfizer)	4 mg/kg IV q12h	315.18
Echinocandin		
Caspofungin Cancidas (Merck)	50 mg IV once	372.68
Azoles (Oral)		
Fluconazole-average generic Diflucan (Pfizer)	200-400 mg PO once	28.77 30.74
Itraconazole Sporanox (Janssen)	200 mg PO bid	39.60
Voriconazole Vfend (Pfizer)	200 mg PO q12h	67.36

*For one day's treatment of a 70-kg patient at the highest usual dosage, according to AWP listings in Red Book 2004 and Update January 2005. Cost may vary among institutions based on formulary contracts.
Adapted from The Medical Letter: Antifungal Drugs. Treatment Guidelines from The Medical Letter 2005;30:7-14.

Other Fungal Infections of the Genitourinary Tract

Aspergillosis

Epidemiology and Predisposing Factors. Aspergillosis is a major cause of morbidity and mortality in immunocompromised patients. *Aspergillus* is recognized as causing a variety of pulmonary illnesses, including asthma, allergic alveolitis, and cavitary aspergillomas. Primary extrapulmonary foci of *Aspergillus* infection is uncommon but may cause cutaneous, naso-orbital, and genitourinary disease (Flechner and McAninch, 1981; Cross, 1987; Rippon, 1988).

The most common infecting species, in decreasing frequency, are *A. fumigatus*, *A. flavus*, *A. terreus*, and *A. niger*. **Aspergilli are ubiquitous in the environment and can be found throughout the world in soil, water, food, and air. Outbreaks of disease have been attributed to contaminated air conditioning systems, surgical theaters, dialysis fluid, and construction dust. Disseminated *Aspergillus* is a major opportunistic fungus in patients compromised by malignancy, diabetes mellitus, AIDS, immunosuppressive agents,**

and organ transplantation (Gallis et al, 1975; Gustafson et al, 1983; Asnis et al, 1988).

Genitourinary Manifestations. Young and coworkers (1970) analyzed postmortem studies of 98 patients with aspergillosis. In most patients, the primary underlying diagnosis was leukemia or lymphoma. Aspergilli infected the pulmonary tract in 92 patients (94%), the gastrointestinal tract in 21 (23%), the brain in 19 (21%), the liver in 12 (13%), and the kidney in 12 (13%). The infected kidneys demonstrated multiple small focal abscesses, vascular occlusion by fungi, and multiple renal infarcts.

Renal aspergillosis may present as flank pain, renal tenderness, and fever. Radiographic studies demonstrate filling defects within the collecting system that are unilateral or bilateral (Fig. 14–18) (Irby et al, 1990). Primary renal aspergillar infection with obstructive uropathy has been associated with diabetes mellitus and intravenous drug abuse (Melchior et al, 1972; Warshawsky et al, 1975; Flechner and McAninch, 1981; Godec et al, 1989). Renal aspergillomas or pseudotumors have developed in AIDS patients (Halpern et al, 1992; Piketty et al, 1993; Viale et al, 1995; Martinez-Jabaloyas et al, 1995).

Prostatic aspergillar infection has been reported in four patients (Abbas et al, 1995). All patients presented with signs and symptoms of bladder outlet obstruction. Predisposing medical conditions included prolonged antibiotic use, diabetes mellitus, chronic corticosteroid use, and indwelling bladder catheter.

Diagnosis and Treatment. Aspergillar infection can be established by identification (with methenamine silver or periodic acid–Schiff [PAS] stain) of the fungus in the urine or in tissue removed from the infected organ. *Aspergillus* species

differ from agents of zygomycosis, which have broader, nonseptate branching hyphae. Tissue or excreted material can also be cultured in Sabouraud's medium or brain-enriched infusion broths (Cross, 1987). Blood cultures are often negative. Finally, immune diffusion or radioimmunoassay serologic studies may be helpful in determining diagnosis (de Repentigny and Reiss, 1984; Rippon, 1988). The use of PCR amplification has provided a more sensitive method to detect *Aspergillus* in blood and urine (Reddy et al, 1993).

The outcome of therapy is extremely poor in invasive aspergillosis, with mortality rates of 40% to 90%. Amphotericin B desoxycholate was traditionally the drug of choice. **Current recommendations are to use either amphotericin in one of its lipid formulations or one of the newer azoles (voriconazole, itraconazole) or an echinocandin (caspofungin)** (see Table 14–4) (Ostrosky-Zeichner et al, 2003; The Medical Letter, 2005).

Cryptococcosis

Epidemiology and Predisposing Factors. *Cryptococcus neoformans* infection most commonly involves the lung and the central nervous system. The skin, eye, prostate, and other organs may also be involved as part of a disseminated infection. **C. neoformans thrives in any environment inhabited by birds and is readily found in old attics, buildings, and barn lofts.** After inhalation, the fungus may cause a pulmonary infection that can be asymptomatic or develop into a virulent respiratory infection that mimics severe bacterial pneumonia. The pulmonary infection may be self-limiting with the formation of residual pulmonary calcification and granulomas. Compromise of the patient's immune system however increases vulnerability for disseminated infection. In a study of 99 immunocompromised patients with fungemia, *C. neoformans* accounted for 22% of positive blood cultures (*C. albicans*, 48%; other *Candida* species and fungi, 30%) (Perduca et al, 1995). AIDS patients are at increased risk to develop disseminated cryptococcal infection (Kovacs et al, 1985; Scully et al, 1987; Chuck and Sande, 1989). The central nervous system is the primary target of hematogenous spread with resultant meningitis and meningoencephalitis.

Genitourinary Manifestations. In a pre-AIDS era postmortem study of 39 patients with disseminated cryptococcal infection, 20 (51%) had renal involvement, whereas 6 of the 23 male patients (26%) had prostatic infection (Salyer and Salyer, 1973). Renal findings revealed focal abscesses confined primarily to the cortex. Cryptococcal prostatic lesions varied from small chronic inflammatory changes to large granulomas with caseation (Salyer and Salyer, 1973). Before the era of AIDS, the clinical diagnosis of prostatic cryptococcal infection was rare (Braman, 1981). Prostatic cryptococcosis has been reported in patients with diabetes mellitus (Huyn and Reyes, 1982), lymphoma (King et al, 1990), and alcohol abuse (Hinchey and Someren, 1981).

In AIDS patients, the prostate has been recognized as a "reservoir" for relapsing cryptococcosis, following successful treatment for cryptococcal meningitis (Fig. 14–19) (Larsen et al, 1989). After 6 weeks of systemic amphotericin B and flucytosine for cryptococcal meningitis, 9 (22%) of 41 AIDS patients developed positive urine cultures. It is now recommended that these AIDS patients be maintained on

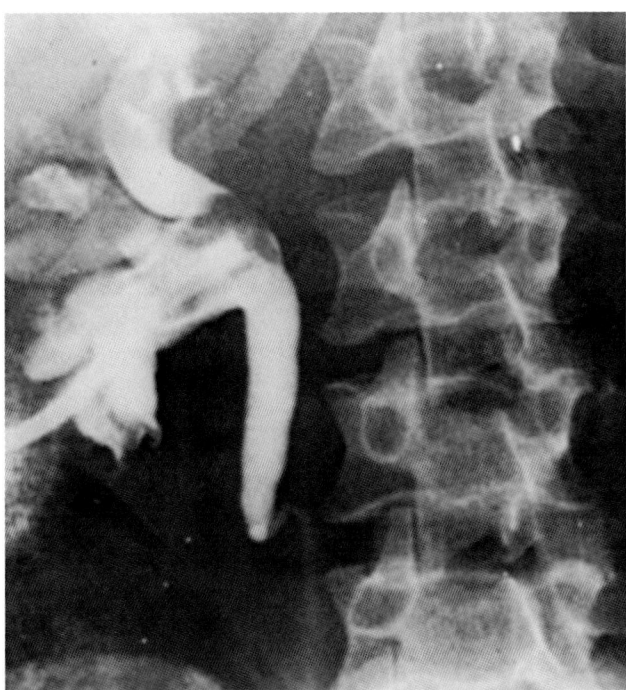

Figure 14–18. Nephrostogram demonstrates an *Aspergillus* bezoar. (From Irby PB, Stoller ML, McAninch JW: Fungal bezoars of the upper urinary tract. J Urol 1990;143:447.)

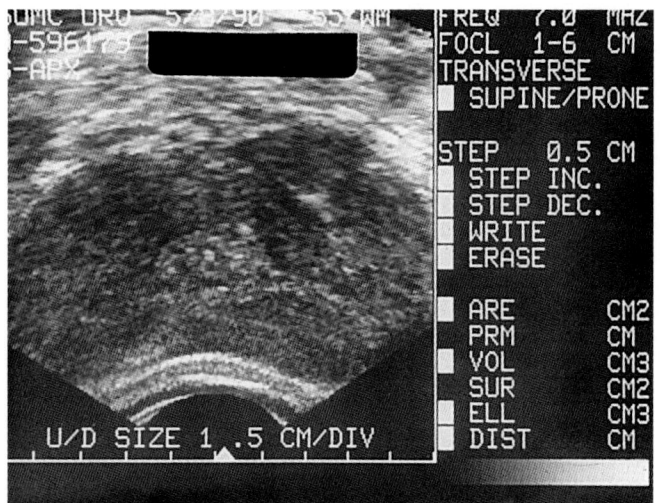

Figure 14–19. Transrectal ultrasonogram demonstrates findings in a prostate with cryptococcosis. (From Adams JR Jr, Mata JA, Culkin DJ, et al: Acquired immunodeficiency syndrome manifesting as prostate nodule secondary to cryptococcal infection. Urology 1992;39:289-291.)

suppressive doses of fluconazole after completing the standard course of therapy (see Table 14–4) (Bozzette et al, 1991; The Medical Letter, 2005).

Unusual manifestations of genital cryptococcal infection have been reported, including epididymo-orchitis and penile lesions (Perfect and Seaworth, 1985; Vapnek and McAninch, 1990; James and Lomax-Smith, 1991). The penile lesions have varied from a glans ulcer to a large exophytic lesion (Concus et al, 1988).

Diagnosis and Treatment. *Cryptococcus* can be cultured from urine, cerebrospinal fluid, or other infected fluid on most fungal and bacterial media. Direct examination of infected fluid with India ink stain may reveal budding yeast with capsule (Rippon, 1988). *C. neoformans* may be identified in tissue by PAS or methenamine silver stain. Latex agglutination and enzyme immunoassay tests are very sensitive and specific in detecting cryptococcal antigen in cerebrospinal fluid and serum (Jaye et al, 1998). Cryptococcal antigen has also been found in urine of patients with AIDS (Chapin-Robertson et al, 1993). **Amphotericin and/or fluconazole are the drugs of choice for cryptococcosis** (see Table 14–4).

Phycomycosis (Mucormycosis, Zygomycosis)

The taxonomic class Zygomycetes contains the family Mucoraceae with the genera *Rhizopus, Rhizomucor, Mucor,* and *Absidia.* Each genus includes species that can cause disease in humans (Rippon, 1988). These fungi have worldwide distribution and can be readily found in the soil and in wild or domestic animals. Disease in humans may cause rhinocerebral infection that involves the sinus, pharynx, meninges, and brain. Pulmonary infection has been associated with hematologic malignancies, whereas gastrointestinal infection has been noted in malnourished children (Scully et al, 1988). The diagnosis is established by demonstrating the organism in tissue.

Renal involvement with and without associated disseminated disease is rare but has been reported (Prout and Goddard, 1960; Langston et al, 1973; Low et al, 1974; Dansky et al, 1978; Sane and Deshmukh, 1988; Davila et al, 1991; Santos et al, 1994). Renal zygomycosis (mucormycosis) may cause acute illness with signs of sepsis, associated with fungus-induced obstructive uropathy and renal infection. Extensive renal involvement with pseudotumor has developed in AIDS patients (Vesa, 1992; Carvalhal et al, 1997; Guardia et al, 2000).

Untreated renal mucormycosis has a mortality rate exceeding 90% (Davila et al, 1991). Treatment with nephrectomy and systemic amphotericin B (see Table 14–4) has resulted in 76% survival. Medical management of renal infection with amphotericin B lipid complex and granulocyte colony-stimulating factor has also been reported (Weng et al, 1998).

Blastomycosis

Epidemiology and Predisposing Factors. The fungus *Blastomyces dermatitidis* is endemic in the basins of the Ohio, Missouri, and Mississippi rivers. It has also been found in the Great Lakes region and Canada; thus, the illness that it causes has been known as North American blastomycosis. Cases, however, have been reported in Africa, the Middle East, and Asia (Rippon, 1988). The North American fungus primarily causes pulmonary infection, and the African isolates cause skin and bone lesions (Blastomycosis, 1989). A different fungus, *Paracoccidioides brasiliensis,* is known for causing a South American blastomycosis.

The natural habitat and ecology of *B. dermatitidis* has not been well defined; however, the fungus has a predilection for moist soil with a high organic content (Rippon, 1988). After inhalation of the fungal spores, a pulmonary infection may develop that is often subclinical and self-limiting. The infection often remains dormant but may disseminate by hematogenous or lymphatic route to extrapulmonary sites, such as the skin, bones, and genitourinary system. Isolated cutaneous lesions have occurred after laboratory accidents or bites by infected animals, particularly canines (Dismukes, 1986).

Blastomycosis has become more prevalent in immunocompromised patients. **Predisposing conditions have included chronic corticosteroid use, hematologic malignancy, solid tumor requiring cytotoxic or radiation therapy, solid organ or bone marrow transplantation, AIDS, end-stage renal or hepatic disease, and pregnancy.**

Genitourinary Manifestations. Genitourinary involvement occurs in 15% to 20% of patients with systemic disease (Malin et al, 1969; Eickenberg et al, 1975; Inoshita et al, 1983; Chapman et al, 2000). In a study of 51 patients with systemic blastomycosis, 11 patients (22%) had genitourinary involvement. Of these 11 patients, the epididymis was infected in 10 (91%), the prostate was infected in 8 (73%); and the kidney, testis, and prepuce each had one lesion (9%) (Eickenberg et al, 1975).

Patients with genitourinary blastomycosis may develop epididymal induration or prostatic symptoms (e.g., urinary frequency, hesitancy, nocturia, or even urinary retention). The patient may have an enlarged or fluctuant prostate. Systemic blastomycosis occurring with prostatic abscess has also been reported (Bergner et al, 1981). Conjugal transmission has been documented, in which a male developed *Blastomyces* infection of the prostate and epididymis and the female consort developed *Blastomyces* infection of the endometrium and fallopian tubes (Craig et al, 1970). Finally, genital blastomycosis has been reported in four female patients who developed tubo-ovarian abscesses caused by undiagnosed pulmonary infection or conjugal transmission (Mouzin and Beilke, 1996).

Diagnosis and Treatment. The diagnosis is established by culture or direct visualization of the organism in tissue, pus, sputum, or other secretions. Changes in chest radiographs and the development of a positive *Blastomyces* skin test are also indicative of infection. The detection of *Blastomyces* A antigen by immunodiffusion is helpful in confirming the diagnosis of prostatic and epididymal *Blastomyces* infection (Seo et al, 1997). Serologic tests utilizing complement fixation, immune diffusion, radioimmunoassay, or enzyme-linked immunosorbent assay are laboratory adjuncts (Rippon, 1988; Areno et al, 1997). The sensitivity of the serologic tests appears to be greatest in patients with the most disseminated disease (Klein et al, 1990). Detection tests for antigen in serum and in urine have also been developed (Wheat et al, 1986).

Genitourinary blastomycosis is a manifestation of disseminated disease that should be treated with amphotericin B (see Table 14–4) (Eickenberg et al, 1975; Inoshita et al, 1983). The azoles (itraconazole, fluconazole) are recommended for mild and moderate disease in immunocompetent patients (Chapman et al, 2000; The Medical Letter, 2005). Chronic therapy has also been advocated for patients with mild to moderate nonmeningeal forms of blastomycosis (Dismukes, 1986).

Coccidioidomycosis

Epidemiology and Predisposing Factors. *Coccidioides immitis* is a fungus indigenous to the semiarid regions of the western United States, Mexico, and Central and South America. The fungus thrives in soil conditions that are inhibitory to competing organisms, namely, high temperature and increased salinity (Rippon, 1988). Outbreaks of coccidioidomycosis have occurred in groups such as construction workers, farmers, and archaeologists exposed to dust containing the fungus. Urban outbreaks have also been attributed to dust storms (Drutz, 1979). An increase in the incidence has been ascribed to changes in the climate such as prolonged drought followed by heavy rain (Jinadu et al, 1994). A significant increase in the prevalence of coccidioidomycosis is attributable, in part, to the increase in the population at risk, the number of aged (>65 years old), and the numbers of immunocompromised patients (AIDS, chemotherapy, neoplastic disease) (CDC, 1996).

Pathogenesis. After inhalation of the arthroconidia, an asymptomatic and transient pulmonary infection develops in a majority of persons. A more virulent infection occurs in some cases, with radiographic changes indicative of pulmonary infiltration or cavitation. This is most common in AIDS patients. An "allergic" reaction may develop in which the patient manifests erythema nodosum, also known as "valley bumps" or "valley fever." Fewer than 1% of patients develop

extrapulmonary disease, principally involving the meninges, bone, joints, skin, and soft tissue. Risk factors for disseminated infection include pregnancy, age younger than 5 years or older than 50 years (Kuntze et al, 1988; Stevens, 1995), corticosteroid use, chemotherapy, malignancy (Einstein and Johnson, 1993), and AIDS (Abrams et al, 1984). Renal transplant patients receiving immunosuppressive therapy have had dormant foci of infection develop into disseminated disease (Schroter et al, 1977).

Genitourinary Manifestations. Postmortem studies in patients with disseminated coccidioidomycosis indicate involvement of the kidney in 30% to 60% of cases, the adrenal gland in 16% to 32%, and the prostate in 6% (Kuntze et al, 1988). The antemortem diagnosis of renal coccidioidal infection is difficult to establish. **Radiographic findings may be similar to those of tuberculosis: "motheaten calyces," infundibular stenosis, and renal calcification** (Conner et al, 1975). Coccidioiduria is not uniformly present in chronic coccidioidomycosis, and the genitourinary pathology may not show the characteristic coccidioidal spherules in the kidney, epididymis, and prostate (Petersen et al, 1976).

Coccidioidomycosis of the male genital tract is very rare. One review describes 30 patients reported since 1943 (Sohail et al, 2005). The disease involved the epididymis (18), prostate (14), and the testis (6). Two thirds of patients had a history of "remote" pulmonary coccidioidomycosis, and 13% had concomitant active pulmonary infection. *C. immitis* was cultured from urine in 63% of cases. Prostatic coccidioidomycosis may cause bladder outflow obstruction, a boggy prostate, or even induration suggestive of neoplasia (Price et al, 1982). Dissemination of infection has been reported to occur in a patient undergoing transurethral resection of the prostate for "benign" disease (Wipf et al, 1983). Genitourinary coccidioidomycosis can cause scrotal swelling, draining sinus, and/or indurated epididymis. Bilateral involvement may also occur. Urethrocutaneous fistula has been reported to occur in a patient with epididymal and prostatic coccidioidal infection (Gottesman, 1974). Finally, coccidioidomycosis of the female genital tract may present as tubo-ovarian disease with peritonitis or as endometritis (Bylund et al, 1986).

Diagnosis and Treatment. The patient's travel or residence in endemic areas or immune suppression should alert the urologist to this infection. Serologic studies (complement fixation, immune diffusion, latex particle agglutination, IgG and IgM antibodies) may provide supportive laboratory evidence of exposure to *C. immitis* (Rippon, 1988; Einstein and Johnson, 1993). Draining sinuses can be cultured for fungi, and tissue obtained by biopsy or at surgery can be stained with PAS or methenamine silver, which facilitates identification of the coccidioidal spherule.

Genitourinary coccidioidal infection is usually a manifestation of multiorgan disease; hence, systemic therapy is advocated. **Effective agents include amphotericin B, fluconazole, and itraconazole** (see Table 14–4) (The Medical Letter, 2005; Galgiani, 1993). The duration of therapy is determined by the location and severity of the disease and can exceed 1 year in severe cases (Rippon, 1988). Isolated lesions, such as epididymal infections, have been treated by surgical excision alone.

Histoplasmosis

Epidemiology and Predisposing Factors. Histoplasmosis occurs throughout the midwestern and southern portions of the United States. *H. capsulatum* thrives in high nitrogen content soil that has been enriched by bird guano. **Outbreaks of the disease have occurred in individuals who work in chicken coops, infested caves, and other bird areas.** Major outbreaks have been reported in association with construction sites and tree removal (Drutz, 1979). In the United States, it has been estimated that 30 to 40 million people have been exposed to the fungus (Rubin et al, 1959; Rippon, 1988).

Inhalation of the fungus may result in asymptomatic, self-limiting pulmonary infection. A small number of exposed individuals (5%) develop symptomatic infection manifested by cough, fever, and hemoptysis. Unless treated, the more virulent pulmonary infection may become chronic. Disseminated invasive disease occurs in children and immunosuppressed individuals. **Disseminated histoplasmosis is a major opportunistic infection in AIDS patients** (Bonner et al, 1984; Wheat LJ et al, 1992; Wheat J, 1997; Mahworter et al, 2000).

Genitourinary Manifestations. The liver, spleen, and lymph nodes are major sites of extrapulmonary histoplasmosis. **The genitourinary tract is infrequently involved in disseminated infection.** In a postmortem study of 17 patients with generalized histoplasmosis, the kidney was infected in 3 patients (18%) and the prostate in 1 (6%) (Rubin et al, 1959).

Renal biopsy of an HIV-infected patient demonstrated both *H. capsulatum* antigens and immune complexes in the mesangium. Disseminated histoplasmosis developed in a female transplant recipient of an infected kidney (Wong and Allen, 1992). Obstructive uropathy was caused by disseminated histoplasmosis that caused sloughed papilla in a renal transplant recipient (Superdock et al, 1994). Percutaneous nephrostomy, long-term amphotericin B, and itraconazole did not control the infection, and the patient required nephrectomy. Superficial penile ulcers have occurred in disseminated infection. Epididymal histoplasmosis has been reported in infected patients with paratracheal lymphadenopathy (Kauffman et al, 1981).

Diagnosis and Treatment. The diagnosis of histoplasmosis is established by culture or smear of tissue, blood, or other body fluids. Culture of sputum, gastric washings, or abscess may yield the putative fungus. *H. capsulatum* can be identified in tissue specimens by methenamine silver or Giemsa stain (Kauffman et al, 1981; Rippon, 1988). In disseminated infection, peripheral blood smears may demonstrate intra-leukocytic budding yeast (Henochowicz et al, 1985). Serologic studies, such as the histoplasmin skin test, are helpful in establishing the diagnosis and monitoring the disease (Rippon, 1988); however, antibody response may be muted in the immunosuppressed patient. The detection of *H. capsulatum* antigen in blood and urine by radioimmunoassay has been shown to be useful in diagnosis (Wheat LJ et al, 1986). Radiographic studies may reveal pulmonary cavitation or nodules and mediastinal lymphadenopathy.

Disseminated histoplasmosis requires systemic therapy with amphotericin or itraconazole (see Table 14–4). Itraconazole is also recommended for long-term suppressive therapy to prevent relapse (Hawkins et al, 1981; Dismukes et al, 1983, Wheat LJ et al, 1992; Drew, 1993). Assessment of serum and urine *Histoplasma* polysaccharide antigen has been a useful marker to assess treatment response in AIDS patients with disseminated histoplasmosis (Wheat LJ et al, 1992).

Antifungal Therapeutic Agents

The treatment of fungal infections has become increasingly complex as new and more effective antifungal agents become available. The present discussion is limited to the major drugs used to treat genitourinary tract infections, namely, amphotericin B and its formulations, the azoles (fluconazole, itraconazole, voriconazole, ketoconazole), caspofungin, and flucytosine. Fungal infections involving the genitourinary tract are frequently one component of a multiorgan systemic disease, often involving an immunocompromised host. **Consultation with infectious diseases experts may provide valuable assistance in the management of these complex patients.**

Amphotericin B

Amphotericin B is a polyene antifungal agent that exerts its fungicidal and fungistatic activity by binding to the ergosterol component of the fungal cell membrane, resulting in disruption of internal cellular components (Medoff and Kobayashi, 1980; Walsh, 1987). **Amphotericin B has been used in the treatment of all of the fungal infections discussed in this chapter** (see Table 14–4).

The intravenous administration of amphotericin B may induce systemic reactions, including rigors, chills, and fever. Pretreatment with ibuprofen, aspirin, or acetaminophen; diphenhydramine; and/or hydrocortisone can decrease the severity of these reactions (Gigliotti et al, 1987). Intravenous meperidine or dantrolene can shorten the duration of rigors (da Camara and Lane, 1987). **Other adverse reactions ascribed to intravenous amphotericin B include generalized pain, headache, convulsions, localized phlebitis, anemia, and thrombocytopenia** (Craven, 1982). Heparin, large-bore intravenous catheters, and rotation of intravenous sites are recommended to minimize the risk of phlebitis.

Amphotericin B nephrotoxicity is the major treatment-limiting side effect (Branch, 1988). **It may also exacerbate the nephrotoxic effects of other agents, such as cisplatin, cyclosporine, tacrolimus, and aminoglycoside antibiotics** (Walsh, 1987; The Medical Letter, 2005). Sodium loading with intravenous saline and hydration may prevent or reduce the severity of the nephrotoxicity (Branch, 1988). Finally, potassium and magnesium wasting due to a mild renal tubular acidosis can commonly accompany amphotericin B administration (Smith et al, 1988).

Amphotericin B lipid formulations provide an effective antifungal agent that has less potential for most of the adverse reactions (Wiebe and Degregorio, 1988; Wong-Beringer et al, 1998). Liposomal amphotericin B preparations have the same spectrum of activity as amphotericin B desoxycholate but less nephrotoxicity (Pathak et al, 1998). Acute infusion reactions, however, may be more severe with some lipid formulations. Furthermore, they have also been associated with hepatic toxicity, an uncommon side effect of conventional amphotericin (Cronin and Barron, 1999). Finally, the higher cost (see Table 14–5) of the lipid formulations often limits their use to patients who cannot tolerate standard (desoxycholate) amphotericin B preparations (Wong-Beringer et al, 1998).

Azoles (Imidazoles and Triazoles)

The imidazoles include the topical drugs clotrimazole and miconazole and the oral agent ketoconazole. The primary mechanism of action of the imidazoles is inhibition of cytochrome P450 that regulates fungal ergosterol metabolism. The triazoles (fluconazole, itraconazole, voriconazole) are similar in chemical structure to the imidazoles, but they have a greater affinity for fungal cytochrome P450 enzymes than the imidazoles (Como and Dismukes, 1994). **There are major drug interactions between the azoles and many commonly used medications** that utilize this pathway (The Medical Letter, 2005). This interaction precludes the use of the azoles in some patients and in certain populations that are genetically deficient in the hepatic enzyme. For example, **the administration of the azoles may result in an increase in serum concentrations of digoxin, cyclosporine, simvastatin, lovastatin, tacrolimus, phenytoin, zidovudine, warfarin, and numerous other drugs.** Concomitant administration of rifampin can reduce the serum levels of fluconazole.

Fluconazole. Fluconazole can be administered orally or intravenously. Oral administration is not affected by the presence of food or gastric acidity. The drug is water soluble and rapidly achieves high levels in plasma, cerebrospinal fluid, and urine. **Fluconazole is efficacious for the treatment of urinary tract infections caused by *Candida* and *Cryptococcus*. Most *Candida* species are sensitive to fluconazole, with the exception of *C. krusei,* which is intrinsically resistant, and many strains of *C. glabrata*. Oral fluconazole (200 mg/day for 7 days) is as effective as bladder irrigations with amphotericin B (50 mg/L for 7 days) in the treatment of bladder candidal infection** (Fan-Harvard et al, 1995). Case studies have reported that fluconazole was effective in the treatment of kidney and collecting system infections (Dave et al, 1989; Corbella et al, 1992). In a study of 164 patients with invasive candidal infection, fluconazole achieved a response rate similar to that of systemic amphotericin B (66% vs. 64%). Adverse events were more frequent with amphotericin B than fluconazole (35% vs. 5%) (Anaissie et al, 1996). Fungal drug resistance to fluconazole has been observed in HIV-infected patients who required long-term treatment for esophageal candidiasis in addition to immunocompetent patients and immunocompromised patients not previously treated with fluconazole (Como and Dismukes, 1994; Goff et al, 1995; Iwen et al, 1995).

Itraconazole. Itraconazole is effective in the treatment of infections caused by *Aspergillus, Blastomyces, Coccidioides,* and *Histoplasma* (Graybill, 1988; Itraconazole, 1993). Absorption is enhanced when the drug is taken with food. The drug is lipophilic and achieves tissue levels two to three times higher than serum. Itraconazole has fewer adverse effects than ketoconazole. The length of therapy is dependent on the extent of infection (Itraconazole, 1993; Como and Dismukes, 1994).

Voriconazole. Voriconazole is similar to itraconazole in its activity and is approved for treatment of invasive aspergillosis and for disseminated *Candida* infections. It is also active against the Zygomycetes and some strains of *C. glabrata* and *C. krusei* that are resistant to the other azoles.

Ketoconazole. Ketoconazole has largely been supplanted by the newer azoles, which have fewer side effects and broader activity. In addition, because of **poor renal excretion,** ketoconazole has low urinary levels that are insufficient to inhibit many fungal species, further limiting its role in the treatment of urinary tract infections (Wise et al, 1985). Ketoconazole's adverse effects include headaches, rashes, elevation of serum triglyceride levels, and abnormal values of liver enzymes.

Caspofungin

Caspofungin is a member of a new class of antifungal agents (the echinocandins) that inhibit synthesis of an essential glycan component of the fungal cell wall (The Medical Letter, 2005). It must be given intravenously. **It has activity against *Candida* and *Aspergillus* species and is well tolerated with few serious side effects.** It also has interactions with other drugs, including efavirenz, nevirapine, dexamethasone, rifampin, and phenytoin, which may decrease caspofungin serum levels.

Flucytosine

Flucytosine is a fluorinated pyrimidine. The antifungal effect of flucytosine is caused by its conversion to 5-fluorouracil by cytosine deaminase that is present in some fungal species but absent or in low concentrations in mammalian cells. The 5-fluorouracil is then converted to 5-fluorodoxyuridine monophosphate, which adversely affects fungal protein and DNA synthesis. It is readily absorbed by the gastrointestinal tract and is excreted unchanged by filtration, achieving high urine levels. In the presence of renal insufficiency, the dosage should be modified in proportion to the degree of renal compromise. **Potentially lethal, dose-related bone marrow toxicity, enterocolitis, and the rapid development of resistance when the drug is used alone sharply limit the use of flucytosine** (The Medical Letter, 2005). Abnormalities in liver function have been noted in 5% of patients (Sande and Mandell, 1985). Primary resistance to the drug may occur in 10% of infections caused by *C. albicans,* but the rate may be as high as 30% with other *Candida* species. Successful management of sensitive urinary candidal infection has been reported to vary from 50% to 90% (Harder and Hermans, 1975).

SECTION IV

KEY POINTS: TUBERCULOSIS AND PARASITIC AND FUNGAL INFECTIONS OF THE GENITOURINARY SYSTEM

■ Renal TB is caused by the activation of a prior bloodborne renal infection.

■ In renal tuberculosis, "sterile pyuria" is the classic urinary finding on routine urinalysis and culture.

■ CT has become more widely available and has arguably replaced IVU as the imaging modality of choice for the diagnosis and evaluation of genitourinary TB.

■ Six-month treatment regimens are effective for most forms of TB, including genitourinary TB.

■ When surgical intervention is mandated for genitourinary TB, it should be delayed until at least 4 to 6 weeks of medical therapy have been administered.

■ The most common sequelae of urinary schistosomiasis result from ureteral involvement causing obstructive uropathy.

■ The symptoms of bancroftian and brugian filariasis range from acute lymphatic inflammation characterized by fever, localized lymphangitis, and transitory lymphadenopathy to chronic lymphatic dilatation with hydrocele, elephantiasis of the limbs, and chyluria.

■ Removal of an indwelling urinary catheter or intravenous line, cessation of antibiotic therapy, and improvement of nutritional status may eliminate candidal colonization or infection.

■ Most *Candida* species are sensitive to fluconazole, with the exception of *C. krusei,* which is intrinsically resistant, and many strains of *C. glabrata.* Oral fluconazole (200 mg/day for 7 days) is as effective as bladder irrigations with amphotericin B (50 mg/L for 7 days) in the treatment of bladder candidal infection.

■ In AIDS patients, the prostate has been recognized as a "reservoir" for relapsing cryptococcosis.

SUGGESTED READINGS

Alexandroff AB, Jackson AM, O'Donnell MA, James K: BCG immunotherapy of bladder cancer: 20 years on. Lancet 1999;353:1689-1694.

Dreyer G, Noroes J, Figueredo-Silva J, Piessens WF: Pathogenesis of lymphatic disease in bancroftian filariasis: A clinical perspective. Parasitol Today 2000;16:544.

Engin G, Acunas B, Acunas G, Tunaci M: Imaging of extrapulmonary tuberculosis. Radiographics 2000;20:471; quiz 529, 532.

Fan-Harvard P, O'Donovan C, Smith SM, et al: Oral fluconazole versus amphotericin B bladder irrigations for treatment of candidal funguria. Clin Infect Dis 1995;21:960-965.

Jorulf H, Linstedt E: Urogenital schistosomiasis: CT evaluation. Radiology 1985;157:745.

Kauffman CA: Candiduria. Clin Infect Dis 2005; 41:S371-S376.

Kauffman CA, Vazquez JA, Sobel JD, et al, and the National Institute of Allergy and Infectious Diseases (NIAID) Mycoses Study Group: A prospective multicenter surveillance study of funguria in hospitalized patients. Clin Infect Dis 2000;30:14-18.

Pappas PG, Rex JH, Sobel JD, et al: Guidelines for treatment of candidiasis. Clin Infect Dis 2004;38:161-189.

Ross A, Bartley P, Sleigh A, et al: Schistosomiasis. N Engl J Med 2002;346:1212.

The Medical Letter: Antifungal drugs. Treatment Guidelines from The Medical Letter 2005;30:7-14.

The Medical Letter: Drugs for parasitic infections. The Medicial Letter on Drugs and Therapeutics 2004;1189:1-12.

The Medical Letter: Drugs for tuberculosis. Treatment Guidelines from The Medical Letter 2004;28:83-88.

Wise GJ, Marella VK: Genitourinary manifestations of tuberculosis. Urol Clin North Am 2003;30:111-121.

SECTION V

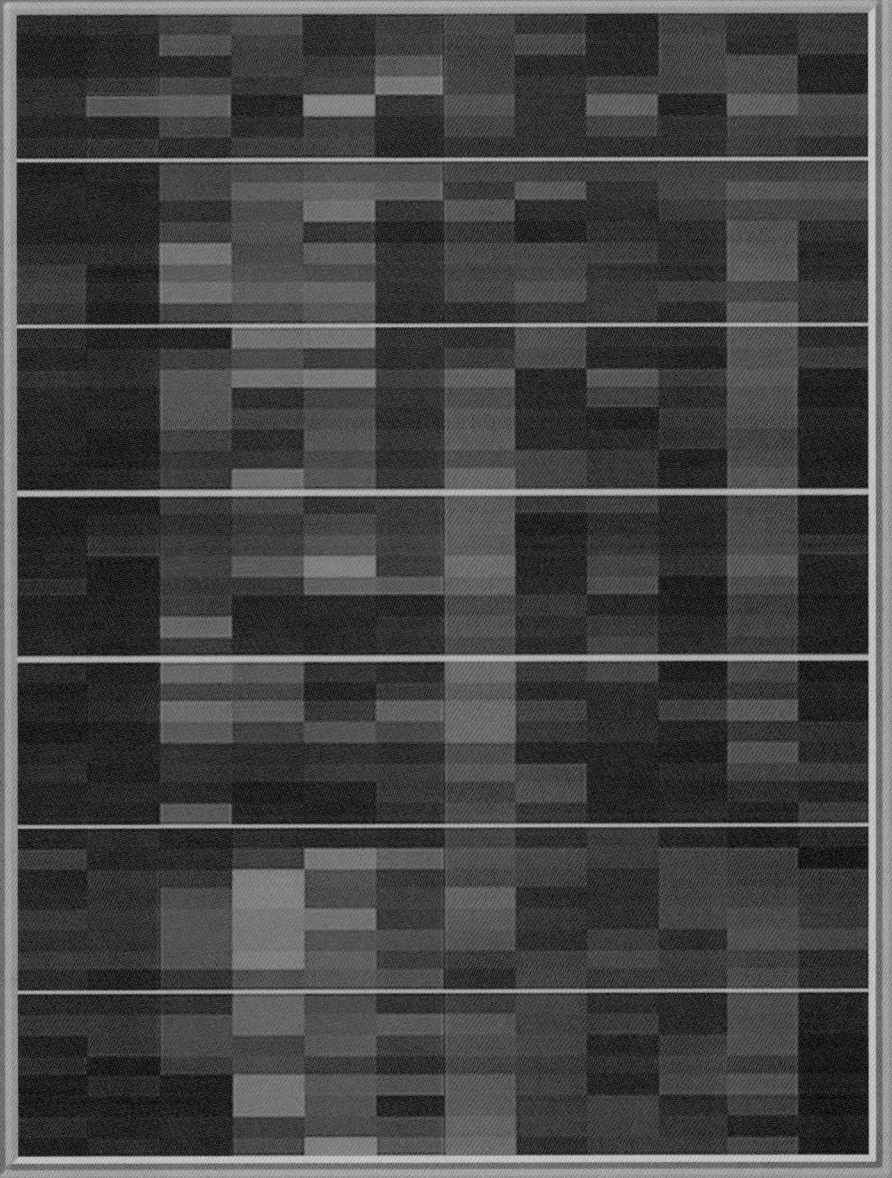

MOLECULAR AND CELLULAR BIOLOGY

15 Basic Principles of Immunology

STUART M. FLECHNER, MD • JAMES H. FINKE, PhD •
ROBERT L. FAIRCHILD, PhD

The immune system is essential for the maintenance of health and for combating disease arising from both internal and external agents. Various immune mechanisms are involved in urologic disorders, including the development and progression of urologic cancer, infections of the urinary tract, the rejection of transplanted organs, the transfusion of blood products, and abnormalities of male reproduction. The immune response, initially catalogued by careful observation, has now been traced to individual cell populations, their secretory and membrane products, and the very intracellular machinery required to unlock these responses. This has come about because of rapid advances in molecular immunology, including the development of monoclonal antibodies, recombinant gene techniques, the ability to place genes into (transfect) or eliminate from (knockout) animals, and the ability to clone cell populations. Nevertheless, the immune response remains identified by unique characteristics that help explain its utility and adaptability against many different foreign invaders. **These include (1) the ability to identify self from non-self, (2) specificity, (3) memory, and (4) rapid amplification.**

INNATE AND ADAPTIVE IMMUNITY

What we characterize as the immune system describes the interplay between two separate biologic responses, those that are **innate** and those that are **acquired**. The innate responses are constitutional and do not improve on repeated contact with the same offending agent (Hoffman et al, 1999). **Innate defense mechanisms represent nonspecific barriers to invaders, which rely primarily on physical barriers, phagocytic cells, natural killer (NK) cells, complement, acute phase proteins, lysozyme, and the interferons.** Innate immunity also lies behind most inflammatory responses; these are triggered in the first instance by macrophages, polymorphonuclear leukocytes, and mast cells through their germline-encoded innate immune receptors. The body's first line of defense includes mechanical, chemical, and biologic barriers that lie external to the basement membrane of the skin and mucous membranes of the respiratory, alimentary, and urinary tract. Hairs and cilia serve to filter and sweep out microbes. The strong periodic flushing of the urinary tract helps to limit bacterial ascension up to the kidneys. Specifically acquired or **adaptive** responses result from repeated exposure to an invader and rely primarily on large populations of lymphocytes, each with its own individual specificity for an invader. **In addition, the clonal expansion of specific lymphocyte populations after first contact with a foreign molecule confers memory and the ability to return a more vigorous response on subsequent exposure to the same foreign molecule.** Recently, the identification of a family of Toll-like receptors (TLRs), which recognize conserved motifs in pathogens, have been recognized as essential in the host defense against microbial pathogens. Individual TLRs can also recognize fungi and viruses and induce upregulation of proinflammatory cytokines, co-stimulatory molecules, and chemokines (Janeway and Medzhitov, 2002). The signaling pathway of *Drosophila* Toll shows remarkable similarity to the mammalian interleukin (IL)-1 pathway, which leads to activation of NFκB, a transcription factor responsible for many aspects of inflammatory and immune responses.

Phagocytosis

Phagocytosis is a nonspecific innate response of circulating neutrophils and macrophages that actively ingest microbes and secrete antimicrobial toxins. Phagocytosis also includes reticuloendothelial cells such as Kupffer cells in the liver and bronchial alveolar macrophages. This process is greatly enhanced by the complement proteins (C3b) and immunoglobulins that bind microbes and act as opsonins to attract these phagocytic cells via surface receptors. The macrophage advances pseudopodia over the opsonized microbe, which is internalized into a phagocytic vacuole that fuses with a lysosomal vacuole. This fusion vacuole results in the degradation of the microbe or particle as digestive enzymes are released. Killing is mediated by reactive oxygen intermediates and hydrogen peroxide (Underhill and Ozinsky, 2002).

Complement

A major component of innate immunity is the collection of about 20 soluble proteins referred to as complement. Complement, once activated, can directly lyse invading bacteria or viruses, and several of its components are important in the regulation of immune responsiveness (Carroll, 1998). **Complement activation results in a cascade phenomenon where the product of one reaction is the enzyme catalyst of the next.** Each component is described by the letter "C" and a number, more closely reflecting the sequence of discovery rather than sequence of action. The split components are called a and b. The most critical component is C3, which has a molecular weight of about 195 kD. Once complement proteins and a target substance interact, a C3 convertase is activated that splits C3 into C3a and C3b fragments (Fig. 15–1). The C3b bound to the target becomes a component of the convertase for C5. The union of C5b with C6-C9 generates the membrane attack complex (MAC), which associates with the lipid bilayer of the target cell. The MAC produces cell membrane lesions that permit loss of potassium and ingress of salt and water, leading to hypotonic lysis.

Not all C3b produced becomes a component of the C5 convertase. Some binds directly to the cell membrane and acts as an **opsonin** for phagocytes such as neutrophils and macrophages that have receptors for C3b. In addition, fragments C3a and C5a serve as powerful **anaphylatoxins** that degranulate mast cells with release of histamine that enhances vascular permeability and smooth muscle contraction. The C5a fragment is also a chemoattractant for polymorphonuclear leukocytes (PMNs) and macrophages.

Multiple substances may trigger the complement system, which has two pathways of activation. **The classical pathway is a mechanism to activate C3 via the serum proteins C1, C4, and C2. The process is initiated when an antigen-antibody complex fixes the first component C1q, which results in the cascade C1qrs, 4, 2, 3, 5, 6, 7, 8, 9 to produce lysis.** Complement fixation requires one IgM or several IgG antibody molecules. **The alternative pathway is non–antibody dependent and does not require C1, C4, C2 to initiate the process.** It is dependent upon bacterial products such as endotoxin and microbial polysaccharides and a serum globulin called properdin, which activates C3 directly. An

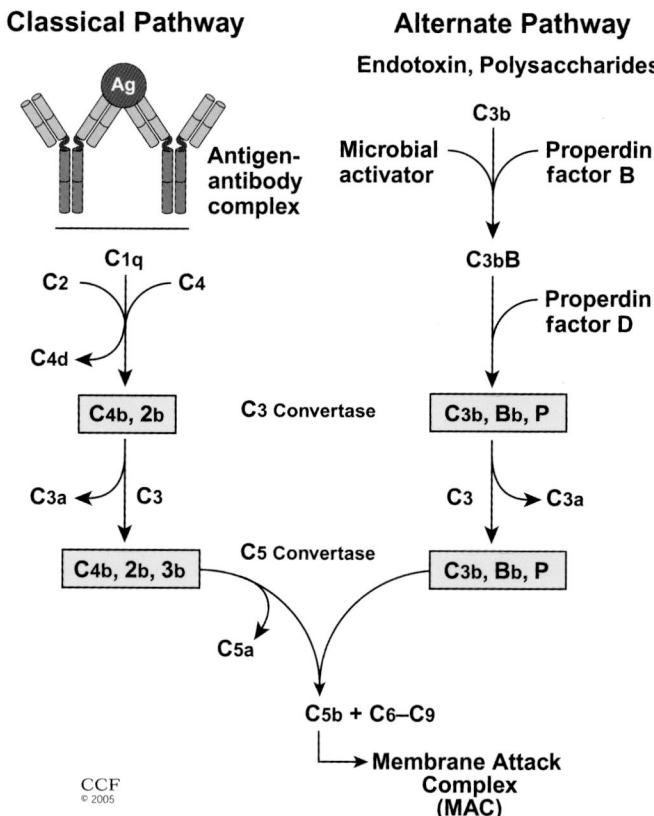

Figure 15–1. The classic and alternative complement pathways. Each component protein labeled "C" acts as an enzyme catalyst for a subsequent product in a ever-expanding cascade. The process can be initiated when an antigen-antibody complex fixes the first component C1q to the cell surface. Alternatively, the cascade can be initiated by microbial products and properdin that can directly activate C3. In addition to forming the membrane attack complex, C3b fragments can function as opsonins and C3a and C5a function as anaphylatoxins.

alternative C3 convertase is formed that triggers the sequence, leading to cell lysis. The complement system is regulated by endogenous inhibitors, which protect the host from continuous activation. These complement regulatory proteins, such as decay accelerating factor (DAF), membrane cofactor protein (MCP, CD46), and CD59, are glycoproteins found on erythrocytes, platelets, neutrophils, and selected mucosal epithelial and endothelial cells. They function by inactivating the C3/5 convertase.

Recently, complement activity has become an important target for immune responses to transplanted organs. The human gene for DAF has been transfected into pigs in an attempt to control complement activation during a pig-to-primate xenograft rejection model. In addition, the complement protein split product C4d has been proposed as a reliable marker for antibody-mediated rejection of renal allografts. Antibody-mediated activation of the classical complement pathway leads to the formation of C4d, which covalently binds to the endothelial surface of the kidney peritubular capillaries, which leaves an imprint of antibody activity that persists for days to weeks (Collins et al, 1999). C4d staining in the kidney correlates with the presence of circulating donor-specific antibody in the recipient.

Lymphoid Organs and Tissues

Although descriptions of immune interactions are often presented as individual events, in vivo they take place within the organized architecture of lymphoid tissue. **Bone marrow stem cells differentiate into immunocompetent T and B cells in the primary lymphoid organs and then colonize the secondary lymphoid tissues where the immune responses take place.** The primary lymphoid organs are the thymus, which is responsible for the selection and education of T cells, and the bone marrow itself, which is responsible for the education of B cells. Secondary or peripheral lymphoid tissue includes the spleen, lymph nodes, and unencapsulated tissue lining the alimentary, respiratory, and urogenital tracts (Fu and Chaplin, 1999). **The spleen filters the blood, the lymph nodes drain local body tissues, and the unencapsulated tissues associated with mucosal surfaces can secrete IgA antibodies.** The lymphoid tissues communicate through a network of lymphoid ducts that drain all the viscera and return via the thoracic duct to the circulation (Fig. 15–2). This communication is maintained by populations of recirculating lymphocytes, which can travel from the blood into the spleen, lymph nodes, and peripheral tissues and return. **This traffic or recirculation of lymphocytes between the peripheral tissues, lymph nodes, and bloodstream enables the immune system to function as a single organ.** Antigen responsive cells can be recruited to peripheral sites for initial activation, and memory cells can be disseminated to these sites to amplify ongoing responses.

Cellular immune traffic is also highly organized and restricted, with certain cell populations directed to specific sites. For example, lymphoblasts and memory cells display tissue-restricted migration to extralymphoid sites such as the skin or mucosal surfaces whereas lymphocytes, neutrophils, and monocytes target and migrate to sites of inflammation in response to local mediators. **Such direction of immune cells is termed** *homing* **and results from the interaction of various homing receptors that recognize their complementary ligands on the surface of specialized vascular endothelium in selected tissues** (Salmi and Jalkanen, 1997). Much of this directional trafficking is directed by two families of G protein–coupled receptors: chemokine receptors and sphingosine-1-phosphate (S1P) receptors (Cyster, 2005). In the spleen, lymphocytes enter the lymphoid area (white pulp) from the arterioles, pass to the sinusoids of the erythroid area (red pulp), and leave by the splenic vein.

IMMUNORESPONSIVE CELL POPULATIONS

Immune mechanisms rely on the interactions between diverse cell populations, which at any point in time are in various stages of differentiation. In contemporary terms, immunity can be divided into two separate responses. **Cell-mediated immune responses describe those primarily directed by cell to cell contact, and humoral immune responses describe those primarily due to the production of antibody (immunoglobulin).** In fact, most responses involve both cellular and humoral events, which are mediated by several different types of immune competent cells. Whereas the small lymphocyte is the backbone of the immune response, several other bone marrow–derived cells are needed for a mature immune response. **These cells "talk" to each other and their surroundings through receptors that they express on their surface, and through cytokines, which are small peptides that they secrete locally** (Clark and Ledbetter, 1994). The receptors are usually glycoproteins that extend off the cell surface as single chains or double chains called dimers, which are often designated α and β. A nomenclature has developed to describe these markers from international workshops comparing several monoclonal antibodies from different laboratories. When a cluster of monoclonal antibodies are found to react with the same surface polypeptide, it is designated a CD number (cluster of differentiation). The number of CD specificities on leukocytes is now in the 100s, and Table 15–1 provides the ones more commonly associated with immune responses. **A cell surface receptor bound by its ligand will often trigger downstream intracellular events, thereby activating the cell to either produce specific cytokines, express other surface markers required for immune interactions, or enter cell cycle progression and proliferation.**

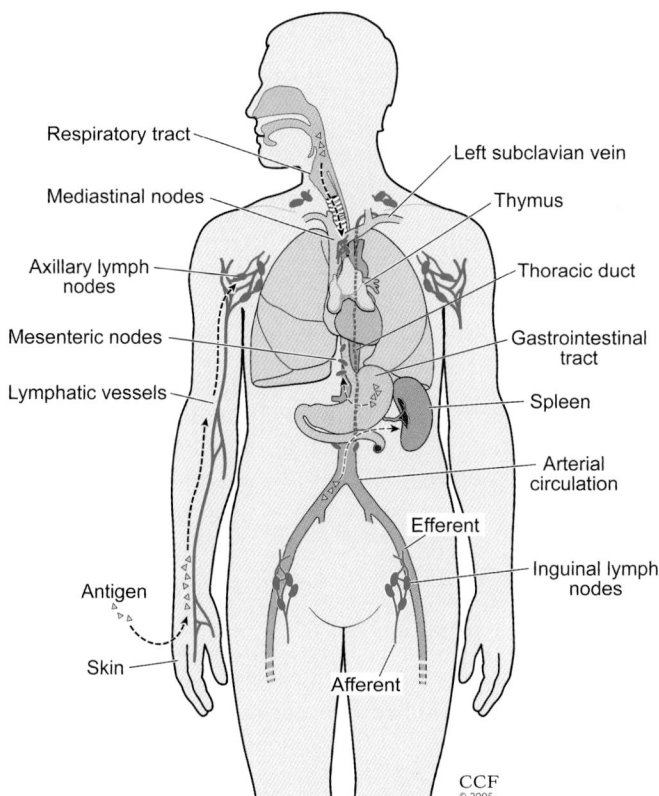

Respiratory tract
Mediastinal nodes
Axillary lymph nodes
Mesenteric nodes
Lymphatic vessels
Antigen
Skin
Left subclavian vein
Thymus
Thoracic duct
Gastrointestinal tract
Spleen
Arterial circulation
Efferent
Inguinal lymph nodes
Afferent
CCF © 2005

Figure 15–2. The lymphatic system. A major function of the lymphatic system is to collect antigens from their portals of entry and deliver them to lymph nodes where they first interact with immunoresponsive cells of the host. Numerous lymphatic capillaries in the periphery absorb and drain interstitial fluid (lymph), which flows into convergent ever-larger central lymphatic vessels. Ultimately the large central thoracic duct drains into the superior vena cava, returning the lymph to the circulation. Lymph nodes are interposed along lymphatic vessels and act as filters that sample the lymph at numerous points before it reaches the circulation. The course of antigens (Δ) entering in the periphery or the gastrointestinal tract are followed. Lymphatic vessels that carry lymph into a lymph node are referred to as afferent, and those that drain lymph from the node are called efferent.

Table 15–1. Some of the Major Cell Surface CD (Cluster of Differentiation) Markers

CD No.	Cellular Association	Membrane Component/Ligand
CD2	T cells	Receptor for LFA3 (CD58), sheep RBC rosettes
CD3	T cells	Component of T-cell receptor, signal transduction
CD4	Helper T cells	Receptor for MHC class II and HIV virus
CD8	Cytotoxic T cells	Receptor for MHC class I
CD16	PMNs, NK, macrophages	Phagocytosis and ADCC
CD18	All leukocytes	Integrin β chain
CD19	B cells	Pan B-cell marker
CD25	Activated T and B cells, macrophages	IL2-receptor, also called Tac
CD28	T cells	Ligand for B7 co-stimulator (CD80)
CD40	B cells, antigen-presenting cells	Receptor for CD40 ligand (CD154) B-cell co-stimulator
CD45	Leukocytes	Leukocyte common antigen, tyrosine phosphatase
CD45RO	Activated and memory T cells, B cells subset, monocytes, macrophages	Isoform of CD45
CD52	T and B cells, some monocytes, macrophages	Campath-1, unknown function
CD54	Dendritic, macrophages, B cells	Leukocyte adhesion, also called intercellular adhesion molecule-1 (ICAM-1)
CD55	Most cells	Decay accelerating factor (DAF), binds C3b
CD56	NK, few T cells	Adhesion
CD62L	B and T cells, monocytes, PMNs	L-Selectin, endothelial adhesion, homing of naive T cells to lymph nodes
CD69	Activated leukocytes	Activation inducer molecule (AIM), signal transduction
CD71	Erythroid cells	Transferrin receptor, iron uptake
CD80	Dendritic, macrophages, B cells	Ligand for CD28, also B7.1, T-cell co-stimulator
CD86	Dendritic, macrophages, B cells, T-cell co-stimulator	Ligand for CD28 and CD152 (CTLA-4), also B7.2
CD152	Activated T cells	Also called CTLA-4; negative regulation of co-stimulation; binds CD80 (B7.1) and CD86 (B7.2)
CD154	Activated CD4+ T cells	CD40 ligand, activates B cells

PMNs, polymorphonuclear leukocytes; NK, natural killer; ADCC, antibody-dependent cell-mediated cytotoxicity.

Lymphocytes

These mononuclear cells are the "linchpin" of the immune system and are sometimes described as small, medium, and large based on their diameter (4 to 15 μm). Once activated they may become lymphoblasts, up to 30 μm in diameter. Morphologically they look similar but may have distinct functions based on their lineage and distinguishing cell surface markers. **Circulating lymphocytes originate from the bone marrow or thymus, the lymph nodes, or the spleen. At any time about 70% of bloodborne lymphocytes are recirculating, traveling to or from the secondary lymphoid organs. The remaining 30% comprise immature short-lived T cells, which remain in the intravascular space or are eliminated.** The circulating lymphocyte pool consists of T cells (60% to 70%) and B cells (10% to 20%), with the remainder NK cells and null cells. Null cells (10% to 20% of circulating lymphocytes) do not manifest any markers (CD or immunoglobulins) for T or B cells and may be undifferentiated stem cells that can mature into T or B cells after appropriate induction or become large granular lymphocytes of the NK cell family.

B Lymphocytes

B cells are responsible for the production of immunoglobulin or antibody. They are so named because they mature in hindgut lymphoid tissue called the bursa of Fabricius in birds. In mammals the bone marrow serves as their point of origin and maturation. Immature B cells express immunoglobulin in their cytoplasm and mature B cells on their cell surface. **Cell surface immunoglobulin, both IgD and IgM, serves as the antigen receptor on B cells. Each B cell has about 10^5 identical antibody molecules on its surface. Once activated by** antigen bound to its surface antibody, B cells mature to become plasma cells, which secrete the specific antibody. That is, a single B cell produces only one antibody specificity that recognizes only one antigenic determinant (epitope). B cells also express receptors for the Fc portion of antibody (FcR), which serves to concentrate antigen-antibody complexes on their cell surface. In addition, B cells also express receptors for the third component of complement (C3R). Plasma cells develop from B cells and are large, ellipsoid with an eccentric nucleus, and 15 to 20 μm in diameter. They are factories for antibody production, although they do not express surface antibody, complement receptors, or CD19 and CD20.

T Lymphocytes

T cells originate in the bone marrow and migrate to the thymus where they undergo a complex process of maturation. Mature T cells are responsible for cell-mediated cytotoxicity, providing help to antibody-producing B cells and delayed-type hypersensitivity and playing specific roles in immune regulation. Stem cells first enter the outer cortical thymus and mature as they pass to the medulla. During this migration the critically important surface TCR genes are rearranged and the CD3, CD4, and CD8 surface molecules appear (Starr et al, 2003). **During maturation CD4– CD8– (double negative) T cells develop into CD4+ CD8+ (double positive), and then become single positive CD4–/CD8+ (cytotoxic/suppressor) or CD4+/CD8– (helper/inducer) T-cell precursors. Each retains the pan–T-cell CD3 marker, which is a signal-transducing component of the TCR.** Thymic T-cell maturation also involves the critical initial process of self-recognition, which is a consequence of the interaction between maturing T cells and the surrounding cortical epithelium. This leads to the selection of those T cells that are to be saved. **Negative selection** occurs when CD4+/CD8+/TCR+ thymocytes recognize self-peptide/MHC complexes on thymic epithelium with high avidity, which leads to apoptosis or deletion of these clones. The majority of cortical thymocytes are killed during the selection process, thus preventing the development of autoimmune T cells. During **positive selection,** CD4+/CD8+/TCR+ thymocytes recognize self-peptide/major histocompatibility complex (MHC) complexes on thymic epithelial cells with low avidity. This saves them from programmed cell death. **The resulting T-cell populations are self-MHC restricted and tolerant to self-antigens but are capable of reacting to foreign antigens.** Cells leaving the thymus migrate to the peripheral lymphoid organs and seed the T cell–dependent regions of lymph nodes, spleen, and lymphoid follicles (Przylepa et al, 1998).

Natural Killer Cells

NK cells are large granular lymphocytes that can destroy various nucleated cells, including tumors and virus-infected cells. **They are an important component of innate immunity and do not require prior contact with antigen, nor are they MHC restricted.** NK cells release cytotoxic factors such as perforin, serine proteases called granzymes, and tumor necrosis factor (TNF)-β. They can also trigger apoptosis in their targets. Interferons seem to augment their activity. They also participate in antibody-dependent cell-mediated cytotoxicity (ADCC) through binding of their cell surface Fc receptor (CD16) to the Fc portion of antibody-coated cells. The precise lineage of NK cells is not known. Characterized by the presence of CD16 and CD56, and the absence of CD3, they have IL-2 receptors and respond to exogenous IL-2. Although their TCR genes are not rearranged, they would seem to be related to T cells in some fashion (Yokoyama et al, 2004).

Granulocytes

The polymorphonuclear leukocyte (PMN) shares a common stem cell precursor with the other formed blood elements and is the predominant cell type, comprising 60% to 75% of the circulating white blood cells. The name derives from its multilobed nucleus, and the cytoplasm is filled with granules. The granules are often lysosomal and contain the enzymes necessary to digest engulfed microorganisms. Based on the histologic appearance of the granules, they are identified as neutrophils, eosinophils, or basophils and are 16 to 18 μm in diameter. **PMNs are phagocytic and can be attracted to a local site by chemotactic factors such as complement C5a.** The eosin-staining granules of eosinophils contain cationic peptides that are toxic to surrounding tissues. Eosinophil levels rise during allergic reactions and during parasitic infestations. Basophil granules stain with basic dyes and contain heparin, histamine, and proteases. Surface receptors bind IgE with high affinity. **Binding of antigens to the surface IgE of basophils causes them to degranulate, resulting in immediate (type I) hypersensitivity. When basophils are fixed in the tissues they are called mast cells.**

Monocytes and Macrophages

Bone marrow–derived mononuclear phagocytic cells circulate in the blood for 1 to 2 days and then migrate and fix into the tissues where they mature and become macrophages. **They usually occupy perivascular areas and can be called Kupffer cells in the liver, alveolar macrophages in the lung, histiocytes in connective tissue, brain microglia, or kidney glomerular mesangial cells.** They are relatively large (15 to 25 μm) and have abundant lysosomes and digestive enzymes required for phagocytosis. These cells have a variety of cell surface receptors that enable them to bind to carbohydrates and protein molecules such as immunoglobulins (Fc receptor) and complement (CR 1 and 3). Mononuclear phagocytes also secrete a rich array of cytokines such as TNF-α, IL-1, IL-6, prostaglandins, and some complement proteins. Activated macrophages can also express cell surface MHC class I and II molecules, which play an important role in antigen presentation.

Antigen-Presenting Cells

An antigen-presenting cell (APC) is a cell that can process a protein antigen, breaking it into peptides and then presenting it in conjunction with MHC molecules on the cell surface where it may interact with appropriate T cell receptors. Macrophages, monocytes, some B cells, Langerhans cells of the skin, dendritic reticulum cells, and vascular endothelium can process and present antigen. The most efficient are the dendritic cells, which have a characteristic starfish shape and line the epithelial layer of exposed surfaces. Once mature, they travel to the periphery to pick up antigen, process it, and present it to naive T cells in the lymphoid tissues. These cells ingest proteins and split them into small peptides in endosomes. The peptides are then transported to the cell surface and assembled in the peptide binding groove on the MHC molecules for presentation (Trombetta and Mellman, 2005). **The peptides presented by APCs must be assembled with self-MHC molecules, which forms the basis of MHC restriction in the immune response.** CD4+ T cells will recognize antigens only in the context of self-MHC class II molecules on the surface of the APCs. Cells that can initiate an immune response such as dendritic cells, macrophages, and some B cells are sometimes referred to as "professional APCs."

Vascular Endothelial Cells

The endothelial cells lining the blood vessels are an active and essential part of the immune response. Once activated by inflammation or antigens (i.e., IL-1 or TNF), they respond by expressing adhesion molecules, selectins, chemotactic factors, and MHC molecules, which are necessary for the recruitment and activation of immune competent cells. Vascular endothelial cells also react to a number of substances that may change their conformation. Permeability factors such as serotonins, histamines, kinins, and leukotrienes can increase the spaces between the capillaries and small vessels, facilitating the loss of proteins and transmigration of cells from the blood into the extravascular fluid.

Antibody Production

While the thrust of this chapter focuses on cell-mediated immunity, a brief description of antibody structure follows. Antibodies are glycoprotein molecules, of the globulin fraction, produced by plasma cells in response to stimulation with an immunogen. They are also called immunoglobulins and constitute 1% to 2% of the total serum proteins. **The term** *antigen* **is used to describe a molecule capable of being recognized by an antibody or a TCR.** The immunoglobulin molecule consists of two identical heavy (H) and two light (L) chains held together by disulfide bonds (Fig. 15–3). **There are five antibody classes termed** *isotypes,* **so named by their different heavy chains and designated IgM, IgG, IgA, IgD, IgE. Two types of light chains, kappa and lambda, are present in all five antibody classes, although only one is present in a specific molecule.** The basic structure is Y-shaped with a hinge region rich in proline, stabilized by the disulfide bridges and noncovalent forces. Both H and L chains have constant amino acid sequences at their carboxyl terminus and variable sequences at their amino terminus (Alzari et al, 1988).

Much has been learned about antibody structure and binding after digestion experiments using the proteolytic enzymes papain and pepsin (see Fig. 15–3). Digestion with papain yields two Fab (antibody binding) and one Fc (crystallizable) fragments. Each Fab fragment has one antibody-binding site. The Fc fragment does not bind antibody but is responsible for fixation to complement and attachment of the molecule to the cell surface. Digestion with pepsin cleaves the

molecule toward the carboxyl terminal side of the disulfide bonds, resulting in a single F(ab')₂ fragment with two antigen-binding sites and a functionless heavy chain segment. **These experiments confirmed that specific antigen binding occurs at the Y limb of the molecule and that the nonspecific functions of each antibody isotype reside in the Fc end** (Harris et al, 1999).

Each antibody H and L chain also conforms to several domains of 110 amino acids residues, which form loops that are linked by disulfide bonds. In a typical IgG molecule an H chain will have four domains and an L chain will have two domains. Three of the H chain domains and one of the L chain domains are usually invariable in amino acid sequences and are called the constant regions. **The amino-terminal domain on the H and L chains contains unique sequences for each molecule and is called the variable region. Several sites within the variable region are even more unique and are referred to as hypervariable. These hypervariable sequences govern both the conformation and specificity of the antigen-binding site of an antibody molecule.** The part of the hypervariable regions on the antibody that contacts the antigen is called the **paratope,** and the part of the antigen that is in contact with the **paratope** is called the **epitope.** Both the variable and constant regions of each antibody molecule are encoded by specific gene sequences. The term **idiotype** is used to describe the unique antigen-binding site of each antibody molecule.

The in-vivo antibody response to an antigen is polyclonal in that many different antibody molecules are generated that will bind to the antigen. Each antibody originates from a specific clone of plasma cells and binds to a different antigenic determinant or epitope. **Monoclonal antibodies are synthesized from a single clone of cells. The identical copies produced contain only one class of H chain and one type of L chain.** They are produced by fusing antigen-primed splenic B cells with an immortal myeloma cell line to create a hybridoma (Kohler and Milstein, 1975). Polyethylene glycol is used to effect the cell fusion. The antibody-producing B cell provides the specificity and the myeloma cell provides the immortality to the hybridoma, which can generate large quantities of the monoclonal antibody.

CELL SURFACE ACTIVATION

The initiation of an immune response occurs as an antigen physically interacts with either an antibody on the surface of B cells or the TCR on the surface of T cells. **In man, a primary immune response (to a previously unseen antigen) takes 7 to 10 days and has a lag period. A secondary response (re-exposure to the same antigen) is both more rapid (1 to 5 days) and often more vigorous.** A paradox of the immune system is that individuals have all of their antigen-specific pre-committed T and B cells shortly after birth and before encounter with a foreign antigen. There are an estimated 10^7 to 10^9 epitopes recognized separately by T and B cells, yet the human body contains "only" 10^9 to 10^{10} lymphocytes. Therefore, a few epitope-specific T lymphocytes must interact with an equally small number of T or B cells. **The immune system answers this paradox by clonally expanding the number of antigen-specific T and B cells on activation, and this accounts for much of the lag phase seen in the development**

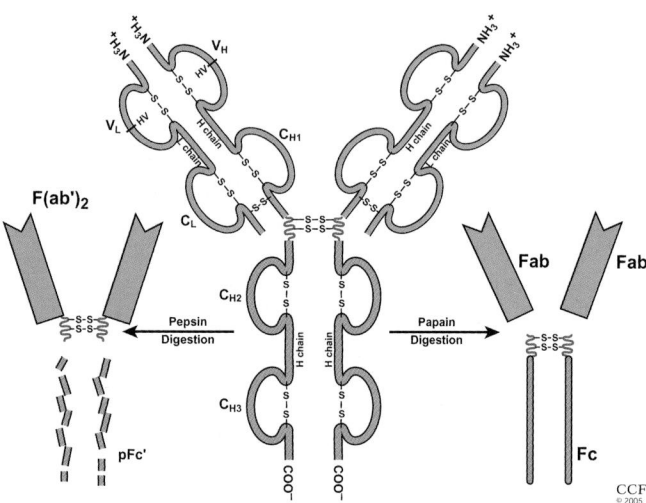

Figure 15–3. Schematic diagram of a typical IgG antibody molecule. Antibodies are dimers of two identical amino acid chains joined by disulfide bonds. These bonds provide the alignment of the two heavy and light chains and the formation of domains. The domains at the carboxyl-terminal ends are generally uniform or constant in sequence. The domains at the amino-terminal ends are variable and unique for each antibody molecule. There are usually three constant domains in heavy chains (C_H) and one in light chains (C_L). The antigen binding sites are formed by the juxtaposition of variable light chain (V_L) and variable heavy chain (V_H) domains. Enzymatic digestion with pepsin results in a divalent antigen binding fragment termed F(ab')₂. Digestion with papain results in three functional fragments: two (Fab) that bind antigen and an Fc that identifies the different antibody isotypes.

of a primary immune response (Burnet, 1957). This clonal expansion of antigen-specific cells serves to increase their numbers and increase the likelihood of an encounter with antigen and decreases the lag time observed when re-exposure takes place. Thus, a secondary response is characterized by a shorter lag phase and a more rapid and prolonged response, which are the hallmarks of immunologic **memory and specificity.**

The surface of the lymphocyte is the site of interaction with antigen. To dissect how antigen interacts with immune competent T and B cells it is important to understand the topography of the cell surface. This requires some background on several important markers on the cell surface, such as the MHC, the TCR, co-stimulatory molecules (B7, CD28), and other T- or B-cell–specific glycoproteins (CD2, CD4, CD8, intercellular adhesion molecule [ICAM]). **As will be apparent, many cell surface markers and receptors are dimers, are similar to antibodies, and constitute the immunoglobulin (Ig) superfamily. They have specific exposed sites, usually the amino terminus, extending off the cell surface where contact with antigen takes place. Changes in the amino acid sequences of these binding areas can alter the types and sizes of the antigens that can be bound.** These changes can also alter the avidity of the binding, which may include electrostatic, hydrogen, hydrophobic, and other intermolecular forces.

The Major Histocompatibility Complex

The MHC describes a region of genes located on chromosome 6 in humans that encode proteins that are responsible for the rejection of tissue between different species or members of the same species. More importantly, these cell surface proteins serve as identity markers on cells interacting with T lymphocytes carrying out specific immune functions. The cell surface MHC markers are called human leukocyte antigens (HLA) because they were first identified on white blood cells. There are two major types of HLA antigens termed class I and class II. Interestingly, a heterogeneous group of protein products that track with the MHC termed class III have immune-related functions and include some complement proteins and TNFs. **Virtually all nucleated cells express HLA class I antigens, whereas class II antigens are primarily found fon B cells, monocytes, macrophages, and APCs.** Many other cells can express class II antigen once activated, such as renal tubular epithelium during kidney allograft rejection. Interferon (IFN) is a cytokine that can upregulate different cells to express class II antigens during activation. **Each individual inherits two class I and one class II antigen from each parent, so six HLA antigens constitute an individual's tissue type (three from each parent).** The HLA molecules are polymorphic, based on multiple alleles (alternative genes at each locus), with over 150 now serologically defined. Therefore, it is very unusual if two unrelated individuals have the same tissue type of six HLA antigens.

Both class I and II molecules are dimers, with an α and a β chain (Fig. 15–4). The class I α chain has three domains of amino acids and a constant β chain called β_2-microglobulin, which is the same in all class I molecules and does not insert into the cell membrane (Bjorkman et al, 1987). The class II molecules have two domains for each chain, and both chains

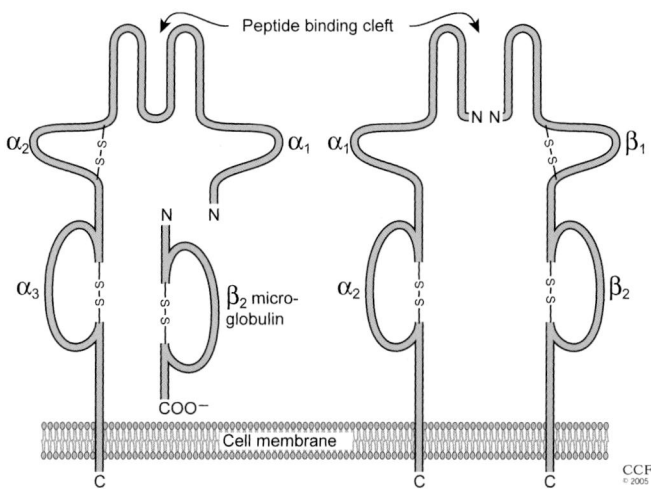

Figure 15–4. Schematic diagram of MHC class I and class II molecules. Both are cell surface glycoprotein dimers with the carboxyl terminus directed toward the plasma membrane. Class I molecules (*left*) have an α chain with three domains and an invariant β chain with a solitary domain. Class II molecules (*right*) have two α- and two β-chain domains. Both molecules have polymorphic Ig-like regions that extend off the cell surface and form a cleft in which small peptides can bind. A peptide residing in an MHC molecule cleft provides signal 1 to the receptor of a naive T cell during activation. The nonpolymorphic Ig-like domains of MHC molecules contain binding sites for the T cell molecules CD4 and CD8.

insert into the cell membrane. **The α1 and α2 domains of class I molecules and the α1 and β1 domains of the class II molecules form a unique antigen peptide-binding cleft that cradles the antigen and is essential for antigen presentation.** Analysis of peptides eluted from the binding groove of MHC class I molecules revealed that a maximum of 8 to 10 amino acids will fit, whereas the groove for the MHC class II molecule is larger and allows a peptide of 12 to 28 amino acids in length. The β_2-microglobulin domain of the class I and the α2β2 domains of the class II molecules are fairly invariant, so the diversity of the different HLA antigen molecules resides in the domains that define the peptide-binding groove.

The T-Cell Receptor

The TCR is that cell surface structure responsible for the initial steps in T-cell activation on encounter with antigen. The TCR is composed of at least seven receptor subunits whose production is encoded by six separate genes that are precisely assembled (Davis and Bjorkman, 1988). The TCR is composed of the clonotypic α and β chains, which are responsible for antigen binding and are noncovalently associated with the invariant CD3-γ, -δ, -ε, and TCR ζ chains. The cytoplasmic tails of the CD3 and TCR ζ chains contain a critical amino sequence known as the immunoreceptor tyrosine-based activation motif (ITAM) that includes two tyrosine residues. The CD3 chains contain one ITAM whereas the TCR ζ chain contains three ITAM sequences (Fig. 15–5). **CD3 is commonly called the pan–T cell marker, present on all T cells.** There are generally two types of TCRs, named TCR1 and TCR2. The TCR1 consists of a γδ heterodimer, appears first in ontogeny, and represents about 5% of circulating T cells in an adult. The TCR2, representing 95% of peripheral blood T

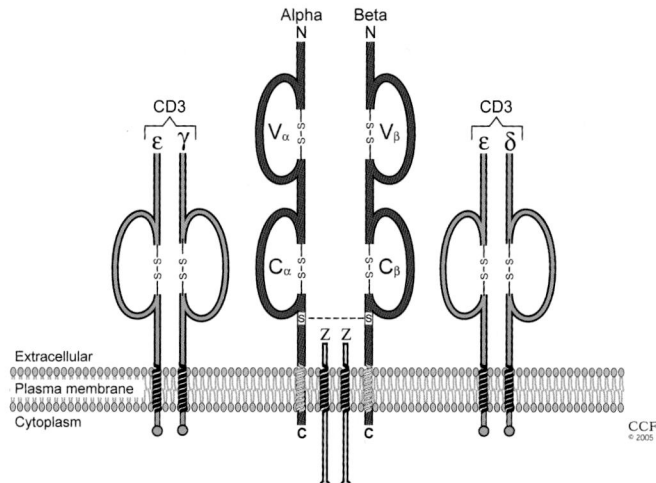

Figure 15–5. Schematic diagram of the T-cell receptor. The receptor is a complex of two main glycoprotein α and β chains (defining an αβ TCR) non-covalently linked to the CD3 proteins (γ, δ, ε) and the ζ chain. As in other Ig superfamily products, disulfide bonds form domains and the carboxyl terminus of each chain is inserted into the plasma membrane. The amino-terminal extracellular domains are variable in amino acid sequence and form the site of recognition of MHC-peptide complexes. The CD3 and ζ chains have intracytoplasmic ends (o) with signaling functions termed *immuno-receptor tyrosine–based activation motifs* (ITAMs). The phosphorylation of the tyrosines in ITAMs represents the initial intracellular signaling events induced by TCR interaction with antigen.

cells, has an αβ heterodimer. Each of the two polypeptides comprising each receptor has a constant and a variable region (similar to immunoglobulin). **Antigen recognition takes place at the variable αβ heterodimer, resembling an antibody Fab antigen-binding fragment.** The relatively invariant transmembrane CD3 complex transmits the signal to the cell interior. Reminiscent of the diversity of antibody molecules through rearrangements of variability, diversity, and joining genes, the TCRs can likewise identify a large number of antigenic specificities, estimated to be 10^{10} to 10^{12} epitopes (Davis et al, 1998).

The Presentation of Antigen

An essential requirement of immunity is that the system cannot be continuously triggered by self-antigens. As described previously, an early process of selection of T cells during maturation in the thymus deletes many offending clones and selects those for future antigen response by utilizing MHC restriction. The TCR2 T cells bearing αβ receptors only respond when the APCs express the same MHC molecules as the host from which the T cells were derived (the MHC molecules that first primed the T cell). The types of responses are also controlled by the specificity of the MHC antigens on the APCs themselves. **Those T cells bearing CD8 that are programmed to be cytotoxic require APCs to present antigen in context of MHC class I molecules, whereas those helper T cells expressing CD4 require antigen to be associated with MHC class II molecules on the APC for activation** (Micelli and Parnes, 1993).

An additional layer of control is also imbedded into this system. Antigen must be processed into smaller pieces (linear

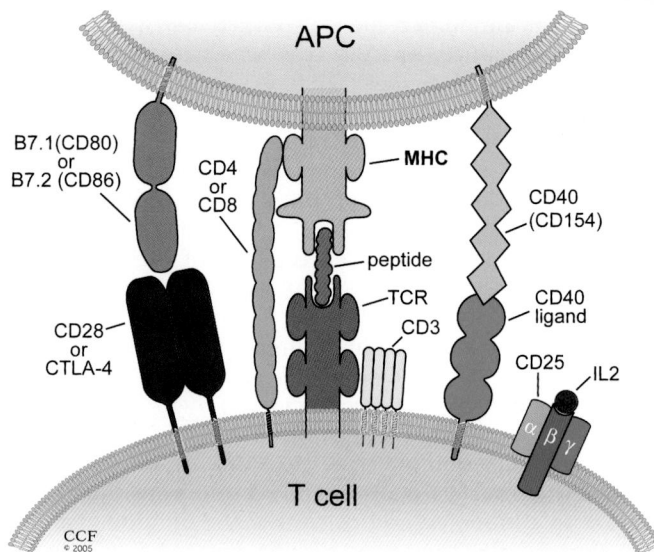

Figure 15–6. T-cell activation requires three signals. Activation is initiated at the cell surface between an antigen-presenting cell (APC) and a T cell bearing a T-cell receptor (TCR). Signal 1 is delivered by an APC via an MHC molecule with peptide bound to a tight-fitting TCR. This interaction is stabilized by a T-cell CD4 during presentation by MHC class II molecules and by a CD8 for presentation by MHC class I molecules. Activation will not proceed without the delivery of a second signal, which is required for further intracellular signal transduction. The second signal may be delivered by one of several glycoproteins such as B7 (CD 80,86) and CD40 to their T cell ligands CD28 and CD40 ligand (CD 154), respectively. The necessary signal 3 is delivered by interleukin-2 and other cytokines (IL-15) to their respective receptors. This leads to activation of various cyclins and the target of rapamycin (TOR), resulting in T-cell proliferation.

8- to 20-amino acid sequences) so it can fit precisely into a groove created by the outermost domains of the class I and class II MHC molecules (Germain, 1994). The result is that the T cell must recognize both MHC and peptide in a particular arrangement for antigen-specific activation to take place (Madden, 1995). **Antigen processing necessitates the conversion of native proteins to peptide/MHC complexes. This involves uptake by the cell, proteolysis, and additional mechanisms for the repackaging and transport of the MHC/peptide complex to the cell surface.** In general, peptides associated with MHC class I are derived from proteins synthesized within the cell on cytosolic ribosomes such as viral and oncogenic products. Those peptides associated with MHC class II molecules often originate from extracellular fluids such as bacterial products and toxins and are taken up by receptor-mediated endocytosis.

Three Signals

T cells become activated when the TCR engages an antigen for which it is specific; however, the TCR must "see" the antigen peptide presented in the groove of an MHC molecule on an APC. The interaction of one TCR and an MHC-peptide is of surprisingly low affinity and must be stabilized by an appropriate co-receptor: CD4 for MHC class II and CD8 for MHC class I molecules (Fig. 15–6). **This initial step is called signal 1.** Although triggering by signal 1 is necessary, it not sufficient for T-cell activation alone. In fact, stimulation by signal 1 alone leads to a state of anergy whereby the T cell becomes unresponsive to antigen. **Activation requires co-stimulation by proteins on the APC that engage specific receptors on the T-cell surface, referred to as signal 2.** The major APC molecules providing signal 2 are B7.1 (CD80) and B7.2 (CD86), but a number of other accessory molecules may support or enhance co-stimulation, such as CD2 engaging leukocyte functional antigen (LFA)-3 (CD58) and LFA-1 engaging ICAM. These molecules engage the T-cell surface glycoprotein CD28, and, when combined with signal 1, lead to activation of the calcium-calcineurin, the mitogen-activated protein (MAP) kinase, and the protein kinase C pathways, which in turn initiate transcription (Halloran, 2004) (see section on signal transduction). **Completion of activation requires the delivery growth factors (IL-2 and 15), via the phosphoinositide-3-kinase (PI-3K) and the target of rapamycin (TOR) pathways, initiating the cell cycle—signal 3.**

Recognition of Alloantigens

The MHC was originally defined by its ability to provoke and sustain the rejection of organs and tissues between members of the same species (the allograft response). This response can be very rapid and intense, because individuals have a very high frequency of potentially alloreactive T cells. **As previously described, only a small fraction of T cells are specific for a single peptide, yet upward of 10% of the T-cell population can react with alloantigens. Why is this so? Alloantigens create a unique potential for T-cell activation because they serve both as immunogens as well as participants in the activation of the immune response in the host.** When an allograft kidney, heart, or liver is transplanted into a recipient it brings with it an array of tissue-bound cell surface class I and II MHC antigens that are foreign to the host. In addition, the grafted organs transport large numbers of "passenger leukocytes," which can be both adherent to the blood vessels as well as within the interstitial tissues. As a "passenger leukocyte," the mononuclear dendritic cell is particularly suited to augment the alloimmune response, because it functions as an APC and can traffic from the graft to recipient secondary lymphoid tissues to interact with immune competent cells. **Remember that the requirements for T-cell activation are dependent on both the presentation of peptide-MHC complexes and the co-stimulatory signals provided by professional APCs.**

The immune response is provided by two distinct pathways for allo-recognition (Gould and Auchincloss, 1999). In the **direct recognition** pathway, recipient T cells engage peptide-MHC molecules expressed on allogeneic cells. **The direct pathway is mainly responsible for the initiation of acute cellular rejection of allografts, and evidence suggests that passenger leukocytes (dendritic cells) play a key role.** These donor APCs must express both MHC class II and the appropriate co-stimulatory molecules, because the depletion of either will prevent an immune response from taking place. The peptides sitting in the MHC groove may be derived from endogenous proteins of either the donor or the recipient. Thus, the foreign MHC molecules presented to the recipient can be a myriad of alloantigens, including the allogeneic MHC molecule itself plus the many different peptides derived from endogenous proteins. There is also evidence that recipient T cells can recognize allo-MHC molecules that are empty, with no peptide in the binding groove. These observations help

explain why so many recipient T cells can become alloreactive and rapidly destroy a graft.

The immune response is also provided by an indirect recognition pathway for alloantigens whereby T cells recognize processed alloantigens presented by recipient APCs in association with self-MHC class II molecules. Mechanistically, this pathway requires the uptake and processing of the donor MHC molecules (to form peptide fragments) by the APCs of the recipient. **The evidence for such an indirect pathway comes from observations that rejection can take place even if donor and recipient share most, if not all, MHC antigens.** During indirect pathway recognition recipient APCs migrate to the graft and take up soluble donor MHC molecules for processing. The actual T-cell activation occurs in recipient secondary lymphoid tissues, similar to activation in the direct pathway. Because the indirect pathway results in T cells that are self-MHC restricted, their numbers are much smaller than those produced from direct pathway recognition, which predominates during the initiation of acute allograft rejection. However, the direct route becomes less important with time as the number of donor APCs diminish by senescence. The ready supply of recipient APCs involved in the indirect pathway is never depleted and can continuously process and present donor antigens. **For this reason indirect recognition is thought to be more closely linked to chronic rejection of an allograft.**

Activation of B Cells

B cells require the help of CD4+ T cells to proliferate and differentiate into plasma cells that synthesize and secrete specific antibody (Parker, 1993). After B cell immunoglobulin receptors react with protein antigens, the antigens are endocytosed, processed, and transported to the cell surface for presentation to resting T cells, only in the context of MHC class II molecules on the surface of the B cell. The helper T cell TCR is engaged and stabilized by its CD4 molecule, which leads to T-cell activation and secretion of lymphokines, including IL-2. These lymphokines promote B-cell growth and differentiation into plasma cells that secrete specific antibodies. **B-cell activation also requires the presence of a second co-stimulatory signal to complete the process. In this case a marker on the B-cell surface, CD40, must be engaged by its ligand CD40L on the surface of the helper T cell** (Foy et al, 1996). **T cells are also required for isotype switching that occurs during some immune responses** (Stavnezer, 1996). Plasma cells often secrete IgM antibodies after primary antigen exposure. Secondary responses (after re-exposure to the same antigen) usually results in the production of IgG or IgA antibodies by B cells with the same antibody-binding variable regions.

B and T cells usually recognize different antigens and/or different epitopes on the same antigen. **B cells usually recognize native proteins, peptides, or denatured proteins through their surface immunoglobulin receptors, whereas T cells are more complex in their recognition system in that smaller peptides are only recognized when processed and presented to T cells by APCs in the context of MHC class I or II molecules.** However, B cells can recognize certain antigens without T cell help. These so-called **T cell–independent antigens** are large macromolecules with repeating segments such as bacterial polysaccharides and lipopolysaccharides that can crosslink many B-cell receptors. These antigens can bypass the second co-stimulatory signal (CD40), elicit a weaker response with poor memory, and usually cause a polyclonal IgM response only. **T cell–dependent antigens** are smaller and more complex and elicit a more specific antibody response with durable memory. All antibody classes can be generated, but this process remains dependent on the delivery of two signals for T-cell help.

CELL SIGNAL TRANSDUCTION

The response of cells to external stimuli typically through surface receptors results in the conversion of that signal into intracellular biochemical events, which ultimately lead to the expression of a variety of genes that are critical for cell function and growth.

TCR Signaling Proximal Events

Activation of T cells is dependent on the signaling events transmitted via the TCR to the nucleus (Fig. 15–7). **Phosphorylation of the tyrosines in ITAMS represents the initial intracellular signaling event after lymphocyte detection of specific antigen** (Van Leeuwen and Samelson, 1999; Kane et al, 2000; Myung et al, 2000). Phosphorylation of ITAMs is

mediated by two Src family kinases: Lck, which constitutively associates with CD8 and CD4 molecules, and Fyn, which interacts with the cytoplasmic domains of the CD3ε and ζ chain after receptor engagement. The phosphotyrosines produced by tyrosine kinases form binding sites for protein domains referred to as SH2 domains (Src homology 2 domains) that are present in a number of signaling molecules. The interaction of SH2 domains with the phosphotyrosines provides an important way for the recruitment of signaling proteins to the activated receptors. TCR signaling can also be negatively regulated by the protein tyrosine kinase Csk, which alters the phosphorylation status of the Src kinases. The kinase domain of the Src kinase contains two tyrosine residues, where one provides an activation signal while the other inactivates the enzyme. In resting cells, the Csk kinase phosphorylates the inhibitory tyrosine that maintains the Src enzymes in an inactive state. The negative effect of Csk on Src kinase function can be reversed by the protein tyrosine phosphatase CD45, which is involved in receptor signaling in T cells. This involves the removal of the phosphate group from the inhibitory tyrosine residue of the Src kinase.

The most effective activation of the TCR requires the interaction with the co-receptor molecules CD4 and CD8 that serves to bring Lck in close proximity to the cytoplasmic domains of the TCR complex (Van Leeuwen and Samelson, 1999; Kane et al, 2000; Myung et al, 2000). Once activated, Lck phosphorylates the tyrosine residues in the ITAMS of the CD3 and TCR ζ chains, which then provide the docking site for the tyrosine kinase ZAP-70. After recruitment to the TCR, ZAP-70 becomes activated as a result of its phosphorylation on multiple tyrosine residues by either Lck or Fyn kinases. Activated ZAP-70 then leads to the activation the adaptor molecules LAT (linker of activation in T cells) and SLP-76. LAT is a transmembrane protein expressed in T cells and NK cells. It is a critical SH-2 domain–binding protein involved in transmitting the signal from the membrane to downstream targets. LAT is essential for coupling the TCR to the PLCγ1-Ca^{2+} and the Ras-signaling pathways. SLP-76 is another adaptor protein that is also important for efficient TCR-induced tyrosine phosphorylation of PLCγ1, inositol phosphate accumulation, Ca^{2+} mobilization, and Ras activation. Thus, the adaptor proteins help to expand the signal from the membrane to the nucleus.

Lipid rafts play an important role in promoting signal transduction via the T-cell receptor. After peptide/MHC class recognition, signaling, adhesion, and cytoskeletal molecules in T cells concentrate at the site of contact with the APCs (Grakour et al, 1999). This immunologic synapse at the contact site represents a specific arrangement of aggregated proteins, which is necessary to initiate intracellular signaling. Lipid microdomains composed of cholesterol and sphingolipid, referred to as lipid rafts (Cherukuri et al, 2001), play a critical role in the localization of signaling proteins to the immunologic synapse. In resting cells the lipid rafts are small (70 nm) but reorganize after stimulation into large aggregates that co-localize with the immunologic synapse. After T-cell activation, the TCR, co-receptors, and the Src kinases Fyn and Lck associate with these lipid rafts as a result of post-translational S-acylation or the addition of GPI proteins (e.g., Lck and LAT) (Bromley et al, 2001). Co-stimulatory molecules appear to play a role in mediating raft aggregation at the site

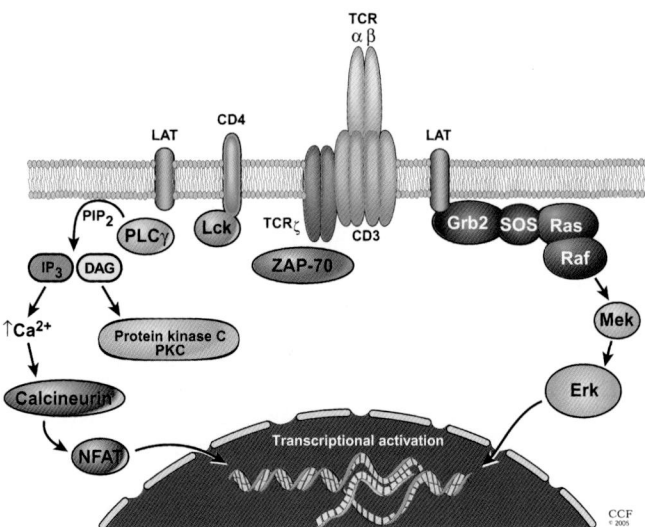

Figure 15–7. Signaling pathway induced by the T-cell receptor. The binding of antigen to the αβ chains of the TCR causes activation of Lck, which in turn results in the phosphorylation of TCR ζ and the recruitment and activation of another tyrosine kinase ZAP-70. This kinase phosphorylates the adaptor molecules LAT and SLP-76 *(not shown)*. LAT then recruits PLCγ to the membrane, where it cleaves its substrate PIP$_2$ into IP$_3$ and diacylglycerol (DAG). IP$_3$ increases Ca^{2+}, which activates the phosphatase calcineurin. Activated calcineurin then dephosphorylates the transcription factor NFAT that then translocates to the nucleus. DAG release leads to the activation of protein kinase-C (PKC). Phosphorylated LAT also binds Grb2 that recruits the guanine-nucleotide exchange factor SOS that activates Ras. Activated Ras then recruits Raf-1 to the membrane where it is activated. Raf-1 then phosphorylates and activates the kinase Mel that then initiates the activation of other kinases in this pathway. The end result is the activation of a number of transcription factors that initiate gene expression.

of synapse (Viola, 1999). Lipid rafts appear to be critical for signaling because disruption of these lipid domains with detergents inhibits T-cell activation. There are also data showing that lipid rafts regulate recruitment of MHC class II and co-stimulatory molecules in dendritic cells and this recruitment is antigen dependent (Meyer zum Bueschenfeld et al, 2004).

Activation of Intracellular Calcium and PKC

Phosphorylation of the enzyme PLC-γ is a critical event in transmitting the activation signal from the membrane downstream (Myung et al, 2000). Once activated, PLC-γ cleaves membrane-bound phospholipid phosphatidylinositol bisphosphate (PIP_2) into two active components, inositol triphosphate (IP_3) and diacylglycerol (DAG). IP_3 induces the release of Ca^{2+} into the cytosol from storage sites within the endoplasmic reticulum, which raises the intracellular levels of Ca^{2+}. This event also leads to the opening of the Ca^{2+} channels in the plasma membrane, which further increases Ca^{2+} levels. **Elevated Ca^{2+} results in the activation of the enzyme calcineurin, which is a cytosolic serine/threonine protein phosphatase that regulates the activation of a family of transcription factors, termed NFAT (nuclear factor of activated T cells).**

NFAT transduces Ca^{2+} signals not only in T lymphocytes but also in B cells, NK cells, monocytes, and nonhematopoietic cells, including those of the cardiac and nervous system (Zhu and McKeon, 2000). Four separate genes are present that encode different NFATs: NFAT1/p, NFAT2.c, NFAT3, and NFAT4. **NFAT along with other transcription factors play a critical role in T cell activation and clonal expansion through their activation of the interleukin-2 gene.** The inactive form of NFAT is retained in the cytoplasm unable to translocate to the nucleus because its nuclear localization sequence (NLS) is phosphorylated on serine/threonine. Calcineurin is composed of a catalytic subunit and a regulator subunit and is activated by the recruitment of Ca^{2+}-bound calmodulin. The association of calmodulin with calcineurin alters the structure of catalytic subunit, leading to activation of its phosphatase activity. Calcineurin then dephosphorylates the NLS of NFAT, allowing the transcription factor to translocate into the nucleus.

NFAT is important for T-cell activation; and because of its role in the regulation of critical genes in this process (e.g., IL-2, proto-oncogenes c-*myc* and cytokine receptors), it is a target for immune suppression in the allotransplant setting (Matsuda and Koyasu, 2000). **The immunosuppressive drugs cyclosporine and tacrolimus function by blocking the NFAT pathway.** Cyclosporine is a small, cyclic, fungus-derived peptide that is immunosuppressive once it has formed a complex with its cytoplasmic receptor, cyclophilin, a ubiquitous cytosolic protein. The activity of tacrolimus also is dependent on binding to its receptor, FK-binding protein 12 (FKBP12). **The active complexes, cyclosporine/cyclophilin and tacrolimus/FKBP12, are known to block NFAT nuclear translocation by binding to the catalytic subunit of calcineurin and inhibiting its phosphatase activity.** The major inhibitory activity of cyclosporine and tacrolimus is thought

to be their suppression of the growth factor IL-2. In addition to the calcineurin/NFAT pathway, it appears that cyclosporine may also block T cell activation by blocking activation of the transcription factor JNK.

The cleavage of the PIP_2 by PLC-γ enzyme also results in the formation of DAG, which remains attached to the inner surface of the plasma membrane (Myung et al, 2000). DAG is involved in the activation of protein kinase C (PKC), a serine/threonine protein kinase that regulates the nuclear translocation of various transcription factors, including NFκB. PKC can be further activated by the rise in Ca^{2+} resulting from the release of IP_3.

Ras Pathway

Another important pathway that results from the activation of the TCR-associated tyrosine kinases involves the small guanosine triphosphate (GTP)-binding protein Ras (Genot and Cantrell, 2000). **Ras proteins are proto-oncogenes that were initially discovered because of their effect on tumor cell growth. However, a decade ago it was found that activated Ras also accumulates in normal lymphocytes after activation. Ras is an essential component of pathways that activate transcription factors involved in cytokine gene induction.** This includes the AP-1 family of transcription factors, which are composed of heterodimers of the oncogenes *fos* and *jun*. Ras also regulates other transcription factors such as NFAT, Elk-1, and the serum response factor (SRF). Ras also mediates TCR signals important to thymocyte and B-cell development. Moreover, defects in the activation of Ras have been linked to the development of T-cell anergy. Ras is a guanine-nucleotide binding protein that rapidly cycles from an inactive guanosine diphosphate (GDP) bound to an active GTP-bound state. Ras has GTPase activity that removes a phosphate group from GTP to leave the inactive GDP-bound form. The activation of Ras involves a guanine-nucleotide exchange factor; and, once activated, it induces a cascade of protein kinases referred to as the mitogen-activated protein kinases (MAP kinase) cascade. One of the best characterized Ras effector pathways is mediated by the MAP kinase Raf-1. Activation through the TCR results in the tyrosine phosphorylation of LAT that binds to Grb2 and recruits the guanine-nucleotide exchange factor SOS that activates the G protein, Ras. Activated Ras recruits Raf-1 to the plasma membrane where Raf-1 is activated. Raf-1 then phosphorylates and activates the kinase Mek, which then activates the MAPKs Erk1 and Erk2. These events ultimately lead to the activation of a variety of transcription factors.

B-Cell Signaling

The receptor on B cells that recognizes antigen and transmits signal to the nucleus for gene expression is composed of a cell surface immunoglobulin containing heavy and light chains with variable regions (Janeway et al, 1999). The immunoglobulin molecule is linked to two proteins (Igα and Igβ) that consist of a single amino-terminal Ig-like domain and a transmembrane domain linked to a cytoplasmic tail. Igα and Igβ are involved in signaling and contain one ITAM each. The Src kinases Fyn, Blk, and Lyn are associated with the B-cell receptor and are responsible for the phosphorylation of the ITAM after antigen engagement. The phosphatase CD45 is likely involved in removing inhibitory phosphates from the Src kinases and thus allowing their activation. Signaling, via the immunoglobulin receptors, is facilitated by co-receptor molecules that include CD19, CD21, and CD81. CD21 is a receptor for complement fragments that can recognize complement associated with antigen bound to the immunoglobulin receptor. These complexes crosslink CD21, which then induces phosphorylation of the cytoplasmic tail of CD19, allowing other Src kinases to bind and thus enhance receptor signaling. The next protein tyrosine kinase involved in the B-cell pathway is Syk, which induces the activation of phospholipase C-γ, leading to an increase in Ca^{2+} levels and activation of PKC. The tyrosine kinases are also responsible for activating the Ras pathway. Activation of these various pathways leads to induction of transcription factors that initiate gene expression required for B-cell proliferation and effector function.

JAK/STAT Signaling Pathway

The Janus family of kinases (Jak kinases) and the STAT (signal transducers and activators of transcription) proteins constitute one of the main signaling pathways that regulate cytokine gene expression (Schindler, 1999; Imada and Leonard, 2000). In mammals there are four Jak kinases, Jak1, Jak2, Jak3, and Tyk2, which are constitutively associated with many different cytokine receptors. However, different cytokines receptors are regulated by select Jak kinases. For example, Jak1 and Tyk2 are required for IFN-α/β signaling whereas IFN-γ is dependent on Jak1 and Jak2. On the other hand, cytokines whose receptors share γc (IL-2, IL-4, IL-7, IL-9, and IL-15) utilize Jak1 and Jak3, except IL-13, which uses Jak1, Jak2, and Tyk2. Cytokines whose receptors share βc (IL-3, IL-5, and granulocyte-macrophage colony-stimulating factor [GM-CSF]) use Jak2. Ligand binding causes dimerization of receptor chains, leading to activation of the Jaks and phosphorylation of the receptors that provide docking sites for the STAT proteins. The recruited STATs are phosphorylated by the Jaks and then translocate to the nucleus, where they initiate transcription. Seven different STAT proteins have been identified. Differences in the SH2 domains of the different STAT proteins determine their selectivity to various cytokine receptors.

The biologic importance of different Jaks and STATs has been revealed by deficiencies in these proteins in both humans and animal models (Imada and Leonard, 2000). **Mutations in Jak3 have resulted in patients having severe combined immunodeficiency (SCID), which is similar to X-linked SCID, which occurs because of a mutation in the common cytokine receptor γ chain.** Mice that are deficient in either Jak1 or Jak2 show perinatal lethality. STAT1-deficient mice demonstrate a significant defect in INF-dependent antiviral and antimicrobial immune responses. STAT4-deficient mice confirm that STAT4 is only activated by IL-12, as illustrated by the fact that T cells from these mice were unresponsive to IL12 and were defective in TH1 development. It has also been noted that STAT6-deficient mice are impaired in the development of a Th2 immune response as predicted because IL-4 and IL-13 activate STAT6.

T-CELL ACTIVATION AND EFFECTOR FUNCTION

After development in the thymus, T cells seed the peripheral lymphoid tissues such as the spleen, the lymph nodes, and the gut-associated lymphoid tissue (GALT). Until they are activated through TCR-mediated engagement of specific antigen/MHC complex on professional APCs, these T cells are immunologically quiescent and do not express immune functions. **Activation of specific T cells and the generation of an immune response requires transport of antigenic components to the lymphoid tissue. For the induction of most T cell–mediated immune responses, the critical APC is the dendritic cell. These cells are interspersed throughout peripheral tissues** (Banchereau and Steinman, 1998). As situated in the peripheral tissues, dendritic cells exist in an immature state and must be activated to perform the immune functions of antigen-processing and presentation and trafficking to the lymphoid tissue.

The immune system has evolved with highly regulated components to control the activation of dendritic cells and the transport of antigenic material to the lymphoid tissue. **Tissue trauma and/or the deposition of antigenic material into peripheral tissues such as a microbial infection, vaccination, or an organ allograft induce a local inflammatory response. This inflammation is initiated by the production of TNF-α and IL-1 in response to tissue trauma and/or recognition of microbial products** (Tracey and Cerami, 1994). An important consequence of this response is that inflammation is stimulatory for antigen capture, processing, and transport to the lymphoid tissues. **Interstitial dendritic cells are activated by TNF-α to become phagocytic cells and ingest pieces of foreign material and tissue debris. The ingested material is processed or degraded within specialized intracellular compartments, and peptides and glycolipids are presented as complexes in association with class I or II MHC-encoded proteins. TNF-α produced during tissue inflammation also stimulates the dendritic cells to downregulate the expression of molecules retaining or tethering dendritic cells in parenchymal tissues and to upregulate expression of receptors for chemoattractant cytokines, or chemokines, that direct trafficking of the dendritic cells through the afferent lymphatic vessels and into the T cell–rich areas of lymphoid tissues draining the tissue site** (Saeki et al, 1999).

After trafficking to the lymphoid tissue, dendritic cells presenting peptide/MHC complexes secrete proteins that attract naive T cells to survey or sample the dendritic cell surface. **During antigen presentation in the lymphoid tissues, T cells expressing receptors with specificity for peptides presented in association with class II MHC molecules (i.e., CD4+ T cells) and/or T cells with specificity for peptides presented in association with class I MHC molecules (i.e., CD8+ T cells) are stimulated to develop into effector cells** (Germain and Margulies, 1993). In addition to TCR engagement of peptide/MHC complexes, activation of naive T cells to functional activity requires other receptor-ligand interactions

(Schwartz, 1992). This co-stimulation is provided by several complementary sets of molecules. During the initial period of T-cell priming, TCR engagement of peptide/class II MHC complexes on the dendritic cell stimulates the CD4+ T cell to express the ligand, CD154, which binds to a co-stimulatory molecule, CD40, constitutively expressed by dendritic cells. Engagement of this ligand-receptor pair stimulates the dendritic cell to upregulate expression of the CD80/B7-1 and/or CD86/B7-2 co-stimulatory molecules that bind to a constitutively expressed molecule, CD28, on the T-cell surface.

CD8+ T cells do not express CD154 during peptide/class I MHC interaction for the generation of many immune responses. However, other co-stimulatory molecules such as 4-BB1 have been identified for CD8+ T cells and these molecules may in some circumstances substitute for the absence of CD154 expression. Similar to the activation of CD4+ T cells, most CD8+ T cell responses are dependent on B7-mediated co-stimulation during priming. **It is also important to note that the generation of many CD8+ T cell–mediated responses requires provision of CD4+ T cell helper signals. The CD4+ T cells' help is not provided through production of cytokines for antigen-specific CD8+ T cell growth but through delivery of signals to the antigen-presenting dendritic cells that "license" the dendritic cell to activate the CD8+ T cell.** CD40-CD154 interactions appear to be important signaling components in dendritic cell licensing to activate CD8+ T cells, and CD4+ T-cell help can be replaced by agonist anti-CD40 antibodies. CD4+ T-cell helper dependent CD8+ T-cell responses include most CD8+ T-cell responses to viruses and to solid organ allografts, whereas CD4+ T cell–independent responses include CD8+ T-cell responses to skin allografts and to contact allergens.

During T-cell priming by dendritic cells in the lymphoid tissues, many regulated events occur that promote the optimal development of T cell–mediated immune responses. These events include the expression of growth factor receptors on the T cell, production of the appropriate growth factors, the expression of molecules that direct trafficking of the primed T cells to inflammatory sites, and production of effector molecules mediating the immune response after T-cell arrival at the peripheral site of inflammation and interaction with cells expressing the target peptide/MHC complex. These immune functions may include the production of various cytokines or the expression of cytolytic functions where target cells expressing the specific peptide/MHC complex are induced to undergo apoptosis during interaction with the primed T cell.

Clonal Expansion of Specific T Cells

Because the frequency of naive T cells for a particular peptide/self MHC complex is very low (e.g., 1 in 10^5-10^6 T cells), the pool of reactive T cells needs to be expanded during priming to mount an effective immune response. **Most naive or quiescent T cells constitutively express the common cytokine receptor γ chain, which is a component of the receptor for many cytokines, including IL-2, IL-4, IL-7, IL-9, and IL-15** (Leonard, 1996). The common γ chain is the target defect in X-linked SCID. In addition to the common γ chain, most naive T cells constitutively express the IL-2 receptor β

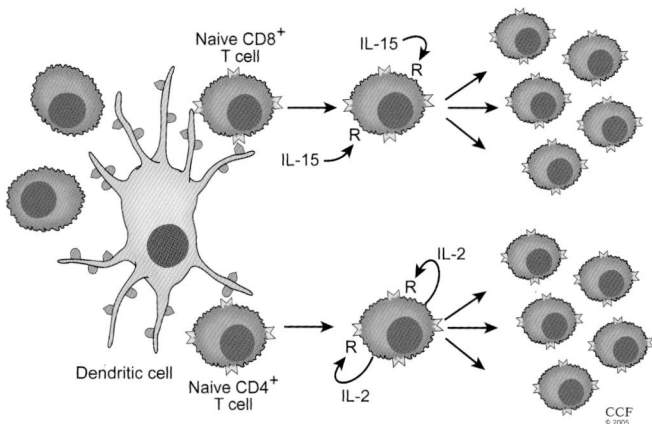

Figure 15–8. Activation of naive CD4+ and/or CD8+ T cells by dendritic cells results in proliferation of the reactive T-cell clones. After emigration from the peripheral tissues to lymphoid tissues, dendritic cells presenting foreign peptides in the context of class I and/or class II MHC molecules activate CD8+ and CD4+ T cells bearing receptors with specificity for the peptide/MHC complex. This activation includes the upregulation of growth factor receptor components that increase the affinity of the growth factor receptor. In addition to the expression of CD25 and high-affinity IL-2 receptors, activated CD4+ T cells produce IL-2, which is utilized in an autocrine manner to drive clonal proliferation of the activated CD4+ T cell. During activation, CD8+ T cells are stimulated to express the α chain of the IL-15 receptor that forms the high-affinity receptor for this growth factor. In contrast to IL-2–mediated expansion of CD4+ T cells, IL-15 is not produced by the CD8+ T cell but is produced by the dendritic cell and stromal cells in the lymphoid tissue.

chain. The combination of the β and γ chains forms a receptor complex with low affinity for IL-2. **TCR engagement of specific ligand with delivery of co-stimulation during CD4+ T-cell priming induces the expression of the IL-2 receptor α chain (CD25) on the T cells. In combination, the α, β, and γ chains constitute the high-affinity IL-2 binding receptor.** TCR engagement plus co-stimulation also stimulates the CD4+ T cells to produce IL-2, which binds to the high-affinity trimer and stimulates clonal proliferation of the CD4+ T cells in an autocrine manner (Fig. 15–8). This series of events results in rapid expansion of the reactive CD4+ T cell pool. Activation of naive CD8+ T cells does not generally induce the IL-2 receptor α chain. **Although CD8+ T cell expansion can be promoted in vitro during culture with IL-2, a different growth factor, IL-15, appears to be critical for naive CD8+ T cell proliferation during antigen priming in vivo** (Kennedy et al, 2000). **For expansion of reactive CD8+ T cells, TCR engagement of peptide/class I MHC complexes stimulates the upregulated expression of the α chain of the IL-15 receptor. Rather than T cells, IL-15 is produced by a number of nonlymphoid cells, including fibroblasts, epithelial cells, and dendritic cells.**

After initial priming and expansion of the peptide/MHC-reactive T-cell pool, T cells develop into cells with effector function. Effector T cells mediate and regulate immune responses through two activities: cytokine production and expression of cytolytic function. These effector functions are then expressed by antigen-primed T cells after interaction with target cells expressing the specific peptide/MHC ligand in peripheral tissues during elicitation of the immune response.

Table 15–2. **Representative Cytokines**

Cytokine	Cellular Source	Major Activities
IL-1	Macrophages, endothelial cells, keratinocytes	Upregulation of adhesion molecule expression, stimulation of chemokine production, activation of macrophages and T cells
IL-2	T cells	Activation of NK cells, T-cell growth factor
IL-4	Type 2 CD4+ and CD8+ T cells	T-cell growth factor, B-cell growth factor, Ig class switching to IgE
IL-5	Type 2 CD4+ and CD8+ T cells	Stimulation of eosinophil development
IL-6	Type 2 CD4+ T cells, macrophages	Stimulation of acute phase proteins, activation of lymphocytes
IL-10	Th2 and Th3 T cells, macrophages	Immunosuppression
IL-12	Macrophages, dendritic cells	Stimulation of IFN-γ production
IL-13	Type 2 CD4+ T cells	Allergic inflammation, upregulation of vascular cell adhesion molecule-1 (VCAM-1) expression
IL-15	Fibroblasts, endothelial cells, dendritic cells	CD8+ T-cell growth factor
TNF-α	T cells, NK cells, macrophages	Upregulation of adhesion molecule expression, stimulation of chemokine production, inflammation
TNF-β	Type 1 CD4+ and CD8+ T cells	Macrophage activation, cytolysis
IFN-γ	Type 1 CD4+ and CD8+ T cells, NK cells	Macrophage activation, upregulation of adhesion molecule expression, production of T-cell chemoattractants, inhibition of Th2 cells
GM-CSF	T cells, NK cells, B cells, macrophages	Stimulation of macrophages and granulocyte development
TGF-β	T cells, B cells, mast cells, macrophages	Immunosuppression

IL, interleukin; TNF, tumor necrosis factor; IFN, interferon; GM-CSF, granulocyte-macrophage colony-stimulating factor; TGF, transforming growth factor.

T-Cell Development of Cytokine-Producing Phenotypes

During antigen priming, CD4+ T cells develop into cells producing type 1 cytokines (e.g., Th1 cells) or into cells producing type 2 cytokines (e.g., Th2 cells) (O'Garra, 1998). Type 1 cytokines include IFN-γ and TNF-β (also called lymphotoxin) and are critical components of cell-mediated immune responses, particularly in responses to intracellular parasites and tuberculin delayed-type hypersensitivity (Table 15–2). The prototypic type 1 cytokine IFN-γ induces a number of proinflammatory events, including stimulating increased class I and class II MHC expression, stimulating production of intracellular molecules required for antigen processing and presentation, and stimulating macrophage proinflammatory activities, such as superoxide and nitrous oxide production, which render macrophages engulfing bacteria competent to kill the bacteria. These inflammatory functions are also important components of many organ-specific autoimmune diseases. Type 2 cytokines include IL-4, IL-5, IL-6, and IL-9 and are critical components of allergic responses and immune responses to extracellular parasites such as helminths. These activities include the stimulation of eosinophil and mast cell growth and function, including the release of histamine and other molecules involved in allergic responses. IL-4 is also an important stimulus of B-cell growth.

The type 1 and type 2 cytokines also influence the isotype of antibody produced by B cells during an immune response. In general, the type 1 cytokines skew antibody responses to those fixing complement and participating in cell-mediated immune responses that are critical for protection against intracellular pathogens such as opsonization. In contrast, type 2 cytokines stimulate IgE production and other antibodies involved in allergic reactions. Obviously, the phenotype of T-cell cytokine production will have an important impact on the course of immune responses to infectious agents, as well as on the sequelae of the response.

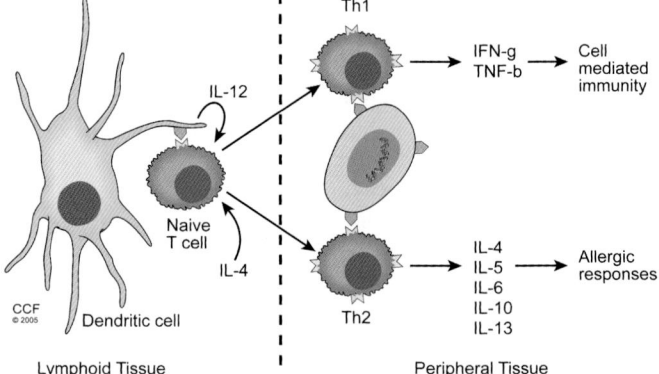

Figure 15–9. The cytokine environment during peptide/class II MHC priming influences skewing of CD4+ T cell development to Th1 or Th2 cells. After emigration from the peripheral tissues to lymphoid tissues, dendritic cells presenting foreign peptide in the context of class II MHC molecules activate specific CD4+ T cells to develop to immune effector T cells. The production of IL-12 by the dendritic cell or the presence of IL-12 during CD4+ T cell priming skews the CD4+ T cells to develop into Th1 cells. On encounter with the specific peptide/class II MHC complex in the periphery, the Th1 cells are activated to produce type 1 cytokines such as IFN-γ or TNF-β during the elicitation of the immune response. The presence of IL-4 in the priming environment skews the CD4+ T cells to develop into Th2 cells. On encounter with the specific peptide/class II MHC complex in the periphery, the Th2 cells are activated to produce type 2 cytokines such as IL-4, IL-5, or IL-13 that promote allergic-type immune responses.

The most important factor influencing the development of CD4+ T cells to Th1 or Th2 cells is the cytokine environment present during priming by the APC (Fig. 15–9). Within 48 hours of initial priming by dendritic cells, CD4+ T cells are polarized to type 1 or type 2 cytokine production (i.e., Th1 or Th2 cells). **Production of the cytokine IL-12 by antigen-presenting dendritic cells is a critical factor in skewing CD4+ T-cell development to the type 1 cytokine producing phenotype** (Gately et al, 1998). IL-12 is a 75-kD disulfide-linked dimer of p35 and p40 subunits. The p35 subunit is constitutively produced by many cells, whereas production of the p40 subunit is restricted to macrophages and dendritic cells. Induction of p40 expression and IL-12 heterodimer production by these cells is stimulated by microbial products and by CD40 ligation during interaction with T cells. In the absence of IL-12 or in the presence of IL-4, CD4+ T-cell development is skewed to the type 2 cytokine-producing phenotype. The source of this IL-4 during priming of the Th2 cells is not clear but may be provided by cells that express at least some properties of NK cells and some properties of T cells, NK T cells. Other factors may also influence CD4+ T-cell development to Th1 versus Th2 cells, including the IL-12–related cytokines IL-23 and IL-27, the antigen dose, and the type of co-stimulation provided during priming.

Antigen priming of CD8+ T cells in vivo usually induces IFN-γ–producing cells. In contrast to CD4+ T cells, CD8+ T-cell development to IFN-γ–producing cells is not dependent on the presence of IL-12 during priming. In vitro, development of CD8+ T cells to type 1 versus type 2 production can be promoted during antigen stimulation in the presence of IL-12 or IL-4, respectively. CD8+ T cells producing IL-4 and IL-5 have been isolated from patients with the tuberculoid form of leprosy or the acquired immunodeficiency syndrome (AIDS), which may indicate that the induction of type 2–producing CD8+ T cells in vivo is limited to certain disease states.

An important facet of the immune system is that type 1 and type 2 cytokines are counterregulatory (Sher and Coffman, 1992). **IFN-γ inhibits IL-4 production as well as the development of CD4+ T cells to the type 2 cytokine–producing phenotype. Similarly, IL-4 inhibits the development of CD4+ T cells to IFN-γ–producing cells.** During T cell/dendritic cell interactions there are many cytokine-mediated regulatory events that occur. For example, the presence of IL-12 induces the production of IFN-γ that, in turn, stimulates increased expression of the inducible IL-12 β_2 receptor component. Alternatively, the presence of IL-4 downregulates the expression of the β_2 receptor subunit and the T-cell development is skewed to the type 2 cytokine–producing phenotype.

In addition, IL-12 stimulates T-cell production of the transcription factor T-Bet, which promotes IFN-γ production, whereas IL-4 stimulates production of the transcription factors c-Maf and GATA-3, which promote IL-4 production. **In addition to the Th1 and Th2 populations of cytokine-producing T cells, a novel population of CD4+ T cells that produce IL-10 and TGFβ has been identified in some experimental systems and in humans** (Groux et al, 1997). **These cytokines, and therefore these T cells, have potent downregulatory activities for Th1- and Th2-mediated responses.**

T Cell–Mediated Cytolysis of Target Cells

The development of CD8+ T cells with cytolytic function is a critical component of many immune responses to tumors, viruses, and other intracellular parasites. Cytolysis of infected target cells is an efficient mechanism for inhibiting the replication of intracellular parasites. **There are two major mechanisms utilized by CD8+ T cells to mediate cytolysis of cells expressing the target peptide/class I MHC complex** (Fig. 15–10). **During priming in the lymphoid tissue, CD8+ T cells may develop into cells containing intracellular granules containing a protein called perforin and a family of serine esterases, of which granzyme B is the prototype enzyme** (Shi et al, 1997). After TCR engagement of the specific peptide/class I MHC complex on a target cell the CD8+ T cell becomes activated to release these granules toward the target cell. The perforin monomers polymerize in the membrane of the target cell, forming a pore. Granzyme B then enters the target cell and enzymatically activates intracellular caspases, such as caspase 10, leading to the induction of apoptosis. Perforin/granzyme B–mediated cytolysis is also an important function expressed by NK cells during innate immune responses and immune surveillance. Another lytic protein in T-cell and NK-cell granules, granulysin, is an

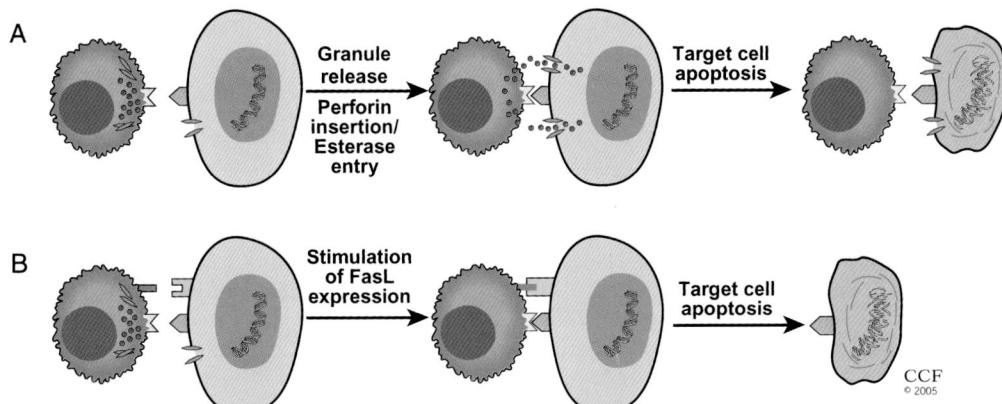

Figure 15–10. Two pathways utilized by CD8+ T cells to mediate cytolysis of target cells. After priming by peptide/class I MHC complexes presented by dendritic cells in the lymphoid tissues, CD8+ T cells enter peripheral tissues and mediate cytolysis of target cells expressing the priming peptide/class I MHC complex. **A,** After recognition of the target complex on target cells, the CD8+ T cell is activated to release cytotoxic granules containing perforin and serine esterases, such as granzymes A and B. The perforin monomers form a complex in the cell membrane of the target cell, allowing the serine esterases to enter the target cell. The enzymes activate caspases, which promote apoptosis of the target cell. **B,** After recognition of the target complex on target cells, the CD8+ T cell is activated to express FasL. The interaction of FasL with Fas on the surface of the target cell stimulates the induction of the apoptotic pathway and the death of the target cell.

important component of CD8+ T cell–mediated responses to intracellular microbial infections (Stenger et al, 1998). **The second major cytolytic mechanism is mediated through expression of Fas ligand (FasL), a member of the TNF family of proteins** (Sabelko-Downes and Russell, 2000). **FasL is induced on T cells after TCR recognition of the specific peptide/MHC complex. Engagement of FasL with the Fas receptor expressed by the target cell transduces apoptotic signaling, resulting in target cell death.** Although cytolytic function has been primarily attributed to CD8+ T cells during immune responses, there is considerable evidence for CD4+ T-cell expression of perforin/granzyme B- and FasL-mediated lytic function, which may be an important component of immune responses to class II MHC–bearing target cells. Expression of mRNA encoding perforin and FasL is observed during rejection of renal allografts and is a reliable indicator of an ongoing acute rejection response.

Phenotypic Changes on T Cells during TCR-Mediated Activation

In addition to alterations in immune function, priming induces many phenotypic changes in T cells. As discussed earlier, the expression of high-affinity receptors for growth factors is necessary for clonal expansion of reactive T cells and for their development to cells with immune effector function. An activation antigen, CD69, is expressed within hours of TCR engagement, and this expression disappears within 18 hours of its initial appearance. **Once T cells have been primed to the specific peptide/MHC complex, it is essential that they be able to get to sites in the peripheral tissue where an immune response is needed. During activation T cells downmodulate expression of CD62L, a receptor that facilitates T cell entry into lymph nodes. Activation also stimulates T cells to express adhesion molecules and chemokine receptors that direct the cells to inflammation in the vascular endothelium.** These molecules and their role in the immune response are discussed in more detail later. Phenotypic analysis of circulating T cells is often used in diagnosis of an ongoing immune response, such as during an infection or autoimmune disease.

Memory Cells

During activation and clonal expansion of specific T cells a portion of the pool develops into a population of memory T cells (Dutton et al, 1998). **In contrast to the effector T cells developing during the course of a primary immune response, the memory T cell population is long lived.** This results in an increased frequency of reactive T cells when compared with the original naive progenitor T cells. Whether memory T cells originate from specific precursor cells or from a set of long-lived primary effector T cells is still not clear and is under investigation in many laboratories. **Phenotypically, memory T cells express a high-molecular-weight form of CD45, CD45ROA, whereas naive T cells express the low-molecular-weight form, CD45RA. In addition to an increased precursor frequency, memory T cells have a lower threshold of activation and require less antigen/MHC**

complex to become activated. After re-encounter with the specific ligand, memory T cells will more quickly expand and develop to effector T cells than naive T cells. In contrast to effector T cells generated during a primary immune response, memory T cells may also express multiple immune effector functions.

Similar to T cells, naive B-cell activation results in the development of a memory B-cell pool. Subsequent activation of memory B cells results in more rapid generation of antibody responses than during primary antibody responses. **In contrast to memory T cells, the antibody produced by memory B cells is of increased affinity that is the result of somatic hypermutation of the V region genes of the memory B cell** (Wagner and Neuberger, 1996). **Furthermore, the isotypes of antibody produced by memory B cells (e.g., IgG and IgA) are different from those produced during primary B cell responses (e.g., primarily IgM with some IgG).** The purpose of vaccination is to induce populations of memory T and B cells so that on infection with the microbial agent a protective immune response is quickly mounted and consists of a broader range of protective effector mechanisms.

APOPTOSIS-PROGRAMMED CELL DEATH
Death Receptor Pathway

Apoptosis is a mechanism by which an organism deletes aged, damaged, and autoimmune cells or cells that are no longer required in subsequent stages of differentiation (Ashkenazi and Dixit, 1998; Scaffidi et al, 1999). There are many stimuli that induce apoptosis, and numerous intracellular pathways that lead from these to the final effector phase of the process. **The proteins responsible for executing the suicide program, the caspases, are essentially common to all the stimuli and pathways and mediate the nuclear and cytoplasmic alterations characteristic of apoptotic cell death.** The specific roles of each member of the caspase cascade are gradually becoming defined, where caspases-3, -6 and -7 have been identified as the terminal effectors mediating DNA fragmentation and chromatin condensation. The caspase cascade has been best defined in the Fas (CD95) and TNFR (CD120a) pathways (Fig. 15–11).

Fas and TNFR1 belong to the TNF receptor gene superfamily and contain a cytoplasmic sequence termed the *death domain*. The death domains enable the death receptors to engage the cells' apoptosis machinery. Interaction between the Fas receptor (Apo-1/CD95) and its ligand (Fas-L/CD95-L) is known to regulate several types of physiologic apoptosis. Fas-L is used by lymphocytes not only as a cytotoxic effector mechanism to induce apoptosis in Fas expressing targets but also to diminish the immune response once the targeted antigen has been eliminated. Fas/Fas-L–mediated induction of apoptosis is also an effective mechanism of T-cell homeostasis whereby self-reactive clones can be eliminated. Fas/Fas-L is also involved in killing of inflammatory cells at immune-privileged sites. The engagement of TNFR1 by its ligand TNF activates the transcription factors NFκB and AP-1, leading to the induction of proinflammatory and immunomodulatory genes that are critical to the development of an immune response. In contrast to Fas, TNF does not induce apoptosis

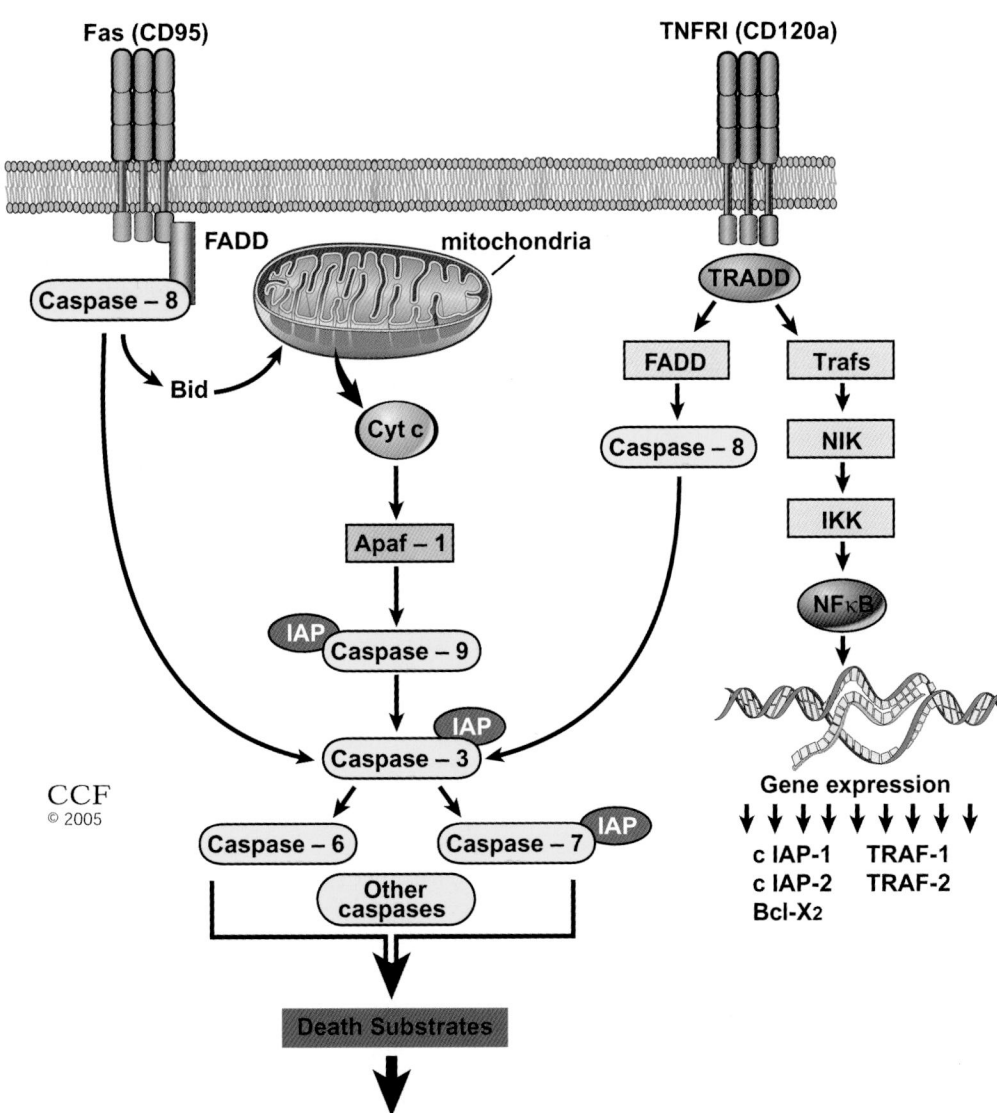

Figure 15–11. Scheme of Fas and TNFR1 activation leading to apoptosis. Ligation of Fas results in FADD binding to the death domains of the Fas receptor. FADD then recruits and activates caspase-8, which in turns activates downstream caspases in this pathway. Caspase-8 can also cleave Bid, which can induce the release of cytochrome *c* from the mitochondria. Cytochrome *c* binding to Apaf-1 results in caspase-9 activation that then initiates the caspase cascade to apoptosis. TNFR1 ligation can also initiate the death pathway through the activation of caspase-8. It also activates the signaling pathway for the activation of the transcription factor NFκB. NFκB regulates the expression of a number of anti-apoptotic genes (e.g., cIAP), some of which can bind to and inhibit the activity of caspases.

via TNFR1 unless protein synthesis is blocked, suggesting that preexisting anti-apoptotic genes can block the apoptotic pathway.

Oligomerization of Fas (or under certain conditions TNFR1) results in the direct or indirect recruitment, respectively, of the Fas-associated death domain (FADD), which in turn activates caspase-8. Using selective inhibitors, a branched protease cascade was revealed in the Fas pathway, in which caspase-8 activates caspases-3 and -7 and caspase-3 activates caspase-6. Caspases-3 and -6 have specific roles in the nuclear changes accompanying apoptosis, whereas caspase-7 was responsible for the mitochondrial permeability transition and cytoplasmic shrinkage.

Mitochondrial Pathway

In many apoptosis scenarios, changes in mitochondria play an integral role in the cell death process (Green and Reed, 1998). Although the caspases can be characterized as the molecules that directly mediate apoptotic cell death, the Bcl-2 family of proteins regulates apoptosis at the mitochondrial level. The anti-apoptotic members of this group (Bcl-2 and Bcl-X_L) buffer some of the signals that initiate the sequence to cell destruction, whereas others in the family (BAD, BAX) are pro-apoptotic (Adams and Cory, 1998). The anti-apoptotic and pro-apoptotic members act by differentially modulating cytochrome *c* release from mitochondria. Binding of cytochrome *c* to Apaf-1 causes a conformational change that results in the interaction of Apaf-1 with procaspase-9 and the ultimate activation of the latter to initiate a caspase cascade. Some pro-apoptotic members of the Bcl-2 family bind and destabilize the mitochondrial membrane directly, whereas others heterodimerize to and antagonize the anti-apoptotic membrane–spanning proteins. In addition to stabilizing the mitochondrial membrane to prevent cytochrome *c* release, Bcl-2 also acts cytoplasmically to inhibit activation of caspase-9. Overexpression of Bcl-2 and Bcl-X_L by gene transfer acts dominantly to prevent the activity of expressed pro-apoptotic Bcl family members. It is also clear that the mitochondria pathway can be induced after activation of the death receptors

(Fas). The linkage between these pathways is the protein Bid, which is inactive in the cytosol but can be cleaved into an active form by caspase-8. The active fragment of Bid travels to the mitochondria and induces cytochrome *c* release, resulting in the activation of downstream effector caspases (Lu et al, 1998).

NFκB Regulation of Apoptosis

The importance of NFκB in host survival has been elucidated from studies using knockout mice having deletions of individual NFκB family members (Barkett and Gilmore, 1999). Cells deficient in RelA are much more sensitive to TNFα-mediated apoptosis as compared with the wild type. This increased sensitivity to apoptosis is reversed by over-expression of RelA. The inhibition of NFκB activation in T cells from mice expressing a dominant/negative form of IκBα also leads to a dramatic increase in apoptosis. Sensitivity to Fas-mediated apoptosis is also enhanced in T cells in which NFκB activation is impaired.

The increased susceptibility to apoptosis in NFκB defective cells probably results from the fact that NFκB regulates the expression of anti-apoptotic genes (Deveraux and Reed, 1999). This includes TRAF-1 and TRAF-2, which associate with the cytoplasmic regions of TNFR family members. TRAF-2 interacts with downstream signal transducers that activate NFκB, while TRAF-1 is required for the recruitment of the NFκB-inducible cellular inhibitors of apoptosis proteins (cIAP-1 and cIAP-2). The cIAPs can directly bind and neutralize caspases-3, -7 and -9, and are thought to have other downstream anti-apoptotic roles as signal transducers. Interestingly, the relative expression levels of these proteins can also impact on cell survival. Once bound, TRAF-2 can recruit either TRAF-1 or cIAP for protective responses or other, pro-apoptotic molecules capable of inhibiting TRAF-2-mediated NFκB activation. Thus, inhibited TRAF-1 expression, notwithstanding abundant TRAF-2 levels, could itself render T cells sensitive to AICD. Overexpression of TRAF-1, TRAF-2, cIAP-1, and cIAP-2 by transfection can together inhibit the apoptosis observed when NFκB activation is suppressed in TNF-sensitive cells. IEX-1L is another NFκB-dependent gene, whose transfection into NFκB-defective mutants also provides protection against apoptosis in some systems.

Other anti-apoptotic molecules with NFκB-dependent expression include Bcl-2, Bcl-X$_L$, and Bfl-1/A1, members of the Bcl family of proteins. While some members of the family are pro-apoptotic, these molecules are known to protect against apoptosis induced by mediators of the mitochondrial permeability transition and also have been found to inhibit the activation of caspase-9. Again, the relative expression levels of pro-apoptotic and anti-apoptotic Bcl-2 family members have a significant impact on cell survival.

LYMPHOCYTE TOLERANCE

The recombinatorial mechanisms generating receptors on T and B lymphocyte precursors results in the appearance of cells expressing receptors with reactivity to self-proteins. If allowed to mature and become activated in peripheral tissues, self-reactive lymphoid cells could cause considerable harm by mediating autoimmune disease. In addition to the generation of T and B cell clones with reactivity to a great number of different antigens, an essential feature of the immune system is the presence of mechanisms to remove or inactivate those cells with specificity for self-peptides. The development of autoimmune disease represents the failure of mechanisms maintaining nonresponsiveness or tolerance to self-proteins. Formally, tolerance may be defined as the inability of the immune system to react to a specific determinant after an initial encounter with that determinant. Thus, the development of tolerance results in the absence of lymphocyte reactivity to receptor reactive ligands that have been encountered previously by the immune system. The immune system has evolved with several mechanisms to circumvent the activation of antigen reactive T and B lymphocytes. As is briefly discussed next, mechanisms mediating tolerance to self-proteins may be manipulated in the design of strategies to induce tolerance to exogenous antigens, such as alloantigens expressed by organ allografts.

Central Tolerance

An important mechanism mediating tolerance to self-proteins is the deletion of self-reactive T cells and B cells during maturation. This mechanism is termed *central tolerance*. Maturation of T cells occurs in the thymus, and those cells that undergo a process termed positive selection are given signals to leave the thymus and seed the peripheral lymphoid tissues, whereas those with high reactivity for self are deleted or negatively selected (Sebzda et al, 1999). These selection processes begin when T-cell precursor cells originating from the fetal liver (in preborn and neonates) and the bone marrow traffic to the thymus. Within the thymic environment the precursor cells receive stimuli to initiate the recombination of TCR α- and β-chain genes, which results in the vast array (approximately 10^8) of different clones of T cells. Immature thymocytes express the α/β receptor as well as both the CD4 and CD8 co-receptors and are termed double-positive (e.g., CD4+/CD8+) T cells at this stage of development. Maturation is completed as the receptor-bearing thymocytes react with class I and class II MHC–bearing cells in the cortex and medulla of the thymus and become single-positive (e.g., CD4+ or CD8+) T cells. Three potential outcomes arise from these interactions. Those T cells expressing receptors that do not engage peptide/MHC complexes in the thymus undergo apoptosis due to the absence of survival signals delivered from the thymic cells. Those T cells expressing receptors with moderate reactivity to self-peptide/MHC complexes receive signals to survive and these are the cells that are positively selected to emigrate from the thymus and seed the peripheral lymphoid tissues to form the peripheral T cell repertoire. In contrast, those T cells expressing receptors with very high reactivity to complexes of self-peptides and MHC molecules receive signals to undergo programmed cell death and are negatively selected or deleted from the repertoire. Animal models have demonstrated that defects in the deletion of self-reactive T cells result in the development of overt autoimmune disease. **Immature B-cell precursors expressing surface immunoglobulin receptors with reactivity to self-proteins are deleted during maturation in the bone marrow in a similar manner as T cells are negatively selected in the thymus** (Nemazee, 2000). Deletion of self-reactive B cells in the bone marrow appears to be dependent on cell-associated rather than soluble antigen.

Peripheral Tolerance

Negative selection does not result in deletion of all self-reactive T and B lymphocytes during maturation. One factor accounting for the incompleteness of this mechanism is that not all self-peptides may be presented with MHC molecules by cells in the thymus. The escape of self-reactive T and B cells from the thymus and the bone marrow imparts the need for mechanisms to mediate tolerance of self-reactive lymphocyte clones in the periphery. Compensating for the incomplete deletion of self-reactive lymphocytes during maturation are mechanisms mediating deletion (e.g., clonal exhaustion and veto cell–mediated deletion) or inactivation (clonal anergy and active suppression) of peripheral T and B cells.

Peripheral Deletion of T Cells

Several mechanisms mediate deletion of antigen-specific T cells in the periphery. **Administration of large antigen doses stimulates the rapid proliferation of reactive T cells, but this is quickly followed by apoptosis of the reactive cells. This form of deletion due to "clonal exhaustion" has been shown experimentally in mouse models using virus infections and is thought to be operative in removing viral antigen-reactive CD8+ T cells during HIV infections** (Moskophidis et al, 1993). Clonal exhaustion is likely to occur in response to the large amount of self-proteins in the periphery, acting as a backup to remove self-reactive T cells that escaped negative selection during maturation in the thymus.

An active mechanism of T cell deletion in the periphery is mediated through cells expressing "veto" function. Veto cells express target peptide/MHC molecules and induce the death of T cells interacting with the expressed complex. Cells mediating veto function also express CD8α chains, and the interaction of this chain with class I MHC α3 domains on the reactive T cell is required to induce the death of the T cell. Cells shown to express veto function include CD8+ T cells, natural killer cells, and CD8α+ dendritic cells.

Clonal Anergy

Clonal anergy of T cells is induced by TCR engagement of peptide/MHC complexes in the absence of co-stimulatory signals (Schwartz, 1997). In the two signal models of naive T cell activation, signal one (e.g., TCR-mediated stimulation) is delivered in the absence of signal two (e.g., B7/CD40 mediated co-stimulation). The major consequence of clonal anergy induction is the inability of the anergized T cell to produce IL-2 in response to subsequent encounter with the specific peptide/MHC ligand. Thus, these T cells are unable to clonally expand and differentiate into effector cells. In at least some experimental model systems, T cells rendered anergic are able to proliferate when provided with exogenous growth factors such as IL-2, and their continued proliferation in the presence of growth factors promotes development to effector function such as IFN-γ production.

Clonal anergy of T cells can be induced by TCR engagement of specific antigen/MHC presented by nonprofessional APCs that do not express co-stimulatory molecules, by resting professional APCs that do not express co-stimulatory molecules, by interaction with chemically fixed APCs, or by blocking mediated co-stimulatory interactions, particularly CD28- and/or CD154-mediated co-stimulation.** In some instances co-stimulation may also be delivered by other receptor ligand interactions during naive priming by professional APCs. Administration of antibodies to adhesion molecules such as ICAM-1 and LFA-1 and to CD45RB during antigen priming induces clonal anergy of specific T cells. The ability to induce clonal anergy using these strategies emphasizes the importance of a highly regulated process of antigen capture, processing, and presentation by professional APCs having the ability to delivery the necessary co-stimulatory signals during T-cell priming. Anergy of B cells is also induced by antigen binding to surface immunoglobulin in the absence of co-stimulatory signals that are required for complete activation and development to antibody-producing cells.

Blockade of co-stimulation delivery during TCR interaction with peptide/MHC complexes results in the alteration of many intracellular biochemical events observed during TCR-mediated activation of T lymphocytes. These events include absence of kinase activation including the Lck and ZAP-70 kinases, absence of phosphorylation of CD3 components, and absence of activation of transcription factors, including AP-1 and NFAT. These intracellular signaling alterations suggest that the induction of clonal anergy is an active process. The ability of many immunosuppressants to block clonal anergy during naive T-cell interaction with peptide/MHC complexes in the absence of appropriate co-stimulation is consistent with clonal anergy induction as an active process.

In addition to the removal or inactivation of autoreactive lymphocytes through TCR engagement in the absence of co-stimulation, it is obvious that this feature of the immune system can be manipulated to induce tolerance and promote the survival of allografts or to ameliorate active autoimmune disease. **The induction of clonal anergy by co-stimulation blockade forms the basis of several immunosuppressive strategies currently under investigation in clinical transplantation and autoimmune disease. Many of these studies have utilized CTLA-Ig, which binds to B7-1 and B7-2 molecules with high affinity and blocks interaction with CD28 expressed by T cells in combination with anti-CD154 monoclonal antibodies** (Larsen et al, 1996). Preclinical studies testing this approach have shown considerable promise in prolonging allografts in nonhuman primate models. In addition, strategies combining co-stimulatory blockade with injection of donor bone marrow at the time of allograft transplantation appear to be effective in inducing recipient tolerance to graft alloantigens.

Regulatory T Cells

An active mechanism of tolerance mediated by T cells with suppressive or downregulatory activities may also be induced to inhibit immune responses to self and exogenous antigens. The concept of T cells with suppressive or downregulatory function was originally conceived by Gershon (1975) in experiments utilizing mouse models. Mice primed with high doses of antigen were not only rendered unresponsive to subsequent challenges with the original antigen but the tolerant state was transferable to naive animals by T cells from the tolerant animals. Treatment with nondepleting anti-CD4 monoclonal antibodies during antigen priming also induces a population of CD4+ T cells that can transfer tolerance to naive animals. More recent studies have identified a population of CD25+/CD4+ T cells that inhibit the activation of peripheral T cells to self antigens. Depletion or removal of these regulatory T cells promotes the development of autoimmune disease in animal models of colitis and diabetes (Salomon et al, 2000). Similar populations of regulatory CD4+ T (also termed Th3 cells) have been identified in humans. The forkhead/winged helix transcription factor FoxP3 is required for the development of CD4+/CD25+ regulatory T cells. and FoxP3 is currently used as a reliable marker of these cells. The immunosuppressive functions expressed by these regulatory T cells appear to be mediated at least in part through production of the immunosuppressive cytokines IL-10 and transforming growth factor-β (TGF-β), which may inhibit APC function during T-cell priming. Other mechanisms are mediated through expression of FasL and deletion of APCs during effector T-cell priming. An important consequence of tolerance mediated by regulatory T cells specific is the ability to inhibit immune responses to an irrelevant antigen when that (irrelevant) antigen and the regulatory T cell–specific antigen are presented by the same APC. This form of so-called linked immunosuppression may be further manipulated in future strategies to inhibit responses to self and allogeneic antigens.

ADHESION MOLECULES AND CONTROL OF LYMPHOCYTE TRAFFICKING

A critical feature of the immune system is the restriction imposed on the migration of T lymphocytes through lymphoid versus peripheral tissues. This restriction is dependent on the stage of T-cell development or activation. As is discussed in detail below, trafficking of naive T cells is restricted to primary lymphoid tissues. It is in these tissues that the chances of encountering dendritic cells presenting foreign peptide/MHC complexes are highest. In contrast, T-cell activation results in the ability of the T cells to recognize and stop at sites of vascular inflammation. This allows the T cells to traverse the endothelium barrier and enter peripheral tissues where the effector functions of primed T cells may be needed during an immune response.

The lymphoid system is organized into primary and secondary lymphoid tissue compartments. The bone marrow and the thymus where T-cell precursors originate and develop, respectively, comprise the primary lymphoid tissues. After maturation in the thymus, T cells seed the secondary lymphoid tissues, comprising the spleen, lymph nodes, Peyer's patches, and gut associated lymphoid tissues (GALT). Similarly, after maturation in the bone marrow B cells seed the secondary lymphoid tissues, where they form follicles.

Trafficking of Naive T Cells

Rather than remain passively in the lymphoid tissues, naive or antigen-inexperienced T cells circulate through the secondary lymphoid tissues using the lymphatic and blood vessels (Picker and Butcher, 1992). From the blood vessels, T cells enter secondary lymphoid tissues using specialized car-

bohydrate binding proteins termed *selectins.* Naive T cells express high levels of L-selectin (CD62L) that mediate binding to its ligand, peripheral lymph node vascular addressin (PNAd). PNAd is expressed by specialized postcapillary venules, the high endothelial venules (HEV), draining the lymphoid node. CD62L-PNAd engagement ceases the circulation of the T cells, allowing the T cells to traverse the HEV barrier and enter the cortical areas of the lymph node. The cortical areas of lymphoid tissues are rich in professional APCs such as macrophages and dendritic cells. As the naive T cells percolate through this area the TCRs on each cell can survey the surface of these APCs for recognition of the specific peptide/MHC ligand, leading to cellular activation. This restricted circulation of naive T cells optimizes the chance of T-cell encounter with dendritic cells presenting the specific ligand and is critical for efficient immune surveillance in light of the low number of T cells specific for any particular antigen/MHC complex (approximately 1 in every 10^5-10^6 cells). Unless the T cell encounters the appropriate activating complex presented by an APC, the naive T cells exit the lymph node via the efferent lymphatics and are eventually carried into the thoracic duct. The thoracic duct drains into the blood vessels, and the pattern of naive T-cell circulation through the secondary lymphoid tissues continues.

Upregulated Adhesion Molecule Expression

TCR engagement of specific ligand in association with appropriate co-stimulation during interaction with APCs leads to T-cell activation. Activation induces two phenotypic changes that alter the migration pattern of the T cell. First, the expression of the lymph node homing receptor CD62L is downregulated. This decreases the ability of the T cells to traffic into the lymph nodes and promotes T-cell circulation through the blood vessels. Second, expression of molecules that facilitate localization of antigen-primed T cells to inflammatory sites in the vascular endothelium is stimulated. T cells and other leukocytes travel through the circulation under extremely high shear forces. **The expression of these adhesion molecules is critical for mediating the arrest of the activated cells on the vascular endothelium under this high shear force and facilitates T cell entry into the peripheral tissues** (Springer, 1994). Complementary sets of receptors on leukocytes and endothelial cells help mediate the arrest of activated T cells and other leukocytes at inflammatory foci on the vascular endothelium. These molecules include the selectins and their ligands, the addressins, and the integrins and their ligands, which are members of the Ig superfamily.

The principal adhesion molecules upregulated during cellular activation of leukocytes are the integrins, a family of noncovalently associated dimers composed of an α chain and a common β chain (Table 15–3). On T cells, antigen-priming stimulates increased expression of CD11a which associates with CD18 to form the integrin LFA-1 or $\alpha_L\beta_2$. T-cell activation also induces expression of the integrin VLA-4 (very late activation antigen-4) or $\alpha_4\beta_1$. **In addition to their adhesive functions, integrin ligation may deliver co-stimulatory signals during T-cell interaction with APCs** (Ni et al, 1999).

Table 15-3. **Representative Integrins**

α/β Chains	Common Name	CD Designation	Ligand
αLβ2	LFA-1	CD11a/CD18	ICAM-1; ICAM-2; ICAM-3
αMβ2	MAC-1	CD11b/CD18	ICAM-1; fibronectin
α4β1	VLA-4	CD49d/CD29	VCAM-1; fibronectin
α5β1	VLA-5	CD49e/CD29	Fibronectin
α4β7	LPAM-1	CD107a	VCAM-1; MAdCAM-1

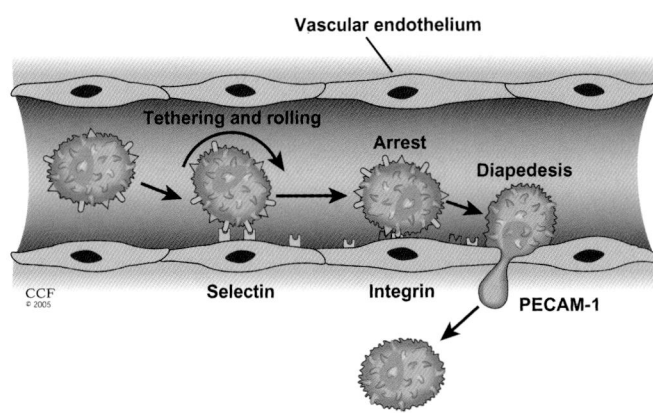

Figure 15–12. Localization of leukocytes to sites of vascular inflammation. During inflammation, vascular endothelial cells are activated to express adhesion molecules such as selectins and ligands for integrins and several different chemokines. Under high shear forces, leukocytes in the circulation are slowed down by selectin-mediated tethering on the endothelium. As the leukocytes are rolling along the vascular endothelial surface, expressed integrins are activated by endothelial chemokines, and the interaction of the integrins with their ligands results in leukocyte arrest. Through the homotypic interactions of PECAM-1 on the leukocyte and endothelial cell surfaces, the leukocyte transmigrates across the vascular endothelial cell barrier.

Integrins also bind to extracellular matrix proteins, and this engagement may augment T-cell effector function during the elicitation of an immune response. Activation of leukocytes including T cells also upregulates expression of a proteoglycan binding receptor, CD44. Macrophages and neutrophils also express LFA-1 as well as CD11b in association with CD18 ($\alpha_M\beta_2$), commonly called Mac-1.

In addition to integrins, T cells and other leukocytes express selectin binding molecules that direct cells to inflammatory sites in the vascular endothelium. **The P-selectin glycoprotein ligand (PSGL-1) is expressed by granulocytes and T lymphocytes and is the major ligand for P-selectin on endothelial cells** (Kansas, 1996). Expression of these ligands may also direct the T cells to distinct tissue sites. Activated T cells that are programmed to traffic to the skin also express cutaneous lymphoid antigen (CLA), which binds to E-selectin. In contrast, T cells trafficking to the gut mucosa are stimulated to express α4β7 during priming.

Adhesion Molecule Expression on Endothelial Cells

Vascular endothelial cells normally express low levels of ligands for integrins and other adhesion molecules. **During tissue inflammation, endothelial cells are activated to produce several cytokines, including TNF-α and IL-1** (Pober et al, 1986). These cytokines stimulate the endothelial cells to express several classes of adhesion molecules. Endothelial cells express two different selectins that facilitate the localization of activated T cells and other leukocytes to the vascular endothelium surface. P-selectin is preformed in specialized vacuoles called Weibel-Palade bodies, and surface expression is mobilized after activation of the endothelial cells. In contrast, endothelial cell activation initiates transcription and expression of E-selectin. During activation, endothelial cell expression of adhesion molecule members of the Ig superfamily is also upregulated. These molecules include ICAM-1 and a very late cell adhesion molecule (VLA-4). Another member of this family, ICAM-2, is constitutively expressed on the endothelial cell surface and is not upregulated by proinflammatory cytokines such as TNF-α and IL-1 during inflammatory processes.

T Cell/Endothelial Cell Interactions

The localization of T cells and other leukocytes in response to inflammation on the vascular endothelium is a highly regulated process (Ebnet et al, 1996). This localization begins with the regulated expression of adhesion molecules and their ligands on the leukocytes and endothelial cells. As the leukocytes are circulating through the vessel, engagement of

selectins tether the cells and slow their movement to rolling along the endothelial surface (Fig. 15–12). **After cell movement is slowed by selectin-mediated tethering, the binding of integrins to Ig superfamily counter receptors mediates the arrest of the T cells on the vascular endothelium. During this process, leukocyte engagement of cytokines produced by endothelial cells including IL-8 and TARC is required to trigger activation of the integrins** (Campbell et al, 1996). Binding of these cytokines through specific G protein–coupled receptors induces a conformational change to a high-affinity binding molecule and mediates arrest of the leukocytes on the vascular endothelium. As leukocyte movement is arrested there is a considerable amount of "crosstalk" between the leukocyte and the endothelial cell. Activation of macrophages, neutrophils, and possibly other leukocytes at the endothelial cell surface stimulates the leukocytes to produce TNF-α, which provides continued stimulation to express increased levels of VCAM-1 and ICAM-1 on the endothelial cell surface. Furthermore, antigen-primed T cell recognition of specific peptide/MHC complexes on the endothelial cell surface stimulates the T cells to express immune function such as cytokine production. T-cell production of IFN-γ stimulates endothelial cells to upregulate expression of MHC molecules and to produce chemoattractant cytokines, which amplifies T-cell recruitment and the immune response to localized areas in the endothelium.

Traversing the Endothelial Barrier

After the arrest of the leukocyte on the vascular endothelium, the cell traverses the endothelial barrier into the peripheral tissue, a process termed *diapedesis*. **Platelet/endothelial cell adhesion molecule-1 (PECAM, CD31) is expressed on endothelial cells and is concentrated at the cell junctions in the vessel** (Muller and Randolph, 1999). This molecule is also expressed on the surface of leukocytes. A critical property of PECAM-1 is the ability to bind to another PECAM-1 molecule, a process called homophilic adhesion. During diapedesis, PECAM-1 on the leukocyte binds to a PECAM-1 molecule at the endothelial cell junction and the leukocyte begins to traverse the endothelial barrier. In addition to these interactions, other molecules including CD99 and JAM (junctional adhesion molecule) are expressed by leukocytes and endothelial cells and coordinate with PECAM-1 interactions to guide the leukocyte through the endothelium and the leukocyte enters the peripheral tissue. After TCR-mediated activation, the T cell expresses immune function such as cytokine production or target cell cytolysis.

CHEMOKINES AND PERIPHERAL TISSUE RECRUITMENT OF LEUKOCYTES

Cytokines with chemoattractant properties, chemokines, are also critical in mediating localization and trafficking of leukocytes to tissue sites during physiologic processes, including inflammation and homeostasis (Rollins, 1997). Chemokines are a superfamily of small (<14 kd), heparin-binding proteins. More than 50 chemokine proteins have been identified and are grouped into four families based on a cysteine motif in the amino terminal area of the protein (Table 15–4). The C-X-C chemokines, in which these cysteines are separated by a single amino acid, are attractant for neutrophils and include IL-8 and GROα. The CXC chemokines also include three members, IP-10 (IFN-γ inducible protein), Mig (monokine induced by IFN-γ), and I-TAC (INF-inducible T-cell α chemoattractant), which are chemoattractant for activated T cells. The C-C chemokines, in which the two cysteines are adjacent, are chemoattractant for a variety of leukocytes including monocytes, eosinophils, T lymphocytes, NK cells, and dendritic cells. Representative C-C chemokines include MIP (macrophage inflammatory protein)-1α, MIP-1β, and monocyte chemoattractant protein-1 (MCP-1). The C family consists of a single cytokine, lymphotactin, which is chemo-

tactic for NK cells and T cells. The C-X$_3$-C family also contains a single chemokine, fractalkine, which is on a membrane-bound mucin stalk and has adhesive and chemoattractant properties for IL-2–activated NK cells and CD8+ T cells.

Under appropriate stimulatory conditions such as inflammation virtually all cells produce specific chemokines. **Chemokine production is primarily regulated by the cytokine environment.** TNFα and IL-1 induce many different cell types to produce neutrophil (e.g., IL-8 and Groα) and macrophage (e.g., MCP-1) chemoattractants. IFN-γ stimulates many different cells to produce the T-cell attractants IP-10, Mig, and ITAC. Cytokines including IL-4, IL-10, and IFN-γ inhibit production of specific chemokines during many processes.

Chemokines play a major role in tissue pathology by directing receptor-bearing leukocytes to tissue sites of inflammation. The hepta-transmembrane spanning chemokine receptors are linked to G-coupled proteins, which transduce intracellular signals after ligand binding. Because chemokines bind to glycosaminoglycans on cell surfaces and to extracellular matrix proteins, leukocytes expressing the appropriate receptors most likely bind chemokines as solid phase, not as soluble, proteins during infiltration into inflammatory tissue sites; and this solid-phase binding may be required or augment intracellular signaling. Chemokine receptors are constitutively expressed by some leukocyte populations, but cellular activation is required for expression of chemokine receptors on other types of cells. The expression of chemokine receptors such as CXCR3, the ligand for IP-10 and Mig, on T cells is induced by antigen priming and/or cytokines. There is considerable experimental and clinical evidence indicating that populations of CD4+ T cells producing type 1 (e.g., Th1 cells) versus type 2 (e.g., Th2 cells) cytokines express unique patterns of chemokine receptors (Bonnechi et al, 1999). TNF-α stimulates the expression of CCR7 on interstitial dendritic cells and directs their migration through the afferent lymphatics into the draining lymphoid tissue, where they prime peptide/MHC-specific T cells.

The critical role of chemokines during inflammatory processes has been clearly demonstrated in animal models where neutralization of specific chemokines results in inhibition of leukocyte infiltration and tissue pathology (Huffnagle et al, 1995; Koga et al, 1999). Chemokines are produced by all renal cell types and promote tubulointerstitial and glomerular pathology (Segerer et al, 2000). **In addition to leukocyte recruitment, many chemokines stimulate other proinflammatory activities, which may amplify the function of target leukocyte populations in vivo and intensify tissue inflammation.** These activities include the ability of specific chemokines to (1) trigger the arrest of monocytes and T lymphocytes rolling on endothelial surfaces under physiologic shear conditions in an adhesion molecule–dependent manner; (2) stimulate increased integrin expression and cell adhesion; (3) stimulate the release of granules by neutrophils and granulocytes; and (4) amplify CD8+ T cell– and NK cell–mediated cytotoxicity. Each of these processes has a critical impact on the intensity and duration of inflammation and is likely to be augmented by specific chemokines.

Chemokines also play a crucial role in immune homeostasis (Cyster, 1999). For example, chemokines such as B-

Table 15–4. Representative Chemokines and Receptors			
Family	**Chemokine**	**Receptor**	**Responsive Leukocyte Populations**
CXC	IL-8	CXCR1, CXCR2	Neutrophils
	Groα	CXCR2	Neutrophils
	IP-10	CXCR3	Activated T cells
	Mig	CXCR3	Activated T cells
	SDF	CXCR4	Naive T cells, B cells, dendritic cells, macrophages
	BLC	CXCR5	B cells
CC	MIP-1α	CCR1, CCR5	T cells, NK cells, macrophages
	MCP-1	CCR2, CCR10	Macrophages
	TARC	CCR4	T cells
	Eotaxin	CXCR3	Eosinophils
	RANTES	CCR1, CCR3, CCR5	T cells, macrophages, NK cells
	MIP-3α	CCR6	Immature dendritic cells
	SLC	CCR7	Mature dendritic cells, T cells
C	Lymphotactin	XCR1	T cells, NK cells
CX$_3$C	Fractalkine	CX$_3$CR1	CD8+ T cells, NK cells

lymphocyte chemoattractant (BLC) direct newly matured B cells to form follicles in the secondary lymphoid tissue. The localization of immature dendritic cells in peripheral tissues where they will function as antigen processing cells and APCs during the initiation of immune responses is also directed by specific chemokines.

TUMOR IMMUNOLOGY

Several important concepts have emerged over the past 2 decades that have shaped the current basic and clinical research efforts in tumor immunology (Sogn, 1998). This includes the fact that most tumors are antigenic. **Although the normal immune system is not a significant barrier to tumor growth and metastasis, manipulation of the immune system can lead to tumor rejection.** The induction of an effective antitumor immune response has been most effectively demonstrated in animal models, with some success in humans. Tumor-induced alterations in the functional status of immune cells may be responsible for the poor development of antitumor immunity in many cancer patients. However, it is hoped that the development of new strategies to activate the immune cells and a better understanding of immune dysfunction and how to prevent it will lead to more effective immunotherapy for the treatment of cancer.

Role of T Cells

The immune system plays a critical role in tumor rejection, and T lymphocytes are central to the generation of an effective tumor immune response (Cheever and Chen, 1997). **In fact, most forms of immunotherapy are centered on the activation of T-cell responses in the tumor-bearing host.** The importance of T cells is demonstrated by the fact that adoptive transfer of T cells with reactivity to a variety of murine tumors has been shown to protect animals from subsequent challenge with the appropriate viable tumor cells and in some instances can mediate the rejection of established tumors. Furthermore, the in-vivo deletion of T cells using antibodies to CD8 and in some cases to CD4 will eliminate antitumor activity normally induced by various forms of immunotherapy.

Generation of the most effective tumor immune response likely depends on the activation of CD8+ T cells that recognize tumor-associated antigens (TAA) presented by MHC class I molecules and CD4+ T cells that respond to TAA presented by MHC class II molecules (Robbins and Kawakami, 1996). Dendritic cells infiltrating the tumor bed and present in the draining lymph nodes are critical for the presentation of processed tumor antigen peptides to the T cells and their subsequent activation (Schuler and Steinman, 1997). Tumor cells are generally considered to be poor stimulators of T cells, owing in part to the lack of expression of MHC class II molecules and their variable expression of MHC class I molecules. After T-cell activation, tumor rejection is thought to occur by several mechanisms that may vary depending on the effectors generated and the sensitivity of the tumors (Kagi et al, 1996). Both CD8+ and CD4+ T cells can destroy tumor cells by the elaboration of cytoplasmic granules containing the pore-forming protein perforin, resulting in plasma membrane disruption, or by the upregulation of Fas ligand that can bind to

Fas (on the tumors) to induce apoptosis. The elaboration of cytokines is also important to tumor rejection. IFN-γ produced by both CD4+ and CD8+ T cells is known to be critical, likely because of its activation of other effectors cells, such as macrophages, that are known to infiltrate the tumor (Brunda et al, 1995). Although IFN-γ production is necessary, it is not sufficient for tumor rejection. Other TH1 cytokines such as IL-2 and IL-12 are involved in antitumor response primarily through their ability to activate effector T cells and induce their clonal expansion (Burke, 1999). The secretion of select chemokines is also necessary for the recruitment of additional T cells and dendritic cells to the tumor site (Tannenbaum et al, 1998).

Tumor Antigens

In the past decade a number of TAAs have been identified for human tumors. The isolation and characterization of genes that encode for TAA and their peptides has involved the transfection of cDNA libraries into cell lines expressing the appropriate MHC class I allele. These transfected cells can present antigen to MHC-restricted T-cell clones, and antigen recognition by the appropriate T cells is detected by the secretion of cytokines such as IFN-γ and TNF-α (Boon et al, 1997). Based on the sequence of the TAA a number of synthetic peptides are generated to define which of the peptide epitopes are actually recognized by the original T-cell clone. Peptides recognized by tumor-specific T cells have also been directly isolated by acid elution of the peptides from the tumor cell MHC complexes. These peptides are sequenced by mass spectroscopy, and a number of these peptides are synthesized and then tested for there ability to reconstitute T-cell recognition when pulsed onto the appropriate target cells (Bellone et al, 1999; Robbins and Kawakami, 1996). Many of the TAAs that have been identified are expressed on melanomas, which is attributable to the ease in which it has been possible to isolate and detect MHC-restricted melanoma-specific T cells from this patient population.

By utilizing these techniques different types of antigens have been identified. **One group of tumor antigens is expressed on a variety of tumors, including melanomas, lung tumors, breast tumors, head and neck tumors, and bladder cancer** (Robbins and Kawakami, 1996; Bellone et al, 1999). These antigens are not expressed by most normal tissue, with the exception of testis and placenta. **Therefore, these antigens appear to be relatively tumor specific and are encoded by a family of genes referred to as *MAGE-1, MAGE-2, BAGE, and RAGE* (Table 15-5).** T cells from melanoma patients also recognize tissue-specific differentiation antigens that are expressed on normal melanocytes but not on other normal tissues. This includes antigens that are encoded by genes such as *MART-1/MelanA* and *gp100.* Tyrosinase, another melanocyte lineage protein that is a key enzyme in pigment synthesis can also serve as a target for melanoma-specific T cells. Most antigenic peptides derived from these differentiation proteins are presented by HLA-A2, but other restricting elements have been found. **There are also a number of TAAs that have resulted from mutation or from overexpression in tumor cells.** Several different cytotoxic T lymphocytes have been shown to recognize antigens that are expressed ubiquitously but are mutated in tumor cells.

Table 15–5. Human Tumor Antigens Recognized by T Cells

	Expressed by RCC
Tumor Specific (widely expressed)	
MAGE-1	
MAGE-3/MAGE-6	+
BAGE	
GAGE-1, -2	
RAGE-1	+
Tissue Specific (melanocyte lineage)	
pg100	
MART-1	
TRP-1 (gp75)	+
Tyrosinase	
Mutated or Overexpressed	
Cyclin-dependent kinase (CDk4)	
B-catenin	
p53	
Carcinoembryonic antigen	
G250	+
Intestinal carboxyl esterase	+
hTERT(mutant HSP-70)	+
Her-2/neu	+
MUC-1 (mucin)	+
PRAME	+
Oncogenic Viral Antigens	
E7, human papillomavirus	

An antigenic mutation in the gene encoding the cyclin-dependent kinase 4 *(CD4K)* has been observed in several different melanomas. Mutation in this cell-cycle–regulating kinase prevented the binding to one of its inhibitors, p16, which is thought to be oncogenic. A point mutation in the widely expressed gene β-catenin can serve as antigen for melanoma. β-Catenin is involved in cell surface adhesion and has been implicated in tumor cell metastasis. Antigens that are overexpressed or mutated are also present on tumors besides melanoma. This includes the p53 protein that appears to be naturally processed and presented on tumor cell surfaces. HER2/neu is another protein that is present in normal tissues at low levels but is overexpressed in some tumors, particularly breast and ovarian carcinomas. Peptides from this oncogene product that appear to represent potential dominant T-cell epitopes have been identified and are being tested as a vaccine. There are other antigens that have been identified that can serve as potential targets for immunotherapy. This includes MUC-1, a cell surface protein composed of multiple tandem repeats that can be recognized by T cells directed against breast, ovarian, and pancreatic tumors. The heavily glycosylated mucin, present in normal cells, is underglycosylated in tumors, which allows recognition of the peptide repeats by the cytotoxic T lymphocytes. The MUC-1 epitopes are predominantly recognized in a non–MHC-restricted manner. The carcinoembryonic antigen that is highly expressed on many colorectal, gastric, and pancreatic cancers can also be recognized by T cells. Proteins produced by certain oncogenic viruses also represent another source of tumor antigens. Recent studies have shown that peptide epitopes from the human papillomavirus type 16 E7 are expressed on most cervical carcinomas and can be presented to cytotoxic T cells by

HLA-A2. Thus, a wide variety of human tumor antigens recognized by T cells have been identified and are currently being evaluated for their ability to stimulate antitumor immune response in cancer patients.

There is strong evidence that renal cell carcinomas have the potential to stimulate an immune response (Bukowski and Novick, 2000). **CD4+ and CD8+ T cell lines and clones have been isolated from patients with renal cell carcinoma that can produce IFN-γ and mediate lysis in response to autologous tumor cells. Renal cell carcinomas have been shown to express a number of antigens that are shared by other tumor types.** This includes RAGE-1, HER2/neu. PRAME, pg75, MUC-1, the heat-shock protein HSP-70, and a protein derived from an alternate reading frame of the intestinal carboxyl esterase gene. However, there is considerable variation in the level of expression and percentage of cells expressing these antigens among renal tumors. For example, RAGE is expressed on 2% to 20% of renal cell carcinomas whereas most renal cell carcinomas (75%) express carboxyl esterase. Recently, MAGE-6 has been shown to be expressed on 30% of renal cell carcinomas whereas the receptor kinase EphA2 is expressed on most renal cell carcinomas (90%) and is associated with a more aggressive phenotype (Tatsumi et al, 2002, 2003; Herrem et al, 2005). The demonstration of TAAs on renal cell carcinomas is an important step toward developing vaccine strategies for this disease.

Role of Innate Immunity

NK cells represent part of the host immune response against neoplastic cells (Basse et al, 2000). NK cells can recognize and destroy some tumors, particularly those of lymphoid origin, without any exogenous activation. However, the lysis of many freshly isolated solid tumors requires activation of these cells by IL-2; thus, NK cells have been referred to as lymphokine-activated killer (LAK) cells. **The destruction of tumor target cells by NK cells does not involve MHC restriction, and in fact these cells are thought to be most effective against tumor cells that express low to no MHC class I. NK cells can also kill tumor targets by antibody-dependent cell-mediated cytotoxicity.** In this setting there is redirected lysis since the specificity of tumor recognition resides in the variable region of the antibody. While the Fab portion of the antibody binds to its tumor antigen, the Fc portion of the immunoglobulin engages the Fc receptor on an NK cell, which in turn activates the cells lytic machinery. **The relevance of NK cells in defense against cancer cells has been demonstrated by the fact that the depletion of this population in some tumor models by anti-NK antibodies reduces or eliminates antitumor activity.** Furthermore, activated NK cells when adoptively transferred into tumor-bearing host along with IL-2 have been shown to have antitumor activity. These LAK cells were most effective against pulmonary metastasis because the majority of adoptively transferred NK cells are trapped in the lungs.

Mechanisms of Tumor Evasion of the Immune System

Whereas most solid tumors, including renal cell carcinomas, express TAAs that can be recognized by T cells and

have a significant infiltrate of lymphocytes, there is little evidence of a local immune response to the malignant cells (Finke et al, 1998; Uzzo et al, 2000). In fact, T cells infiltrating tumors are functionally impaired, as demonstrated by reduced ability to proliferate to a variety of stimuli and decreased cytotoxic activity. **There are also reports that dendritic cells within the tumor are impaired in antigen-presenting function, which may contribute to the immune dysfunction noted in the tumor microenvironment.** In patients with advanced disease there is evidence that immune dysfunction is present even within peripheral blood T cells. Recent studies have found that tumor-specific CD4+ T cells in the peripheral blood of renal cell carcinoma and melanoma patients with active disease are predominately Th2 type cells, because they produce IL-5 in response to dendritic cells pulsed with peptides to either MAGE-6 or EphA2. However, these was no or only minimal production of IFN-γ (Th1 cells) by either MAGE-6-specific or EphA2-specific CD4+ T cells from these same patients. In contrast, renal cell carcinoma patients who have no evidence of disease do express Th1 MAGE-6-specific and EphA2-specific IFN-γ–producing T cells (Tatsumi et al, 2002, 2003). These findings suggest that the tumor microenvironment may shift the balance from a Th1 cytokine response, which is known to be important for the rejection of tumors in animal models, to a Th2 cytokine response, which is primarily effective at promoting a humoral immune response.

The functional defects are accompanied by alterations in select signal transduction pathways in T cells from cancer patients. This includes reduced expression of the TCR ζ chain and TCR-associated protein tyrosine kinases, Lck and Fyn. The activation and nuclear translocation of the transcription factor NFκB is also impaired in T cells from some cancer patients. Increased sensitivity to apoptosis also contributes to the immune dysfunction observed in T cells from cancer patients, including those with renal cell carcinoma, melanoma, and squamous cell carcinoma of the head and neck (Gastman et al, 2000). Thus, the tumor environment has a negative influence on cells of the immune system, which may represent a barrier to the development of an effective antitumor immune response.

Mechanisms of Tumor Escape

Impaired Antigen Presentation

The recognition of tumor cells by T cells may be impaired owing to defective antigen processing and presentation (Pawelec et al, 1997; Seliger et al, 1997). Reduced or loss of MHC class I and class II expression by tumors, including renal cell carcinomas, has been well documented. In some tumors there is also decreased expression of transporter proteins associated with antigen processing (TAP proteins), as well as deficient levels of LMP proteosomal complexes. A reduction in mRNA and protein levels of these molecules appears more pronounced in renal cell carcinoma cells that have acquired metastatic potential, suggesting that the process of malignant transformation may include progressive loss of TAP and LMP. Increasing the levels of TAP in tumors, either by stimulating with IFN-γ or by transfection with TAP-1 cDNA, results in higher expression of MHC class I molecules on the tumor cell surface and enhanced tumor-specific, class I–restricted cytotoxic T-cell recognition.

Secretion of Immunosuppressive Products

A number of molecules with known immunosuppressive activity are increased in expression within the tumor microenvironment (Fig. 15–13). These products may be secreted by the tumor cells themselves or by surrounding mononuclear inflammatory infiltrates (Pawelec et al, 1997). **Among the best-studied immunosuppressive molecules overexpressed in the tumor microenvironment is the TH2 cytokine IL-10** (Pawelec et al, 1997; Uzzo et al, 2000). **The primary inhibitory effect of this cytokine is related to its ability to downregulate MHC class II expression on monocytes/dendritic cells, resulting in reduced antigen presentation.** IL-10 may also directly block T-cell growth and prevent the release of monocyte-derived reactive oxygen intermediates. It may further reduce antitumor immunity by inhibiting the production of other proinflammatory cytokines, such as IL-1, IL-6, IL-8, and TNF-α. The immunosuppressive properties of IL-10 may be partly attributable to its ability to inhibit activation of the transcription factor NFκB, which regulates a number of genes important to tumor immunity development. Although it is clear that IL-10 is immunosuppressive, its impact on the generation of an antitumor immune response is complex. In knockout mice deficient in IL-10, tumor growth is either reduced or prevented when compared with tumor growth in IL-10–producing mice. However, tumor cells genetically modified to overexpress IL-10 are found to be less tumorigenic than wild-type tumors (Halak et al, 1999).

TGF-β is also thought to contribute to the suppression of tumor immunity (Pawelec et al, 1997). **TGF-β is produced by a variety of tumors, including renal cell carcinoma, and increased levels of this cytokine have been reported in the serum of patients with kidney tumors. TGF-β is a potent inhibitor of IL-2–dependent T-cell proliferation affecting both helper and cytotoxic lymphocyte populations.** TGF-β appears to suppress T-cell growth by blocking TCR- and IL-2R–mediated tyrosine phosphorylation, thereby impairing downstream signaling events central to the control of cell cycle progression.

T-reg cells (CD4+, CD25High, FoxP3+) have emerged as another mechanism that may promote immune suppression in a tumor-bearing host by inhibiting the proliferation of CD4+ T helper cells as well as their ability to produce the cytokines IFN-γ and IL-2 (Curiel et al, 2004). T-reg cells appear to preferentially migrate to and accumulate in tumors and ascites of cancer patients. The expression of T-regs in cancer patients may have a negative impact on clinical outcome. A recent study has shown that the number of tumor T-regs is a significant predictor of increased risk for death and for reduced survival for patients with ovarian cancer. It also appears that the cytokine IL-2 produced by T-helper cells may promote the growth of T regulatory cells (Antony and Restifo, 2005).

Prostaglandin E$_2$ (PGE$_2$) is frequently present in the tumor bed and is known to inhibit T cell activation (Uzzo et al, 2000). PGE$_2$ may block T-cell proliferation by several mechanisms, which include increasing the levels of the intracellular second messenger, cyclic adenosine monophosphate, inhibiting the

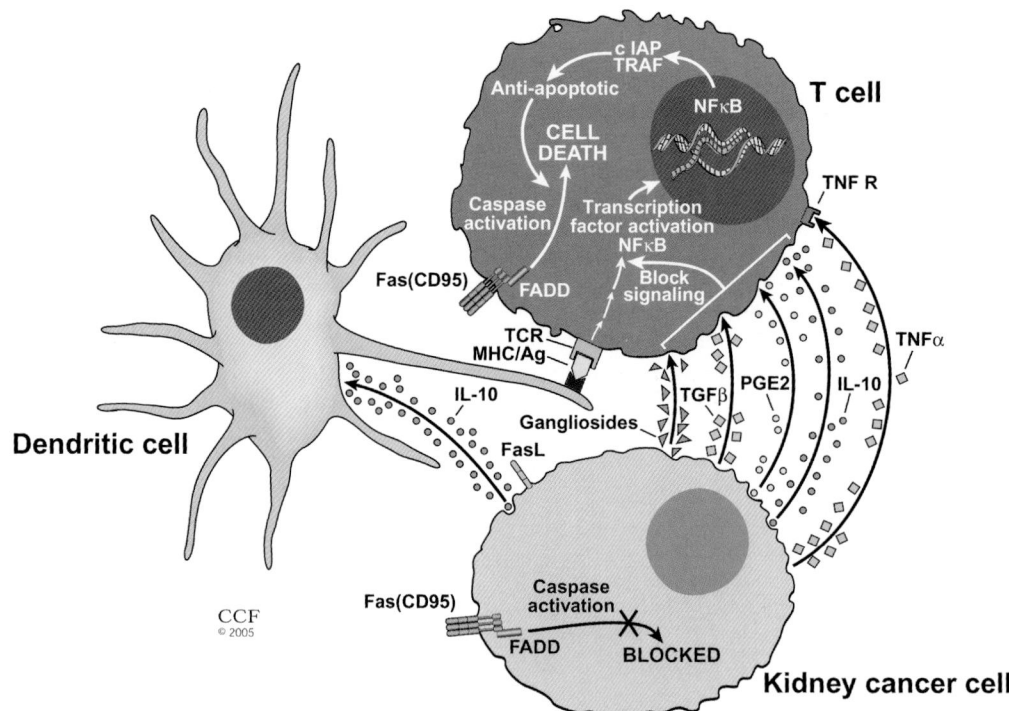

Figure 15–13. Scheme showing the mechanisms by which tumor cells can induce immune dysfunction in T cells and dendritic cells. Tumor cells can produce a variety of immunosuppressive products that include IL-10, gangliosides, transforming growth factor-β, and prostaglandins. These products can affect T-cell signaling, including the suppression of transcription factor activation such as NFκB. Blocking NFκB may also reduce expression of certain anti-apoptotic genes that would then make cells more sensitive to apoptosis. IL-10 can also inhibit the antigen-presenting function of dendritic cells. Moreover, some tumors express Fas ligand (FasL) that can induce apoptosis in T cells that express Fas receptor. However, some tumor cells may be protected from apoptosis induced by FasL expression on the activated T cells. Certain tumors express Fas but have reduced expression of molecules such as caspase that are essential for activating the pathway leading to apoptosis.

DNA binding activity of NFκB, and blocking IL-2–dependent G1-S transition. This latter defect may be due to downregulation of Jak3 expression, resulting in impaired phosphorylation and DNA binding activity of STAT5 (signal transducer and activator of transcription). Prostaglandins may also adversely affect the function of NK cells.

Gangliosides are structurally diverse acidic glycosphingolipids present in the outer leaflet of the plasma membrane (Deng et al, 2000) that are involved in cell-cell interactions and membrane receptor modulation. Importantly, they also act as inhibitors of the host immune response. Gangliosides contribute to the immune suppression observed in tumor-bearing hosts. Select gangliosides are increased in expression and shed into the tumor microenvironment. For example, in malignant melanomas and neuroblastomas there is overexpression of GD3, GD2, and GM2 (Hakomori, 1996). Rapid progression of tumor and lower survival rate was related to higher GD2 levels in patients with neuroblastoma. Recent findings also show increased expression of GD1a, GM1, and GM2 in renal cell carcinomas as compared with normal kidney tissue. Gangliosides isolated from different tumor types, such as neuroblastoma, lymphoma, and melanoma, all can inhibit immune responses. **Gangliosides have been shown to interfere with proliferation, antigen presentation, cytotoxic effector function, and IL-2 and IFN-γ production by T cells, without affecting production of the Th2 cytokine IL-10.** Animal studies have shown that the administration of tumor-derived GM1b inhibits the in-vivo development of antitumor immu-

nity (McKallip et al, 1999). Thus, mediators within the tumor environment may diminish effective antitumor immunity through a number of mechanisms that result from select alterations in signal transduction pathways critical for normal T-cell activation.

Tumor Induction of Apoptosis in T Cells

Recent evidence suggests that the downregulation of antitumor immunity may be due in part to the induction of the Fas apoptotic pathway in T cells (Gastman et al, 2000). Malignant cells from a number of solid tumors, including renal cell carcinoma, have been shown to express FasL, and tumor-infiltrating lymphocytes (T-TIL) are potential targets for the FasL-expressing tumor cells. In-vitro experiments have shown that when activated T cells expressing Fas come in contact with FasL-positive tumor cells they undergo apoptosis. T-cell death can be partially prevented by adding blocking antibodies to FasL. However, the importance of FasL expression on tumor cells as a mechanism for inducing apoptosis in T cells is not clear and may not be operative with some tumor types. **A second mechanism whereby T-cell deletion may occur is through activation-induced apoptosis (AICD).** T cells from some patients with renal cell carcinoma undergo apoptosis after stimulation that is not observed with T cells from normal individuals (Uzzo et al, 2000). This heightened sensitivity to apoptosis likely contributes to the immune dysfunction observed in T cells from these patients and has recently been observed in T cells from patients with melanoma and squamous cell carcinoma of the head and neck (Saito et al, 2000). AICD may be due to the upregulation of FasL and Fas expression of T cells, with the resulting interaction between ligand and receptor inducing apoptosis. **Thus, T cells that are stimulated by tumor antigen may undergo cell death rather than cell activation.** Recent studies suggest that gangliosides expressed by renal cell tumor lines can induce apoptosis of T cells in co-culture experiments, suggesting that perhaps they may contribute to the tumor-induced apoptosis of lymphocytes in vivo (Thornton et al, 2004).

Immunotherapy

Adoptive Cell Therapy

The transfer of tumor reactive T cells has been shown to protect animals from tumor challenges and to cause rejection of established tumors (Cheever and Chen, 1997). **T-cell transfer has been used for the treatment of metastatic melanoma and renal cell carcinoma. This has included the administration of tumor-infiltrating lymphocytes (TIL) that had been expanded ex vivo with IL-2** (Rosenberg et al, 1994). TIL containing melanoma-specific T cells did display some antitumor, but the adoptive transfer of TIL was no more effective than IL-2 alone. Others have shown that T cells expanded from draining lymph nodes of patients with renal cell carcinoma vaccinated with irradiated autologous tumor plus GM-CSF have antitumor activity in a small subset of patients even in the absence of IL-2 administration (Plautz et al, 1999). Melanoma-specific CD8+ MHC class I restricted T-cell clones or groups of clones have been employed in adoptive transfer and have demonstrated their ability to home to metastatic sites (Riddell et al, 2000). An improvement in tumor regression using tumor reactive–expanded tumor-infiltrating lymphocytes when combined with IL-2 administration was observed when patients underwent lymphodepletion conditioning with cyclophosphamide and fludarabine before cell transfer (Dudley, 2002).

Cytokines and Interferons

Subsets of patients have benefited from cytokine therapy (Bukowski and Novick, 2000). **The use of natural and recombinant cytokines has been investigated over the past 2 decades, with IFN-γ and IL-2 being the only agents appearing to at least reproducibly cause tumor regressions in 10% to 15% of patients with renal cell carcinoma. Responses to IFN-γ occur most frequently in patients with pulmonary metastases and good performance status, where the median response duration is between 6 to 10 months** (Bukowski and Novick, 2000). Randomized trials in metastatic disease comparing IFN-γ with other therapeutic approaches do suggest IFN-γ may enhance survival in patients with metastatic RCC, but the effect is only modest at best. IL-2 is currently the only immunotherapeutic agent approved for use in renal cell carcinoma by the U.S. Food and Drug Administration on the basis of demonstrated safety and efficacy in clinical studies involving 255 patients. The cumulative experience with high-dose IL-2 therapy has demonstrated approximately a 15% objective response rate (both complete and partial responses), mostly in patients with good clinical performance status. However, toxicity, including hypotension, dyspnea, thrombocytopenia, malaise, and disorientation, associated with high-

dose IL-2 treatment represents a serious obstacle to this single-agent therapy.

A number of studies have tested whether combining IL-2 with IFN-γ would improve the therapeutic activity over either agent alone. This combination of cytokines caused only a modest increase in response rates and no effects on survival were evident. Other combinations are currently being tested in phase I/II trials, and this includes IL-12 combined with IFN-γ and the triple combination of IL-2, GM-CSF, plus IFN-γ. It is clear from these and other studies that a subset of individuals with metastatic renal cancer do respond favorably to cytokine therapy; however, they represent a minority of patients (<15% response rate).

Cancer Vaccines

Several different vaccine approaches are underway to stimulate the immune response in patients with existing tumors. **One approach that has shown promise in animal tumor models involves the injection of irradiated tumors genetically engineered to secrete various immunostimulatory cytokines such as IL-2, IL-4, IFN-γ, IL-12, and GM-CSF** (Sogn, 1998; Burke, 1999). A variety of different chemokines (e.g., IP-10 and MIG) have also been expressed in tumors as a means of attracting T cells as well as APCs into the tumor microenvironment. Many of the chemokines and cytokines secreted by the tumor cells decreased tumorigenicity, and some could protect animals from subsequent challenge with the parental tumor. The inhibition in tumor growth occurred through a variety of mechanisms, including, in some cases, the generation of an antitumor T-cell response. Tumors deficient in expression of the co-stimulatory molecules B7.1 and B7.2 have been transfected with these genes to improve their immunogenicity. Although the transfer of this technology to cancer patients has been difficult, some clinical trails using gene-modified tumor cells have been used as vaccines. This included immunizing renal cell carcinoma patients with autologous tumors expressing GM-CSF. Technical problems that have hindered the use of gene therapy in cancer patients thus far include the low efficiency of transfections, the safety issues of infecting with retroviral vectors, and the development of antiviral responses to adenoviral constructs that may compromise the immune response generated to the tumor.

Synthetic peptides corresponding to defined TAAs (e.g., MART-1) have been used as vaccines in cancer patients, including those with melanoma, lung carcinoma, pancreatic cancer, and prostate carcinoma (Robbins and Kawakami, 1996; Bellone et al, 1999). The defined peptides have been given in the absence and presence of adjuvants or pulsed on autologous monocytes or dendritic cells. In some cases, vaccination with defined TAAs has led to induction of a TAA peptide–specific T-cell response in cancer patients. **After immunization, increases in peptide-specific CD8+ T cells from the peripheral blood and draining lymph nodes have been detected by their binding to MHC class I tetramer complexes containing the appropriate TAA peptide. Increases in antigen-specific cytokine-secreting T cells have been detected by the use of ELISPOT assays. However, typically there has been a poor correlation between induction of specific T cells and the clinical responses.** Moreover, the increase in TAA-specific T cells after vaccination has not always been equated with potent effector function, since in some patients T-cell anergy has been observed in the peptide-specific population (Lee et al, 1999). **A drawback to immunization with a single TAA is the potential to generate antigen loss variants that are not recognized by the specific T cells. To circumvent this problem some studies are utilizing combinations of peptides that should evoke a broader range of tumor-reactive T cells.** Another approach is to use tumor cell lysates that contain a wide variety of peptides for the pulsing of dendritic cells. Indeed, antitumor responses have been seen in melanoma and renal cell carcinoma patients immunized with dendritic cells pulsed with whole tumor cell lysates. Another method of immunizing patients with multiple peptides has been to electrofuse dendritic cells with tumors to generate dendritic-tumor hybrids. One group has had promising results in kidney cancer patients using allogeneic dendritic cells fused to autologous tumor cells as a vaccine (Kugler et al, 2000), although this was not observed by others. Another approach to vaccine treatment that is early in the developmental stage is the use of autologous dendritic cells that have been fused with tumor cells to activate T cells (Avigan, 2004).

Allogeneic Bone Marrow Transplantation

The employment of allogeneic bone marrow transplantation (BMT) to induce graft versus leukemia (GVL) mediated by donor lymphocytes is being tested in a variety of hematologic malignancies. There has been an increasing appreciation for the therapeutic contribution made by the transplanted allogeneic bone marrow cells (Khouri et al, 1998). Investigators have found that donor leukocytes infused into patients who have experienced relapse after allogeneic BMT may, independent of any chemotherapy or radiation therapy, generate immunologic responses that lead to clinical remissions. In patients with chronic myelogenous leukemia relapsing after allogeneic BMT, the infusion of donor leukocytes results in clinical remission rates of 60% that are often durable. It is now believed that the GVL effect is the primary mechanism by which some patients undergoing allogeneic BMT are cured (Khouri et al, 1998). Recently, nonmyeloablative allogeneic BMT/peripheral blood progenitor cell transplantation has been utilized for various leukemias (Childs et al, 2000) with only minimal levels of chemotherapy and radiation provided to prevent rejection of the donor cells. The advantage of nonmyeloablative allogeneic transplantation is that the early toxicity associated with high doses of chemotherapy is minimized. Furthermore, because renal cell carcinoma is known to respond to several immunologic therapies but is resistant to chemotherapy, testing the GVL effect in patients with renal cell carcinoma while avoiding myeloablative doses of chemotherapy is rational. Indeed, a recent study demonstrated that significant numbers of patients with metastatic renal cell carcinoma exhibited objective clinical responses to nonmyeloablative allogeneic BMT that appeared to correlate to the onset of complete donor T-cell chimerism (Childs et al, 2000). This study raised the possibility that appropriately activated T cells could sustain effector function and withstand the immunosuppressive environment typically associated with advanced renal cell carcinoma.

Monoclonal Antibodies

There is also renewed interest in monoclonal antibodies for the treatment of select tumors. Antibodies to CD20 have produced meaningful responses in a number of patients with B cell lymphoma patients who were refractory to chemotherapy (Maloney et al, 1997). The FDA has also approved an antibody to HER-2/neu for the treatment of patients with breast cancer. The development of genetic-engineered antibodies should improve results using this form of immunotherapy.

IMMUNITY TO INFECTIONS

The immune system provides protection against the ubiquitous numbers of infectious microbes that surround us at all times. They can range in size from 10^{-4}-mm viruses to 10^3-mm worms. **The initial barrier to these pathogens is the skin and external body fluids described as innate immunity, which is rapid but does not expand with repeated exposure** (Brandtzeg, 1995). If penetration occurs, organisms can be killed by soluble factors such as lysozyme, which is an antibacterial enzyme present in the tears, saliva, and phagocytic cells that digests peptidoglycans in bacterial cell walls. **Neutrophils and macrophages provide the first line of defense of the innate immune system by phagocytosing, killing, and digesting bacteria and fungi.** Killing is accomplished by digestive enzymes and by oxygen free radicals and other reactive oxygen species generated by the NADPH oxidase and oxidized halides produced by myeloperoxidase. The oxidase pumps electrons into the phagocytic vacuole, which produce conditions conducive to microbial killing and digestion by enzymes released into the vacuole from the cytoplasmic granules. **This process is greatly enhanced by the complement proteins that not only are cytotoxic but also are attractants for phagocytic cells and facilitate inflammation and cell adhesion.** The combination of innate and adaptive immunity is required for complete eradication of the offending organisms (Janeway and Medzhitov, 2002). However, the burden of invading microbes may be large and overwhelm immune mechanisms, so that drainage or (surgical) removal and the use of antimicrobial drugs to diminish replication may be required for complete elimination of the invading organisms.

Bacterial Infections

Extracellular bacteria are susceptible to killing by phagocytosis and complement. However, bacteria try to evade these mechanisms by surrounding themselves with capsules that do not readily adhere to phagocytic cells, by secreting exotoxins that can impede host responses, or by proliferating in relatively inaccessible locations. For example, some gram-positive bacteria have developed capsules that do not favor stable binding of the complement C3 convertase or prevent the insertion of the lytic C5b-9 membrane attack complex. Circulating antibodies can override some of these mechanisms by directly binding to bacterial exotoxins and "neutralizing" them. They can also bind to the encapsulated bacteria, which will permit ingestion by polymorphs and macrophages. **These coated bacteria become "opsonized" as the Fc portion of the antibody permits binding to high-affinity receptors on**

phagocytes and can fix complement as well. In addition, secretory IgA (and some IgM) antibodies can afford protection in the tears, saliva, gut, vaginal mucosa, and lung by preventing bacterial adherence to these epithelial surfaces. Opsonized bacteria too large for phagocytosis can also be killed because the Fc portion of antibody can attract "killer" lymphocytes by ADCC.

Some bacteria such as the bacilli that cause tuberculosis, leprosy, listeriosis, and brucellosis try to escape the immune system by growing within macrophages (Schaible et al, 1997). They defy the innate killing mechanisms by blocking macrophage activation, scavenging oxygen radicals, or inhibiting lysosomal fusion with the phagocytic vacuole. These organisms develop strong lipid outer coats and can escape from the phagosome into the cytoplasm of the macrophage and proliferate. **Clearance of these intracellular microbes is directly dependent on T cells, which in turn must activate the infected macrophages. Specifically primed T cells react with processed antigen derived from the intracellular bacteria in association with MHC class II on the macrophage surface.** The subsequent T-cell release of lymphokines, such as IFN-γ and other macrophage-activating factors, upregulate the macrophage killing mechanisms. These include the formation of nitric oxide and other reactive oxygen intermediates within the macrophage.

Chronic Inflammation

The character of the immune response can change during persistent infections or when the immune response is ineffective or unable to clear the offending microbe. In these instances the site of infection becomes dominated by macrophages in various stages of activation. These cells may fuse and appear as "giant cells" or line up in arrays called "epithelioid cells." Macrophages bearing bacterial antigens on their surface may actually become targets of cytotoxic T cells and be destroyed. Lymphocytes in various stages of activation will also be present. This combination of immune-activated cell types is also associated with proliferating fibroblasts and areas of necrosis. **This reaction represents an attempt by the body to wall off a site of persistent infection and is referred to as a granuloma. Such a response can also arise from the persistence of undigested inorganic materials or antigen-antibody complexes.**

Viral Infections

Viruses are subject to the same mechanisms of immune clearance as other microbes but attempt to avoid the immune system by altering their surface antigens. **Minor change in surface antigens due to point mutations in the viral genome is referred to as antigenic drift, whereas major change arising from exchanges of large portions of the viral genome with other viruses is called antigenic shift. Influenza viral epidemics often result from such antigenic shifts, which act like new infections and bypass host immune memory and recall.** Viruses can use certain host receptors (the CD4 molecule by HIV) to gain entry into the host cell. Altered viral epitopes can inhibit the triggering of the host TCRs, block complement components, and prevent antigen processing by APCs. The viral genome may encode proteins similar to host

cytokines and their receptors, which subvert immune activation (Watts and Bertram, 2004). **As with bacterial infection, host antibody is essential for eliminating extracellular viral particles, and cell-mediated responses are necessary for those that are intracellular.** Antibodies can neutralize viruses by blocking their surface receptors, activating the classical complement pathway, and clumping or aggregating the viral particles for enhanced phagocytosis. These responses are especially effective when the virus has to travel in the bloodstream to reach its target such as the poliovirus, which enters via the gut and travels to the nervous system. When the target organ is at the portal of entry such as the gut or lung, rapid release of local interferon and recruitment of NK cells is essential for immune clearance.

Toll-like Receptors and Microbial Killing

Toll receptors were originally identified as transmembrane receptors required for the establishment of polarity in the developing *Drosophila* embryo but also were shown to have a role in host defenses. The mammalian counterpart, a family of 10 structurally similar proteins, has been identified and named Toll-like receptors (TLRs 1-10) (Takeda et al, 2003). Most tissues express at least one TLR, but phagocytes in particular show abundant expression of all known TLRs. The mRNA of TLRs has been found in monocytes and macrophages, dendritic cells, mast cells, B cells, and epithelial cells of the respiratory and intestinal tract. The first mammalian TLR identified, TLR-4, was shown to cause induction of the genes for several inflammatory cytokines and co-stimulatory molecules. Therefore, it was anticipated that the TLRs might be involved in immune responses, especially in the activation of innate immunity. TLR-4 was then shown to be involved in the recognition of lipopolysaccharide (LPS), a major cell wall component of gram-negative bacteria. Subsequently, other members of the TLR family have been shown to be essential for the recognition of a wide range of microbial components, including double-stranded RNA, flagellin, taxol, fibrinogen, peptidoglycan, and various other viral and fungal envelope proteins and products (Table 15–6). TLRs also recognize some endogenous ligands such as heat-shock proteins. A wide variety of stressful conditions such as heat shock, ultraviolet radiation, and viral and bacterial infection induce the increased synthesis of heat-shock proteins, which can activate macrophages and dendritic cells to secrete proinflammatory cytokines and to express co-stimulatory molecules.

Expression of TLRs is modulated by a variety of factors such as microbial invasion, microbial components, and cytokines such as colony-stimulating factor-1 and macrophage migration inhibitory factor (MIF). On recognition of their cognate ligands, TLRs induce the expression of a variety of host defense genes. These include inflammatory cytokines and chemokines, antimicrobial peptides, co-stimulatory and MHC molecules, and other effectors necessary to arm the host cell against the invading pathogen. The pathways that transduce TLR signals in mammals are highly homologous to that of the IL-1R family and ultimately lead to the activation of two distinct signaling pathways: JNK and NFκB. Once freed from inhibitors, NFκB translocates into the nucleus and turns on

Table 15-6. Toll-like Receptors and Their Ligands

TLR Family	Ligands (Origin)
TLR1	Tri-acyl lipopeptides (bacteria, mycobacteria)
	Soluble factors (*Neisseria meningitidis*)
TLR2	Lipoprotein/lipopeptides (a variety of pathogens)
	Peptidoglycan (gram-positive bacteria)
	Lipoteichoic acid (gram-positive bacteria)
	Lipoarabinomannan (mycobacteria)
	A phenol-soluble modulin (*Staphylococcus epidermidis*)
	Zymosan (fungi)
	HSP70 (host)
TLR3	Double-stranded RNA (virus)
TLR4	LPS (gram-negative bacteria)
	Taxol (plant)
	Fusion and envelope protein (RSV)
	HSP60 and HSP70 (*Chlamydia*, host)
	Type III domain A of fibronectin (host)
	Oligosaccharides of hyaluronic acid (host)
	Polysaccharide fragments of heparan sulfate (host)
	Fibrinogen (host)
TLR5	Flagellin (bacteria)
TLR6	Di-acyl lipopeptides (*Mycoplasma*)
TLR7	Synthetic compounds
TLR9	CpG DNA (bacteria)
TLR8 and 10	??

transcription of target genes. Not surprisingly, NFκB is critical in the function and development of dendritic cells. Both TLR and IL-1R interact with an adaptor protein MyD88, which is critical to the production of inflammatory cytokines induced by the TLR family. Indeed, no activation of NFκB was observed in macrophages of MyD88-deficient mice, which were found to be susceptible to infection by *Staphylococcus aureus*.

Recognition of microbial components by TLRs triggers activation of not only innate immunity but also adaptive immunity, which is largely provided by dendritic cells. Immature dendritic cells residing in the periphery have a high capacity for endocytosis, which facilitates antigen uptake. They are activated by various microbial components to undergo maturation and express many of the TLRs. TLR-mediated recognition of microbial components by dendritic cells induces the expression of co-stimulatory molecules such as CD80/CD86 and production of inflammatory cytokines such as IL-12. Once matured, dendritic cells lose their capacity for endocytosis and migrate into the draining lymph nodes. Here they present microorganism-derived peptide antigens expressed on the cell surface with MHC class II antigen to naive T cells, thereby initiating an antigen-specific adaptive immune response. In addition to controlling the development of adaptive immunity, activation of TLRs appears to be directly involved in antimicrobial activity. TLR-2 activation leads to nitric oxide–dependent and nitric oxide–independent killing of intracellular *Mycobacterium tuberculosis* in macrophages. TLR-2 confers LPS and lipoprotein-induced apoptosis of macrophages, indicating the possible involvement of TLRs in infection-induced cell death.

Passive and Acquired Immunity

Protection against a specific infection can be passively transferred from one individual to another via serum containing preformed antibodies. This type of passive immunity is generally short lived because the half-life of immunoglobulins is generally 1 to 2 weeks. Patients with immunodeficiency diseases may actually be sustained by regular treatments with pooled nonspecific human gamma globulin treatments. High-titered pooled specific antibodies to agents such as cytomegalovirus can be given as prophylaxis or treatment of the viral infection. Equine globulin raised against diphtheria and tetanus toxin has also been effective, although globulin from nonhuman species tends to be more toxic and runs the risk of serum sickness. Passive immunity is also transferred from mother to child via the placental transfer of IgG during gestation and the intestinal absorption of secretory IgA in the mother's milk.

The most durable form of protection from infection results from active immunization. This can arise from an acquired infection that results in host immunity or vaccination by intentional exposure to either killed or attenuated live organisms. **Attenuated organisms, which cause only a very mild form of the natural disease yet retain the antigenic specificity of the organism, are most effective.** Attenuated organisms replicate, which provides for a larger dose, and the immune response is produced at the site of natural infection. The objective is to provide effective immunity by establishing adequate levels of antibody and a primed population of memory cells, which can rapidly expand on rechallenge with the offending agent. Successful immunization requires a combination of specific-antibody, macrophage-activating cell-mediated immunity and the generation of cytotoxic T cells to be most effective.

MOLECULAR IMMUNOLOGY

During the past decade the first version of the complete human genome has been sequenced and published (http://www.ncbi.nlm.nih.gov), which has unlocked a remarkable potential for discovery in human biology and medicine. In parallel, recent advances in molecular biologic techniques have permitted the profiling of the global mRNA transcript, which encompasses the cell's transcription of activated genes that drive the subsequent events of protein translation, modification, and metabolism, creating the complex functions of any biologic system. **These emerging technologies have set the stage for the "omics" era of biology in which cellular events are described in terms of the transcriptome (mRNA transcripts); the proteome (proteins); the metabolome (metabolic products); and glycomics (carbohydrate modifications to proteins), etc.** The immense potential of these technologies lies in the fact that they provide a global view of changes in gene expression in the tissue or organ studied. The changes can be profiled to identify normal or healthy from disease states. This genome-wide approach can describe both the expression of known genes and mechanistic pathways as well as the discovery of as yet unknown genes and pathways. These newly identified genes and proteins may provide the key targets for future therapies. Such genomic profiling can also identify prognostic biomarkers to diagnose, classify, and guide the treatment of disease. Several clinical fields related to urology have begun to explore these technologies, including oncology, immunology, and transplantation biology. The initial foray into these technologies has been the analysis of gene expression profiles using DNA microarrays.

The Gene Chip

Whereas earlier estimates suggested that the linear sequence of 3 billion base pairs in human DNA encoded over 100,000 genes, these numbers have now been downsized by more than half. High-throughput technologies are now in place to identify most of the known genes that have been previously identified and annotated. **The basic principle involves the "spotting" of a sequence of nucleotides on a glass support that represent a particular gene (a probe) to which a complementary sequence of nucleotides (a target) will hybridize according to molecular attraction (A-T and G-C). The probe is generally a piece of complementary DNA several hundred nucleotides in length that is generated as a PCR product from a known cDNA library. More recently, machine-synthesized oligonucleotides of between 25- to 75-mer length have been used as probes. When thousands of these probes are spotted they are described as a DNA microarray or a DNA gene chip.** The target can come from any tissue or cell type of interest by first extracting its total RNA, then labeling the mRNA fraction with a fluorescent isotope. The relative amount of labeled target that hybridizes to the DNA on the chip gives off a signal captured by a laser scanner that reflects the expression level of the corresponding gene. By using the current version of a commercially produced DNA microarray (the U133A plus, Affymetrix, Santa Clara, CA), about 38,000 genes can be screened on one chip. Once such large volume of raw data is generated, computerized bioinformatics is necessary to identify relationships. A commonly used technique is hierarchical clustering of upregulated or downregulated genes comparing experimental groups to controls.

Gene Expression Profiling in Urologic Oncology

At the present time DNA microarray analysis is expensive, labor intensive, and cumbersome. However, a number of initial experiences provide exciting future possibilities. **Gene expression profiling has the potential to significantly advance the diagnosis and classification, the prognosis, and the treatment of kidney cancers.** Such profiling has been used to distinguish the various histologic subtypes of renal cell carcinoma, each with a unique molecular signature. For example, microarrays identified strong α-methylacyl coenzyme A racemase staining, found in 41/41 papillary renal cell carcinomas, including 6 with metastases, whereas this gene was only weakly found in less than 15% of all others renal cancers tested (Tretiakova et al, 2004). Clear cell renal cancers commonly express glutathione-S-transferase-α, whereas carbonic anhydrase II is upregulated in chromophobe renal cancers. For these reasons it has been suggested that gene expression profiling may someday permit the use of renal biopsy to accurately diagnose radiographic renal masses as cancers. Two studies reported a 40-gene and a 45-gene cluster associated with poor cause-specific survival for clear cell renal cell carci-

noma and suggested that VCAM-1 may be a useful prognostic marker (Takahashi et al, 2001; Vaselli et al, 2003). Gene expression profiling can also identify targets for therapeutic intervention. Topoisomerase II, identified as being highly upregulated in aggressive Wilms' tumors, has also been found in renal medullary cancers, making it an early molecular target for therapeutic interventions.

Gene Expression Profiling in Transplantation

Another area explored with DNA microarray technology has been renal transplantation, in particular the gene profiles associated with allograft rejection and renal dysfunction. By using a spotted cDNA array consisting of about 12,440 selected genes created at Stanford University, 67 pediatric renal allograft biopsies were profiled. **Hierarchical clustering of gene expression demonstrated three patterns of acute rejection that also correlated with 2-year graft survival and suggested a previously unknown correlation with genes linked to B cell–mediated immunity** (Sarwal et al, 2003). Two reports describe the use of high-density oligonucleotide arrays to define molecular signatures for transplant kidney biopsies as well as peripheral blood lymphocytes (PBL). Affymetrix HG-U95Av2 GeneChips (over 22,600 genes) were used in four groups of transplant patients: normal donors, recipients with well-functioning kidneys, patients with acute rejection, and patients with renal dysfunction but no rejection. Distinct gene expression profiles were identified for both kidney biopsies as well as PBL that correlated and classified each of the four groups of patients (Flechner et al, 2004). **Interestingly, the genes upregulated in the PBL did not overlap with the biopsies associated with acute rejection, suggesting that the PBL and the transplanted kidney represent two distinct compartments with respect to the immune mechanisms involved.** In another study the same group compared the gene expression profiles from 2-year kidney biopsies in recipients treated with or without a calcineurin inhibitor (CNI) drug. The authors showed that the patients on the CNI-free immunosuppressive protocol had better renal function and a significantly diminished prevalence of chronic allograft nephropathy by histology. **Gene expression profiles of kidneys that were graded with higher Banff scores for chronic allograft nephropathy showed a marked upregulation of genes that were involved in immune/inflammation and tissue injury/remodeling and fibrosis** (Flechner et al, 2004). In addition, cDNA microarrays were used to study specific mechanisms of renal transplant physiology by comparing the gene expression profiles from laparoscopically removed donor kidneys (Kurian et al, 2005) and from the glomeruli and tubulointerstitium obtained by microdissection of biopsies from both deceased and live donor kidneys (Kainz et al, 2004). One can see that several hours of pneumoperitoneum and laparoscopic surgery causes a specific signature of upregulated and downregulated genes compared with controls (Fig. 15–14). **Such expression patterns can be used to identify which compartments in the kidney may be most susceptible to ischemia and which biologic products may be targets to help minimize injury.**

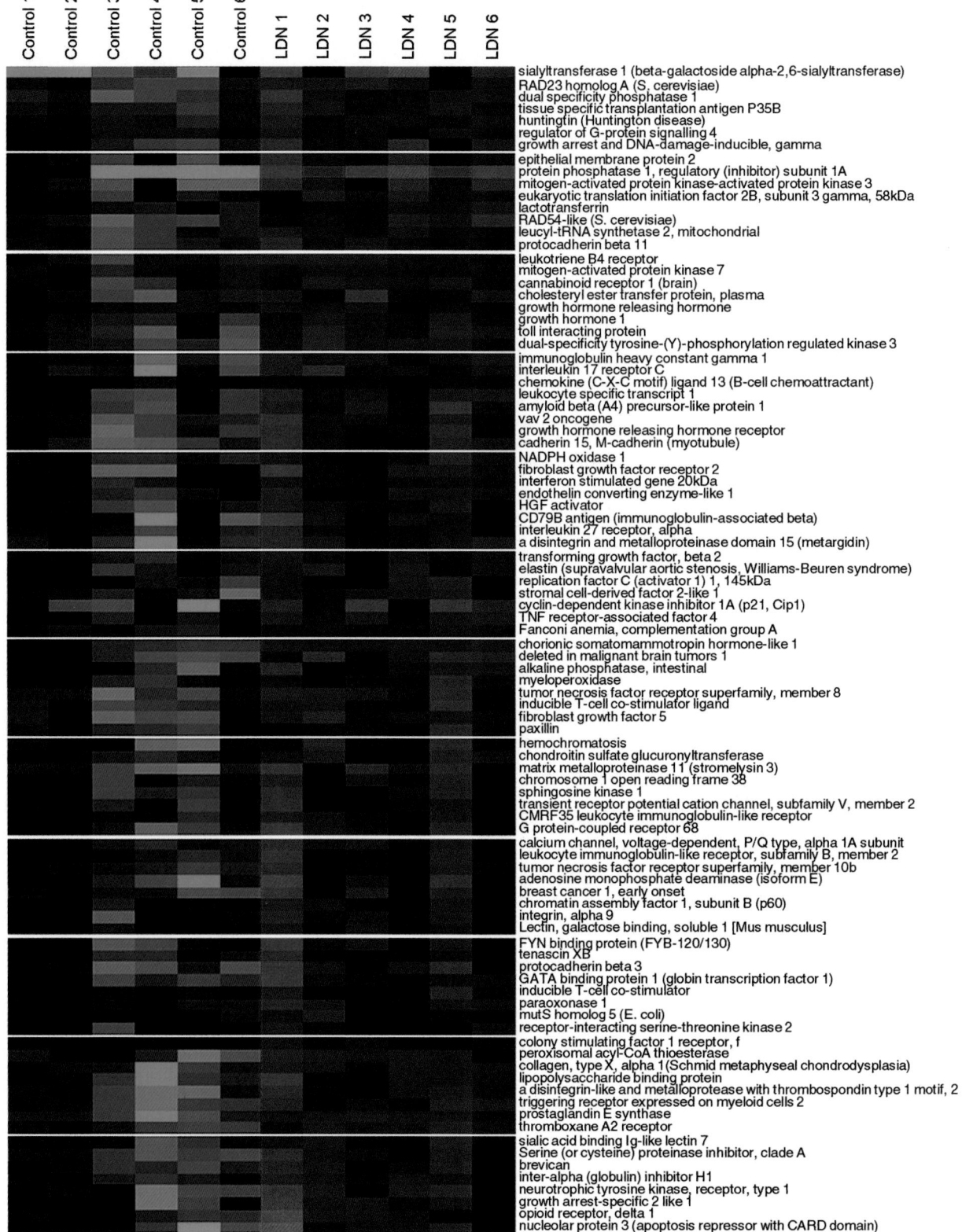

Figure 15–14. Heat map representing the relative signal intensities of a subset of 95 differentially expressed genes selected from a class comparison of the gene expression profiles between control and laparoscopic donor kidneys. Control biopsies were obtained from open nephrectomies before surgical manipulation. Genes were selected based on association with ischemia, tissue injury, and stress from a literature search using publicly available databases.

KEY POINTS: BASIC PRINCIPLES OF IMMUNOLOGY

■ The immune response remains identified by unique characteristics that include (1) the ability to identify self from non-self; (2) specificity; (3) memory; and (4) rapid amplification.

■ What we characterize as the immune system describes the interplay between two separate biologic responses: those that are innate and those that are acquired.

■ Bone marrow stem cells differentiate into immunocompetent T and B cells in the primary lymphoid organs and then colonize the secondary lymphoid tissues where the immune responses take place.

■ Whereas the small lymphocyte is the backbone of the immune response, several other bone marrow–derived cells are needed for a mature immune response. These cells "talk" to each other and their surroundings through receptors that they express on their surface and through cytokines, which are small peptides that they secrete locally.

■ A primary immune response (to a previously unseen antigen) takes 7 to 10 days and has a lag period. A secondary response (re-exposure to the same antigen) is both more rapid (1 to 5 days) and often more vigorous.

■ A cell surface receptor bound by its ligand will often trigger downstream intracellular events, thereby activating the cell to either produce specific cytokines, express other surface markers required for immune interactions, or enter cell cycle progression and proliferation.

■ An antigen presenting cell (APC) is a cell that can process a protein antigen, breaking it into peptides and then presenting it in conjunction with MHC molecules on the cell surface where it may interact with appropriate T-cell receptors (TCRs).

■ The MHC describes a region of genes located on chromosome 6 in humans that encode proteins that are responsible for the rejection of tissue between different species or members of the same species.

■ T cells become activated when the TCR engages an antigen for which it is specific; however, the TCR must "see" the antigen peptide presented in the groove of an MHC molecule on an APC, referred to as signal 1.

■ Activation requires co-stimulation by proteins on the APC that engage specific receptors on the T-cell surface, referred to as signal 2.

■ Completion of activation requires the delivery growth factors (IL-2 and IL-15) for initiating the cell cycle, referred to as signal 3.

■ Activation of T cells is dependent on the signaling events transmitted via the TCR to the nucleus. Phosphorylation of the tyrosines in immunoreceptor tyrosine-based activation motifs (ITAMS) represents the initial intracellular signaling event after lymphocyte detection of specific antigen. This event also leads to increased Ca^{2+} levels, which results in the activation of the enzyme calcineurin, which regulates the activation of a family of transcription factors, termed NFATs (nuclear factor of activated T cells).

■ Apoptosis is a mechanism by which an organism deletes aged, damaged, and autoimmune cells or cells that are no longer required in subsequent stages of differentiation.

■ Cytokines with chemoattractant properties called chemokines are critical in mediating localization and trafficking of leukocytes to tissue sites during physiologic processes, including inflammation and homeostasis.

■ Because most tumors are antigenic, the immune system plays a critical role in tumor rejection. Generation of the most effective tumor immune response depends on the activation of T cells that recognize tumor-associated antigens. The elaboration of cytokines is also important to tumor rejection, especially IFN-γ, owing to its activation of other effectors cells, such as macrophages that are known to infiltrate the tumor.

■ Although most solid tumors including renal cell carcinoma express tumor-associated antigens that can be recognized by T cells and have a significant infiltrate of lymphocytes, there is little evidence of a local immune response to the malignant cells. This is because tumors can evade host immune mechanisms. Malignant cells from a number of solid tumors have been shown to express FasL and can induce apoptosis of tumor-infiltrating lymphocytes.

■ Extracellular bacteria are susceptible to killing by phagocytosis and complement. Phagosomes in neutrophils and macrophages release digestive enzymes and oxygen free radicals and other reactive oxygen species. Bacteria try to evade these mechanisms by surrounding themselves with capsules and by secreting exotoxins that can impede host responses.

■ Toll-like receptors found in monocytes and macrophages, dendritic cells, mast cells, B cells, and epithelial cells are triggers for a variety of host defense genes. They can recognize a wide range of microbial components.

■ Protection against a specific infection can be passively transferred from one individual to another via serum containing preformed antibodies, but the most durable form of protection from infection results from active immunization.

■ DNA microarrays can be made by "spotting" of a sequence of nucleotides on a glass support that represent a particular gene (a probe) to which a complementary sequence of nucleotides (a target) will hybridize according to molecular attraction (A-T and G-C).

SUGGESTED READINGS

Antony PA, Restifo NP: CD4+CD25+ T regulatory cells, immunotherapy of cancer and interleukin-2. J Immunother 2005;28:120-128.

Ashkenazi A, Dixit VM: Death receptors: Signaling and modulation. Science 1998;281:1305-1308.

Banchereau J, Steinman RM: Dendritic cells and the control of immunity. Nature 1998;392:245-252.

Boon T, Coulie PG, Van den Eynde B: Tumor antigens recognized by T cells. Immunol Today 1997;18:267-268.

Cyster JG: Chemokines and cell migration in secondary lymphoid organs. Science 1999;286:2098-2102.

Flechner SM, Kurian SM, Solez K, et al: De novo kidney transplantation without use of calcineurin inhibitors preserves renal structure and function at 2 years. Am J Transplant 2004;4:1776-1785.

Gould DS, Auchincloss H: Direct and indirect recognition: The role of MHC antigens in graft rejection. Immunol Today 1999;20:77-82.

Halloran PF: Immunosuppressive drugs for kidney transplantation. N Engl J Med 2004;351:2715-2729.

Imada K, Leonard WJ: The Jak-STAT pathway. Mol Immunol 2000;37:1-11.

Janeway CA, Medzhitov R: Innate immune recognition. Annu Rev Immunol 2002;20:197-216.

Kohler G, Milstein C: Continuous cultures of fused cells secreting antibody of predefined specificity. Nature 1975;256:495-497.

Kugler A, Stuhler G, Walden P, et al: Regression of human metastatic renal cell carcinoma after vaccination with tumor cell-dendritic cell hybrids. Nat Med 2000;6:332-336.

Schwartz RH: T-cell clonal anergy. Curr Opin Immunol 1997;9:351-357.

Sebzda E, Mariathasan S, Ohteki T, et al: Selection of the T cell repertoire. Annu Rev Immunol 1999;17:829-874.

Starr TK, Jameson SC, Hogquist KA: Positive and negative selection of T cells. Annu Rev Immunol 2003;21:139-176.

Takeda K, Kaisho T, Akira S: Toll-like receptors. Annu Rev Immunol 2003;21:335-376.

Trombetta ES, Mellman I: Cell biology of antigen processing in vitro and in vivo. Annu Rev Immunol 2005;23:975-1028.

Vaselli JR, Shih J, Iyengar SR, et al: Predicting survival in patients with metastatic kidney cancer by gene expression profiling in the primary tumor. Proc Natl Acad Sci U S A 2003;100:6958-6963.

16 Molecular Genetics and Cancer Biology

ADAM S. KIBEL, MD • ROBERT E. REITER, MD

DNA

Throughout the diverse manifestations of life, all organisms and many viruses share a common molecule that determines their structure and function: deoxyribonucleic acid (DNA) provides the blueprint for the character of life for past, present, and future generations. Within this simple series of repeating chemicals is the code that guides not only normal growth and development but also many diseases. Our under-standing of DNA and the biology surrounding it, known as molecular biology, has grown exponentially since its discovery 5 decades ago (Watson and Crick, 1953). Recently, the entire human genome has been sequenced, and eventually a reading of an individual's DNA sequence may be as common a diagnostic tool as cholesterol screening (Pennisi, 2003). The keys to our understanding of health, disease, and, soon, treatment lie in this exquisite molecule (Table 16–1).

In a rudimentary form, DNA is the fusion of three different elements: a base (either a pyrimidine or a purine), a sugar (in the case of DNA called 2-dioxyribose, for RNA called ribose), and a phosphate (which links individual nucleotides together) (Fig. 16–1). The repeating connections between the phosphates and the sugars provide the backbone from which the information-carrying bases protrude. In its "resting" or nonreplicating form, this chain of elements forms a helix of two strands called a double helix. The helix consists of one strand of bases ordered in one direction and the other strand of complementary bases ordered in the opposite direction (Fig. 16–2). The two strands are held together by the hydrogen bonds. Based on the connection of a phosphate to a sugar, each strand will end with part of the sugar ring exposed: this open position is denoted as 5' or 3'. By convention, the leading strand runs from 5' to 3', and the complementary strand runs from 3' to 5'.

When DNA is replicated, each strand of the double helix provides a template to order the bases of the new strand. The physical chemistry of the bases requires that a purine form a specific hydrogen bond with a pyrimidine: the purine adenine (A) always binds to the pyrimidine thymine (T), and the purine guanine (G) always binds to the pyrimidine cytosine (C) (Watson and Crick, 1953). Therefore, when the parent strand exposes the bases in the order AGCT the new daughter strand must order the bases as TCGA. This requirement of precisely pairing A with T and C with G (Fig. 16–3) ensures that the code contained within the repeating base pairs (bps) can be replicated precisely. In fact, one parent strand joining a new daughter strand to form a double helix is called semiconservative replication (Meselson and Stahl, 1958). It has been argued—perhaps only to emphasize the importance of DNA—that perpetuating DNA though replication is the ultimate reason for life: the expression of DNA, although crucial for the manifestations of life, primarily facilitates the propagation of DNA from one generation to the next.

Table 16–1. Molecular Biology: Glossary of Terms

Allele: An alternative form of a gene.
Amplification: Additional copies of a chromosomal sequence; these sequences may include genes.
Aneuploid: Deviation in chromosomal number from the usual diploid state.
Annealing: The pairing of two single strands of complementary DNA sequences to form a double helix.
Alternative splicing: A mechanism by which variations in the incorporation of a gene's coding regions leads to the production of multiple related forms of a gene.
Base pair: The physical relationship between adenine/thymidine and guanine/cytosine within the double helix of DNA. Abbreviated as bp, it provides the unit of measurement for DNA.
cDNA: A segment of DNA complementary to an RNA sequence.
Chromosome: A distinct segment of DNA expressing a large number of genes. In humans there are 23 such segments.
Codon: Three sequential nucleotides that specify a particular amino acid or a stop signal.
Deletion: The removal of a segment of DNA, with rejoining of the ends.
Diploid: A set of chromosomes containing two complete copies of DNA.
Dominant: Allele determining the expression of a gene.
Endonuclease: An enzyme that cuts DNA or RNA within the chain.
Exon: A sequence of DNA that is represented with a complementary RNA sequence, also known as the coding sequence.
Expression vector: A vector designed to encode a particular DNA sequence or gene for transcription and translation into protein.
Epigenetic: Nongenetic information, such as methylation or acetylation, that modifies gene expression.
Frameshift mutation: A deletion or insertion of DNA that shifts the normal codons into a different order for translation into protein.
Gene: A segment of DNA that contributes to the formation of a protein, including both the introns (noncoding regions) and the exons (coding regions) as well as the regions preceding and the following the coding regions.
Genetic code: The correspondence between triplets of DNA or RNA (codons) and amino acids making up proteins.
Genotype: The genetic makeup of an organism as reflected in its DNA sequence.
Haplotype: A group of alleles in relative close proximity on a chromosome that are inherited together.
Hemizygote: Having only one copy of a gene owing, for example, to the loss of chromosomal material.
Heterozygote: Having two different copies (alleles) of a gene.
Homozygote: Having two identical copies (alleles) of a gene.
Hybridization: The physical pairing of complementary RNA and DNA.
Intron: A segment of DNA that is transcribed but is removed by the splicing together of the exons on either side; part of the noncoding sequences of a gene.
Karyotype: All the chromosomes within a cell.
Linkage: The tendency for genes in proximity to one another on a chromosome to be inherited together.
Locus: The position of a particular gene on a particular chromosome.
Methylation: The addition of a methyl group to the nucleotide cytosine; DNA methylation is often associated with decreased transcription of genes.
Mutation: Any change in the sequence of genomic DNA.
Northern blotting: A technique of transferring RNA from an agarose gel to a nitrocellulose filter for hybridization with a complementary DNA.
Oncogenes: Genes that encode for proteins that have the ability to transform normal cells into cancerous cells.
Polymerase chain reaction (PCR): A technique using sequential temperature cycles favoring denaturation, annealing of primer sequences, and extension with DNA polymerase to amplify a large number of copies of a particular sequence of DNA. This technique can be used to detect very small amounts of DNA by creating a huge number of identical copies.
Phenotype: The appearance or function of an organism, reflecting the contributions of the genotype and the environment.
Ploidy: The number or copies of chromosomes within a cell; diploid has two copies, triploid has three copies, and tetraploid has four copies.
Point mutation: A change in a DNA sequence involving a single base pair.
Polymorphism: A difference in normal DNA sequence between individuals. It can be a repetitive element or a single nucleotide polymorphism (SNP).
Promoter: The region of DNA in the binding of RNA polymerase and gene transcription. This region is often the sequence of DNA 100 to 500 base pairs immediately before the initiation site.
Recessive: An allele that is not expressed in the presence of a dominant allele.
Reporter gene: A gene encoding for a new or foreign protein that can easily be detected. For example, the luciferase gene, encoding the light-producing proteins of the firefly, is introduced into cells that do not express this gene.
Restriction enzyme: Recognizing specific short sequences of DNA, these enzymes cut the DNA at a particular location.
Silent mutation: An alteration in a DNA sequence that does not change the product of the gene.
Southern blotting: A technique of transferring denatured DNA from an agarose gel to a nitrocellulose filter for hybridization with complementary DNA.
Splicing: The removal of introns (spliced out) and the connection of exons (spliced together) in RNA.
Transcription: Synthesis of RNA on a DNA template.
Transfection: The addition of DNA sequences to a cell.
Transgenic animals: Animals created by the introduction of new DNA into the germ line (into the egg).
Translation: Synthesis of protein from the messenger RNA template.
Vector: A plasmid, bacteriophage, or virus that carries new DNA into a cell. Vectors are often designed to produce large amounts of protein encoded by the gene within the host cell.

Expression

The genetic code contained within DNA determines, in part, what we are and how we function. However, the genetic code is only the beginning. **The expression of the information carried with the sequences of DNA requires two additional processes, known as transcription and translation.** The physical locations of the genetic code (DNA) and the manifestation of that code (protein synthesis) are separate: DNA is in the nucleus and protein synthesis is cytoplasmic. To bridge this gap, copies of the DNA (mRNA transcripts) are made in the nucleus. The mRNA transcripts are then transported to the cytoplasm where they are translated into proteins (Meselson and Stahl, 1958). One of the remarkable aspects of

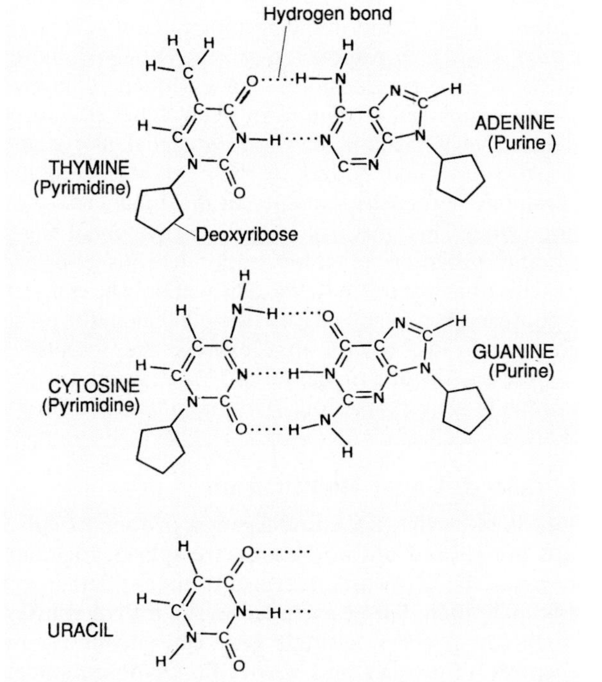

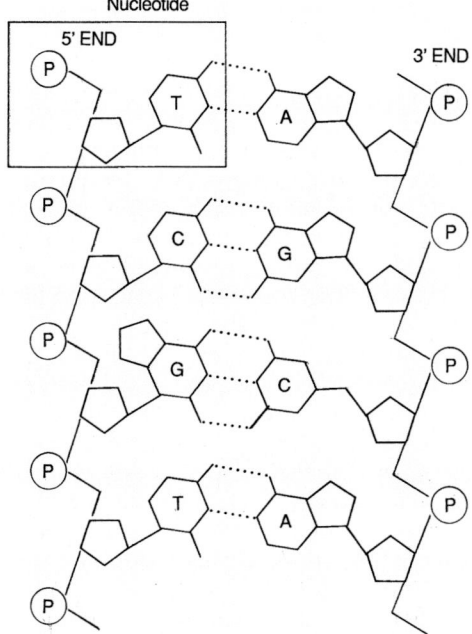

Figure 16–1. The alphabet consists of four bases: the purines adenine (A) and guanine (G) and the pyrimidines thymine (T) and cytosine (C). Uracil (U) is substituted for thymine in the case of RNA. The combination of a base and a sugar (deoxyribose) is referred to as a *nucleoside*.

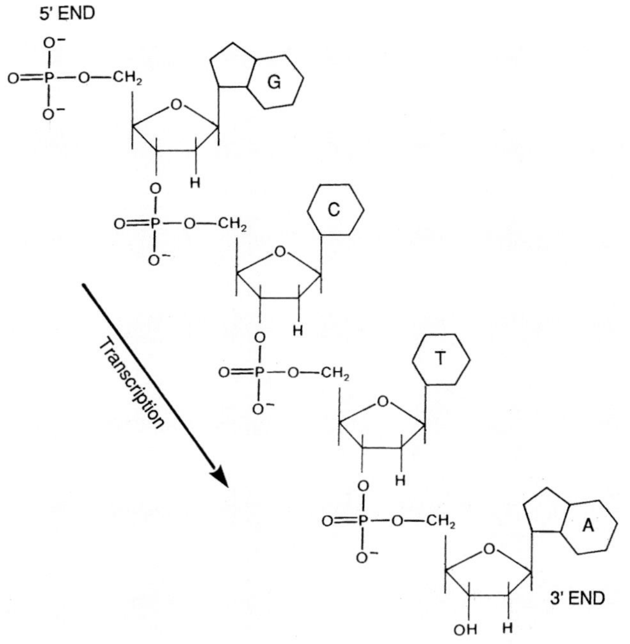

Figure 16–3. During transcription, DNA is used as a template for messenger RNA. This always occurs in a 5′ to 3′ direction.

Figure 16–2. The combination of a sugar phosphate group and a base constitutes a *nucleotide*. The double helix is made from two polynucleotide chains, each of which consists of a series of 5′- to 3′-sugar phosphate links that form a backbone from which the bases protrude. The double helix maintains a constant width because purines always face pyrimidines in complementary A-T and G-C base pairs, respectively.

the genetic code is its use of simplicity. When unwound, DNA is a linear structure: nucleotides follow nucleotides in a single-file manner. **In the process of transcription, linear DNA is converted to linear mRNA. In the process of translation, linear mRNA is converted to a linear set of amino acids, as the first step in the formation of functional proteins** (Fig. 16–4) (Sanger, 1988).

Transcription

Transcription is the first step in converting DNA to protein; a single strand of RNA is copied from one of the strands of DNA. Structurally, RNA is very similar to DNA: in RNA, the sugar element is ribose and the pyrimidine uracil substitutes for thymine. The enzyme RNA polymerase II is responsible for synthesizing the first copy of RNA, which is a complementary replica of the template DNA. In eukaryotic cells, this primary strand of RNA, called heterogeneous nuclear RNA, contains both the coding sequences of the DNA, known as exons, and noncoding or silent sequences of DNA, known as introns. Because introns contain sequences not necessary for protein production, they are spliced out and the exons are spliced together to make the condensed functional message, known as messenger RNA (mRNA). **By definition, therefore, exons are the sequences of DNA that have corresponding sequences in the mRNA and introns are the regions of DNA not represented in mRNA** (Witkowski, 1988).

In eukaryotic cells, mRNA undergoes modification before it is transported to the cytoplasm: on the end of the mRNA first to be synthesized, the 5′ end, a guanine is added leading to the formation of a methylated cap (Perry, 1981); on the 3′ end, last to be synthesized, a chain of approximately 200 adenines are added, called the poly(A) tail (Jackson and Standart, 1990). This modification may provide increased stability to the mRNA.

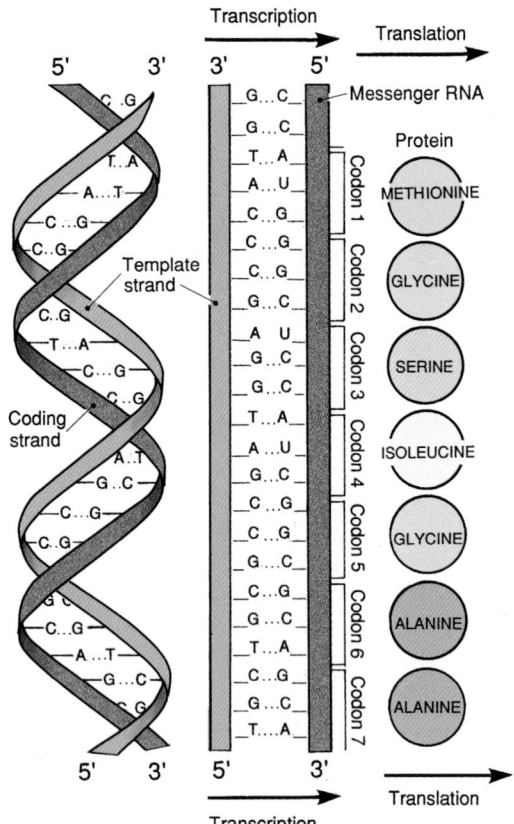

Figure 16–4. During transcription, the coding strand conveys its message through the template strand to make messenger RNA that is eventually translated into polypeptides by ribosomes. The relationship between DNA sequence and corresponding protein is called the *genetic code,* which is read in triplets or codons.

Transcriptional Regulation

With the exception of germ cells, every cell in our bodies has the same DNA and, potentially, could make any particular transcript. However, regulation of expression ensures that genes are only produced in specific tissues at specific points in time. For example, prostate-specific antigen (PSA) is produced by prostate epithelium and not by the brain whereas testosterone is produced by Leydig cells and the adrenal cortex but not by the ureter. If the process of gene transcription were a random event, then the cells of our bodies would behave like teratocarcinomas, expressing ectoderm, mesoderm, and endoderm without organization. Transcription must be regulated to ensure that proteins are produced in a specific tissue at a specific point in development. **Transcriptional regulation of gene expression is primarily controlled at the initiation of RNA transcription** (Maniatis et al, 1987).

There are two general components involved in transcriptional regulation: (1) specific sequences within the DNA and (2) proteins that interact with those sequences (Mitchell and Tjian, 1989). **DNA not only contains genetic information but also provides specific docking sites for proteins that control the expression of the genetic information. This is accomplished by altering the activity of the transcriptional machinery.** For example, the gene regulatory protein Sp1 specifically recognizes and binds to the nucleotide sequence

GGGCGG (Kadonaga et al, 1987, 1988). Other specific sequences of DNA found in the promoter or enhancer regions of a gene, known as response elements, act to promote the initiation of gene transcription. These sequences, known as consensus sequences, are found in many genes that respond in a coordinated fashion to a specific signal. For example, glucocorticoids when bound to their receptor recognize a 15-nucleotide consensus sequence in the enhancer region of specific genes. This, in turn, leads to activation of the promoter and initiation of transcription (Evans and Arriza, 1989). This does not mean that a gene will only be transcribed in response to glucocorticoids, but simply that, in the presence of glucocorticoids, tissues that express the receptor will express these genes at a higher level. This allows the organism to coordinate gene expression in multiple tissues throughout the body.

Post-transcriptional Modification

As described earlier, RNA undergoes a process of splicing: introns are spliced out and exons are spliced together. In many genes, the RNA can undergo alternate splicing: certain exons can be included or excluded in the mRNA transcript. Through this process, a single gene can encode for many polypeptide sequences and a specific DNA sequence can encode a gene that has different functions (Perry, 1981; Sharp, 1987). For example, the fibroblast growth factor receptor gene encodes for a single pre-mRNA but through extensive alternative splicing a large number of different mRNA transcripts and, hence, protein isoforms of the receptor are produced (Chellaiah et al, 1994). Errors in splicing can predispose cells to malignant degeneration (Venables, 2004). In a prostate cancer model, deregulation of this splicing accompanies the transition from well-differentiated, androgen-dependent cells to more aggressive, androgen-independent cells (Carstens et al, 1998).

RNA Interference

A major advance in our understanding of gene regulation has been recently discovered—RNA interference. In this process, cells can modulate transcription not only by the expression of regulatory transcription factors but also post-transcriptionally by the expression of noncoding RNAs (ncRNA). These ncRNAs have the capacity to bind to and degrade messenger RNAs. These ncRNAs are collectively called RNAi, or RNA interference (Ishikawa et al, 1991; Medema, 2004; Schutze, 2004; Barik, 2005; Karagiannis and El-Osta, 2005; Rao and Sockanathan, 2005; Tan and Yin, 2005; Wheeler et al, 2005). Although RNAi were first discovered in the experimental model system *C. elegans,* they are now known to exist in virtually all species, including humans. They are also a mechanism by which invading pathogens can control host cell transcription. They have also become a powerful tool by which scientists can control target gene expression and are being explored as novel therapeutics.

RNAi are double-stranded RNA species transcribed from cellular genes or infecting pathogens. This initial double-stranded RNA species is diced by a specialized ribonuclease (RNAse) III-like enzyme, named Dicer, into 21- to 23-bp products with two-nucleotide 3′ overhangs, known as small or short interfering RNA (siRNA). In the execution phase of the

RNAi, the antisense strand of the siRNA is incorporated into the "RNA-induced silencing complex" (RISC), which then engages the target RNA of the complementary sequence. An RISC-associated "slicer" RNAse belonging to the Ago2 gene family then cleaves the target in the middle of the homologous gene segment, leading to its degradation.

A variation on this theme generates microRNAs, instead of siRNA. Long microRNAs contain self-complementary regions that result in the formation of a hairpin, which is sequentially cleaved by two RNAse III-like enzymes. The first enzyme, called Drosha, trims the long hairpin to generate a short hairpin RNA (shRNA). The shRNA is then processed by cytoplasmic Dicer to produce double-stranded miRNA capable of binding target genes for destruction, as described earlier.

Although the precise molecular biology of RNAi is not of obvious relevance to the practicing urologist, its application in the laboratory and clinic is of utmost relevance. In the laboratory, the concept of RNAi has been exploited to the utmost to study gene function. Generation of synthetic siRNA and shRNA has led to the ability to knockdown specific gene expression in a highly exacting manner. This has enabled scientists to evaluate the effect that loss of a single gene has on cell function. In the case of oncology, this has made it possible for scientists to evaluate the relevance of single gene products on tumor biology. For example, a major question in prostate cancer biology is the role of the androgen receptor (AR) in hormone-refractory prostate cancer progression. By using shRNA against the androgen receptor, Chen and colleagues could knockdown AR expression in hormone-refractory prostate cancer xenografts and cell lines and demonstrate that AR is necessary and sufficient for tumor growth, implicating continued AR function as the underlying cause of both hormone-dependent and hormone-independent prostate cancer growth (Chen et al, 2004). Not only has RNAi led to an explosion of molecular knowledge, but it has also catalyzed the development of an entire new biotechnology sector, one focused on translation of this technique into therapies. One obvious example that many groups are working on is to target the AR itself for RNAi knockdown in patients. Although the technology to do this in humans is still complex, it can be expected that new drugs based on RNAi technology will eventually hit the marketplace, just as antisense technology and monoclonal antibody technology have now reached the clinic as a means of specific gene targeting.

Nuclear Matrix

One characteristic common to all cancer cells is abnormal nuclear shape. In fact, these alterations are so prevalent in cancer cells they are commonly used as a pathologic marker of malignancy. Nuclear shape reflects the internal nuclear structure and processes and is determined, at least in part, by the nuclear matrix (Pienta et al, 1989). The nuclear matrix consists of approximately 10% of the nuclear proteins and is virtually devoid of lipids, DNA, and histones (Fey et al, 1991). **It has a central role in the regulation of important cellular processes, such as DNA replication and transcription** (Getzenberg, 1994). The nuclear matrix is the framework or scaffolding of the nucleus, consisting of an internal ribonucleic protein network, residual nucleoli, and the peripheral lamins and pores complexes (Berezney and Coffey, 1974).

The structural components of the nucleus have a central role in the specific topologic organization of DNA. This topologic organization contributes to control of gene expression; genes are physically positioned within the nucleus to permit the expression of both housekeeping and cell type–specific genes. The average mammalian somatic cell nucleus holds a linear equivalent of 2 meters of DNA: this is packed by a 200,000-fold linear condensation into a 10-μm nucleus. With the use of in-situ hybridization (McNeil et al, 1991), there is direct evidence for specific three-dimensional organization of the DNA within the nucleus (Carter and Lawrence, 1991; Haaf and Schmid, 1991). Importantly, this appears to have functional significance because distinct cell types have a specific pattern of interphase chromosome three-dimensional organization (Manuelidis and Borden, 1988). For example, comparing the chromosomal topography of human lymphocytes, amniotic fluid cells, fibroblasts, and human cerebral/cerebellar samples demonstrates topologic DNA organization is cell type specific (Arnoldus et al, 1989; Emmerich et al, 1989).

Tissue-specific gene expression is in part based on this higher-order structure of DNA. The nuclear matrix is the site of mRNA transcription. Active genes are associated with the nuclear matrix only in cell types in which they are expressed (Getzenberg, 1994). The association of active genes with the nuclear matrix is based on a DNA loop anchorage site in the enhancer regions or intronic sequences of several genes (Roberge and Gasser, 1992). In addition, because transcription factors are localized or sequestered on the nuclear matrix, genes to be expressed in a particular tissue are topographically placed in close proximity to enzymes critical for transcription (van Wijnen et al, 1993; Nardozza et al, 1996). In contrast, genes not expressed are sequestered from transcription factors. For example, DNA-binding nuclear matrix proteins in the seminal vesicles are involved in the tissue-specific regulation of genes encoding seminal vesicle secretory proteins (Horton and Getzenberg, 1999). The nuclear matrix also plays a central role in RNA processing and is the site of attachment for products from RNA cleavage and for RNA processing intermediates (Carter et al, 1993).

Whereas all cell types share the majority of known nuclear matrix proteins (NMPs), some NMPs appear to be unique to certain cell types. Therefore, the protein composition of the nuclear matrix is tissue specific and can serve as a fingerprint of each cell and/or tissue type (Getzenberg et al, 1990). Furthermore, cell proliferation and differentiation alter the composition of nuclear matrix proteins and structure (Stuurman et al, 1989; Dworetzky et al, 1990). Differences in NMP composition are found also in a number of human cancers, including prostate cancer (Getzenberg et al, 1991; Partin et al, 1993), renal cell carcinoma (Konety et al, 1998), and transitional cell carcinoma (Getzenberg et al, 1996). In bladder cancer, antibodies raised against one of the unique nuclear matrix proteins (BLCA4) have been used as a biomarker of transitional cell carcinoma. In preliminary studies, BLCA4 was a very sensitive (96.4%) and specific (100%) marker for bladder cancer (Konety et al, 2000).

Translation

The translation of the mRNA message consisting of four bases (the nucleotides A, U, C, G) into 20 amino acids uses a

functional set of three adjacent nucleotides, called a codon (Crick et al, 1961; Crick, 1970). Reading the code in groups of three nucleotides results in 64 unique codons, which is more than the total number of amino acids. This results in redundancy; more than one codon encodes for each amino acid. For example, the codons CAA and CAG both encode for glutamine. Three codons, UAA, UAG, and UGA, do not encode for any amino acids but instead function as STOP codons; they signal for chain termination. There are several important consequences of codons. First, a single base insertion or deletion results in a shift in the reading frame leading to a frame-shift mutation. This type of mutation results in a nonfunctioning protein product. In contrast, single-base substitutions may or many not result in a change in amino acid sequence and therefore may have minimal to no functional significance.

In the process of translation, two other forms of RNA are important. Transfer RNA (tRNA) is a small (75 to 85 bases long) adapter molecule that is covalently linked to a single amino acid at one end and an anticodon in the middle of the chain. This anticodon is a triplet of nucleotides complementary to the codon representing a particular amino acid. Ribosomal RNA (rRNA), which constitutes about 80% of the RNA within a cell, makes up part of the ribosome, the cytoplasmic structure integral in protein synthesis. In eukaryotic cells, the ribosome is composed of large (60S) and small (40S) subunits (the designation "S" refers to their rate of sedimentation in an ultracentrifuge): within the larger subunit are 28S rRNA, 5.8S rRNA, and 5.0S rRNA; within the smaller subunit is 18S rRNA. Because 28S and 18S rRNA are so abundant, they are used as convenient markers in Northern blot analysis of mRNA. The ribosome has three binding sites for RNA: two for tRNA (called P and A) and one for the mRNA.

Protein synthesis has three major stages. Initiation is the first, and often rate-limiting, step of translation (Hunt, 1980; Merrick, 1992). The 40S ribosome binds to the mRNA and forms an initiation complex that binds a tRNA with an amino acid attached: because the initiation codon is AUG, all new proteins start with methionine. **The second stage, called elongation, is the most rapid: amino acids are added to the peptide chain one at a time, with the ribosome moving along the mRNA chain, similar to beads on a string.** For any given mRNA transcript, multiple ribosomes are simultaneously moving along the chain, actively making new polypeptide chains (Rich, 1963). **Termination, the last stage of protein synthesis, is signaled by one of the three STOP codons** (Tate and Brown, 1992). A cytoplasmic protein, called the release factor, binds to the stop codon, catalyzing the hydrolysis of the aminoacyl linkage and in doing so releases the carboxyl end of the polypeptide chain (Merrick, 1992). Therefore, the amino terminal is the first amino acid of a polypeptide and the carboxyl terminal is the last amino acid of the chain. After termination, the ribosome releases from the mRNA and dissociates into its two subunits, making the ribosome available to begin the process of translation again.

Ubiquitination

Ubiquitin is a small protein that when linked to a wide variety of cellular proteins is involved in such diverse cellular processes as endocytosis, chromatin remodeling, and transcriptional activation (Marx, 2002; Muratani and Tansey, 2003; Kao et al, 2004). **However, the primary cellular role for ubiquitin is to mark proteins for active destruction** (Ciechanover et al, 1981).

In the absence of an efficient mechanism to dispose of proteins, ongoing protein production would quickly overwhelm the cell. Therefore, active, controlled, precise protein degradation is critical to cell survival. For example, certain proteins, such as cell cycle proteins, act as potent stimulators or inhibitors and therefore can only be present at a precise point in time to properly function (Koepp et al, 2001). These proteins need to be rapidly degraded once they are no longer necessary. Other cases in which ubiquitination is useful are when proteins are inadvertently produced in excess, when they fail to fold into the correct configuration, or when they are damaged by normal cellular activity. If these irregular or extra proteins were allowed to persist the cell would not be able to function. **To identify and degrade these proteins, a small protein called ubiquitin is covalently linked to the protein, tagging it for destruction** (Ciechanover et al, 1981). **Additional ubiquitin moieties are added, forming a polyubiquitin chain** (Chau et al, 1989).

The actual destruction of this protein-polyubiquitin complex takes place in the proteasome (Peters, 1994). This large protein complex, visible by electron microscopy, has a cylinder-like configuration (Peters et al, 1993). The inner walls contain many proteases that degrade the protein into small peptides. Targeted inhibition of proteasome function has emerged as novel antitumor strategy. For example, blocking proteasome degradation of the cell cycle inhibitor CDKN1A leads to intracellular accumulation of CDKN1A, limiting cell cycle progression, and, eventually, leading to apoptosis (Adams et al, 1999). Others have demonstrated induction of programmed cell death with proteasome inhibition (Herrmann et al, 1998). In prostate cancer, the cell death–promoting protein BAX levels were inversely related to Gleason score and the activity of proteasome-mediated BAX degradation increased with higher-grade disease (Li and Dou, 2000). In other words, higher-grade cancers appear to degrade this signal for cell death at an increased rate. In doing so, the cancer cells inhibit apoptosis and enhance their own survival.

KEY POINTS: DNA

- DNA encodes each individual's genetic information.
- With the exception of germ cells, all cells in an individual have the same DNA.
- The DNA is organized in the nuclear matrix, and this organization influences gene expression.
- The information in DNA has to be transcribed into RNA and then translated into protein.
- Transcription of RNA is tightly regulated and is tissue specific.
- RNAi is a newly discovered process by which cells can also regulate gene transcription.
- Once proteins have performed their task, they are actively degraded in a process called ubiquitination.

DYSREGULATION

With all the complex biology discussed earlier, it is a wonder that DNA is decoded into functional proteins. Often, the message is damaged; and when this happens, a cell must decide if it can be fixed and, if not, the cell undergoes programmed cell death (see sections on "DNA Repair" and "Apoptosis"). Unfortunately, some cells continue to divide despite errors in the DNA and/or altered reexpression of the critical proteins. Cancer cells actually exploit this dysregulation by producing proteins that assist with survival and spread.

Mutation

The DNA sequence can be changed or mutated in a variety of ways (Fig. 16–5). A point mutation is a single base pair substituted by another nucleotide. If this occurs in the coding region of a gene, it can produce a change in the codon, resulting in an amino acid substitution or a termination signal. A deletion is a loss of DNA sequence. If the deletion is large, it can result in a truncated form of a protein. Alternatively, a smaller deletion of even one base pair can result in a frame-shift mutation, where the normal triplet of nucleotides is shifted to a new reading frame. This usually results in a truncated protein product, as a stop codon occurs eventually by chance in the new reading frame. Insertions, the addition of DNA sequence, can result in the same frame shift and ensuing truncated protein product. Lastly, translocations, moving DNA sequences from one part of the genome to another, can have similar effects as simple insertions or deletions; however, they can also create fusion proteins that promote cancer. This is classically exemplified by the exchange between the long arms of chromosomes 9 and 22, producing the so-called Philadelphia chromosome of chronic myelogenous leukemia (Nowell and Hungerford, 1960; Groffen et al, 1984). This translocation results in a formation of a fusion protein, BCR-ABL, in which the tyrosine kinase activity of ABL is constantly active. In

addition, the BCR-ABL fusion protein is trapped in the cytoplasm of the cell, where it stimulates proliferation and inhibits apoptosis (Schwartz, 2002).

The contribution of a mutation to carcinogenesis and tumor progression requires it be heritable: that is, the change in DNA must be passed to the daughter cells (Nowell, 1976). Many mutations, therefore, are of no real threat; the alteration is either silent (occurring in a nonencoding region of a gene or not altering the final polypeptide sequence) or, in altering some critical gene product, results in the death of the cell. Considering all the possible genes within human DNA, the mutations linked with cancers occur in a relatively few genes and frequently those associated with promoting or inhibiting cell proliferation. **When the growth-promoting genes (or proto-oncogenes) are mutated and become hyperactive, they are called oncogenes** (Heldin and Westermark, 1984). **Mutation and inactivation of a growth-inhibiting gene can have the same net effect: if the gene is no longer inhibiting growth, cellular growth is unchecked, much like the loss of brakes on an automobile do not cause the car to go faster but prevent it from stopping. These tumor suppressor genes are defined by their absence in a malignancy and are best characterized by the hereditary cancers** (Marshall, 1991).

Oncogenes

Oncogenes are the mutated form of normal genes (proto-oncogene) often associated with cell proliferation (Cross and Dexter, 1991). Many oncogenes were first identified through their presence in a class of RNA viruses, known as retroviruses, capable of inducing the malignant transformation of normal cells (Martin, 1970). These *viral* genes, designated by the prefix *v-* (as in *v-SRC*) induce tumor formation in animals; their *cellular* counterparts, designated by the prefix *c-*, have been identified in human tumors. For example, the retrovirus (MC29) responsible for avian myelocytomatosis carries the oncogene *v-MYC*. The proto-oncogene, *MYC*, encodes an early-response gene product (activation within 15 minutes of exposure to a growth factor) called MYC: this transcription factor regulates cell proliferation. The oncogene *c-MYC* is overexpressed in many cancers (Wong et al, 1986).

In another example, hepatocyte growth factor (also known as scatter factor) acts through a receptor encoded by the proto-oncogene c-*MET* (Bottaro et al, 1991). Hepatocyte growth factor has diverse action on the kidney: it appears to have a role in normal renal development, acts as a potent mitogen for renal tubular cells, and induces tubulogenesis of renal cells in vitro (Stoker et al, 1987; Montesano et al, 1991; Santos and Nigam, 1993). In renal cell carcinoma, c-*MET* immunoreactivity was detected in the majority of tumors and was more common in higher-grade cancers (Pisters et al, 1997). In hereditary renal cell carcinoma, characterized by a predisposition to multiple, bilateral papillary renal tumors, missense mutations of the *MET* proto-oncogene appear to lead to constitutive activation of the MET protein in these tumors (Schmidt et al, 1997). In squamous cell carcinomas of the head and neck, mutations in the *MET* proto-oncogene appear to be selected for in metastatic lesions: transcripts of mutant alleles are highly represented in metastases but not in primary tumors (Di Renzo et al, 2000). As this example demonstrates,

```
        M     A     L     T     R     @
A     ATG   GCT   CTG   ACT   AGG   TAG

        M     A     L     T     R     @
B     ATG   GCA   CTG   ACT   AGG   TAG

        M     G     L     T     R     @
C     ATG   GGT   CTG   ACT   AGG   TAG

        M     G     S     D     @
D     ATG   GGC   TCT   GAC   TAG   GTA G

        M     L     &
E     ATG   GCTC  TGA   CTA   GGT   AG
```

Figure 16–5. Examples of mutations. **A,** Wild-type. **B,** Point mutation that does not result in amino acid change. **C,** Point mutation that results in amino acid change. *Note:* only one amino acid changes and the result is often a protein with some function. **D,** Insertion that results in frame shift and premature termination of protein. **E,** Deletion that results in frame shift and premature termination of protein.

a normal cellular receptor, associated with growth and differentiation, can become abnormally activated, thereby contributing to carcinogenesis and tumor progression.

There are at least three ways a proto-oncogene can be converted into an oncogene. First, a mutation can occur within the coding sequence, producing a permanently activated form of the gene. If the gene regulates cell proliferation, the cell will get a continuous signal to proliferate, leading to uncontrolled growth. The proto-oncogene *ERBB* encodes for the epidermal growth factor receptor (EGFR) (Downward et al, 1984). Mutations of *ERRB* can lead to overexpression of a constitutively active form of the receptor. One of the members of the EGFR family, known as ERBB2 (or HER2/NEU) is overexpressed in a subset of breast cancers: a humanized anti-HER2/NEU antibody (trastuzumab [Herceptin]), directed against this target, is used in the treatment of these tumors (Slamon et al, 2001). Because EGFR family members are overexpressed in a variety of cancers, it is hoped that inhibition will control other diseases, including urologic malignancies (Grunwald and Hidalgo, 2003). For example, in preclinical animal models of prostate cancer, ERBB2 inhibition has showed significant growth inhibition (Agus et al, 1999; Sirotnak et al, 2000; Wakeling et al, 2002).

A second mechanism converting a proto-oncogene into an oncogene is through gene amplification. Genes often become amplified through errors in chromosomal replication, a common manifestation of cancer known as aneuploidy. In this process, the number of copies of a gene increase at the DNA level; the DNA templates produce many mRNA transcripts and the result is overproduction of protein. For example, c-*MYC* overexpression in a subset of bladder cancers is secondary to this mechanism (Christoph et al, 1999). As a result, MYC protein levels, studied by immunohistochemical staining, are overexpressed in more than half of the papillary (58%) and invasive bladder cancers (59%) (Schmitz-Drager et al, 1997). **A third mechanism of oncogene formation is through chromosomal rearrangement,** such as the translocation described earlier producing the Philadelphia chromosome of chronic myelogenous leukemia.

The relevance of oncogene mutations to cancer has been brought to increasing prominence recently with the advent of novel small molecule and antibody drugs that can bind to and inhibit oncogene signaling. Mutations have been determined both to predict susceptibility of given tumors to targeted agents and to predict resistance to these drugs. Iressa, for example, is a small molecule antagonist of the epidermal growth factor receptor (EGFR), a prominent member of the EGF receptor family. Clinical trials of Iressa in patients with lung cancer revealed that approximately 10% of patients have dramatic responses characterized by prolonged survival. Of note, investigators found that response rates were particularly high in subsets of patients, particularly in Asians with lung cancer. Subsequent studies showed that patients who responded had specific mutations of the EGFR kinase, or active, domain (Lynch et al, 2004; Paez et al, 2004). These mutations are more common in Asians with lung cancer and explain at the molecular level why some patients respond and others do not. Tests to identify EGFR kinase mutations are now available to select appropriate patients for treatment with Iressa. Knowledge of point mutations in oncogenes may also

lead to advances in the treatment of patients with chronic myelogenous leukemia. Gleevec is a small molecule antagonist of the *BCR-ABL* oncogene in chronic myelogenous leukemia. Whereas most patients respond dramatically to this drug, some go on to develop acute myelogenous leukemia. Patients in blast crisis also frequently develop resistance to Gleevec. Research has now shown that resistance is caused by the acquisition of novel point mutations in the *BCR-ABL* oncogenes (Gorre et al, 2002; Roumiantsev et al, 2002; Talpaz et al, 2002). New drugs that suppress mutated *BCR-ABL* are now being tested in resistant patients, and combinations of drugs are contemplated to reduce the emergence of resistant cells, similar to cocktail therapy for human immunodeficiency virus (HIV) infection.

Tumor Suppressor Genes

Unlike oncogenes, which generally act as dominant accelerants for tumor growth, tumor suppressor genes are defined by the consequence of their absence (Marshall, 1991). **Also, unlike oncogenes, which can be active with only one allele expressed, classically both copies of tumor suppressor genes need to be inactivated to permit carcinogenesis** (see discussion, "Inherited Susceptibility to Cancer"). Recently, it has become apparent that in some cases loss of one copy of a tumor suppressor gene, particularly in concert with other genetic events, is sufficient for malignant degeneration. This is called haploinsufficiency and is discussed later in the chapter in more detail (Fero et al, 1998; Di Cristofano et al, 2001).

As their name implies, many tumor suppressor genes normally act to regulate cell growth and, therefore, function normally in the regulation of cell cycle. Others play critical roles in DNA repair and cell signaling. Classic tumor suppressor genes discussed later in this chapter are the retinoblastoma gene *(RB)* and *TP53* (see "The Cell Cycle").

Hypermethylation

Mutations, defined broadly as a change in DNA sequence, are called genetic changes. There are other classes of changes in which the DNA sequence integrity is preserved yet gene expression is altered, resulting in an altered phenotype: these are known as epigenetic changes. Hypermethylation of DNA is one such example. DNA methylation occurs exclusively on cytosine nucleotides in the dinucleotide sequence **CG.** Within the genome, if one assumes random distribution of the dinucleotides, the nucleotide cytosine followed by the nucleotide guanine should occur, on average, once every 16th dinucleotide. In fact, the dinucleotide CG occurs only about 20% of that expected by random distribution and, when expressed, are often clustered in regions of increased density known as CpG islands. These stretches of DNA have about a 60% density of CG dinucleotides, compared with the rest of the DNA (Razin and Kafri, 1994) and are often found in the 5′ promoter regions of genes. **Somatic methylation of CpG dinucleotides in these regulatory regions has been frequently associated with diminished transcriptional activity** (Bird, 1986). **In other words, DNA methylation can regulate which genes are active (or transcribed) and those which are not.**

It is important to recognize that methylation is a normal process and that gene silencing by methylation is an important normal regulatory mechanism. For example, imprinting is a specific form of epigenetic modification in which a paternally or maternally derived allele is silenced by methylation. As a result, only one parental allele is expressed in an individual. In fact, loss of imprinting, which leads to expression of both alleles, can predispose the individual to disease such as Wilms' tumor (Klein, 2005).

In cancer, CpG island methylation may result in the inactivation of a tumor suppressor gene (Baylin et al, 1991; Jones, 1996). For example, methylation of the tumor suppressor *CDKN2A* results in decreased transcription and contributes to carcinogenesis (Little, et al, 1995; Merlo et al, 1995). In prostate cancer, several genes that have undergone methylation have been identified. In fact, one of the most common alterations found in prostate cancer is methylation of the 5′ CG island region of the pi-class glutathione S-transferase gene, occurring in up to 91% of tumors studied (Lee et al, 1994, 1997). In a second example, the 5′ CG island of the endothelin B receptor gene is methylated in 70% of the tumors studied (Nelson et al, 1997). Given the frequency with which methylation occurs at these sites in prostate cancer—but not in normal tissues—it is possible methylation status could be used as an effective biomarker of the disease. Less frequently methylated genes, such as the androgen receptor gene (Jarrard et al, 1998; Kinoshita et al, 2000) and the neutral endopeptidase gene (Usmani et al, 2000), are associated with loss of protein expression common in prostate cancer progression.

Because DNA methylation is an epigenetic change and not an alteration to the DNA sequence itself, reversal of methylation, known as demethylation, could result in the reexpression of a normal gene: if a tumor suppressor gene is silenced by methylation, then demethylation and reexpression could be an effective strategy for the treatment of cancer.

It is not surprising that loss of methylation can also predispose patients to cancer. As outlined previously, one important role for methylation is imprinting. Loss of imprinting (LOI) is the loss of methylation in the normally methylated allele,

leading to aberrant activation of the normally silent copy of a growth-promoting gene (Feinberg, 2004). The best example of LOI is the human insulin-like growth factor-2 gene *(IGF2)*. Activation of the normally silent maternally inherited allele of *IGF2* occurs in many common cancers but appears to have the strongest association with colorectal neoplasia (Woodson et al, 2004; Sakatani et al, 2005).

KEY POINTS: DYSREGULATION

- Mutations in DNA can lead to changes in protein function or expression that increase the risk of cancer initiation, progression, or metastasis.
- Oncogenes are genes that promote cell growth. Their increased expression contributes to cancer.
- Tumor suppressor genes are genes that inhibit growth. Their loss of expression contributes to cancer.
- An alternative method of dysregulation is alteration in methylation of gene promoters.
- Methylation of normally unmethylated genes can suppress gene expression.
- Loss of methylation of normally methylated genes can increase gene expression.

INHERITED SUSCEPTIBILITY TO CANCER

A strong family history of malignancy has long been recognized as a risk factor for developing cancer. The increased risk can be due to either a shared genetic heritage or a shared environmental exposure. Identifying patients with a hereditary predisposition to a particular malignancy has proven to be a powerful tool to identify genes responsible for not only hereditary tumor syndromes but also sporadic malignancies (Tables 16–2 and 16–3). So although only 1% of

Table 16–2. Tumor Syndromes Associated with Genitourinary Malignancies

Syndrome	Tumor	Chromosome	Gene	Function
Wilms' tumor	Wilms' tumor	11p13	WT1	Transcriptional repressor
Beckwith-Wiedemann	Wilms' tumor	11p15	CDKN1C	Cell cycle regulator
Von-Hippel-Lindau	Clear cell renal carcinoma Pheochromocytoma	3p25	VHL	Transcriptional elongation and ubiquitination
Hereditary papillary renal cell carcinoma	Papillary renal carcinoma	7q31	MET	Receptor tyrosine kinase
Birt-Hogg-Dubé	Papillary renal carcinoma Oncocytoma	17p11.2	FLCN	Unknown
Multiple endocrine neoplasia type II	Pheochromocytoma	10q11	RET	Receptor tyrosine kinase
Hereditary nonpolyposis colorectal cancer	Upper tract transitional cell carcinoma	2p22, 3p21.3, 2p16, 2q31-q33, 7p22, 14q24.3	MSH2, MLH1, MSH6, PMS1, PMS2, MLH3	DNA mismatch repair
Hereditary prostate cancer	Prostate cancer	1q24-25, 1p36, 1q42-43, 8p22-23, 17p11, 20q13, Xq27-28	RNASEL, MSR1, ELAC2	Endoribonuclease, macrophage specific receptor, cell cycle regulator

Table 16–3.   **Selected Tumor Syndromes Not Associated with Genitourinary Malignancies**

Syndrome	Primary Tumor	Chromosome	Gene	Function
Familial retinoblastoma	Retinoblastoma	13q14	RB	Transcriptional regulation
Li-Fraumeni	Sarcoma, breast carcinoma	17p13	TP53	Transcription factor
		22q12	hCHK2	Serine kinase
Familial adenomatous polyposis	Colorectal carcinoma	5q21	APC	Regulates β-catenin activity
Familial breast carcinoma	Breast carcinoma	17q21, 13q12	BRCA1, BRCA2	DNA double strand break repair
Cowden's disease	Breast carcinoma	10q23	PTEN	Phosphatase
Multiple endocrine neoplasia type I	Pancreatic islet cell carcinoma	11q13	MEN1	Transcription factor

cancer cases are estimated to be inherited (Fearon, 1997), the identification of the genes responsible for that 1% has illuminated the molecular cause of many sporadic malignancies and expanded our understanding of cancer in general.

To identify the gene responsible for a hereditary tumor syndrome, it is necessary to find patients with the syndrome. This is relatively easy if a rare cancer affects multiple family members, from different generations living in different environments. Examples of diseases like this are retinoblastoma and Wilms' tumor (Van Heyningen and Hastie, 1992). Identification of patients with a hereditary predisposition to more common malignancies is also relatively easy if the tumors are linked to a familial syndrome with a clear phenotype involving multiple stigmata. Two examples are von Hippel-Lindau disease (VHL) and hereditary nonpolyposis colon cancer (HNPCC), which provided clues as to the cause of sporadic renal cell and colon carcinomas, respectively (Fishel et al, 1993; Linehan et al, 1995).

Identification of genes responsible for more common malignancies such as prostate or breast carcinoma, which are not part of any classic familial tumor syndromes, has proven to be more difficult. One reason for this is that without additional clinical characteristics to distinguish the hereditary cancer the difference between a hereditary and sporadic case within a family is not obvious. If there is a high risk that a given patient within a family developed the malignancy by chance and not because of a genetic predisposition, linkage analysis, the methodology employed to identify such genes, is not robust enough to overcome the problems that these phenocopies present.

Clues to Cancer

The first insight that hereditary tumor genes provide into sporadic cancer is that often the gene responsible for the hereditary form of the disease is the same gene responsible for the sporadic form as well. Knudson (1971) proposed that the only difference between sporadic and hereditary disease was that the patient with hereditary cancer was born with one of the two copies of the tumor suppressor gene already malfunctioning. Therefore, a mutation in the remaining copy of the gene is all that is required for tumor formation. The sporadic tumors on the other hand require mutations to occur in *both* copies of the gene before the malignant phenotype can be produced (Fig. 16–6). Clinically, the inherited form of the disease differs from the sporadic form in that it tends to be multifocal, to be bilateral, and to affect younger patients. The key element to this hypothesis is that the same gene is responsible for sporadic and hereditary disease.

KNUDSON'S HYPOTHESIS

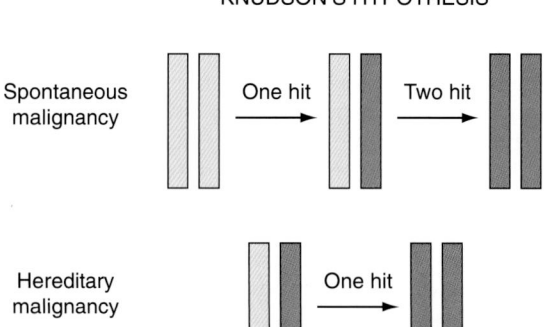

Figure 16–6. Knudson's hypothesis was that inactivation of the same gene was responsible for both sporadic and hereditary malignancies. Patients with sporadic tumors had two normal copies of the gene, and therefore the sporadic tumors required inactivation of both copies of the gene. Patients with hereditary tumor syndromes were born with only one functioning copy of the gene of interest, and therefore the hereditary tumors required inactivation of only one copy.

The second insight is that genetic inactivation of the hereditary tumor gene may provide clues as to the cellular pathway disrupted in sporadic disease. Colon carcinoma provides the best example of this. Familial adenomatous polyposis (FAP) accounts for less than 1% of colon carcinomas and yet mutations in the gene responsible for FAP, the *APC* gene, have been identified in more than 70% of adenomatous polyps and carcinomas of the rectum and colon (Kinzler and Vogelstein, 1996). In addition, since the primary function of *APC* is to regulate β-catenin activity, it is not surprising that mutations of β-catenin have been identified in intestinal tumors that do not harbor *APC* mutations (Fearon, 1997).

Lastly, genes responsible for hereditary disease often play important roles in malignancies that were not part of the tumor syndrome originally studied. The best example of this is *RB*. Although *RB* was originally identified by studying hereditary retinoblastoma, mutations have been linked to other tumors, including genitourinary malignancies (Friend et al, 1986; Bookstein et al, 1990; Horowitz et al, 1990). A second example is HNPCC, also called Lynch syndrome. HNPCC stigmata are not limited to colon carcinoma; there is an increased risk for malignancy at several extracolonic sites, particularly the endometrium, ovary, stomach, small bowel, hepatobiliary tract, pancreas, ureter, and renal pelvis (Watson and Lynch, 1993). In contrast to FAP, the defect in HNPCC affects tumor aggression by targeting the genome guardian function of DNA repair. Initial work demonstrated that

HNPCC was in large part caused by mutations in *MLH1* (Papadopoulos et al, 1994). Subsequent work has identified other DNA mismatch repair genes *(MLH1, MSH2, MSH6, PMS1,* and *PMS2)* (Lynch and de la Chapelle, 1999). Most importantly, *MLH1* and related DNA repair genes have subsequently been implicated in a wide variety of malignancies, and the concept of genomic integrity has become central to our understanding of malignant transformation (see "DNA Repair").

The genes responsible for hereditary tumors are identified most commonly by linkage analysis using a genome-wide scan. This is performed by identifying families that, on the basis of a careful family history, have a high likelihood of having the hereditary tumor syndrome of interest. A pedigree for each family is developed (Fig. 16–7). Normal DNA is collected from both affected and unaffected family members and is analyzed for known polymorphic markers that are evenly spaced throughout the genome. Alleles of polymorphic loci that are near the hereditary tumor gene will be more likely to co-segregate with the disease, that is, be passed on to the offspring who develop the disease, than alleles at loci that are far away for the disease gene. Linkage analysis does not identify genes but simply regions of the genome that are statistically likely to contain a gene. After linkage analysis is complete, individual genes in the region are identified and then screened for disease-associated alterations in family members with the tumor syndrome (Latif et al, 1993).

Genitourinary Syndromes

Von Hippel-Lindau Disease

VHL is a hereditary tumor syndrome that predisposes patients to clear cell renal carcinoma, retinal angiomas, pheochromocytomas, hemangiomas of the central nervous system (CNS), epididymal cystadenomas, and pancreatic islet cell tumors (Linehan et al, 1995). von Hippel first described the retinal lesions in 1904 and the link between the retinal lesions and other stigmata of the syndrome was made by Lindau in 1927.

The disease affects approximately 1 in 36,000 live births. Of the nonurologic stigmata, the most common are retinal angiomas, which affect 60% of patients and can lead to blindness, and CNS hemangiomas, which also affect 60% of patients and can lead to neurologic deficits. The urologic cancer manifestations include clear cell renal carcinoma, pheochromocytoma, and epididymal cystadenomas. Each affects approximately 40%, 18%, and 10% of patients, respectively. Clear cell renal carcinoma and pheochromocytoma both have malignant potential and therefore need to be excised. Renal cell carcinoma occurs at a mean age of 39 years and frequently recurs (Linehan et al, 1995). It therefore is generally managed with serial partial nephrectomies (Walther et al, 1999). Epididymal cystadenomas are benign but can be a rare cause of infertility (Linehan et al, 1995).

Chromosome 3 has been implicated as the location of the gene responsible for VHL since the late 1970s when karyotypic abnormalities involving that chromosome were identified in VHL families (Cohen et al, 1979; Pathak et al, 1982). Subsequent analysis identified 3p as a region of frequent chromosomal loss in primary sporadic clear cell tumors and renal carcinoma cell lines, providing strong evidence that the gene responsible for von Hippel-Lindau disease was also responsible for sporadic clear cell renal carcinoma (Zbar et al, 1987; Anglard et al, 1991). **Linkage analysis of affected and unaffected VHL family members was then used to identify a small region on 3p24 that proved to contain the VHL tumor suppressor gene** (Latif et al, 1993).

True to Knudson's hypothesis, the VHL tumor suppressor was found to be genetically altered in close to 80% of sporadic clear cell renal carcinomas (Gnarra et al, 1994; Herman et al, 1994). The gene functions as a classic tumor suppressor because reintroduction of the gene into renal tumor cells suppresses tumor formation in nude mice (Iliopoulos et al, 1995). The VHL protein forms a stable complex with elongin B, elongin C, cullin-2, and rbx-1 (Kamura et al, 1999). This complex targets various substrates for ubiquitin-mediated degradations. Loss of VHL results in decreased degradation of important substrates. Of particular importance, loss of VHL increases the cellular levels of HIFα, which in turn leads to the increased expression of cellular factors critical to renal tumor formation such as vascular endothelial growth factor (VEGF) (angiogenesis), GLUT1 (glucose transport), and transforming growth factor-α (TGF-α) (growth factor) (Iliopoulos et al,

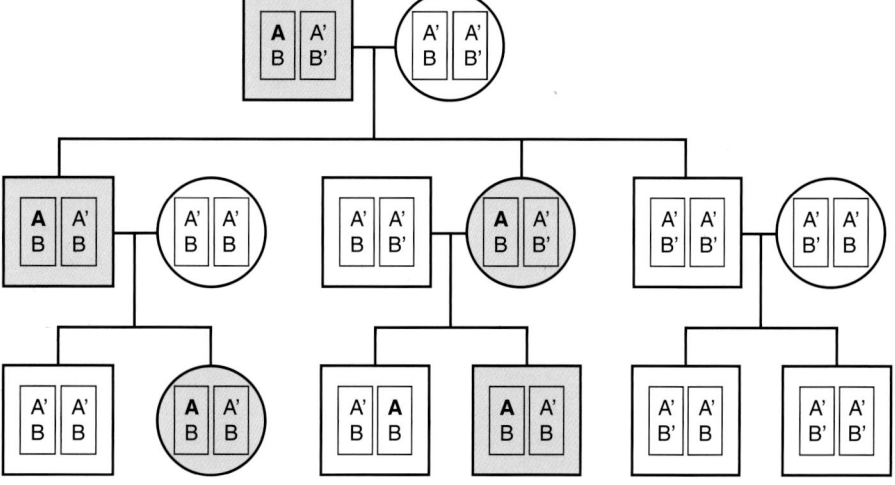

Figure 16–7. The familial tumor syndrome is passed from generation to generation. Genotyping demonstrates that the polymorphic marker A *(marked in red)* is passed also from generation to generation in concert with the phenotypic disease. Presumably a gene responsible for the syndrome is located near marker A. Linkage analysis is complicated by incomplete penetrance (not all members of the family with the allele get the disease), phenocopies (family members who have sporadic disease), inability to get DNA from all family members, and the large number of markers being simultaneously analyzed.

1996; Kamura et al, 2000; Ohh et al, 2000; de Paulsen et al, 2001).

Hereditary Papillary Renal Cell Carcinoma

HPRCC was originally described by Zbar and associates in 1994. **It is an inherited kidney cancer syndrome characterized by a predisposition to develop multiple, bilateral papillary renal tumors.** Linkage analysis mapped the gene(s) responsible for HPRCC to several different loci, including *PRCC* at 1q21, *TFE* at Xp11, *MET* at 7q31, and *RCC17* at 17q25 (Sidhar et al, 1996; Schmidt et al, 1997; Heimann et al, 2001). **The gene with the strongest evidence is *MET*. Once linkage analysis identified *MET* as the candidate gene at this locus, mutation analysis of *MET* identified mutations in HPRCC families** (Schmidt et al, 1997).

Interestingly, unlike *VHL*, *MET* does not appear to play as strong a role in sporadic papillary renal carcinoma. Whereas trisomy 7 is commonly associated with sporadic papillary renal cell carcinomas (Kovacs et al, 1991), only 13% of sporadic papillary tumors have *MET* mutations (Schmidt et al, 1999), suggesting that sporadic and hereditary disease may develop by different mechanisms.

Birt-Hogg Dubé Syndrome

BHD syndrome was first described in 1977 in a kindred that exhibited skin lesions, fibrofolliculomas, trichodiscomas, and acrochordons on the face, neck, and upper trunk (Birt et al, 1977). This hereditary tumor syndrome is currently characterized by hair follicle hamartomas, kidney tumors, spontaneous pneumothorax, and colonic polyps (Nickerson et al, 2002; Khoo et al, 2003). After its initial description in 1977, Roth and associates (1993) linked the disease to renal carcinomas. Unlike the other familial renal tumor syndromes, BHD is not limited to one histologic subtype. Families have been described with oncocytomas, chromophobe renal carcinomas, and papillary renal carcinomas. Molecular analysis demonstrated that these patients did not have germline mutations in the known renal carcinoma tumor suppressor genes *VHL* or *MET* (Toro et al, 1999) and therefore linkage analysis was used to search for the responsible tumor suppressor gene. Schmidt and coworkers (2001) identified 33 families with BHD skin lesions and associated renal tumors, lung cysts, or pneumothorax and using linkage analysis mapped the gene to 17p12-q11.2. Eventually the region of interest was narrowed to a 700-kb segment on 17p11.2, and by positional cloning they identified a novel gene in this region encoding a protein called folliculin (FLCN), which was mutated in BHD families (Nickerson et al, 2002). The function of this gene is unknown.

Hereditary Prostate Carcinoma

HPC has been defined as either a cluster of three affected relatives within a nuclear family or the occurrence of prostate cancer in three generations or two affected relatives who both developed prostate cancer when younger than 55 years of age (Carter et al, 1993). Segregation analysis of HPC families demonstrated a pattern of inheritance most consistent with an autosomal dominant pattern, and the carriers of this high-risk allele are predisposed to an earlier onset of prostate cancer. So while the inherited form of prostate cancer is estimated to be responsible for only 9% of all prostate cancer, it is implicated in 43% of disease diagnosed before age 55 (Carter et al, 1992).

Linkage analysis of HPC families has been used to identify at least seven loci that potentially contain genes important in the development of hereditary prostate carcinoma: 1q24-25 *(HPC1)*, 17p11 *(HPC2)*, 8p22-23, Xq27-28 *(HPCX)*, 1p36 *(CAPB)*, 20q13 *(HPC20)*, and 1q42-43 *(PCAP)* (Smith et al, 1996; Berthon et al, 1998; Xu et al, 1998, 2001b; Gibbs et al, 1999; Berry et al, 2000; Tavtigian et al, 2001). **The multiple genomic loci implicated and the inability to confirm linkage in some populations reflects (1) the different inclusion criteria in different studies, (2) the different populations studied, and (3) the high likelihood that several genes may be responsible for hereditary prostate carcinoma. In addition, whereas three candidate genes have been identified *(RNAEL, ELAC2, MSR1)*, in all cases confirmatory studies have not clearly validated these genes in HPC.**

The first published study by Smith and associates (1996) demonstrated evidence of linkage on chromosomes 1, 4, 5, 7, 13, and X, with the strongest association at 1q24-25 *(HPC1)*. Subsequent analysis revealed that families linked to this locus had earlier mean age at diagnosis and larger number of affected family members (Gronberg et al, 1997). The linkage was particularly strong in families with early age at onset and male-to-male transmission. *RNASEL* is the primary candidate gene in this region based on its position within the HPC1 region (1q24-25) and the identification of variants segregating with hereditary prostate cancer families (Carpten et al, 2002). It is an endoribonuclease that has both antiviral and proapoptotic activity (Hassel et al, 1993; Castelli et al, 1998).

Tavtigian and colleagues (2001) performed a genome-wide scan on Utah families and found linkage to 17p *(HPC2)*. Mutational analysis of candidate genes implicated *ELAC2* as the HPC gene at this locus. ELAC2 is a novel protein that may have a role in regulation of cell cycle progression (Korver et al, 2003; Takaku et al, 2003). At the current time it is unclear if *ELAC2* is an HPC susceptibility gene. Subsequent studies have failed to identify linkage between 17p11 and HPC (Xu et al, 2001b) nor mutations in *ELAC2* in HPC families (Rokman et al, 2001; Wang et al, 2001).

The most recently identified gene linked to prostate cancer susceptibility is the macrophage scavenger receptor 1 *(MSR1)* gene located at 8p22-23. Allelic loss and homozygous deletions at 8p22 are one of the most common genetic abnormalities in prostate cancer cells (Bova et al, 1993). More recently, linkage studies in HPC families have implicated 8p22-23 in HPC (Xu et al, 2001c; Wiklund et al, 2003). Subsequent work identified germline mutations in *MSR1* in HPC families (Xu et al, 2002a); however, additional studies in the United States and Europe have failed to demonstrate as strong an association between *MSR1* and HPC (Seppala et al, 2003; Wang et al, 2003b).

The role of these genes in nonhereditary prostate carcinoma is unclear at the current time. Somatic mutations of these genes in sporadic prostate carcinoma are rare (Nupponen et al, 2004). Although some studies have implicated common polymorphic variants in sporadic disease (Rebbeck et al, 2000; Casey et al, 2002; Xu et al, 2003), confirmatory studies in additional patient populations often failed to validate initial findings (Suarez et al, 2001; Wang et al, 2002, 2003b).

Hereditary Nonpolyposis Colorectal Cancer (HNPCC)

HNPCC, also known as Lynch syndrome, predominantly increases the risk of colon carcinoma and endometrial carcinoma. The syndrome is caused by mismatch repair enzyme defects, and there are six different types based on which mismatch repair gene is mutated. Types 1 to 6 are caused by mutations in *MSH2, MLH1, PMS1, PMS2, MSH6,* and *MLH3*, respectively. *MSH2* was the first gene linked to this disease (Fishel et al, 1993). Subsequently, Papadopoulos and colleagues (1994) identified *MLH1* as a second susceptibility allele in this disease and proposed *PMS1* and *PMS2* as possible additional susceptibility genes. Nicolaides and coworkers (1994) demonstrated germline mutations in both *PMS1* and *PMS2* in HNPCC cohorts without *MLH1* or *MSH2* mutations (Nicolaides et al, 1994). MSH6, is less well characterized than the other types but is believed to predispose patients to endometrial carcinoma (Wijnen et al, 1999). Mutation analysis of the most recently identified gene, *MLH3*, in 39 HNPCC families and in 288 patients suspected of having HNPCC identified 10 different germline *MLH3* variants (Xu et al, 2001b; Wiklund et al, 2003).

Although this tumor syndrome was originally believed to be associated with an increased risk of transitional cell carcinoma of the bladder, it has become apparent that it only increases the risk of upper tract transitional carcinoma (Watson and Lynch, 1993). This, however, does not mean that these enzymes do not play an important role in sporadic genitourinary malignancies. Mismatch repair enzyme defects have been implicated in sporadic prostate (Boyer et al, 1995; Dahiya et al, 1997) and bladder carcinoma (Christensen et al, 1998; Jin et al, 1999).

Hereditary Wilms' Tumor

Hereditary Wilms' tumor accounts for approximately 1% of Wilms' tumor cases (Van Heyningen and Hastie, 1992). **The classic disease was first described by Fitzgerald and Hardin in 1955 and is characterized by bilateral and multicentric tumors. Wilms' tumor can also occur as part of the more complex tumor syndromes, WAGR syndrome, Denys-Drash syndrome, and Beckwith-Wiedemann syndrome (BWS).**

WAGR syndrome is characterized by Wilms' tumor, aniridia, genitourinary abnormalities, gonadoblastoma, and mental retardation and was first described by Miller and associates in 1964. Denys-Drash syndrome is characterized by Wilms' tumor, genitourinary abnormalities, pseudohermaphroditism, and nephropathy and was first described in 1967 (Denys et al, 1967). **Both of these syndromes along with hereditary Wilms' tumors are caused, at least in part, by genetic abnormalities in the same gene, *WT1*.**

WT1 **was isolated using positional cloning to 11p13. It encodes a zinc finger protein that is believed to function as a transcriptional regulator** (Call et al, 1990). During development the gene is expressed primarily in kidney, genital ridge, developing gonad, and mesothelium (Pritchard-Jones et al, 1990), and it is therefore not surprising that mutations in this gene cause abnormalities in these organs. Consistent with Knudson's hypothesis, subsequent analysis has demonstrated mutations in *WT1* in sporadic Wilms' tumors, although this is not common (Coppes et al, 1993).

WAGR is a contiguous gene syndrome caused by genetic abnormalities in *WT1* and adjacent genes. It is likely that aniridia and mental retardation are caused not by genetic abnormalities in *WT1* but by abnormalities in genes located in the vicinity (Davis et al, 1988). Denys-Drash syndrome appears to be caused solely by mutations in *WT1*. Greater than 95% of patients with the Denys-Drash syndrome carry constitutional *WT1* mutations (Little and Wells, 1997). The special characteristics of the disease appear to be due to mutations that specifically affect the ability of WT1 to bind to DNA (Little et al, 1995).

Wilms' tumor is also associated with Beckwith-Wiedemann syndrome. BWS, first characterized in 1964 by a German pediatrician, is characterized by exomphalos, macroglossia, and gigantism in the neonate (Wiedemann, 1964). Patients can also develop hemihypertrophy and are at increased risk for malignancy, particularly Wilms' tumor and adrenocortical carcinoma (Tank and Kay, 1980). Linkage analysis identified 11p15.5, a region distinct from *WT1*, as the locus for BWS (Koufos et al, 1989).

The gene most closely linked to BWS is the cell cycle regulator *CDKN1C*. Decreased expression of *CDKN1C* has been identified in BWS (Algar et al, 1999). Whereas mutations in this gene have been identified in a subset of patients with BWS and a small minority of sporadic Wilms' tumors (Lam et al, 1999), it appears that BWS results from a disruption of imprinted gene expression. This LOI results in abnormal silencing of *CDKN1C* and the development of BWS (Fitzpatrick et al, 2002). Importantly, *CDKN1C* is not the only gene at 11p15.5 whose expression is altered by LOI. This has led to the hypothesis that alterations in expression of several genes at 11p15.5, such as *IGF2* and *H19*, play a role in BWS (Ramesar et al, 1993; Lee et al., 1999). Recently, *NSD1* has been implicated in BWS. This tumor suppressor gene is responsible for Sotos' syndrome, which shares many of the physical stigmata of BWS. Baujat and colleagues (2004) identified two patients with BWS who had mutations in *NSD1* and speculated that *NSD1* could be responsible for a subset of patients with BWS.

Polymorphisms and Cancer

As outlined in the previous section, the study of cancer genetics has, until the recent past, focused on the identification of major cancer susceptibility genes, such as *VHL* and *WT1*. The paradigm held that identification of a hereditary genetic defect would elucidate the cause of the more common sporadic disease. Although identification of these genetic defects has provided important insights into the molecular basis of cancer, these germline mutations are rare and account for increased cancer risk in only a small segment of the population. With the cloning of the human genome it has become apparent that genetic anomalies are not limited to high-risk individuals; over 10 million common genetic variants exist (as of 2005). This has raised the possibility that these common variants, called polymorphisms, could be used to assess hereditary risk of disease.

There are two types of polymorphic variants: (1) microsatellite repeats and (2) single nucleotide polymorphisms (SNP) (Fig. 16–8). Microsatellite repeats are repetitive DNA sequences that are of variable lengths. One of the best

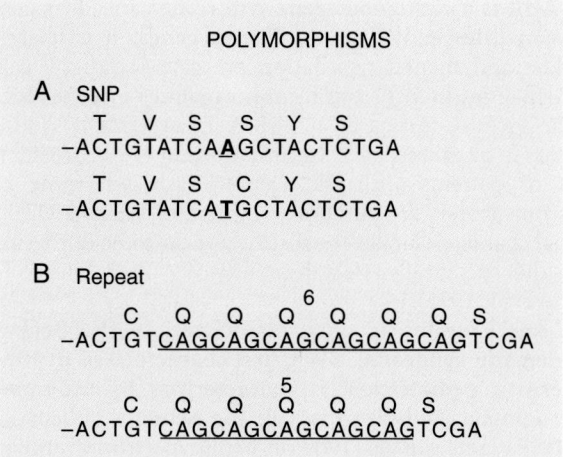

POLYMORPHISMS

A SNP

```
      T   V   S   S   Y   S
  -ACTGTATCAAGCTACTCTGA
      T   V   S   C   Y   S
  -ACTGTATCATGCTACTCTGA
```

B Repeat

```
                        6
      C  Q  Q  Q    Q  Q  Q  S
  -ACTGTCAGCAGCAGCAGCAGCAGTCGA
                     5
      C  Q  Q  Q   Q  Q  S
  -ACTGTCAGCAGCAGCAGCAGTCGA
```

Figure 16–8. Types of polymorphisms. **A,** Single nucleotide polymorphism—a single base pair change that can result in a change in amino acid sequence. **B,** Microsatellite repeat—a variation in a repeating sequence of nucleotides that can result in a change in amino acid sequence.

characterized is the CAG repeat in the androgen receptor. Shorter CAG repeats have been demonstrated to increase androgen receptor activity (Chamberlain et al, 1994).

An SNP is a base pair within the genome that varies between two or more nucleotides. SNPs can alter gene function in a variety of ways: nonsynonymous variants alter function by changing the amino acid sequence of a gene (Makridakis et al, 1997), variants within the promoter can alter transcription of a gene (Amirimani et al, 1999), and variants in close proximity to intron-exon boundaries can alter splicing (Sawa et al, 1998).

The vast majority of polymorphic variants have no functional significance, but the few that do can influence tumor development or progression. Importantly, because many of these minor susceptibility variants are common in the population at large, they have the potential to influence disease progression in a large percentage of the population. Polymorphisms are present in germline DNA and are different than mutations. As such, the genomic revolution has provided an exciting opportunity to both elucidate the genetic causes of cancer and potentially develop screening tools for common cancers.

Prior Study of Polymorphic Variants

A review of all polymorphic variants implicated in urologic malignancies is beyond the scope of this chapter. However, prostate cancer provides the best example in genitourinary malignancies and illustrates approaches to studying variants in cancer. For most of the genes studied, there has been a biologic rationale, such as the androgen axis. Polymorphisms within the androgen axis have been extensively studied as risk modifiers of developing prostate carcinoma. The rationale for studying androgen metabolism variants is based on the fact that steroid hormones appear to play a critical role in prostate malignancy (Gann et al, 1996) and certain polymorphic variants of genes in this pathway appeared to increase androgen activity (Chamberlain et al, 1994). The gene that has been most extensively studied is the androgen receptor *(AR).* Studies have demonstrated an association between CAG

microsatellite repeats and prostate carcinoma (Giovannucci et al, 1997; Ingles et al, 1997). Several other genes involved in this pathway have been studied in less depth, such as the steroid 5α-reductase type II *(SRD5A2)* (Jaffe et al, 2000), cytochrome P450 family members (Haiman et al, 2001), and UDP-glucuronosyltransferase members (MacLeod et al, 2000).

To date, most studies have examined genes in isolation and not as part of a pathway. Because genes do not function in isolation, it is not surprising that only by examining all the genes within a pathway that the true risk of a particular SNP can be best determined. The best example of an integrated pathway is the glutathione S-transferase (GST) family of genes. The GSTs function to detoxify the products of reactive oxygen species such as organic epoxides, hydroperoxides, and aldehydes (Hayes and McLellan, 1999). Polymorphisms with *GSTP1, GSTM1,* and *GSTT1* have functional significance (Seidegard et al, 1988; Zimniak et al, 1994) and the *GSTP1* variant has been linked to an increased risk of prostate carcinoma in some studies. Whereas *GSTT1* and *GSTM1* variants were not associated with increased risk, several authors have found that carrying more than one putative high-risk allele in the GST family was associated with an even higher risk of prostate carcinoma (Kote-Jarai et al, 2001; Nakazato et al, 2003). For example, Kote-Jarai and colleagues (2001) found not only that the *GSTP1* I105V variant increased the risk of prostate carcinoma with an odds ratio of 1.8 (95% CI, 1.11 to 2.91), but in conjunction with additional high-risk GSTM and T alleles the odds ratio increased to 2.48 (95% CI, 1.22 to 5.04). By integrating multiple SNP signatures into a risk assessment tool, we may be able to dramatically improve our ability to identify individuals at risk for urologic malignancies.

In summary, multiple groups are examining variants in an effort to improve our understanding of malignancies in general and urologic cancers specifically. By looking at multiple variants within one pathway more robust associations between variants and disease can be identified.

THE CELL CYCLE

The cell cycle refers to the unidirectional process that allows an ordered replication of each cell's genome followed by division into two daughter cells. The fundamental role of this highly ordered process is the accurate replication of the cell's genome. Whereas cell cycle dysregulation can result in rapid cellular proliferation, it is the loss of ability to pass an unaltered copy of the genome to the daughter cell that makes cell cycle abnormalities a hallmark of cancer (Sherr, 1996). Cell cycle arrest gives the cell the opportunity to repair the DNA damage (see "DNA Repair") or proceed to programmed cell death (see "Apoptosis"). A loss of cell cycle control allows mutations that result in a growth advantage to be transmitted to daughter cells. Therefore, loss of cell cycle control underlies the evolution of a tumor toward a more locally aggressive and eventually metastatic phenotype (Bartek et al, 1999).

The cycle is described in four steps (Fig. 16–9). G_1 (for gap 1) is when the cell prepares to duplicate its DNA; S phase is when the cell duplicates its DNA; G_2 (for gap 2) is when the cell prepares to divide; and M phase (for mitosis phase) is when the cell divides. Cells that are quiescent are described

CDKN2A. Cdk inhibitors then block cell cycle progression by inhibiting cyclins. Cyclins therefore cannot perform their normal function of activating proteins critical for DNA replication and cell division. The following sections will outline the G_1S, S, and G_2M checkpoint cascade in more detail and emphasize the role that key regulatory elements, such as *TP53* and *RB,* have in controlling cell division.

G_1S Checkpoint

As the cell progresses from G_1 to S phase, it must (1) receive a signal from the organism that the cell should divide, (2) ensure that it is in the appropriate environment (i.e., nutrient and oxygen rich), (3) ensure that the DNA is not mutated, and (4) initiate the DNA synthesis process.

TP53 is a Critical Regulator of G_1S Checkpoint

The critical protein in the cell's response to DNA damage or extracellular growth regulatory signals is the transcription

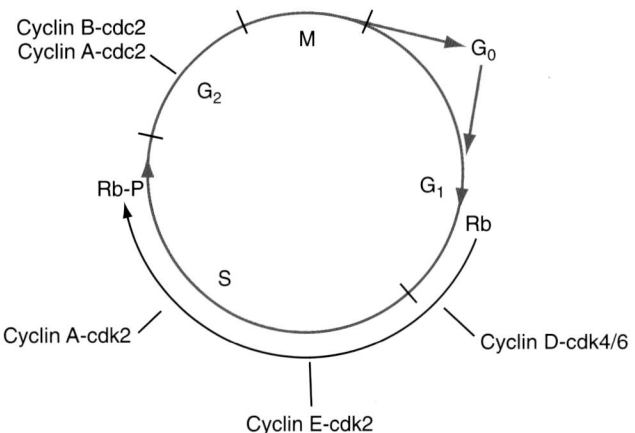

Figure 16–9. A schematic drawing of the cell cycle. Sequential activation of cyclin-cdk complexes is critical to the orderly progression of the cell's replication.

as being in G_0 (Elledge, 1996). **The two main points of control are the G_1S and G_2M checkpoints.**

The checkpoints are controlled by a cascade of positive and negative regulatory elements. The cascade for the G_1S checkpoint is outlined in Figure 16–10. Briefly, intracellular and extracellular signals, such as hypoxia or DNA damage, activate cyclin-dependent kinase (cdk) inhibitors, such as CDKN1A or

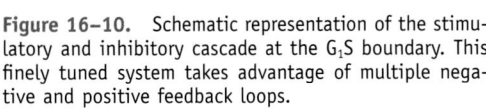

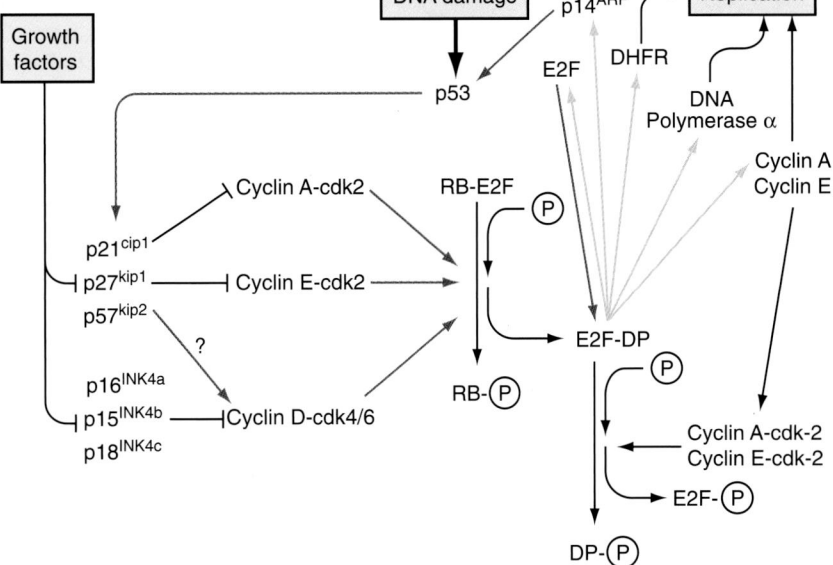

Figure 16–10. Schematic representation of the stimulatory and inhibitory cascade at the G_1S boundary. This finely tuned system takes advantage of multiple negative and positive feedback loops.

factor TP53. **Active TP53 binds to the promoter region of TP53-responsive genes and stimulates the transcription of genes responsible for cell cycle arrest, repair of DNA damage, and apoptosis** (Elledge, 1996). TP53 responds to DNA damage by inducing cell cycle arrest CDKN1A and then transcriptionally activating DNA repair enzymes. If the cell cannot arrest growth and/or repair the DNA, TP53 induces apoptosis (Levine, 1997). Expression of these TP53-dependent genes ensures that an accurate replica of the genome is passed on to both daughter cells (Elledge, 1996).

TP53 activity is altered by a variety of stimuli (Fig. 16–11) and is regulated by a variety of post-transcriptional mechanisms, including phosphorylation and acetylation (Giaccia and Kastan, 1998). These post-translational modifications either alter TP53 activity directly by decreasing the affinity for associated proteins or indirectly by modifying TP53 stability. Radiation exposure stimulates the activity of *ATM* kinase, which in turn increases TP53 activity by phosphorylation. Phosphorylated TP53 no longer binds *MDM2,* a proto-oncogene that inactivates TP53, and therefore TP53 remains in an active state (Momand et al, 1992). In this manner, *ATM* increases TP53 activity, which translates into cell cycle arrest and increased transcription of DNA repair enzymes (Kastan et al, 1992).

TP53 activity can also be controlled by altering the activity of TP53 regulatory proteins. The best example of this is p14^{ARF}. p14^{ARF} was originally identified as an alternative splice variant of the cdk inhibitor CDK2A (Stone et al, 1995). It has been demonstrated that p14^{ARF} functions not as a cdk inhibitor but by degrading MDM2 (Zhang et al, 1998b). Because degraded MDM2 is unable to bind TP53, TP53 activity increases. Because p14^{ARF} is primarily increased in response to cellular division, this p14^{ARF}/TP53 negative feedback loop is critical to arrest a cell that is dividing too rapidly, that is, proceeding toward a malignant phenotype.

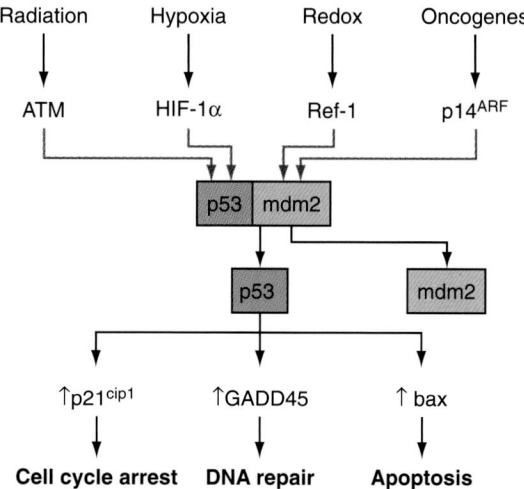

Figure 16–11. TP53 plays a central role in the cell's response to extracellular stimuli. Radiation, hypoxia, redox reactions, and oncogenes can all increase TP53 activity through different mechanisms. In response, the cell initially stops dividing and then attempts to repair the DNA damage. If it fails to repair the DNA, it undergoes apoptosis or programmed cell death. These functions are mediated through transcriptional activation of a variety of genes, some examples of which are indicated in the figure.

Lastly, TP53 also regulates itself thorough autofeedback. Two of TP53's transcriptional targets are MDM2 and cyclin G. TP53 increases expression of both of these regulatory proteins by binding to their promoters. Cyclin G then activates MDM2, which in turn targets TP53 for degradation. In this manner, increased levels of TP53 contribute to its own downregulation (Okamoto et al, 2002; Grossman et al, 2003).

TP53 in Urologic Malignancies

Given the pivotal role that *TP53* plays in DNA repair, cell cycle arrest, and apoptosis, it is not surprising that it is the most commonly mutated gene in human tumors, including genitourinary malignancies. Close to 50% of all tumors have *TP53* mutations (Hollstein et al, 1991).

Mutational inactivation of *TP53* is a particularly frequent event in bladder carcinoma and has been associated with high-grade muscle invasive disease (Sidransky et al, 1991; Fujimoto et al, 1992). Most published studies in bladder cancer examine the level of TP53 protein expression by immunohistochemistry. These studies are based on the strong correlation between increased immunoreactivity for TP53 and presence of *TP53* mutations (Esrig et al, 1993). TP53 accumulation in the transitional cell carcinoma cell nuclei, as detected by immunohistochemistry, predicts risk of recurrence and death independent of stage, grade, and lymph node status in some (Sarkis et al, 1993; Esrig et al, 1994) but not all studies (Underwood et al, 1996). The difference in results may be due to lack of staining protocol standardization or of uniform interpretation of results (McShane et al, 2000).

TP53 status in primary tumors may not only predict likelihood of recurrence but also whether patients will respond to bacillus Calmette-Guérin (BCG) or to chemotherapy. It is unclear at the current time if TP53 expression in the primary tumor predicts response to BCG. Although initial studies demonstrated a clear association (Caliskan et al, 1997; Ick et al, 1997), a recent review of the literature failed to demonstrate a clear association between TP53 expression and response (Saint et al, 2003). It does appear, however, that TP53 overexpression in tumors after BCG therapy is a predictor of progression (Lacombe et al, 1996). TP53 expression also appears to predict response to chemotherapy. Cote and colleagues (1997) found no advantage to adjuvant chemotherapy after cystectomy in patients without TP53 abnormalities but did find a 3.0-fold decreased risk of recurrence and a 2.6-fold decreased risk of death in patients with TP53 abnormalities in the primary tumor.

TP53 does hold tremendous promise not only as a marker of tumor aggression but also as a therapeutic target. Because the majority of bladder carcinomas have lost TP53, reintroduction of wild-type TP53 into bladder cancer cells lacking TP53 has the potential to treat the cancer at the molecular level. Bladder cancer is a particularly attractive target because of the high frequency of *TP53* mutations and because the vector can be placed in direct contact with the cancer cell transvesically (Slaton et al, 2001).

TP53 mutations in prostate cancer were first identified in cell lines and one clinical specimen (Isaacs et al, 1991). Subsequent studies have confirmed that *TP53* mutations occur in primary and metastatic tumors, although there appears to be a clear trend toward increased mutation rates with advanced disease (Chi et al, 1994). **Mutations in prostate specimens** range from 10% to 35% in untreated primary tumors to 40% to 50% in hormone-refractory metastatic disease (Heidenberg et al, 1996).

Aberrant TP53 expression by immunohistochemistry has been extensively studied as a diagnostic tool for aggressive prostate carcinoma and again demonstrated that increased TP53 expression was associated with advanced disease (Navone et al, 1993; Aprikian et al, 1994). Unfortunately, immunohistochemistry has not always outperformed stage, grade, and PSA in predicting survival (Kibel and Isaacs, 2000).

Other urologic malignancies also have been linked to TP53 abnormalities. Mutations in TP53 occur in renal cell carcinoma, particularly metastatic lesions (Reiter et al, 1993). Patients with abnormal expression in primary tumors may have an increased risk of progression, particularly in conventional renal cell carcinoma (Uhlman et al, 1994; Zigeuner et al, 2004). These results suggest that, although the disease gene for kidney cancer is VHL, abnormalities of TP53 occur and may be involved in progression. Although initial work did not conclusively link penile carcinoma to TP53 mutations (Leis et al, 1998), more recent work has demonstrated an association between TP53 immunoreactivity and lymph node metastasis (Lopes et al, 2002).

Cyclin–Cyclin-Dependent Kinase Complexes

Expression of other proteins is also important in the regulation of the G₁S checkpoint. **Passage through the cell cycle requires the sequential activation of cyclin-cdk complexes. The extent and particularly the timing of cyclin-cdk activation is tightly regulated by phosphorylation and protein interaction. Common G₁S cyclin-cdk complexes are cyclin A-cdk2, cyclin E-cdk2, cyclin D-cdk4, and cyclin D-cdk6** (Sherr, 1996; Massague, 2004). These cyclin-cdk complexes are required for cells to traverse G₁ and enter S phase. Overexpression of cyclin-cdk complexes shortens G₁S arrest, whereas decreased expression arrests the cells in G₁ (Resnitzky et al, 1994). This ability to control the G₁S checkpoints has implicated the cyclins and cdks as potentially important oncogenes (Strauss et al, 1995).

Cyclin D expression is critical at the G₁S checkpoint. Expression is mitogen dependent, meaning it normally occurs only in response to an extracellular signal (Matsushime et al, 1991). Integration of positive regulatory signals (e.g., growth factors) and negative regulatory signals (e.g., nutrient-poor environment) through the cyclin D family members leads the cell to commit to cellular replication. After the restriction point is passed, the cell no longer requires growth factors to complete DNA synthesis (Pardee, 1989).

Cyclin-cdk complexes primarily function at the G₁S checkpoint to phosphorylate the retinoblastoma protein (RB) (Sherr, 1996). Since loss of RB function has been found to be critical to tumor formation, it is not surprising that cyclin-cdk activity is closely regulated at multiple levels. Activity can be controlled by both inducing expression and post-transcriptional modification (Morgan, 1995; Sherr, 1995; Diehl et al, 1998). However, the primary point of control is through controlled degradation (ubiquitination) and by the binding of positive and negative regulatory elements, such as proliferating cell nuclear antigen (PCNA) and cdk inhibitors (Pagano et al, 1995; King et al, 1996; Sherr, 1996).

Cyclin-Dependent Kinase Inhibitors

The activity of the G₁S cyclin-cdk complexes is in large part controlled by members of the cip-kip and INK4 families of cdk inhibitors (Sherr, 1996). Cdk inhibitors accumulate in response to a variety of signals, including DNA damage, cell-cell contact, cytokine release, and hypoxia. The INK4 (inhibit cdk4) family members specifically bind cdk4 and cdk6, whereas the cip/kip family members bind most cyclin-cdk complexes (Clurman and Porter, 1998). **By binding to cyclin-cdk complexes, both families inhibit RB phosphorylation and thereby arrest the replicative machinery.**

INK4 Function. The INK4 family of cdk inhibitors directly inhibits the assembly of cyclin D with cdk4 and cdk6 by blocking the phosphorylation of the cyclin D-cdk4/6 complex. This phosphorylation is necessary for activation of the complex (Kato et al, 1994). **The family has four members: CDKN2A, CDKN2B, CDKN2C, and CDKN2D** (Sherr and Roberts, 1999). **Inactivating mutations and abnormal methylation of CDKN2A and CDKN2B have been strongly implicated in cancer in general** (Kamb et al, 1994; Hirama and Koeffler, 1995) **and specifically in genitourinary malignancies** (Cairns et al, 1995; Herman et al, 1995).

The best studied is CDKN2A. The gene was initially found to demonstrate mutations and deletions in a wide variety of tumors including bladder and kidney (Kamb et al, 1994). Subsequent analysis has demonstrated that inactivation often occurs by hypermethylation, an alternative method of gene inactivation (Merlo et al, 1995). CDKN2B lies adjacent to CDKN2A on chromosome 9p and therefore was deleted in many of the same tumors and cell lines that lost CDKN2A (Hannon and Beach, 1994). However, CDKN2B does not appear to play as strong a role in tumorigenesis as CDKN2A (Stone et al, 1995).

The CDKN2A gene inactivation in bladder carcinoma appears to be predominantly secondary to deletion. Cairns and colleagues (1995) identified homozygous deletions of CDKN2A in 44% of bladder cancers. A similar study by Williamson and coworkers (1995) confirmed that deletion was the primary method of inactivation. Importantly, both studies excluded CDKN2B as the primary tumor suppressor at this site because it was not within the deletion. A study by Orlow and colleagues (1999) found that deletion and methylation of CDKN2A occurred frequently in superficial bladder carcinoma, but only those deletions that affect both CDKN2A and p14^ARF correlated with a decrease in disease-free survival.

Mutational inactivation of INK4 family members appears to be rare in prostate carcinoma. Komiya and associates (1995) identified a mutation of CDKN2A in only 1% of clinical specimens. Park and associates (1997) examined primary prostate carcinomas for mutations in CDKN2A, CDKN2B, and CDKN2C and identified one mutation in CDKN2A. In contrast, inactivation of CDKN2A by hypermethylation has been strongly implicated in prostate cancer. Herman and associates (1995, 1996) demonstrated hypermethylation of CDKN2A in 60% of prostate cancer cell lines whereas CDKN2B was rarely inactivated.

Cip/Kip Function. Members of the cip/kip (CDKN1A, CDKN1B (p27), CDKN1C) family of cdk inhibitors are strong negative regulators of cyclin-cdk complexes (Sherr, 1996). By binding to cyclin A-cdk2 and cyclin E-cdk2 complexes, they prevent the phosphorylation of RB and maintain cell cycle arrest. *CDKN1A* and *CDKN1B (p27)* also bind to cyclin D-cdk4 complexes, but this actually functions to indirectly activate cyclin E-cdk2; in the presence of mitogenic stimulation, cyclin D-cdk4 sequesters *CDKN1A* and *CDKN1B*, thereby releasing cyclin E-cdk2 and indirectly inactivating RB. *CDKN2A* contributes to cell cycle arrest not only by binding and inactivating cyclin D-cdk4 but also by releasing *CDKN1A* and *CDKN1B* from cyclin D-cdk4 repression (Sherr, 2001).

Despite the critical role that cip/kip family members play in G₁S cell cycle arrest, they are rarely mutated in a wide variety of malignancies, including genitourinary tumors, and there are no reports of hypermethylation (Shiohara et al, 1994; Kawamata et al, 1995). However, expression of this family of cdk inhibitors plays an important role in cancer (Catzavelos et al, 1997; Loda et al, 1997; Yatabe et al, 1998) in general and, in particular, in genitourinary carcinoma. Stein and associates (1998) found increased expression of *CDKN1A* in 64% of bladder tumors and that increased expression was associated with decreased probability of tumor recurrence and improved patient survival. Decreased *CDKN1B* expression has also been linked to increasing tumor grade, pathologic stage, and poor survival in bladder carcinoma (Del Pizzo et al, 1999).

The expression of CDKN1A in prostate cancer has not demonstrated a clear correlation with advanced disease or poor outcome (Kibel and Isaacs, 2000). However, altered expression of *CDKN1B (p27)* has been implicated in aggressive disease in multiple studies. Cordon-Cardo and colleagues (1998) examined radical prostatectomy specimens and found that absent or low expression by immunohistochemistry was an independent risk factor for disease-free survival by multivariate analysis. Cote and coworkers (1998) found that decreased *CDKN1B (p27)* nuclear staining not only correlated with decreased disease-free survival but also overall survival in radical prostatectomy patients. Loss of *CDKN1B (p27)* expression has also been correlated with decreased survival in men with locally advanced prostate cancers. Thomas and associates (2000) showed that loss of *CDKN1B (p27)* expression could be detected in prostate biopsy samples, raising the possibility that it may be a useful molecular marker at the time of prostate cancer diagnosis. Recently, Freedland and colleagues (2003) found that *CDKN1B (p27)*-positive cells in the prostate needle biopsy specimen had a 2.5-fold increased risk of biochemical recurrence.

The relevance of *CDKN1B (p27)* to prostate cancer is also supported by studies of mouse models. For example, mice deficient in *Cdkn1B (p27)* develop prostate hyperplasia, confirming the potential importance of this gene in prostate homeostasis (Cordon-Cardo et al, 1998). More excitingly, recent studies by Di Christofano and colleagues (2001) have shown that mice deficient in both *Cdkn1B* and *Pten* have a high incidence of prostate cancer. These results provide the best proof yet that *CDKN1B*, together with additional tumor suppressor genes (e.g., *PTEN*) and oncogenes, plays a critical role in the molecular etiology of prostate cancer.

Retinoblastoma Protein

Yet another key regulatory element at the G₁S checkpoint is RB. *RB* was initially identified as the gene responsible for familial and sporadic retinoblastoma (Friend et al, 1986).

Cyclin-cdk complexes phosphorylate *RB* or its family members, *RBL1* and *RBL2*. Phosphorylated *RB* disrupts can no longer bind to members of the E2F family of transcription factors. Free E2F heterodimerizes with DP-1 or DP-2 and transcriptionally activates genes important in DNA replication, such as DNA polymerase-α, and the cell cycle, such as E2F-1 (Sherr, 1996). By activating both sets of genes, E2F activity links DNA replication to advancing the cell cycle. Once the cycle is complete, *RB* returns to the hypophosphorylated state until the cell is ready to divide again (Ludlow et al, 1993).

This is the simple model of RB function. A more complex model recognizes that there are at least six different E2F family members identified to date that each bind different RB family members and transcriptionally activate or inactivate different proteins (Dyson, 1998). In addition, RB-E2F-DP complexes appear to bind histone deacetylase and in doing so actively interfere with gene transcription (Lai et al, 1999). Although the complexity of the model is increasing, the underlying concept remains unchanged; phosphorylation of RB induces cell division, and loss of RB function leads to uncontrolled cell division.

Recent data have implicated RB in other cellular processes critical to malignant transformation. RB appears to maintain heterochromatin in its inactive state. This raises the possibility that RB is not only a transcriptional repressor of specific target genes but may nonselectively repress gene expression by maintaining DNA in a repressive state (Gonzalo et al, 2005).

Retinoblastoma Protein and Genitourinary Malignancies. Mutational analysis has identified *RB* mutations in a variety of sporadic tumors, particularly lung and bladder carcinoma. Mutations have been identified in approximately one third of bladder tumors (Horowitz et al, 1990) and reintroduction of the *RB* gene into bladder carcinoma cell lines has been found to inhibit cell growth and tumor formation (Takahashi et al, 1991). Altered expression of RB has been also identified in approximately one third of bladder carcinomas (Logothetis et al, 1992) and altered expression has been correlated with higher-stage disease and decreased patient survival (Cordon-Cardo et al, 1992).

Prostate carcinoma has not been as strongly linked to *RB*. Although *RB* mutations are identified in 10% to 30% of prostate cancer specimens (Bookstein et al, 1990; Kubota et al, 1995), decreased RB expression is not consistently identified with high-risk patients or recurrent disease (Kibel and Isaacs, 2000). Ittmann and Wieczorek (1996) found no correlation between expression and grade or stage, but Theodorescu and associates (1997) demonstrated that low RB expression did correlate with decreased disease-specific survival in univariate and multivariate analysis.

Renal carcinoma has not been clearly linked to RB. RB is rarely inactivated in renal carcinoma cell lines or tumors (Ishikawa et al, 1991), and analysis of clinical specimens has not demonstrated a clear association between prognosis and RB expression (Lipponen et al, 1995).

Progression through S Phase

As the cell progresses through the G₁S checkpoint, E2F accumulates. E2F-DP heterodimers increase the transcription of cell cycle proteins, which further drives the cell cycle. This positive feedback loop needs to be terminated once the cell has completed S phase. This is believed to be accomplished by phosphorylation of E2F and DP family members by cyclin A-cdk2 (see Fig. 16–10). Phosphorylation of the E2F-DP heterodimer inhibits its DNA-binding activity and therefore its transcriptional activity. This leads to cell cycle arrest (Dynlacht et al, 1994). A second negative feedback loop is mediated by E2F increasing levels of p14[ARF]. As outlined earlier, this increases TP53 activity by targeting MDM2 for degradation. This leads to cell cycle arrest and even apoptosis in a cell dividing too rapidly.

Whereas cell cycle control during S phase is not as important as during G$_1$S and G$_2$M, the cell does maintain the ability to arrest the cell and repair DNA damage through two mechanisms both mediated through ATM. In response to genotoxic insults, CDC25A is ubiquinated through an ATM-dependent cascade, resulting in rapid decrease in CDC25A levels. Because CDC25 family members normally activate CDK2, the loss of CDC25A function then maintains CDK2 in its inactive form. Inactive CDK2 prevents CDC45 from recruiting DNA polymerase. This cascade maintains the cell in S phase (Bartek and Lukas, 2003; Bartek et al, 2004).

The second mechanism mediated by ATM is phosphorylation of DNA repair enzymes such as NBS1 and SMC1 (see "DNA Repair"). These two parallel pathways highlight the interaction between DNA repair and checkpoint control. It is not surprising that S-phase control has been documented in response to DNA-damaging agents because it is the last opportunity to repair DNA damage before replication (Falck et al, 2002; Pichierri and Rosselli, 2004). It is important to note that the cascade does not appear to be mediated by TP53 and therefore is an intriguing target for therapy in the future (Kastan and Bartek, 2004).

G$_2$M Checkpoint

The G$_2$M checkpoint is a second major point of control for cell division. Loss of function allows inappropriate division to occur. Unlike the G$_1$S checkpoint, which responds to a variety of extracellular signals in addition to DNA damage, G$_2$M appears to be similar to S-phase arrest and respond only to DNA damage. It therefore serves as an important point of control for replication errors (Weinert, 1997; Bartek et al, 1999).

Once the cell has replicated its genome, it must separate the two copies of each chromosome. Cyclin-cdk complexes coordinate this separation in a manner similar to those employed at the G$_1$S checkpoint. The cyclin-cdk complexes with greatest activity at the G$_2$M checkpoint, cyclin B-cdc2 and cyclin A-cdc2, phosphorylate proteins critical to coordinating spindle assembly and chromatin modification (Li et al, 2004; Li and Zheng, 2004).

DNA damage secondary to radiation is believed to induce G$_2$M arrest through ATM and the protein kinases CHK1 and CHK2. ATM activates CHK1/2 in response to DNA damage and then CHK1/2 inactivates the CDC25 family proteins through phosphorylation. CDC25A primarily functions at G$_1$M and S phase checkpoints as outlined previously whereas CDC25B and CDC25C primarily function at the G$_2$M check-

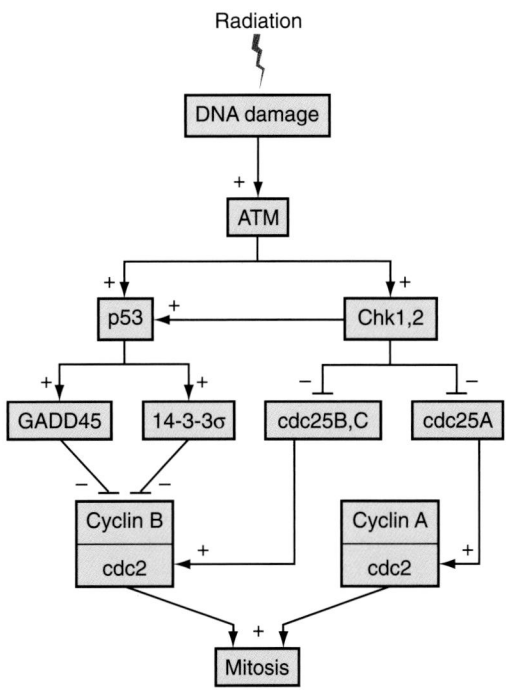

Figure 16–12. Schematic representation of the cascade at the G$_2$M checkpoint in response to genotoxic events such as radiation. Increased ATM activity eventually leads to inhibition of cyclin B through TP53 and decreased stimulation of cdc2 though chk1 and chk2. This leads to cell cycle arrest.

point. Because CDC25B/C functions to activate CDC2, CDC25B/C phosphorylation inactivates CDC2 and, therefore, the cyclin B-cdc2 and cyclin A-cdc2 complexes (Fig. 16–12) (Mailand et al, 2002; Donzelli and Draetta, 2003).

It has become apparent that at least in part G$_2$M arrest may also be mediated by *TP53* and *BRCA1* (Bunz et al, 1998; Xu et al, 2001). Transcriptional upregulation of cell cycle inhibitors (e.g., CDKN1A, GADD45, and 14-3-3) by *TP53* maintains the cell in G$_2$M arrest (Nyberg et al, 2002). **As a result, it appears that *TP53* mediates both G$_1$S and G$_2$M arrest, consistent with its critical role in preserving genomic integrity.**

Therapeutic Implications

It is important to recognize that defects in this point of control carry implications not only for the initiation and progression of cancer but also for the cell's ability to respond appropriately to chemotherapy and radiation therapy, therapeutic modalities that depend in large part on DNA damage. Cancer cells with defects in the G$_2$M checkpoint are unable to repair damaged DNA, which is deleterious to the cancer cells' survival, while surrounding normal cells retain the ability to appropriately repair the damage (Hartwell et al, 1997).

In summary, genetic alterations in cell cycle proteins occur in genitourinary malignancies. Genetic alterations in cell cycle proteins appear to be important in the development of bladder carcinoma in particular and, to a lesser extent, prostate carcinoma. Integration of the cell cycle and DNA repair machinery is critical to the cellular response to genotoxic exposures. As more recently identified cell cycle genes are being evaluated, such as E2F family members and *MDM2,* a clearer picture of the role of cell cycle dysregulation in cancer initiation and progression will emerge.

KEY POINTS: THE CELL CYCLE

- The cell cycle allows the ordered replication of each cell into two daughter cells.

- Primary points of cell cycle controls are G_1S and G_2M.

- Expression of TP53 results in cell cycle arrest and repair of DNA damage. If the DNA damage cannot be repaired, TP53 stimulates cell death (apoptosis)

- *TP53* is the most commonly mutated gene in cancer and plays a prominent role in genitourinary malignancies.

- Cyclin–cyclin-dependent kinase complexes function by activating the machinery that allows the cell to replicate its DNA.

- Cyclin-dependent kinase inhibitors such as *CDKN2A* and *CDKN2B* stop the cell from replicating its DNA response to a variety of signals, including DNA damage, cell-cell contact, cytokine release, and hypoxia.

- Mutations in *RB* are common in urologic malignancies.

- *ATM* plays a central role in sensing DNA damage, inducing S phase and G2M phase arrest, and DNA repair.

DNA REPAIR

A second hallmark of cancer is mutational activation or inactivation of genes. Through the accumulation of genetic events, the cell acquires the ability to grow more rapidly, die less easily, invade surrounding tissue, and eventually kill the host organism. DNA damaging agents are a constant threat to produce mutations and, in doing so, a cancerous cell. Foods (Ames et al, 1995), the environment (Shields and Harris, 1990), and even the body's own metabolism (Loeb, 1989) produce DNA-damaging agents. An antioxidant defense system composed of enzymes and scavengers (e.g., superoxide dismutase and glutathione peroxidase) helps prevents DNA damage by neutralizing these agents (Finkel and Holbrook, 2000). Even if DNA damage occurs, it does not often lead to malignancy because the cell possesses multiple mechanisms to repair the DNA.

The integration of the cell cycle and DNA repair cannot be overemphasized. In response to DNA damage, the first step is to arrest the cell so that the DNA can be repaired. It is therefore not surprising that there is substantial overlap between the initiators of DNA repair and cell cycle arrest (Kastan and

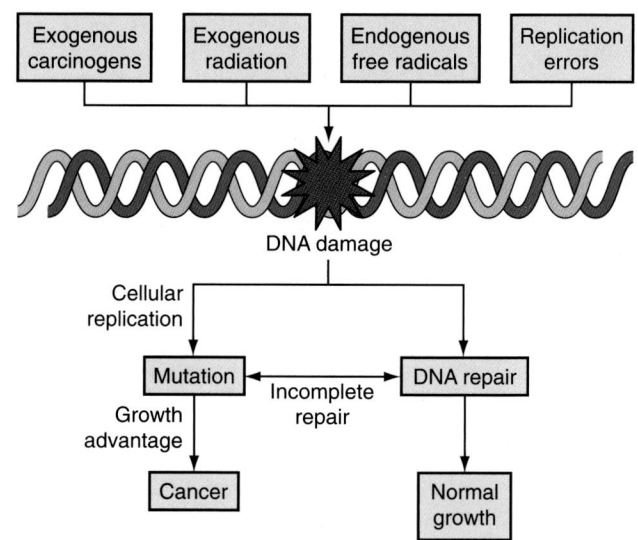

Figure 16–13. The cell is subjected to DNA damage from a variety of exogenous and endogenous sources. Failure to correct the damage can produce a malignant cell.

Bartek, 2004). For example, ATM and ATR are both activated in response to DNA damage. Both activate TP53, CHK1, and other proteins critical to cell cycle arrest (Bartek and Lukas, 2003). In addition, both recruit and activate DNA repair enzymes, such as NBS1, BRCA1, and RPA to the sites of damage (Zou and Elledge, 2003; Kitagawa et al, 2004).

Because DNA repair mechanisms play such an important and constant role in protecting the genome, it is not surprising that loss of these repair mechanisms is critical to the development of the cancer cell (Fig. 16–13) (Loeb and Loeb, 2000). **Loss of DNA repair mechanisms increases the mutation rate of the cell. The cell develops a "hypermutable" phenotype, which significantly increases the likelihood that additional tumor-promoting mutations will occur.** By the time the tumor is clinically detectable, it may contain thousands of mutations, some of which may provide a growth advantage. Clinically, this translates to a more aggressive tumor (Loeb and Loeb, 2000). In addition, cells with a "hypermutable" phenotype are often more difficult to treat because the selection pressure of therapy may rapidly select tumor cells with mutations conferring resistance (Tlsty et al, 1989).

Given the importance of DNA repair in protecting the cell from DNA changes that have the potential to transform the cell, it is not surprising that individuals with an inherited defect in DNA repair have a 1000-fold increase in the risk of developing cancer. Xeroderma pigmentosum (Sancar, 1996), HNPCC (Modrich,1994), and hereditary breast cancer (Patel et al, 1998) have been linked to defects in genes critical to DNA repair. Analysis of these DNA repair genes in sporadic malignancies, including genitourinary tumors, has identified deficiencies (Jin et al, 1999; Yuan et al, 1999). **Whereas defects in DNA repair appear to be important to the development of malignancy, it is important to recognize that failure to accurately repair DNA does not directly cause tumor formation but increases the likelihood that a gene critical for tumor formation and/or progression will be mutated.**

DNA repair is not one system but at least four: nucleotide excision repair (NER), base excision repair (BER), mismatch repair (MMR), and double-stranded break repair (DSBR) (Fig. 16–14). Each of these systems provides an important barrier to malignant transformation.

Nucleotide Excision Repair

NER is a major defense against DNA damage caused by ultraviolet radiation and chemical exposure. NER acts on a wide range of alterations that result in large local distortions in DNA, by recognizing distortions in the DNA helix, excising the damaged DNA, and replacing it with the correct sequence (Krokan et al, 1997; Wood, 1997).

Study of three syndromes—xeroderma pigmentosum, Cockayne's syndrome, and trichothiodystrophy—associated with inborn defects in proteins essential to NER has been critical to expanding our understanding of this pathway (Hoeijmakers, 2001). Patients with xeroderma pigmentosum have a risk of skin cancer that approaches 100% by 20 years of age. The increased cancer risk is linked to exposure to ultraviolet radiation. The fact that these patients are at such a profound risk for developing malignancies demonstrates the fundamental importance of NER in protecting DNA from mutation (Kraemer, 1997). In contrast, skin cells of patients with Cockayne's syndrome and trichothiodystrophy are particularly sensitive to lesion-induced apoptosis. The result is accelerated aging but no predisposition to cancer (Hoeijmakers, 2001).

NER requires six enzymes in humans: RPA, XPA, XPC, TFIIH, XPG, and XPF (Mu et al, 1997; Sancar et al, 2004). DNA damage that produces a substantial distortion in the DNA helix is recognized by XPA, which binds to the damaged DNA and recruits the other enzymes critical for DNA repair. XPA forms a complex with replication protein A

(RPA) and then recruits the transcription complex TFIIH. This protein complex has helicase activity, which allows the complex to unwind the damaged DNA. A 24- to 32-bp segment of DNA is then excised by exonucleases, and the excised sequence is replaced by DNA polymerase δ or ε. The newly synthesized DNA is then ligated into place (Wood, 1997; Sancar et al, 2004).

Base Excision Repair

The BER pathway repairs damage caused by a variety of events including spontaneous deamination of bases, radiation, oxidative stress, alkylating agents, or replication errors. In particular, the pathway is critical for repair of oxidative lesions caused by reactive oxygen species (ROS). Because ROS are a normal byproduct of metabolism, loss of BER repair is detrimental in the fidelity of DNA. ROS react with DNA to produce DNA base modifications. The modified bases often mispaired during DNA replication, resulting in mutations (Croteau and Bohr, 1997).

As the name implies, the initial step in BER is the removal of a base rather than a nucleotide. The key element of the repair is the recognition of the modified bases by a glycosylase, a family of over 20 different enzymes that recognize DNA modifications. Many DNA glycosylases are nonspecific and remove several structurally different damaged bases. Others have specific substrates. Each glycosylase identifies the damaged base, cleaves the N-glycosidic bond between the target base and the deoxyribose, and, in doing so, releases the damaged base and leaves an apurinic/apyrimidinic nucleotide (Wyatt et al, 1999; Bruner et al, 2000).

There are two forms of BER: short patch repair and long patch repair. In a short patch repair of one nucleotide, the 5′ endonuclease APE1 and the 3′ phosphodiesterase activity of

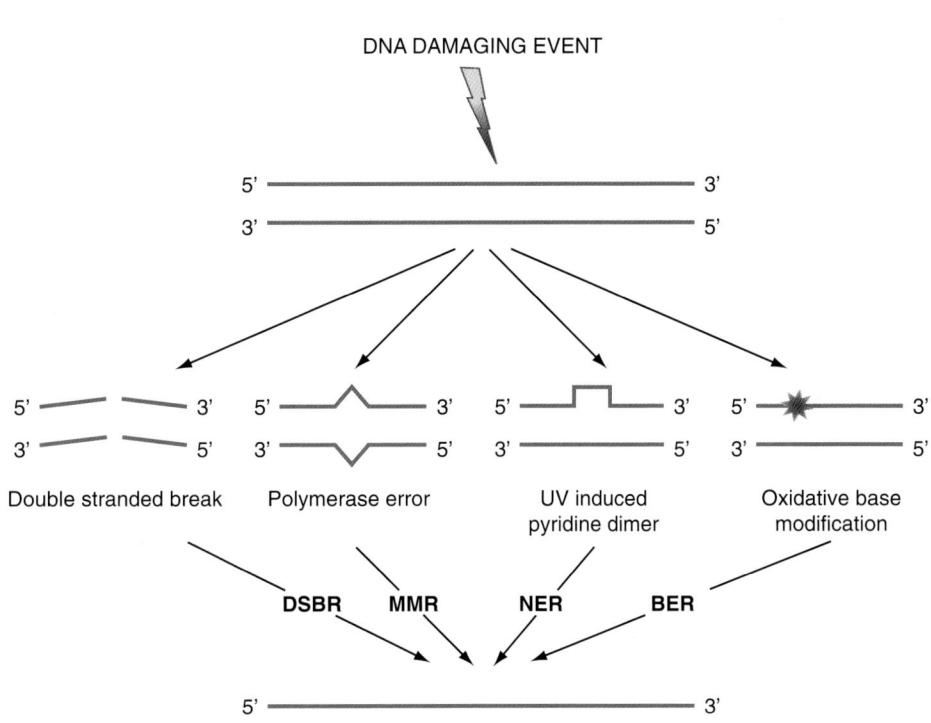

Figure 16–14. Model of different DNA damaging events and repair mechanisms.

DNA polymerase β excise the glycosylated nucleotide and then DNA polymerase β fills the single nucleotide gap (Beard and Wilson, 2000). Lastly, Lig3/XRCC1 complex ligates the inserted nucleotide (Cappelli et al, 1997). An alternative BER mechanism is a long patch repair. This allows insertion of a 2- to 10-bp sequence beginning at the damaged nucleotide. It is most useful in cases in which the damaged moiety is refractory to polymerase β excision (Gary et al, 1999). APE1 again makes a 5′ incision next to the damaged nucleotide, but in this case recruits DNA polymerase δ/ε, PCNA, and FEN1. A 2- to 10-bp patch is then synthesized, which displaces the damaged nucleotide along with adjacent nucleotides and then is ligated by Lig1 (Klungland and Lindahl, 1997; Levin et al, 1997).

Whereas oxidative damage has clearly been linked to an increased risk of cancer, there had been no human genetic disorders attributed to BER defects until recently. Al Tassan and colleagues found that the mutations in the MUTYH glycosylase are associated with colorectal carcinoma. This glycosidase functions with OGG1 to correct A/G and A/C mismatches (Al-Tassan et al, 2002). Interestingly, polymorphic variants of OGG1 have been implicated in genitourinary malignancies (Xu et al, 2002).

Mouse models provide some insight into associations between components of the BER pathway and cancer risk. Whereas loss of some glycosylases can increase the risk of developing malignancies when exposed to mutagens (Elder et al, 1998), in general loss of individual glycosylases does not cause an overt phenotype, probably owing to overlapping function (Hoeijmakers, 2001). On the other hand, core BER enzymes appear to be essential because inactivation in knockout mice are embryonic lethal (Friedberg et al, 1998).

Mismatch Repair

MMR removes nucleotides mispaired by DNA polymerases and insertion/deletion loops (ranging from 1 to 10 or more bases) that result from slippage during replication of repetitive sequences or during recombination.

The MMR pathway functions primarily to reverse errors made by DNA polymerase. Defects in MMR dramatically increase mutation rates. Although DNA polymerases have the ability to identify and correct their own errors, some mistakes are not identified. Several of the proteins responsible for MMR (MSH2, MSH3, MLH1, PMS1, PMS2, and MSH6) have been identified through the study of HNPCC (see "Inherited Susceptibility to Cancer"). The MMR process has been elucidated in large part by studying the proteins responsible for MMR in bacteria (Modrich, 1997).

Once an error has been detected, it is critical for the MMR proteins to distinguish the newly synthesized strand of DNA, that is, the strand that contains the error, from the template. The mechanism for strand distinction has not been well elucidated in eukaryotes, but in *Escherichia coli* the parental strand is methylated, which allows identification of the daughter strand (Modrich, 1997).

The MMR proteins form heterodimers, each of which is responsible for detecting specific DNA replication errors. The MSH2/MSH3 heterodimer (MutSβ) mediates repair of insertions and deletions whereas the MSH2/MSH6 heterodimer (MutSα) recognizes the single nucleotide mismatches in addition to insertions and deletions. Once the error has been detected, MutSα and MutSβ complexes with the MLH1/PMS2 heterodimer (MutLα) to direct the repair process. The newly synthesized strand containing the incorrect base(s) is degraded along with surrounding nucleotides. DNA polymerase then replaces the degraded DNA using the parental strand as a template (Kolodner and Marsischky, 1999; Jiricny, 2000).

The MutSα and MutSβ complexes have also been found to play a role in cell cycle arrest (Meyers et al, 1997) and apoptosis (Tominaga et al, 1997). This is a further example of the integration that exists between cell cycle arrest, DNA repair, and apoptosis that is critical to protecting the fidelity of the DNA.

The critical role of MMR in protecting the cell from mutations that may lead to tumorigenesis is highlighted by their role in HNPCC, studies of sporadic tumors, and evidence from knockout mice. Inherited mutations in MSH2, MLH1, PMS1, PMS2, and MSH6 have all been linked to an increased risk of malignancy (Fishel et al, 1993; Nicolaides et al, 1994; Papadopoulos et al, 1994; Wijnen et al, 1999). Genetic inactivation of MMR genes, particularly *MLH1*, is a frequent event in sporadic colon carcinoma (Veigl et al, 1998) and has been implicated in prostate (Boyer et al, 1995; Dahiya et al, 1997) and bladder carcinoma (Christensen et al, 1998; Jin et al, 1999). The finding that MMR knockout mice are cancer prone provides additional evidence that defects in MMR repair contribute substantially to tumorigenesis (Friedberg et al, 1998).

Double-Stranded Break Repair

DSBs arise from ionizing radiation or x-rays, free radicals, chemicals, and during replication of a single-strand break. After DSB detection, a complex cascade of reactions is triggered that halts the cell cycle machinery and recruiting repair factors (Kastan and Bartek, 2004). **Double-stranded breaks have the potential to be the most disruptive form of DNA damage. If they are not repaired, the cell will undergo apoptosis. This process of apoptosis in cells with double-stranded DNA breaks is the basis of radiation therapy and many chemotherapeutic agents because both function primarily by inducing double-strand breaks.** Incorrectly repaired DNA can lead to DNA mutations, rearrangements, and even chromosomal translocations. There are two methods of DSBR: homologous recombination and nonhomologous enjoining (Sancar et al, 2004).

The Ku protein is a heterodimer that initiates the nonhomologous end-joining repair by binding to the broken end of the DNA (Falzon et al, 1993). Ku complexes with DNA-dependent protein kinase (DNA-PK) and in doing so activates DNA-PK's kinase activity (Anderson, 1993). Active DNA-PK phosphorylates a large number of proteins, including Ku. The phosphorylated Ku is a helicase that unwinds the damaged DNA and allows the ligase 4/XRCC4 heterodimer to repair the break (Nick McElhinny et al, 2000; Tuteja et al, 1994).

Homologous recombination involves the transfer of genetic information between sister chromosomes. While it plays a critical role in meiotic recombination, it is becoming apparent that it also plays an important role in DNA repair. Essentially, homologous repair allows the normal undamaged sister chromatid to act as a template to allow precise repair of a damaged segment of DNA (Johnson et al, 1999).

The first step is ATM recruitment to the site of DNA damage. ATM then phosphorylates genes critical to chromatin remodeling, such as *H2AX* (Lukas et al, 2003) and DSBR, such as *NBS1, BRCA1,* and *SMC1* (Kitagawa et al, 2004). Chromatin remodeling by *H2AX* allows access for DNA repair machinery (Bassal and El-Osta, 2005). The activated NBS1-MRE11-RAD50 complex can then bind to RAD52 and the broken chromosomal ends (Lobachev et al, 2004). *RAD51* along with the breast cancer susceptibility genes, *BRCA1/2,* and *BRCA1*-associated-RING-domain 1 *(BARD1)* then replicate the undamaged region from the sister chromosome template (Welcsh et al, 2000; Sancar et al, 2004).

Similar to other DNA repair mechanisms, defects in DSBR have clearly been linked to malignancy. *BRAC1* and *BRAC2* are associated with familial breast and ovarian cancer (Miki et al, 1994; Tavtigian et al, 1996). Patients with Nijmegen breakage syndrome have mutation in *NBS1* and are predisposed to leukemia, lymphoma, and breast carcinoma (Varon et al, 1998). Patients with mutations in *MRE11* are also predisposed to cancer (Stewart et al, 1999). Whereas knockout mice with defective repair mechanisms are characterized by a high rate of embryonic lethality, survivors are sensitive to DNA damaging agents (Friedman et al, 1998).

KEY POINTS: DNA REPAIR

- DNA damage does not often lead to malignancy because the cell possesses multiple repair mechanisms.

- Defects in DNA repair allow the cell to accumulate the mutations critical for tumor formation and progression.

- Nucleotide excision repair (NER) is a major defense against DNA damage caused by ultraviolet radiation and chemical exposure.

- Base excision repair (BER) repairs damage caused by spontaneous deamination of bases, radiation, oxidative stress, alkylating agents, and replication errors.

- Mismatch repair (MMR) removes nucleotides mispaired by DNA polymerase.

- Double-stranded break repair (DSBR) is a major defense again DNA damage caused by ionizing radiation, free radicals, and chemicals.

APOPTOSIS

The next barrier against malignant transformation is the apoptotic cascade. If a normally functioning cell is unable to induce cell cycle arrest or repair damaged DNA, apoptosis (programmed cell death) is triggered. Apoptosis clearly is an advantageous response to DNA damage if DNA repair fails, because it allows multicellular organisms to eliminate potentially harmful cells. Eliminated cells can be replaced from the organism's pool of undamaged cells. Depending on the location, environment, or extent of damage apoptosis may even be the primary response (Evan and Littlewood, 1998). Therefore,

it is not surprising that aberrations of apoptosis can be detrimental and that failure of dividing cells to initiate apoptosis after sustaining severe DNA damage contributes to cancer (Ashkenazi and Dixit, 1998).

The cell cycle, DNA repair, and apoptosis pathways are integrated at multiple levels. Whereas TP53 is commonly recognized as playing an important role in all three (May and May, 1999), it is not the only apoptotic regulator that has been implicated in cell cycle arrest. Members of the BCL2 family have been implicated in G_1S arrest (Brady et al, 1996), and the apoptotic protein survivin has been implicated in the G_2M checkpoint (Li et al, 1998).

It is also important to recognize that apoptosis is not simply a protective mechanism for DNA damage. It also plays a vital role in normal development, tissue homeostasis, and defense against pathogens (Ashkenazi and Dixit, 1998). Abnormalities in the apoptotic machinery therefore have implications for malignancy beyond an individual cell's ability to respond appropriately to DNA damage. First, the apoptosis cascade is critical to the immune system's ability to eliminate cancer cells (Nagata, 1997). This has clear implications for both the organism's intrinsic immunosurveillance for malignancy and the tumor's response to extrinsic immunotherapy. Second, because cytotoxic cancer therapies depend in large part on inducing apoptosis, defects in the cascade can profoundly influence tumor response to chemotherapy and radiotherapy (Thornberry and Lazebnik, 1998).

Death Receptor–Induced Apoptosis

The initiation phase of apoptosis involves the integration of intracellular and/or extracellular signals to trigger cell death via caspases. Extracellular signals are transmitted to the apoptotic machinery via death receptors (Fig. 16–15). These receptors belong to the tumor necrosis factor superfamily and contain a ligand specific extracellular domain and an intracellular death domain. The death domain allows the receptor to bind to intracellular adaptor proteins that also contain a death domain. In addition to a death domain, the adaptor proteins have a death effector domain that allows the adaptor protein to bind to the caspase recruitment domain (CARD) of initiator caspases (caspases 2, 8, 9, 10) (Ashkenazi and Dixit, 1998). Once bound, the initiator caspases undergo self-cleavage and are then capable of activating effector caspases, such as caspase 7, or pro-apoptotic members of the BCL2 family (Li et al, 1998; Muzio et al, 1998).

The best characterized death receptor is CD95, or FAS, which appears to play an important role in cancer immunosurveillance (Ashkenazi and Dixit, 1998). The ligand CD95L forms a trimer that binds three CD95 receptors (Nagata, 1997). The clustering of CD95 allows the adaptor protein FADD to bind to CD95 via their death domains. In turn, procaspase 8, or FLICE, binds to FADD via the death effector domain. Procaspase 8 oligomerization promotes autoactivation to caspase 8 (Muzio et al, 1998). Other initiator procaspases, such as procaspase 10, are activated through similar mechanisms (Vincenz and Dixit, 1997). Negative regulatory molecules, such as FLIP, bind to FADD and in doing so inhibit procaspase 8 binding and therefore apoptosis (Irmler et al, 1997).

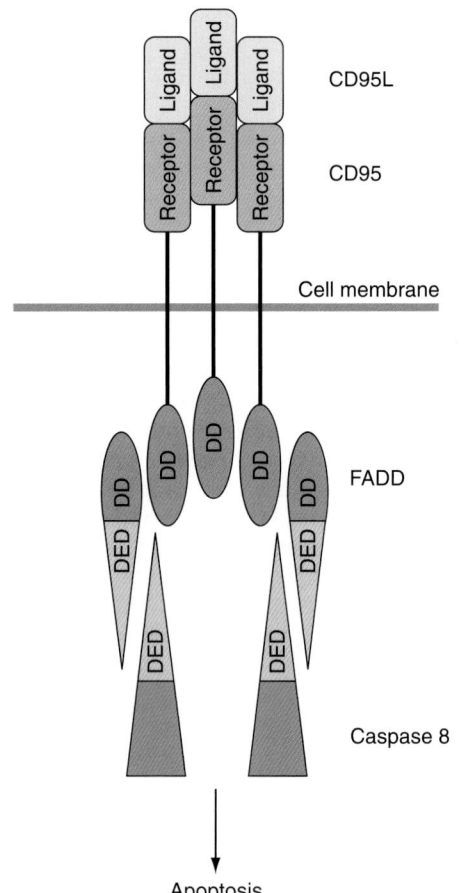

Figure 16–15. Example of death receptor–mediated activation of initiator caspases.

A second important TNF family member that also triggers apoptosis in tumor cell lines is TRAIL (Mariani et al, 1997). In contrast to CD95L, which is predominantly expressed on activated T lymphocytes, and natural killer cells (Nagata, 1997), TRAIL's receptors DR4 and DR5 are expressed in many human tissues, including the prostate. Similar to CD95L-mediated apoptosis, TRAIL induces cell death through caspase activation. Again, negative regulatory elements, such as the decoy receptor TRID, play an important role in modifying the ligand's activity. TRID binds to TRAIL, but because it lacks a death domain it is unable to bind adaptor proteins and therefore blocks the pathway (Pan et al, 1997).

Death Receptors and Ligands as Targets for Cancer Therapy

The death receptor pathway does not appear to have a direct role in the etiology of cancer. Patients with hereditary defects in this system and knockout mice are both characterized by T-cell abnormalities and fatal autoimmune syndromes, not hereditary tumor syndromes (Nagata, 1997). **However, the identification of ligand-dependent apoptosis receptors may have a profound impact on therapy. Most cancer therapies (i.e., chemotherapy and external-beam radiation therapy) depend on *TP53* to induce apoptosis in the cancer cell. Because *TP53* is mutated in over half of malignancies**

(Hollstein et al, 1991), ***TP53*-independent pathways for apoptosis are of great clinical interest. Because the ligand-dependent apoptosis described earlier is independent of *TP53*, this makes these receptors and ligands attractive novel treatment targets.** Unfortunately at the current time compounds that bind to the receptors are extremely toxic (Nagata, 1997). It is hoped that novel compounds will have improved toxicity profiles.

TP53-Induced Apoptosis

The mechanism by which TP53 decides whether to induce cell cycle arrest or apoptosis is still not well understood, but in both cases recognition of DNA damage triggers TP53 activation (Sabbatini et al, 1995; Attardi et al, 1996). **TP53-induced apoptosis is mediated by transcriptional activation of genes that initiate the apoptotic cascade and inhibition of genes that block the cascade** (Miyashita et al, 1994; Miyashita and Reed, 1995; Oda et al, 2000). TP53-induced apoptosis is dependent of the APAF1/caspase 9 activation pathway (Fig. 16–16) (Soengas et al, 1999). Whereas the BCL2 family member BAX has been implicated as the primary factor responsible for TP53 induction of this cascade (Miyashita and Reed, 1995), BAX is not essential for TP53-dependent apoptosis (Knudson et al, 1995). It is possible that inhibition of BCL2 (Miyashita et al, 1994) or upregulation of the pro-apoptotic BCL2 family member noxa, may allow cells lacking BAX to still undergo TP53-dependent apoptosis (Oda et al, 2000).

Cell Survival and BCL2 Family Members

TP53-induced apoptosis is mediated through BCL2 family members. Dysregulation of this apoptotic pathway has direct relevance to the etiology of cancer. BCL2 family members can be divided into pro- and anti-apoptotic members. The pro-apoptotic group includes BAX, BAK, BOK, BIK, BAD, BID, and BIM and the anti-apoptotic BCL2 family members include BCL2, BCLX$_L$, BCLW, and MCL1 (Adams and Cory, 1998). All members contain BCL2 homology domains (BH1 to BH4) that allow members of the family to heterodimerize. BCL2 family members regulate each other's function through these BH domains (Chittenden et al, 1995; Cheng et al, 1996).

Whereas each pro-apoptotic BCL2 family member responds to different stimuli, the principal mechanism by which they induce cell death is by increasing mitochondrial membrane permeability (Kroemer and Reed, 2000). This leads to the release of cytochrome C (Jurgensmeier et al, 1998), which induces APAF-1 dimerization and in doing so exposes the APAF-1 CARD. Procaspase 9 binds to the CARD, oligomerizes, and then autoactivates. This initiator caspase can then activate the executioner caspases, such as caspase 3 and 7. Anti-apoptotic BCL2 family members block apoptosis by inhibiting the pro-apoptotic family members and, in doing so, decreasing mitochondrial permeability (see Fig. 16–16) (Li et al, 1997b; Srinivasula et al, 1998).

BAX is the most well studied pro-apoptotic BCL2 family member. It is transcriptionally activated in response to TP53. Once activated, BAX dimerizes at the mitochondrial

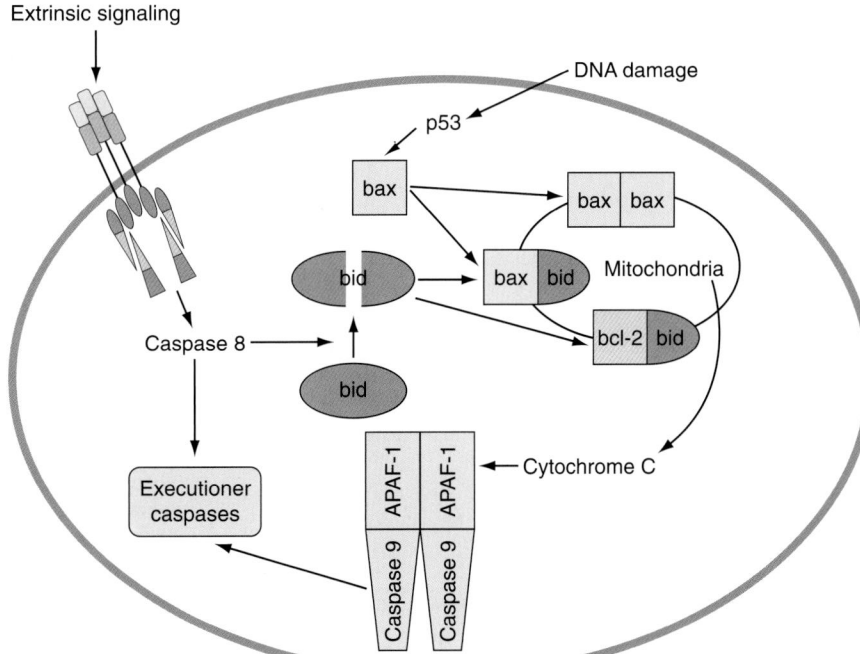

Figure 16–16. Cascade of extrinsic and intrinsic mechanisms of apoptosis. The extrinsic system depends on ligand-induced activation of executioner caspases whereas the intrinsic system depends on the dimerization of BCL2 family members to alter mitochondrial membrane permeability.

membrane. The dimer forms a channel that facilitates the release of cytochrome C from the mitochondria. BCL2 is the best studied anti-apoptotic BCL2 family member. It functions by binding to BAX and, in doing so, blocks bax-induced permeability (Miyashita et al, 1994; Adams and Cory, 1998).

Other pro-apoptotic family members are activated by a variety of stimuli. Often they function not by inducing mitochondrial permeability directly but by activating or inhibiting other BCL2 family members. The first example is BID. BID is regulated by initiator caspases. Cytosolic BID is activated by caspase 8 (see Fig. 16–16). This allows dimerization of BID with either BAX and BCL2. This dimerization activates BAX activity and inhibits BCL2. The net result is pro-apoptotic (Li et al, 1998b). Because BID is activated by caspases, it provides a link between the ligand-induced apoptotic machinery and BCL2 family members.

A second example is BAD. BAD is not regulated by transcription or by cleavage but by phosphorylation. BAD is tonically inactivated by Akt-dependent phosphorylation. In tumors with activation of the PI3 kinase pathway via loss of the tumor suppressor *PTEN* or signaling through one of a number of tyrosine kinase receptors, the resulting Akt activation leads to BAD phosphorylation and is pro cell survival. In contrast, removal of growth factors has been demonstrated to deactivate Akt, which leads to dephosphorylation of BAD. BAD can then bind to and inactive BCL2. The net result is again pro-apoptotic (Kroemer and Reed, 2000).

Cell Death

Executioner caspases initiate the process of cell death by targeting multiple cellular proteins critical for cell survival for degradation. In doing so, the cell's ability to survive is systematically destroyed. The initial target of executioner caspases is the apoptotic machinery itself. Cleavage of pro-apoptotic proteins, such as procaspase 8, activates them and accelerates the apoptotic process. Cleavage of anti-apoptotic proteins, such as BCL2 and BCLX$_L$, not only destroys their anti-apoptotic function but actually releases pro-apoptotic carboxyl-terminal fragments, which further stimulates cell death (Wolf and Green, 1999).

Executioner caspases then target proteins critical to cell survival, from DNA to the extracellular matrix. Cleavage of DNA repair and replication proteins, such as DNA-PK$_{CS}$ and replication factor C, leads to nuclear dysregulation. Nuclear structural proteins, such as lamins NuMa and SAF-A, are fragmented, contributing to dissolution of the nucleus and nuclear condensation. Proteolysis of cytoskeletal proteins such as fodrin, keratin, and actin lead to destruction of the internal structural integrity of the cell. Lastly, cleavage of proteins critical to cell-cell interaction, such as β-catenin and focal adhesion kinase (FAK), complete the destruction of the cell (Orth et al, 1996; Wen et al, 1997; Wolf and Green, 1999). **The end result is a stereotypical death in which the cytoplasm shrinks, cell membrane blebs, and the nuclear chromatin condenses. The entire process can be completed in 60 minutes** (Thornberry and Lazebnik, 1998).

Apoptosis and Genitourinary Malignancies

Because a tumor cell's inability to undergo apoptosis appropriately is a hallmark of malignancy, multiple groups have attempted to characterize the apoptotic response of genitourinary malignancies. Because cells undergoing apoptosis undergo a stereotypical death, global analysis of apoptosis is possible using assays designed to detect the fragmented DNA characteristic of the process, as well as assays designed to detect abnormalities in specific apoptotic proteins.

Global Defects in Apoptosis

Both high-grade prostatic intraepithelial neoplasia (HGPIN) and prostate carcinoma actually have significantly higher levels of apoptosis than normal prostatic epithelium. The level of apoptotic activity is relatively low compared with other malignancies and is balanced by increased replication. Prostate cancer cells can be induced to undergo apoptosis in response to androgen withdrawal (Kyprianou et al, 1990; Tu et al, 1996). As the tumor progresses to androgen independence, it is unclear if the androgen-resistant cells have an increased or decreased rate of apoptosis, because studies have demonstrated both in hormone-refractory disease (Berges et al, 1995; Koivisto et al, 1997). The conflicting data may reflect both the tumor's dynamics and the effect of therapy. There is a clear survival advantage for the advanced cancer cell that can protect itself from apoptosis. However, a rapidly growing, infiltrative, advanced tumor, which is outgrowing its blood supply and mutating its DNA, may have a high apoptotic rate in spite of protective mechanisms the tumor's cells have acquired.

Studies of apoptosis in bladder carcinoma have demonstrated an association with aggressive high-grade advanced disease but not with decreased disease-free survival (Lipponen and Aaltomaa, 1994; King et al, 1996a). External-beam radiation therapy has been associated with a modest improvement in survival for tumors with high apoptotic rates. This may reflect the fact that external-beam radiation therapy requires an intact apoptotic mechanism to be effective (Rodel et al, 2000).

Assessment of Individual Members of the Apoptotic Machinery

Individual members of the apoptotic machinery have been frequently studied. All studies suffer from an inability to assay all elements of the apoptotic machinery simultaneously and therefore to globally assess the tumor's ability to undergo programmed cell death.

TP53 **mutations and abnormalities in expression are among the most frequent in cancer and have been identified in prostate, bladder, and renal cancers** (Hollstein et al, 1991; Sidransky et al, 1991; Esrig et al, 1993; Reiter et al, 1993). Abnormalities in *TP53* cause dysregulation of the cell cycle and DNA repair mechanisms in addition to apoptosis and are covered in more detail in the section "The Cell Cycle."

BCL2 family members have been studied in genitourinary malignancies. **Elevated levels of BCL2 have been identified in the majority of hormone-refractory prostate tumors, reflecting the tumor's relative resistance to apoptosis in the advanced state** (McDonnell et al, 1992; Colombel et al, 1993). Both increased and decreased levels of BCL2 have been identified in localized prostate tumors, and few studies have found a correlation with grade, stage, and progression (Byrne et al, 1997; Lipponen and Vesalainen, 1997; Theodorescu et al, 1997; Johnson et al, 1998). Other anti-apoptotic members of the BCL2 gene family, *BCLX* and *MCL1*, may also be linked to prostate carcinoma (Krajewska et al, 1996). Analysis of bladder carcinoma has demonstrated similar results. BCL2 levels are higher in more aggressive bladder carcinoma, but expression of BCL2 had no effect on treatment outcome (King

et al, 1996; Rodel et al, 2000). As noted earlier, phosphorylation of BAD by Akt can also tilt the scales toward cell survival, especially in concert with elevated levels of BCL2. Akt activation is commonly seen in many urologic malignancies and can result from loss of the tumor suppressor *PTEN*, mutation and constitutive activation of PI3 kinase, and/or activation of tyrosine kinase receptors such as HER2/NEU, EGFR, and insulin-like growth factor receptor (IGFR).

Other BCL2 family members have not been as well studied. Loss of BAX expression is not a common mechanism for the development of prostate carcinoma (Krajewska et al, 1996; Johnson et al, 1998) but may play a role in progression of localized bladder carcinoma (Ye et al, 1998).

In summary, deficiencies in signal transduction pathways leading to apoptosis clearly play a role in the initiation and progression of malignancy. It is unclear if expression analysis of the apoptotic machinery will provide additional prognostic information from traditional histochemical analysis. However, it is clear that effective chemotherapy and radiation therapy is in large part dependent on apoptosis. In addition, in the future the apoptotic machinery may be manipulated using novel ligands that bind to death receptors and promote TP53-independent cancer cell death.

Alternative Regulators of Apoptosis in Genitourinary Malignancies

In addition to the classic regulators of apoptosis, a number of other pathways for cell survival and death have been uncovered that play key roles in urologic cancer. Some of these pathways are being actively explored as targets for cancer therapy. The Vancouver group has mapped out a detailed gene profile of prostate tumors treated with neoadjuvant hormonal ablation therapy to identify key regulators of cell death and survival after castration. In addition to BCL2, which is upregulated in surviving cancer cells, they have also reported on *clusterin* and Hsp27. **Clusterin, or TRPM2 (testosterone repressed prostate message-2), is upregulated both in patient samples after hormone ablation as well as in the Shionogi and CWR-22 xenograft models of hormone-sensitive tumors. Although its precise function is not known, a large body of evidence suggests that clusterin is induced by stress and functions to stabilize the cell during periods of stress.** In this model, clusterin is believed to act like heat shock proteins, whose role as a protein chaperone is also to stabilize client proteins. Clusterin is activated by heat shock protein-1 (HSP1). Functional evidence of clusterin's role comes from studies in which clusterin is either overexpressed or knocked down using antisense strategies. In the first scenario, clusterin expression promotes hormone-refractory cell growth and prevents androgen withdrawal–induced apoptosis. In the second scenario, treatment of hormone-refractory cells with antisense clusterin promotes apoptosis. **These findings are being translated into clinical trials using antisense clusterin for the treatment of hormone-refractory prostate cancer** (Miyake et al, 2000, 2004; July et al, 2002; Gleave and Miyake, 2005). This same group of investigators has also reported that the heat shock protein HSP27 is also frequently overexpressed in hormone-refractory prostate cancers. Similar experiments using overexpression and antisense strategies have suggested that targeting HSP27 may influence the course of hormone-refractory cancers, in particular in combination with cytotoxic chemotherapies (Rocchi et al, 2004).

Another family of cellular signaling molecules that play a role in the regulation of cell survival and apoptosis is the sphingolipids. Sphingolipids are one of three major constituents of the cell membrane, alongside phospholipids and cholesterol. Sphingolipid generation is regulated by a large cast of enzymes, notably the sphingomyelinases, ceramide synthase, and the ceramidases. Ceramide is produced from sphingomyelin by sphingomyelinase and from sphinganine by ceramide synthase. Ceramidases, on the other hand, degrade ceramide and lead to formation of sphingosine and sphingosine-1-phosphate. Ceramide is a potent pro-apoptotic molecule that can promote apoptosis through the classical mitochondrial activation of caspases or through a nonclassical caspase-independent form of apoptosis. Sphingosine-1-phosphate, in contrast, is a powerful anti-apoptotic molecule that may modulate the degree of apoptosis like a rheostat.

The importance of ceramide to genitourinary tumors is that it appears to be a key modulator of radiation-induced tissue damage and apoptosis. As with clusterin and other heat shock proteins, ceramide appears to be a critical mediator of stress response in cells, in this case promoting apoptosis as opposed to cell survival. Studies supporting ceramide's role in radiation-induced apoptosis are manifold, including studies demonstrating the direct cell death signal induced by exogenous treatment of cells with ceramide, studies of radiation response in mouse knockout models, and studies of radiation response in the presence and absence of inhibitors of sphingolipid metabolism. It is hoped that therapeutics that increase ceramide production and promote apoptosis can be developed. The role of sphingolipid-1-phosphate has also emerged from these studies, and recent work suggests that this molecule is a promising target for cancer therapy (Gulbins and Kolesnick, 2003; Kester and Kolesnick, 2003; Perry and Kolesnick, 2003).

KEY POINTS: APOPTOSIS

■ Apoptosis stands for programmed cell death, a natural process by which cells die after specific signals and stress of DNA damage.

■ Apoptosis is tightly integrated with DNA repair and the cell cycle.

■ Apoptosis plays a vital role in normal development.

■ Cancer is characterized by interruptions in the normal process of apoptosis, resulting in cell survival.

■ BCL2 is a classic inhibitor of the mitochondrial pathway of apoptosis and is overexpressed in some genitourinary malignancies.

■ Novel agonists and antagonists of apoptosis, such as ceramide and clusterin, may successfully be controlled to combat cancer.

TELOMERASE

Once a cancer cell has developed the ability to grow without the constraints of the cell cycle or apoptotic mechanisms, it must still acquire the ability to divide an unlimited number of times (Harley et al, 1990). Most cells in the body can only replicate a finite number of times before they lose the ability to divide. A malignant cell only capable of a finite number of divisions is of questionable clinical significance. The ability to replicate repeatedly is most commonly accomplished by expressing the gene telomerase. Telomerase is normally only expressed in cells that need to divide an unlimited number of times, such as gametes or stem cells. Whereas other normal tissues do not express telomerase, nearly all human tumors express active telomerase (Kim et al, 1994).

Telomerase immortalizes cells by maintaining the ends of the chromosomes, or telomeres, which normally shorten with each cell division. Telomerase is necessary because DNA polymerase cannot replicate DNA in a 3′ to 5′ direction. Because DNA is only copied at the replication fork, it is only possible to replicate one strand continuously. The other strand must be replicated discontinuously. The polymerase replicates the other strand in short sequences in a 5′ to 3′ direction and ligates the sequences together (Fig. 16–17). RNA primers are used to initiate these short strands of DNA, and the RNA primers are then degraded as the strand extends. Although this effectively replicates the DNA, a consequence of this strategy is that when the RNA primer at the telomere is degraded, that portion of the chromosome is lost. This limits the number of replications that a cell can undergo. Telomerase solves this problem by extending the 3′ end of the parental strand and preserving telomer length (Levy et al, 1992).

Whereas active telomerase appears to be critical to survival of the malignant cell (Kim et al, 1994), and telomerase can immortalize normal cells (Bodnar et al, 1998), expression of telomerase alone does not appear to induce the malignant phenotype (Jiang et al, 1999). Malignant transformation requires oncogene activation and/or tumor suppressor gene inactivation in addition to telomerase (de Lange and DePinho, 1999).

Genitourinary malignancies appear to be similar to all other cancers and express high levels of telomerase in almost all tumors. Increased activity has been identified in prostate carcinoma and prostatic intraepithelial neoplasia (Zhang et al, 1998a), testicular tumors (Albanell et al, 1999),

KEY POINTS: TELOMERASE

■ Each cycle of cellular division results in loss of a chromosomal end (telomere).

■ This limits the number of cellular divisions a cell can undergo.

■ Telomerase maintains the chromosomal length by rebuilding the telomere and is necessary for a cell that is to undergo unlimited cellular divisions.

■ Telomerase activity does not cause cancer and is present in selected normal cells such as gametes and stem cells.

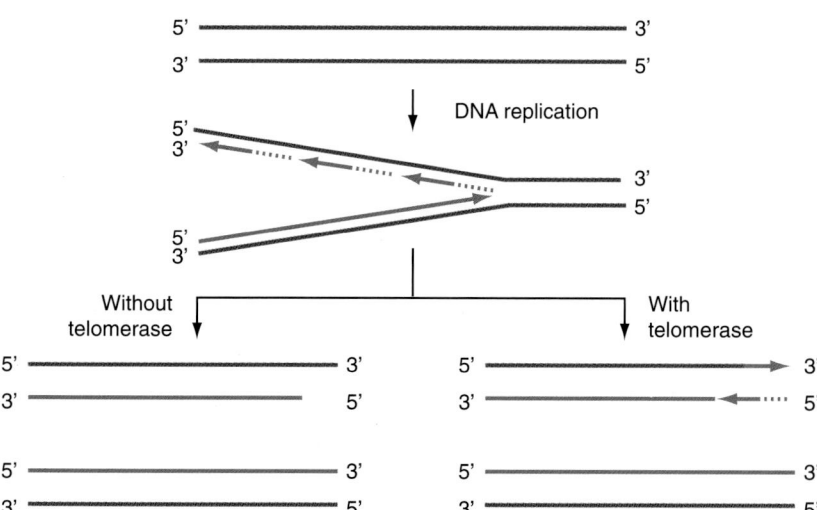

Figure 16–17. One strand of the DNA is replicated continuously and the other discontinuously. The degradation of the RNA primer leaves the telomere of the discontinuous strand unreplicated. The unreplicated portion of the strand is then degraded, thereby shortening the chromosome. Telomerase extends the parent strand and in doing so allows complete replication of the parent strand.

renal carcinoma (Mehle et al, 1996), and bladder carcinoma (Yoshida et al, 1997). Its use as an independent marker of aggressive disease is limited by the fact that it is expressed in almost all tumors, irrespective of grade or stage. However, the fact that it is rarely, if ever, expressed by normal somatic tissue makes it an attractive diagnostic and therapeutic target in a wide variety of malignancies (Yoshida et al, 1997; Buys, 2000).

STEM CELLS AND CANCER

One key to unraveling the etiology of cancer is to understand the cell type(s) from which it arises. Study of this target cell(s) may lead to new insights into the molecular origins of cancer.

Most epithelial organs in the body are believed to contain stem cells capable of multilineage differentiation. **Common properties of stem cells include immortality, the ability both to self-renew and spawn progeny, their localization within specialized niches, and their ability to give rise to all cell types within the organ.** Recently, there has been considerable progress in identifying the presence of stem and progenitor cells in the prostate, given this organ's unique ability to regress and regenerate after castration and androgen-addback (Isaacs and Coffey, 1989; Bui and Reiter, 1998; De Marzo et al, 1998). Prostatic stem cells are believed to reside within the basal epithelium and give rise to a hierarchy of progenitor cells committed to differentiate into secretory or neuroendocrine cells. Xin and associates (2005) and Burger and colleagues (2005) have published papers demonstrating the presence of SCA-1–positive cells in the proximal ducts of the mouse prostate that have stem cell properties. SCA-1 is a glycosyl phosphatidylinositol–anchored (GPI) membrane protein commonly used as a marker of stem cells in the hematopoietic system. SCA-1–positive cells in the prostate were able to give rise to new prostates when co-cultured with urogenital mesenchyme and placed under the kidney capsule of mice. SCA-1–negative prostate cells could not regenerate the prostate. The regenerated prostates from SCA-1–positive cells contained both basal cell and luminal cell layers and contained both SCA-1–positive and SCA-1–negative cells, indicating multipotential differentiation. As predicted, the percentage of SCA-1–positive cells was low in adult prostates but was increased after castration. **These studies suggest that a population of cells expressing SCA-1 may have stem cell properties.** Other markers of these cells include nuclear p63, cytokeratin 5/14, and BCL2. In addition to these studies, a number of investigators have also identified progenitor cells within the prostate that have more limited proliferative potential and are intermediate in differentiation. Markers of these cells include the cytokeratins 5/14/18, prostate stem cell antigen (PSCA), and c-*MET* (Verhagen et al, 1992; Tran et al, 2002). The temporal and spatial regulation of these intermediate cells in the prostate has also been studied using mouse models (Watabe et al, 2002).

Recent studies in multiple cancer types suggest that cancers are caricatures of normal tissue development and likely arise from and are dependent on a small population of stem cells. This stem cell hypothesis argues that cancers arise from transformation of stem or progenitor cells capable of multilineage differentiation. The cancer stem cell accounts for only a small percentage of any given tumor, but this small population is critical for tumor survival. Indeed, only cancer stem cells are believed to have the capability to give rise to tumors. Initial evidence for this model came from the field of leukemia. However, a number of studies now show that breast and neurologic cancers are also characterized by the presence of cancer stem cells with the expected characteristics. For example, Al-Hajj and colleagues (2003, 2004) reported that the CD44+/CD24low/– population of cells in primary breast tumors are capable of forming tumors when engrafted into nude mice but the remaining cells were not, thereby identifying this population of cells as the breast cancer stem cell (Dontu et al, 2003). Similar reports in glioblastoma have pointed to a CD133-positive population as the putative stem cell (Singh et al, 2003, 2004; Dirks, 2005).

To date no such cells have been identified in any urologic cancer, although significant evidence points to the existence of such cells. In the prostate, for example, the paper by Xin and associates (2005) showed that only the SCA-1–positive population was easily transformed by oncogenic Akt. Also, prostate cancers in mice had an increased percentage of SCA-1– and PSCA-positive cells. Additional work is necessary to pinpoint the prostate cancer stem cell and to identify its normal correlate (Burger et al, 2005; Xin et al, 2005).

Why is the stem cell hypothesis important? The primary reason is that if true it may totally change the paradigm by which we identify tumor targets and treat cancer. It suggests that we need not target the entire tumor for annihilation but rather focus our energies on the cancer-causing and sustaining stem cell. The model predicts that tumors recur because we do not kill the stem cell but only its progeny. To treat cancer successfully, we must identify the markers of the stem cell and understand its regulation. Telomerase, discussed previously, is one such possible target, because it is expressed by all stem cells in the body and most likely by the cancer stem cell as well. Telomerase inhibition may abrogate the immortality characteristic of the cancer stem cell and lead to improved outcomes.

KEY POINTS: STEM CELLS AND CANCER

- Stem cells are defined by their capacity to differentiate along multiple lineages and their immortality.
- Cancer is believed to be a stem cell disease in which a small population of cancer stem cells maintains the larger tumor.
- The cancer stem cell is capable of multilineage differentiation.
- New evidence supports the hypothesis that prostate cancer is a stem cell disease.
- Prostate stem cells in mice can be identified using the SCA-1 antigen.
- Cancer ultimately may be eradicated by targeting only the cancer stem cell.

CELLULAR SIGNALING

Cancers are masters of exploiting their environment. For example, malignant cells use signals normally active in homeostasis, wound healing, angiogenesis, and vasoconstriction to enhance their ability to survive and proliferate. In this section, we review oncogenes and tumor suppressor genes that normally function in cellular signaling but have been coopted by cancer cells to promote initiation and/or progression malignancy. In addition, we discuss the concept of haploinsufficiency, which states that complete loss of function or expression is not required for cancer predisposition but rather that partial or haploinsufficient loss alone of a tumor suppressor gene may be sufficient to cause cancer.

PTEN

Loss of heterozygosity (LOH) at chromosome 10q is a frequently observed genetic alteration in prostate cancer. Unlike LOH at chromosome 8p, loss at 10q is associated with advanced disease, suggesting that the gene(s) harbored at this locus are associated with prostate cancer progression. Rubin and colleagues (2000), for example, found that 43% of lymph

node–positive tumors have LOH at 10q23 compared with only 14% without lymph node involvement.

Recently, the *PTEN/MMAC* tumor suppressor gene was identified and mapped to chromosome 10q23. *PTEN* encodes a protein/lipid phosphatase that is mutated or deleted in a large number of human cancers, including glioblastoma and endometrial cancer (Li et al, 1997; Steck et al, 1997). Interestingly, alterations of *PTEN* are also associated with Cowden's disease, a familial cancer syndrome characterized by the development of skin, thyroid, breast, and endometrial tumors (Liaw et al, 1997).

Alterations of *PTEN* have been identified in both localized and metastatic prostate tumors. Consistent with the LOH data, 10% to 20% of organ-confined and approximately half of advanced tumors contain mutations in or loss of *PTEN* alleles (Cairns et al, 1997a, 1998). Loss of *PTEN* function has also been reported to occur through loss of expression. Whang and associates (1998) reported that 50% of advanced human prostate cancer xenografts had low or absent *PTEN* expression despite the absence of inactivating mutations or allelic loss. Demethylation restored *PTEN* expression, indicating that hypermethylation of *PTEN* regulatory sequences can inactivate this gene. Similarly, a recent immunohistochemical study of *PTEN* expression suggested that loss of *PTEN* expression might be more common than mutation or LOH (McMenamin et al, 1999).

A number of studies have shown that *PTEN* is a negative regulator of the PI3 kinase/Akt signaling pathway (Wu et al, 1998). PI3 kinase is a downstream target of a number of growth factors implicated in prostate cancer development and progression, including EGFR, IGFR, and HER2/NEU. **Activation of PI3 kinase via these and other signals leads to activation of *Akt*, a known oncogene that then can lead to proliferation and/or inhibition of apoptosis.** *PTEN*'s normal function is to dephosphorylate and inactivate PI3 kinase. Loss of *PTEN* in prostate cancer leads to constitutive activation of PI3-kinase and, in turn, *Akt* and its downstream signals. Consistent with this model, Wu and colleagues showed a perfect inverse correlation between loss of *PTEN* and activation of *Akt* in a series of prostate cancer xenografts (Wu et al, 1998).

Current work has focused on identifying the downstream targets of *PTEN* loss that are essential for prostate cancer progression. One pathway that has received significant attention is the Akt-mTOR-S6 kinase signaling cascade involved in protein translation (Nave et al, 1999; Sekulic et al, 2000). This pathway is particularly exciting because of the existence of rapamycin, a known inhibitor of mTOR activity (Nave et al, 1999; Sekulic et al, 2000). Neshat and coworkers (2001) have shown that *PTEN* null tumors upregulate mTOR and its downstream target S6 kinase. Inhibition of this pathway with rapamycin or rapamycin analogs leads to dramatic growth arrest of *PTEN* null tumors, suggesting that the Akt-mTOR pathway is critical for prostate cancer growth. These studies have been confirmed by others, most notably in animal models in which investigators have shown that *PTEN*- and *Akt*-dependent carcinogenesis is absolutely dependent on mTOR (Grunwald et al, 2002; Majumder et al, 2004; Tolcher, 2004; Wu et al, 2005). mTOR blockade by rapamycin or rapamycin analogs abrogates tumor growth in these models and reverts prostate epithelium back to normal. These exciting studies in the laboratory have now led to successful clinical trials of the rapamycin analog CCI-779 in men with high-risk and advanced prostate cancer and again show the inherent promise of molecular genetics to treat cancer rationally.

A notable property of *PTEN* is that complete loss of expression is not necessary for cancer causation. Rather, partial loss of *PTEN* is sufficient to induce cancer. Using mouse models with varying doses of *PTEN* in the prostate, Trotman and colleagues (2003) were able to show the exquisite dose sensitivity of *PTEN* both in cancer development and cancer latency. The greater the loss of *PTEN*, the more aggressive the resulting cancer. These studies are particularly relevant to the human disease, because partial loss of *PTEN* is commonly seen in human samples (Thomas et al, 2004). These studies suggest that in human cancer even partial *PTEN* loss may play an important role, a fact that has important implications for rational cancer therapy using rapamycin analogs even in tumors without complete loss of *PTEN* expression.

NKX3-1

LOH on chromosome 8p is the earliest and most common genetic abnormality in prostate cancer. The actual gene involved in prostate tumorigenesis at chromosome 8p is not known. One excellent candidate gene is *NKX3-1*, an androgen regulated and prostate specific gene located at chromosome 8p21 (He et al, 1997; Prescott et al, 1998). ***NKX3-1* belongs to a larger family of homeobox genes, which play important roles in the development and homeostasis of organs.** Aberrant expression of homeobox genes has been implicated in a number of tumors, suggesting that *NKX3-1* might play a role in prostate tumorigenesis. **Bhatia-Gaur and colleagues (1999) demonstrated that mice deficient in *Nkx3-1* (via gene targeting) have significant defects in prostate ductal morphogenesis and secretory protein production** (Oda et al, 2000). **Most intriguingly, aging *Nkx3-1*–deficient mice developed dysplastic changes and even cancer.** Of importance, these investigators noted that loss of a single *Nkx3-1* allele (e.g., in heterozygous mice) was sufficient to result in this dysplasia, suggesting that haploinsufficiency may be enough to lead to cancer (Bhatia-Gaur et al, 1999). Haploinsufficiency of *NKX3-1* for HGPIN development was also reported by Magee and colleagues (2003). These investigators also provided functional evidence of the role of *NKX3-1*, showing that loss of this gene led to increased proliferation in the prostate ductal epithelium. This was particularly notable during regeneration of the prostate after castration and androgen-addback. These results suggest that any loss of *NKX3-1* can lead to hyperproliferation and the increased accumulation of mutations resulting in cancer. Finally, Gelmann and coworkers (2003) studied human prostate cancers and have shown that indeed there is significant loss of *NKX3-1* in most prostate cancers, providing correlative evidence for the importance of this gene in the initiation of prostate cancer.

Epidermal Growth Factor

Originally isolated from mouse submandibular glands by the Nobel laureate Stanley Cohen (Heimberg et al, 1965), epidermal growth factor (EGF) and its family members, notably transforming growth factor-α (TGF-α), act through the EGF receptor, a receptor tyrosine kinase (Hackel et al, 1999; Moghal et al, 1999). **EGF induces cell proliferation across a broad set of cell types, including those derived from all three embryonic tissues: ectoderm, mesoderm, and endoderm** (Massague, 1990). It is not surprising, therefore, to find EGF acting as an inductive signal in embryogenesis.

The role of EGF in progression of urologic malignancies has been the subject of extensive investigation. In prostate cancer, both androgen-sensitive and androgen-insensitive prostate cancer cell lines produce TGF-α (Steiner, 1995). In response to androgen, TGF-α and EGF receptor production increases in androgen-sensitive cell lines, suggesting both an autocrine loop and a potential mechanism for androgen stimulation of cell proliferation (Connolly et al, 1990; Liu et al, 1993). Indeed, the androgen receptor demonstrates a certain promiscuity to growth factors, such as EGF, keratinocyte growth factor (KGF), and insulin growth factor (IGF-1). In a prostate cancer cell line with no androgen receptor, DU145, an artificially placed (or transfected) androgen receptor responded to those growth factors (Culig et al, 1994). In the presence of an androgen-depleted environment, continued prostate cancer growth—synonymous with the lethal form of the disease—may use an androgen-signaling chain activated by these peptide growth factors. In kidney cancer, there is overexpression of TGF-α and EGFR, reminiscent of expression patterns seen in the embryo (Mydlo et al, 1989). A promising strategy to block EGF activity in cancer is the use of an antibody directed against EGFR (Mendelsohn, 1997). This monoclonal antibody (Mab 225), Erbitux, has been approved for treatment of colon cancer and works both by blocking activation of the receptor tyrosine kinase and recruiting the host immune system. This antibody appears to act synergistically with classic chemotherapeutic agents. Two small molecule antagonists of EGFR have also been approved recently, Tarceva and Iressa. As was discussed earlier in this chapter, Iressa leads to dramatic responses in a small subset of non–small lung cancer patients with activating mutations in the EGFR kinase domain.

Transforming Growth Factor-β

If members of the broad family of peptide growth factors have personalities, then TGF-β could be considered the most bipolar. **TGF-β is a positive regulator of stromal cell growth, stimulates extracellular matrix production, simultaneously induces cell cycle arrest in epithelial and hematopoietic cell populations, and is a potent immunosuppressant** (Massague, 1998). TGF-β was first isolated from human platelets and subsequently cloned. It is part of the superfamily bearing its name, including bone morphogenetic proteins (BMPs), growth and differentiation factors, TGF-β2 and TGF-β3, activin, inhibin, and müllerian inhibiting factor. Consistent with the well-known role of the last factor in genitourinary tract development, almost all members of the TGF-β superfamily are involved in embryogenesis.

TGF-β is produced by the cell as a precursor that although cleaved before secretion remains latent (or inactive) through noncovalent interactions with this latency-associated peptide (Gentry et al, 1987). In this latent form, TGF-β cannot bind to the TGF-β receptor. Furthermore, a glycoprotein known as latent TGF-β–binding protein has been implicated as a mediator of extracellular matrix storage of TGF-β.

TGF-β is produced by many malignancies, including prostate and kidney cancers. In many cases, the malignant cells—derived from epithelial cells that are normally growth inhibited by TGF-β—are no longer sensitive to TGF-β in this way. In fact, **TGF-β may promote tumor progression in a variety of ways: TGF-β enhances angiogenesis, which is crucial for nutrient support of the growing tumor mass; it also suppresses the immune system, limiting the ability of the host's best defense system to eliminate tumor cells; by stimulating the production and turnover of extracellular matrix, tumor-derived TGF-β provides both the physical and invasive support for malignant growth and progression** (Steiner, 1995).

Insulin-like Growth Factor

Sharing functional and sequence similarities to insulin, insulin-like growth factors 1 and 2 (IGF-1, IGF-2) stimulate cell proliferation (Daughaday et al, 1989). Unlike the endocrine actions of insulin, however, IGF-1 and IGF-2 are produced and appear to act at the local tissue level. For example, IGFs are secreted by prostatic stromal cells and act as mitogens for prostatic epithelial cells (Cohen et al, 1994). The activities of IGF-1 and IGF-2 are modulated by a set of IGF-binding proteins that inhibit their interaction with the IGF receptors.

Plasma concentrations of IGF-1 have been associated with the risk of developing prostate cancer. From 14,916 physicians enrolled in the Physicians' Health Study, 152 cases of prostate cancer were matched with 152 controls; plasma obtained at the start of the study was assayed of IGF-1 concentrations (Chan et al, 1998). A positive association between initial IGF-1 levels and eventual prostate cancer was observed: by univariate analysis, men in the highest quartile for IGF-1 levels had a relative risk of 2.4 (95% CI 1.2 to 4.7) for the disease compared with men in the lowest quartile for plasma IGF-1 concentrations. The major IGF-binding protein, IGFBP-3, has growth-inhibitory properties and may reduce the bioactivity of IGF: the authors hypothesized that high-level IGFBP-3 may be inversely related to risk. After correcting for IGFBP-3 levels, the risks of developing prostate cancer were approximately 4.5 times greater between the highest and lowest quartiles for plasma IGF-1 concentrations. Although these findings have been confirmed, in part, by other groups (Wolk et al, 1998), others have found no significant association between IGF serum levels and prostate cancer (Cutting et al, 1999; Kurek et al, 2000), and even a negative correlation (Baffa et al, 2000).

As with EGF, a promising method to block IGF is to inhibit its receptor IGF-1R. A number of important recent studies have shown that monoclonal antibodies targeting IGF-1R can inhibit tumor growth (Burtrum et al, 2003; Gao et al, 2004). These molecules are heading toward the clinic in the near future and hold particular promise for prostate cancer. Another method to block IGF that is receiving attention is to neutralize it with IGFBP3. This is particularly appealing because of the diverse roles IGFBP3 appears to play. Not only can it neutralize IGF, but it also has direct pro-apoptotic effects on cancer cells (Shim et al, 2004; Kwok et al, 2005; Lee et al, 2005). Recombinant IGFBP3 is in preclinical trials.

G Protein–Coupled Ligands

The small bioactive peptides bombesin, endothelin-1 (ET-1), and neurotensin act through specific, high-affinity heptahelical, G protein–coupled receptors (Kitabgi et al, 1985; Spindel et al, 1990; Cyc et al, 1991). There is increasing evidence for the role of these small peptides in carcinogenesis and disease progression. In prostate cancer, the enzyme responsible for the degradation of these peptides, endopeptidase 24.11, is decreased in androgen-independent disease (Papandreou et al, 1998): loss of local peptide degradation may enhance the local concentrations of these bioactive peptides and enhance cancer progression.

Endothelin-1

Endothelin-1 is the most potent endogenous vasoconstrictor known (Yanagisawa et al, 1988). The endothelin family contains several 21 amino acid members: ET-1, ET-2, and ET-3 and the sarafotoxins (isolated from the venom of the Israeli burrowing asp *Atractaspis engaddensis*) (Inoue et al, 1989; Kitazumi et al, 1990). These ligands bind to the endothelin receptors ET_A and ET_B with varying affinity. Endothelin-1 is produced by many different cell types (Rubanyi et al, 1994), including prostatic epithelium (Langenstroer et al, 1993): almost all the secretory columnar epithelium produces ET-1. The concentrations of immunoreactive ET-1 are highest in seminal fluid, reported to be approximately 500 times greater than the concentration in circulation (Casey et al, 1992). Every prostate cancer cell line tested produces ET-1 mRNA and protein, and a majority of men with androgen-refractory prostate cancer had abnormally elevated plasma ET-1 concentrations (Nelson et al, 1995). Every primary prostate cancer and 14 of 16 prostate cancer metastases were uniformly positive for ET-1 expression by immunohistochemistry (Nelson et al, 1996).

ET-1 synergized the proliferative effects of other peptide growth factors in certain prostate cancer cell lines (Nelson et al, 1996). The effects of ET-1 on prostate cancer cells appear to be mediated through the ET_A receptor subtype exclusively: the addition of an ET_A receptor antagonist blocked the growth promoting effects of ET-1 (Nelson et al, 1996). ET-1 also acts as a survival factor for cells exposed to a cytotoxic agent: in prostatic smooth muscle cells, paclitaxel-induced apoptosis was significantly reduced in the presence of ET-1 (Wu-Wong et al, 1997, 2000).

Whereas benign prostatic epithelium expresses the ET_B receptor subtype predominantly (Kobayashi et al, 1994), in prostate cancer cells the ET_B receptor is not expressed; in both primary and metastatic prostate tumors, expression of the ET_B receptor is reduced (Nelson et al, 1996). The ET_B receptor gene *(EDRNB)* contains a CpG in the promoter region, and in 70% of the prostate cancers studied the CpG island of the *EDNRB* gene is methylated (Nelson et al, 1997).

ET-1 is a mitogen for osteoblasts and has been shown to inhibit osteoclast function. In prostate cancer, ET-1's effect on bone is believed to play a major role in the evolution of osteoblastic lesions. In a matrix-induced bone-forming system, ET-1 increased alkaline phosphatase activity (used as an index of new formation) (Nelson et al, 1995). By using another osteoblastic model system, stable transfection of an ET-1 overexpression vector increased the area of new bone formation and chronic administration of an ET_A receptor antagonist decreased new bone formation (Nelson et al, 1999). This exciting paper demonstrated that treatment of mice bearing osteoblastic lesions with the ET-1 receptor antagonist atrasentan restored the bone surrounding tumor deposits to normal. Collectively, these data support a potential role of ET-1 in the osteoblastic response of bone to metastatic prostate cancer and provide the rationale for ET-1 receptor antagonists in the treatment of metastatic prostate cancer to bone.

Atrasentan (ABT-627), a highly potent and selective ET_A receptor antagonist, was studied in men with progressive, hormone-refractory prostate cancer. In the phase I studies, ABT-627 was very well tolerated, with mild to moderate headache being the most common side effect. In 70% (7/10) of patients with pain requiring a narcotic, ABT-627 reduced pain (as measured by the Visual Analog Scale), and in several patients narcotic use declined. In 68% (15/22) of men, PSA dropped, ranging from less than 5% to 90%. In a randomized, double-blind, placebo-controlled phase II study, atrasentan significantly prolonged time to clinical progression in men with hormone-refractory prostate cancer (Jimeno and Carducci, 2005). Phase III studies have now been completed and show a delay in prostate cancer clinical progression in bone and a reduction in opiate needs. Another phase III study has been completed in men with nonmetastatic hormone-refractory prostate cancer. Results of this trial are pending. Atrasentan is under review by the U.S. Food and Drug Administration.

KEY POINTS: CELLULAR SIGNALING

- Cells communicate by transmission of signals one to another.

- Classically, signals are transmitted through cell surface or cytoplasmic receptors and generate a cascade of downstream events that are tightly regulated.

- In cancer, cell signaling is co-opted to support the survival and proliferation of the cancer cell.

- Overexpression or mutation of growth factor receptors, such as EGFR and IGFR, is common in urologic cancers.

- The PTEN lipid and protein phosphatase is a negative regulator of the PI3 kinase pathway that leads to constitutive activation of the Akt oncogene. It is frequently mutated or lost in urologic cancers, such as bladder and prostate cancer.

- Cancer signaling is a major target for therapeutic intervention that is revolutionizing the treatment of cancer. Already, a number of small molecular and antibody drugs have entered standard clinical practice.

RECEPTORS AND THE CELL SURFACE

Quite literally, every connection we have with the outside world is dependent on the integrity and function of the cell surface. This humble 5-nm-thick film also provides the orga-

nizational structure to how we respond to both our internal and external environment, how we physically hold ourselves together, and how we tell us from everything else. It is far from hyperbole to claim our lives depend on the cell surface.

All of this is based on a simple structure that exploits the different polarities of phospholipids to water: the hydrophilic polar ends (sticking out) and the hydrophobic tails (sandwiched within) will form bilayers, even under artificial conditions (Singer et al, 1972). This structure will, within limits, shrink and expand to seal the inside from the outside and spring back into shape when torn, as the hydrophobic tails seek to avoid the water world in which they are immersed. The lipid bilayer is also used to form lysosomes, endoplasmic reticulum, and mitochondria. The major classes of phospholipids (phosphatidylcholine, sphingomyelin, phosphatidylserine, and phosphatidylethanolamine) are joined by inositol phospholipids, a smaller but crucial component for cell signaling. Embedded within the lipid bilayer are molecules that stabilize and maintain its permeability, like cholesterol, or interact with the extracellular domain, like the glycolipids (Yeagle, 1985). Perhaps the most important structures embedded in the cell membrane are proteins, which are key in cell signaling and linking the cytoskeleton to the surface.

Receptors

Whatever the form of the signal, large proteins, peptides, steroids, fatty acids, or even gases, such as nitric oxide, the recipient cell's first response is through a specific receptor. The specificity of the response is usually regulated by a very small amount of a molecule or ligand binding to a receptor with very high affinity for the ligand. **Most receptors are bound to the cell surface, with an extracellular ligand binding in the extracellular space and the receptor activating pathways within the cell. Notable exceptions are the intracellular receptors, such as the androgen receptor, which binds to the small, lipid diffusible ligand testosterone.** In general terms, the nature of a signaling pathway is described in terms of where the signal arose: the autocrine signaling loop implies a cell produces the signal that acts back on the same cell. Signals produced locally, like those existing between the stroma and epithelial components of a tissue, are called paracrine signaling. When the signal, like leutinizing hormone, is produced remotely and reaches target cells—in this case Leydig cells—through systemic circulation it is considered an endocrine signal.

There are three general classes of membrane-bound receptors (Alberts et al, 1994). **The ion channel–linked receptors,** such as the acetylcholine receptors active in the neuromuscular junction, are characterized by a rapid on/off signal, ideal for conducting nervous impulses to muscle. **Enzyme-linked receptors,** such as growth factor receptors, bridge the cell membrane and activate an intracellular enzyme in response to an extracellular ligand. **G protein–linked receptors,** all characterized by seven pass transmembrane (heptahelical) proteins, activate G proteins after ligand binding and, with over 100 members in mammals, represent the largest family of cell surface receptors.

The steroid hormone receptor superfamily is characterized by direct interaction of the receptor-ligand complex with DNA, regulating the transcription of particular genes

(Evans, 1988). A host of structurally diffuse ligands, such as the steroid hormones testosterone, estradiol and cortisol, thyroxine, retinoids, and vitamin D, share a similarly small size, are hydrophobic, and easily diffuse directly across the plasma membrane. The steroid receptors bind to ligand in the cytosol and then bind to target DNA sequences to stimulate or repress gene transcription (Yamamoto, 1985).

Enzyme-Linked Receptors

Because many of the growth factors implicated in carcinogenesis and progression bind to enzyme-linked receptors, this group of receptors has received intense study in oncologic research. As the name implies, **these receptors are linked to cytoplasmic enzymes—either intrinsically or intimately associated—that are activated in response to extracellular ligand binding.** There are five classes of enzyme-linked receptors: (1) receptor tyrosine kinases, like the EGF receptor; (2) tyrosine-kinase-associated receptors, like the IL-2 receptor; (3) receptor serine/threonine kinases, like receptors of the TGF-β superfamily; (4) receptor tyrosine phosphatases; and (5) receptor guanylyl cyclases (Alberts et al, 1994).

Receptor Tyrosine Kinases. Many of the growth factors studied in cancer progression act through receptor tyrosine kinases, including EGF, VEGF, NGF, FGF, IGF-1, and PDGF. Although the receptors differ in both their extracellular binding domains, in every case the receptor initiates intracellular signaling by phosphorylating (or activating) themselves (Ullrich et al, 1990). This is accomplished either by receptor dimerization, and autophosphorylation within the two halves of the pair, or by inducing an allosteric interaction between the two halves. Activated receptor tyrosine kinases bind a host of other intracellular proteins, which, in turn, activate other signaling pathways. Common to many of these binding proteins are highly conserved domains, known as SH2 and SH3, which allow binding to the activated receptor tyrosine kinases (Koch et al, 1991). The SH2 and SH3 domains are named for their homology to the chicken sarcoma virus proto-oncogene Src. Another heavily studied family of receptor tyrosine kinase–binding proteins are the RAS proteins (Hall A, 1993). Mutations in the *RAS* gene, resulting in cell proliferation in the absence of growth factor binding, occur in about 30% of human cancers. The *ERBB* oncogene *(HER2/NEU)* encodes for a constitutively active form of the EGF receptor. A subset of breast cancers, shown to express ERBB, responds clinically to an antibody (Herceptin) directed against the receptor (Pegram et al, 1999).

Tyrosine Kinase–Associated Receptors. Unlike the tyrosine receptor kinases, which have an intracellular activating domain covalently linked to the extracellular binding domain, the tyrosine kinase–associated receptors work through associated proteins, such as the Src family of proteins and the Janus family (JAK1, JAK2) (Argentsinger et al, 1993). Ligands activating these receptors include prolactin; growth hormone; many cytokines, such as erythropoietin and granulocyte-macrophage colony-stimulating factor; and many interleukins.

Receptor Serine/Theonine Kinases. The TGF-β superfamily, including the bone morphogenetic proteins, activin, inhibin, and müllerian inhibiting substance, all act through receptor serine/threonine kinases (Massague, 1992). Type I TGF-β receptors phosphorylate the SMAD proteins. As is the

case with receptor tyrosine kinases, the TGF-β receptors also form complexes with each other: because the bioactive form of TGF-β are dimers, the ligand/receptor complex is heterotetrameric (Massague, 1998).

One of the effects of TGF-β on target cells and, in particular, epithelial cells, is as a negative regulator of cell proliferation. It is not surprising, therefore, that defects in TGF-β receptors have been detected in epithelial-derived cancers. For example, in prostate cancer, loss of TGF-β receptor type I expression has been shown to significantly associate with increasing Gleason score, clinical tumor stage, short-term survival, and biochemical recurrence after radical prostatectomy (Kim et al, 1996, 1998).

G Protein–Coupled Receptors

As the name implies, **this group of receptors activates intracellular responses through trimeric guanosine triphosphate (GTP)-binding proteins or, simply, G proteins, and represents the largest family of cell-surface receptors** (Linder et al, 1992). These receptors often work through "rapid" secondary messengers, such as Ca^{2+} and cyclic adenosine monophosphate (AMP): through the activity of adenylase cyclase, concentrations of cyclic AMP can increase manyfold within seconds. Likewise, given the large concentration gradients of Ca^{2+} between the endoplasmic reticulum, the extracellular space, and the cytosol, swift Ca^{2+} fluxes can occur. It is not surprising, therefore, to find G protein–coupled receptors mediating the effects of proteins known for quick responses, such as epinephrine or norepinephrine acting through the β-adrenergic receptor or as mediators of the sense of sight and smell.

Adhesion Molecules

The connection of cells to the surrounding matrix is not only required to hold us together but also for cells to sense their relationship to each other and the outside world. Indeed, the **loss of normal cell-to-cell contact behavior often defines cancer:** in culture, normal cells will stop proliferating when a particular cell density is achieved whereas cancer cells will continue to proliferate, having lost this contact inhibition. In this section we address two of the important proteins in the relationship of the cells to the extracellular matrix and each other: integrins and E-cadherin.

Integrins

Bridging the gap between the extracellular matrix and the cytoskeleton are the integrins, which act not only as structural elements but also as a type of receptor (Clark et al, 1995). At a basic level, **the integrins are heterodimers, made of two proteins known as the α and β chains:** owing to alternative splicing of integrin mRNA there are a large number of integrin combinations with differing affinities to extracellular matrix and cellular proteins (Keely et al, 1998). For example, β1 chains combine with α chains to mediate cell-matrix adhesion: α6β1 and α6β4 are laminin receptors, whereas αvβ3 is a receptor for a large number of extracellular ligands, including vitronectin, fibronectin, thrombospondin, and osteopontin. Many of the integrins recognize the amino acid sequence arginine-glycine-aspartate (RGD sequence) present on many extracellular ligands such as fibronectin (Eliceiri et al, 1999).

The β2 chains are expressed on white blood cells and mediate cell-cell adhesion (Porter et al, 1998). The cytoplasmic tail of the β chain is attached to the actin cytoskeleton by linker proteins, such as talin, α-actinin, paxillin, and vinculin.

Integrins have been shown to regulate cell proliferation, survival, and differentiation (Ruoslahti at al, 1994). When integrins bind to extracellular ligands and undergo clustering (Kornberg et al, 1991), a process that occurs with the formation of adhesive contacts, there is activation and autophosphorylation of the tyrosine kinase focal adhesion kinase (FAK) (Dogic et al, 1998). FAK is important in regulating the cytoskeleton, cell motility, and tumor invasion. It also activates other proliferation pathways, such as the Src-family of kinases and mitogen-activated (MAP) kinases. The interactions of integrins with the extracellular matrix activates FAK and suppresses apoptosis in diverse cell types (Xu et al, 1996; Kyle et al, 1997). For example, inhibition of integrin function leads to loss of cell-cell adhesion and apoptosis, and **loss of interactions between normal epithelial cells and the extracellular matrix also leads to apoptosis, a process known as "anoikis"** (Frisch et al, 1994).

In many carcinomas, the overall expression of integrins is reduced (Boudreau et al, 1998). The alternatively spliced variant of the β1 subunit containing an unique 48 amino acid carboxyl-terminus sequence called β1c is expressed in normal prostate epithelium but is reduced in prostate cancer (Fornaro et al, 1999). When β1c is expressed in mouse fibroblasts there is a marked inhibition of DNA synthesis: it is possible that loss of this negative regulator of cell proliferation accompanies carcinogenesis (Meredith et al, 1995). In some cases integrin expression is increased (such as high αvβ3 expression in melanoma progression) or changes its normal distribution (such as loss of basolateral expression of α6β1 and α6β4 in normal cells to a more diffuse pattern in cancer) (Nip et al, 1995). There is a correlation between invasion and metastatic spread and αvβ3, perhaps through an interaction with matrix-degrading proteases such as urokinase plasminogen activator.

E-Cadherin

Whereas the integrins primarily mediate adhesion and interactions with the extracellular matrix, the cadherins are responsible for cell-cell adhesion and tissue integrity. E-cadherin (present on epithelial cells) is also known as uvormorulin, a glycoprotein identified in the embryonic compaction of the mouse morula (Peyriras et al, 1983). The Ca^{2+}-dependent homophilic interaction (binding to the same protein on other cells) of E-cadherin is dependent on its interaction with the catenins (α, β, γ) linking E-cadherin to the actin cytoskeleton (Christofori et al, 1999). Therefore, disruptions of any of the elements in this chain of proteins will lead to loss of adhesion. Although such disruptions could result in loss of tissue integrity, these are precisely the kinds of changes observed in cancer.

There is considerable evidence for a central role of E-cadherin pathway perturbations in tumor progression and metastases. Early work showed that antibodies directed against E-cadherin produced benign canine kidney cells with invasive properties and viral transformation of those benign cells produced invasive cells with no expression of E-cadherin (Behrens et al, 1989). Likewise, in the normal rat prostate and in the noninvasive sublines of the rat prostate Dunning tumor E-cadherin is expressed, but in the invasive sublines there is no E-cadherin mRNA or protein expression (Bussemakers et al, 1992). In human tumors, loss of E-cadherin or α-catenin expression is associated with more aggressive and metastatic disease: in prostate cancer, increasing Gleason grade and cancer-specific death rates were significantly associated with reduced or absent E-cadherin expression (Morton et al, 1993; Umbas et al, 1994; Richmond et al, 1997). Similar correlations have been made in bladder cancer (Imao et al, 1999) and renal cell carcinoma (Shimazui et al, 1998), although there is redundant expression of other cadherin family members in renal cell carcinoma (Shimazui et al, 1996).

In many tumors, the loss of E-cadherin is associated with a concomitant gain in expression of N- and P-cadherins. These mesenchymal cadherins are believed to promote invasion and metastasis. **The process by which cells acquire more mesenchymal properties is called epithelial to mesenchymal transition and is thought to be a major mode whereby tumors become metastatic** (Gao et al, 2004; Karreth and Tuveson, 2004). Current studies suggest that this is a common property of both bladder and prostate cancers (Rieger-Christ et al, 2004; Kwok et al, 2005). A number of transcription factors that regulate this process have also been discovered, including TWIST and SNAIL (Gao et al, 2004; Kang and Massague, 2004; Karreth and Tuveson, 2004).

Caveolin

Caveolins (caveolin-1, -2, and -3) are proteins that are the major constituents of the plasma membrane structure called caveolae: these "little caves" are 50- to 100-nm non–clathrin-coated vesicles that are critical transport mechanisms for many proteins and appear to be extensively involved in cell signaling (Lisanti et al, 1994). Caveolae have been shown to transport albumin, low density lipoproteins, ceramide, and cholesterol, as well as act as a site for binding of many extracellular ligands. For example, the potent vasoconstrictor endothelin-1, implicated in the pathophysiology of prostate cancer, binds to the endothelin receptor subtype A within caveolae, leading to rapid endocytosis of the receptor/ligand complex (Chun et al, 1994). Caveolae are also associated with intercellular signaling proteins, such as Src-like kinase, GPI-linked proteins, G proteins, as well as protein kinase C, gelsolin, actin, and osteopontin.

Caveolae, which resemble satellite dishes both structurally and functionally, are abundant in endothelium, smooth muscle, and fibroblasts. Although caveolin expression is rare in prostatic epithelium, it is increased in prostate cancer metastatic to lymph nodes (Yang et al, 1998). Caveolin expression is also positively correlated with increasing Gleason score, extraprostatic extension, and time to disease progression (Yang et al, 1999). Unlike a positive association between caveolin and prostate cancer progression, researchers have shown reduced caveolin expression in androgen-independent clones of androgen-sensitive prostate cancer cells and reduced expression of caveolin in oncogenically transformed mouse fibroblasts (Koleske et al, 1995; Pflug et al, 1999). Some have proposed caveolin may act as a tumor suppressor, perhaps as a general kinase inhibitor (Engelman et al, 1998). Although at present its role in carcinogenesis and progression is far from clear, caveolin and its intercepting pathways merit continued attention (Nelson, 1998).

KEY POINTS: RECEPTORS AND THE CELL SURFACE

■ The cell surface of cancer cells is characterized by the presence of an amazing variety of receptors, enzymes, adhesion molecules, and membrane microdomains containing important signaling molecules.

■ These cell surface components all play major roles in a cell's ability to transmit signals and regulate its extracellular environment.

■ Corticosteroid receptors are not present on the cell surface and transmit signals by binding their ligand in the cytoplasm, then shuttling to the nucleus where they interact directly with DNA to stimulate or block transcription.

■ Adhesion molecules such as integrins and cadherins regulate cellular attachment and motility. Abnormalities in cellular attachment and motility are central to normal development as well as cancer metastasis.

■ Membrane microdomains such as cholesterol rafts and caveolae are believed to be platforms of cell signaling critical to normal homeostasis and cancer progression.

VIRUSES

Viral infections are believed to be causally related to approximately one in seven human malignancies. They induce tumor formation through a variety of mechanisms, including expression of viral oncogenes (Rous, 1911), inducing the abnormal expression of host oncogenes (Hayward et al, 1981), or alternating the immune status of the host (Howley et al, 1997). It is important to emphasize that no human viruses have been found to cause malignancy independent of other genetic events in keeping with the multistep model for tumorigenesis (Bishop, 1990).

RNA Viruses

There are two groups of RNA retroviruses that cause transformation. The acutely transforming retroviruses transform virtually all infected cells. This type of virus was first described in chicken sarcomas (Rous, 1911). The virus causing the malignant transformation, Rous sarcoma virus, was eventually found to contain the oncogene v-src, which had been captured by the virus from the avian genome. Other retroviruses have been found to contain other oncogenes. These viral oncogenes are believed to have originated in the host but have been incorporated by the retrovirus in the distant past (Stehelin et al, 1976). More than 70 different viral proto-oncogenes have been identified. These genes encode a variety of cellular elements that all act in a dominant fashion to promote cell growth. The proto-oncogene products include growth factors, cell cycle regulators, protein kinases, and transcriptional regulators (Slamon, 1987).

A second mechanism by which viruses can contribute to malignant transformation is through genomic insertion. The virus does not contain transforming genes but instead contributes to malignancy by activating a host organism's oncogene or inactivating a tumor suppressor gene. The virus inserts into the host genome in a location that affects transcriptional activation of the gene. The prototype virus in this class is the avian leukosis virus, which often integrates in the vicinity of the c-MYC oncogene and in doing so activates it (Hayward et al, 1981).

The retrovirus family found to cause malignancy in humans is the human T-cell leukemia viruses (HTLV). HTLV-1 is believed to cause adult T-cell leukemia by viral-induced changes in the host genome (Hinuma et al, 1981). Another member of this family of retroviruses, HTLV-2, has been linked to hairy cell leukemia, although it is unclear how it is the causative agent (Poeschla and Wong-Staal, 1997). HTLV-3, more commonly known as human immunodeficiency virus (HIV-1), has been linked to an increased risk of malignancy, but this is believed to be secondary to altered immunosurveillance, not to genomic changes in the cancer cell. At the current time no genitourinary malignancies have been directly linked to retroviruses.

DNA Viruses

DNA viruses are believed to play much more of a role in human tumorigenesis than RNA viruses, with hepatitis B and papillomaviruses responsible for 80% of virus-induced malignancies (zur Hausen, 1991). Included in this group of viruses is papillomaviruses, the only viruses conclusively linked to common urologic malignancy.

The first virus linked to human tumor formation was Epstein-Barr virus (EBV), which was found to be associated with Burkitt's lymphoma in 1964 (Epstein and Barr, 1964). EBV is believed to induce tumor formation through two mechanisms. The first is that the virus causes B-lymphocyte proliferation in most patients. If the patient becomes immunosuppressed, the fastest growing B-lymphocyte clones emerge as a lymphoproliferative disease. An alternative method of tumor formation, which occurs in patients with normal immune function, is translocation of the c-MYC oncogene. This leads to unregulated expression of this oncogene and unregulated growth (Howley et al, 1997).

Hepatitis B virus (HBV) is a DNA virus that has been linked to hepatocellular carcinoma, one of the world's most common malignancies (Beasley, 1988). The chronic infection causes hepatocellular injury, and the injury triggers a proliferative response. It is believed that this proliferative response increases the opportunity for genetic errors and therefore the risk of malignancy (Howley et al, 1997)

The DNA viruses that have been most convincingly linked to genitourinary malignancies are the human papillomaviruses (HPV). More than 70 different HPV subtypes have been described of which at least 30 have been linked to intraepithelial neoplasia or carcinoma (de Villiers, 1994; Howley et al, 1997). HPV-16, 18, 31, 33, and 35 are the subtypes most commonly linked to invasive carcinoma (Griffiths and Mellon, 1999). Because of the strong association between HPV and malignancy, the mechanism of action has been more fully elucidated than other malignancies.

The HPV subtypes linked to malignancy are capable of immortalizing normal primary human cells in culture. Although these immortalized cells do not have all the characteristics of transformed cells, they resemble intraepithelial neoplasia (Durst et al, 1987). **The viral genes responsible for immortalization are E6 and E7** (Hawley-Nelson et al, 1989). **Both E6 and E7 inactivate cell cycle regulatory and apoptosis proteins. E6 appears to primarily function by targeting TP53 for ubiquitin-mediated degradation. Inactivation of TP53 blocks both cell cycle arrest and apoptosis and in doing so promotes the malignant phenotype** (Scheffner et al, 1990). **E7 functions by inactivating RB. This promotes the release of E2F and activates the transcriptional machinery** (Scheffner et al, 1990) (see "Apoptosis" and "The Cell Cycle"). The E6 and E7 proteins clearly provide a survival advantage for the virus, because they allow the virus to replicate in a cell with active transcriptional machinery and thus is unable to undergo programmed cell death. A byproduct of the inactivation of TP53 and RB is that the infected cell is predisposed to malignancy.

HPV infection with high-risk subtypes has been linked to penile carcinoma. HPV has been detected in 15% to 80% of penile lesions (Griffiths and Mellon, 1999). **HPV-16 appears to be the dominant subtype and has been identified in up to 90% of HPV-positive lesions** (Cupp et al, 1995). HPV-11, 18, and 33 have also been identified in penile tumors (Villa and Lopes, 1986; Amerio et al, 1998; Dianzani et al, 1998). The detection of HPV virus in carcinoma in situ supports the conclusion that HPV contributes to the malignant phenotype early in the transformation process. Although HPV is commonly detected in normal penile tissue, these commonly are not the high-risk subtypes (Griffiths and Mellon, 1999).

Evidence supporting the role of HPV in prostate, bladder, renal, and testis tumor is lacking, and it is unlikely that HPV is an important factor. Whereas some studies have detected HPV in these malignancies, the findings have not been confirmed. Therefore, the positive results may have been an artifact of the collection process or a consequence of an overly sensitive polymerase chain reaction (PCR) assay (Griffiths and Mellon, 2000).

KEY POINTS: VIRUSES

■ The first oncogenes discovered were viruses.

■ Viruses are believed to play a central role in cancer causation.

■ Human papillomavirus is a cause of cervical cancer.

ANGIOGENESIS

In solid tumors, an adequate supply of oxygen and nutrients is required for cell survival and growth. Based on this simple biologic principle, the field of angiogenesis has exploded over that past decade, with the identification of a host of endothelial cell growth factors and inhibitors. In both the scientific and lay press, the promise of agents directed against tumor neovascularity had been reported with almost unwavering ebullience until practical concerns about drug stability and

large-scale production arose (Cohen, 1999). Whether agents of anti-angiogenesis will make a difference in the treatment of cancer is unknown, but there are certainly reasons for optimism.

Given the physical limitations of oxygen diffusion in solid tissue, which is limited to about 200:M, the growth of a tumor over 2 mm requires a supporting vasculature (Tomlinson et al, 1955). The term *angiogenesis,* coined in 1935 to describe the growth of new blood vessels in the placenta, now includes a complex set of positive and negative angiogenic factors whose balance determines vascularization. In normal adult tissues, the inhibitors of angiogenesis predominate, but in developing tissues, in wound healing, and in cancer, inducers of angiogenesis gain the upper hand and new vessels are formed.

Angiogenesis Activators

There are a host of factors identified as stimulating angiogenesis that are secreted by the tumors themselves or by infiltrating immune cells leading to new blood vessel formation (Campbell, 1997). **Many angiogenesis activators, such as fibroblast growth factor-2 (FGF-2, also known as basic fibroblast growth factor [bFGF]), are also sequestered in the extracellular matrix, bound to heparin sulfate: degradation of the matrix by tumor-derived proteases releases these factors and stimulates endothelial cell proliferation** (Folkman et al, 1987). Two of the best studied angiogenesis activators are FGF-2 and vascular endothelial growth factor (VEGF).

FGF-2

FGF-2 is a potent angiogenic factor and stimulates endothelial proliferation, migration, and formation of differentiated microvasculature (Esch et al, 1985; Abraham et al, 1986). Capillary endothelial cells produce and release active FGF-2, raising the possibility of an autocrine loop, where endothelial cells produce a factor that, in turn, stimulates them (Schweigere et al, 1987). **Endothelial cells also store FGF-2 in two ways: it is either sequestered within the cell or is secreted and becomes incorporated into the surrounding extracellular matrix** (Vlodavsky et al, 1987). This incorporation within the extracellular matrix can have tumor-promoting effects. For example, urine obtained from patients with bladder cancer can have levels of FGF-2 100-fold higher than normal individuals, yet expression of FGF-2 by the tumor itself is generally less than normal bladder tissue. It appears the increased FGF-2 levels result from degradation of extracellular matrix by the tumor (O'Brien et al, 1997). The release of this potent angiogenic factor is precisely what a growing tumor would need.

VEGF

Unlike FGF-2, which acts on a variety of cell types, VEGF, also known as vascular permeability factor (VPF), may function only to regulate angiogenesis (Leung et al, 1989; Senger et al, 1986, 1993). **As its two names imply, VEGF/VPF acts as both an inducer of endothelial cell proliferation and as a potent permeability factor.** In fact, VPF was first isolated from tumor ascites fluid from guinea pigs, hamsters, and mice (Senger et al, 1983). There are four species of VEGF, containing 121,

165, 189 and 206 amino acids (Ferrara et al, 1991). **The expression of VEGF can be induced by hypoxia, a common condition at the leading edge of a growing mass or within a solid tumor** (Shweiki et al, 1992; Liu et al, 1995). In tumors, it appears tumor necrosis induces the expression of VEGF, which, acting as a paracrine factor, leads to the sprouting of new tumor vessels. **Interestingly, VEGF/VPF levels within seminal plasma are very high and prostate and seminal vesicle tissues are labeled strongly for VEGF/VPF mRNA and protein** (Brown et al, 1995). Concentrations of VEGF in prostatic fluid—often measured in the milligram per milliliter range—were fourfold to fivefold higher than the levels in seminal vesicle fluid (Joseph et al, 1997). In a model of prostate cancer, highly metastatic variants had greater expression of VEGF and flk-1 (a VEGF receptor) coupled with high microvessel density compared with slightly metastatic or nonmetastatic variants (Balbay et al, 1999).

Angiogenesis Inhibitors

Broadly defined, angiogenesis inhibitors include both endogenous substances and exogenous compounds or treatments not typically considered anti-angiogenic, such as chemotherapy and radiation therapy. Anti-angiogenic qualities are found in cytotoxic agents such as methotrexate, paclitaxel, and bleomycin; antibiotics such as linomide, fumagillin, and suramin; anticancer treatments, such as hyperthermia and radiotherapy; or otherwise unrelated compounds such as aspirin, captopril, and thalidomide. **There are four general mechanisms through which angiogenesis inhibitors act** (Campbell, 1997): **(1) prevention of tumor cell production of angiogenesis factors, such as interferons α and β blocking the production of bFGF; (2) neutralizing angiogenesis factors, such as the VEGF neutralizing antibody Avastin; (3) blocking the response of endothelial cells to angiogenic factors, such as the activity of thrombospondin or angiostatin on endothelial cells or small molecule antagonists of VEGF receptor; and (4) interference with the matrix degradation required for vessels to sprout and grow through solid tissues, such as the matrix metalloproteinase inhibitor BB-94.** The new angiogenesis inhibitors have created unique challenges in clinical translation. For example, the timing of therapy is not established: in a transgenic mouse model of pancreatic islet cell carcinogenesis, different anti-angiogenic drugs had distinct efficacy profiles depending on when in tumor progression they were applied (Bergers et al, 1999). Furthermore, the classic measures of clinical response may not apply for agents that are tumor static.

Chemotherapeutic Agents. The chemotherapeutic agents **bleomycin and vincristine are strong inhibitors of angiogenesis,** which, in one study, approached the activity of the standard anti-angiogenic agent fumagillin (AGM-1470) (Schirner et al, 1998). Interestingly, the effects of these agents on angiogenesis were observed in fast-growing, but not slow-growing, xenografts. Methotrexate inhibits angiogenesis in arthritis and corneal inflammation models, and paclitaxel inhibits angiogenesis in vitro and in vivo at noncytotoxic doses (Belotti et al, 1996; Joussen et al, 1999). The partial estrogen antagonists tamoxifen, nafoxidine, and clomiphene and the pure antiestrogen ICI 182,780 significantly inhibited endothelial cell growth stimulated by bFGF and VEGF in vitro and inhibited angiogenesis in vivo (Gagliardi et al, 1993, 1996). This angiostatic activity was not altered by excess estrogen, suggesting a mechanism other than the inhibition of estrogen action.

Antibiotics. Linomide, a quinolone (roquinimex), selectively inhibits true angiogenesis, or new blood vessel formation, but does not affect established vessels, as demonstrated by a reduction in blood flow within a tumor but not in a variety of non–tumor-bearing organs (Vukanovic et al, 1993). In animal models of prostate cancer, linomide was effective as a chemopreventive for tumor formation and reduced tumor blood vessel density (Joseph et al, 1996; Hartley-Asp et al, 1997). Linomide also inhibits secretion of angiogenesis inducers, such as tumor necrosis factor-α, by tumor-infiltrating macrophages (Vukanovic et al, 1995; Joseph et al, 1996). Finally, the reduction in the VEGF secretion by prostate cancer that follows castration is potentiated by linomide (Joseph et al, 1997).

Fumagillin is a naturally occurring inhibitor of endothelial cell proliferation secreted from *Aspergillus fumigatus fresenius*. It was first isolated from a fungus contaminating a culture of capillary endothelial cells (Ingber et al, 1990). The small molecule derivatives of fumagillin, AMG-1470 and TMP-470, inhibit neovascularization via endothelial cell cycle arrest in late G_1 phase (Abe et al, 1994). TPM-470 covalently binds to the intracellular enzyme methionine aminopeptidase-2 (Sin et al, 1997), one of the two enzymes responsible for the removal of the initiator methionine during protein translation (Bradshaw et al, 1998). The cell cycle inhibition by TMP-470 is dependent on activation of the TP53 pathway, inducing accumulation of the G_1 cdk inhibitor CDKN1A (Zhang et al, 2000). TMP-470 has also been shown to inhibit the growth and metastasis of hormone-independent rat (AT6.1) and human (PC-3) prostatic carcinoma cell lines, in part through a direct inhibition of prostate cancer cell growth (Yamaoka et al, 1993; Miki et al, 1998). Interestingly, in clinical trials of TNP-470 for prostate cancer, increases in serum PSA have been observed, despite predicted antitumor effects, with reversal after removal of the drug; in vitro, increased PSA transcription and protein levels were observed after TNP-470 exposure (Horti et al, 1999).

Agents that disrupt the remodeling of extracellular matrix required for blood vessel growth inhibit angiogenesis. For example, minocycline, a semi-synthetic tetracycline with anticollagenase properties, decreased tumor-induced angiogenesis severalfold in vivo (Tamargo et al, 1991). The matrix metalloproteinase inhibitors appear to have a similar profile of activity (see later). Finally, suramin, an antiparasitic compound originally developed nearly 75 years ago for use as a trypanocidal agent, is a potent antitumor agent (La Rocca et al, 1990). Suramin inhibits binding of a large number of growth factors to their receptors, including angiogenic factors such as bFGF (Stein, 1993). Suramin and its analogs have anti-angiogenic properties both in vitro and in vivo (Gagliardi et al, 1998; Bocci et al, 1999).

Proteolytic Products of Inactive Molecules. Growth inhibition of metastases by the primary tumor has been observed both in animal models and anecdotally in human tumors. Based on this observation, a potent angiogenesis

inhibitor call angiostatin was isolated from the urine of mice bearing the murine Lewis lung carcinoma (O'Reilly et al, 1994). **This 38-kD protein is a cleaved internal fragment of the first four kringle domains of plasminogen** (Cao et al, 1996). Human prostate cancer cell lines PC-3, DU145, and LNCaP express enzymatic activity capable of cleaving bioactive angiostatin from plasminogen (Gately et al, 1996); in addition to this serine proteinase activity, a macrophage metalloelastase and matrix metalloproteinase 3 (MMP-3 or stomelysin) can catalyze the cleaving of angiostatin from plasminogen (Dong et al, 1997; Lijen et al, 1998). By rendering endothelium refractory to angiogenic stimuli, systemically administered angiostatin inhibited primary tumor growth with no obvious toxicity or tumor resistance (O'Reilly et al, 1996). Although the precise mechanism whereby angiostatin inhibits endothelial cell migration and proliferation is unknown, binding studies reveal a site distinct from plasminogen binding. Surprisingly, angiostatin was found to bind to the α/β subunits of adenosine triophosphate synthase, and antibodies directed against the α subunit reduced angiostatin binding by 50% and reduced angiostatin's inhibition of endothelial cell growth by 90% (Moser et al, 1999). Among the implications of this observation is the potential that endothelial cells—which must survive in oxygen-poor tumor environments—may be capable of producing ATP in a process that does not require oxygen (Barinaga, 1999).

Using the same rationale—tumors produce inhibitors of angiogenesis—another proteolytic product of an inactive molecule was identified by the same group who isolated angiostatin: **endostatin, a 20-kD carboxyl-terminal fragment of collagen XVIII, was isolated from conditioned media from a murine hemangioendothelioma cell line** (O'Reilly et al, 1997). **Endostatin inhibited endothelial cell proliferation and induced regression of established tumors to microscopic dormancy.** Endostatin induces G_1 arrest in endothelial cells and treatment of bovine endothelial cells caused apoptosis, with a reduction in anti-apoptotic protein BCL2 and $BCLX_L$ expression (Dhanabal et al, 1999). Endostatin dose-dependently inhibited VEGF-induced endothelial cell migration (Yamaguchi et al, 1999), and, using an adenoviral vector to express large quantities of endostatin in vivo, tumor growth and metastases were significantly inhibited (Sauter et al, 2000). Like angiostatin, enzymatic cleavage of endostatin from collagen XVIII results from the activities of cathepsin L (Felbor et al, 2000) and several members of the elastase family (Wen et al, 1999).

Endogenous Angiogenesis Inhibitors. The interferons (α, β, and γ) are a pleiotropic family of glycoproteins, first identified based on antiviral activities, which influence a host of cellular functions and the immune system and have antitumor effects in a few, but not most, malignancies (Grander et al, 1998). **Interferons (INF) inhibit angiogenesis** (Sidky et al, 1987). In renal cell, bladder, and prostate carcinoma cell lines, bFGF expression and protein production were downregulated by IFN-α and IFN-β but not IFN-γ (Singh et al, 1995; Dinnet et al, 1998). Similarly, IFN-β and IFN-γ inhibited the induced expression of IL-8, an important factor in angiogenesis (Oliveira et al, 1992). The angiogenesis, tumorigenicity, and metastasis of a highly metastatic clone of an androgen-independent prostate cancer cell line, PC-3M, was significantly inhibited after those cells were transfected with murine IFN-β cDNA and constitutively produced high levels of IFN-β (Dong et al, 1999).

One of the first demonstrations that inhibitors of angiogenesis could act as tumor suppressors was made when a 140-kD protein was identified in the conditioned media of hamster cells and hamster-human hybrids that possessed potent anti-angiogenic qualities (Rastinejad et al, 1989). This protein was identified as thrombospondin (Good et al, 1990), the ubiquitous adhesive glycoprotein, of which several protein fragments retained anti-angiogenic qualities (Tolsma et al, 1993). **Thrombospondin inhibits neovascularization in vivo and endothelial cell migration in vitro** (Volpert et al, 1995) **and induces apoptosis in endothelial cells** (Jimenez et al, 2000). Similiar to the suppression of metastases by a primary tumor leading to the isolation of angiostatin, high levels of circulating thrombospondin also appear to inhibit angiogenesis: in a fibrosarcoma tumor model that produces large quantities of thrombospondin, the metastatic growth of a highly metastatic melanoma line (B16/F10) was suppressed (Volpert et al, 1998).

Protease Inhibitors. **The proteolytic degradation of extracellular matrix by "invading" endothelial cells and vessels is a critical step in establishing neovascularity.** Matrix metalloproteinases (MMPs) are a family of metal-dependent enzymes with substrate-specific proteolytic activity: for example, MMP-1, MMP-8 and MMP13 are collagenases, MMP-2 is a gelatinase A, and MMP-9 is a gelatinase B. **Balancing the activity of these proteases are endogenous inhibitors, known as tissue inhibitors of metalloproteinase (TIMPs), which bind tightly in a noncovalent fashion to the MMPs** (Moses, 1997). The observation that certain tissues, like cartilage, are resistant to vascular invasion has lead to the isolation of inhibitors of MMPs and neovascularity (Moses et al, 1990, 1991, 1992). Polyamines, such as spermine and spermidine, induce angiogenesis in chick embryos; this effect is blocked by TIMP-1 and TIMP-2 (Takigawa et al, 1990). TIMP-1 also inhibits the endothelial cell response to bFGF, in part through inhibition of endothelial cell migration (Johnson et al, 1994). Other inhibitors of angiogenesis have been isolated from cartilage, such as the contractile protein troponin (Moses, 1999). A synthetic, low-molecular-weight, MMP inhibitor batimastat (BB-94) has been shown to decrease tumor burden and increase survival in a number of xenograft models (Davies et al, 1993), including models of prostate cancer invasion (Knox at al, 1998) and local tumor growth (Lein et al, 2000).

Plasmin, a protease with a broad spectrum of substrate activity, is cleaved from plasminogen by urokinase plasminogen activator (u-PA), with generation of plasmin being most pronounced when u-PA is bound to its receptor. There is a good correlation between the amount of plasmin bound to the tumor cell surface and the extent to which a basement membrane substrate is degraded (Cohen et al, 1991). **Inhibitors of u-PA action, such as high-affinity inhibitors of the u-PA receptor, can significantly reduce angiogenesis in vitro and in vivo** (Min et al, 1996). In a model of metastatic prostate cancer, expression of a mutant u-PA that retains receptor binding but not proteolytic activity results in a reduction in tumor growth, metastases, and microvessel density (Evans et al, 1997).

Thalidomide. The potent teratogen thalidomide produces dysmelia, or stunted limb growth, in humans. Originally developed as a seemingly safe sedative, an association between limb defects and maternal thalidomide use was reported (McBride, 1961). It is now known that thalidomide has potent anti-angiogenic qualities, which may be the cause of limb growth abnormalities. Thalidomide inhibits FGF-2–induced angiogenesis in vivo (D'Amato et al, 1994). Vessels that did form in experimental animals exposed to thalidomide were immature, with poorly formed cell junctions and an incomplete basement membrane.

Exploiting this anti-angiogenic quality, clinical trials of thalidomide in hormone-refractory prostate cancer are underway (Figg et al, 1999). In particular, a phase III trial combining thalidomide and docetaxel (Taxotere) with docetaxel alone is being conducted. Interestingly, thalidomide has been shown to increase PSA expression for the prostate cancer cell line LNCaP (Dixon et al, 1999).

Avastin. Avastin is a humanized monoclonal antibody that neutralizes the angiogenic factor VEGF (Ferrara et al, 2005; van Spronsen et al, 2005). Avastin is the first clearly anti-angiogenic agent to be approved for the treatment of cancer. Randomized clinical trials have shown that Avastin can prolong survival of patients with metastatic colon and breast cancers when combined with conventional chemotherapies for these malignancies. In kidney cancer, as discussed earlier in this chapter, Avastin was shown to delay progression in patients with metastatic disease (Yang et al, 2003). Studies comparing standard chemotherapy regimens to chemotherapy plus Avastin are now ongoing or planned for prostate and bladder cancers.

Small Molecules. A large number of tyrosine kinase receptor antagonists are being developed for the treatment of cancer. Among these, a number have been developed with specific affinity for the VEGF receptor. Recently, studies of two of these drugs, sorafenib (BAY-43-9006) and Sutent (SU11248), have demonstrated significant antitumor activity in renal cell carcinoma, a cancer driven in large part by VEGF. Both drugs have been found to lead to significant disease remissions and prolonged stable disease and survival. Although both drugs act on a number of tyrosine kinase receptors expressed by both tumor and endothelium, such as PDGFR and raf kinase, the major mechanism of action is thought to take place at the endothelial level via antagonism of VEGFR1. Both drugs are nearing approval and are expected to revolutionize the treatment of advanced kidney cancer.

MOUSE MODELS OF MALIGNANCY

Recent advances in molecular biology have led to the identification of gene alterations specific to malignancies. There is now a critical need to decode the functional significance of the alterations identified. **Whereas analysis on the cellular level provides insight into gene function, cancer grows, progresses, and metastasizes within an organism, not in cell culture. It is therefore necessary to study genetic changes in the context of an entire organism to understand the genetic events that predispose to the cell's malignant trans-**

formation and metastasis. Once the cellular pathways are understood within the context of an entire organism attempts can be made to manipulate those same pathways to prevent or cure the disease. The mouse has been an important experimental tool for research in general and cancer research specifically for many years. Recent advances in molecular biology have made the mouse model increasingly valuable. Currently these models are being exploited to understand cancer biology, to characterize cancers based on specific genetic changes, and to test novel targeted therapies.

Xenografts and Mutagenesis

Xenografting cancer cells into immunologically compromised mice has been used extensively, particularly in studying prostate carcinoma. Tumor cells are injected subcutaneously into athymic or SCID mice. As the cancer cells grow into a tumor, they are supported by mouse stromal elements. Because the mice are immunodeficient, they do not reject the xenografts and subcutaneous tumors form (Pretlow et al, 1993; Ellis et al, 1996; Klein et al, 1997).

Although xenografts allow the study of human tumors in an environment that more closely matches that seen in nature, there are several important disadvantages to this experimental design. First, xenografts do not allow the study of tumor development, because the cells initially implanted are already genetically advanced. This limits the model's ability to illuminate initial tumorigenic events. Second, the immunodeficient host was chosen because it is unable to mount an effective immune response against the tumor. Therefore, this model does not recapitulate the host/cancer interaction in most individuals, which are not immunodeficient. This not only has implications for studying cancer growth and metastasis but also in using the model to evaluate treatment modalities (Klausner, 1999).

A second experimental design better recapitulates the initiating events in tumor formation by exposing mice to carcinogens (Hitotsumachi et al, 1985). The mice that develop cancer are then studied in an effort to identify the genetic cause for the malignancy. This approach was used successfully to identify animals at increased risk for intestinal neoplasms secondary to mutations in the *Apc* gene (Su et al, 1992). While this mouse, the min mouse, is an excellent genetic model for human intestinal neoplasia, the induction of the mutation was not a controlled event and therefore not easily reproducible in other organ systems.

Recent advances in genetic engineering allowed researchers to move toward the controlled manipulation of the mouse genome. Targeting a specific gene of interest, which has already been implicated in tumorigenesis, allows researchers to understand the role of a specific gene in malignant transformation.

Advances in Genetic Engineering

In the early 1980s, methods were developed to introduce or delete genes of interest from mouse germlines. This allowed researchers to express oncogenes or delete tumor suppressor genes in an entire organism for the first time.

Transgenic mice were developed by introducing foreign DNA into a mouse oocyte by pronuclear injection. The fertilized oocyte would be screened for expression of the gene of interest and a phenotype could be identified (Bedell et al, 1997).

At the same time, the ability to culture pluripotent murine embryonic stem cells (ES cells) provided the cellular material for developing knockout mice (Evans and Kaufman, 1981; Bradley et al, 1984). Genes of interest could be deleted from ES cells in culture by exploiting the process of homologous recombination and then reintroduced into a developing mouse blastocyst. This produced a chimeric mouse. The ES cell populates all tissues in the growing mouse, including the gametes. The altered genome can then be passed onto subsequent generations through conventional breeding and mice could be selected that were entirely populated by the manipulated cells. The same technology used to "knock out" genes could also be used to "knock in" a gene of interest, providing an alternative to conventional transgenic models in which a gene is inserted into its proper chromosomal location.

Both transgenic and knockout mice allow the targeted manipulation of the murine genome in the otherwise intact host, producing an inherited genetic defect (Majzoub and Muglia, 1996). **The result is that a causal relationship between expression of a gene and tumor development could be studied in the context of a whole animal.**

Oncogene-Induced Tumorigenesis

Early experiments addressed the effect of introducing oncogenes. By selecting the appropriate promoter, it was possible to have tissue-specific expression of the gene of interest (Clarke, 2000). The SV40 large tumor T antigen was one of the earliest and most extensively studied oncogenes. It induces transformation by inhibiting the activity of both Tp53 and Rb (Lane and Crawford,1979; DeCaprio et al, 1988). When over-

expressed in a tissue-specific manner in mice, it was found to predispose cells to tumorigenesis in the choroid plexus (Palmiter et al, 1985). Similar experiments have confirmed these findings in other tissues such as pancreas and prostate (Ornitz et al, 1987; Greenberg et al, 1995). Transgenic experiments have not been confined to SV40. Other oncogenes, such as c-*Myc,* have been expressed in a tissue-specific manner and been found to induce neoplasia (Leder et al, 1986). In the case of genitourinary tumors, SV40, *Myc,* and *Akt* have all been shown to cause either HGPIN or frank cancer in multiple transgenic model systems (Gingrich et al, 1996; Ellwood-Yen et al, 2003; Majumder et al, 2004). In bladder cancer, SV40 and *Ras* have been shown to lead to invasive cancer versus superficial tumors, respectively (Bratt et al, 1999; Zhang et al, 2001; Gao et al, 2004).

Knockout Mice

Knockout mice are similar to transgenic mice except that the gene of interest is removed from the mouse genome instead of introduced. Mouse homologs of human tumor suppressor genes are deleted from ES cells, and the mouse is bred to produce a mouse hereditary tumor syndrome. The individual mice can then be bred to carry one copy of the normal gene (heterozygous knockout) or no copies of the gene (homozygous knockout). This experimental design has been useful in elucidating the role of some, but not all, tumor suppressor genes (Majzoub and Muglia, 1996).

The first tumor suppressor gene studied was *Tp53* (Donehower et al, 1992). Not only were the homozygous and heterozygous knockout mice predisposed to tumor formation, but the tumor types observed (soft tissue sarcomas, osteosarcomas, and lymphomas) also are often seen in Li-Fraumeni families (Malkin, 1994). In contrast to *Tp53, Rb* knockout mice have not recapitulated the human tumor syndrome; the mice develop pituitary adenomas, not retinoblastoma (Jacks et al, 1992). Interestingly, mice that have lost both *Rb* and a related tumor suppressor gene, *Rbl1,* have been found to develop retinal lesions (Lee et al, 1996). *Rbl1* has not been implicated in human hereditary retinoblastoma. This difference between mice and humans highlights the potential difficulty in extrapolating findings in murine to human malignancies.

In the case of genitourinary tumors, a number of knockout models have been instructive in elucidating the complex interaction between different genes implicated. For example, experiments examining knockout mice of *Cdkn1B (p27), Nkx3-1,* and *Pten* have been informative in understanding the phenotype associated with loss of gene function. Knockout of *CDKN1B (p27)* leads to prostate hyperplasia but not cancer (Gao et al, 2004; Gary et al, 2004), whereas loss of NKX3-1 leads to prostate dysplasia and HGPIN (Oda et al, 2000; Kim et al, 2002; Magee et al, 2003). On the other hand, *Pten* knockouts do develop prostate cancer but at an advanced age (Di Cristofano et al, 2001; Kwabi-Addo et al, 2001). Crosses of *Cdkn1B (p27)* with either *Nkx3-1* or *Pten* knockouts lead to acceleration of HGPIN and cancer, indicating that while *Cdkn1B (p27)* does not cause cancer alone, in conjunction with other genetic defects it may be permissive (Di Cristofano et al, 2001).

Conditional Knockout Mice

The phenotypic differences between mice and humans are only one of the limitations identified. Many genes with roles in tumorigenesis play important roles in development. Therefore, loss of these genes often leads to early developmental lethality, which precludes analysis of gene function in the adult. This is often secondary to loss of gene expression in an organ that is of questionable significance in studying the tumor suppressor.

Von Hippel-Lindau disease is an example of this limitation. Patients with von Hippel-Lindau disease develop multiple neoplasms. The tumor syndrome is caused by genetic defects in the *VHL* gene (see "Inherited Susceptibility to Cancer"). However, mice heterozygous for the *Vhl* gene have a normal phenotype. The homozygote knockout mice die during the second week of gestation because of inadequate vasculogenesis in the placenta or defects in fibronectin matrix assembly (Gnarra et al, 1997; Ohh et al, 1998). Although these findings are clearly important in understanding the function of the *VHL* tumor suppressor gene in development, it would be useful to elucidate the effect of gene loss after the animal has reached adulthood.

Selective deletion of genes once the mouse reached maturity became possible in 1988 when Sauer and Henderson demonstrated that the cre protein isolated from bacteriophage could be used to induce recombination events in mammalian cells at genetically engineered sites. This allowed the mouse to develop normally until exposed to the cre protein, at which point the cells exposed would delete the gene of interest. Conditional knockouts of the *Apc* gene are allowed to develop normally until adulthood. Exposure of the colonic mucosa to cre leads to loss of the *Apc* gene in some cells and the development of colon carcinoma. This more closely recapitulates the chain of events that leads to colon carcinoma (Shibata et al, 1997). A number of conditional knockouts of the prostate have been made using a Probasin-cre mouse model. Conditional knockout of both *Pten* alleles in the prostate leads to rapid and completely penetrant prostate cancer, which is androgen dependent and progresses to androgen independence and metastasis (Wang et al, 2003). A conditional *Nkx3-1* knockout was also made, in which HGPIN is seen, but without some of the morphologic changes seen when *Nkx3-1* is knocked out during fetal life (Magee et al, 2003).

Future Directions

The mouse models described in the preceding sections are now being used to study cancer gene signatures using the latest genomic and proteomic tools. These signatures are then being correlated with human cancers to categorize individual tumors better. For example, certain cancers appear to be driven by *Myc* and have a distinct gene expression profile. Others are dependent on loss of *Pten*. Better categorization will enable better prognostication and better treatment selection using modern targeted drugs. Mouse models are also being used to test drug efficacy. One example is the use of mTOR inhibition to treat tumors generated by activated Akt or loss of *Pten*. One study showed that mTOR is required for Akt-driven HGPIN and that treatment with the mTOR antagonist rapamycin prevented HGPIN development (Majumder

et al, 2004). Markers of drug activity are also being explored using these mouse models to provide a manner for clinicians to follow the effects of drug treatment. For example, at the University of California at Los Angeles, investigators have shown that S6 kinase can be used to determine if mTOR activity has been shut down using rapamycin (Thomas et al, 2004). This is now being tested in a clinical trial of the rapamycin analog CCI-779 in men undergoing radical prostatectomy for high-risk prostate cancer.

KEY POINTS: MOUSE MODELS OF MALIGNANCY

- Mouse models of cancer provide an experimental platform to understand and treat cancer.

- Transgenic mice are created by introducing an exogenous gene into the mouse genome. These genes can cause cancer and provide a model to study the role of a single gene in cancer causation and progression. An example is the role of the *Myc* oncogene in the causation of prostate cancer.

- Knockout mice are created by removing a specific gene in the mouse through homologous recombination in embryonic stem cells and provide the means to study the effect of loss of genetic function in cancer. An example is the role of the *PTEN* tumor suppressor in prostate cancer causation.

- Conditional transgenic and knockout mice allow the investigator to control gene expression in specific organs. This is particularly necessary for genes that are toxic to specific organs or necessary for embryonic development.

- Transgenic models can be used to test new drugs preclinically.

MOLECULAR DIAGNOSIS IN ONCOLOGY

Pathologic examination is a cornerstone of diagnosis and treatment of malignancy. Information derived from gross and microscopic histopathologic analysis allows clinicians not to just determine the type of tumor but also to choose additional therapy and predict the patient's response. The standard of practice remains microscopic interpretation of hematoxylin and eosin–stained tissue sections; however, the field has not been static over the past 40 years. Special adjuvant techniques, such as immunohistochemistry and cytogenetics, are often useful in establishing a diagnosis. In the future, molecular techniques may allow more accurate identification of tumor subtypes and prediction of prognosis (Jones and Fletcher, 1999).

Immunohistochemistry

Immunohistochemical analysis is clearly the most widespread use of molecular analysis. This is for several reasons. First, it is the most similar to conventional light microscopy, which allows the technique to be more rapidly disseminated. Second, it can be rapidly adapted to new markers. Once a novel marker is identified an antibody can be rapidly developed and used for staining. Third, the antigen of interest can be localized to specific cells by simple visual inspection. Many of the newer techniques cannot easily separate normal from tumor.

Immunohistochemistry is performed by designing monoclonal antibodies that bind to a molecule of interest. Formalin-fixed, paraffin-imbedded tissue can be then stained with the monoclonal antibody to assess for expression to the protein of interest.

Immunohistochemistry has several important uses in oncology. Immunohistochemistry is crucial to the accurate identification of tumors of uncertain origin, if conventional light microscopy cannot identify the tumor (Jones and Fletcher, 1999). Poorly differentiated neoplasms can be difficult to identify the cell of origin. This can be crucial for instituting proper therapy. For example, PSA staining has proven to be a useful adjunct to identify adenocarcinomas of uncertain origin as prostatic (Harper et al, 1996). A second example is the use of α-methylacyl-coenzyme-A racemase (AMACR) in identification of small foci of prostate carcinoma in the prostate. AMACR mRNA expression in malignant prostate specimens is approximately ninefold higher than in normal prostate tissues and by immunohistochemical staining is overexpressed in prostate cancer and HGPIN. Because of the high sensitivity and specificity of AMACR for prostate cancer, it has become a common addition to the pathologist's armamentarium in diagnosing prostate cancer. Cancer markers are not limited to prostate cancer. For example, they have also proven extremely useful in determining if adenocarcinomas presenting in the bladder are primary or metastatic lesions (Torenbeek et al, 1998).

A second use of immunohistochemistry is to stain for prognostic biomarkers. The subclassification of tumors into aggressive and indolent on the basis of the molecular profile has the potential to radically change practice (Golub et al, 1999). For example, prostate cancers of identical stage and grade can have variable clinical courses. The ability to identify patients who have a poor prognosis and/or those that will respond to a particular treatment independent of grade and stage would be of significant clinical utility. Although still experimental, *TP53* in bladder cancer is emerging as a potential independent indicator of aggressive disease and may prove to be useful in stratifying patients for neoadjuvant chemotherapy (Esrig et al, 1994; Cote et al, 1997).

Lastly, molecular identification of tumor targets for therapy will become increasingly prevalent in the near future. The best example of this is the use of immunohistochemistry to identify the presence of HER2/NEU receptors in breast cancer. The HER2/NEU receptor not only provides prognostic information in breast cancer, but if the receptor is present it also provides a molecular target for antibody therapy. Preliminary data have demonstrated that the antibody Herceptin is effective in treating patients whose tumors express the receptor (Lebwohl and Canetta, 1999).

Molecular Genetics

The search for meaningful molecular prognostic markers has not been limited to immunohistochemistry. Karyotypic or cytogenetic information can be used to identify tumor types and predict outcome. It has been most widely used in hematopoietic neoplasms. Karyotyping allows the identification of abnormalities of chromosome number and translocations. Chronic myeloid leukemia (CML) is one of the best examples of the use of karyotypic analysis. The Philadelphia chromosome, a fusion of chromosomes 9 and 22, is found in 90% of CML patients. The translocation gives rise to chimeric genes or fusion proteins that are believed to contribute to the malignancy (Thijsen et al, 1999). Karyotypic analysis of other hematopoietic neoplasms has also been found to contribute prognostic information independent of morphologic features (Jones and Fletcher, 1999), and analysis of tumor-specific translocations in pediatric tumors has become the standard of care in many centers (Pui, 1995).

Conventional karyotyping has several disadvantages. Because cytogenetic analysis has to be performed on actively dividing cells, it is more difficult to perform on tumors that are not rapidly dividing. In addition, because karyotyping can only be performed on fresh tissue, the need for a karyotype has to be known before the tissue is fixed. Technical advances have circumvented these problems to a certain degree. Reverse transcriptase polymerase chain reaction (RT-PCR) and fluorescent in-situ hybridization (FISH) allow the study of genetic abnormalities in cells that are formalin-fixed, embedded in paraffin, and not actively dividing. RT-PCR uses the PCR for rapid amplification of RNA of specific translocations. It is particularly useful in studying fusion proteins and has been used to provide prognostic information in leukemia and sarcoma (Huang et al, 1993; Kawai et al, 1998). FISH allows the labeling of specific regions of DNA, using sequence specific oligonucleotides to identify chromosomal aberrations. It has been used to identify translocations in sarcomas and the 12p isochromosome in testis tumors (Nagao et al, 1996; Blough et al, 1998).

Karyotypic abnormalities have been identified in a wide range of urologic malignancies. Multiple gains and losses have been identified in prostate carcinoma (Bova and Isaacs, 1996), and karyotypic abnormalities at 3p were instrumental in identifying the *VHL* tumor suppressor gene in clear cell renal carcinoma (Cohen et al, 1979; Pathak et al, 1982). **Still, the urologic malignancy most closely linked to a karyotypic abnormality is testicular cancer. A 12p isochromosome was first identified in testis tumors in the 1980s** (Atkin and Baker, 1982), **and experimentally this cytogenetic hallmark of testicular tumors has diagnostic and prognostic value** (Geurts van Kessel et al, 1993).

Differential Display Technology and the PCA3 Story

An early application of molecular genetics to cancer was to define genes expressed in cancer versus normal tissue. One such technology, differential display, involved comparing displayed mRNA species from cancer and normal alongside each other, then picking bands present in cancer and not normal and vice versa. This technology led to the early identification of numerous differentially expressed genes, including *PSCA*. One interesting gene identified in this manner was called *DD3*, because it was differentially expressed in prostate cancer (de Kok et al, 2002; Hessels et al, 2003; Tinzl et al, 2004). *DD3* encodes a nontranslated mRNA that is present 10- to 100-fold higher in prostate cancer than normal. It does not correlate with cancer stage or grade. Recently this discovery has been applied to prostate cancer diagnosis. In this assay, prostate cells shed into the urine after prostate massage are collected, converted to RNA, and subjected to quantitative PCR for PSA and *DD3* (now called *PCA3*). The presence of *PCA3* transcripts in PSA-producing cells implies the presence of prostate cancer. Two early reports suggest that this new assay has sensitivities ranging from 60% to 80% in the PSA 2.5 to 10 range, with specificities of 80% to 90%. One issue that needs to be addressed relates to data interpretability, because only 80% of patients had evaluable specimens; that is, prostate cells were shed in only approximately 80% of patients. Nevertheless, this test promised to add to the diagnostic armamentarium, particularly in men with negative biopsies at high suspicion for prostate cancer. If these patients are *PCA3* positive, it is likely they need additional biopsies to identify a probable cancer (de Kok et al, 2002; Hessels et al, 2003; Tinzl et al, 2004).

Microarray Technology

Advances in basic science research now allow the simultaneous analysis of thousands of genes. The integration of computers with gene or protein arrays has made it possible to identify tumors based solely on their molecular characteristics (Golub et al, 1999; Alizadeh et al, 2000). It is important to recognize that at the current time these methods of analysis are only beginning to make inroads into clinical practice and significant technical barriers still exist to the routine clinical application of this technology.

DNA microarrays contain thousands of DNA sequences organized in an area no larger than a microscope slide. They can contain upward of 40,000 genes, roughly half of the predicted number of genes in the human genome. To determine the expression profile of interest, RNA transcripts are isolated from the cells of interest, labeled with a fluorescent dye, and allowed to bind to the DNA on the microarray. Alternatively, to identify DNA sequence mutations or polymorphisms, DNA from the cell of interest can be labeled and allowed to bind. An automated image-capturing device then uses the intensity of the signal for each of the genes on the array, to quantitate expression (Diehn et al, 2000).

DNA microarray technology has revolutionized the laboratory and promised to revolutionize clinical medicine. Already, genes identified by microarray technology have entered clinical practice. One example is *AMACR*, which was discussed earlier. *AMACR* was identified by multiple groups as being expressed by a majority of prostate cancers using microarray technology. *AMACR* is now a common criterion for a diagnosis of prostate cancer. Microarrays have also been used in the laboratory to understand gene function. By cataloguing every gene whose expression is upregulated or downregulated by a single genetic manipulation, the function of said gene can be deduced. Our understanding of the *MYC* oncogene, for example, has been fundamentally changed by the ability to measure all genes affected by MUC overexpression in cultured cells.

In the field of prognosis, microarray technology has multiple uses. First, it can help categorize tumors at the genetic level. For example, clear cell and papillary renal cancers have vastly different, easily definable expression array signatures (Liou et al, 2004; Kosari et al, 2005; Maina et al, 2005; Yang et al, 2005). Many leukemias and lymphomas are subtyped by microarray technology. Breast cancers cans be categorized according to cell of origin (basal or luminal) using gene expression microarrays. In addition to simple categorization, gene expression microarrays promise to improve our ability to predict the clinical course of individual tumors. Already a plethora of manuscripts have identified combinations of genes that predict for poor or good outcome (Latil et al, 2003; Glinsky et al, 2005). Recently, a number of papers have found common signatures of metastatic tumors that can be identified in the primary cancer (Glinsky et al, 2005; Minn et al, 2005; O'Donnell et al, 2005). Although few of these discoveries have yet made it to the clinic, it is likely that gene arrays will be a common platform for cancer diagnosis, prognosis, and treatment planning over the next decade. In particular, they will be used for selection of targeted drugs and for entry into clinical trials.

Other potential applications include the screening of tumor DNA for specific mutations (Hacia, 1999) and genotyping of polymorphisms affecting disease susceptibility (Sapolsky et al, 1999). Once it is possible to identify high-risk individuals on the basis of their genotype, aggressive screening or prophylactic measures can be instituted in these individuals.

Proteomics and Epitomics

Microarray technology allows the analysis of multiple molecular targets. Unfortunately, expression analysis is limited to mRNA, which is imprecise because it may or may not reflect actual protein expression or activity. Proteomics is emerging as a field to rapidly identify protein expression. Proteins isolated from body fluids or cells are ionized by matrix-assisted laser desorption ionization (MALDI) or electrospray ionization (ESI). This produces gas phase ions, which produce a reproducible pattern when analyzed by a mass spectrometer. Comparing the pattern produced to a database of known patterns identifies the protein of interest (Yates, 2000). As tumor-specific patterns of protein expression are identified, antibodies for microarray can be developed that can be used to isolate the proteins of interest for analysis. This will have an immense impact on clinical diagnosis in the coming years.

One interesting new offshoot related to proteomics has been called "epitomics." In this technology, investigators take advantage of the host's B cell response to cancer epitopes to aid diagnosis. For example, AMACR is pathognomonic for prostate cancer. Detection of autoantibodies that recognize *AMACR* in an individual's blood may signal the presence of prostate cancer (Sreekumar et al, 2004). Thousands of proteins are arrayed on slides and a patient's serum is added to them. Individual spots, such as that for *AMACR*, can then be scored. This technology may also be used to identify potential new targets and therapeutics for cancer.

New Modalities Not Ready for Routine Clinical Use

Although these new diagnostic modalities hold promise for a new era in applying molecular biology to the routine care of patients, it is important to recognize that these techniques are not the standard of care. Currently, for urologic malignancies, there is not a single tissue marker, detectable by any means, that has entered routine clinical practice as a prognostic marker. Only immunohistochemistry has entered routine clinical practice and then only for the diagnosis of tumors, not to stratify patient prognosis. It is hoped that molecular profiling of genitourinary malignancies will eventually prove to be of prognostic value and will become routine clinical practice.

KEY POINTS: MOLECULAR DIAGNOSIS IN ONCOLOGY

- Advances in molecular biology have led to new diagnostic modalities in pathology, including immunohistochemical and cytogenetic diagnosis.

- One example includes the ability to diagnosis prostate cancer based on expression of the gene *AMACR*.

- cDNA microarray refers to the ability to screen for expression of thousand of genes simultaneously on silicon chips. This technology has revolutionized the categorization of individual tumor types based on differences in gene expression.

- Proteomics is a new technology that can distinguish thousands of proteins simultaneously.

RATIONAL DRUG DEVELOPMENT

Perhaps the best way to understand rational drug development is to consider how drugs were discovered in the past. Many of the most effective anticancer drugs are the result of serendipity. Consider, for example, the discovery of cisplatin, the chemotherapeutic agent that has transformed testicular carcinoma from a disease with an ominous prognosis to one in which cure is expected. In 1961, Barnett Rosenberg at Michigan State University was studying the effects of electrical fields on the behavior of *Escherichia coli*. He found cell division was inhibited but not cell growth: the *E. coli* grew in long filamentous forms. The platinum-containing electrodes produce a soluble platinum salt that, when isolated, produced the same effects on the *E. coli* in the absence of an electrical current (Rosenberg et al, 1967). Further work identified the *cis* configuration of these platinum-containing compounds that inhibited cell division with minimal cell toxicity, an ideal attribute for an anticancer agent. By applying this compound to animal tumors, it was found that cisplatin could cure estab-

lished tumors (Rosenberg et al, 1969). Based on the success of cisplatin clinically, second-generation agents with less toxicity have been designed: these new agents, such as carboplatin, build from the basic structure of cisplatin. As can be seen in this example, a serendipitous discovery leads to a widely used chemotherapeutic agent with second-, third- and fourth-generation compounds being developed. It was not known until much later that cisplatin damages DNA, producing major adducts and leading to unwinding of the duplex: in fact, it appears to be a specific cisplatin-DNA-protein complex that is required for the anticancer activity of this drug (Ohndorf et al, 1999).

Unlike classic drug discovery, **rational drug discovery seeks to identify and exploit specific targets in a biochemical pathway. This may be through blocking particular receptor/ligand interaction, through inhibiting the enzyme activity of a particular kinase or phosphatase or altering the final protein product of a gene.** For example, the oncogene *RAS* is mutated in many cancers: in one study of pancreatic cancer, *KRAS* was mutated in every tumor (Rozenblum et al, 1997). *RAS* is a small GTP-binding protein that transduces signals from the cell surface to the nucleus, ultimately leading to cell division. Mutations in *RAS* lead to unregulated and continuous signals for cell division. Although this target has been known for some time, inhibitors of *RAS* were not forthcoming. In order for *RAS* to be become functional, however, a particular post-translational modification is required—the addition of a farnesyl group to a specific cysteine at the carboxyl terminus of the protein. The enzyme responsible for this addition is known as farnesyl transferase (Scharovsky et al, 2000). Specific inhibitors of farnesyl transferase and, ultimately, functional *RAS*, are emerging as novel anticancer agents: early clinical trial results hint at clinical activity of these agents (Adjei et al, 2000).

As can be seen in the two previous examples of drug discovery, there are clear differences between medicinal approaches and rational drug development. In the former, a general target is identified, such as cell division. Lead compounds are chosen, based on activity in other systems or on a history as a folk remedy, such as paclitaxel being extracted from the yew tree (Mann, 1994). Successful approaches may require serendipity, the screening of a large number of compounds with little or no bias for potential activity. Advances are incremental, like the development of carboplatin from cisplatin. Screening for activity is often nonspecific: does this agent produce reduction in the size of an animal tumor? In rational drug development, on the other hand, a specific enzyme (in the case of farnesyl transferase), receptor, or signaling pathway is targeted, with a clear understanding of the expected endpoint. Screening for drug activity is often more precise: does this receptor antagonist block binding of the ligand? With the increased understanding of the nuances within the biology of cancer, many more targets for this rational approach will be identified and exploited. Many have already been explored in this chapter: rapamycin to antagonize the PTEN/Akt/mTOR pathway, Iressa and Erbitux to block EGFR activation, Avastin to neutralize VEGF, atrasentan to block endothelin receptor, and Herceptin to block *HER2/NEU*. This is the future of molecular medicine and urologic cancer!

- Advances in our understanding of the molecular biology of cancer have led to the concept of rational drug development based on the individual and shared characteristics of tumors.

- The process involved target identification and then the design of drugs, both small molecular and antibody, that bind to and activate or inactivate the target.

- Gleevec and Herceptin are among the first rationally designed drugs that target the *BCR-ABL* and *HER2/NEU* genes, respectively.

- In urologic cancers, examples include Avastin targeting VEGF and atrasentan targeting the endothelin receptor.

GENE THERAPY

Gene therapy compromises a large and diverse set of therapeutic interventions unified by one common element: DNA. **Whereas standard medical approaches to disease use drugs, in gene therapy, DNA is the drug.** The theory behind gene therapy is straightforward. In many hereditary diseases, such as cystic fibrosis, characterized by a mutation in a specific gene, the correct copy of that gene is replaced (Whitsett et al, 1992). In cancers known for mutations in *TP53*, for example, a correct (or wild type) copy of the *TP53* gene can lead cells out a proliferating pathway into a programmed cell death. **Another approach is to express a foreign gene within a cell that, when exposed to an otherwise harmless drug, produces a toxin that kills the cell. For example, the herpes simplex thymidine kinase gene encodes an enzyme not normally expressed by mammalian cells. After exposure to the antiviral drug ganciclovir, cells expressing the enzyme will undergo cell death** (Moolten et al, 1990; Culver et al, 1992). **This "suicide gene" approach is also used when the bacterial enzyme cytosine deaminase is artificially expressed in mammalian cells, which will metabolize innocuous 5-fluorocytosine to the toxin 5-fluorouracil** (Mullen et al, 1992). One of the benefits of this approach is the so-called bystander effect: not only is the cell expressing the gene killed, but a great number of neighboring cells are killed as well (Pierrefite-Carle et al, 1999). In fact, the amplification of cell death may be 100- to 1000-fold greater than the original number of cells expressing the gene (Steiner et al, 2000). Although the precise mechanism of this effect is still unknown, it may involve gap junctions between neighboring cells (Mesnil et al, 2000).

Although the theory behind gene therapy may be simple, the practice and application of gene therapy is not. **Although the insertion of genes into cells outside the body, or ex vivo, is relatively easy** (Sanda et al, 1994), **insertion of those genes into the specific target cells in the body is not. One approach to overcome this problem is the use of tissue-specific promoters and enhancers.** As mentioned earlier, in the section on transcriptional regulation, while the entire DNA sequence is present in every somatic cell in the body, only certain genes are expressed by certain cells. This is the reason why PSA is

prostate specific. By physically linking the gene to be expressed with a promoter specifically recognizing the tissue, one can get expression of the gene only in the cell of interest. There is tremendous variability in the activities of a promoter/enhancer to drive the transcription of a particular gene: some viral promoters are quite active, but many tissue-specific promoters are not.

The largest obstacle to systemic in-vivo gene therapy is the lack of an effective gene transfer, or, put simply, getting the gene both to and into the target cells (Rodriguez et al, 1999). Local injection approaches have been widely used to overcome the delivery problems (Herman et al, 1999), but in the presence of widely metastatic disease this strategy is clearly inadequate. **Vectors are the vehicles to get genes into cells** (Steiner et al, 2000). Our bodies are designed to limit the entry of foreign DNA or RNA into cells, which is precisely what viruses are designed to do. Viral vectors are commonly employed in clinical trials of gene therapy. **Retroviruses integrate into the DNA of a cell, leading to stable expression, but transduce only dividing cells, thus limiting efficient gene transfer** (Miller, 1992). **Adenoviruses, on the other hand, infect both dividing and nondividing cells, leading to more efficient gene transfer: gene expression is transient, limiting expression. Adenoviruses are also very immunogenic, limiting repeat dosing.**

The adenovirus usually used for introducing genes into cells has been neutered: the parts of the genome responsible for viral replication have been removed and, although the adenovirus can infect cells, it is unable replicate and induce cell lysis. By using an adenovirus that retains the ability to replicate (so-called replication competent adenovirus), cells that are infected will yield large numbers of virus and, in the process, undergo cell lysis. In the absence of cell specificity, such a virus is not unlike the "garden variety" adenovirus responsible for the common cold: any infected cell could potentially undergo lysis. **To specifically target prostate cancer cells, a replication competent adenovirus has been designed that will only replicate in cells making PSA. This virus (CN706) can eliminate established PSA-producing prostate cancer tumors (LNCaP) in a mouse model** (Rodriguez et al, 1997). By injecting this virus directly into the prostate, it is anticipated many cells in the gland will become infected but only those cells (benign and malignant) that make PSA will allow replication and cell lysis.

- Gene therapy is another form of rational drug development in which genes are transferred directly to tumors.

- Multiple strategies have been used or are envisioned. Examples include delivery of toxic genes directly into tumor tissue and replacement of absent tumor suppressors directly into tumor cells.

- The promise of gene therapy still awaits fulfillment. Difficulties include adequate gene delivery as well as controlled gene delivery. Many exciting developments, such as conditional promoters to control gene delivery, provide hope that gene therapy will someday become a reality.

SECTION V

SUGGESTED READINGS

Fearon ER: Human cancer syndromes: Clues to the origin and nature of cancer. Science 1997;278:1043-1050.

Feinberg AP: The epigenetics of cancer etiology. Semin Cancer Biol 2004;14:427-432.

Guttmacher AE, Collins FS: Genomic medicine—a primer. N Engl J Med 2002;347:1512-1520.

Kastan MB, Bartek J: Cell-cycle checkpoints and cancer. Nature 2004;432:316-323.

Massague J: G1 cell-cycle control and cancer. Nature 2004;432:298-306.

Rebbeck TR, Spitz M, Wu X: Assessing the function of genetic variants in candidate gene association studies. Nat Rev Genet 2004;5:589-597.

Sancar A, Lindsey-Boltz LA, Unsal-Kacmaz K, et al: Molecular mechanisms of mammalian DNA repair and the DNA damage checkpoints. Annu Rev Biochem 2004;73:39-85.

Watson J, Crick F: Molecular structure of nucleic acids: A structure for deoxyribose nucleic acid. Nature 1953;171:737-738.

tion to form a leading edge of the new capillary; (4) generation of the capillary lumen and formation of a tubelike structure; (5) basement membrane synthesis; and (6) recruitment of pericytes and vascular smooth muscle cells.

When converting to the angiogenic stage, endothelial cells will capture new properties that enable them to neovascularize the tissue (Hanahan and Folkman, 1996). When the new vessels are in place and the vascular network matures, the neovascular endothelial cells resume their quiescent phenotype (Darland and D'Amore, 1999). Several growth factors serve as stimuli for endothelial cell conversion to the angiogenic phenotype (Battegay, 1995). Vascular endothelial growth factor and fibroblast growth factor are two well-characterized and important angiogenic molecules that have a direct effect on endothelial cells.

The understanding of the angiogenic process and the isolation of potent and specific angiogenic growth factors have encouraged the use of these factors therapeutically (Isner and Asahara, 1998; Henry, 1999). Efforts have been aimed at incorporating the knowledge acquired in angiogenesis of ischemic tissues into practical approaches to vascularize bioengineered tissues.

Bioengineered tissues are usually supported by scaffolds of biocompatible matrices made from natural or artificial sources (Hubbel, 1995). Successful vascularization is dependent on the porosity of the supporting matrix. A positive correlation between the pore size of poly-L-lactic acid (PLLA) implants and the rate of vascularization has been observed (Mikos et al, 1993; Rotter et al, 1998).

Three approaches have been used for vascularization of bioengineered tissue: (1) incorporation of angiogenic factors in the bioengineered tissue; (2) seeding endothelial cells with other cell types in the bioengineered tissue; and (3) prevascularization of the matrix before cell seeding. Angiogenic growth factors may be incorporated into the bioengineered tissue before implantation to attract host capillaries and to enhance neovascularization of the implanted tissue. Angiogenic growth factors can be embedded in specific biomaterials and can be controlled to be released slowly (Eiselt et al, 1998). Cells can also be genetically engineered to secrete high levels of angiogenic proteins (Springer et al, 1998).

Another approach for enhancing angiogenesis employed cultured endothelial cells, which are incorporated into the bioengineered tissue before implantation. Human penile corpus cavernosum–derived smooth muscle cells and endothelial cells were seeded on biodegradable polymer scaffolds to reconstruct penile corporal tissue in vitro and in vivo (Park et al, 1999). The use of endothelial cells improved the formation of the engineered tissue. In another study, the addition of both endothelial cells and angiogenic growth factors (vascular endothelial growth factor) accelerated the formation of engineered muscle tissue (De Coppi et al, 2005). An alternative direction in vascularization of bioengineered tissue is the prevascularization of the supporting polymer before cell seeding. In this manner, the bioengineered tissue will be organized around the vascular network, providing sufficient tissue perfusion (Fontaine et al, 1995).

Despite the successes in bioengineering tissues consisting of thin layers of cells such as skin, a major challenge for tissue engineering in the future is the production of larger organs with more complex structures like the kidney. Tissues with a large mass of cells will require a vascular network of arteries, veins, and capillaries to deliver nutrients to each cell. The development of efficient methods to vascularize bioengineered tissues is critical for a successful outcome. There are many obstacles to be overcome before large entire tissue-engineered solid organs are produced. Recent developments in angiogenesis research may provide important knowledge and essential materials to accomplish this goal.

TISSUE ENGINEERING OF UROLOGIC STRUCTURES
Urethra

Various strategies have been proposed over the years for the regeneration of urethral tissue. Woven meshes of PGA without cells (Bazeed et al, 1983; Olsen et al, 1992) or with cells (Atala et al, 1992b) were used to regenerate urethras in various animal models. Naturally derived collagen-based materials such as small intestinal submucosa (Kropp et al, 1998), a bladder-derived acellular submucosa (Chen et al, 1999), and an acellular urethral submucosa (Sievert et al, 2000) have also been tried experimentally in various animal models for urethral reconstruction.

The bladder submucosa matrix (Chen et al, 1999) proved to be a suitable graft for repair of urethral defects in rabbits. The neourethras demonstrated a normal urothelial luminal lining and organized muscle bundles. These results were confirmed clinically in a series of patients with a history of failed hypospadias reconstruction wherein the urethral defects were repaired with human bladder acellular collagen matrices (Atala et al, 1999). The neourethras were constructed by anastomosis of the matrix in an onlay fashion to the urethral plate. The size of the neourethra ranged from 5 to 15 cm. After a 3-year follow-up, three of the four patients had a successful outcome in regard to cosmetic appearance and function (Fig. 17–3). One patient who had a 15-cm neourethra developed a subglanular fistula. The acellular collagen-based matrix eliminated the necessity of performing additional surgical procedures for graft harvesting, and both operative time and the potential morbidity from the harvest procedure were decreased. Similar results were obtained in pediatric and adult patients with urethral stricture disease by use of the same collagen matrices (Kassaby et al, 2000). **More than 120 pediatric and adult patients with urethral disease have been successfully treated in an onlay manner with a bladder-derived collagen-based matrix. One of its advantages over nongenital tissue grafts used for urethroplasty is that the material is "off the shelf."** This eliminates the necessity of additional surgical procedures for graft harvesting, which may decrease operative time, as well as the potential morbidity due to the harvest procedure.

These techniques, using nonseeded acellular matrices, were applied experimentally and clinically in a successful manner for onlay urethral repairs. However, when tubularized urethral repairs were attempted experimentally, adequate urethral tissue regeneration was not achieved and complications ensued, such as graft contracture and stricture formation (De Filippo et al, 2002a, 2002b). Autologous rabbit bladder epithelial and smooth muscle cells were grown and seeded onto

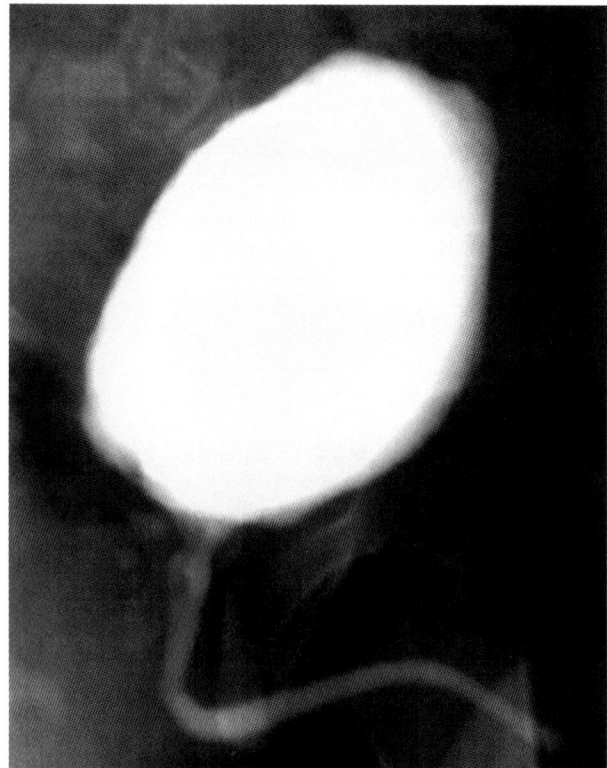

Figure 17–3. Urethrogram 6 months after surgery in a patient who had a portion of his urethra replaced by tissue engineering techniques.

preconfigured tubular matrices. Entire urethra segments were resected, and urethroplasties were performed with tubularized collagen matrices either seeded with cells or without cells. The tubularized collagen matrices seeded with autologous cells formed new tissue that was histologically similar to native urethra. The tubularized collagen matrices without cells led to poor tissue development, fibrosis, and stricture formation. These findings were recently confirmed clinically. A clinical trial using tubularized nonseeded small intestinal submucosa for urethral stricture repair was performed in eight evaluable patients. Two patients with short inflammatory strictures maintained urethral patency. Stricture recurrence developed in the other six patients within 3 months of surgery (le Roux, 2005).

The normal wound healing response to injury is well known, and this knowledge has been helpful in maximizing success for the engineering of tissues. At the time of tissue injury, cell ingrowth is initiated from the wound edges to cover the tissue defect. The cells from the edges of the native tissue are able to traverse short distances without any detrimental effects. If the wound is large, more than a few millimeters in distance or depth, increased collagen deposition, fibrosis, and scar formation ensue. Matrices implanted in wound beds are able to lengthen the distances that cells can traverse without initiating an adverse fibrotic response. However, these distances are also limited. The maximum distance that adjacent cells from the wound edge have to travel to form normal tissue over a biologic matrix is approximately 1 cm. Tissue defects greater than 1 cm that are treated with a matrix alone, without cells, usually have increased collagen deposition, increased fibrosis, and scar formation. Cell-seeded matrices implanted in wound beds are able to further lengthen the distance for normal tissue formation, without initiating an adverse fibrotic response. Studies in the field of tissue engineering have shown that very large defects, greater than 30 cm, can be successfully treated by use of cell-seeded scaffolds. This explains the described experimental and clinical results noted with urethral repair. Nonseeded matrices are able to replace urethral segments when they are used in an onlay fashion because of the short distances required for tissue ingrowth. However, if a tubularized urethral repair is needed, the matrices need to be seeded with autologous cells to avoid the risk of stricture formation and poor tissue development.

Bladder

Currently, gastrointestinal segments are commonly used as tissues for bladder replacement or repair. However, gastrointestinal tissues are designed to absorb specific solutes, whereas bladder tissue is designed for the excretion of solutes. **When gastrointestinal tissue is in contact with the urinary tract, multiple complications may ensue, such as infection, metabolic disturbances, urolithiasis, perforation, increased mucus production, and malignancy** (McDougal, 1992; Atala et al, 1993b; Kaefer et al, 1997, 1998). Because of the problems encountered with the use of gastrointestinal segments, numerous investigators have attempted alternative reconstructive procedures for bladder replacement or repair. These include autoaugmentation (Fig. 17–4) (Cartwright and Snow, 1989a, 1989b; Snow and Cartwright, 1999) and ureterocystoplasty (Bellinger, 1993; Churchill et al, 1993; Adams et al, 1998). In addition, alternative methods for bladder reconstruction have been explored, such as tissue expansion and tissue engineering with cell transplantation.

Tissue Expansion for Bladder Augmentation

A system of progressive dilation for ureters and bladders has been proposed but has not yet been attempted clinically (Lailas et al, 1996; Satar et al, 1999). In an animal experiment, rabbits underwent unilateral ureteral ligation at the ureterovesical junction. A catheter was threaded into the proximal ipsilateral ureter and connected to an injection port, which was secured subcutaneously. A saline-antibiotic solution was injected daily subcutaneously into the injection port. After 1 month of daily saline-antibiotic solution injections, the ureteral units were dilated at least 10-fold, and the diameter exceeded that of adjacent colon in each instance (Fig. 17–5). Augmentation cystoplasty was performed with the reconfigured dilated ureteral segment, resulting in an increased bladder capacity ranging from 190% to 380% (Lailas et al, 1996). In a similar system, a dilating indwelling catheter was used to dilate ureteral tissue in pigs (Ikeguchi et al, 1998).

A system for the progressive expansion of native bladder tissue has also been used for augmenting bladder volumes (Satar et al, 1999). Beagle dog bladders were divided horizontally into two segments, a superior bladder neoreservoir and an intact smaller bladder inferiorly with both ureters left intact and draining. A Silastic catheter was threaded into the newly formed, superiorly located neoreservoir and connected to an

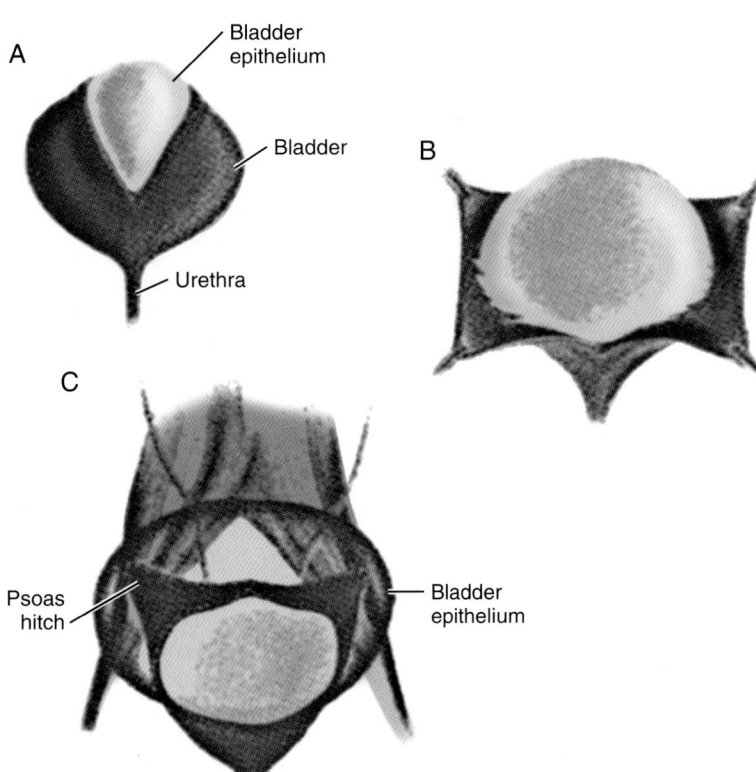

Figure 17–4. Autoaugmentation is performed by incising the detrusor (**A**) and stripping it from intact bladder epithelium (**B**), which allows the urothelial layer to bulge with bladder filling (**C**). (From Cartwright PC, Snow BW: Bladder autoaugmentation: Early clinical experience. J Urol 1989;142:505.)

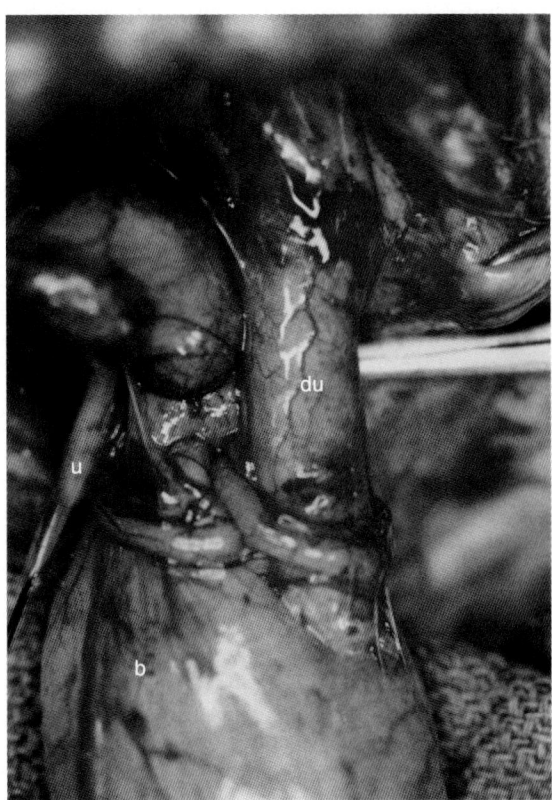

Figure 17–5. Progressive dilation can be performed in a normal-caliber ureter, which can subsequently be used for ureterocystoplasty. After placement of a ureteral dilation device, comparison is made of progressively dilated ureter (du) and native undilated ureter (u) coming off the bladder (b).

injection port, which was secured subcutaneously. Four weeks after surgery, a saline-antibiotic solution was injected daily into the palpable injection port, dilating the neoreservoir through the Silastic catheter. Within 30 days after progressive dilation, the neoreservoir volume was expanded at least 10-fold (Fig. 17–6). Urodynamic studies showed normal compliance in all animals, and microscopic examination of the expanded neoreservoir tissue showed a normal histologic pattern. A series of immunocytochemical studies demonstrated that the dilated bladder tissue maintained normal phenotypic characteristics (Satar et al, 1999).

Ideally, bladder tissue expansion could be performed with an indwelling dilation catheter, similar to a Foley catheter with a large balloon. In the future, one could foresee placement of a dilating catheter intravesically in a patient who requires augmentation, either in an intermittent fashion (e.g., four times daily) or left indwelling. An expanding balloon within the catheter could then be filled progressively, with either continuous or intermittent filling until the desired bladder volume is achieved.

Matrices for Bladder Regeneration

During the last few decades, several bladder wall substitutes have been attempted with both synthetic and organic materials. Synthetic materials that have been tried in experimental and clinical settings include polyvinyl sponge, Teflon, collagen matrices, Vicryl (PGA) matrices, and silicone. Most of the these attempts have failed because of mechanical, structural, functional, or biocompatibility problems. **Usually, permanent synthetic materials used for bladder reconstruction succumb to mechanical failure and urinary stone forma-**

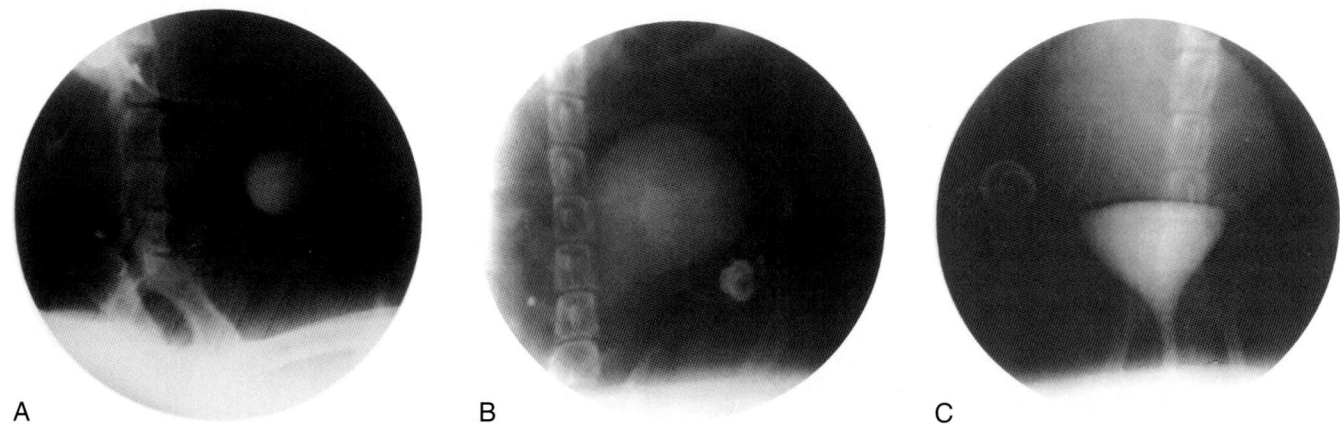

Figure 17–6. Progressive bladder dilatation can be performed with adequate increases in capacity. Cystography of bladder neoreservoir before progressive dilatation (**A**) is compared with cystography results after progressive dilatation (**B**) and with cystogram showing dilated neoreservoir and intact bladder segment (**C**).

tion, and use of degradable materials leads to fibroblast deposition, scarring, graft contracture, and a reduced reservoir
volume over time (Atala, 1995, 1998).

There has been a resurgence in the use of various collagen-based matrices for tissue regeneration. Nonseeded allogeneic acellular bladder matrices have served as scaffolds for
the ingrowth of host bladder wall components. The matrices
are prepared by mechanically and chemically removing all cellular components from bladder tissue (Sutherland et al, 1996;
Probst et al, 1997; Piechota et al, 1998; Yoo et al, 1998b). The
matrices serve as vehicles for partial bladder regeneration, and
relevant antigenicity is not evident.

Cell-seeded allogeneic acellular bladder matrices were used
for bladder augmentation in dogs (Yoo et al, 1998b). The
regenerated bladder tissues contained a normal cellular organization consisting of urothelium and smooth muscle and
exhibited a normal compliance. Biomaterials preloaded with
cells before their implantation showed better tissue regeneration than did biomaterials implanted with no cells, in
which tissue regeneration depended on ingrowth of the surrounding tissue. The bladders showed a significant increase
(100%) in capacity when augmented with scaffolds seeded
with cells compared with scaffolds without cells (30%).

Small intestinal submucosa, a biodegradable, acellular,
xenogeneic collagen-based tissue-matrix graft, was first used
in the early 1980s as an acellular matrix for tissue replacement
in the vascular field. It has been shown to promote regeneration of a variety of host tissues, including blood vessels and
ligaments (Badylak, 2002). The matrix is derived from pig
small intestine in which the mucosa is mechanically removed
from the inner surface and the serosa and muscle layer are
removed from the outer surface. Animal studies have shown
that the nonseeded small intestinal submucosa matrix used for
bladder augmentation is able to regenerate in vivo (Kropp et
al, 1996a, 1996b). On histologic evaluation, the transitional
layer was the same as that of the native bladder tissue, but as
with other nonseeded collagen matrices used experimentally,
the muscle layer was not fully developed. A large amount of
collagen was interspersed among a smaller number of muscle
bundles. A computer-assisted image analysis demonstrated a

decreased muscle-to-collagen ratio with loss of the normal
architecture in the small intestinal submucosa–regenerated
bladders. In vitro contractility studies performed on the small
intestinal submucosa–regenerated dog bladders showed a
decrease in maximal contractile response by 50% from normal
bladder tissues. Expression of muscarinic, purinergic, and
α-adrenergic receptors and functional cholinergic and
purinergic innervation were demonstrated (Kropp et al,
1996b). Cholinergic and purinergic innervation also occurred
in rats (Vaught et al, 1996).

Bladder augmentation by laparoscopic techniques was
performed on minipigs with porcine bowel acellular tissue
matrix, human placental membranes, or porcine small intestinal submucosa. At 12 weeks postoperatively, the grafts had
contracted to 70%, 65%, and 60% of their original sizes,
respectively, and histologically the grafts showed predominantly only mucosal regeneration (Portis et al, 2000). The
same group evaluated the long-term results of laparoscopic
hemicystectomy and bladder replacement with small intestinal submucosa with ureteral reimplantation into the small
intestinal submucosa material in minipigs. Histopathologic
studies after 1 year showed muscle at the graft periphery and
center, but it consisted of small fused bundles with significant
fibrosis. Nerves were present at the graft periphery and center,
but they were decreased in number. Compared with primary
bladder closure after hemicystectomy, no advantage in bladder
capacity or compliance was documented (Landman et al,
2004). More recently, bladder regeneration has been shown to
be more reliable when the small intestinal submucosa was
derived from the distal ileum (Kropp et al, 2004).

In multiple studies using various materials as nonseeded
grafts for cystoplasty, the urothelial layer was able to regenerate normally, but the muscle layer, although present, was
not fully developed (Kropp et al, 1996b; Sutherland et al,
1996; Probst et al, 1997; Yoo et al, 1998b). Studies involving
acellular matrices that may provide the necessary environment to promote cell migration, growth, and differentiation
are being conducted. With continued bladder research in this
area, these matrices may have a clinical role in bladder
replacement in the future.

Tissue Engineering of Bladders with Cell Transplantation

Tissue engineering with selective cell transplantation may provide a means to create functional new bladder segments (Atala, 1997). The success of cell transplantation strategies for bladder reconstruction depends on the ability to use donor tissue efficiently and to provide the right conditions for long-term survival, differentiation, and growth.

Formation of Bladder Tissue Ex Situ. Human urothelial and muscle cells can be expanded in vitro, seeded onto the polymer scaffold, and allowed to attach and form sheets of cells. The cell-polymer scaffold can then be implanted in vivo. Histologic analysis indicated that viable cells were able to self-assemble back into their respective tissue types and would retain their native phenotype (Atala et al, 1993b). Cell-polymer composite implants of urothelial and muscle cells, retrieved at extended times (50 days), showed extensive formation of multilayered urothelial and muscle constructs. These experiments demonstrated, for the first time, that composite layered tissue-engineered structures could be created de novo. Before this study, only nonlayered type structures had been created in the field of tissue engineering.

Formation of Bladder Tissue In Situ. To determine the effects of implanting engineered tissues in continuity with the urinary tract, animal models of bladder augmentation were used (Yoo et al, 1998b). Partial cystectomies were performed in dogs. The animals were divided into two experimental groups. One group had the bladder augmented with a non-seeded bladder-derived collagen matrix, and the second group had the bladder augmented with a cell-seeded construct. The bladders augmented with matrices seeded with cells showed a 100% increase in capacity compared with bladders augmented with cell-free matrices, which showed only a 30% increase in capacity (Fig. 17–7).

Most of the free grafts (without cells) used for bladder replacement in the past were able to show adequate histology in terms of a well-developed urothelial layer, but they were associated with an abnormal muscle layer that varied in terms of its full development (Atala, 1995, 1998).

It has been well established for decades that the bladder is able to regenerate generously over free grafts. Urothelium is associated with a high reparative capacity (De Boer et al, 1994). Bladder muscle tissue is less likely to regenerate in a normal fashion. Both urothelial and muscle ingrowth are believed to be initiated from the edges of the normal bladder toward the region of the free graft (Baker et al, 1955; Gorham et al, 1989). Usually, however, contracture or resorption of the graft has been evident. The inflammatory response toward the matrix may contribute to the resorption of the free graft. It was hypothesized that building the three-dimensional structure constructs in vitro, before implantation, would facilitate the eventual terminal differentiation of the cells after implantation in vivo and would minimize the inflammatory response toward the matrix, thus avoiding graft contracture and shrinkage. The dog study demonstrated a major difference between matrices used with autologous cells (tissue-engineered matrices) and those used without cells (Yoo et al, 1998b). **Matrices implanted with cells for bladder augmentation retained most of their implanted diameter, as opposed to matrices implanted without cells for bladder augmentation, in which**

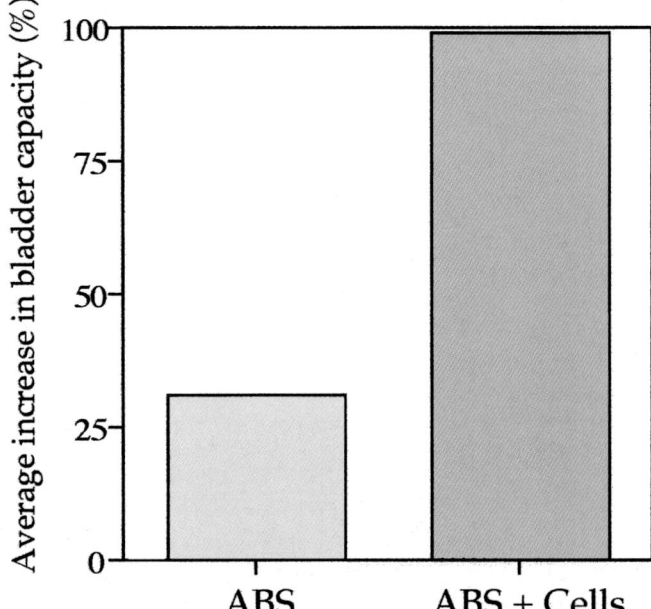

Figure 17–7. Bladders augmented with a collagen matrix derived from bladder submucosa seeded with urothelial and smooth muscle cells (ABS + cells) showed a 100% increase in capacity compared with bladders augmented with the cell-free allogeneic bladder submucosa (ABS), which showed only a 30% increase in capacity within 3 months after implantation.

graft contraction and shrinkage occurred. The histomorphology demonstrated a marked paucity of muscle cells and a more aggressive inflammatory reaction in the matrices implanted without cells. Of interest, the urothelial cell layers appeared normal, even though the underlying matrix was significantly inflamed. It was further hypothesized that having an adequate urothelial layer from the outset would limit the amount of urine contact with the matrix, therefore decreasing the inflammatory response, and that the muscle cells were also necessary for bioengineering, because native muscle cells are less likely to regenerate over the free grafts. Further studies confirmed this hypothesis (Oberpenning et al, 1999; Master et al, 2003). Epithelial mesenchymal signaling is important for the differentiation of bladder smooth muscle. Smooth muscle development is facilitated by the placement of epithelia onto the surface of the matrix. **The presence of both urothelial and muscle cells on the matrices used for bladder replacement is important for successful tissue bioengineering.**

Bladder Replacement by Tissue Engineering

The results of initial studies showed that the creation of artificial bladders may be achieved in vivo; however, it could not be determined whether the functional parameters noted were caused by the augmented segment or by the intact native bladder tissue. To better address the functional parameters of tissue-engineered bladders, an animal model was designed that required a subtotal cystectomy with subsequent replacement with a tissue-engineered organ (Oberpenning et al, 1999).

Cystectomy-only and nonseeded controls maintained average capacities of 22% and 46% of preoperative values, respectively. An average bladder capacity of 95% of the

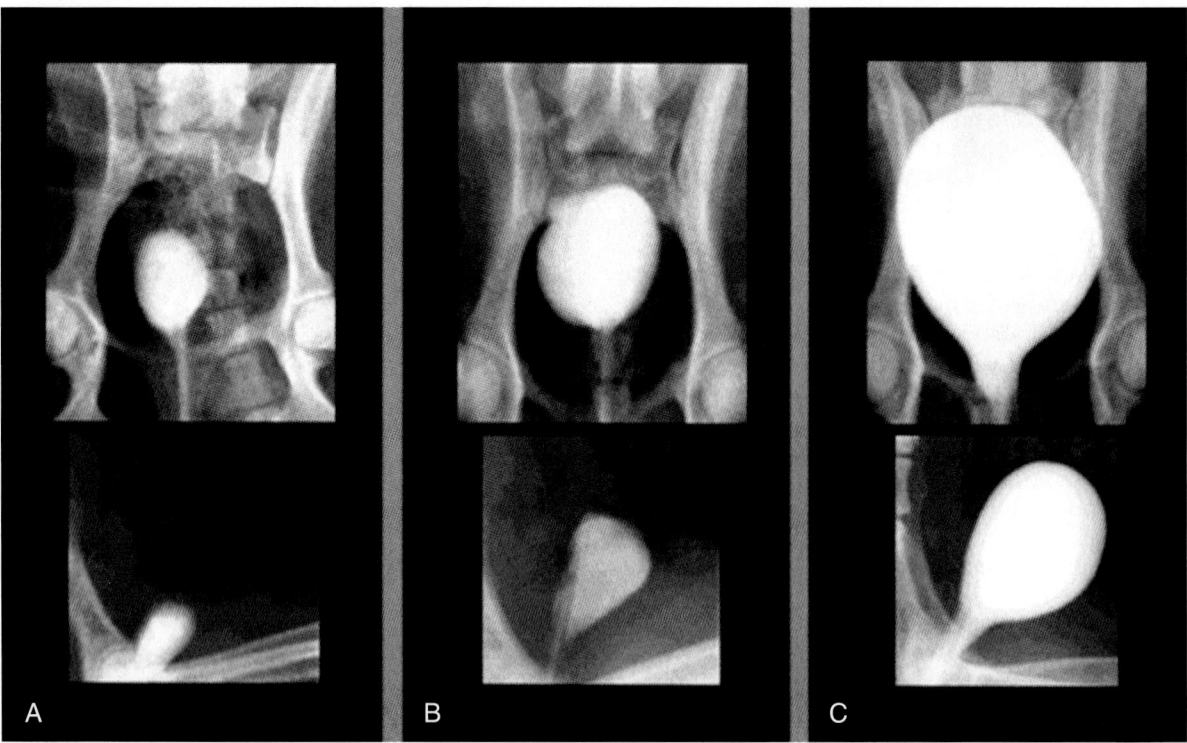

Figure 17–8. Radiographic cystograms in beagles 11 months after subtotal cystectomy without reconstruction (**A**), with reconstruction by a polymer without cells (**B**), and with reconstruction by a polymer and cell-seeded tissue-engineered organ (**C**). Organs after trigone-sparing cystectomy retained a small reservoir. Tissue-engineered neobladders showed a normal configuration and a larger capacity than the trigones grafted with polymer only.

original precystectomy volume was achieved in the cell-seeded tissue-engineered bladder replacements. These findings were confirmed radiographically (Fig. 17–8). The subtotal cystectomy reservoirs that were not reconstructed and the polymer-only reconstructed bladders showed a marked decrease in bladder compliance (10% and 42% total compliance). The compliance of the cell-seeded tissue-engineered bladders showed almost no difference from preoperative values that were measured when the native bladder was present (106%). On histologic examination, the nonseeded scaffold bladders presented a pattern of normal urothelial cells with a thickened fibrotic submucosa and a thin layer of muscle fibers. The retrieved tissue-engineered bladders showed a normal cellular organization, consisting of a trilayer of urothelium, submucosa, and muscle (Fig. 17–9). Immunocytochemical analyses confirmed the muscle and urothelial phenotype. S-100 staining indicated the presence of neural structures (Oberpenning et al, 1999). Preliminary clinical trials for the application of this technology have been performed and the initial results are promising; further expanded studies are being established (Atala et al, 2006).

An area of concern in the field of tissue engineering in the past was the source of cells for regeneration. The concept of creating engineered constructs involves initially obtaining cells for expansion from the diseased organ. How can one be assured that the cell population that is obtained and being expanded for later autologous implantation is normal and will lead to normal tissue formation? For example, if one is dealing with a patient, will the cells obtained from a neuropathic bladder lead to the engineering of another neuropathic bladder? A study showed that cultured neuropathic

bladder smooth muscle cells possess and maintain characteristics different from those of normal smooth muscle cells in vitro, as demonstrated by growth assays, contractility, and adherence tests in vitro (Lin et al, 2004). However, when neuropathic smooth muscle cells were cultured in vitro and seeded onto matrices and implanted in vivo, the tissue-engineered constructs showed the same properties as the tissues engineered with normal cells (Lai et al, 2002). **The progenitor cells, which reside within stem cell niches within each organ, are responsible for new cell differentiation and tissue formation during the normal process of tissue regeneration due to natural turnover, aging, and tissue injury. It is known that genetically normal nonmalignant progenitor cells, which are the reservoirs for new cell formation, are programmed to give rise to normal tissue, regardless of whether the niche resides in either normal or diseased tissues** (Faris et al, 2001; Lai et al, 2002; Haller et al, 2005). Therefore, although the mechanisms for tissue self-assembly and tissue engineering are not fully understood, it is known that the progenitor cells are able to "reset" their program for normal cell differentiation. The stem cell niche and its role in normal tissue regeneration remain a fertile area of ongoing investigation.

From these studies, it is evident, as with the urethral studies, that cell-seeded matrices are superior to nonseeded matrices for the creation of engineered bladder tissues. Although advances have been made with the engineering of bladder tissues, many challenges remain. Current research in many centers is aimed at the development of biologically active and "smart" biomaterials that may improve tissue regeneration.

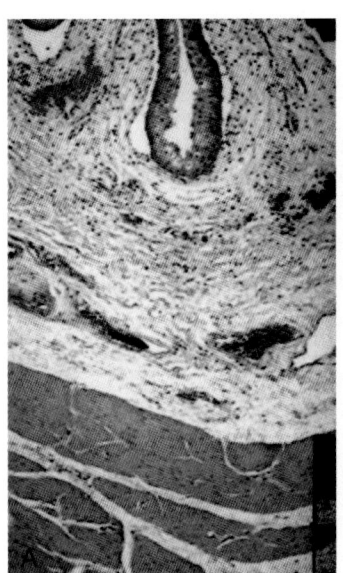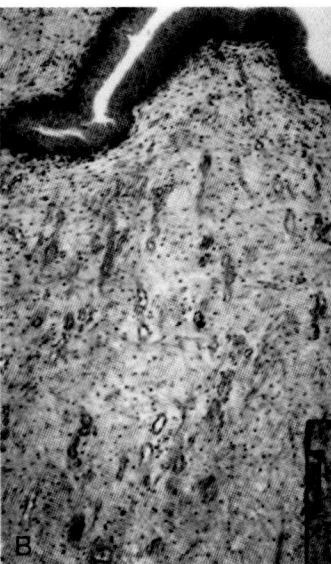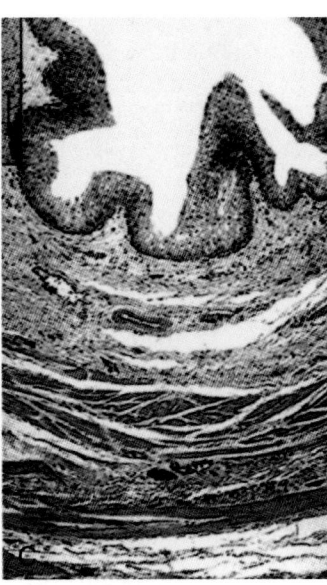

Figure 17–9. Hematoxylin and eosin staining shows histologic results 6 months after surgery (original magnification, ×250). **A,** Normal canine bladder. **B,** The dome of the bladder reconstructed with cell-free polymer consists of normal urothelium over a thickened layer of collagen and fibrotic tissue; only scarce muscle fibers are apparent. **C,** The tissue-engineered neo-organ has a histomorphologically normal appearance. A trilayered architecture consisting of urothelium, submucosa, and smooth muscle is evident.

Ureters

Nonseeded collagen tubular sponges have been used to transplant bladder cells for replacement of ureteral segments in dogs. The study showed severe stricture formation and papillary mucosal thickening at the anastomotic sites. In addition, muscle regeneration into the collagen grafts was not evident. In a urine exposure test, severe salt deposits were noted (Tachibana et al, 1985).

Ureteral nonseeded matrices were used as a scaffold for the ingrowth of ureteral tissue in rats. The matrices were prepared by removing cell and lipid components from ureters. On implantation, the acellular matrices promoted the regeneration of the ureteral wall components (Dahms et al, 1997). Laparoscopic segmental ureteral replacement with cell-free biodegradable grafts was performed in minipigs (Shalhav et al, 1999). A segment of the upper ureter was excised and laparoscopically replaced by a stented tube graft made of acellular matrix prepared from minipig ureters, from domestic pig ureters, and from minipig small intestinal submucosa. In three control animals, the ureteral gap was bridged only by an indwelling stent. The stent was removed at 6 weeks. At 12 weeks, all animals had complete obstruction at the level of the replacement, with fibrosis with or without bone formation at the level of the stricture. Regeneration of urothelium occurred in the ureteral segments, but functional replacement was not possible. Ureteral replacement with polytetrafluoroethylene (Teflon) grafts was attempted in dogs, also with poor functional results (Baltaci et al, 1998). In a more recent study, nonseeded ureteral collagen acellular matrices were tubularized and used to replace 3-cm segments of canine ureters. At the time of sacrifice, there was moderate to marked hydroureteronephrosis above the level of the new tube in all dogs. Marked graft shrinkage was observed with significant narrowing of the ureteral lumen, up to complete occlusion. At 8 weeks, histopathologic examination showed extensive fibro-

sis. The authors concluded that a nonseeded acellular matrix tube is not able to replace a 3-cm segment of the canine ureter (Osman et al, 2004).

Cell-seeded biodegradable polymer scaffolds have been used as cell transplantation vehicles to reconstruct ureteral tissues. In one study, urothelial and smooth muscle cells isolated from bladders and expanded in vitro were seeded onto PGA scaffolds with tubular configurations and implanted subcutaneously into athymic mice. After implantation, the urothelial cells proliferated to form a multilayered luminal lining of tubular structures; the smooth muscle cells organized into multilayered structures surrounding the urothelial cells. Abundant angiogenesis was evident. The degradation of the polymer scaffolds resulted in the eventual formation of natural urothelial tissues (Atala et al, 1993b). This study suggested that it was possible to engineer urologic tissues containing multiple cell types. This approach was expanded to replacement of ureters in dogs by transplantation of smooth muscle cells and urothelial cells on tubular polymer scaffolds (Yoo et al, 1995). The limitations of transferring this technology to humans are the small number of patients requiring this type of tissue and the large investment that would be required for regulatory approval.

Genital Tissues

Reconstructive surgery is required for a wide variety of pathologic penile conditions, including penile carcinoma, trauma, severe erectile dysfunction, and congenital conditions such as ambiguous genitalia, hypospadias, and epispadias. One of the major limitations of phallic reconstructive surgery is the availability of sufficient autologous tissue. Nongenital autologous tissue sources have been used for decades. Phallic reconstruction was initially attempted in the late 1930s, with rib cartilage used as a stiffener for patients

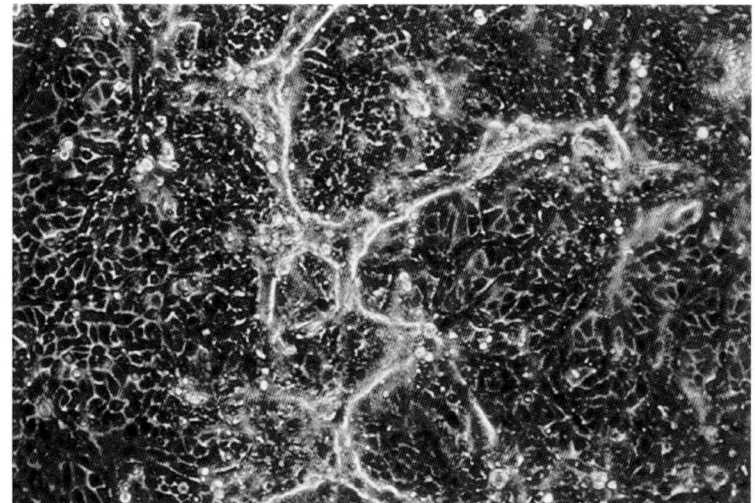

Figure 17–10. Human corporal cavernosal endothelial cells form capillary-like structures in vitro (original magnification, ×100).

with traumatic penile loss (Frumpkin, 1944; Goodwin and Scott, 1952). This method, involving multiple staged surgeries, was soon discouraged because of the unsatisfactory functional and cosmetic results. Silicone rigid prostheses were popularized in the 1970s and have been used widely (Small et al, 1975; Bretan, 1989). However, biocompatibility issues have been a problem in selected patients (Thomalla et al, 1987; Nukui et al, 1997). Tissue transfer techniques with flaps from various nongenital sources such as the groin, dorsalis pedis, and forearm have been used for genital reconstruction (Jordan, 1999). However, operative complications such as infection, graft failure, and donor site morbidity are not negligible. Phallic reconstruction with autologous tissue, derived from the patient's own cells, may be preferable in selected cases.

Reconstruction of Corporal Tissues

Reconstruction of Corporal Smooth Muscle. One of the major components of the phallus is corporal smooth muscle. The creation of autologous functional and structural corporal tissue de novo would be beneficial. Initial experiments showed that cultured human corporal smooth muscle cells may be used in conjunction with biodegradable polymers to create corpus cavernosum tissue de novo (Kershen et al, 1998). **When grown on collagen, corporal cavernosal endothelial cells formed capillary structures that created complex three-dimensional capillary networks** (Fig. 17–10). In a subsequent study, the possibility was investigated of developing human corporal tissue in vivo by combining smooth muscle and endothelial cells (Park et al, 1999). Primary normal human corpus cavernosum smooth muscle cells and human endothelial cells were seeded on biodegradable scaffolds and implanted in the subcutaneous space of mice. The ratio of muscle to endothelial tissue was 2 to 1, approximately equivalent to the ratio of muscle to endothelial cell seeding before implantation. These experiments showed that human corporal smooth muscle cells and endothelial cells seeded on biodegradable polymer scaffolds are able to form vascularized cavernosal muscle when implanted in vivo. Endothelial cells are able to act in concert with the native vasculature.

A naturally derived acellular corporal tissue matrix that possesses the same architecture as native corpora was developed (Fig. 17–11). Acellular collagen matrices were derived

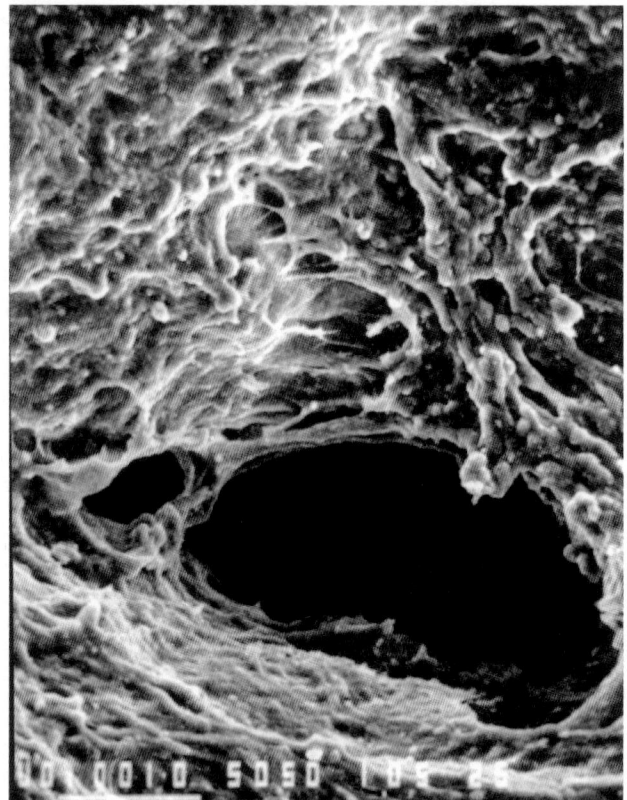

Figure 17–11. Scanning electron microscopy of human cavernosal smooth muscle and endothelial cells seeded on acellular matrices.

from processed donor rabbit corpora by cell lysis techniques. Human corpus cavernosal muscle and endothelial cells were derived from donor penile tissue, and the cells were expanded in vitro and seeded on the acellular matrices (see Fig. 17–10). The matrices were covered with the appropriate cell architecture 4 weeks after implantation (Falke et al, 1999). This study demonstrated that **human cavernosal smooth muscle and endothelial cells seeded on acellular corporal tissue matrices are able to form vascularized corporal structures in vivo.** The use of these tissue matrices as cell delivery scaffolds allowed the development of adequate structural constructs.

To look at the functional parameters of the engineered corpora, acellular corporal collagen matrices were obtained from donor rabbit penis and autologous corpus cavernosal smooth muscle and endothelial cells were harvested, expanded, and seeded on the matrices. An entire cross-sectional segment of protruding rabbit phallus was excised, leaving the urethra intact, and the cell-seeded matrices were interposed into the excised corporal space. Functional and structural parameters (cavernosography, cavernosometry, mating behavior, and sperm ejaculation) were followed, and histochemical, immunocytochemical, and Western blot analyses were performed up to 6 months after implantation. The engineered corpora cavernosa achieved adequate structural and functional parameters (Kwon et al, 2002). This technology was further confirmed when the entire rabbit corpora were removed and replaced with the engineered scaffolds. The experimental corporal bodies demonstrated intact structural integrity by cavernosography and showed similar pressure by cavernosometry compared with the normal controls. The control rabbits without cells failed to show normal erectile function throughout the study period. Mating activity in the animals with the engineered corpora appeared normal by 1 month after implantation. The presence of sperm was confirmed during mating, and sperm was present in all the rabbits with the engineered corpora. The female rabbits mated with the animals implanted with engineered corpora and also conceived and delivered healthy pups. Animals implanted with the matrix alone were unable to demonstrate normal mating activity and failed to ejaculate into the vagina. On gross examination, the corporal implants with cells showed continuous integration of the graft into native tissue. On histologic examination, sinusoidal spaces and walls, lined with endothelium and smooth muscle, were observed in the engineered grafts. Grafts without cells contained fibrotic tissue and calcifications with sparse corporal elements. Each cell type was identified immunocytochemically and by Western blot analyses. The engineered corporal tissues were able to contract and relax in response to electric field and pharmacologic stimulation, and the contractile response reached levels similar to normal corpora by 6 months after implantation (Chen et al, 2005).

This series of studies demonstrates that penile corpora cavernosa tissue can be engineered. The engineered tissue is able to achieve adequate structural and functional parameters sufficient for erection, copulation, ejaculation, conception, and delivery in rabbits. Further studies will be needed to confirm the long-term functionality of these organs. In addition, further studies are needed to show that human structures can also be engineered.

Engineered Penile Prostheses. Although silicone is an accepted biomaterial for penile prostheses, biocompatibility is a concern (Thomalla et al, 1987; Nukui et al, 1997). The use of a natural prosthesis composed of autologous cells may be advantageous. A feasibility study for creating natural penile prostheses made of cartilage was performed initially (Yoo et al, 1998a).

Cartilage, harvested from the articular surface of calf shoulders, was isolated, grown, and expanded in culture. The cells were seeded onto preformed cylindrical polyglycolic acid polymer rods and implanted in mice. At retrieval, all of the polymer scaffolds seeded with cells formed milky-white, rod-shaped, solid cartilage structures, maintaining their preimplantation size and shape (Fig. 17–12). In a subsequent study using an autologous system, the feasibility of applying the engineered cartilage rods in situ was investigated (Yoo et al, 1999). Autologous chondrocytes harvested from rabbit ear were grown and expanded in culture. The cells were seeded onto biodegradable PLLA-coated polyglycolic acid polymer rods and implanted into the corporal spaces of rabbits. Examination at retrieval showed the presence of well-formed, milky-white cartilage structures within the corpora at 1 month. The animals were able to copulate and impregnate their female partners without problems.

Female Genital Tissues

Congenital malformations of the uterus may have profound implications clinically. Patients with cloacal exstrophy and intersex disorders may not have sufficient uterine tissue present for future reproduction. The possibility of engineering functional uterine tissue with autologous cells was investigated (Wang et al, 2003). Autologous rabbit uterine smooth muscle and epithelial cells were harvested, then grown and expanded in culture. These cells were seeded onto preconfigured uterine-shaped biodegradable polymer scaffolds, which were then used for subtotal uterine tissue replacement in the corresponding autologous animals. On retrieval 6 months after implantation, histologic, immunocytochemical, and Western blot analyses confirmed the presence of normal

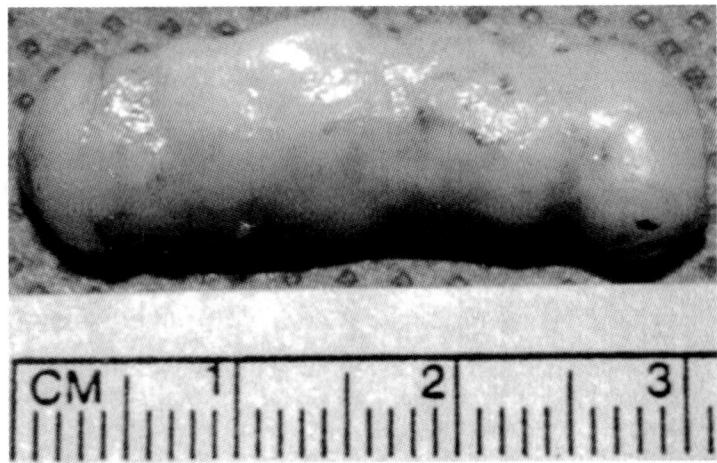

Figure 17–12. Cylindrical polymer scaffolds seeded with chondrocytes and implanted in vivo formed milky-white, rod-shaped, solid cartilaginous structures.

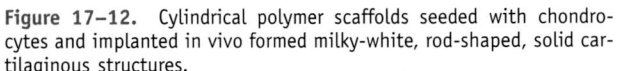

uterine tissue components. Biomechanical analyses and organ bath studies showed that the functional characteristics of these tissues were similar to those of normal uterine tissue. Breeding studies using these engineered uteri are currently being performed.

Similarly, several pathologic conditions, including congenital malformations and malignant disease, can adversely affect normal vaginal development or anatomy. Vaginal reconstruction has traditionally been challenging because of the paucity of available native tissue. The feasibility of engineering vaginal tissue in vivo was investigated (De Filippo et al, 2003a). Vaginal epithelial and smooth muscle cells of female rabbits were harvested, grown, and expanded in culture. These cells were seeded onto biodegradable polymer scaffolds, and the cell-seeded constructs were then implanted into nude mice for up to 6 weeks. Immunocytochemical, histologic, and Western blot analyses confirmed the presence of vaginal tissue phenotypes. Electrical field stimulation studies in the tissue-engineered constructs showed functional properties similar to those of normal vaginal tissue. When these constructs were used for autologous total vaginal replacement, patent vaginal structures were noted in the tissue-engineered specimens, whereas the non–cell-seeded structures were noted to be stenotic (De Filippo et al, 2003b).

Formation of Renal Structures

Although the kidney was the first organ to be substituted by an artificial device and the first successfully transplanted organ (Murray et al, 1955), current modalities of treatment are far from satisfactory. Renal transplantation is currently the preferred method for treatment of end-stage renal disease. A major problem with transplantation therapy is the shortage of suitable organs. In addition to the inherent shortage of transplant organs, complications associated with renal transplantation are yet to be resolved. Short-term side effects of immunosuppressive therapy, chronic allograft failure due to chronic rejection, increased incidence of cardiovascular disease, infections, increased frequency of cancer, osteoporosis, osteomalacia, and bone disease secondary to hyperparathyroidism are still prevalent (Julian et al, 1993; Cohen et al, 1994; Raine, 1994).

The kidney is probably the most challenging organ in the genitourinary system to reconstruct by tissue engineering techniques because of its complex structure and function.

The greatest challenge for the evolving discipline of tissue engineering is the generation of whole organs. Emerging concepts for a bioartificial kidney are currently being explored. Some investigators are pursuing the replacement of isolated kidney function parameters with the use of extracorporeal units; others are aiming at the replacement of total renal function by tissue-engineered bioartificial structures.

Creation of Functional Renal Structures In Vivo

An approach toward the achievement of improved renal function involves the augmentation of renal tissue with kidney cell expansion in vitro and subsequent autologous transplantation. The feasibility of achieving renal cell growth, expansion, and in vivo reconstitution with the use of tissue engineering techniques was explored. Isolated rabbit renal

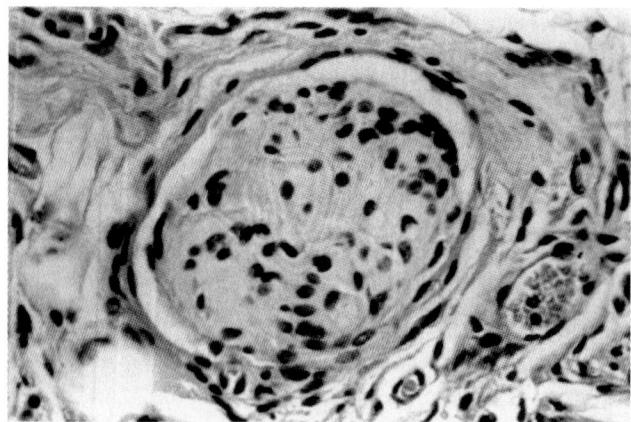

Figure 17–13. Retrieved tissue-engineered renal units demonstrate formation of glomeruli (hematoxylin and eosin stain; original magnification, ×400).

cells were expanded in vitro, seeded onto biodegradable scaffold, and implanted in nude mice. The cells replicated and organized into nephron segments as the polymer scaffolds, which acted as cell delivery vehicles, underwent biodegradation (Atala et al, 1995).

The renal tubular reconstitution process was also studied (Fung et al, 1996). When in vitro conditions that produced minimal epidermal growth factor receptor expression were used, renal epithelial cells seeded in a form of a single-cell suspension were found to reconstitute into tubular structures.

An attempt was made to harness the reconstitution of renal epithelial cells for the generation of functional nephron units. Renal cells were harvested and expanded in culture. The cells were seeded onto a tubular device constructed from a polycarbonate membrane, connected at one end with a Silastic catheter that terminated into a reservoir (Fig. 17–13). The device was implanted in athymic mice. Histologic examination of the implanted devices over time revealed extensive vascularization with formation of glomeruli and highly organized tubule-like structures. Immunocytochemical staining confirmed the renal phenotype. Yellow fluid was collected from inside the implant, and the fluid retrieved was consistent with the makeup of dilute urine in its creatinine and uric acid concentrations (Yoo et al, 1996). The results of these studies demonstrate that **renal cells can be successfully harvested, expanded in culture, and implanted in vivo.** The single cells form multicellular structures and become organized into functional renal units that are able to excrete high levels of solutes through a urine-like fluid. Further studies, described later in the section "Therapeutic Cloning," were performed. The studies showed the formation of renal structures in cows with use of nuclear transfer techniques (Lanza et al, 2002). Challenges await this technology, including the expansion of this system to larger, three-dimensional structures.

OTHER APPLICATIONS OF GENITOURINARY TISSUE ENGINEERING
Fetal Tissue Engineering

The prenatal diagnosis of fetal abnormalities is now more prevalent. Prenatal ultrasonography allows a thorough survey of fetal anatomy. For example, the absence of bladder filling, a mass of echogenic tissue on the lower abdominal wall, or a low-set umbilicus on prenatal sonographic examination may suggest the diagnosis of bladder exstrophy. These findings and intraluminal intestinal calcifications suggest the presence of a cloacal malformation.

The natural consequence of the evolution in prenatal diagnosis was the use of intervention before birth to reverse potentially life-threatening processes. However, the concept of prenatal intervention itself is not limited to this narrow group of indications. A prenatal rather than a postnatal diagnosis of urologic conditions such as exstrophy may be beneficial under certain circumstances. There is now renewed interest in single-stage reconstruction surgery for some patients with bladder exstrophy. Limiting factors for choosing a single- or multiple-stage approach may include the finding of a small, fibrotic bladder patch without either elasticity or contractility and the finding of a hypoplastic bladder.

There are several strategies that may be pursued, using today's technologic and scientific advances, to facilitate the future prenatal management of patients with urologic disease. Having a ready supply of urologic-associated tissue for surgical reconstruction at birth may be advantageous. Theoretically, once the diagnosis of the pathologic condition is confirmed prenatally, a small tissue biopsy specimen could be obtained under ultrasound guidance. These biopsy materials could then be processed and the various cell types expanded in vitro. With tissue engineering techniques, reconstituted structures in vitro could then be readily available at the time of birth for reconstruction (Fig. 17–14).

Toward this end, a series of experiments was conducted on fetal lambs (Fauza et al, 1998a, 1998b). Bladder exstrophy was created in fetal lambs, and a bladder biopsy specimen was

processed and the cells expanded and seeded on biodegradable scaffolds. After delivery, the bladders were surgically closed by use of the tissue-engineered bladder tissue. Histologic analysis of the engineered tissue showed a normal histologic pattern and good compliance. Similar prenatal studies were performed in lambs with engineering of skin for reconstruction at birth (Fauza et al, 1998a).

With tissue engineering techniques, the bladder exstrophy complex could be managed not only in utero but also after birth in a similar manner, whenever a prenatal diagnosis is not certain. In these instances, bladder tissue biopsy specimens could be obtained at the time of the initial surgery. Various tissues could be harvested and stored for future reconstruction, if necessary. A tissue bank for patients with exstrophy complex could preserve the different cell types.

Injectable Therapies

Both urinary incontinence and vesicoureteral reflux are common conditions affecting the genitourinary system for which injectable bulking agents can be used for treatment. There are definite advantages to endoscopic treatment of urinary incontinence and vesicoureteral reflux. The method is simple and can be completed in less than 15 minutes; it has a low morbidity, and it can be performed on an outpatient basis. The goal of several investigators has been to find alternative implant materials that are safe for human use (Kershen and Atala, 1999). **The ideal substance for endoscopic treatment of reflux and incontinence should be injectable, nonantigenic, nonmigratory, volume stable, and safe for human use.** Toward this goal, long-term studies were conducted to determine the effect of injectable chondrocytes in vivo (Atala et al, 1993a). It was initially determined that alginate, a liquid

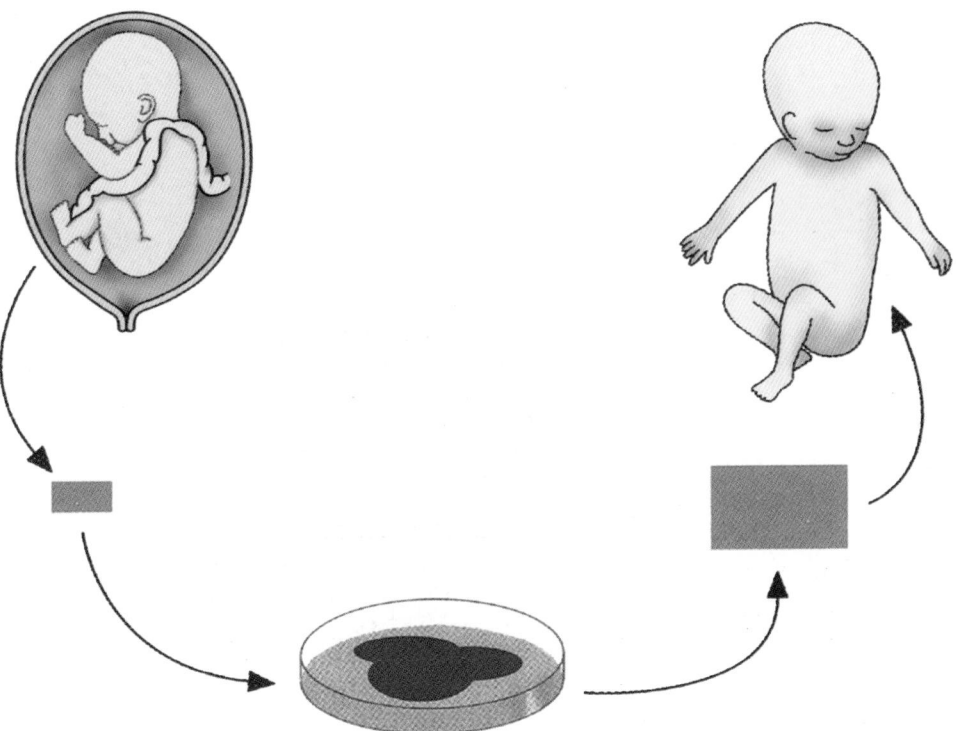

Figure 17–14. In utero tissue engineering strategy. Certain conditions, such as bladder exstrophy, can be diagnosed prenatally. Bladder, cartilage, skin, and other tissues can be retrieved by fetoscopy or percutaneously under ultrasound guidance. Cells can be harvested, expanded in vitro, and reconstituted into tissue structures. Tissue is then readily available at the time of birth for reconstruction.

solution of glucuronic and mannuronic acid, embedded with chondrocytes, could serve as a synthetic substrate for the injectable delivery and maintenance of cartilage architecture in vivo. A biopsy of the ear could be easily and quickly performed, followed by chondrocyte processing and endoscopic injection of the autologous chondrocyte suspension for the treatment of reflux. In mouse models, the cartilage matrix replaced the alginate as the polysaccharide polymer underwent biodegradation. This system was adapted for the treatment of vesicoureteral reflux in a porcine model (Atala, 1994). Miniswine underwent bilateral creation of reflux. Chondrocytes were harvested from the left auricular surface of each animal and expanded. The animals underwent endoscopic repair of reflux with the injectable autologous chondrocyte solution on the right side only. These studies showed that chondrocytes can be easily harvested and combined with alginate in vitro, the suspension can be easily injected cystoscopically, and the elastic cartilage tissue formed is able to correct vesicoureteral reflux without any evidence of obstruction (Atala, 1994).

The first human application of cell-based tissue engineering technology for urologic applications occurred with the injection of chondrocytes for the correction of vesicoureteral reflux in children (Fig. 17–15) and for urinary incontinence in adults. Two multicenter clinical trials were conducted by use of the engineered chondrocyte technology. Patients with urinary incontinence secondary to intrinsic sphincter deficiency were treated endoscopically with injected chondrocytes at three different medical centers. Phase 1 trials showed an approximate success rate of 80% at both 3 and 12 months postoperatively (Bent et al, 2001). Patients with vesicoureteral reflux were treated at 10 centers throughout the United States. The patients had a success rate similar to that with other injectable substances in terms of cure. The overall success rate in 29 children (47 ureters) was 86%. At 1-year follow-up, reflux correction was maintained in 70% of the ureters. Chondrocyte formation was not noted in patients who had treat-

ment failure (Diamond and Caldamone, 1999; Caldamone and Diamond, 2001).

With cell therapy techniques, the use of autologous smooth muscle cells was explored for both urinary incontinence and vesicoureteral reflux applications (Cilento and Atala, 1995). In vivo experiments were conducted in minipigs, and reflux was successfully corrected. The potential use of injectable, cultured myoblasts for the treatment of stress urinary incontinence has also been investigated (Yokoyama et al, 1999; Chancellor et al, 2000). Labeled myoblasts were directly injected into the proximal urethra and lateral bladder walls of nude mice with a microsyringe in an open surgical procedure. Tissue harvested up to 35 days after injection contained the labeled myoblasts as well as evidence of differentiation of the labeled myoblasts into regenerative myofibers. The authors reported that a significant portion of the injected myoblast population persisted in vivo. Similar techniques of sphincter-derived muscle cells have been used for the treatment of urinary incontinence in a pig model (Strasser et al, 2004). The same authors treated 42 patients (29 women and 13 men) with urinary stress incontinence. Myoblasts were injected into the rhabdosphincter. A cure was reported by 35 patients, and 7 had marked improvement. No side effects or complications were encountered postoperatively (Strasser et al, 2004).

The use of injectable muscle precursor cells has also been investigated in the treatment of urinary incontinence due to irreversible urethral sphincter injury or maldevelopment. Muscle precursor cells are the quiescent satellite cells found in each myofiber that proliferate to form myoblasts and eventually myotubes and new muscle tissue. Intrinsic muscle precursor cells have previously been shown to play an active role in the regeneration of injured striated urethral sphincter (Yiou et al, 2003a). In a subsequent study, autologous muscle precursor cells were injected into a rat model of urethral sphincter injury, and both replacement of mature myotubes and restoration of functional motor units were noted in the regenerating sphincteric muscle tissue (Yiou et al, 2003b). This is

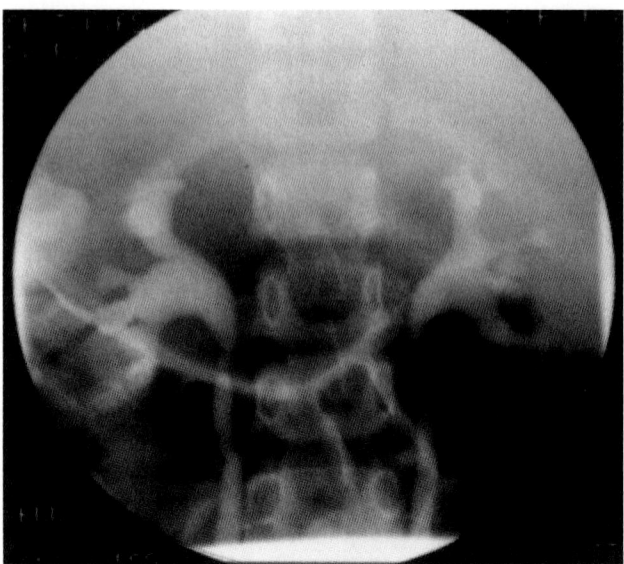 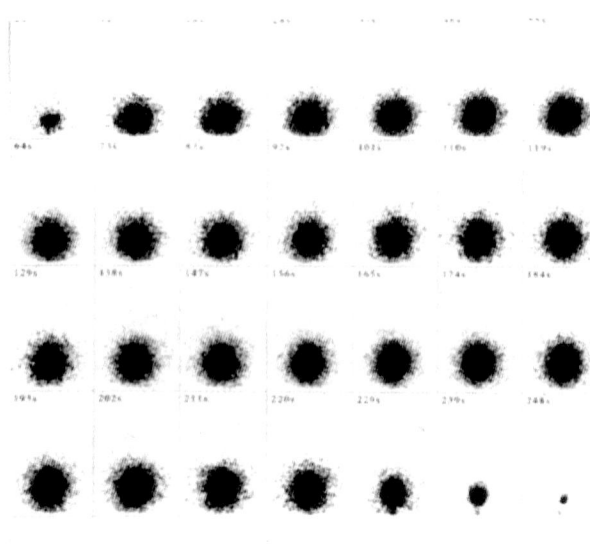

Figure 17–15. *Left,* Preoperative voiding cystourethrogram of a patient showing bilateral reflux. *Right,* Postoperative radionuclide cystography sequence of the same patient 6 months after the injection of autologous chondrocytes.

the first demonstration of the replacement of sphincter muscle tissue and its innervation by the injection of muscle precursor cells. As a result, muscle precursor cells may be a minimally invasive solution for urinary incontinence in patients with irreversible urinary sphincter muscle insufficiency.

In addition, injectable muscle-based gene therapy and tissue engineering were combined to improve detrusor function in a bladder injury model and may potentially be a novel treatment option for urinary incontinence (Huard et al, 2002). Highly purified muscle-derived cells that display stem cell characteristics were genetically engineered to express the gene encoding β-galactosidase, then injected into the bladder walls of mice. The injectable cells were able to survive in the lower urinary tract and improve the contractility of the bladder after the induced injury as well as to become innervated into the bladder as early as 2 weeks after injection. These findings may be useful in the setting of urinary incontinence; these muscle-derived cells may help bulk up the urethral wall, enhance coaptation, and improve the urinary sphincter muscle.

Testicular Hormone Replacement

Leydig cells are the major source of testosterone production in males. Patients with testicular dysfunction require androgen replacement for somatic development. Conventional treatment of testicular dysfunction consists of periodic intramuscular injections of chemically modified testosterone or, more recently, skin patch applications. However, long-term nonpulsatile testosterone therapy is not optimal and can cause multiple problems, including erythropoiesis and bone density changes.

A system was designed wherein Leydig cells were microencapsulated for controlled testosterone replacement. **Microencapsulated Leydig cells offer several advantages, such as serving as a semipermeable barrier between the transplanted cells and the host's immune system, as well as allowing the long-term physiologic release of testosterone.**

Purified Leydig cells were isolated and encapsulated in an alginate–poly-L-lysine solution (Fig. 17–16). The encapsulated Leydig cells were injected into castrated animals, and serum testosterone was measured serially; the animals were able to maintain testosterone levels in the long term (Machluf et al, 1998). These studies suggest that microencapsulated Leydig cells may be able to replace or to supplement testosterone when anorchia or testicular failure is present.

Stem Cells for Tissue Engineering

Most current strategies for tissue engineering depend on a sample of autologous cells from the diseased organ of the host. However, for many patients with extensive end-stage organ failure, a tissue biopsy specimen may not yield enough normal cells for expansion and transplantation. In other instances, primary autologous human cells cannot be expanded from a particular organ, such as the pancreas. In these situations, pluripotent human embryonic stem cells are envisioned as a viable source of cells because they can serve as an alternative source of cells from which the desired tissue can be derived. Combining the techniques learned in tissue engineering during the past few decades with this potentially endless source of versatile cells could lead to novel sources of replacement organs.

Embryonic stem cells exhibit two remarkable properties: the ability to proliferate in an undifferentiated but pluripotent state (self-renew) and the ability to differentiate into many specialized cell types (Brivanlou et al, 2003). They can be isolated by immunosurgery from the inner cell mass of the embryo during the blastocyst stage (5 days after fertilization). These cells have demonstrated longevity in culture by maintaining their undifferentiated state for at least 80 passages when grown by current published protocols (Thomson et al, 1998).

Human embryonic stem cells have been shown to differentiate into cells from all three embryonic germ layers in vitro, including ectoderm (skin and neurons), mesoderm (blood, cardiac cells, cartilage, endothelial cells, and muscle), and endoderm (liver, pancreas). In addition, as further evidence of their pluripotency, embryonic stem cells can form embryoid bodies, which are cell aggregations that contain all three

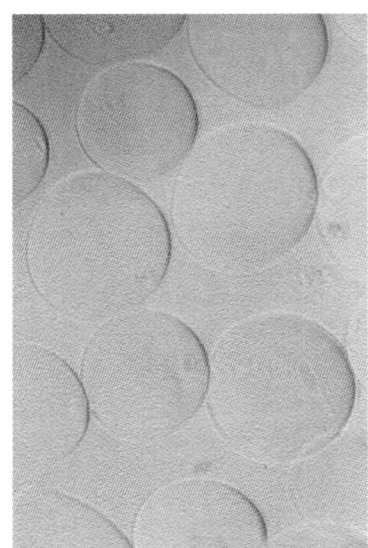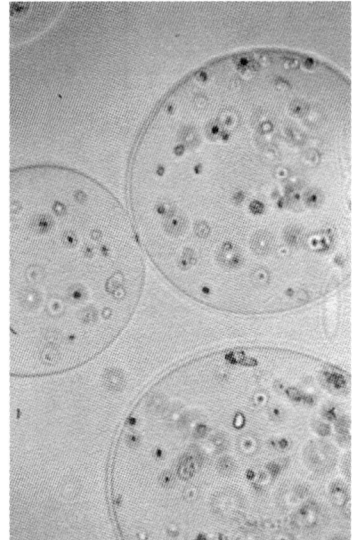

Figure 17–16. *Left,* Hydrogel microcapsules without cells. *Right,* Leydig cells encapsulated in hydrogel microcapsules secrete testosterone in vitro and in vivo.

embryonic germ layers, while in culture, and they can form teratomas in vivo (Itskovitz-Eldor et al, 2000). **The ability of the pluripotent embryonic stem cells to form teratomas is consistent with their ability to also transdifferentiate into an aneuploid state. All 22 human embryonic stem cell lines currently available for research through the U.S. federal government are aneuploid.** Therefore, systems to ensure that embryonic cells do not transdifferentiate to a malignant phenotype need to be established before these cells can be used therapeutically. **In addition, human embryonic cells are immunocompetent and would require immunosuppression if used clinically. Nonetheless, these cells do hold promise for advances in the field of regenerative medicine, for both research and therapy.**

Adult stem cells have the advantage of avoiding some of the ethical issues associated with embryonic cells, and also they do not transdifferentiate spontaneously to a malignant phenotype. The use of adult stem cells is limited for clinical therapy because of the difficulties encountered with cell expansion to large quantities. The main source of adult stem cells is bone marrow, but their collection requires a bone marrow biopsy, which is often difficult and painful. The possibility of deriving stem cells from postnatal mesenchymal tissue from the same host, from an easily accessible site such as skin, and inducing their differentiation in vitro and in vivo was investigated. Stem cells were isolated from human foreskin–derived fibroblasts (Fig. 17–17). Stem cell–derived muscle, fat, and bone cells were obtained through a cell-specific lineage process. The cells were grown, expanded, seeded onto biodegradable scaffolds, and implanted in vivo, where they formed mature tissue structures. This was the first demonstration that stem cells can be derived from postnatal connective tissue and can be used for engineering tissues in vivo ex situ (Bartsch et al, 2005).

Fetal stem cells derived from amniotic fluid and placentas have been described and represent a novel source of stem cells. The cells express markers consistent with human embryonic stem cells, such as OCT4 and SSEA-4, but do not form teratomas and do not spontaneously transdifferentiate to a malignant phenotype. The cells are multipotent and are able to differentiate into all three germ layers. In addition, the cells have a high replicative potential and could be stored for future self-use, without the risks of rejection, and without ethical concerns (Siddiqui and Atala, 2004).

Therapeutic Cloning

Nuclear cloning, which has also been called nuclear transplantation and nuclear transfer, involves the introduction of a nucleus from a donor cell into an enucleated oocyte to generate an embryo with a genetic makeup identical to that of the donor. Whereas there has been tremendous interest in the field of nuclear cloning since the birth of Dolly in 1997, the first successful nuclear transfer was reported more than 50 years ago by Briggs and King (Briggs and King, 1952). Cloned frogs, which were the first vertebrates derived from nuclear transfer, were subsequently reported by Gurdon in 1962 (Gurdon, 1962), but the nuclei were derived from nonadult sources. In the past 6 years, tremendous advances in nuclear cloning technology have been reported, indicating the relative immaturity of the field. Dolly was not the first cloned mammal to be produced from adult cells; in fact, live lambs were produced in 1996 by nuclear transfer and differentiated epithelial cells derived from embryonic disks (Campbell et al, 1996). The significance of Dolly was that she was the first mammal to be derived from an adult somatic cell by nuclear transfer (Wilmut et al, 1997). Since then, animals from several species have been grown by nuclear transfer tech-

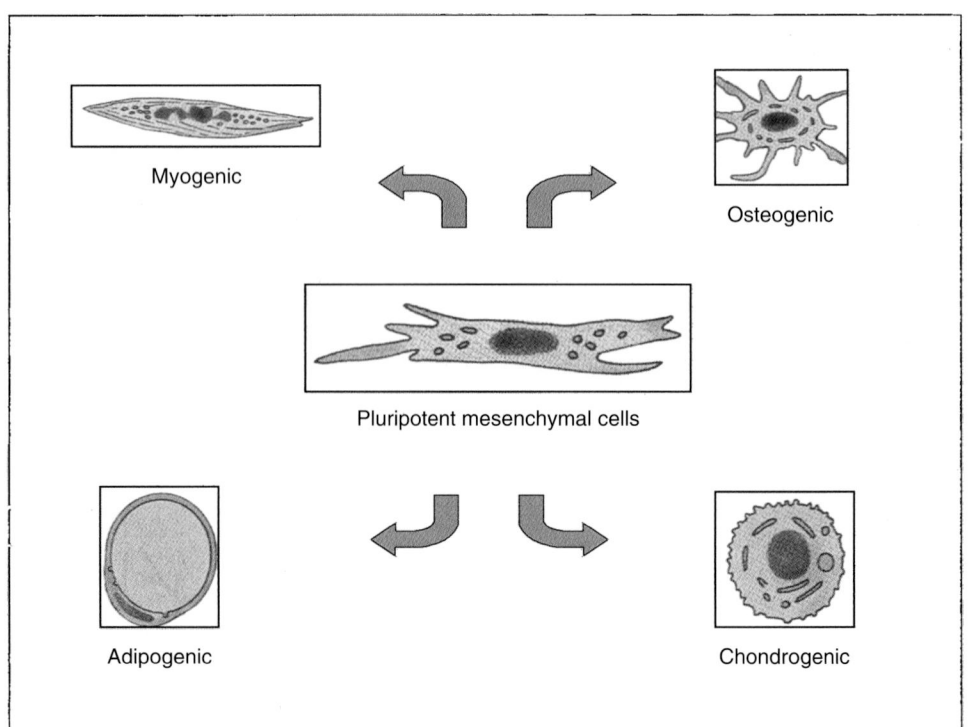

Figure 17–17. Schematic diagram of pluripotential stem cell lineages that can be derived from postnatal tissue.

Myogenic

Osteogenic

Pluripotent mesenchymal cells

Adipogenic

Chondrogenic

nology, including cattle, goats, mice, and pigs (Atala and Koh, 2004).

Two types of nuclear cloning, reproductive cloning and therapeutic cloning, have been described, and a better understanding of the differences between the two types may help alleviate some of the controversy that surrounds these revolutionary technologies. Banned in most countries for human applications, **reproductive cloning is used to generate an embryo that has the identical genetic material as its cell source. This embryo can then be implanted into the uterus of a female to give rise to an infant that is a clone of the donor.** On the other hand, **therapeutic cloning is used to generate early-stage embryos that are explanted in culture to produce embryonic stem cell lines whose genetic material is identical to that of its source. These autologous stem cells have the potential to become almost any type of cell in the adult body and thus would be useful in tissue and organ replacement applications** (Hochedlinger and Jaenisch, 2003). Some useful applications would be in the treatment of diseases, such as end-stage kidney disease, for which there is limited availability of immunocompatible tissue transplants.

Therefore, therapeutic cloning, which has also been called somatic cell nuclear transfer, provides an alternative source of transplantable cells that theoretically may be limitless. Figure 17–18 shows the strategy of combining therapeutic cloning with tissue engineering to develop tissues and organs. According to data from the Centers for Disease Control and Prevention, it has been estimated that approximately 3000 Americans die every day of diseases that could have been treated with embryonic stem cell–derived tissues. With current allogeneic tissue transplantation protocols, rejection is a frequent complication because of immunologic incompatibility, and immunosuppressive drugs are usually administered to treat and, it is hoped, prevent host-versus-graft disease (Hochedlinger and Jaenisch, 2003). The use of transplantable tissue and organs derived from therapeutic cloning may lead to the avoidance of immune responses that typically are associated with transplantation of nonautologous tissues. As a result, with therapeutic cloning, the variety of serious and potentially life-threatening complications associated with immunosuppressive treatments may be avoided.

The principles of both tissue engineering and therapeutic cloning (nuclear transfer) were applied in an effort to produce genetically identical renal tissue in a large animal model, the cow *(Bos taurus)*. Single bovine skin fibroblast donor cells were isolated and microinjected into the perivitelline space of donor enucleated oocytes (nuclear transfer). From the resulting stem cells, cloned renal cells were seeded on scaffolds consisting of three collagen-coated cylindrical polycarbonate membranes (Fig. 17–19A). The ends of the three membranes of each scaffold were connected to catheters that terminated into a collecting reservoir. This created a renal neo-organ with a mechanism for collecting the excreted urinary fluid (Fig. 17–19B). These scaffolds with the collecting devices were transplanted subcutaneously into the same steer from which the genetic material originated and then retrieved 12 weeks after implantation (Lanza et al, 2002).

Chemical analysis of the collected urine-like fluid, including urea nitrogen and creatinine levels, electrolyte levels, specific gravity, and glucose concentration, revealed that the implanted renal cells possessed filtration, reabsorption, and secretory capabilities.

Histologic examination of the retrieved implants revealed extensive vascularization and self-organization of the cells into glomeruli- and tubule-like structures. A clear continuity between the glomeruli, the tubules, and the polycarbonate membrane was noted that allowed the passage of urine into the collecting reservoir (Fig. 17–19C). Immunohistochemical analysis with renal-specific antibodies revealed the presence of renal proteins, reverse transcription–polymerase chain reaction analysis confirmed the transcription of renal-specific RNA in the cloned specimens, and Western blot analysis confirmed the presence of elevated renal-specific protein levels.

Oocyte-derived mitochondrial DNA was thought to be a potential source of immunologic incompatibility in the cloned renal cells. A possible T-cell response to the cloned renal devices was evaluated by delayed-type hypersensitivity testing in vivo and ELISPOT analysis of interferon-γ–secreting T cells in vitro (Fig. 17–19D). Both analyses revealed that the cloned renal cells showed no evidence of a T-cell response, suggesting that rejection will not necessarily occur in the presence of oocyte-derived mitochondrial DNA. This finding may

Figure 17–18. Therapeutic cloning strategy and its application to the engineering of tissues and organs.

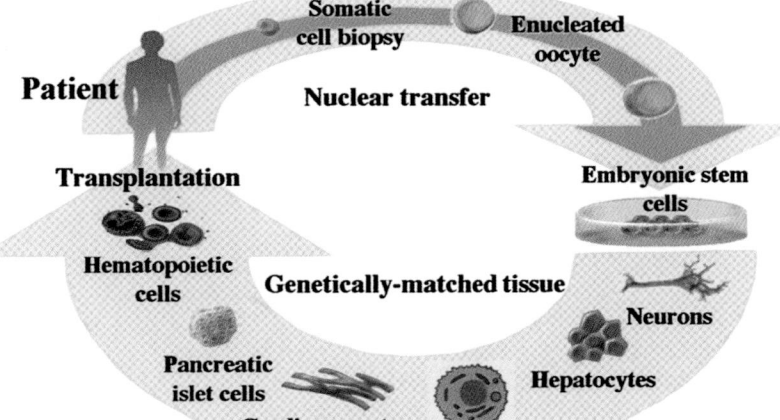

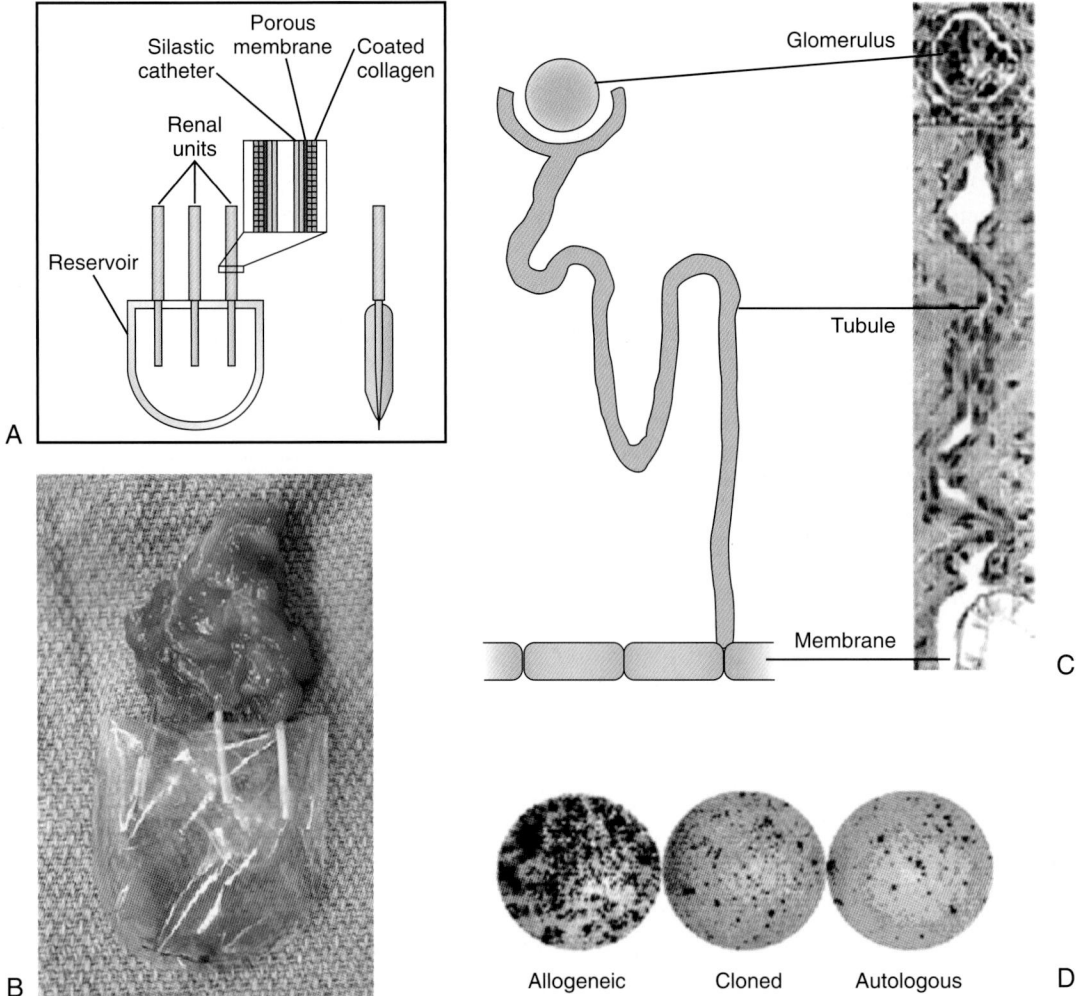

Figure 17–19.   Production of kidney tissue by therapeutic cloning and tissue engineering. **A,** Illustration of the tissue-engineered renal unit. **B,** Renal unit seeded with cloned cells, 3 months after implantation, showing the accumulation of urine-like fluid. **C,** There was a clear unidirectional continuity between the mature glomeruli, their tubules, and the polycarbonate membrane. **D,** ELISPOT analyses of the frequencies of T cells that secrete interferon-γ after primary and secondary stimulation with allogeneic renal cells, cloned renal cells, or nuclear donor fibroblasts.

represent a step forward in overcoming the histocompatibility problem of stem cell therapy (Lanza et al, 2002).

These studies demonstrated that cells derived from nuclear transfer can be successfully harvested, expanded in culture, and transplanted in vivo with the use of biodegradable scaffolds on which the single suspended cells can organize into tissue structures that are genetically identical to the host. These studies were the first demonstration of the use of therapeutic cloning for regeneration of tissues in vivo.

SUMMARY

Tissue engineering efforts are currently being undertaken for every type of tissue and organ within the urinary system. Most of the effort expended to engineer genitourinary tissues has occurred within the last decade. **Tissue engineering techniques require a cell culture facility designed for human** application. **Personnel who have mastered the techniques of cell harvest, culture, and expansion as well as polymer design are essential for the successful application of this technology. Before these engineering techniques can be applied to humans, further studies need to be performed in many of the tissues described. Recent progress suggests that engineered urologic tissues and cell therapy may have clinical applicability.**

KEY POINTS: TISSUE ENGINEERING

- New advances in the ability to expand cells in vitro, smart biomaterials, and new techniques for vascularization are allowing more complex organs to be engineered.

- Tissue injury can be repaired with minimal fibrosis by the natural wound healing response for small defects, by the use of nonseeded matrices for defects up to 1 cm from any edge, and by the use of cell-seeded matrices for defects greater than 1 cm.

- Stem cells may provide large repositories of different cell types for tissue and organ repair.

- Embryonic stem cells may transdifferentiate to a malignant phenotype and require immunosuppression. Adult stem cells usually do not replicate readily. Fetal stem cells replicate readily and do not transdifferentiate.

- Nuclear transfer can be used either for reproductive cloning or for therapeutic cloning.

SUGGESTED READINGS

Atala A, Cima LG, Kim W, et al: Injectable alginate seeded with chondrocytes as a potential treatment for vesicoureteral reflux. J Urol 1993;150:745-747.
Chancellor MB, Yokoyama T, Tirney S, et al: Preliminary results of myoblast injection into the urethra and bladder wall: A possible method for the treatment of stress urinary incontinence and impaired detrusor contractility. Neurourol Urodynam 2000;19:279-287.
Dahms SE, Piechota HJ, Dahiya R, et al: Composition and biochemical properties of the bladder acellular matrix graft: Comparative analysis in rat, pig and human. Br J Urol 1998;82:411-419.
Diamond DA, Caldamone AA: Endoscopic correction of vesicoureteral reflux in children using autologous chondrocytes: Preliminary results. J Urol 1999;162:1185-1188.
Kassaby EA, Yoo J, Retik A, Atala A: A novel inert collagen matrix for urethral stricture repair. J Urol 2000;308S:70.
Kropp BP, Rippy MK, Badylak SF, et al: Small intestinal submucosa: Urodynamic and histopathologic evaluation in long term canine bladder augmentations. J Urol 1996;155:2098-2104.
Lanza RP, Chung HY, Yoo JJ, et al: Generation of histocompatible tissues using nuclear transplantation. Nat Biotechnol 2002;20:689-696.
Oberpenning F, Meng J, Yoo J, Atala A: De novo reconstitution of a functional urinary bladder by tissue engineering. Nat Biotechnol 1999;17:149-155.
Strasser H, Marksteiner R, Margreiter E, et al: Stem cell therapy for urinary incontinence. Urologe A 2004;43:1237-1241.
Yiou R, Yoo JY, Atala A: Restoration of functional motor units in a rat model of sphincter injury by muscle precursor cell autografts. Transplantation 2003;76:1053-1060.

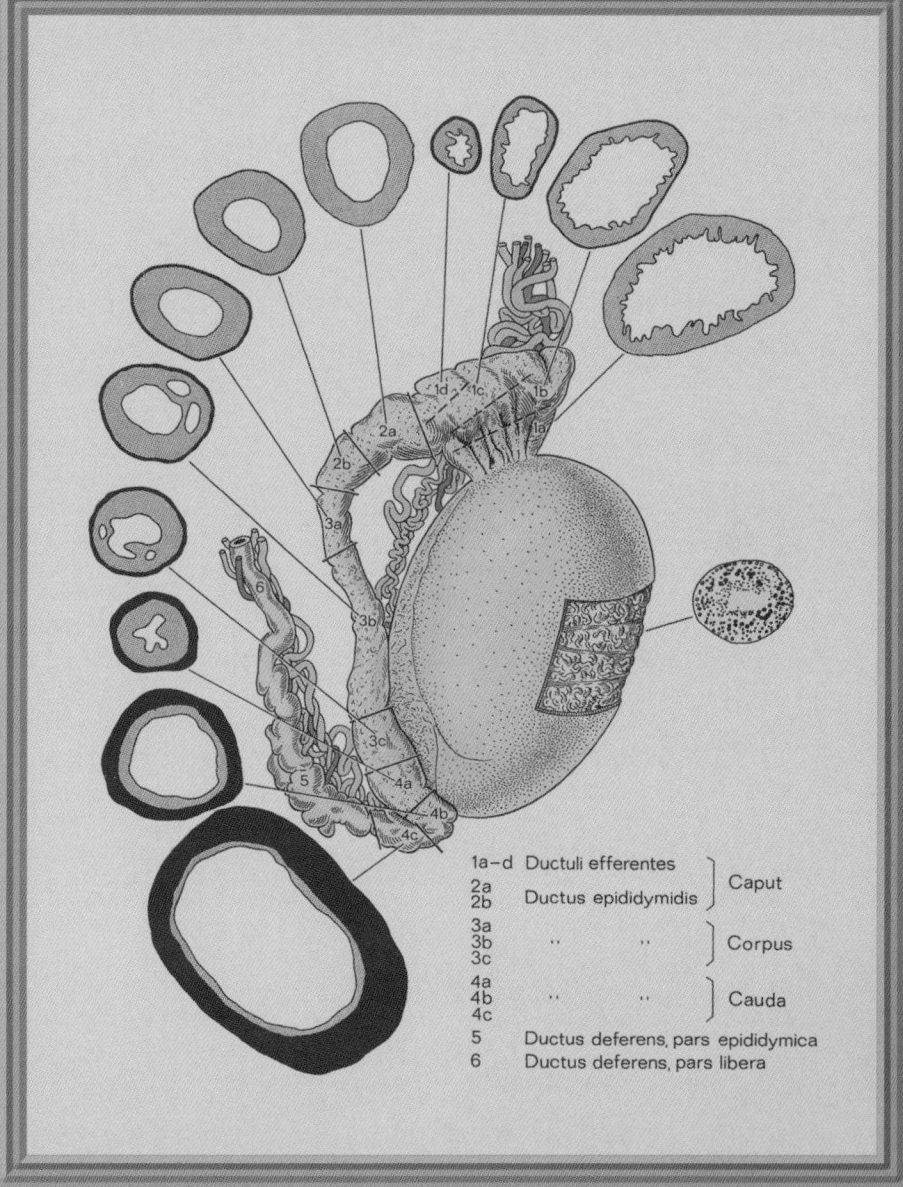

1a–d	Ductuli efferentes	
2a	Ductus epididymidis	} Caput
2b		
3a		
3b	״ ״	} Corpus
3c		
4a		
4b	״ ״	} Cauda
4c		
5	Ductus deferens, pars epididymica	
6	Ductus deferens, pars libera	

REPRODUCTIVE AND SEXUAL FUNCTION

18 Male Reproductive Physiology

PETER N. SCHLEGEL, MD • MATTHEW P. HARDY, PhD • MARC GOLDSTEIN, MD

THE MALE REPRODUCTIVE AXIS

Male reproductive function is controlled by the reproductive axis, which has three tiers of organization: the hypothalamus of the brain, the pituitary gland, and the testis. In this chapter we broadly review the preeminent features of reproductive axis physiology. Each of the two upper tiers of the axis produces an endocrine signaling molecule that acts as a secretogogue for hormone secretion at the next lower level. Thus, hypothalamic neurons located in the preoptic area with axons projecting to the median eminence secrete gonadotropin-releasing hormone (GnRH) into a portal system of blood vessels leading to the pituitary, the hypothalamohypophysial shunt. The anterior pituitary gland (or adenohypophysis) contains gonadotropes, or cells that are specialized for the secretion of gonadotropins. Secretory activity of the gonadotropes is stimulated by GnRH. The two gonadotropins secreted by pituitary gonadotropes are luteinizing hormone (LH) and follicle-stimulating hormone (FSH). In addition to GnRH, local production within the pituitary of the dimeric peptide activin selectively stimulates FSH secretion (de Kretser et al, 2000). **The two gonadotropins then enter the bloodstream and are borne to the testis, where LH stimulates testosterone production by Leydig cells in the interstitium while FSH, through stimulation of Sertoli cells, supports spermatogenesis in the seminiferous epithelium.** The rates of testosterone secretion and sperm production are fine tuned by a network of negative feedback relationships between the testis and the upper levels of the reproductive axis. Testosterone and its metabolite, estradiol, suppress secretory activity by GnRH neurons and gonadotropes.

Inhibin, a 32-kD glycoprotein hormone secreted primarily by Sertoli cells, suppresses FSH secretion by gonadotropes. The form of inhibin that is secreted by human Sertoli cells, inhibin B, is so named because it is a heterodimer composed of α and β subunits and has the B variant of the β subunit (i.e., $\alpha\beta_B$, [de Kretser and Robertson, 1989]). Inhibin B selectively suppresses FSH secretion in gonadotropes by inhibiting transcription of the gene encoding the β subunit of FSH (Clarke et al, 1993). The clinical use of inhibin B as a marker of impaired testicular function has been controversial (Kolb et al, 2000). Whereas some have proposed that inhibin B is an independent predictor of the presence of spermatozoa within the testis, others have suggested that inhibin B levels are more sensitive than FSH. Both inhibin B and FSH have been suggested to be predictors of the presence of sperm in the testes of infertile men (von Eckardstein et al, 1999). An additional dimension of control for FSH secretion is created by the production of 30-kD proteins that are closely related to inhibin called activins, which are also secreted in the testis primarily by Sertoli cells and are composed of heterodimers and homodimers of β subunits (i.e., $\beta_A\beta_A$, $\beta_A\beta_B$, and $\beta_B\beta_B$, with the last being predominant). Activins stimulate transcription of the FSH β subunit and are in turn negatively regulated by the binding protein follistatin (de Kretser et al, 2000). Figure 18–1 shows the feedback relationships between the brain, pituitary, and testis.

Hypothalamus

The GnRH neurons receive input from neurons in other parts of the brain, including the amygdala and both the olfactory and visual cortex. The output of GnRH is influenced by three types of rhythmicity: seasonal, on a time scale of months and peaking in the spring; circadian, resulting in highest testosterone levels during the early morning hours; and pulsatile, with peaks occurring every 90 to 120 minutes on average. **The neurons that comprise the GnRH pulse generator have not been identified, but the seasonal and circadian rhythms are modulated by melatonin signaling from, respectively, the pineal gland and neural connections arising**

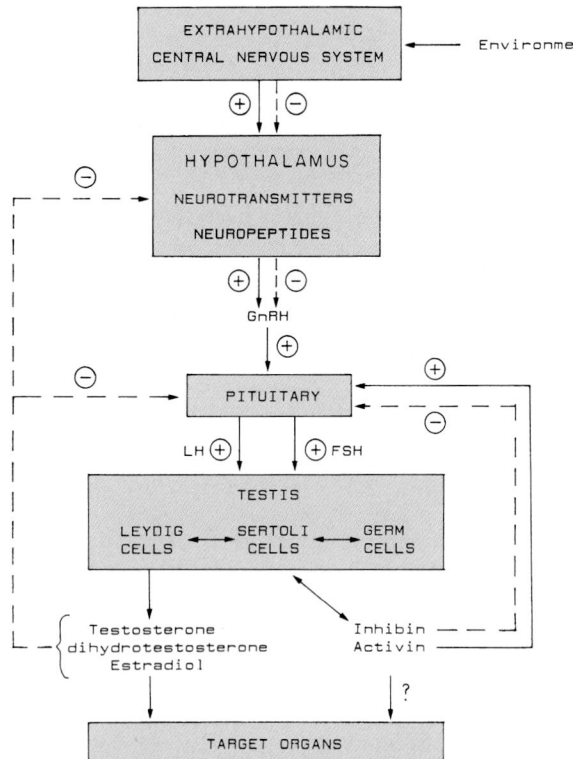

Figure 18–1. Diagram of the hypothalamic-pituitary-testis axis. LH, luteinizing hormone; FSH, follicle-stimulating hormone. (From Swerdloff RS, Wang C: Physiology of hypothalamic-pituitary function. In Walsh PC, Wein AJ, Retik AB, Vaughan ED [eds]: Campbell's Urology, 7th ed. Philadelphia, WB Saunders, 1997, pp 1239-1253.)

from the suprachiasmatic nucleus, which is the internal 24-hour clock in mammalian species. **The precursors of GnRH neurons migrate to their positions in the hypothalamus from the olfactory placode during embryonic development.** In Kallman's syndrome, a condition of congenital hypogonadotropic hypogonadism, the GnRH precursor neurons fail to migrate normally and the capacity for hypothalamic secretion of GnRH is not developed. Presentation of olfactory deficiency (anosmia) or other midline defects together with hypogonadotropic function is diagnostic of Kallman's syndrome.

Pituitary

The pituitary has two lobes: posterior and anterior. The posterior lobe, or neurohypophysis, is formed during development as a ventral outpocket of the hypothalamus (Fig. 18–2). The secretion of the two neurohypophysial hormones, oxytocin and vasopressin, is driven by neural stimuli. In contrast, the anterior pituitary or adenohypophysis is a glandular structure regulated by bloodborne factors. **LH and FSH are secreted by gonadotropes within the anterior pituitary.** In addition to the gonadotropes, the anterior pituitary contains cells that are specialized for secretion of other glycoprotein hormones: corticotropes secrete adrenocorticotropic hormone (ACTH); lactotropes secrete prolactin (PRL); somatotropes secrete growth hormone (GH); and thyrotropes

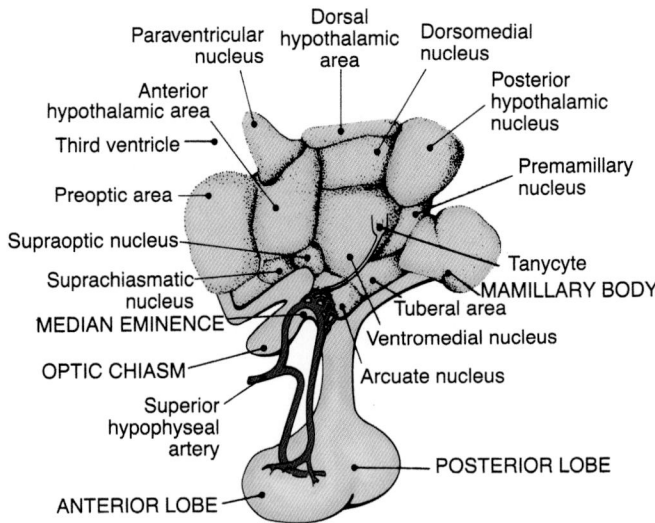

Figure 18–2. Organization of the hypothalamus and pituitary. (From Swerdloff RS, Wang C: Physiology of hypothalamic-pituitary function. In Walsh PC, Wein AJ, Retik AB, Vaughan ED [eds]: Campbell's Urology, 7th ed. Philadelphia, WB Saunders, 1997, pp 1239-1253.)

secrete thyroid-stimulating hormone (TSH). These four other glycoprotein hormones have significant effects on male reproductive function. The natural function of ACTH in the male reproductive system has yet to be defined. In mice, a stimulatory effect of ACTH on fetal Leydig cell steroidogenesis has been observed and interpreted as an indication that adrenocortical and Leydig cells share a common embryonic origin from mesenchymal stem cells in the mesonephros (O'Shaughnessy et al, 2003). Four of the glycoprotein hormones—LH, FSH, PRL, and GH—have significant effects on male reproductive function. This can be seen in instances of pituitary adenomas resulting in chronic oversecretion of prolactin, for example, that suppresses spermatogenesis (Mazzi et al, 1996).

In normal men, pulses of LH are secreted at an average frequency of once every 2 hours, with each pulse having an amplitude of 6 IU/L. The tonic level of LH in the bloodstream is 10 IU/L, which maintains testosterone levels at 5 ng/mL (Hayes and Crowley, 1988).

Steroid Feedback on the Hypothalamus and Pituitary

Negative feedback suppression of the release of GnRH is exerted by testosterone through androgen receptors present in hypothalamic neurons and in the pituitary. Testosterone is not necessarily the active steroid in the target cells: testosterone can be further metabolized by aromatase and 5α-reductase to estradiol and dihydrotestosterone (DHT), respectively. Genetic mutations resulting in partial or complete loss of function in the receptors for androgen (AR) and estrogen (ER) result in increased pituitary release of LH, indicating that both sex steroids participate in negative feedback (Brown, 1995; Shupnik and Schreihofer, 1997). Evidence for the involvement of 5α-reductase in negative feedback is seen in men with a genetic deficiency in 5α-reductase activity who are found to have higher than normal serum LH levels

(Canovatchel et al, 1994). Other studies, however, suggest that 5α-reductase may play a role in metabolic inactivation of testosterone through the subsequent conversion of DHT to a weak androgen, androstanediol (Uygur et al, 1998). Therefore, it seems likely that steroid negative feedback results from AR binding primarily to testosterone, with a contribution from ER binding to estradiol. Testosterone acts primarily to feedback at the level of the hypothalamus, whereas estrogens provide feedback to the pituitary to modulate the gonadotropin secretion response to each GnRH surge (Santen, 1975). In the male, differential regulation of gonadotropin secretion exists for different steroids. Whereas the negative effect of testosterone on LH secretion is mediated primarily by the androgen itself, negative effects of testosterone on FSH secretion are mediated primarily by the aromatized form of testosterone, estradiol (Hayes et al, 2001). Therefore, estradiol is the predominant regulator of FSH secretion in the male. Alternate isoforms of the steroid hormone receptors exist, conferring another level of complexity. The estrogen receptor ERβ is apparently not required for the negative feedback effects of estradiol (Korach et al, 1996). Also, the ligand binding and transcriptional activation properties of the A and B forms of AR differ, but it is not yet known whether they are differentially expressed in the hypothalamus (Gao and McPhaul, 1998).

Development of the Male Reproductive Axis

Developmental commitment to the male body plan is determined at the time of fertilization by the combination of a Y chromosome from the father's sperm with an X chromosome from the mother's oocyte. During embryogenesis, gonadal differentiation in male and female embryos occurs in discrete steps, and the embryonic ovary and testis are at first morphologically indistinguishable. The gonad starts as a thickening (or placode) of the coelomic epithelium on the surface of the primitive kidney (mesonephros). The placode grows into a gonadal ridge, and primordial germ cells subsequently move into the epithelium.

The primordial germ cells migrate into the genital ridge from the yolk sac (allantois) by pseudopodial motion using chemotactic signals and tracks of extracellular matrix proteins to locate their correct positions within the embryo. The gonadal ridge then, during the indifferent gonad stage, develops medullary cords of epithelial tissue. **The first identifiable step separating the ovarian and testicular pathways of differentiation is the movement of primordial germ cells into the medullary cords, at about 7 weeks after conception.** The primordial germ cells, enveloped by Sertoli cell precursors, are thereafter referred to as seminiferous cords, and this transition creates two compartments within the testis: seminiferous and interstitial.

The morphogenetic events of early testis differentiation are controlled by the *SRY* (*Sex-determining Region on the Y* chromosome) gene. **The *SRY* gene product, a nuclear transcription factor, acts in concert with other transcription factors, including WT-1, SOX-9, and DAX-1 to initiate male sexual differentiation** (Parker et al, 1999; de Santa Barbara et al, 2000). Identification of the *SRY* gene product as the testis-

determining factor came from studies showing that males with Y chromosome deletions involving *SRY* were phenotypically female and, conversely, that translocation of the *SRY* gene into an X chromosome is sufficient to confer a male phenotype in a genetic XX female. Further studies have shown that *SRY* is not always required for testicular development. Approximately 10% of 46,XX males have no detectable *SRY* gene (*SRY*–). These men probably have activation of factors normally induced by the transcription factor SRY, despite the absence of the *SRY* gene.

The morphogenetic events corresponding to the onset of *SRY*-mediated signaling are currently under investigation. Migration of cells from the mesonephros into the testis provides a source of mesenchymal stem cells that will later differentiate into Leydig cells. **The Sertoli cell precursors secrete müllerian inhibiting substance (also known as anti-müllerian hormone) that causes the anlagen of the female reproductive tract structures to regress** (Lee and Donahoe, 1993). **Secretion of testosterone by the fetal Leydig cells induces differentiation of the wolffian duct system, which later elaborates into the epididymides, vas deferens, and sex accessory glands.** Steroidogenic factor-1 (SF-1), another transcription factor produced under the direction of *SRY,* induces expression of the cytochrome P450 steroidogenic enzymes in Leydig cells, and also promotes differentiation of Sertoli cells and pituitary gonadotropes (Ikeda, 1996).

Endocrinology of the Testis

For many years, the hormonal control of testis function could be conceptualized simply, with a two-compartment model in which **FSH stimulates Sertoli cells to nurture germ cells through the process of spermatogenesis and LH stimulates Leydig cells to secrete testosterone.** With respect to Leydig cells, this simplification remains applicable, but genetic data on mutations resulting in decreased FSH action have led to the hypothesis that FSH is not essential for spermatogenesis. Male mice with knockout mutations in the FSH and FSH receptor genes remain fertile (Levallet et al, 1999), as do some men with defective FSH receptors, although sperm output is quantitatively reduced for these men (Tapanainen et al, 1997). Recent studies have suggested that failing testes have increased conversion of testosterone to estradiol, reflected by increased testosterone/estradiol ratio. This anomaly is treatable with an aromatase inhibitor that minimizes the conversion of testosterone to estradiol (Pavlovich et al, 2001). Meanwhile, other mutations identified in studies of transgenic mice have revealed factors that are clearly essential for spermatogenesis in this rodent model, such as stem cell factor (Blume-Jensen et al, 2000; Kissel et al, 2000). Stem cell factor operates as a local, or paracrine, signaling agent in the testis; it is secreted by the Sertoli cells and binds to cell surface receptors in spermatogonia, spermatocytes, and round spermatids. Thus, the endocrine control of spermatogenesis is complex because of the intricate cell-cell interactions that underlie germ cell differentiation within the seminiferous tubules. The cellular organization of the testis is reviewed next to provide a context for these endocrine and paracrine controls.

The testis, epididymis, and ductus deferens are responsible for producing and transporting the highly specialized male gamete to the ejaculatory duct. Production of spermatozoa requires many weeks from the initial mitotic divisions through the myriad changes readying it for ejaculation and fertilization. Highlights of this incredible transformation include (1) the initial mitotic divisions that produce either a set of stem cells relatively resistant to external injury or a population of rapidly proliferating germ cells destined to become spermatozoa; (2) meiosis, within a unique intratesticular environment created in part by Sertoli and interstitial cells, which results in the formation of the haploid gamete; and (3) the dramatic differentiation of the prospective gamete into a specialized cell ideally suited for transit through the female reproductive tract and, ultimately, fertilization.

Although the spermatozoon resulting from this complex process assumes its final shape and size in the testis, it normally achieves the ability to fertilize as well as the capacity for motility, only after passing through some portion of the epididymis. Newer techniques of assisted reproduction have been applied to spermatozoa and their precursors that would be unlikely to effect fertilization of an oocyte without assistance (Kimura and Yanagimachi, 1995; Palermo et al, 1994; Tesarik et al, 1995). The success of these interventions with intact spermatozoa and the potential applications of immature male gamete micromanipulation have increased the importance of understanding the contribution of a male gamete to fertilization and subsequent embryo development (Cummins and Jequier, 1994; Schatten, 1994).

During in utero development of the male fetus, Leydig cells differentiate from mesenchymal precursor cells in the connective tissue stroma of the testis between the seminiferous tubules. This process occurs by the seventh week of gestation and is associated with the appearance of androgens in circulation. The activation of Leydig cell steroidogenesis correlates with the onset of androgen-dependent differentiation of the male reproductive system. The placenta secretes an LH-like gonadotropin, human chorionic gonadotropin (hCG), that is thought to provide a sufficient stimulus for the development of fetal Leydig cells, based on the observation that these cells differentiate even in abnormal, anencephalic fetuses in which there is no internal secretion of LH. Studies in rats have established that the onset of steroidogenic enzyme gene expression in fetal Leydig cells is independent of stimulation by gonadotropin (El-Gehani et al, 1998; Majdic et al, 1998). It is probable that local factors secreted in the testis act in concert with gonadotropin to effect complete differentiation of the Leydig cells and to coordinate that process with developmental events in the seminiferous tubules.

The fetal Leydig cells regress after birth without continued stimulation by hCG, but, at 2 to 3 months after birth, a second wave of Leydig cell differentiation occurs, briefly elevating testosterone levels in male infants. This second peak in circulating androgen occurs in response to gonadotropin production from the pituitary of the neonate, since maternal hCG is no longer present. Androgen produced during the first 2 to 6 months of a male neonate's life is thought to hormonally imprint the hypothalamus, liver, and prostate such that they respond appropriately to androgen stimulation later in life. Imprinting of the phallus and scrotum is also thought to occur during this period of time; the absence of an androgen surge in the newborn male may prevent normal development in affected males (Main et al, 2000). The Leydig cells of the early infant then regress, and the testis remains in a state of dormancy during childhood.

The hypothalamic capacity to generate pulses of GnRH arises at puberty, usually initiating around the 12th year. The pubertal onset of GnRH pulses typically occurs at night, due in part to a gradual decrease in nocturnal melatonin secretion by the pineal gland. When the mature pattern of GnRH pulsatility is developed, the pulses continue to be more frequent at night than during the day. The "gonadostat" hypothesis for puberty holds that, in addition to the abatement of the inhibition by melatonin, androgen negative feedback is delayed until steroidogenic capacity of the testes is developed. This is achieved through metabolism of testosterone by 5α-reductase and 3α-hydroxysteroid dehydrogenase to androgens, such as androstanediol, that have a weak affinity for ARs.

Puberty is also influenced by the growth rate and nutritional status of the body. Growth hormone and its paracrine mediator, insulin-like growth factor-1 (IGF-1), have pronounced stimulatory effects on reproductive function (Bartke, 1999). The adipocyte hormone leptin is now thought to affect the timing of puberty (Clement et al, 1998). Leptin is the body's regulatory signal governing the size of the fat stores. A human population of individuals with early onset of obesity was found to have a gene defect causing a truncation in the leptin receptor. Puberty is delayed in these individuals, and there is increasing evidence that leptin modulates hypothalamic and pituitary activity (Caprio et al, 1999; Kiess et al, 1999; Quinton et al, 1999). As with the hypothesized gonadostat, a neural mechanism, or ponderostat, may exist to set the threshold value of leptin stimulation informing the body that nutritional resources are sufficient for reproduction. The mechanism by which leptin controls reproduction remains under investigation. Stimulatory effects of leptin on gonadotropin secretion have been reported (Dearth et al, 2000), but leptin receptors are also present in the testis, where the effects of this peptide appear to be inhibitory (Tena-Sempere et al, 2000).

Aging of the Hypothalamic and Pituitary Axis

As men age beyond 50 years serum testosterone levels decline. Declining health status in older men may contribute to the decreased output of testosterone, but there is also a specific effect of aging. The basal levels of LH in the blood increase in older men, but LH pulsatility is blunted, indicating an effect of aging on the GnRH pulse generator. In addition, Leydig cell steroidogenic capacity decreases. Studies in the brown Norway rat suggest that Leydig cell aging may result from defects in Leydig cell proteins caused by oxygen free radicals that are byproducts of steroidogenesis (Zirkin et al, 1997; Zirkin and Chen, 2000). High testicular concentrations of testosterone are required to maintain spermatogenesis, and men older than age 40 years have lower fecundity, measured as a 50% lower probability of achieving a pregnancy with their partners within 1 year, compared with men younger than age 25 (Ford et al, 2000). Thus, the age-related decline in Leydig cell steroidogenesis has potential implications for male fertility.

TESTIS
Gross Structures and Vascularization

In healthy young men the ovoid testis measures 15 to 25 mL in volume (Prader, 1966) **and has a longitudinal length of 4.5 to 5.1 cm** (Tishler, 1971; Winter and Faiman, 1972). The testicular parenchyma is surrounded by a capsule made up of three layers: the outer visceral layer of the tunica vaginalis, the tunica albuginea, and the innermost layer of the tunica vasculosa. The tunica albuginea contains large numbers of branching smooth muscle cells that course through the predominantly collagenous tissue (Langford and Heller, 1973). These smooth muscle cells may impart a contractile capability to the human testicular capsule because contractions have been elicited in the isolated testicular capsule from humans (Rikmaru and Shirai, 1972) and other species (Davis and Langford, 1969; Davis, 1970) by electrical stimulation and specific autonomic drugs. In humans and several other species, **capsular smooth muscle tone or contractions may affect blood flow into the testis** (Schweitzer, 1929), because the testicular artery traverses the capsule at an oblique angle. Whether capsular smooth muscle contraction plays a significant role in promoting the flow of seminiferous tubule fluid out of the testis (Davis and Horowitz, 1978) is uncertain because some fluid flow from the rat rete testis is maintained after removal of the capsule (Free et al, 1980). **The testicular arteries penetrate the tunica albuginea and then travel inferiorly along the posterior surface of the testicular parenchyma, with branches passing anteriorly in a variable transverse fashion over the testicular parenchyma.** Major testicular artery branches also travel over the inferior pole of the testis, passing anteriorly and branching out over the surface of the testis. The location of these vessels is clinically important, because they may be injured during orchiopexy or testis biopsy procedures (Jarow, 1991; Schlegel and Su, 1997). **The medial and lateral midsection of the testis has fewer vessels compared with anterior or inferior sections of the testis** (see also Fig. 3–44). Individual arteries to tubules travel within the septa that contain each seminiferous tubule.

Within the capsule, the testis is divided into compartments separated by septa of the testis. Each septum separates seminiferous tubules and contains at least one centrifugal artery. Within each septum are individual seminiferous tubules, which contain the developing germ cells, as well as interstitial tissue. Interstitial tissue is composed of Leydig cells, mast cells, and macrophages as well as nerves and blood and lymph vessels. **In humans, interstitial tissue takes up 20% to 30% of the total testicular volume** (Setchell and Brooks, 1988). The relationship between seminiferous tubules and interstitial tissue is demonstrated in Figure 18–3.

The seminiferous tubules are long, highly coiled, and looped, both ends of which usually terminate in the rete testis. Lennox and Ahmad (1970) estimated that **the combined length of the 600 to 1200 tubules in the human testis is approximately 250 meters. The rete testis coalesces to form the 6 to 12 ductuli efferentes, which act as conduits to carry testicular fluid and spermatozoa into the caput epididymis** (Fig. 18–4). Roosen-Runge and Holstein (1978) suggested that the rete testis topography acts as a "valve" with a built-in

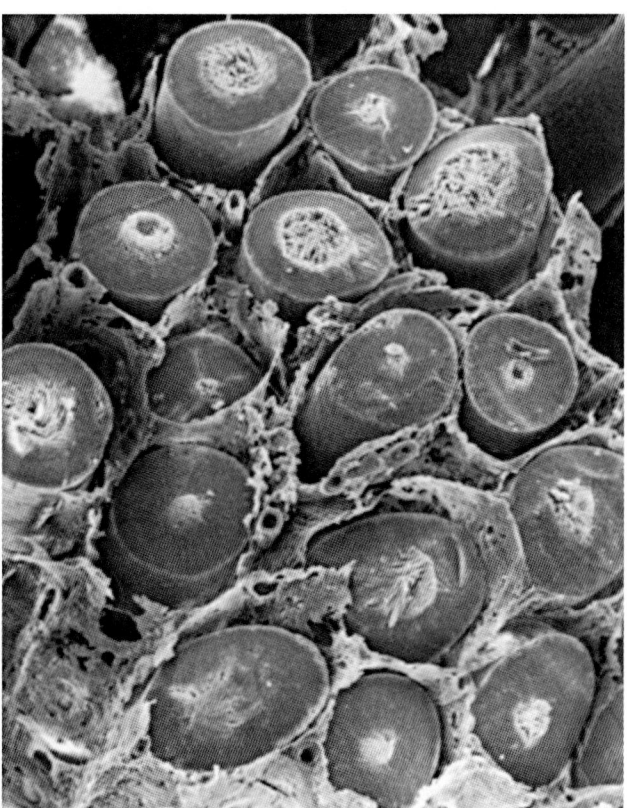

Figure 18–3. Scanning electron micrograph of the cut surface of the human testis. Note the relationship of interstitial tissue to seminiferous tubules. (From Christensen AK: Leydig cells. In Greep RO, Astwood EB [eds]: Handbook of Physiology. Washington, DC, American Physiology Society, 1975, pp 57-94.)

mechanism for activating the flow of fluid and spermatozoa toward the epididymis.

The testis has no somatic innervation but receives autonomic innervation primarily from the intermesenteric nerves and renal plexus (Mitchell, 1935). These nerves run along the testicular artery to the testis. Baumgarten and colleagues (1968) found that the testicular adrenergic innervation is restricted primarily to small blood vessels supplying clusters of Leydig cells. Studies in rats point to a regulatory role of the innervation in controlling Leydig cell steroidogenesis: in the brain, intraventricular administration of the immune system cytokine interleukin causes profound reductions in testosterone (Turnbull and Rivier, 1997). Because androgen inhibits immune function, interleukins acting in the brain during infection could, by rapid suppression of Leydig cells, potentiate an appropriate immune response. Other studies suggest that vascular tone in the testis appears to be at least partially under nervous control (Linzell and Setchell, 1969). (See Hodson [1970] for a complete discussion of testicular and epididymal innervation.) The functional importance of testicular innervation in humans, however, remains to be defined.

The human testicular parenchyma is provided with approximately 9 mL of blood per 100 g of tissue per minute (Pettersson et al, 1973). Fritjofsson and associates (1969) claimed that in humans blood flow to the left testis varies from 1.6 to 12.4 mL/100 mg/min, whereas that to the right testis

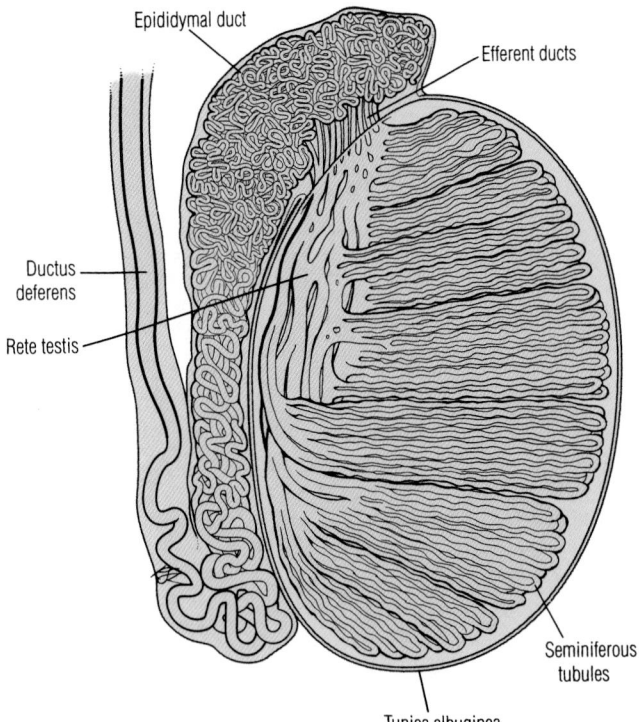

Epididymal duct

Efferent ducts

Ductus deferens

Rete testis

Seminiferous tubules

Tunica albuginea

Figure 18–4. Drawing of the human testis showing the seminiferous tubules, epididymis, and ductus deferens. (Illustration based on Hirsh AV: The anatomical preparations of the human testis and epididymis in the Glasgow Hunterian Collection. Hum Reprod Update 1995;1:515-521.)

ranges from 3.2 to 38.5 mL/100 g/min. The significance of this variation in testicular blood flow is unknown.

The vasculature of the mammalian testis has been thoroughly discussed in three excellent reviews (Gunn and Gould, 1975; Free, 1977; Setchell and Brooks, 1988). **The arterial supply to the human testis and epididymis is derived from three sources: the internal spermatic testicular artery, the deferential vasal artery, and the external spermatic or cremasteric artery** (Harrison and Barclay, 1948). The spermatic artery arises from the abdominal aorta just below the renal artery, becomes a component of the spermatic cord above the internal inguinal ring, and is intimately associated with a network of anastomotic veins that eventually form the pampiniform plexus. The vascular arrangement in the pampiniform plexus, with the counterflowing artery and veins separated only by the thickness of their vascular wall in some areas (Harrison, 1949b), facilitates the exchange of heat and small molecules. For example, testosterone is transported from the vein to the artery via a concentration-limited, passive diffusion process in men (Bayard et al, 1975). **The counter-current exchange of heat in the spermatic cord provides blood to the testis that is 2°C to 4°C lower than rectal temperature in the normal individual** (Agger, 1971). This results in intratesticular temperatures that are 3°C to 4°C lower than rectal temperatures in normal men (Kurz and Goldstein, 1986). A loss of the temperature differential is associated with testicular dysfunction in humans with idiopathic infertility, as well as varicocele (Mieusset et al, 1987; Goldstein and Eid, 1989) and cryptorchidism (Marshall and Edler, 1982).

Leaving the pampiniform plexus and extending to the mediastinal area of the testis the spermatic artery becomes highly coiled and branches before entering the testis. Extensive interconnections, especially between the internal spermatic and deferential arteries (Fig. 18–5), allow maintenance of testicular viability even after division of the internal spermatic artery in some males. Kormano and Suoranta (1971) completed an angiographic study of the arterial pattern of 78 human autopsy testes and observed that **a single artery enters the testis in 56% of cases; two branches enter in 31% of cases; and three or more branches enter in 13% of cases.** From a practical standpoint it is important to consider the number of testicular arteries that are present in the spermatic cord at the inguinal level. Jarow and colleagues (1992) found an average of 2.0 arteries during intraoperative dissection with loupes, but 2.4 arteries in the inguinal region could be identified in cadaveric dissections. Another intraoperative dissection study of over 100 spermatic cords identified a single internal spermatic artery at 10 to 15 times magnification in 50% of cases, with two arteries in 30% of spermatic cords and three arteries for 20% (Beck et al, 1992). Breaching of the testicular artery most commonly occurs during its course through the inguinal canal (Hopps et al, 2003). Within the testis, the artery divides into a series of centrifugal arteries that penetrate the testicular parenchyma. Subsequent branches give rise to a dual set of arterioles that supply blood to individual intertubular and peritubular capillaries (Muller, 1957). In some men, up to 90% of testicular blood supply derives from the testicular artery. In these men, interruption of the testicular blood supply may result in testicular atrophy (Silber, 1979). The capillaries inside the columns of interstitial tissue are called the intertubular capillaries, whereas the rope ladder–like capillaries running near the seminiferous tubule are called the peritubular capillaries.

Testicular blood flow appears to be regulated at several levels. Autoregulation of flow through the testicular artery may involve myogenic mechanisms in the subcapsular region of the artery, at least in the rat (Davis et al, 1990). In addition, **although total testicular blood flow is relatively constant, the regional distribution of flow within the testis is thought to vary significantly based on local metabolic needs.** Local peptide effectors, such as atrial natriuretic peptide, which increases blood flow in rat testes (Collin et al, 1997), afford one means of selective control. In addition, there is evidence for assisted transport of systemic effectors, such as LH, across the vascular endothelium. Transport of LH may be achieved by a receptor-mediated mechanism, because vascular endothelial cells have been shown to express LH receptors on their luminal surfaces (Milgrom et al, 1997). In rats, the concentration of LH in the interstitial fluid is only about one tenth that in the blood (Setchell et al, 2002). The timing of LH action on rat Leydig cells appears to precede its delivery to the interstitium (Turner, 1995), which may be achieved through rapid release of cytokines by the endothelial cells on binding to LH. Testosterone produced in the interstitium emerges from the testis predominantly in testicular venous effluent, not in lymph (Desjardins, 1989). Finally, differential dilation and constriction of terminal arterioles allow capillary units to be perfused selectively. Taken together, these observations suggest a highly specialized function for the microvasculature

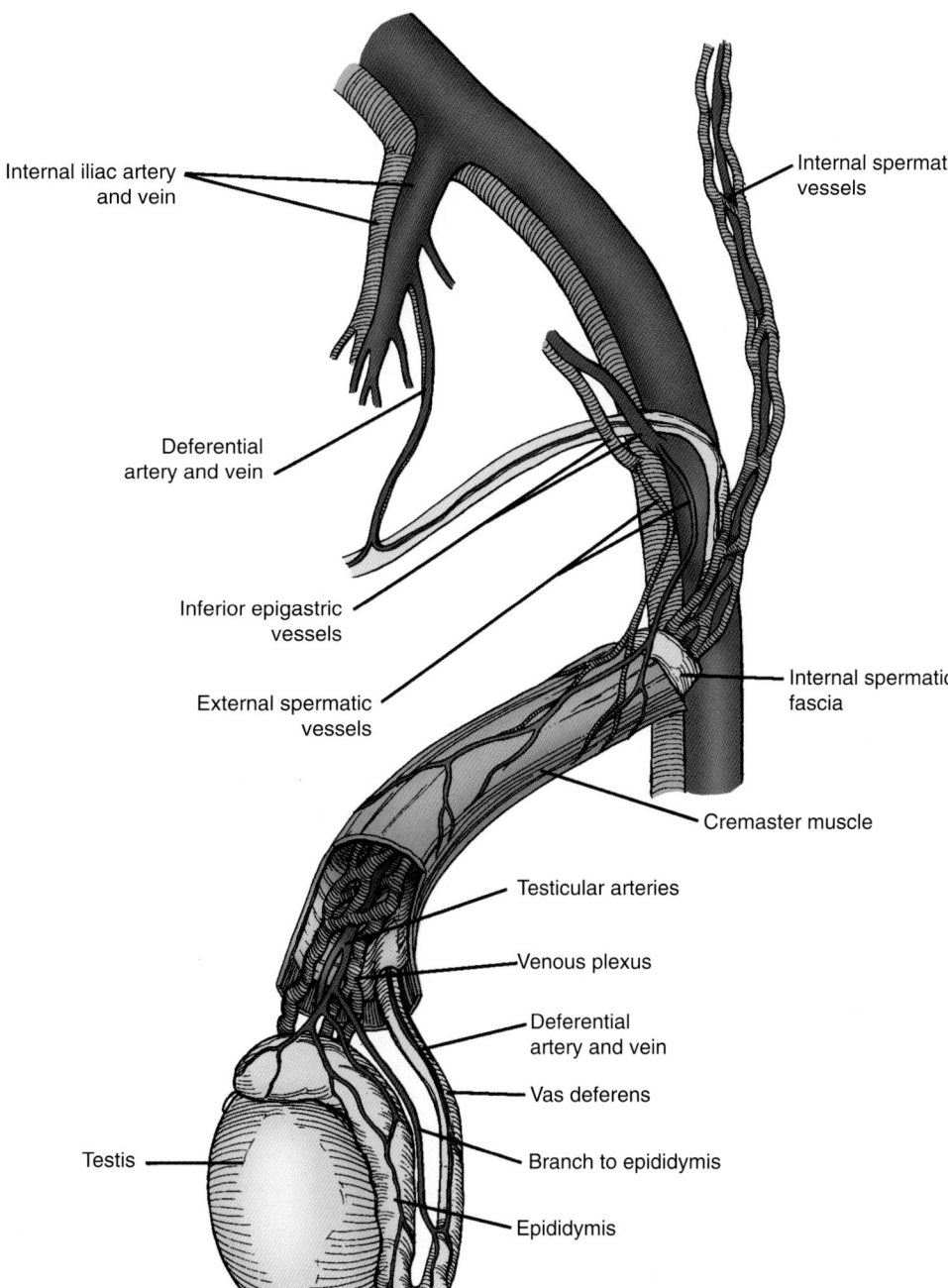

Figure 18–5. Schematic illustration of the interconnections between internal spermatic, external spermatic (cremasteric), and deferential vessels in the peritesticular region and schematic cord.

of the testis. (See Desjardins [1989] and Ergun and associates [1977] for an excellent discussion of testicular microcirculation.)

The veins within the testis are unusual in that they do not run with the corresponding intratesticular arteries. The small veins in the parenchyma empty into either the veins on the surface of the testis or into one of a group of veins near the mediastinum that travel toward the region of the rete (Setchell and Brooks, 1988). These two sets of veins join together with deferential veins to form the pampiniform plexus. Ishigami and associates (1970) stated that blood in this venous system tends to stagnate because the spermatic vein is thin walled, is

poorly muscularized, and lacks effective valves except at the inflow points into the inferior vena cava or the renal vein. This issue remains controversial.

There are prominent lymphatic ducts in the spermatic cord of the human testis (Wenzel and Kellermann, 1966; Hundeiker, 1971). The lymph capillaries that give rise to these lymph ducts originate within the intertubular spaces and do not penetrate the seminiferous tubules. Obstruction of the lymphatic ducts in the spermatic cord invariably is followed by dilatation of the interstitium but not the seminiferous tubules, suggesting that although the extracellular space of the interstitium is drained via the lymphatics, the seminiferous tubules are not. Obstruction of the lymphatics can also result in hydrocele formation, a common complication on non-microscopic varicocelectomy (Goldstein, 1997). In some species, testicular lymph flow is transported to the ipsilateral epididymis (Setchell and Brooks, 1988), suggesting an effect of testicular lymph on epididymal function. Whether there is a testis-epididymis lymphatic system in humans is not known.

The extracellular fluid bathing the Sertoli cells and germinal cells flows from the seminiferous tubules into the rete to form rete testis fluid, which is transported into the caput epididymis. Originally, it was thought that the fluid probably originates both from primary secretions within the seminiferous tubules and from epithelial secretions directly into the rete (Tuck et al, 1970; Kormano and Suoranta, 1971; Levine and Marsh, 1971). However, Setchell and Brooks (1988) suggested that "the majority of the fluid leaving the rete, originates in the tubules." Whatever its origin, rete testis fluid is a dilute suspension of spermatozoa in a fluid isosmotic with plasma. Reabsorption of fluid within the rete testis and efferent ductules is regulated by estrogen action. Estrogens appear to regulate this reabsorption of fluid in the rete testis and efferent ducts. Rodents with estrogen receptor knockouts (ERKO) have faulty reabsorption of intratubular fluid leaving the testis, with subsequent accumulation of fluid inside the seminiferous tubules that results in significant focal seminiferous tubular dysfunction (Lee et al, 2000).

Setchell and Waites (1975) reported that in the ram the ion composition and the carbohydrate, amino acid, and protein content of rete testis fluid are markedly different from those in blood plasma or lymphatics. They correctly pointed out that **"differences in composition between the fluid inside the seminiferous tubules and excurrent ducts of the testis and blood plasma or testicular lymph make it clear that substances do not diffuse freely into and out of tubules."** Extrapolation of this idea led to the concept of a blood-testis barrier, which exists to a greater or lesser extent in numerous species (Setchell and Waites, 1975), including man (Koskimies et al, 1973). This topic is discussed in detail later in this chapter.

Cytoarchitecture and Function of the Testis

Interstitium

The interstitium contains blood vessels, lymph vessels, fibroblastic supporting cells, macrophages, mast cells, and Leydig cells (Fig. 18–6). Recently, testicular macrophages have been shown to be involved in the regulation of parenchymal cells within the testis, including Leydig cells (Hutson et al, 1994). Resting macrophages normally facilitate testosterone biosynthesis by secreting the steroid precursor 25-hydroxycholesterol (Nes et al, 2000). In contrast, activation of testicular macrophages during disease is associated with release of proinflammatory cytokines, such as interleukin-1, that inhibit Leydig cell function (Hales et al, 1999). Stereologic analysis (Kaler and Neaves, 1978) showed that a human testis from a 20-year-old man contained approximately 700 million Leydig cells. Leydig cells alone account for 5% to 12% of the total volume of the human testis (Christensen, 1975; Kaler and Neaves, 1978). The mechanisms by which Leydig cells develop and mature were reviewed by Huhtaniemi and Pelliniemi

(1992). Evidence obtained after ablation of Leydig cells from mature rat testes with ethane dimethyl sulfonate (EDS) suggests that paracrine factors within the testis and pituitary LH influence the differentiation of Leydig cells from precursor cells (Keeney et al, 1990; Teerds and Dorrington, 1993). Recently, it has been shown that precursors of mouse and rat Leydig cells begin to express steroidogenic enzymes before they become sensitive to LH (O'Shaughnessy et al, 1998; Teerds et al, 1998). Therefore, IGF-1 and other paracrine factors may be particularly important for the induction of LH sensitivity (Le Roy et al, 1999).

The Leydig cell is responsible for the bulk of testicular steroid production. Testosterone, synthesized from the steroid precursor cholesterol, is the principal steroid produced by the human testis (Lipsett, 1974), although numerous C_{18}, C_{19}, and C_{21} steroids are also produced (Lipsett, 1974; Ewing and Brown, 1977). It is unclear whether the bulk of cholesterol used for testosterone biosynthesis is derived from blood plasma (Anderson and Dietschy, 1977) or from de novo biosynthesis (Charreau et al, 1981). In either event, Figure 18–7 shows that cholesterol from the metabolically active pool must be transported into the mitochondria, where the cholesterol side-chain cleavage enzyme converts it to pregnenolone and the C6 fragment isocaproaldehyde. Movement of cholesterol to the inner membrane of the mitochondrion is conducted by two transport proteins: steroid acute regulatory protein (StAR) and peripheral benzodiazepine receptor (PBR).

LH binding elicits new protein synthesis in the Leydig cell, and the newly-synthesized StAR contains a signal sequence that enables the protein to be threaded through the outer mitochondrial membrane (Stocco, 2000). It is unclear, however, that the signal sequence is required for the cholesterol transport function of StAR. The PBR forms a channel for cholesterol in the mitochondrial membrane (Culty et al, 1999). Whether the two proteins interact or function independently has not been established, although a recent analysis of cells in which the two proteins were fluorescently labeled indicates that they form a close association (West et al, 2001). Pregnenolone must then be transported out of the mitochondrial membrane into the smooth endoplasmic reticulum, where it is converted into testosterone. The four major enzymes participating in testosterone biosynthesis are, therefore, cholesterol side-chain cleavage enzyme, 3β-hydroxysteroid dehydrogenase, cytochrome P450 17α-hydroxylase/C_{17-20}-lyase, and 17β-hydroxysteroid dehydrogenase. Details of the enzymology, human chromosomal locations, and molecular genetics these enzymes have been reviewed (see Payne and Hales [2004]). Mutations in the genes encoding these enzymes have been described (Miller, 2002), although it is noted that disorders of androgen biosynthesis are a relatively rare cause of sexual ambiguity in normal XY males. Once synthesized, testosterone probably diffuses across the cell membrane and is trapped in the extracellular fluid and blood plasma by steroid-binding macromolecules. This biosynthetic process is schematically demonstrated in Figure 18–7.

The control of Leydig cell steroidogenesis has been reviewed exhaustively (Rommerts et al, 1974; Christensen, 1975; Eik-Nes, 1975; Catt and Dufau, 1976; Dufau and Catt, 1978; Hall, 1979; Ewing, 1983; Payne and Youngblood, 1995). Suffice it to say that the primary, acute, regulation of testosterone

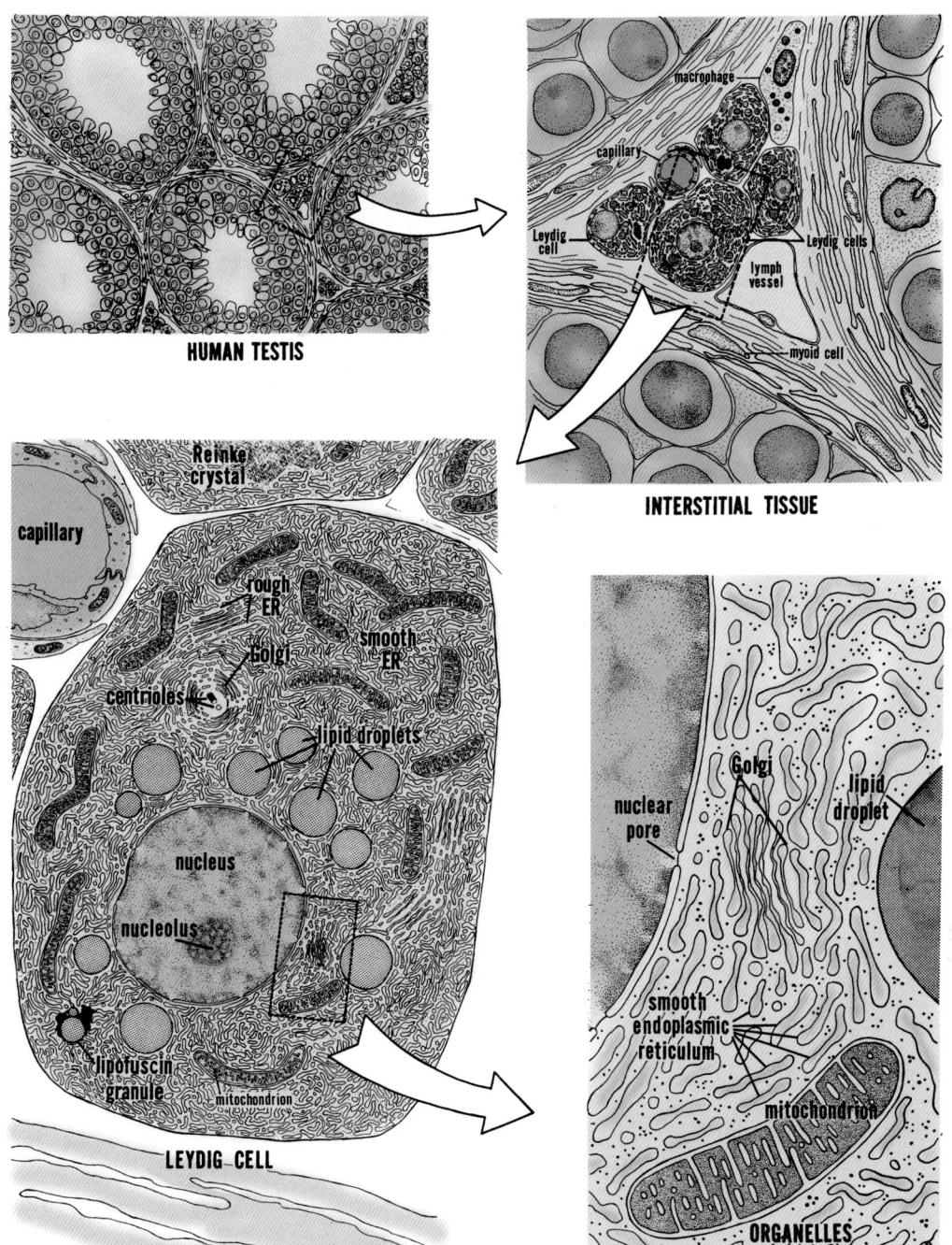

Figure 18–6. Location and fine structure of human Leydig cells. Leydig cells occur in clusters in the interstitial tissue between the seminiferous tubules *(upper left)*. Interstitial tissue *(upper right)* contains macrophages and fibroblasts as well as capillaries and lymph vessels. Seminiferous tubules are surrounded by a boundary layer of myoid cells. The most abundant organelle within the cytoplasm of the Leydig cell is the smooth endoplasmic reticulum *(lower left)*. Some of the organelles are seen in greater detail in a selected area of cytoplasm *(lower right)*. (From Christensen AK: Leydig cells. In Greep RO, Astwood WB [eds]: Handbook of Physiology, Section 7. Endocrinology. Baltimore, Williams & Wilkins, 1975. Copyright 1975, The American Physiological Society, Bethesda, MD.)

production is dependent on LH. LH binding, through generation of cyclic adenosine monophosphate (AMP) and several other intracellular events, initiates transport of cholesterol into the mitochondria. Efflux of chloride ions (Cooke, 1996), influx of calcium (Cooke, 1996), and release of arachidonic acid from phospholipids (Wang et al, 1999) all play a role in the acute stimulation of steroidogenesis. Pituitary peptides other than LH (e.g., FSH and PL) have also been shown to

modify the LH-stimulated increase (see Ewing [1983]). Nonpituitary factors capable of altering the production of steroids by Leydig cells include LH releasing hormone (LHRH) (Sharpe, 1984), inhibin and activin (Bardin et al, 1989), the growth factors epidermal growth factor (EGF), IGF-1, and transforming growth factor-β (TGF-β) (Ascoli and Segaloff, 1989; Saez et al, 1991) prostaglandins (Eik-Nes, 1975a), and adrenergic stimulation (Eik-Nes, 1975a). Most of

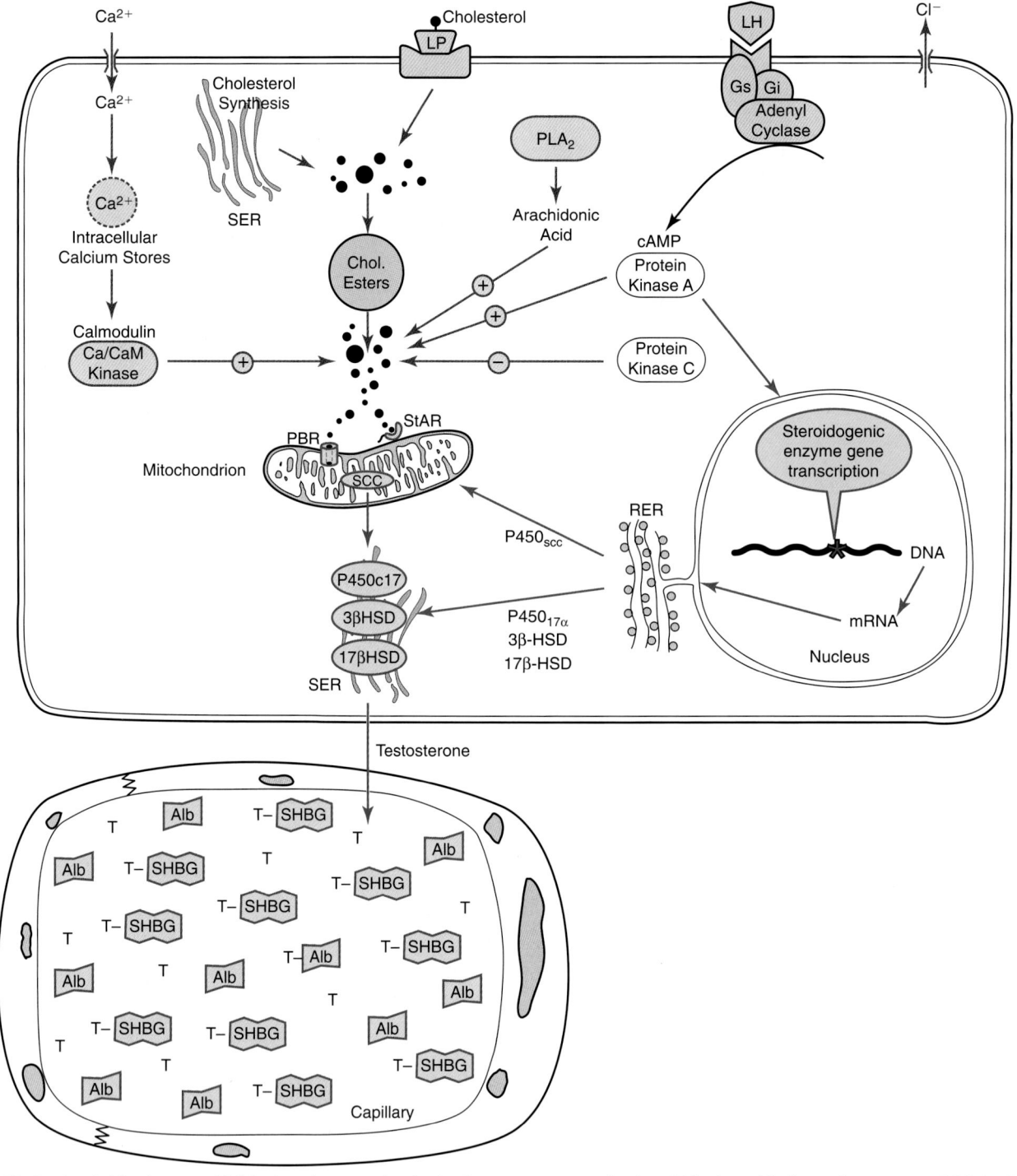

Figure 18–7. Luteinizing hormone (LH) is the primary tropic stimulus for testosterone production. LH is shown binding to its receptor. Highlighted in *red* are the events associated with the acute regulation of steroidogenesis, namely, mobilization of the initial substrate for testosterone biosynthesis, cholesterol. These events occur within minutes of LH binding. The *green arrows* denote chronic events triggered by LH, which include increased transcription and translation of the genes encoding the steroidogenic enzymes. LH stimulation also increases the number and size of Leydig cell organelles that are involved in steroidogenesis, such as the mitochondria and smooth endoplasmic reticulum (SER) membranes. These events are chronic and require several hours, to days, before they become evident. The LH receptor *(in yellow)* has seven membrane-spanning domains and is coupled to G proteins that modulate its activation of adenylate cyclase. Cyclic adenosine monophosphate (cAMP) stimulates protein kinase A. LH binding also initiates several other events in parallel: calcium influx leading to calmodulin activation of a calcium/calmodulin kinase; arachidonic acid mobilization from phospholipase A_2 activity; and efflux of chloride ions *(all shown in red)*. The net effect of these changes is to make more substrate cholesterol available for steroidogenesis. The three main sources of cholesterol in the Leydig cell are (1) externally, from bloodborne lipoprotein and internalization of cholesterol/lipoprotein receptor complexes, (2) from de novo synthesis from acetate, and (3) from stored cholesterol esters in lipid droplets. Maintenance of cholesterol stores is part of the normal resting function of the Leydig cell; LH stimulation evokes cholesterol mobilization through cholesterol esterase activity. The free cholesterol then associates with steroid acute regulatory protein (StAR) for transport to the inner membrane of the mitochondrion. A key part of the transport mechanism is the signal sequence *(depicted as a blue threadlike tail)* that enables StAR protein to pass through mitochondrial membranes. Peripheral benzodiazepine receptor (PBR) forms a channel in the mitochondrial membranes and also facilitates cholesterol entry. The cholesterol side-chain cleavage enzyme (cytochrome $P450_{scc}/\Delta^{5-4}$ isomerase, $P450_{scc}$) cleaves cholesterol at C21 to form pregnenolone. This and subsequent steps of steroidogenesis are shown in *blue*. Pregnenolone diffuses out of the mitochondrion to the SER. In the Δ^5 pathway of human Leydig cells, the ordering of steroidogenic enzymes in the SER is as shown: cytochrome P450 17α-hydroxylase/C_{17-20} lyase (P450c17) → 3β-hydroxysteroid dehydrogenase (3β-HSD) → 17β-hydroxysteroid dehydrogenase (17β-HSD). Rodent Leydig cells have a different ordering of these enzymes, with 3β-HSD acting first (the Δ^4 pathway). Testosterone diffuses out of the Leydig cell and associates quickly with binding proteins, including albumin (Alb) and, primarily, sex hormone binding globulin (SHBG), in the circulation.

this information, however, is derived from in vitro experiments using laboratory animals, and the role of these factors in normal testicular function in humans is uncertain. Other yet poorly understood autocrine and paracrine effectors of Leydig cell function also have been proposed (for reviews of this literature see Hedger and de Kretser [2000], Saez [1994], and Skinner [1990]). Finally, direct inhibition of Leydig cell steroidogenesis via estrogens and androgens may exist (Darney et al, 1996; Ewing, 1983).

Testosterone concentrations in peripheral blood of men change dramatically during the life cycle. Figure 18–8 shows that a peak of testosterone occurs in the blood of the human fetus between 12 and 18 weeks of gestation. Another testosterone peak occurs at approximately 2 months of age. Testosterone reaches a maximal concentration during the second or third decade of life, then reaches a plateau, and declines thereafter. Additionally, annual and daily rhythms (see Fig. 18–8, insets A and B) in testosterone concentration occur. Superimposed on these rhythms are irregular fluctuations in testosterone concentration in peripheral blood (see Fig. 18–8, inset C). See the review by Ewing and associates (1980) for a thorough discussion of this subject.

In those species that have been studied thoroughly, **the major epochs in testosterone production represent an orderly sequence of temporal signals that cause the following: (1) the differentiation and development of the fetal reproductive tract; (2) the neonatal organization or "imprinting" of androgen-dependent target tissues, ensuring their appropriate response later in puberty and adulthood; (3) the masculinization of the male at puberty; and (4) the maintenance of growth and function of androgen-dependent organs in the adult.** In part, these temporal changes in testosterone production reflect a complex interaction between the pituitary gland and the testis. For a thorough discussion of this latter topic see the works of DiZerga and Sherins (1981), Faiman and associates (1981), Santen (1981), and Swerdloff and Heber (1981).

Seminiferous Tubules

The seminiferous tubules, with their germinal elements and supporting cells, provide a unique environment for the production of germ cells. The supporting cells include the sustentacular cells of the basement membrane and the Sertoli cells. The germinal elements comprise a population of epithelial cells, including a slowly dividing primitive stem cell population, the rapidly proliferating spermatogonia, spermatocytes undergoing meiosis, and the metamorphosing spermatids. The following sections describe the components of the seminiferous tubule as well as the environment formed by "the blood-testis barrier" in the seminiferous tubule.

Peritubular Structures

The seminiferous tubule is surrounded in the human by several layers of peritubular tissue (Fig. 18–9; Hermo et al, 1977). Separating the interstitial tissue from the tubule is an outer adventitial layer of fibrocytes. The next layer consists of myoid cells interspersed with connective tissue lamellae. A third peritubular layer is present immediately adjacent to the

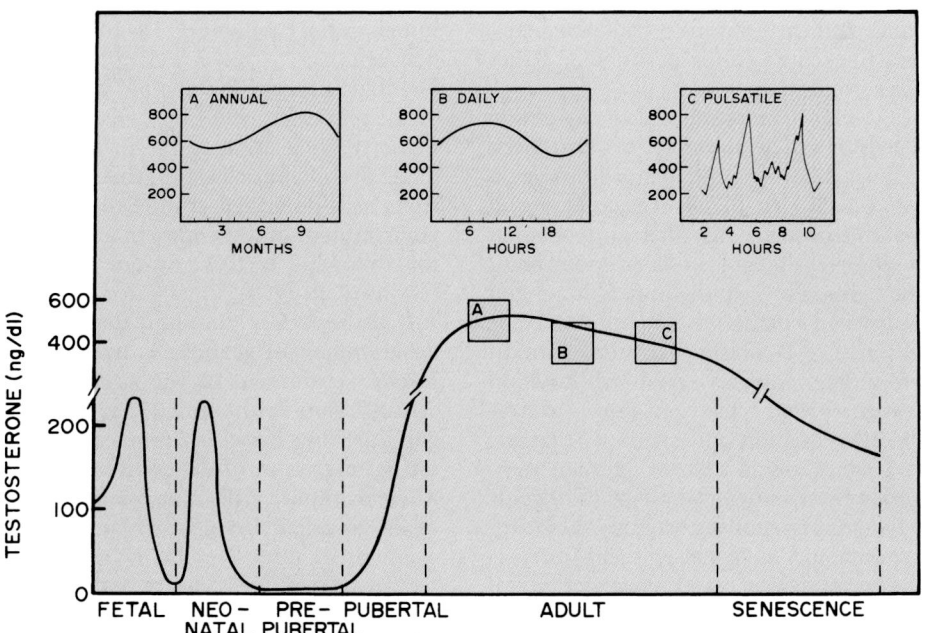

Figure 18–8. Concentration of testosterone in peripheral blood of the human male at different times of the life cycle. The peak of testosterone in the peripheral blood of the fetus occurs between 12 and 18 weeks of gestation *(lower left corner; gestational age not shown)*. The peak of testosterone in the peripheral blood of the neonate occurs at approximately 2 months of age. Testosterone declines to low levels during the prepubertal period. The pubertal increase in testosterone concentration in peripheral blood occurs between 12 and 17 years of age. Testosterone concentration in the adult reaches its maximum during the second or third decade of life and then declines slowly through the fifth decade. Testosterone concentration in peripheral blood declines dramatically during senescence. Inset A shows the annual rhythm in testosterone concentration in peripheral blood of the human male. The peak and nadir occur in the fall and spring, respectively. Inset B shows the daily rhythm in testosterone concentration in peripheral blood of the adult human male. The peak and nadir occur in the morning and evening, respectively. Inset C shows the frequent and irregular fluctuations in testosterone concentration in peripheral blood of the human male. (From Ewing LL, Davis JC, Zirkin BR: Regulation of testicular function: A spatial and temporal view. In Greep RO [ed]: International Review of Physiology. Baltimore, University Park Press, 1980, p 41.)

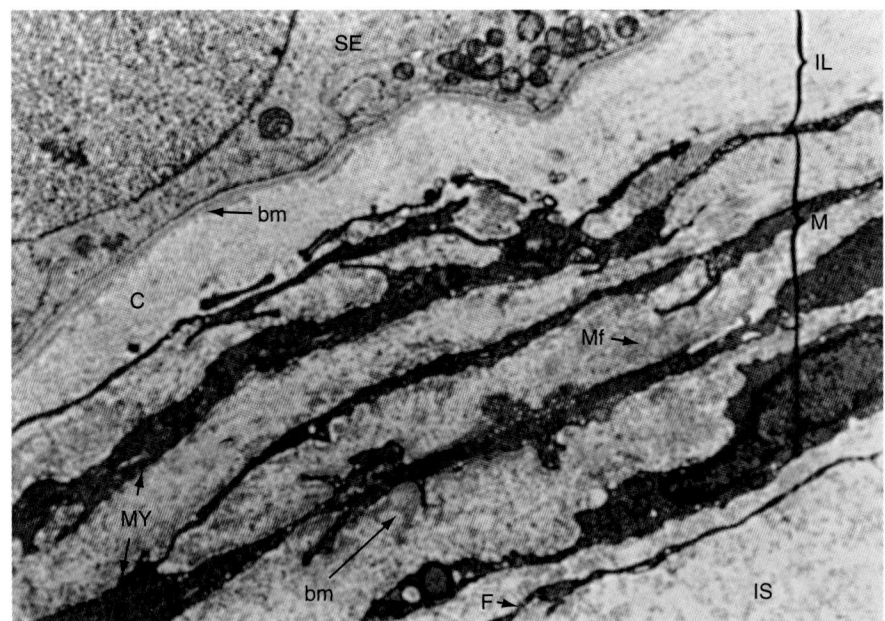

Figure 18–9. Low-power electron micrograph of the peritubular tissue in a human testis. Peritubular tissue lies between the basement membrane (bm) of the seminiferous epithelium (SE) and the interstitial tissue (IS). Three zones are present in peritubular tissue: the inner lamella (IL); the myoid layer (M), containing myoid cells (MY) with abundant microfibrils (Mf); and an adventitial layer containing fibroblasts (F). (From Hermo L, Lalli M, Clermont Y: Arrangement of connective tissue elements in the walls of seminiferous tubules of man and monkey. Am J Anat 1977;148:433-446.)

basement membrane underlying the seminiferous epithelium. This thick inner lamella contains a large amount of collagen.

In humans the peritubular myoid cells are thought to primarily have a contractile function (Toyama, 1977). In the rat, the contractile function of these cells has been shown to be very sensitive to their thermal and endocrine environment; the contractions disappear within 5 days of the establishment of experimental cryptorchidism (Suvanto and Kormano, 1970), with subsequent thickening of the peritubular structures as spermatogenesis is affected.

Tung and colleagues (1984) have demonstrated the ability of peritubular myoid cells to secrete a number of substances, including the extracellular matrix components fibronectin and collagen type I. It is likely that these peritubular myoid cells synthesize much of the substance that makes up the inner collagenous layer that separates the myoid cells from the basement membrane of the seminiferous epithelium. Skinner and coworkers (1988) have isolated a paracrine factor produced by peritubular myoid cells, named P-Mod-S (peritubular modifies Sertoli), that profoundly modulates Sertoli cell function and differentiation in vitro. P-Mod-S has been shown to have effects on Sertoli cell differentiation and synthesis that are more profound than FSH effects in culture. Human peritubular cells in vitro have been shown to have steroidogenic functions, including the secretion of testosterone, associate with Sertoli cells in a specific mesenchymal-epithelial interaction, and exert regulatory influences on secretory activity of Sertoli cells (Cigorraga et al, 1994). Further evidence for the profound effect of peritubular structures on spermatogenesis is the observation that Sertoli cells in culture will form cords reminiscent of seminiferous tubules after the addition of specific components of extracellular matrix (Hadley et al, 1985; Richardson, 1990).

The Sertoli Cell

The morphologic and ultrastructural characteristics of the human Sertoli cell have been well described (Kerr and deKretser, 1981; Nistal et al, 1982; Bardin et al, 1994). The Sertoli cell is characterized by its irregularly shaped nucleus, prominent nucleolus, low mitotic index, Sertoli-germ cell connections, and unique tight junctional complexes between adjacent Sertoli cell membranes. **The Sertoli cell rests on the basement membrane of the seminiferous tubule and extends filamentous cytoplasmic ramifications toward the lumen of the tubule** (Fig. 18–10). Germinal cells are arranged between these Sertoli cell cytoplasmic projections. The undifferentiated spermatogonia are near the basement membrane of the seminiferous tubule, whereas the more advanced spermatocytes and spermatids are arranged at successively higher levels in this epithelium. In this respect, **the Sertoli cell functions as a polarized epithelium, with its base in a plasma environment and its apex in an environment, described in the following section, unique to the seminiferous tubule** (Ewing et al, 1980).

It is generally thought that Sertoli cells support the development of germ cells by (1) creating the specialized microenvironment of the adluminal compartment of the seminiferous epithelium, (2) supporting germ cells through gap junctions between Sertoli and germ cells, and (3) facilitating migration of differentiating germ cells in the seminiferous tubule. This microenvironment is one of the levels of the so-called blood-testis barrier. The blood-testis barrier exists at multiple levels within the testis. The junctions between Sertoli cells are remodeled to allow "opening" and "closing" that facilitates continuous interaction of germ cells with Sertoli cells as well as migration of the germ cells to the adluminal surface (Mruk and Cheng, 2004). Sertoli cell functions obviously encompass physical contact with sperm cells, phagocytosis, fluid secretion and production, and secretion of a variety of molecules.

Androgen-binding protein (ABP) was one of the first Sertoli cell secretory products identified (Hansson and Djoseland, 1972; Ritzen et al, 1981). ABP is an intracellular carrier of androgen within the Sertoli cell. In addition, it may serve

Germ cells

**Supporting cells
(Sertoli cells)**

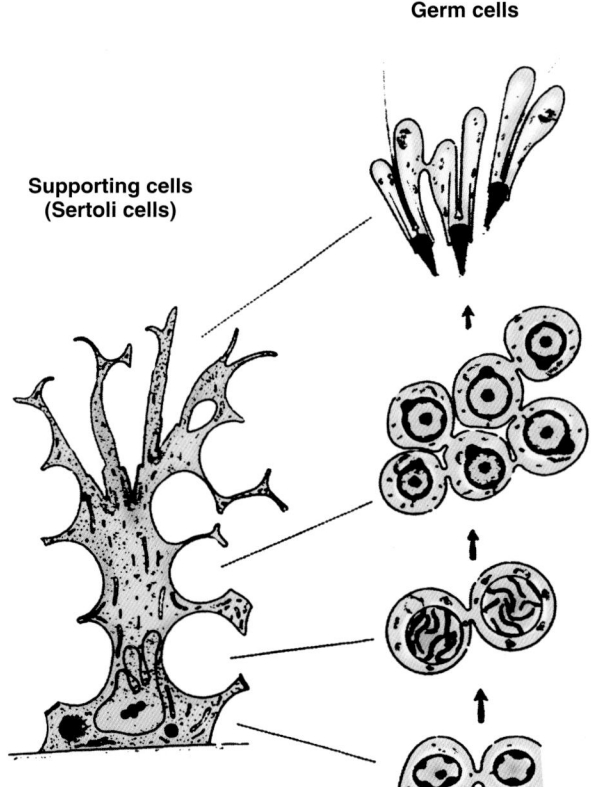

Figure 18–10. Diagrammatic representation of Sertoli and germ cells composing the seminiferous epithelium,. The Sertoli cells represent a fixed population of nondividing support cells. The proliferating germ cells move upward along the sides of the Sertoli cells as they differentiate into spermatozoa. (From Fawcett DW: The cell biology of gametogenesis in the male. Perspect Biol Med 1979;Winter:S56-S73.)

as a reservoir of androgenic hormones for the seminiferous tubule and possibly the epididymis as well. ABP production has proven to be an excellent marker to test the hormonal regulation of Sertoli cell function in vitro. However, the measurement of ABP or other Sertoli cell product as a marker of Sertoli cell function is yet to have a demonstrable role in the evaluation of male infertility (Chan et al, 1986).

Other Sertoli cell secretory products include extracellular matrix components (lamin, collagen type IV, and collagen type I) and numerous proteins such as ceruloplasmin, transferrin, glycoprotein 2, plasminogen activator, somatomedin-like substances, T proteins, inhibin, H-Y antigen, clusterin, cyclic proteins, growth factors, somatomedin, and androgen-binding protein (for a review of Sertoli cell function see Mruk and Cheng [2004]). Steroids, such as DHT, testosterone, androstenediols, 17β-estradiol, and numerous other C_{21} steroids (Ewing et al, 1980; Mather et al, 1983) have also been shown to be produced by Sertoli cells. Although their specific functions remain to be fully elucidated, further studies on these Sertoli cell products promise to provide important insight into the role of Sertoli cells in creating the microenvironment in which spermatogenesis occurs.

The consensus (Ewing et al, 1980; Means et al, 1980; Ritzen, 1983; Griswold et al, 1988; Maddocks and Setchell, 1988) is that FSH and testosterone play an important role in the regulation of Sertoli cell function, including ABP production.

Feedback inhibition of FSH secretion is predominantly provided by the Sertoli cell product inhibin B in the human male. The clinical value of inhibin B analysis as well as the molecular forms of inhibin are discussed in the beginning of this chapter. Mather and associates (1983) suggested that in addition to testosterone and FSH, multiple agents including progesterone, hydrocortisone, insulin, EGF, transferrin, and vitamins A and E are required for maximal ABP secretion by Sertoli cells cultured in vitro. Finally, as discussed previously, Sertoli cell function is stimulated in vitro by substances secreted by testicular peritubular cells (Skinner and Fritz, 1985; Lubahn et al, 1993). Unfortunately, the physiologic role of these effector molecules and the mechanism by which they regulate Sertoli cell function remain to be elucidated.

KEY POINTS: GENETICS AND DEVELOPMENT

- The product of the SRY gene on the Y chromosome, a nuclear transcription factor, acts together with other transcription factors such as DAX-1 to initiate male sexual differentiation.

- The AZFa and AZFb regions of the Y chromosome are critical to completion of spermatogenesis.

- From 7 to 9 years of life, mitotic activity of gonocytes is detectable, giving rise to spermatogonia that populate the base of the seminiferous tubule.

- The hypothalamic capacity to generate pulses of GnRH arises at puberty, usually beginning around the 12th year. The pubertal onset of GnRH pulses typically occurs at night.

- The blood-testis barrier functionally develops at the onset of spermatogenesis, but the presence of germ cells is not necessary for the development of the barrier.

The Blood-Testis Barrier

It has been observed that many substances injected into the bloodstream will rapidly appear in testicular lymph but not in rete testis fluid (Fawcett, 1979). From this observation and others, the concept of a "blood-testis barrier" was formed. Ultrastructural studies demonstrated that specialized junctional complexes between adjacent Sertoli cells subdivide the seminiferous epithelium into a basal compartment and adluminal compartment in many species (Flickinger, 1967; Dym and Fawcett, 1970), including man (Chemes et al, 1977). It has been shown (Dym and Fawcett, 1970; Dym, 1973) that the Sertoli-Sertoli tight junctions prevent the deep penetration of electron opaque tracers into the seminiferous epithelium from the testicular interstitium. The blood-testis barrier appears to have three different levels within the testis. The primary level is formed by tight junctions between Sertoli cells and segregates pre-meiotic germ cells (spermatogonia) from other germ cells. Two additional levels of blood-testis barrier exist at the level of the endothelial cells in capillaries as well as at the level of the peritubular myoid cells.

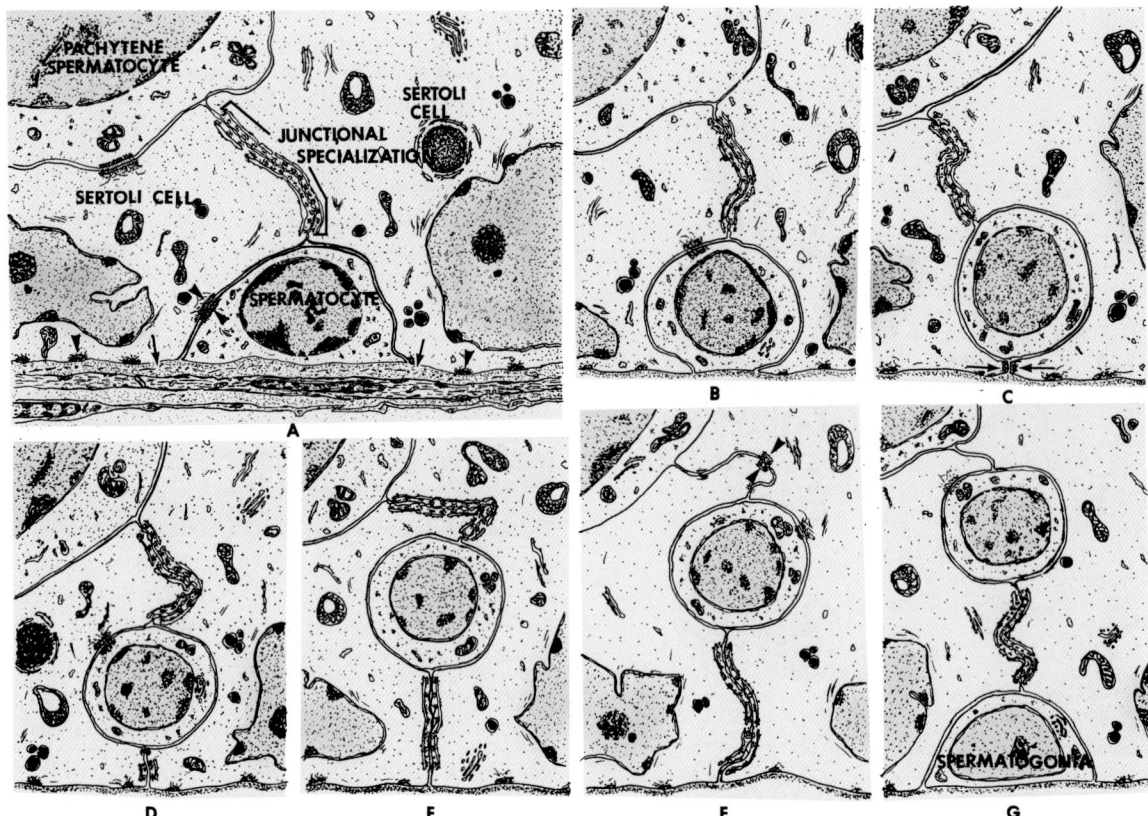

Figure 18–11. Diagram of the steps required to transfer rat primary spermatocytes from the basal to the adluminal compartment of the seminiferous tubule. Initially (**A, B**) the Sertoli cells are attached to each other above the spermatocytes by tight junctions. Next (**C** to **E**), Sertoli cells form new junctions below the spermatocytes, isolating the spermatocytes in an intermediate compartment, above and below which are tight junctions. The junctions above the spermatocytes then break down (**F, G**), and the spermatocytes enter the adluminal compartment. (From Russell L: Desmosome-like junctions between Sertoli cells and germ cells in the rat testis. Am J Anat 1977;148:313.)

Spermatogonia and young spermatocytes are outside the blood-testis barrier in the basal compartment, whereas mature spermatocytes and spermatids are sequestered above the barrier in the adluminal compartment. It is during the extended meiotic prophase (leptotene, zygotene, pachytene) that the spermatocytes move out from the basal compartment and migrate into the adluminal compartment of the seminiferous tubule. This migration (Fig. 18–11) was described elegantly for the rat testis by Russell (1980), who stated that the adluminal-to-luminal migration begins when "Sertoli cell processes undermine the young spermatocytes to separate them from the basal lamina, and as the processes meet they form junctions impermeable to substances from the blood" (see Fig. 18–11C to E). Consequently, "in those stages where young spermatocytes (leptotene, zygotene) move toward the lumen, these germ cell types are noted in regions where occluding junctions exist both above and below the germ cell." Russell designated the region with tight junctions above and below the germ cell the "intermediate compartment" (Fig. 18–12) and suggested that it represents "a transit chamber in which cells may move from one compartment to another without disrupting the integrity of the blood-testis barrier."

The blood-testis barrier functionally develops at the onset of spermatogenesis (Kormano, 1967). **However, the presence of germ cells is not necessary for the development of the barrier** (Tindall et al, 1975). Other factors controlling formation of the blood-testis barrier are poorly understood except that the administration of gonadotropins is associated with formation of inter-Sertoli cell junctions in men with hypogonadotropic hypogonadism (de Kretser and Burger, 1972).

We can only speculate as to the importance of such a blood-testis barrier, because the functional significance of this barrier remains to be proved. This barrier could be important for meiosis, because the fluid bathing the germinal cells is more stable than and quite different from that in the compartments outside the barrier. In addition, the blood-testis barrier may isolate the haploid male gamete, which is not recognized as "self" by the male immune system. The clinical importance of the blood-testis barrier is only realized after puberty, because "antigens"—on the germ cells advancing through meiosis—are only present after initiation of puberty. So, a testicular insult, such as biopsy, torsion, or trauma, will not induce antisperm antibodies if the insult occurs before puberty. However, a similar insult that results in physical disruption of the blood-testis barrier and exposure of the immune system to advancing germ cells could lead to formation of an immune reaction to germ cell-associated (including sperm) antigens. A practical consideration is the possibility of differential drug access to the cells sequestered behind the barrier, including limited ability to treat

Figure 18–12. A diagrammatic representation of the tree-shaped Sertoli cell with a thickened central portion, or "trunk," and more delicate processes, or "limbs." The diagram is split vertically to allow the presentation of major configurational changes that occur during the spermatogenic cycle. Note the basal, intermediate, and adluminal compartments of the seminiferous epithelium. Spermatogonia and early spermatocytes share a position on the basal lamina and are overreached by one surface of adjacent Sertoli cells that join to form occluding junctions (site of blood-testis barrier) (A). Sertoli cells form junctional complexes both above and below leptotene-zygotene spermatocytes in the process of being translocated from the basal to the adluminal compartment (B). The spermatocytes enter the adluminal compartment of the seminiferous epithelium when the higher Sertoli junctions dissociate (C). The elongating spermatid becomes situated within a narrow recess of the trunk of the Sertoli cell (D). As the spermatid elongates further, the cell becomes lodged within the body of the Sertoli cell (E). The advanced spermatid moves toward the lumen of the seminiferous epithelium in preparation for spermiation. Only the head region remains in intimate contact with the Sertoli cell. Specialized cell-to-cell contracts: *Asterisks,* desmosome-gap junction complex; *arrowheads,* ectoplasmic specializations; *isolated arrows,* tubulobulbar complexes. (From Russell L: Sertoli-germ cell interactions: A review. Gamete Res 1980;3:179.)

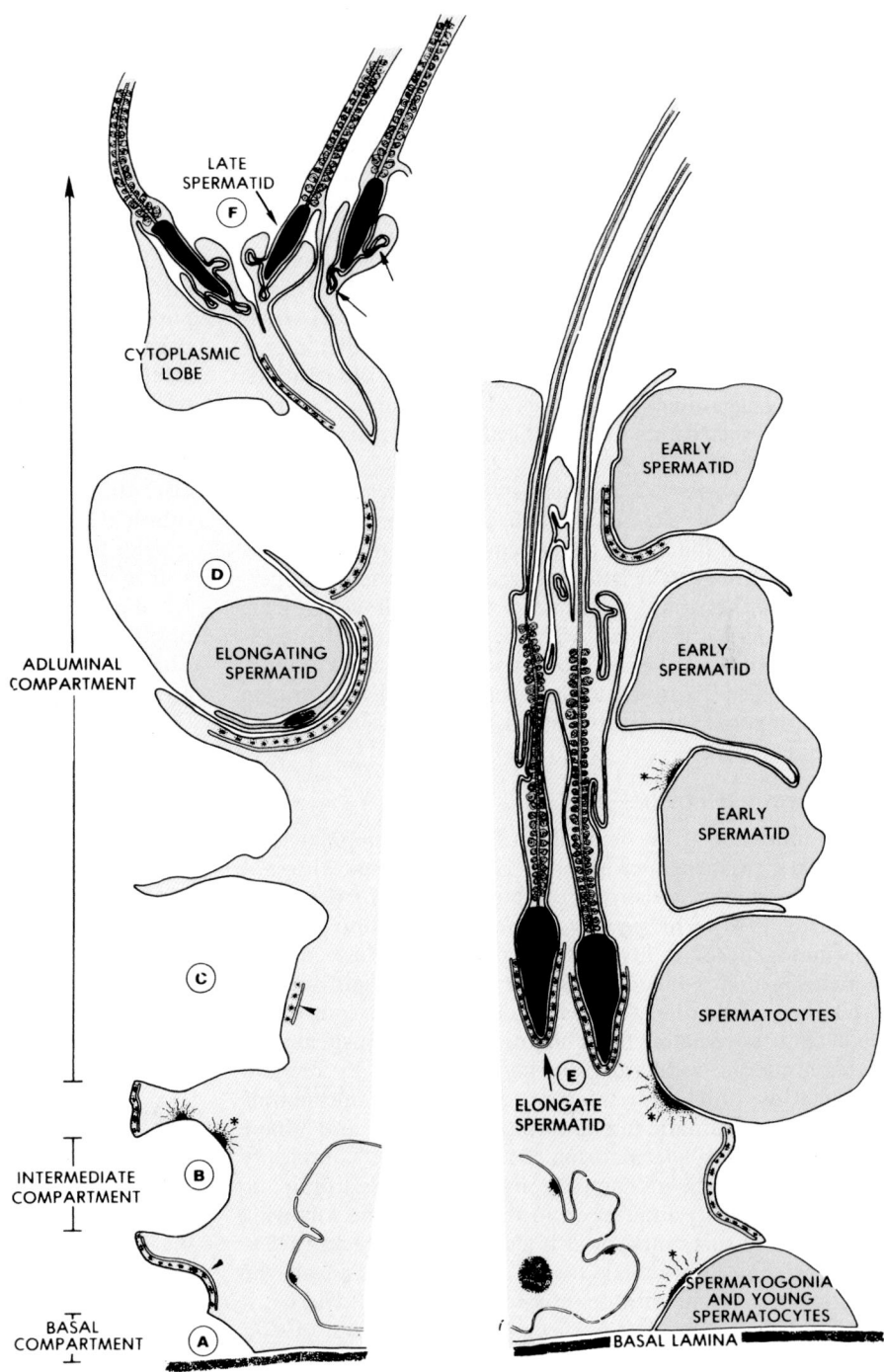

neoplastic cells within the seminiferous tubule with chemotherapeutic agents.

Sertoli Cell–Germ Cell Associations

Studies on laboratory animals revealed a complex network of cell-cell interactions within the testis: between Leydig cells and Sertoli cells; between Leydig cells and peritubular cells; between Sertoli and peritubular cells (see previous discussion on peritubular structures); and between Sertoli cells and germinal cells. The reader is referred to an excellent review by Skinner (1995) for a summary of these complex interactions, including a discussion of the paracrine factors that drive them.

Because of space limitations and because most of these testicular cell-cell interactions are at present not well characterized, the discussion here will focus on Sertoli cell–germ cell associations.

It was once thought that specialized junctions between Sertoli cells and germ cells did not exist (Fawcett, 1974). Now it is widely accepted that several types of Sertoli cell–germ cell associations are present in mammalian testes (Connell, 1974; Kaya and Harrison, 1976; Russell and Clermont, 1976; Russell, 1977; Romrell and Ross, 1979). This topic has been well reviewed (Russell and Malone, 1980, Parvinen et al, 1986, Skinner, 1995).

Figure 18–12 is a diagram of the Sertoli cell and its configurational relationship with germ cells. Russell and Malone (1980) stated that "desmosome-like contacts function as attachment devices that maintain the integrity of the seminiferous epithelium and at the same time ensure that germ cells are transported in an orderly fashion, toward the tubular lumen by virtue of configurational changes of the Sertoli cell." They further stated that "ectoplasmic specializations are complex surface specializations that appear to hold elongated spermatids within deep recesses of the Sertoli cell." Finally, they stated that "both the Sertoli cell and spermatid participate in the formation of tubulobulbar complexes that appear in the few days preceding sperm release." These observations led to the suggestion that the bulk of cytoplasm is lost from condensing spermatids by Sertoli cell phagocytosis of tubulobulbar complexes.

In summary, physical contact between the Sertoli cell and the germ cell may play some role in propelling the germ cell upward toward the lumen of the seminiferous tubule. Moreover, the intimate association between the condensing spermatid and the apical portion of the Sertoli cell during spermiogenesis is associated with the casting off of the residual cytoplasm from the developing spermatid. Lastly, the junctional complexes between adjacent Sertoli cells clearly form an important component of the blood-testis barrier with all its consequences.

The Germinal Epithelium

The epithelium of the seminiferous tubule is populated by cells that give rise to approximately 123×10^6 (range: 21 to 374 $\times 10^6$) spermatozoa daily in the human male (Amann and Howards, 1980). **This process of sperm production is called spermatogenesis. It involves a proliferative phase during which spermatogonia divide either to replace their number (stem cell renewal) or to produce daughter cells committed to become spermatocytes, a meiotic phase when spermatocytes undergo reduction division, resulting in haploid spermatids; and a spermiogenic phase when spermatids undergo a dramatic metamorphosis in size and shape to form mature spermatozoa.** Because of the complexity of the topic, lack of complete information regarding the human, and space limitations in this chapter, the following discussion of spermatogenesis is general in nature and references are not always made to original research. Instead, the discussion rests heavily on excellent reviews by Clermont (1972), Steinberger (1976), Ewing and associates (1980), DiZerga and Sherins (1981), and de Kretser and Kerr (1988).

Histologic examination of the human testis with the aid of the light microscope revealed large numbers of germ cells arrayed among Sertoli cells and extending from the basement membrane to the lumen of the seminiferous tubule. Morphologic analysis (Clermont, 1963; Heller and Clermont, 1964) revealed the presence of at least 13 recognizable germ types in the human testis (Fig. 18–13). These cells were thought to represent different steps in the developmental process. **Proceeding from the least to the most differentiated, they were named dark type A spermatogonia (Ad); pale type A spermatogonia (Ap); type B spermatogonia (B); preleptotene primary spermatocytes (R); leptotene primary spermatocytes (L); zygotene primary spermatocytes (z); pachytene**

primary spermatocytes (p); secondary spermatocytes (II); and Sa, Sb1, Sb2, Sc, Sd1, and Sd2 spermatids.

Spermatogonial Development

Prenatal development of the testis involves migration of primordial germ cells to the gonadal ridge and association of these precursors with Sertoli cells to form primitive testicular cords (Witschi, 1948). In many species, a period of mitotic activity subsequently occurs in the fetal testis that increases germ cell numbers, but they remain the minority cell population within the testis (de Kretser and Kerr, 1988). **The primitive germ cells of the undifferentiated gonad are referred to as gonocytes after the gonad differentiates into a testis by forming seminiferous cords. At this time, the gonocytes are located within the seminiferous cords in a central position. They are classified subsequently as spermatogonia after the gonocytes have migrated to the periphery of the tubule** (Gondos and Hobel, 1971).

Prior to birth, from the 8th to the 22nd week of pregnancy, a steep increase in the number of germ cells per tubule (from 1.1 to 3.5) occurs. Thereafter, a slight decrease in the number of germ cells per Sertoli cell occurs until 4 months after birth. This relative decrease in germ cells is due to proliferative activity of immature Sertoli cells during this period of time (Hilscher and Engemann, 1992). Until approximately 7 years of life there appears to be very little morphologic change of the human testis. **From 7 to 9 years of life, mitotic activity of gonocytes is detectable, with spermatogonia populating the base of the seminiferous tubule in numbers equal to those of the Sertoli cells** (Muller and Skakkebaek, 1983). There appears to be little further morphologic change in spermatogonia until spermatogenesis begins at the time of puberty. Further observations regarding the maturation of gonocytes and their migration to the base of the seminiferous tubule, including the factors that may be responsible for these changes, may provide greater insight into clinical problems affecting the testis, including cryptorchidism.

Spermatogonial Proliferation and Stem Cell Renewal

Pale type A spermatogonia are located in the basal compartment of the seminiferous tubule that is formed by overreaching Sertoli-Sertoli cell tight junctions. These Ap spermatogonia divide at 16-day intervals in the human (Clermont, 1972) to form B spermatogonia, which are committed to become spermatocytes. Interestingly, the spermatogonial cytoplasm generally does not separate completely when the nuclei divide after mitosis. Therefore, cytoplasmic bridges are formed between adjacent spermatogonia. Evidently this process continues during meiosis, because cytoplasmic bridges have been observed between all classes of germ cells (Ewing et al, 1980). Although the functional significance of cytoplasmic bridges remains unknown, their presence could be important for the synchronization of cellular proliferation, differentiation, and possibly the control of gene expression in haploid cells.

Periodically the population of undifferentiated spermatogonia must be replenished (stem cell renewal). The mechanisms by which spermatogonia both replenish their population and generate precursors for spermatogenesis are not completely clear. Evidence has suggested that a growth factor/receptor called the kit ligand/c-kit receptor system is

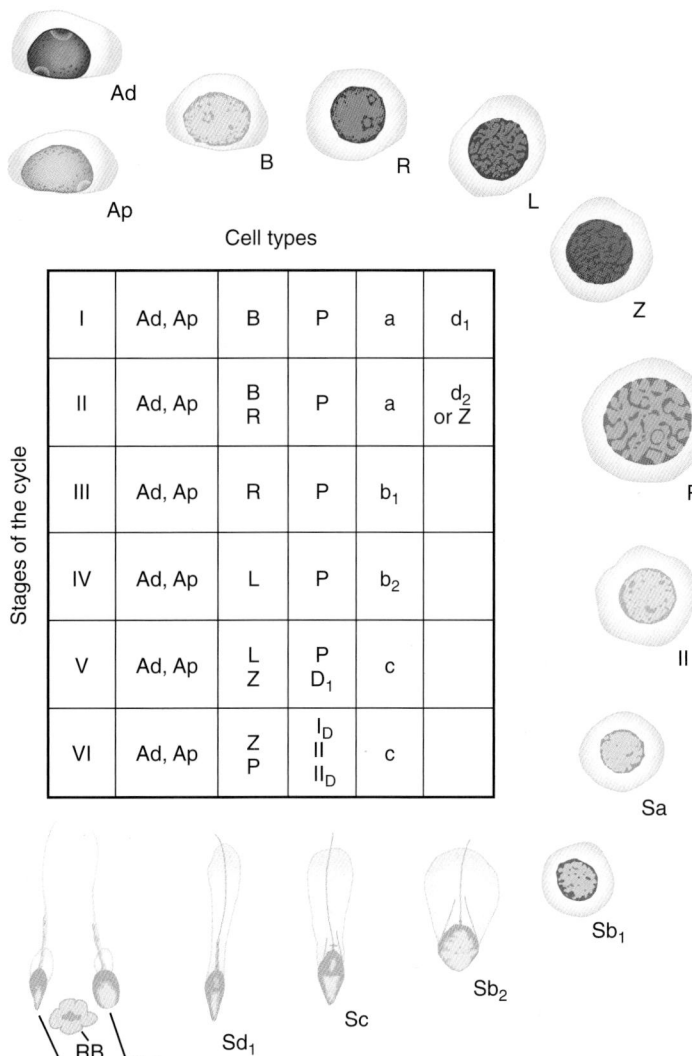

Figure 18–13. The steps of spermatogenesis in man. Ad, dark type A spermatogonium; AP, pale type A spermatogonium; B, type B spermatogonium; R, resting or preleptotene primary spermatocyte; L, leptotene spermatocyte; Z, zygotene spermatocyte; P, pachytene spermatocyte; II, secondary spermatocyte; Sa(a), Sb1(b1), sb2(b2), Sc(c), sd1(d1), Sd2(d2), spermatids; Rb, residual body. The table shows the cells that make up the six stages of the cycle of the seminiferous epithelium (I to VI): D1, diakenesis; ID and IID, first and second maturation divisions of spermatocytes. (Modified from Clermont Y: Renewal of spermatogonia in man. Am J Anat 1966;118:509.)

Cell types

Stages of the cycle

I	Ad, Ap	B	P	a	d_1
II	Ad, Ap	B R	P	a	d_2 or Z
III	Ad, Ap	R	P	b_1	
IV	Ad, Ap	L	P	b_2	
V	Ad, Ap	L Z	P D_1	c	
VI	Ad, Ap	Z P	I_D II II_D	c	

involved in spermatogonial stem cell self-renewal. In fact, the c-kit receptor is a marker for type A cells in rats (reviewed by Dym [1994]). The result of this process is that some type A_4 spermatogonia differentiate into intermediate and then type B spermatogonia that proceed through spermatogenesis, in a c-kit–dependent process, whereas other A_4 spermatogonia renew the stem cell population of type A_1 spermatogonia (Yoshinaga et al, 1991). One unresolved issue is why and how approximately two thirds of all spermatogonia undergo programmed cell death (Allan et al, 1992; Print and Loveland, 2000).

Meiosis

Type B spermatogonia interconnected by cytoplasmic bridges divide mitotically to form primary spermatocytes that will undergo meiosis. This process has been described in general by Ewing and associates (1980) and for the human by Kerr and de Kretser (1981). **Chains of interconnected mature spermatocytes are therefore found in the adluminal compartment of the seminiferous tubule behind the blood-testis barrier created by the Sertoli-Sertoli cell tight junctions.** The spermatocytes complete the subsequent meiotic di-

visions. In most organisms a reductional division is followed by an equatorial division, resulting in the production of daughter cells with the haploid chromosome number and, as a consequence of recombination, with different genetic information. The result of this process in the human is the round Sa spermatid (see Fig. 18–13).

Spermiogenesis

During spermiogenesis the products of meiosis, the round Sa spermatids, metamorphose into mature spermatids (see Fig. 18–13). During this metamorphosis, extensive changes occur in both the spermatid cytoplasm and the nucleus but cell division is not required. These changes have been described in detail by Kerr and de Kretser (1981) and include loss of cytoplasm, formation of the acrosome, formation of the flagellum, and migration of cytoplasmic organelles to positions characteristic of the mature spermatozoon. If the human is similar to the rat, then the clone of spermatids are connected to each other via cytoplasmic bridges and to Sertoli cells via ectoplasmic specializations.

The entire spermatogenic process in humans requires approximately 64 days (Clermont, 1972). **If spermatogenesis**

is viewed from a fixed point in a seminiferous tubule, six recognizable cellular associations (stages of the cycle of the seminiferous epithelium) occur one after another in a predictable and constant fashion during this 64-day interval (Heller and Clermont, 1964; Fig. 18–14). Accordingly, the proliferative phase of spermatogenesis (differentiation of Ap to B spermatogonia) is initiated four times (every 16 days) during the period required for an Ap spermatogonium to differentiate into a spermatozoon. The result is that the adult human testis is populated by one or two cohorts of spermatogonia, one or two cohorts of spermatocytes, and one or two cohorts of spermatids. This stage-specific production of spermatogonia allows the efficient production of millions of spermatozoa a day.

In rodents, the stages of spermatogenesis occur more or less consecutively from the first to the last stage along a given segment of the tubule in repeating sequences. One complete series of segments representing the recognized cellular associations (stages) is called the wave of the seminiferous epithelium. It has long been claimed (Roosen-Runge and Barlow, 1953; Heller and Clermont, 1964; Leidl and Waschke, 1970) that man does not exhibit a wave of the seminiferous epithelium. Instead, the stages occupy only a portion of the circumference of the tubule, thus forming a mosaic rather than a well-defined linear array of succeeding stages of spermatogenesis. This concept has been challenged by Schulze (1989) who, using computer-aided three-dimensional imaging, reported an orderly sequence of stages in oblique orientation

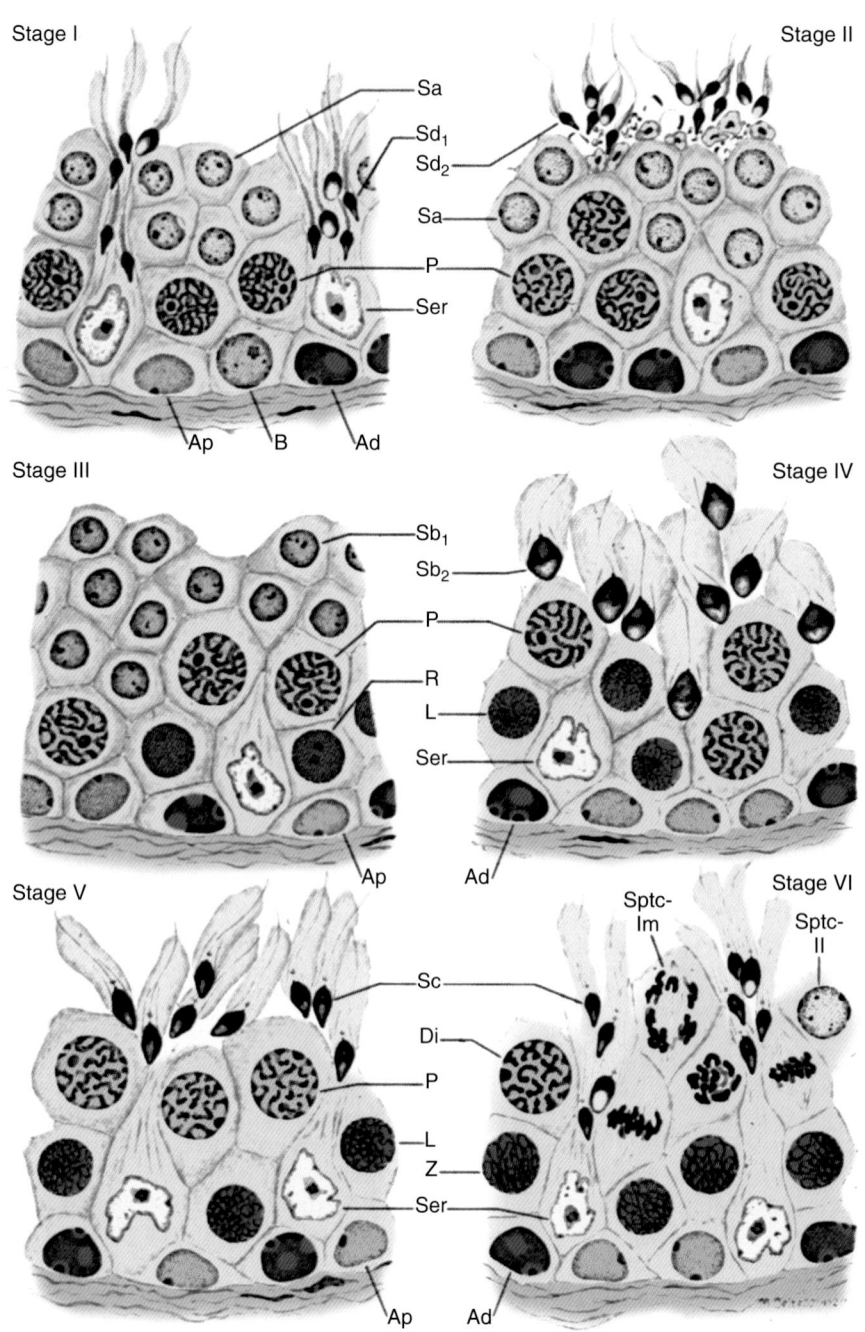

Figure 18–14. Cellular composition of the six cellular associations (stages I to VI) found in human seminiferous tubules. Ser, Sertoli nuclei; Ad and Ap, dark and pale type A spermatogonia; B, type B spermatogonia; R, resting (preleptotene) primary spermatocytes; L, leptotene spermatocytes; Z, zygotene spermatocytes; P, pachytene spermatocytes; Di, diplotene spermatocytes; Sptc-Im, primary spermatocytes in division; Sptc-II, secondary spermatocytes in interphase; Sa, Sb, Sb2, Sc, Sd1, Sd2, spermatids at various steps of spermatogenesis. (Modified from Heller CG, Clermont Y: Kinetics of the germinal epithelium in man. Rec Prog Horm Res 1964;20:545.)

that implies a helical arrangement of stages of the seminiferous tubule in humans (Fig. 18–15). The exact configuration of the spermatogenic wave in the human testis remains to be confirmed.

Hormonal Regulation of Spermatogenesis

Testosterone levels in the testis of man and other mammals are often nearly 100-fold greater than that seen in peripheral circulation (Sealey et al, 1988; Jarow et al, 2005). The maintenance of peripheral circulating testosterone levels with exogenous androgen treatment with the marked suppression of spermatogenesis, and often azoospermia, support the importance of high intratesticular testosterone levels for human males. Consistent with this observation, 20% to 30% of men with infertility have low peripheral testosterone levels (Lombardo et al, 2005). The use of testosterone (or GnRH agonists) as a male contraceptive has been somewhat limited by the failure of these treatments to completely inhibit FSH production by the pituitary. In a primate model, testosterone-induced inhibition of spermatogenesis is more closely related to suppression of FSH than to testicular androgen levels (Weinbauer et al, 2001).

Hypophysectomy results in testicular atrophy in numerous species (Steinberger, 1971), including humans (Mancini et al, 1969, 1972; Mancini, 1973). In the rat, "hypophysectomy apparently produces several lesions: a block in spermatid

maturation, severe damage to the meiotic prophase, and partial interference with the quantitative formation of type A spermatogonia" (Steinberger, 1971). Testes of hypophysectomized men are characterized by Leydig cell atrophy, peritubular hyalinization, and germinal depletion that vary from tubules containing only spermatogonia to those with scattered spermatocytes (Mancini et al, 1969). The return of nearly normal spermatogenesis with the intratesticular injection of testosterone microspheres in GnRH agonist–treated rats supports the importance of high intratesticular testosterone levels to spermatogenesis (Turner et al, 1990).

The hormonal regimen required to restore spermatogenesis after hypophysectomy depends on whether spermatogenesis is to be maintained immediately after hypophysectomy or reinitiated after the germinal epithelium has been allowed to regress completely. Moreover, the amount of hormone required depends on the desired endpoint: production of a few advanced spermatids (qualitative) or complete restoration of spermatid numbers (quantitative). Testosterone regulates spermatogenesis probably via an effect on the Sertoli cell (Lyon et al, 1975). **Testosterone will initiate and qualitatively maintain spermatogenesis in humans.** This was demonstrated by Steinberger and colleagues (1973), who reported a case of a 6-year-old boy in whom there was active spermatogenesis in the testicular tissue containing an androgen-producing Leydig cell tumor, in the absence of gonadotropin

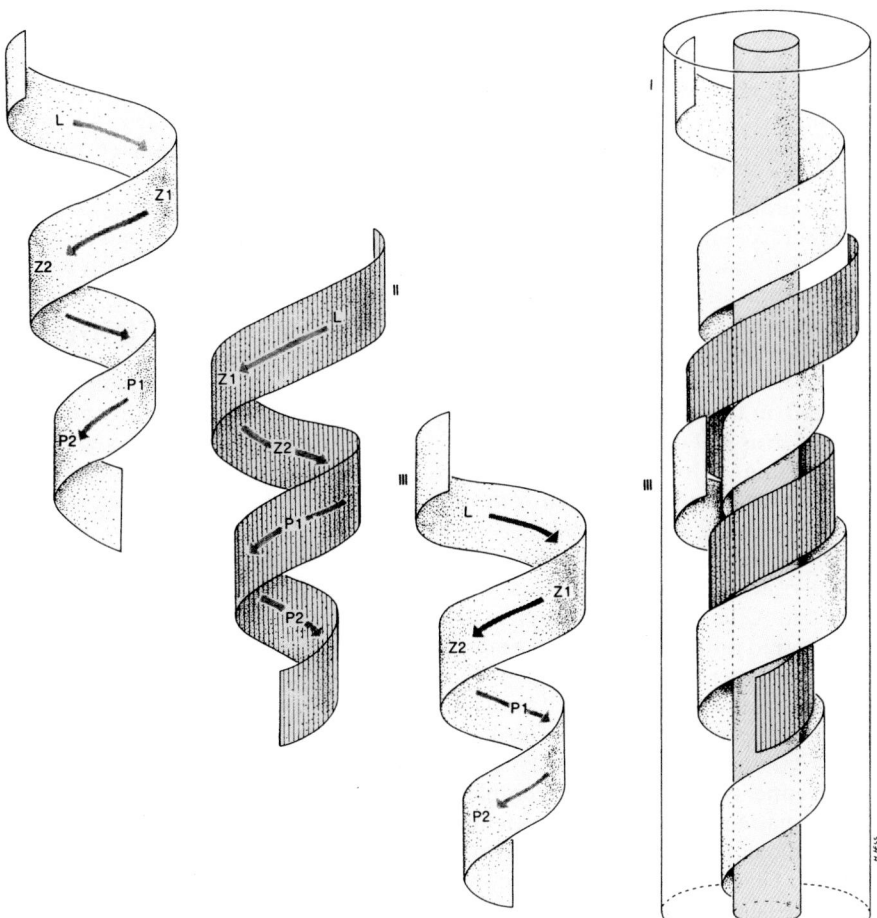

Figure 18–15. Helical configuration of stages of the seminiferous tubule epithelium in man. (From Schulze W, Rehder U: Organization and morphogenesis of the human seminiferous epithelium. Cell Tissue Res 1984;237:395-407.)

production. The fact that spermatogenesis was absent in the contralateral testis, which was free of steroid-producing tumor tissue, suggested that spermatogenesis was initiated and maintained by the androgenic steroids produced by the tumor. Quantitative maintenance of spermatogenesis in the human male has not been achieved to date, probably because of the difficulty in achieving a high enough blood level of testosterone.

The effect of pituitary gonadotropins on spermatogenesis has been reviewed (Steinberger, 1971; Ewing et al, 1980; DiZerga and Sherins, 1981; Simoni et al, 1999). There is little evidence at present to suggest that LH acts other than by stimulating endogenous testosterone production.

The role of FSH in spermatogenesis has been more controversial. Human males with defects of the FSH receptor that nearly ablate its function have been reported to be fertile, although testicular volume, sperm concentration, and morphology is severely impaired (Tapanainen et al, 1997). Studies of hypogonadal men have also demonstrated fertility in the absence of FSH (Bremner et al, 1981). It has been suggested that FSH, by some poorly understood mechanism, facilitates the initiation of spermatogenesis in pubertal males and reinitiates spermatogenesis in hypophysectomized animals after the germinal epithelium regresses following hypophysectomy (Steinberger, 1971; Ewing et al, 1980; DiZerga and Sherins, 1981). Although FSH is not required for initiation of spermatogenesis in human males with hypogonadotropic hypogonadism, optimal quantitative and qualitative spermatogenesis requires FSH treatment. Although some sperm production occurs in testes in the absence of FSH, only the combination of FSH and testosterone supports a qualitatively and quantitatively fully normal level of spermatogenesis (Simoni et al, 1999).

Genetic Basis of Spermatogenesis

The localization of specific genes that are critical for spermatogenesis remains the subject of active investigation. The detection of microdeletions of a region of the Y chromosome referred to as interval 6 in 5% to 10% of azoospermic men has focused attention on this area as the site for a critical factor (**Azoospermic** Factor) important for spermatogenesis (Chandley and Cooke, 1994; Girardi et al, 1997). **One gene localized on the long arm of the Y chromosome in a region referred to as AZFc (Azoospermic Factor) is _DAZ_ (deleted in azoospermia). One study of men with nonobstructive azoospermia identified 12 men with deletions of the AZFc region involving the gene _DAZ_** (Reijo et al, 1995). Other regions of the Y chromosome that are commonly deleted in azoospermic men, but not normal men, are referred to as AZFa and AZFb. **Men with complete deletions of the entire AZFa region uniformly have had azoospermia with a Sertoli cell–only pattern on testis biopsy.** The gene in the AZFa region that is deleted in all patients with severe impairments of spermatogenesis is _DBY_, a DEAD-box protein that is a transcriptional regulator (Foresta et al, 2000). **The AZFb region appears to be critical to completion of spermatogenesis. No patients with complete deletion of the AZFb region have had completely developed spermatozoa present within the testis** (Brandell et al, 1998). Other testicular autocrine and paracrine factors are probably involved, directly or indirectly, in the regulation of spermatogenesis: seminiferous growth

factor (SGF), basic fibroblast growth factor (bFGF), IGF-1, Sertoli cell–secreted growth factor (SCSGF), transforming growth factor-α (TGF-α), interleukin-1, chalones, meiosis-inhibiting substances, and meiosis-preventing substances. The reader is referred to excellent reviews on these topics (Saez et al, 1987; Bellve and Zheng, 1989; Skinner, 1995).

Recent work has suggested that components of the male gamete may have significant importance for embryonic development. Significant interspecies variability of embryonic growth potential has been identified. **In humans, however, the mitotic activity of embryos appears to be organized normally by the paternally derived centrosome** (Schatten, 1994; Simerly et al, 1995). Observations of human embryos supports the finding that the male gamete provides not only genetic material but that normal mitotic activity is derived from the centrosome provided by the male gamete. In the absence of this contribution from a male gamete, mitotic activity of the human embryo is chaotic, and a viable embryo is not produced (Palermo et al, 1994). Further observations and experiments will be necessary to delineate exactly which components of the male gamete are necessary to facilitate embryo development.

Summary

Human spermatogenesis can be summarized as follows: Given the proper hormonal environment, a new cohort of spermatogonia (type Ap-B) is started through spermatogenesis every 16 days at any one site in the seminiferous epithelium. At this juncture, a few primitive spermatogonia (Ap-Ap) are set aside by an equivalent mitosis to provide stem cells for a later cohort of differentiating spermatogonia. Because the first cohort of germ cells requires 64 days to differentiate into Sd2 spermatids, four cohorts of differentiating sperm cells are observed in the seminiferous epithelium. The simultaneous differentiation of these different cohorts of cells over concurrent 64-day periods includes six stages of spermatogenic cycle that can be observed on examination of histologic specimens of human testis.

EPIDIDYMIS

Normally, testicular spermatozoa do not display progressive motility and are incapable of fertilizing ova. After traversing the epididymis, spermatozoa are motile and capable of fertilizing oocytes. With excurrent ductal obstruction, however, testicular spermatozoa can acquire progressive motility (Jow et al, 1993). Even in unobstructed systems, testicular spermatozoa can display twitching motility and will fertilize ova when intracytoplasmic sperm injection is utilized. The bulk of evidence from studies of laboratory and domestic animals as well as the limited information on humans suggest that the functional capacity of spermatozoa is realized after epididymal transit. Unfortunately, the mechanisms by which the epididymis exerts these changes on the traversing spermatozoon remain largely unknown. Moreover, the physiology of the human reproductive tract in the presence, and after the release of, obstruction is also not well understood. The following sections describe the structures and functions of the epididymis and discuss the physiologic and biochemical events associated with sperm epididymal maturation.

Gross Structures

In men, the epididymal tubule is 3 to 4 meters in length (Turner et al, 1978). The entire length of the epididymal tubule is coiled and encapsulated within the sheath of connective tissue of the tunica vaginalis (Lanz and Neuhauser, 1964). Extensions from this connective tissue sheath enter the interductal spaces, forming septa that divide the duct into histologically similar regions (Kormano and Reijonen, 1976). A loose network of tissue arises from the septa, supporting the ducts and their associated vascular supply and innervation. Anatomically, the epididymis is divided into three regions: the caput, the corpus, and the cauda epididymis (Fig. 18–16). On the basis of histologic criteria, each of these regions can be subdivided into distinct zones separated by transition segments. **The human caput epididymis consists of 8 to 12 ductuli efferentes and the proximal segment of the ductus epididymis. The lumen of the ductuli efferentes is large and somewhat irregular in shape near the testis, becoming narrow and oval near the junction with the ductus epididymis.** Distal to this junction the diameter of the duct increases slightly and thereafter remains relatively constant throughout the corpus, or body, of the epididymis. In the bulky cauda epididymis the diameter of the duct enlarges substantially and the lumen acquires an irregular shape. Progressing distally, the duct gradually assumes the characteristic appearance of the ductus deferens.

Contractile Tissue

External to the basal lamina of the ductuli efferentes and the epididymal tubule are contractile cells of varying architecture and quantity (Baumgarten et al, 1971). In the ductuli efferentes, the distal regions of the caput epididymis, and the proximal segments of the corpus epididymis, the contractile cells form a loose layer two to four cells deep around the tubule. These cells contain myofilaments and are connected by numerous nexus-like junctions. In the distal regions of the corpus epididymis, other contractile cells are present. These cells are much larger than the contractile cells in the more proximal regions, have fewer nexus-like intracellular junctions, and resemble thin smooth muscle cells. In the cauda epididymis, the thin contractile cells decrease in number and are replaced by thick smooth muscle cells that form three layers—the outer two layers oriented longitudinally and the

Figure 18–16. Schematic drawing of the human epididymis showing regionalization of the ductal epithelium and muscle layer. Locations of epididymal segments shown in cross sections are identified by number. (From Baumgarten HG, Holstein AF, Rosengren E: Arrangement, ultrastructure, and adrenergic innervation of smooth musculature of the ductal efferentes, ductus epididymidis, and ductus deferens in man. Z Zellforsch Mikrosk Anat 1971;120:37.)

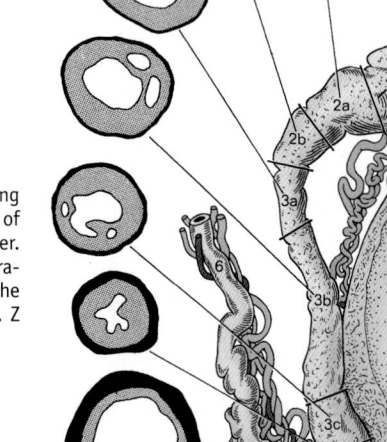

1a–d	Ductuli efferentes	} Caput
2a	Ductus epididymidis	
2b		
3a	" "	} Corpus
3b		
3c		
4a	" "	} Cauda
4b		
4c		
5	Ductus deferens, pars epididymica	
6	Ductus deferens, pars libera	

central layer circularly. This contractile layer increases in thickness distally and ultimately joins the ductus deferens.

Innervation

The innervation of the human epididymis is derived primarily from the intermediate and inferior spermatic nerves, which, in turn, arise from the superior portion of the hypogastric plexus and from the pelvic plexus, respectively (Mitchell, 1935). The ductuli efferentes and the proximal segments of the ductus epididymis are sparsely innervated by sympathetic fibers (Baumgarten and Holstein, 1967; Baumgarten et al, 1968). In these regions the fibers are present in a peritubular plexus and are principally associated with blood vessels. The number of nerve fibers rises significantly at the level of the mid-corpus epididymis and progressively increases distally along the epididymis, coincident with the appearance and proliferation of smooth muscle cells (Baumgarten et al, 1971). The differential distribution of the contractile cells and the sympathetic nerves within the epididymis may be responsible for the rhythmic peristaltic movements of the ductuli efferentes and the initial segments of the epididymis, as well as the intermittent contractile activity of the normally quiescent cauda epididymis and the ductus deferens during emission and ejaculation (Risely, 1963). The significance of these physiologic events to the movement of spermatozoa through the epididymis is discussed in a later section.

Vascularization

In humans, the caput and the corpus epididymis receive arterial blood via a single branch from the testicular artery, which divides into the superior and inferior epididymal branches (MacMillan, 1954). **The blood supply to the epididymis is also derived from branches of the deferential arteries, so a collateral series of vessels connect from the deferential arterial system to the testicular blood supply.** The cauda epididymis is supplied by branches from the deferential artery (artery of the vas deferens), which also communicates with the arteries of the caput epididymis. The deferential vasal and cremasteric arteries serve as collateral sources to the epididymis in the event that the main testicular artery is obstructed or ligated.

The arterial branches leading to the epididymis enter along the septa formed by the connective tissue sheath. Once having entered the epididymis these vessels become extensively coiled before transforming into the straight vessels of the microvascular bed (Kormano and Reijonen, 1976). The microvascularization varies significantly along the length of the ductus epididymis, with the proximal segments of the caput epididymis containing a dense subepithelial capillary network and the degree of vascularization decreasing distally along the epididymal duct.

Studies using experimental animals demonstrated that the capillary network within the epididymis is under hormonal control. For example, in rabbits, bilateral castration results in progressive deterioration and eventual disappearance of the epididymal capillary network (Clavert et al, 1981). It is not clear whether vascularization in the human epididymis is also under hormonal control.

According to MacMillan (1954), venous drainage from the corpus and cauda epididymis join to form the vena marginalis epididymis of Haberer. The capital veins communicate with the pampiniform plexus or the vena marginalis, the latter then joining the vena marginalis testis, the pampiniform plexus, the cremasteric vein, or the deferential vein.

Lymphatic drainage of the epididymis occurs through two routes (Wenzel and Kellermann, 1966). Lymph from the caput and corpus epididymis is removed via the same vessels draining the testis. These vessels follow the internal spermatic vein through the inguinal canal and ultimately terminate in the preaortic nodes. Lymph vessels from the cauda epididymis join those draining the ductus deferens and terminate in the external iliac nodes.

Epithelial Histology

The epithelium of the human epididymis exhibits regional differences along the length of the duct. The junction of the rete testis and the ductuli efferentes is characterized by a distinct transition from a low to a high cuboidal epithelium. The epithelium in the ductuli efferentes consists of ciliated cells and two types of nonciliated cells (Holstein, 1969). The ciliated cells are interdispersed throughout the epithelium. Nonciliated cells with protruding apices, suggesting secretory activity, predominate in the proximal region of the ductuli efferentes. These cells are often present in shallow areas of the epithelium, thereby forming intraepithelial glands (Vendrely, 1981). Other nonciliated cells possessing microvilli, which suggest resorptive activity, predominate in the distal region of the ductuli efferentes. Both the nonciliated and the ciliated cells are joined apically through junctional complexes. In laboratory animals, similar junctions between epithelial cells within the caput epididymis are thought to form a blood-epididymis barrier analogous to the blood-testis barrier (Suzuki and Nagano, 1978; Hoffer and Hinton, 1984). **The blood-epididymis barrier probably extends from the caput into the cauda epididymis. Howards and associates** (1976) **demonstrated that the barrier in the hamster cauda epididymis is permeable to low-molecular-weight substances, such as water and urea, but impermeable to inulin, a compound with a molecular weight of 5000 daltons.** As discussed later, the blood-epididymis barrier may play an important role in influencing the composition of fluid present within different segments of the epididymal lumen (Turner, 1979).

The histology of the human ductus epididymis has been reviewed by Holstein (1969) and Vendrely (1981). The epithelium consists of two major cells types: principal cells and basal cells (seen at low ultrastructural magnification in Fig. 18–17). Principal cells vary in height and length of stereocilia, generally being tall (120 μm), with long stereocilia in the proximal regions of the epididymis, and small (50 μm), with short stereocilia in the more distal regions. The nuclei in these cells are elongated and often possess large clefts and one or two nucleoli. The presence of numerous coated pits, micropinocytotic vesicles, multivesicular bodies, and irregularly shaped membranous vesicles near the apex of these cells, in addition to an extensive Golgi apparatus, suggests that principal cells carry out both absorptive and secretive processes. In humans, the amounts of coated pits and vesicles, multivesicular bodies, and Golgi body in principal cells vary quantitatively along the

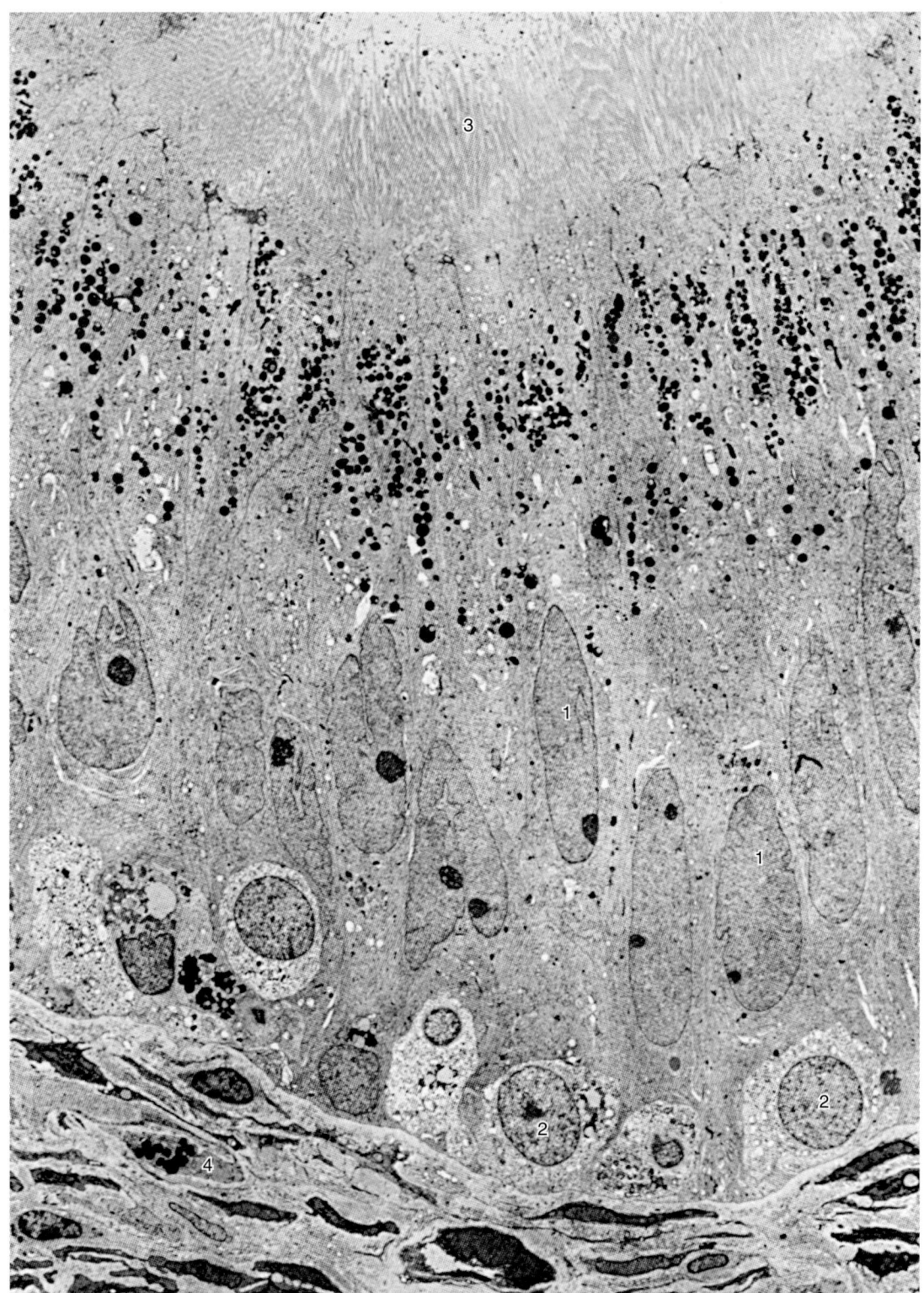

Figure 18–17. Electron micrograph of a cross section through the human ductus epididymis. Major components of the luminal epithelium are principal cells (1), basal cells (2), stereocilia (3), and myofilaments (4). (Magnification approximately ×1800.) (From Holstein AF in Hafez ESE [ed]: Human Semen and Fertility Regulation in Men. St. Louis, CV Mosby, 1976.)

epididymis, suggesting that these cells possess a differential ability for absorption and secretion along the length of the duct (Vendrely and Dadoune, 1988). Basal cells are dispersed among the more numerous principal cells within the epithelium. These tear-shaped cells rest on the basal lamina and extend approximately 25 μm toward the lumen, their apices forming threads between adjacent principal cells. Basal cells are thought to be derived from macrophages. The morphology of basal cells remains relatively constant throughout the epididymal duct.

Functions of the Epididymis

Regional differences in (1) the anatomic structures of the epididymal tubule, (2) the innervation and vascularization of the duct, and (3) the histology of the epithelium suggest that the epididymis is actually a succession of different tissues (Vendrely, 1981). The following sections describe the functions of this complex system, specifically, sperm transit and storage and sperm fertility and motility maturation. Additional information concerning epididymal function can be obtained from reviews by Cosentino and Cockett (1986), Robaire and Hermo (1988), and Moore and Smith (1988).

Sperm Transport

Depending on the measurements employed, **sperm transport through the human epididymis has been observed to require anywhere from 2 to 12 days** (Rowley et al, 1970; Amann, 1981; Johnson and Varner, 1988). Sperm transit time through the caput-corpus portion of the epididymis is roughly similar to the transit time through the cauda epididymis. Amann (1981) suggested that sperm epididymal transit time is influenced by daily testicular sperm production rate rather than by a direct influence of age. This hypothesis was confirmed by Johnson and Varner (1988), who found no difference in sperm epididymal transit time between groups of men aged 20 to 49 and 50 to 79 years. Moreover, they observed that sperm epididymal transit time averaged only 2 days in men with high daily sperm production rate (137 million per testis), compared with an average of 6 days in men with low daily sperm production rate (34 million per testis). With respect to sexual activity, Amann (1981) reported that whereas sperm transit time through the caput and corpus epididymis is not affected, "recent emissions" reduce transit time through the cauda epididymis by 68%.

Because it is generally accepted that, in unobstructed systems, human spermatozoa are immotile within the epididymal lumen, other mechanisms must be involved in the movement of the spermatozoa through the epididymis. These mechanisms may be inferred from the results of animal studies (Bedford, 1975; Courot, 1981; Hamilton, 1977; Jaakkola and Talo, 1982; Jaakkola, 1983). Initially, spermatozoa are carried into the ductuli efferentes by rete testis fluid; the flow of the fluid is facilitated by the resorption of water by ductal epithelial cells. As noted earlier, this reabsorption is mediated by action of the estrogen receptor. Motile cilia and the contraction of the myoid cells surrounding the ductuli efferentes may also assist the movement of spermatozoa into the epididymis. **The principal mechanism responsible for moving spermatozoa through the epididymis is probably the spontaneous rhythmic contractions of the contractile cells surrounding the epididymal duct.** The regionalization of the smooth muscle cells, and the adrenergic innervation within the epididymis described earlier, serve to optimize the ability of the epididymal duct to transport spermatozoa to the ductus deferens.

Sperm Storage

After migrating through the caput and corpus epididymis, spermatozoa are retained in the cauda epididymis for varying lengths of time, depending on the degree of sexual activity. Amann (1981) observed that in a group of men 21 to 55 years of age, an average of 209 to 155 million spermatozoa were present in each epididymis. Similar observations concerning epididymal sperm storage in men were made by Johnson and Varner (1988). **In humans, approximately half of the total number of epididymal spermatozoa are stored in the caudal region.**

As discussed in the following sections, spermatozoa stored in the cauda epididymis are capable of undergoing progressive motility and have the capacity to fertilize eggs. The length of time that spermatozoa can be stored within the epididymis in this potentially fertile state is uncertain. Early studies using experimental animals demonstrated that spermatozoa can be maintained in a viable state for several weeks within the cauda epididymis after ligation of the ductus deferens (Hammond and Asdell, 1926; Young, 1929). More recent studies, however, showed that rabbit (Cooper and Orgebin-Crist, 1977) and rat (Cuasnicu and Bedford, 1989) sperm fertility, measured in vivo, diminished when spermatozoa were retained in the epididymis for longer than normal times. Johnson and Varner (1988) speculated, without presenting data, that in humans the aging of sperm as a result of extended epididymal transit time (prolonged storage) "may contribute to reduced fertility." This interesting hypothesis requires further study.

The fate of unejaculated epididymal spermatozoa in humans is unknown. Studies using experimental animals suggest a variety of sperm-removal mechanisms. In the rat and guinea pig, spermatozoa are lost via spontaneous seminal discharge and oral self-cleaning (Martan, 1969). Rams lose approximately 90% of their daily production of 7 billion spermatozoa into urine (Lino et al, 1967), whereas bulls may lose about 50% of the spermatozoa produced by the testis owing to resorption in the epididymis (Amann and Almquist, 1961). In humans, phagocytosis of spermatozoa by macrophages within the lumen of the epididymis is observed after ligation of the ductus deferens (Phadke, 1964; Alexander, 1972). However, removal of large numbers of spermatozoa from the epididymis of unvasectomized men by spermiophages, spontaneous emission, or epididymal resorption has not been reported. Spermiophagy in the ampullary region of the vas deferens is discussed in a later section.

Maturation of Spermatozoa

Studies in laboratory and domestic animals suggest that beyond serving as a mere conduit and storage depot for spermatozoa, the epididymis sustains maturation processes that support the acquisition of progressive motility and fertility by spermatozoa. Several reports suggest that similar processes also occur in humans. The following sections discuss sperm epididymal maturation, with reference to human studies where appropriate. The possible effects of reproductive tract obstruction on sperm epididymal maturation will also be discussed.

Sperm Motility Maturation. Human spermatozoa develop an increased capacity for motility as they migrate through the epididymis. This process of motility maturation is expressed as a change in the pattern of sperm motility, as well as in an increase in the percentage of spermatozoa exhibiting more "mature" motility patterns. Bedford and coworkers (1973) observed that the majority of spermatozoa taken from the ductuli efferentes and resuspended in culture medium are immotile or exhibit only weak tail movements. A few spermatozoa from these samples have "immature" tail movements characterized by wide arcs of "thrashing" beats that result in little forward progression. The number of spermatozoa possessing this immature motility pattern increases in the initial segment of the epididymis. More distally, in the mid-corpus region, the proportion of spermatozoa exhibiting the immature motility decreases, with a corresponding increase in the number of spermatozoa possessing a "mature" motility pattern characterized by high-frequency, low-amplitude beats that result in progressive motility (Fig. 18–18). In the cauda epididymis, more than 50% of spermatozoa possess the mature motility pattern when diluted in culture medium, the remainder of the spermatozoa being immotile or having the immature motility forms observed in the proximal regions of the epididymis. **Moore and colleagues (1983) confirmed the observations regarding the increased capacity of human spermatozoa for progressive forward motility during epididymal transit.** When diluted in physiologic buffer, 0%, 3%, 12%, 30%, or 60% of spermatozoa were motile when taken from the efferent ducts, caput, proximal corpus, distal corpus, or cauda epididymis, respectively (Fig. 18–19).

Studies involving experimental animals indicate that motility maturation may be, in part, an intrinsic sperm process that occurs independent of specific interactions with the epididymis. Although hamster and rabbit spermatozoa are generally immotile in the caput epididymis, motile spermatozoa were found in this region after ligation of the duct at the level of the corpus epididymis (Horan and Bedford, 1972; Orgebin-Crist, 1969). However, the time required for the development of motility in the spermatozoa entrapped proximally by the ligature was much longer than that required for the maturation of motility when spermatozoa were allowed to migrate through the epididymal duct. In addition, the motility observed in caput epididymal sperm after ligation of the corpus did not persist for more than a very brief period (see Bedford [1975]). These data suggest that **spermatozoa are inherently able to develop some degree of motility based on their duration of contact with proximal epididymal epithelia but that normally the maturation of sperm motility is potentiated through interaction with the epididymis during migration into more distal regions of the duct.**

Whether, and to what degree, epididymal sperm motility maturation in humans is dependent on specific epididymal regions is not clear. Data from studies of patients with congenital absence of the vas deferens or with epididymal obstruction frequently report poor motility in spermatozoa aspirated from the distal epididymis, with optimal sperm quality in the proximal epididymis (Schoysman and Bedford, 1986; Jardin et al, 1988; Silber, 1989; Matthews et al, 1995). However, these observations may reflect an alteration or decrement in epididymal function in these patients, rather

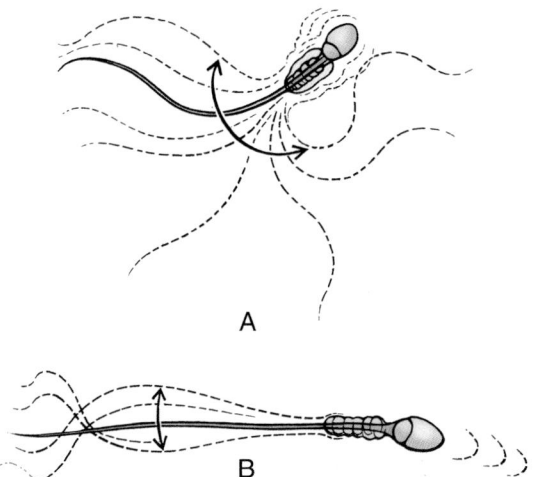

Figure 18–18. Patterns of tail movement in human epididymal spermatozoa. **A,** The pattern shown by spermatozoa taken from proximal regions of the epididymis is characterized by a high-amplitude, low-frequency beat producing little forward movement. **B,** In contrast, tail movement in a large proportion of spermatozoa from the cauda epididymis is characterized by low-amplitude, rapid beats that result in forward progression. (From Bedford JM, Calvin HI, Cooper GW: The maturation of spermatozoa in the human epididymis. J Reprod Fertil 1973;18:199-213.)

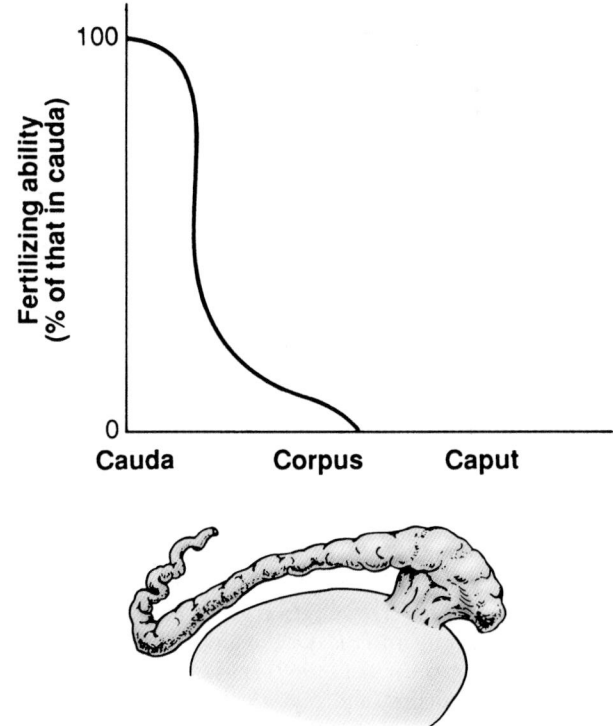

Figure 18–19. Sperm fertility maturation in the human epididymis. Sperm fertilizing ability was assessed using zona pellucida–free hamster eggs and by changes in motility, which increases in the distal regions of the human epididymis. (From Bedford JM: The bearing of epididymal function in strategies for in vitro fertilization and gamete intrafallopian transfer. Ann N Y Acad Sci 1988;541:284-291.)

than intrinsic sperm processes. Unquestionably, the process of sperm motility maturation in the human epididymis requires additional investigation.

KEY POINTS: HORMONAL AND SPERMATOGENETIC FUNCTION OF THE TESTIS

- The scrotal temperature is lower because a counter-current exchange of heat occurs in the spermatic cord and provides blood to the testis that is 2°C to 4°C below rectal temperature in the normal individual.

- Androgen synthesis in testicular Leydig cells requires that cholesterol be transported, assisted by steroid acute regulatory protein and peripheral benzodiazepine receptor, into the mitochondria, where the cholesterol side-chain cleavage enzyme converts it to pregnenolone.

- Testosterone will initiate and qualitatively maintain spermatogenesis in humans.

- The extracellular fluid bathing the Sertoli cells and germinal cells flows from the seminiferous tubules into the rete to form rete testis fluid, which is transported into the caput epididymis. This fluid has a different composition than blood plasma or testicular lymph.

- In the human testis, the seminiferous tubules have a combined length of approximately 250 meters. The rete testis coalesces to form the 6 to 12 ductuli efferentes, which act as conduits to carry testicular fluid and spermatozoa into the caput epididymis.

- Sperm fertility maturation in humans is, in most part, achieved at the level of the distal corpus or proximal cauda epididymis.

- The oval sperm head consists principally of a nucleus that contains highly compacted chromatin material and an acrosome that contains the enzymes required for penetration of the outer vestments of the egg prior to fertilization.

Sperm Fertility Maturation. Convincing evidence from experimental studies demonstrated that testicular spermatozoa are incapable of fertilizing eggs (Orgebin-Crist, 1969; Bedford, 1974), unless they are delivered into the egg by intracytoplasmic sperm injection (Yanagimachi, 2005). In most animals the ability to fertilize eggs is gradually acquired as the spermatozoa migrate into the distal regions of the epididymis. For example, Orgebin-Crist (1969) showed that spermatozoa from the caput, corpus, and cauda epididymis of the rabbit are able to fertilize 1%, 63%, and 92% of exposed rabbit eggs, respectively. Evidence has also been presented for epididymal sperm fertility maturation in humans. Using zona pellucida–free hamster eggs to assess the fertilizing capacity of human epididymal spermatozoa, Hinrischsen and Blaquier (1980) demonstrated that while spermatozoa from the proximal regions of the epididymis are able to bind to the zona-free

eggs, only spermatozoa from the cauda epididymis are able to both bind and penetrate the eggs. Essentially the same observations were made by Moore and coworkers (1983). Taken together, **these studies suggest that sperm fertility maturation in humans is, in most part, achieved at the level of the distal corpus or proximal cauda epididymis.**

More recent studies, however, have questioned whether sperm fertility maturation in humans requires sperm migration into the distal regions of the epididymis. In these studies, patients with ductal obstruction or with congenital absence of the vas deferens were able to achieve pregnancies after vasoepididymostomy up to the level of the ductuli efferentes (Schoysman and Bedford, 1986; Silber, 1989). The probability for fertility was greater when the anastomoses was performed lower in the epididymis. Additional studies using spermatozoa aspirated from men with congenital absence of the vas deferens and in-vitro fertilization confirmed that the fertilizing capacity of spermatozoa is improved when a greater length of epididymis is present (Schlegel and Goldstein, unpublished results). Taken together, these studies demonstrate that in patients with ductal obstruction or with congenital absence of the vas deferens, some degree of sperm fertility maturation occurs in the caput epididymis but that sperm-fertilizing capacity is enhanced with further migration through the epididymis.

The apparent discrepancy between the studies using zona pellucida–free hamster eggs and those on patients with ductal obstruction in localizing the site of fertility maturation in the human epididymis may be explained by earlier studies on laboratory animals. These studies showed that after ductal obstruction by surgical ligation of the epididymis or vas deferens, the normal pattern of fertility maturation along the epididymal duct is "skewed" proximally (see Bedford [1967, 1988] and Orgebin-Crist [1969]). In addition, a report by Turner and Roddy (1990) demonstrated that after surgical obstruction, the flow of fluid through the lumen of the rat epididymis was reduced significantly, even after the reestablishment of ductal patency. At present it is uncertain whether, in humans, epididymal function with respect to sperm fertility maturation is also altered with ductal obstruction or congenital absence of the vas deferens. Clearly, additional studies are required to address this question and to determine the site of sperm maturation in the normal human epididymis.

Controversy exists concerning the outcome of fertilization by spermatozoa that have just acquired fertilizing capacity in the proximal regions of the epididymis. Overstreet and Bedford (1976) reported that embryonic mortality in the rabbit is not increased after fertilization with spermatozoa taken from the distal corpus epididymis. However, other studies using rabbits (Orgebin-Crist, 1969; Orgebin-Crist and Jahad, 1977; Brackett et al, 1978), sheep (Fournier-Delpech et al, 1979), and rats (Paz et al, 1978) indicated that fertilization using immature or young spermatozoa from proximal regions of the epididymis results in a higher rate of embryonic mortality compared with fertilization using ejaculated spermatozoa or mature spermatozoa from the distal epididymis. Because of the occurrence of high vasoepididymostomies using microsurgical techniques and the use of caput epididymal spermatozoa for in-vitro fertilization and other assisted reproductive technologies, this controversy and its relevance to humans must be resolved by future studies.

Biochemical Changes in Spermatozoa during Epididymal Maturation. Spermatozoa undergo a myriad of biochemical and molecular changes as they pass through the epididymis. The topic of sperm modification in the epididymis has been reviewed extensively (see Brooks [1983], Moore and Bedford [1979], Olson and Orgebin-Crist [1982], and Jones [1989]). Although information from human studies is sparse, it is apparent that sperm surface membranes assume an increasingly negative net charge during epididymal transit (Bedford et al, 1973). In addition, sperm membrane sulfhydryl groups undergo oxidation to disulfide bonds (Reyes et al, 1976), as do the sulfhydryl groups in the sperm head and sperm tail structures (Bedford et al, 1973). Bedford and associates (1973) suggested that the formation of intracellular disulfide bonds may provide the sperm tail and head with structural rigidity necessary for progressive motility and successful penetration of eggs.

Studies on laboratory animals described yet other sperm membrane changes associated with sperm epididymal migration, including the post-testicular modification of membrane components, the addition of new membrane components, and the loss of sperm membrane components of testicular origin (see reviews in Hammerstedt and Parks [1987] and Jones [1989]). Specific modifications include alterations in sperm lectin-binding properties (Nicholson et al, 1977; Courtens and Fournier-Delpech, 1979; Olson and Danzo, 1981), phospholipid and lipid content (Dacheux and Laporte, 1977; Nikolopoulou et al, 1985), glycoprotein composition (Fournier-Delpech et al, 1977; Olson and Danzo, 1981; Brown et al, 1983), immunoreactivity (Killian and Amann, 1973; Brooks and Tiver, 1983; Tezon et al, 1985), and iodination characteristics (Nicholson et al, 1979; Olson and Danzo, 1981). Orgebin-Crist and Fournier-Delpech (1982) demonstrated that in the rat, sperm membrane modifications during epididymal passage result in an increased ability to adhere to the zona pellucida of the egg. More recently, Blobel and coworkers (1990) reported that a guinea pig sperm integral membrane glycoprotein (PH-30) is modified during epididymal transit and suggested that the modified protein functions as a sperm-egg fusion molecule during fertilization. This exciting observation provides important insight into the maturation of sperm fertility in the epididymis.

Spermatozoa also undergo numerous metabolic changes during epididymal transit (see reviews by Voglmayr [1975] and Dacheux and Paquignon [1980]). **Studies using experimental animals describe the acquisition of an increased capacity for glycolysis** (Hoskins et al, 1975), **changes in intracellular pH and calcium content, modification of adenylate cyclase activity** (Casillas et al, 1980), **and alterations in cellular phospholipid and phospholipid-like fatty acid content** (Voglmayr, 1975). Whether similar modifications occur in human spermatozoa during epididymal migration is unknown.

Factors Involved in Epididymal Function

Although the mechanisms by which the epididymis carries out its functions of sperm transport, sperm maturation, and sperm storage are unclear, the consensus is that these processes are influenced by the fluids and secretions within the epi-

didymal lumen (for reviews see the works of Brooks [1979], Cooper [1986], and Blaquier and associates [1989]). The constituents of this fluid have been reviewed by Turner (1979), Waites (1980), Orgebin-Crist (1981), and Robaire and Hermo (1988). Studies using laboratory animals demonstrated that the biochemical composition of epididymal fluid not only differs from that of blood serum but also undergoes regional changes within the epididymis. For a thorough discussion of the regionalization of epididymal fluid the reader is referred to excellent reviews by Turner (1979) and by Robaire and Hermo (1988). Suffice it to say that the osmolarity, electrolyte content, and protein composition of luminal fluid varies significantly from region to region in the epididymis. This fluid compartmentalization may reflect the multifunctional nature of the epididymis and is probably the consequence of the differential vascularization along the epididymal tubule, the semipermeability of the blood-epididymis barrier, and the selective absorption and differential secretion of fluid constituents along the length of the duct. In this regard, several studies have described regionalized protein synthesis (Junera et al, 1988) and differential gene expression (Brooks et al, 1986; Ghyselinck et al, 1989; Garrett et al, 1990; Kirchhoff et al, 1990) within specific regions of the epididymis.

Specific constituents of epididymal fluid identified in laboratory studies include glycerylphosphorylcholine (GPC), carnitine, and sialic acid. In addition, epididymal fluid contains proteins that have physiologic effects on spermatozoa in vitro. Examples of these proteins are forward motility protein (Brandt et al, 1978), sperm survival factor (Morton et al, 1978), progressive motility sustaining factor (Sheth et al, 1981), sperm motility–inhibiting factor (Turner and Giles, 1982), acidic epididymal glycoprotein (Pholpramool et al, 1983) and the EP2-EP3 proteins that induce sperm binding to zona pellucida (Cuasnicu et al, 1984; Blaquier et al, 1988). Other proteins are secreted into specific regions of the epididymis and subsequently become associated with spermatozoa (Kohane et al, 1980; Orgebin-Crist, 1981; Cornwall et al, 1990).

Control of Epididymal Function

Testosterone and DHT are found at very high concentrations within the human epididymis. There does not appear to be a gradient of androgen levels in different regions of the epididymis (Leinonen et al, 1980). The relative enrichment of DHT and the high levels of 5α-reductase in the epididymis support this androgen as being important in epididymal function. From animal studies it is clear that the functions of the epididymis are androgen dependent (see reviews by Orgebin-Crist and colleagues [1975], Turner and associates [1979], and Brooks and Tiver [1983]). Clearly, the synthesis of some, but not all, epididymal proteins is androgen regulated (Jones et al, 1980; Brooks and Tiver, 1983; Charest et al, 1989; Toney and Danzo, 1989). Bilateral castration results not only in the loss of androgen-dependent epididymal proteins but also in the loss of epididymal weight, in the perturbation of luminal histology, and in changes in the synthesis and secretion of epididymal fluid components including GPC, carnitine, and sialic acid. Ultimately, the epididymis loses the ability to sustain the processes of sperm motility and fertility maturation and sperm storage. Most of these degenerative processes can be reversed by androgen replacement therapy. However, the effects of androgen on the initial segments of the epididymis are thought to be mediated by testosterone bound to androgen-binding protein and possibly other testicular factors. If the testis is separated from the epididymis, preventing transport of the typically very high levels of testosterone and androgen-binding protein, then exogenous (or implanted testosterone) is limited in its ability to reverse the adverse effects of loss of the rich testicular source of testosterone (Brooks, 1979). The importance of androgen levels on epididymal function is supported by the observation that alterations in sperm function are observed within days after exogenous estrogen treatment, independent of an effect on spermatogenesis (Kaneto et al, 1999).

Studies using laboratory animals indicated that, compared with the accessory sex glands, the epididymis requires higher levels of androgen for maintenance of its structure and functions (Prasad and Rajalakshmi, 1976). The regulatory effects of androgen on the epididymis appear to be mediated through DHT, the primary androgen in epididymal tissue extracts (Vreeburg, 1975, Pujol et al, 1976) and/or 5α-androstane-3α,17β-diol (3α-diol) (Lubicz-Nawrocki, 1973; Orgebin-Crist et al, 1975). The enzymes Δ^4-5α-reductase, which catalyzes the formation of DHT from testosterone, and 3α-hydroxysteroid dehydrogenase, which converts DHT to 3a-diol, are present in the epididymis and have been localized within the subcellular fractions of epididymal homogenates from humans (Kinoshita et al, 1980; Larminat et al, 1980) and experimental animals (Robaire et al, 1977; Scheer and Robaire, 1983).

Studies in the rat demonstrated that epididymal functions are also influenced by temperature (Foldesy and Bedford, 1982; Wong et al, 1982). Abdominal placement of the epididymis, resulting in exposure to body temperature, causes the loss of sperm storage and electrolyte transport functions. Whether the functions of the human epididymis are similarly affected by body temperature is unknown. The potential influence of temperature on epididymal function in humans may be an important consideration in investigating the relationships between varicocele or cryptorchidism and male infertility.

Recent evidence from studies in the rat have suggested also that ability of the epididymis to store spermatozoa may be influenced by the sympathetic nervous system. Surgical partial denervation of the epididymis resulted in an abnormal accumulation of spermatozoa within the cauda epididymis and a decrease in the curvilinear and straight-line swimming speed of the retained spermatozoa (Billups et al, 1990). These results suggest that chemical or surgical sympathetic denervation, or nerve trauma, may have an adverse affect on subsequent fertility.

SPERMATOZOA

For reviews of sperm structure and function the reader is referred to Fawcett (1979), Tash and Means (1988), Garbers (1989), Lindemann and Kanous (1989), and Majumder and associates (1990). Mature spermatozoa stored within the cauda epididymis and the ductus deferens are highly differentiated cells (Fig. 18–20). The human spermatozoon is approximately 60 μm in length (Flechon and Hafez, 1976). **The oval sperm head, about 4.5 μm long and 3 μm wide, consists principally of a nucleus, which contains the highly compacted chromatin material, and an acrosome, a membrane-bound**

organelle that contains the enzymes required for penetration of the outer vestments of the egg before fertilization (Chang and Hunter, 1975; Yanagimachi, 1978). The middle piece of the spermatozoon is a highly organized segment consisting of helically arranged mitochondria surrounding a set of outer dense fibers and the characteristic 9 + 2 microtubular structure of the sperm axoneme. The outer dense fibers, rich in disulfide bonds, are thought to provide the sperm tail (having a length of about 60 μm) with the rigidity necessary for progressive motility (Bedford et al, 1973; Oko and Clermont, 1990). The sperm mitochondria contain the enzymes required for oxidative metabolism and for the production of adenosine triphosphate (ATP), the primary energy source for the cell. The sperm axoneme contains the enzymes and structural proteins necessary for transduction of the chemical energy of ATP into the mechanical movement resulting in motility. The outer dense fibers and axonemal structures present in the middle piece continue, with slight modification, through the principal piece of the spermatozoon, which is surrounded by a fibrous sheath. At the distal end of the principal piece the outer dense fibers terminate, leaving the axonemes as the primary structure in the end-piece region. Except for the end-piece region, the spermatozoon is enveloped by a highly specialized plasma membrane that regulates the transmembrane movement of ions and other molecules (Friend, 1989). Moreover, as shown in studies with mice, the plasma membrane covering the sperm-head region contains specialized proteins that participate in sperm-egg interactions during the early stages of fertilization (for reviews see Dietl and Rauth [1989] and Saling [1989]). In particular, carbohydrate-binding proteins on the sperm membrane interact with the species-specific ZP3 protein in the egg zona pellucida, with the interaction resulting first in sperm binding to the zona and subsequently in the induction of the acrosome reaction (see Dietl and Rauth [1989], O'Rand [1988], Shabanowitz [1990], and Wassarman [1988]). Another sperm membrane protein, PH30, was described by Primakoff (1987). This protein is present on testicular sperm, is modified into an active form during sperm migration through the epididymis, and functions as a fusion protein between the sperm and egg plasma membranes during fertilization (Blobel et al, 1990).

The functionally competent spermatozoon is a result of the complex processes of spermatogenesis and epididymal maturation. Because of its highly specialized morphology and physiology the resulting spermatozoon is marvelously suited for its single purpose, reproduction.

Effects of Sex Accessory Gland Secretions on Spermatozoal Function

The variability of sex accessory gland structure in different mammals is impressive. Whereas cats and dogs have no seminal vesicles, rodents have well-developed seminal vesicles, coagulating glands, and prostates. For each species, an effective mode for trapping spermatozoa within the vagina exists. In dogs, swelling of a penile bulb results in the penis being "locked" into the vagina, effectively trapping the ejaculate in the vagina by mechanical means. Although this is feasible for a carnivore, rodents have developed the capacity to produce

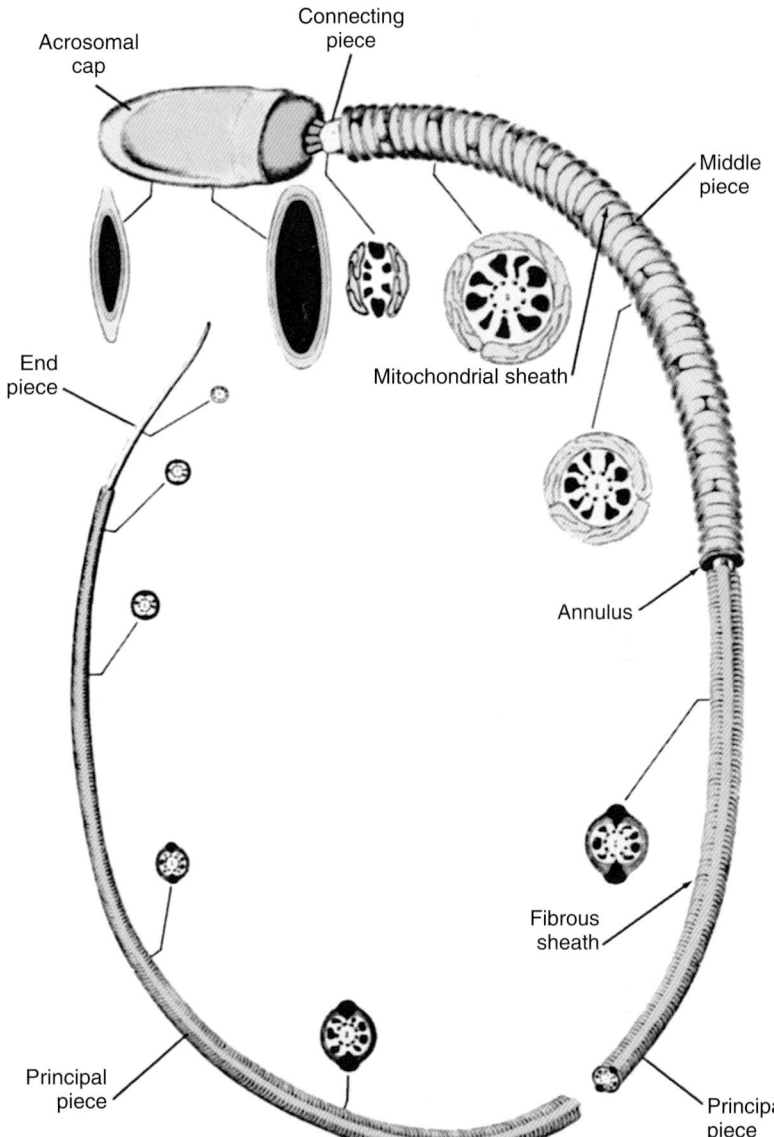

Figure 18-20. Diagram of a typical mammalian spermatozoon. The plasma membrane is omitted in order to illustrate the major components of the spermatozoon. Cross-sectional insets show the orientation of the internal cell structures. (From Fawcett DW: The mammalian spermatozoon. Dev Biol 1975;44:394-436.)

an effective copulatory plug that does not require male and female animals to remain attached after coital activity but maintain spermatozoa in the vagina above the plug (in juxtaposition to the cervix.)

The human ejaculate maintains an ability to coagulate initially and is subsequently liquefied by proteases produced by the prostate, primarily prostate specific antigen. It is not clear what mechanical assistance the coagulum of the human ejaculate provides to maintain spermatozoa within the vagina. After ejaculation, spermatozoa must pass into and through the cervical mucus and subsequently transit the uterus to enter the oviduct, where fertilization naturally occurs. Uterine transport in the woman takes 5 to 68 minutes (Harper, 1982). During residence in the female reproductive tract, spermatozoa must undergo a process referred to as capacitation prior to oocyte fertilization. Capacitation occurs at different rates for individual spermatozoa. During capacitation, a number of changes occur from a structural and biochemical standpoint, but the most obvious notable changes are the acrosome reac-

tion and development of hyperactivated motility (see Yanagimachi [1994]). It is not clear if prostatic or seminal vesicle secretions contribute to the process of capacitation. For additional reviews of sperm function during fertilization—egg binding and the acrosome reaction—see the work of Garbers (1989), Dietl and Rauth (1989), and Saling (1989).

Biochemical properties of the ejaculate that support spermatozoal function have not been well elucidated. Fructose, produced in the seminal vesicles, will provide an energy source for ejaculated spermatozoa. Macromolecules, including albumin, help to support and stimulate spermatozoa (White et al, 1987). The best-elucidated function of human semen appears to be its ability to provide antioxidative protection to spermatozoa that are very sensitive to the effects of oxidants (Jones et al, 1979). Semen is rich in antioxidant enzymes including glutathione peroxidase, superoxide dismutase, and catalase (Yeung et al, 1998). In addition, the antioxidant molecules taurine, hypotaurine, and tyrosine are present at high concentrations in semen (Holmes et al, 1992; van Overveld et al, 2000). Oxidative effects on spermatozoa may result in lower sperm motility and increased damage to sperm DNA (Fraga et al, 1996). Not surprisingly, separation of spermatozoa from semen, for example during sperm centrifugation or other processing techniques, may expose sperm to an increased risk of oxidative damage.

DUCTUS VAS DEFERENS

The ductus deferens is a tubular structure derived embryologically from the mesonephric (wolffian) duct. **In humans, the ductus deferens is 30 to 35 cm in length; it begins at the cauda epididymis and terminates in the ejaculatory duct near the prostate gland.** Lich and colleagues (1978) stated that "the ductus deferens may be divided into five portions: (1) the sheathless epididymal portion contained within the tunica vaginalis, (2) the scrotal portion, (3) the inguinal division, (4) the retroperitoneal or pelvic portion, and (5) the ampulla." In cross section, the ductus deferens consists of an outer adventitial connective tissue sheet that contains blood vessels and small nerves, a muscular coat that is made up of a middle circular layer surrounded by inner and outer longitudinal muscle layers, and a mucosal inner layer made up of an epithelial lining (Neaves, 1975). **The outer diameter of the vas deferens varies from 2 to 3 mm in diameter, and the lumen of the unobstructed tubule varies from 300 to 500 μm in diameter.**

Vascularization and Innervation

The ductus deferens receives its blood supply from the deferential artery via the inferior vesicle artery (Harrison, 1949a). Kormano and Reijonen (1976) discovered that the microvascularization of the sheathless portion of the human ductus deferens is divided into an outer network within the adventitial layer and an inner subepithelial capillary network.

The ductus deferens of the human receives nerve fibers from both the sympathetic and the parasympathetic nervous system (Sjostrand, 1965). The cholinergic supply is of minor importance in the motor activity of the ductus deferens (Baumgarten et al, 1975). In contrast, **the human ductus deferens has a rich supply of sympathetic adrenergic nerves** (Sjostrand, 1965; Alm, 1982; McConnell et al, 1982) derived from the hypogastric nerves via the presacral nerve (Batra and Lardner, 1976). Interestingly, the ductus deferens receives a special type of short adrenergic nerve (Sjostrand, 1965). McConnell and coworkers (1982) reported that adrenergic nerve fibers were observed in all three layers of the tunica muscularis, with the greatest concentration in the outer longitudinal layer. Neurons containing other neurotransmitter substances have been identified (Alm, 1982; McConnell et al, 1982). However, it remains to be proved whether these other neurotransmitters are important in the physiologic functions of the ductus deferens.

Cytoarchitecture of the Ductus Deferens

There have been numerous studies in experimental animals describing the cytoarchitecture of the ductus deferens (for a review see Hamilton [1975]). Similar detailed descriptions of the human ductus deferens at the light and electron micro-scopic level have been presented (Popovic et al, 1973; Friend et al, 1976; Hoffer, 1976; Paniagua et al, 1981; Riva et al, 1982). Paniagua and colleagues (1981) observed that the ductus deferens was lined by pseudostratified epithelium, that the epithelial height decreased along the length of the ductus, that the longitudinal folds of the epithelium were simple in the proximal region and became more complex toward the distal segments, and that the thickness of the entire muscle layer gradually decreased along the length of the ductus deferens. Hoffer (1976) and Paniagua and colleagues (1981) report that the pseudostratified epithelium lining the lumen of the ductus deferens is composed of basal cells and three types of tall thin columnar cells. The latter, which extend from the base of the epithelium to the lumen, include principal cells, pencil cells, and mitochondrion-rich cells. All of these cells show stereocilia and irregular convoluted nuclei. According to Paniagua and colleagues (1981), principal cells are the most frequent cell type in the proximal portion of the ductus deferens. In contrast, the portion of both pencil cells and mitochondrion-rich cells increases toward the distal end of the ductus deferens.

The complexity of the muscular layers, the specialized and rich adrenergic innervation, the variety of epithelial cells in the mucosal layer, and the changing structural characteristics from the proximal to the distal end suggest strongly that the ductus deferens in humans is more than a passive conduit for the transport of sperm from the cauda epididymis to the urethra.

Function of the Ductus Deferens
Spermatozoal Transport

These are numerous theories to explain the transport of spermatozoa through the ductus deferens in humans (Gunha et al, 1975; Neaves, 1975; Batra and Lardner, 1976). Unfortunately, data supporting these theories are fragmentary and the issue remains unresolved. However, several pertinent observations have been made. Apparently, the human ductus deferens exhibits a spontaneous motility (Ventura et al, 1973). Also, the human ductus deferens has the capacity to respond when stretched (Bruschini et al, 1977). Finally, the contents of the ductus can be propelled into the urethra by strong peristaltic contractions that are elicited either by electrical stimulation of the hypogastric nerve (Bruschini et al, 1977) or by adrenergic neurotransmitters (Ventura et al, 1973; Bruschini et al, 1977; Lipshultz et al, 1981). **Immediately before emission, rapid and effective transport of spermatozoa from the distal epididymis and proximal vas deferens occurs, apparently related to sympathetic stimulation. This efficient transport of spermatozoa reflects the observation that the ductus deferens has the greatest muscle-lumen ratio (~10:1) of any hollow viscus in the human body.**

In the human male, epididymal reserves of spermatozoa total approximately 182 million spermatozoa with 26% in the caput, 23% in the corpus, and 52% in the cauda. Transit times of spermatozoa through the caput, corpus, and cauda epididymis have been estimated at 0.7, 0.7, and 1.8 days, respectively. Spermatozoal reserves in the ductus deferens have been estimated at approximately 130 million spermatozoa. Therefore, a significant proportion of spermatozoa in the human ejaculate appear to be stored in the ductus deferens, with slightly less than half of the spermatozoa in each ejaculate stored in the cauda epididymis (Amann and Howards, 1980). The effect of frequency of ejaculation on these estimates has not been reliably evaluated.

Prins and Zaneveld (1979, 1980a, 1980b) have obtained interesting results regarding the transport of spermatozoa through the ductus deferens at sexual rest, after sexual stimulation, and after ejaculation. Using the rabbit as a model, they showed that **"during the sexual rest, epididymal contents were transported distally through the vas deferens into the urethra in small amounts and at irregular intervals,"** supporting the idea that urethral disposal is a mechanism for ridding the epididymis of excess spermatozoa. Furthermore, they showed that when rabbits were sexually stimulated, spermatozoa were transported from the cauda epididymis and proximal ductus deferens toward the distal ductus deferens. If ejaculation occurred, spermatozoa were propelled into the urethra.

After sexual stimulation and/or ejaculation, an interesting phenomenon occurred. The contents of the ductus deferens were propelled back toward the proximal epididymis and even into the cauda epididymis because the distal portion of the ductus deferens contracted with greater amplitude, frequency, and duration than did the proximal portion of the ductus deferens (Prins and Zaneveld, 1980a). Importantly, this process was reversed on prolonged sexual rest, and the excess cauda epididymal spermatozoa that derived from daily spermatozoa production were once again transported distally. These results were interpreted to mean that the ductus deferens of the rabbit played an important role not only in sperm transport during sexual activity but also in the maintenance of epididymal sperm reserves. It remains to be seen whether similar mechanisms are at work in sperm transport through the human ductus deferens.

Absorption and Secretion

Based on morphologic criteria, it has been suggested that the human ductus deferens may have both absorptive and secretory functions (Hoffer, 1976; Paniagua et al, 1981). Unfortunately, inadequate experimental results in the human exist to confirm this idea.

Hoffer (1976) and Paniagua and colleagues (1981) reported that the principal cells of the human ductus deferens have characteristics typical of cells that are capable of synthesizing and secreting glycoproteins. This is in keeping with reports by Gupta and associates (1974) and Bennett and coworkers (1974) that the rat ductus deferens synthesizes and secretes glycoproteins into the tubular lumen.

The stereocilia, apical blebbing, and primary and secondary lysosomes of principal cells in the human ductus deferens are also characteristic of cells involved in absorptive functions (Hoffer, 1976; Paniagua et al, 1981; Murakami et al, 1988). Protein absorption from the tubular lumen of the rat ductus deferens has been observed (Friend and Farquhar, 1967). Cooper and Orgebin-Crist (1977) have shown that the terminal region and gland of the rat ductus deferens have the capacity to phagocytose and absorb spermatozoa. Using scanning electron microscopy, Murakami and coworkers (1988) reported spermiophagy by epithelial cells in the ampullary region of the ductus deferens in men and monkeys. Whether the amount of spermiophagy in the ampulla and in other regions of the excurrent duct is sufficient for the removal of excess spermatozoa in men remains to be seen.

The structure and function of the ductus deferens probably depends on androgen stimulation because (1) the human ductus deferens converts testosterone to DHT (Dupuy et al, 1979); (2) castration causes atrophy of—and testosterone treatment, restoration of—monkey vas (Dinakar et al, 1977); and (3) spontaneous as well as α- and β-adrenergic stimulated contractions of the rat ductus deferens are altered by castration and/or testosterone treatment (Borda et al, 1981).

SUMMARY

The hypothalamo-pituitary-gonadal axis provides pulsatile secretion of GnRH and subsequently LH and FSH release from the pituitary to stimulate spermatogenesis and testosterone production. GnRH pulses are released every 90 to 120 minutes. Diurnal variation of testosterone results in higher morning levels of testosterone than that observed in the afternoon and evening. The testis is a specialized structure that functions optimally 2°C to 4°C below body temperature. Spermatogenesis is less efficient in humans than in most other animals. The process of spermatogenesis and spermiogenesis takes approximately 64 days in humans and results in a haploid germ cell that acquires natural ability to fertilize oocytes during epididymal transport. Spermatogenesis is an androgen-dependent process that optimally occurs with very high intratesticular levels of testosterone. Spermatozoa exiting the testis are immotile and have limited capacity to fertilize an oocyte unless assisted reproductive techniques are applied. After epididymal transit (that takes 2 to 11 days), sperm are typically motile and capable of fertilization without assistance. Immediately before emission, spermatozoa are rapidly and efficiently transported to the ejaculatory ducts from the distal epididymis. Spermatozoal function does not stop at the time of fertilization; sperm-derived spindles even drive embryo development.

KEY POINTS: SPERMATOZOA AND FERTILITY

- The middle piece of the spermatozoon consists of helically arranged mitochondria surrounding a set of outer dense fibers and the characteristic 9 + 2 microtubular structure of the sperm axoneme.

- The sperm tail has outer dense fibers, rich in disulfide bonds, that are thought to provide the rigidity necessary for progressive motility.

- In humans, the mitotic activity of embryos normally appears to be organized by the paternally derived centrosome.

- The entire spermatogenic process in humans requires approximately 64 days.

- High testicular concentrations of testosterone are required to maintain spermatogenesis, and men older than age 40 years have lower fecundity compared with men younger than age 25 years.

SUGGESTED READINGS

Levallet J, Pakarinen P, Huhtaniemi IT: Follicle-stimulating hormone ligand and receptor mutations, and gonadal dysfunction. Arch Med Res 1999;30:486-494.

Lombardo F, Sgro P, Salacone P, et al: Androgens and fertility. J Endocrinol Invest 2005;28:51-55.

Payne AH, Hales DB: Overview of steroidogenic enzymes in the pathway from cholesterol to active steroid hormones. Endocr Rev 2004;25:947-970.

Reijo R, Lee T-Y, Salo P, et al: Diverse spermatogenic defects in humans caused by Y chromosome deletions encompassing a novel RNA-binding protein gene. Nat Genet 1995;10:383-393.

Yanagimachi R: Fertilization and developmental initiation of oocytes by injection of spermatozoa and pre-spermatozoal cells. Ital J Anat Embryol 2005;110:145-150.

19 Male Infertility

MARK SIGMAN, MD • JONATHAN P. JAROW, MD

The past decade has seen refinement in reproductive techniques but not major advances in the ability to improve impaired spermatogenesis. The use of spermatozoa recovered from the testes of patients with nonobstructive azoospermia for intracytoplasmic sperm injection (ICSI) has now become routine. Unfortunately, the development of effective treatments has been hampered by a lack of knowledge of the etiology of many cases of male infertility. The past several years have seen steady gains in the understanding of the multiple factors that may adversely affect male fertility—ranging from an increasing variety of genetic abnormalities to environmental and lifestyle gonadotoxins. As we gain an understanding of the underlying causes of infertility, treatment options should improve with the development of therapies designed for specific defects.

Because of the success of the assisted reproductive techniques (ART), the evaluation of the man is often ignored. The physician should not forget the fact that many causes of male infertility such as varicocele, ductal obstruction, and infections are easily and effectively treated. In addition, without a full evaluation, significant diseases such as testicular cancer, pituitary tumors, and neurologic disease may be overlooked (Jarow, 1994b). Finally, as greater inroads into the genetic causes of male infertility have been made there has been increased importance placed on the proper evaluation and counseling for the male partner before beginning the ART.

The chance of a normal couple conceiving is estimated to be 20% to 25% per month, 75% by 6 months, and 90% by 1 year (Spira, 1986). Fertility rates are at their peak in men and women at age 24; beyond that age, fertility rates begin to decline with age in both sexes (Noord-Zaadstra et al, 1991; Ford et al, 2000). Studies of couples of unknown fertility status that are attempting to conceive have demonstrated that although most couples achieve conception within 1 year, approximately 15% of couples are unable to do so (Hull et al, 1985; Greenhall and Vessey, 1990; Thonneau et al, 1991). Approximately 20% of cases of infertility are due entirely to a male factor, with an additional 30% to 40% of cases involving both male and female factors (Mosher and Pratt, 1991; Thonneau et al, 1991). Therefore, a male factor is present in one half of infertile couples. Of infertile couples without treatment, 25% to 35% will conceive at some time by intercourse alone (Collins et al, 1983). Within the first 2 years 23% will conceive, whereas an additional 10% will do so within 2 more years (Aafjes et al, 1978). This baseline pregnancy rate of 1% to 3% per month (in non-azoospermic couples) must be kept in mind while managing infertile couples and evaluating the results of therapy. Although infertility is often not considered to exist until after 12 months of attempted conception (Guidelines, 2004b), with the advancing age of infertile couples, we do not recommend deferring an initial evaluation. A basic, simple, cost-effective evaluation of both the male and female partners should be initiated at the time of presentation.

The approach to the evaluation of the infertile man should be similar to that used to evaluate other medical problems. A thorough history should be obtained, with particular attention to those areas that may affect fertility. This should be followed by a physical examination. An initial series of laboratory tests completes the basic evaluation. The results of the history, physical examination, and initial laboratory testing are used to formulate a differential diagnosis that may lead to more specific testing. Many tests are available to evaluate different aspects of male infertility, but not all patients require all tests.

The goals of the evaluation of the infertile man are to identify (1) reversible conditions; (2) irreversible causes that may be managed by ART using the male partner's sperm; (3) irreversible conditions that may not be managed by the above techniques and where the couple should be advised to pursue donor insemination or adoption; (4) significant underlying medical pathology; and (5) genetic and/or chromosomal abnormalities that may affect either the patient or his offspring. Ideally, the evaluation of the infertile man should result in the identification of the specific abnormality responsible for infertility. Although this is possible in some instances, many men have abnormal semen analyses for which no etiology can be identified. When possible, specific treatment is directed toward a specific etiology. However, both empirical therapies and ART such as intrauterine insemination (IUI) and in-vitro fertilization (IVF) may be of value in the absence of known etiologic factors. Therapeutic donor insemination and adoption are treatment alternatives. The infertile couple should be made aware of these options, with the physician playing a counseling role to avoid excessively prolonged, futile treatments.

HISTORY

The evaluation of the male partner of an infertile couple should include a thorough medical and reproductive history exploring all aspects that may be related to fertility (Table 19–1) (Sharlip et al, 2002). The duration of infertility, details of prior pregnancies initiated, methods of birth control utilized in the past, the couple's frequency of sexual intercourse, as well as the timing of coitus should be recorded. It should be determined whether the couple realizes that ovulation occurs during the middle of the menstrual cycle and that the female is only fertile during this time. Sexual relations at any other time of the menstrual cycle will not result in a pregnancy. The timing of sexual intercourse does not have to coincide exactly with ovulation since sperm remain viable within the cervical mucus and crypts for 48 hours or longer. Studies have shown that conception may occur when sexual relations take place up to 5 days before ovulation but, owing to the short life span of oocytes, will not occur if sexual relations are performed the day after ovulation (Wilcox et al, 1995b). **Although there is some controversy, most experts advise vaginal intercourse every 2 days near the time of ovulation, which ensures that viable sperm are present during the 12- to 24-hour period in which the oocyte is within the fallopian tube and is capable of being fertilized.** Intercourse that is too frequent may result in inadequate numbers of sperm being deposited in the vaginal vault and, similarly, the ovulatory period may be missed if sexual activity is too infrequent. The timing of intercourse, relative to ovulation, has no relation to the sex of the child (Wilcox et al, 1995b).

Erectile and ejaculatory function should be assessed. In addition, the use of any vaginal lubricants during intercourse should be noted. Most of the commonly used lubricants, such as Astroglide, Lubafax, K-Y Jelly, Keri Lotion, Surgilube, and saliva, adversely affect sperm motility (Tagatz et al, 1972; Goldenberg and White, 1975; Tulandi et al, 1982; Boyers et al, 1987; Kutteh et al, 1996). Lubricants that do not impair in-vitro sperm motility include peanut oil, safflower oil, vegetable oil, and raw egg white. In general, a couple should be advised to use a lubricant only if necessary and to use a minimal amount of one that does not impair sperm function.

The developmental history of the patient should also be explored. **Unilateral cryptorchidism slightly decreases fertility, and bilateral cryptorchidism results in a significant reduction in fertility** (Cendron et al, 1989). There is both experimental and clinical evidence that the timing of orchidopexy does not appear to affect the findings of spermatogenic abnormalities in these testes as long as the testes were

Table 19–1. Components of the History in Evaluation of the Infertile Male

Sexual History

Duration of sexual relations with and without birth control
Methods of birth control
Sexual technique: potency, use of lubricants (some are spermicidal)
Frequency and timing of coitus

Past History

Developmental
  History of cryptorchidism
  Age at puberty
  Gynecomastia
  Congenital abnormalities of urinary tract or central nervous system

Surgical
  Orchidopexy
  Pelvic, scrotal, inguinal, or retroperitoneal surgery
  Herniorrhaphy
  Sympathectomy
  Vasectomy
  Scrotal trauma
  Spinal cord injury
  Testicular torsion

Medical
  Urinary infections
  Sexually transmitted diseases
  Viral orchitis
  Renal disease
  Diabetes
  Radiotherapy
  Recent febrile illness
  Epididymitis
  Tuberculosis or other chronic diseases
  Anosmia
  Midline defects (cleft palate)

Drugs
  Complete list of all past and present medications. Many drugs interfere with spermatogenesis, erection, or ejaculation.
Occupation and Habits
  Exposure to chemicals and heat, hot baths, steam baths, radiation, cigarettes, alcohol, illicit drugs, and anabolic steroids
Past Reproductive History (including pregnancies and offspring with other partners)
Previous Infertility Evaluation and Treatment

Family History

Hypogonadism
Cryptorchidism
Congenital midline defects
Cystic fibrosis

Female Reproductive History

Past history including pregnancies and offspring with other partners
Menstrual history
Infertility evaluation to date

brought down before puberty (Lipshultz et al, 1976; Cendron et al, 1989; Pryor et al, 1989; Lerchl et al, 1993). A history of delayed or absent puberty may be associated with an endocrinopathy or androgen receptor abnormality (Kulin, 1997). A history of gynecomastia may be associated with either testis cancer, hyperprolactinemia, or estrogen abnormalities (Limone et al, 1989).

The patient's past surgical history may be of particular importance. Pelvic or retroperitoneal surgery may affect erectile and ejaculatory function. Bladder neck surgery may result in retrograde ejaculation. Retroperitoneal lymph node dissection for testis cancer may injure the sympathetic nerves, resulting in failure of emission or retrograde ejaculation. Modifications of this surgery by either a template method or nerve sparing have resulted in preservation of the sympathetic nerves responsible for ejaculation, allowing the retention of ejaculatory function in most patients (Jewett, 1990; Donohue et al, 1993). The vas deferens may be inadvertently injured or stripped of its blood supply during a herniorrhaphy. Likewise, any scrotal surgery, such as hydrocelectomy, may result in injury to either the vas deferens and/or epididymis. Testicular trauma or torsion may result in testicular atrophy; such patients may also be predisposed to the development of antisperm antibodies, although the evidence for this is not strong (Cerasaro et al, 1984; Heidenreich et al, 1994).

The patient should be questioned for a history of urinary tract infections or sexually transmitted diseases. A history of prostatitis and/or pyospermia should be noted, although there is no convincing evidence that these conditions actually cause infertility (Weidner et al, 1999). Mumps does not appear to affect the testis when it occurs in a prepubertal child; however, mumps orchitis and other forms of viral orchitis may develop if the patient has passed puberty. Ten to 30 percent of pubertal infected patients develop mumps orchitis (Erpenbach, 1991). Bilateral involvement is seen in 20% to 60%.

A history of absent or low volume ejaculate suggests the possibility of retrograde ejaculation, hypogonadism, ejaculatory duct obstruction, or congenital hypoplasia or absence of the vas deferens and seminal vesicles (Jarow, 1996c). Systemic illnesses may have an adverse effect on male fertility. Ejaculatory dysfunction or erectile abnormalities may develop in patients with diabetes mellitus or multiple sclerosis. Infertility is common in patients with end-stage renal disease. **Oligospermia is identified in approximately 60% or more of testicular cancer and lymphoma patients at the time of diagnosis** (Carroll et al, 1987; Nijman et al, 1987; Rustin et al, 1987). Chemotherapy or radiation therapy may further impair testicular function. Spermatogenesis may take up to 4 to 5 years to return after radiation therapy or chemotherapy (Orecklin et al, 1973; Rustin et al, 1987; Costabile, 1993). The initial depression in spermatogenesis after chemotherapy is due to direct cytotoxicity to rapidly dividing germ cells. Various agents affect different steps in spermatogenesis, and permanent azoospermia may result from irreversible stem cell damage. The prognosis can be predicted if the details of the chemotherapeutic regimen including the specific agents, the doses, and the duration of treatment are known (Costabile, 1993). **After a febrile illness, spermatogenesis may be impaired for up to 3 months** (Buch and Havlovec, 1991). **In patients with abnormal semen analyses and a history of a systemic illness within 3 months of the evaluation, additional semen analysis should be obtained over a 3- to 6-month period to adequately assess the patient's baseline fertility status.** Azoospermia in a patient with a history of bilateral epididymitis suggests the presence of epididymal obstruction. There are three male infertility conditions associated with chronic upper respiratory infections. Immotile cilia syndrome, or *Kartagener's syndrome*, should be suspected in patients with immotile sperm, a history of frequent respiratory tract infections, and situs inversus (Wilton et al, 1986). Almost all male patients with clinical cystic fibrosis have bilat-

eral congenital absence of the vas deferens (Kaplan et al, 1968; Taussig et al, 1972). Conversely, the majority of men with congenital bilateral absence of the vas deferens (CBAVD) have a mutation in the cystic fibrosis transmembrane conductance regulator gene *(CFTR)* (Patrizio and Leonard, 2000). Azoospermia associated with a history of frequent respiratory infections also suggests the possibility of Young's syndrome (Wilton et al, 1991). In these patients, epididymal obstruction due to inspissation of secretions accounts for azoospermia. A history of severe headaches, galactorrhea, or impaired visual fields should raise the possibility of a pituitary tumor. *Kallmann syndrome* is a congenital form of hypogonadotropic hypogonadism associated with midline defects such as anosmia. Many medications and drugs, including nitrofurantoin, cimetidine, sulfasalazine, cocaine, nicotine, and marijuana have been implicated as impairing spermatogenesis (Kolodny et al, 1974; Van Thiel et al, 1975; Abel et al, 1989; Berul and Harclerode, 1989; Marshburn et al, 1989; Benoff et al, 1994). Spermatogenesis and/or sperm function may return to normal after cessation of these agents.

Anabolic steroid abuse by athletes has been increasing. Hypogonadotropic hypogonadism may result from the androgenic component of the steroids. Normal hormonal function usually returns after these agents are discontinued, but this is not always the case (Jarow and Lipshultz, 1990). Exposure to environmental toxicants such as pesticides should be noted, because these may be gonadotoxic. Testicular temperatures are normally 1°F to 2.5°F below body temperature. Impaired semen quality and spermatogenesis have resulted from experimental hyperthermia. Similarly, the frequent use of hot tubs has been found to result in a 10% decrease in sperm motility (Procope, 1965). Therefore, the use of saunas and hot tubs should be discontinued in those patients with suboptimal semen analyses. There is no evidence that the type of underwear worn affects spermatogenesis (Wang et al, 1997).

The effect of cigarette smoking on spermatogenesis is unclear. A meta-analysis of 21 studies on the effect of cigarette smoking on semen quality revealed that smoking lowered sperm density by 13% to 17%, although 14 of the studies did not document an effect (Vine et al, 1994). However, smoking may serve as a cofactor for patients with other causes of male infertility (Peng et al, 1990). Androgen receptor abnormalities should be suspected in patients with a family history of intersex disorders. Many of the genes that affect male reproduction, including the androgen receptor gene, are located on the X chromosome. Therefore, family history should focus on the phenotype of the maternal uncles. In-utero exposure to diethylstilbestrol (DES) causes an increased incidence of epididymal cysts, a slightly increased frequency of cryptorchidism, but little or no effect on semen quality in those men who do not have a history of undescended testis (Wilcox et al, 1995a). Finally, the physician should be aware of the results of the female partner's fertility evaluation.

THE EVALUATION OF THE FEMALE PARTNER

Abnormalities in the woman are involved in approximately three-fourths of infertile couples. Ovulatory disorders are present in approximately 30% of cases, with fallopian tube abnormalities in 25%, endometriosis in 4% to 5%, and cervical mucus abnormalities and hyperprolactinemia each found in approximately 4% of cases (Thonneau et al, 1991; Collins, 1995). The approach to the evaluation of the female partner is similar to that of the male partner, consisting of a thorough history and physical examination followed by appropriate testing (Smith et al, 2003; Practice Committee of the American Society for Reproductive Medicine, 2004).

Evaluation of Ovulation and the Luteal Phase

There are several methods used to evaluate ovulatory function. Most often, combinations of different methods are used over several cycles to determine the adequacy and consistency of ovulation.

- **Menstrual history: Regular menstrual cycles of 21 to 35 days suggest the presence of ovulation, whereas irregular, short (<21 days), or excessively long (>35 days) menstrual cycles suggest ovulatory dysfunction.**
- **Basal body temperature charting:** A normal biphasic basal body temperature chart demonstrates an increased temperature of at least 0.4°F for 12 to 15 days after ovulation. A temperature drop before the rise correlates with the time of ovulation but is more difficult to detect before ovulation. Because of this, **basal body temperature charting can document ovulation but it is not used to predict ovulation.**
- **Midluteal phase serum progesterone:** Adequate progesterone levels require ovulation and corpus luteum function. **Levels of greater than 3.0 ng/mL suggest ovulation, whereas levels greater than 10 ng/mL also indicate a normal luteal phase.**
- **Urinary or plasma LH levels:** Plasma and urinary LH levels increase just before ovulation. **Over-the-counter urinary ovulation predictor kits are convenient and accurate methods of detecting the LH surge.** Measurement of plasma LH levels is often performed when using ovulation-induction medications.
- **Endometrial biopsy: This is usually performed several days before the time of expected menstruation and is used to diagnose a luteal phase defect and to confirm ovulation.** Luteal phase defects are characterized by a sustained increase in temperature lasting less than 11 days, out-of-phase endometrial biopsy, or low midluteal progesterone levels (less than 10 ng/mL). Currently there is controversy about the utility of the endometrial biopsy as well as the relationship between luteal phase defects and female infertility (Balasch et al, 1992).
- **Ovarian ultrasound: Transvaginal ultrasonography is a very effective method of predicting ovulation.** It is used before ovulation to evaluate follicular development and oocyte release. Ovarian ultrasonography is often used in combination with urinary LH testing to predict the time of ovulation.
- **Follicle-stimulating hormone: An FSH level performed on menstrual cycle day 3 of greater than 10 mIU/mL suggests poor ovarian reserve.** These patients may respond poorly to ovulation-induction regimens.

The choice of treatment for ovulatory disorders is dependent on the underlying etiology for the disorder. The most common treatment strategies employ ovulation-induction agents such as clomiphene citrate or gonadotropins.

Evaluation of the Fallopian Tubes

Tubal disease may be caused by pelvic inflammatory disease, endometriosis, prior abdominal inflammation, or surgery.

- **Hysterosalpingography (HSG) is performed by injecting contrast medium through the cervix to outline the uterine cavity and tubal lumens. It determines the patency of the fallopian tubes as well as the normality of the uterine cavity.** It is usually performed in the early follicular phase of the menstrual cycle to prevent radiation exposure to a fertilized ovum. Both oil-based and water-based contrast agents are used. Although there are limited data suggesting higher pregnancy rates with intercourse after oil-based hysterosalpingographic studies, this remains controversial (de Boer et al, 1988; Rasmussen et al, 1991). Proximal tubal obstruction is often mimicked by cornual spasm on these studies. Because laparoscopy is often performed to further evaluate tubal obstruction, two separate hysterosalpingograms should be performed before confirming this diagnosis.
- **Laparoscopy** combined with transcervical injection of a diluted dye may be performed to confirm tubal disease.
- **Tubal cannulation** with fluoroscopic or hysteroscopic guidance can help confirm tubal occlusion and may be used to treat proximal tubal obstruction.
- **Sonohystography** combines ultrasonographic imaging with the transcervical injection of contrast medium. Recent evidence indicates that it is superior to HSG for detecting tubal and uterine abnormalities (Kodaman et al, 2004).

Treatment of tubal pathology involves either surgical repair or IVF.

Evaluation of the Uterus

Anatomic or functional abnormalities of the uterus may cause female infertility but are not common. Methods to determine the status of the uterus include the following:

- Hysterosalpingography
- Ultrasonography
- Hysteroscopy

Evaluation of the Peritoneal Cavity

The female history or physical examination may suggest the presence of peritoneal factors such as endometriosis or tubal or ovarian adhesions that may impair fertility. Although ultrasonography may demonstrate some abnormalities, laparoscopy is the most sensitive and specific diagnostic modality for the detection of peritoneal factors.

For most women, in the absence of evidence of peritoneal disease (tubal disease, adhesions, or endometriosis), laparoscopy is not necessary (Opsahl et al, 1993).

Because the just-mentioned tests and procedures are usually performed during particular periods of the menstrual cycle, the evaluation of the woman takes longer than that of the man. It is important to take the age of the woman into consideration when recommending therapy. **Conception rates drop more rapidly in the 35- to 39-year-old age group. Thus, it is common to recommend more aggressive therapy in couples in which the woman is approaching 40 years old and to take a slower stepwise approach in younger couples.** With a basic understanding of the evaluation of the female partner, the urologist is better able to counsel the couple as to which treatments are most appropriate given both the female and male infertility factors.

KEY POINTS: HISTORY

■ Fifteen percent of couples suffer from infertility, with 50% involving a male factor.

■ Pregnancy rates in normal fertile couples are 20% to 25% per cycle compared with 1% to 3% in infertile couples.

■ A thorough medical and reproductive history should be obtained on all men presenting with infertility.

■ The female partner should be questioned about key aspects of her fertility evaluation.

PHYSICAL EXAMINATION

The physical examination should be directed toward identifying abnormalities that may be associated with infertility. The patient's habitus as well as the pattern of virilization should be noted. Abnormalities of the secondary sex characteristics may indicate whether there is a congenital endocrine disorder such as a eunuchoid appearance associated with Klinefelter's syndrome. Lack of temporal pattern balding and fine wrinkles on the face may be indicative of an acquired androgen deficiency. **Gynecomastia is suggestive of either an estrogen/androgen imbalance or an excess of prolactin.** Situs inversus raises the possibility of Kartagener's syndrome associated with immotile cilia and thus immotile sperm.

Genital Examination

Specific attention should be directed toward the genital examination. The penis should be examined for evidence of hypospadias and severe chordee. Both of these may interfere with proper deposition of semen in the deep vagina near the cervix. **The scrotal contents should be examined with the patient standing in a warm room to allow for relaxation of the cremaster muscle.** The testes should be carefully palpated to determine consistency and to rule out the presence of an intratesticular mass. **Because the majority of the testicular volume (~80%) consists of seminiferous tubules and germinal elements, a reduction in the number of these cells is typically manifested by a reduction in testicular volume or testicular atrophy.**

The dimensions of the testes should be measured. This may be performed using calipers, an orchidometer, or sonography (Takihara et al, 1983). The normal adult testis is greater than 4 × 3 cm in its greatest dimensions or greater than 20 mL in

Table 19–2. Comparisons of Testicular Dimensions (Length × Width) and Volume for Prepubertal, Pubertal, and Normal Adult Men

Clinical Status	Volume (mL)	Length (cm) × width (cm)
Prepubertal	1	1.6 × 1.0
2	2.0 × 1.2	
3	2.3 × 1.4	
4	2.5 × 1.5	
5	2.7 × 1.6	
6	2.9 × 1.8	
Pubertal	8	3.1 × 2.0
10	3.4 × 2.1	
12	3.7 × 2.3	
15	4.0 × 2.5	
Adult*	20	4.5 × 2.7
25	5.0 × 3.0	
30	5.5 × 3.2	

*Normal adult testicular size 24 ± 4 (SD) mL (n = 44).

volume for whites and African Americans (Table 19–2) (Carney and Tuttle, 1960). Asian men normally have smaller testes. Decreased testicular size, whether unilateral or bilateral, correlates with impaired spermatogenesis (Lipshultz and Corriere, 1977). Careful palpation of the epididymis should determine the presence of the head, body, and tail. The possibility of epididymal obstruction is suggested by the presence of induration or cystic dilation of the epididymis. Spermatoceles and epididymal cysts are common findings and do not indicate the presence of obstruction. Palpation of the vas deferens is performed to ensure its presence as well as to rule out areas of atrophy.

Examination of the spermatic cords should be performed to identify the presence of a varicocele. Small varicoceles (grade I) are palpable only during the Valsalva maneuver. Moderate-sized varicoceles (grade II) are palpable with the patient in the standing position, whereas large varicoceles (grade III) are visible through the scrotal skin and are palpable when the patient is in the standing position. Asymmetry of the spermatic cords, accentuated by the Valsalva maneuver, suggests the presence of a small varicocele. In patients with strong cremasteric reflexes, or in those with high-riding testes, slight traction on the testes during the Valsalva maneuver allows for a more accurate examination of the spermatic cords. Thickening and asymmetry of the spermatic cords that persists in the supine position suggests the possibility of a lipoma of the cord or caval obstruction due to a retroperitoneal or renal tumor. Varicoceles decrease in size when the patient is in the recumbent position. Similarly, bilateral thickening of the cords, resolving with the patient in the supine position, suggests the presence of bilateral varicoceles.

Many diagnostic methods have been employed to identify subclinical varicoceles, those that are not palpable by physical examination. Venography has been used for many years and is considered by some to be a gold standard. However, venography is invasive and is not without complications (Seyferth et al, 1981). The results of venography are affected by the position of the catheter tip, pressure of injection, and judgment of the examiner. The presence of a venous rushing sound that increases with Valsalva maneuver is used to identify the presence of a varicocele with the Doppler stethoscope (Greenberg et al, 1979). Both real-time scrotal ultrasonography and duplex scrotal ultrasonography have been used to visualize dilated spermatic veins in the scrotum. The presence of multiple veins with at least one larger than 3 mm in diameter is believed to be indicative of a subclinical varicocele (McClure and Hricak, 1986; Eskew et al, 1993), whereas a diameter of 3.5 mm by ultrasound is more predictive of a clinical varicocele (Meacham et al, 1994; Jarow et al, 1996b). Increased scrotal temperature detected by contact scrotal thermography is believed to correlate with the presence of a varicocele (WHO, 1985; Comhaire, 1991; Trum et al, 1996). However, all of these techniques are too sensitive; and in the absence of a universally agreed-upon "gold" standard diagnostic test it is difficult to determine their specificity. With the use of these diagnostic methods, up to 91% of patients with idiopathic infertility have been identified as having subclinical varicoceles, bilateral varicoceles have been demonstrated in up to 58% of patients, whereas only 10% of patients are identified as having bilateral varicoceles by clinical examination alone (Perrin et al, 1980; Narayan et al, 1981; Gonzalez et al, 1983). **There have been no controlled studies demonstrating improved pregnancy rates after the diagnosis and treatment of subclinical varicoceles. We therefore do not recommend evaluating patients for the presence of subclinical varicoceles.**

Finally, many experts recommend that a careful rectal examination should be done to evaluate the prostate as well as the areas above the prostate for evidence of cystic dilatation of the seminal vesicles. Significant prostatic tenderness raises the possibility of prostatic infection. However, many abnormalities of the prostate and seminal vesicles observed with transrectal ultrasonography are not detected by routine rectal examination (Jarow, 1993).

INITIAL BASIC LABORATORY EVALUATION

After the history and physical examination, the male partner of an infertile couple should have appropriate laboratory testing performed. **All patients should have at least two or three semen analyses** (American Urologic Association and the American Society of Reproductive Medicine, 2001).

Semen Analysis

The semen analysis remains the cornerstone of the laboratory evaluation of the infertile man. Despite this, it is important to realize that the measurement of semen parameters does not necessarily constitute a measure of fertility. **Except in cases of azoospermia, the semen analysis does not allow for the definitive separation of patients into sterile and fertile groups. As semen parameters decrease in quality, the statistical chance of conception decreases but does not reach zero.** Nevertheless, an accurately performed semen analysis remains an important tool for the evaluation of the infertile man.

Collection

To compare different semen samples from the same patient with accuracy, it is important to maintain consistency in the duration of sexual abstinence before collection of the spec-imen. Changes in the intervals between ejaculations will affect the results of the semen analysis. Increases in sperm concentration of 25% per day of abstinence for the first 4 days have been reported (Carlsen et al, 2004). Increases in seminal volume and therefore total sperm count also increased with increased days of abstinence, but motility and morphology were unaffected. Of note, ejaculation in the 7 days before the beginning of the abstinence period also resulted in lower sperm concentrations. Even with this precaution, the results of semen analyses are often inconsistent and therefore multiple analyses are indicated in equivocal or difficult situations. Clean, wide-mouthed containers should be used for specimen collection. These containers should be obtained from the physician because residual chemicals in other containers may injure sperm. The specimen may be collected in the physician's office or at home and brought to the office by placing the container in a shirt pocket next to the body to keep it warm during transit.

Most specimens are obtained by masturbation. In those cases in which the patient objects to collecting the specimen through masturbation, special condoms designed for semen collection may be used, allowing the couple to have intercourse. Ordinary latex condoms should not be used since they interfere with the viability of spermatozoa and often contain spermicides. While coitus interruptus may be used as an alternative method for obtaining specimens, this is not an ideal method since the initial portion of the ejaculate may be lost and bacteria and acidic vaginal secretions may contaminate the specimen. The specimen should be examined in the laboratory within 1 to 2 hours of collection. A label on the container should state the patient's name, the date, the time of collection, and the abstinence period. **In most cases, two or three specimens examined over a period of several weeks will give an adequate assessment of baseline spermatogenesis** (Carlsen et al, 2004). **In those occasional cases in which parameters differ markedly in the initial semen specimens, additional specimens, collected over a 2- to 3-month period, may be obtained.**

Methodology

Physical Characteristics. Freshly ejaculated semen is a coagulum that liquefies over a 5- to 25-minute period. The seminal vesicles secrete the substance responsible for coagulation. **Patients with congenital bilateral absence of the vas usually have absent or hypoplastic seminal vesicles. Semen in these patients does not coagulate, is acidic, and has a low volume.** Secretions from the testis, epididymis, bulbourethral glands (Cowper's glands), glands of Littre (periurethral glands), prostate, and seminal vesicles compose the normal seminal fluid. The fluid is released from the glands in a specific sequence during ejaculation. Before the ejaculation of the major portion of the ejaculate, a small amount of fluid from the glands of Littre and the bulbourethral glands is secreted. This is followed by a low viscosity opalescent fluid from the prostate containing a few sperm. The principal portion of the ejaculate contains the highest concentration of sperm, along with secretions from the testis, epididymis, and vas deferens, as well as some prostatic and seminal vesicle fluids. The last fraction of the ejaculate consists of seminal vesicle secretions. The secretions from Cowper's glands account for 0.1 to 0.2 mL, prostatic secretions account for 0.5 mL, and the secretions from the seminal vesicles account for 1.5 to 2.0 mL. The majority of ejaculated sperm come from the distal epididymis, with a small contribution from the ampulla of the vas. The unobstructed seminal vesicle is not normally a reservoir for sperm. Semen liquefaction is due to prostatic derived proteases, including prostate-specific antigen and plasminogen activator. Failure of liquefaction should be differentiated from semen that remains hyperviscous after liquefaction. Nonliquefied semen remains a coagulum and does not change consistency after ejaculation. Hyperviscous liquefied semen becomes less of a coagulum after ejaculation; however, its consistency remains thicker than normal. The effect that semen nonliquefaction has on male fertility remains unclear. Some patients with nonliquefying semen have normal postcoital test (PCT) results. In addition, sperm may be found in the cervical mucus before semen liquefaction (Santomauro et al, 1972). Although liquefaction of semen may be induced by the addition of seminin (a seminal protease) or α-amylase, there is no evidence that treatments with these agents increase fertility (Syner et al, 1975; Wilson and Bunge, 1975). Liquefied semen should be able to be poured drop by drop, whereas hyperviscous semen forms thick strands instead of drops. The cause of semen hyperviscosity remains unclear, but recent evidence suggests disulfide bonds between seminal proteins are involved (Mendeluk et al, 2000). Whereas in the past semen hyperviscosity has been thought to be due to genital tract infection, recent studies do not support this (Munuce et al, 1999). **In those cases in which the semen demonstrates nonliquefaction or hyperviscosity, a PCT may be performed. If the results are normal, demonstrating adequate numbers of motile sperm in the cervical mucus, the consistency of the semen may be disregarded. The consistency of the seminal fluid may be of significance if the PCT demonstrates few sperm with good quality mucus. Although a cross-mucus hostility test or an in-vitro cervical mucus-sperm interaction test may be employed in these cases, semen processing and IUI using the male partner's sperm (artificial insemination with husband's sperm [AIH]) will likely be indicated whether the results indicate a cervical mucus or semen viscosity problem.**

Small volume ejaculates may be produced in patients with obstruction of the ejaculatory ducts, androgen deficiency, retrograde ejaculation, sympathetic denervation, absence of the vas deferens and seminal vesicles, drug therapy, or bladder neck surgery.

The significance of high-volume ejaculates remains unclear. While sperm density may be decreased in high-volume samples, sperm motility remains unchanged (Dickerman et al, 1989). For those cases in which high-volume ejaculates are thought to cause significant low sperm densities, therapeutic insemination of the female partner has been recommended. However, not all investigators agree on this approach. A normal PCT result strongly suggests that a high-volume ejaculate is not a factor in infertility. If high seminal volume is believed to be the etiologic factor, semen processing with concentration of sperm and IUI may be employed.

Sperm Count. A sperm count refers to the concentration of sperm within the seminal plasma. Most methods of sperm count determination utilize counting chambers wherein sperm are counted within a grid pattern. There are multiple chambers currently in use. Comparison of methods has revealed significant differences between chambers (Imade et al, 1993; Mahmoud et al, 1997). Because of this and a lack of quality control in many laboratories, results of semen analyses from different laboratories may be quite disparate (Keel, 2004). Detailed description of semen analysis techniques are available from several sources (WHO, 1999). Specimens in which no sperm are identified should be centrifuged and the pellet examined for the presence of sperm.

Motility. Motility is the percent of sperm that demonstrate flagellar motion. The evaluation is ideally performed within 1 to 2 hours of ejaculation and the specimen kept at room or body temperature to avoid a decrease in sperm motility. An assessment of the quality of forward movement of the sperm should be noted. One commonly used method rates the sperm movement on a five-point scale. A rating of zero signifies no motility; 1 denotes sluggish or nonprogressive movement; 2 refers to sperm moving with a slow, meandering forward progression; 3 signifies sperm moving in a reasonably straight line with moderate speed; and 4 indicates sperm moving in a straight line with high speed (Amelar et al, 1973). The most common category of sperm movement is reported. An alternate system places the sperm into four categories. "A" signifies rapid progressive motility; "B," slow or sluggish progressive motility; "C," nonprogressive motility; and "D," no motility. In this system, the percent of sperm falling into each category is reported (WHO, 1999). It is unnecessary and of no proven prognostic value to determine motility parameters at repeated time points after seminal collection. This is a nonphysiologic measurement because sperm leave the semen and enter the cervical mucus within minutes of deposition within the vaginal vault (MacLeod, 1965). Occasional clumps of agglutinated sperm are of no consequence. **However, frequent sperm agglutination is abnormal and suggests the presence of antisperm antibodies.** Notation should be made of the presence of other cell types. **In the unstained, wet mount semen specimen, white blood cells (WBCs) and immature germ cells are similar in appearance and are known as round cells.** An estimate of the number of these cells per high-power field (HPF) should be made. Special stains are used to differentiate WBCs from immature germ cells. (See "Leukocyte Staining.") **Cases in which the semen sample demonstrates all non-motile sperm or less than 5% to 10% motility may be due to ultrastructural defects, in which case the sperm are alive but have defects in the flagella. Although immotile, these sperm may appear morphologically normal. Alternatively, non-motile sperm may be dead, in which instance the patient is said to demonstrate necrospermia.**

Morphology

The morphologic examination of spermatozoa is a sensitive indicator of the quality of spermatogenesis and of fertility (Talbot and Chacon, 1981; Kruger et al, 1988). Whereas some gross morphologic abnormalities can be identified with brightfield or phase-contrast microscopy of unstained semen, these are very insensitive determinations. Proper morphologic examination involves the use of stained semen specimens. **There is no consensus among laboratories as to the classification system of sperm morphology with multiple systems currently in use.** Observation of spermatozoa recovered from postcoital cervical mucus or from the surface of zona pellucida have been used to define the appearance of normal spermatozoa (Fredricsson and Bjork, 1977; Mortimer et al, 1982; Menkveld et al, 1990; Liu and Baker, 1992). Older systems have classified the sperm into one of several categories, such as normal (oval head), amorphous (irregular head), tapered head, large- and small-headed, and immature (Fig. 19–1) (MacLeod, 1965). These systems would classify borderline forms as normal and define normal specimens as containing 60% or more normal forms with less than 3% immature forms. **Most laboratories currently use more rigid criteria for the definition of a normal sperm** (Fig. 19–2). **Borderline forms are considered abnormal** (Katz et al, 1986; Kruger et al, 1986). **Using these criteria, Kruger and associates (1988) found that in a group of men with sperm densities greater than 20 million/mL and motility greater than 30%, fertilization rates during IVF were 37% for those with less than 14% normal sperm by strict criteria and 81% to 91% for those with greater than 14% normal sperm. A second study demonstrated that those men with less than 4% normal forms had a fertilization rate of 7.6% whereas those with 4 to 14% normal forms had a fertilization rate of 63%.** In most subsequent studies similar results have been reported (Coetzee et al, 1998). **There have been limited studies examining the relationship between strict morphology and conception by IUI or intercourse. Most studies demonstrate**

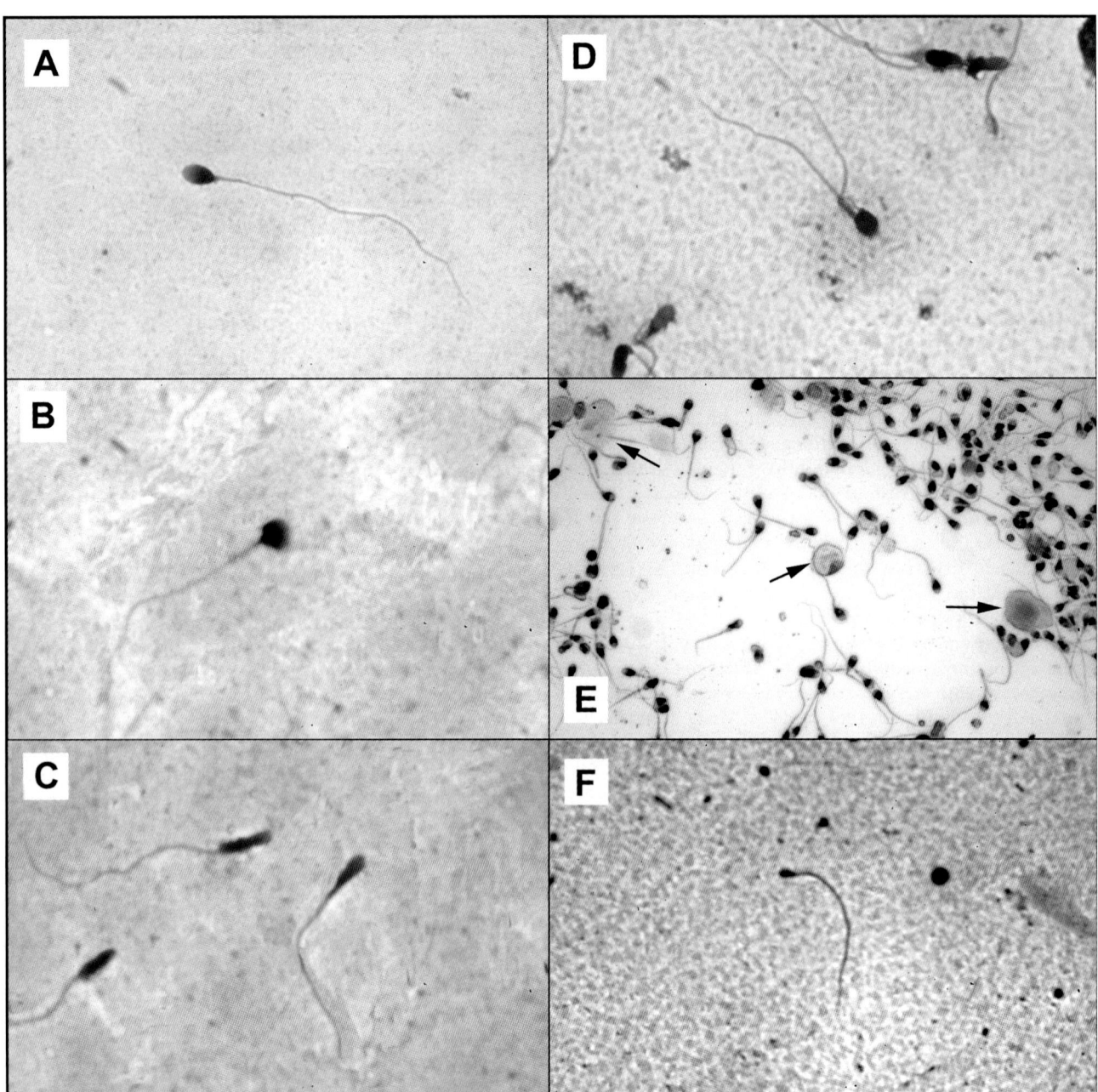

Figure 19–1. Patterns of sperm morphology. **A**, Normal. **B**, Large-headed sperm. **C**, Tapered sperm. **D**, Double-tailed sperm. **E**, Immature germ cells *(arrows)*. **F**, Pinhead sperm.

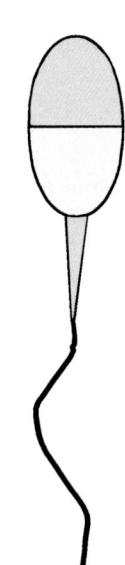

Head
Length: 5–6 μm
Width: 2.5–3.5 μm

Acrosome: 40%–70% of head

Midpiece
Width ≤ 1 μm
Length 1.5 x head length

Tail
Approximately 45 μm long
Uniform
Thinner than midpiece
Uncoiled
Free from kinks

Cytoplasmic droplets
Less than one half of head area
In midpiece only

Figure 19–2. Criteria for normal sperm morphology by rigid criteria.

lower pregnancy rates after IUI when sperm morphology is less than 4% (Van Waart et al, 2001). **Studies of pregnancies by intercourse in fertile and infertile couples also indicate lower pregnancy rates in those with the lowest morphology scores, but the morphology ranges are less clear** (Kruger et al, 2004). **Experience with morphology has indicated pregnancies are still possible with low morphology scores, and therefore morphology scores should not be utilized in isolation from other parameters.** Some investigators have found the determination of the percent of sperm with normal acrosomes (the acrosome index) useful in the population of patients with less than 5% normal forms by strict criteria. Those patients with less than 5% normal forms and an acrosome index of greater that 5% to 15% will fertilize over 50% of ova during IVF, whereas those with an acrosome index of less than 5% to 15% perform poorly (Menkveld, 2004).

Computer-Assisted Sperm Analysis

Computer-assisted sperm analysis (CASA) refers to a semi-automated technique used to individualize and digitalize static and dynamic sperm images. Most systems employ video with multiple frames that when played back creates moving images. The computerized systems are able to determine parameters not measurable manually. Curvilinear velocity is the average distance per unit time between successive positions of an individual sperm. Straight-line velocity is the speed of a sperm in a forward direction. This is a measure of forward progression and can be correlated with manual methods of forward progression measurement (Yeung et al, 1997). Linearity is determined by dividing straight-line velocity by curvilinear velocity. Additional measurements include lateral head displacement, flagellar beat frequency, and circular movement analysis. Hyperactivation is a state of motility that sperm attain after capacitation in which large-amplitude movements

of the head and tail of the sperm are coupled with a slow or nonprogressive motility (Yanagimachi, 1970). Although over 20 different parameters may by measured by CASA devices, the clinical utility of most of these is limited (Amann and Katz, 2004). The advantages of CASA include the ability to get quantitative objective data and the potential for standardization of semen analysis procedures. However, the equipment is expensive, the technique remains without standardization, and the results can be affected by many factors (Keel et al, 2000). **When used clinically, CASA has not been documented to give a more accurate prognosis or to affect treatment as compared with a manual semen analysis** (Davis and Katz, 1993; Krause, 1995; Amann and Katz, 2004).

Additional Semen Parameters

The pH of normal semen is 7.2 or more (WHO, 1999). **Semen pH is due to a balance between acidic prostatic secretions and alkaline seminal vesicle secretions. Low ejaculate volume with normal pH may be normal for some patients but may also indicate incomplete collection or retrograde ejaculation, whereas low ejaculate volume with an acidic pH suggests ejaculatory duct pathology or absent seminal vesicles.** The seminal vesicles produce fructose in an androgen-dependent process. Normal semen fructose concentrations range from 120 to 450 mg/dL. Inflammation of the seminal vesicles, androgen deficiency, partial obstruction of the ejaculatory ducts, or incomplete ejaculation may result in fructose concentrations below 120 mg/dL. In cases of absent seminal vesicles, fructose is usually absent from the semen. **Patients with obstructed seminal vesicles or congenital absence of the seminal vesicles, which is usually associated with bilateral absence of the vas deferens, demonstrate azoospermic, acidic, fructose-negative semen that does not coagulate. In addition, their ejaculate volume is low (<1.0 mL).** Transrectal ultrasonography is currently more commonly used to diagnose absence or obstruction of the seminal vesicles and ejaculatory ducts than fructose determinations. Measurements of many other seminal plasma components such as citrate, carnitine, α-glucosidase, fructose, granulocyte elastase, zinc, prostate-specific antigen (PSA), glucose, pepsinogen C, insulin-like growth factor, binding protein-3, and prostaglandin D synthase (PGDS) have been performed. Although levels of certain compounds may correlate with spermatogenic activity, these determinations are currently not clinically useful (Diamandis et al, 1999; Chia et al, 2000b; Zopfgen et al, 2000).

Interpretation of the Semen Analysis

To properly interpret a semen analysis, the clinician must understand the difference between average semen parameters of a population of normal men and minimal levels of adequacy for normal fertility. **Studies of populations of fertile or presumably fertile men report median sperm densities of 70 to 100 million sperm per milliliter** (Irvine et al, 1996; Saidi et al, 1999; Jensen et al, 2000). Considerable controversy has resulted from the publication of a meta-analysis of past studies on sperm counts, which reported a decrease in sperm counts over the past 50 years (Carlsen et al, 1992). Regional variation in semen parameters has been demonstrated (Jorgensen et al, 2001; Swan et al, 2003a). Thus, further evaluation of the meta-analysis data has suggested that the reported decline in sperm counts may be due to geographic differences in the populations studied (Fisch and Goluboff, 1996). Recent analyses of U.S. studies have found no evidence of a decrease in sperm densities over time. Additional studies of European populations have found evidence supporting (Auger et al, 1995; Irvine et al, 1996; Bonde et al, 1998) and refuting (Gyllenborg et al, 1999) a drop in sperm counts over time. Because of the multitude of possible confounding variables in 50-year-old studies, further prospective studies will be required to determine if sperm counts are truly declining worldwide.

The normal range of most diagnostic tests in medicine is determined by using the mean plus or minus 2 standard deviations. Whereas this may be used to determine "normal" from "abnormal" this does not separate fertile from infertile men. When semen parameters from populations of fertile and infertile men are compared, there is a large amount of overlap between the two groups (Guzick et al, 2001). **This occurs because fertility is dependent on more than just one semen parameter and on factors affecting both partners.** Whereas a count of 70 million is considered normal, a patient with 70 million sperm per milliliter but absent motility will be infertile. **Studies of couples attempting to conceive have found decreasing probabilities of conception with decreasing sperm counts.** Smith and colleagues reported a 44% pregnancy rate in couples in whom the male partner had counts between 12.5 and 25 million sperm per milliliter as compared with a 25% pregnancy rate in those in which the male partner had counts less than 12.5 million sperm per milliliter (Smith et al, 1977). Others have found sperm motility and/or morphology to be equally if not more important than sperm count (Mayaux et al, 1985; Bostofte et al, 1990). In addition, conception is dependent on the fertility status of both partners. **Although azoospermic patients are sterile, the majority of infertile men have some motile sperm in their semen and therefore should be considered subfertile rather than sterile.**

The reference ranges used to interpret the semen analysis are more accurately defined as minimal levels of adequacy. The finding of parameters below these levels is suggestive of infertility, whereas the finding of parameters above these levels is suggestive of fertility. There are clearly fertile patients with semen parameters below these levels and infertile patients with parameters above these levels. **The World Health Organization defines the following reference values** (WHO, 1999):

Volume: 2.0 mL or more
pH: 7.2 or more
Sperm concentration: 20×10^6 or more spermatozoa/mL
Total sperm number: 40×10^6 or more spermatozoa per ejaculate
Motility: 50% or more with grade "a + b" motility or 25% or more with grade "a" motility
Morphology: 15% or more by strict criteria
Viability: 75% or more of sperm viable
WBCs: Less than 1 million/mL

It should be realized that levels that may constitute requirements for natural conception do not apply to ART, wherein fertilization may occur with suboptimal semen specimens. Similarly, with the advent of the ability to inject individual sperm into individual ova, it has become clear that the bulk semen parameters do not predict the fertility of individual spermatozoa.

Hormonal Evaluation

The purpose of the hormonal evaluation of an infertile male patient is to identify endocrinologic disorders that adversely affect male reproduction and to gain prognostic information. **Although male reproductive function is critically dependent on endocrinologic control, less than 3% of infertile men have a primary hormonal etiology** (Sigman and Jarow, 1997a). The most common hormonal abnormality detected on routine testing of infertile men is an elevated serum FSH. In the presence of normal spermatogenesis, FSH secretion is regulated by negative feedback inhibition by the hormone inhibin, which is produced by the Sertoli cells. FSH is often but not always elevated in patients with abnormal spermatogenesis (Turek et al, 1995). **Therefore, an elevated serum FSH is indicative of a significant problem with spermatogenesis whereas a normal serum FSH does not guarantee intact spermatogenesis.** Patients with complete testicular failure have inadequate Leydig and Sertoli cell function that results in elevated gonadotropin levels associated with normal or low testosterone levels (Table 19–3). Patients with either hypothalamic or pituitary dysfunction have both low serum gonadotropin and testosterone levels as well as absent spermatogenesis (hypogonadotropic hypogonadism).

Gonadotropin-releasing hormone (GnRH) is secreted in a pulsatile fashion, and, as a result, gonadotropin hormones are secreted episodically, particularly luteinizing hormone (LH). Some clinicians believe that a proper hormonal assessment requires routinely measuring pooled samples consisting of individual samples taken at 15-minute intervals. **Despite the inaccuracies of single determinations, it is rare for a patient's clinical endocrine status to be inaccurately determined by a single measurement. We recommend a pooled blood sample only when the results of one hormonal determination do not fit the clinical situation** (Bain et al, 1988).

Throughout early childhood, gonadotropin and testosterone levels remain low. LH and FSH levels begin increasing from 6 to 8 years of age (Conte et al, 1975). Testosterone levels begin increasing at 10 to 12 years of age (Rifkind et al, 1967). During the reproductive years, gonadotropin and testosterone levels remain relatively constant. Later in life, testosterone levels, particularly free testosterone levels, decrease and gonadotropin concentrations rise (Tenover et al, 1987).

There is no agreement as to what should constitute the initial endocrine evaluation of infertile men. **We recommend that all men with an indication in the history or physical**

Table 19–3. Hormonal Status as a Function of Clinical Diagnosis

Clinical Status	FSH (mIU/mL)	LH (mIU/mL)	Testosterone (ng/dL)
Normal men or obstruction	Normal	Normal	Normal
Isolated spermatogenic failure	↑	Normal	Normal
Testicular failure	↑	↑	Normal or ↓
Hypogonadotropic hypogonadism	↓	↓	↓

examination or a sperm density less than 10 million/mL have serum FSH and morning testosterone levels measured because endocrine abnormalities are rarely present when the sperm concentration is greater than 10 million/mL (Sigman and Jarow, 1997a). If these preliminary screening tests are abnormal, further testing with repeat testosterone, prolactin, and LH is indicated. However, some experts believe that all infertile men should undergo endocrine testing and others recommend a more comprehensive panel of tests, including serum LH, prolactin, and thyroid function tests on preliminary screening.

If an isolated serum testosterone level is low or borderline and the LH is not elevated, we recommend a morning testosterone and bioavailable testosterone, since morning levels of testosterone are higher and bioavailable testosterone levels are useful in equivocal cases. A serum prolactin test and pituitary magnetic resonance imaging should be obtained if the repeat testosterone level is low (see later). Impaired visual fields or severe headaches suggest the presence of a central nervous system tumor. Prolactin determination should be performed in these patients. However, not all pituitary tumors are functional and serum prolactin concentration may be normal. Most prolactin-secreting tumors in men are macroadenomas (tumors greater than 1 cm) because men tend to present late in the course of the illness (Carter et al, 1978). Prolactin levels in these patients are typically higher than 50 ng/mL, and both gonadotropin and serum testosterone levels are depressed. Mild elevations of prolactin (<50 ng/mL) are more frequently discovered in infertile patients, and their clinical significance is questionable. Imaging often fails to identify a tumor in these patients, and they often have normal gonadotropin and testosterone levels. Potential causes for mild prolactin elevation include stress, renal failure, medications, chest wall irritation, and thyroid dysfunction. We do not recommend treatment of isolated mild hyperprolactinemia because, in our experience, this has not resulted in improved spermatogenesis. However, these patients should undergo an evaluation to rule out a pituitary tumor.

The GnRH stimulation tests may be abnormal in men with suboptimal semen quality, demonstrating an exaggerated pituitary response. However an abnormal GnRH test does not alter treatment. Therefore, we do not advocate routine GnRH stimulation testing. Likewise, the human chorionic gonadotropin (hCG) stimulation test used to assess Leydig cell function rarely provides diagnostic information beyond routine hormonal tests and is not recommended for routine clinical practice.

Male infertility secondary to congenital adrenal hyperplasia (CAH) is very rare. These patients may have a history of precocious puberty, a family history of CAH, short stature due to premature closure of the epiphyseal plates, and testicular enlargement that may be indicative of adrenal rest tumors of the testis. Plasma 17-hydroxyprogesterone levels are elevated in these patients. The infertility of male patients with CAH is due to feedback inhibition of gonadotropin secretion by excessive adrenal androgens that results in suppression of testicular function. Interestingly, many male patients with CAH are fertile (Urban et al, 1978). Partial, late-onset CAH has been found in some cases of male infertility but is uncommon (Augarten et al, 1991). We do not advocate routine screening for CAH.

Estrogen excess may be endogenous or exogenous. Measurement of estradiol in men is complicated by the fact that the assay is not very reliable at the low concentrations found in normal men. Testosterone-estradiol ratios have been proposed as a method to detect estrogen excess, but normal values for this have not been well established (Pavlovich et al, 2001). Patients with estrogen excess often have bilateral gynecomastia, erectile dysfunction, and atrophic testes. One of the most common causes of estrogen excess is morbid obesity because fat cells contain the enzyme aromatase that converts testosterone to estradiol (Schneider et al, 1979). Estradiol normally stimulates hepatic production of sex steroid hormone binding globulin (SHBG), which would lower the amount of bioavailable testosterone. Yet many patients with morbid obesity also have hepatic dysfunction and their SHBG levels may be depressed (Glass et al, 1977). Normal levels of plasma FSH, LH, and testosterone are usually found in patients with mildly elevated serum estradiol levels. Thyroid function studies do not need to be determined because these are generally normal unless there is clinical evidence of thyroid disease.

DIAGNOSTIC ALGORITHMS BASED ON THE INITIAL EVALUATION

Based on the initial history, physical exam, and laboratory studies, a differential diagnosis may be developed (Table 19-4). Furthermore, more specific testing allows the physician to place the patient into an etiologic category. The frequency of semen abnormalities and etiologic categories in a group of our patients are listed in Tables 19-5 and 19-6.

Absent or Low-Volume Ejaculate

Absent ejaculation may be due to either retrograde ejaculation or failure of emission (no expulsion of semen through the vas deferens into the posterior urethra) (Fig. 19-3). The complete absence of seminal fluid is called aspermia, and this disorder should be differentiated from azoospermia, which is absence of sperm within the seminal fluid. **The most common cause of ejaculatory failure is spinal cord injury.** Other neurologic disorders such as diabetes mellitus and multiple sclerosis are frequent causes. Medications no longer used for the treatment of hypertension (ganglionic blockers) caused retrograde ejaculation in the past but are no longer clinically relevant. Retroperitoneal surgery may injure the sympathetic ganglia that control ejaculation, but current methods of nerve-sparing retroperitoneal lymph node dissection avoid this complication in the majority of patients (Foster et al, 1994; Klein, 2000). Another cause of aspermia is psychologic disturbances associated with an inability to obtain orgasm. The most common cause of low ejaculate volume is incomplete collection of the specimen. Thus, repetitive testing is warranted to rule out a collection problem. The other main cause is partial retrograde ejaculation, which may be due to neurologic disorders, medications, or bladder neck surgery or may be idiopathic.

Because the majority of seminal fluid is contributed by the seminal vesicles, in the absence of retrograde ejaculation, a low-volume ejaculate suggests the lack of seminal vesicle contribution. Partial or complete ejaculatory duct obstruction may also cause low-volume ejaculate (Jarow, 1996c). Likewise,

Table 19–4. Classification of Male Infertility Status by Criteria of Semen Analysis

I. Low Ejaculate Volume
   A. Drugs
   B. Retroperitoneal or bladder neck surgery
   C. Ejaculatory duct obstruction
   D. Diabetes mellitus
   E. Spinal cord injury
   F. Psychologic disturbances
   G. Idiopathic
   H. Incomplete collection
II. Azoospermia
   A. Hypogonadotropic hypogonadism
      1. Kallmann syndrome
      2. Pituitary tumor
   B. Spermatogenic abnormalities
      1. Chromosomal abnormalities
      2. Y-chromosome microdeletions
      3. Gonadotoxins
      4. Varicocele
      5. Viral orchitis
      6. Torsion
      7. Idiopathic
   C. Ductal obstruction
III. Oligoasthenoteratospermia (OAT)
   A. Varicocele
   B. Cryptorchidism
   C. Idiopathic
   D. Drugs, heat, toxins
   E. Systemic infection
   F. Endocrinopathy
IV. Normal But Infertile
   A. Gynecologic abnormality
   B. Abnormal coital habits
   C. Acrosomal defects
   D. Antisperm antibodies
   E. Unexplained
V. Asthenospermia
   A. Spermatozoal structural defects
   B. Prolonged abstinence
   C. Idiopathic
   D. Genital tract infection
   E. Antisperm antibodies
   F. Varicocele
   G. Partial obstruction

Table 19–5. Distribution of Patients Presenting with Infertility by Findings on Semen Analysis

Semen Pattern	No. Patients	%
Normal	297	14
Azoospermia	299	14
Multiple parameters abnormal	1040	49
Single abnormal parameter		
Asthenospermia	127	6
Teratospermia	85	4
Oligospermia	83	4
Low volume	149	7
Pyospermia	42	2

Table 19–6. Distribution of Patients by Diagnostic Category after Full Evaluation

Category	No. Patients	%
Varicocele	806	38
Idiopathic	482	23
Obstruction	271	13
Normal	197	9
Cryptorchidism	73	3
Testicular failure	54	3
Antisperm antibodies	42	2
Ejaculatory dysfunction	49	2
Gonadotoxin*	43	2
Endocrinopathy	25	1
Pyospermia	22	1
Genetic/chromosomal[†]	11	0.5
Torsion	11	0.5
Erectile dysfunction	8	0.4
Testis cancer	9	0.4
Ultrastructural	7	0.3
Viral orchitis	7	0.3
Systemic illness	4	0.2
Hypospadias	1	0.05

*Includes exposure to chemotherapeutic agents and radiation, heat, drugs, etc.
[†]Includes chromosomal abnormalities such as Klinefelter's syndrome and genetic abnormalities such as CFTR mutations.

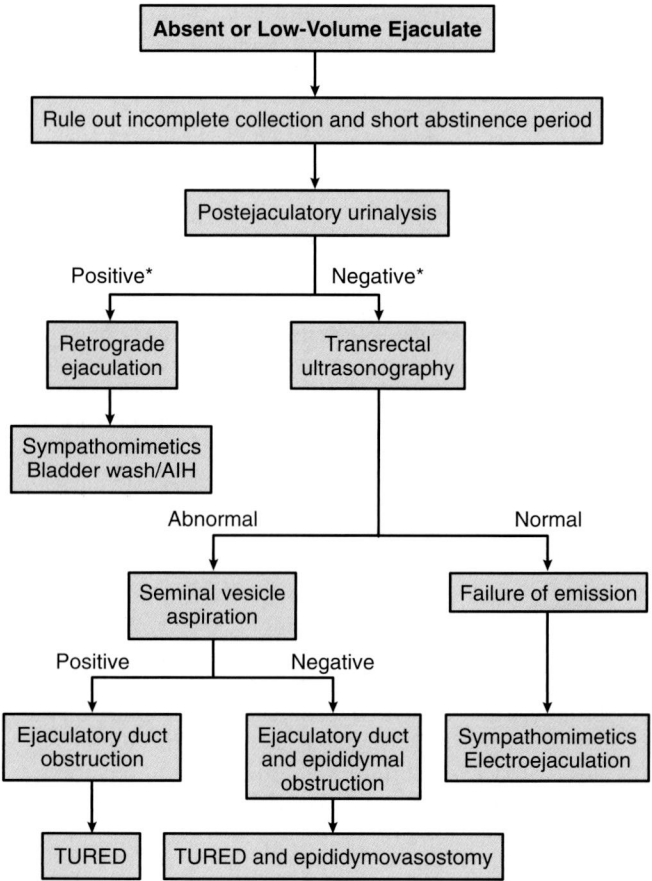

Figure 19–3. Algorithm for the evaluation of the patient with low-volume or absent (aspermia) ejaculate. AIH, artificial insemination using husband's sperm; TURED, transurethral resection of the ejaculatory ducts.*See text.

vasal agenesis, which is often associated with seminal vesicle agenesis, will present as low ejaculate volume azoospermia (Goldstein and Schlossberg, 1988). Finally, the seminal vesicles and prostate are under androgen control for the production of their secretions. Androgen deficiency will therefore result in reduction of seminal volume. However, all of these causes also produce azoospermia and are discussed in further detail in the next section. Some men produce low-volume ejaculates when masturbating into a container but produce normal volumes when ejaculation is accomplished by intercourse. Collection of a specimen with intercourse using a seminal collection condom will identify these cases. Finally, incomplete specimen collection should be ruled out as well as a decreased abstinence period. All cases of absent ejaculation and low-volume ejaculation (<1.5 mL) should be evaluated with a repeat semen analysis and post-ejaculate urine specimen. The post-ejaculate urine specimen is evaluated by centrifuging the urine for 10 minutes at 300 g or more. The pellet should then be inspected and interpreted in relationship to the patient's clinical findings. In patients with absent ejaculation, the finding of greater than 10 to 15 sperm/HPF indicates retrograde ejaculation. In patients with low-volume ejaculates, the finding of more sperm in the urine than in the antegrade specimen suggests a significant component of retrograde ejaculation. Finally, in patients with azoospermia, the finding of any sperm in the post-ejaculate urine rules out complete bilateral ductal obstruction. In the absence of sperm in the post-ejaculate urine, ejaculatory duct obstruction should be suspected. Although fructose and pH determinations were traditionally used to evaluate the presence or absence of seminal vesicle contributions to the ejaculate, transrectal ultrasonography (TRUS) is most commonly employed now (Belker and Steinbock, 1990). Patients with normal TRUS and low ejaculate volume azoospermia are evaluated like any other patient with azoospermia (see later). Testicular biopsy should be performed if the serum FSH is in the normal range. Ductal obstruction is present if spermatogenesis is intact on testicular biopsy. To identify the location of the obstruction, a scrotal exploration with vasogram and sampling of vasal fluid is performed at the time of anticipated reconstructive surgery. In low-volume oligospermic patients there is generally very little reason to perform a testis biopsy because spermatogenesis must be present. In some of these cases, evidence of ejaculatory duct obstruction may be suggested by TRUS but partial ejaculatory duct obstruction is an investigative diagnosis at this time. Cases of true partial ejaculatory duct obstruction are extremely rare (Beiswanger et al, 1998).

Azoospermia

Azoospermia may be due to inadequate hormonal stimulation (hypogonadotropic hypogonadism), spermatogenic abnormalities, or obstruction. **The evaluation of the azoospermic patient should be geared toward determining whether azoospermia is due to abnormal spermatogenesis or ductal obstruction** (Fig. 19–4). The initial step should be to centrifuge the semen specimen. The presence of any sperm in the pellet rules out bilateral ductal obstruction, and the patient should be evaluated for oligospermia (Corea et al, 2005). Although numerous findings on history and physical examination may be predictive of the cause of azoospermia, the main features utilized to determine the etiology of normal

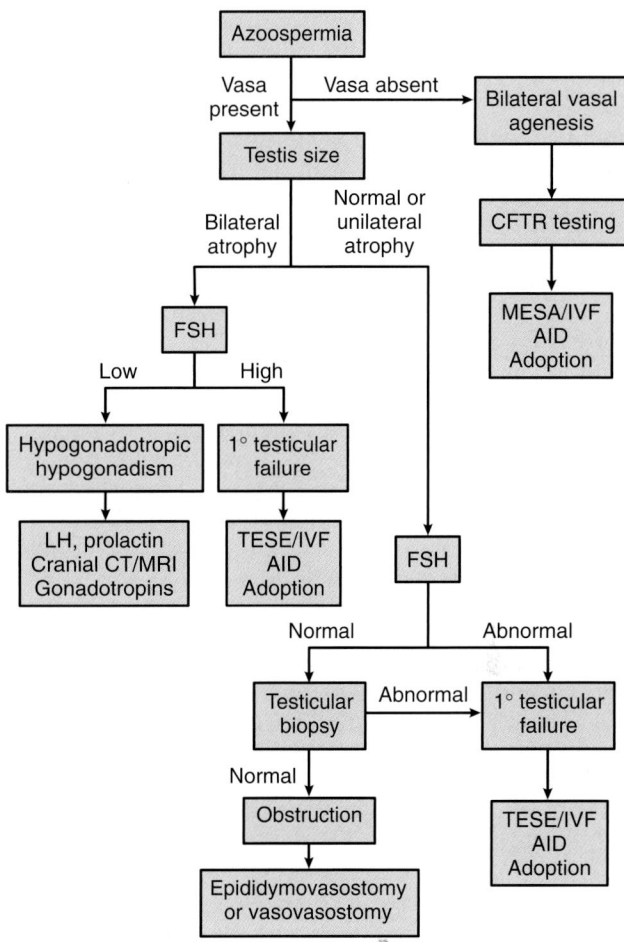

Figure 19–4. Algorithm for the evaluation of the patient with azoospermia. AID, artificial insemination using donor sperm; CFTR, cystic fibrosis transmembrane conductance regulator gene; FSH, follicle-stimulating hormone; IVF, in-vitro fertilization; LH, luteinizing hormone; MESA, microsurgical epididymal sperm aspiration; TESE, testicular sperm extraction.

ejaculate volume azoospermia include presence of the vasa deferentia, testicular size, and serum FSH (Jarow et al, 1989).

The first step is to determine whether the vasa are present because congenital bilateral absence of the vasa deferentia (CBAVD) is a common cause of obstructive azoospermia. CBAVD is a clinical diagnosis based on physical examination and is due to an abnormality in the cystic fibrosis transmembrane conductance regulator (CFTR) gene (Anguiano et al, 1992; Oates and Amos, 1994). Further radiologic imaging is not routinely necessary, although a small percentage of these patients have upper tract abnormalities and an abdominal ultrasound may be obtained (Schlegel et al, 1996; de la Taille et al, 1998). The vast majority of these patients have normal spermatogenesis such that screening with a serum FSH test alone in the presence of normal testicular volume is sufficient prior to management. A testicular biopsy may be performed if the history, physical examination, or laboratory studies suggest an abnormality of spermatogenesis.

Patients with small (atrophic) testes have either primary or secondary testicular failure. Serum hormone testing including testosterone, LH, FSH, and prolactin is done to differentiate between the two as well as to identify both functioning and nonfunctioning pituitary tumors. **Patients with small testes** and FSH concentrations greater than two to three times normal have severe germ cell failure, and the prognosis for natural conception is poor. A testicular biopsy should only be performed in these patients if testicular sperm retrieval combined with IVF is being considered, and this is often performed in conjunction with egg retrieval in the spouse. Patients with azoospermia due to testicular failure should be offered genetic testing to rule out chromosomal abnormalities such as Klinefelter's syndrome and microdeletions of the Y chromosome. Patients with secondary testicular failure may be treated with hormone therapy, whereas primary testicular failure is almost always irreversible.

Finally, patients with vasa present, normal testicular volume, and normal serum FSH require testicular biopsy to differentiate between spermatogenic abnormalities and ductal obstruction (Jarow et al, 1989). Scrotal exploration with vasography should be performed at the time of reconstructive surgery and not at the time of testicular biopsy. Patients with a normal-sized testis on one side and an atrophic or absent testis on the contralateral side should undergo testicular biopsy even if the FSH is mildly elevated because they may have normal spermatogenesis in the larger testis. Patients with unilateral ductal obstruction typically have a normal sperm count and fertility potential. However, this may not be the case if significant antisperm antibodies have developed owing to exposure to sperm antigens. There are rare patients with unilateral obstruction and an abnormal unobstructed contralateral testis who have oligospermia on semen analysis (Matsuda et al, 1992b).

Oligospermia

Oligospermia refers to sperm densities of less than 20 million sperm/mL. Isolated oligospermia with normal motility and morphology parameters is uncommon. In cases with less than 10 million sperm/mL, testosterone and FSH levels should be determined. If these levels are abnormal, a complete endocrine evaluation should be obtained as outlined earlier in the section "Hormonal Evaluation." However, further endocrinologic evaluation is not necessary in oligospermic patients with an isolated elevation of serum FSH because this indicates abnormal spermatogenesis and is not a true endocrine abnormality. Endocrine abnormalities should be treated appropriately as described in this chapter. Oligospermia as an isolated abnormality is uncommon and most often due to either androgen deficiency or, more often, is idiopathic. Whereas varicoceles are the most common identifiable etiology for oligospermia there are usually abnormalities in other semen parameters as well. Evaluation and treatment of these disorders is discussed later in the section on "Multiple Defects in Seminal Parameters." Treatment options for patients with idiopathic oligospermia include empirical medical therapy and assisted reproductive technology.

Asthenospermia

Defects in sperm movement (asthenospermia) refer to low levels of motility or forward progression, or both. Spermatozoal structural defects, prolonged abstinence periods, genital tract infection, antisperm antibodies, partial ductal obstruction, varicoceles, and idiopathic causes may be

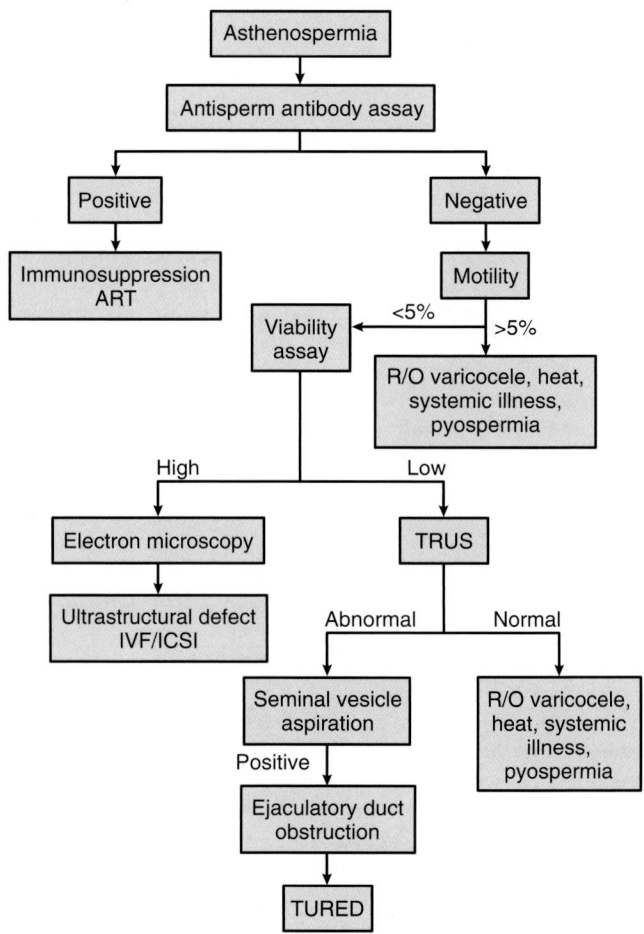

Figure 19–5. Algorithm for the evaluation of the patient with asthenospermia. ART, assisted reproductive technology; ICSI, intracytoplasmic sperm injection; IVF, in-vitro fertilization; R/O, rule out; TRUS, transrectal ultrasonography; TURED, transurethral resection of the ejaculatory ducts.

responsible for these cases (Fig. 19–5). The finding of asthenospermia or significant sperm agglutination raises the possibility of immunologic infertility. An antisperm antibody assay, preferably a direct assay, should be performed. Patients with antisperm antibodies are most commonly directed toward ART. While success with immunosuppressive regimens has been reported, their overall efficacy is low and there is a risk of serious side effects such as aseptic hip necrosis. Hormonal studies are not indicated for isolated asthenospermia. Infection should be suspected if increased numbers of round cells have been reported in the semen analysis. In these instances, a study to differentiate immature germ cells from WBCs, such as the Endtz test or immunohistochemical staining, may be considered. Semen cultures for *Mycoplasma genitalium* or urine DNA testing for *Chlamydia trachomatis* may be performed to further evaluate true pyospermia. In addition, urinalysis should be performed to rule out the presence of a urinary tract infection. Semen cultures may be performed but are often contaminated by distal urethral organisms (Kim and Goldstein, 1999).

A varicocele is the most common surgically correctable abnormality found in infertile men and may be responsible for sperm motility defects as well as defects in sperm count and shape. Partial ejaculatory duct obstruction may be suspected in asthenospermic patients, particularly in the presence of low ejaculate volume and low viability. TRUS may be performed in these instances; and when the test is abnormal, further evaluation for ejaculatory duct obstruction should be performed. **Complete absence of sperm motility or cases with motilities less than 5% to 10% should be evaluated by a sperm viability assay. Necrospermia exists when the nonmotile sperm are not viable. The finding of a high fraction of viable sperm in the presence of low or absent sperm motility suggests an ultrastructural abnormality, such as that found in primary ciliary dyskinesia (PCD, formerly called immotile cilia syndrome) and Kartagener's syndrome (PCD associated with situs inversus).** Patients with classic PCD typically have a history of chronic respiratory tract infections. This is due to a lack of dynein arms in the axoneme of the cilia of the respiratory tract and in the flagella of the spermatozoa. Situs inversus is present in approximately 50% of these patients (see "Ultrastructural Abnormalities of Sperm"). Electron microscopic evaluation of spermatozoa identifies these cases. Other ultrastructural defects such as dysplasia of the fibrous sheath may also be identified by electron microscopy. The genetically based conditions retinitis pigmentosa and Usher's syndrome are also associated with severe motility defects. Occasionally, excessively prolonged abstinence periods may result in severely depressed motility. Finally, toxic contaminants in the collection container or exposure of the specimen to hot or cold environments may also account for low motility.

Teratospermia

Defects in morphology are termed *teratospermia* and are found more commonly with the increased utilization of rigid criteria for the evaluation of sperm morphology. Teratospermia is often associated with both oligospermia and asthenospermia. Temporary insults to spermatogenesis and varicoceles are potential causes. Rarely, patients may have round-headed sperm due to absence of the acrosome.

Multiple Defects in Seminal Parameters

Combined defects in sperm density, motility, and morphology are known as *oligoasthenoteratospermia* (OAT) and are most frequently due to a varicocele effect. Varicoceles are diagnosed by physical examination and are graded as small, medium, and large. Diagnostic testing for a varicocele, other than physical examination, is not indicated in the routine patient, but scrotal ultrasonography, thermography, or venography may be utilized in patients who are difficult to examine due to either obesity or vasovagal response to physical examination of the scrotum (Sharlip et al, 2002). Venography is the best method to confirm the presence of a persistent varicocele after surgical treatment in a patient with suspicious results after examination. Other causes of multiple sperm defects include cryptorchidism, temporary insults to spermatogenesis such as heat, drugs, or environmental toxins, or idiopathic causes. A heat effect may be either environmental or endogenous due to a fever. If a temporary insult is suspected, several semen analy-

ses over one to two spermatogenic cycles (3 to 6 months) should be obtained once the inciting agent is removed (Buch and Havlovec, 1991). As mentioned previously, partial ejaculatory duct obstruction may be a cause of low seminal volume associated with multiple defects in semen parameters (Meacham et al, 1993). TRUS and seminal vesicle aspiration have been advocated to diagnose this disorder (Jarow, 1994a). However, this diagnosis is very difficult to document and many patients who are thought to have partial obstruction likely have idiopathic infertility. Partial ejaculatory duct obstruction should be considered an investigational diagnosis at this time.

Normal Semen Parameters

Normal semen analyses in infertile couples suggest the possibility of a female factor as well as immunologic infertility or incorrect coital habits. A postcoital test (PCT) should be obtained in these instances. If no sperm are identified, the couple must be questioned about their coital technique. The presence of a shaking motion of sperm in the cervical mucus suggests the presence of antisperm antibodies. If the evaluation of both partners is normal, the couple is labeled as having "unexplained infertility." In these instances both partners should be evaluated for the presence of antisperm antibodies. A direct assay is preferred in the male while an indirect one is performed in the female. The female should also be carefully evaluated to rule out significant female factors. Rarely, men with normal semen parameters have a functional defect that prevents their sperm from fertilizing eggs in vivo and in vitro. Sperm function testing by either the sperm penetration assay or acrosome reaction test may be performed in the male partner of a couple with unexplained infertility. Abnormal sperm function testing results should instigate a reevaluation of the male looking for correctable abnormalities. If no abnormalities are detected, then IVF with ICSI should be considered.

ADDITIONAL TESTING

Based on the initial evaluation and the differential diagnosis suggested by this evaluation, additional, more specific testing may be indicated, as outlined in the algorithms presented earlier. The purpose of these additional tests is to rule in or out specific causes for male infertility. It is important to keep in mind that there are specific indications for each of these tests and that they do not need to be performed on a routine basis.

Antisperm Antibodies

A blood-tissue barrier exists in the testis and ductal system that prevents the immune system from coming in contact with sperm surface antigens that are present on postmeiotic germ cells. In the testis, as spermatogenesis begins in the pubertal male, tight junctions develop between Sertoli cells in the seminiferous tubules, forming a critical component of the blood-testis barrier.

Risk factors for the development of antisperm antibodies include conditions that may disrupt the blood-testis barrier. Obstruction of the ductal system is clearly associated with

the development of antisperm antibodies. **After vasectomy, approximately 60% of men develop antisperm antibodies** (Ansbacher, 1971; Fuchs and Alexander, 1983) **whereas approximately one third of patients with CBAVD are found to have antisperm antibodies** (Patrizio et al, 1992). Although many conditions have been reported to be associated with the presence of antisperm antibodies, the evidence is often conflicting. Thus, most studies have not found testicular torsion to be a risk factor for the presence of antisperm antibodies (Henderson et al, 1985; Puri et al, 1985; Hagen et al, 1992). Conflicting data also exist for cryptorchidism (Mirilas et al, 2003), varicoceles (Oshinsky et al, 1993), and testicular biopsy (Steele et al, 2001). **Abnormal postcoital tests, particularly when immotile sperm with a shaking motion are noticed, are highly suggestive of the presence of antisperm antibodies** (Matson et al, 1988; Menge and Beitner, 1989; Pretorius and Franken, 1989; Kremer and Jager, 1992). **Couples with unexplained infertility as well as cases with impaired sperm motility or sperm agglutination have also been reported to have a higher incidence of antisperm antibodies** (Menge and Beitner, 1989; Omu et al, 1999; Cimino et al, 1993).

Immunoglobulins may enter the genital tract through the seminiferous tubules, epididymis, or prostate. Immunoglobulin A (IgA) and immunoglobulin G (IgG) may both passively diffuse into the genital tract; however, IgA is also actively secreted. Because immunoglobulins may be secreted locally in the genital tract, it is not surprising that there may be antisperm antibodies present on the sperm surface that are not found in the serum. There are many assays to test for the presence of antisperm antibodies. **Direct assays detect the presence of antisperm antibodies on the patient's sperm. Indirect assays measure antisperm antibodies in the patient's serum** and generally require antisperm antibody negative donor sperm. Because it is the sperm that reach the female reproductive tract, not serum, direct assays have an advantage of only detecting sperm-bound immunoglobulins. The presence of antisperm antibodies in the serum is not always associated with the presence of these antibodies on sperm (Hellstrom et al, 1988). In addition, IgM class antibodies that may be present in serum do not usually make it to the semen. In general, the higher the titer of antibodies in the serum, the more likely there will be antibodies in semen. Most

investigators believe that only antibodies present on the spermatozoal surface are clinically significant. Thus, most recent investigations have been aimed at direct assays determining the presence of sperm-bound antibodies instead of the indirect detection of serum antisperm antibodies (Table 19–7). The immunobead assay and the mixed agglutination reaction (MAR) are commonly used for the detection of antisperm antibodies. These assays utilize synthetic beads or red blood cells that will bind to antibodies bound to the sperm surface. Scoring is based on the percentage of motile sperm with bead or red blood cell binding (Ayvaliotis et al, 1985; Clarke et al, 1985a). Most laboratories consider a sample positive for the presence of antisperm antibodies if more than 20% to 50% of the sperm demonstrate binding. An indirect assay may be performed by using patient's serum with donor sperm.

Antisperm antibodies can affect sperm function at several different levels.
- Motility (Bohring and Krause, 2003)
- Cervical mucus penetration (Jager et al, 1980).
- Capacitation (Benoff et al, 1993)
- Acrosome reaction (Francavilla et al, 1997)
- Binding to and penetration of the zona pellucida (Mahony et al, 1991)
- Oolemma binding (Liu et al, 1991)

Antisperm antibodies may consist of mixtures of antibodies directed against different antigens. In addition, antibodies in different patients may be directed against different antigens. It is likely that the variable effects of antisperm antibodies may, in part, depend on which antigen the antibody is directed against. Presently we do not know the majority of antigens or which antibodies adversely affect fertility. Current clinically used antisperm antibody assays do not identify specific antigens and therefore cannot determine if the antisperm antibodies will result in infertility. The identification of specific antigens may, in the future, allow for differentiation between clinically significant and insignificant antisperm antibodies (Bohring and Krause, 2003).

Antisperm antibodies are detected in approximately 10% of males presenting with infertility as opposed to 2% or less of fertile men (Clarke et al, 1985b; Sinisi et al, 1993). In general, there is a direct relationship between the amount (titer) of antisperm antibody activity and the effect on fertil-

Table 19–7. Antisperm Antibody Assays				
Assay	**Type**	**Measurement**	**Advantage**	**Disadvantage**
Mixed antiglobulin reaction (MAR)	Direct or indirect	Anti-human Ig-coated RBC bind to sperm	Quick—uses unwashed semen Determines % of sperm coated with Ig	Titer not determined Only detects IgG
Sperm MAR	Direct or indirect	Anti-human Ig-coated latex particles bind to sperm	Quick—uses unwashed semen Determines % of sperm coated with Ig	Titer not determined. Only detects IgG
Immunobead test	Direct or indirect	Anti-human Ig-coated polyacrylamide beads bind to sperm	Determines Ig class (IgA, IgG, IgM) and location of Ig on sperm as well as % of sperm coated with Ig	Must wash sperm Titer not determined
Tray agglutination test (TAT) Gelatin agglutination test (GAT)	Indirect	Sperm agglutination	Determines titer	Does not determine amount of AB on sperm surface or class of Ig
Sperm immobilization assay (SIT)	Indirect	Immobilization of sperm	Determines titer	Only detects complement-fixing Ig
Enzyme-linked immunosorbent assay (ELISA)	Direct or indirect	Color change of solution	Can determine quantity and class of Ig	Uses fixed sperm that exposes intracellular, clinically irrelevant antigens

ity. Similarly, low concentrations of antibodies seem to have little effect on fertility (Ayvaliotis et al, 1985; Rumke et al, 1974). While assays such as the immunobead assay determine the percent of sperm with antibody bound to their surface, they do not give a measurement of the amount of antibody bound to the sperm. Indirect assays yield this information, and therefore some have suggested direct assays be used as a screening test (because of their high specificity), followed by indirect assays to determine serum titers (Hjort, 1999).

Fertility may also be impaired in the presence of antisperm antibodies in the female. Of necessity, indirect assays must be used on females and therefore are subject to the same problems as indirect assays in the male. Although serum is easier to work with, antisperm antibodies in the cervical mucus are more clinically significant; however, this substance is technically difficult to work with.

We believe that patients with the previously mentioned risk factors, those demonstrating impaired sperm motility, sperm agglutination, and abnormal PCT findings, and couples with unexplained infertility should be tested for the presence of antisperm antibodies. Because the presence of serum antisperm antibodies does not affect the decision to proceed with vasectomy reversals, we do not recommend preoperative testing in these patients. Testing may be performed on patients with patent anastomoses after reversals who are not able to impregnate their partners within 1 year.

Leukocyte Staining

Both immature germ cells (spermatocytes) and leukocytes appear similar under wet mount microscopy and are known as round cells. These two cell types cannot usually be differentiated without special stains—which are not generally used during the performance of a semen analysis. Semen analysis reports that list numbers or concentrations of WBCs should be viewed with skepticism. Unless special stains are performed, the reports should list these cells as round cells. The presence of greater than 1 million WBCs/mL is considered abnormal and raises the possibility of a genital tract infection or inflammation. There remains considerable controversy about the significance of pyospermia. Although infertile couples tend to have greater concentrations of WBCs than fertile populations (Wolff and Anderson, 1988), not all studies of patients with increased numbers of leukocytes in the semen report decreased fertility rates (Tomlinson et al, 1993). Although both infection and infertility have been associated with pyospermia (Caldamone et al, 1980; Berger et al, 1982; Maruyama et al, 1985), the presence of bacteria in semen has not always correlated with the presence of pyospermia (Rodin et al, 2003). **Many patients with pyospermia do not have genital tract infections.** Most studies suggest detrimental effects of leukocytes on sperm function and semen parameters (Yanushpolsky et al, 1996; Aziz et al, 2004). The concentration of immature germ cells is proportional to the concentration of sperm. Many men with poor semen quality have a higher percentage of immature cells than fertile men, but the patient-to-patient variation is considerable and is of unclear significance (Wolff et al, 1990). **Approximately one third of the cases demonstrating increased numbers of round cells will be found to have true pyospermia, with the remainder of cases having increased numbers of immature germ cells** (Sigman and Lopes, 1993).

There are several techniques available to differentiate round cells from leukocytes. Traditional staining techniques, such as the Papanicolaou stain, may be used; however, these methods necessitate a highly trained observer. Immunohistochemical techniques utilizing monoclonal antibodies directed against WBC surface antigens detect all leukocyte types (Homyk et al, 1990) but are labor intense. A relatively simple technique relying on the presence of peroxidase within the WBCs underestimates the number of leukocytes within semen since monocytes do not contain this enzyme (Endtz, 1974). **We recommend some type of WBC staining of semen in patients with more than 10 to 15 round cells/HPF or more than 1 million round cells/mL. If the majority of cells are WBCs and their concentration is greater than 1 million cells/mL, the patient should be evaluated for a genital tract infection.** The management of pyospermia, in the absence of genital tract infection, has included anti-inflammatory medication, empirical antibiotic therapy, frequent ejaculations, and prostatic massage. However, these therapies lack proven efficacy (Yanushpolsky et al, 1995). Semen processing to remove the WBCs combined with IUI or IVF should be considered in these cases.

Semen Cultures

Genital tract infections are uncommon causes of male infertility, and the role of asymptomatic genital tract infection in male infertility is controversial. Many organisms, including aerobic and anaerobic organisms, as well as *Mycoplasma*, have been cultured from human semen (Swenson et al, 1980; Lewis et al, 1981; Busolo et al, 1984b; Upadhyaya et al, 1984; Naessens et al, 1986). Although studies have found that bacteria may be spermicidal (Paulson and Polakoski, 1977), others have found no consistent effect on fertility (Makler et al, 1981; Berger et al, 1982). **In the presence of a culture-positive genitourinary infection with clinical symptoms—such as cystitis, urethritis, or prostatitis—appropriate treatment should be instituted. However, routine genital tract bacterial cultures are not indicated in the absence of clinical symptoms or documented pyospermia.**

Mycoplasmas are aerobic bacteria of the family Mycoplasmataceae, which includes the genera *Mycoplasma* and *Ureaplasma*. These bacteria bind to the cell membranes of the head and midpiece of spermatozoa and do not stain with Gram's stain. Both *Mycoplasma hominis* and *Ureaplasma urealyticum* have been associated with nongonococcal urethritis in humans (Bowie et al, 1977), but recent evidence suggests that these may colonize the genital system but may not be pathogenic in men (Uuskula and Kohl, 2002). In contrast, **most current evidence suggests that *Mycoplasma genitalium* is a common cause of urethritis** (Jensen, 2004). Whereas some studies have reported decreased motility and membrane changes in semen samples with *Ureaplasma* (Nunez-Calonge et al, 1998), others have found no differences in semen parameters between culture-positive and culture-negative men (Busolo et al, 1984a; Soffer et al, 1990; Andrade-Rocha, 2003). In addition, recent studies found no evidence of inflammatory reactions in the semen of men culture positive for *M. hominis* or *U. urealyticum* (Pannekoek et al, 2000). This strongly suggests that **the presence of *M. hominis* and *U. urealyticum* in semen represents colonization and not infection.** Although *M. genitalium* is clearly pathogenic in men, studies evaluating the role of it in male infertility are lacking.

C. trachomatis is one of the most common sexually transmitted diseases; however, its role as a causative agent in male infertility is unclear. The organism is an obligate intracellular bacterium and a frequent cause of epididymitis and nongonococcal urethritis. *Chlamydia* has been cultured from semen, prostatic secretions, and urine (Thompson and Washington, 1983), and the organism appears to bind to spermatozoa (Wolner-Hanssen and Mardh, 1984). Although epididymal obstruction from chlamydial epididymitis may occur, in the absence of obstruction, past infection does not seem to affect semen parameters (Ness et al, 1997). In-vitro studies have demonstrated toxic effects of *Chlamydia* on sperm due to lipopolysaccharide (Eley et al, 2005). However, clinical studies on men with infection have not generally demonstrated effects on semen quality or sperm function (Eley et al, 2005).

We recommend only evaluating patients for infection if they have clinical evidence of an inflammatory or infectious process. These patients may be tested for *M. genitalium* and *C. trachomatis* infections. First-void urine testing by polymerase chain reaction techniques have higher sensitivity than culturing and are less uncomfortable for patients than the use of urethral swabs (Maeda et al, 2004). Bacterial cultures of semen frequently yield low concentrations of multiple organisms due to distal urethral contamination. Antibacterial skin preparation and voiding before ejaculation decreases the incidence of, but does not eliminate, false-positive cultures (Kim and Goldstein, 1999). Urine cultures should also be obtained in those patients with evidence of cystitis or urethritis.

Chromatin/DNA Integrity Testing

Sperm chromatin consists of DNA and specialized proteins. During spermatogenesis and epididymal transport, sperm chromatin undergoes specific changes involving the replacement of histones with protamines and the formation of crosslinking disulfide bonds. This results in a tightly organized, condensed chromatin that is relatively resistant to genetic damage. After fertilization, the sperm nucleus (termed the *male pronucleus*) undergoes decondensation (Tesarik and Kopecny, 1989a). There is evidence of some paternal (sperm) DNA transcription at this stage, but most paternal gene expression begins at the four cell embryonic stage (Tesarik and Kopecny, 1989b). Evidence has been increasing that defects in chromatin organization may lead to infertility in men. Although sperm DNA damage repair may occur within the egg after fertilization, it may be overwhelmed by a large amount of damage. **Risk factors for abnormal sperm DNA or chromatin include smoking** (Potts et al, 1999), **exposure to industrial toxicants** (Spano et al, 1998; Lemasters et al, 1999), **air pollution** (Selevan et al, 2000), **cancer** (Evenson et al, 1984; Fossa et al, 1997; Kobayashi et al, 2001), **fever** (Evenson et al, 2000), **as well as male infertility.**

Abnormal chromatin organization or DNA damage may occur through several possible mechanisms. During normal nuclear maturation, single-strand nicks occur in DNA and are repaired. Defects in the repair process may lead to sperm with increased amounts of nicked DNA (Manicardi et al, 1995). Abnormal protamine function or content may result in deficient chromatin structure (de Yebra et al, 1998). Apoptosis is a normal physiologic process during spermatogenesis that involves double-stranded DNA breaks that ultimately lead to a cascading process of programmed cell death. This process regulates the number of spermatozoa that reach final maturity. If abnormalities in the apoptotic pathway prevent these cells from dying, mature sperm with DNA breaks will be produced (Sakkas et al, 2002). Finally, oxidative stress due to reactive oxygen species (ROS) may induce DNA damage in spermatozoa (Aitken and Krausz, 2001).

A variety of methods have been employed to measure the extent of chromatin abnormalities or DNA damage in sperm. The TUNEL (terminal deoxyribonucleotidyl transferase-mediated dUTP nick-end labeling) assay labels sites of DNA breaks with deoxyuridine triphosphate (dUTP) attached to a marker. The amount of dUTP labeling correlates with the amount of DNA nicks (Lopes et al, 1998). Depending on the label, measurement may be performed by flow cytometry, fluorescent microscopy, or light microscopy. The percent of sperm with fragmented DNA can then be determined. In the comet assay, sperm are placed on an agarose gel, lysed, subjected to electrophoresis, and treated with a fluorescent DNA-binding dye. The resultant fluorescent pattern looks like a comet with a tail. Increased DNA strand breaks result in increased tail fluorescence (Hughes et al, 1996) and tail length (Singh and Stephens, 1998). The initial comet assay used alkaline conditions to denature the DNA. This may have identified single-strand DNA breaks that were not clinically relevant. Recent studies utilizing neutral conditions for the comet assay may improve the specificity of this test (Singh and Stephens, 1998; Trisini et al, 2004). The sperm chromatin structure assay (SCSA) does not directly measure DNA breaks as do the TUNEL and comet assays. This assay is based on the finding that damaged sperm chromatin will easily denature when subjected to an acid environment whereas normal chromatin will not. Acridine orange binds to denatured DNA, fluorescing green when the DNA is double stranded (immature or damaged chromatin) and red if single stranded (fragmented DNA). Thus, abnormal chromatin will demonstrate a high amount of staining and, if fragmented, a preponderance of red fluorescence as opposed to green (Evenson et al, 2002). The fluorescence of 5000 to 10,000 sperm is measure by flow cytometry. The reported parameters include the percent of sperm with an increased ratio of red/(red plus green) fluorescence (termed the *DNA fragmentation index* [DFI]) and the percent of sperm with green staining (termed the *high DNA-stainable [HDS] fraction*). Other less commonly employed methods include the in-situ nick translation assay (Manicardi et al, 1995), the acridine orange test (Tejada et al, 1984; Hoshi et al, 1996), and the sperm chromatin dispersion test (Fernandez et al, 2003).

There is considerable controversy about the role of DNA and chromatin integrity assays in the evaluation and management of the infertile male. Most data suggest a loose, but significant, correlation with semen parameters. Patients with abnormal semen parameters will often have abnormal DNA integrity testing whereas some patients with normal semen parameters may also have abnormal results (Agarwal and Said, 2003). Studies examining the relationship between DNA integrity and pregnancy rates by intercourse have usually shown a relationship (Agarwal and Said, 2003). By using the SCSA assay in a group of 165 couples without known fertility problems who where trying to conceive by intercourse, thresholds for DFI were derived. Of all pregnancies that occurred during the 12 months of the study, 75% occurred in those with 0% to 15% DFI, in 22% with more than 15% to 30% DFI, but in only 3% with more than 30% DFI (Evenson et al, 1999). Utilizing the threshold of more than 30% DFI as a positive (abnormal) result to predict miscarriage or no pregnancy, the sensitivity was 15% with a specificity of 96%. **As might be expected, these data suggest that whereas a high degree of chromatin damage makes pregnancy unlikely, normal chromatin is not sufficient to ensure pregnancy.**

Much interest in DNA and chromatin integrity assays derives from the potential to employ the results to direct the appropriate use of IUI, IVF, and ICSI. Lower IUI pregnancy rates have been reported when the sperm contain high amounts of DNA fragmentation, as determined by TUNEL (Duran et al, 2002) and SCSA (Bungum et al, 2004) assays. Most recent studies have examined the relationship between DNA or chromatin damage and IVF or ICSI results. Studies of couples with more than 30% DFI scores after SCSA testing report conflicting results ranging from no IVF pregnancies in those couples with high DFI values (Larson-Cook et al, 2003) through decreased (28% vs. 47%) pregnancy rates (Virro et al, 2004) to no effect of high DFI (Bungum et al, 2004; Gandini et al, 2004). Similar contradictory results have been reported when using the TUNEL assay (Benchaib et al, 2003; Henkel et al, 2003, 2004; Seli et al, 2004; Tesarik et al, 2004). Of interest, some studies suggest that sperm DNA abnormalities do not affect fertilization or early embryo development but become evident later in embryonic development, affecting pregnancy and miscarriage rates (Tesarik et al, 2004). This might be predicted since the spermatozoal DNA is not greatly activated until the embryo reaches the four cell stage. Others have suggested that much of the DNA/chromatin damage occurs outside of the testis and have reported lower DNA fragmentation and higher pregnancy rates with ICSI using testicular sperm instead of ejaculated sperm (Greco et al, 2005).

Proposed indications for these assays include unexplained infertility, repeated IVF failure, recurrent miscarriage, and risk factors in the male for DNA damage. Whereas most studies employing the SCSA have used similar, but not always identical, techniques and ranges, there has been very little consistency between studies utilizing the other DNA integrity assays. Until universal standards are developed, widespread acceptance of these assays will be hindered.

Ultrastructural Evaluation

Light microscopic examination of stained spermatozoa is a routine part of the semen analysis. Gross tail abnormalities such as bent or coiled tails as well as some acrosomal defects including vacuoles, large or small acrosomes, and complete absence of the acrosome may be identified in this manner. However, other ultrastructural abnormalities, such as defects of the mitochondria, outer dense fibers, or microtubules, require electron microscopy for detection. These defects generally result in absent or extremely low motility but will not affect sperm density. In these cases, a sperm viability assay

should be performed to differentiate dead sperm from live nonmotile sperm. Most sperm in samples with ultrastructural abnormalities will be viable. **Electron microscopy should be considered for patients with sperm samples with motility of less than 5% to 10% associated with reasonably high viability.**

Radiologic Evaluation

The main purpose of the radiologic evaluation of the genital system of the infertile male is to identify evidence of either complete or partial ductal obstruction. A patient with complete obstruction of the excurrent ductal system typically has azoospermia, whereas patients with partial obstruction can have a variety of seminal findings, including oligospermia, asthenospermia, and/or early demise of sperm after ejaculation. **It is extremely difficult to differentiate partial ductal obstruction from other causes of male infertility, particularly idiopathic oligospermia.** The currently available radiologic imaging studies cannot provide a definitive diagnosis for partial obstruction. Thus, the diagnosis and management of partial ductal obstruction continues to be investigational.

Vasography

The traditional and most commonly employed radiologic imaging study for the evaluation of the vasal and ejaculatory duct patency is vasography. **Vasography is indicated to determine the site of obstruction in azoospermic patients that have active spermatogenesis documented by testis biopsy.** Vasography is best performed in conjunction with reconstructive surgery because this procedure carries an inherent risk of vasal injury that could complicate future reconstructive surgery if performed separately (Poore et al, 1997). A retrograde method employing endoscopic canalization of the ejaculatory ducts is no longer utilized because of both technical difficulties and the risk of epididymitis when contrast medium is injected in a retrograde fashion. Vasography is most commonly performed at the level of the scrotal vas deferens by either direct puncture or through a transverse vasotomy. The site of obstruction is determined by the combination of injection of an agent distally and microscopic inspection of the intravasal fluid to determine epididymal patency. Injection of saline or saline combined with a colored dye is utilized initially to document distal patency. However, if the saline does not flow easily, injection of dilute nonionic contrast agent or passage of a 2-0 monofilament suture is necessary to determine the site of obstruction. A normal vasogram is documented when contrast agent is visualized throughout the length of the vas deferens, seminal vesicles, ejaculatory duct, and bladder (Fig. 19–6). **Proximal patency of the epididymis is documented by microscopic (400×) visualization of sperm in the intravasal fluid.** This procedure is discussed in greater detail in Chapter 20. Vasography may also be indicated in the severely oligospermic patient in whom there is reason to suspect a unilateral vasal obstruction (e.g., from a hernia repair) with an abnormal contralateral testis (Matsuda et al, 1992b). An alternative approach to detect ejaculatory duct obstruction is seminal vesiculography (see Fig. 19–6). However, there is a significant risk of introducing infection into a closed system, particularly if seminal vesicle puncture is performed transrectally rather than transperineally.

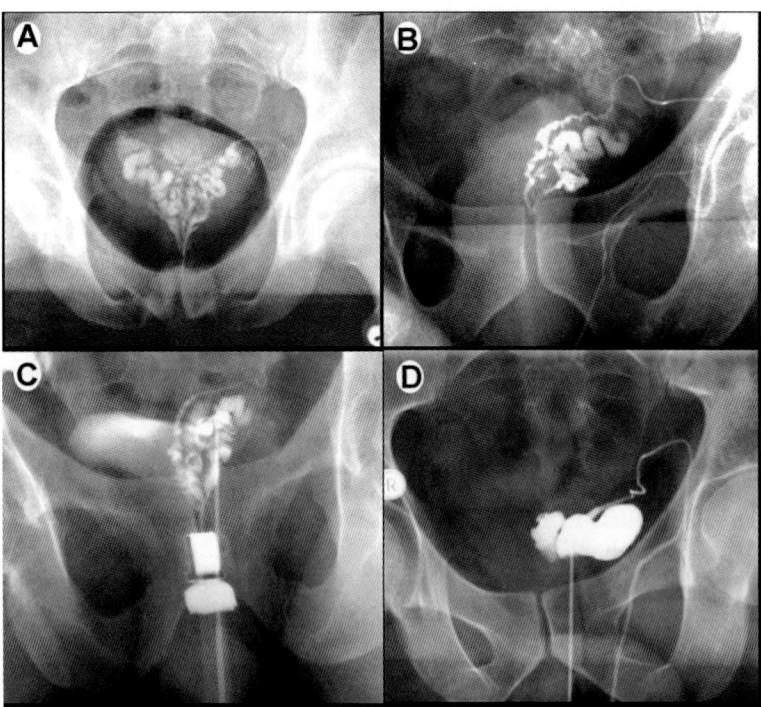

Figure 19–6. Examples of vasography and seminal vesiculography. **A,** Normal vasogram; note contrast agent in bladder. **B,** Vasogram depicting left ejaculatory duct obstruction. **C,** Normal seminal vesiculogram, again note contrast agent in bladder. **D,** Seminal vesiculogram demonstrates complete left ejaculatory duct obstruction.

Therefore, it is best to perform this diagnostic procedure at the time of intended relief of obstruction. Seminal vesiculography can also be utilized in patients with suspected obstruction of the inguinal portion of the vas deferens but should not be used to evaluate the scrotal vas deferens because of the risk of epididymitis if contrast agent enters the epididymis (Riedenklau et al, 1995). Vasography should not be performed on oligospermic patients who do not have a history or physical examination suggestive of unilateral obstruction (i.e., history of hernia repair and asymmetrical testicular volume).

Transrectal Ultrasonography

Transrectal ultrasonography allows for the anatomic visualization of the prostate, seminal vesicles, and ampullary portion of the vas deferens (Fig. 19–7). **TRUS is indicated in azoospermic patients suspected of having ejaculatory duct obstruction.** The typical seminal findings in patients with complete ejaculatory duct obstruction include low ejaculate volume (<1 mL), acidic pH, absent fructose, and failure to coagulate due to the absence of seminal vesicle secretions. The differential diagnosis for these seminal findings includes both ejaculatory duct obstruction and vasal agenesis associated with seminal vesicle agenesis or hypoplasia. Obstruction of the ejaculatory ducts is suggested by the presence of dilated seminal vesicles. **The normal diameter of the seminal vesicles on transverse imaging behind the bladder is up to 1.5 cm** (Carter et al, 1989). Hypoplasia or absence of the seminal vesicles is easily diagnosed, but some patients with complete ejaculatory duct obstruction do not have dilated seminal vesicles (Jarow, 1996b). Either vasography or seminal vesicle aspiration may be necessary to establish the diagnosis of ejaculatory duct obstruction in patients with equivocal ultrasonographic

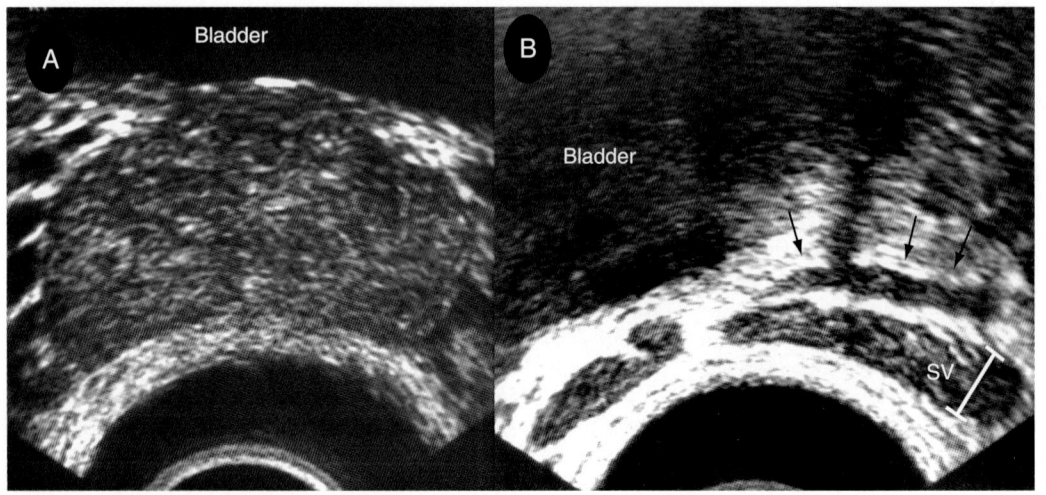

Figure 19–7. Normal transrectal ultrasound (TRUS) of the prostate and seminal vesicles. **A,** Transverse view of the mid prostate. **B,** Transverse view of seminal vesicles (SV) and vas deferens *(arrowheads)*. The seminal vesicles are measured in anteroposterior diameter as depicted.

findings. Seminal vesicle aspiration is performed under transrectal ultrasonography using a 30-cm or longer 20-gauge needle. The presence of millions of sperm in the seminal vesicle aspirate of an azoospermic man is diagnostic of ejaculatory duct obstruction (Jarow, 1996a). Moreover, the presence of sperm in these patients obviates the need for testicular biopsy to confirm the presence of active spermatogenesis and rules out the presence of concomitant epididymal obstruction (Silber, 1980).

It has been suggested by some investigators that select infertile patients have partial ejaculatory duct obstruction (Hellerstein et al, 1992; Goluboff et al, 1995; Beiswanger et al, 1998). The clinical findings that are thought to be consistent with partial ejaculatory duct obstruction include normal or low normal semen volume, reduced motility, and early demise of sperm in vitro in patients with normal hormonal profiles and normal-sized testes (Hellerstein et al, 1992). Whereas dilated seminal vesicles greater than 1.5 cm associated with a dilated ejaculatory duct are suggestive of ejaculatory duct obstruction, these findings are not diagnostic. In addition, it has been suggested that the finding of intraprostatic cysts and hyperechoic lesions within the prostate are associated with ejaculatory duct obstruction. Yet, hyperechoic lesions of the prostate are frequently seen in fertile volunteers and intraprostatic cysts can be an incidental finding (Jarow, 1993; Poore and Jarow, 1995). It has also been suggested that the finding of a large number of motile sperm in a seminal vesicle aspirate is consistent with partial ejaculatory duct obstruction, but this assertion remains unproved (Jarow, 1994b). The indications for TRUS in patients with suspected partial ejaculatory duct obstruction as well as the ultrasonographic criteria to diagnose this condition remain quite controversial, and treatment of these patients should be considered investigational.

Venography

Internal spermatic vein venography is utilized to both detect and potentially treat varicoceles. Venography is performed using a Seldinger technique via either a right femoral venous or right internal jugular venous approach. The femoral vein approach is generally preferred, but the internal jugular approach is superior if embolization of the right side or bilateral varicoceles is being contemplated. It is important that diagnostic venography be performed under low pressure and, for the left side, with the catheter tip positioned inside the renal vein lateral to the junction with the internal spermatic vein to avoid a false-positive study (Fig. 19–8). Regrettably, there are many false-positive and false-negative results with venography because of technical errors and anatomic variations. **The valves of the internal spermatic veins are often located very close to the ostium, and a false-positive result may be obtained if the vein is cannulated or extreme pressures are used during injection of contrast material** (Nadel et al, 1984). In addition, there are frequently multiple openings of the internal spermatic veins at their origin. Both of these features may lead to a false-positive diagnosis of a varicocele by venography. Conversely, a false-negative study may occur if the patient is not studied in the reverse Trendelenburg position or if the reflux is due to collateral veins not visualized during the study (Wishahi, 1991). Although there is considerable controversy regarding the role of venography in the management of varicoceles, many clinicians utilize venography for patients with a suspected recurrence after varicocele repair to both document the recurrence and embolize the persistent veins.

Scrotal Ultrasonography

The main application of scrotal ultrasonography in male infertility has been for the diagnosis of varicoceles. Varicoceles are normally detected by physical examination, but some patients may be difficult to examine or have an equivocal examination. Color duplex scrotal ultrasonography has been applied as a noninvasive alternative to internal spermatic vein venography in an attempt to objectively diagnose varicoceles. Other noninvasive tests for varicoceles include the Doppler

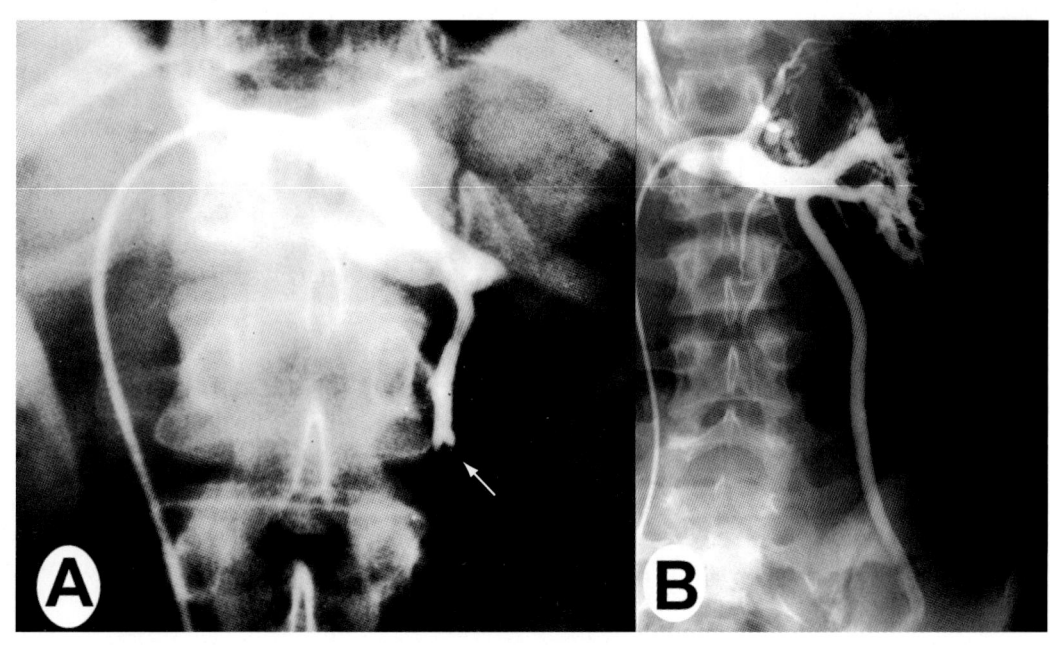

Figure 19–8. Percutaneous venography used for the evaluation of varicoceles. **A,** Normal left-sided venogram demonstrates an intact venous valve of the left internal spermatic vein (*arrowhead*). **B,** Venogram demonstrates reflux through incompetent venous valves of the left internal spermatic vein consistent with a varicocele.

stethoscope, thermography, and radionuclide studies (WHO, 1985). The initial criteria developed to diagnose a varicocele include the presence of numerous large veins (>3 mm) and reversal of blood flow with Valsalva maneuver (McClure and Hricak, 1986). However, further studies have shown that the accuracy of color duplex ultrasonography diagnosis of varicoceles is only 60% when compared with both physical examination and venography (Eskew et al, 1993). Moreover, there is little evidence that repair of subclinical varicoceles has any positive effect on male fertility (Jarow et al, 1996b; Yamamoto et al, 1996). Therefore, there is limited value in routinely utilizing scrotal ultrasonography for the detection of varicoceles in subfertile men. **Imaging studies should not be utilized to search for varicoceles in men with normal and adequate physical examinations.** Color duplex scrotal ultrasonography should be reserved for those patients with an inadequate physical examination due to either obesity or testicular sensitivity. A venous diameter of 3.5 mm or greater should be utilized as the criteria to diagnose a clinical varicocele in these patients (Eskew et al, 1993; Meacham et al, 1994). The other application of scrotal ultrasonography in the subfertile patient is to rule out the presence of testicular tumors. Subfertility is sometimes a presenting symptom of testicular germ cell neoplasia, and scrotal ultrasonography is the best radiologic imaging modality for this entity (Honig et al, 1994; Hopps and Goldstein, 2002). In addition, Leydig cell tumors are often not palpable and should be suspected in subfertile men with a high serum testosterone and/or estradiol level or gynecomastia (Horstman et al, 1994; Lemack et al, 1995). **The use of scrotal ultrasonography to detect testicular tumors should be restricted to patients with suggestive findings of histories, physical examinations, or hormonal values. It should not be utilized as a routine examination to screen all infertile men.**

Abdominal Ultrasonography

Abdominal ultrasonography is used to assess the kidneys in patients with absence of the vas deferens. The vas deferens and ureter share a common embryologic origin in the mesonephric duct. Hence, patients with congenital absence of the vas deferens are also at risk for renal agenesis. **Ipsilateral renal anomalies are present in up to 80% of men with unilateral absence of the vas deferens, with the most common anomaly being renal agenesis** (Donohue and Fauver, 1989). In contrast, congenital bilateral absence of vasa deferentia appears to occur through a different mechanism and the risk for renal anomalies is much lower (Schlegel et al, 1996). **Therefore, abdominal ultrasonography should be considered to rule out renal agenesis in patients with a nonpalpable vas deferens. It is not mandatory to perform abdominal ultrasonography in those patients with absence of the vas deferens due to a proven mutation upon cystic fibrosis genetic testing.**

Sperm Function Testing

Sperm–Cervical Mucus Interaction

For conception to occur after intercourse, sperm must travel through the cervical mucus. The PCT assesses this interaction. The examination should be performed just before ovulation, at which point the cervical mucus becomes clear and thin. A drop of cervical mucus is examined under a microscope (Moghissi, 1976). Although the test has been used for more than 60 years, there is no agreement as to how the test should be performed, the timing of the test, or the grading system.

A normal test result is usually defined as one in which more than 10 to 20 sperm/HPF (400×) are identified. Progressive motility should be present in the majority of sperm. Most investigators agree that in the presence of normal postcoital findings a cervical factor or semen deposition abnormality is not involved in the couple's infertility. However, abnormal PCTs may result from many causes. Inappropriate timing of the PCT is the most common cause for an abnormal result. Other causes include anatomic abnormalities, semen or cervical mucus antisperm antibodies, inappropriately performed intercourse, and abnormal semen. The ability of the PCT to aid in the prediction of infertility or subsequent pregnancy has been examined in prospective studies with conflicting results (Jette and Glass, 1972; Lyon et al, 1982; Collins et al, 1984; Oei et al, 1998). A recent study used logistical analysis to determine the contribution of the medical history, semen analysis, and PCT results to a model to predict pregnancy. The authors concluded that the PCT was useful in approximately 50% of couples (van der Steeg et al, 2004).

In an attempt to standardize the cervical mucus interaction, a variety of in-vitro cervical mucus tests have been developed (Morgan et al, 1977; Gaddum-Rosse et al, 1980; Alexander, 1981; Mangione et al, 1981; Moghissi et al, 1982; Eggert-Kruse et al, 1989; Papp and Vajna, 1989; Farhi et al, 1995). Despite the additional information that may be obtained from these assays, they are not commonly used in most couples.

Because of the lack of standardization and reproducibility, the utility of the PCT as part of the routine evaluation of the infertile couple has come into question (Glatstein et al, 1995; Smith et al, 2003). **The PCT test is indicated if the results will influence the management of the couple** (Practice Committee of the American Society for Reproductive Medicine, 2004). **This may include cases of hyperviscous semen, unexplained infertility, and low volume semen specimens with normal total sperm counts. Because patients with very poor quality semen invariably have poor PCTs, it is not necessary to perform PCTs in this group of patients. A persistently abnormal PCT in the presence of reasonably good semen parameters should lead the physician to question the quality of the cervical mucus.** The quality of the mucus is rated by inspecting its ferning and spinnbarkeit. The gynecologist usually performs this at the time of the PCT. If the mucus quality is reported to be good, then poor timing relative to the time of ovulation is not likely to be involved. If no sperm are seen in good quality cervical mucus, the couple should be questioned about their coital technique and the physician should be sure that the patient does not have hypospadias, which would lead to a sperm deposition problem. The finding of good quality mucus and few or nonmotile sperm or immobilized sperm demonstrating a shaking motion should lead to the evaluation of both the male and female partners for the presence of antisperm antibodies. **After an abnormal PCT, some would recommend an in-vitro cervical mucus interaction test to further localize the source of the defect. However, because the results of these tests will not usually affect management and because of the success of the ART, we recom-**

mend proceeding with IUI rather performing additional diagnostic tests.

Acrosome Reaction

Sperm must undergo capacitation and the acrosome reaction to attain the ability to fertilize ova. Whereas the gross appearance of the acrosome is apparent during the performance of normal sperm morphology evaluation, differentiation of acrosome-reacted sperm from acrosome intact sperm requires specialized techniques (Zeginiadou et al, 2000). Transmission electron microscopy remains the gold standard but is an expensive, labor-intensive procedure that is not practical for routine clinical use. Many other techniques including differential staining, fluorescence microscopy with labeled lectins or anti-acrosomal antibodies, and polyacrylamide beads coated with anti-acrosomal antibodies have also been developed (Talbot and Chacon, 1981; Kallajoki et al, 1986; Lee et al, 1987; Mortimer et al, 1987; Cross and Meizel, 1989; Sharma et al, 1997). After capacitation, sperm may be induced to undergo the acrosome reaction by exposing them to acrosome-inducing agents. Acrosome reaction assays may determine the percent of cells in the semen sample that have spontaneously undergone the acrosome reaction as well as the percent of cells that may be induced to undergo the acrosome reaction after capacitation and exposure to an inducing agent. Assays may employ artificial acrosome inducers such as the ionophore A23187 or natural agents such as zona pellucida. The results of assays with different inducers may not correlate (Liu and Baker, 1996). **In general, normal semen samples demonstrate spontaneous acrosome reaction rates of less than 5% and induced acrosome reaction rates of 15% to 40%. Samples from infertile populations have demonstrated high spontaneous rates of acrosome-reacted sperm and low rates of induced acrosome reactions** (Fenichel et al, 1991). **Although acrosome reaction assays are not widely available, they may be considered in patients with unexplained poor fertilization rates obtained in IVF or in cases of unexplained infertility. If an acrosome reaction defect is identified, IVF with ICSI is indicated.** Because normal penetration in a sperm penetration assay (SPA) requires the sperm to undergo the acrosome reaction, an SPA may be performed if an acrosome reaction assay is not available.

Sperm Penetration Assay

The zona pellucida is a glycoprotein layer that surrounds the ovum of most species and prevents cross-species fertilization. The removal of this layer allows human sperm to fuse with hamster oocytes. Scoring is performed by determining the percent of ova that have been penetrated or by calculating the number of sperm that have penetrated each ovum. Thus, this assay requires sperm to be able to undergo (1) capacitation, (2) the acrosome reaction, (3) fusion with the oolemma, and (4) incorporation into the ooplasm. Since the zona has been removed, this test will not detect abnormalities of sperm-zona interaction. Samples are commonly believed to be normal if the sperm penetrate between 10% and 30% of ova. Unfortunately, the assay is a bioassay with variable results and is not standardized. Therefore, there are conflicting results and significant controversies as to its interpretation. A modification of the SPA procedure, involving incubation of the sperm in a more potent capacitating media, results in the majority of oocytes being penetrated. Scoring for these assays is based on the number of penetrations per ova. SPA results using this approach have correlated well with pregnancies after intercourse in male factor couples with a positive predicted value of 77.8% and a negative predicted value of 92.3% (Gattuccio et al, 1988). Others have found similarly good correlations between the results of the SPA and fertilization and pregnancy rates by conventional IVF (Shibahara et al, 1998; Smith et al, 1987). For proper interpretation of the SPA, the physician must be familiar with the laboratory that is performing the assay and should be aware of what correlations have been documented between the results of the assay and actual human fertilization. Couples with semen samples with very poor parameters will usually be directed toward ICSI instead of regular IVF and will not benefit from an SPA. **We believe that an SPA may be considered in those patients with semen parameters good enough for regular IVF but low numbers of morphologically normal sperm to rule out a fertilization defect. Some clinicians also obtain SPAs in couples with unexplained infertility. Those couples with abnormal SPA results should consider IVF with ICSI as opposed to IUI or conventional IVF** (Shibahara et al, 1998).

Other Sperm Function Tests

Hemizona Assay. In the hemizona assay, the human zona pellucida is microscopically divided in half. Each half is then incubated with either patient sperm or sperm from a fertile donor. A hemizona index is then calculated by counting the number of sperm bound to each zona half and dividing the number of sperm bound from the patient by the number of sperm bound from the donor. Most male patients who do not fertilize human ova in vitro demonstrate a hemizona index of less than 0.60 (Burkman et al, 1988). Because this assay requires a source of human ova and significant micromanipulation skills, it has not gained widespread use. Both zona pellucida derived from cadavers and failed IVF cycles have been utilized to increase the availability of zona for this assay (Franken, 1998; Henkel et al, 1999). This test will determine if a zona-sperm interaction defect is present in cases in which IVF has not resulted in fertilization in the presence of a normal SPA. Patients demonstrating defects in the hemizona assay should be referred for IVF with ICSI. However, with the availability of ICSI, this test has become unnecessary and is not often performed.

Sperm Viability Assays. **In most instances nonmotile sperm are dead, but in some cases they may be viable but lack the ability to move. The finding of sperm motility of less than 5% to 10% suggests the presence of ultrastructural defects. To differentiate these two states, sperm viability assays are utilized.** Traditional viability assays expose sperm to dyes, which may penetrate dead sperm but are excluded from live sperm with intact cell membranes. Eosin Y and trypan blue stains are commonly employed. Dead sperm are stained while live sperm remain unstained. This assay is indicated in samples with absent motility or very low (less than 5% to 10%) motility. The hypo-osmotic sperm-swelling test (HOST) is based on the principle that live sperm with intact membranes will be able to maintain an osmotic gradient. When placed in a hypo-osmotic solution, water will flow into viable cells, causing the membrane to bulge, which is particularly noticeable in the sperm tails. Nonviable sperm will not maintain an osmotic gradient and therefore will not swell (Jeyendran et al, 1984). The results of this assay generally correlate well with the results of standard sperm viability staining (Avery et al, 1990; Jeyendran et al, 1992; Buckett, 2003). The HOST may be utilized to select viable sperm to be injected during IVF with ICSI when the sperm are nonmotile. In these instances, sperm that demonstrate swelling under hypo-osmotic conditions are viable and may be utilized for ICSI (Casper et al, 1996; Barros et al, 1997; Liu et al, 1997).

Reactive Oxygen Species Testing. The production of various ROS such as superoxide radicals (O_2^-), hydrogen peroxide (H_2O_2), and the hydroxyl radical (OH^-) is a normal cellular occurrence. Small amounts of ROS are required for processes such as sperm hyperactivation and capacitation (de Lamirande and Gagnon, 1993; Ford, 2004). In higher concentrations, ROS may cause sperm cell damage through lipid peroxidation of the plasma membrane, single- and double-stranded DNA breaks (Agarwal and Said, 2003), as well as the induction of germ cell apoptosis (Rao and Shaha, 2000). This may result in detrimental effects on sperm metabolism, morphology, motility, and fertilizing capacity (Alvarez and Storey, 1982; Aitken and Clarkson, 1987; Aitken et al, 1989; Rao et al, 1989). Current evidence suggests that both spermatozoa and WBCs in semen produce ROS, although WBCs produce far more than do sperm. A greater proportion of infertile men demonstrate elevated levels of seminal ROS as compared with populations of fertile men (Iwasaki and Gagnon, 1992; Mazzilli et al, 1994; Agarwal et al, 2003). ROS are constantly inactivated by antioxidant scavengers that break the chain reactions induced by these compounds. Seminal plasma contains significant amounts of antioxidants, and lower levels of these compounds have been reported in semen from infertile men (Chen et al, 2001). The term *oxidative stress* is used to indicate an excess of ROS relative to antioxidant capacity. The balance between ROS production and total antioxidant capacity (TAC) of semen has been measured by an ROS-TAC score (Sharma et al, 1999). It has been suggested that an ROS-TAC score of less than 30 is abnormal and associated with infertility (Agarwal et al, 2003). Although there is clear evidence that ROS are detrimental to sperm function there is no consensus on the indications for ROS testing, and these assays are not yet routinely available.

Genetic Testing

Genetic causes for male infertility include karyotypic abnormalities (structural or numerical chromosomal abnormalities), Y chromosome microdeletions, and gene mutations. Genetic testing consists of karyotype, Y chromosome microdeletion analysis, and specific gene mutation testing. The frequency of abnormal findings for these tests in the general subfertile population is low, but the absence of a positive finding does not rule out the presence of currently unknown genetic abnormalities. Chromosomal abnormalities may involve large or small amounts of chromatin. The karyotype analysis detects both numerical and structural chromosome abnormalities involving large amounts of DNA. Small deletions will not be identified by this technique but require microdeletion analysis. **Approximately 6% of infertile men are found to have chromosome abnormalities detected by karyotype analysis. The prevalence of abnormalities increases as the sperm count decreases. The highest prevalence is found in azoospermic patients, with 10% to 15% of patients demonstrating abnormalities of the karyotype** (Hendry et al, 1975; Chandley, 1979; Retief et al, 1984; Bourrouillou et al, 1985; Bourrouillou et al, 1992). **The prevalence falls to 4% to 5% in oligospermic patients and 1% in normospermic patients** (Matsuda et al, 1992a). This is significantly higher than the approximately 0.4% prevalence of chromosome abnormalities in newborns. Sex chromosomal abnormalities predominate in azoospermic men, whereas autosomal abnormalities predominate in oligospermic men. The most common chromosomal abnormality among azoospermic men is the sex chromosome aneuploidy Klinefelter's syndrome. This is associated with sterility, but testicular sperm that can be utilized for IVF using ICSI are found in approximately 50% of these men (Friedler et al, 2001). Individual counseling of these patients is important because of the medical risks associated with Klinefelter's syndrome, such as breast cancer.

Microdeletions of sections of the long arm of the Y chromosome have been identified in approximately 13% of azoospermic men and 3% to 7% of oligospermic men (Reijo et al, 1995; Nakahori et al, 1996; Seifer et al, 1999). Approximately 7% of infertile men have been found to have Y chromosome microdeletions (Girardi et al, 1997; Pryor et al, 1997; Kleiman et al, 1999). The Y chromosome was first found to be involved with spermatogenesis when in 1976 six azoospermic men were missing the long arm of the Y chromosome on karyotype (Tiepolo and Zuffardi, 1976). The region contained in this arm came to be known as AZF (azoospermia factor). Microdeletion analysis of this region became possible with advances in molecular technology, and the AZF region is now divided into three subregions labeled AZFa, AZFb, and AZFc. A variety of genes have been identified in this region, including testis-specific RNA-binding motifs such as *DAZ* (the deleted in azoospermia gene) (Saxena et al, 1996). In general, the size of the microdeletion in the AZF region is inversely proportional to spermatogenic activity. There also appears to be some prognostic information regarding location of the deletions within the AZF, with large lesions involving AZFa and AZFb carrying a poor prognosis for sperm retrieval for IVF (Hopps et al, 2003). Currently, genetic causes of male infertility are not curable; however, many of these patients are candidates for IVF combined with ICSI. **Patients with either severe oligospermia (less than 5 million sperm/mL) or nonobstructive azoospermia who are considered candidates for the ART should be offered genetic screening with both karyotype and Y chromosome microdeletion analysis.**

Genetic testing also includes mutation analysis of specific genes based on phenotypic suspicion. The most common setting is CBAVD. Mutations of *CFTR*, which is the causative agent of cystic fibrosis, are associated with absence of the vas deferens. The vast majority of males with cystic fibrosis are azoospermic due to absence of the vas deferens. Most men with azoospermia due to CBAVD harbor mild mutations in the *CFTR* gene even though they do not have clinical cystic fibrosis. The carrier rate among partners of northern European extraction is quite high, approximately 1 in 20. Thus, genetic testing and counseling for both partners is important in this clinical setting. It is important to consider the fact that most panels for mutation analysis only test for the most common mutations, and thus a negative test may not be a true negative. A variety of other gene mutations may affect male reproductive function, including sperm motility (Kartagener's syndrome) and endocrine function (androgen insensitivity and Kallmann syndrome) (Maduro et al, 2003). A myriad of genes may affect male fertility and have yet to be described or fully understood. Therefore, it is important to counsel infertile couples that the use of ART may propagate unrecognized genetic abnormalities of the parents into the offspring despite negative testing for the known genetic causes of infertility.

Testicular Biopsy

There are two types of testicular biopsy. The first is a diagnostic testicular biopsy utilized to differentiate obstructive from nonobstructive causes of azoospermia. The second is a testicular biopsy performed to harvest sperm to be used during IVF. **Diagnostic testicular biopsy is performed only on azoospermic patients. Most clinicians perform bilateral testicular biopsy, but in patients with discrepant testicular volume some physicians perform a biopsy on the larger testis only.** Patients with clinical findings that are pathognomonic for either obstruction, such as bilateral absences of the vasa or testicular failure, do not require a testicular biopsy to establish the cause of their azoospermia. Clinical findings pathognomonic for testicular failure include bilateral small testes and/or a markedly elevated serum FSH. Thus, a diagnostic testicular biopsy is only needed in those patients in whom ductal obstruction is suspected based on the presence of a relatively normal serum FSH and testicular volume (Jarow et al, 1989). The other role of testicular biopsy is in the management of patients with nonobstructive azoospermia who are considering sperm retrieval and IVF. In this setting a testicular biopsy may be performed to obtain prognostic information, but this assessment is of limited value because sperm may be found with more extensive dissection in men with all histopathologic types and the presence of sperm on one biopsy does not guarantee finding sperm on future biopsies (Schlegel, 1999). Therefore, one might consider the possibility of cryopreserving sperm for later use in IVF in patients undergoing a diagnostic testicular biopsy. Testicular biopsy is not indicated in patients with oligospermia, because the results will not alter therapy. A biopsy is rarely performed to rule out partial ductal obstruction in patients with severe oligospermia, normal-sized testes, and normal FSH values. Partial ductal obstruction is suggested in these cases if the biopsy specimen demonstrates normal spermatogenesis. The details of the technique of testicular biopsy are discussed at length in Chapter 20.

The interpretation of testicular biopsies is subjective and suffers from a lack of uniformity of the systems of classification. Objective methods to quantify spermatogenesis are reproducible but rarely add to the clinical management and are thus used primarily in research studies (Johnsen, 1970; Silber and Rodriguez-Rigau, 1981). The most commonly employed classification patterns are based on the appearance of spermatogenesis ranging from normal to Sertoli cell–only pattern with maturation arrest and hypospermatogenesis in between. The examination should evaluate the size and

number of seminiferous tubules, the thickness of the seminiferous tubule basement membrane, the relative number and types of germ cells within the seminiferous tubules, the degree of fibrosis in the interstitium, as well as the presence and condition of Leydig cells. Very commonly, more than one pattern is identified in a single biopsy specimen. This has contributed to some of the inconsistencies in classification systems. The following classification scheme is commonly used and clinically practical.

Normal Testes

The bulk of the volume of the normal testis is made up of seminiferous tubules that are separated by a thin layer of loose interstitium-containing Leydig cells, blood vessels, lymphatics, and connective tissue (Fig. 19–9A). Leydig cells are acidophilic, round to polygonal cells found in groups and may contain crystalloids of Reinke. Sertoli cells and spermatogonia line the basement membrane of the seminiferous tubule. The steps of spermatogenesis include mitotic division of the stem cells (spermatogonia), meiotic division of the germ cells (primary and secondary spermatocytes), and spermiogenesis or the development of a spermatozoon (spermatids). Germ cells in all steps of spermatogenesis should be seen within the seminiferous tubules. However, not all tubules contain all stages of spermatogenesis. Unlike most other mammalian testes that exhibit the stages of spermatogenesis in a wave along the tubule, the human has a patchwork pattern. Normal testicular biopsy specimens are found in azoospermic patients with ductal obstruction. However, because there is distal obstruction, overcrowding of the tubule lumens and disorganization are common (Levin, 1979). In addition, the seminiferous tubules become dilated and their walls thickened with long-term obstruction (Jarow et al, 1985).

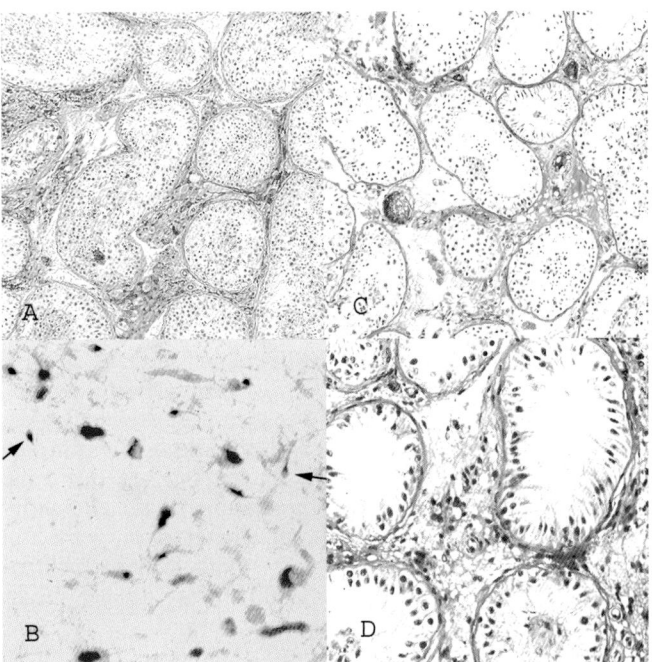

Figure 19–9. Diagnostic findings on testicular biopsy. **A,** Normal. **B,** Normal touch preparation demonstrating mature spermatozoa. **C,** Complete early maturation arrest. **D,** Sertoli cell–only pattern.

Hypospermatogenesis

A reduction in the number of all germinal elements within the seminiferous tubule is present in cases of hypospermatogenesis. Thus, histologic examination reveals thinner layers of germ cells within the seminiferous tubules. The organization of the germinal epithelium may be disrupted, and immature germ cells may be found in the lumen in some instances. The interstitium and Leydig cells are normal. Patients with hypospermatogenesis often have oligospermia but in severe cases may be azoospermic. A certain level of sperm production must be reached before spermatozoa produced by the testis are seen in the ejaculate.

Maturation Arrest

Histologic examination of these testes reveals spermatogenesis proceeding normally through a specific stage at which point no further maturation of germ cells is identified. The arrest may occur at the primary spermatocyte, secondary spermatocyte, or spermatid stage. In a given patient, the block is typically consistent throughout the testis. Cases of late maturation arrest are often difficult to differentiate from normal spermatogenesis without the use of a testicular touch preparation (Kim et al, 1996). Mature spermatozoa are present on a testicular touch preparation in patients with normal spermatogenesis and absent in cases of complete late maturation arrest (see Fig. 19–9B). Patients with complete maturation arrest at any stage exhibit azoospermia, whereas patients with partial maturation arrest have varying degrees of oligospermia. It is common to see a mixture of maturation arrest and hypospermatogenesis in the same testis.

Germ Cell Aplasia

This condition is also known as Sertoli cell–only syndrome. Testicular histology reveals seminiferous tubules containing Sertoli cells with a complete absence of all germ cells. The diameter of the seminiferous tubules is reduced, and the interstitium is usually minimally altered. **Patients with Sertoli cell–only syndrome have small to normal-sized testes associated with normal or elevated levels of FSH** (Turek et al, 1995). There is no effective treatment for this condition. However, many patients with a Sertoli cell–only pattern on a diagnostic biopsy have low levels of spermatogenesis in other areas of the testis. This condition should also be differentiated from end-stage testes, which is a sclerotic testis with some tubules containing only Sertoli cells.

End-Stage Testes

Tubular and peritubular sclerosis is characteristic of an end-stage testis. Germ cells are absent from the sclerotic seminiferous tubules. Sertoli cells may or may not be present. Leydig cells may be absent or decreased in number within the sclerotic interstitium. Clinically, these testes are bilaterally atrophic and firm. A gradual decrease in spermatogenic activity leads to a reduction and disappearance of all germ and Sertoli cells in the testes of patients with Klinefelter's syndrome. Tubular sclerosis and hyalinization usually result. Clumping of Leydig cells may be apparent.

Other Patterns

In cases of hypogonadotropic hypogonadism, seminiferous tubules remain very small, demonstrating an absence of germ cells, with the exception of immature spermatogonia, and Leydig cells. This is the pattern of a 7-month-old fetus. In cases of isolated LH deficiency (fertile eunuchs), normal spermatogenesis or hypospermatogenesis may be present. However, Leydig cell numbers may be reduced. Testicular atrophy, manifested as normal-sized seminiferous tubules with a depletion of germ cells, is found in hypophysectomized adult males who were sexually mature at the time of gonadotropin depletion. Leydig cells may be depleted or absent in these specimens.

The testicular biopsy is rarely pathognomonic of a single etiology. In addition, several patterns may be present in an individual biopsy specimen. Thus, in most cases, a testicular biopsy does not result in the identification of a specific etiologic factor of a patient's infertility.

Percutaneous fine needle aspiration cytology has been used to determine the presence of spermatogenesis (Cohen et al, 1984). This technique may be performed in the office without anesthesia but requires a highly skilled cytologist. The interpretation is similar to that of a testicular touch preparation. Flow cytometry may be combined with fine-needle aspiration, and the ploidy patterns correlated with the state of spermatogenesis (Chan et al, 1984; Kaufman and Nagler, 1987). Although published clinical studies have documented the efficacy of these techniques, the requirement for specialized skills or equipment has limited their popularity.

KEY POINTS: LABORATORY EVALUATION

- After a thorough history and physical examination, almost all patients should have two to three properly collected semen analyses performed.

- Semen analysis is a difficult and subjective test; because of this, the physician should only utilize laboratories proficient in the performance of this test.

- Additional laboratory studies should judiciously be utilized to further define the possible causes of a male infertility factor.

TREATMENT OVERVIEW

Based on the results of the history, physical examination, and laboratory studies, the physician should place the patient into an etiologic category. The clinician is then faced with three potential management options. The first option is to improve the fertility potential of the male partner by either correcting the underlying abnormalities or utilizing empirical therapies. The second is to improve the odds of conception without altering the male partner's fertility status through the use of assisted reproductive technology. The third option is to bypass the male partner completely by utilizing donor sperm or adoption. **We believe that as a general rule, it is preferable to treat the male to improve his fertility status whenever possible rather than ignore the male factor and use high-cost advanced ART, which places the burden of treatment and risk on the female partner for a male problem.** On the other hand, it is often not possible to improve spermatogenesis or attempted treatment may fail. In addition, there may be a concomitant female factor that requires treatment with ART. In these instances it is appropriate to proceed directly to ART. These two management approaches are not mutually exclusive, and some couples may choose to treat the male concurrently with utilization of the ART. This more aggressive approach may be used in the older couple when the female's reproductive potential is diminishing because of age. Finally, couples should be counseled on both donor insemination and adoption as alternatives.

DIAGNOSTIC CATEGORIES

The results of the history, physical examination, and laboratory testing allow the clinician to place the patient into a diagnostic classification. These categories may imply an etiology for the subfertility, although a significant percentage of patients still fall into the idiopathic category.

Endocrine Causes

Endocrine causes of male infertility are often referred to as *pretesticular causes*. Impairment of fertility in these cases is secondary to either hormone deficiency, hormone excess, or receptor abnormality.

Pituitary Disease

Pituitary function may be affected in cases of pituitary surgery, infarction, tumors, radiation, or infectious diseases. Patients with prepubertal onset of pituitary disease are usually diagnosed before a fertility evaluation as a result of growth retardation, delayed puberty, or adrenal and thyroid deficiency. Infertility, erectile dysfunction, visual field disturbances, and severe headaches may be presenting symptoms in the adult male with pituitary tumors. Normal male secondary sexual characteristics are usually present in those patients with postpubertally acquired pituitary disease. Patients with congenital pituitary disease typically undergo adrenarche with development of small amounts of straight pubic hair, unless concomitant adrenal insufficiency exists. The testes are small and soft. In contrast, the testes of patients with acquired primary testicular failure are small and firm, presumably secondary to fibrosis. Plasma testosterone levels are typically low or low normal, and gonadotropin levels are low in most patients with pituitary disease. However, the normal range for gonadotropins, particularly LH, goes quite low. Thus, a normal LH value associated with a very low serum testosterone value should be considered suspicious and further evaluation of the pituitary gonadal axis is required. Most patients with borderline low serum testosterone levels associated with a normal or low LH value ultimately have normal endocrine function on further testing (Sigman and Jarow, 1997a). Evaluation of other pituitary hormones and endocrine functions, adrenal and thyroid, should be performed only if there is clinical evidence of a specific endocrinopathy.

Isolated Hypogonadotropic Hypogonadism

Gonadotropin deficiency may occur in the presence of otherwise normal pituitary function. **This condition may be due to** *Kallmann syndrome* **(congenital hypogonadotropic hypogonadism associated with anosmia) or idiopathic hypogonadotropic hypogonadism.** Kallmann syndrome is a genetically heterogeneous disorder that may be inherited in an X-linked, autosomal dominant or autosomal recessive pattern (Duke et al, 1995; Maya-Nunez et al, 1998). The most prevalent is an X-linked form that maps to the *KAL1* gene that encodes for a neuron adhesion molecule thought to be responsible for guiding migration of LH–releasing hormone-secreting neurons to the medial basal hypothalamus (Dacou-Voutetakis, 1992; Lutz et al, 1993). Complete or partial anosmia is a consistent finding in these patients. Cryptorchidism and gynecomastia are common, and micropenis occurs in approximately 50% of affected males. The primary hormonal defect is a failure of GnRH secretion by the hypothalamus, leading to secondary testicular failure (Hoffman and Crowley, 1982).

Multiple other congenital anomalies such as craniofacial asymmetry, cleft palate, harelip, color blindness, congenital deafness, and renal anomalies may be associated with this syndrome (Danish et al, 1980). A delay in pubertal development is the hallmark of the syndrome and most commonly causes the patient to present for medical evaluation. The diagnosis may occasionally be made in early childhood because of the presence of cryptorchidism or micropenis. As a result of a delay in the androgen-dependent closure of the epiphyseal plates, the length of the arms and legs may be greater than that of the trunk. In addition, the testes are prepubertal, usually being smaller than 2 cm in diameter. In the prepubertal male, differentiating between Kallmann syndrome and delayed sexual maturation can be difficult (Whitcomb and Crowley, 1993). The presence of a family history of Kallmann syndrome or of somatic midline defects such as anosmia may help in the prepubertal diagnosis of Kallmann syndrome.

The first sign of puberty is testicular growth. Thus, if the testes are enlarged, the patient is experiencing delayed puberty rather than hypogonadotropic hypogonadism. Normal males experiencing delayed puberty will demonstrate LH pulses if frequent blood samples are obtained. These pulses are not present in patients with Kallmann syndrome (Boyar et al, 1972). GnRH stimulation testing of these patients results in an absent or blunted rise in gonadotropins. However, repeated GnRH injections prime the pituitary gland, resulting in rises of both gonadotropins. This pattern of response may also be found in prepubertal boys (Snyder et al, 1979). Finally, following doses of 5000 IU of hCG, prepubertal and pubertal boys demonstrate larger rises in testosterone levels than patients with Kallmann syndrome. **Androgen replacement with testosterone is adequate treatment for the virilization of adolescents with Kallmann syndrome. Treatment with exogenous androgens inhibits spermatogenesis; thus, other forms of therapy are necessary when the patient desires fertility.** Prior treatment with androgens does not impair subsequent testicular response to gonadotropin therapy (Ley and Leonard, 1985). Testosterone replacement therapy is currently available in four forms: oral, parenteral, transdermal, and buccal. Androgen therapy has been most commonly given in parenteral form as testosterone enanthate or cypionate owing to decreased cost. Intramuscular injections of 200 mg every other week are usually sufficient to induce full virilization in most patients. Although oral androgens are available as fluoxymesterone and 17-methyltestosterone, they are less potent, owing to erratic absorption and hepatic metabolism, and result in a higher incidence of hepatic abnormalities. Reversible intrahepatic cholestasis resulting in elevations of plasma transaminase, lactate dehydrogenase (LDH), and bilirubin may be noted. Transdermal testosterone by either patch or gel is both effective and has fewer side effects than parenteral administration. The topical forms have less variation in levels from day to day, and polycythemia rarely occurs (Basaria and Dobs, 2003). The major disadvantage is cost. In addition, there has been a significant risk of dermatitis with some of the transdermal patches.

Gonadotropin therapy is required for the initiation of spermatogenesis. Given as 2000 IU subcutaneously three times per week, hCG initiates spermatogenesis in most patients with acquired hypogonadotropic hypogonadism. **However, the completion of spermatogenesis in patients with congenital forms of hypogonadotropic hypogonadism usually requires the addition of FSH.** FSH may be given in the form of human menopausal gonadotropin (hMG), which contains 75 IU of FSH and 75 IU of LH per vial. The alternative to hMG is recombinant human FSH, which has pure FSH activity (Kliesch et al, 1995; Liu et al, 1999). The intramuscular administration of FSH at a dose of 37.5 IU ($^1/_2$ vial) to 75 IU (1 vial) three times per week is most commonly started after 3 to 6 months of hCG therapy and usually results in the completion of spermatogenesis (Finkel et al, 1985). Stimulation of the testes with FSH and LH results in testicular growth, although the final testis volume often remains below normal. Although the semen motility and morphology parameters are usually quite good, oligospermia with counts below 10 million sperm/mL are common. In contrast to patients with idiopathic oligospermia who are often infertile with sperm densities below 20 million/mL, many patients with treated hypogonadotropic hypogonadism are able to conceive despite very low sperm densities (Burris et al, 1988a).

GnRH supplied via intermittent subcutaneous injections or via a pulsatile infusion pump with 90-minute pulses is an alternative to treatment with gonadotropin therapy in patients with hypogonadotropic hypogonadism who have intact pituitary glands. **GnRH therapy is only effective in patients with an intact native pituitary gland because it is ultimately dependent on pituitary secretion of gonadotropins.** Therefore, GnRH therapy is contraindicated in patients with acquired hypogonadotropic hypogonadism due to pituitary tumors, pituitary surgery, or head trauma. Studies have shown that pulsatile infusion is superior to intermittent injections of GnRH (Shargil, 1987), but direct comparison of pulsatile infusion GnRH therapy to gonadotropin therapy has not shown a significant difference to justify the increased expense and inconvenience of GnRH therapy (Liu et al, 1988). Previous therapy with testosterone does not affect subsequent response to therapy (Ley and Leonard, 1985), and the best predictor is baseline testicular volume (Burris et al, 1988b). **We usually use hCG followed by recombinant human FSH as the initial treatment and reserve infusion pump therapy for those patients who do not respond adequately.**

Fertile Eunuch Syndrome

Isolated LH deficiency occurs rarely in patients with normal FSH levels. These men demonstrate a eunuchoid habitus, large testes, and small-volume ejaculates that may contain a few spermatozoa (Faiman et al, 1968). Plasma testosterone and LH levels are low, but FSH levels are within the normal range. Testicular biopsy demonstrates maturation of the germinal epithelium. However, Leydig cells may not be apparent because of insufficient LH stimulation. A rise in serum testosterone after hCG therapy documents normal Leydig function in these patients. Sufficient intratesticular testosterone appears to be produced to support a minimal degree of spermatogenesis. However, inadequate peripheral androgen levels result in a lack of virilization.

Isolated FSH Deficiency

Patients with this rare disorder demonstrate normal virilization, normal LH and testosterone levels, and normal-sized testes. Because of a lack of FSH, oligospermia or azoospermia is present. **Administration of hMG has been shown to effectively stimulate spermatogenesis in these patients** (Al Ansari et al, 1984). Recombinant human FSH is the preferred treatment today.

Other Congenital Syndromes

The Prader-Willi syndrome consists of obesity, hypotonic musculature, mental retardation, small hands and feet, short stature, and hypogonadism. There is a familial tendency. The locus for Prader-Willi syndrome has been mapped to chromosome 15q11-q13. The cause of the syndrome is a deletion or uniparental disomy. The DNA probe PW71 can be utilized to establish the diagnosis (Lerer et al, 1994). Patients with Prader-Willi syndrome have LH and FSH deficiencies due to a lack of GnRH secretion. Treatment is identical to that for Kallmann syndrome. As a result of the multiple anomalies in these patients, however, infertility is often not a clinical problem (Bray et al, 1983). A similar clinical picture is found in patients with Laurence-Moon-Bardet-Biedl syndrome, which consists of hypogonadotropic hypogonadism, retinitis pigmentosa, polydactyly, and hypomnesia.

Androgen Excess

Gonadotropin production is inhibited by negative feedback by both estrogens and androgens at the level of the hypothalamus and pituitary. A hypogonadal state, therefore, may be induced by androgen excess, whether it is due to exogenous sources such as anabolic steroid abuse or to endogenous production, such as a metabolic abnormality or an androgen-producing tumor. **The intratesticular testosterone concentration is 100-fold higher than serum levels owing to local production** (Jarow et al, 2001). Thus, when androgen synthesis takes place in the Leydig cells the seminiferous tubules are normally exposed to extremely high levels of testosterone. Introduction of sex steroids into the circulation from either an extragonadal source or a focal tumor within one testis has an inhibitory effect on spermatogenesis because of the resultant reduction of both intratesticular testosterone and FSH through feedback inhibition on the pituitary gland. **Thus, exogenous testosterone (including anabolic steroids) is a male contraceptive.**

Congenital adrenal hyperplasia is the most common cause of endogenous androgen excess. A congenital deficiency of 21-hydroxylase is the most common of the five enzyme defects responsible for this syndrome. The diagnosis can be established in the first trimester of pregnancy by DNA analysis of biopsies of the chorionic villi (New, 1994). Enzyme defects such as a deficiency of 21-hydroxylase result in a decrease in cortisone synthesis. Pituitary production and secretion of adrenocorticotropic hormone (ACTH) increase owing to the lack of feedback inhibition by cortisol. Elevated levels of ACTH result in hyperstimulation of the adrenal gland and an increased production of adrenal androgens. The resultant serum excess of adrenal androgens has a negative feedback effect on pituitary gonadotropin secretion. These patients often have short stature and may develop precocious puberty. As a result of androgen stimulation, premature enlargement of the penis may occur; however, because of a lack of gonadotropin stimulation, the testes remain small. Basal plasma 17-hydroxyprogesterone levels are often elevated 50 to 200 times above normal levels. In addition, elevated urinary 17-ketosteroid and pregnanetriol levels may occur. Not all patients with this syndrome demonstrate fertility abnormalities. Urban and coworkers (1978) studied 20 patients with CAH who were identified in adulthood. Almost all patients demonstrated normal serum gonadotropin and testosterone levels. Two patients were untreated, and 3 had been poorly treated; however, 4 of these patients had children. Of the 15 treated patients, 8 were able to initiate conception. In some patients, the adrenal androgen production may not be sufficient to interfere with the normal hypothalamic-pituitary-gonadal axis, explaining the fertility of these patients. **Glucocorticoid therapy results in a reduction of ACTH levels, which induces a decrease in peripheral adrenal androgens, thus stimulating endogenous gonadotropin secretion and testicular steroidogenesis.** This approach has been successfully employed in the treatment of men with infertility secondary to CAH (Augarten et al, 1991). Testicular adrenal rest tumors may develop unilaterally or bilaterally in patients with CAH. These tumors often resolve with hormonal therapy (Cutfield et al, 1983). However, patients with 21-hydroxylase deficiency, complicated by adrenal rest tumors, may be permanently infertile due to testicular fibrosis. Men with a partial 21-hydroxylase deficiency may remain undiagnosed into adulthood if there is sufficient glucocorticoid production and the mild elevation of adrenal androgens does not lead to precocious puberty. There have been case reports of infertile men with partial 21-hydroxylase deficiencies; however, most of these men would be expected to be fertile.

Excess androgen production may also occur in patients with either adrenal or testicular tumors. This results in the failure of testicular development when present in prepubertal patients. Tubular and peritubular sclerosis may occur in the postpubertal patient and may be irreversible. Leydig cell tumors are not always evident on physical examination. Therefore, imaging studies of the adrenal gland, either by magnetic resonance imaging or computed tomography and testicular ultrasonography, should be obtained as part of the evaluation of patients with androgen excess.

Estrogen Excess

Peripheral estrogens normally suppress pituitary gonadotropin secretion. A state of secondary testicular failure may be induced by estrogen-secreting tumors in the adrenal cortex or in the testis. Testicular Sertoli cell tumors or interstitial cell (Leydig cell) tumors may produce estrogen. Excess peripheral estrogens may also result from hepatic dysfunction or obesity. **Peripheral adipose tissue contains aromatase, an enzyme that converts androgen into estrogen.** Elevated estrogen levels have been identified in morbidly obese patients; however, not all investigators have confirmed this finding (Hargreave et al, 1988; Jarow et al, 1993). **Erectile dysfunction, gynecomastia, and testicular atrophy may be present in patients with estrogen excess.** Hormonal studies demonstrate low levels of FSH, LH, and testosterone in the presence of elevated serum estrogens. Urinary 17-ketosteroid levels may also be elevated. Treatment is directed at the underlying condition. Some infertile men, particularly those with Klinefelter's syndrome, have a nonspecific imbalance in their testosterone to estradiol ratio. It has been proposed that these individuals' semen parameters improved with aromatase inhibitor therapy, but this observation has not been confirmed with controlled studies (Raman and Schlegel, 2002).

Prolactin Excess

Hyperprolactinemia may be caused by a pituitary tumor, stress, medications, medical illness, or idiopathic causes. **Both erectile dysfunction and male infertility are associated with hyperprolactinemia.** Routine screening of infertile men for hyperprolactinemia has not been shown to be useful (Eggert-Kruse et al, 1991; Sigman and Jarow, 1997a). In patients with prolactin-secreting pituitary adenomas, gonadotropin and testosterone levels are depressed whereas prolactin levels are markedly elevated. A small percentage of men with prolactin-secreting pituitary adenomas have borderline normal serum testosterone levels (Carter et al, 1978; Spark et al, 1982). Men with prolactin-secreting pituitary adenomas are typically diagnosed later in the course of their disease than women and have larger tumors with higher serum prolactin levels. Patients with an elevated prolactin level should undergo imaging of the pituitary gland, preferably magnetic resonance imaging with gadolinium contrast. In addition, because thyrotropin-releasing hormone stimulates prolactin secretion, hypothyroidism should be ruled out. **Although surgery and radiation therapy were used in the past to treat patients with prolactin-secreting pituitary tumors, the vast majority of patients respond to medical therapy.** The two most commonly used agents today are bromocriptine and cabergoline. Cabergoline has replaced bromocriptine since it has fewer side effects, requires less frequent dosing, and is just as effective (De Rosa et al, 1998). Patients with idiopathic hyperprolactinemia are treated with medication as well, which may be withdrawn yearly to determine whether hyperprolactinemia persists (Dollar and Blackwell, 1986; Wang et al, 1987). We do not recommend treatment of patients with isolated mild hyperprolactinemia because, in our experience, this has not resulted in improved spermatogenesis.

Thyroid Abnormalities

Although hyperthyroidism has been associated with male infertility, patients with thyroid disorders rarely present with infertility as their chief complaint (Clyde et al, 1976; Kidd et al, 1979). Despite the high prevalence of thyroid diseases in the general population, male reproductive function in patients with thyroid disease has been the subject of only a few studies. Hyperthyroidism appears to cause alterations in the sex steroid hormone metabolism as well as in spermatogenesis that reverses after restoration of euthyroidism (Abalovich et al, 1999; Krassas et al, 2002). Testicular and pituitary abnormalities as well as elevated levels of circulatory estradiol have been identified in patients with hyperthyroidism. In addition, maturation arrest patterns have been identified on testicular biopsy specimens. Radioiodine therapy for hyperthyroidism or thyroid cancer may cause transient reductions in sperm count and motility, but there appears to be little risk of permanent effects provided that the cumulative dose is less than 14 MBq (Hyer et al, 2002). The effects of hypothyroidism on male reproduction appear to be more subtle than those of hyperthyroidism and reversible. Severe, prolonged hypothyroidism in childhood may be associated with permanent abnormalities in gonadal function. It is extremely rare for a male patient with thyroid disease to present with infertility.

Glucocorticoid Excess

Glucocorticoid excess may suppress LH secretion, resulting in androgen deficiency and testicular dysfunction. Glucocorticoid excess may be secondary to endogenous production as in Cushing's syndrome or secondary to exogenous intake from medical therapy. Hypospermatogenesis or maturation arrest patterns have been found on testicular biopsy specimens of patients with Cushing's syndrome (Gabrilove et al, 1974). However, this is rarely a problem in patients receiving therapeutic dosages of corticosteroids. Therapy is directed at correction of the underlying glucocorticoid abnormality.

Abnormalities of Androgen Action

Androgen abnormalities may involve a deficiency in androgen synthesis, a deficiency in conversion of testosterone to dihydrotestosterone (5α-reductase deficiency) or androgen receptor abnormalities. Both defects in androgen synthesis and 5α-reductase deficiency commonly result in ambiguous genitalia and are therefore discussed in Chapter 128. **The androgen insensitivity syndrome (AIS) is an X-linked genetic disorder caused by mutations in the androgen receptor gene.** The androgen receptor mediates the effects of the androgens testosterone and dihydrotestosterone. **The majority of circulating testosterone is bound to hepatic-derived sex hormone–binding globulin and albumin. Once testosterone reaches a target cell it diffuses into the cytoplasm, where it may remain unchanged, be metabolized into a more active androgen (dihydrotestosterone), aromatized into estradiol, or converted into a weaker androgen.** After activation by androgen binding, the androgen receptor translocates to the nucleus and binds to androgen response elements in the promoter regions of androgen-responsive genes, thereby affecting specific gene transcription. Abnormalities of the androgen receptor result in resistance to androgens proportional to the severity of the defect despite the presence of elevated testosterone levels. **These patients are 46,XY males with phenotypes ranging from pseudohermaphroditism to a normal male phenotype with infertility.** Androgen insensitivity syndromes have been identified in phenotypically normal men with azoospermia and severe oligospermia (Giwercman et al, 2001). **The endocrine findings of patients with partial androgen insensitivity include elevated serum testosterone and LH levels.** FSH levels are typically normal or elevated. Select series have documented partial androgen insensitivity in phenotypically normal infertile men with the

characteristic hormonal pattern described earlier (Aiman et al, 1979; Schulster et al, 1983), but this condition is not found very often in an unselected infertile patient population (Griffin and Wilson, 1980). Moreover, more recent molecular studies of the androgen receptor gene have not found a high incidence of mutations in infertile men (Puscheck et al, 1994). **Because the androgen receptor gene is located on the X chromosome at Xq11-12, this syndrome is inherited as an X-linked recessive trait.** Several investigators have observed expansion of the polymorphic CAG repeat located on exon 1 in infertile men, which purportedly decreases the activity of the androgen receptor (Dowsing et al, 1999; Yoshida et al, 1999). However, other investigators could not reproduce these findings (Dadze et al, 2000). **Androgen receptor abnormalities resulting in partial androgen insensitivity should be suspected in patients with elevated serum testosterone and LH levels but is extremely rare.**

Disorders of Spermatogenesis

Chromosomal Disorders

Klinefelter's Syndrome. The presence of an extra X chromosome is the genetic hallmark of Klinefelter's syndrome. Nondisjunction of the meiotic chromosomes of the gametes of either parent leads to pure Klinefelter's syndrome, whereas nondisjunction during mitotic cell division of the developing embryo leads to mosaicism. This syndrome is identified in 1 of every 600 male births (Paulsen et al, 1968; Nielsen and Wohlert, 1991). **A phenotypic male with small firm testes, gynecomastia, and elevated gonadotropins characterizes the classic form of Klinefelter's syndrome** (Klinefelter et al, 1942). More recent studies have confirmed the presence of testicular atrophy in the vast majority of patients; however, gynecomastia and a female escutcheon pattern may be observed in less than half of patients (Okada et al, 1999). In addition, up to 50% of the patients may have normal testosterone concentrations, although gonadotropins are usually elevated even in these cases (Okada et al, 1999). Although secondary sexual characteristics begin developing at the appropriate time, the completion of puberty is often delayed, at which point eunuchism, gynecomastia, or sexual dysfunction may be noted. Virilization may be complete, and the diagnosis is often delayed until adulthood, when the patient may present with infertility. Mental retardation and various psychiatric disturbances have been identified in some of these patients (Becker et al, 1966; Theilgaard, 1984). Azoospermia is typically present. Seminiferous tubular sclerosis is commonly identified on testicular biopsy, but occasional tubules with Sertoli cells and spermatozoa may be found (Vernaeve et al, 2004). Plasma FSH levels are usually markedly elevated as a result of the severe seminiferous tubular injury, whereas LH levels can be elevated or normal. Total plasma testosterone levels are decreased in 50% to 60% of patients (Paulsen et al, 1968; Okada et al, 1999). The physiologically active free testosterone concentrations are usually decreased. In addition, plasma estradiol levels are usually increased, stimulating increased levels of sex hormone–binding globulin and resulting in a decreased testosterone-to-estrogen ratio, which is believed to be responsible for the gynecomastia observed in these individuals (Chopra et al, 1973; Wang et al, 1975). Barr body analysis provides a quick and reliable screening test, with high sensitivity (82%) and specificity (95%) (Kamischke et al, 2003). **Karyotypes by chromosome analysis in lymphocytes confirms the diagnosis of Klinefelter's syndrome, demonstrating 47,XXY or, less commonly, a mosaic pattern of 46,XY/47,XXY.** Less severe abnormalities are present in patients with the mosaic form of Klinefelter's syndrome and occasional patients are fertile (Foss and Lewis, 1971; Laron et al, 1982). In addition, more than one extra X chromosome may uncommonly occur in this syndrome. There have been many reports of various cancers developing in patients with Klinefelter's syndrome. A 50-fold higher risk of breast cancer development has been reported in these patients (Hultborn et al, 1997). However, not all studies have noted an overall increase in cancer development (Hasle et al, 1995).

There is no therapy to improve spermatogenesis in Klinefelter's syndrome. For the patient with mosaic Klinefelter's syndrome and severe oligospermia, ICSI combined with IVF is a possibility (Harari et al, 1995). Recently, testicular sperm extraction has been performed in patients with azoospermia and nonmosaic Klinefelter's syndrome. Retrieved sperm have been successfully used for IVF with ICSI, resulting in the birth of normal children (Palermo et al, 1998; Reubinoff et al, 1998; Ron-El et al, 1999). There remains concern that the use of spermatozoa from these patients may result in transmission of this karyotypic abnormality to their offspring. Recent studies examining the chromosomal complement of the sperm cells from patients with mosaic and nonmosaic Klinefelter's syndrome have revealed an increased prevalence of abnormal chromosomal complements in sperm from these patients. Interestingly, despite this, the majority of sperm have been found to have normal chromosomal complements, which may account for why the few live births that have been reported have had normal karyotypes (Estop et al, 1998; Foresta et al, 1998; Tachdjian et al, 2003). It is strongly recommended that men with Klinefelter's syndrome undergo genetic counseling, because they have increased medical risks for diseases such as diabetes, cardiovascular disease, and cancer and there is an increased risk for chromosomal abnormalities in their offspring (Lanfranco et al, 2004).

XX Male. Findings similar to those of Klinefelter syndrome's are found in patients with the XX male syndrome (sex reversal syndrome). **These patients demonstrate small firm testes, frequent gynecomastia, small to normal-sized penises, and azoospermia.** Testicular biopsy may demonstrate seminiferous tubule sclerosis, resulting in elevated gonadotropins and decreased testosterone levels (Perez-Palacios et al, 1981). Unlike typical patients with Klinefelter's syndrome, these individuals have shorter than normal average heights, show no higher prevalence of mental deficiency, and have an increased prevalence of hypospadias (de la Chapelle, 1981). **Karyotypes reveal 46,XX chromosomal complements.** Although it has been presumed that portions of the Y chromosome are present, molecular studies have not always demonstrated this. Some patients have been found to have the testis-determining gene *(SRY)*. This has not been demonstrated in all patients (Lopez et al, 1995). Recently the duplication of another Y chromosome gene to an autosome has been identified in an *SRY*-negative XX male (Huang et al, 1999). This demonstrates that XX males are genetically heterogeneous. Because these

patients do not have any of the AZF regions present it is presumed that attempts at sperm retrieval will be unsuccessful, and, as of yet, there have been no reports of sperm being isolated from these patients.

XYY Syndrome. Patients with the XYY syndrome are characteristically tall, and semen analyses typically reveal severe oligospermia or azoospermia. Although this karyotype has been linked to aggressive and criminal behavior (Jacobs et al, 1965; Walzer and Gerald, 1975; Freyne and O'Connor, 1992), the cause for this finding is controversial. Some have believed that these behaviors are secondary to tall stature, which may predispose individuals to these behaviors (Hook, 1973), whereas others have suggested it may be related to lower intelligence (Gotz et al, 1999). The XYY karyotype occurs in 0.1% to 0.4% of newborns (Balodimos et al, 1966; Price et al, 1966; Walzer and Gerald, 1975). As has been found in Klinefelter's syndrome, an increased prevalence of chromosomal abnormalities involving the sex chromosomes has been found in the sperm from these patients (Han et al, 1994; Blanco et al, 1997; Lim et al, 1999). Testicular biopsy specimens reveal patterns ranging from maturation arrest to complete germinal aplasia, as well as occasional cases demonstrating seminiferous tubule sclerosis (Santen et al, 1970; Skakkebaek et al, 1973b; Baghdassarian et al, 1975). Sporadic patients have been fertile (Stenchever and Macintyre, 1969). Plasma gonadotropins and testosterone levels are most often within the normal range in these patients (Lundberg and Wahlstrom, 1970). Elevations of plasma FSH levels may be found in association with more severe patterns of testicular dysfunction. Although there is no treatment to improve spermatogenesis, these patients are candidates for ART. Genetic counseling should be offered before beginning this form of therapy.

Noonan's Syndrome. The phenotypic appearance of patients with this syndrome is similar to that found in Turner's syndrome (XO). Thus, these patients have short stature and demonstrate hypertelorism, webbed neck, low-set ears, cubitus valgus, ptosis, and cardiovascular abnormalities (Collins and Turner, 1973). Chromosomal analysis reveals a 46,XY karyotype. Cryptorchidism and testicular atrophy are commonly present, with associated elevations of gonadotropins. Of interest, females may be affected with this disorder carrying a karyotype of XX and are usually fertile. Although most cases of Noonan's syndrome are sporadic, familial transmission has been reported. In addition, a gene on chromosome 12 has been linked to this defect (Ogata et al, 1998). Although androgens may be given to complete virilization, there is no treatment for the fertility abnormality in these patients.

Y Chromosome Microdeletions. The majority of Y chromosome microdeletions that have been associated with azoospermia or severe oligospermia occur in one of three nonoverlapping regions of the long arm of the Y chromosome designated as AZFa (proximal), AZFb (middle), and AZFc (distal) (Vogt et al, 1996). The vast majority of these deletions occur de novo and are not inherited from the parents. Rare vertical transmission from father to son has been reported (Stuppia et al, 1996; Chang et al, 1999). Although most studies have examined patients with idiopathic azoospermia or severe oligospermia, a 7% prevalence of Y chromosome microdeletions has been reported in patients with nonidiopathic severe male factor infertility (Krausz et al, 1999). Patients with these microdeletions are phenotypically normal, with the only apparent abnormality being a defect in spermatogenesis. There is no strict correlation between the deletion and histologic phenotype on testis biopsy. Patients, with what appear to be similar deleted intervals, may have different testicular histologies. This may be due to the many genes involved in these intervals and the fact that many of the genes are present in multiple copies. **Deletions in AZFc are the most frequently identified microdeletions in azoospermic and severely oligospermic men. The deletion in the azoospermia gene** *(DAZ)* **is thought to be responsible for spermatogenic defects in patients with deletions in this interval.** *DAZ* is expressed exclusively in the testes and seems to produce an RNA-binding protein (Menke et al, 1997; Habermann et al, 1998). Sperm have been reported to be retrieved in over 50% of men with azoospermia and Y chromosome microdeletions limited to AZFc undergoing testicular sperm extraction (Brandell et al, 1998; Silber et al, 1998). **A gene called** *RBMY* **(RNA-binding motif, Y chromosome; also called** *RBM* **for RNA-binding motif) is thought to be the candidate spermatogenic gene in the AZFb region.** There are multiple copies of this gene, which is germ cell specific (Ma et al, 1993; Elliott et al, 1997). This gene produces an RNA-binding protein localized to germ cell nuclei. Some have reported a decreased likelihood of finding sperm on testicular sperm retrieval in patients with AZFb deletions (Brandell et al, 1998), but all authors have not reported this (Ferlin et al, 1999). **It appears that larger deletions involving more than one AZF region are more likely to yield Sertoli cell–only histology and a lower likelihood of sperm retrieval** (Silber et al, 1998; Ferlin et al, 1999). Deletions in AZFa are less common than the other deletions. At least three genes have been identified in this region: *USP9Y* (also known as *DFFRY*), *DBY,* and *UTY.* Recent evidence suggests that most deletions in this region that affect spermatogenesis involve *DBY,* with a lesser number involving *USP9Y.* Deletions limited to *UTY* may not affect spermatogenesis (Foresta et al, 2000). **There is currently no treatment to improve spermatogenesis in patients with Y chromosome microdeletions; however, these patients are candidates for IVF with ICSI.** Sperm from semen may be used in oligospermic patients, whereas attempts at testicular sperm extraction may be employed in azoospermic patients. **It is important to realize that these deletions will be transmitted to male offspring** (Jiang et al, 1999; Page et al, 1999). **Couples in whom the husband has Y-chromosome microdeletions should be offered genetic counseling before embarking on a course of ART** (Sharlip et al, 2002).

Other Chromosomal Abnormalities. Various other chromosomal abnormalities have been identified in infertile patients. These include Robertsonian translocations, ring chromosomes, and isodicentric chromosomes (Plymate et al, 1976; Sarto and Therman, 1976; Chandley, 1979). In addition, testicular biopsy specimens of oligospermic men have demonstrated meiotic abnormalities of the germ cells but with normal peripheral karyotypes (Hulten et al, 1970; Pearson et al, 1970; Skakkebaek et al, 1973a; Koulischer and Schoysman, 1974). Karyotypic abnormalities have been identified in the male partners of women who have recurrent abortions (Blumberg et al, 1982; Fortuny et al, 1988). **Therefore, kary-**

otype analysis should be offered to male partners of women with recurrent miscarriages. Several syndromes with a genetic component are associated with male infertility. Prune belly syndrome is associated with absence of the abdominal wall musculature, cryptorchidism, and urogenital tract abnormalities, and an autosomal dominant inheritance pattern is suggested (Riccardi and Grum, 1977). The Prader-Willi and Laurence-Moon-Biedl syndromes also have a genetic basis and are associated with infertility.

Bilateral Anorchia

Also known as vanishing testis syndrome, bilateral anorchia is found in genetic XY males with nonpalpable testes. Patients demonstrate prepubertal male phenotypes, indicating that testicular tissue, secreting both androgens and müllerian inhibiting substance, must have been present in utero. It is thought that the testes may have been lost in utero secondary to infection, vascular injury, or testicular torsion. Molecular analysis of DNA from these patients has shown no abnormalities in the testis-determining regions of the Y chromosome (*SRY* gene) (Lobaccaro et al, 1993). Low plasma testosterone and elevated gonadotropin levels are present in these males (Aynsley-Green et al, 1976). These patients require exogenous testosterone for virilization at puberty and lifetime maintenance. In the absence of any testicular tissue their infertility is not treatable.

Cryptorchidism

Cryptorchidism is present in 3% to 4% of full-term boys (Scorer and Farrington, 1971). By 1 year of age, 1% to 1.6% of boys demonstrate undescended testes (Scorer and Farrington, 1971; Cryptorchidism..., 1992). After 6 months of age the undescended testis is unlikely to descend on its own. Two thirds of cases are unilateral, whereas one third of cases are bilateral. **Sperm concentrations below 12 to 20 million/mL are found in 50% of patients with bilateral cryptorchidism and in approximately 25% of patients with unilateral cryptorchidism** (Lipshultz, 1976; Lipshultz et al, 1976; Okuyama et al, 1989). Testicular biopsy of the cryptorchid testis reveals decreased numbers of Leydig cells. Within the first 6 months of life, the number of germ cells in the cryptorchid testis is within the normal range; however, the normal increase in germ cell numbers seen in early infancy does not occur. By 2 years of age, 38% of unilateral and bilaterally cryptorchid testes will have lost germ cells. The descended testis, in cases of unilateral cryptorchidism, may also demonstrate abnormalities with lower numbers of germ cells. **In general, there is a direct relationship between testicular position and fertility potential; the higher the cryptorchid testis, the more severe the testicular dysfunction. Absence of germ cells is found in 20% to 40% of inguinal testes in contrast to 90% of intra-abdominal testes** (Hadziselimovic et al, 1984). Both mechanical and hormonal etiologic factors have been suggested to explain the mechanism of cryptorchidism. Increasing evidence points to a defect in the hypothalamic-pituitary-gonadal axis in patients with cryptorchidism (Canlorbe et al, 1974), but underlying testicular abnormalities in both the cryptorchid and the normally descended contralateral testis are frequently seen. It is important to differentiate the cryptorchid testis from both retractile testis, which is caused by a hyperactive cremasteric reflex, and an ectopic testis. The latter two cases are not typically associated with testicular dysfunction. The finding of histologic changes in cryptorchid testis within the first year of life has led to therapy directed at correction of cryptorchidism by 1 to 2 years of age as well as administration of hormonal therapies to restore normal testicular development (Hadziselimovic et al, 1984; Hadziselimovic and Herzog, 1997). Retrospective studies report fertility rates from 78% to 92% in patients with surgically corrected unilateral cryptorchidism (Puri and O'Donnell, 1988; Cendron et al, 1989; Kumar et al, 1989). The fertility rate for men with corrected bilateral cryptorchidism is significantly lower, 30% to 50% (Chilvers et al, 1986).

Testicular Torsion

Testicular torsion occurs most commonly during adolescence with an incidence that has been estimated to be 1 in 4000 males younger than age 25 years (Barada et al, 1989). It is thought that testicular torsion is due to an anatomic abnormality of a narrow mesenteric attachment from the spermatic cord onto the testis. However, there may be an underlying abnormality of these testes as well. **Biopsies of the uninvolved contralateral testis in boys with unilateral testicular torsion suggest the presence of an underlying testicular abnormality that may affect fertility** (Hadziselimovic et al, 1986; Dominguez et al, 1994; Hadziselimovic et al, 1998). In fact, most follow-up studies of patients who had torsion reveal reduced testicular exocrine function even in the uninvolved testis (Thomas et al, 1984; Anderson et al, 1992). The severity of the semen abnormalities appears to be directly related to the duration of testicular torsion. Several investigators had reported abnormalities in the normal contralateral testis of animals undergoing experimental unilateral testicular torsion, suggesting the presence of a humoral factor (Nagler and White, 1982; Heindel et al, 1990). Yet, other investigators fail to identify any abnormality in the contralateral testis even after prolonged torsion in animal models (Turner, 1987). In fact, clinical experience does not support either inherent bilateral testicular abnormalities or a humoral effect adversely affecting the contralateral testis in patients with unilateral torsion since the fertility of adults with prepubertal testicular torsion does not appear to be reduced (Puri et al, 1985). The incidence of testicular torsion is so low and the time so remote from attempted paternity that study of this problem has been close to impossible. Therefore, firm conclusions regarding the role of unilateral testicular torsion in adult male infertility are not available. On the other hand, bilateral testicular torsion is a cause of testicular failure.

Varicocele

A varicocele is an abnormal tortuosity and dilatation of the testicular veins within the spermatic cord. A clinical varicocele exists when these dilated veins are palpable on physical examination, whereas a subclinical varicocele is present when these dilated veins are only detectable by ancillary techniques. Varicoceles are rarely detected before the age of 10, with the prevalence increasing to approximately 15% by early adulthood. In contrast, the prevalence of varicoceles in men presenting with infertility is 20% to 40% (Dubin and Amelar, 1977; Cockett et al, 1979; Aafjes and van der Vijver, 1985; Marks et al, 1986). **The varicocele is the most common correctable cause of male infertility. Approximately 90% of varicoceles are left sided. Whereas most studies report an approximately 10% prevalence of bilateral varicoceles, a few have reported a higher prevalence of bilaterality.** Some studies have reported a significantly higher prevalence of varicoceles in patients with secondary infertility as compared with primary infertility (Gorelick and Goldstein, 1993; Witt and Lipshultz, 1993; Jarow et al, 1996b). Differences in the venous drainage patterns of the right and left testicular veins may account for this left-sided predominance. The left testicular vein normally drains directly into the left renal vein, whereas the right testicular vein drains into the inferior vena cava. In addition, an absence of the venous valves is more commonly found on the left side than on the right (Ahlberg et al, 1966). Finally, the left renal vein may be compressed between the superior mesenteric artery and the aorta. This "nutcracker phenomenon" may result in increased pressure in the left testicular venous system (Coolsaet, 1980). Unilateral right-sided varicoceles are uncommon and raise the possibility of thrombosis or occlusion of the vena cava (as with a right-sided renal tumor with vena caval thrombosis) or situs inversus (Grillo-Lopez, 1971). **Varicoceles due to venous occlusion will not collapse with the patient in the supine position.** The mechanism by which varicoceles affect testicular function remains unclear (Howards, 1995). Intratesticular temperatures decrease by 0.5°C in men without varicoceles when they rise from a supine to a standing position as opposed to an increase of 0.78°C in men with varicoceles (Yamaguchi et al, 1989). In addition, oligospermic patients with varicoceles have been found to have intrascrotal temperatures of 0.6°C higher than oligospermic patients without varicoceles (Zorgniotti and MacLeod, 1973). Other studies have found that elevated intratesticular temperatures are common in oligospermic patients regardless of the cause of the spermatogenic defect (Mieusset et al, 1989). Not all investigators have found an association between higher intratesticular temperatures and varicoceles (Tessler and Krahn, 1966; Stephenson and O'Shaughnessy, 1968).

Other suggested causes for the detrimental effect of varicoceles have included reflux of renal and adrenal metabolites from the renal vein (Comhaire and Vermeulen, 1974), decreased blood flow (Saypol et al, 1981), and hypoxia (Chakraborty et al, 1985). Experimental animal models have demonstrated that following production of unilateral varicoceles, bilateral increases in testicular blood flow and temperature occur. Thus, it may be that an increase in blood flow leads to a secondary increase in testicular temperature, resulting in an impairment of spermatogenesis (Saypol et al, 1981). Subsequent repair of these experimental varicoceles has resulted in a normalization of blood flow and temperature (Green et al, 1984). These data may explain the bilateral effect of unilateral varicoceles. Other factors may influence the effect of varicoceles on spermatogenesis. Several studies have demonstrated that smoking in the presence of a varicocele has a greater adverse effect than either factor alone (Klaiber et al, 1987; Peng et al, 1990). **Varicoceles are associated with smaller ipsilateral testes in both adolescents and adults. In addition, ipsilateral testicular growth is often impaired in adolescents with varicoceles** (Lyon et al, 1982; WHO, 1992b). **Semen samples from infertile men with varicoceles have demonstrated decreased motility in 90% of patients and sperm concentrations less than 20 million sperm/mL in 65%**

of patients. In addition, specific abnormalities in sperm morphology have been described as a stress pattern consisting of increased numbers of amorphous cells and immature germ cells, as well as more than 15% tapered forms (MacLeod, 1965). This pattern is not unique to varicoceles and has been found in infertile patients without varicoceles (Rodriguez-Rigau et al, 1981; Portuondo et al, 1983; Ayodeji and Baker, 1986). Thus, the presence of tapered forms is not adequate to make the diagnosis of a varicocele. Of note, with current utilization of strict morphology, the presence of tapered forms may no longer be noted on the semen analysis report. **Varicocele repair has been demonstrated to result in catch-up growth in adolescents with varicoceles and ipsilateral loss of testicular volume** (Kass and Belman, 1987; Paduch and Niedzielski, 1997). **In addition, an improvement in semen parameters as well as testicular volume has been reported after repair of adolescent varicoceles** (Okuyama et al, 1988). Finally, high fertility rates were found in a small population of adults patients who had undergone varicocele repair as adolescents (Salzhauer et al, 2004). Infertile patients with varicoceles and testicular atrophy have worse semen parameters than those with varicoceles without atrophy (Sigman and Jarow, 1997b). **Varicocele repair should be considered in adolescents with grade II or III varicoceles associated with ipsilateral testicular growth retardation.** Men with large varicoceles tend to have lower sperm counts and motility than those with smaller varicoceles (Steckel et al, 1993; Sigman and Jarow, 1997b). Not all investigators have found a relationship between the size of the varicocele and semen quality (Dubin and Amelar, 1977). **It is quite clear that varicoceles are detrimental to testicular growth and spermatogenesis. However, the majority of men with varicoceles are fertile because the effect is modest or they started with a high spermatogenic potential and remained within the fertile range despite the adverse effect of the varicocele.** Normal gonadotropin and testosterone levels are usually found on hormonal studies, whereas elevations of FSH may be found in some patients (Swerdloff and Walsh, 1975). Abnormal GnRH stimulation tests are often present in both adolescents and subfertile men with varicoceles (Hudson et al, 1981). Although it has been suggested that abnormal GnRH stimulation tests predict an improvement in semen parameters after varicocele repair, a recent study has found no predictive value to this test (O'Brien et al, 2004). Treatment of varicoceles is directed at ligation or occlusion of the dilated testicular veins. Surgical, radiographic, and laparoscopic techniques have been used toward this end and are discussed in depth in a later chapter. Although medical therapy has been proposed, there are no well-designed studies demonstrating a role for this approach (Netto Junior et al, 1984). **Improvement in seminal parameters is demonstrated in approximately 70% of patients after surgical varicocele repair.** Improvements in motility are most common, occurring in 70% of patients, with improved sperm densities in 51% and improved morphology in 44% of patients.

Conception rates have averaged 40% to 50% (Tulloch, 1955; Brown, 1976; Glezerman et al, 1976; Dubin and Amelar, 1977; Cockett et al, 1979; Marks et al, 1986; Marmar and Kim, 1994). Most studies examining the effect of the varicocele on fertility have been uncontrolled. A review of randomized and nonrandomized controlled studies reported an average pregnancy rate of 33% in the varicocele repair group compared with 16% in the control group (Schlegel, 1997). An early study by Nilsson and colleagues (1979) reported no effect of varicocele repair, but this study reported extremely low pregnancy rates in both the treated and nontreated groups, suggesting the presence of significant untreated female factors. Another negative study reported a 29% pregnancy rate in the treatment group and a 25.4% pregnancy rate in the nontreated group over a 12-month observation period (Nieschlag et al, 1998). Of note, the nontreatment arm was not a true control because the spouse's gynecologist was requested to optimize female reproductive functions and the couples were counseled on a regular basis. Two additional prospective randomized studies have reported a significant positive effect of varicocele repair on fertility. Madgar and colleagues (1995) reported a 60% pregnancy rate at 1 year in the treated group as opposed to a 10% pregnancy rate in the nontreated group. After 1 year of observation, varicocele repair was performed on the patients in the nontreatment arm of the study whose partners had not conceived. In this group, a 44% pregnancy rate was reported within 12 months after varicocele repair. A large study by the World Health Organization reported a 1-year pregnancy rate of 34.8% in the treatment group as compared with a 16.7% in the nontreatment group (Hargreave, 1997). The presence of a varicocele alone is not an indication for varicocele repair because the majority of men with varicoceles are fertile. The presence of a clinically detectable varicocele associated with an abnormal semen analysis in an infertile couple is an appropriate indication for treatment after the female partner has been evaluated (Report on varicocele . . . , 2004). Azoospermic patients will generally not obtain normal semen parameters after varicocele repair. However, significant numbers of these patients may develop low sperm densities in their semen after repair (Mehan, 1976; Matthews et al, 1998; Kim ED et al, 1999). Despite this, after surgery most of these patients do not have enough viable sperm in their semen and will still require testicular sperm extraction to proceed with IVF with ICSI (Schlegel and Kaufmann, 2004).

Sertoli Cell–Only Syndrome

The testes of patients with Sertoli cell–only syndrome (SCOS) reveal seminiferous tubules containing Sertoli cells but an absence of germ cells. The term *Sertoli cell only* has been used to describe two histologic patterns. Some have defined idiopathic or pure SCOS as a congenital condition due to a lack of germ cell migration from the yolk sac into the seminiferous cords during embryogenesis. The only difference between these testes and normal testes is the absence of germ cells. A second category with a Sertoli cell–only pattern consists of those cases in which the condition is acquired, due to loss of germ cells. This pattern, also called mixed SCOS, is considered a degenerative form (Anniballo et al, 2000). Numerous differences between the two conditions have been described (Table 19–8). This has gained added significance with reports of successful testicular sperm retrieval in up to 50% of patients with SCOS (Tournaye et al, 1997). Unfortunately, reports of sperm retrieval often do not differentiate between the two types and further studies are needed to determine if the noted differences allow prediction of the success of sperm retrieval. There are various causes of SCOS, with some patients having defined Y chromosome microdeletions

Table 19–8. **Proposed Differences between Pure SCOS and Acquired SCOS**

	Pure (Congenital) SCOS	Mixed (Acquired) SCOS
Cytokeratin	Absent	Present
Telomerase	Absent	May be present
Sertoli cells' morphology	Normal	Abnormal
Basement membranes	Thin (normal)	Thickened or edematous
Hyalinization of tubules	Absent	Often present
Seminiferous tubule size	Normal	Small and variable
Cytoplasmic lipid granules in Sertoli cells	Rare	Common
Immature germ cells found in semen	Never	Possible
Spermatogenesis present in some sections of the testes	Never	Sometimes

or karyotypic abnormalities and others having apparently normal genetic evaluations (Kamp et al, 2001). SCOS has also been associated with cryptorchidism, orchitis, chemotherapy, radiation therapy, or estrogen treatment, but in most patients the condition is idiopathic (Rothman et al, 1982; Talati and Sheikh, 1991). Patients usually present with small- to normal-sized testes and azoospermic semen specimens. Phenotypically, these patients are normally virilized males. Plasma FSH levels are often, but not invariably, elevated because of the absence of germ cells, whereas plasma testosterone and LH levels are normal.

Orchitis

Mumps may be associated with orchitis in 30% of patients, if contracted after puberty. The orchitis is bilateral 10% to 30% of the time (Beard et al, 1977). **Permanent testicular atrophy may develop within several months to several years after infection.** Pathologically, there is intense interstitial edema and mononuclear infiltration (McKendrick and Nishtar, 1966). This may result in atrophy of the seminiferous tubules. Severe bilateral orchitis may result in hypergonadotropic hypogonadism and gynecomastia. The entity has become uncommon since the advent of a mumps vaccine, although it is still a causative agent in developing countries (Casella et al, 1997; Bayasgalan et al, 2004;). A randomized study demonstrated a quick recovery and absence of permanent testicular atrophy with treatment with interferon-α 2b during the orchitis (Ku et al, 1999). Treatment with the long-acting GnRH analog has also been reported effective (Vicari and Mongioi, 1995). Testicular sperm extraction combined with IVF and ICSI may be attempted in patients made azoospermic by mumps orchitis (Lin et al, 1999). Orchitis may also develop in patients with syphilis, gonorrhea, leprosy, and mononucleosis.

Myotonic Dystrophy

Myotonic dystrophy causes myotonia, which is a condition of delayed muscle relaxation after contraction. Patients may also demonstrate posterior subcapsular cataracts, cardiac conduction defects, premature frontal baldness, and mental retardation. Testicular atrophy develops in up to 80% of patients during adulthood (Drucker et al, 1963). Leydig cells

typically are uninvolved, with biopsy specimens demonstrating severe tubular sclerosis. Serum FSH levels are elevated (Mahler and Parizel, 1982). Of interest, before the development of testicular atrophy, some patients with apparently normal semen parameters are sterile. Defects in the ability of sperm from these patients to undergo capacitation and the acrosome reaction have been reported (Hortas et al, 2000). The disease is transmitted as an autosomal dominant trait with variable penetrance. Myotonic dystrophy is due to an expansion in the number of CTG repeats in a protein kinase gene on chromosome 19 (Buxton et al, 1992; Jansen et al, 1994). The severity of the myotonic dystrophy is directly related to the number of repeats. It has been proposed that the higher the number of CTG repeats the greater the likelihood of azoospermia, but this is controversial (Pan et al, 2002; Kunej et al, 2004). There is no therapy to prevent the testicular atrophy in these patients. Preimplantation genetic diagnosis has been applied to embryos from IVF cycles involving men with myotonic dystrophy, to avoid implanting those embryos with the genetic defect (Harper et al, 2002).

Chemotherapy

The majority of chemotherapeutic agents adversely affect spermatogenesis (Parvinen et al, 1984). Cells most susceptible to the adverse effects of chemotherapy are those most actively dividing and consist of spermatogonia and spermatocytes up to the preleptotene stage. The specific combination of drugs used for therapy, the dose administered, and the age of the patient at the time of treatment are the major determinants of the specific effect on the gonads. Studies of large groups of patients who survived cancers in childhood have demonstrated that fertility rates of patients treated with alkylating agents were 60% lower than controls. As single drugs, alkylating agents and procarbazine seem to result in the greatest amount of testicular damage (Waxman, 1983). The use of multidrug chemotherapeutic regimens has made it difficult to determine which specific agents are responsible for specific defects. Permanent sterility occurs in 80% to 100% of patients with Hodgkin's disease treated with MOPP and COPP regimens (Roeser et al, 1978; Kreuser et al, 1987). More recent protocols such as with mitoxantrone (Novantrone), vincristine (Oncovin), vinblastine, and prednisone (NOVP) have resulted in fertility being restored to pretreatment levels in Hodgkin's disease patients (Meistrich et al, 1997). Less severe effects on fertility have also been found after treatment of non-Hodgkin's lymphoma and leukemia, conditions in which less toxic chemotherapeutic regimens are used (Bokemeyer et al, 1994). **During chemotherapy, most patients demonstrate elevations of serum FSH levels that correlate with the development of azoospermia. Those patients in whom FSH levels decline demonstrate a return of spermatogenesis, whereas those in whom FSH levels remain elevated are unlikely to recover** (Kader and Rostom, 1991). Of interest, patients with leukemia and lymphoma often have some degree of spermatogenic impairment before treatment, with Hodgkin's lymphoma patients having the lowest pretreatment semen quality (Lass et al, 1998; Hallak et al, 1999). **Preexisting spermatogenic defects in the contralateral testis are found in 25% of testicular cancer patients** (Berthelsen et al, 1983). These defects tend to be worse than in patients with nontesticular malignancies (Lass et al, 1998). **Although many** patients have transient azoospermia, resumption of spermatogenesis occurs in 50% to 60% of these patients with the use of chemotherapeutic agents such as PVB, PVP-16, and POMP/ACE (Drasga et al, 1983; Hendry et al, 1983; Fossa et al, 1985; Kreuser et al, 1987; Nijman et al, 1987; Rustin et al, 1987). The cumulative dose of cisplatin determines whether spermatogenesis is impaired irreversibly by chemotherapy (Pont and Albrecht, 1997). **With cisplatin-based chemotherapy, most patients will become azoospermic; however, the majority will recover spermatogenesis within 4 years** (Ohl and Sonksen, 1996). **There appears to be no increased risk of birth defects in children born to patients after chemotherapy** (Senturia et al, 1985). Of note, sex chromosomal and autosomal aneuploidy has been noted in human sperm during chemotherapy (Robbins et al, 1997). **Thus, patients should bank sperm before but not during chemotherapy. In addition, contraception should be used during and for a period of time (6 to 24 months) after chemotherapy.** Attempts to protect spermatogenesis during chemotherapy have been disappointing. Downregulation of spermatogenesis with GnRH agonists has not been successful (Johnson et al, 1985; Waxman, 1987; Shetty and Meistrich, 2005). Future attempts may focus on cryopreservation and in-vitro culture of testicular tissue before therapy and germ cell transplantation (Avarbock et al, 1996).

Radiation Exposure

Because of the high rate of cell division, the germinal epithelium is very radiosensitive. Spermatids are more resistant than spermatogonia or spermatocytes. **Leydig cells are reasonably radioresistant; therefore, testosterone levels usually remain normal after radiation exposure.** Serum FSH levels increase after irradiation but may revert to normal after a return of spermatogenesis. Azoospermia usually results from doses of over 65 cGy (Sandeman, 1966; Hahn et al, 1982). After dosages less than 100 cGy, recovery takes 9 to 18 months; with doses of 200 to 300 cGy, recovery may take 30 months; and at dosages of 400 to 600 cGy, more than 5 years may be required for spermatogenesis to return (Rowley et al, 1974). Because radiation directed at the abdomen scatters and affects the testes, most centers use gonadal shielding. Hahn and associates estimated the gonadal exposure at 78 cGy in the presence of gonadal shielding. Sperm counts decreased into the oligospermic range between 1 and 4 months after irradiation. Most men were azoospermic between 2.5 and 7.5 months after irradiation (Hahn et al, 1982). **Semen quality will usually return to baseline within 2 years after radiation therapy for seminoma** (Ohl and Sonksen, 1996). **Approximately one fourth of patients may become permanently infertile from such radiation treatment** (Fossa et al, 1989). **After radiation therapy most patients are advised to avoid conception a minimum of 6 to 24 months. Pregnancies after treatment have revealed no evidence of an increase in the prevalence of congenital anomalies in the offspring of these patients** (Senturia et al, 1985; Nygaard et al, 1991).

Heat

There is human and animal experimental evidence that heat exposure may be detrimental to spermatogenesis (MacLeod and Hotchkiss, 1941). Heat exposure through the use of saunas (Brown-Woodman et al, 1984; Saikhun et al, 1998), hot baths (Lue et al, 2002), or temporary placement of the testes into the inguinal canal during the day (Mieusset et al, 1987) has been shown to have a detrimental effect on semen parameters. A review of publications examining the relationship between fertility and occupations in which heat exposure occurs reported a detrimental effect on sperm morphology and time to conception (Thonneau et al, 1998). Occupations that have been reported to be associated with heat exposure and infertility include bakers, drivers (industrial machinery, taxis, trucks), ceramic oven operators, welders, and workers in submarines (Velez de la Calle et al, 2001). In addition, a dysfunction of testicular thermoregulation has been suggested to occur in paraplegic men in wheelchairs (Brindley, 1982). A very small prospective randomized study found lower sperm counts in those wearing tight underwear as opposed to loose boxer shorts (Tiemessen et al, 1996); however, a larger study has demonstrated no effect (Wang et al, 1997). **We currently recommend men wear whatever underwear they feel comfortable in but avoid the use of saunas, Jacuzzis, or hot tubs while fertility remains an issue.**

Environmental Toxins and Occupational Exposures

Spermatogenesis has been shown to be adversely effected by exposure to lead, mercury, arsenic, hydrocarbons, cadmium, amebicide soil fumigants, as well as 2-bromopropane, a substitute for chlorofluorocarbons (Lancranjan et al, 1975; Toth, 1979; Van Thiel et al, 1979; Lipshultz et al, 1980; Kim Y et al, 1999; De Celis et al, 2000; Telisman et al, 2000). Exposure to a variety of agricultural pesticides has also been linked to impaired semen quality (Swan et al, 2003b). Men with exposure to organic solvents have been reported to have elevated serum FSH levels as compared with unexposed workers (Luderer et al, 2004) as well as impaired semen parameters (Cherry et al, 2001). **Patients thought to have high exposure to heavy metals, such as lead or mercury, should have serum levels measured if possible.** Most controversial is the theory that sperm counts in men are declining over time, and the reason for this decline is prenatal exposure to environmental toxicants (endocrine disruptors) that have estrogenic effects on the embryo (Sharpe and Skakkebaek, 1993). It is suggested that prenatal exposure to endocrine disruptors cause a testicular dysgenesis syndrome leading to increased rates of cryptorchidism, hypospadias, testicular cancer, as well as infertility (Aitken et al, 2004). Recent research has demonstrated that chemicals may act as antiandrogens, inhibitors of steroidogenic pathways as well as estrogens or anti-estrogens (Fisher, 2004). There currently are insufficient data to support or refute this theory, but much research is ongoing.

Drugs, Medications, and Other Gonadotoxins

Drugs. Decreased serum testosterone levels, gynecomastia, a decrease in sperm concentration, and pyospermia have been demonstrated in patients with heavy marijuana use (Harmon and Aliapoulios, 1972; Hembree et al, 1976; Close et al, 1990). Cocaine use has been correlated with decreased sperm counts (Bracken et al, 1990).

Medications. Antihypertensive medications have frequently been associated with sexual dysfunction but, other than erectile dysfunction, most do not affect fertility. However, some have been associated with infertility. Spironolactone, an aldosterone antagonist that has been associated with sexual dysfunction also may be detrimental to semen quality through its antiandrogen activity (Tidd et al, 1978). There is evidence that calcium channel blockers cause a reversible functional defect in sperm, interfering with the ability of sperm to fertilize eggs but otherwise not interfering with sperm production or standard semen analysis parameters (Benoff et al, 1994). Although this effect may be reversible after cessation of the medication (Hershlag et al, 1995), not all investigators have found detrimental effects with calcium channel blockers (Katsoff and Check, 1997). A higher prevalence of epididymal cysts and cryptorchidism has been noted in patients with prenatal exposure to DES (Coscrove et al, 1977). Of significance, follow-up studies of men with prenatal DES exposure have revealed no adverse effects on fertility or sexual function (Wilcox et al, 1995a). Although finasteride at a dose of 5 mg/day for obstructive voiding symptoms causes decreased ejaculate volumes, young men taking 1 mg/day as given for hair loss were found to have no changes in semen parameters (Overstreet et al, 1999). Many common antibiotics have the potential to adversely affect male fertility (Schlegel et al, 1991). Early maturation arrest at the primary spermatocyte stage may be induced by chronic high doses of nitrofurantoin (Nelson and Steinburger, 1952; Nelson and Bunge, 1957), although short-term, low-dose therapy is not likely detrimental. Whereas erythromycin, tetracycline, and gentamicin have the potential to adversely affect fertility, documentation of in-vivo detrimental affects is lacking (Hargreaves et al, 1998). Sulfasalazine treatment for ulcerative colitis induces reversible defects in sperm concentration and motility (Birnie et al, 1981; Toovey et al, 1981). Patients with ulcerative colitis should be treated with 5-aminosalicylic acid, which does not affect semen parameters (Riley et al, 1987). Cimetidine has been found to cause degeneration of germ cells while ranitidine did not (Gill et al, 1991). Long-term use of colchicine in patients with Behçet's disease has been associated with oligospermia, but short-term use in healthy males was not detrimental to semen parameters (Sarica et al, 1995; Haimov-Kochman and Ben Chetrit, 1998). It is unclear if the spermatogenic defects are due to long-term colchicine use or to the underlying disease. The immunosuppressant cyclosporine has been associated with impaired fertility in rats (Srinivas et al, 1998), but human data are lacking. While there has been concern about the effects of the cholesterol lowering hydroxyl-methyl-glutaryl coenzyme A (HMG-CoA) reductase inhibitors ("statins"), physiologic doses in animal studies have not been detrimental to fertility (Niederberger, 2005). Chronic oral as well as intrathecal opioid use has been clearly documented to cause hypogonadotropic hypogonadism, with low serum testosterone and gonadotropins levels (Daniell, 2002; Roberts et al, 2002). Sexual dysfunction is commonly reported in patients using these medications for chronic pain as well as those on methadone maintenance; however, no studies have examined effects of chronic opioid use on fertility.

Alcohol. Both the testes and the liver are directly affected by ethanol. Testicular atrophy is commonly found in chronic alcoholics. Testicular specimens demonstrate peritubular fibrosis and a reduction in the number of germ cells. Free testosterone levels are often decreased, whereas total testosterone levels may be within the normal range secondary to elevated levels of sex hormone–binding globulin. Patients, therefore, may demonstrate erectile dysfunction and gynecomastia as well as a decrease in general virilization (Mendelson et al, 1977). Gonadotropin levels may or may not be increased, because pituitary function may be suppressed. Studies on the acute consumption of alcohol in nonalcoholics demonstrate decreased testosterone levels with ingestion of alcohol (Gordon et al, 1976). No correlation has been found between sperm count or motility and the level of ethanol consumption in groups of infertile men (Marshburn et al, 1989; Dunphy et al, 1991). In addition, the chance of couples conceiving (fecundity) has not been found to be associated with alcohol consumption in men (Goverde et al, 1995; Curtis et al, 1997; Olsen et al, 1997). **Thus, there is no evidence that moderate alcohol consumption impairs male fertility.** Of interest, one study did find an association between female alcohol consumption and fecundity whereas most studies have not (Jensen et al, 1998c).

Cigarettes. **The data on the effect of cigarette smoking on semen parameters and fertility is conflicting; however, increasing evidence suggests detrimental effects.** DNA binding carcinogens from cigarette smoke have been found in spermatozoa of smokers as well as in the embryos formed during IVF cycles using the sperm from these men (Zenzes et al, 1999). The heavy metal cadmium and the toxic alkaloid nicotine are present in increased amounts in the semen of smokers (Zenzes, 2000). Studies have correlated smoking with adverse effects on parameters such as seminal volume, sperm count, motility, morphology, and increased numbers of WBCs in the semen (Evans et al, 1981; Marshburn et al, 1989; Close et al, 1990; Vine et al, 1996; Merino et al, 1998; Chia et al, 2000a). Other studies, however, have found no influence of cigarette smoking on semen parameters (Rodriguez-Rigau et al, 1982; Dikshit et al, 1987; Dunphy et al, 1991; Osser et al, 1992; Goverde et al, 1995). Recent publications have reported increased seminal oxidative stress in smokers (Saleh et al, 2002). Smoking has been found to have an adverse effect on female fecundity, whereas the effects on male fecundity are conflicting (Goverde et al, 1995; Bolumar et al, 1996; Jensen et al, 1998a). A recent robust analysis reported a delay in conception when the male smoked and evidence of a delay in conception when the nonsmoking female was passively exposed to cigarette smoke (Hull et al, 2000). In addition, a decreased success of IVF was reported when the male was a smoker (Zitzmann et al, 2003). Of note, a study by Jensen while finding no adverse effect of current smoking on male fecundity did demonstrate an adverse effect of prenatal smoke exposure on subsequent male fertility in the offspring (Jensen et al, 1998b). We believe the evidence is strong enough that smoking should be considered a risk factor for infertility and patients should be strongly encouraged to discontinue this habit.

Caffeine. It has been suggested that caffeine affects sperm density and shape; this has not been confirmed (Fraser, 1984). Studies examining fecundity have not consistently demonstrated a direct effect of caffeine (Jensen et al, 1998a). Of note, caffeine applied to sperm in vitro results in increased sperm motility. **We do not recommend that our patients eliminate caffeine from their diet.**

Idiopathic Infertility

Despite the advancements in diagnostic methodology, up to 25% of patients exhibit abnormal semen analyses for which no cause can be identified. This condition is referred to as *idiopathic male infertility* and is likely associated with a multitude of causes. Not unexpectedly, semen parameters of these patients demonstrate a wide range of abnormalities. Although often referred to as idiopathic oligospermia, the vast majority of these patients have abnormalities of all semen parameters or oligoasthenoteratospermia (OAT). Isolated abnormalities of sperm concentration, motility, and morphology are much less common (see Table 19–5). History and physical examination are generally unremarkable, and hormonal determinations are typically normal. Patients with mild elevations of FSH levels are also included, because this hormonal abnormality is a result rather than a cause of abnormal spermatogenesis.

In the absence of an identifiable or correctable etiology, patients with idiopathic male infertility are managed with either empirical medical therapy or assisted reproductive technology. A variety of medical therapies have been recommended to treat this group of patients, but, with few exceptions, none of these therapies has been shown to be effective in repeated controlled trials. **A meta-analysis of all controlled studies for idiopathic male infertility has failed to reveal significant efficacy of currently available treatments** (O'Donovan et al, 1993). Yet, because of isolated case reports and small patient series demonstrating efficacy of some of these agents there is continued hope that they may be effective in select subpopulations of men with idiopathic infertility. **There is a significant background pregnancy rate (26%) for untreated couples with abnormal semen parameters independent of treatment** (Collins et al, 1983). Because of the variability in semen analyses as well as the occurrence of treatment-independent pregnancies in couples, placebo-controlled, randomly assigned, double-blinded, crossover studies are required to determine the therapeutic efficacy of empirical medical therapies (Collins et al, 1983).

ART, which offer hope to these patients, are discussed later in the chapter. These techniques include semen processing associated with IUI, IVF, and related technologies as well as micromanipulation of sperm and/or ova. For the majority of patients, initial attempts are directed at improving the quality of semen through treatment of specific abnormalities. **If empirical pharmacologic therapy is going to be used, it should be administered for a minimum of a 3- to 6-month period so that at least one full spermatogenic cycle will be incorporated.** If this is unsuccessful, ART are often employed. In view of the limited efficacy of empirical therapy, many couples proceed with ART alone or a combination of both approaches simultaneously, which emphasizes the need for individualized therapy.

Gonadotropin-Releasing Hormone

Several investigators have tested gonadotropin-releasing hormone therapy for idiopathic oligospermia with disappointing results. LH is normally released by the pituitary gland in a pulsatile fashion. Aulitzky and associates (1988), in an uncontrolled study, selected 14 men with idiopathic infertility who had an abnormal pulse pattern in their LH secretion. They observed an improvement in sperm count in 8, and the partners of 3 became pregnant. Although GnRH therapy is efficacious in the treatment of patients with Kallmann syndrome, two controlled studies failed to find efficacy in patients with idiopathic infertility (Badenoch et al, 1988; Crottaz et al, 1992). Therefore, we do not recommend GnRH therapy in patients with idiopathic infertility owing to its high cost and lack of efficacy.

Gonadotropins

The two gonadotropins FSH and LH stimulate spermatogenesis and steroidogenesis, respectively. Historically, these hormones were only available as hMG and hCG, which were purified from the urine of menopausal and pregnant women, respectively. Now more purified as well as recombinant forms of these gonadotropins are available. Numerous uncontrolled studies have been performed with hCG and significantly less with hMG in men with idiopathic oligospermia. These studies have revealed limited efficacy while the only published controlled study failed to find any efficacy over placebo (Knuth et al, 1987). As with GnRH, these treatments are expensive and of limited efficacy. We do not currently recommend these therapies in men without a demonstrable hormonal abnormality.

Clomiphene Citrate and Tamoxifen

Antiestrogen agents are the most commonly used medical therapy for idiopathic oligospermia. **Antiestrogens increase pituitary gonadotropin secretion by blocking feedback inhibition, thus increasing both serum FSH and LH levels as well as the testicular production of testosterone.** Clomiphene citrate (25 mg/day) is the standard recommended treatment. Higher doses may cause downregulation of the system, although they are occasionally indicated. There are many uncontrolled studies reporting a high percentage of patients with improved semen quality and impressive pregnancy rates among their partners. **However, the majority of investigators have found pregnancy rates lower than 30%.** There have been nine published controlled studies of clomiphene citrate dating back to the early 1970s, and the majority failed to identify any efficacy over placebo (Foss et al, 1973; Paulson, 1979; Rönnberg, 1980; Abel et al, 1982; Micic and Dotlic, 1985; Sokol et al, 1988; WHO, 1992a). Two more recent studies did reveal a positive effect on both sperm counts and pregnancy rates (Wang et al, 1983; Check et al, 1989). Controlled studies using tamoxifen (10 to 20 mg/day) have all had negative results (Willis et al, 1977; Török, 1985; AinMelk et al, 1987; Krause et al, 1992). Antiestrogens are relatively inexpensive and safe oral medications for the treatment for idiopathic male infertility, which explains their popularity. Because their efficacy is in doubt, prolonged courses of empirical therapy should not be used as a substitute for more effective modes of management.

Testolactone

Testolactone is an aromatase inhibitor that has a similar effect to an antiestrogen because it blocks the conversion of testosterone to estradiol. This oral agent is very expensive and has not been widely studied. A single controlled study failed to find a significant effect on fertility over placebo (Clark and Sherins, 1989). There is a theoretical basis to recommend either this agent or antiestrogens in men with low testosterone-estradiol ratios, such as obese men or men with Klinefelter's syndrome, but this has never been formally studied (Raman and Schlegel, 2002).

Androgens

Various androgens have been utilized in the treatment of idiopathic male infertility in one of two protocols: high-dose testosterone rebound therapy and low-dose continuous therapy. In the presence of an intact hypothalamic-pituitary-gonadal axis, the effect of androgen administration is to lower the concentration of testosterone in the testis (Coviello et al, 2004).

Testosterone rebound therapy involves large doses of exogenous testosterone, which are administered parenterally to suppress the activity of the patient's pituitary gland. Suppression of pituitary release of LH, in turn, reduces the intratesticular level of testosterone. The androgen therapy is then stopped in the hope that the system will rebound and improved spermatogenesis will result. There has been only one controlled study of this approach, and it did not demonstrate efficacy (Wang et al, 1983). There is currently no role for testosterone rebound therapy, because there are other methods that are equally good or better and because some patients have persistent azoospermia after treatment.

Low-dose continuous androgen therapy attempts to supplement androgen stimulation of spermatogenesis. Mesterolone is a synthetic androgen widely used in Europe to treat idiopathic male infertility in doses ranging from as low as 2 mg/day up to 150 mg/day. The World Health Organization sponsored a double-blind study of men who received placebo or 75 or 150 mg of mesterolone daily (WHO, 1989). This, as well as four other controlled studies, failed to show a positive effect of this drug on fertility (Aafjes et al, 1983; Wang et al, 1983; Comhaire, 1990; Gerris et al, 1991). **Just as with testosterone rebound therapy, continuous androgen administration has a contraceptive effect on men by lowering intratesticular testosterone concentration and should never be used in the treatment of infertility** (Anderson and Wu, 1996).

Miscellaneous Treatments

A variety of vitamins, nutritional supplements, and anti-inflammatory agents have been used in the empirical therapy for male infertility. Thyroxine, arginine, corticosteroids, antibiotics, zinc, methylxanthines, bromocriptine, and vitamins A, E, and C have all been shown to be of little or no benefit in the treatment of infertile men without evidence of a specific deficiency. Controlled studies of kallikrein, indomethacin, and glutathione have shown mixed results but nothing sufficient to promote their use (Barkay et al, 1984; Glezerman et al, 1993; Lenzi et al, 1993). The basis of therapy for some of these agents is their antioxidant activity. Reactive oxygen species have been shown to be associated with a variety of causes of male infertility as well as sperm chromatin denaturation (Sharma and Agarwal, 1996). Yet, in the absence of evidence that there is an excessive amount of reactive oxygen species and that these systemically administered agents concentrate to a degree necessary within the male reproductive tract, all of these therapies must be considered "empirical" and

have not been shown to be efficacious in controlled studies (Silver et al, 2005).

L-Carnitine is an essential molecule involved in mitochondrial metabolism, controlling the transport of acetyl and acyl groups across the mitochondrial inner membrane. Carnitine and acetylated carnitine are found in high concentrations in the epididymis. Their exact role in the epididymis is unknown, but they are believed to protect against oxidative damage. Both L-carnitine and L-acetyl-carnitine are now available as an over-the-counter nutritional supplement for the treatment of idiopathic male infertility. Studies have not shown a direct relationship between semen L-carnitine levels and fertility or that orally administered carnitine increases levels within the epididymis (Soufir et al, 1984). Uncontrolled studies demonstrate improvement in semen parameters but not fertility (Vitali et al, 1995). There have been two controlled studies of the efficacy of L-carnitine therapy of men with idiopathic infertility. In the first study, men with idiopathic OAT were treated for 2 months with 2 g/day of oral L-carnitine supplementation (Lenzi et al, 2003). Statistically significant seminal improvement could only be achieved by excluding outliers, and fertility was not assessed. In the second placebo-controlled study, 30 men completed 6 months of therapy with a combination of L-carnitine and L-acetyl-carnitine (Lenzi et al, 2004). No statistically significant improvement of semen parameters was observed with therapy, and fertility was not assessed by pregnancy rates. At this time there is little evidence that carnitine therapy has any benefit.

Sperm Delivery Disorders

Ductal Obstruction

Genital duct obstruction is a potentially surgically curable cause of male infertility. Obstruction of the ductal system is found in 7% to 12% of all infertile men and is much more common in azoospermic men (Dubin and Amelar, 1971; Greenberg et al, 1978; Jarow et al, 1989). Obstruction may be bilateral or unilateral and may occur at multiple locations. For instance, concomitant epididymal obstruction may be present in patients with either vasal or ejaculatory duct obstruction, presumably owing to a back-pressure phenomenon (Silber, 1979, 1980). Unilateral ductal obstruction should not adversely affect fertility except when there is a contralateral testicular pathologic process, such as torsion, varicocele, or cryptorchidism. However, unilateral obstruction may be a risk factor for the development of antisperm antibodies. Detection of unilateral ductal obstruction in a patient with oligospermia requires a high degree of clinical suspicion (Matsuda et al, 1992b). The etiology of ductal obstruction may be congenital, because of malformation or absence of ductal structures such as in CBAVD, or acquired secondary to infection, iatrogenic injury, or vasectomy.

Congenital bilateral absence of the vas deferens is the most common cause of obstructive azoospermia in patients who have not undergone elective sterilization (Jarow et al, 1989). Careful physical examination reveals a range of epididymal findings, but the most common finding is the presence of the caput epididymis without the remainder of the epididymis or the vas deferens being present. The seminal vesicles are often absent or hypoplastic in these patients (Goldstein and Schlossberg, 1988). Renal anomalies including agenesis has also been observed in patients with CBAVD (McCallum et al, 2001) but is more common in patients with unilateral vasal agenesis due to wolffian duct anomalies (Mickle et al, 1995; Schlegel et al, 1996). As noted previously, low-volume azoospermic acidic ejaculates are characteristic of these patients. Testicular biopsies generally demonstrate normal spermatogenesis. Surgical treatment with either alloplastic (Belker et al, 1986) or natural spermatoceles (Wen et al, 1993) has resulted in extremely low pregnancy rates of 0 to 4% and is not currently recommended. The development of ICSI for IVF has greatly improved the treatment of couples with infertility due to this condition. Temple-Smith and colleagues (1985) were the first to report a pregnancy after IVF using sperm aspirated from the epididymis of a patient with obstructive azoospermia. Subsequent reports revealed that this same technique could be used in men with obstructive azoospermia due to congenital absence of the vas deferens (Silber et al, 1990). However, the poor fertilization rates achieved using standard IVF with epididymal sperm limited the overall success of this treatment until ICSI was introduced (Schlegel et al, 1995). The epididymis is not the only potential source of sperm in these patients. Sperm retrieval can be achieved by either open surgical or percutaneous aspiration from either the testis or epididymis (Meniru et al, 1997; Dohle et al, 1998). If there is no epididymis or viable epididymal sperm are not identified, testicular biopsy with sperm harvesting may be utilized. **The currently recommended management of couples with infertility due to CBAVD is sperm retrieval combined with IVF using ICSI after appropriate genetic testing and counseling of the couple regarding the risk of cystic fibrosis.**

Bilateral complete ejaculatory duct obstruction has pathognomonic clinical findings of acidic, fructose-negative, low-volume ejaculate azoospermia. The main differential diagnosis for these findings is CBAVD, which can easily be distinguished by the presence of vasa on physical examination. In contrast, the diagnosis of partial ejaculatory duct obstruction is much more difficult to establish. Some authors believe that partial obstruction of the ejaculatory ducts can cause poor motility, poor forward progression, and decreased sperm count (Nagler et al, 2002). However, this is still a controversial diagnosis and further investigation is required (Jarow, 1996c). If partial or unilateral obstruction is suspected because of a low volume ejaculate in an oligospermic patient or, because of a normal volume ejaculate with low motility and poor forward progression, TRUS can be used to identify dilated seminal vesicles. TRUS alone has poor specificity, and more dynamic tests such as seminal vesiculography or chromotubation may be more helpful in patients with suspected ejaculatory duct obstruction (Purohit et al, 2004). The diagnosis of ejaculatory duct obstruction is traditionally established by the combination of testicular biopsy and vasography. However, TRUS is currently the imaging modality of choice for the evaluation of patients with suspected ejaculatory duct obstruction (Belker and Steinbock, 1990). The presence of dilated seminal vesicles is suggestive of ejaculatory duct obstruction, which can then be confirmed by finding numerous sperm in aspirates from the seminal vesicles (Jarow, 1994b). The current standard treatment for ejaculatory duct obstruction is transurethral resection of the ejaculatory ducts (TURED). Balloon dilation of the ejaculatory ducts has been

reported but remains investigational (Jarow and Zagoria, 1995).

Ductal obstruction may also be present in either the epididymis or vas deferens. The most common cause is elective sterilization. Semen volume is typically normal in these patients because the testis and epididymis contribute less than 5% to the ejaculate volume. A variety of biochemical tests have been employed to detect the presence of epididymal constituents such as carnitine in the ejaculate, but have generally not aided in the differentiation of obstructive from nonobstructive azoospermia (Zopfgen et al, 2000). The diagnosis of either vasal or epididymal obstruction is established at the time of scrotal exploration for intended reconstruction in azoospermic patients with intact spermatogenesis documented on a prior testicular biopsy. Patients with epididymal or vasal obstruction can be managed by either surgical reconstruction or sperm retrieval combined with IVF using ICSI (Pavlovich and Schlegel, 1997; Donovan et al, 1998).

Ejaculatory Problems

Any process that interferes with the peristaltic function of the vas deferens and closure of the bladder neck may result in either failure of emission or retrograde ejaculation. Ejaculatory dysfunction should be suspected in any patient with low volume (<1.0 mL) or absent ejaculate and should be distinguished from anorgasmia. Retrograde ejaculation is diagnosed by examining the post-ejaculate urine for sperm. Although exact criteria have not been established for a positive post-ejaculate urinalysis, the finding of greater than 10 to 15 sperm/HPF confirms the presence of retrograde ejaculation. In contrast, sperm will not be present in the urine of a patient with failure of emission, a diagnosis established by clinical suspicion alone.

The causes of ejaculatory dysfunction are divided into anatomic and functional because these categories determine effective management. Patients with retrograde ejaculation due to anatomic causes including bladder neck surgery and transurethral resection of the prostate do not respond to medical therapies. In contrast, patients with ejaculatory dysfunction due to neurologic abnormalities such as diabetes mellitus, multiple sclerosis, and retroperitoneal surgery may respond to medical intervention. **Pharmacologic therapy for retrograde ejaculation is only likely to be effective in patients who do not have surgical changes of the bladder neck and for patients with failure of emission.** Phenylpropanolamine (75 mg bid), ephedrine (25 to 50 mg qid), pseudoephedrine (60 mg qid), and imipramine (25 mg bid) may induce ejaculation secondary to an increase in the sympathetic tone of the internal sphincter and vas deferens. Some patients with failure of seminal emission may be converted to retrograde ejaculation by oral medical sympathomimetic therapy. Medical therapy for ejaculatory dysfunction is administered on a cyclical basis timed to the partner's ovulatory cycle. These medications are more effective if given for a period of at least 7 to 10 days before planned ejaculation, and tolerance may develop if administered continuously over several cycles. Success is unlikely if no effect is observed within 2 weeks of treatment. **Those patients with retrograde ejaculation unresponsive to medical therapy or due to ablation of the bladder neck may be treated by recovery of sperm from the bladder urine combined with IUI (Meacham, 2005;**

Shangold et al, 1990). The urine pH and osmolarity should be optimized for sperm survival in the urine by adjusting the patient's fluid intake and by the administration of sodium bicarbonate (650 mg qid), acetazolamide (250 mg qid) or baking soda (2 tablespoons the night before and 2 hours before ejaculation). This may take several attempts before the best combination is found. Sperm are recovered from the urine by gentle centrifugation and then washed in an appropriate insemination media (Zhao et al, 2004). Deposition of pH-adjusted media into the bladder before ejaculation will lessen the toxic effect of urine and may be used as an adjunct to protect the sperm if the other methods are not successful. Surgical reconstruction of the bladder neck had been attempted in the past (Abrahams et al, 1975), but with the advancement in semen processing techniques, this surgery is not indicated today.

Spinal cord injury (SCI) is a common cause of ejaculatory dysfunction (failure of emission), and these patients rarely respond to oral medical therapy. **Penile vibratory stimulation results in ejaculation in approximately 70% of spinal cord–injured men** (Ohl et al, 1996; Brackett et al, 1998). Although specially designed equipment with specific vibration frequency and amplitudes are available, many practitioners have found good results using readily available vibrators intended for general use. **This approach works best in patients with upper motor neuron lesions such as spinal cord injuries above T10. Patients with spinal cord injuries involving the lower spinal cord or peripheral neural lesions, such as after retroperitoneal surgery, are not likely to respond to vibratory ejaculation.** Predictors for response to penile vibratory stimulation include cervical levels of injury, injury at T1-T6 with at least one reflex present (bulbocavernosus and hip reflexes), and injury at T7-T12 with either both reflexes or only the bulbocavernosus reflex present (Bird et al, 2001). Electroejaculation involves the application of pulsed electrical current applied to the periprostatic plexus with the use of either a rectal probe or needle electrodes. The ejaculation has been successfully induced in patients after spinal cord injury, retroperitoneal lymph node dissections, multiple sclerosis, transverse myelitis, and diabetes mellitus. **Rectal probe ejaculation produces an ejaculation in approximately 75% of patients** (Brindley, 1981; Ohl et al, 1989; Shaban et al, 1988). In spinal cord–injured patients with complete cord lesions, the procedure may be performed in an office setting without anesthesia. However, in patients with incomplete cord lesions, or with intact pelvic sensation, general anesthesia is required (Bennett et al, 1987). **Electroejaculation should be attempted in only those patients who are not candidates for or have failed to respond to penile vibratory stimulation.** The results of electroejaculation may be optimized by simultaneous collection of bladder urine since retrograde ejaculation frequently occurs and by eradication of any urinary tract infections or colonization. Autonomic dysreflexia may occur during either vibratory stimulation or electroejaculation. This occurs primarily in patients with lesions above the T4 level. Pretreatment of these patients with 20 mg of sublingual nifedipine 15 minutes before the procedure will usually allow the procedure to be performed safely (Steinberger et al, 1990).

The typical ejaculate obtained from patients with failure of emission has large numbers of poor quality sperm. Initial studies suggested that the electroejaculation process itself might be harmful to the sperm (Rajasekaran et al, 1994; Sikka et al, 1994). However, more recent studies have not supported this theory and similar quality sperm is obtained after penile vibratory stimulation or regular ejaculation (Witt et al, 1992; Ohl et al, 1994; Hovav et al, 2002). Another potential explanation is testicular changes after spinal cord injury due to either a heat effect or a chronic infection (Hirsch et al, 1991; Elliott et al, 2000). Yet the most likely explanation may be the simplest, that is, stasis within the genital tract due to a lack of peristalsis (Ohl et al, 1999), particularly since there appears to be improvement in semen quality with repeated electroejaculation (Giulini et al, 2004). Pregnancies have been achieved through the combination of penile vibratory stimulation (for patients with spinal cord lesions above T10) or electroejaculation and IUIs on a sporadic basis. However, the majority of couples do not conceive through IUI and require IVF using ICSI (Shieh et al, 2003).

Sperm Function Disorders
Immunologic Infertility

Two approaches have been used for the treatment of immunologically mediated infertility. In the first, an attempt is made to suppress antibody formation. The second approach uses the spermatozoa, with or without semen processing to remove antibodies or select those spermatozoa not bound by antibodies, for the ART.

Corticosteroids have been the most commonly employed medications used to attempt to suppress antisperm antibody formation (Shulman, 1976). Although corticosteroids are effective as suppressants of inflammation, they are not particularly effective as suppressants of antibody formation. Regimens have included high-dose cyclic therapy, in which the male takes the medication for 1 week during each menstrual cycle of the female partner, as well as intermediate- and low-dose, long-term therapy. Changes in antibody titers, semen parameters, and pregnancy rates have been inconsistent (Kremer et al, 1978; Dondero et al, 1979; Haas and Manganiello, 1987; Sharma et al, 1995). Most studies have been uncontrolled and report pregnancy rates of 30% to 40%. A double-blind crossover trial by Hendry using an intermittent intermediate dose regimen reported a 31% pregnancy rate in the corticosteroid-treated group as compared with a less than 10% pregnancy rate in those receiving placebo (Hendry et al, 1990). A double-blind placebo-controlled study by Haas and associates found no effect of corticosteroid therapy on pregnancy rates (Haas and Manganiello, 1987). **It appears that in some patients, corticosteroid treatment may result in improved fertility; however, this does not occur in the majority of patients.** The vast majority of pregnancies have occurred in partners of men with normal sperm densities. The chance of success must be weighed against the possible complications, the most devastating of which is aseptic necrosis of the hip, which appears to be a dose-dependent complication of corticosteroid treatment. Semen processing techniques have not been able to completely remove antibodies from the surface of spermatozoa (Lenzi et al, 1988). Chymotrypsin has been used to digest off the Fc portion from the spermatozoa. Pregnancy rates utilizing chymotrypsin-processed sperm for IUI were higher than when utilizing standard semen processing (Bollendorf et al, 1994). Attempts to select sperm without antibody binding have not been successful. IVF has been used in the management of couples with antisperm antibodies, and decreased fertilization rates have been documented when high levels of antisperm antibodies are present (Lahteenmaki, 1993). ICSI used in conjunction with IVF is a highly effective treatment for these couples (Clarke et al, 1997). With ICSI there is no need to remove antibodies or choose sperm without bound antibodies. While the pregnancy rate per cycle is higher with ICSI than IUI combined with chymotrypsin processing, because of the lower cost a trial of IUI is reasonable before proceeding with ICSI (Check et al, 2004). The advantages and risks of prednisone therapy should be weighed against the chances of pregnancy through IUI or IVF with ICSI. **Although we present the patient the option of corticosteroid treatment, we encourage couples to consider IUI or ICSI if their semen is of adequate quality. For couples wishing to proceed with immunosuppressive therapy, we recommend an intermediate-cyclic corticosteroid regimen such as the one used by Hendry and coworkers (1990).**

Ultrastructural Abnormalities of Sperm

Electron microscopy allows for the identification of ultrastructural abnormalities of spermatozoa. Defects in outer dense fibers, microtubules, mitochondria, connecting piece, and acrosome may be detected (Carbone et al, 1998; Chemes and Rawe, 2003). The flagellum is a common site of abnormalities affecting sperm motility (Turner, 2003). The axoneme normally contains microtubules in a 9 + 2 pattern with inner and outer dynein arms attached to each of the nine outer doublets. Defects in this pattern are commonly found in patients with immotile but viable sperm. **The most common of these defects involves a complete absence of both inner and outer dynein arms.** Other patterns consist of absence of either the inner or outer arms, absence of the radial spokes or abnormal central doublets, or abnormal positions of the microtubules. In addition, in some cases, not all spermatozoa demonstrate the same defects. Complete absence of the axonemal elements is rare. **Ultrastructural axonemal defects are commonly associated with identical defects in the cilia of the respiratory tract. This condition is known as the primary ciliary dyskinesia or immotile cilia syndrome** (Eliasson et al, 1977). This syndrome is heterogeneous and motility may be maintained by some spermatozoa (Sturgess et al, 1979; Jouannet et al, 1983). Chronic sinus infections and bronchiectasis are common in these patients. **When these clinical findings are combined with situs inversus, which is present in 50% of these cases, the patient has Kartagener's syndrome.** Primary ciliary dyskinesia (and Kartagener's syndrome) has an autosomal recessive inheritance pattern. In a minority of these patients, defects in genes that encode components of the dynein arms have been identified (Guichard et al, 2001).

While the axoneme is present throughout the entire flagellum, the fibrous sheath is present only in the principal piece that lies under the plasma membrane and surrounds the outer dense fibers and the axoneme (Eddy et al, 2003). Dysplasia of the fibrous sheath (DFS) is associated with absent or low sperm motility. Both complete and partial forms of DFS occur, with 20% to 30% of sperm being normal in the partial form. Because the affected sperm display thick, short flagella

often with irregular shapes, this condition is often referred to as "stump tail syndrome." Electron microscopy reveals hypertrophy and disorganization of the fibrous sheath (Rawe et al, 2001). Defects of the axoneme are often present as well. Although this condition is thought to have a genetic basis, the specific genes involved have not been identified. Abnormalities in the outer dense fibers have been reported to result in dyskinetic sperm with flagella movement that is not normal (Feneux et al, 1985). Defects in the sperm head have also been identified by electron microscopy. Round-headed sperm (globozoospermia) are characterized by an absence of the acrosome as well as absence of a cytoskeletal protein (calicin). Two types of this condition have been identified. Type I is characterized by a complete absence of the acrosome and acrosomal contents. This is the classic form of this disease in which sperm lack the ability to fertilize human ova. Sperm with the type II defect, referred to as acrosomal hypoplasia, contain remnants of the acrosome and may retain some ability to fertilize ova (Singh, 1992). The inheritance pattern for these conditions remains unclear. Although there have been a few pregnancies reported with ICSI of round-headed spermatozoa, most attempts have failed. Finally, abnormalities of the connecting piece may be identified. Separation of the head from the tail is occasionally seen on the semen analysis wherein headless motile flagella are noted. Although these are often referred to pin-headed sperm, there is no nuclear material attached to the tails and they are more accurately referred to as acephalic sperm. Ultrastructural defects in the region of the junction of the sperm tail to the head have been identified; however, the genetics behind this remain unknown (Toyama et al, 2000). **Although there is no cure for these ultrastructural conditions, the sperm may be used for IVF with ICSI. Caution should be exercised when recommending this treatment in this population because some of these conditions have a genetic basis.**

ASSISTED REPRODUCTIVE TECHNIQUES

Assisted reproductive techniques have become increasingly utilized for the management of infertile couples. These techniques involve the manipulation of sperm or ova or both in an attempt to improve the chance of conception and resultant live birth rates. Most ART are referred to by abbreviations rather than their full descriptive names (Table 19–9). ART is frequently indicated in idiopathic male infertility, unexplained infertility, or in cases in which no therapy is available or has effectively resulted in conception. The range of techniques varies from those that involve only manipulation of sperm to more sophisticated procedures involving the manipulation of sperm, ova, and/or embryos. Fertilization may occur inside the woman (in vivo) or in vitro. Controlled ovarian hyperstimulation, also referred to as superovulation, involves hormonal stimulation of the female to induce the simultaneous development of multiple ova and plays a critical role in most forms of ART. Commonly used medications are clomiphene citrate (an oral medication) or gonadotropins given parenterally (usually subcutaneously). Because of the growth in the number of centers offering ART and the ability to perform IVF with ICSI in cases of severe male factor infertility, there has been a trend to pursue IVF as a first-line therapy. This approach either does not treat the male or ignores simpler,

Table 12–9. Assisted Reproductive Techniques and Abbreviations	
Technique	**Abbreviation**
Intrauterine insemination	IUI
In-vitro fertilization	IVF
Intracytoplasmic sperm injection	ICSI
Microsurgical epididymal sperm aspiration	MESA
Percutaneous sperm aspiration	PESA
Testicular sperm extraction	TESE
Testicular sperm aspiration	TESA

less-expensive management options. Economic analyses of the cost per live birth have not supported this approach (Shin and Honig, 2002). **Varicocele repair has been demonstrated to be more cost effective than IVF with ICSI** (Schlegel, 1997). **Similarly, for patients after vasectomy, vasectomy reversal is more cost effective than IVF with ICSI; for patients who have failed one vasectomy reversal, a repeat vasectomy reversal has been found more cost effective than IVF with ICSI; and for patients with epididymal obstruction, vasoepididymostomy has been demonstrated to be more cost effective than IVF with ICSI** (Kolettis and Thomas, 1997; Pavlovich and Schlegel, 1997; Donovan et al, 1998; Heidenreich et al, 2000). **In addition, IVF as an initial treatment for infertile couples in general is less cost effective than more standard approaches such as IUI** (Van Voorhis et al, 1997; Guzick et al, 1998; Karande et al, 1999; Goverde et al, 2000). These data make it clear that ART should be used in appropriate settings and not as broad cure-all techniques. For many couples in which infertility is due to a mild to moderate male factor, IUI or IVF are viable options. Because of the significantly lower cost of IUI, this is often the initial treatment, and couples failing to conceive may proceed to IVF. If there is reason to believe the sperm may not fertilize ova without assistance, then IVF with ICSI may be the initial treatment. Such cases include severe male factor infertility in which inadequate numbers of motile sperm are available for regular IVF or IUI. In addition, cases with abnormal sperm function testing, such as a zero score on the SPA, may proceed with IVF rather than IUI. If an initial IVF cycle demonstrates fertilization but pregnancy does not ensue, the couple may consider proceeding with IUI in lieu of further IVF cycles.

Semen Processing

Semen must be processed before use for ART. A variety of procedures are used, including simple sperm washing, swim-ups (allowing pelleted sperm to swim up into the supernatant), sedimentation, and centrifugation through density gradients (Pousette et al, 1986; Adeghe, 1987; Pardo et al, 1988; Tanphaichitr et al, 1988; McClure et al, 1989; Joshi et al, 1998). Seminal plasma is removed in all of these procedures, whereas other methods select motile sperm by removing nonmotile sperm and leukocytes.

Intrauterine Insemination

Intrauterine insemination involves using a small catheter to inject processed sperm through the cervix into the uterine cavity. It is hoped that by bypassing the cervical mucus, higher numbers of motile sperm will be able to reach the fallopian tubes, thus increasing the chances of conception. The injection of raw semen is contraindicated because seminal prostaglandins may cause severe uterine cramping and pelvic infection may be induced by bacterial contamination of the seminal fluid. **Male factor infertility, unexplained infertility, cervical mucus abnormalities, and anatomic abnormalities interfering with the deposition of sperm at the cervical os (severe hypospadias, retrograde ejaculation, and in some cases erectile dysfunction) are all indications for IUI.** Female factors such as cervical factor infertility, anatomic abnormalities interfering with vaginal intercourse such as dyspareunia, or psychogenic sexual dysfunction are also indications for IUI. Women undergoing IUI may be allowed to ovulate naturally (natural cycle IUI) or may be given medication to induce maturation of multiple ova (superovulation or controlled ovarian hyperstimulation [COH]). **Natural cycle IUI is indicated primarily in cases in which proper deposition of semen into the vagina is not possible (hypospadias, ejaculatory dysfunction, sexual dysfunction). It is also indicated when using cryopreserved sperm that demonstrated normal semen parameters before cryopreservation. This is the case with donor insemination or the use of sperm cryopreserved before chemotherapy or radiation therapy. Natural cycle insemination is not effective when the male has abnormal semen parameters, but when IUI is combined with COH pregnancy rates are clearly increased** (Cruz et al, 1986; Bolton et al, 1989; Evans et al, 1991; Kirby et al, 1991; Ho et al, 1992; Nulsen et al, 1993; Arici et al, 1994; Ombelet et al, 2003). **Pregnancy rates may increase with increasing motile sperm counts up to 10 to 20 million sperm/mL but appear to plateau beyond that point** (Berg et al, 1997; Centola, 1997). **It is our policy to offer IUI to couples with at least 1 million to 3 million motile sperm after semen processing. Because semen processing has yields of only 10% to 50%, semen samples usually have at least 5 million to 10 million motile sperm before processing.** Complications of IUI include uterine cramping, which is generally self limited, pelvic infections in less than 0.5% of patients, and rare allergic reactions to the insemination media (Corson et al, 1989; Sonenthal et al, 1991). Although the addition of ovulation induction has improved pregnancy rates, it has also resulted in multiple gestations in 15% to 30% of pregnancies. Approximately 80% of multiple gestations involve twins, with approximately 12% involving triplets and 7% involving more than three gestational sacs (Schenker et al, 1981; Dickey et al, 1992). Occasionally, HIV-negative females inquire about conceiving with their HIV-positive male partners. HIV is present in WBCs in semen and free in seminal plasma. Select centers have reported successful IUI after semen processing to remove viral particles. This approach requires the ability to test semen and the processed sperm for the presence of viral RNA. IUI in this setting has gained popularity in Europe with no maternal HIV conversions reported after 4989 IUI cycles resulting in the birth of more than 500 children (Semprini and Fiore, 2004). IVF with ICSI has also been used for these couples. A similar approach has been reported for men with hepatitis C (Garrido et al, 2004). The long-term serologic follow-up of these women is incomplete, and these approaches have not yet become popular in the United States.

In-Vitro Fertilization

IVF has become increasingly used to treat infertile couples, with over 45,000 infants born in the United States in 2002 (CDC, 2004). Most centers utilize gonadotropin COH to recruit multiple oocytes each cycle. Follicular development is monitored ultrasonically, and ova are harvested before ovulation with the use of ultrasound-guided needle aspiration. In-vitro insemination is performed by mixing processed sperm with recovered oocytes. In standard IVF, when fertilization occurs, the developing embryos are incubated for 2 to 3 days in culture and then placed transcervically into the uterus. Only 20% to 30% of transferred embryos will implant and produce clinical pregnancies. Recently, embryos have been cultured for 5 days to transfer them at the blastocyst stage. It appears that implantation rates may be higher with blastocyst transfer as compared with standard day 3 embryo transfer, but fewer embryos survive in culture until day 5 (Gardner et al, 1998). Current evidence suggests no improvement in overall pregnancy rates with this approach, but fewer embryos are transferred, decreasing the risk of multiple gestations (Blake et al, 2004; Kolibianakis et al, 2004). Weakening of the zona pellucida (assisted hatching) has also been used to improve implantation rates, which may benefit a subgroup of IVF patients (De Vos and Van Steirteghem, 2000; Role of assisted hatching . . . , 2004). More than 90% of inseminated oocytes are routinely fertilized when sperm function is normal. However, fertilization rates are reduced significantly when a male factor is present. With IVF combined with ICSI, single sperm are injected into individual ova. This allows for fertilization with extremely low numbers of sperm (Van Steirteghem et al, 1993). IVF with ICSI is indicated in cases of severe male factor infertility, in couples with prior failed or poor fertilization during regular IVF cycles, or in cases in which the sperm demonstrate significant fertilizing ability defects. Clinical pregnancy refers to pregnancies in which at least one gestational sac is present within the uterus, as documented by ultrasonography. This is in contrast to biochemical pregnancies, which may never reach the clinical pregnancy stage. Clinical pregnancy rates should be used when reporting IVF results. The clinical pregnancy rates by IVF and ICSI average 20% to 37% per initiated cycle. There is a significant effect of the female age on pregnancy rates with IVF or ICSI. For instance, the Centers for Disease Control and Prevention's survey for IVF and ICSI cycles in 2002 reported pregnancy rates of 36.9% in women younger than age 35 years and 10.7% in women older than age 40 years (CDC, 2004). It should be realized that pregnancy rates are not live birth rates because not all cycles in which women begin ovarian stimulation result in retrieval of oocytes and transfer of embryos, and miscarriages are common. Among women younger than 34 years of age, miscarriages occur in 14% of cycles whereas the miscarriage rate in women 40 years old is 30%. Current recommendations suggest transferring no more than two to four embryos for IVF or ICSI cycles and even fewer if embryos are transferred at the blastocyst stage (Guidelines . . . , 2004a). Multiple gestations occur in 45% of pregnancies. Although the majority

are twins, 7% are triplet or higher multiple gestations (CDC, 2004).

Sperm Retrieval

IVF with ICSI still requires the presence of viable sperm. In those cases with azoospermia or only nonviable sperm in the semen, sperm retrieval may be considered. This may be employed in patients with either obstructive azoospermia or nonobstructive azoospermia. Both percutaneous and open techniques are currently used. For patients with obstructive azoospermia, sperm may be retrieved from the ductal system or from the testicular parenchyma. In contrast, only testicular sperm retrieval is applicable for patients with nonobstructive azoospermia. Microsurgical epididymal sperm aspiration (MESA) is commonly employed to retrieve sperm out of the ductal system in cases with obstructive azoospermia such as CBAVD (Silber et al, 1988). Some have advocated percutaneous epididymal sperm aspiration (PESA) as a less invasive technique that does not require microsurgical skills (Craft et al, 1995). Pregnancy rates are likely comparable between open and percutaneous sperm retrieval techniques for patients with obstruction; however, many more sperm are retrieved by MESA as opposed to PESA (Sheynkin et al, 1998). Because excess sperm may be cryopreserved and used for subsequent IVF cycles, patients are likely to only need one MESA procedure whereas they may require multiple PESA procedures for subsequent cycles. **In men with obstructive azoospermia, there is no difference in pregnancy rates by ICSI between frozen and fresh epididymal sperm** (Nicopoullos et al, 2004). Other techniques that have been employed for retrieval of sperm in cases of obstructive azoospermia include seminal vesical aspiration and vasal aspiration (Hovatta et al, 1996; Jarow, 1996d). These techniques are limited to those patients with either distal obstruction or anejaculation. Testicular sperm retrieval techniques may be utilized in cases of obstructive as well as nonobstructive azoospermia. **For obstructive azoospermia, there appears to be no significant difference in pregnancy rates regardless of the sperm retrieval technique employed, and sperm are usually retrieved with any of the techniques; however, open techniques tend to retrieve more sperm than percutaneous techniques.** This is not the case for those with nonobstructive azoospermia. **In patients with nonobstructive azoospermia, open surgical testicular sperm extraction techniques retrieve sperm in a greater percent of patients and yield higher numbers of sperm than percutaneous techniques** (Friedler et al, 1997b; Ostad et al, 1998; Schlegel, 1999). Some have found the use of an operating microscope useful to identify larger seminiferous tubules that are more likely to contain sperm in patients with nonobstructive azoospermia. Use of this approach for open testicular sperm extraction resulted in an increase in the percent of patients in which sperm are retrieved from 45% to 63% (Schlegel, 1999). Recent experience suggests this approach is most useful in patients with heterogeneous seminiferous tubule diameter, whereas it may have no advantage over multiple open biopsies in those cases with homogeneous tubule diameter (Tsujimura et al, 2002). **For patients with nonobstructive azoospermia, we recommend open testicular sperm extraction.** Pregnancy rates in cases of nonobstructive azoospermia appear to be less than in cases of obstructive azoospermia (Palermo et al, 1999). It remains unclear whether pregnancy rates are the same for cryopreserved and fresh testicular sperm in cases of nonobstructive azoospermia (Friedler et al, 1997a; De et al, 1998; Habermann et al, 2000). Current data suggest that if motile sperm are identified in the thawed sample, pregnancy rates are likely the same for fresh or frozen testicular sperm (Nicopoullos et al, 2004). For those cases of nonobstructive azoospermia in which no spermatozoa are retrieved, attempts have been made to use elongated spermatids as well as round spermatids. Elongated spermatids have been successfully utilized in several centers. However, the use of round spermatids is controversial because of several unresolved issues. Accurate identification of round spermatids is difficult; there are potential detrimental effects on the embryonic centrosome (possibly impaired oocyte activation) and unknown risks of genetic abnormalities in the offspring (Round spermatid nucleus injection . . . , 2004). Reported pregnancy rates are low, and this approach should be considered experimental (Al Hasani et al, 1999; Ghazzawi et al, 1999; Gianaroli et al, 1999; Prapas et al, 1999; Schoysman et al, 1999; Zech et al, 2000).

Although this technology represents a major advance in the management of the infertile male, it must be remembered that these techniques are relatively new and their long-term safety has yet to be determined. There is evidence of an increase in sex chromosomal abnormalities in children born from ICSI cycles (Tarlatzis and Bili, 2000). Although some studies have reported delayed mental development in children conceived through ICSI, a recent analysis of published data suggests ICSI itself is not a risk factor (Bowen et al, 1998; Sutcliffe et al, 1999; Leslie, 2004). Additional evidence questioning increases in major congenital malformation rates remains highly controversial (Kurinczuk and Bower, 1997; Bonduelle et al, 1998; Hawkins et al, 1999; Givens, 2000). Although these techniques offer the possibility of parenthood to many couples with otherwise untreatable infertility, there remain unresolved issues of safety. The physician must understand the appropriate role of these techniques as well as the potential risks to be able to properly manage these patients.

SUGGESTED READINGS

Agarwal A, Saleh RA, Bedaiwy MA: Role of reactive oxygen species in the pathophysiology of human reproduction. Fertil Steril 2003;79:829-843.
American Urologic Association and the American Society of Reproductive Medicine: Report on the Optimal Evaluation of the Infertile Male, 2001.
American Urologic Association and the American Society of Reproductive Medicine: Report on the Varicocele and Infertility, 2001.
Centers for Disease Control and Prevention: 2002 Assisted Reproductive Technology Success Rates: National Summary and Fertility Clinic Reports (www.cdc.gov/art/art02), 2004.

KEY POINTS: TREATMENT

- There are three options to deal with a male infertility factor:

  Treat the male partner to improve his fertility status.

  Utilize the male's sperm for use in assisted reproductive techniques.

  Bypass the male's gametes through the use of donor sperm or adoption.

- Current technology often allows for paternity for men previously labeled sterile.

- Genetic testing and counseling should be considered in appropriate cases, because genetic factors may impact both the patient and his potential offspring.

- In general, if possible, it is preferable to improve the male's fertility potential and allow the couple to conceive by intercourse.

Collins JA, Wrixon W, Janes LB, Wilson EH: Treatment-independent pregnancy among infertile couples. N Engl J Med 1983;309:1201-1206.
de la Chapelle A: The etiology of maleness in XX men. Hum Genet 1981;58:105-116.
de la Taille A, Rigot JM, Mahe P, et al: Correlation between genito-urinary anomalies, semen analysis and CFTR genotype in patients with congenital bilateral absence of the vas deferens. Br J Urol 1998;81:614-619.
De Rosa M, Colao A, Di Sarno A, et al: Cabergoline treatment rapidly improves gonadal function in hyperprolactinemic males: A comparison with bromocriptine. Eur J Endocrinol 1998;138:286-293.
Dubin L, Amelar RD: Varicocelectomy: 986 cases in a twelve-year study. Urology 1977;10:446-449.
Girardi SK, Mielnik A, Schlegel PN: Submicroscopic deletions in the Y chromosome of infertile men. Hum Reprod 1997;12:1635-1641.
Guzick DS, Overstreet JW, Factor-Litvak P, et al: Sperm morphology, motility, and concentration in fertile and infertile men. N Engl J Med 2001;345:1388-1393.
Honig SC, Lipshultz LI, Jarow J: Significant medical pathology uncovered by a comprehensive male infertility evaluation. Fertil Steril 1994;62:1028-1034.
Jarow JP: Diagnosis and management of ejaculatory duct obstruction. Tech Urol 1996c;2:79-85
Palermo GD, Schlegel PN, Hariprashad JJ, et al: Fertilization and pregnancy outcome with intracytoplasmic sperm injection for azoospermic men. Hum Reprod 1999;14:741-748.
Thonneau P, Marchand S, Tallec A, et al: Incidence and main causes of infertility in a resident population (1,850,000) of three French regions (1988-1989). Hum Reprod 1991;6:811-816.
World Health Organization: WHO Laboratory Manual for the Examination of Human Semen and Sperm-Cervical Mucus Interaction, New York, Cambridge University Press, 1999.

20 Surgical Management of Male Infertility

LARRY I. LIPSHULTZ, MD • ANTHONY J. THOMAS, JR., MD • MOHIT KHERA, MD, MBA, MPH

DIAGNOSTIC PROCEDURES

PROCEDURES TO IMPROVE SPERM PRODUCTION

PROCEDURES TO IMPROVE SPERM DELIVERY

SPERM RETRIEVAL

SURGICAL MANAGEMENT OF EJACULATORY DUCT OBSTRUCTION

TREATMENT OF ANATOMIC, CONGENITAL, AND ORGANIC CAUSES OF INFERTILITY

GENETIC ABNORMALITIES RELATED TO AZOOSPERMIA

IN VITRO FERTILIZATION WITH INTRACYTOPLASMIC SPERM INJECTION

Surgical management of male infertility has advanced significantly during the past 10 years. This improvement in operative intervention is due in part to advancements in assisted reproductive technologies and associated new sperm retrieval techniques, an increased awareness among vasectomized men that they may still have their own biologic offspring after a vasectomy reversal, and a more scientific understanding of the effects of varicoceles on spermatogenesis as well as the introduction of innovative techniques in their surgical repair.

Approximately 12% of men aged 20 to 39 years in the United States have had a vasectomy, making this operation the most commonly performed urologic procedure (Massey et al, 1984; Forste et al, 1995). At least 500,000 vasectomies are performed every year, with 72% of these procedures being performed by a urologist. A study by the National Center for Health Statistics found that 43% of first marriages end in separation or divorce within 15 years; predictably, a large number of men will have had vasectomies and after divorce may change their minds about permanent sterility. **In fact, up to 6% of vasectomized men ultimately will desire a reversal.**

Furthermore, 6% of men who suffer iatrogenic injuries to the vas deferens, such as those associated with a hernia repair, may also require a vasovasostomy (Sheynkin et al, 1998). Thus, vasovasostomy and epididymovasostomy procedures are being performed with increased frequency in the United States. These microsurgical procedures, however, are among the most technically challenging operations performed by urologists and require specialized skills and expertise.

Varicoceles are now recognized as the most surgically correctable cause of male infertility. They are present in 15% of the normal male population and in up to 40% of patients with male infertility (Nagler and Martinis, 1997). **Approximately 70% of patients with secondary infertility have been found to have a varicocele as an underlying cause** (Witt and Lipshultz, 1993). Furthermore, varicocele repair has been shown not only to improve spermatogenesis but also to retard further damage to testicular function, to increase serum testosterone (Kass and Belman, 1987; Cayan et al, 1999), and even to facilitate the return of sperm in the ejaculate of azoospermic men. Numerous studies have shown that when it is indicated, varicocele repair remains the most cost-effective procedure in helping a subfertile man establish a pregnancy (Schlegel, 1997; Penson et al, 2002).

The advancement of assisted reproductive technologies, particularly the introduction of intracytoplasmic sperm injection (ICSI), has revolutionized the field of male infertility and now offers reproductive options to men who could not have initiated a pregnancy just 12 years ago. With the increased popularity and success of assisted reproductive techniques, there has been an increased demand for sperm retrieval procedures. For example, testis biopsy is no longer performed for diagnostic purposes alone but is also used as a therapeutic procedure for sperm retrieval and combined with in vitro fertilization (IVF) and ICSI. Developments in open surgical approaches for sperm retrieval, such as microscopic testicular sperm extraction, have increased the options urologists now have for retrieval of sperm.

Surgical treatments of male infertility can be divided into three main categories: diagnostic procedures, procedures to improve sperm production, and procedures to improve sperm delivery. Diagnostic procedures include testis biopsy, seminal vesicle aspiration, and vasography. Procedures to improve sperm production are mainly focused on varicocele repair. Procedures to improve sperm delivery include vasovasostomy and epididymovasostomy, usually after a vasectomy, as well as surgical treatments of anatomic, congenital, and organic causes of infertility, such as hypospadias repair, electroejaculation for anejaculation, and treatment of Peyronie's disease. These topics are discussed in detail in this chapter.

DIAGNOSTIC PROCEDURES
Indications for Testicular Biopsy

A biopsy of the testis should be performed only when the information obtained will help direct future therapy or enable sperm retrieval. Before a testicular biopsy, the patient should undergo a comprehensive physical examination with particular attention to the size and consistency of the testes and the presence and normalcy of the vas deferens and epididymides. Patients with congenital absence of the vas deferens, normal gonadotropin levels, and normal-sized testes will have normal spermatogenesis on testicular biopsy (Goldstein and Schlossberg, 1988). Therefore, a diagnostic testis biopsy is not indicated in these patients.

Since the introduction of ICSI, a testis biopsy is now indicated for therapeutic as well as for diagnostic purposes. **Azoospermia is usually attributable to one of three causes: obstruction; a complete defect in spermatogenesis; or a defect that is incomplete, having foci of mature sperm.** A diagnostic testicular biopsy is indicated when an azoospermic man has normal levels of follicle-stimulating hormone (FSH) and testes of normal size and consistency. A biopsy in this instance can determine whether a patient's azoospermia is due to obstruction or spermatogenic failure. **Whereas a normal FSH level in an azoospermic patient does not ensure active spermatogenesis, an elevated FSH level is most likely indicative of impaired spermatogenesis. An azoospermic patient with an elevated FSH level, especially if it is combined with bilateral small (<15 cm^3) testes, usually has nonobstructive azoospermia.** Such patients who desire to proceed with attempted sperm retrieval and IVF with ICSI should undergo a testis biopsy for both diagnostic and therapeutic purposes (see the section on sperm retrieval). Taking biopsy specimens from multiple sites or microscopic sperm extraction should be reserved for patients with nonobstructive azoospermia when a physician is actively searching for sperm to be cryopreserved or used fresh for IVF-ICSI.

Results of a single biopsy of one testis may not be indicative of the spermatogenic process in the remainder of that testis or the contralateral testis (Skakkebaek et al, 1973; Kahraman et al, 1996; Yoshida et al, 1997). A study by Kahraman and associates found that if only a single testis had been sampled, successful sperm recovery would be missed in 25% of cases. **Other investigators have shown that the percutaneous testis biopsy with one pass through the testis failed to provide adequate tissue for a correct diagnosis in approximately 8% of patients** (Kessaris et al, 1995). Thus, multiple biopsies or microscopic sperm extraction from *both* testes should be performed in patients with nonobstructive azoospermia.

In the **azoospermic patient in whom an obstruction is highly suspected,** a biopsy can be performed as a separate procedure or combined with corrective surgery. If the testes

are normal and equal in size, a single biopsy of one testis should be sufficient to determine if there is complete spermatogenesis. If there is a discrepancy in size, biopsy of the larger, more normal testis should be performed first, as it is more likely to reveal the most favorable histologic features; the smaller testis can then be tested. An otherwise normal, obstructed testis should reveal active spermatogenesis in any randomly chosen site that is sampled. It is best to choose a site that is least vascular, such as the upper medial portion of the testis.

Open Testicular Biopsy (Diagnostic): Surgical Technique

An open testicular biopsy can be performed with local, spinal, or general anesthesia. **Although local anesthesia with a cord block is effective, one must be cautious not to inadvertently injure the testicular artery or to cause a cord hematoma.** One method that may minimize the chance of injury to an artery or vein in the cord is to isolate the vas deferens medial to the cord structures as if one were going to grasp the vas through the skin for a vasectomy. Instead, once the vas is isolated from the cord, 1 mL of a one-to-one mixture of 1% lidocaine HCl and 0.25% bupivacaine is injected in the skin over the vas with a 30-gauge needle. The needle is then advanced beneath the skin to the area of the vas, and another 1 or 2 mL of the local anesthetic is injected (Fig. 20–1).

The anterior scrotal skin is then stretched over the testis while the testis is lifted up. The position of the epididymis, posterior and lateral, is confirmed. The scrotal skin and tunica vaginalis are then infiltrated with 2 mL of 1% lidocaine with a 30-gauge needle. A 1- to 2-cm transverse incision is made to the parietal tunica vaginalis through the anesthetized region. Hemostasis is achieved by bipolar electrocautery. Held in the grasp of toothed forceps, the tunica vaginalis is then opened with scissors, and the edges are grasped and held apart with two small hemostats or a small self-retaining eyelid retractor. Lidocaine (2 to 3 mL) is dripped onto the exposed tunica albuginea to anesthetize the testicular surface where the biopsy specimen will be taken (Fig. 20–2). The tunica

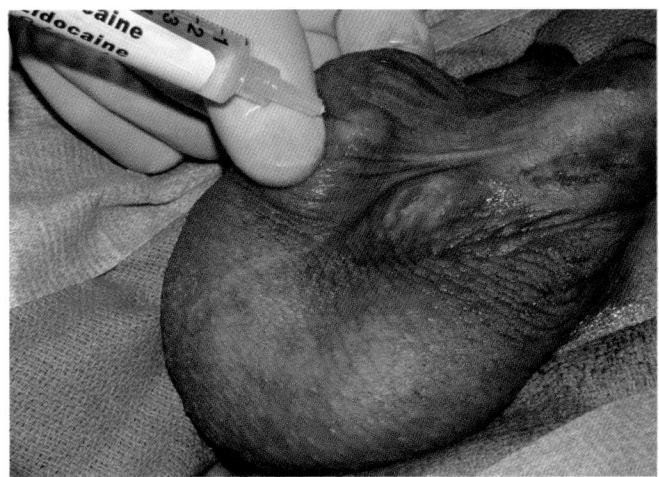

Figure 20–1. Method of skin and perivasal nerve block in preparation for testis biopsy.

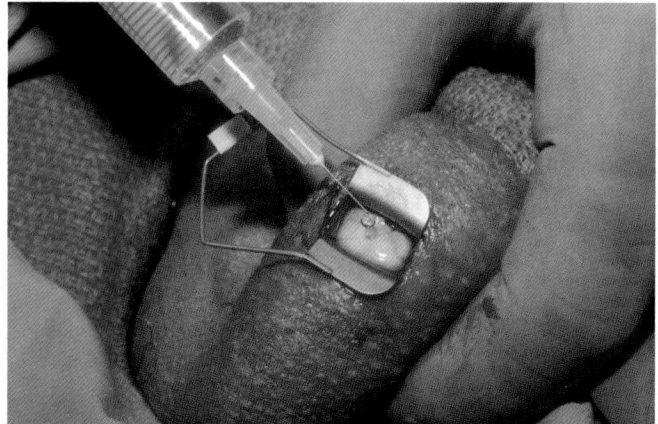

Figure 20–2. Lidocaine HCl (1%) is dripped over the exposed surface of the tunica albuginea before suture placement and incision.

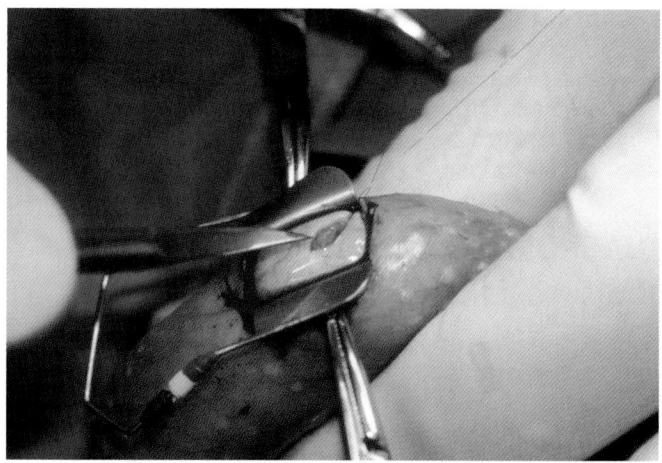

Figure 20–3. A fine iris scissors is used to excise the extruded seminiferous tubules. Forceps are not used to pick up the tissue because they will crush and distort the biopsy specimen.

albuginea is carefully inspected for the least vascular area for the incision. A 5-0 Prolene suture is passed at one end of the proposed site of incision in the testis. It is tied and the tail kept long and tagged with a hemostat. The suture remains intact and will be used to close the incision. The point of the needle end is placed in the needle holder and placed away from the surgical site. A 4- to 5-mm incision is made in the tunica albuginea by use of a No. 11 scalpel or a microknife, allowing extrusion of the seminiferous tubules. Further extrusion of the seminiferous tubules is achieved by applying gentle pressure to the testis. **With the "no-touch" technique, fine, sharp iris scissors are used to carefully excise the extruded tubules** (Fig. 20–3). The specimen is then placed in Zenker's, Bouin's, or buffered glutaraldehyde solution. **The testicular specimen should not be placed in formalin;** this solution will distort the histologic features, making fine detail more difficult to read. If corrective surgery is planned, the status of sperm production should be established immediately. There are several methods for quick identification of mature sperm.

A cytologic smear, or "touch imprint," can be completed at the time of the biopsy to identify the presence of sperm. A sterile microscope slide is blotted onto the cut surface of the testis several times. Alternatively, a second piece of testicular tissue is excised from the biopsy site, and the specimen is gently and repeatedly touched or moved across a sterile microscope slide. The slide is immediately immersed in 95% ethanol or sprayed with a cytofixative solution and then stained with Papanicolaou stain or just simply methylene blue. The cytofixative must be applied to the slide quickly as the cellular architecture becomes distorted if the slide air dries. The specimen is then viewed under the microscope for the presence or absence of sperm with tails.

An intraoperative "wet preparation" can also be employed by placing a small portion of the tissue on a sterile microscope slide covered with a drop or two of normal saline or lactated Ringer's solution. Teasing the tissue apart with a fine forceps or needles as well as covering and compressing it with a coverslip will thin out the tissue for adequate examination (Fig. 20–4). Microscopic examination of the slide can rapidly assess whether sperm are present (Fig. 20–5). It is not uncommon to see some motile sperm.

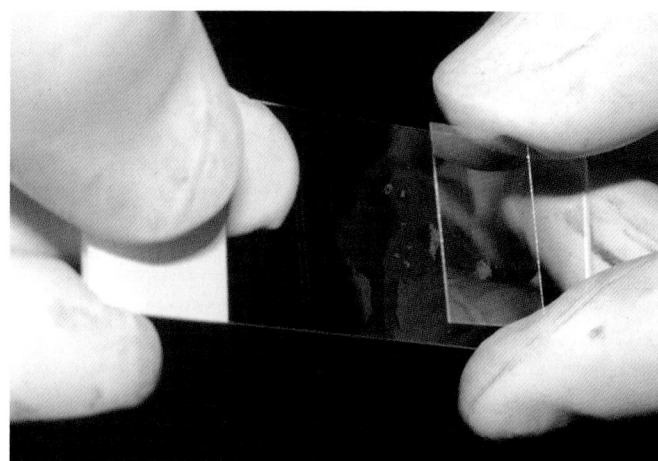

Figure 20–4. Coverslip is pressed firmly over the small piece of testicular tissue to be examined for sperm.

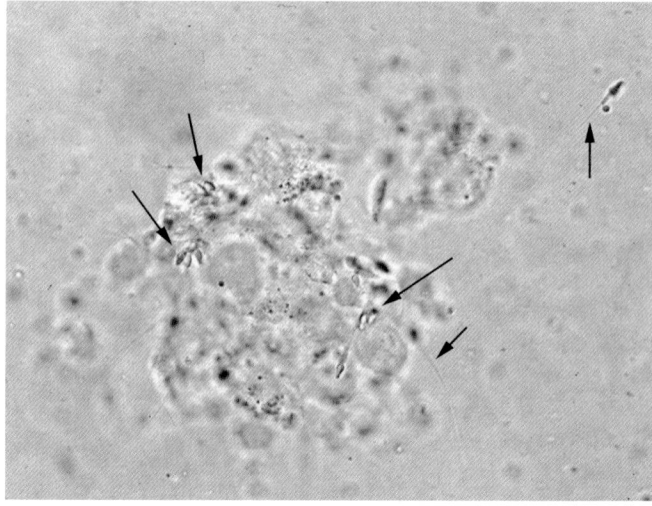

Figure 20–5. Tissue from a testis with normal spermatogenesis readily demonstrates multiple sperm *(arrows)*.

In a comparative study of touch imprint cytology, wet preparation, and testicular histopathology, Kahraman and associates (2001) found that touch imprint cytology was more predictive than wet preparation in the evaluation of spermatogenesis. Kim and colleagues (1996) demonstrated that the **touch imprint is able to differentiate between late spermatids and mature spermatozoa as well as to identify other spermatogenic elements.** These authors concluded that the touch imprint is an extremely important adjunct to the open testis biopsy because of its ability to identify whole sperm quickly and accurately.

If sperm are found and cryopreservation of testicular tissue is to be done, additional testicular tissue can be taken from the same site and placed in appropriate medium in individual Eppendorf tubes for processing by the andrology laboratory.

The incision is then closed with the previously placed 5-0 Prolene suture. The tail of the suture, which was left long and tagged with a hemostat, acts as a "handle" to pull the biopsy site back to the incision if the testis slips or moves during the examination. The use of a nonabsorbable suture minimizes the scarring and adhesion formation to the inner aspect of the tunica vaginalis. **It is important to close the tunica vaginalis over the testis with absorbable suture, such as 4-0 chromic or Vicryl.** Leaving the tunica vaginalis open or turning it around the testis, as with a hydrocele, leads to much more extensive scarring and prolongs the healing phase. Of perhaps greater importance is the degree of difficulty one would have in reoperating in the scrotum if this were necessary. Similarly, the dartos muscle should be approximated with an absorbable suture separate from the skin. A simple subcuticular skin closure is performed, and light gauze dressing and a scrotal support are applied.

Percutaneous Testicular Biopsy

Percutaneous testicular biopsy can be performed with local anesthesia in an office-based setting, and it is generally associated with less pain and morbidity than an open testicular biopsy. However, this technique has several potential disadvantages, including an increased risk of injury to the testicular artery or epididymis due to the blind insertion of the biopsy needle and the fact that a needle biopsy offers fewer seminiferous tubules for examination. A study by Kessaris and associates (1995), however, demonstrated a high correlation between percutaneous and open surgical biopsy specimens. A 95% correlation was described between percutaneous needle and open biopsy techniques in 24 testes when both techniques were applied. **Because the percutaneous testis biopsy may be performed in an office setting and, if done properly, correlates with open biopsy results, it is useful as a diagnostic tool, as long as sufficient material is available for a proper diagnosis to be made.** In men with obstructive azoospermia and normal spermatogenesis, this technique can also be used for sperm retrieval for ICSI. **Patients who have previously undergone scrotal surgery and have extensive scarring are probably not good candidates for this procedure because of the increased risk of inadvertent cord or epididymal injury.**

The Biopty gun, used for prostate biopsies, offers an effective and simplified means of obtaining a testis needle biopsy specimen. Before the biopsy is performed, the skin is punctured with a scalpel to prevent inclusion of scrotal skin with the specimen. To avoid injury to the epididymis and the surgeon's hand, the point of the needle insertion should be from the lower pole toward the upper pole (Fig. 20–6).

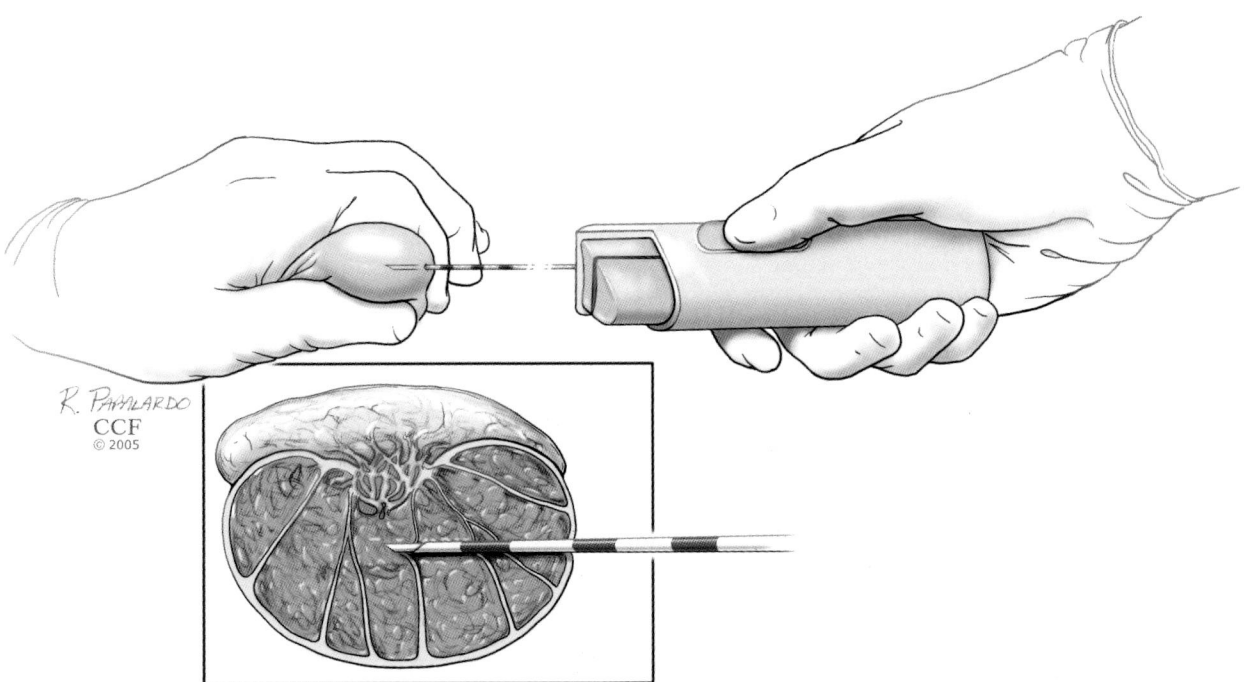

Figure 20–6. Biopsy needle is inserted from the lower pole toward the upper pole, keeping both the epididymis and the surgeon's fingers well away from the point of the needle.

Testicular Sperm Aspiration

Fine-needle aspiration of the testis is the least invasive and least painful technique possible for sperm retrieval. **However, this procedure provides only cytologic, not histologic, information about the testis.** It involves insertion of a 21- to 23-gauge needle into the testis and aspiration with a 10- to 20-mL syringe. **It is recommended that at least three separate sites be aspirated because of the heterogeneity of the testis and the small amount of material that is obtained.** Gottschalk-Sabag and colleagues (1995) demonstrated that fine-needle aspirates taken from three different sites in 13 patients had a wide deviation in cytologic results from each of the different sites.

Nevertheless, fine-needle aspiration is slowly gaining acceptance because of its accuracy in assessing different histologic patterns in the testis. A study by Meng and coworkers (2001) demonstrated that when 87 men underwent both diagnostic fine-needle aspiration mapping and open testis biopsy, there was a 94% correlation between biopsy specimen results. **Others have used fine-needle aspiration testis mapping as an adjunct to open testicular biopsy to help locate sperm** (Turek et al, 1997, 2000; Meng et al, 2000).

Complications

The most common complications after testis biopsy are bleeding and formation of hematomas (Beierdorffer and Schirren, 1979). In general, this problem is related to a missed, cut vessel in the dartos muscle or the tunica vaginalis. A hematocele can form if the tunica albuginea is not hemostatically closed. Testicular atrophy is, fortunately, a rare complication of testis biopsy but has been reported. Dardashti and colleagues reported a scrotal hematoma requiring surgical drainage in 3 of 119 patients and testicular atrophy in 1 of 119 patients (Dardashti et al, 2000). The investigators performed an additional 107 testis biopsies using a microscope and did not encounter any complications with postoperative testicular atrophy or scrotal hematoma. The authors concluded that **the use of an operating microscope for testicular biopsy makes it possible to identify and to avoid testicular vessels and thus minimize complications.**

Inadvertent biopsy of the epididymis has also been reported as a complication of open biopsy. This is more likely to occur when the patient has previously undergone scrotal surgery or has had inflammation, either of which can distort the testis and associated structures. **If the position of the epididymis and cord is at all difficult to identify, it is best to deliver the testis from the scrotum before entering the tunica vaginalis so that the important structures can be palpated or visualized and avoided.**

PROCEDURES TO IMPROVE SPERM PRODUCTION

Varicocele Repair

Varicoceles are present in 15% of the normal male population and in up to 40% of patients with male infertility (Nagler and Martinis, 1997). **In approximately 70% of patients with secondary infertility, a varicocele is an under-**lying cause (Witt and Lipshultz, 1993). In a series of 9034 infertile men, **the World Health Organization reported that varicoceles were found in 25.4% of men with abnormal semen parameters compared with 11.7% of men with normal semen** (World Health Organization, 1992). **The World Health Organization concluded that varicoceles are clearly associated with impairment of testicular function and infertility.**

Varicoceles have been associated with impaired semen quality and decreased Leydig cell function, and this impairment has been shown to be progressive in nature. However, varicocele repairs have been shown to improve not only spermatogenesis but also Leydig cell function (Dubin and Amelar, 1977; Su et al, 1995). A varicocele is now recognized as the most surgically correctable cause of male infertility, and a varicocele repair is the most commonly performed surgical procedure in treatment of male infertility.

Diagnosis

Patients with a varicocele should undergo a detailed medical and reproductive history, a physical examination, and at least two semen analyses. The physical examination is the most important part of the diagnosis and should be performed with the patient in both the recumbent and standing positions. The examination is best performed if the patient is relaxed and the scrotum is warm. There are three grades of varicoceles (Table 20–1). Grade I varicoceles are palpable only with the Valsalva maneuver. Grade II varicoceles are large enough to be palpably detected without the Valsalva maneuver. Grade III varicoceles are visible through the scrotal skin when the patient is at rest.

The success of a varicocele repair depends in part on the preoperative grade of the varicocele. **The larger the varicocele, the more likely that it is associated with impairment in semen quality. Repair of larger varicoceles results in significantly greater improvement in semen quality than does repair of smaller varicoceles** (Steckel et al, 1993; Jarow et al, 1996).

The diagnosis of varicoceles can also be achieved radiographically, but the physical examination remains the "gold standard." Radiographic tests such as real-time scrotal ultrasonography and color Doppler ultrasonography, spermatic venography, radionuclide scanning, and thermography have been used to diagnose varicoceles. **Typically, an ultrasound examination demonstrating veins 3.5 mm or larger in diameter, with reversal of venous flow after the Valsalva maneuver, is consistent with the diagnosis of a varicocele** (Figs. 20-7 and 20-8) (McClure and Hricak, 1986; Hoekstra and Witt, 1995).

Subclinical varicoceles are those that are not palpable or suspected on physical examination but are diagnosed radiographically. The need to treat subclinical varicoceles and the

Table 20–1.	**Grading of Varicoceles**
Grade	*Findings*
I (small)	Palpable only with the Valsalva maneuver
II (moderate)	Palpable without the Valsalva maneuver
III (large)	Visible through the scrotal skin

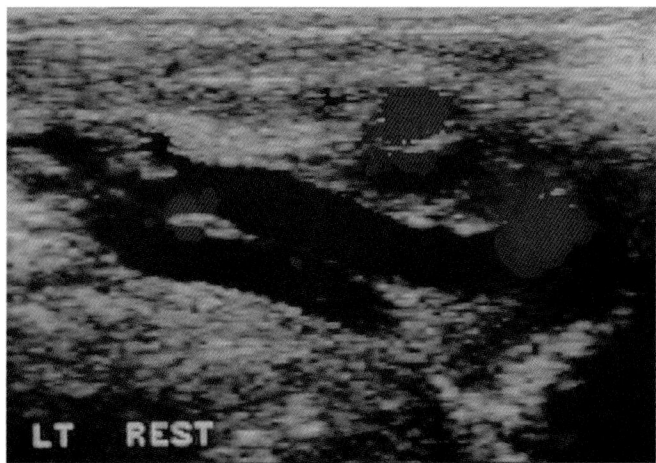

Figure 20–7. Dilated testicular vein at rest.

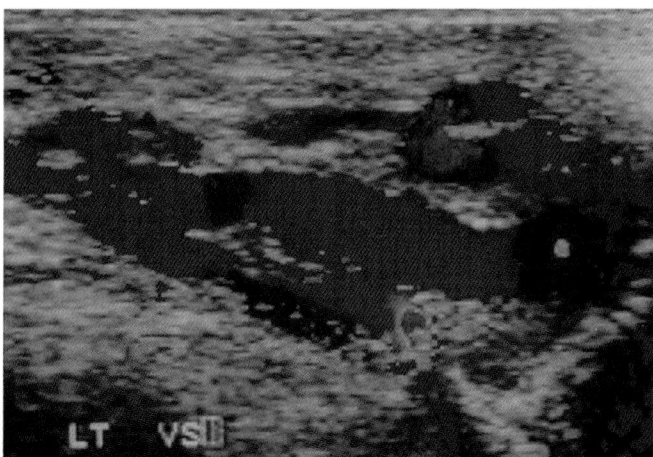

Figure 20–8. Reversal of flow seen in varicocele during Valsalva maneuver.

direct effect these vascular lesions have on male infertility have been debated. **Studies have demonstrated that subclinical varicoceles have no impact on fertility and that repair of subclinical varicoceles does not improve fertility rates** (Jarow et al, 1996). The other concern with the radiographic diagnosis of varicoceles is that untrained radiologists can go past the small tenuous valves in the proximal internal spermatic vein and describe a false positive. **Therefore, radiographic testing to diagnose varicoceles should be used only when the presence of a varicocele is uncertain on physical examination or recurrence is suspected or persistent.**

Indications for Treatment

An infertile adult man with a varicocele should be considered a candidate for a varicocele repair if all of the following four conditions are met: the couple has known infertility; the female partner has normal fertility or a potentially treatable cause of infertility; the varicocele is palpable on physical examination, or if it is suspected, the varicocele is corroborated by ultrasound examination; and the male partner has an abnormal semen analysis (Report on Varicocele and Infertility, 2004). Adult men with a varico-

cele and abnormal semen parameters who may wish to conceive not now but in the future could also be considered for a varicocele repair.

Adolescent men with varicoceles should be presumed to be candidates for a varicocele repair if there is a reduction in volume of the ipsilateral testis. If there is no reduction in ipsilateral testicular volume, these young men can be observed with annual physical examinations or a semen analysis if they are psychosexually mature.

Surgical Approaches

Scrotal Approach. The scrotal approach was one of the first used for varicocele repairs. Early techniques involved external clamping of varicoceles as well as radical resection of the scrotum, as first described by Hartmann in 1904 (Noske and Weidner, 1999). **The scrotal approach has now become virtually obsolete because of the increased risk of injury to the testicular artery and the high rate of failure related to the complexity of the scrotal pampiniform plexus.** In the scrotum, the pampiniform plexus has multiple sites of division and a complex anastomotic network that makes a successful repair extremely challenging.

Retroperitoneal Approach. Palomo (1948) was one of the first to describe high ligation of the entire spermatic cord above the internal inguinal ring. The retroperitoneal approach involves ligation of the internal spermatic vein as it exits the inguinal canal and preservation of the internal spermatic artery.

A transverse abdominal incision is made at the level of the internal inguinal ring, approximately two fingerbreadths medial to the anterior superior iliac spine (Fig. 20–9). The incision is carried down to the external oblique aponeurosis, which is incised in the direction of its fibers. The internal oblique muscle is bluntly split and the transversus abdominis muscle incised. The peritoneum is reflected medially, and the muscles are retracted cephalad to expose the internal spermatic vessels. The internal spermatic vein is then ligated and divided, proximal to its insertion into the left renal vein. To more easily identify and ligate any collateral vessels, the dissection may be carried cephalad toward the left renal vein. Some surgeons have advocated the use of intraoperative venography to better delineate these collateral vessels.

A common complication of the retroperitoneal approach is varicocele recurrence or persistence, estimated to be between 11% and 15% (Homonnai et al, 1980; Rothman et al, 1981; Niedzielski and Paduch, 2001). **A possible explanation for varicocele recurrence is that this approach does not allow ligation of the external gonadal (cremasteric) vessels, which have been thought to cause recurrent or persistent varicoceles** (Sayfan et al, 1980; Murray et al, 1986). The recurrence rate with this approach is higher in children than in adults, and is estimated to be between 15% and 45% (Gorenstein et al, 1986; Levitt et al, 1987; Reitelman et al, 1987; Lemack et al, 1998; Minevich et al, 1998). However, Kass and Marcol (1992) reported that in children and adolescents, the recurrence can be significantly reduced by intentional ligation of the testicular artery. This is thought to ensure ligation of the periarterial veins and thus to prevent recurrence.

Laparoscopic Approach. The laparoscopic varicocele repair, which should be performed by an experienced laparoscopic

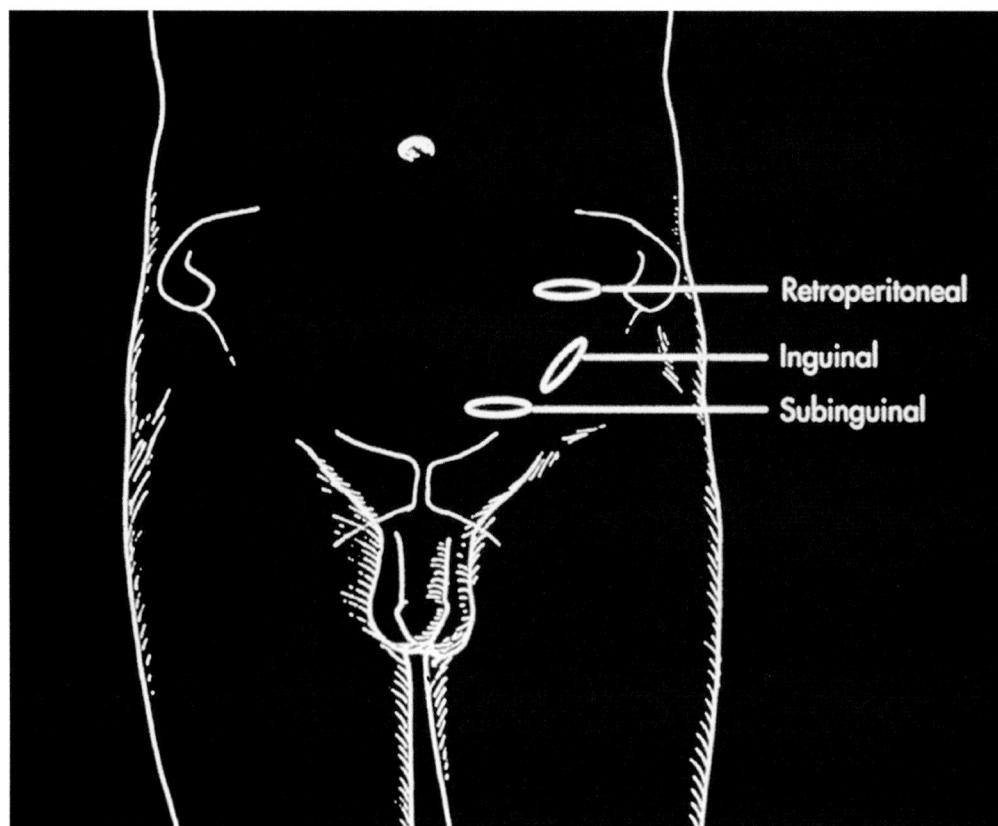

Figure 20–9. Different incision sites for each type of varicocele repair.

surgeon, is essentially the same as the retroperitoneal procedure. This type of repair is rarely used to treat varicoceles in adults because it generally involves ligation of the testicular artery, which can lead to testicular atrophy, and it is excessively invasive for what should be a minor outpatient procedure.

A Foley catheter and a nasogastric tube are placed at the beginning of the operation. To create a pneumoperitoneum, a Veress needle or 10-mm trocar (under direct vision) is placed just below the umbilicus. Another 10-mm port is placed on the contralateral side just lateral to the rectus muscle and below the umbilicus. Next, a 5-mm port is placed to the left of the umbilicus. The table should be rotated away from the surgical side and the patient placed in the Trendelenburg position. With the camera through the umbilical port, the iliac vessels, the spermatic cord, the median umbilical ligament, the internal ring, and the vas deferens should be easily identified (Fig. 20–10).

Initially, the parietal peritoneum is incised just lateral to the spermatic cord. The testicular artery and veins are dissected and isolated. Pulling on the testis can help identify the vessels. Furthermore, the use of a Doppler probe or of vasodilators, such as papaverine or lidocaine, can aid in identification of the testicular artery. Once the veins are isolated, they are clipped both proximally and distally with titanium endoclips, and these vessels are then transected. After hemostasis is achieved, the ports are removed under direct vision and the fascia is closed with No. 1 synthetic absorbable suture. Finally, the subcuticular layer is closed with a 4-0 synthetic absorbable suture.

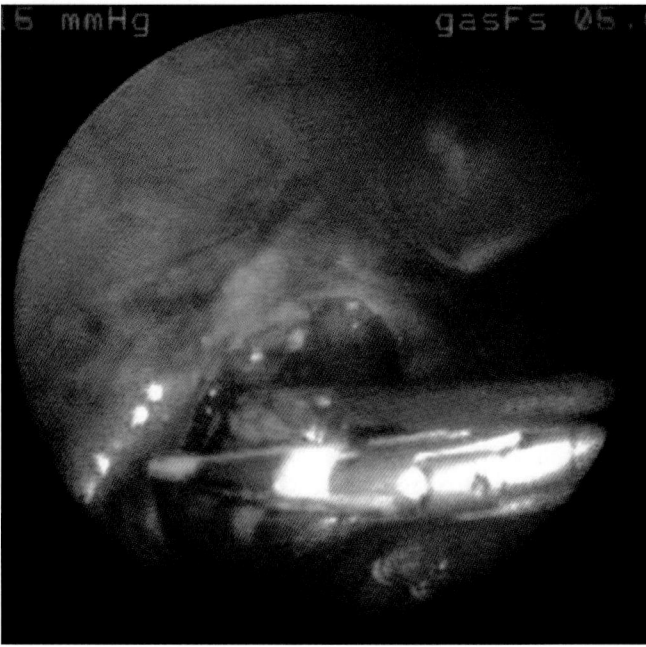

Figure 20–10. Laparoscopic view during varicocele repair illustrating the spermatic cord and the vas deferens.

Laparoscopic dissection of the spermatic veins and artery can be challenging, and some authors have advocated ligation of all of the vessels, including the testicular artery, during the procedure. The argument is that the collateral blood supply to the testis, namely, through the

cremasteric and vasal arteries, is sufficient to prevent testicular atrophy.

In addition to general complications associated with laparoscopic surgery, **laparoscopic varicocele repairs have been associated with a recurrence rate of less than 2% and formation of hydroceles in 5% to 8% of patients** (Esposito et al, 2001; Nyirady et al, 2002; Itoh et al, 2003; Koyle et al, 2004; McManus et al, 2004). In a series of 62 laparoscopic varicocele repairs, 4.8% of patients experienced transient numbness of the ipsilateral anterior thigh, which resolved or improved in an average of 8.0 months. It was believed that cautery or harmonic dissection of the peritoneum overlying the spermatic cord and excessive traction on the tissues surrounding the cord could have resulted in nerve injury (Chrouser et al, 2004).

Inguinal and Subinguinal Approaches. Surgical repairs by most urologic reproductive surgeons involve microsurgical techniques to preserve the internal spermatic arteries and lymphatics. The inguinal and subinguinal approaches are the preferred approaches. However, there are certain specific indications for each.

Marmar and Kim (1994) showed that there was less morbidity associated with the subinguinal (infrainguinal) approach than with the laparoscopic and inguinal approach because of the preservation of the muscle layers and the inguinal canal. **However, a greater number of internal spermatic veins and arteries lie below the external ring, making this procedure technically more challenging** (Hopps et al, 2003). In one series, investigators found that internal spermatic arteries at the subinguinal level were more than three times as likely to be surrounded by a network of adherent veins as those identified at the inguinal level (Hopps et al, 2003).

Inguinal Approach (Modified Ivanissevich). A 3- to 4-cm oblique incision, two fingerbreadths above the symphysis pubis and just above the external ring, is carried laterally along Langer's lines (Fig. 20–11). The incision is carried down to the external oblique aponeurosis, which is incised in the direction of its fibers. Care is taken to identify and to preserve the ilioinguinal nerve. Next, the spermatic cord is mobilized near the pubic tubercle, and a Penrose drain is passed beneath the cord. The Penrose drain is used to elevate the cord and bring it through the incision.

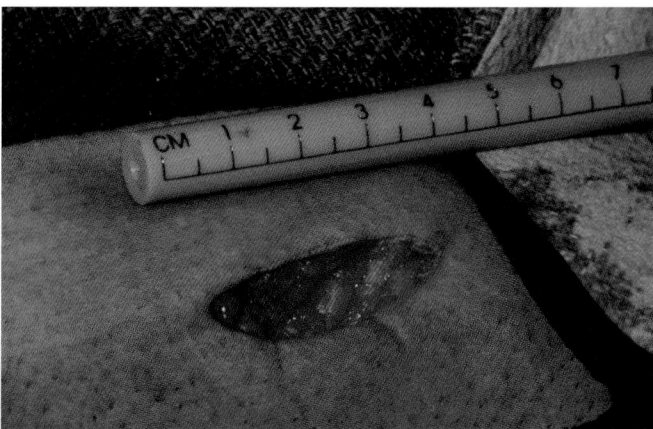

Figure 20–11. Incision for inguinal varicocele repair.

For the microsurgical technique, the microscope is now brought into the operating field (Fig. 20–12). The internal and external spermatic fasciae are incised, and the dilated veins are identified. Varicoceles generally appear with a typical vascular pattern in which the artery is next to or adherent to several veins, and there is a separate isolated vein nearby (Fig. 20–13). In approximately 50% of cases, the testicular artery is adherent to the undersurface of a large vein (Beck et al, 1992). A Doppler probe as well as vasodilators, such as papaverine or lidocaine, may be used to help identify the testicular artery. We recommend use of a 1-mm Doppler microprobe to help identify the testicular artery (Fig. 20–14). Once the dilated veins are isolated, they are doubly ligated with either 2-0 silk sutures or small titanium surgical clips (Fig. 20–15). A Jacobson instrument is useful in isolating these testicular veins (Fig. 20–16). With the microsurgical technique, the lymphatic channels can be clearly visualized, and these should be preserved to prevent postoperative hydrocele formation. The floor of the inguinal canal, near the external ring, should also be inspected to identify and ligate any external cremasteric veins. These veins drain into the external pudendal vein and have been shown to be responsible for varicocele recurrence.

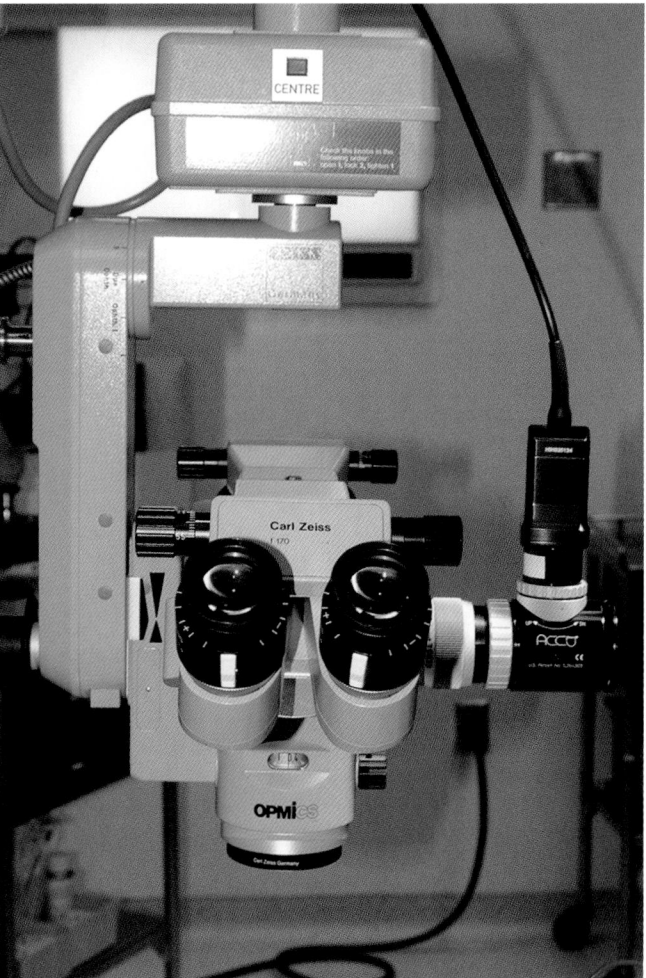

Figure 20–12. Surgical microscope used for microsurgical varicocele repair.

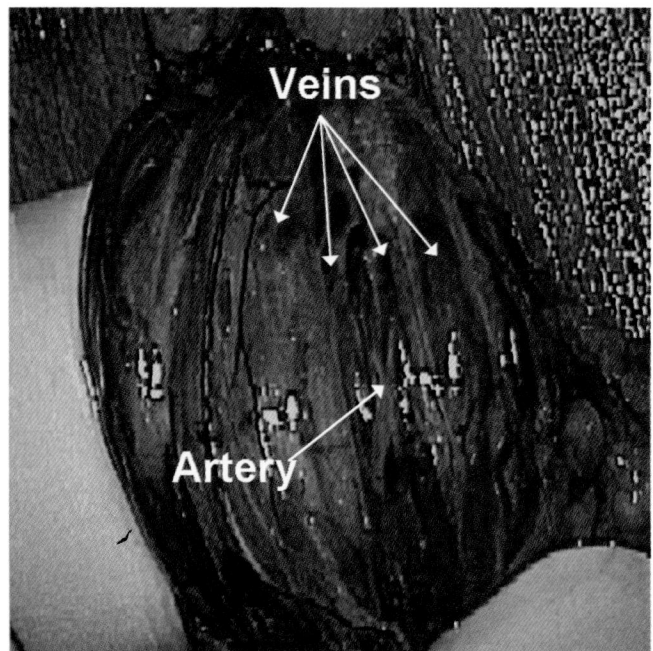

Figure 20–13. Typical pattern of artery and veins during varicocele repair. Several veins are next to or adherent to the testicular artery, and there is a nearby isolated vein.

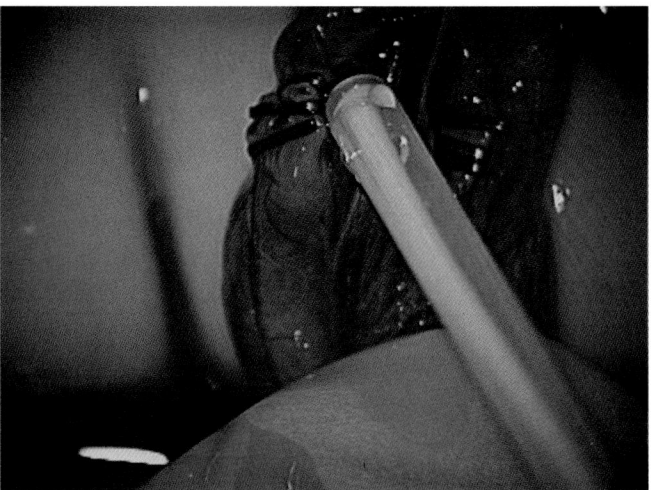

Figure 20–14. Doppler microprobe used to ensure that the artery is not inadvertently ligated.

If it is needed, hemostasis can be achieved with bipolar electrocautery.

The cord is placed back into the canal, and the external oblique fascia is closed with a 3-0 Vicryl suture. The subcutaneous layer is reapproximated with a 3-0 plain catgut suture, and the subcuticular layer is closed with a 4-0 Monocryl suture. The incision is infiltrated with 1% lidocaine mixed with an equal amount of 0.5% bupivacaine.

Subinguinal Approach. A 2- to 3-cm transverse incision is made at the level of the external ring (see Fig. 20–9). The incision is carried down to the external oblique fascia, which is not incised. The spermatic cord is then identified as it exits the external ring. The cord is mobilized at the external ring and brought out of the wound, and a Penrose drain is placed beneath it. Care must be taken to identify and to ligate any posterior cremasteric veins to prevent varicocele recurrence. For the microsurgical approach, the microscope is now brought into the operating field. The remainder of the operation is similar to the inguinal approach.

Microsurgical Versus Nonmicrosurgical Approaches. The main advantage of the microsurgical over the nonmicrosurgical technique is the significant reduction in postoperative complications, such as testicular artery injury, hydrocele formation, and varicocele recurrence. The complication rates for hydrocele formation with the nonmicrosurgical technique range from 3% to 39% (Szabo and Kessler 1984; Amelar, 2003), whereas hydrocele formation is rarely reported in association with a microsurgical technique (Goldstein et al, 1992). These improved results are thought to be due to the greater ability to identify and preserve individual lymphatics. The recurrence rate for microscopic inguinal varicocelectomy has been reported between 1% and 2%, compared with 9% and 16% for nonmicroscopic inguinal

varicocele repair (Goldstein et al, 1992; Marmar and Kim, 1994; Cayan et al, 2000). **The recurrence rate for nonmicroscopic subinguinal varicocele repair is reported to be 5% to 20%** (Szabo and Kessler, 1984; Marmar et al, 1985). Whereas most male infertility surgeons now use the microsurgical approach, varicocele repairs still can be achieved with successful results and minimal complications without microsurgery as long as they are carefully performed.

Delivery of the Testicle. Delivery of the testis to identify and ligate scrotal collaterals, such as gubernacular veins, has also been described (Goldstein et al, 1992). The testis is delivered through a 2- to 3-cm inguinal incision, and all external spermatic and gubernacular veins are ligated. The testis is then returned to the scrotum, and the standard inguinal or subinguinal varicocele repair is completed. This technique, thought to prevent varicocele recurrence, is not performed as frequently as the subinguinal or inguinal procedure in which the testis is not delivered.

Percutaneous Embolization

In 1978, the first reports of transvenous sclerotherapy for the ablation of varicoceles were published (Lima et al, 1978). **Today, embolization of the spermatic veins can be accomplished with coils, balloons, or sclerotherapy.** The placement of coils or balloons is performed with local anesthesia and involves a cut-down incision over the femoral or internal jugular vein. A catheter is passed to the internal spermatic veins, and the balloon or coils are deployed. Sclerotherapy allows occlusion of smaller collateral veins (Comhaire and Kunnen, 1985), but use of this technique can be a tedious process.

Complications associated with percutaneous embolization include balloon deflation and migration (Formanek et al, 1981; Kaufman et al, 1983), **varicocele recurrence, and failure of initial attempted procedures.** Pryor and Howards (1987) summarized the success rates of percutaneous embolization and found that 73% were successful at the time of the procedure. They also found the recurrence rate after the time of embolization to be approximately 5%. **Thus, the**

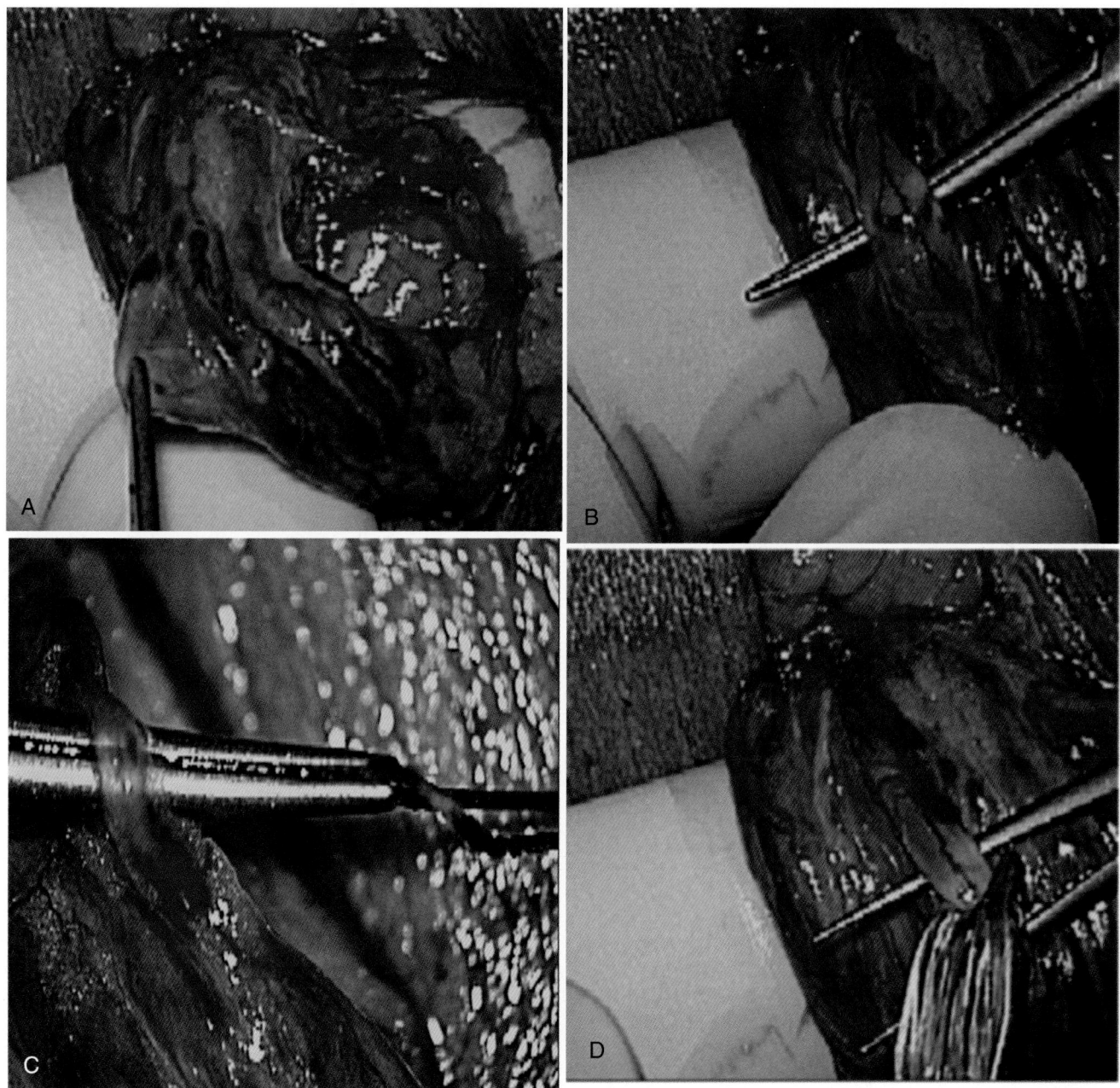

Figure 20–15. Dilated veins are first identified (**A**), the vein is mobilized (**B**), and a 2-0 silk suture is passed beneath the dilated vein (**C**) or the vein is occluded with hemoclips (**D**).

overall success rate in this series, taking into account the failed first attempts and the recurrence rate, was 68% (Pryor and Howards, 1987). Other investigators have found the recurrence rate of varicocele balloon embolization to be between 4% and 11% (Kaufman et al, 1983; Murray et al, 1986; Matthews et al, 1992). **Percutaneous varicocele embolization is especially useful in a recurrent or persistent varicocele, when the anatomy causing the varicocele needs to be radiographically clarified.**

Outcomes

Varicoceles have also been associated with a progressive and duration-dependent decline in testicular function (Lipshultz and Corriere, 1977; Chehval and Purcell, 1992; Gorelick and Goldstein, 1993; Witt and Lipshultz, 1993). **However, studies have shown that repair of varicoceles can retard further damage to testicular function** (Kass and Belman, 1987).

Most of the literature supports an improvement in fertility rates after varicocele repair (Madgar et al, 1995), but only a limited number of prospective randomized controlled trials have looked at the effectiveness of varicocele repairs in infertile men. The two most widely quoted, prospective randomized controlled trials revealed a statistically significant improvement in sperm density after varicocele repair, and one of these studies demonstrated a statistically significant

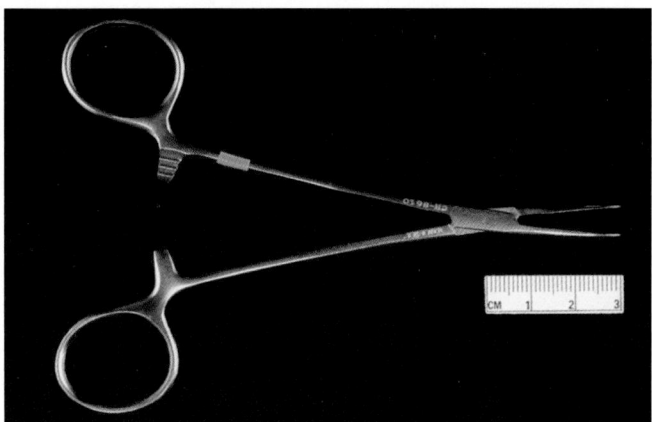

Figure 20–16. Jacobson instrument used to dissect and isolate varicocele veins.

improvement in pregnancy rate (Madgar et al, 1995; Nieschlag et al, 1998).

In a study by Madgar and colleagues (1995), 10% of men with varicoceles randomized to "no therapy" were able to achieve spontaneous pregnancies in 1 year, compared with 60% of men who underwent a varicocele repair. A review of 12 controlled studies found a pregnancy rate of 33% in couples after varicocele repair compared with 16% in untreated couples observed for 1 year (Schlegel, 1997). **In a series of 1500 microsurgical varicocele repairs, Goldstein and coworkers (1992) reported that 43% of couples were pregnant in the first year and 69% at 2 years, when couples with female factor were excluded.**

The improvement in spontaneous pregnancy rates can largely be attributed to the improvement in semen parameters. A study by Marks and colleagues (1986) showed improvement of approximately 41% in sperm motility and morphologic features and 21% in sperm forward progression. **A review of the literature by Pryor and Howards (1987) demonstrated that the overall rate of improvement in semen parameters after varicocelectomy ranged from 51% to 78%. These authors also reported the overall pregnancy rate after varicocele repair to be 24% to 53%.** A meta-analysis of more than 2000 patients found that approximately 50% to 60% of patients experienced an improvement in semen variables and 30% to 40% of patients initiated a pregnancy after varicocele repair (Nagler and Martinis, 1997). Investigators have also demonstrated a return of sperm in the ejaculate of azoospermic men after microsurgical varicocelectomy. Kim and associates (1999) demonstrated that varicocele repair can result in sperm in the ejaculate of azoospermic men when severe hypospermatogenesis or late maturation arrest is identified histologically; that is, when spermatids are identified. Similarly, Matthews and coworkers (1998) found that 55% of men with azoospermia and 69% of men with zero motile sperm before surgery had motile sperm in their ejaculate after varicocele repair. However, other investigators have found that men with nonobstructed azoospermia will rarely have adequate sperm in their ejaculate after varicocele repair undertaken to avoid testicular sperm extraction (Schlegel and Kaufmann, 2004).

Correction of varicoceles has also been shown to improve not only semen motility, density, and morphologic features but also serum FSH and testosterone levels (Su et al, 1995; Cayan et al, 1999). Cayan and associates (1999) reported a significant increase in serum free testosterone levels after varicocelectomy as well as a significant improvement in sperm concentration and motility. These investigators also reported **a significant *decrease* in mean FSH level from 15.2 mIU/mL before surgery to 10.8 mIU/mL after varicocele repair.** Su and coworkers (1995) demonstrated that after a varicocele repair, the mean serum testosterone level significantly increased from a preoperative level of 319 ± 12 to 409 ± 23 ng/dL. These investigators further demonstrated that men with at least one firm testis preoperatively had a significantly greater increase in serum testosterone concentration.

Studies have shown that laparoscopic varicocelectomy offers no advantage over open microsurgical repair. Enquist and colleagues (1994) compared patients who underwent laparoscopic and subinguinal varicocelectomy and found that operative times and mean number of days of analgesic use in the two groups were similar. However, the complication rate and the number of days off required after the procedure were significantly greater in the laparoscopic group. Other studies have also concluded that the laparoscopic technique has no advantage over an open repair as measured by days of work missed and the degree of postoperative pain (Ross and Ruppman, 1993).

Predicting Successful Repairs

Recent literature reveals much interest in identifying predictive indicators to assess which male patients would most benefit from varicocele repair. **Several investigators have found significantly higher spontaneous post-repair pregnancy rates in couples in whom the man's initial sperm concentration was greater than 5 million sperm/mL** (Kamal et al, 2001; Matkov et al, 2001). Kamal and associates found that men with more than 5 million sperm/mL had a spontaneous pregnancy rate of 61% after varicocele repair compared with men with less than 5 million sperm/mL, who had a spontaneous pregnancy rate of 8% after varicocele repair.

Marks, McMahon, and Lipshultz were able to identify four preoperative factors associated with an increased likelihood of postoperative pregnancy (Marks et al, 1986). **These factors included lack of testicular atrophy, sperm density greater than 50 million per ejaculate, sperm motility of 60% or more, and serum FSH values less than 300 ng/mL (normal, 50 to 300 ng/mL).** In this series, 56% of patients with normal testicular size established pregnancy compared with 33% of patients with testicular atrophy. Thirty percent of patients with preoperative sperm motility of less than 60% initiated pregnancies, whereas 60% of patients with normal preoperative sperm motility were able to achieve pregnancy. Forty-six percent of patients with normal FSH levels achieved pregnancy compared with 25% of patients whose FSH level was above 300 ng/mL.

Previous reports have suggested that the gonadotropin-releasing hormone (GnRH) stimulation test may be useful in predicting clinical outcomes after microsurgical varicocelectomy. Studies have shown that FSH and luteinizing hormone responses to GnRH stimulation are exaggerated in those men who respond well to varicocelectomy with improved semen

Table 20-2. **Complication Rates Associated with Different Varicocele Repairs**			
Technique	Artery Preserved	Hydrocele (%)	Recurrence (%)
Retroperitoneal	No	7	11-15
Conventional inguinal	No	3-39	9-16
Laparoscopic	Yes	5-8	<2
Radiographic	Yes	0	4-11
Microscopic inguinal or subinguinal	Yes	0	<2

parameters, regardless of the degree of oligospermia (Hudson and McKay 1980; Atikeler et al, 1996; Segenreich et al, 1998). However, more recent data suggest that GnRH does not predict improvement in semen parameters or unassisted pregnancy outcomes in couples in whom the man undergoes a varicocelectomy (O'Brien et al, 2004). Conflicting data in the literature suggest an explanation for infrequent use of this test in clinical practice.

Complications

Complication rates for the various varicocele repair techniques can be found in Table 20-2.

Hydrocele. The most common complication after non-microsurgical varicocelectomy is hydrocele formation, occurring in 3% to 39% of cases (Szabo and Kessler, 1984; Amelar, 2003). These formations arise presumably because of the difficulty in clearly identifying the lymphatic vessels without magnification and hence failure to complete their ligation. Lymphatic obstruction is a more likely cause of hydrocele formation than is venous obstruction because the average protein content of a post-varicocelectomy hydrocele is between 5 and 6 g/100 mL, rather than the less than 1.5 g/100 mL that would be expected with a venous obstruction (Szabo and Kessler, 1984). Szabo and Kessler (1984) demonstrated that the rate of hydrocele occurrence subsequent to retroperitoneal varicocele repair is about 7%. A study of complication rates in 139 men undergoing microsurgical varicocelectomy found that none of the men developed hydroceles (Carbone and Merhoff, 2003). Similarly, percutaneous venous balloon occlusion has not been shown to cause hydrocele formation (Walsh and White, 1981).

Recurrence. The recurrence or, perhaps, persistence rate for varicoceles is highly contingent on the type of procedure and technique used. For example, whereas the recurrence rate for microscopic inguinal varicocelectomy has been reported to be between 1% and 2%, for nonmicroscopic inguinal varicocele repair, it has been reported to be between 9% and 16% (Goldstein et al, 1992; Marmar and Kim, 1994; Cayan et al, 2000). The recurrence rates for high retroperitoneal varicocele repairs have been reported to be between 11% and 15% (Homonnai et al, 1980; Rothman et al, 1981; Niedzielski and Paduch, 2001). For retroperitoneal varicocele repairs, Niedzielski and Paduch (2001) have advocated the use of intraoperative venography to identify the nonligated vessels and the left-to-right cross-communicating vessels. These authors found that this intraoperative procedure reduced the rate of recurrence from 11% to 2.8% in patients undergoing

varicocele repair by the high retroperitoneal approach, sparing the testicular artery.

Furthermore, it is important that all internal and external spermatic veins be ligated to prevent varicocele recurrence. Sayfan and associates (1980) demonstrated through phlebography that three of four patients who had a varicocele recurrence had dilated external spermatic veins in the presence of completely ligated internal spermatic veins. One advantage of the inguinal and subinguinal approaches is the better visualization of external spermatic veins (93% versus 74% in the inguinal dissection) (Hopps et al, 2003). The recurrence rate associated with radiographic balloon occlusion techniques has been reported to be between 4% and 11% (Kaufman et al, 1983; Murray et al, 1986; Matthews et al, 1992).

Testicular Artery Injury. The rate of testicular artery injury also depends on the surgical technique used. However, **the more distal the incision down the inguinal canal, the more likely the occurrence of injury to the testicular artery, particularly because the arterial collaterals in the inguinal region are limited in number** (Silber, 1979). Chan and Goldstein (2005) reported that in a series of 2102 cases, 19 (0.9%) experienced testicular artery injury during microsurgical varicocelectomy; subsequent testicular atrophy occurred in only one patient. Thus, the overall risk of testicular atrophy was well below 1%. Kumar and associates (2003) actually identified and repaired a testicular artery injury during a microsurgical varicocelectomy procedure. **Injury to the testicular artery does not always result in testicular atrophy because of the presence of other spermatic cord arteries, such as the vasal and cremasteric arteries.**

Cost-Effectiveness

Recent literature supports the concept that varicocele repair is far more cost-effective than IVF-ICSI as first-line therapy in assisting the infertile patient to establish a pregnancy. A meta-analysis by Penson and coworkers (2002) demonstrated that the probability of a live birth after a varicocelectomy was 29.7% versus 25.4% after IVF-ICSI, yet the cost of performing IVF-ICSI was substantially greater. **Schlegel reported in 1997 that the cost per delivered baby was $26,268 after varicocelectomy compared with $89,091 with IVF-ICSI.** Although the success of IVF-ICSI has increased since 1992, the cost difference remains significant.

Follow-up

A semen analysis should be performed 4 months after varicocele repair. Semen should be monitored regularly for at least 1 year or until pregnancy is achieved. If the varicocele persists or recurs, internal spermatic venography can be performed to localize the site of persistently refluxing veins.

PROCEDURES TO IMPROVE SPERM DELIVERY
Vasectomy Reversal

It is estimated that approximately 6% of men who have undergone vasectomy will subsequently request a vasectomy reversal (Potts et al, 1999). The reason most frequently given by men requesting a reversal is divorce and remarriage with a desire to have children with their new spouse. A significantly smaller number of men requesting a reversal may still be married to their same spouse and, for a variety of reasons, wish to have more children. Fewer yet request vasectomy reversal for personal or religious reasons, thinking they may have done something against their current beliefs in undergoing the vasectomy in the first place and wishing to rectify the situation.

When a man having had a vasectomy wishes to have his own biologically related children, his choices are to have a vasectomy reversal or to have sperm extraction (see the section on sperm acquisition) in conjunction with IVF and ICSI. These choices plus the options of donor sperm, adoption, and remaining without children should be discussed with the couple. Whereas many couples will have an idea of what actions they want to take to have children, some may have learned about the different methods for conception available to them from Internet sites, which may or may not present a balanced account of the different procedures in terms of risk-benefit, costs, and ease of performance. Similarly, Internet-reported success of vasectomy reversal or IVF-ICSI cannot be interpreted as universal for all physicians and centers performing these procedures; these data are individual or center specific, and patients should be properly advised to avoid misconceptions.

The initial consultation with the individual or couple should offer the opportunity to obtain a concise health and reproductive history of both the patient and his partner and to examine the man. Chances for success (patency or pregnancy) based on the personal experience of the surgeon, the patient's health history, and the results of examination of the man and the age and reproductive potential of his partner are discussed. **It is recommended that the man's partner consult with her gynecologist to be comfortable that there are no significant impediments that may prevent conception.**

Some men requesting a vasectomy reversal will require vasoepididymostomy rather than vasovasostomy because of a secondary obstruction in the epididymis. **Epididymal obstruction appears, in most instances, to be a time-related phenomenon; the longer the time from vasectomy, the greater the chances of an epididymal obstruction** (Silber, 1979, 1981, 1984; Potts et al, 1999; Fuchs and Burt, 2002; Chawla et al, 2004). This possibility of a need for a vasoepididymostomy should be discussed with the patient along with a candid discussion of the surgeon's experience in performing this more complex procedure.

A review (unpublished) of 483 men who underwent vasectomy reversal at one center described the requirement for vasoepididymostomy on one or both sides as being related to time of obstruction (Thomas and Parekattil, 2004). **Fuchs and Burt (2002) reported that 62% of patients who underwent reversal 15 years or more after their vasectomy required either a unilateral or a bilateral vasoepididymostomy.** The criteria for deciding to perform a vasoepididymostomy are not always clear. **The decision to perform a vasoepididymostomy is based, in large part, on the quality of fluid found in the proximal (testicular) vas deferens at the time of reversal.** Fluid obtained from the proximal vas lumen is placed on a sterile glass slide covered with a few drops of saline or lactated Ringer's solution to dilute it and make it easier to examine. The slide is examined under 400× magnification with a light

microscope. **Vasoepididymostomy should be considered in the following instances: when the material coming from the proximal vas lumen is thick, pasty, and devoid of sperm; if the fluid is creamy, containing only debris; and if there is no fluid whatsoever when the vas is milked toward the cut end and if irrigation of the proximal vas with 0.1 to 0.2 mL of saline with a 24-gauge plastic angiocatheter attached to a tuberculin syringe fails to wash out any sperm.**

Preparation for Vasectomy Reversal

With rare exceptions, the results of microsurgical vasectomy reversal are superior to results of nonmicrosurgical techniques in terms of patency and pregnancy. Therefore, training and experience in microsurgical technique are necessary to obtain the best results in performing either vasovasostomy or vasoepididymostomy. **Patency and pregnancy rates do not appear to be significantly different if a multilayer anastomosis is performed as opposed to a modified single-layer technique** (Belker et al, 1991), **but the success is physician-dependent.**

Instruments for Microsurgical Reconstruction

When Silber and Owen independently reported their results with microsurgical vasectomy reversal in the mid-1970s, there were no specific instruments made just for urologists (Owen, 1977; Silber, 1977a, 1977b). Most surgeons who adopted these techniques borrowed the instruments from ophthalmologists, since they had been doing microsurgery for years. Many companies now manufacture a variety of instruments for urologic and plastic microsurgery. Suture manufacturers have likewise responded to the needs of the microsurgeon with specific sutures and needles that make the performance of these often tedious procedures less burdensome.

The number and type of instruments one chooses to use for vasectomy reversals need not be extensive but should be chosen carefully to fit both the hands and the needs of the surgeon. Duplicates of important instruments, such as needle holders, microforceps, and scissors, are critical in the event that one of these delicate instruments is accidentally dropped or the tips bent. Figure 20–17 shows some of the essential instruments that one of the authors finds useful in performing vasectomy reversals. A variety of sutures can be used. Two sutures used by one of the authors appear to work well for both vasovasostomy and vasoepididymostomy. The 10-0 suture ($\frac{3}{8}$ circle 135 M.E.T., Sharpoint microneedle, Surgical Specialties Corporation) is 2.5 cm in length and is double-armed with a sharp 70-μm needle, ideal for approximating vas-to-vas lumen or the opened epididymal tubule to the vas lumen. The 9-0 suture (9-0 Ethilon, VAS100-4 single needle manufactured by Ethicon) is a tapered needle that is strong enough to pass easily through the thicker muscularis and adventitia.

Regardless of the site of vasal obstruction, certain basic principles need to be followed to optimize the chance for success. There should be sufficient mobilization of both ends of the vas deferens to prevent any tension on the anastomosis. The perivasal adventitia must remain intact. **Stripping away the adventitia surrounding the cut ends of the vas risks excising an important blood supply to the vas and may lead to ischemia and ultimate narrowing and occlusion of the anastomosis.** Precise approximation of the cut lumens is mandatory to avoid sperm leakage with formation of a sperm

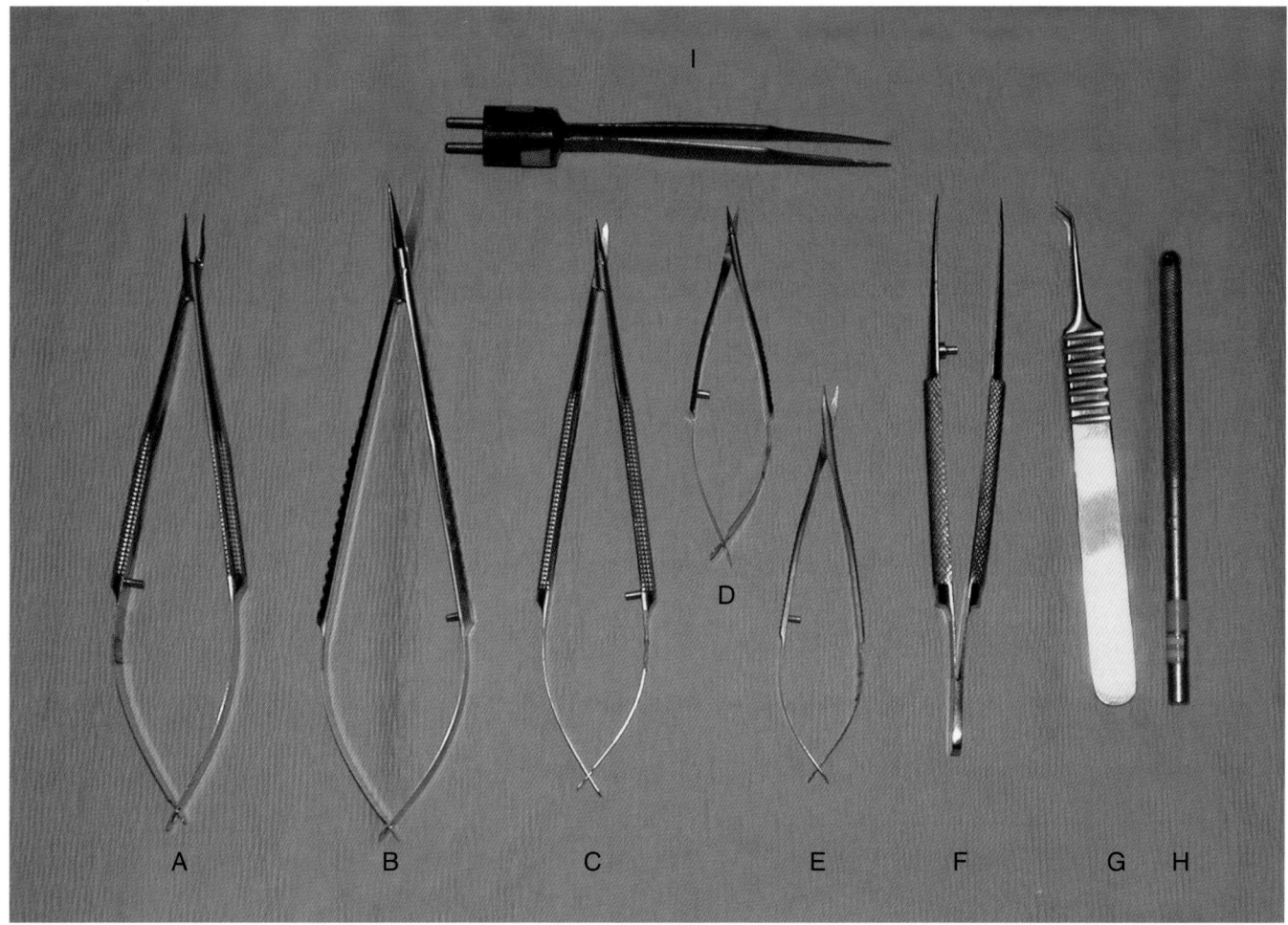

Figure 20–17. A modest array of good-quality microsurgical instruments is needed to perform vasovasostomy or vasoepididymostomy. **A,** Nonlocking needle holder. **B,** Suture scissors. **C,** Dissecting scissors. **D** and **E,** Very fine pointed and round-tipped scissors. **F,** Round-handled platform forceps. **G,** Curved dilating forceps. **H,** Round-handled small knife blade holder. **I,** Microtip bipolar cautery.

granuloma that may disrupt the lumen and result in a failed procedure.

Anesthetic Considerations

Depending on the comfort level of the surgeon and the patient, many men can undergo vasectomy reversal with local anesthesia (a one-to-one mixture of 1% lidocaine HCl and 0.25% bupivacaine HCl) combined with intravenous sedation; other patients may prefer general anesthesia in a day surgery setting. Some men may have specific medical problems that dictate the need for a certain type of anesthesia. If the procedure is prolonged (>3 hours), the level of the patient's anxiety is high, the anatomy of the vas and epididymis is difficult to feel through a thickened or tight scrotum, or extensive vasal or epididymal mobilization is needed, a general or epidural anesthetic may be more appropriate.

Preparing the Vas for Anastomosis

With the patient supine, the vas deferens is grasped between the surgeon's thumb and forefinger above the vasectomy site. When local anesthesia is used, a skin wheal is raised over the vas by use of a 30-gauge needle. The vas is grasped with a towel clamp (Fig. 20–18) or vas clamp, and additional local anesthetic is injected in the skin, after which a 1- to 1.5-cm-long incision is made directly over the vas.

Once the vas itself is isolated, 2 mL of the anesthetic mixture is injected into the vasal sheath, and the vas is dissected both proximally and distally to the vasectomy site. The length of vas freed from its surrounding tissue should be sufficient to allow the freshly cut ends of the vas to slightly overlap one another once they are positioned for anastomosis. Once the vas deferens is dissected free on both sides of the vasectomy site, a towel clamp placed around the vas secures its position above the skin. The opposite side is isolated in a similar fashion. When both vasa have been dissected free, the vasa can be held with the towel clamp above skin level and held well out of the skin incision for the anastomosis by placement of 6-0 Prolene sutures through the muscular wall of each end of the vas at the level where the vas exits the skin. Once the decision is made to perform a vasovasostomy, these sutures can be tacked outward to the drapes to hold the cut ends of the vas in a position so that the anastomosis can be performed more easily. Some surgeons prefer to use a vas

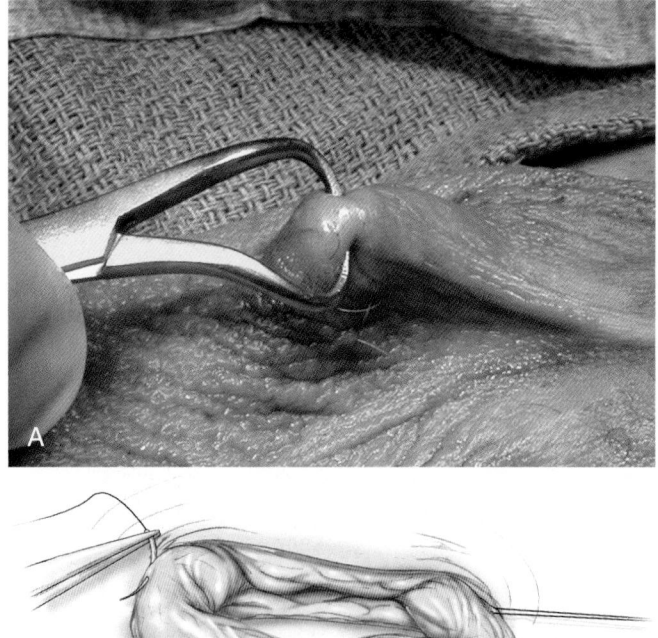

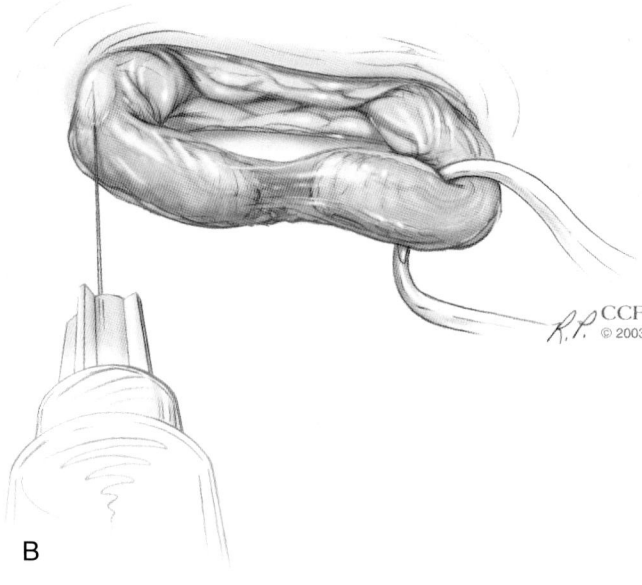

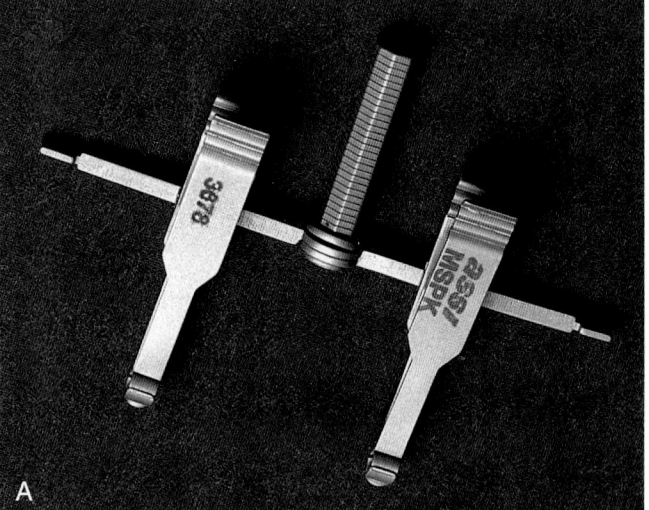

Figure 20–18. A, Vas grasped through skin above the vasectomy site. **B,** Once the vas is exposed, injection of a mixture of 0.5% bupivacaine and 1% lidocaine into the distal perivasal sheath will provide sufficient anesthetic coverage for the vasal anastomosis to be performed. **C,** Placement of 6-0 Prolene sutures just into the muscularis holds the vas above the incision and make it easily accessible for anastomosis.

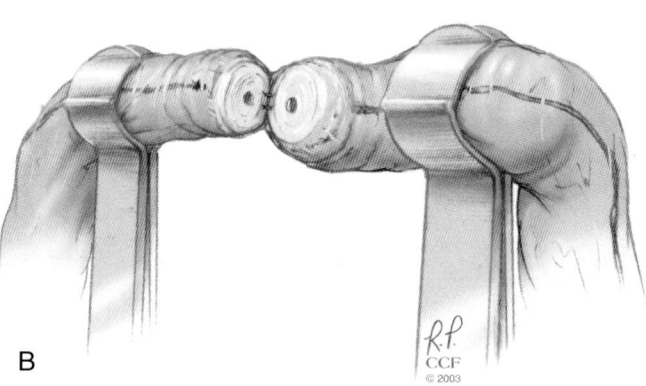

Figure 20–19. A and **B,** Microspike approximator clamp can also be used to hold the ends of the vas deferens close together for anastomosis.

clamp* rather than the suture method to hold the vas deferens in position for suturing (Fig. 20–19). Whichever method is preferred, sufficient length of the vas with its associated blood supply needs to be isolated on both ends so that the surgery can be performed without tension.

The vas above and below the vasectomy site should be transected with use of the operating microscope to examine the vas; a supple, normal area of the vas is chosen to be cut and anastomosed. Once the point of the vas that is to be cut is chosen, the vasal vessels are secured with 7-0 Prolene sutures just proximal to the point of transection. Some experienced microsurgeons prefer to cut the vas deferens through the groove of a nerve-holding forceps* to ensure a straight cut (Fig. 20–20). After the vas is cut, the ends should be inspected

---

*Microspike approximator clamp, ASSI.MSPK-3678, Accurate Surgical and Scientific Instruments, Westbury, NY.

*ASSI.NHF-2.5 from Accurate Surgical and Scientific Instruments, Westbury, NY.

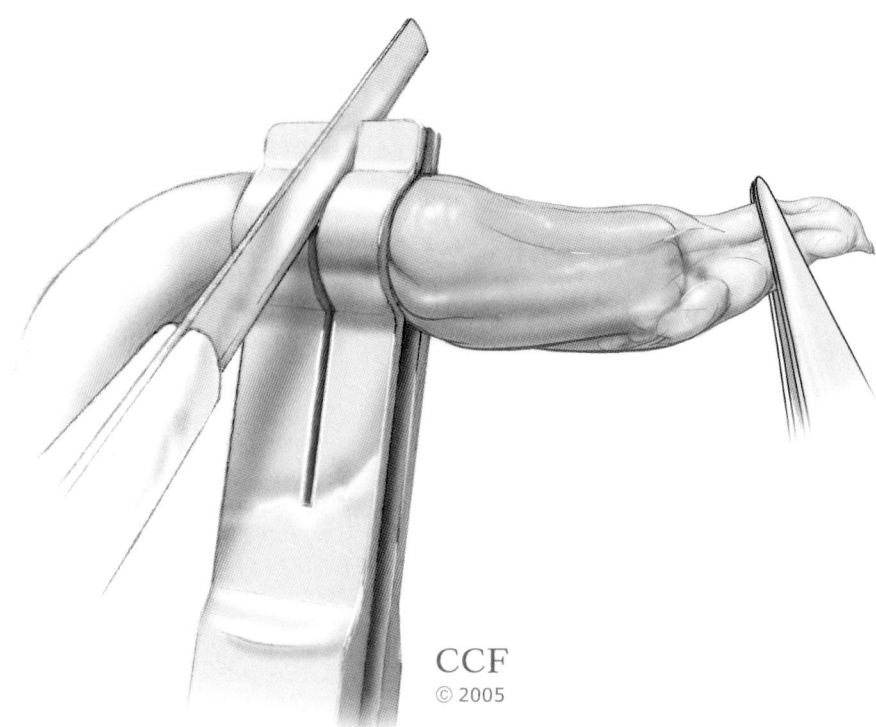

Figure 20-20. Nerve-holding forceps are used to facilitate making a straight cut of the ends of the vasa.

CCF
© 2005

and gently dilated with forceps. **No attempt is made to dilate the lumen progressively with lacrimal duct probes as this may tear or otherwise traumatize the delicate vas lumen.** The proximal vas lumen generally is dilated and without discernible layers of muscle; on the abdominal side, the muscle groups are readily visible.

A few drops of fluid from the testicular end of the vas lumen are placed on a sterile glass slide and examined by light microscopy. **If there are sperm or sperm parts (sperm heads, sperm with partial tails) in large numbers or the fluid is clear and copious with no visible sperm, vasovasostomy is generally indicated. If the fluid is thick, pasty, and devoid of sperm or contains only a few sperm heads, vasoepididymostomy should be considered.**

Multilayer Vasovasostomy

Once the cut ends of the vas deferens are positioned next to one another, the anastomosis is begun by passing a 9-0 suture through the muscularis and the adventitia at the 5- and 7-o'clock positions of each side of the vas deferens. A double-armed 10-0 suture is passed through the lumen at the posterior 6-o'clock position and tied (Fig. 20-21). The next sutures are placed in the wall of the lumen on either side of the first. These sutures are tied after both are in place. Three to five more sutures are placed equidistant from one another to close the remainder of the lumen but are left untied until all the sutures have been placed (Fig. 20-22). They are tied alternatively with the more lateral suture toward the one positioned at 12-o'clock. Once the anastomosis of the lumen has been completed, the 9-0 suture is again used to bring the muscularis together. A suture is placed at the 12-o'clock position first, then sequentially around the cut end of the vas until the first two sutures are reached (Fig. 20-23). The adventitia is

brought together over the muscularis suture line with interrupted 9-0 sutures to further enhance the blood supply at the level of the anastomosis (Fig. 20-24). If a vasovasostomy is to be done on both sides, the procedure is completed on one side before the other side is approached.

Modified Single-Layer Vasovasostomy

Some investigators have reported that with respect to patency and pregnancy, a modified single-layer microsurgical anastomosis is as effective as the multilayer anastomosis. Some surgeons prefer this method because it is simpler, uses fewer sutures, and requires less microsurgical skill. Nevertheless, this single-layer technique should still be carried out in the same exacting fashion as the multilayer anastomosis to maximize success.

With the ends of the vas visible with the operating microscope, a double-armed 10-0 suture is passed full thickness through the edge of the proximal and distal lumen at the 6-o'clock position. Two more sutures are placed, full thickness, at the 4- and 8-o'clock positions and tied. Three more full-thickness sutures are passed at the 10-, 12-, and 2-o'clock positions and then tied (Fig. 20-25). It is important when these sutures are placed that only a small edge of the lumen be incorporated in the suture to prevent the lumen from becoming compressed and its size compromised. The anastomosis is completed by closing the muscularis and adventitia to the opposite side, placing two 9-0 sutures between each of the 10-0 full-thickness sutures (Fig. 20-26).

Inguinal Vasovasostomy

Obstruction of the vas deferens within the inguinal canal is most often related to a direct injury to the vas during the

Text continued on p. 675.

SECTION VI

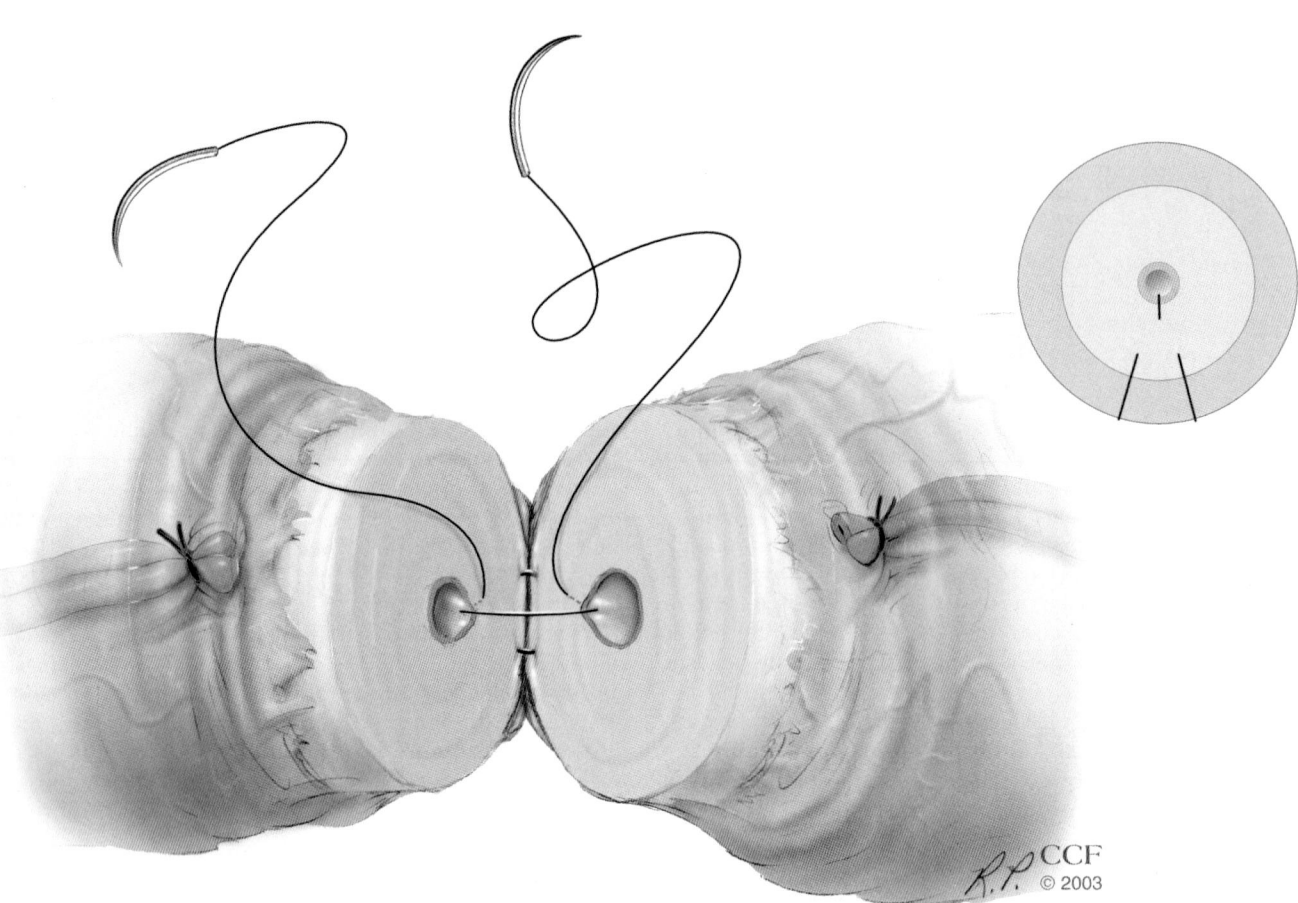

Figure 20–21. First mucosal suture placed at 6-o'clock position.

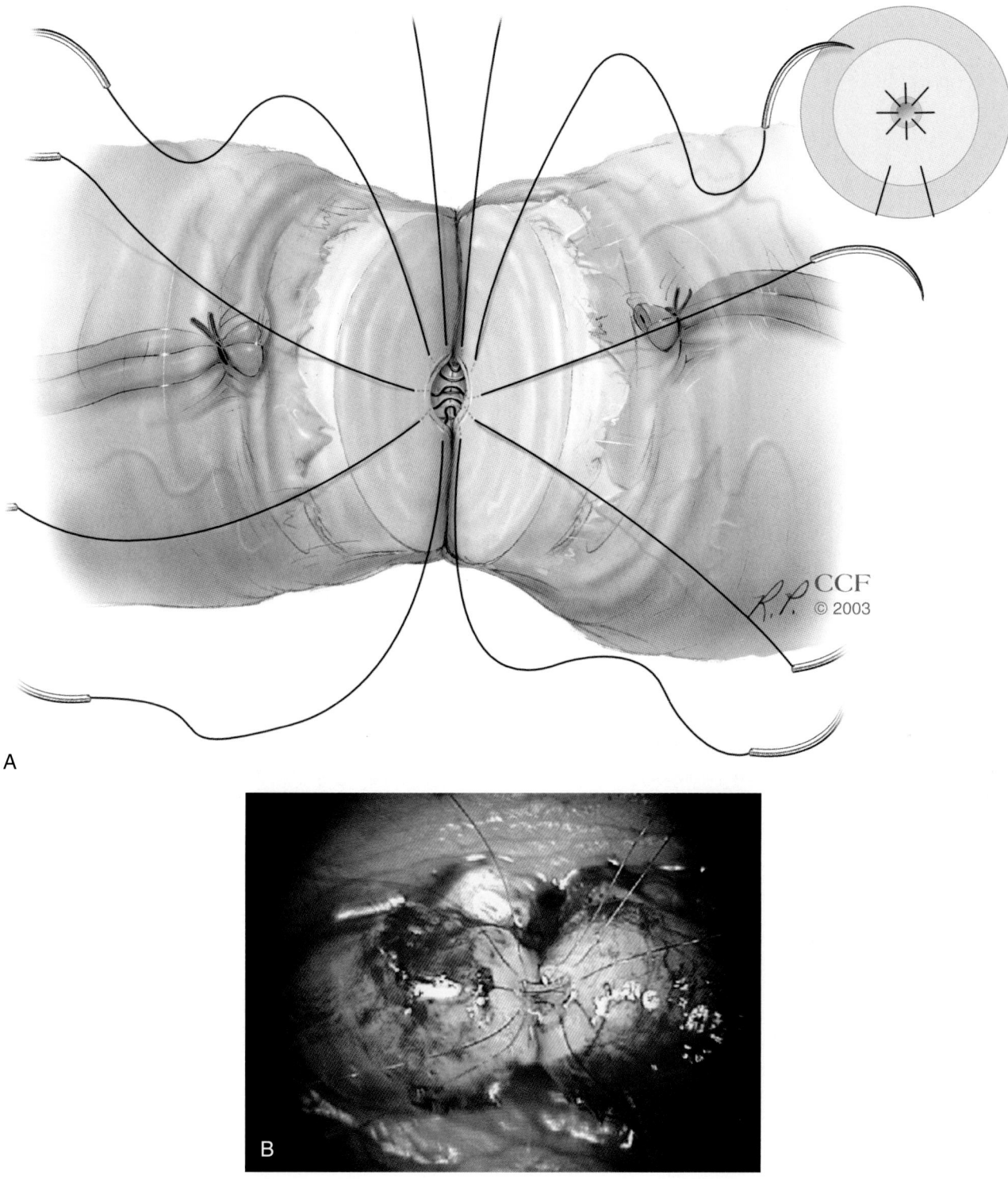

A

B

Figure 20–22. **A** and **B,** All anterior sutures are placed in the edge of the vas lumen, incorporating a small amount of muscularis.

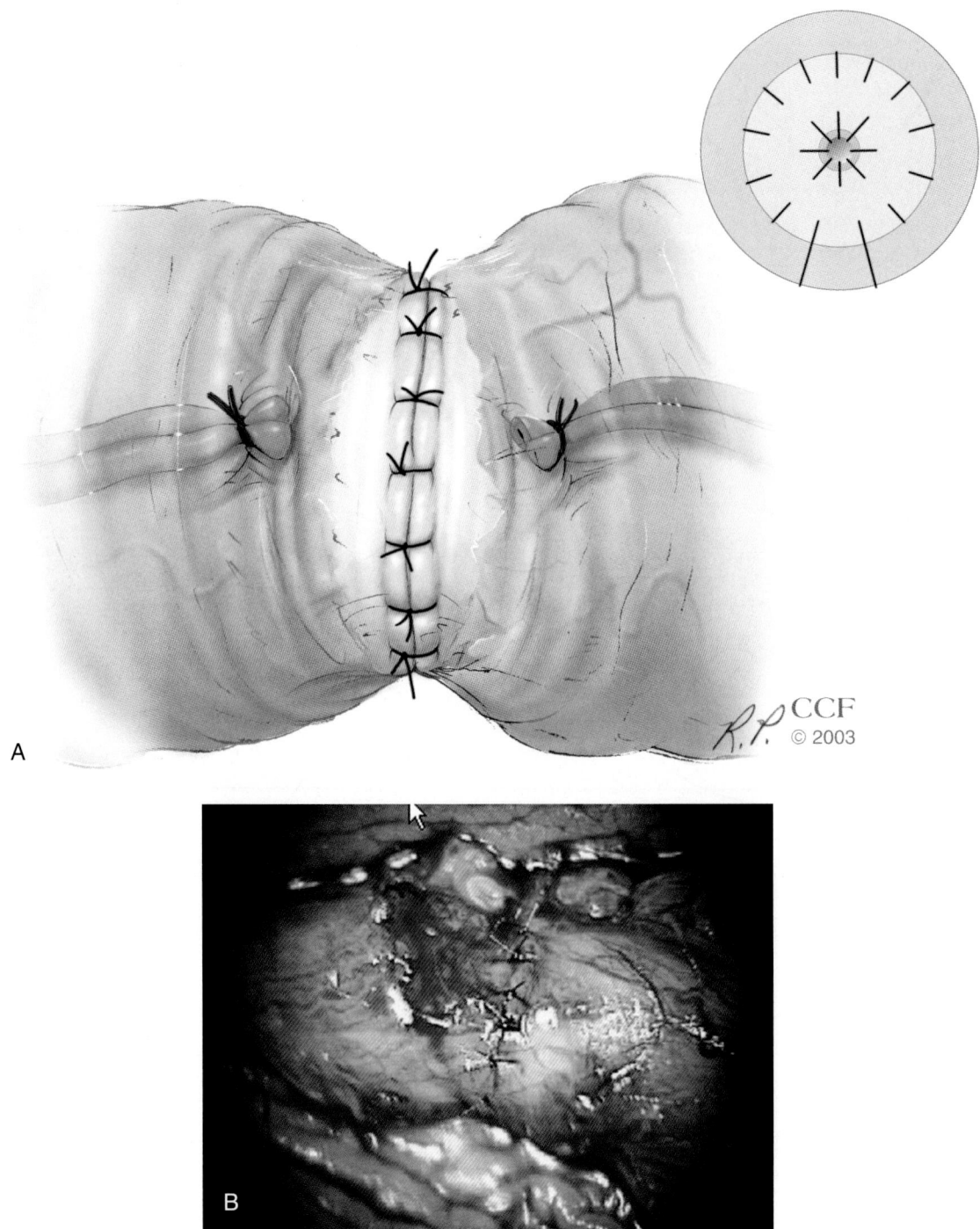

A

B

Figure 20–23. **A** and **B**, Muscularis has been approximated with 9-0 nylon suture.

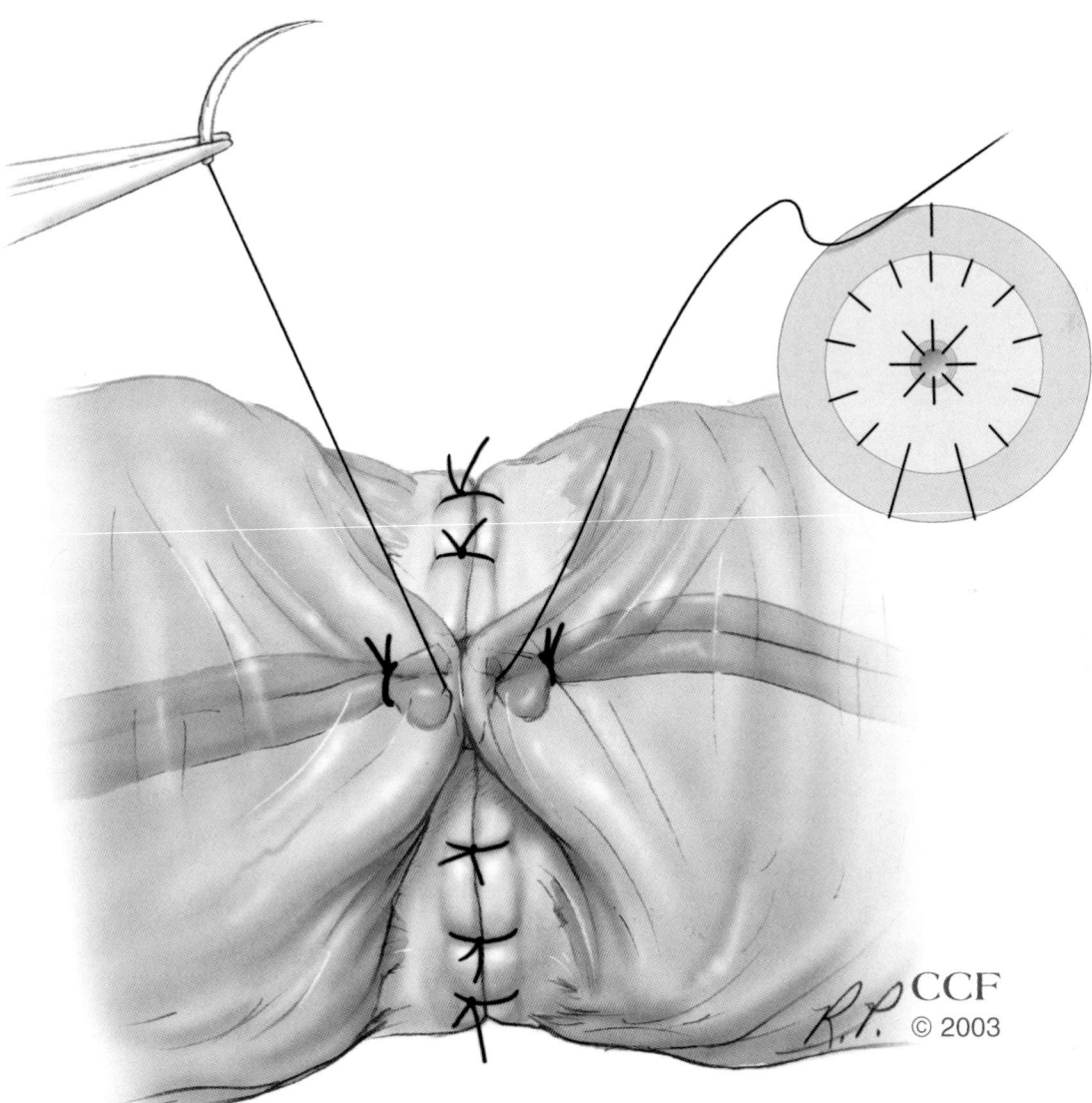

Figure 20-24. Closure of the adventitial "third layer."

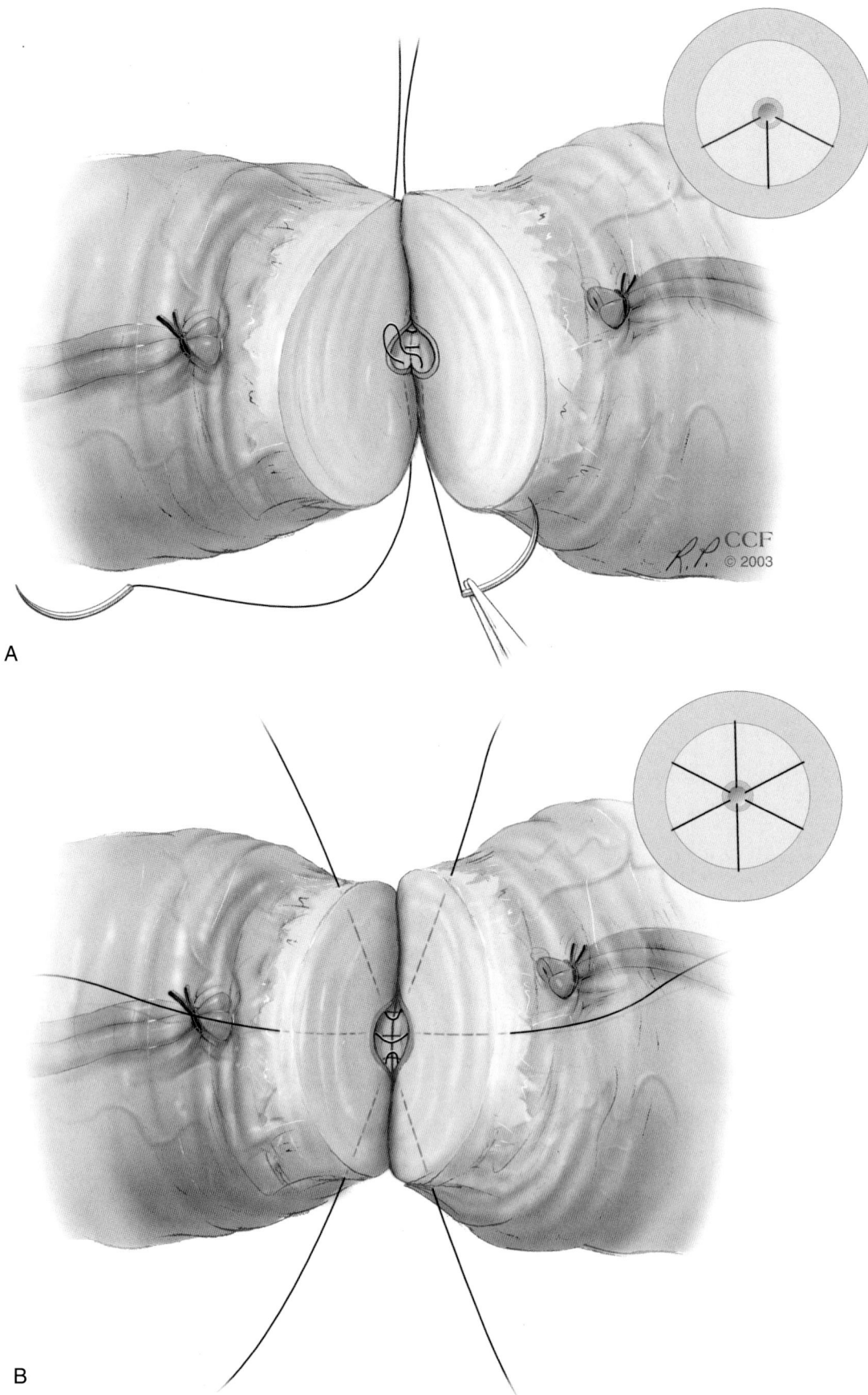

Figure 20–25. **A** and **B**, Placement of first three full-thickness sutures.

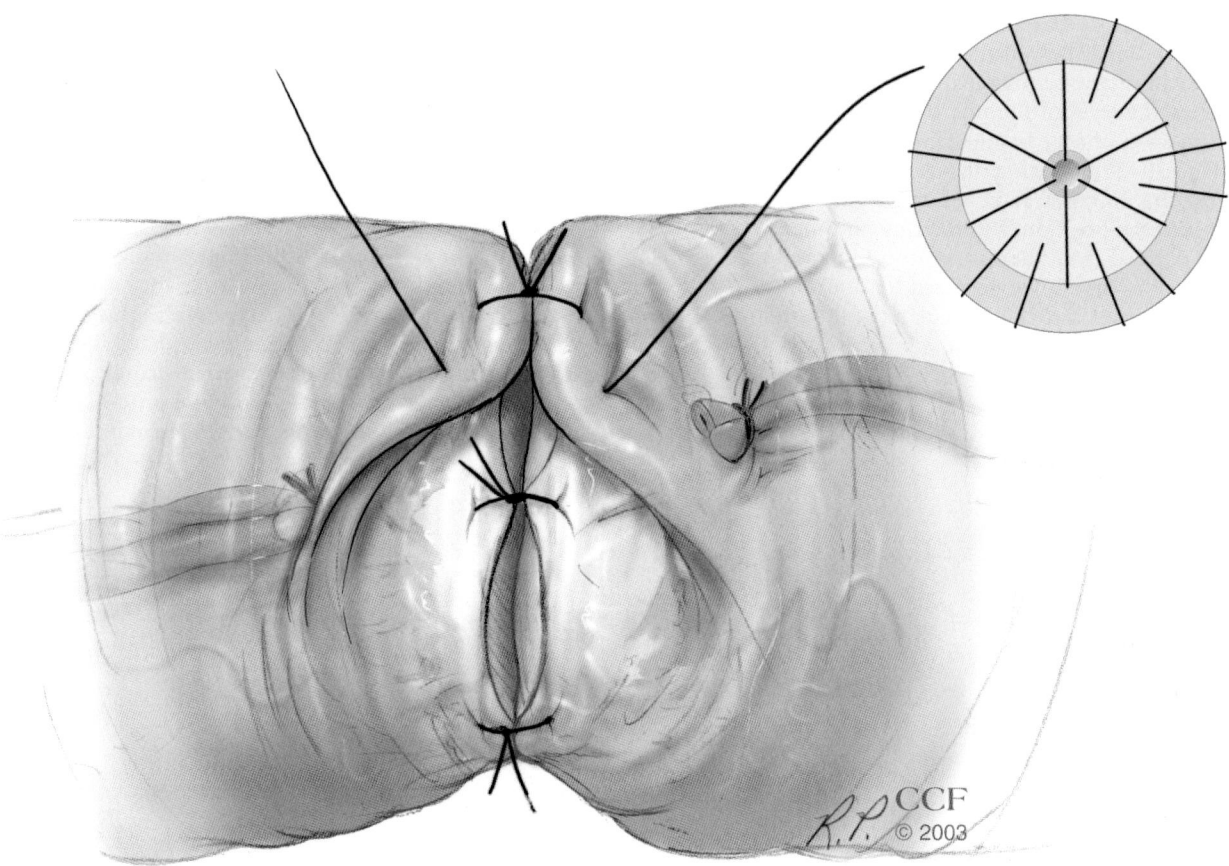

Figure 20–26. Anterior three full-thickness sutures are all placed before they are tied.

repair of a hernia. It is most likely to be the result of a pediatric hernia repair, when the cord structures are small and more susceptible to trauma. The possibility of an inguinal vasal obstruction should be considered in any infertile man who gives a history of an infant hernia repair (Partrick et al, 1998; Sheynkin et al, 1998; Matsuda, 2000; Ridgway et al, 2002). Examination of individuals with inguinal vas obstruction may reveal the testis to be normal size, the epididymis full and firm, and the vas thickened with the convoluted portion more prominent to palpation. Synthetic mesh commonly placed within hernia repairs has the potential to cause an inflammatory response that could affect the integrity of the vas lumen. In some instances, obstruction or narrowing of the vas may result from an inflammatory reaction associated with the use of mesh, inserted through the groin during open surgery or placed laparoscopically (Silich and McSherry, 1996; Uzzo et al, 1999; Meacham, 2002; Berndsen et al, 2004) to strengthen the hernia repair. In one multi-institutional study, 14 men had obstructions in the area of polypropylene mesh used in hernia repair; 9 had bilateral vasal obstructions, and 5 had unilateral obstruction with contralateral testis atrophy or epididymal obstruction (Shin et al, 2005). It would be difficult to determine how many men may have obstructed vasa secondary to implantation of mesh if only one vas is affected and the contralateral side is functioning normally. Whenever there is a history of hernia repair, of whatever type, the possibility of obstruction should at least be suspected. Whereas physical examination can suggest an obstruction of the

inguinal vas, vasography can confirm that suspicion. The vas lumen is dilated, and the contrast material stops somewhere within the inguinal canal or just beyond it (Fig. 20–27).

When an obstruction is identified after hernia repair, a high inguinal incision usually allows adequate exposure of the inguinal canal, where the testicular vas can be isolated and a

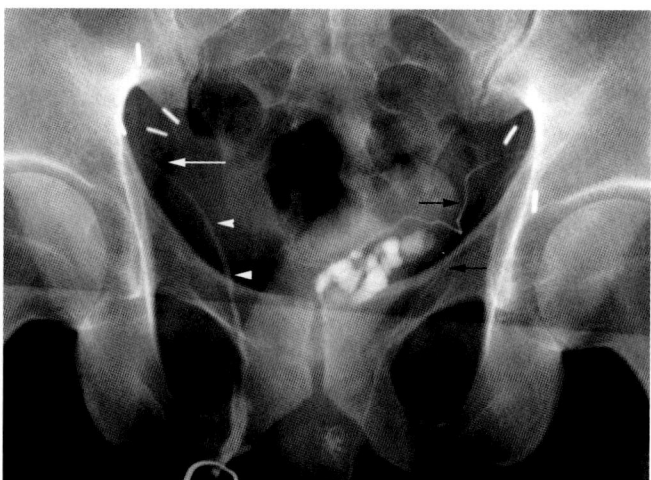

Figure 20–27. Bilateral vasogram demonstrates an obstructed vas on the left at the level of the internal inguinal ring *(white arrow)*. On the opposite side, the normal patent vas lumen is thin *(black arrows)* as opposed to the more dilated obstructed lumen on the left *(arrowheads)*.

vascular loop passed around it and used for traction. If mesh was not used or if the vas may have been injured during the course of an infant hernia repair, the distal vas is often found just below the level of the internal inguinal ring. There may be a thin strip of scar tissue connecting the two ends of the vas (Fig. 20–28). Tracing the testicular vas cephalad and opening the internal inguinal ring inferiorly allow small retractors to be positioned in the ring and the distal vas to be identified, freed from the tissues around it, and then brought out, above the ring, to be prepared for anastomosis. Two stay sutures are passed into the muscularis of the abdominal vas to hold it out of the incision for an easier anastomosis (Fig. 20–29).

If mesh was used in the hernia repair, the testicular side of the vas may be found stuck to the floor of the canal where the mesh was placed. The vas can be traced to the point where the vas and cord dip into a dense, fibrotic mass of tissue. If separation of the distal vas from the mesh risks injury to the vascular cord structures, it may be easier to extend the incision superiorly above the mesh and enter the retroperitoneum superior to the vas, freeing it at the level where it exits the floor of the canal and transposing it inferiorly to be brought out directly through the external ring, where there is no mesh and where the anastomosis can be done more easily. Once the proximal and distal ends are isolated, the vasovasostomy can be performed as described before with a modified single or multilayer technique. **Some men who have a vas obstructed in the groin may, like other men after scrotal vasectomy, have developed a concomitant epididymal obstruction as well. If there are no sperm coming from the proximal vas lumen, it**

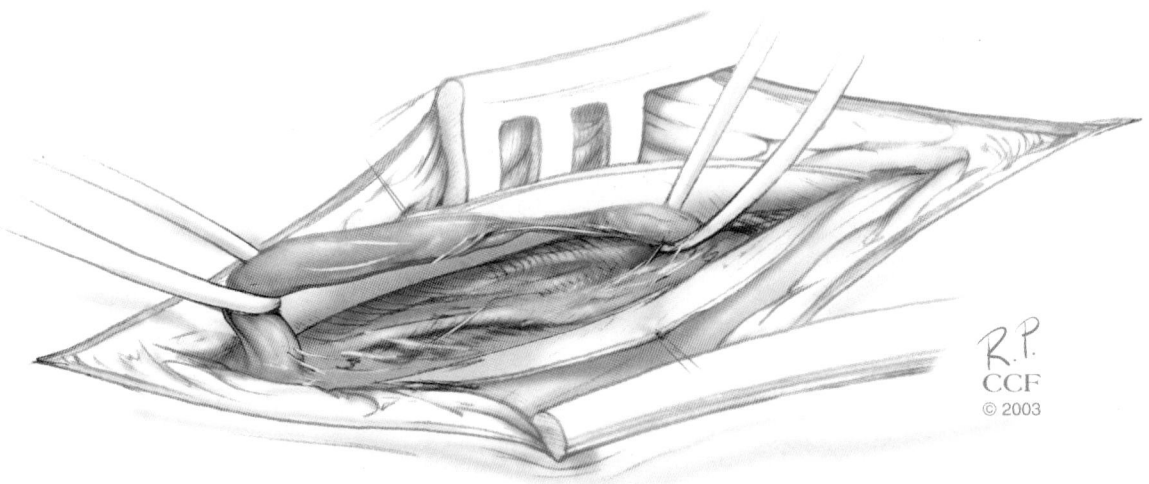

Figure 20–28. In the absence of synthetic mesh at the hernia repair site, the distal vas may still be attached to the proximal (testicular) end by a strand of connective tissue.

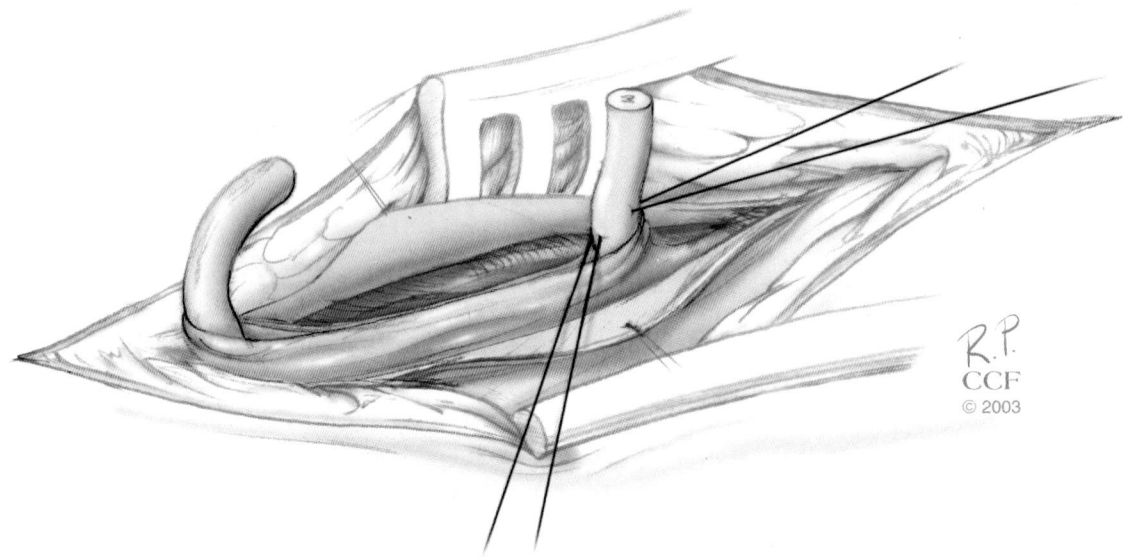

Figure 20–29. Once it is isolated and freed from surrounding tissue, the abdominal end of the vas deferens is held in position for anastomosis by two 6-0 Prolene sutures.

is reasonable to repair the inguinal obstruction first, and if sperm do not appear in the semen after 6 months, the patient should be offered vasography and possible vasoepididymostomy. There are reports of simultaneous vaso-vasostomy and ipsilateral vasoepididymostomy, but if the procedures are to have a chance of succeeding, the blood supply must be preserved at both ends of the vas. Another option that should always be borne in mind is the possibility of using the contralateral nonobstructed vas deferens if the contralateral testis is less functional than the one that has the obstruction. These "crossover procedures" are often more successful than inguinal vasovasostomies. **The vas deferens from the small, poorly functional testis can be cut and brought through the scrotal raphe in a gentle curve to be anastomosed to the proximal vas on the opposite side or to the epididymis as is indicated in Figure 20–30** (Lizza et al, 1985; Sabanegh and Thomas, 1995).

Sperm Retrieval for Cryopreservation at the Time of Vasovasostomy

Some physicians suggest simultaneous sperm retrieval and cryopreservation when a vasectomy reversal is performed so that sperm will be available in the event that the operation is unsuccessful. Some patients are in favor of doing this during the vasectomy reversal; however, in many instances, motile sperm are not found coming from the proximal vas. At times, when motile sperm are seen, the quantity is small, and saving it may take extra time in the operating room that may increase the cost to the patient. **Studies have reported that only 8% to 14% of individuals use their sperm cryo-**

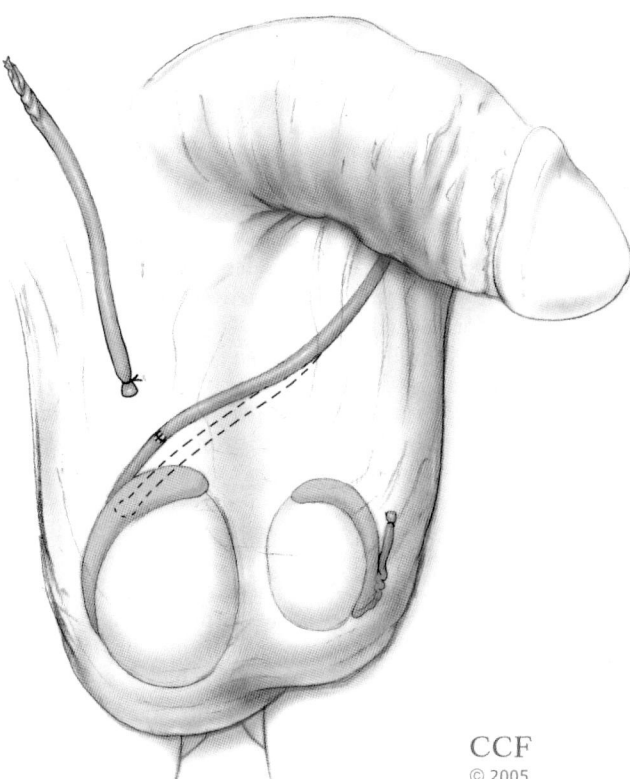

Figure 20–30. "Crossover" vasovasostomy or vasoepididymostomy.

CCF
© 2005

preserved at the time of vasectomy reversal (Glazier et al, 1999; Schrepferman et al, 2001). **If there is an overall patency rate of at least 86% and all patients banked their sperm, less than 15% would have a need to use it, and only if they wished to pursue IVF-ICSI.** Later sperm retrieval for men with vasal or epididymal obstruction can usually be easily accomplished by percutaneous aspiration or simple open biopsy when sperm are needed for IVF-ICSI. Some patients will still want their sperm saved. **If motile sperm are not found in the vas fluid, a testis biopsy and sperm extraction should be done to obtain sufficient sperm without jeopardizing the vasovasostomy** (see the section on sperm retrieval).

Postoperative Care

Following vasovasostomy, the patient is told to moderate his activity for the first week after surgery and to refrain from heavy exercise and sexual activity for 3 weeks. Examination of the semen occurs at 1 month and every 3 months in the year after surgery. Most patients will have sperm in their semen within 4 weeks after vasovasostomy. Some will take longer. If sperm are not present by 6 months, the operation is considered a failure. Repeated surgery or sperm retrieval and IVF-ICSI may be offered.

Complications of Vasovasostomy

Major complications after vasovasostomy are rare. Scrotal ecchymosis and small hematomas are not uncommon. Most significant hematomas can be prevented by meticulous dissection and attention to the many small vessels attached to the vas that need to be occluded with bipolar cautery as the dissection is being done. Infection is rare, as it is our practice to give patients a preoperative dose of a cephalosporin a half-hour before surgery. **On occasion, a large granuloma is present at the site of vasectomy. If it is adherent to the adjacent cord structures, excision potentially could injure the arterial supply to the testis and result in atrophy. It is better to cut the vas on either side of the granuloma, bringing the vas ends together around it, leaving the granuloma and the intact cord structures untouched.**

Secondary obstruction and consequent azoospermia after initially successful vasovasostomy have been reported to occur in 3% to 12% of men (Glazier et al, 1999; Kolettis et al, 2002). One of the initial signs is often a marked decrease in motility and the appearance of sperm heads along with some normal sperm. This has led some to recommend that patients consider sperm cryopreservation once motile sperm return to their semen.

Patency and Pregnancy Rates after Vasovasostomy

Men undergoing inguinal vasovasostomy after accidental injury to the vas deferens generally have a lower success rate than do those men having scrotal vasovasostomy after purposeful vasectomy. This difference could be the result of a longer period of obstruction. Even in reversal of an elective vasectomy, the duration of obstruction appears to be important, as does the age of the female partner.

The largest series of patients undergoing thorough analysis after vasovasostomy was that described in 1991 by members of the Vasovasostomy Study Group. Five experienced micro-

SECTION VI

Years of Obstruction	Patency (%), Sperm Present	Pregnancy (%)
<3	86/89 (97)	56/74 (76)
3–8	525/600 (88)	253/478 (53)
9–14	205/261 (79)	92/209 (44)
≥15	32/45 (71)	11/37 (30)

From Belker AM, Thomas AJ Jr, Fuchs EF, et al: Results of 1,469 microsurgical vasectomy reversals by the Vasovasostomy Study Group. J Urol 1991;145:505-511.

surgeons pooled their data and carefully analyzed it. The patency and pregnancy rates related to time are shown in Table 20–3. Their average patency rate was 86%, and 52% of the couples achieved a pregnancy (Belker et al, 1991). **In this report, the pregnancy rate was 30% when men had had obstructions for more than 15 years.** The authors also noted that too few vasoepididymostomies were performed in this series to support comment on its effectiveness. **More recent studies indicate that men who have had obstructions for more than 15 years will require vasoepididymostomy to increase patency and pregnancy rates.** The age of the female partner has also been more carefully investigated as it pertains to a successful pregnancy after vasectomy reversal. As expected, as women approach or pass the age of 40 years, chances of becoming pregnant are reduced (Fuchs and Burt, 2002; Kolettis et al, 2002, 2003; Thomas and Parekattil, 2004).

Many investigators have reported patency and pregnancy rates after microsurgical vasovasostomy. **Most studies with large numbers of patients have generally found patency rates of 75% to 85% and pregnancy rates of 45% to 70%** (Owen and Kapila, 1984; Silber, 1989; Belker et al, 1991; Fox, 1994; Boorjian et al, 2004; Chan and Goldstein, 2004). Sharlip (1993) carefully culled out the patients who had "achieved completely and consistently normal postoperative semen analyses" and reported the best rate of pregnancy to be 61% to 67%. A review of the largest number of patients to undergo vasectomy reversal by a single surgeon reported that 94% had sperm in their ejaculate after vasovasostomy. Unfortunately, only half the patients who underwent vasovasostomy were available to be followed up for pregnancy. Of these 801 men, 741 reported that they had established a pregnancy (Silber and Grotjan, 2004).

Couples seeking advice as to the best means of establishing a pregnancy when the male partner has had a vasectomy should be counseled openly about their options, risks, and costs. **Men who have failed a first attempt at vasectomy reversal can be offered another try, which, in experienced hands, has led to pregnancy rates ranging between 27% and 57%** (Fox, 1997; Hernandez and Sabanegh, 1999; Paick et al, 2003).

Most reports comparing the success of initial vasectomy reversal with that of sperm retrieval and IVF-ICSI clearly demonstrated that reversal of the vasectomy was superior with respect to cost and at least equal to and in many instances better than IVF-ICSI regarding pregnancy (Kolettis and Thomas, 1997; Pavlovich and Schlegel, 1997). One of the

major issues with respect to costs is the additional burden of multiple births and the attendant risks associated with assisted reproduction and IVF-ICSI. As reproductive endocrinologists improve their ability to successfully transfer fewer embryos, this difference will disappear. Nonetheless, fair assessment based on the years of vasal obstruction, the age and reproductive condition of the female partner, and the personal experience of the surgeon is needed so that the couple can make an informed choice of their reproductive options.

Vasoepididymostomy

In 1901, Dr. Edward Martin, Professor of Surgery at the University of Pennsylvania, reported the first human vasoepididymostomy (Martin et al, 1902). It was performed in a side-to-side method with four fine silver wires to attach the splayed open vas lumen to an opened epididymal tubule in the hope that a patent fistula would be created and remain patent (Fig. 20–31). Several years later, he reported on a series of 14 men who underwent side-to-side vasoepididymal anastomosis. Six men (43%) subsequently had sperm in their semen, and three men (21%) fathered children (Martin, 1909).

A quarter century later in 1936, Hagner reported on a larger series of patients who underwent epididymovasostomy by Martin's technique. Sixty-five men underwent surgery, but Hagner found a patent vas deferens and sperm in the epididymis in only 33 of them. Of these 33 men, 21 (64%) ultimately had sperm in their semen, and 16 (48%) established one or more pregnancies. **With a few exceptions and some modification, the side-to-side method of anastomosis of the epididymis to the vas deferens stood as the standard for the surgical correction of epididymal obstruction until Silber's 1978 description of a microsurgical anastomosis of the vas lumen to a transversely end-cut epididymal tubule.** It was soon apparent that the side-to-side "fistula" anastomosis would not be comparable to a precise microsurgical anastomosis in terms of either patency or pregnancy rates.

Although Silber is often credited with the first report of a microsurgical vasoepididymal anastomosis, his was not the first description of a single tubule anastomosis to the vas lumen. In 1918, V. D. Lespinasse described a "direct vasoepididymostomy." Careful examination shows that this technique, performed without optical magnification, microsutures, or microinstruments, is actually the precursor to the more recently described intussusception method of vasoepididymal anastomosis (see later). A portion of the epididymal tubule was exposed from beneath the tunic after a small longitudinal incision had been made in the vas deferens opposite the dilated epididymis. A 6-0 silk suture on a straight needle was passed through the longitudinal axis of the tubule and then through the opening in the vas deferens, pulling the loop into the vas lumen (Fig. 20–32). The vas was stabilized to the epididymal tunic with four sutures and the luminal silk suture brought out through the skin of the scrotum. Erosion of the invaginated side of the epididymal loop had occurred by 2 weeks, and the suture was extracted from the skin and epididymis by gentle traction. One patient was described, and sperm appeared in his semen (Lespinasse, 1918).

At present, there are three variations of the microsurgical technique for accurate anastomosis of the lumen of the vas

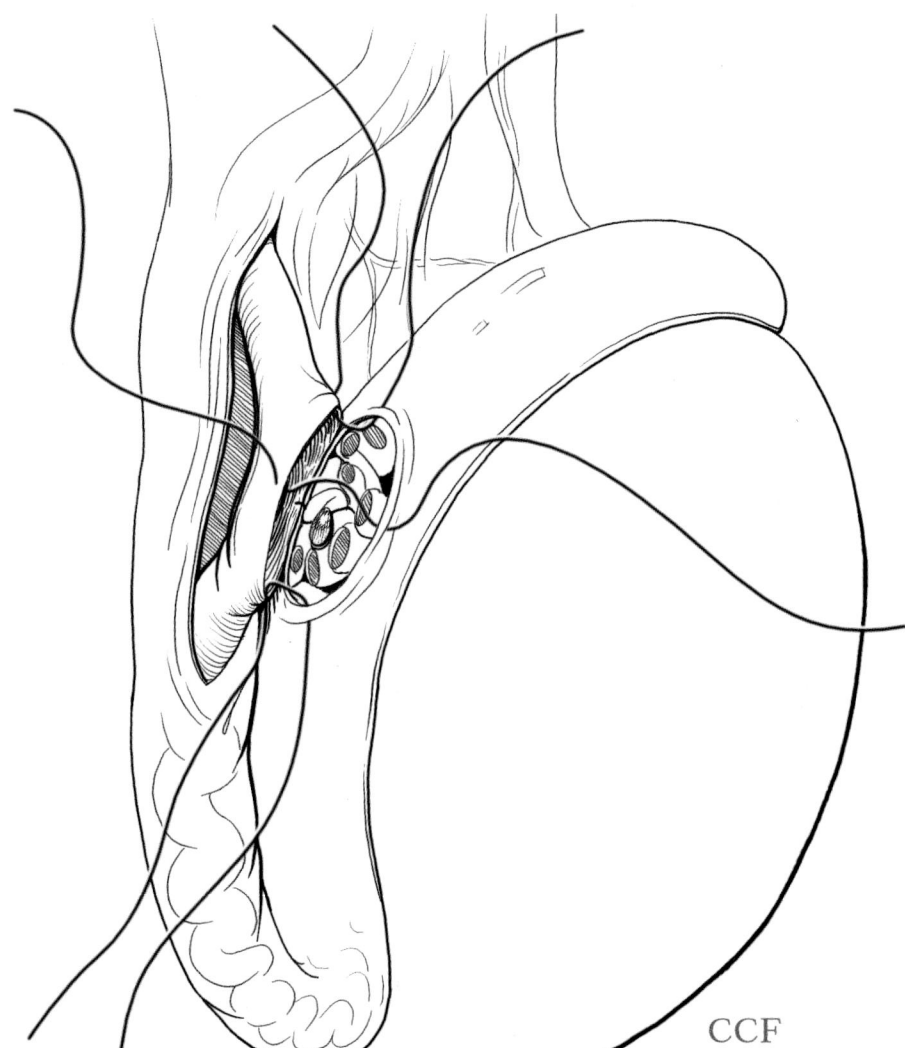

Figure 20–31. Martin's classic side-to-side vasoepididymal anastomosis.

deferens to the single tubule of the epididymis: direct end-to-end, end-to-side, and end-to-side intussusception technique. Performance of all three procedures requires excellent microsurgical skills.

Diagnosis of Epididymal Obstruction

The diagnosis of epididymal obstruction (except in post-vasectomy patients) can be suspected when a man presents with azoospermia, normal gonadotropin levels, semen volume of more than 1.5 mL, normal-feeling vasa deferentia, normal-sized testes, and palpably full or indurated epididymides. Testicular biopsy will reveal presence or absence of active spermatogenesis.

The cause of epididymal obstruction is often obscure. Post-gonococcal epididymitis, which was one of the most common causes of obstruction in Martin and Hagner's time, is rare today because of effective antibiotic therapy. **More subtle causes of epididymal obstruction are a previous injury, congenital abnormalities between vas and epididymis (e.g., in patients with cystic fibrosis mutations), and nonspecific inflammatory events, long forgotten by the time a man presents with azoospermia.**

Vasectomy is certainly one of the most common known causes of epididymal obstruction (Uzzo et al, 1999; Meacham, 2002; Ridgway et al, 2002). **The incidence of epididymal obstruction is time related to the vasectomy. Epididymal obstruction rarely occurs within 4 years of a vasectomy but can occur in 60% or more of patients on one or both sides after 15 years of vasal obstruction** (Fuchs and Burt, 2002). The epididymal obstruction is presumed to occur when pressure within the epididymis exceeds the integrity of the delicate epididymal tubule and results in extravasation of sperm with consequent epididymal obstruction. **A preoperative sign of epididymal obstruction is palpable fullness of the epididymis more than 4 to 5 years after vasectomy.** Parekattil and coworkers (2004) attempted to predict the possibility of epididymal obstruction after vasectomy by use of a mathematical formula based on the patient's age and years of obstruction. This computer model, which included all men who would require a vasoepididymostomy, was of limited specificity and included some who required only a vasovasostomy on the basis of characteristics of fluid from the proximal vas at the time of surgery. Such a model, despite limitations, suggests to a urologist who is not comfortable performing the

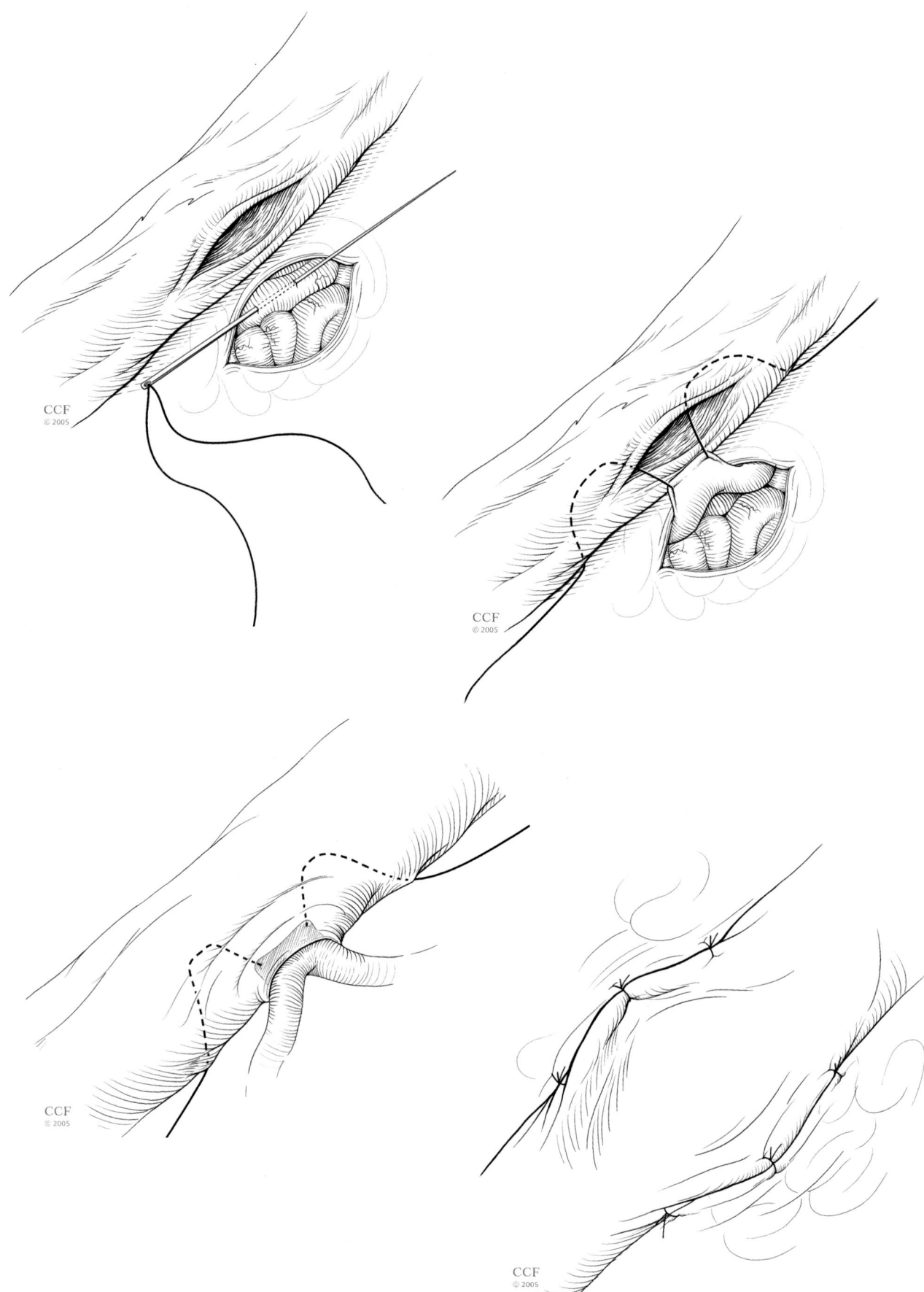

Figure 20–32. Lespinasse single-tubule, nonmicrosurgical intussuscepted vasoepididymal anastomosis.

technically more demanding vasoepididymostomy the need to refer patients likely to require a vasoepididymostomy to someone with appropriate expertise and experience (Thomas, 2004).

A set of criteria that indicate the need to consider vasoepididymostomy is described in the section on vasovasostomy. **The actual decision to perform a vasoepididymostomy is based primarily on the quality of fluid found at the proximal (testicular) vas deferens.** If fluid can be obtained from the proximal vas lumen, it is placed on a sterile glass slide with a few drops of saline or lactated Ringer's solution to dilute the vasal fluid, and it is immediately examined under 200× and 400× magnification with a light microscope. **Vasoepididymostomy should be considered in the following instances: when the material coming from the proximal vas lumen is thick, pasty, and devoid of sperm; if the fluid is creamy and contains only debris and perhaps a few sperm heads; when there is no fluid with milking of the vas; and when irrigation of the proximal vas with 0.1 to 0.2 mL of saline with a 24-gauge plastic angiocatheter attached to a tuberculin syringe fails to wash out any sperm.**

Preoperative Considerations

When there is no clear-cut inflammatory or iatrogenic cause of the presumed epididymal obstruction, the patient should be evaluated for a cystic fibrosis gene mutation, sometimes associated with epididymal obstruction (Mak et al, 1999). If the test result is positive, the patient's wife should also be tested and appropriate genetic counseling given before surgery is performed.

The possibility and advisability of cryopreserving sperm harvested from testis tissue or from the epididymis at the time of surgery should be discussed with the couple. **Because these procedures may take between 3 and 6 hours, depending on their complexity, previous surgery, scarring, or the need to mobilize long segments of the vasa or epididymides, use of a general anesthetic or continuous epidural anesthesia with intravenous sedation works well.**

In counseling patients as to the type of procedure that will most likely be performed (i.e., vasovasostomy versus vasoepididymostomy), the presence of a sperm granuloma or a long testicular vasal remnant (>2.7 cm) will predict the greater likelihood of performing a vasovasostomy (Witt et al, 1994). Except in those men who have had a vasectomy, if one suspects an epididymal obstruction, testis biopsy (if it has not been done previously), vasography, and vasoepididymostomy can be performed as a single operative event.

Operative Procedures

Regardless of the method chosen for the vasoepididymal anastomosis, a few preparatory steps are common to all.

Once the patient is anesthetized, his position and comfort are critical; these can be prolonged procedures, and undue pressure or overextension of the arms can lead to significant morbidity in a young, otherwise healthy man. The operating table should have a soft padding that allows support but also provides cushion to the torso and legs. The patient's arms are positioned comfortably at a 45- to 60-degree angle from the body with the elbows slightly flexed and supinated to prevent undue pressure at the antecubital joint or pressure against the ulnar nerve. A soft blanket roll or small pillow is placed

beneath the knees, and sequential compression stockings are routinely used to minimize the chance of venous thrombosis. A soft doughnut pad beneath the patient's head and occasional shifting of the head position by the anesthesiologist can prevent the pressure-related alopecia that can occur in prolonged operations.

A vertical incision in the scrotum is made for each testis; this allows the incisions to be extended into the groin if more extensive mobilization of the vas is needed. **If a testis biopsy has not been performed previously, a 2-cm vertical incision is made over the anterior surface of the testis, exposing the tunica albuginea, and the biopsy is carried out as described earlier in this chapter.** A segment of testis tissue is sent for frozen section analysis, or the tissue is examined in the operating room as previously detailed. If there is a light microscope in the operating room, a small fragment of seminiferous tubules can be placed on a sterile glass slide and teased apart with a microforceps and a 22-gauge needle (Fig. 20–33). One or two drops of lactated Ringer's solution are placed over the tissue, and a coverslip is pressed against the tissue to spread it out and make examination for sperm under 200× and 400× magnification easy and quick. If spermatogenesis is normal, numerous sperm will easily be seen floating in the fluid or attached to the tissue at the periphery of the teased ends. Frequently, motile sperm can be seen (Jarow et al, 1995).

Once spermatogenesis is confirmed, the incision is enlarged and the testis delivered out of the scrotum and examined. In most instances, the epididymis will be visibly dilated, even without optical magnification (Fig. 20–34). Vasography is performed in the manner described later with a 30-gauge needle or partial vasotomy. If vasal patency is confirmed from the junction of the straight and convoluted vas where the needle was placed or the vas incised, it is likely that any obstruction in the convoluted vas proximal to the needle would be grossly visible; therefore, the obstruction must be in the epididymis or the efferent ducts. **Some surgeons prefer to transect the vas at the junction of the straight and convoluted vas both to check the fluid (if any) that may come from the proximal vas and to use the more muscular straight vas for the anastomosis. Others will use the distal convoluted**

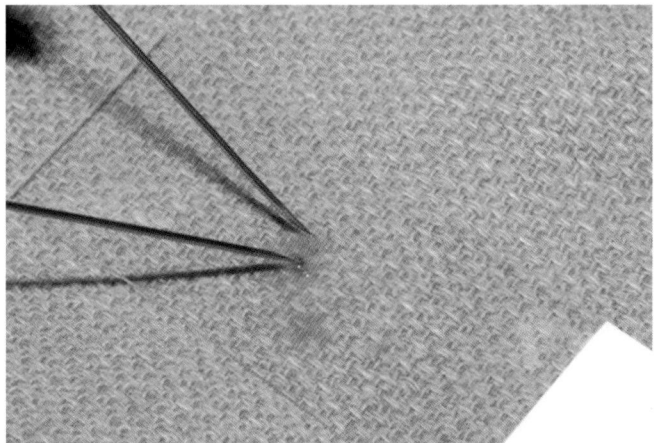

Figure 20–33. Two needles are used to tease apart a small fragment of seminiferous tubules for intraoperative examination for sperm.

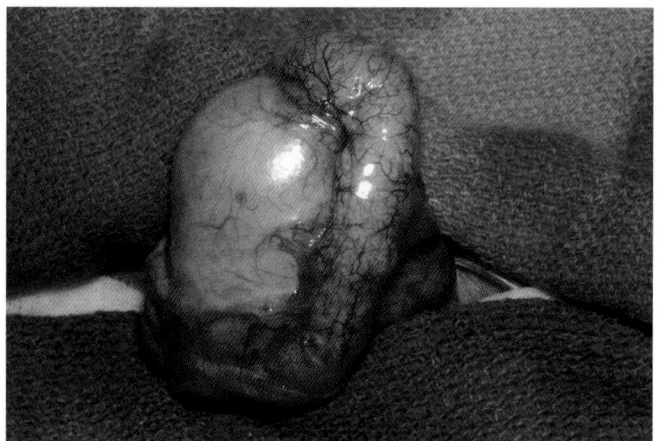

Figure 20–34.   Grossly dilated epididymis resulting from an obstruction at the level of the cauda epididymis.

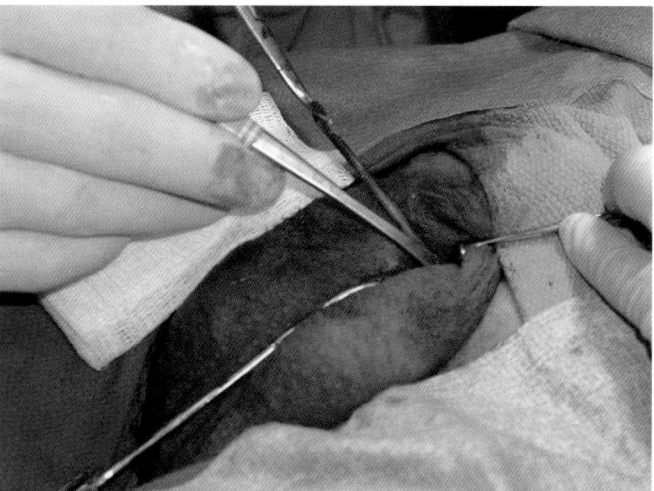

Figure 20–35.   Penfield elevator used to push away the loose connective tissues attached to the vas deferens to gain vasal length in preparation for a vasoepididymostomy.

vas to gain extra length without the need for extensive mobilization.

Before the vas is cut, the vessels are ligated in two places a few millimeters apart with 6-0 nylon at the point of planned transection. The vas is cut between the two sutures and the proximal end tied off or simply cauterized to avoid bleeding. A 5-0 Prolene suture can be passed 0.5 cm from the end of the cut distal vas to act as a holding suture; the vas is freed from the cord, and sufficient length is obtained to allow it to cover the midepididymis without tension.

In the patient requiring a vasoepididymostomy after prior vasectomy, adequate length of the distal vas may be a problem, depending on the level of the vasectomy. Length may be gained with a few simple maneuvers, but always keeping in mind the need to preserve the blood supply to the vas and epididymis.

With the vas on mild traction by the 5-0 Prolene holding suture or a hemostat, the loose tissue attaching it to the cord is teased away, and small vessels are cauterized with a bipolar microcautery. The incision can be extended cephalad to the level of the pubic tubercle and the vas, further exposing the vas by holding back the skin and cord with small right-angled retractors. The vas can then be freed further by pushing away the adherent tissue with a small, blunt, Penfield periosteal elevator or similar blunt instrument (Fig. 20–35). If further length is needed, the incision can be extended to the level of the internal inguinal ring, and the external oblique fascia is incised to expose and free more of the vas.

On the other end, the tail and proximal body of the epididymis can be freed up as well to provide some additional length. **Often, carefully inverting the testis while keeping the spermatic cord from kinking or twisting makes it possible to place the vas in proximity to the epididymis without tension or torsion.**

Once sufficient vasal length has been achieved, the operating microscope is brought into position to examine the epididymis and identify the most distal, patent portion at which the anastomosis can be performed.

Methods of Anastomosis

End-to-End Technique. Silber described this method of anastomosis in 1978. It was a purposeful, carefully thought

out and performed approximation of the cut end of the patent epididymal tubule and the vas lumen. The rationale for the anastomosis is that the body and tail of the epididymis are a single, continuous, convoluted tubule. If it is cut transversely, only the cut end of the tubule above the level of the obstruction will exude sperm.

Some surgeons have found that the end-to-end method of anastomosis is best suited for distal epididymal obstruction because the epididymal tubule is larger and the wall a bit thicker than the corpus or caput. The epididymal tail can be dissected free from the inferior aspect of the testis and the epididymis transected at its distal end (Fig. 20–36). When the epididymis is cut proximal to the obstructed area, there will be a continuous flow of sperm-laden fluid from one opened epididymal tubule. The presence of sperm is confirmed by irrigation of the cut surface, aspiration of fluid from the end of the open tubule with a small capillary tube, and examination of the fluid by light microscopy. **If no sperm are found, another transecting cut is made approximately 0.5 cm higher, toward the head of the epididymis, until the patent portion of the tubule is identified by the presence of normal-appearing motile or nonmotile sperm.**

The lumen of the vas deferens is anastomosed to the cut, open tubule exuding sperm. The first step is to secure the cut end of the abdominal vas to the epididymal tunic with two 9-0 nylon sutures passed through the edge of the epididymal tunic and into the adventitia and muscularis of the vas deferens at the 5- and 7-o'clock positions. Four equally spaced double-armed 10-0 sutures are placed into the edge of the epididymal tubule, inside out, and then carried through the vas lumen, beginning at the 6-o'clock position. The first suture is tied, but the sutures at the 3-, 9-, and 12-o'clock positions are not tied until all are placed (Fig. 20–37). Once the vas lumen and the opened tubule are brought together, the muscularis and adventitia of the vas deferens are secured to the tunic of the epididymis with interrupted 9-0 sutures (Fig. 20–38).

End-to-Side Technique. The rationale for the end-to-side techniques, whether directly sewn (Fogdestam and Fall,

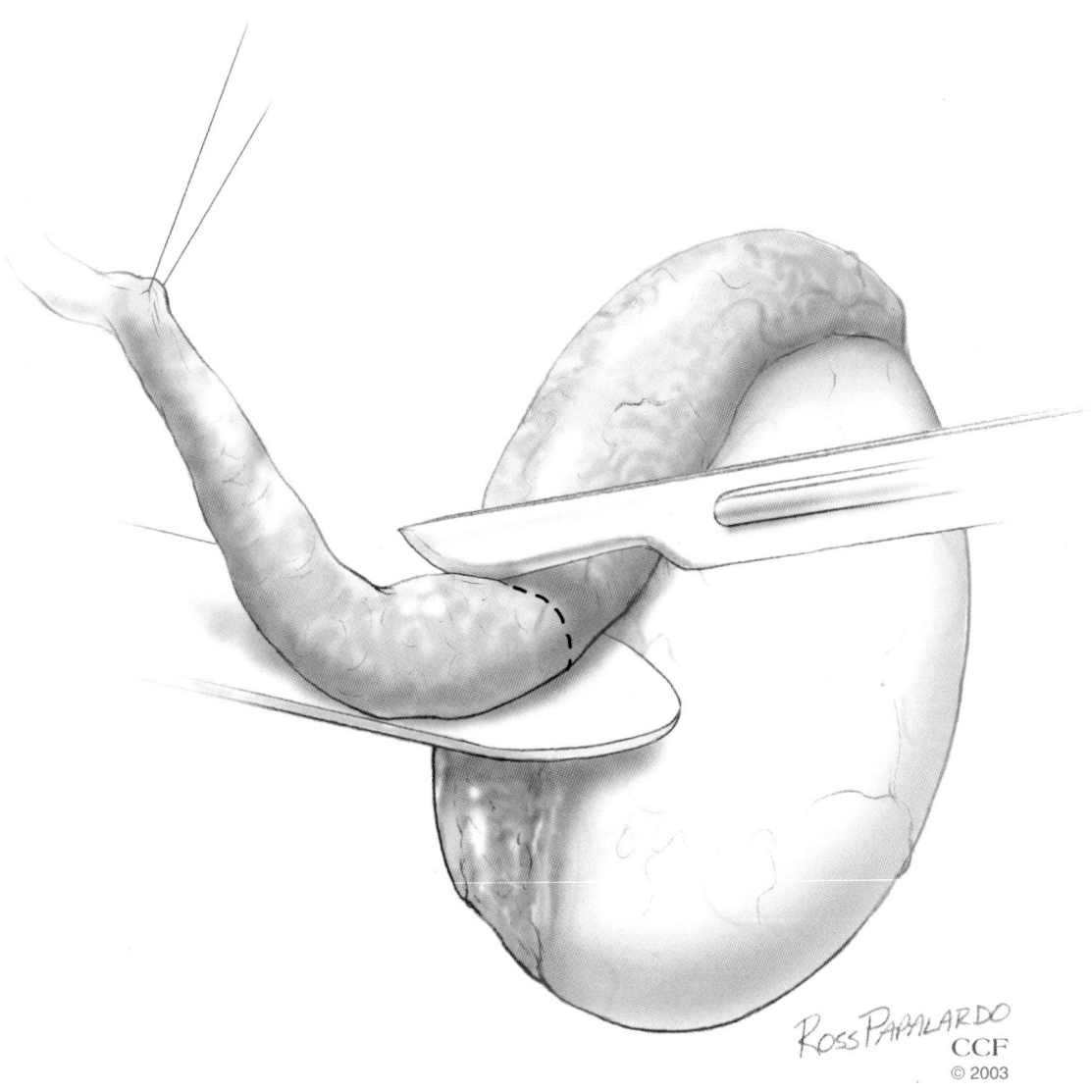

Figure 20–36. Transection of the tail of the epididymis in preparation for an end-to-end vasoepididymostomy.

1983; Thomas, 1987) **or intussuscepted, is that there is far less dissection required, less troublesome bleeding from the transected epididymis, and therefore a clearer field in which to perform this delicate anastomosis.**

Once the vas is prepared in the manner described before, the epididymis is examined under the operating microscope. Beginning at the level of the cauda, a 0.5-cm incision is made in the tunic of the epididymis, pushing the tubule toward the tunic surface by compressing the tubule with thumb and forefinger (Fig. 20–39). Once the tunic is opened, a small window is made in the tunic, exposing the loops of the intact epididymal tubule below. The loops will bulge through the opened tunic, and a single loop is carefully isolated from its surrounding connective tissue. The anterior surface of this loop is incised along its longitudinal axis (Fig. 20–40) with a microknife, making an opening of approximately 0.5 mm. The fluid exuding from this loop is aspirated, placed on a glass slide, and examined for sperm. If normal-appearing sperm (motile or nonmotile) are present, the anastomosis is per-

formed with this opened tubule. If no sperm or only sperm parts (heads, heads with partial tails) are found in the fluid, the tunic is incised more cephalad, and the same procedure is repeated until normal-appearing spermatozoa are identified. Once the patent loop is identified and opened, three 10-0 double-armed sutures are placed (inside-out) in a triangular fashion equidistant from one another (Fig. 20–41). If sperm are motile and are to be cryopreserved, they are aspirated with a 24-gauge angiocatheter attached to a tuberculin syringe as they flow from the opened loop. The fluid is placed in an appropriate medium and sent for cryopreservation.

The vas deferens is brought through the uppermost portion of the tunica vaginalis and either beneath or over the spermatic cord to the lateral aspect of the testis close to the opened portion of the epididymal tunic. Two 9-0 nylon sutures are used to hold the muscularis and adventitia of the vas deferens to the opened epididymal tunic. The previously placed 5-0 Prolene holding suture can then be removed. The apical suture

Text continued on p. 689.

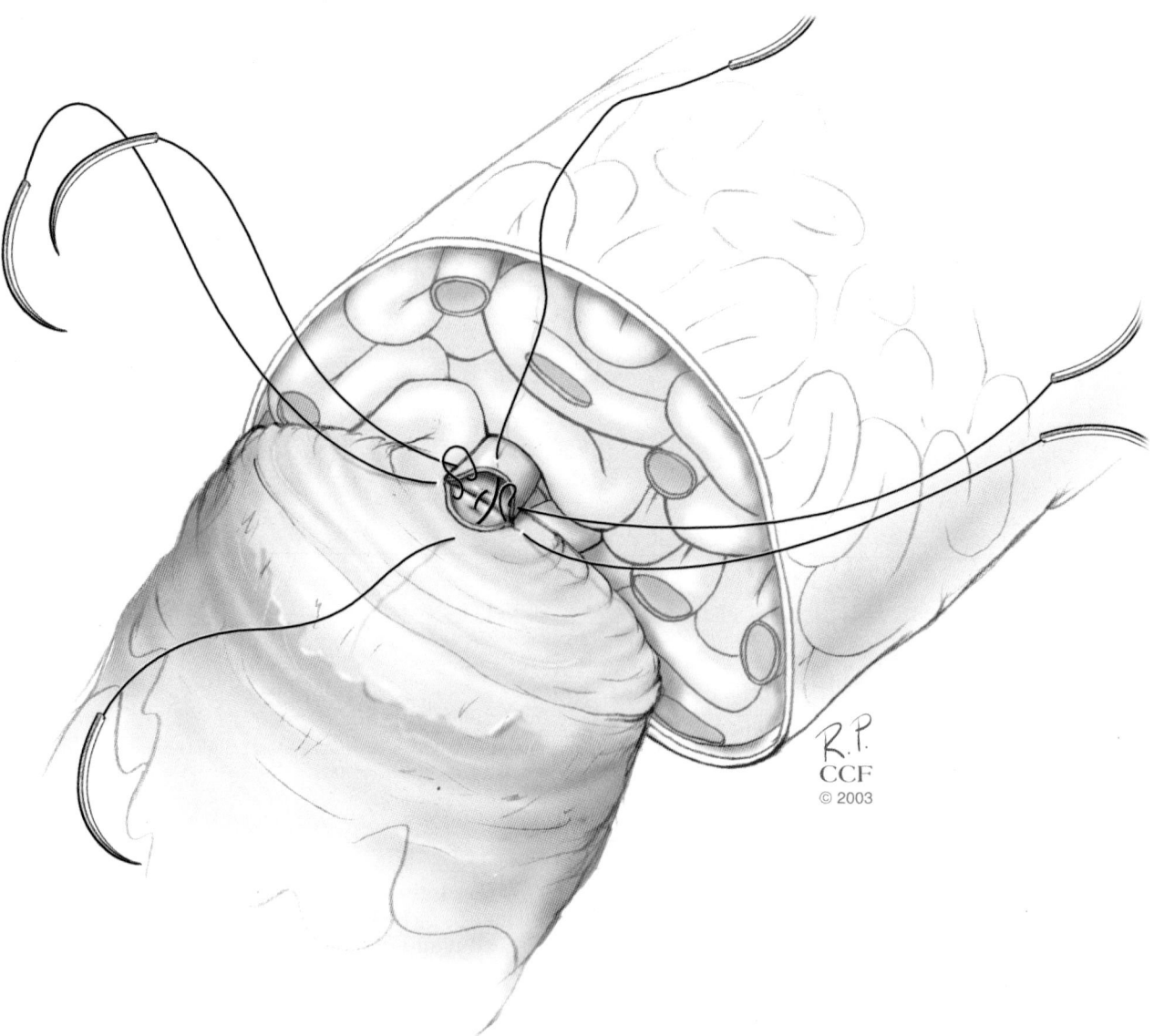

Figure 20–37. The sutures at the 3-, 12-, and 9-o'clock positions are all placed, then tied to approximate the lumens of the vas and epididymis.

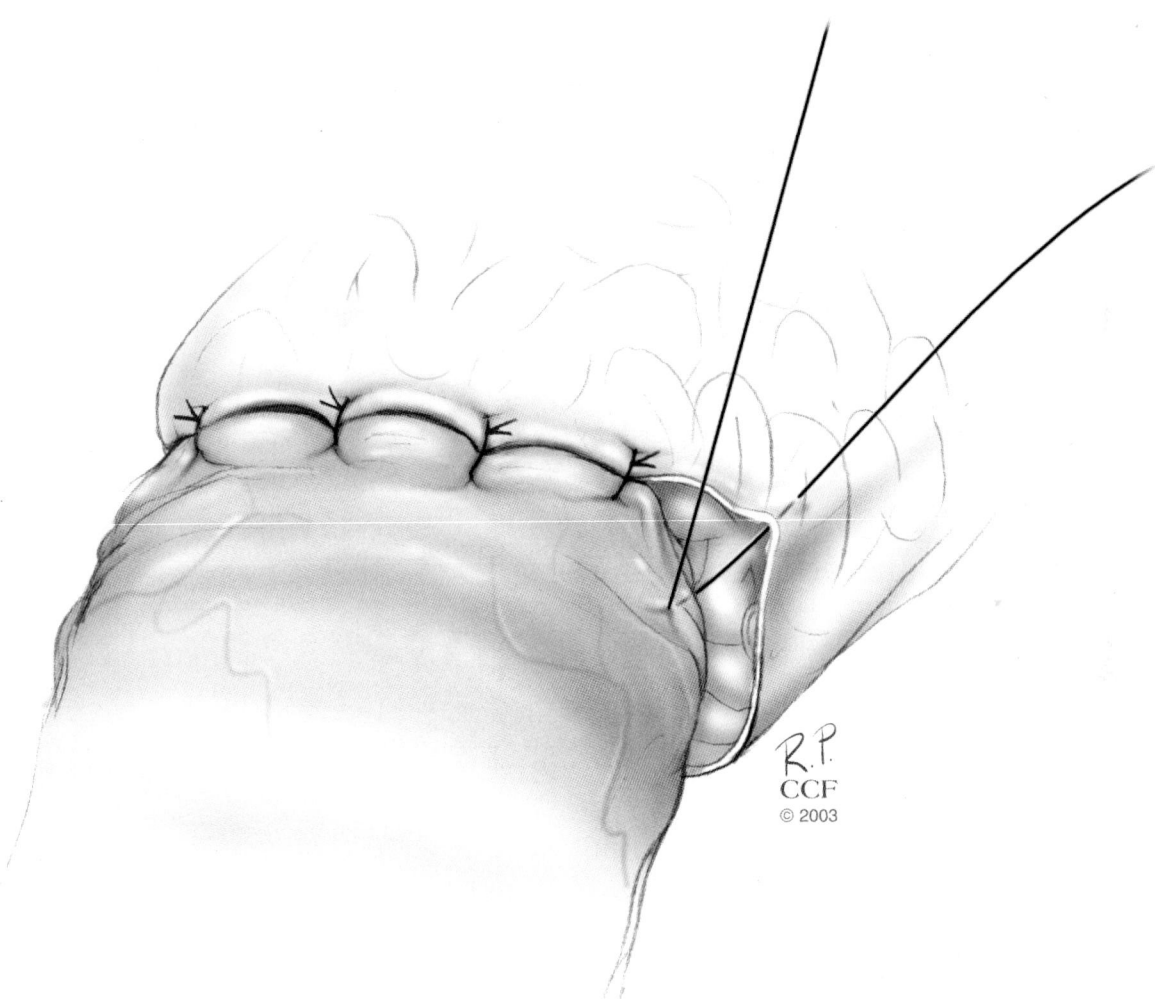

Figure 20–38. The adventitia and muscularis of the vas are approximated to the epididymal tunic.

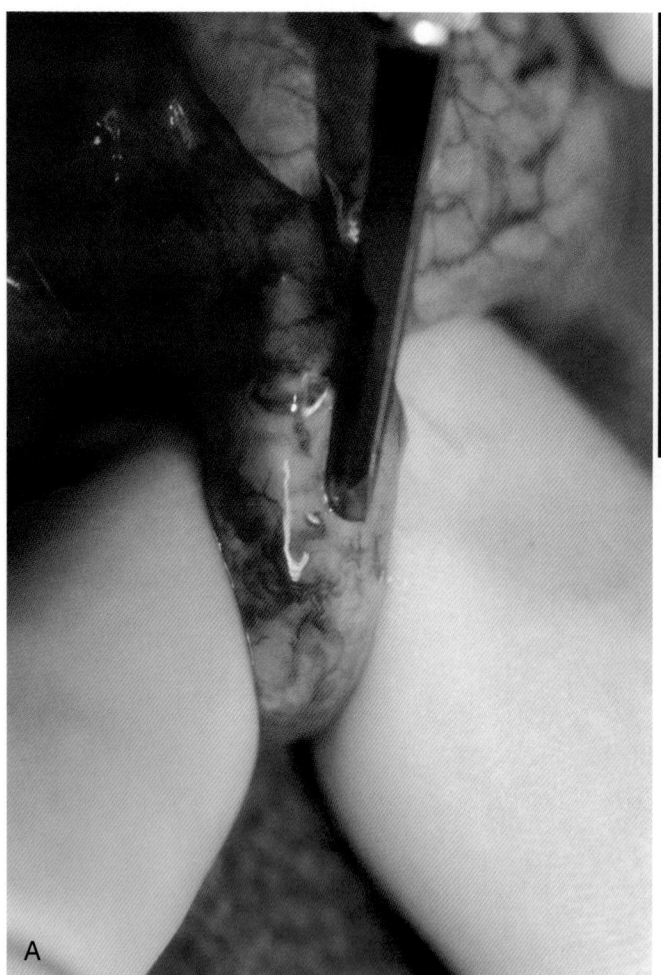

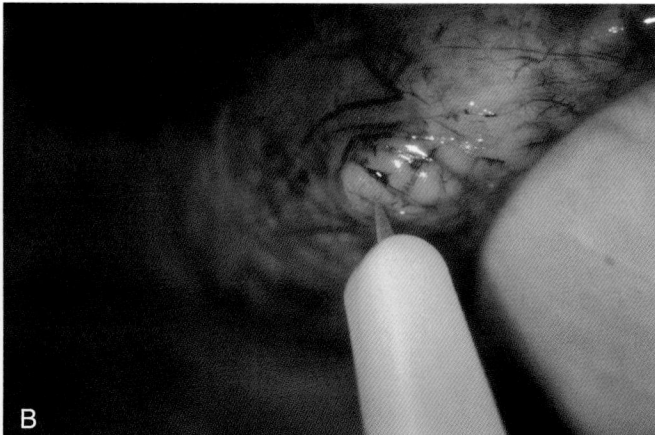

Figure 20–39. **A** and **B,** The epididymal tunic is incised by a round-tipped blade, with care taken not to enter the epididymal tubule beneath.

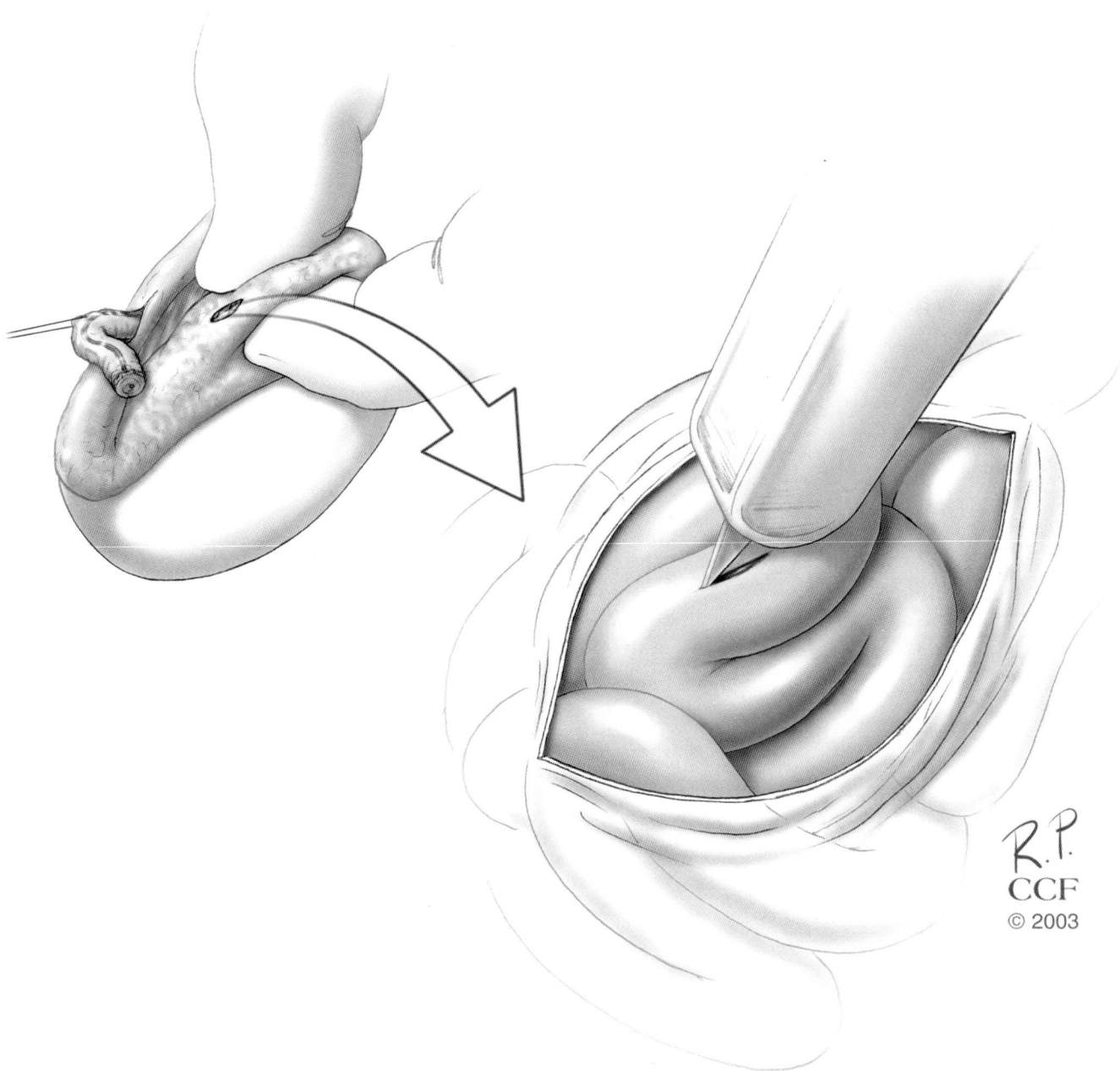

Figure 20–40. A window in the tunic having been made, the chosen epididymal loop is opened with a 1.5-mm microknife.

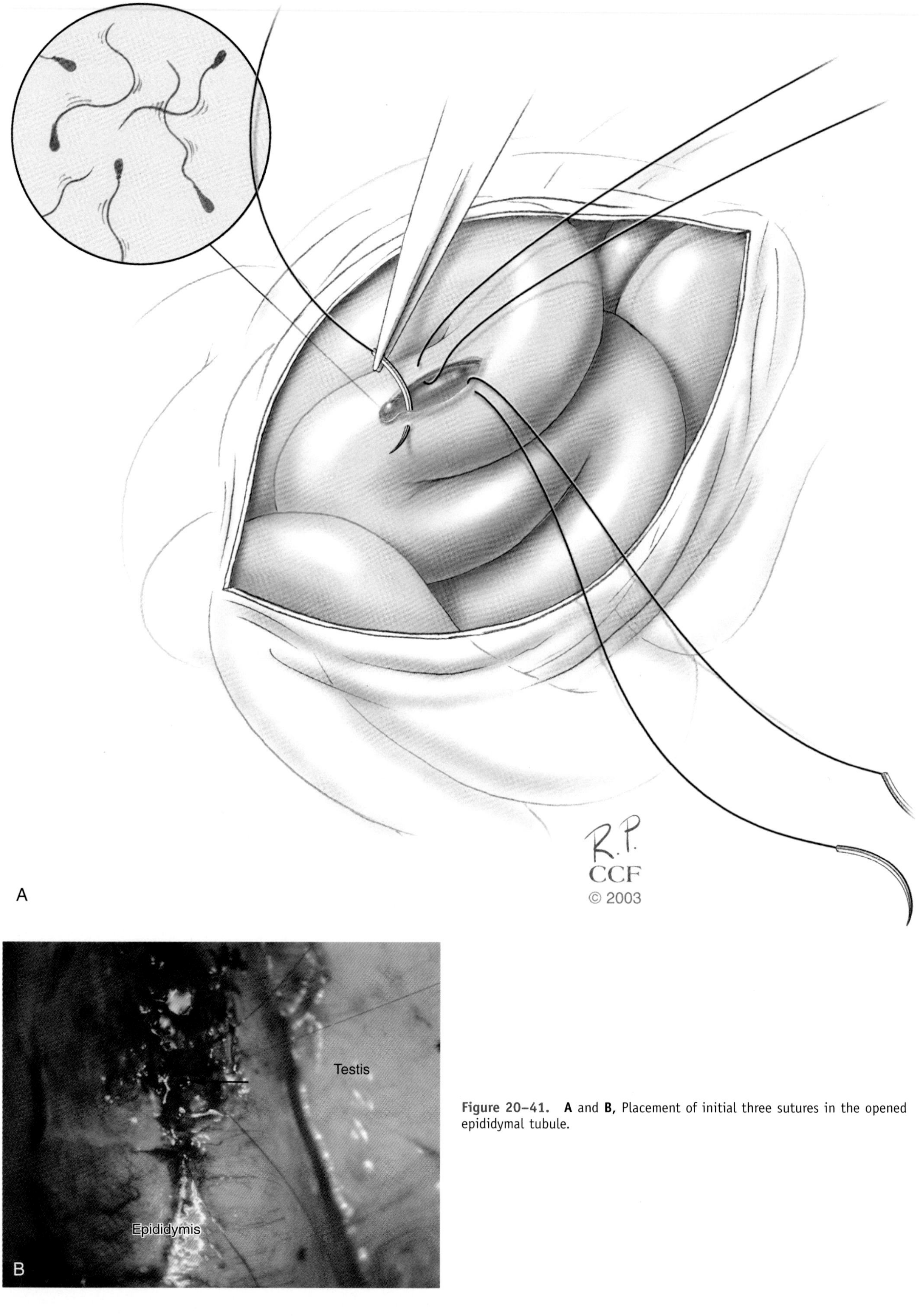

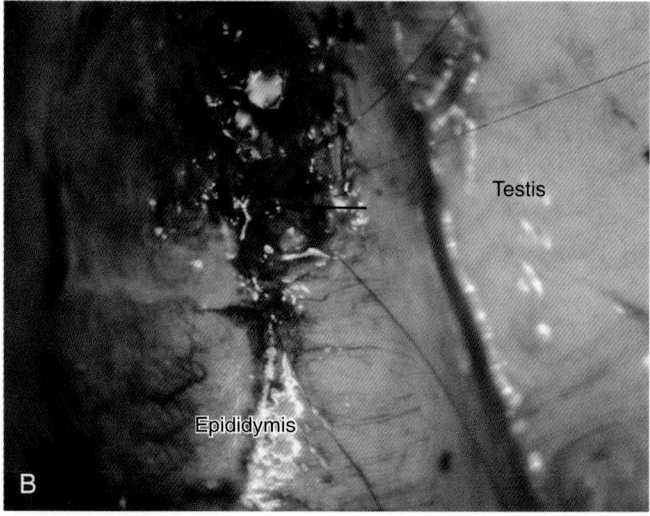

A

B

Testis

Epididymis

Figure 20–41. **A** and **B,** Placement of initial three sutures in the opened epididymal tubule.

that was passed into the epididymal lumen is now passed into the lumen of the vas deferens and secured (Fig. 20–42). The other two sutures are passed through the lumen but not tied. Mild traction on these sutures opens up the epididymal lumen and allows easier passage of two new sutures at the 4- and 8-o'clock positions into the epididymal lumen and the vas (Fig. 20–43). Once properly placed, they are tied. A sixth suture is passed directly opposite the first, and the last three sutures are tied (Fig. 20–44).

The muscularis and adventitia of the vas deferens are approximated to the epididymal tunic, in a circumferential fashion, with eight to ten 9-0 sutures (Fig. 20–45). Bolstering sutures are placed along the side of the vas, attaching it to the visceral tunic. These sutures prevent stress on the anastomosis when the testis is placed back in the scrotum.

Intussusception Technique. This technique differs from the end-to-side technique in that the lumen is opened after

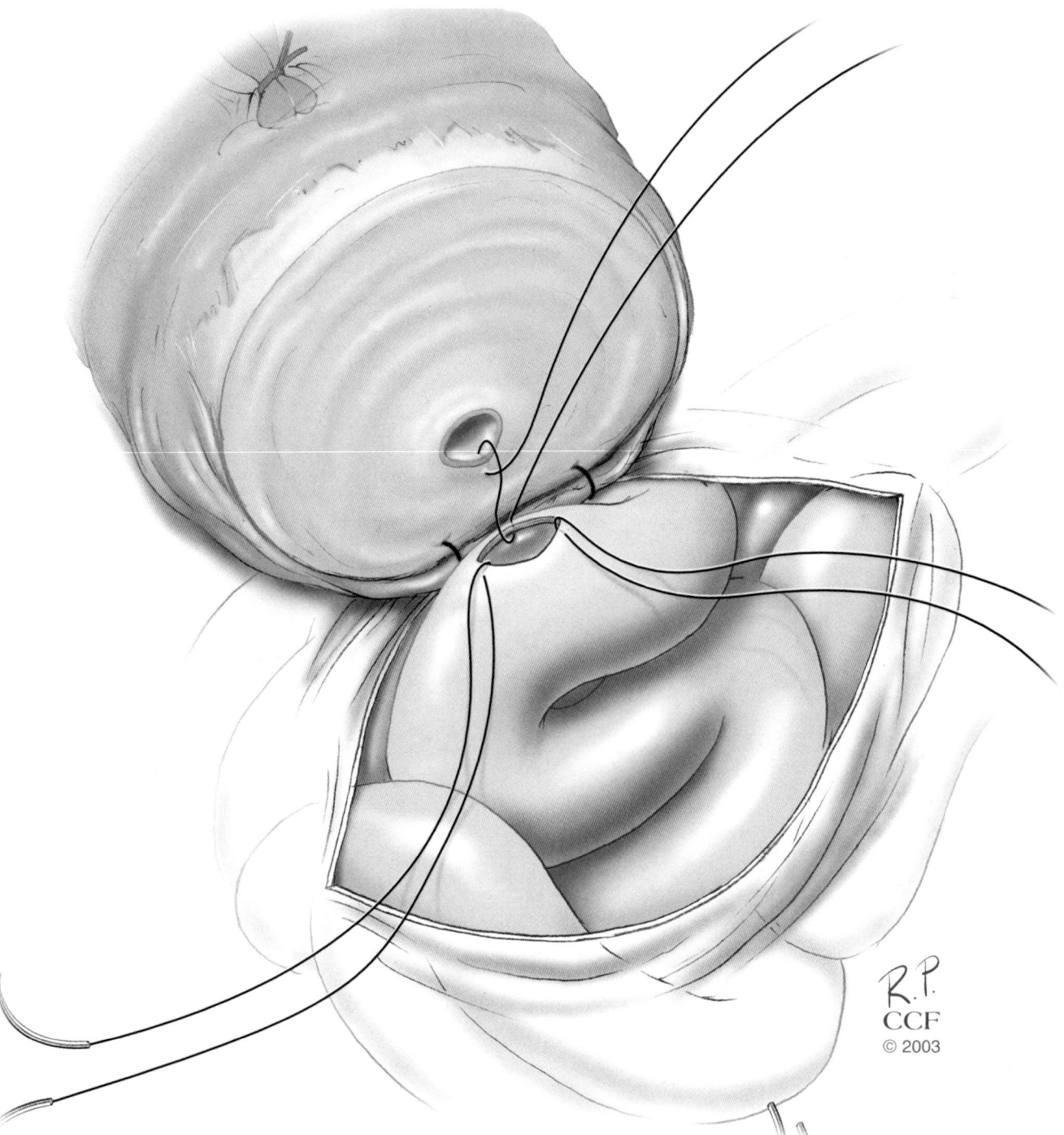

Figure 20–42.   First vasoepididymal suture placed at most inferior position.

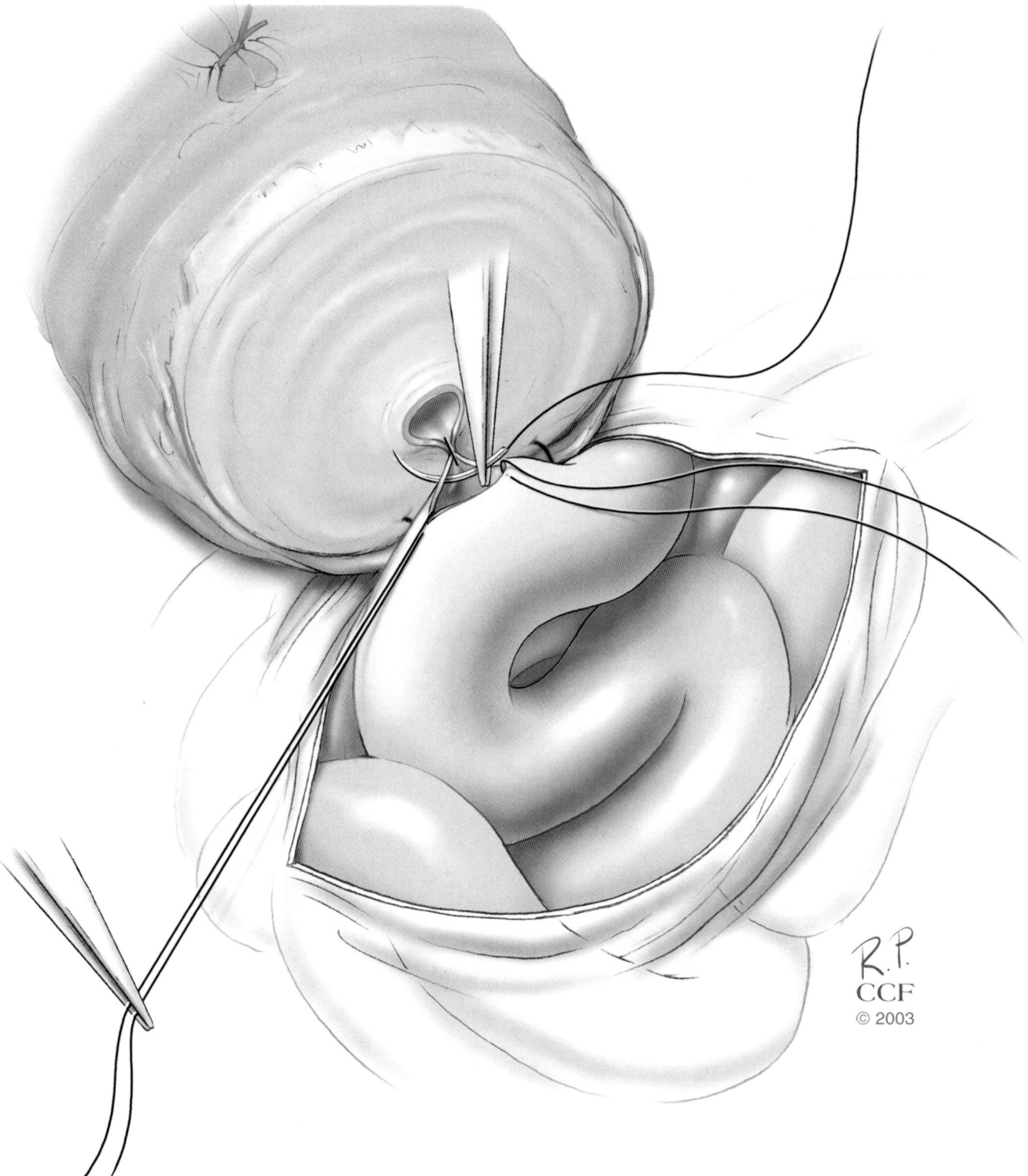

Figure 20–43. By placement of a small amount of traction on the second and third epididymal sutures, the edge of the tubule becomes easy to see for passage of another suture next to the first tied suture.

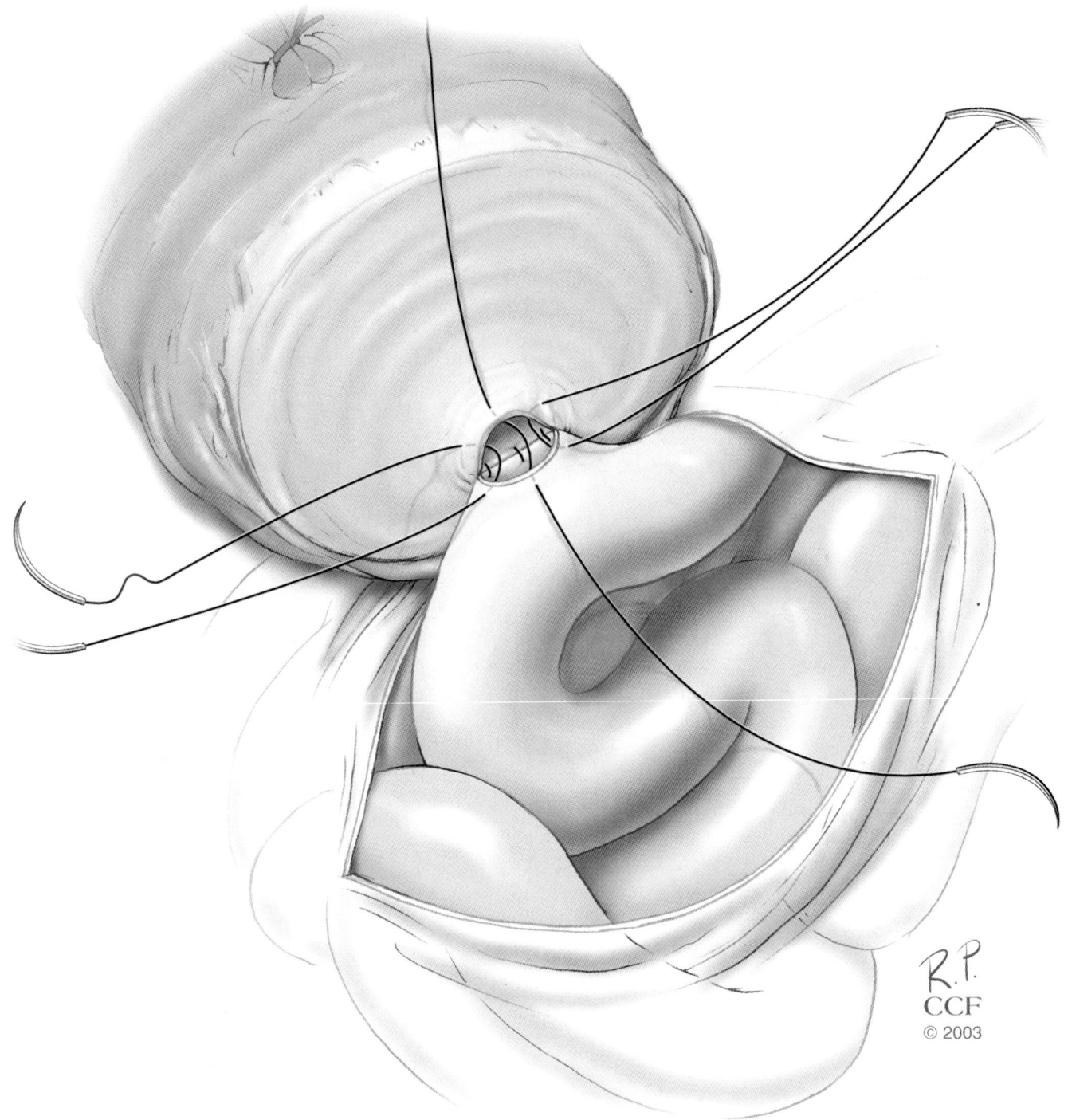

Figure 20–44. The three anteriorly placed sutures are passed into the wall of the vas lumen and then tied.

R.P.
CCF
© 2003

the sutures are positioned in the epididymal loop. Once the lumen is opened, the loop is drawn into the vasal lumen with the sutures rather than approximated to it (Berger, 1998). For this anastomosis to be performed more easily, the epididymal loop has to be freed from the connective tissue around it so that it can be pulled into the vasal lumen without tension. A small window is made in the epididymal tunic as with the end-to-side anastomosis. The dilated loops are freed from the over-

lying tissues, and an appropriate loop is chosen. The cut end of the distal vas is approximated to the lower portion of the opened tunic. Three double-armed 10-0 sutures are placed in a triangular fashion, leaving the center open for incision (Fig. 20–46). When the needles are placed, an incision is made between the three needles, and the fluid that exudes is examined. If sperm are found, the needles are drawn through and the sutures left intact. If there are no sperm, the needles are

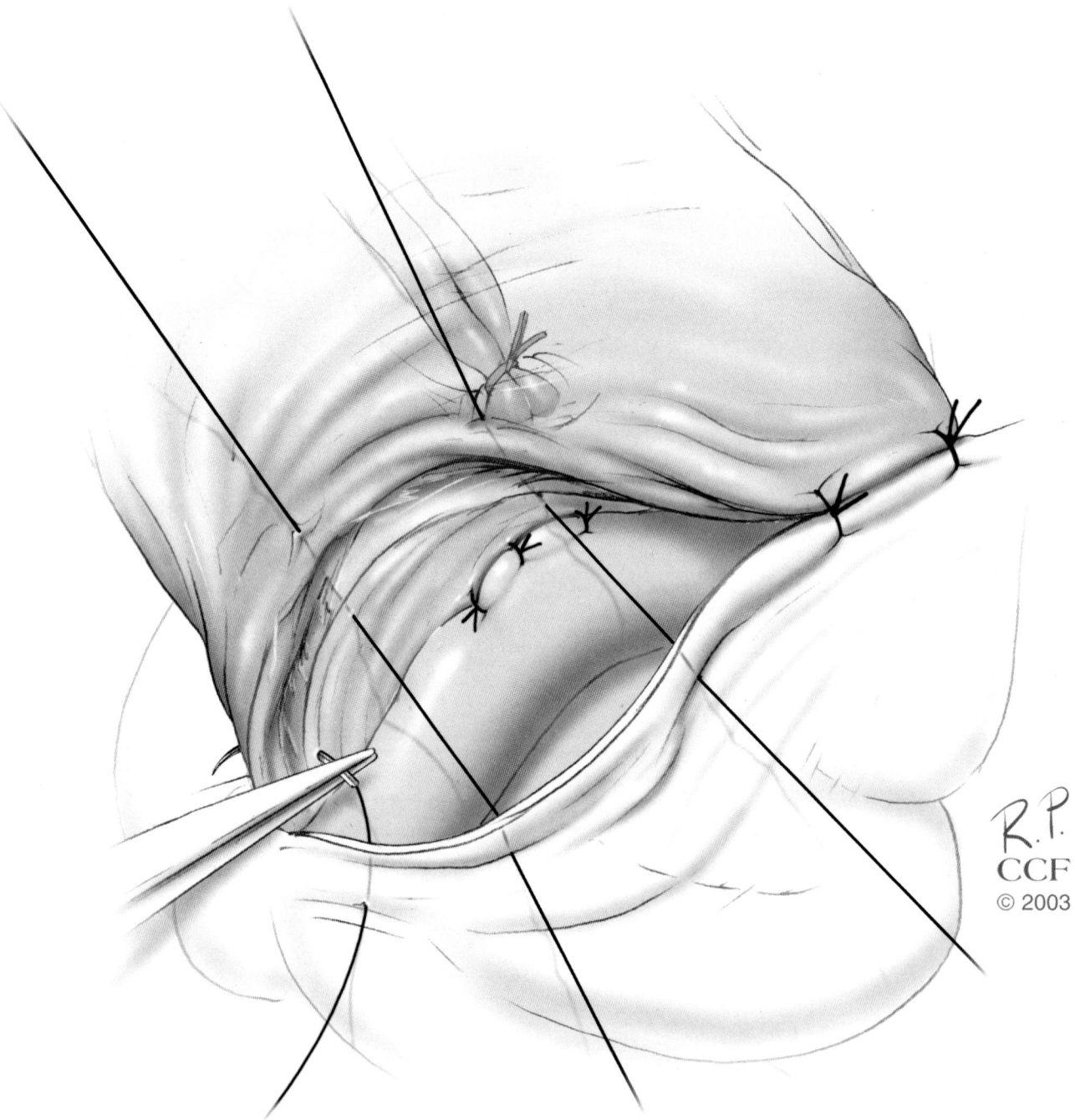

R.P.
CCF
© 2003

Figure 20–45. The adventitia and muscularis are secured to the edge of the window made in the epididymal tunic.

backed out from the loop and used again in a more cephalad loop. The two needles (Fig. 20–47, a and a′) attached to the suture closest to the vas are passed into the vas lumen and brought out just through the muscularis. The other two sutures (Fig. 20–47, b and b′, c and c′) are passed sequentially in a similar fashion. The initially passed suture is tied first, then the other two. When the sutures are tied, the opened lumen is pulled into the vas lumen. The adventitia and muscularis of the vas deferens are sutured to the tunic of the epididymis with interrupted 9-0 nylon sutures (Fig. 20–48).

As with most surgical techniques, modifications have been made in an effort to make the procedure easier and more successful. **To this end, Marmar described a two-suture intussusception model; a vertical rather than a horizontal epididymal tubule incision has been suggested** (Marmar, 2000; Chan et al, 2003).

In the two-suture modification, once the dilated epididymal loop is identified and the end of the vas brought in close to the epididymal loop, it is secured to the tunic with a single 9-0 suture, and *two* parallel sutures are passed into the tubule

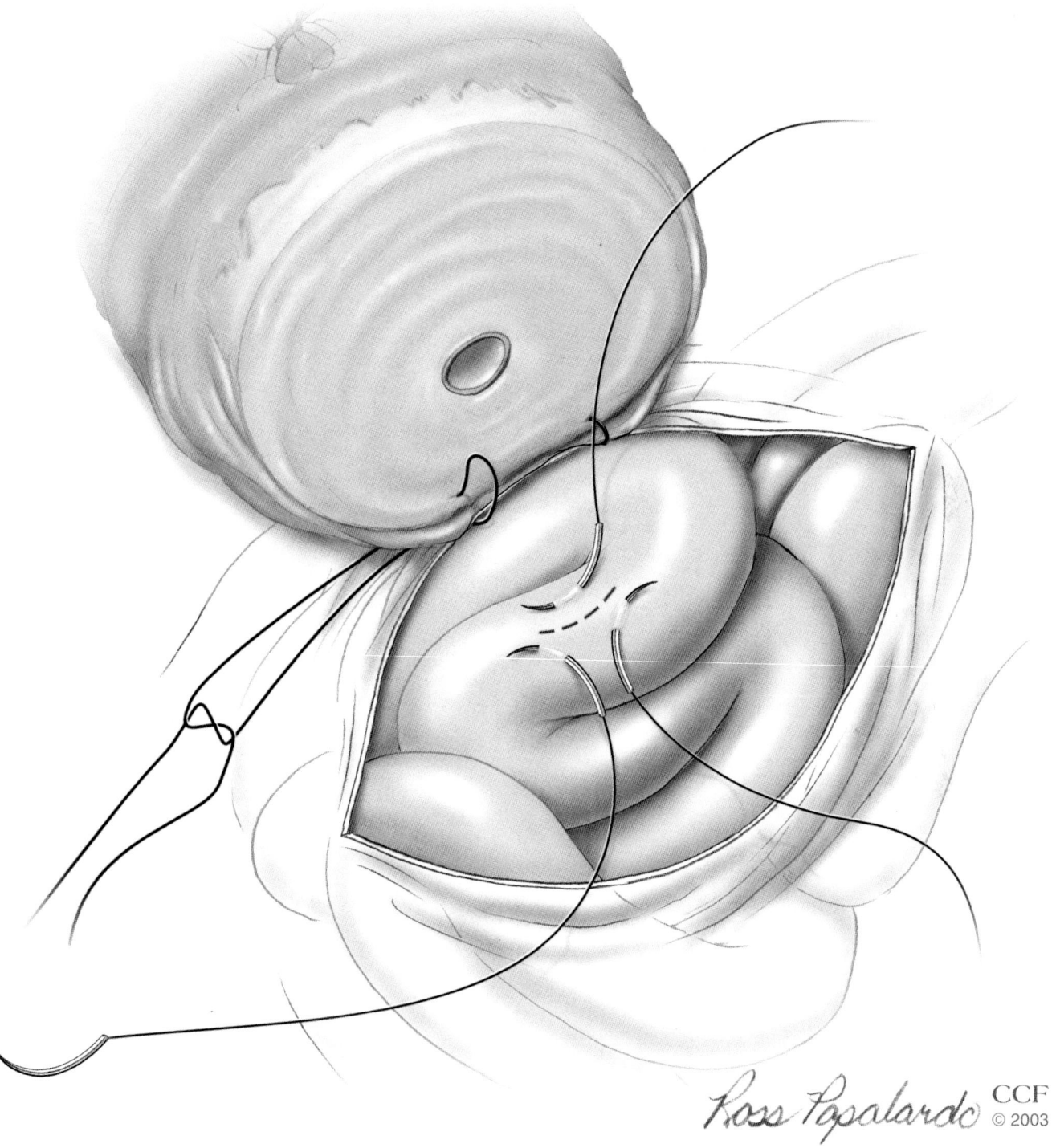

Figure 20–46. Placement of the three needles for the intussusception method of vasoepididymostomy.

and left in position (Fig. 20–49). A small incision is made between the two needles, and the exuded fluid is examined. If sperm are found, the two sutures are passed into the vasal lumen, beginning with the suture closest to the vas lumen. When each is tied, the lumen is drawn into the vasal lumen, and then the muscularis and adventitia are secured to the epididymal tunic. **With all procedures, the anastomosis should be within the tunica vaginalis, which can be closed over the testis at the end of the procedure.**

Potential Complications

Possible complications resulting from this surgery are related to the length of the procedure, the possibility of

Text continued on p. 698.

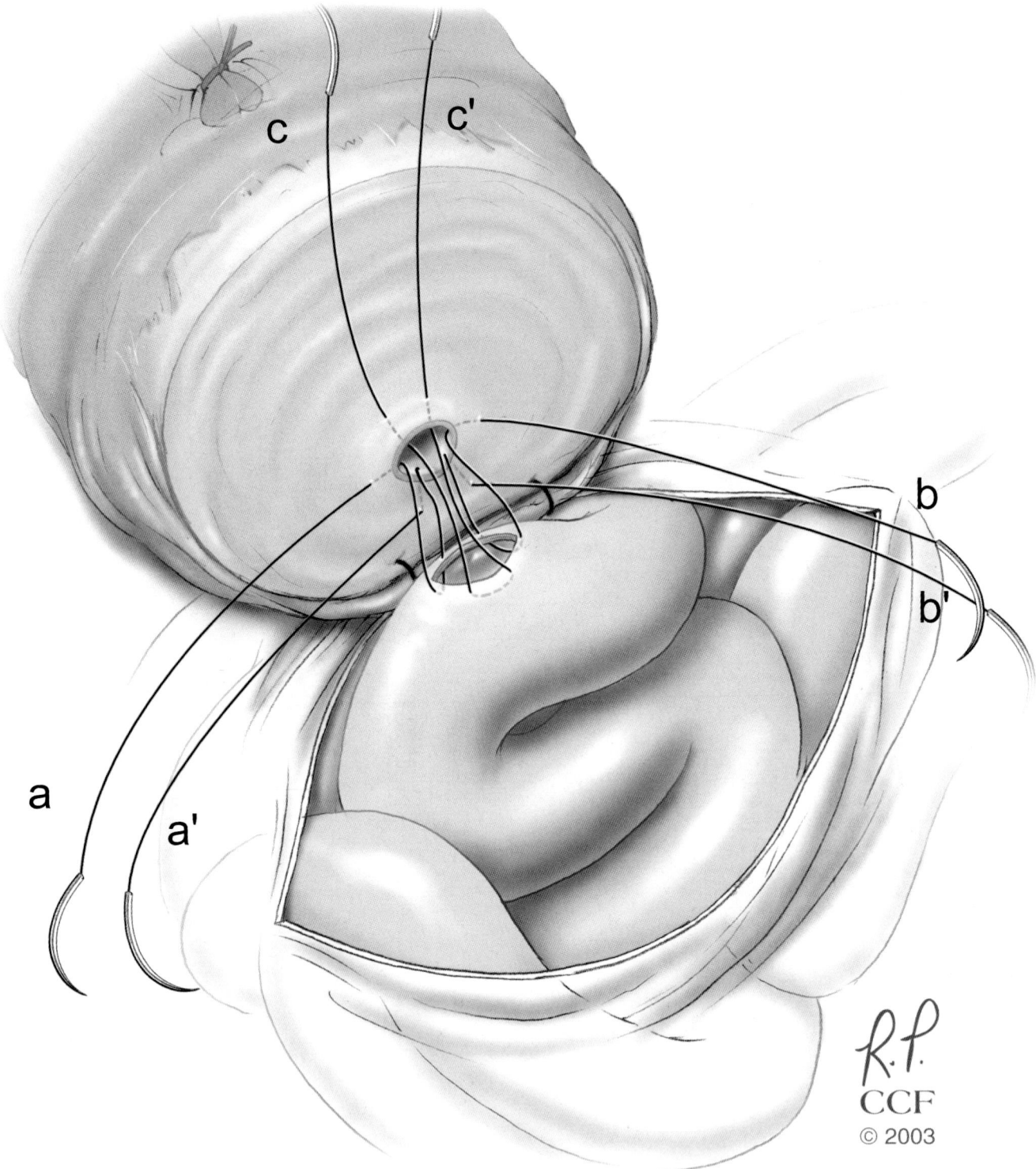

Figure 20–47. The double-armed sutures are passed through the vas lumen as shown.

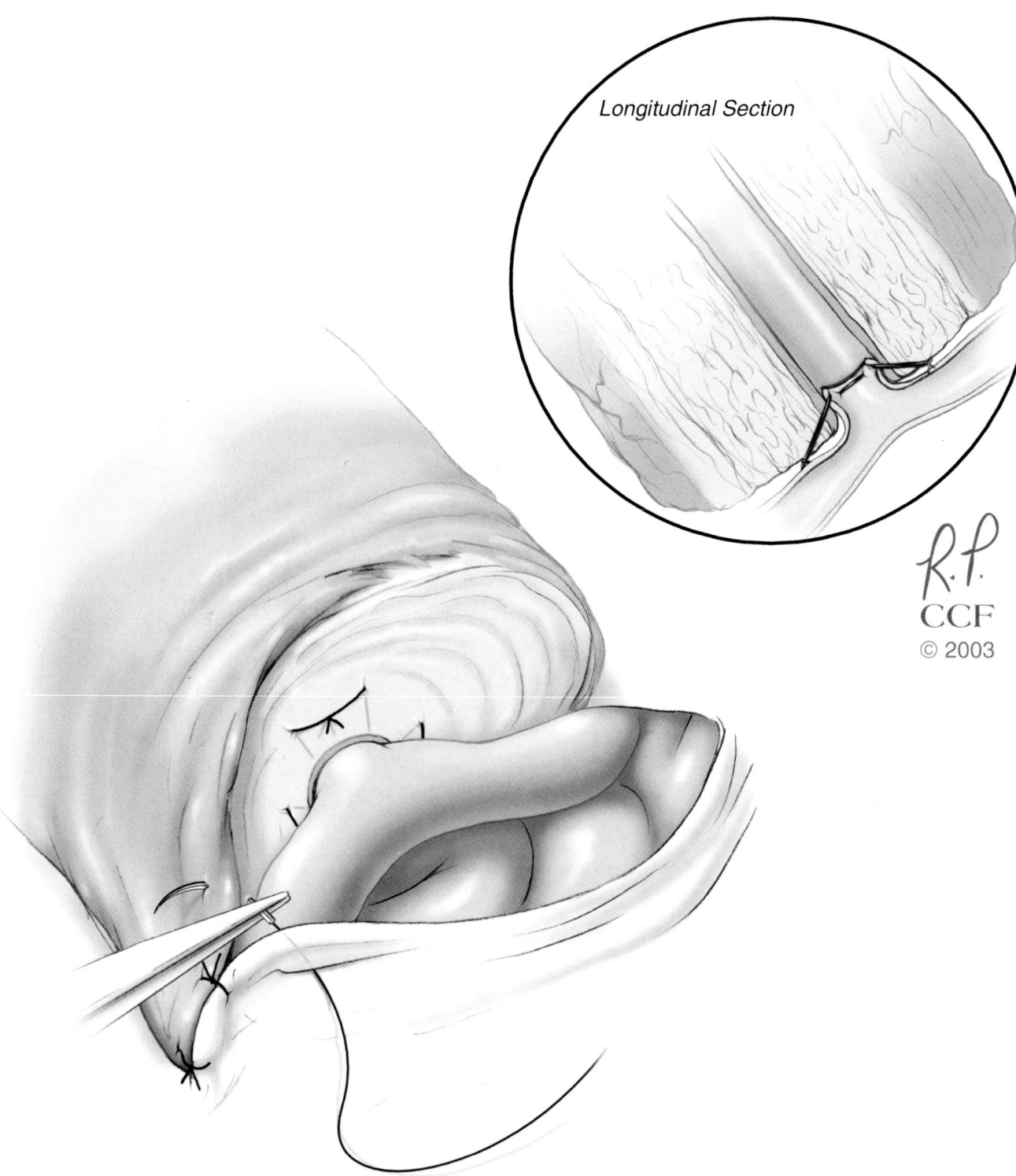

Longitudinal Section

R.P.
CCF
© 2003

Figure 20–48. When the sutures are tied, the epididymal lumen gets pulled into the lumen of the vas, and then the muscularis and adventitia can be closed to the epididymal tunic with interrupted 9-0 sutures, as was done in the end-to-side anastomosis.

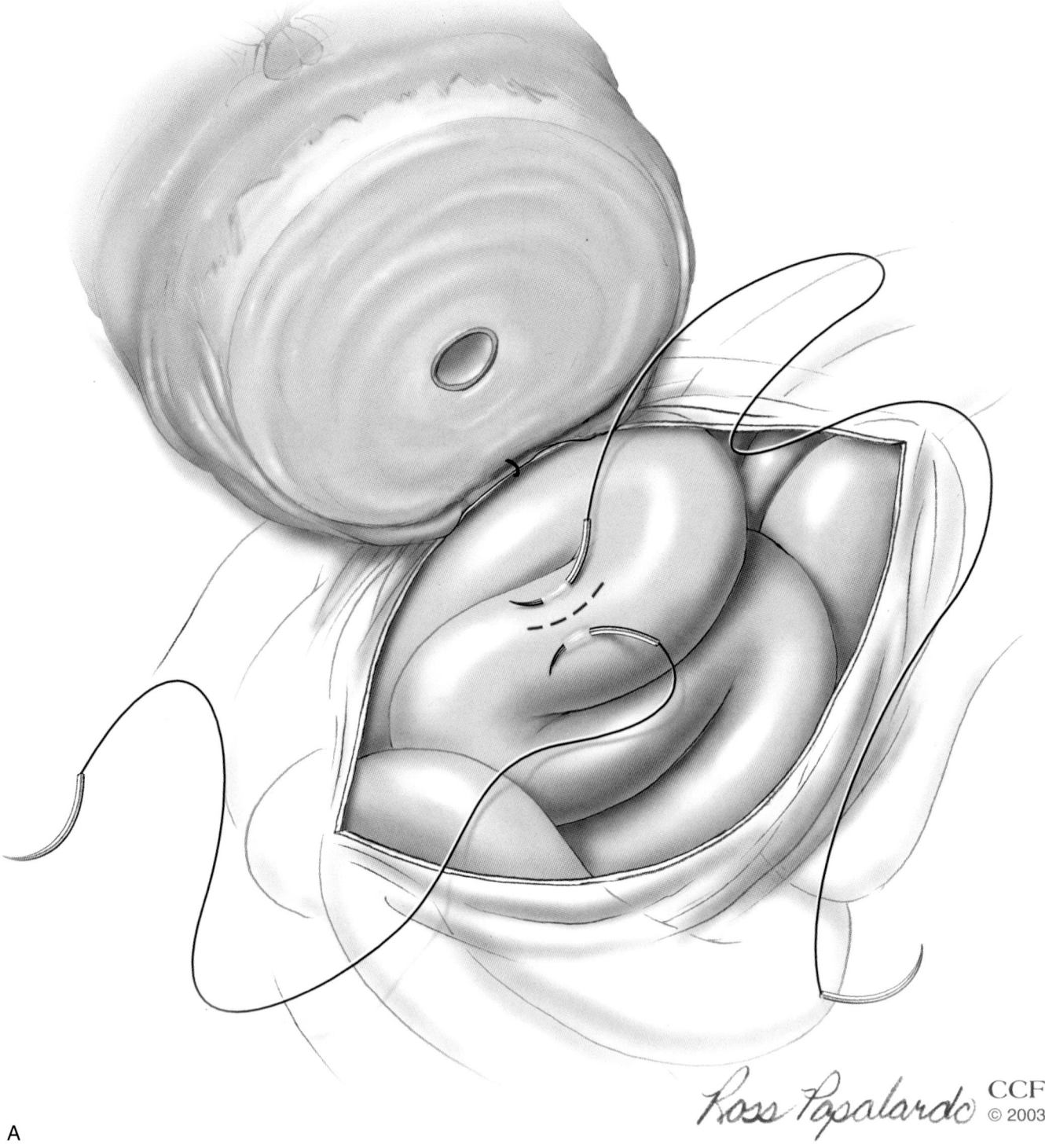

A

Figure 20–49. **A** and **B,** The two-suture method of intussuscepting the epididymal tubule into the vas lumen is a bit simpler than the three-suture technique. If the epididymal opening is made too large, the loop may not fully pull into the vas lumen, potentially causing a sperm leak and failed anastomosis. *Continued*

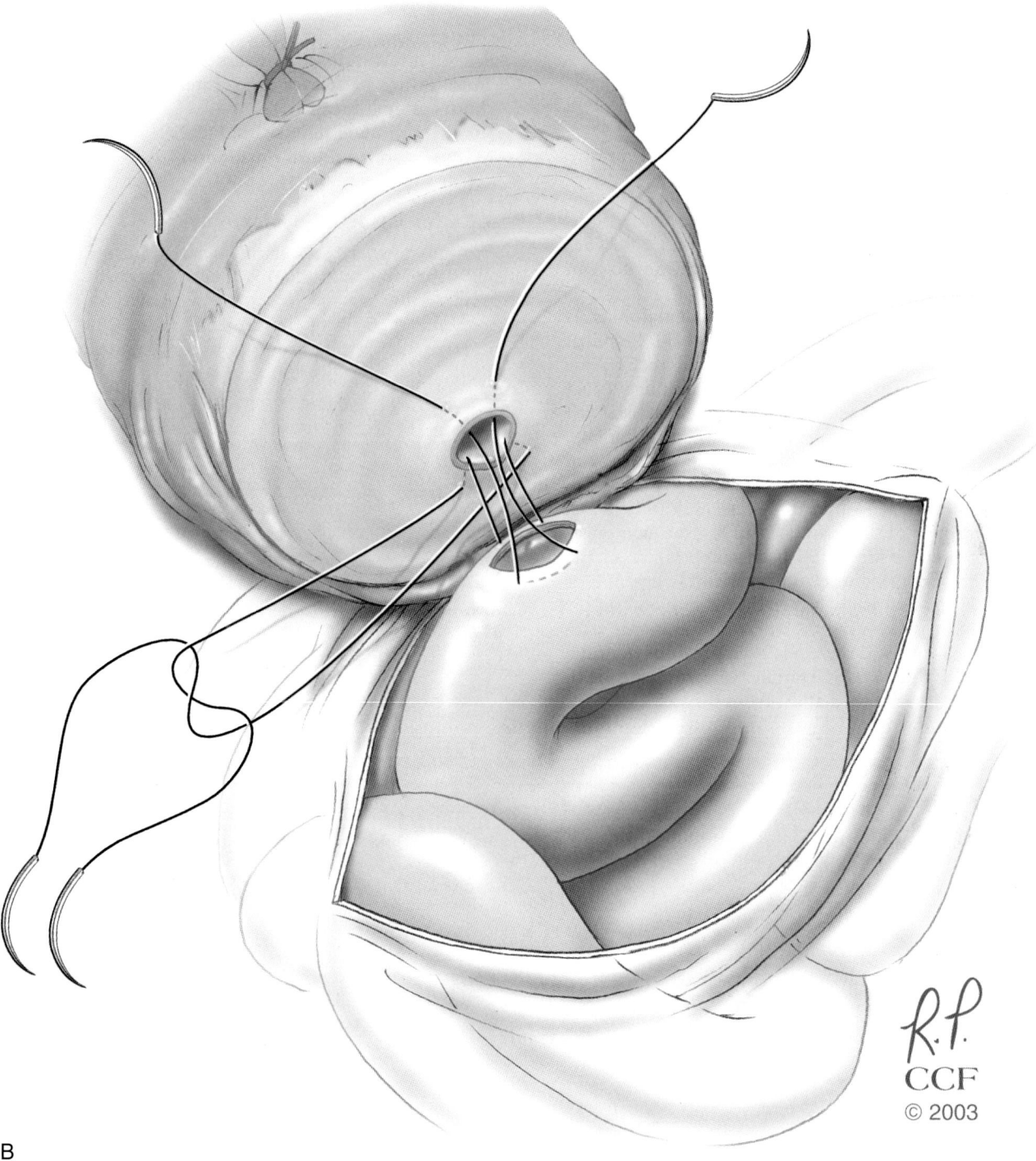

B

Figure 20–49, cont'd.

infection and hematoma formation, and the potential for injury to the arterial blood supply to the testis. Because these procedures can take 2 to 4 hours or longer, depending on the complexity of the dissection, the amount of scar tissue resulting from earlier surgery or inflammation, or the need to manipulate the vas to have sufficient length, there is a risk of venous thrombosis, as with any surgical procedure. It is prudent, therefore, to supply compressive stockings to patients undergoing these procedures. Since they ambulate early after surgery and are generally healthy men, the risk of this complication is relatively small. Infection is likewise a rare phenomenon. It is reasonable but not mandatory to give an antibiotic 30 minutes before surgery.

Bleeding, with subsequent formation of hematomas, is perhaps the most common complication that can be minimized, although not totally avoided, by paying meticulous attention to hemostasis throughout the procedure. Most hematomas are small and will resolve on their own, if left alone. It is rare that a second procedure is needed to drain the hematoma unless significant swelling and pain occur soon after surgery.

Injury to the testicular blood supply can result in ischemia and ultimate atrophy of the testis. It is an unusual complication that may occur if there has been compromise of the vasculature during a prior vasectomy, varicocele ligation, or hernia repair. If the vasal artery is then the major blood supply to the testis, cutting it with the vas will compromise the arterial integrity of the testis. **If there has been previous inguinal surgery, it is advisable to use a Doppler ultrasonic probe to identify the artery in the cord apart from the vas.**

Postoperative Care

The instructions are simple and straightforward. They are similar for vasovasostomy and vasoepididymostomy.

- **Keep an ice pack over the scrotal area for the first 12 hours after surgery.**
- **Avoid strenuous activity for 3 weeks.**
- **Avoid intercourse and ejaculation for 3 weeks.**
- **Wear supportive briefs for at least 2 weeks.**

Results for Vasoepididymostomy

Patency and pregnancy results after vasoepididymostomy vary greatly, depending on the surgical technique used, the level of obstruction, the age and reproductive capacity of the female partner, and the skill of the surgeon. Tables 20-4 and 20-5 summarize the results from both nonmicrosurgical and

Table 20–4. Results of Nonmicrosurgical Vasoepididymostomy

Author	Year	No. of Patients	No. with Sperm Present (%)	No. Pregnant (%)
Martin	1909	11	7 (64)	3 (27)
Lespinasse	1918	1	1 (100)	Not reported
Hagner	1936	33	21 (64)	16 (48)
Kar and Phadke	1975	281	137 (49)	40 (14)
Schoysman	1981	261	134 (51)	40 (14)
Lee	1987	97	30 (31)	12 (12)

Table 20–5. Results of Microsurgical Vasoepididymostomy

Author	Year	No. of Patients	No. with Sperm Present (%)	No. Pregnant (%)	Method of Anastomosis
McLoughlin	1982	23	Not reported	9 (39)	End-to-end End-to-side
Dubin and Amelar	1984	46	18 (39)	6 (13)	End-to-end
Fogdestam et al	1986	41	35 (85)	15 (37)	End-to-side
Lee	1987	158	58 (37)	32 (20)	Side-to-side
Silber	1989	139	(78)	(56)	End-to-end
Fuchs	1991	39	(60)	(36)	End-to-end
Thomas	1992	137	108 (79)	47 (50)*	End-to-side
Schlegel and Goldstein	1993	107	64 (70)	28 (35)†	End-to-end End-to-side
Matsuda et al	1994	24‡	21 (81)	10 (42)	End-to-end End-to-side
Matthews et al	1995	100	(65)	(21)	End-to-end End-to-side
Jarow et al	1995	89	(56)	Not reported	End-to-side
Dewire and Thomas	1995	137	108 (79)	47 (50)*	End-to-side
Boeckx and Van Helden	1996	31	11 (35)	3 (10)	End-to-end End-to-side
Kolettis and Thomas	1997	55§	(85)	20 (44)	End-to-side
Berardinucci et al	1998	49	(61)	Not reported	End-to-side
Berger	1998	12	11 (92)	Not reported	Intussusception
Hibi et al	2000	24	13 (54)	4 (17)	End-to-side
Marmar	2000	9	7 (78)	2 (22)	Intussusception
Schrepferman et al	2001	18	9 (50)	2 (13)	End-to-side Intussusception
Schoor et al	2002	32	10 (31)	Not reported	End-to-side Intussusception

*Based on 94 patients with a follow-up of 1 year or longer.
†Reported on 81 couples without female factor infertility and observed for longer than 1 year.
‡Two men had repeated procedures for 26 operations.
§All patients had prior vasectomy.

microsurgical reports. It is apparent that there is wide variation in the results achieved by many good surgeons, further emphasizing the technical difficulty in performing this procedure.

SPERM RETRIEVAL
Sperm Retrieval for Obstructive Azoospermia

When a man has obstructive azoospermia, for whatever reason, there are numerous methods by which sperm can be obtained. Even when men choose to have corrective surgery, some will request that sperm be obtained for cryopreservation at the time of their reconstructive surgery. Other patients either are not candidates for reconstruction or simply choose to have sperm retrieved for use with assisted reproductive techniques without corrective surgery.

Vasal Aspiration of Sperm

Aspiration of motile sperm from the vas deferens is an option for men whose lack of ejaculation has a neurologic cause. If the patient has normal neurologic sensation (e.g., anejaculation secondary to diabetes or muscular sclerosis), local anesthesia is used as for a vasectomy. Once the vas is grasped and exposed, the anterior wall is hemitransected with a 1.5-mm microknife, and fluid exuding from the proximal vas is aspirated while the distal epididymis and proximal vas are gently compressed (Fig. 20–50). When sufficient fluid (sperm) has been obtained and sperm motility quantitated microscopically, the vas is closed with interrupted 9-0 nylon sutures and dropped back into the scrotum. The skin is closed with one or two absorbable sutures. The sperm obtained are often sufficient to be used fresh for intrauterine insemination or can be cryopreserved and used for IVF-ICSI at a later date.

Epididymal Aspiration of Sperm

Sperm can be obtained from an obstructed epididymis by either percutaneous aspiration or open microsurgical aspiration. **The two most common requirements for one of these procedures are prior vasectomy with no wish for reversal and congenital bilateral absence of the vas deferens.**

Percutaneous Epididymal Sperm Aspiration

This method of obtaining sperm for cryopreservation or fresh IVF-ICSI is relatively quick and inexpensive compared with microsurgical open aspiration. **One criticism of the method is that frequently insufficient sperm are obtained for cryopreservation.** This may occur when there is minimal dilation of the caput epididymis because fewer sperm are aspirated when the efferent tubules are not distended. These infertile men may be better served with open aspiration or testis biopsy for sperm recovery. If there is moderate or marked fullness of the epididymis, however, there is a better possibility of passing the needle into the tubules and obtaining better numbers of motile sperm.

The equipment needed for percutaneous epididymal sperm aspiration is readily available and inexpensive: a 23-gauge butterfly needle, a 10-mL syringe, a 3-mL syringe with a 30-gauge needle, a small hemostat, two 1-mL Eppendorf tubes, 5 mL of 1% lidocaine HCl, and 5 mL of sperm nutrient medium.

After the genitalia are washed and draped in a sterile fashion, a cord block can be performed, as previously described, but it is not needed in many cases. The epididymis to be aspirated is held in the surgeon's nondominant hand; the head of the epididymis is held between thumb and forefinger with the scrotal skin snug against the epididymis. It is sometimes helpful for an assistant to hold the bottom of the testis with his or her nondominant hand to stabilize it. A small wheal of 1% lidocaine is raised in the skin at the point between thumb and forefinger, where the aspirating needle will be inserted into the caput epididymis (Fig. 20–51A). A 23-gauge butterfly needle attached to the 10-mL syringe previously flushed with just enough sperm nutrient medium to moisten the needle is inserted into the caput along its long axis (Fig. 20–51B). The assistant pulls back on the syringe to produce and hold 5 mL of negative pressure. **The needle is moved back and forth a few millimeters within the epididymal head while the sides of the epididymis are gently compressed to "encourage" the sperm into the needle.** When aspirated fluid is seen in the clear tubing just above the needle hub, the tubing is clamped with the hemostat to hold the fluid in place, and the negative pressure in the syringe is slowly released. After the needle is withdrawn from the epididymis, mild pressure is placed on the puncture site to prevent a hematoma. The needle is placed in the Eppendorf tube, and the tubing and needle are flushed with 0.5 mL of sperm nutrient medium. An aliquot of the aspirate is examined immediately to determine if there are sufficient motile sperm to be cryopreserved or used fresh for ICSI (Fig. 20–51C). If the sperm are insufficient, the process can be repeated but with limited attempts based on the patient's comfort. If sperm are not obtained, open aspiration or testis biopsy is recommended.

Microsurgical Epididymal Sperm Aspiration

This technique is appropriate for men who have an epididymal or vasal obstruction. Microsurgical epididymal sperm aspiration enables the surgeon to collect large numbers of motile sperm for cryopreservation. The disadvantage of this method is that it involves a surgical procedure requiring an operating microscope and consequently increases the cost for a couple who also require IVF-ICSI.

The epididymis is exposed and examined under the operating microscope to identify a point where the epididymal tubule is dilated. The epididymal tunic is incised, exposing the tubules below. A microknife is used to open a single loop of the epididymal tubule, and the fluid exuding from it is aspirated with a 24-gauge angiocatheter connected to a 1-mL tuberculin syringe primed with 0.1 mL of buffer (Fig. 20–52). The fluid is examined to be certain there are motile sperm present. If not, another loop of an epididymal tubule is chosen more cephalad, and the procedure is repeated until motile sperm are identified. The aspirate is put in 1-mL Eppendorf tubes mixed with sperm nutrient medium, such as Quinn's sperm washing medium or other appropriate medium. After sufficient sperm are collected, the tubule and the tunic are closed with 10-0 and 9-0 nylon suture, respectively.

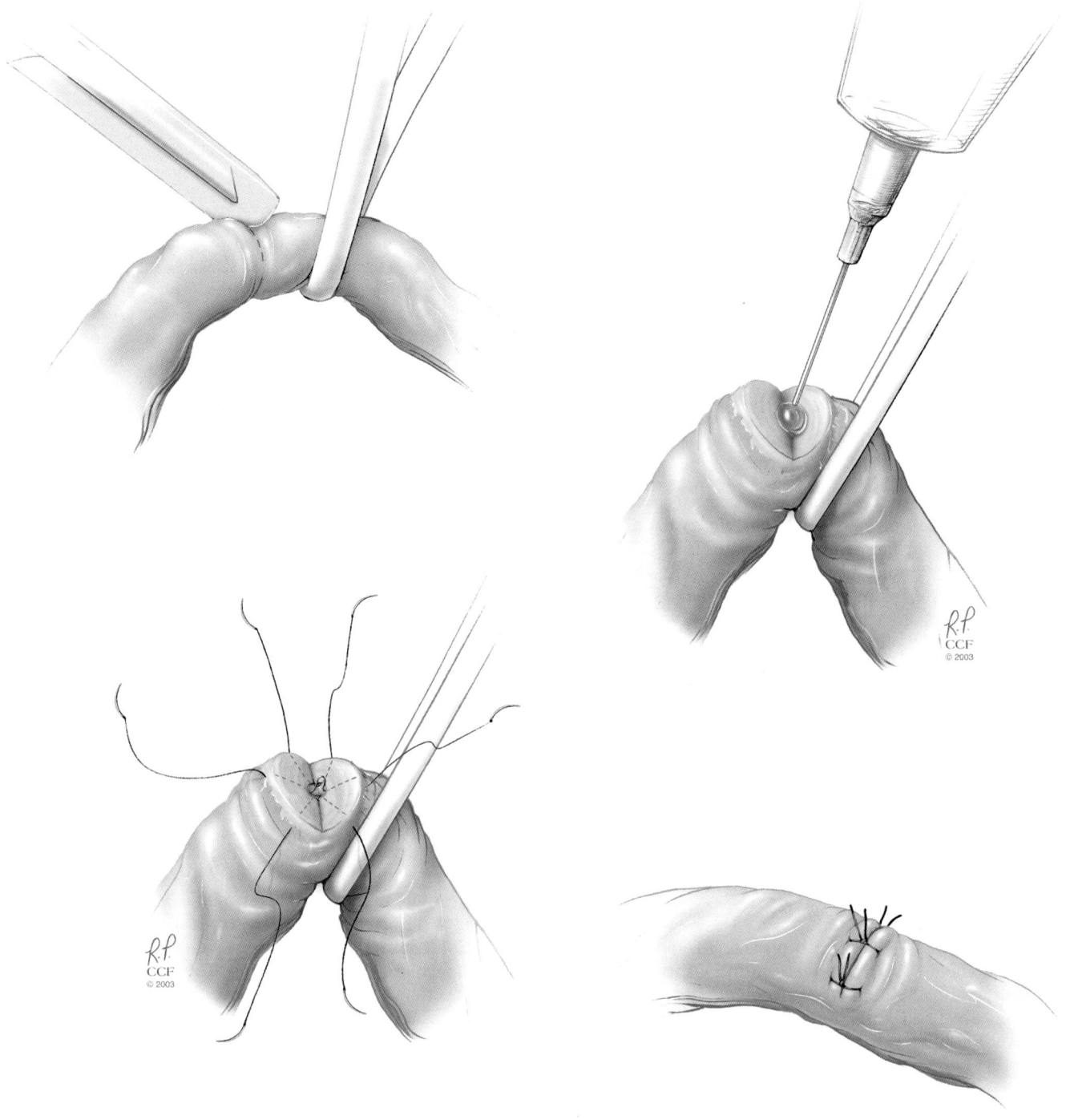

Figure 20–50. Vasal aspiration of sperm.

Open Testis Biopsy

Open biopsy of the testis is described earlier in this chapter. The only difference from a simple, single, diagnostic biopsy is that therapeutic sperm retrieval requires the removal of four to six small pieces of testicular tissue from the same incision that are placed in separate containers with sperm nutrient medium. Sperm can readily be extracted from normal tissue and either used immediately for IVF-ICSI or cryopreserved.

Testis Sperm Aspiration and Needle Biopsy

Sperm can also be obtained by needle aspiration of the testis. The sperm numbers are less likely to be adequate for standard cryopreservation but are often sufficient for fresh cycle IVF-ICSI. **The major advantage, as with percutaneous epididymal sperm aspiration, is that both cost and morbidity are low.**

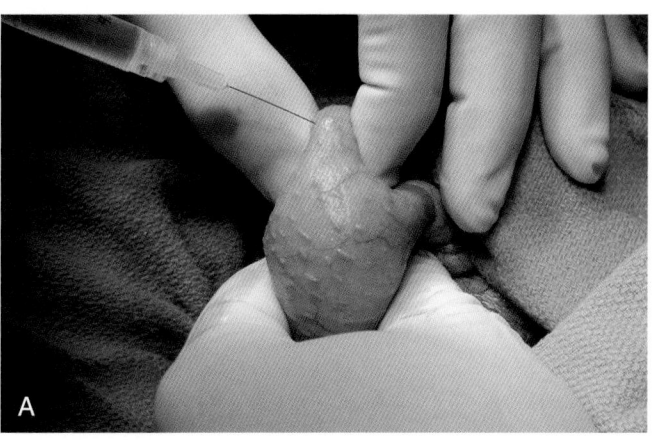

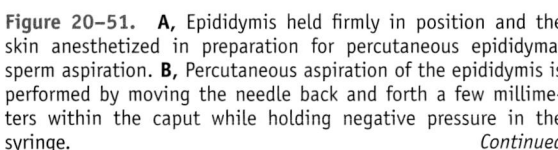

Figure 20–51. **A,** Epididymis held firmly in position and the skin anesthetized in preparation for percutaneous epididymal sperm aspiration. **B,** Percutaneous aspiration of the epididymis is performed by moving the needle back and forth a few millimeters within the caput while holding negative pressure in the syringe. *Continued*

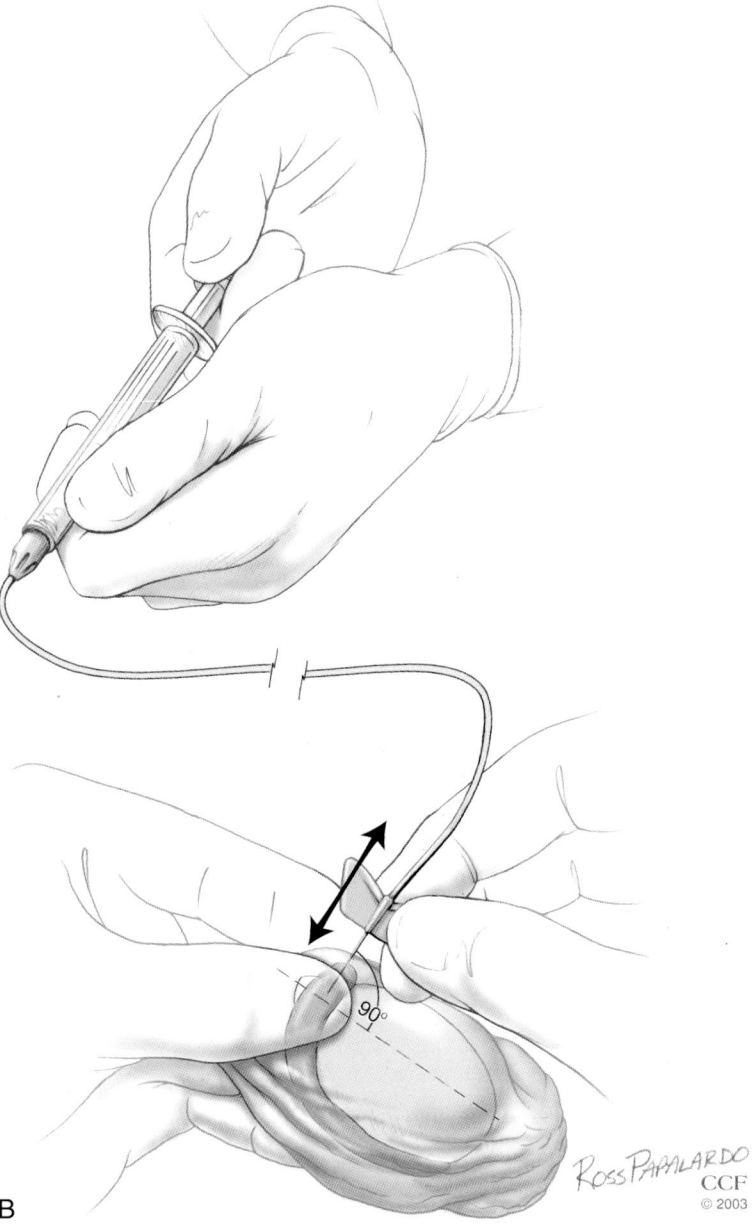

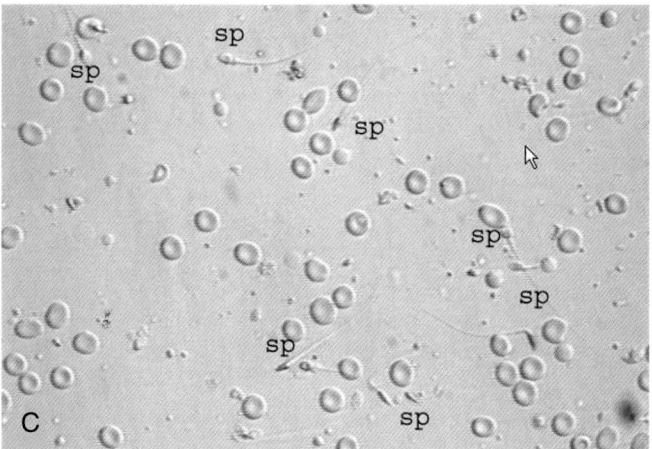

Figure 20–51, cont'd. C, Diluted epididymal aspirate showing numerous sperm (sp) for ICSI or cryopreservation.

Belker and associates (1998) described an effective method of aspirating sperm from the testis in men with both obstructive and nonobstructive azoospermia. They had more success with men who had obstructions (100% sperm retrieved) than with those with nonobstructive azoospermia (27%). A 1.5-inch, 20-gauge needle attached to a 20-mL syringe connected to the appropriately sized pistol-grip device (Cameco syringe holder) to hold the syringe is recommended. **Most men can undergo the procedure with only local anesthesia, although some may require an oral or intravenous sedative.**

After testes are appropriately prepared and draped, a cord block is performed. The testis is held by the surgeon in the nondominant hand with the scrotal skin pulled back tightly against the anterior surface of the testis; 1 mL of 1% lidocaine HCl is infiltrated into the skin where the needle will puncture (Fig. 20–53). With the aspirating device held in the dominant hand, the testis is punctured, and negative pressure is exerted on the syringe by pulling the pistol grip as far back as it will go. Holding continuous negative pressure, the surgeon moves

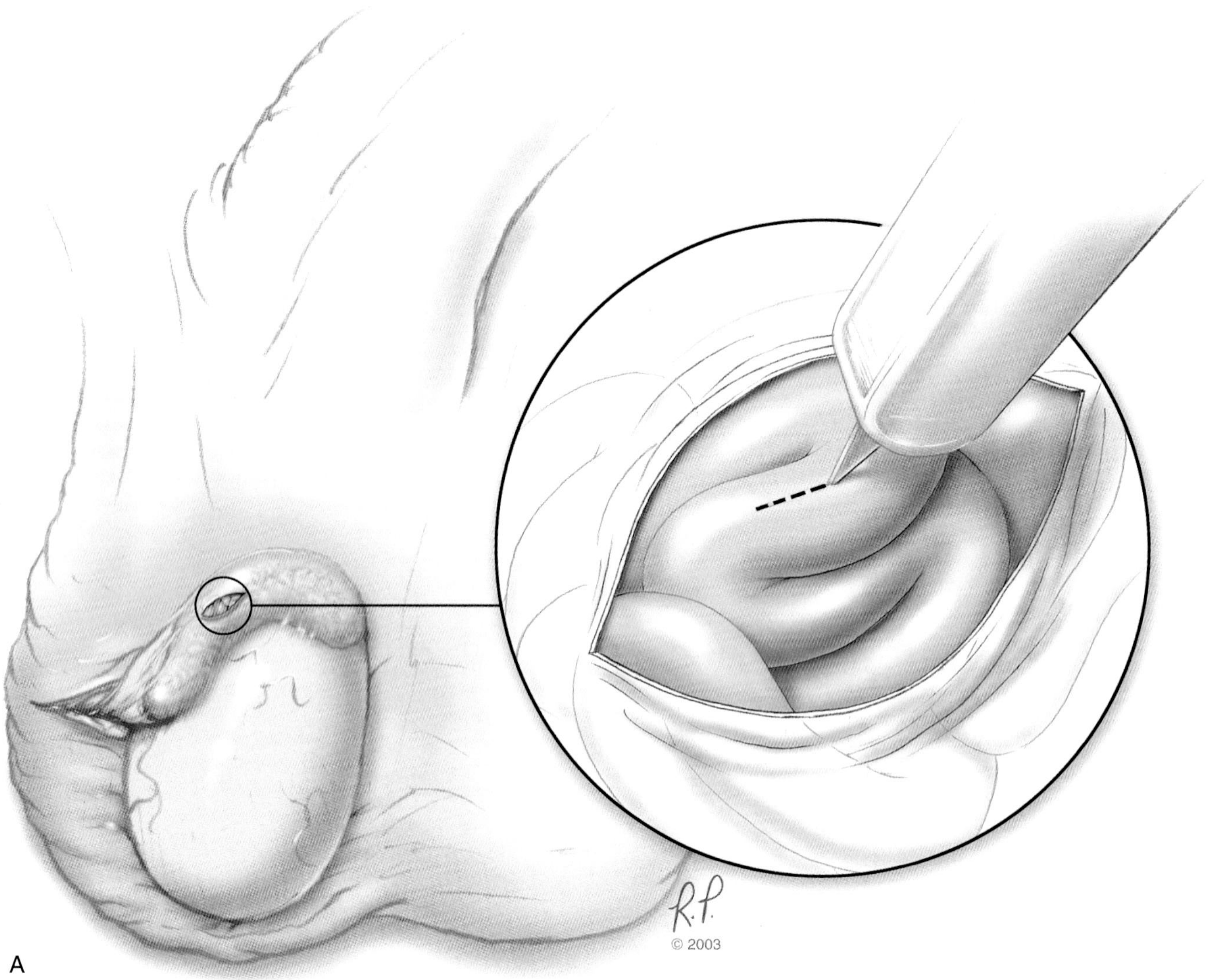

A

Figure 20–52. A and **B,** Method for microsurgical epididymal sperm aspiration.

Continued

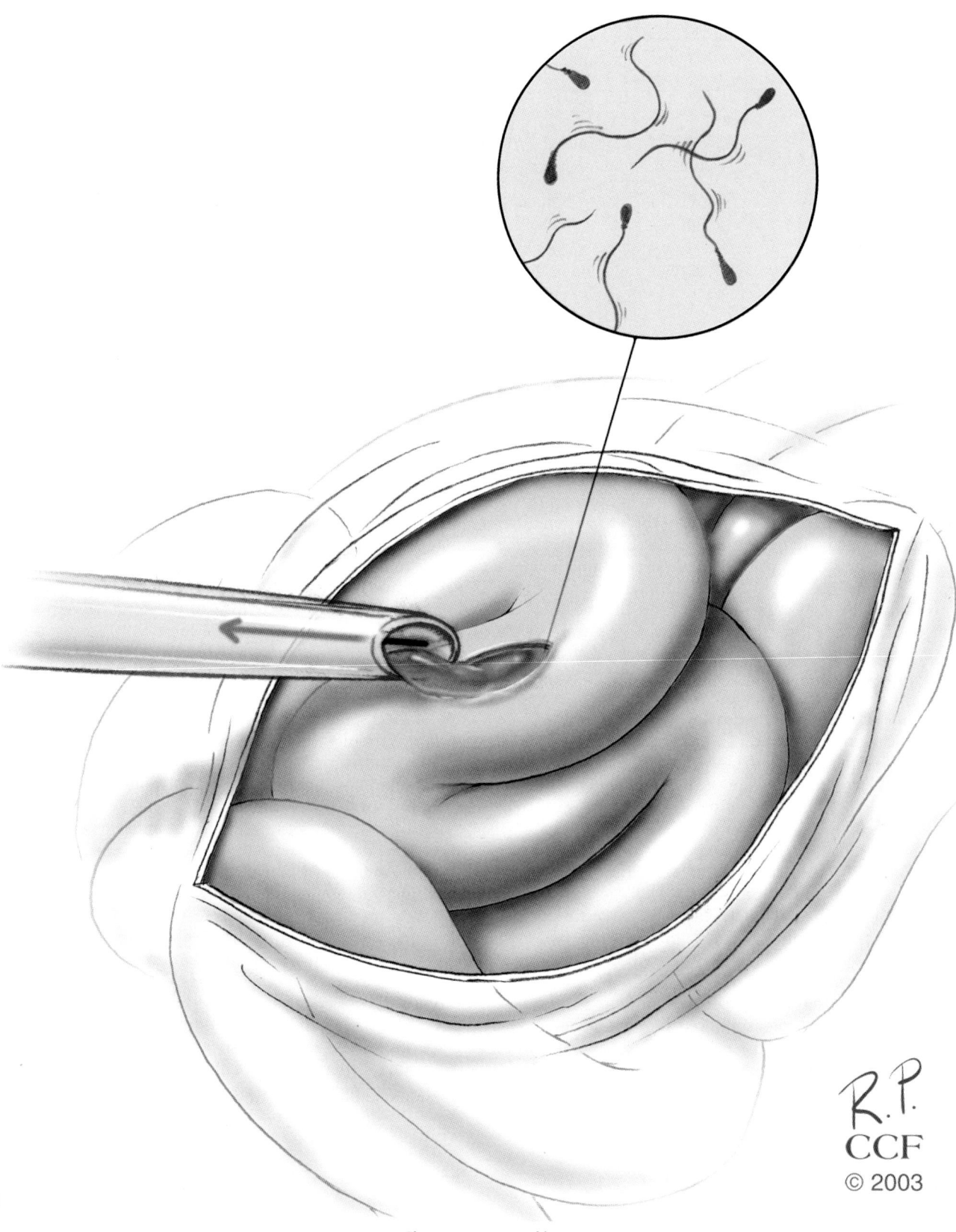

B

Figure 20–52, cont'd.

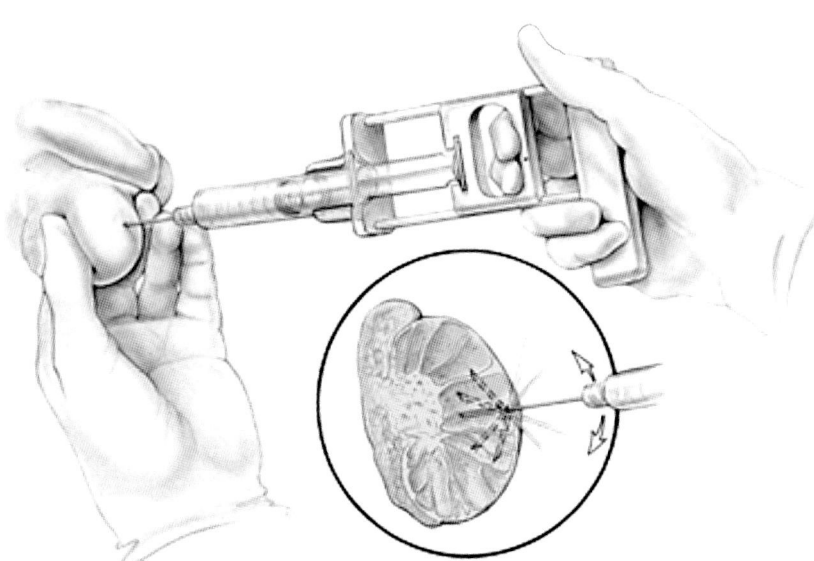

Figure 20–53. Testicular sperm aspiration performed with a Cameco syringe holder to create and hold negative pressure within the testis.

the needle back and forth four or five times in different directions without removing the needle from the site of puncture. The negative pressure in the syringe is reduced by allowing the plunger to return to its original neutral position during a period of 30 to 60 seconds. This slow release minimizes the possibility for the aspirated tissue to be flushed from the needle back into the testis. When there is no pressure in the syringe, the needle is withdrawn from the testis, and any tubules protruding from the puncture site are cut off and transferred to a 1-mL Eppendorf tube prefilled with sperm nutrient medium. Gentle manual pressure on the puncture site is used to minimize the risk of bleeding. The needle is removed from the 20-mL syringe and attached to a 10-mL syringe prefilled with air. The needle is flushed with the air into an Eppendorf tube containing 50 μL of sperm nutrient medium. An aliquot of the fluid is examined for sperm.

Fine-needle mapping for patients with nonobstructive azoospermia has been described by Turek and colleagues (2000) as a means of locating the area of the testis where sperm may be identified by open biopsy. This technique has the advantage of minimizing testis biopsy sites. However, negative results may be obtained when adjacent areas may have sperm.

Needle core biopsies of the testis can be done with preparation similar to that for aspiration, but instead of a fine needle, a spring-loaded biopsy needle is used to remove thin pieces of tissue. Most urologists are familiar with the biopsy needle that is more often used for prostate biopsies (refer to the earlier section on testis biopsy). When it is used to obtain testis tissue, the skin at the puncture site should be nicked with the point of a No. 11 knife blade to minimize the chance of dragging skin in with the needle and the sampled tissue.

Microsurgical Testicular Sperm Extraction

Use of the operating microscope to identify wider caliber seminiferous tubules that may contain sperm in a patient with nonobstructive azoospermia is thought by some clinicians to have several advantages over the process of random biopsy of the testis. **Clinicians who favor this technique report, first,**

that it allows more meticulous opening of the tunica albuginea, possibly avoiding cutting across blood vessels that may be critical to testis survival; second, that less tissue needs to be extracted and therefore more of the testis is preserved; and, finally, that there appears to be a higher rate of sperm retrieval for use with ICSI (Schlegel, 1999). The seminiferous tubules of men with Sertoli cell–only syndrome, sclerosis associated with Klinefelter's syndrome, testicular atrophy, cryptorchidism, or prior orchitis are generally smaller than tubules with active spermatogenesis. With use of the operating microscope to carefully examine the seminiferous tubules, those that are fuller may possibly be identified and individually extracted.

A horizontal incision is made at midtestis approximately two thirds of the circumference of the testis. Arteries and large veins are carefully preserved, but the smaller vessels encountered are cauterized with bipolar cautery. Once the bleeding from the incision is controlled, the testis is gently spread open, exposing the lobules of seminiferous tubules. High magnification is used in a systematic search for prominent tubules that may contain mature sperm. Most of the testis can be explored through this single incision. Any larger, fatter tubules thought to contain sperm are teased away from the thinner tubules and placed in a collecting well containing sperm nutrient medium (Fig. 20–54). This is immediately examined by an embryologist or technician, who teases the tissue apart to determine if sperm are present. If sperm are found or if adequate sampling has not resulted in identification of sperm, the procedure is terminated and the incision in the tunic is closed with 5-0 Prolene suture.

Schlegel (1999) initially described this method. **He reported an increase in the number of men who produced sperm from 45% (10 of 22 men) to 63% (17 of 27 men), including six men who had undergone biopsy without findings of sperm.** Furthermore, the amount of tissue removed with microdissection averaged 9.4 mg as opposed to 750 mg in the nonmicrosurgical group. Subsequent reports from this author and his co-investigators have continued to demonstrate high yields for sperm retrieval in patients with various

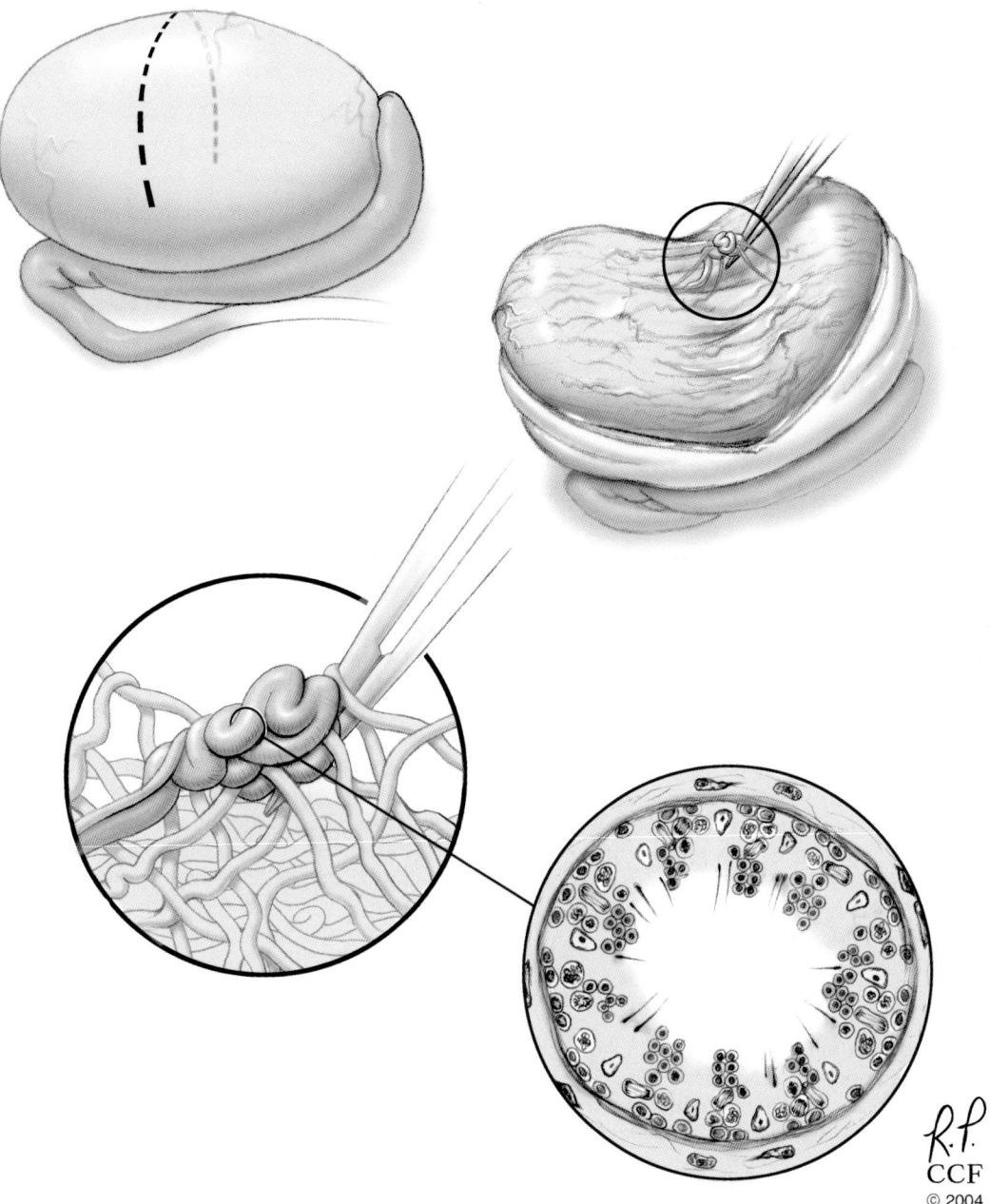

Figure 20–54. Microsurgical testicular exploration for sperm in nonobstructive azoospermia depends on identification of the larger caliber seminiferous tubules that may contain all elements of complete spermatogenesis for sperm retrieval.

causes of their nonobstructive azoospermia (Chan et al, 2001; Raman et al, 2003). Whereas some other investigators have also found the method better with respect to sperm retrieval, a comparative study of microtesticular sperm extraction and standard multiple biopsies reported by Tsujimura and coworkers (2002) found that the differences were marginal and did not reach statistical significance.

Nonmicrosurgical Testicular Sperm Extraction

If one chooses not to use the operating microscope, it is still possible to find sperm in some men with nonobstructive azoospermia by taking multiple mini–biopsy specimens from the testis, being cautious to avoid major vessels and making only horizontal incisions in the tunica albuginea. Starting in the center of the testis, the initial incision is made and the expressed tissue is sharply excised and placed in medium for teasing and examination. If no sperm are found, a biopsy specimen of the tissue just below the first incision is taken and placed in sperm nutrient medium. Each biopsy specimen contains approximately 50 mg of tissue. This biopsy process is repeated in the areas shown in Figure 20–55. Each of the biopsy sites is subsequently closed with 5-0 Prolene suture.

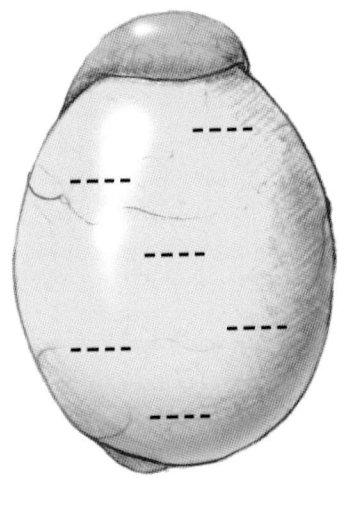
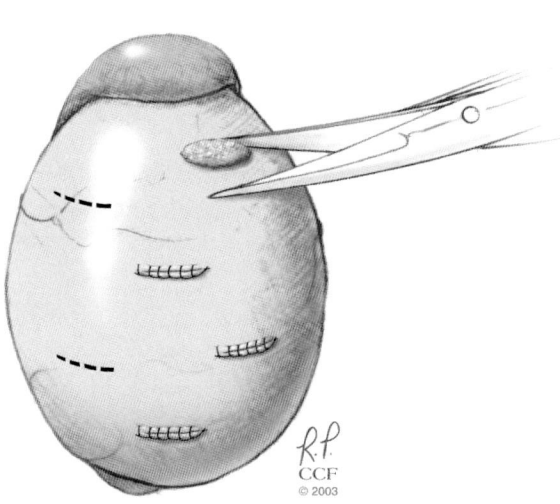

Figure 20–55. As an alternative to microsurgical exploration, multisite biopsy can be performed in the hope of identifying some seminiferous tubules with mature spermatozoa.

SURGICAL MANAGEMENT OF EJACULATORY DUCT OBSTRUCTION

Ejaculatory duct obstruction is diagnosed in 1% to 5% of infertile men (Pryor and Hendry, 1991). Ejaculatory duct obstruction can be either congenital or acquired, partial or complete. Congenital causes include utricular, müllerian, and wolffian duct cysts as well as congenital atresia or stenosis of the ejaculatory ducts. Acquired causes include infection, calculus formation (Hellerstein et al, 1992), trauma, and cyst formation associated with prior instrumentation (Mayersak, 1989).

Diagnosis

The diagnosis and evaluation of patients with suspected ejaculatory duct obstruction are discussed in Chapter 19 "Male Infertility". *Complete* ejaculatory duct obstruction should be suspected in patients with azoospermia and decreased ejaculatory volume (<1.0 mL) in the presence of acidic semen lacking fructose. Serum testosterone and gonadotropin levels are usually within normal limits. On occasion, rectal examination will reveal a palpable midline mass or dilated seminal vesicles. Jarow and colleagues (1989) reported that 37% of infertile patients with azoospermia have some form of ductal obstruction and that 6% of azoospermic men have ejaculatory duct obstruction.

Partial ejaculatory duct obstruction has highly variable signs and symptoms and can be found in infertile patients who have significantly low sperm motility and oligospermia despite normal testicular size and normal hormone profile (FSH, luteinizing hormone, testosterone) (Hellerstein et al, 1992). In some men with partial ejaculatory duct obstruction, some of the semen parameters approach normal (Meacham et al, 1993). Partial ejaculatory duct obstruction leads to entrapment of sperm at the point of obstruction, and the increased body temperature at this location as well as sperm stasis is thought to cause unique impairment in sperm motility.

We suggest that transrectal ultrasonography be used to evaluate infertile patients with low ejaculatory volume (<1.0 mL), low sperm motility (<30%), or oligospermia (<20 million sperm/mL) when findings on physical examination are normal and serum gonadotropin and testosterone are within normal ranges.

The many methods used to diagnose ejaculatory duct obstruction can be subdivided into static tests and dynamic tests (Purohit et al, 2004). Static tests include transrectal ultrasonography, magnetic resonance imaging, and seminal vesicle aspiration (Orhan et al, 1999); dynamic tests include vasography and seminal vesiculography. In a comparative study of dynamic and static tests for the diagnosis of ejaculatory duct obstruction, Purohit and colleagues (2004) found that transrectal ultrasonography used alone had a poor specificity for diagnosis of ejaculatory duct obstruction. When dynamic tests were incorporated into the diagnostic evaluation, the rate of unnecessary duct resections was significantly decreased.

Transrectal Ultrasonography

Transrectal ultrasonography has become the standard modality for diagnosis of ejaculatory duct obstruction. It should be performed with the patient in the lateral decubitus position with a high-resolution, 7-MHz probe in both the longitudinal and transverse planes. Ejaculatory duct obstruction is suspected in the presence of a cystic midline structure within the prostate as well as dilated seminal vesicles (Fig. 20–56). Seminal vesicles are considered dilated when their axial diameters are greater than 1.5 cm (Littrup et al, 1988; Jarow, 1993). However, it is possible that partial ejaculatory duct obstruction can exist when the axial diameters of seminal vesicles are normal (Jarow, 1993).

Vasography and Seminal Vesicle Aspiration

Historically, vasography was the gold standard for diagnosis of ejaculatory duct obstruction (Ford et al, 1982; Pryor and Hendry, 1991; Jarow, 1993). However, the risk of vasal injury and subsequent vasal occlusion has limited its use. Vasography is now used to help confirm equivocal

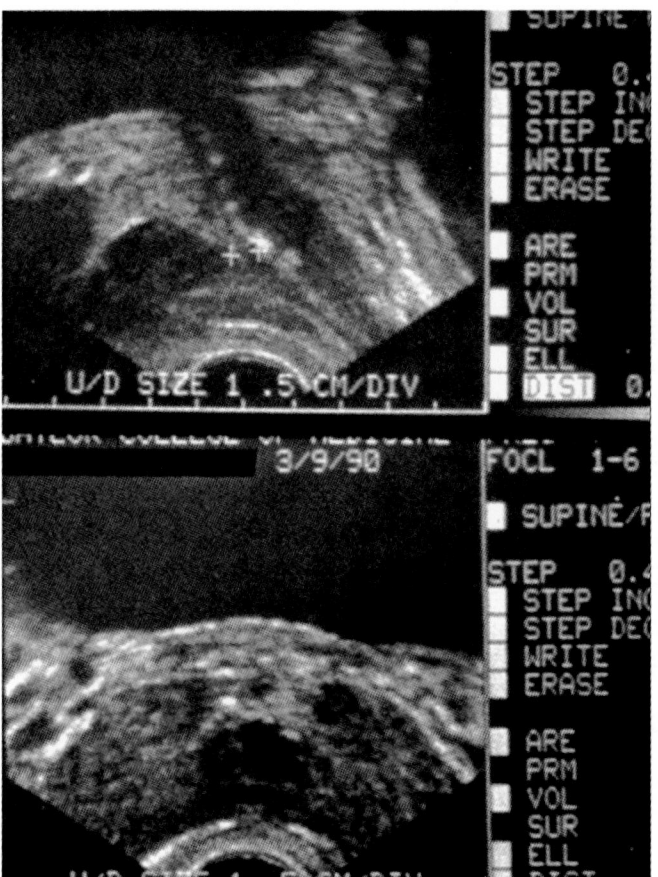

Figure 20–56. Cystic midline prostatic structure seen on ultrasound examination.

transrectal ultrasonography findings. **Vasography is also necessary if no sperm are found on seminal vesicle aspiration.** Vasography, with instillation of methylene blue dye or indigo carmine, can be used instead of seminal vesiculography to guide in the resection of the ejaculatory ducts. **It is important to document sperm production as well as patency of the seminal vesicles, especially in patients with partial ejaculatory duct obstruction, before initiating surgical correction. Therefore, transrectal ultrasonography–guided aspiration of the seminal vesicles should be performed before surgery.** (For detailed description of these procedures, see "Vasography" and "Seminal Vesicle Aspiration and Seminal Vesiculography" sections later in this chapter.)

Treatment

Transurethral Resection of the Ejaculatory Duct

Transurethral resection of the ejaculatory duct, first described by Farley and Barnes in 1973, is the primary treatment of ejaculatory duct obstruction. A 24 French resectoscope is placed into the urethra, and resection is carried out at the level of the verumontanum. An O'Connor drape is used with a finger in the rectum to allow better depth perception and visualization of the posterior prostate. **If an ejaculatory duct cyst is present, it is usually deep and just posterior to the verumontanum.** Therefore, the verumontanum is deeply

resected with care not to injure the rectum (Fig. 20–57). Real-time ultrasonography can be used concurrently to visualize the resection of the ejaculatory cyst. **Once efflux from the ejaculatory ducts of copious cloudy material or indigo carmine, if present, is identified, the resection is complete.** If the cyst still is not unroofed, a Collings knife is used to make bilateral incisions just lateral to the base of the resected verumontanum. These incisions make it possible to open obstructed ejaculatory ducts that may have been missed during the initial midline incision. **Electrocautery is used judiciously to avoid occlusion of the newly opened ejaculatory ducts. Care is taken at all times to protect the bladder neck and external sphincter from injury that might result in retrograde ejaculation and urinary incontinence.** A urethral catheter is left in place overnight and removed the next day.

Transurethral Balloon Dilation of the Ejaculatory Ducts

An alternative approach to the treatment of ejaculatory duct obstruction that involves balloon dilation of the ejaculatory ducts has also been described (Schlegel, 1997). In this procedure, the verumontanum is at least partially resected, and the ejaculatory ducts are cannulated and dilated with a 4-mm-wide and 2-cm-long balloon. The undilated balloon catheter is 0.04 inch in diameter and is usually passed easily into the strictured ejaculatory ducts. The overall success rates and long-term patency rates of this procedure are yet to be determined. However, certain patients with an extraprostatic or partial obstruction of the ejaculatory ducts may benefit from this approach (Jarow, 1996b).

Other Techniques

Although some have reported success with antegrade seminal vesicle lavage to relieve ejaculatory duct obstruction (Colpi et al, 1995), others have found forced vasal lavage to be unsuccessful (Paick et al, 2000). Some have advocated laser drilling of the ejaculatory ducts as well as their transurethral incision (Halpern and Hirsch, 2000; Fuse et al, 2003). Both of these innovative procedures are associated with a high rate of restenosis and are not recommended.

Complications

A common complication of transurethral resection of the ejaculatory duct is the reflux of urine into the ejaculatory ducts and subsequently into the seminal vesicles, vas deferens, or even the epididymis. This reflux into the epididymis can lead to acute or chronic epididymitis. Other complications include retrograde ejaculation secondary to bladder neck injury, incontinence secondary to external sphincter injury, and, although rare, rectourethral fistula secondary to rectal injury (Vazquez-Levin et al, 1994; Goluboff et al, 1995a, 1995b). Postoperative bleeding, bladder neck contractures, and erectile dysfunction are also known complications. Large defects within the prostate can allow mixing of semen and urine, which can further impair sperm quality.

Outcomes

Results of studies treating infertile men with ejaculatory duct obstruction are shown in Table 20–6. Overall results from surgical correction of ejaculatory duct obstruction show a

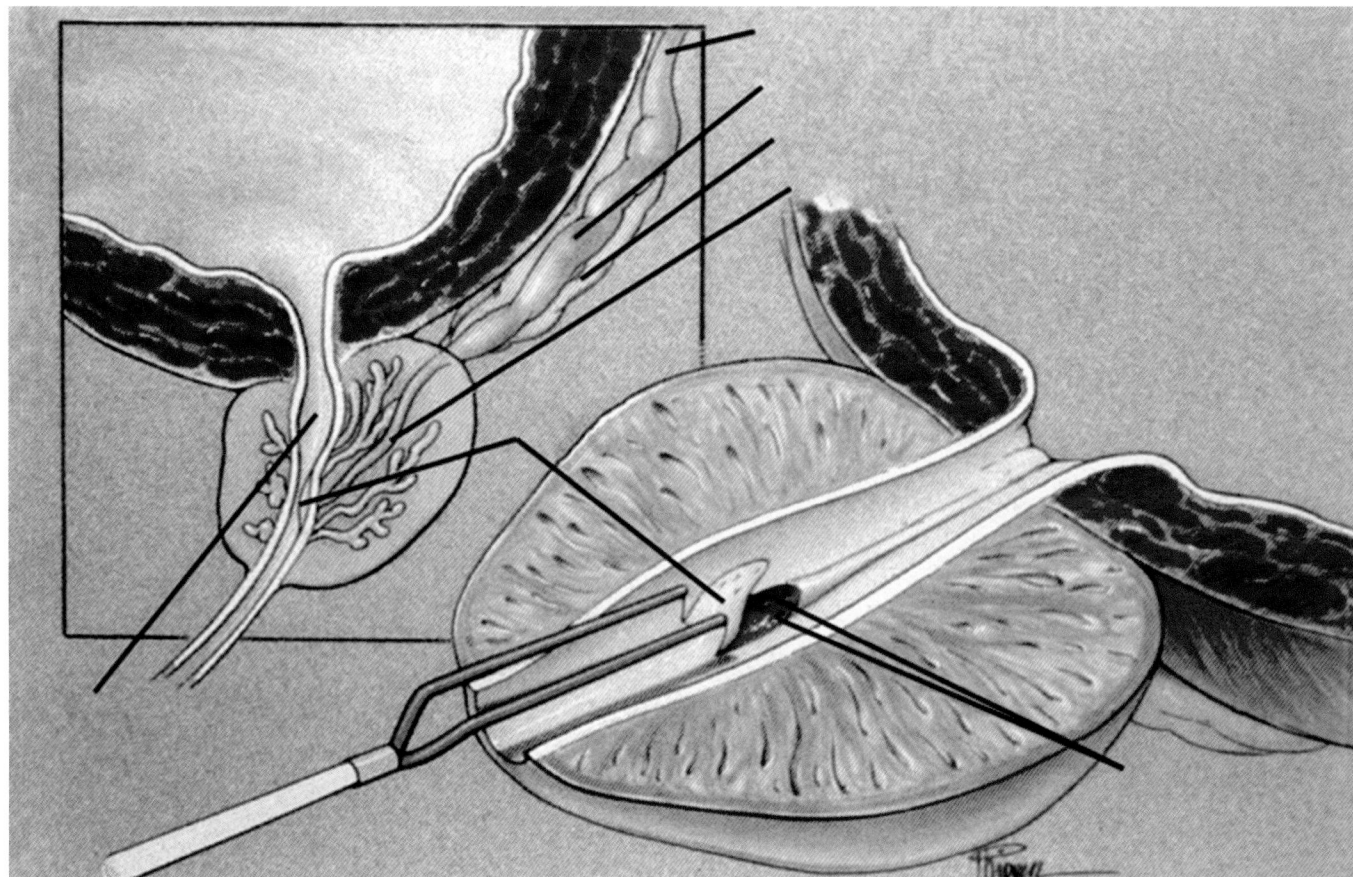

Figure 20–57. Transurethral resection of the ejaculatory duct. The resection is started deep and posterior to the verumontanum to ensure complete resection of the ducts.

Table 20–6. Results of Treatment of Ejaculatory Duct Obstruction in Infertile Men

Date	Author	No. of Patients	No. of Surgical Procedures	Improved Semen Quality	No. of Pregnancies
1978	Hassler and Weber	1	1	1	1
1978	Porch	1	1	1	1
1980	Weintraub	4	4	2	1
1980	Silber	4	4	1	0
1982	Amelar and Dubin	6	6	2	1
1983	Vicente et al	9	9	3	1
1984	Carson	4	4	3	1
1985	Goldwasser et al	1	1	1	1
1986	Dunetez and Krane	1	1	1	1
1991	Pryor and Hendry	87	31	18	8
1992	Hellerstein et al	2	2	2	2
1992	Hendry and Pryor	26	26	12	7
1993	Meacham et al	24	26	12	7
1998	Netto et al	14	14	10	5
1998	Popken et al	8	8	6	0
2003	Fuse et al	10	10	7	3
	Total	202	148	82 (55%)	40 (27%)

55% improvement in semen parameters and a 27% pregnancy rate.

The type (partial versus complete), location, and etiology of ejaculatory duct obstruction can have an impact on surgical outcomes. Kadioglu and associates (2001) reported that after surgical treatment of ejaculatory duct obstruction, improvement of semen parameters was greater in patients with partial obstruction (94%) than in patients with complete obstruction (59%). Others have shown that patients with midline cysts treated by transurethral resection tend to have better outcomes than do patients with other causes of ejaculatory duct obstruction (Kendirci et al, 2004). Finally, Netto and coworkers (1998) demonstrated in their series that after treatment, 83% of patients with congenital ejaculatory duct obstruction had an improved sperm count, and pregnancy was achieved through sexual intercourse by 66% of the patients. Of those with acquired ejaculatory duct obstruction, 37.5% had improved semen quality after transurethral resection of the ejaculatory duct, and 12.5% achieved pregnancy by sexual intercourse. **Thus, patients with partial, congenital, and midline cystic causes of ejaculatory duct obstruction tend to have the best surgical outcomes.**

Seminal Vesicle Aspiration and Seminal Vesiculography

Seminal vesicle aspiration can be a useful diagnostic tool in assessing ejaculatory duct obstruction (Jarow, 1994; Orhan et al, 1999). Some investigators have also used this technique as an alternative to vasography to diagnose distal vasal obstruction (Riedenklau et al, 1995). If transrectal ultrasonography shows that the seminal vesicles are dilated or that a midline (müllerian duct) cyst is present in a man with obstructive azoospermia or severe oligospermia and decreased motility with a normal testicular size and a normal FSH value, seminal vesicle aspiration and seminal vesiculography should be performed to help confirm the diagnosis of obstructive azoospermia.

Before seminal vesicle aspiration is performed, the patient is instructed to ejaculate the day before the procedure to decrease the likelihood of retrograde ejaculation into the seminal vesicles as a result of prolonged abstinence (Jarow, 1996a). Before the procedure, the patient should also undergo a standard bowel preparation and receive antibiotics similar to those used for a transrectal prostate biopsy. Under ultrasound guidance, the size and location of the seminal vesicles as well as the presence of any midline prostatic structures are noted (Fig. 20–58). The seminal vesicles are then aspirated with a Chiba biopsy needle and a syringe (Fig. 20–59). When the aspirated fluid is examined under a microscope, a finding of three or more motile sperm per high-power field is indicative of ejaculatory duct obstruction, and after centrifugation, the fluid can be cryopreserved (Fig. 20–60). **The presence of sperm indicates that at least one vas and epididymis are patent. If no sperm are found on seminal vesicle aspiration, sperm production should be confirmed with a testis biopsy. If the biopsy finding is normal, the possibility of ejaculatory duct obstruction or epididymal obstruction should be discussed with the patient.** Vasography should be performed, if indicated, at the time of reconstruction (see later). **If epididymal obstruction is identified in the presence of ejaculatory duct obstruction, it is appropriate first to relieve the distal obstruction and after 1 to 2 months, if the semen volume has increased, to consider confirmatory vasography and vasoepididymostomy. If there is persistent obstruction, these patients should be considered for microsurgical epididymal sperm aspiration and subsequent IVF with ICSI.** The success rate with simultaneous transurethral resection of the ejaculatory duct and epididymovasostomy is difficult to evaluate since so little information is available.

Seminal vesiculography involves injection of contrast material, which can be mixed with indigo carmine, into the seminal vesicles. This procedure can help assess the feasibility of surgical resection of an ejaculatory duct obstruction (i.e., to more accurately assess the depth of the obstructing cyst) as well as the distance between the obstructing entity and the rectum. Approximately 1.5 mL of indigo carmine is diluted with 8.5 mL of 50% water-soluble contrast medium and then injected into the seminal vesicle. Using a total of 10 mL provides enough contrast for visualization in the bladder. The instillation of indigo carmine is useful in later transurethral resection of the obstructed ducts to indicate when the obstructed system has been opened.

Vasography

Vasography should answer the question of whether sperm are present in the vasal fluid and whether the vas is obstructed. Vasography is indicated in the azoospermic man who is found to have many mature spermatozoa on testicular biopsy and who also has at least one palpable vas.

Copious vasal fluid containing many sperm indicates vasal obstruction or ejaculatory duct obstruction, and formal contrast vasography is performed to document the exact location of the obstruction. **Copious, thick, white fluid without sperm in a dilated vas indicates secondary epididymal obstruction in addition to a potential vasal obstruction or ejaculatory duct obstruction.** Vasography with radiographic contrast medium and intraoperative radiography are rarely indicated. There is no need to perform vasography at the time of testicular biopsy for azoospermia unless immediate reconstruction is planned and the touch or wet preparation biopsy reveals mature sperm with tails. **If it is performed carelessly, vasography can cause stricture or even obstruction at the vasography site, which can complicate subsequent reconstruction** (Howards et al, 1975; Poore et al, 1997). In addition, because the majority of non–vasectomy-related obstructions are epididymal, vasography is of no value in making the diagnosis.

Technique

Vasography can be performed either by insertion of a fine needle through the wall of the vas deferens or by open vasotomy with a microsurgical technique. **Blind insertion of a needle into the vas is not only technically challenging but also associated with potential complications, such as perivasal bleeding and vasal injury with subsequent vasal obstruction.** However, if it is performed by a skilled surgeon comfortable with this technique and if the vasal lumen is enlarged from distal obstruction, this transvasal approach can be used. This technique involves exposure of a straight portion of the vas, insertion of a 30-gauge lymphangiogram needle attached to Silastic tubing and a syringe into the vasal lumen, and, finally, injection of 50% water-soluble contrast medium to confirm patency radiographically (Dewire and Thomas, 1995). **It is often difficult to obtain sufficient vasal sperm for cryopreservation with this fine-needle vasography.**

Open vasotomy involves isolating the vas deferens within the scrotal skin and delivering it through a small scrotal incision. A straight clamp or flat instrument is placed beneath the vas to serve as a platform. A hemivasotomy is made with use of high-powered magnification and a microknife (Fig. 20–61). If any fluid is present in the vasal lumen, it is mixed with saline solution and examined under a microscope. If no sperm are present, repeated samples can be taken while milking the

SECTION VI

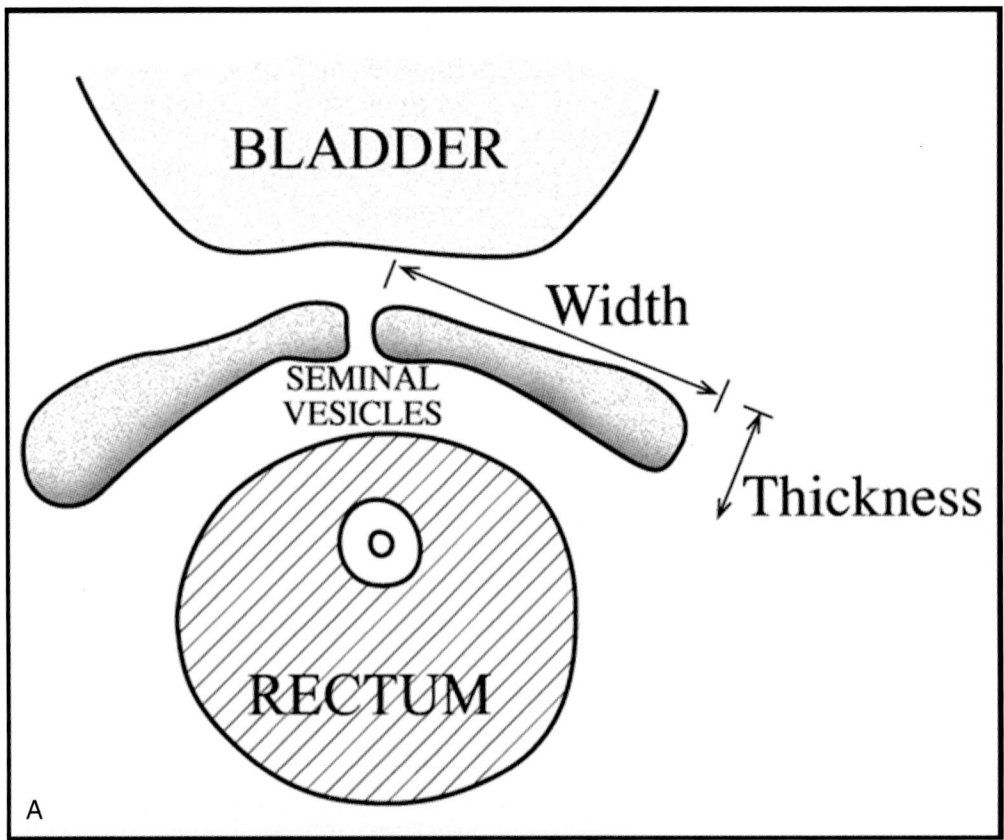

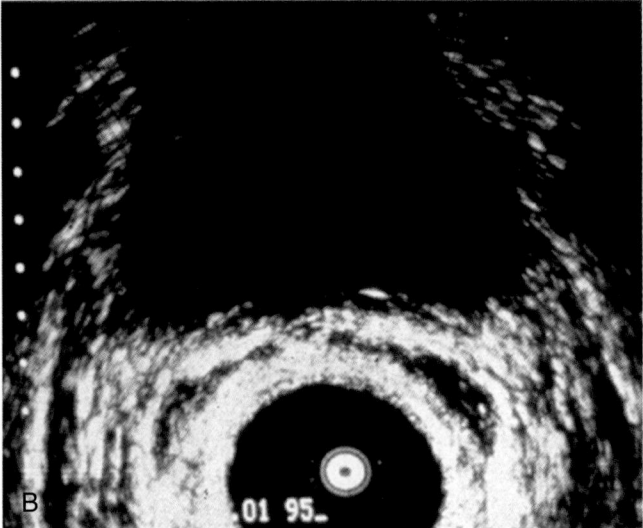

Figure 20–58. Illustration (**A**) and correlating ultrasound image (**B**) of the anatomic relationship of the seminal vesicles, rectum, and bladder.

epididymis and convoluted vas. **If no sperm are present on these repeated samples, epididymal obstruction is highly suspected.** A 24-gauge angiocatheter can be inserted in the distal end of the vas, and 10 mL of lactated Ringer's solution is injected to confirm patency. Formal vasography is not needed if the solution passes easily. If the solution does not pass easily, contrast material or indigo carmine can be injected in the direction of the ejaculatory ducts (Fig. 20–62). Contrast material should not be injected in the direction of the epididymis because of the risk of epididymal injury associated

with this procedure. Furthermore, indigo carmine should be used instead of methylene blue because methylene blue has the potential to impair sperm motility (Sheynkin et al, 1999; Wood et al, 2003). A Foley catheter should be placed in the bladder and the balloon filled with air to help identify the bladder neck on radiography. The presence of blue dye in the catheter confirms the patency of the vas deferens. Once the patency of the vas has been confirmed and if epididymal obstruction is suspected, the vas is completely transected, and a vasoepididymostomy is performed.

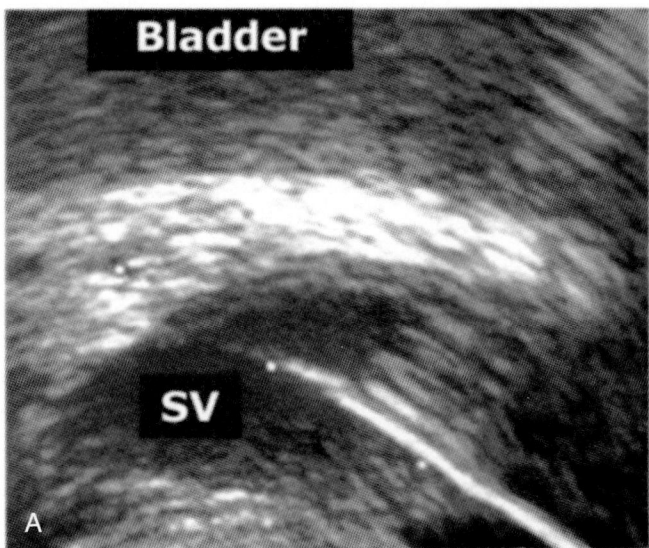

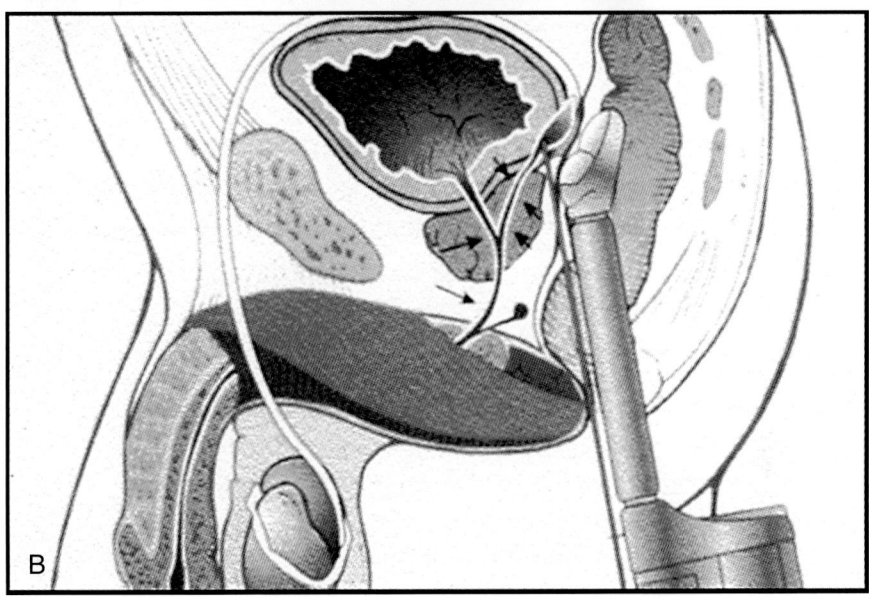

Figure 20–59. Seminal vesicle (SV) aspiration (**A**) and illustration of the relationship of probe and needle to nearby surrounding structures (**B**).

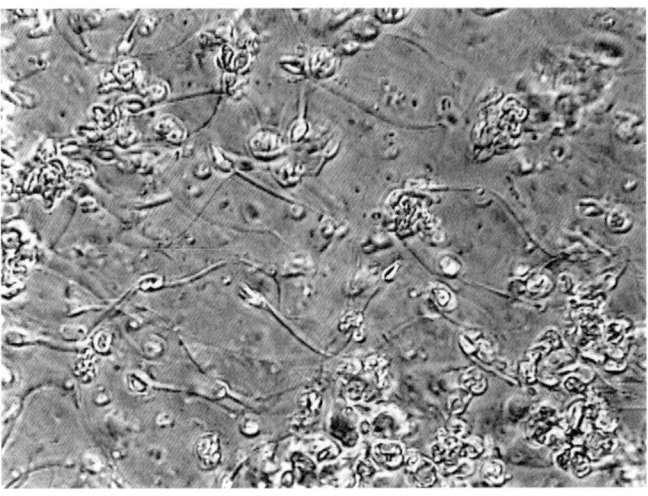

Figure 20–60. Seminal vesicle aspirate demonstrating numerous sperm.

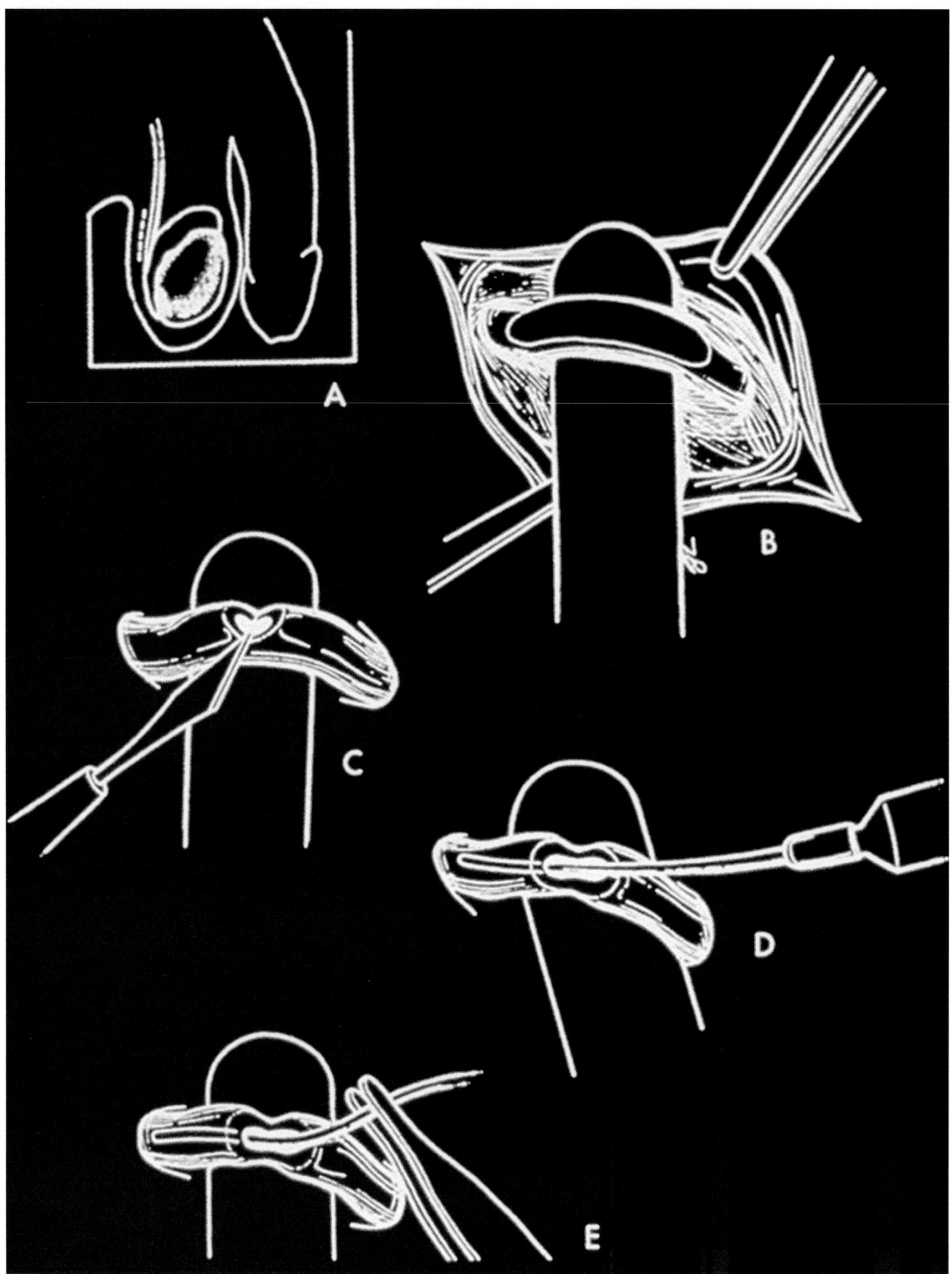

Figure 20–61. Open vasotomy technique. **A,** The vas is palpated within the scrotum. **B,** The vas is brought up through the scrotal incision. **C,** A hemivasotomy is made with a microknife. **D,** A 24-gauge angiocatheter can be inserted in the distal end of the vas, and 10 mL of lactated Ringer's solution is injected to confirm patency. **E,** A Prolene suture can be passed also to confirm vasal patency.

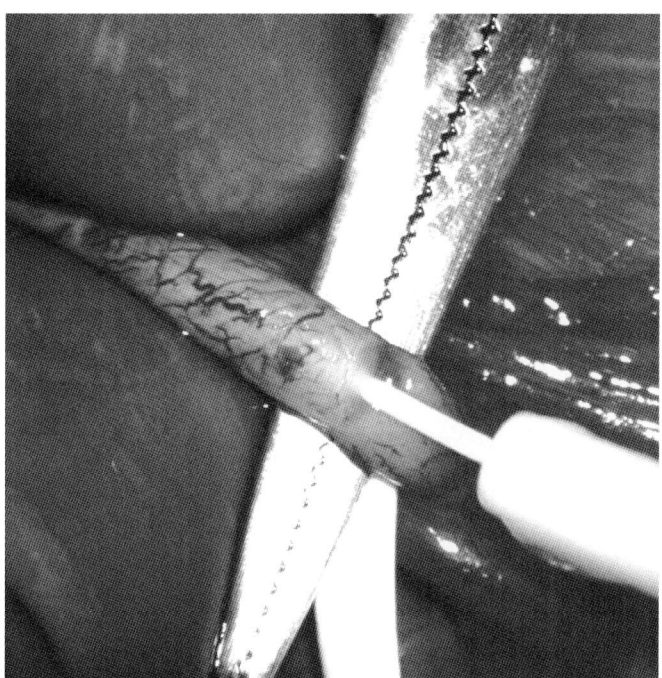

Figure 20–62. Cannulation of vasal lumen with a 24-gauge Angiocath sheath.

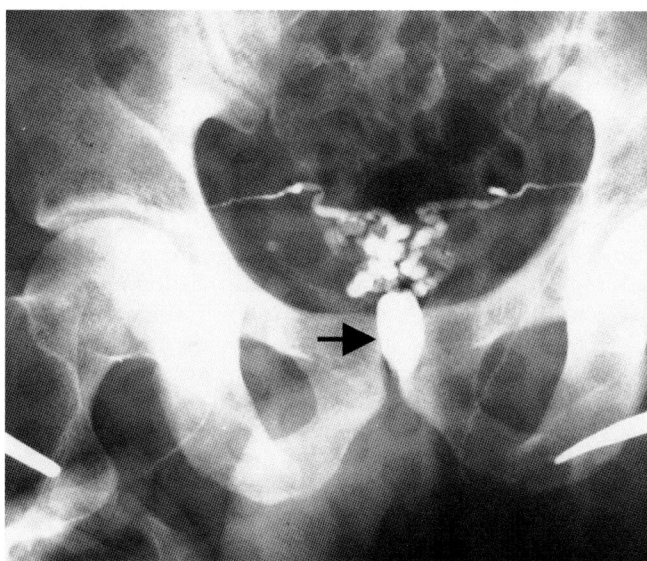

Figure 20–63. Both vasa are visualized after injection of contrast medium into the right vas only. The vasa empty into a common cavity, probably a midline ejaculatory duct cyst *(arrow)*.

If sperm are identified in the vasal fluid, this indicates that the obstruction is more distal, that is, toward the ejaculatory ducts. A 1-0 Prolene suture is passed into the vasal lumen toward the ejaculatory ducts. A hemostat is placed on the suture once it no longer advances, and the suture is withdrawn from the vasal lumen. By measuring the length of suture placed, the surgeon can assess the distance to the obstruction. Vasography, if it is still considered necessary, can then be performed by passing a 24-gauge angiocatheter needle toward the ejaculatory ducts and injecting water-soluble contrast material. If an obstruction is identified in the ejaculatory ducts, transurethral resection of the ejaculatory duct is performed. On occasion, both vasa deferentia are visualized after only one injection, indicating that they both empty into a single cavity, such as an ejaculatory duct cyst (Fig. 20–63). Indigo carmine can be injected into both vasa during the transurethral resection of the ejaculatory duct to help determine when the resection has been completed.

On completion of vasography, the hemivasotomy is closed in two layers with interrupted 10-0 nylon suture for the inner mucosal layer and 9-0 nylon suture for the outer adventitial layer.

Complications

Vasography is associated with several complications, such as hematoma, stricture, sperm granuloma, and vascular injury to the vas deferens. Whereas these complications are more commonly seen with fine-needle transvasal vasography, they have also been described in association with the open technique. **Stricture formation is usually due to granuloma formation, perivasal bleeding, or submucosal injection of contrast material. Stricture formation can also be a result of a poor vasotomy closure** (Poore et al, 1997) **or vascular injury to the vas deferens.**

TREATMENT OF ANATOMIC, CONGENITAL, AND ORGANIC CAUSES OF INFERTILITY

There are many anatomic, congenital, and organic causes of male infertility. Among them are hypospadias, Peyronie's disease, and erectile and ejaculatory dysfunction, all of which are examined in detail in other chapters in this text. We discuss these topics briefly as they pertain to male infertility and surgical management to improve sperm delivery.

Hypospadias Repair

Hypospadias represents an anatomic cause of infertility since it can impair delivery of sperm into the female reproductive tract. Pregnancies can be achieved by surgical correction of the hypospadias or through intrauterine insemination. Hypospadias has been associated with abnormal sperm morphologic features and function in the fathers of hypospadiacs in addition to endogenous endocrine abnormalities, such as impaired testosterone biosynthesis and androgen insensitivity. **Thus, it is believed that there are other factors, in addition to the anatomic abnormalities, contributing to infertility in these patients** (Fritz and Czeizel, 1996; Sasagawa et al, 2002; Silver, 2004).

Plication for Peyronie's Disease

Peyronie's disease, first described in 1743 by François Gigot de la Peyronie, is characterized by the acquired formation of fibrous plaques within the tunica albuginea of the corpora cavernosa of the penis (Peyronie, 1743). These plaques can result in a significant curvature of the penis, painful intercourse, painful erections, and early loss of erections; the inability to have intercourse may be due to erectile dysfunction, the penile deformity, or pain. Peyronie's disease has a prevalence of 0.4% to 3.2% and occurs in men between 40 and 70 years of age (Lindsay et al, 1991; Schwarzer et al, 2001).

Peyronie's disease is initially managed conservatively with nonsurgical treatments. Gelbard and colleagues (1990) have shown that **14% of patients have complete, spontaneous resolution of their disease and 40% of patients experience progression of their disease within 1 year. Thus, it is important to wait at least 1 year until the fibrotic process has stabilized and there are no clinical signs of improvement before proceeding with interventional procedures, including surgical correction.** There are certain characteristics that have been associated with lack of spontaneous resolution of Peyronie's disease. These include calcification of plaques, penile curvature greater than 45 degrees, symptoms lasting more than 2 years, and associated Dupuytren's contractures (Gholami et al, 2003).

The surgical treatment of Peyronie's disease can be divided into three main categories: penile shortening procedures, penile lengthening procedures, and penile prosthesis implantation. Penile shortening procedures involve plication techniques, such as the Nesbit procedure. Penile lengthening procedures involve excision or incision of the plaque with subsequent grafting. A wide array of grafts are currently available: autografts (tunica vaginalis, fascia lata), allografts (cadaveric pericardium), xenografts (porcine small intestine submucosa), and synthetic grafts (Dacron mesh, polytetrafluoroethylene). Insertion of a penile prosthesis is reserved for those patients with Peyronie's disease and concomitant erectile dysfunction. After insertion and inflation of the penile prosthesis, the plaque is incised and patched, if needed, or the penis is bent in the opposite direction of the curvature, thus breaking the plaque. **This technique, described as modeling, has resulted in long-term satisfaction rates of up to 90%** (Wilson and Delk 1994; Wilson et al, 2001).

Erectile Dysfunction

Erectile dysfunction is defined as the persistent inability to achieve and to maintain an erection sufficient for intercourse. **Feldman and associates (1994)** have shown that in the general population, *complete* impotence increases from 5% among men 40 years of age to 15% among men 70 years and older.** Thus, a significant number of men, particularly in their later reproductive years, are infertile because of erectile dysfunction. Erectile dysfunction can be managed medically or surgically. Surgical treatments for erectile dysfunction include insertion of a penile prosthesis and revascularization procedures, both of which are discussed in another chapter.

Ejaculatory Dysfunction

Ejaculatory dysfunction affects approximately 2% of infertile men, and it can be caused by retrograde ejaculation or anejaculation (Dubin and Amelar, 1971). Anejaculation may be due to nerve damage, neurologic disease, or psychogenic etiology. Initially, stimulation of the sympathetic nerves T10 to L2 produces emission of semen into the posterior urethra. Ejaculation is then caused by a reflex stimulated by distention of the posterior urethra by seminal fluid. Antegrade ejaculation is achieved by the sympathetically induced closure of the

bladder neck; somatic efferents (S2 to S4), arising from the motor division of the pudendal nerve, induce contractions of the striated pelvic floor and periurethral muscles. The diagnosis and treatment of erectile dysfunction are further discussed in detail in Chapter 19, "Male Infertility".

Retrograde Ejaculation

Retrograde ejaculation is defined as the propulsion of seminal fluid from the posterior urethra into the bladder, and it can be either complete or incomplete. A review of 206 patients with retrograde ejaculation revealed that the most common cause of retrograde ejaculation was a retroperitoneal lymph node dissection, followed by diabetes mellitus, bladder neck surgery, unknown trauma, medications, urethral strictures, spinal cord injury, and transurethral resection of the prostate (Kamischke and Nieschlag, 2002). The α blockers used to treat benign prostatic hyperplasia, such as tamsulosin, have also been shown to cause retrograde ejaculation (Mann et al, 2000; Schulman, 2003).

Some patients with retrograde ejaculation can be treated medically with the goal of closing the bladder neck or by retrieval of sperm from their postejaculate urine. Common pharmacologic agents used to treat retrograde ejaculation include α agonists (milodrin, pseudoephedrine, ephedrine) and antihistamines (brompheniramine) (Kamischke and Nieschlag, 2002). Sympathomimetics, such as pseudoephedrine and ephedrine, are known to close the bladder neck and enhance antegrade ejaculation. Imipramine, a tricyclic antidepressant with both anticholinergic and sympathomimetic properties, has been widely used to treat retrograde ejaculation (Kamischke and Nieschlag, 2002). In one study, of the 264 patients treated with α agonists, anticholinergics, and antihistamine drugs for retrograde ejaculation, 133 (50%) were able to achieve antegrade ejaculation (Kamischke and Nieschlag, 2002). **If medications fail, sperm can be retrieved from an alkalinized postejaculate urine specimen and used for intrauterine insemination or IVF cycles. Postejaculate urine examination also should be performed when a man has an ejaculatory volume of less than 1 mL to rule out incomplete retrograde ejaculation.**

Anejaculation

Anejaculation is defined as the absence of seminal emission into the posterior urethra. Anejaculation should be suspected in patients with complete absence of antegrade ejaculation as well as a fructose-negative, sperm-negative, nonviscous postorgasmic urinalysis (Murphy and Lipshultz, 1987). **In a review of 560 patients diagnosed with anejaculation, the most common cause of anejaculation was spinal cord injury, followed by retroperitoneal lymph node dissection** (Kamischke and Nieschlag, 2002). **These two causes were responsible for almost 90% of all cases of anejaculation.** A psychological cause of anejaculation should be considered for any patient who suddenly is unable to ejaculate, especially if he can masturbate to completion and if no other causes of ejaculatory dysfunction can be identified.

Anejaculation can be treated medically or by use of penile vibratory stimulation or electroejaculation. Medical treatment of anejaculation includes the use of α agonists. However, there have been only a few case reports of spontaneous pregnancy in partners of patients with anejaculation being treated with α agonists (Goldwasser et al, 1983; Schill, 1990). Some investigators have shown that bupropion (Wellbutrin) is also effective in treating anejaculation (Modell et al, 2000).

Ejaculation can be induced in many neurologically impaired men with penile vibratory stimulation, which involves placing a vibrator on the frenulum of the glans penis. For vibratory stimulation to induce ejaculation, the ejaculatory reflex arc in the thoracolumbar spinal cord must be intact. Therefore, spinal cord–injured patients with lesions above T10 are more likely to benefit from vibratory stimulation than are those with lesions below T10 (Sonksen and Ohl, 2002).

If penile vibratory stimulation is unsuccessful, electroejaculation can be attempted. Electroejaculation involves use of a rectal probe to stimulate the perirectal, periprostatic sympathetic nerves electrically (Fig. 20–64). Patients without a spinal cord injury or those with low or incomplete spinal cord lesions will require general anesthesia. **During electroejaculation, spinal cord–injured patients with lesions above T6 or a history of autonomic dysreflexia should have blood pressure monitored frequently for signs of autonomic dysreflexia and severe hypertension. These patients also should be given 10 to 30 mg of nifedipine sublingually 10 minutes before the procedure.**

The patient should be placed in the lateral decubitus or lithotomy position and a digital rectal examination performed. Anoscopy is performed before and after the procedure to look for any preexisting or iatrogenic pre-procedural rectal trauma. Pretreatment preparation of the patient includes pseudoephedrine (Sudafed) for 7 to 10 days to facilitate ejaculation; potassium citrate (Urocit-K), 10 mEq three times a day to alkalinize the urine; and a Fleet enema to optimize the electrical stimulation. **Initially, the bladder should be catheterized to empty the urine, and 30 mL of an alkalinizing medium (Ham's F-10, 20 mmol of HEPES buffer, and 1% human serum albumin) is placed inside the bladder. Mineral oil is used when the Foley catheter is inserted because commonly used lubricants are spermicidal.** A rectal probe is inserted with the electrodes facing anteriorly and pressed firmly against the prostate and seminal vesicles (Fig. 20–65). In the event that the patient becomes hypertensive during the procedure, the probe is removed and the procedure terminated. Electrical stimulation is administered initially at 5-volt increments and then increased by 1-volt increments until ejaculation is achieved. The probe temperature is simultaneously measured during the procedure and should not exceed 40°C. In the event that the probe temperature rises rapidly or the temperature rises above 40°C, the procedure is suspended until the probe has time to cool. On ejaculation, the antegrade ejaculate is collected in a sterile container, and any retrograde ejaculate is obtained by catheterization of the patient. The antegrade and retrograde specimens should be processed separately.

There are several differences between penile vibratory stimulation and electroejaculation. First, electroejaculation requires general anesthesia and is thus much more expensive than vibratory stimulation. A study by Ohl and coworkers (2001) found that if general anesthesia is required to perform electroejaculation, it is usually more cost-effective to perform IVF subsequently rather than intrauterine insemination. Intrauterine insemination after electroejaculation was cost-effective only in patients with spinal cord injuries who did not require general anesthesia.

Several investigators have also found differences in quality of semen obtained by the two procedures. **Sperm obtained from electroejaculation have been shown to be of poor quality, exhibiting poor motility and viability, decreased ability to penetrate cervical mucus, and impaired fertilizing capacity** (Denil et al, 1992; Buch and Zorn, 1993; Chung et al, 1995; Brackett et al, 1997; Ohl et al, 1997; Brackett and Lynne, 2000). Consequently, it is not surprising that investigators have found low pregnancy rates in patients undergoing electroejaculation and subsequent intrauterine insemination (Buch and Zorn, 1993; Chung et al, 1996). **A study by Schatte and colleagues (2000) demonstrated that pregnancy rates per couple were significantly lower in patients who underwent electroejaculation with ICSI than in patients with ejaculated specimens and subsequent ICSI (29% versus 47%, respectively).** However, these techniques remain controversial.

Several novel approaches to the treatment of anejaculation have been described in the literature. Some investigators have

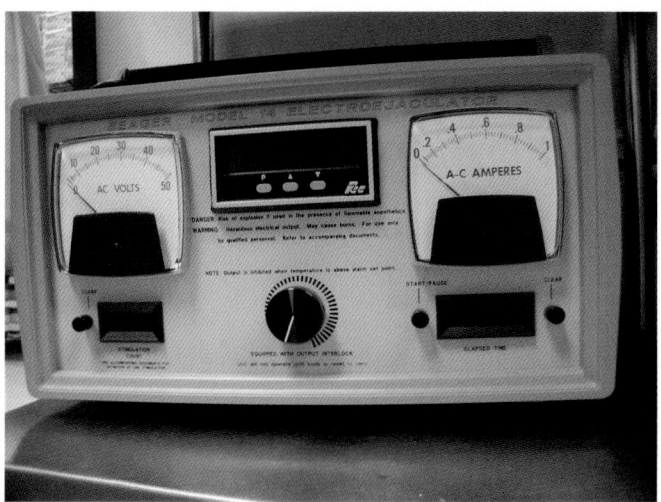

Figure 20–64. A Seager Model 14 electroejaculation machine.

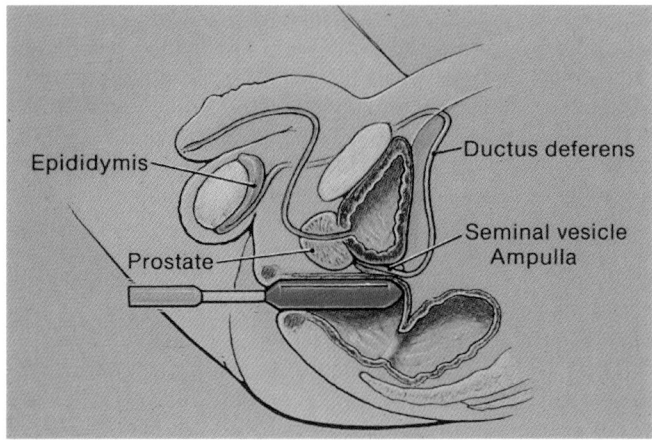

Figure 20–65. Illustration of rectal probe and its relation to nearby surrounding structures.

reported use of prostatic massage to successfully treat both psychogenic and neurogenic causes of anejaculation (Fahmy et al, 1999; Marina et al, 1999; Hovav et al, 2000; Okada et al, 2001). Qiu and associates (2003) have shown that infertile men with anejaculation can also be treated with percutaneous vasal sperm aspiration and intrauterine insemination. These investigators performed 34 percutaneous vasal aspirations and intrauterine inseminations in 26 men with anejaculation and were able to achieve a pregnancy rate of 73.1%.

GENETIC ABNORMALITIES RELATED TO AZOOSPERMIA

Azoospermia can be divided into two categories, obstructive and nonobstructive. Both types may carry some genetic risk to the offspring, depending on the cause of the azoospermia. These genetic risks need to be assessed and explained to the patient if he and his partner are to make an informed decision regarding their desire to have their own biologic offspring.

The patients with obstruction can be subdivided into those for whom the cause of the azoospermia is known, such as prior vasectomy, epididymitis, or testicular trauma, and those for whom the cause of the obstruction is unknown or is a known congenital cause. With a known cause, there is no indication to pursue genetic testing unless something else in the medical history becomes apparent. **If a man has congenital absence of the vas deferens or a vasal or epididymal obstruction with no apparent cause, testing for mutations in the cystic fibrosis transmembrane conductance regulator gene (*CFTR*) is indicated. The incidence of *CFTR* mutations in the nonaffected general population of men and women is approximately 4%. Comparatively, approximately 70% of men with bilateral congenital absence of the vas deferens and 21% of men with idiopathic epididymal obstruction will have at least one mutation of *CFTR*** (Mak et al, 1999; Sokol, 2001; Cuppens and Cassiman, 2004). Identification of a gene mutation in either the man or possibly his partner should prompt a referral for genetic counseling to discuss their risk of having a child who may be a carrier of a mutated gene or even have cystic fibrosis.

Approximately 12% of nonobstructive azoospermic men will have an abnormal karyotype. The most common karyotypic abnormality is an extra X chromosome (47,XXY), a condition commonly known as Klinefelter's syndrome (Klinefelter et al, 1942; Johnson, 1998; Cruger et al, 2003; Foresta et al, 2005). Approximately 10% of men with Klinefelter's syndrome have a mosaic genetic pattern (46,XY/47,XXY). A few of these patients are severely oligospermic, and all have hypergonadotropic hypogonadism. Sperm can be retrieved from some of these men after testicular sperm extraction, but the data are mixed about whether the majority of offspring will possess a normal karyotype (Friedler et al, 2001; Madgar et al, 2002; Hopps et al, 2002; Staessen et al, 1976; Lanfranco et al, 2004; Vernaeve et al, 2004).

There are other non–sex chromosome–related abnormalities found more commonly in azoospermic and severely oligospermic men. Translocations of whole or partial arms of one chromosome into another may be the cause of a man's infertile condition and carry a risk of genetic transmission to

his offspring if sperm are found and used with ICSI. **Pregnancies resulting from the use of chromosomally unbalanced gametes may have a higher rate of spontaneous abortion; or, if pregnancy continues, offspring may carry significant genetic abnormalities** (Veld et al, 1997; Antonelli et al, 2000; Egozcue et al, 2000; Dohle et al, 2002).

In the mid-1970s, Tiepolo and Zuffardi identified a relationship between a deletion in the region of Yq11 and male factor infertility (Tiepolo and Zuffardi, 1976). This locus is now known as the AZF (azoospermia factor) region. There have been three important loci identified, simply referred to as AZFa, AZFb, and AZFc. Deletions in these regions are associated with azoospermia or severe oligospermia. **Four percent of men with oligospermia have Y chromosome microdeletions. This increases to 14% in men with sperm concentrations less than 5 million/mL and 11% to 18% in men with nonobstructive azoospermia** (Brugh et al, 2003; Foresta et al, 2005). Studies have indicated that if there is a complete absence of AZFa to AZFc, sperm will not be found in the testes. If AZFa or AZFb is completely absent, mature sperm are not likely to be found. **Men with an AZFc deletion may be severely oligospermic; if they are azoospermic, some may have foci of mature sperm in their testes** (Oates et al, 2002; Hopps et al, 2003). Studies suggest that fertilization and pregnancy rates are not affected by a microdeletion in the AZFc region if sperm are found. However, because there may be other, yet unrecognized phenotypic expressions of these microdeletions, it is imperative that affected men and their partners understand these potential implications (Choi et al, 2004). **All nonobstructed azoospermic as well as severely oligospermic (<5 million sperm/mL) men should be advised to be screened for Y chromosome microdeletions if they are trying or will try to establish a pregnancy.**

Use of penile vibratory stimulation and electroejaculation for the purpose of sperm retrieval from some men with spinal cord injuries, sympathetic nerve impairment due to diabetic neuropathy, multiple sclerosis, or non–nerve-sparing retroperitoneal lymph node dissection has been addressed previously.

Another method by which sperm can be obtained from men with ejaculatory dysfunction is by direct aspiration of the seminal vesicle guided by transrectal ultrasonography. This is thoroughly described earlier in the section entitled "Seminal Vesicle Aspiration and Seminal Vesiculography."

IN VITRO FERTILIZATION WITH INTRACYTOPLASMIC SPERM INJECTION

IVF combined with the assisted fertilization technique of ICSI is a highly successful treatment of otherwise untreatable severe male factor infertility (Palermo et al, 1992; Van Steirteghem et al, 1993). However, the availability of assisted reproductive technology does not obviate the need of a proper workup to diagnose the cause of male infertility and to provide a proper and specific treatment to reverse the underlying cause of testicular failure and obstruction. Rather, these assisted reproductive techniques offer the opportunity for urologists to assist men who would not have been candidates for any therapeutic interventions just 15 years ago to father their own biologic children.

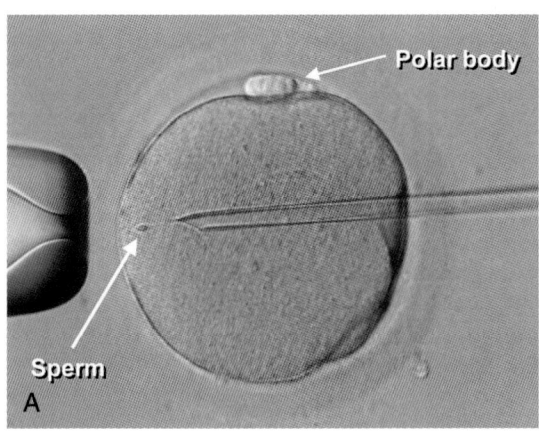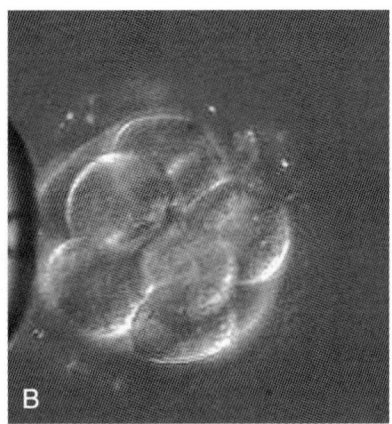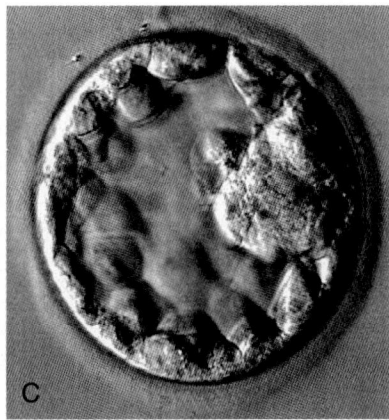

Figure 20–66. **A,** Intracytoplasmic sperm injection. **B,** Multicellular embryo 2 to 3 days after fertilization. **C,** Blastocyst at 5 days after fertilization.

Examples of these pathophysiologic paradigms, as discussed earlier in this chapter, include the following:

- Men with surgically unreconstructible obstruction, such as congenital bilateral absence of the vas deferens.
- Men with few viable sperm in the ejaculate.
- Azoospermic men with varicoceles. Forty percent of these men will respond to varicocelectomy with return of enough sperm to ejaculate to achieve pregnancy by IVF with ICSI (Matthews et al, 1998).
- Men with nonobstructive azoospermia.

With ICSI, viable sperm are injected directly into an oocyte (Fig. 20–66A) after the sperm tail is immobilized. Only one viable sperm is needed for each oocyte retrieved. **In experienced hands** (Van Steirteghem et al, 1993), **fertilization rates are in the range of 70%, and delivery rates per retrieval are currently 50% in the more than 1000 couples treated with ICSI.** The rate of oocyte damage should be less than 10%. The incidence of major fetal abnormalities is 3.2% compared with 1.6% in natural conception. IVF with ICSI is now the treatment of choice for severe uncorrectable male factor infertility. ICSI is costly ($12,000 to $15,000 for a single attempt) and usually not covered by health insurance. It also involves putting the female partner through a month of intramuscular injections, frequent sonographic monitoring, and measurement of blood hormone levels, culminating in the transvaginal retrieval of multiple oocytes under sedation or general anesthesia. Embryos that cleave and continue to develop are transferred to the uterus transvaginally 3 to 5 days after fertilization (Fig. 20–66B and C).

Aside from the cost and discomfort, each IVF-ICSI attempt is an "emotional roller coaster" for the couple. These procedures should not be recommended indiscriminately. Every attempt should be made to treat both male and female infertility issues and enable the couple to conceive as naturally as possible. Most couples prefer natural conception. Although IVF-ICSI may be the most rational approach to advanced maternal age or irreversible tubal occlusion, specific treatments of male factor infertility, such as microsurgical vasovasotomy, with a better than 50% natural pregnancy rate, and varicocelectomy, with a natural pregnancy rate of 40% to 70%, are more cost-effective than IVF with ICSI (Pavlovich and Schlegel, 1997) and should be the first level of therapy.

KEY POINTS: SURGICAL MANAGEMENT OF MALE INFERTILITY

- Azoospermia is attributable to an obstruction, a complete defect in spermatogenesis, or an incomplete defect with foci of mature sperm.

- Repair of a subclinical varicocele does not improve fertility rates.

- Pregnancy rates are not significantly different between multilayer and single-layer vasovasostomy reconstructions.

- The longer the time from vasectomy, the greater the chance of epididymal obstruction.

- Although microsurgical epididymal sperm aspiration is a surgical procedure, it enables the collection of large numbers of motile sperm for men with obstructive azoospermia.

- Congenital absence of the vas deferens calls for cystic fibrosis screening.

SUGGESTED READINGS

Kahraman S, Ozgur S, Aksoy S, et al: High implantation and pregnancy rates with testicular sperm extraction and intracytoplasmic sperm injection in obstructive and non-obstructive azoospermia. Hum Reprod 1996;11:673-676.

Kolettis PN, Thomas AJ Jr: Vasoepididymostomy for vasectomy reversal: A critical assessment in the era of intracytoplasmic sperm injection. J Urol 1997;158:467-470.

Murphy JB, Lipshultz LI: Abnormalities of ejaculation. Urol Clin North Am 1987;14:583-596.

Palermo G, Joris H, Devroey P, Van Steirteghem AC: Pregnancies after intracytoplasmic injection of single spermatozoon into an oocyte. Lancet 1992;340:17-18.

Schlegel PN: Is assisted reproduction the optimal treatment for varicocele-associated male infertility? A cost-effectiveness analysis. Urology 1997; 49:83-90.

Silber SJ, Grotjan HE: Microscopic vasectomy reversal 30 years later: A summary of 4,010 cases by the same surgeon. J Androl 2004;25:845-859.

Steckel J, Dicker AP, Goldstein M: Relationship between varicocele size and response to varicocelectomy. J Urol 1993;149:769-771.

Physiology of Penile Erection and Pathophysiology of Erectile Dysfunction

TOM F. LUE, MD

PHYSIOLOGY OF PENILE ERECTION

PATHOPHYSIOLOGY OF ERECTILE DYSFUNCTION

PERSPECTIVES

"The penis does not obey the order of its master, who tries to erect or shrink it at will. Instead, the penis erects freely while its master is asleep. The penis must be said to have its own mind, by any stretch of the imagination."

Leonardo da Vinci

PHYSIOLOGY OF PENILE ERECTION
Historical Aspects

The first description of erectile dysfunction (ED) dates from about 2000 BC and was set down on Egyptian papyrus. Two types were described: natural ("the man is incapable of accomplishing the sex act") and supernatural (evil charms and spells). Later, Hippocrates reported many cases of male impotence among the rich inhabitants of Scythia and ascribed it to excessive horseback riding. (The poor were not affected because they traveled by foot.) Aristotle stated that three branches of nerves carry spirit and energy to the penis and that erection is produced by the influx of air (Brenot, 1994). His theory was well accepted until Leonardo da Vinci (1504) noted a large amount of blood in the erect penis of hanged men and cast doubt on the concept of the air-filled penis. His writings, however, were kept secret until the beginning of the 20th century (Brenot, 1994). Nevertheless, in 1585, in *Ten Books on Surgery* and the *Book of Reproduction*, Ambroise Paré gave an accurate account of penile anatomy and the concept of erection. He described the penis as being composed of concentric coats of nerves, veins, and arteries and of two ligaments (corpora cavernosa), a urinary tract, and four muscles.

"When the man becomes inflamed with lust and desire, blood rushes into the male member and causes it to become erect." The importance of retaining blood in the penis was stressed by Dionis (1718; quoted by Brenot, 1994), who attributed this to the muscles cramping the veins at the proximal end, and by Hunter (1787), who thought that venous spasm prevented the exit of blood.

Many theories have since been added to explain the hemodynamic events during erection and detumescence. In the 19th century, venous occlusion was thought to be the main factor in achieving and maintaining erection (Bochdalek, 1854; Waldeyer, 1899), but later investigators (Deysach, 1939; Christensen, 1954; Newman et al, 1964; Dorr and Brody, 1967) stressed the importance of increased arterial blood flow; and Newman and associates (1964), in human cadavers and volunteers, showed that erection could be induced by saline solution perfusion alone without venous constriction. However, radioactive xenon washout and cavernosography studies in human volunteers exposed to audiovisual sexual stimulation yielded conflicting results: Shirai and associates (1978) concluded that, although venous flow is increased, the markedly increased arterial flow overwhelms it; Wagner (1981) also showed increased arterial flow but concluded that venous drainage is decreased.

Even more controversial than the hemodynamics of erection is its anatomic mechanism. Various theories have been proposed to explain the erectile process: arterial polsters (Von Ebner, 1900; Kiss, 1921), arterial and venous polsters (Conti, 1952), a sluice mechanism (Deysach, 1939), an arteriovenous shunt (Newman et al, 1964; Wagner et al, 1982), and contraction of the cavernous smooth muscles (Goldstein et al, 1982).

Much of the current understanding of erectile physiology was gained in the 1980s and 1990s. In addition to the role of smooth muscle in regulating arterial and venous flow, the three-dimensional structure of the tunica albuginea and its role in venous occlusion were elucidated. An important breakthrough in the understanding of neural influences was the identification of nitric oxide (NO) as the major neurotransmitter for erection and of phosphodiesterases (PDEs) for detumescence. The role of endothelium in regulating smooth muscle tone and of the intercellular links effected by gap junctions has been uncovered. Furthermore, the importance of ion channels (potassium and calcium) and Rho/Rho kinase pathways in contraction and relaxation of smooth muscle has been shown. In pathophysiology, changes in smooth muscle, nerve endings, endothelium, and the fibroelastic framework associated with disease have been identified. These developments are discussed in detail in this chapter.

Functional Anatomy of the Penis

The penis is composed of three cylindrical structures, the paired corpora cavernosa and the corpus spongiosum (which houses the urethra), covered by a loose subcutaneous layer and skin. Its flaccid length is controlled by the contractile state of the erectile smooth muscle and varies considerably, depending on emotion and outside temperature. In one study, penile length, measured from the pubopenile junction to the meatus, was 8.8 cm flaccid, 12.4 cm stretched, and 12.9 cm erect, with neither age nor the size of the flaccid penis accurately predicting erectile length (Wessells et al, 1996). In another study, the author concluded that about 15% of men have a downward curve during erection, erect angle is below horizontal in one quarter, and shorter erect lengths (from 4.5 to 5.75 inches) occur in 40% of men (Sparling, 1997). Since then, more studies have been reported from several countries (Awwad et al, 2005) (Table 21–1). Regarding penile morphology and erection, one study showed that, during erection, the penile buckling forces are dependent not only on intracavernous pressures but also on penile geometry and erectile tissue properties. The authors concluded that, in patients with normal penile hemodynamics but without adequate rigidity, structural causes should be investigated (Udelson et al, 1998).

Tunica Albuginea

The tunica affords great flexibility, rigidity, and tissue strength to the penis (Hsu et al, 1992) (Fig. 21–1). **The tunical covering of the corpora cavernosa is a bilayered structure with multiple sublayers. Inner-layer bundles support and contain the cavernous tissue and are oriented circularly.** **Radiating from this inner layer are intracavernous pillars that act as struts to augment the septum and provide essential support to the erectile tissue. Outer-layer bundles are oriented longitudinally, extending from the glans penis to the proximal crura; they insert into the inferior pubic rami but are absent between the 5 and 7 o'clock positions. In contrast, the corpus spongiosum lacks an outer layer or intracorporeal struts, ensuring a low-pressure structure during erection.**

The tunica is composed of elastic fibers that form an irregular, latticed network on which the collagen fibers rest (Fig. 21–2). The detailed histologic composition of the tunica varies with anatomic location and function. Emissary veins run between the inner and outer layers for a short distance, often piercing the outer bundles obliquely. However, the cavernous artery and the branches of the dorsal artery that give additional blood supply to the corpus cavernosum take a more direct route and are surrounded by a periarterial soft tissue sheath, which protects the arteries from occlusion by the tunica albuginea during erection.

The outer tunical layer appears to play an additional role in compression of the emissary veins during erection. It also determines, to a large extent, the variability in tunical thickness and strength (Hsu et al, 1992). Between the 6 and 7 o'clock positions, the tunical thickness is 0.8 ± 0.1 mm; at the 9 o'clock position, 1.2 ± 0.2 mm; and at the 11 o'clock position, 2.2 ± 0.4 mm. At the 3, 5 to 6, and 1 o'clock positions, the measurements are nearly identical in mirror-image fashion. (Differences at specific locations have been found to be statistically significant.)

The stress on the tunica before penetration has been measured as $1.6 \pm 0.2 \times 10^7$ N/m^2 between the 6 and 7 o'clock positions, $3.0 \pm 0.3 \times 10^7$ N/m^2 at the 9 o'clock position, and $4.5 \pm 0.5 \times 10^7$ N/m^2 at the 11 o'clock position. **The strength and thickness of the tunica correlate in a statistically significant fashion with location. The most vulnerable area is located on the ventral groove (between the 5 and 7 o'clock positions), where the longitudinal outer layer is absent; most prostheses tend to extrude here** (Hsu et al, 1994).

The tunica albuginea is composed of fibrillar collagen (mostly type I, but also type III) in organized arrays interlaced with elastin fibers. Although collagen has a greater tensile strength than steel, it is unyielding. In contrast, elastin can be

Table 21–1.	**Penile Length in Adults**					
First Author	Year of Report	Number of Subjects	Age in Years (range)	Flaccid Length (cm)	Stretched (S) or Erect (E) Length (cm)	Country
Kinsey	1948	2770	20-59	9.7	15.5 (E)	United States
Bondil	1992	905	17-91	10.7	16.74 (S)	France
Da Ros	1994	150	NA	NA	14.5 (E)	Brazil
Wessells	1996	80	21-82	8.85	12.45 (S), 12.89 (E)	United States
Ponchietti	2001	3300	17-19	9	12.5 (S)	Italy
Ajmani	1985	320	17-23	8.16	NA	Nigeria
Schneider	2001	111	18-19	8.6	14.48 (E)	Germany
		32	40-68	9.22	14.18 (E)	
Awwad	2003	271 (N)	17-83	9.3	13.5 (S)	Jordan
		109 (ED)	22-68	7.7	11.6 (S)	

E, erect length; ED, erectile dysfunction; N, normal; NA, not available; S, stretch length.
Modified from Awwad Z, Abu-Hijleh M, Basri S, et al: Penile measurements in normal adult Jordanians and in patients with erectile dysfunction. Int J Impot Res 2005;17:191-195.

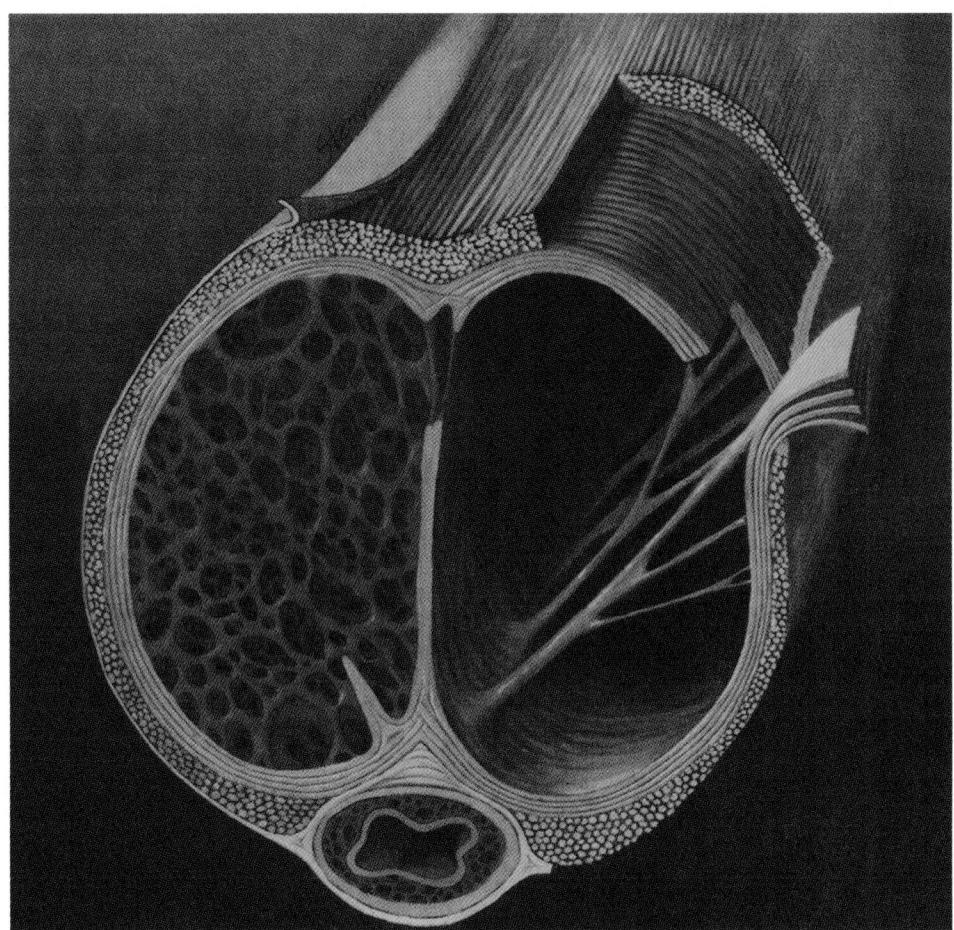

Figure 21–1. Artist's cross-sectional drawing of the penis, depicting the inner circular and outer longitudinal layers of the tunica albuginea as well as the intracavernous pillars. The longitudinal layer is absent in the ventral groove housing the corpus spongiosum. (From Lue TF, Akkus E, Kour NW: Physiology of erectile function and dysfunction. Campbell's Urology Update, 1994;12:1-10.)

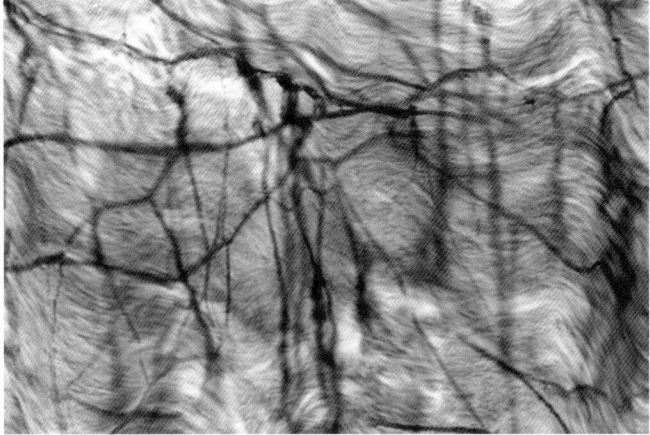

Figure 21–2. Micrograph of the human tunica albuginea, showing the interwoven elastic fibers and the finer collagen fibers. (Hart stain, ×100.)

stretched up to 150% of its length. It is the elastin content that allows tunical expansion and helps to determine stretched penile length.

External penile support consists of two ligamentous structures: the fundiform and suspensory ligaments. The fundiform ligament arises from Colles' fascia and is lateral, superficial, and not adherent to the tunica albuginea of the corpora cavernosa. The suspensory ligament arises from

Buck's fascia and consists of two lateral bundles and one median bundle, which circumscribe the dorsal vein of the penis. Its main function is to attach the tunica albuginea of the corpora cavernosa to the pubis, and thus it provides support for the mobile portion of the penis (Hoznek et al, 1998). In patients with congenital deficiency or in whom this ligament has been severed in "penile elongation" surgery, the erect penis may be unstable or droop.

Corpora Cavernosa, Corpus Spongiosum, and Glans Penis

The corpora cavernosa comprise two spongy, paired cylinders contained in the thick envelope of the tunica albuginea. Their proximal ends, the crura, originate at the undersurface of the puboischial rami as two separate structures but merge under the pubic arch and remain attached up to the glans. **The septum between the two corpora cavernosa is incomplete in men but is complete in some species, such as the dog.**

The corpora cavernosa are supported by a fibrous skeleton that includes the tunica albuginea, the septum, the intracavernous pillars, the intracavernous fibrous framework, and the periarterial and perineural fibrous sheath (Goldstein and Padma-Nathan, 1990; Hsu et al, 1992). Bitsch and coworkers (1990) believed that the intracavernous framework adds significant strength. Within the tunica are the interconnected sinusoids separated by smooth muscle trabeculae surrounded by elastic fibers, collagen, and loose areolar tissue. The terminal cavernous nerves and helicine arteries are intimately associated with the smooth muscle. Each corpus cavernosum is a conglomeration of sinusoids, larger in the center and smaller in the periphery. In the flaccid state, the blood slowly diffuses from the central to the peripheral sinusoids and the blood gas levels are similar to those of venous blood. During erection, the rapid entry of arterial blood to both the central and the peripheral sinusoids changes the intracavernous blood gas levels to those of arterial blood (Sattar et al, 1995).

The structure of the corpus spongiosum and glans is similar to that of the corpora cavernosa except that the sinusoids are larger; the tunica is thinner in the spongiosum (with only a circular layer [see earlier]) and is absent in the glans.

Arteries

The source of penile blood is usually the internal pudendal artery, a branch of the internal iliac artery (Fig. 21–3A). In many instances, however, accessory arteries exist, arising from the external iliac, obturator, vesical, and femoral arteries, and they may in some men constitute the dominant or only arterial supply to the corpus cavernosum (Breza et al, 1989). In a study of 20 fresh human cadavers, Droupy and colleagues (1997) reported three patterns of penile arterial supply: type I arising exclusively from internal pudendal arteries (3 of 20), type II arising from both accessory and internal pudendal arteries (14 of 20), and type III arising exclusively from accessory pudendal arteries (3 of 20). Careful preservation of the accessory pudendal artery during radical retropubic prostatectomy has been shown to support and hasten the recovery of sexual function (Rogers et al, 2004).

The internal pudendal artery becomes the common penile artery after giving off a branch to the perineum. The three branches of the penile artery are the dorsal, bulbourethral, and cavernous. Distally, they join to form a vascular ring near the glans. The dorsal artery is responsible for engorgement of the glans during erection. The bulbourethral artery supplies the bulb and corpus spongiosum. The cavernous artery effects

KEY POINTS: PENILE COMPONENTS AND THEIR FUNCTION DURING ERECTION

■	Corpora cavernosa	Support corpus spongiosum and glans
■	Tunica albuginea (of corpora cavernosa)	Contains and protects erectile tissue Promotes rigidity of the corpora cavernosa Participates in veno-occlusive mechanism
■	Smooth muscle	Regulates blood flow into and out of the sinusoids
■	Ischiocavernosus muscle	Pumps blood distally to hasten erection Provides additional penile rigidity during rigid erection phase
■	Bulbocavernosus muscle	Compresses the bulb to help expel semen
■	Corpus spongiosum	Pressurizes and constricts the urethra lumen to allow forceful expulsion of semen
■	Glans	Acts as a cushion to lessen the impact of the penis on female organs Provides sensory input to facilitate erection and enhance pleasure Facilitates intromission because of its cone shape

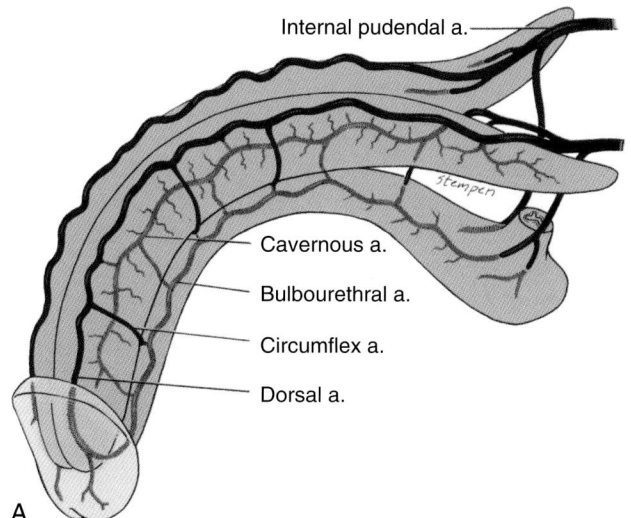

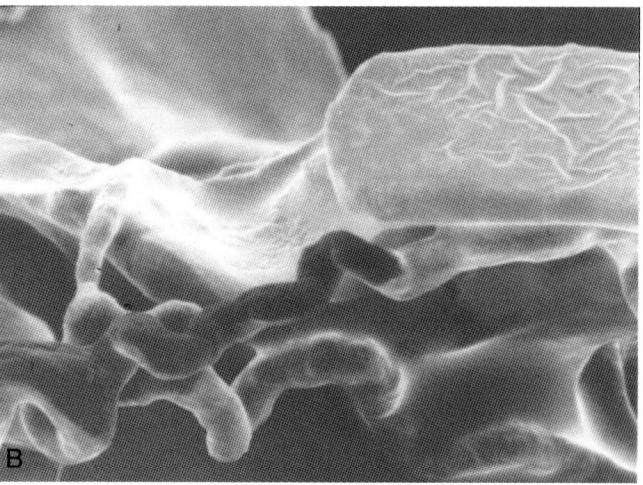

Figure 21–3. **A,** Penile arterial supply. **B,** Scanning electron micrograph of a human penile cast showing helicine arteries opening directly into the sinusoids without intervening capillaries.

tumescence of the corpus cavernosum and enters it at the hilum of the penis, where the two crura merge. Along its course, it gives off many helicine arteries, which supply the trabecular erectile tissue and the sinusoids (Fig. 21–3B). These helicine arteries are contracted and tortuous in the flaccid state and become dilated and straight during erection.

Veins

The venous drainage from the three corpora originates in tiny venules leading from the peripheral sinusoids immedi- **ately beneath the tunica albuginea. These venules travel in the trabeculae between the tunica and the peripheral sinu- soids to form the subtunical venous plexus before exiting as the emissary veins** (Fig. 21–4A). Outside the tunica albu- ginea, venous drainage is as follows.

The Skin and Subcutaneous Tissue. Multiple superficial veins run subcutaneously and unite near the root of the penis to form a single (or paired) superficial dorsal vein, which in turn drains into the saphenous veins. Occasionally, the super- ficial dorsal vein may also drain a portion of the corpora cavernosa.

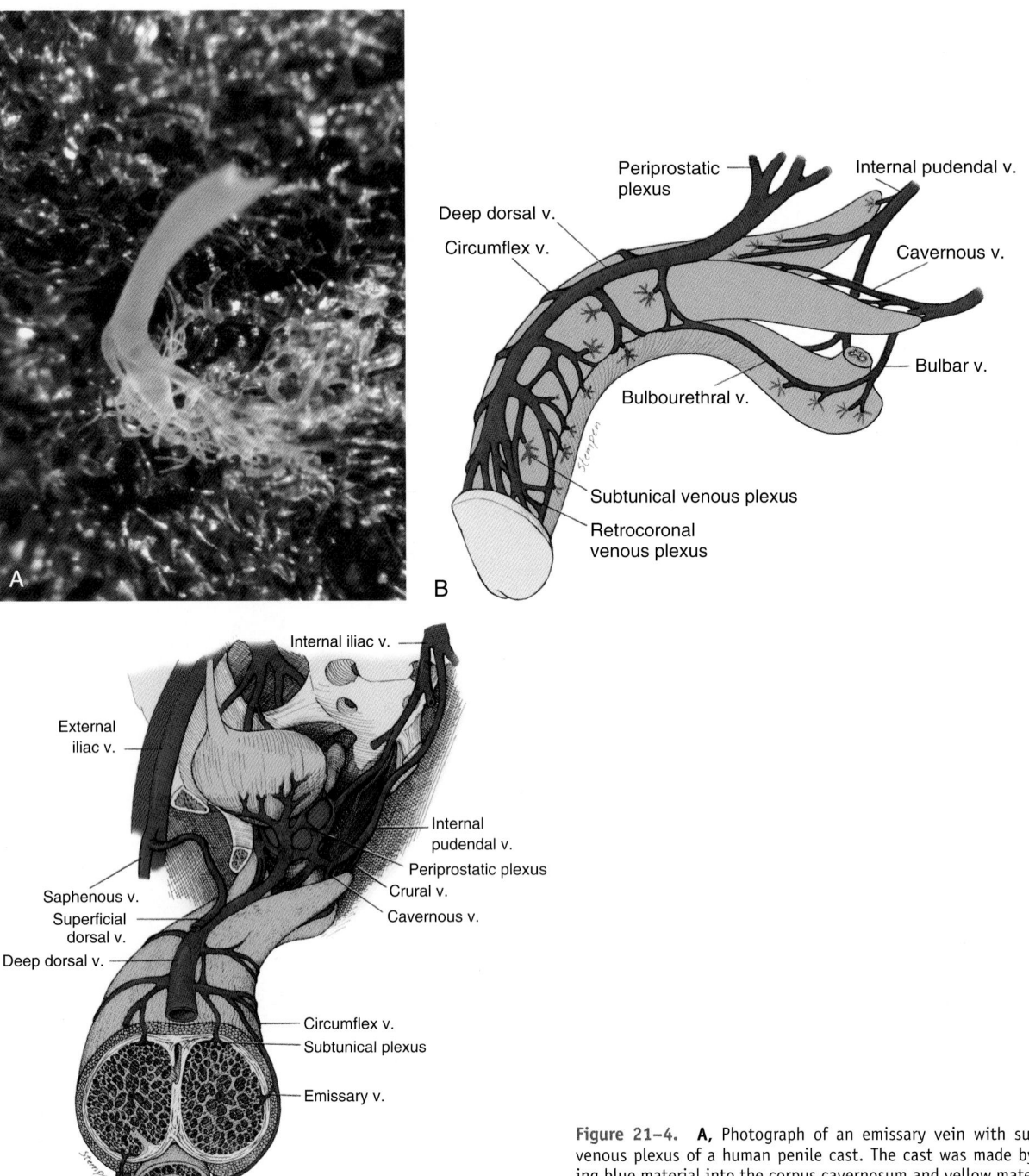

Figure 21–4. **A,** Photograph of an emissary vein with subtunical venous plexus of a human penile cast. The cast was made by inject- ing blue material into the corpus cavernosum and yellow material into the deep dorsal vein. The skin and tunica albuginea were then digested away with KOH solution. **B** and **C,** Penile venous drainage.

The Pendulous Penis. The emissary veins from the corpus cavernosum and spongiosum drain dorsally to the deep dorsal, laterally to the circumflex, and ventrally to the periurethral veins. Beginning at the coronal sulcus, multiple venous channels coalesce to form the deep dorsal vein, which is the main venous drainage of the glans penis and distal two thirds of the corpora cavernosa. Usually a single vein, but sometimes more than one deep dorsal vein, runs upward behind the symphysis pubis to join the periprostatic venous plexus. There are also small venous channels accompanying the paired dorsal artery. In addition, many veins travel longitudinally within the layers of the tunica albuginea to join the dorsal vein or Santorini's plexus proximally (Hsu et al, 2003). These become enlarged after the deep dorsal vein is ligated and may be the cause of recurrent leakage in venogenic ED (Chen et al, 2005).

The Infrapubic Penis. Emissary veins draining the proximal corpora cavernosa join to form cavernous and crural veins. These join the periurethral veins from the urethral bulb to form the internal pudendal veins.

The veins of the three systems communicate variably with each other. Indeed, variations in the number, distribution, and termination of these venous systems are common (Fig. 21–4B and C).

Hemodynamics and Mechanism of Erection and Detumescence

Corpora Cavernosa

The penile erectile tissue, specifically the cavernous smooth musculature and the smooth muscles of the arteriolar and arterial walls, plays a key role in the erectile process. **In the flaccid state, these smooth muscles are tonically contracted, allowing only a small amount of arterial flow for nutritional purposes.** The blood partial pressure of oxygen (PO_2) is about 35 mm Hg (Sattar et al, 1995). The flaccid penis is in a moderate state of contraction, as evidenced by further shrinkage in cold weather and after phenylephrine injection.

Sexual stimulation triggers release of neurotransmitters from the cavernous nerve terminals. **This results in relaxation of these smooth muscles and the following events** (Fig. 21–5): **(1) dilation of the arterioles and arteries by increased blood flow in both the diastolic and systolic phases; (2) trapping of the incoming blood by the expanding sinusoids; (3) compression of the subtunical venous plexuses between the tunica albuginea and the peripheral sinusoids, reducing venous outflow; (4) stretching of the tunica to its capacity, which occludes the emissary veins between the inner circular and outer longitudinal layers and further decreases venous outflow to a minimum; (5) an increase in PO_2 (to about 90 mm Hg) and intracavernous pressure (around 100 mm Hg), which raises the penis from the dependent position to the erect state (the full-erection phase); (6) a further pressure increase (to several hundred millimeters of mercury) with contraction of the ischiocavernosus muscles (rigid-erection phase).**

The angle of the erect penis is determined by its size and attachment to the puboischial rami (the crura) and the anterior surface of the pubic bone (the suspensory and funiform ligaments). In men with a long heavy penis or a loose suspensory ligament, the angle is usually not greater than 90 degrees, even with full rigidity.

Three phases of detumescence have been reported in an animal study (Bosch et al, 1991). The first entails a transient intracorporeal pressure increase, indicating the beginning of smooth muscle contraction against a closed venous system. The second phase shows a slow pressure decrease, suggesting a slow reopening of the venous channels with resumption of the basal level of arterial flow. The third phase shows a fast pressure decrease with fully restored venous outflow capacity.

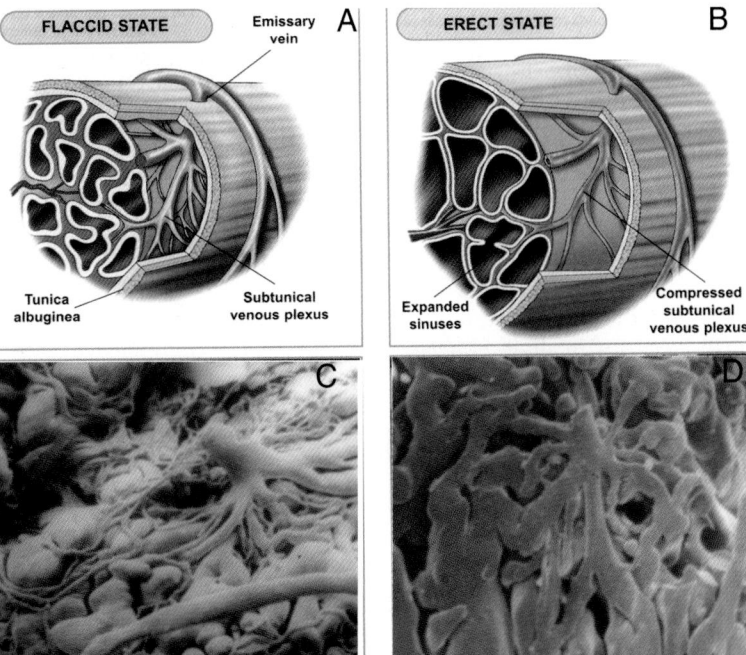

Figure 21–5. The mechanism of penile erection. **A,** In the flaccid state, the arteries, arterioles, and sinusoids are contracted. The intersinusoidal and subtunical venous plexuses are wide open, with free flow to the emissary veins. **B,** In the erect state, the muscles of the sinusoidal wall and the arterioles relax, allowing maximal flow to the compliant sinusoidal spaces. Most of the venules are compressed between the expanding sinusoids. The larger venules are sandwiched and flattened between the distended sinusoids and the tunica albuginea. This effectively reduces the venous capacity to a minimum. **C** and **D,** Scanning electron micrographs of casts of a canine subtunical venous plexus in the flaccid and erect states, respectively. **(B,** From Lue TF, Giuliano F, Khoury S, Rosen R: Clinical Manual of Sexual Medicine: Sexual Dysfunction in Men. Paris, France, Health Publications, 2004.)

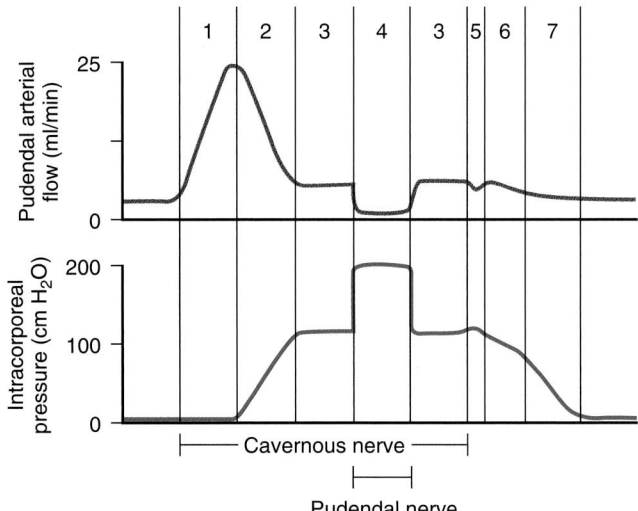

Figure 21–6. Blood flow and intracavernous pressure changes during the seven phases of penile erection and detumescence: **0**, flaccid; **1**, latent; **2**, tumescence; **3**, full erection; **4**, rigid erection; **5**, initial detumescence; **6**, slow detumescence; **7**, fast detumescence.

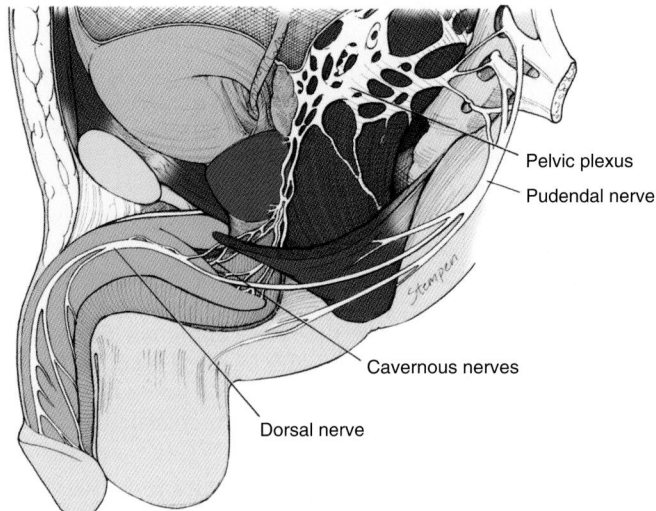

Figure 21–7. Penile neuroanatomy.

Erection thus involves sinusoidal relaxation, arterial dilation, and venous compression (Lue et al, 1983). The importance of smooth muscle relaxation has been demonstrated in animal and human studies (Saenz de Tejada et al, 1989a; Ignarro et al, 1990). To summarize the hemodynamic events of erection and detumescence, seven phases have been observed in animal experiments that reflect the changes in and the relationship between penile arterial flow and intracavernous pressure (Fig. 21–6).

Corpus Spongiosum and Glans Penis

The hemodynamics of the corpus spongiosum and glans penis are somewhat different from those of the corpora cavernosa. **During erection, the arterial flow increases in a similar manner; however, the pressure in the corpus spongiosum and glans is only one third to one half that in the corpora cavernosa because the tunical covering, which is thin over the corpus spongiosum and virtually absent over the glans, ensures minimal venous occlusion.** During the full-erection phase, partial compression of the deep dorsal and circumflex veins between Buck's fascia and the engorged corpora cavernosa contributes to glanular tumescence, although the spongiosum and glans essentially function as a large arteriovenous shunt during this phase. In the rigid-erection phase, the ischiocavernosus and bulbocavernosus muscles forcefully compress the spongiosum and penile veins, resulting in further engorgement and increased pressure in the glans and spongiosum.

Neuroanatomy and Neurophysiology of Penile Erection

Peripheral Pathways

The innervation of the penis is both autonomic (sympathetic and parasympathetic) and somatic (sensory and motor) (Fig. 21–7). From the neurons in the spinal cord and peripheral ganglia, the sympathetic and parasympathetic nerves merge to form the cavernous nerves, which enter the corpora cavernosa and corpus spongiosum to effect the neurovascular events during erection and detumescence. The somatic nerves are primarily responsible for sensation and the contraction of the bulbocavernosus and ischiocavernosus muscles.

Autonomic Pathways. The sympathetic pathway originates from the 11th thoracic to the 2nd lumbar spinal segments and passes through the white rami to the sympathetic chain ganglia. Some fibers then travel through the lumbar splanchnic nerves to the inferior mesenteric and superior hypogastric plexuses, from which fibers travel in the hypogastric nerves to the pelvic plexus. In humans, the T10 to T12 segments are most often the origin of the sympathetic fibers, and the chain ganglia cells projecting to the penis are located in the sacral and caudal ganglia (de Groat and Booth, 1993).

The parasympathetic pathway arises from neurons in the intermediolateral cell columns of the second, third, and fourth sacral spinal cord segments. The preganglionic fibers pass in the pelvic nerves to the pelvic plexus, where they are joined by the sympathetic nerves from the superior hypogastric plexus. **The cavernous nerves are branches of the pelvic plexus that innervate the penis.** Other branches innervate the rectum, bladder, prostate, and sphincters. The cavernous nerves are easily damaged during radical excision of the rectum, bladder, and prostate. A clear understanding of the course of these nerves is essential to the prevention of iatrogenic ED (Walsh et al, 1990). Human cadaveric dissection has revealed medial and lateral branches of the cavernous nerves (the former accompanying the urethra and the latter piercing the urogenital diaphragm 4 to 7 mm lateral to the sphincter) and multiple communications between the cavernous and dorsal nerves (Fig. 21–8) (Paick et al, 1993).

Stimulation of the pelvic plexus and the cavernous nerves induces erection, whereas stimulation of the sympathetic trunk causes detumescence. This clearly implies that the sacral parasympathetic input is responsible for tumescence and the thoracolumbar sympathetic pathway is responsible for detumescence. In experiments with cats and rats, removal of

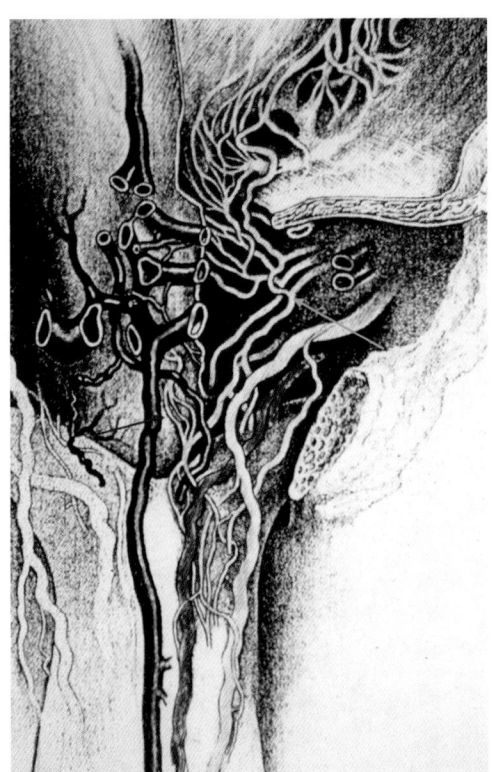

Figure 21–8.   Drawing from a human cadaveric dissection shows the medial *(red arrow)* and lateral *(green arrow)* bundles of the cavernous nerve distal to the prostate. (From Paick JS, Donatucci EF, Lue TF: Anatomy of cavernous nerves distal to prostate: Microdissection study in adult male cadavers. Urology 1993;42:145-149, with permission from Exerpta Medica, Inc.)

the spinal cord below L4 or L5 reportedly eliminated the reflex erectile response, but placement with a female in heat or electrical stimulation of the medial preoptic area (MPOA) produced marked erection (Root and Bard, 1947; Courtois et al, 1993). Paick and Lee (1994) also reported that apomorphine-induced erection is similar to psychogenic erection in the rat and can be induced by means of the thoracolumbar sympathetic pathway in case of injury to the sacral parasympathetic centers. In man, many patients with sacral spinal cord injury retain psychogenic erectile ability even though reflexogenic erection is abolished. These cerebrally elicited erections are found more frequently in patients with lower motoneuron lesions below T12 (Bors and Comarr, 1960); no psychogenic erection occurs in patients with lesions above T9. The efferent sympathetic outflow is thus suggested to be at levels T11 and T12 (Chapelle et al, 1980). These authors have also reported that, in patients with psychogenic erections, lengthening and swelling of the penis are observed but rigidity is insufficient.

It is therefore possible that, for rigid-erection production in normal men, cerebral impulses travel as follows: through the sympathetic pathway, inhibiting norepinephrine release; through the parasympathetic, releasing NO and acetylcholine; and through the somatic, releasing acetylcholine. In patients with a sacral cord lesion, the cerebral impulses can still travel by means of the sympathetic pathway to inhibit norepinephrine release, and NO and acetylcholine can still be released through synapse with postganglionic parasympathetic and

somatic neurons. Because the number of these synapses is less than in men with an intact sacral spinal cord, the resulting erection is not as strong.

Somatic Pathways.   The somatosensory pathway originates at the sensory receptors in the penile skin, glans, and urethra and within the corpus cavernosum. In the human glans penis are numerous afferent terminations: free nerve endings and corpuscular receptors in a ratio of 10:1. The free nerve endings are derived from thin myelinated A_δ and unmyelinated C fibers and are unlike any other cutaneous area in the body (Halata and Munger, 1986). The nerve fibers from the receptors converge to form bundles of the dorsal nerve of the penis, which joins other nerves to become the pudendal nerve. The latter enters the spinal cord through the S2-S4 roots to terminate on spinal neurons and interneurons in the central gray region of the lumbosacral segment (McKenna, 1998). Activation of these sensory neurons sends messages of pain, temperature, and touch by means of spinothalamic and spinoreticular pathways to the thalamus and sensory cortex for sensory perception.

The dorsal nerve of the penis used to be regarded as purely somatic; however, nerve bundles testing positive for NO synthase (NOS), which is autonomic in origin, have been demonstrated in the human by Burnett and colleagues (1993) and in the rat by Carrier (1995). Giuliano and associates (1993) have also shown that stimulation of the sympathetic chain at the L4-L5 level elicits an evoked discharge on the dorsal nerve and that stimulation of the dorsal nerve evokes a reflex discharge in the lumbosacral sympathetic chain of rats. These findings clearly demonstrate that the dorsal nerve has both somatic and autonomic components that enable it to regulate both erectile and ejaculatory functions.

Onuf's nucleus in the second to fourth sacral spinal segments is the center of somatomotor penile innervation. These nerves travel in the sacral nerves to the pudendal nerve to innervate the ischiocavernosus and bulbocavernosus muscles. **Contraction of the ischiocavernosus muscles produces the rigid-erection phase. Rhythmic contraction of the bulbocavernosus muscle is necessary for ejaculation.** In animal studies, direct innervation of the sacral spinal motoneurons by brain stem sympathetic centers (A5-catecholaminergic cell group and locus ceruleus) has been identified (Marson and McKenna, 1996). This adrenergic innervation of pudendal motoneurons may be involved in rhythmic contractions of perineal muscles during ejaculation. In addition, oxytocinergic and serotonergic innervation of lumbosacral nuclei controlling penile erection and perineal muscles in the male rat has been demonstrated (Tang et al, 1998).

Depending on the intensity and nature of genital stimulation, several spinal reflexes can be elicited (Table 21–2). The best known is the bulbocavernosus reflex, which is the basis of genital neurologic examination and electrophysiologic latency testing. Although impairment of bulbocavernosus and ischiocavernosus muscles may impair erection, the significance of obtaining a bulbocavernosus reflex in overall sexual dysfunction assessment is controversial.

Supraspinal Pathways and Centers

Studies in animals have identified the MPOA and the paraventricular nucleus (PVN) of the hypothalamus and

Table 21–2. **Spinal Reflexes Involved in Stimulation of Penile Dorsal Nerve**

Stimulation	Spinal Center	Efferent	Effect
Noxious, abrupt stimulation	Sacral motor neurons	Pudendal nerve (motor)	Bulbocavernous reflex
Low-intensity continuous (e.g., vibratory, manual)	Sacral parasympathetic neurons and interneurons	1. Pelvic nerves 2. Cavernous nerve	1. Bladder inhibition and closure of bladder neck 2. Penile erection
High-intensity continuous	Sacral motor and parasympathetic Thoracolumbar sympathetic neurons	Pudendal, pelvic, and cavernous nerves	Ejaculation

Table 21–3. **Brain Centers Involved in Sexual Function**

Level	Region	Function
Forebrain	Medial amygdala Stria terminalis	Control sexual motivation
	Pyriform cortex	Inhibits sexual drive (hypersexuality when destroyed)
	Hippocampus	Involved in penile erection
	Right insula and inferior frontal cortex Left anterior cingulate cortex	Increased activity during visually evoked sexual stimulation (sexual arousal)
Hypothalamus	Medial preoptic area (MPOA)	Ability to recognize a sexual partner, integration of hormonal and sensory cues
	Paraventricular nucleus (PVN)	Facilitates penile erection (through oxytocin neurons to lumbosacral spinal autonomic and somatic efferents)
Brain stem	Nucleus paragigantocellularis	Inhibits penile erection (through serotonin neurons to lumbosacral spinal neurons and interneurons)
	A5-catecholaminergic cell group Locus ceruleus	Noradrenergic innervation of anterior horn motor neurons to perineal striated muscles
Midbrain	Periaqueductal gray	Relay center for sexually relevant stimuli

hippocampus as important integration centers for sexual function and penile erection (Sachs and Meisel, 1988; Marson et al, 1993) (Table 21–3): electrostimulation of this area induces erection, and lesions limit copulation. Marson and associates (1993) injected pseudo-rabies virus into the rat corpus cavernosum and traced labeled neurons from major pelvic ganglia to neurons in the spinal cord, brain stem, and hypothalamus. Mallick and coworkers (1994) also showed that stimulation of the dorsal nerve in the rat influenced the firing rate of about 80% of the neurons in the MPOA but not in other areas of the hypothalamus. Efferent pathways from the MPOA enter the medial forebrain bundle and the midbrain tegmental region (near the substantia nigra). Pathologic processes in these regions, such as Parkinson's disease or cerebrovascular accidents, are often associated with ED. Axonal tracing in monkeys, cats, and rats has shown direct projection from hypothalamic nuclei to the lumbosacral autonomic erection centers. The neurons in these hypothalamic nuclei contain peptidergic neurotransmitters, including oxytocin and vasopressin, which may be involved in penile erection (Sachs and Meisel, 1988). Several brain stem and medullary centers are also involved in sexual function. The A5-catecholamine cell group and locus ceruleus have been shown to provide adrenergic innervation to the hypothalamus, thalamus, neocortex, and spinal cord. Projections from the nucleus paragigantocellularis, which provides inhibitory serotonergic innervation, have also been demonstrated in the hypothalamus, limbic system, neocortex, and spinal cord.

Central Neural Activation during Arousal. Positron emission tomography (PET) and functional magnetic resonance imaging (fMRI) have allowed a greater understanding of brain activation during human sexual arousal by demonstrating increases in regional cerebral blood flow or changes in regional cerebral activity during a particular moment in time. Generally, in young heterosexual men sexual arousal is triggered with sexually explicit pictures or videos. Scanned brain images taken during arousal are compared with images taken in response to sexually neutral media (e.g., documentaries or humorous video clips). Centers of activation and deactivation can be demonstrated. Although the simplicity of these study designs is elegant, multiple factors are involved in sexual arousal—especially when triggered by visual clues. The authors of these studies have placed many necessary conditions in an attempt to standardize the methods and participants; however, the complexity of human emotion and sexual response is extremely difficult to regulate.

In 1999, Stoleru and associates studied eight healthy right-handed heterosexual men with PET during visually evoked sexual arousal. Regions of brain activation were correlated with testosterone plasma levels and penile tumescence. Significant activation was seen in the bilateral inferior temporal cortices, right insula, right inferior frontal cortex, and left anterior cingulate cortex. From this landmark study a tentative model was introduced, suggesting that visually evoked sexual arousal has three components associated with neuroanatomic regions: (1) a perceptual-cognitive component that recognizes the visual stimuli as sexual and is processed in the bilateral inferior temporal cortices; (2) an emotional-motivational component that integrates sensory information with motivational states and is processed in the right insula, right inferior frontal cortex, and left cingulate cortex (paralimbic areas); and (3) a physiologic component that coordinates the endocrine and autonomic functions and is processed in the left anterior cingulate cortex.

Further investigations have been done with visual sexual stimuli and PET scanning. Bocher and coworkers (2001) demonstrated increased activation in the inferior lateral occipital cortex, bilateral posterior temporal cortices (right greater than left), right inferior lateral prefrontal cortex, left postcentral gyrus, bilateral inferior parietal lobules, left superior parietal lobules, frontal pole (Brodmann area 10), left prefrontal cortex, and midbrain regions. They also noted deactivation in the medial frontal and anterior cingulate, contrary to Stoleru's report. Again, visual association centers were noted to be activated, in particular the posterior temporal cortices and postcentral gyrus. Interestingly, the midbrain activation seen in this study correlates with the location of the dopaminergic neurons. It was not demonstrated in other studies, but that may owe to these authors' use of prolonged provocation: the visual sexual stimulus was a 30-minute continuous video clip, whereas other studies used brief visual stimuli (2 to 10 minutes).

Park and associates studied 12 healthy men with fMRI (Park et al, 2001) in response to erotic and noneretic film clips. With the former, regional brain activation was generally seen in the inferior frontal lobe, cingulate gyrus, insular gyrus, corpus callosum, thalamus, caudate nucleus, globus pallidus, and inferior temporal lobes. Some activation regions were similar to those in other studies, in particular the inferior frontal lobes, inferior temporal lobes, and insular gyrus.

In a well-designed study with fMRI and visual stimuli, correlated with penile turgidity, Arnow and coworkers demonstrated a significant region of activation in the right subinsular/insular region, including the claustrum (Arnold et al, 2002), a response also seen in previous studies with PET (Stoleru et al, 1999; Redoute et al, 2000). This region has been associated with sensory processing, and this activation may represent somatosensory processing and recognition of erection. Other brain regions activated during visual sexual stimuli were the right middle gyrus, right temporal gyrus, left caudate and putamen, bilateral cingulate gyri, right sensimotor, and premotor regions. Also, a lesser activation was seen in the right hypothalamus. (Dopamine is projected to the hypothalamus, and the evidence that dopamine facilitates male sexual behavior is substantial.) The activation of the right middle temporal gyrus is probably associated with visual processing.

In 2003, Mouras and associates studied eight men with fMRI. Video clips were not used; rather, still photographs (neutral and sexually arousing) were shown quickly. The authors believed that, by using shorter visual sexual stimuli, early neural responses would be generated instead of responses to the perception of penile tumescence. Again, activation of the middle and inferior occipital gyri was demonstrated, most likely linked to the visual stimuli but not necessarily to the sexual component. In addition to multiple brain centers that showed activation with visual sexual stimuli (bilateral parietal lobules, left inferior parietal lobule, right postcentral gyrus, right parieto-occipital sulcus, left superior occipital gyrus, bilateral precentral gyrus), the cerebellum demonstrated activation in three subjects and deactivation in four. As many other reports have demonstrated activation of

the cerebellum in response to erotic films and pictures of love partners (Bartels and Zeki, 2000; Garavan et al, 2000; Beauregard et al, 2001), visual sexual stimuli probably promote activation in regions within the cerebellum.

With the advances with fMRI, detailed comparisons of brain activation in response to visual sexual stimuli have been performed on varied groups. Stoleru and colleagues (2003) compared healthy men with men with hypoactive sexual desire disorder (HSDD) and reported that the left gyrus rectus, a portion of the medial orbitofrontal cortex, remained activated in the latter group in contrast to its deactivation in healthy men. This region is believed to mediate inhibition of motivated behavior, and its continued activation may help explain the pathophysiology of HSDD. Montorsi and coauthors (2003) compared men with psychogenic ED and potent control subjects after the administration of apomorphine. During visual sexual stimulation, the former group evidenced extended activation of the cingulate gyrus, frontal mesial, and frontal basal cortex, suggesting an underlying organic cause for psychogenic ED. However, their fMRI images after apomorphine were similar to those of the potent controls. Apomorphine caused additional activation of foci in the psychogenic ED patients (seen in the nucleus accumbens, hypothalamus, and mesencephalon), and it was significantly greater in the right hemisphere than in the left. This greater right-sided activation is a common finding in sexually evoked brain activation studies.

Brain scanning with PET and fMRI has become a powerful tool in the study of central activation of sexual arousal, with many brain regions of activation demonstrated in these reports (Table 21–4). Psychogenic ED, premature ejaculation, sexual deviations, and orgasmic dysfunction are just a few conditions that may accompany alterations in higher brain function and perhaps now can be studied. As we begin to understand brain function with normal sexual response and arousal, the causes of dysfunction may be elucidated.

The structures discussed previously are responsible for the three types of erection: psychogenic, reflexogenic, and nocturnal. Psychogenic erection is a result of audiovisual stimuli or fantasy. Impulses from the brain modulate the spinal erection centers (T11-L2 and S2-S4) to activate the erectile

Table 21–4. Common Brain Activation Regions with Visual Sexual Stimuli*

Brain Activation Regions	Functional Association
Bilateral inferior temporal cortex (right > left)	Visual association area
Right insula	Processes somatosensory information with motivational states
Right inferior frontal cortex	Processes sensory information
Left anterior cingulate cortex	Controls autonomic and neuroendocrine function
Right occipital gyrus	Visual processing
Right hypothalamus	Male copulatory behavior
Left caudate (the striatum)	Processes attention and guides responsiveness to new environmental stimuli

*These regions demonstrate activation with visual sexual stimuli in multiple studies.

process. Reflexogenic erection is produced by tactile stimulation of the genital organs. The impulses reach the spinal erection centers; some then follow the ascending tract, resulting in sensory perception, whereas others activate the autonomic nuclei to send messages through the cavernous nerves to the penis to induce erection. This type of erection is preserved in patients with upper spinal cord injury. Nocturnal erection occurs mostly during rapid-eye-movement (REM) sleep. PET scanning of humans in REM sleep shows increased activity in the pontine area, the amygdalae, and the anterior cingulate gyrus but decreased activity in the prefrontal and parietal cortex. The mechanism that triggers REM sleep is located in the pontine reticular formation; the cholinergic neurons in the lateral pontine tegmentum are activated, and the adrenergic neurons in the locus ceruleus and the serotonergic neurons in the midbrain raphe are silent. This differential activation may be responsible for these nocturnal erections.

Neurotransmitters

Peripheral Neurotransmitters and Endothelium-Derived Factors

Flaccidity and Detumescence. α-Adrenergic nerve fibers and receptors have been demonstrated in the cavernous trabeculae and surrounding the cavernous arteries, and norepinephrine has generally been accepted as the principal neurotransmitter to control penile flaccidity and detumescence (Hedlund and Andersson, 1985; Diederichs et al, 1990). Receptor binding studies have shown the number of α adrenoceptors to be 10 times higher than the number of β adrenoceptors (Levin and Wein, 1980). Currently, it is suggested that sympathetic contraction is mediated by activation of postsynaptic α_{1a}- and α_{1d}-adrenergic receptors (Christ et al, 1990; Traish et al, 1995) and modulated by presynaptic α_2-adrenergic receptors (Saenz de Tejada et al, 1989b).

Endothelin, a potent vasoconstrictor produced by the endothelial cells, has also been suggested to be a mediator for detumescence (Holmquist et al, 1990; Saenz de Tejada et al, 1991a). Endothelin-1 is a member of a family of three peptides and is a potent constrictor synthesized by the sinusoidal endothelium (Holmquist et al, 1990; Saenz de Tejada et al, 1991a). Its presence in human cavernous tissue suggests the participation of this peptide in the regulation of trabecular smooth muscle. Endothelin also potentiates the constrictor effects of catecholamines on trabecular smooth muscle (Christ et al, 1995b). Two receptors for endothelin, ETA and ETB, mediate the biologic effects of endothelin in vascular tissue. The mechanism of intracellular transduction for both receptors is the activation of the degradation of inositol phosphate (IP), with release of intracellular calcium and activation of protein kinase C (PKC). Endothelin has also been suggested to regulate smooth muscle proliferation in the penis (Giraldi et al, 1998).

Several constrictor prostanoids, including prostaglandin I₂ (PGI₂), PGF₂α, and thromboxane A₂ (TXA₂), are synthesized by the human cavernous tissue. In vitro studies have demonstrated that prostanoids are partly responsible for the tone and spontaneous activity of isolated trabecular muscle (Christ et al, 1990). Functional characterization of prostanoid receptors in human trabecular and arterial penile smooth muscle has revealed that only thromboxane prostanoid (TP) receptors

mediate contractile effects of prostanoids in these tissues (Angulo et al, 2002). Also, it has been observed in vitro that constrictor prostanoids, simultaneously released with NO, attenuate the dilator effect of the latter (Azadzoi and Goldstein, 1992; Minhas et al, 2001).

The renin-angiotensin system may also play a significant role in the maintenance of penile smooth muscle tone. Angiotensin II has been detected in endothelial and smooth muscle cells of human corpus cavernosum (Kifor et al, 1997) and evokes contraction of human (Becker et al, 2001a) and rabbit (Park et al, 1997) corpus cavernosum in vitro. This contractile effect is mediated by interaction with AT-I subtype receptors (Park et al, 1997). These are G protein–coupled receptors and involve Gq stimulation, which activates phospholipase C, promoting generation of inositol triphosphate (IP₃) and subsequent intracellular calcium increase (Berry et al, 2001). Intracavernous injection of angiotensin II reverses spontaneous erections in dogs, and the AT-I receptor antagonist losartan increases the intracavernous pressure (Kifor et al, 1997). Finally, intracavernous blood levels of angiotensin II, which are higher than levels in systemic peripheral blood, increase in the detumescence phase (Becker et al, 2001b) Thus, local production of angiotensin II may increase penile smooth muscle contractility by way of AT-I receptors, facilitating penile detumescence.

The current consensus holds that the maintenance of the intracorporeal smooth muscle in a semicontracted (flaccid) state probably results from three factors: intrinsic myogenic activity (Andersson and Wagner, 1995), adrenergic neurotransmission, and endothelium-derived contracting factors such as angiotensin II, PGF₂α, and endothelins. On the other hand, **detumescence after erection may be a result of cessation of NO release, the breakdown of cyclic guanosine monophosphate (cGMP) by phosphodiesterases, or sympathetic discharge during ejaculation.**

Erection. Acetylcholine has been shown to be released with electrical field stimulation of human erectile tissue (Blanco et al, 1988). Traish and coworkers (1990) reported the density of muscarinic receptors in cavernous tissue to range from 35 to 65 fmol/mg protein and in endothelial cell membrane from 5 to 10 fmol/mg protein. However, intravenous or intracavernous injection of atropine has failed to abolish erection induced in animals by electrical neurostimulation (Stief et al, 1989) and in men by erotic stimuli (Wagner and Uhrenholdt, 1980). Although acetylcholine is not the predominant neurotransmitter, it does contribute indirectly to penile erection by presynaptic inhibition of adrenergic neurons and stimulation of NO release from endothelial cells (Saenz de Tejada et al, 1989a).

Most researchers now agree that NO released from nonadrenergic, noncholinergic neurotransmission and from the endothelium is the principal neurotransmitter mediating penile erection. NO increases the production of cGMP, which in turn relaxes the cavernous smooth muscle (Ignarro et al, 1990; Holmquist et al, 1991; Kim N et al, 1991; Pickard et al, 1991; Burnett et al, 1992; Knispel et al, 1992; Rajfer et al, 1992; Trigo-Rocha et al, 1993a, 1993b). The emerging consensus is that NO derived from neuronal NOS (nNOS) in the nitrergic nerves is responsible for the initiation and majority of the smooth muscle relaxation whereby NO from endothelial NOS (eNOS) contributes to the maintenance of the erection (Hurt et al, 2002). (For a fuller discussion of NO, see specific "Nitric Oxide" sections.)

Other investigators believe that vasoactive intestinal polypeptide (VIP) may be one of the neurotransmitters responsible for erection, and other potential candidates include a relaxing factor working through a K^+ channel (Okamura et al, 1998), a non-NO, cGMP-dependent pathway (Reilly et al, 1997b), and prostaglandins (Adaikan et al, 1988; Saenz de Tejada et al, 1989b).

Interactions among Nerves and Neurotransmitters. Acetylcholine, by acting on the presynaptic receptors on adrenergic neurons, has been shown to modulate the release of norepinephrine (Saenz de Tejada et al, 1989b), which can also be inhibited by PGE_1 (Molderings et al, 1992). In the human corpus cavernosum, noradrenergic responses are under nitrergic control. Conversely, adrenergic neurons, through prejunctional α_2 receptors, can also regulate the release of NO.

Several studies have demonstrated that the interaction between the two systems also occurs in the smooth muscle (Brave et al, 1993; Angulo et al, 2001a). The NO-cGMP-cGMP-dependent protein kinase type I (cGKI) pathway can lead to inhibition at several sites on the noradrenergic contractile pathway in the vascular smooth muscle, impairing IP_3 production by phospholipase C (Hirata et al, 1990), IP_3 receptor activity (Schlossmann et al, 2000), and the RhoA/Rho kinase pathway (Sauzeau et al, 2000). However, interaction sites have not yet been identified in penile smooth muscle. A nitrergic-noradrenergic imbalance owing to defective nitrergic neurotransmission has been implicated in penile tissue from patients and in animal models with ED (Christ et al, 1995a; Cellek et al, 1999). Similar to the interaction between nitrergic and noradrenergic pathways, vasoconstrictive actions of endothelin have been shown to be inhibited by NO during erection (Mills et al, 2001).

A number of factors have been reported to increase both NOS activity and NO release. These include molecular oxygen, androgen, chronic administration of L-arginine, and repeated intracavernous injection of PGE_1 (Kim N et al, 1993; Escrig et al, 1999; Marin et al, 1999). Decreased NOS activity has been associated with castration, denervation, hypercholesterolemia, and diabetes mellitus. Interaction of different types of NOS may also occur. For example, nNOS activity has been to shown to decrease and inducible NOS (iNOS) levels to increase after injection of transforming growth factor (TGF)-β1 into the penis (Bivalacqua et al, 2000), and eNOS levels are reportedly significantly higher in nNOS knockout mice (Burnett et al, 1996).

Central Neurotransmitters and Neural Hormones. A variety of neurotransmitters (dopamine, norepinephrine, 5-hydroxytestosterone [5-HT], and oxytocin) and neural hormones (oxytocin, prolactin) have been implicated in regulation of sexual function. It is suggested that dopaminergic and adrenergic receptors may promote sexual function and 5-HT receptors inhibit it (Foreman and Wernicke, 1990).

Dopamine. There are many dopaminergic systems in the brain with ultrashort, intermediate, and long axons. The cell bodies are located in the ventral tegmentum, substantia nigra,

and hypothalamus. One of these dopaminergic systems, the tuberoinfundibular system, secretes dopamine (DA) into the portal hypophysial vessels to inhibit prolactin secretion (Ganong, 1999a). Five different DA receptors have been cloned (D1 to D5), and several of these exist in multiple forms (Ganong, 1999b). **In men, apomorphine, which stimulates both D1 and D2 receptors,** induces erection that is unaccompanied by sexual arousal (Danjou et al, 1988). In male rats, Hull and associates (1992) have found that low levels of dopaminergic stimulation through the D1 receptor increase erection; higher levels or prolonged stimulation produces seminal emission through D2 receptors. The erectile response induced by injection of apomorphine into the paraventricular area can be suppressed by blockers of both DA and oxytocin receptors (Melis et al, 1989). Injection of oxytocin into the paraventricular area also induces erection, but this cannot be blocked by DA receptor blockers. These findings suggest that dopaminergic neurons activate oxytocinergic neurons in the paraventricular area and that the release of oxytocin produces erection (Melis et al, 1992).

In general terms, DA is supportive of copulation and 5-HT is inhibitory. DA is released in the MPOA at the time of ejaculation (5-HT is not), and changes in DA and 5-HT in different areas of the brain may promote copulation and sexual satiety, respectively (Hull et al, 1999). Testosterone enhances DA release in the MPOA at rest and with sexual challenge, possibly by upregulating NOS, which increases NO and thereby increases DA release. The same pattern of copulatory activity promoting DA release in the MPOA and the enhanced effect of the presence of sex hormones is seen in female rats. Longer lasting changes may be seen through the postcopulatory effects of gene expression and this expression increases with increased sexual experience—effectively changing the phenotype of certain cells in sexually experienced animals. Cells of the MPOA have high densities of α_2-noradrenergic receptors as well as DA receptors, and the effects of DA in the MPOA are most likely facilitated by the activation of α_2 (inhibition) and α_1 (excitation) adrenoceptors owing to cross talk within central nervous system (CNS) catecholamine systems (Cornil et al, 2002).

DA agonists (apomorphine and pergolide) and DA uptake inhibitors (nomifensine and bupropion) have been reported to enhance sexual drive in patients (Jeanty et al, 1984). In animal studies, selective activation of D2-dopaminergic receptors by the systemic administration of agonists such as apomorphine and quinelorane increases sexual behavior, and this effect can be counteracted by centrally acting antagonists.

Serotonin. Neurons containing 5-HT have their cell bodies in the midline raphe nuclei of the brain stem and project to a portion of the hypothalamus, the limbic system, the neocortex, and the spinal cord (Ganong, 1999a). Currently, 5-HT receptors 1 to 7 have been cloned and characterized. Within the 5-HT1 group are the 5-HT1 A, B, D, E, and F subtypes. Within the 5-HT2 group are the 5-HT2 A, B, and C subtypes. There are two 5-HT5 subtypes, 5-HT5 A and B (Ganong, 1999b). **General pharmacologic data indicate that 5-HT pathways inhibit copulation but that 5-HT may have both facilitory and inhibitory effects on sexual function, depending on the receptor subtype, the receptor location, and the species investigated** (de Groat and Booth, 1993). Andersson and Wagner (1995) have summarized the results of administration of selective agonists and antagonists as follows: 5-HT1 A receptor agonists inhibit erectile activity but facilitate ejaculation; stimulation of 5-HT2 C receptors causes erection; 5-HT2 agonists inhibit erection but facilitate seminal emission and ejaculation. Steers and de Groat (1989) have also shown increased firing of the cavernous nerve and erection when *m*-chlorophenylpiperazine, a 5-HT2 C receptor agonist, is given to rats. Stimulation of both 5-HT2 and 5-HT2 C receptors also has been reported to increase oxytocin secretion (Bagdy et al, 1992). In addition, 5-HT may affect the spinal reflex because Marson and McKenna (1992) have reported that endogenous 5-HT may act in the lumbar cord to inhibit sexual reflexes.

5-HT is believed to be an inhibitory transmitter in the control of sexual drive (Foreman et al, 1989). Suppressed libido has been reported in patients taking fenfluramine, a 5-HT–releasing agent, but elevated libido in patients taking buspirone, a 5-HT neuron suppressor (Buffum, 1982).

Norepinephrine. The cell bodies of the norepinephrine-containing neurons are located in the locus ceruleus and the A5-catecholaminergic cell group in the pons and medulla. The axons of these noradrenergic neurons ascend to innervate the paraventricular, supraoptic, and periventricular nuclei of the hypothalamus, the thalamus, and neocortex. They also descend into the spinal cord and the cerebellum. **Central norepinephrine transmission seems to have a positive effect on sexual function.** In both humans and rats, inhibition of norepinephrine release by clonidine, an α_2-adrenergic agonist, is associated with a decrease in sexual behavior, and yohimbine, an α_2-receptor antagonist, has been shown to increase sexual activity (Clark et al, 1985). Beta blockers have also been implicated in sexual dysfunction, probably because of their central side effects such as sedation, sleep disturbances, and depression.

γ-Aminobutyric Acid. γ-Aminobutyric acid (GABA) activity in the PVN provides a mechanism to balance (inhibit) proerectile signaling (Melis et al, 2001). Agonism for the type A receptor for GABA in the PVN can reduce both pharmacologically (apomorphine) and physiologically induced erections.

Opioids. Endogenous opioids are known to affect sexual function, but the mechanism of action is far from clear. Injection of small amounts of morphine into the MPOA facilitates sexual behavior in rats. Larger doses, however, inhibit both penile erection and yawning induced by oxytocin or apomorphine. It is suggested that endogenous opioids may exert an inhibitory control on central oxytocinergic transmission (Argiolas, 1992).

Oxytocin. Oxytocin is a neural hormone secreted by the neurons into the circulation. These are found in the posterior pituitary gland, but, because they are also found in the neurons projecting from the PVN to the brain stem and spinal cord, oxytocin can also function as a neurotransmitter. The blood level is increased during sexual activity in humans and animals and, when injected into the paraventricular area in rats, oxytocin produces yawning and penile erection. Calcium has been suggested as the second messenger mediating oxytocin-induced penile erection. Because neurons in the paraventricular area have been shown to contain NOS and NOS inhibitors prevent apomorphine- and oxytocin-induced erec-

tion, it is suggested that oxytocin acts on neurons whose activity is dependent on certain levels of NO (Vincent and Kimura, 1992; Melis and Argiolas, 1993).

Nitric Oxide. NO is a gaseous molecule produced from various tissues, in particular the endothelium and nerve. It mediates penile erection at the level of the PVN (Melis et al, 1998) and at other levels of the neural pathway supporting the sexual response. The presence of NO and the soluble guanylyl cyclase needed to generate cGMP is seen throughout the human brain. The NO/cGMP pathway (see later) is affected by aging in the brain and offers a potentially significant but unexplored site for mediating the deleterious effects of age on sexual function (Ibarra et al, 2001). Testosterone or its metabolite dihydrotestosterone (DHT) downregulates NOS activity and messenger RNA (mRNA) expression and the number of nNOS-containing neurons (Singh et al, 2000). Direct evidence of the importance of NO in central signaling related to erectile function resulted from a series of experiments designed to alter CNS NO activity (Sato et al, 2001): manipulation of NO or cGMP levels altered MPOA-triggered intracavernous pressure response through CNS, not peripheral, mechanisms.

Melanocortins. Melanocortin-4 receptor (MC4R), implicated in the control of food intake and energy expenditure, also modulates erectile function and sexual behavior. Evidence supporting this notion is based on several findings: (1) a highly selective nonpeptide MC4R agonist augments erectile activity initiated by electrical stimulation of the cavernous nerve in wild-type, but not MC4R-null, mice; (2) copulatory behavior is enhanced by administration of a selective MC4R agonist and is diminished in mice lacking MC4R; (3) reverse transcriptase polymerase chain reaction (RT-PCR) and non–PCR-based methods demonstrate MC4R expression in the rat and human penis and rat spinal cord, hypothalamus, brain stem, and pelvic ganglion (major autonomic relay center to the penis) but not in rat primary corpus cavernosum smooth muscle cells; and (4) in situ hybridization of glans tissue from the human and rat penis reveals MC4R expression in nerve fibers and mechanoreceptors in the glans. Collectively, these data implicate MC4R in the modulation of penile erectile function and provide evidence that MC4R-mediated proerectile responses may be activated through neuronal circuitry in spinal cord erectile centers and somatosensory afferent nerve terminals of the penis (Van der Ploeg et al, 2002). Small-molecule analogs active at the MC4R are currently in clinical trials.

Prolactin. **Increased levels of prolactin suppress sexual function in men and experimental animals. In rats, high levels of prolactin decrease the genital reflex and disturb copulatory behavior. It is suggested that the mechanism of prolactin's action is through inhibition of dopaminergic activity in the MPOA and decreased testosterone. In addition, prolactin may have a direct effect on the penis through its contractile effect on the cavernous smooth muscle** (Ra et al, 1996).

Smooth Muscle Physiology

Spontaneous contractile activity of cavernous smooth muscle has been recorded in vitro and in vivo. In isolated strips of rabbit corpus cavernosum, Mandrek (1994) demonstrated spontaneous mechanical activity with a frequency of 6 to 30 contractions per minute accompanied by fluctuations in membrane potential. Stimulation of the tissue with tetraethyl-ammonium chloride and norepinephrine produced strong tonic contractions with relative electrical silence. In a human study, Yarnitsky and colleagues (1995) found two types of electrical activity recorded from the corpus cavernosum: spontaneous and activity induced. Levin and coworkers (1994) reported that in vitro spontaneous contractile activity is correlated with a phasic increase in intracellular calcium and a biphasic change in the NADH/NAD ratio, suggesting an initial increase and then a decrease of intracellular energy. Italiano and coworkers (1998) suggested that phasic contraction of the penis is through the enzyme sodium-potassium adenosine triphosphatase (ATPase) and the resting tone is mediated by the endothelium through the release of $PGF_{2\alpha}$. Field stimulation results in a decrease in tension and intracellular calcium at low frequencies and an increase in tension and intracellular calcium at high frequencies. In general, the response to pharmacologic agents correlates with the change in intracellular calcium; for example, phenylephrine produces muscle contraction and an increase in intracellular calcium, whereas nitroprusside causes the opposite.

In a study of myosin isoforms in smooth muscle cells in the corpus cavernosum, DiSanto and associates (1998) reported their overall composition to be between those in aorta and bladder smooth muscles, which generally express tonic- and phasic-like characteristics, respectively. Further studies of isoform changes may elucidate the increased contractility or

impaired relaxation of the cavernous smooth muscle in pathologic conditions.

Molecular Mechanism of Smooth Muscle Contraction and Relaxation

Smooth muscle contraction and relaxation are regulated by cytosolic (sarcoplasmic) free Ca^{2+}. Norepinephrine from nerve endings and endothelins and $PGF_{2\alpha}$ from endothelium activate receptors on smooth muscle cells to increase IP_3 and diacylglycerol, resulting in release of calcium from intracellular stores, such as sarcoplasmic reticulum, or the opening of calcium channels on the smooth muscle cell membrane, leading to an influx of calcium from extracellular space, or both. This triggers a transient increase in cytosolic free Ca^{2+} from a resting level of 120 to 270 nM to 500 to 700 nM (Walsh, 1991). At the elevated level, Ca^{2+} binds to calmodulin and changes the latter's conformation to expose sites of interaction with myosin light-chain kinase. The resultant activation catalyzes phosphorylation of myosin light chains and triggers cycling of myosin crossbridges (heads) along actin filaments and the development of force. In addition, phosphorylation of the light chain activates myosin ATPase, which hydrolyzes ATP to provide energy for muscle contraction (Fig. 21–9).

When the cytosolic Ca^{2+} returns to basal levels, the calcium-sensitizing pathways take over. One such mechanism is through activation of excitatory receptors coupled to G-proteins, which can also cause contraction by increasing calcium sensitivity without any change in cytosolic Ca^{2+}. This pathway involves RhoA, a small, monomeric G-protein that

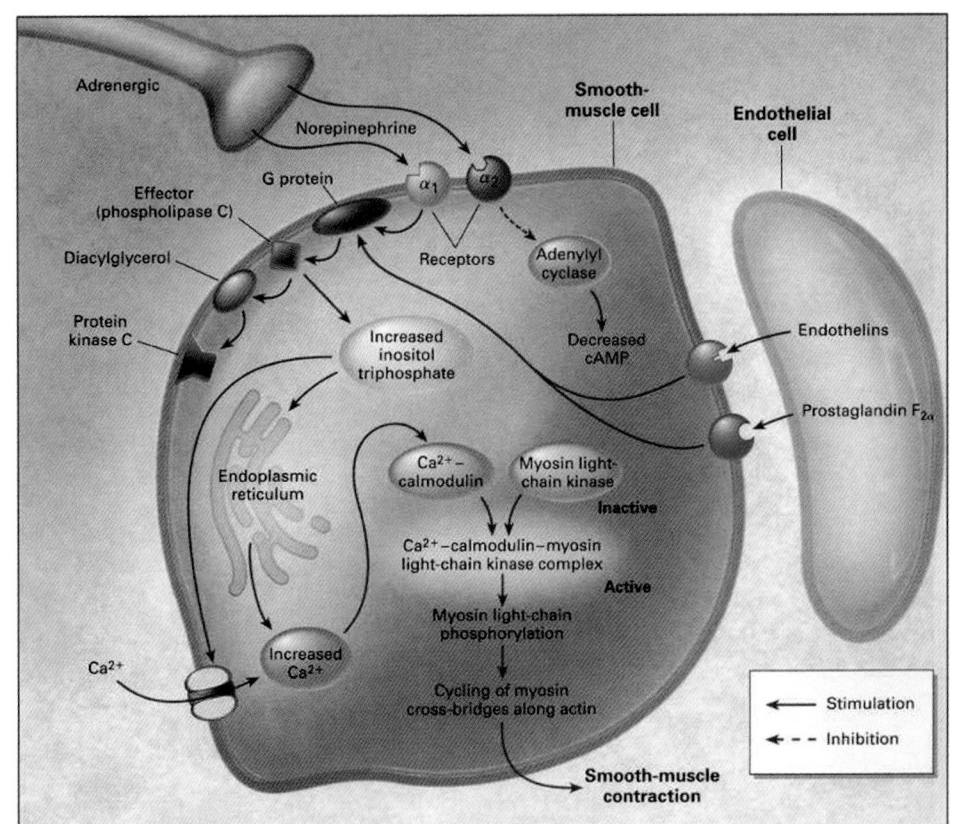

Figure 21–9. Molecular mechanism of penile smooth muscle contraction. Norepinephrine from sympathetic nerve endings and endothelins and prostaglandin $F_{2\alpha}$ from the endothelium activate receptors on smooth muscle cells to initiate the cascade of reactions that eventually result in elevation of intracellular calcium concentrations and smooth muscle contraction. Protein kinase C is a regulatory component of the Ca^{2+}-independent, sustained phase of agonist-induced contractile responses. (From Lue TF: Erectile dysfunction. N Engl J Med 2000;342:1802-1813. Copyright © 2000 Massachusetts Medical Society.)

activates Rho kinase. Activated Rho kinase phosphorylates and thereby inhibits the regulatory subunit of smooth muscle myosin phosphatase, preventing dephosphorylation of myofilaments, thus maintaining contractile tone (Fig. 21–10) (Somlyo and Somlyo, 2000).

RhoA and Rho kinase have been shown to be expressed in penile smooth muscle (Rees et al, 2002; Wang et al, 2002). Interestingly, the amount of RhoA expressed in the cavernous smooth muscle is 17-fold that in vascular smooth muscle (Wang et al, 2002). A selective inhibitor of Rho kinase has been shown to elicit relaxation of human corpus cavernosum in vitro and to induce erection in animal models (Chitaley et al, 2001; Rees et al, 2001). Anesthetized rats transfected with dominant negative RhoA exhibited elevated erectile function when compared with control animals (Chitaley et al, 2002). The emerging consensus is that phasic contraction of penile smooth muscle is regulated by an increase in cytosolic Ca^{2+} and that tonic contraction is governed by the calcium-sensitizing pathways (Cellek et al, 2002)

In addition to the central role of myosin phosphorylation in smooth muscle contraction, other mechanisms may modulate or fine-tune the contractile state. For example, caldesmon may be involved in the latch state in which the force of contraction is maintained at a low level of myosin phosphorylation and with a low energy expenditure.

Relaxation of the muscle follows a decrease of free Ca^{2+} in the sarcoplasm. Calmodulin then dissociates from myosin light-chain kinase and inactivates it. Myosin is dephosphorylated by myosin light-chain phosphatase and detaches from the actin filament, and the muscle relaxes (Walsh, 1991) (Fig. 21–11). Others suggest that the NO-cGMP inhibitory pathway in corpus cavernosum smooth muscle is not simply a reversal of excitatory signal transduction mechanisms but that an unidentified mechanism may contribute to relaxation by decreasing the rate of crossbridge recruitment through phosphorylation (Chuang et al, 1998).

Cyclic adenosine monophosphate (cAMP) and cGMP are the second messengers involved in smooth muscle relaxation. They activate cAMP- and cGMP-dependent protein kinases, which in turn phosphorylate certain proteins and

ion channels, resulting in (1) opening of the potassium channels and hyperpolarization, (2) sequestration of intracellular calcium by the endoplasmic reticulum, and (3) inhibition of voltage-dependent calcium channels, blocking calcium influx. The consequence is a drop in cytosolic free calcium and smooth muscle relaxation.

Cyclic AMP–Signaling Pathway. Cyclic AMP–signaling molecules include adenosine, calcitonin gene–related peptides (CGRPs), prostaglandins, and VIP.

Adenosine. Adenosine is released from a variety of cells as a result of increased metabolic rates, and its actions on the vasculature are most prominent when oxygen demand is high (Tabrizchi and Bedi, 2001). However, the vascular response to the action of adenosine can be either relaxation or constriction, depending on which type of adenosine receptor is activated. Currently four AR subtypes (A1, A2$_A$, A2$_B$, and A3) belonging to the gene protein–coupled receptor (GPCR) superfamily have been recognized (Tabrizchi and Bedi, 2001). In general, the A1 receptor is believed to be coupled to G$_i$ and G$_o$ proteins, and its activation results in inhibition of adenylyl cyclase (AC) and activation of phospholipase C, both of which lead to vasoconstriction. The A2 receptors are coupled to the G$_s$ proteins, and their activation stimulates AC and thus vasorelaxation. The A3 receptor is coupled to G$_i$ and G$_q$ proteins, and its activation results in the activation of phospholipase C/D and the inhibition of AC, leading to vasoconstriction. The differential distribution of these adenosine receptor subtypes largely determines whether a particular vessel relaxes or contracts as a result of adenosine stimulation (Tabrizchi and Bedi, 2001). Whether adenosine plays a role in physiologic erection is unclear. Its intracavernous injection in the dog has been shown to induce full erection (Takahashi et al, 1992), and the A2$_A$ receptor has been shown to mediate the relaxation effects of adenosine in human and rabbit corpus cavernosum (Filippi et al, 2000). However, the adenosine receptor inhibitor 8-SPT had no effect on pelvic nerve stimulation–induced tumescence in anesthetized dogs (Noto et al, 2001), suggesting lack of involvement of adenosine or its receptors in physiologic erection.

Calcitonin Gene–Related Peptide Family. CGRP, amylin, and adrenomedullin are members of the CGRP family. These short-chain peptides are potent vasodilators released from perivascular nerve fibers. They act through the calcitonin receptor–like receptor (CRLR), which belongs to the GPCR superfamily (Conner et al, 2002).

In aging rats, the CGRP levels in the penis, bladder, kidney, testis, and adrenal gland were found to increase gradually up to maturity and then rapidly decline (Wimalawansa, 1992). In ED patients given CGRP intracavernously, a dose-related increase in penile arterial inflow (and erection) occurred (Stief et al, 1991b). Adenovirus-mediated gene transfer of CGRP also enhanced erectile responses in aged rats, apparently through an increase of cAMP levels in the corpora cavernosa (Bivalacqua et al, 2001). Intracavernous administration of adrenomedullin also results in cavernous relaxation; however, the effect is through an NO-cGMP, rather than cAMP, pathway (Nishimatsu et al, 2001).

Prostaglandins. Prostaglandins (PGs) are a family of eicosanoids capable of initiating numerous biologic functions. The prime mode of PG action is through specific PG recep-

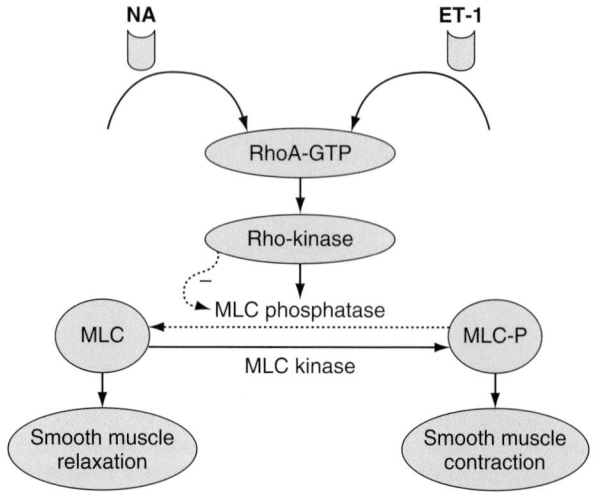

Figure 21–10. RhoA/Rho kinase pathway: the calcium sensitization pathway. ET-1, endothelin receptor 1; GTP, guanosine triphosphate; MLC, myosin light chain; MLC-P, phosphorylated myosin light chain; NA, noradrenalin.

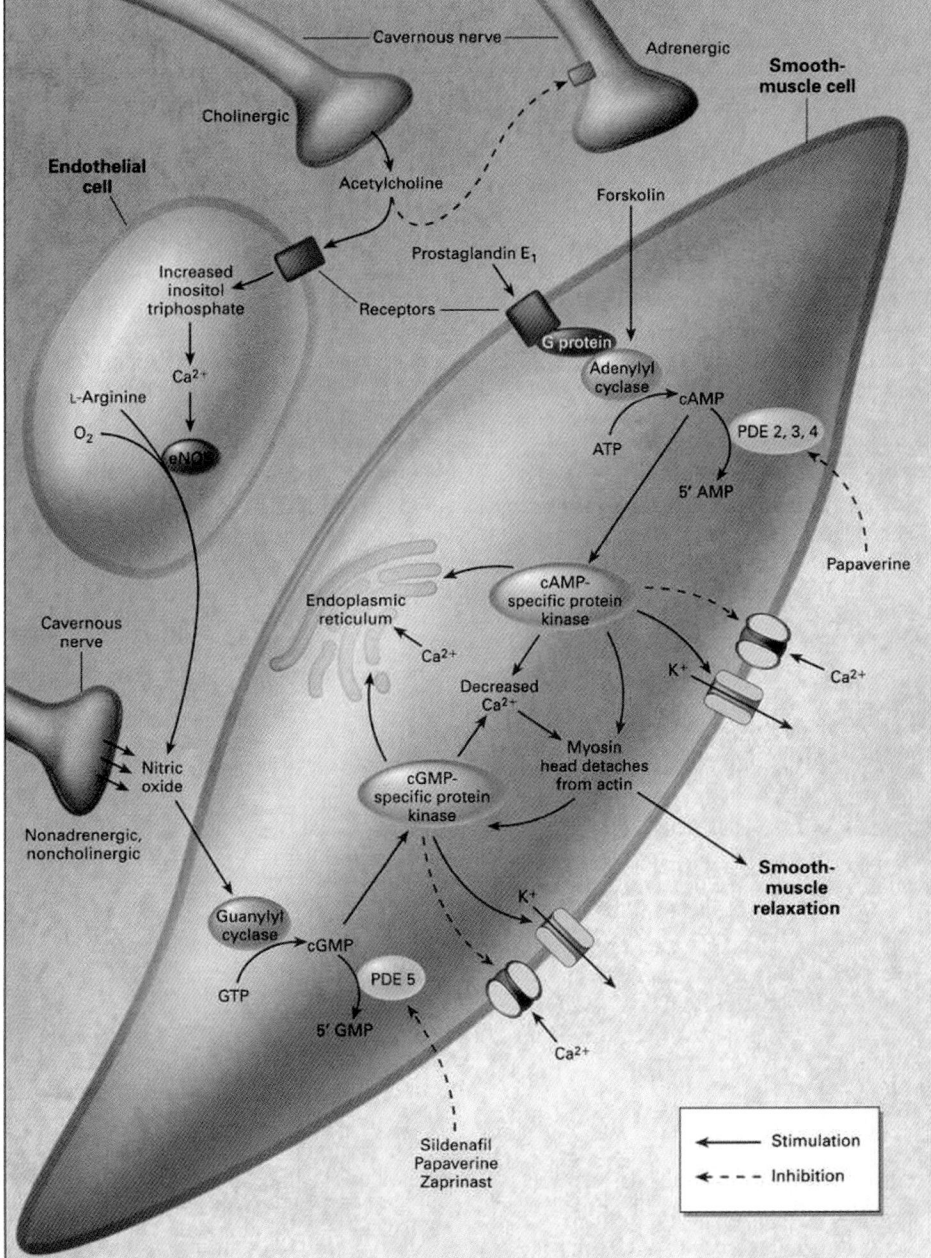

Figure 21–11. Molecular mechanism of penile smooth muscle relaxation. The intracellular second messengers mediating smooth muscle relaxation, cyclic adenosine monophosphate (cAMP) and cyclic guanosine monophosphate (cGMP), activate their specific protein kinases, which phosphorylate certain proteins to cause opening of potassium channels, closing of calcium channels, and sequestration of intracellular calcium by the endoplasmic reticulum. The resultant fall in intracellular calcium leads to smooth muscle relaxation. Sildenafil inhibits the action of phosphodiesterase 5 (PDE5) and thus increases the intracellular concentration of cGMP. Papaverine is a nonspecific phosphodiesterase inhibitor. eNOS, endothelial nitric oxide synthase; GTP, guanosine triphosphate. (From Lue TF: Erectile dysfunction. N Engl J Med 2000;342:1802-1813. Copyright © 2000 Massachusetts Medical Society.)

tors that all belong to the GPCR family. There are at least nine known PG receptor subtypes in mice and humans, as well as several additional splice variants with divergent carboxyl termini (Narumiya and FitzGerald, 2001). Four of the subtypes (EP1 to EP4) bind PGE_2, two (DP1 and DP2) bind PGD_2, and the other three subtypes (FP, IP, and TP) bind PGF_{2a}, PGI_2, and TXA_2, respectively. On the basis of signaling attributes, the PG receptors are classified into three types. The "relaxant" receptors IP, DP1, EP2, and EP4 are coupled to an α_s-containing G-protein and therefore are capable of stimulating AC to increase intracellular cAMP. The "contractile" receptors EP1, FP, and TP are coupled to an α_q-containing G-protein, which activates phospholipase C instead of AC. These contractile receptors therefore do not signal through the cAMP pathway and their signaling outcome is an increase of

intracellular calcium. The EP3 receptor is also a contractile receptor, but it is coupled to an α_i-containing G-protein that inhibits AC to result in a decrease of cAMP formation.

Animal and human corpora cavernosa produce several PGs, including PGF_{2a}, PGE_2, PGD_2, PGI_2, and TXA_2 (Moreland et al, 2001). In studies in isolated human penile tissue, different PGs have been shown to elicit different effects in human corpus cavernosum, corpus spongiosum, and cavernous artery (Hedlund and Andersson, 1985). Whereas PGF_{2a}, PGI_2, and TXA_2 contract the corpus cavernosum and corpus spongiosum, PGE_1 and PGE_2 (but not PGI_2) relax the corpus cavernosum and spongiosum that have been precontracted with noradrenaline or PGF_{2a}. Likewise, PGE_1, but not PGI_2, increases the arterial blood flow when injected into monkey corpus cavernosum (Bosch et al, 1989). Therefore, although

PGI$_2$ is the predominant vasorelaxant in blood vessels, its action in the erectile tissue is either contractile or neutral. This disparity in the action of PGI$_2$ between blood vessels and the erectile tissue and the difference between the effects of PGI$_2$ and PGE$_{1/2}$ in the erectile tissue most likely owe to differences in the distribution of PG receptors. Indeed, studies have shown that, in the corpus cavernosum, the relaxant effects of prostanoids are mediated by EP2 or EP4 receptors (for PGE$_1$ and PGE$_2$), or both, but not IP receptor (for PGI$_2$) (Angulo et al, 2002).

Although the production of PGs and the expression of PG receptors in the erectile tissue have been clearly demonstrated, their roles in physiologic erection are yet to be defined. On the other hand, the erectogenic effects of PGE$_1$ as a pharmaceutical agent have been extensively documented. First described in 1998, intracavernous injection of PGE$_1$ is one of the safest and most effective treatments for ED (Stackl et al, 1988). Transurethral application is an effective alternative.

Vasoactive Intestinal Peptide. The human or animal penis is richly supplied with nerves containing VIP (Andersson, 2001). The primary structure of VIP is closely related to pituitary AC-activating polypeptide (PACAP) and, to a much lesser extent, to secretin, glucagon, gastric inhibitor polypeptide, and helodermin-like peptides. Two subtypes of VIP receptors, VPAC1 and VPAC2, belonging to the GPCR family have been cloned from human and rat tissues. VPAC2 but not VPAC1 mRNA has been identified in cultured rat cavernous smooth muscle cells (CSMCs) (Guidone et al, 2002). In the dog, intracavernous VIP injection has been found to induce penile erection (Juenemann et al, 1987b); in men, it has not produced rigid erection but can improve success rates when combined with papaverine and phentolamine (Kiely et al, 1989). However, it has been shown that VIP release is not essential for neurogenic relaxation of human cavernous smooth muscle (Pickard et al, 1993), and VIP failed to stimulate cAMP production in cultured human CSMCs (Palmer et al, 1994).

Adenylyl Cyclase. Signaling molecules in the cAMP pathway bind to and activate specific cytoplasmic membrane receptors, which, through their coupled G-proteins, activate ACs. To date, nine membrane-bound isoforms and one soluble form of mammalian AC have been cloned and characterized (Patel et al, 2001). The structure of a membrane-bound AC includes a short variable amino terminus, followed by six transmembrane spans, a large cytoplasmic domain, a second set of six transmembrane regions, and another large cytoplasmic domain that includes the carboxyl terminus. The overall similarity among the different ACs is roughly 60%; the most conserved sequences (from 50% to 90%) are located in the two cytoplasmic domains. Although different membrane-bound ACs are regulated differently, they are all stimulated by the guanosine triphosphate (GTP)-bound form of the G$_s$ subunit and are all (except AC9) stimulated by forskolin. Moreover, all membrane-bound ACs are inhibited by P-site analogs, which are essentially adenine nucleoside 3'-polyphosphates.

In rabbits with alloxan-induced diabetes, cAMP formation in the corpus cavernosum in response to forskolin has been shown to be reduced, suggesting impaired AC function in diabetes mellitus (Sullivan et al, 1998).

Protein Kinase A. Protein kinase A (PKA), also called cAMP-dependent kinase (cAK), is the principal receptor for cAMP, and it mediates the vast majority of the cellular effects of cAMP by phosphorylating a wide variety of downstream targets in both the cytoplasmic and nuclear compartments (Johnson et al, 2001). PKA is composed of two regulatory (R) and two catalytic (C) subunits that form a tetrameric holoenzyme R$_2$C$_2$. Binding of cAMP to the R subunits causes the holoenzyme to dissociate into an R$_2$(cAMP)$_4$ dimer and two free catalytically active C subunits. The C subunits are encoded by three different genes, C$_\alpha$, C$_\beta$, and C$_\gamma$, and the regulatory subunits are expressed from four different genes, RI$_\alpha$, RI$_\beta$, RII$_\alpha$, and RII$_\beta$. Two forms of the PKA holoenzyme exist: type I formed by RI$_\alpha$ and RI$_\beta$ dimers and type II by RII$_\alpha$ and RII$_\beta$ dimers. These isozymes may form from either homo- or heterodimers of the R subunits, yielding holoenzyme complexes of PKA with a number of configurations including RI$_{\alpha2}$C$_2$, RI$_{\beta2}$C$_2$, RII$_{\alpha2}$C$_2$, RII$_{\beta2}$C$_2$, and RI$_\alpha$RI$_\beta$C$_2$. The presence of multiple C subunit genes further adds to the diversity and complexity of the various holoenzyme complexes, which differ in biochemical and functional properties as well as patterns of expression and localization. These differences among the isozymes contribute to the broad specificity of PKA in a wide variety of physiologic processes in response to cAMP signaling.

PKA Substrates. More than 100 different cellular proteins have been identified as physiologic substrates of PKA, with more than 90% (135 of 145) being phosphorylated at serine and the remainder at threonine (Shabb, 2001). The predominant target sequence (>50%) is Arg-Arg-X-Ser, in which Ser is the phosphate acceptor. Three PKA substrate proteins have been identified in penile tissue: PDEs, cAMP-responsive element–binding protein (CREB), and ATP-sensitive potassium (K$_{ATP}$) channel.

Cyclic GMP-Signaling Pathway. Signaling molecules in the cGMP pathway include natriuretic peptides and NO, which activate pGC and sGC, respectively.

Natriuretic Peptides. The natriuretic peptide family is involved in the regulation of cardiovascular homeostasis and consists of atrial (ANP), brain (BNP), and C-type (CNP) natriuretic peptides (Matsuo, 2001). Whereas ANP and BNP are ligands for the NPR-A receptor, CNP is a ligand for the NPR-B receptor. Both receptors are members of the guanylyl cyclase (GC) family and are therefore also called GC-A and GC-B.

The effects of ANP, BNP, and CNP on cGMP production and smooth muscle relaxation in isolated human and animal corpus cavernosum and in cultured CSMCs have been investigated (Kim et al, 1998; Guidone et al, 2002; Kuthe et al, 2003). The results indicate that CNP is the most potent natriuretic peptide and that it relaxes the isolated cavernous smooth muscle by binding to NPR-B. However, whether CNP and NPR-B play a role in physiologic erection remains to be seen.

Nitric Oxide. NO, because of its small size, can diffuse inside its target cell, where it interacts with molecules that contain iron in either a heme or iron-sulfur complex. The most physiologically relevant receptor for NO is sGC, and the NO-sGC-cGMP pathway is responsible for the vasorelaxing effect of many endothelium-dependent vasodilators, including histamine, estrogens, insulin, corticotrophin-releasing hormone, nitrovasodilators, and acetylcholine. This pathway is also principally responsible for erection.

Synthesis of NO is catalyzed by NOS, which converts L-arginine and oxygen to L-citrulline and NO. NOS exists as three isoforms in mammals: nNOS and eNOS are preferentially expressed in neurons and endothelial cells, respectively, and iNOS in virtually all cell types. All three NOS isoforms have been identified in the corpus cavernosum, with nNOS and eNOS being considered responsible for initiating and sustaining erection, respectively (Hurt et al, 2002). Downregulation of nNOS expression has been found in the corpus cavernosum of aging rats (Carrier et al, 1997), a model in which corpus cavernous smooth muscle relaxation is impaired (Cartledge et al, 2001). Despite its secondary role in erectile function, the endothelium-dependent cavernous smooth muscle relaxation is attenuated in the aging rabbit, and this age-related defect is paradoxically accompanied by upregulated eNOS expression in both the endothelium and cavernous smooth muscle (Haas et al, 1998; Bakircioglu et al, 2001). A contradictory observation, however, was made in another study, which showed downregulation of eNOS in the corpus cavernosum of aging rats (Rajasekaran et al, 2002).

Gene transfer of nNOS or eNOS to the penis has been shown to augment erectile responses in aging rats (Champion et al, 1999; Magee et al, 2002), and gene transfer of iNOS has enhanced intracavernous pressure (Chancellor et al, 2003). However, despite these encouraging results, it should be noted that mice with disrupted nNOS or eNOS genes have normal erectile function (Burnett et al, 1996; Burnett et al, 2002). Compensatory mechanisms, alternative splicing of the disrupted gene (Ferrini et al, 2003), or other unknown mechanisms are possibly involved in the preservation of erectile function in the NOS knockout mice.

Guanylyl Cyclase. In mammals, seven membrane-bound (particulate) GC isoforms (GC-A to GC-G) and one soluble isoform (sGC) have been identified (Andreopoulos and Papapetropoulos, 2000). Based on their ligand specificity, the particulate GCs (pGCs) have been classified as (1) natriuretic peptide receptors (GC-A and GC-B), which are activated by natriuretic peptides, including ANP, BNP, and CNP; (2) intestinal peptide receptor (GC-C), which is activated by intestinal peptides including guanylin, uroguanylin, and lymphoguanylin; and (3) orphan receptors (GC-D, -E, -F, and -G). Although the membrane-bound GC system is not known to play a role in physiologic erection, expression of GC-B in human and rat corpus cavernosum and induction of cavernous smooth muscle relaxation by CNP (ligand for GC-B) have been demonstrated (Guidone et al, 2002; Kuthe et al, 2003).

The soluble isoform sGC plays a pivotal role in erectile function because it provides the link between NO and cGMP, which represent the extra- and intracellular signaling molecules, respectively, in physiologic erection (Andersson, 2001). A heterodimeric protein, sGC consists of α and β subunits, each of which exists in two isoforms (α1, α2, and β1, β2) that are encoded by two separate genes (Andreopoulos and Papapetropoulos, 2000). Messenger RNAs of these four subunits have been detected in human corpus cavernosum (Behrends et al, 2000). In animal studies, sGC activator YC-1 has been

shown to cause erectile responses (Mizusawa et al, 2002). However, immunohistochemical examination has found sGC expression to be similar in the corpus cavernosum of potent and impotent patients (Klotz et al, 2000).

Protein Kinase G. Protein kinase G (PKG), also called cGMP-dependent kinase (cGK), is the principal receptor and mediator for cGMP signals. In mammals, PKG exists in two major forms, PKG-I and PKG-II, which are encoded by two separate genes. PKG-I, which is important for regulating cavernous smooth muscle tone, exists as α and β isoforms that arise through alternative splicing of the N-terminal region. The two isoforms are often coexpressed; whether they perform different physiologic functions has not been determined.

The PKG-I polypeptide contains three functional domains: the N-terminal, the regulatory, and the catalytic. The N-terminal domain has three functions: dimerization, autoinhibition, and localization. It contains a leucine zipper that holds two PKG-I molecules together as homodimers, it inhibits the catalytic domain in the basal state, and it interacts with specific cellular proteins that anchor PKG-I to different subcellular locations. The regulatory domain contains two tandem cGMP binding sites, and the catalytic domain catalyzes the transfer of the γ phosphate from ATP to a serine/threonine residue of the substrate protein. Binding of cGMP to the regulatory domain induces a conformational change that releases the autoinhibition of the catalytic domain by the N-terminal domain. Deletion of the N-terminal and regulatory domains results in a constitutively active PKG-I, which retains substrate specificity, requires no cGMP for activation (Boerth and Lincoln, 1994), and translocates to the nucleus (Collins and Uhler, 1999). This translocation is reminiscent of the well-established nuclear translocation of the PKA catalytic subunits. Indeed, the PKG-I catalytic domain has been shown to activate CRE-dependent gene transcription (Collins and Uhler, 1999). However, whether the intact PKG-I is capable of nuclear translocation remains controversial (Feil et al, 2002).

Cavernous smooth muscle strips from PKG-I knockout mice cannot be relaxed by agents that raise cGMP levels, and these mice have a low ability to reproduce, presumably owing to ED (Hedlund et al, 2000). Interestingly, the AC activator forskolin has been shown to raise cAMP levels and subsequently relax cavernous smooth muscle strips in PKG-I knockout mice. These observations further affirm the essential role of the cGMP/PKG-I pathway in physiologic erectile function.

PKG Substrates. When compared with PKA substrates, far fewer PKG substrates have been identified and the majority are also phosphorylated by PKA. Some PKG substrates relevant to vascular or cavernous smooth muscle functions are as follows:

Inositol 1,4,5-trisphosphate (IP_3) receptor
IP_3 receptor–associated PKG substrate (IRAG)
Phospholamban (PLB)
Calcium-activated potassium (K_{Ca}) channel
Phosphodiesterase 5 (PDE5)
Heat shock–related protein (HSP20)
Myosin phosphatase (MP)
Phosphatase inhibitor-1 (PPI-1)
GTPase RhoA

Cross-Activation. Cross-activation of PKG by cAMP has been shown in various vascular tissues, including rat aorta, pig coronary artery, and lamb pulmonary artery (Jiang et al, 1992; Eckly-Michel et al, 1997; Dhanakoti et al, 2000). They also overlap substantially in their ability to regulate CO_2-induced cerebral vasodilation of adult rat pial arteries (Wang et al, 1999). Agents that stimulate cAMP production also activate PKG in vascular smooth muscle cells of coronary and pulmonary arteries (White et al, 2000; Barman et al, 2003). Transfected PKG-I_a or PKG-I_β in COS-7 fibroblasts is similarly activated by cAMP and cGMP (Lin et al, 2001a). PKG-I in either aortic or cavernous SMCs has been found to be activated at similar levels by cAMP and cGMP, with the exception that, in old rats, PKG-I in cavernous SMC is less activated by cGMP than by cAMP (Lin et al, 2001a, 2002). An earlier study showed that PKG was activated by cAMP in rat aortic SMCs, leading to a reduction in intracellular Ca^{2+} (Lincoln et al, 1990). Overexpression of NOS, which leads to increased levels of NO and cGMP, was also shown to result in cross-activation of PKA (Lincoln et al, 1995).

Whether cross-activation of PKA and PKG plays a physiologic role has been questioned in a study with PKG-I–deficient mice in which cGMP-induced relaxation in aortic rings was impaired but cAMP-induced relaxation was not (Pfeifer et al, 1998). Furthermore, these mice were hypertensive, implying that PKG-I is the specific mediator of cGMP effects in regulating vascular muscle tone. However, in a more recent study with the same PKG-I–deficient mice, NO was able to relax vascular smooth muscle by increasing sGC activity and cGMP production with subsequent activation of PKA (Sausbier et al, 2000). Thus, the newer data once more support the notion that PKA can be activated by cGMP and this can lead to vasorelaxation.

Phosphodiesterase. In each episode of cyclic nucleotide signaling, the increase of intracellular cAMP or cGMP concentration is typically two to three times the baseline (Francis et al, 2001). Decline occurs rapidly and often during the continued presence of the signaling hormone (Francis et al, 2001). Termination of cyclic nucleotide signals is principally carried out by PDEs, which catalyze the hydrolysis of cAMP and cGMP to AMP and GMP, respectively. Feedback mechanisms that increase PDE activities or expression, or both, by the increased cyclic nucleotide level facilitate cyclic nucleotide degradation (Corbin et al, 2000; Lin et al, 2001b, 2001c).

The superfamily of mammalian PDEs consists of 11 families (PDE1 to PDE11) that are encoded from 21 distinct genes (Lin et al, 2003; Montorsi et al, 2004). Each PDE gene usually encodes more than one isoform through alternative splicing or from alternate gene promoters. PDE1, PDE3, PDE4, PDE7, and PDE8 are multigene families, and PDE2, PDE5, PDE9, PDE10, and PDE11 are unigene families. PDE1, PDE2, PDE3, PDE10 and PDE11 hydrolyze both cAMP and cGMP; PDE4, PDE7, and PDE8 hydrolyze cAMP; and PDE5, PDE6, and PDE9 are specific for cGMP.

With the exception of PDE6, which is specifically expressed in photoreceptor cells, all PDEs have been identified in the corpus cavernosum (Kuthe et al, 2001). **However, there is ample evidence that PDE5 is by far the principal PDE for the termination of cavernous cGMP signaling** (Fig.

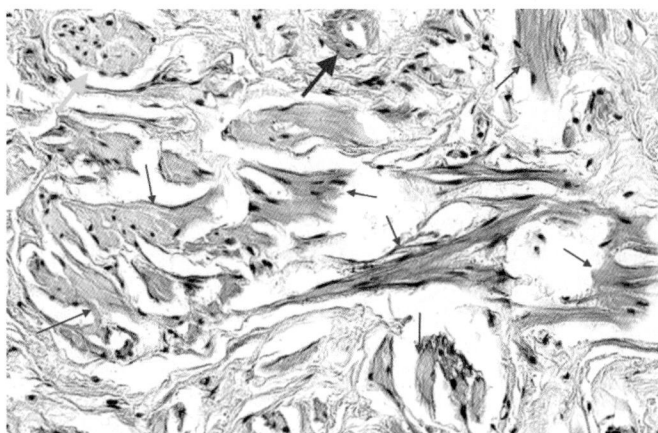

Figure 21–12. Immunohistochemistry of human penile tissue, showing positive phosphodiesterase 5 (PDE5) staining of cavernous smooth muscle fibers *(small blue arrows)*, nerve *(yellow arrow)*, and blood vessel wall *(red arrow)* (×100).

21–12); **for example, inhibition of the cGMP-catalytic activity of PDE5 by specific inhibitors has been shown to be highly effective in treating ED** (Eardley et al, 2002).

PDE3 also appears to play a role in erection, as demonstrated by the erectogenic effect of a PDE3-specific inhibitor, milrinone (Kuthe et al, 2002). Furthermore, although direct inhibition of PDE5 is the main mechanism through which sildenafil exerts its erectogenic effect, it has been shown that sildenafil also significantly increases cAMP concentration in isolated human cavernous tissue strips (Stief et al, 2000). This effect is thought to involve PDE3 because cGMP, which is accumulated as a result of PDE5 inhibition by sildenafil, is capable of preventing cAMP degradation by competing for the same catalytic sites on the PDE3 molecules (Francis et al, 2001). This attenuating effect of cGMP on the cAMP-catalytic activity of PDE3 is also believed to explain why inhibition of PKG could suppress the relaxing effect of forskolin in isolated human cavernous smooth muscle (Uckert et al, 2004).

In a study in which cultured human CSMCs were incubated with forskolin or PGE_1, cGMP accumulation was significantly enhanced (Kim et al, 2000). Because forskolin and PGE_1 are direct and indirect activators, respectively, of AC, their effect on cGMP accumulation was surprising. By showing that cAMP acted as a competitive inhibitor for PDE5, the authors hypothesized that forskolin- or PGE_1-induced cGMP accumulation was the result of inhibition of PDE5 by increased cAMP in response to AC activation. Although it is clear that cAMP does not interact with PDE5 in an allosteric fashion, the mechanism through which cAMP inhibits PDE5 remains to be elucidated.

Ion Channels. In general, there are four major types of ion channels: (1) external ligand-gated, which open to a specific extracellular molecule (e.g., acetylcholine); (2) internal ligand-gated, which open or close in response to an intracellular molecule (e.g., ATP); (3) voltage-gated, which open in response to a change in membrane potential (e.g., sodium, potassium, and calcium channels); and (4) mechanically gated, which open in response to mechanical pressure.

Smooth muscle has neither a T-tubule system nor a well-developed sarcoplasmic reticulum. Therefore, extracellular calcium plays an important role, and calcium must enter the cytoplasm through the plasma membrane during an action potential. Three transmembrane proteins are known to regulate calcium inflow and outflow: calcium channels are the major inflow regulators, whereas the calcium-sodium exchanger and calcium ATPase regulate calcium exit from muscle cells. The presence of voltage-dependent L-type calcium channels (long-duration current, slow calcium channel) in isolated cavernous smooth muscle and cultured muscle cells has been documented. Christ and coworkers (1993b) have reported that both calcium influx through calcium channels and mobilization of intracellular calcium stores are involved during phenylephrine- and endothelin-induced contraction, but only calcium channel influx is apparent for potassium chloride–induced contraction.

Studies have shown at least four potassium channel subtypes in the cavernous smooth muscle: (1) the calcium-sensitive potassium channel (e.g., maxi-K), (2) the metabolically regulated potassium channels (K_{ATP}), (3) the delayed rectifier, and (4) the fast transient A current (I_A) (Christ et al, 1993a; Fan et al, 1995). The calcium-sensitive potassium channels may be involved in cAMP-mediated smooth muscle relaxation. Decreased intracytosolic potassium and altered potassium conductance have been shown to occur in acetylcholine- and sodium nitroprusside–treated corpus cavernosum smooth muscle (Seftel et al, 1996). A stretch-sensitive chloride channel has also been demonstrated in CSMCs (Fan et al, 1999).

Hyperpolarization of the Smooth Muscle Cells. Hyperpolarization causes closure of voltage-dependent calcium channels, a decrease in the intracellular free calcium concentration, and relaxation of the smooth muscle. One of the hyperpolarization mechanisms involves the opening of potassium channels; the opening of ATP-sensitive K^+ channels (K_{ATP}) and Ca^{2+}-activated K^+ channels (K_{Ca}) causes hyperpolarization and relaxation of vascular smooth muscle. These two types of channels are present in human corpus cavernosum smooth muscle (Christ et al, 1993a), and pharmacologic stimulation of K_{ATP} channels induces penile smooth muscle relaxation (Venkateswarlu et al, 2002). Furthermore, PNU-83757, an opener of K_{ATP} channels, has been shown to induce erection when given intracavernously to patients with ED (Vick et al, 2002) The opening of large-conductance K_{Ca} channels, also known as maxi-K, has been found to hyperpolarize and relax human corpus cavernosum (Spektor et al, 2002). The opening of K^+ channels can be stimulated by PKA, PKG, or cGMP.

Hyperpolarization of penile smooth muscle is also important in endothelium-dependent relaxation of human penile arteries, where a significant relaxation remains despite blockade of NO and PG synthesis (Angulo et al, 2003b). This activity has been attributed to the endothelium-derived hyperpolarizing factor (EDHF), which opens K_{Ca} channels and produces hyperpolarization and vasodilation. The nature of EDHF remains undetermined.

Molecular Oxygen as a Modulator of Penile Erection. The PO_2 level of cavernous blood in the flaccid state is similar to that of venous blood (~35 mm Hg). During erection, the large inflow of arterial blood raises PO_2 to approximately 90 mm Hg (Sattar et al, 1995). Molecular oxygen is a substrate, together with L-arginine, for the synthesis of NO by NOS. In the flaccid state, the low oxygen concentration inhibits NO synthesis; during erection, the higher level of substrate induces NO synthesis. It has been estimated that the minimal concentration of oxygen in the cavernous bodies necessary to reach full NOS activity is 50 to 60 mm Hg (Kim et al, 1993).

Similarly, prostaglandin H synthase is also an oxygenase (cyclooxygenase) and uses oxygen as substrate for the synthesis of prostanoids. Production of PGE_1 has been shown to be inhibited in flaccidity and stimulated during erection. Endothelin synthesis is also modulated by oxygen: a low oxygen concentration promotes production, whereas a high concentration inhibits it.

Intercellular Communication. During erection and detumescence, communication should exist among cavernous smooth muscles to mediate synchronized relaxation and contraction (Christ et al, 1991). Although the electromyographic activity in the cavernous tissue of patients with normal erectile function is synchronous (Stief et al, 1991a), the relatively sparse neuronal innervation of cavernous smooth muscle cannot explain this. **Several studies have demonstrated the presence of gap junctions in the membrane of adjacent muscle cells. These intercellular channels allow exchange of ions such as calcium and second-messenger molecules** (Christ et al, 1992). The major component of gap junctions is connexin-43, a membrane-sparing protein of less than 0.25 μm that has been identified between smooth muscle cells of human corpus cavernosum (Campos de Calvalho et al, 1993). Cell-to-cell communication through these gap junctions most likely explains the synchronized erectile response, although their pathophysiologic impact is still unclear.

KEY POINTS: PENILE SMOOTH MUSCLE RELAXATION CAUSES ERECTION

- Relaxation of the cavernous smooth muscle is the key to penile erection.
- Nitric oxide released by nNOS contained in the terminals of the cavernous nerve initiates the erection process, and nitric oxide released from eNOS in the endothelium helps maintain erection.
- Upon entering the smooth muscle cells, NO stimulates the production of cGMP.
- Cyclic GMP activates protein kinase G, which in turn opens potassium channels and closes calcium channels.
- Low cytosolic calcium favors smooth muscle relaxation.
- The smooth muscle regains its tone when cGMP is degraded by phosphodiesterase.

PATHOPHYSIOLOGY OF ERECTILE DYSFUNCTION

Incidence and Epidemiology

The increasing incidence of impotence with age was noted by Kinsey and coworkers in 1948: only 1 in 50 men at age 40 years but 1 in 4 by age 65. In 1990, Diokno and associates reported that 35% of married men aged 60 years and older suffer from erectile impotence.

Modern probability sampling techniques were used by two surveys obtaining prevalence data of ED in the United States: the Massachusetts Male Aging Study (MMAS) and the National Health and Social Life Survey (NHSLS). The MMAS consisted of 1709 noninstitutionalized men between the ages of 40 and 70 years living in the greater Boston area first surveyed between 1987 and 1989 and resurveyed between 1995 and 1997 (Feldman et al, 1994; Johannes et al, 2000). Extensive physiologic measures, demographic information, and self-reported ED status (nine items related to potency on a questionnaire) were components of this report. The MMAS was the first cross-sectional, community-based, random-sample, multidisciplinary epidemiologic survey on ED and its physiologic and psychosocial correlates in men in the United States. **From the prevalence rates reported in the MMAS study, between the ages of 40 and 70 years, the probability of complete ED increased from 5.1% to 15%, moderate dysfunction increased from 17% to 34%, and mild dysfunction remained constant at about 17%.**

The NHSLS was a national probability survey of men ($N = 1410$) and women between the ages of 18 and 59 years living in households in the United States in 1992 (Laumann et al, 1999) and was principally a broad-ranging inquiry into sexual practices and beliefs within that age group. Therefore, the survey collected only limited information on sexual function broadly defined. The following prevalence rates for ED were reported (responses to questions regarding obtaining and maintaining erection): 7% for ages 18 to 29 years, 9% for ages 30 to 39, 11% for ages 40 to 49, and 18% for ages 50 to 59.

Regarding the worldwide prevalence of ED, 24 international studies were reported between 1993 and 2003. All that were stratified by age showed a rising prevalence of ED. Before age 40 the rate was 1% to 9%; from 40 to 59 it ranged from 2% to 9% to as high as 20% to 30%, with some studies showing marked differences between the 40 to 49 and the 50 to 59 groups. The 50- to 59-year groups showed the greatest range of reported prevalence rates. For the group from 60 to 69 years, most of the world showed a rather high rate (20% to 40%), with some increasing after age 65, except for the Scandinavian reports, in which the 70s and older were the time of major rate change. Almost all of the reports showed high prevalence rates for men in their 70s and 80s, ranging from 50% to 75%.

Incidence Studies

The MMAS (Johannes et al, 2000) is the only longitudinal study conducted in the United States (1987 to 1989 and 1995 to 1997). Analyses were performed on 847 of the 1297 men without ED at baseline (1987 to 1989) and with follow-up information in 1995 to 1997. The average age of these men at baseline was 52.2 years (range, 40 to 69 years). **From this group of patients, the crude incidence rate of impotence in white men in the United States was 25.9 cases per 1000 man-years (95% confidence interval [CI], 22.5 to 29.9). The annual incidence rates increased with each decade (per 1000 man-years): 12.4 cases for 40 to 49 years, 29.8 cases for 50 to 59 years, and 46.4 cases for 60 to 69 years. Age-adjusted risk (per 1000 man-years) of ED was higher for men with diabetes mellitus (50.7 cases), treated heart disease (58.3 cases), and treated hypertension (42.5 cases). By using these data and the known population of the United States, it was estimated that, for white men, the new cases in the 40- to 69-year age group would be 617,715 per year (Lewis et al, 2000). Rates reported from Europe and Brazil also suggest an incidence of 25 to 30 per 1000 man-years (Moreira et al, 2003; Schouten et al, 2005).**

Risk Factors

Common risk factor categories associated with sexual dysfunction include the following: general health status, diabetes mellitus, cardiovascular disease, concurrence of other genitourinary disease, psychiatric or psychologic disorders, other chronic diseases, and sociodemographic conditions. For ED, smoking, medications, and hormonal factors also serve as well-defined risk factor–associated conditions. In men, diabetes has been associated with a greater prevalence of decreased desire and orgasmic dysfunction as well as ED. A higher odds ratio is seen with insulin-dependent diabetes mellitus; diabetes present for over 10 years; fair or poor control based on glycosylated hemoglobin; management by means other than diet; a history of diabetes-related arterial, renal, or retinal disease and neuropathy; and concurrent cigarette smoking. Endothelial dysfunction is a condition present in many cases of ED, and thus there are common etiologic pathways for other vascular disease states (Lewis et al, 2004).

Classification

Many classifications have been proposed (Fig. 21–13). Some are based on the cause (diabetic, iatrogenic, traumatic) and some on the neurovascular mechanism (failure to initiate

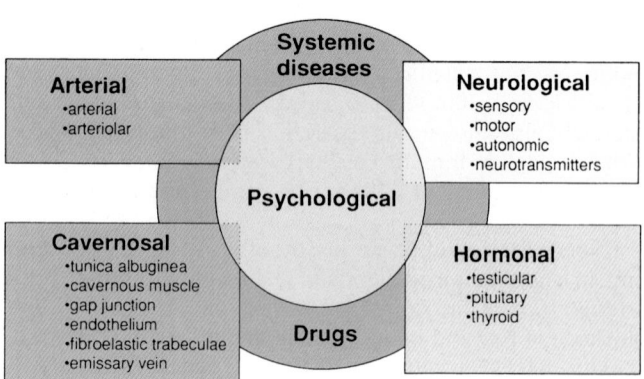

Figure 21–13. A functional classification of impotence. Note that it is unlikely for an individual patient's impotence to derive solely from one source. Most cases have a psychogenic component of varying degree, and systemic diseases and pharmacologic effects can be concomitant and causative. (Modified from Carrier S, Brock G, Kour NW, Lue TF: Pathophysiology of erectile dysfunction. Urology 1993;42:468-481, with permission of Exerpta Medica, Inc.)

Table 21–5. Classification of Male Erectile Dysfunction

Organic
I.   Vasculogenic
     Arteriogenic
     Cavernosal
     Mixed
II. Neurogenic
III. Anatomic
IV. Endocrinologic

Psychogenic
I.   Generalized
     A. Generalized unresponsiveness
        1. Primary lack of sexual arousability
        2. Aging-related decline in sexual arousability
     B. Generalized inhibition
        1. Chronic disorder of sexual intimacy
II. Situational
     A. Partner-related
        1. Lack of arousability in specific relationship
        2. Lack of arousability owing to sexual object preference
        3. High central inhibition owing to partner conflict or threat
     B. Performance-related
        1. Associated with other sexual dysfunction/s (e.g., rapid ejaculation)
        2. Situational performance anxiety (e.g., fear of failure)
     C. Psychological distress- or adjustment-related
        1. Associated with negative mood state (e.g., depression) or major life stress (e.g., death of partner)

[neurogenic], failure to fill [arterial], and failure to store [venous] [I. Goldstein, personal communication, 1990]). A classification recommended by the International Society of Impotence Research is shown in Table 21–5 (Lizza and Rosen, 1999).

Psychogenic

Previously, psychogenic impotence was believed to be most common, thought to affect 90% of impotent men (Masters and Johnson, 1970). This belief has given way to the realization that ED is usually a mixed condition that may be predominantly functional or physical.

Sexual behavior and penile erection are controlled by the hypothalamus, the limbic system, and the cerebral cortex. Therefore, stimulatory or inhibitory messages can be relayed to the spinal erection centers to facilitate or inhibit erection. **Two possible mechanisms have been proposed to explain the inhibition of erection in psychogenic dysfunction: direct inhibition of the spinal erection center by the brain as an exaggeration of the normal suprasacral inhibition** (Steers, 1990) **and excessive sympathetic outflow or elevated peripheral catecholamine levels, which may increase penile smooth muscle tone to prevent its necessary relaxation.** Animal studies demonstrate that the stimulation of sympathetic nerves or systemic infusion of epinephrine causes detumescence of the erect penis (Diederichs et al, 1991a, 1991b). Clinically, higher levels of serum norepinephrine have been reported in patients with psychogenic ED than in normal control subjects or patients with vasculogenic ED (Kim and Oh, 1992).

Bancroft and Janssen theorized that the male sexual response depends on the balance between excitatory and inhibitory impulses within the CNS. They are testing sexually inhibitory and excitatory questionnaires that may help determine whether psychotherapy or pharmacologic treatment will aid an individual patient (Bancroft, 2000).

Neurogenic

It has been estimated that 10% to 19% of ED is neurogenic (Abicht 1991; Aboseif et al, 1997). If one includes iatrogenic causes and mixed ED, the prevalence is probably much higher. The presence of a neurologic disorder or neuropathy does not exclude other causes, and confirming that ED is neurogenic can be challenging. Because erection is a neurovascular event, any disease or dysfunction affecting the brain, spinal cord, and cavernous or pudendal nerves can induce dysfunction.

As discussed earlier, the MPOA, the PVN, and the hippocampus have been regarded as important integration centers for sexual drive and erection (Sachs and Meisel, 1988), **and pathologic processes in these regions, such as Parkinson's disease, stroke, encephalitis, or temporal lobe epilepsy, are often associated with ED. Parkinsonism's effect may result from the imbalance of the dopaminergic pathways** (Wermuth and Stenager, 1992). Other brain lesions associated with ED are tumors, dementias, Alzheimer's disease, Shy-Drager syndrome, and trauma.

In men with a spinal cord injury, its nature, location, and extent largely determine erectile function. In addition to ED, they may have impaired ejaculation and orgasm. **Reflexogenic erection is preserved in 95% of patients with complete upper cord lesions but in only about 25% of those with complete lower cord lesions** (Eardley and Kirby, 1991). **Sacral parasympathetic neurons are important in the preservation of reflexogenic erection, although the thoracolumbar pathway may compensate for sacral loss through synaptic connections** (Courtois et al, 1993). In these patients, minimal tactile stimulation can trigger erection, albeit of short duration and requiring continuous stimulation. Other disorders at the spinal level (e.g., spina bifida, disk herniation, syringomyelia, tumor, transverse myelitis, and multiple sclerosis) may affect the afferent or efferent neural pathway in a similar manner.

Because of the close relationship between the cavernous nerves and the pelvic organs, the incidence of iatrogenic impotence resulting from various pelvic surgical procedures is reportedly high: radical prostatectomy, 43% to 100% (Veenema et al, 1977; Finkle and Taylor, 1981; Walsh and Donker, 1982); perineal prostatectomy for benign disease, 29% (Finkle and Taylor, 1981); abdominal perineal resection, 15% to 100% (Weinstein et al, 1977; Yeager and Van Heerden, 1980); and external sphincterotomy at the 3 and 9 o'clock positions, 2% to 49% (McDermott et al, 1981).

An improved understanding of the neuroanatomy of the pelvic and cavernous nerves (Walsh and Donker, 1982) has resulted in modified surgery for cancer of the rectum, bladder, and prostate, producing a lower incidence of iatrogenic impotence. For example, the introduction of nerve-sparing radical prostatectomy has reduced the incidence of impotence from nearly 100% to 30% to 50% (Catalona and Bigg, 1990; Quinlan et al, 1991). Recovery of erectile function after radical pelvic surgery can take 6 to 24 months. Early treatment with intracavernous alprostadil or oral sildenafil has been shown to improve recovery (Montorsi et al, 1997; Padma-Nathan et al,

2004), as the pharmacologically induced erections prevent the structural tissue changes associated with few or no erections during the nerve recovery period.

In cases of pelvic fracture, ED can be a result of cavernous nerve injury or vascular insufficiency or both. In diabetics, impairment of neurogenic and endothelium-dependent relaxation results in inadequate NO release (Saenz de Tejada, 1989a). Because autonomic penile innervation cannot be tested directly, clinicians should be cautious in diagnosing neurogenic ED. In a study in penile biopsy specimens (Brock et al, 1993), NADPH diaphorase staining of the nonadrenergic, noncholinergic nerve fibers has been proposed as an indicator of neurogenic status, as has single-potential analysis of cavernous nerve electrical activity (Stief et al, 1991a). Further studies are needed before these tests can be used routinely in clinical practice.

Bemelmans and colleagues (1991) performed somatosensory evoked potential and sacral reflex latency studies on impotent patients with no clinically overt neurologic disease and found that 47% had at least one abnormal neurophysiologic measurement and that frequency was greater with age. A decrease in penile tactile sensitivity with increasing age was also reported by Rowland and coworkers (1993). Sensory input from the genitalia is essential to achieve and maintain reflexogenic erection, and the input becomes even more important when older people gradually lose psychogenic erection. Therefore, sensory evaluation should be an integral part of the evaluation for ED in all patients with or without an apparent neurologic disorder.

Endocrinologic

Hypogonadism is a not-infrequent finding in the impotent population. Androgens influence the growth and development of the male reproductive tract and secondary sex characteristics; their effects on libido and sexual behavior are well established. In a review of published articles from 1975 to 1992, **Mulligan and Schmitt** (1993) **concluded that testosterone (1) enhances sexual interest, (2) increases the frequency of sexual acts, and (3) increases the frequency of nocturnal erections but has little or no effect on fantasy-induced or visually stimulated erections.** Granata and coworkers (1997) have reported that the threshold level of testosterone for normal nocturnal erections is about 200 ng/dL. However, exogenous testosterone therapy in impotent men with borderline-low testosterone levels reportedly has little effect (Graham and Regan, 1992).

The mechanism of androgen's effect has been examined by several investigators. Beyer and Gonzales-Mariscal (1994) have reported that testosterone and DHT are responsible for male pelvic thrusting and estradiol or testosterone for female pelvic thrusting during copulation. In rats, castration has been reported to decrease arterial flow, induce venous leakage, and reduce the erectile response to stimulation of the cavernous nerve by about 50% (Mills et al, 1994; Penson et al, 1996). Treatment with flutamide, estradiol, or a gonadotropin-releasing hormone antagonist in addition to castration further depresses the erectile response. Although penile NOS activity is reduced in these animals, nNOS and eNOS are not significantly reduced by this treatment (Mills et al, 1994; Penson et al, 1996). Castration also increases the α-adrenergic responsiveness of penile smooth muscle, increases apoptosis in the

corpus cavernosum in rats, and reduces the trabecular smooth muscle content in rabbits (Reilly et al, 1997b; Shabsigh, 1997; Traish et al, 1999). Clinically, many men receiving long-term androgen ablation therapy for prostate cancer have reported poor libido and ED.

Any dysfunction of the hypothalamic-pituitary axis can result in hypogonadism. Hypogonadotropic hypogonadism can be congenital or caused by a tumor or injury; hypergonadotropic hypogonadism may result from a tumor, injury, surgery, or mumps orchitis.

Hyperprolactinemia, whether from a pituitary adenoma or drugs, results in both reproductive and sexual dysfunction. Symptoms may include loss of libido, ED, galactorrhea, gynecomastia, and infertility. Hyperprolactinemia is associated with low circulating levels of testosterone, which appear to be secondary to inhibition of gonadotropin-releasing hormone secretion by the elevated prolactin levels (Leonard et al, 1989).

ED may also be associated with both hyper- and hypothyroidism. The former is commonly associated with diminished libido (which may be caused by the increased circulating estrogen levels) and less often with ED. In hypothyroidism, low testosterone secretion and elevated prolactin levels contribute to ED.

Diabetes mellitus, although the most common endocrinologic disorder, causes ED through its vascular, neurologic, endothelial, and psychogenic complications rather than through hormone deficiency per se. A detailed discussion is given later in this chapter.

Arteriogenic

Atherosclerotic or traumatic arterial occlusive disease of the hypogastric-cavernous-helicine arterial tree can decrease the perfusion pressure and arterial flow to the sinusoidal spaces, thus increasing the time to maximal erection and decreasing the rigidity of the erect penis. In the majority of patients with arteriogenic ED, the impaired penile perfusion is a component of the generalized atherosclerotic process. Michal and Ruzbarsky (1980) found that the incidence and age at onset are parallel for coronary disease and ED. **Common risk factors associated with arterial insufficiency include hypertension, hyperlipidemia, cigarette smoking, diabetes mellitus, blunt perineal or pelvic trauma, and pelvic irradiation** (Goldstein I et al, 1984; Levine et al, 1990; Rosen et al, 1990). Shabsigh and associates (1991) reported that abnormal penile vascular findings increased significantly as the number of risk factors for ED increased. On arteriography, bilateral diffuse disease of the internal pudendal, common penile, and cavernous arteries has been found in impotent patients with atherosclerosis. **Focal stenosis of the common penile or cavernous artery is most often seen in young patients who have sustained blunt pelvic or perineal trauma** (Levine et al, 1990). **Long-distance cycling is also a risk factor for vasculogenic and neurogenic ED** (Andersen and Bovim, 1997; Ricchiuti et al, 1999).

In one report, diabetic men and older men had a high incidence of fibrotic lesions of the cavernous artery, with intimal proliferation, calcification, and luminal stenosis (Michal and Ruzbarsky, 1980). Nicotine (see section on "Tobacco and Alcohol") may adversely affect erectile function not only by decreasing arterial flow to the penis but also by blocking corporeal smooth muscle relaxation and thus preventing normal venous occlusion (Juenemann et al, 1987a; Rosen et al, 1991).

ED and cardiovascular disease share the same risk factors, such as hypertension, diabetes mellitus, hypercholesterolemia, and smoking (Martin-Morales et al, 2001; Feldman et al, 1994). Lesions in the pudendal arteries are much more common in impotent men than in the general population of similar age (Virag et al, 1985). Therefore, ED can be a manifestation of generalized or focal arterial disease (Sullivan et al, 1999).

Atherosclerosis/Hyperlipidemia. The effect of hypercholesterolemia on erectile function has been studied in different experimental models. In hypercholesterolemic rabbits, examination of the corpus cavernosum ultrastructure revealed an early atherosclerotic process in the sinusoids (Kim et al, 1994b). Although the endothelial NO/cGMP pathway is impaired in this model, neuronal vasodilation does not appear affected (Azadzoi et al, 1998). The NO/cGMP pathway effect is probably due to increased superoxide production (Kim et al, 1997) or endogenous NOS inhibitors such as N^G-monomethyl-L-arginine monoacetate (L-NMMA) and asymmetrical dimethylarginine (ADMA). L-Arginine supplementation reverses endothelium-dependent relaxation impairment (Azadzoi et al, 1998).

In a more severe ischemic experimental model, rabbits underwent balloon de-endothelization of the iliac arteries followed by a high-cholesterol diet (Azadzoi et al, 1992). They developed both penile arterial insufficiency and venoocclusive dysfunction owing to decreased expandability of the cavernous smooth muscle (Azadzoi et al, 1997; Nehra et al, 1998). Changes in iliac and penile vasculature were noted, associated with decreased NOS activity and reduced endothelium-dependent and neurogenic NO-mediated relaxation of the cavernous tissue (Azadzoi et al, 1999). As a result of the impaired NO activity, production of contractile thromboxane and PG increased, leading to potentiation of neurogenic contractions of the cavernous smooth muscle (Azadzoi et al, 1998, 1999).

The risk of developing ED in patients taking statins for hyperlipidemia or coronary arterial disease is a controversial topic and is discussed later (see "Drug-Induced Erectile Dysfunction").

In large arteries in rabbits, oxidized low-density lipoproteins (ox-LDLs) inhibited endothelium-dependent NO-mediated relaxation (Kugiyama et al, 1990), but this has not been found in small systemic arteries (Simonsen et al, 1991) or cavernous smooth muscle (Ahn et al, 1999). Oxidized LDL-induced contractions are probably mediated by elevation of intracellular IP and calcium but not by inhibition of the NO/cGMP pathway (Morita et al, 1989).

Hypertension. Hypertension is an independent risk factor for ED (Feldman et al, 1994; Burchardt et al, 2000; Johannes et al, 2000), **and its consequent cardiovascular complications such as ischemic heart disease and renal failure are associated with even higher ED prevalence** (Feldman et al, 1994; Kaufman et al, 1994; Johannes et al, 2000). **However, in hypertension, the increased blood pressure itself does not impair erectile function; rather, the associated arterial stenotic lesions are thought to be the cause** (Hsieh et al, 1989).

The ED seen in hypertensive men is probably multifactorial. In 32 hypertensive and 78 normotensive impotent men, potential determinants for ED were evaluated: age, body mass index (BMI), hormonal profile, penile arterial flow, arterial risk factors, and neurologic and psychologic abnormalities (Jaffe et al, 1996). The overall analysis showed little difference with the exception that hypertensive men had a marginally higher rate of ischemic heart disease ($P = 0.06$) and lower testosterone levels (Jaffe et al, 1996).

In an animal model of spontaneously hypertensive rats (SHRs), intracavernous pressure was decreased in two studies when expressed as a percentage of mean arterial pressure (Behr-Roussel et al, 2002; Dorrance et al, 2002). However, the absolute increases in intracavernous pressure did not appear different.

Mechanism of Vascular Erectile Dysfunction

Structural Changes. In arteriogenic ED, oxygen tension in corpus cavernosum blood is less than that in psychogenic ED (Tarhan et al, 1997). Formation of PGE_1 and PGE_2 is oxygen dependent, and, in rabbit and human corpus cavernosum, increased oxygen tension was associated with elevation of PGE_2 and suppression of TGF-β1–induced collagen synthesis (Moreland et al, 1995; Nehra et al, 1999). A decrease in oxygen tension may diminish cavernous trabecular smooth muscle content and lead to diffuse venous leakage (Saenz de Tejada et al, 1991; Nehra et al, 1998).

A narrowed lumen or increased wall-to-lumen ratio in the arteries contributes to increased peripheral vascular resistance in hypertension (Mulvany, 2002). Increased resistance has also been found in the penile vasculature of SHRs—an alteration ascribed to structural changes of the arterial and erectile tissue (Okabe et al, 1999; Toblli et al, 2000; Hale et al, 2001). The increase in extracellular matrix expansion affects both interstitium and neural structures of the penis (Toblli et al, 2000).

Vasoconstriction. Enhanced basal and myogenic tone has been observed in arteries from hypertensive rats (Schubert and Mulvany, 1999). Enhanced sympathetic nerve activity accompanying hypertension has also been reported in both men and animals (Norman and Dzielak 1986; Mancia et al, 1999). Enhanced vasoconstriction of the penile vasculature in SHRs seen in response to phenylephrine infusion has been attributed to hypertrophy of the vascular wall (Okabe et al, 1999) but not to an alteration of sympathetic neurotransmitters.

Impaired Endothelium-Dependent Vasodilation. In patients with essential hypertension, endothelium-dependent vasodilation in response to flow or infusion of agonists such as acetylcholine or bradykinin is diminished (Panza et al, 1990; Taddei et al, 1998; Cai and Harrison, 2000). There is evidence indicating that profound endothelial dysfunction in the coronary circulation can predict major coronary events (Schachinger et al, 2000; Suwaidi et al, 2000). Endothelial dysfunction measured as blunted acetylcholine-induced vasorelaxation is evident in small arteries from patients with renovascular hypertension (Rizzoni et al, 1996, 1998). However, penile endothelial function in hypertensive men has not been investigated specifically.

In SHRs, the relaxing effect of acetylcholine is blunted in both large and small arteries (Konishi and Su, 1983), and endothelial dysfunction appears to develop with hypertension. The same blunted relaxation has also been shown in corporeal strips from SHRs and found to be restored with indomethacin (Behr-Roussel et al, 2002). Impairment of endothelium-dependent relaxation in arteries from SHRs could be ascribed to angiotensin II (Rajagopalan et al, 1996; Heitzer et al, 1999), thromboxane, and superoxide (Cosentino et al, 1998; Yang et al, 2002) or to high blood pressure per se (Paniagua et al, 2000).

Cavernous (Venogenic)

Failure of adequate venous occlusion has been proposed as one of the most common causes of vasculogenic impotence (Rajfer et al, 1988). **Veno-occlusive dysfunction may result from a variety of pathophysiologic processes: degenerative tunical changes, fibroelastic structural alterations, insufficient trabecular smooth muscle relaxation, and venous shunts.**

Degenerative changes (Peyronie's disease, old age, and diabetes) or traumatic injury to the tunica albuginea (penile fracture) can impair the compression of the subtunical and emissary veins. In Peyronie's disease, the inelastic tunica albuginea may prevent the emissary veins from closing (Metz et al, 1983). Iacono and coworkers (1994) have postulated that a decrease in the elastic fibers of the tunica albuginea and an alteration in its microarchitecture (Iacono et al, 1993) may contribute to impotence in some men. Changes in the subtunical areolar layer may impair the veno-occlusive mechanism, as occasionally seen in patients after surgery for Peyronie's disease (Dalkin and Carter, 1991).

Structural alterations in the fibroelastic components of the trabeculae, cavernous smooth muscle, and endothelium may result in venous leakage. Insufficient trabecular smooth muscle relaxation, causing inadequate sinusoidal expansion and insufficient compression of the subtunical venules, may occur in anxious individuals with excessive adrenergic tone or in patients with inadequate neurotransmitter release. It has been shown that alteration of an α adrenoceptor or a decrease in NO release may heighten smooth muscle tone and impair relaxation in response to endogenous muscle relaxant (Christ et al, 1990).

Acquired venous shunts—the result of operative correction of priapism—may cause persistent glans/cavernosum or cavernosum/spongiosum shunting.

Fibroelastic Component. Loss of compliance of the penile sinusoids associated with increased deposition of collagen and decreased elastic fiber may be seen in diabetes, hypercholesterolemia, vascular disease, penile injury, or old age (Cerami et al, 1987; Hayashi et al, 1987). Sattar and coworkers (1994) have reported significant differences in the mean percentage of penile elastic fibers: 9% in healthy men, 5.1% in patients with venous leakage, and 4.3% in patients with arterial disease. In an animal model of vasculogenic ED, Nehra and associates (1998) demonstrated that cavernous expandability correlates with smooth muscle content and may be used to predict trabecular histology. Moreland and colleagues (1995) have shown that PGE_1 suppresses collagen synthesis by TGF-β1 in human cavernous smooth muscle, which implies that intracavernous injection of PGE_1 may be beneficial in preventing intracavernous fibrosis.

Smooth Muscle. Because corporeal smooth muscle controls the vascular events leading to erection, a change in smooth muscle content and ultrastructure can be expected to affect erectile response. In a study of human penile tissue, Sattar and associates (1996) demonstrated a significant difference between the mean percentage of cavernous smooth muscle in normal potent men, stained with antidesmin (38.5%) or antiactin (45.2%), and that in a venogenic group (antidesmin, 27.4%; antiactin, 34.2%) or arteriogenic group (antidesmin, 23.7%, antiactin, 28.9%). An in vitro biochemical study has shown impaired neurogenic and endothelium-related relaxation of penile smooth muscle in impotent diabetic men (Saenz de Tejada et al, 1989a). In vasculogenic and neurogenic ED, the damaged smooth muscle can be a key factor, exacerbating the primary cause (Mersdorf et al, 1991). Pickard and coworkers (1994) have also shown impairment of nerve-evoked relaxation and α-adrenergic–stimulated contraction of cavernous muscle as well as reduced muscle content in men with venous or mixed venous/arterial impotence.

Ion channels are intimately involved in the biochemical events of muscle function. Fan and associates (1995) reported an alteration of the maxi-K^+ channel in cells from impotent patients and suggested that this might contribute to decreased hyperpolarizing ability, altered calcium homeostasis, and impaired smooth muscle relaxation. In animal studies, Juenemann and associates (1991) showed significant smooth muscle degeneration with loss of cell-to-cell contact in rabbits fed a high-cholesterol diet for 3 months. In a rabbit model of vasculogenic impotence, Azadzoi and associates (1997) demonstrated that veno-occlusive dysfunction could be induced by cavernous ischemia. Cavernous nerve injury may also affect cavernous smooth muscle relaxation, as demonstrated in neurotomized dogs (Paick et al, 1991).

Gap Junctions. These intercellular communication channels are responsible for synchronization and coordination of the erectile response, although their pathophysiologic impact has yet to be clarified (Christ et al, 1991; Lerner et al, 1993). In severe arterial disease, the presence of collagen fibers between cell membranes reduces or abolishes their contact (Persson et al, 1989). Thus, a malfunction or loss of gap junctions may alter coordinated smooth muscle activity.

Endothelium. By release of vasoactive agents, the endothelium of the corpus cavernosum can modify the tone of adjacent smooth muscle and affect the development or inhibition of erection. NO, PGs, and the polypeptide endothelins have been identified in endothelial cells (Ignarro et al, 1990; Saenz de Tejada et al, 1991a, 1991b). Activation of cholinergic receptors on endothelial cells by acetylcholine or the cells' expansion as a result of increased blood flow may elicit underlying smooth muscle relaxation through the release of NO (Saenz de Tejada et al, 1988; Rubanyi et al, 1989). Diabetes and hypercholesterolemia have been shown to alter the function of endothelium-mediated relaxation of the cavernous muscle (Azadzoi and Saenz de Tejada, 1991) and impair erection.

Drug-Induced Erectile Dysfunction

ED is common among older men and therefore inevitably coexists with other conditions that are themselves risk factors for ED, such as depression, diabetes, and cardiovascular disease (Feldman et al, 1993). In addition, sexual symptoms related to medication can involve a combination of complaints concerning desire, arousal, and orgasm rather than being limited to impaired function. Self-reported and questionnaire data concerning ED as a side effect of medication should be interpreted with caution.

Antihypertensive Agents. Current recommendations for treatment of hypertension suggest thiazide diuretics and β-adrenergic antagonists as first-line agents, with calcium channel antagonists, angiotensin-converting enzyme (ACE) inhibitors, and α-adrenergic antagonists as second-line agents (Joint National Committee, 1997). All drugs have ED listed as a potential side effect, but well-designed controlled clinical trials give conflicting results (Barksdale and Gardner, 1999). Animal studies do suggest possible mechanisms (Andersson and Wagner, 1995).

Diuretics. This class of drug has been extensively studied because early trials showed a high prevalence of self-reported ED. Appropriate controlled studies with ED as an endpoint give consistent results, despite trends toward lower dosages. Older treatment regimens with higher thiazide doses showed a significant increase in ED when compared with placebo (Chang et al, 1991). Addition of a thiazide to treatment with propranolol or methyldopa also increased the prevalence of ED, but this effect did not occur when thiazide was added to an ACE inhibitor (Croog et al, 1988). Data from a large trial in the United Kingdom showed that twice as many men taking thiazides for mild hypertension reported ED than men treated with propranolol or placebo—the most common reason for withdrawal from the bendrofluazide arm of the study (Medical Research Council, 1981).

Similar findings were documented from the Treatment of Mild Hypertension Study (TOMHS), in which the prevalence of ED at 2 years in men taking low-dose thiazide was twice that of those taking placebo or alternative agents (Grimm et al, 1997). Interestingly after 4 years of treatment, the prevalence of ED in the placebo group approached that of the thiazide group, a finding not fully explained by dropouts. It may be that thiazide therapy, rather than causing ED directly, unmasks it at an earlier stage. A study comparing sexual side effects of thiazide, placebo, or atenolol in hypertensive patients also found a higher rate of ED in the thiazide group, although this was ameliorated by weight loss (Wassertheil-Smoller et al, 1991). The mechanism of diuretic-induced ED remains to be elucidated.

β-Adrenergic Blockers. Receptor studies show that only 10% of adrenoceptors in the penile tissue are of the β type, and their stimulation is thought to mediate relaxation (Andersson and Wagner, 1995). This response is attenuated in vitro by nonselective drugs such as propranolol, possibly by a β_2-receptor effect (Srilatha et al, 1999), but not by cardiac-selective agents such as practolol, which selectively inhibits β_1 receptor. The β antagonists also exert an inhibitory effect within the CNS, perhaps leading to lowered sex hormone levels (Suzuki et al, 1988). In the early trials noted previously (Medical Research Council, 1981; Croog et al, 1988), nonselective drugs such as propranolol were associated with a higher prevalence of ED than placebo or ACE inhibitor. Later trials with newer agents with higher selectivity for the β_1 adrenoceptor, such as acebutolol, have shown a substantial reduction in ED, with no difference being found when compared with the placebo and ACE inhibitor groups (Grimm et al, 1997).

α-Adrenoceptor Blockers. Animal studies have demonstrated a positive effect on erection for α antagonists, particularly those acting on the α_1 receptor, by increasing or prolonging the relaxant response of cavernous smooth muscle (Andersson and Wagner, 1995). In addition, prejunctional α_2-receptor activation modulates the release of noradrenaline, suggesting a putative relaxant role for α_2 blockers. In clinical observations, drugs such as doxazosin, used to treat hypertension (Grimm et al, 1997) or lower urinary tract symptoms (Flack, 2002), were not associated with complaints of ED and indeed resulted in lower rates than in placebo groups. Not surprisingly, drugs stimulatory to the α_2 receptor such as clonidine do result in diminished erectile function, both clinically and experimentally, by peripheral and central mechanisms (Hogan et al, 1980; Srilatha et al, 1999). The centrally acting drug methyldopa has also been associated with ED in controlled trials comparing it with placebo and other antihypertensive agents (Croog et al, 1988), and it may act by antagonizing hypothalamic α_2 adrenoceptors.

Angiotensin-Converting Enzyme Inhibitors. These drugs lack any easily appreciated peripheral or central effect that would interfere with sexual function. An in vivo experiment showed that the ACE inhibitor captopril did not cause any significant adverse effect on sexual function in awake normotensive rats (Srilatha et al, 1999). In three clinical studies of hypertension treatment comparing an ACE inhibitor with other agents and placebo, all found either no difference from placebo or improved sexual function over baseline when compared with other agents (Croog et al, 1988; Suzuki et al, 1988; Grimm et al, 1997). An early report also showed that the newest antihypertensive agents, angiotensin II receptor antagonists, have a beneficial effect on existing sexual dysfunction at baseline and no adverse sexual effects over 12 months of treatment (Llisterri et al, 2001).

Calcium Channel Blockers. Clinical studies have demonstrated no adverse effect on erection; ejaculatory complaints, which may owe to decreased force of bulbocavernous muscles, seem short lived (Suzuki et al, 1988). In the TOMHS study there was no ED increase over placebo in the amlodipine group (Grimm et al, 1997). Another study also showed no increase in the prevalence of ED when hypertension was treated with diltiazem alone or in combination with an ACE inhibitor (Cushman et al, 1998).

Summary. Treatment of mild to moderate hypertension requires agents with an acceptable side effect profile to minimize noncompliance. Thiazide diuretic is associated with higher rates of ED, although this may be reduced by combination therapy and weight loss. The α_1 blockers and angiotensin II receptor blockers both tend to improve sexual functioning during treatment and may therefore be useful when commencing antihypertensive therapy in men with pre-existing ED (Khan et al, 2002) (Table 21–6).

Psychotropic Medications. As with hypertension, the underlying disorder may be more relevant for ED than the medication. On the other hand, receptor complexity and interrelation of pathways within the CNS make it extremely likely that neurons and ganglia involved in sexual functioning will be affected by psychotropic drugs, leading to functional changes that may be positive or negative. One example is the loss of sexual desire among nonmedicated patients with schiz-

Table 21-6. Effect of Antihypertensive Agents on Sexual Function

Agent	Effect	Mechanism
Diuretics	ED (twice as placebo)	Unknown
β blocker (nonselective)	ED	Prejunctional α_2-receptor inhibition
β_1 blocker (selective)	None	
α_1 blocker	Decreases ED rate but may cause retrograde ejaculation	Relaxation of internal urinary sphincter
α_2 blocker	ED	Inhibition of central α_2 receptor
ACE inhibitor	None	
Angiotensin II receptor blocker	Decreases ED rate	
Calcium channel blocker	None	

ACE, angiotensin-converting enzyme; ED, erectile dysfunction.

ophrenia; those receiving antipsychotic drugs have shown greater desire but increased erectile and ejaculatory disturbance (Aizenberg et al, 1995).

Antipsychotics. Members of this class of drug have many effects on CNS receptors and may also act peripherally. Their therapeutic effect is thought to be related to dopaminergic receptor blockade within the limbic and prefrontal areas of the brain. Their unwanted effects owe to β-adrenergic blockade and anticholinergic properties as well as to antidopaminergic actions within the basal ganglia, causing extrapyramidal side effects that commonly produce sexual symptoms (Sullivan and Lukoff, 1990).

The occurrence of extrapyramidal effects differentiates the older "typical" antipsychotics, with which they are frequent, from the newer "atypical" antipsychotics, with which they are less common. This difference is probably related to differential affinities for particular classes of receptor (Strange, 2001) or avidity for particular areas of the cerebral cortex (Westerink, 2002). An additional effect of DA blockade, hyperprolactinemia, which also alters sexual function by reducing DA release in permissive cerebral centers, is more common with older typical agents (Smith and Talbert, 1986).

Animal experiments, chiefly in the rat, show that D1 receptor activation in the MPOA of the hypothalamus facilitates erection through intermediary oxytocinergic and spinal cholinergic pathways. It is also possible that activation of D2 receptors in this area has the opposite effect (Zarrindast et al, 1992). Older agents such as haloperidol and flupenthixol have been shown to reduce apomorphine-induced erections in experimental animals by means of D1 receptor antagonism (Andersson and Wagner, 1995). In addition, systemic administration of antipsychotic agents in the rabbit produced erection by a local nondopaminergic action, possibly involving antagonism of α_1 adrenoceptors (Naganuma et al, 1993). Therefore, the clinical effect of antipsychotics on sexual function varies according to their affinity for particular receptors.

In a nonrandomized comparative study of antipsychotic medications, the prevalence of sexual dysfunction ranged from 40% to 70% (Wirshing et al, 2002). Newer agents such as clozapine showed a lower reduction in sexual desire, and the group taking risperidone had the greatest decrease in erectile frequency. An earlier study found that thioridazine, an atypical agent, caused ejaculatory problems rather than ED (Kotin et al, 1976).

Antidepressants. Sexual side effects in both men and women are varied but are important factors governing compliance because these drugs are commonly prescribed to younger and middle-aged adults.

Tricyclics act by inhibiting the reuptake of norepinephrine and serotonin in the CNS. Their sexual side effect profile is thought to be related to peripheral anticholinergic and β-adrenergic effects. It is also possible that they antagonize 5-HT receptors. Controlled clinical studies suggest that orgasmic disorders in both sexes are frequent, explaining the use of these drugs as inhibitors of ejaculation (Harrison et al, 1986; Monteiro et al, 1987).

Monoamine oxidase inhibitors are associated with higher rates of orgasmic dysfunction in controlled trials (Harrison et al, 1986), but the nature of the central or peripheral mechanisms involved is uncertain.

Selective serotonin reuptake inhibitors (SSRIs) are the class of drug commonly used to treat depression at the present time. They inhibit the reuptake of 5-HT into CNS neurons and can therefore produce stimulatory effects on various 5-HT receptors. It is estimated that up to 50% of patients taking these drugs experience a change in sexual function (Rosen et al, 1999; Keltner et al, 2002). Possible mechanisms include stimulation of 5-HT2 and 5-HT3 receptors, which may inhibit erectogenic pathways within the spinal cord (Tang et al, 1998), decreased DA release in the MPOA (Maeda et al, 1994), and inhibition of NOS. A controlled clinical study suggested that the improvement in sexual function resulting from SSRIs' alleviation of clinical depression outweighed any negative effect (Michelson et al, 2001). However, another placebo-controlled randomized study revealed increased sexual dysfunction, mainly anorgasmia, in the SSRI-treated group (Labbate et al, 1998; Croft et al, 1999). Further studies have suggested that these adverse effects can be modified by cotreatment with other drugs such as sildenafil (Nurmberg et al, 2003) or mianserin (Aizenberg et al, 1997).

SSRIs differ in their ability to cause ED. A high incidence has been observed in patients treated with paroxetine (Kennedy et al, 2000), and a lesser impact has been reported with citalopram (Mendels et al, 1999). This suggests that a mechanism or mechanisms other than inhibition of serotonin reuptake may be involved, which is supported by a report that acute or chronic paroxetine, but not citalopram, caused ED in rats by inhibiting NO production (Angulo et al, 2001b). Indeed, the inhibitory effects induced by acute paroxetine on erectile function in the rat can be prevented by inhibition of PDE5 with vardenafil (Angulo et al, 2003a) or by coadministration of the NOS substrate L-arginine (Angulo et al, 2003b). On the other hand, venlafaxine, a mixed inhibitor of serotonin and norepinephrine reuptake, produced ED in rats by increasing norepinephrine levels, as its inhibitory effects on erectile responses were prevented by phentolamine (Angulo et al, 2003b). Thus, the ability to produce ED and the mechanism by which SSRIs cause ED may differ with the specific SSRI compound.

Newer Antidepressants. Animal experiments suggest that stimulation of 5-HT1 receptors within the CNS modulates sexual function, with the 5-HT1 A subtype increasing ejaculation and the 5-HT1 C subtype improving erection. Recently developed antidepressants such as mirtazapine and nefazodone tend to have beneficial effects on sexual function, possibly by activating the 5-HT1 C receptor, which augments sexual response (Stancampiano et al, 1994), although they may also antagonize the 5-HT2 C receptor (Millan et al, 2000). The isolated reports of priapism seen with a prototype agent, trazodone, may be related to the 5-HT1 C erectogenic effect seen with its primary metabolite, *m*-chlorophenylpiperazine, in experimental animals (Andersson and Wagner, 1995). In a clinical study, trazodone was shown to increase nocturnal erectile activity, despite reducing REM sleep (Ware et al, 1994).

Anxiolytics. Although not previously associated with ED, anxiolytics have been implicated in sexual problems by the MMAS study (Derby et al, 2001). Benzodiazepines are thought to potentiate the action of GABA in the reticular and limbic system, but they may also affect the serotonin and dopaminergic pathways. Experimental studies suggest that GABAergic drugs inhibit erection induced by apomorphine, a DA agonist (Zarrindast and Farahvash, 1994). A controlled clinical study demonstrated that a combination of lithium and benzodiazepine was associated with a significantly higher rate of sexual dysfunction than treatment with lithium alone (Ghadirian et al, 1992). More recent anxiolytic agents such as bupropion, acting mainly by inhibiting DA reuptake, and buspirone, acting on 5-HT1 A receptors, were not associated with sexual side effects in placebo-controlled trials (Coleman et al, 2001) and can be used to alleviate sexual symptoms caused by other antidepressant medication (Gitlin et al, 2002).

Antiandrogens. These drugs cause partial or near-complete blockade of androgen's action by inhibiting production of or antagonizing the androgen receptor (AR). (Androgens are believed to modify sexual behavior by modulating AR within the CNS.) The effects of androgen deficiency on sexual activity are variable, ranging from complete loss to normal function. Experimental studies in humans suggest that nocturnal erections during REM sleep are androgen dependent, whereas erections in response to visual sexual stimulation are independent (Andersson and Wagner, 1995). An additional peripheral effect has been suggested from animal experiments in which castration decreased NOS activity within the rat corpus cavernosum, leading to reduced erectile activity. Testosterone restored NOS activity, but treatment with finasteride prevented this recovery, suggesting that DHT may be the important androgen in penile tissue (Lugg et al, 1995).

Indeed, the 5α-reductase inhibitor finasteride is the antiandrogen with the least effect on circulating testosterone. In randomized placebo-controlled studies of patients given finasteride (5 mg daily) for prostatic symptoms, approximately 5% complained of decreased desire and ED compared with 1% in the placebo group (Gormley et al, 1992). At the lower dose used to treat male-pattern alopecia (1 mg daily), no sexual dysfunction was seen (Tosti et al, 2001).

More complete androgen ablation is achieved by competitive antagonism at the AR, thus preventing signal transduction of testosterone and DHT. Nonsteroidal drugs such as flutamide and bicalutamide have relatively pure effects on the AR, and the steroidal antiandrogen cyproterone acetate also has inhibitory effects on the hypothalamus. These drugs are used in the palliative treatment of locally advanced and metastatic prostate cancer, either alone or in combination with a luteinizing hormone–releasing hormone (LHRH) agonist. When used alone, nonsteroidal antiandrogens are associated with a rise in serum testosterone levels; when combined with an LHRH agonist, they reduce testosterone to the castrate range. The main effect is a reduction of sexual desire, which occurs in up to 70% (Iversen et al, 2001).

In a clinical trial with a larger sample size and longer duration, treatment with bicalutamide alone resulted in a lesser decrease in sexual desire than did castration (Iversen et al, 2000). However, in another large controlled trial, treatment with either flutamide or cyproterone resulted in a gradual loss of sexual desire over 2 to 6 years in approximately 80% (Schroder et al, 2000). In a placebo-controlled study, half the patients receiving bicalutamide therapy suffered loss of erectile function, even at a low dose of 50 mg (Eri and Tveter, 1994).

The near-complete androgen deprivation achieved by medical castration with LHRH agonists results in a profound loss of sexual desire, which is usually accompanied by ED (Basaria et al, 2002). This was objectively confirmed by nocturnal penile tumescence (NPT) monitoring before and after initiation of therapy in a small study (Marumo et al, 1999).

Miscellaneous Drugs. Many other drugs are suggested as having sexual side effects, in particular that of ED in men, but these contentions are usually based on anecdotal case reports or postmarketing drug alerts rather than controlled trials.

Digoxin. In an experimental in vitro study with isolated human corpus cavernosum tissue, digoxin attenuated the relaxant response to acetylcholine and intrinsic nerve stimulation; this was linked to findings of reduced penile rigidity not seen in men given a placebo after visual sexual stimulation (Gupta et al, 1998). A randomized clinical study confirmed a negative effect on general sexual functioning linked to a decrease in plasma testosterone (Neri et al, 1987).

Statins. Statins are used to lower lipid levels and thus are mainly used in the aging male population likely to have established risk factors for sexual dysfunction, particularly ED (Schachter, 2000); for example, the MMAS revealed that low levels of high-density lipoprotein cholesterol were an independent risk factor for ED (Feldman et al, 1994). In animal models of hyperlipidemic states, supraphysiologic total cholesterol concentrations resulted in reduced neural and endothelium-dependent relaxation of the cavernous smooth muscle. The responses were partly restored by the NO substrate L-arginine and cholesterol reduction consequent to dietary change (Kim et al, 1994b; Azadzoi et al, 1998). In a single placebo-controlled trial, the rate of ED was twice as high (12% versus 6%) in men taking a statin, despite improvement in other parameters of hyperlipidemic endothelial dysfunction (Bruckert et al, 1996). Not surprisingly, this unexpected association has been questioned (Pedersen and Faergemann, 1999).

In a crossover study of 22 men with hypercholesterolemia randomly assigned to placebo, simvastatin, or lovastatin,

Kostis and colleagues (1994) reported an increase in nocturnal tumescence after 2 weeks, although it was not significant after 6 weeks. In the large Scandinavian simvastatin survival study, 4444 patients with coronary arterial disease were randomly assigned to treatment with simvastatin or placebo for up to 6 years. ED was found in 28 placebo-treated patients (8 resolved) and in 37 simvastatin-treated patients (14 resolved) (Pedersen and Faergemann, 1999). Therefore, in patients treated with statins, the underlying disease process appears to be the cause of ED, instead of the drug.

In patients with hypercholesterolemia, lipid-lowering therapy has been shown to improve endothelium-dependent vasodilation (measured in the forearm), probably owing to increased NO bioavailability (John et al, 1998). This result suggests that the dysfunction of the endothelial NO/cGMP pathway in hypercholesterolemia is reversible. In a study of 18 men whose increased cholesterol was determined to be their only risk factor for ED, erectile function was significantly improved after 2 to 5 months of treatment with atorvastatin (Saltzman et al, 2004).

Histamine H2 Receptor Antagonists. Cimetidine and ranitidine were widely prescribed for prophylaxis and treatment of peptic ulcer disease. Case reports suggested that cimetidine was associated with ED, and postulated mechanisms included anticholinergic effects and androgen inhibition (Gwee and Cheah, 1986). A single in vitro animal study suggested that H2 receptor stimulation causes cavernous relaxation, possibly through endothelial release of NO (Andersson and Wagner, 1995).

Opiates. Long-term intrathecal administration of opiates results in hypogonadotropic hypogonadism and associated sexual dysfunction that can be restored with appropriate supplementation (Abs et al, 2000). However, administration of opioid antagonists to older men with ED was not found to improve erectile function measured objectively by NPT monitoring (Billington et al, 1990). Opioids do have a generalized depressant effect on sexual function when directly administered to the MPOA in rat brain, but treatment with the opioid receptor antagonist naloxone had no sexual effect on healthy male volunteers (Andersson and Wagner, 1995).

Retroviral and Chemotherapeutic Agents. A single retrospective cohort study suggested that the prevalence of ED in men taking protease inhibitors was approximately twice that of matched control subjects, the highest rate being observed with ritonavir (Colson et al, 2002). Many of the anticancer drugs can be associated with a progressive loss of libido, peripheral neuropathy, azoospermia, and erectile failure.

Tobacco and Alcohol. Cigarette smoking may induce vasoconstriction and penile venous leakage because of its contractile effect on the cavernous smooth muscle (Juenemann et al, 1987a). In an NPT study in cigarette smokers, Hirshkowitz and colleagues (1992) reported an inverse correlation between nocturnal erection (both rigidity and duration) and the number of cigarettes smoked per day: men who smoked more than 40 had the weakest and shortest nocturnal erections.

Alcohol in small amounts improves erection and sexual drive because of its vasodilatory effect and suppression of anxiety; however, large amounts can cause central sedation, decreased libido, and transient ED. Chronic alcoholism may also result in liver dysfunction, decreased testosterone and increased estrogen levels, and alcoholic polyneuropathy, which may also affect penile nerves (Miller and Gold, 1988). In an in vitro study of rabbits given 5% alcohol for 6 weeks, Saito and coworkers (1994) reported augmented smooth muscle contraction and relaxation to both electrical field stimulation and vasoconstrictors such as phenylephrine and potassium chloride but not to sodium nitroprusside, suggesting changes in neurovascular function.

Aging, Systemic Disease, and Other Causes

A number of studies have indicated a progressive decline in sexual function in "healthy" aging men. Masters and Johnson (1977) noted a number of changes in older men, including greater latency to erection, less turgidity, loss of forceful ejaculation and decreased volume, and a longer refractory period. Decreased frequency and duration of nocturnal erection with increasing age was reported in a group of men who had regular intercourse (Schiavi and Schreiner-Engel, 1988). Other research has also indicated a decrease in penile tactile sensitivity with age (Rowland et al, 1989). A heightened cavernous muscle tone may also contribute to the decreased erectile response in older men (Christ et al, 1990). In one study, a decrease in testosterone in aging impotent men in association with relatively normal gonadotropins was reported, suggestive of hypothalamic-pituitary dysfunction (Kaiser et al, 1988). In animal studies, Garban and coworkers (1995) reported a decrease in NOS activity in the penile tissue of senescent rats. In an in vitro study of aging rabbit penile tissue, Ragazzi and associates (1996) reported increased contractility to norepinephrine and increased relaxation to adenosine and ATP but decreased relaxation to acetylcholine; they concluded that aging selectively affects endothelium-mediated NO release from cholinergic stimulation. Haas and associates (1998) proposed that the defect is at the level of calcium-eNOS interaction.

Diabetes Mellitus. Diabetes mellitus is a common chronic disease, affecting 0.5% to 2% worldwide. The prevalence of ED is three times higher in diabetic men (28% versus 9.6%) (Feldman et al, 1994), occurs at an earlier age, and increases with disease duration, being approximately 15% at age 30 and rising to 55% at 60 years (McCulloch et al, 1980, 1984). ED among men with diabetes is more frequent in those with coexisting neuropathy. The prevalence of coronary arterial disease (20%) and peripheral vascular disease (5%) among men with diabetes is far higher than in the general population. Diabetes mellitus may cause ED by affecting one or a combination of the following: psychologic function, CNS function, androgen secretion, peripheral nerve activity, endothelial cell function, and smooth muscle contractility (Dunsmuir and Holmes, 1996).

In 12% of diabetic men, deterioration of sexual function can be the first symptom. Duplex ultrasonography after intracavernous injection has revealed a high prevalence (>75%) of penile arterial insufficiency among diabetic men with ED (Wang et al, 1993). Pathologic changes in the cavernous arteries (Michal and Ruzbarsky, 1980), ultrastructural changes in the cavernous smooth muscle (Mersdorf et al, 1991), and impaired endothelium-dependent relaxation of the corporeal smooth muscle (Saenz de Tejada et al, 1989a) have also been noted in penile specimens from diabetic men with ED. Hirshkowitz and associates (1990) reported that impotent men with diabetes have fewer sleep-related erections, shorter tumescence time, diminished penile rigidity, decreased heart rate response to deep breathing, and lower penile blood pressure than age-matched nondiabetic men.

A number of streptozotocin- and alloxan-induced diabetic animal models have been used to study the mechanism of diabetes-induced ED. In general, diabetes causes endothelial cell dysfunction, which results in an increased prevalence of vascular disease in both type 1 and type 2 diabetes. Particularly important effects are reduced activity of eNOS, a diminished

effect of released NO, and the presence of oxidative free radicals including advanced glycosylation end-products (AGEs). Summaries of mechanistic studies in humans and animal models, derived from the committee report of the Second International Consultation of Sexual Medicine (Saenz de Tejada et al, 2004), are shown in Tables 21–7 and 21–8.

Chronic Renal Failure. Sexual dysfunction has been reported in 20% to 50% of men with chronic renal failure (Carson and Patel, 1999). A cross-sectional study demonstrated a 45% prevalence of self-reported severe ED among men receiving hemodialysis (Rosas et al, 2001). The risk

Table 21–7. Summary Findings of Studies in Diabetic Patients

Focus	Finding
Anatomic	More atheromatic lesions in large vessels and stenosis in pudendal and iliac arteries
Functional	Decreased number and rigidity of nocturnal erections
	Lower penile rigidity after intracavernous injection of vasodilators
	High prevalence of penile arterial insufficiency studied with duplex ultrasonography
Cavernous tissue studies	
Ultrastructural	Decreased smooth muscle content, increased collagen, thickening of basal lamina, and loss of endothelial cells (more severe in men with diabetes)
Functional	Reduced endothelial and neurogenic NO-mediated penile smooth muscle relaxation but not nitroprusside-induced relaxation (suggesting impaired NO release or synthesis)
	Increased advanced glycation end products (AGEs) in cavernous tissue
	Contractile response to α-adrenergic agonist is higher in type 1 but not type 2 diabetics.
	In human penile arteries, EDHF-mediated endothelium-dependent relaxation is significantly reduced in penile resistance arteries from diabetic patients.
	Exposure to hyperglycemia induces increased expression of collagen, decreased proliferation, and increased programmed cell death (apoptosis). Expression of tumor necrosis factor α is also increased.
	Insulin is thought to enhance NOS activity by increasing transport of L-arginine into the cell and furnishing greater quantities of the essential cofactor NADPH. These effects are reversed in insulin deficiency or insulin resistance in diabetes.
	The inducible form (arginase II) of arginase, an enzyme that competes with NOS for the substrate L-arginine, is overexpressed in corpus cavernosum from diabetic patients, where inhibition of arginase restores NOS activity.

EDHF, endothelium-derived hyperpolarizing factor; NOS, nitric oxide synthase.

Table 21–8. Summary Findings of Studies in Diabetic Animal Models

Model	Finding
Streptozotocin-induced diabetic rats or mice	Increased activity of AC and GC, resulting in production of more cAMP and cGMP in response to PGE_1 and nitroprusside, respectively
	Decreased endothelial and neurogenic NO-mediated cavernous muscle relaxation
	Increased prostacyclin synthesis
	Increased cavernous muscle tone owing to upregulation of endothelin ETA receptors
	Increased contractile prostaglandins and free oxygen radicals in hyperglycemic state, resulting in reduced response to acetylcholine (reversed by indomethacin and antioxidants)
	Increased levels of oxygen free radicals and oxidative stress injury. Preventive treatment with an antioxidant prevented the appearance of endothelial dysfunction in cavernosal tissue; restorative treatment with same antioxidant only partially reversed the impairment of endothelium-dependent relaxation
	Increased glycated hemoglobin, which impairs endothelium-dependent relaxation in aorta and corpus cavernosum from diabetic rats. This effect is reversed by superoxide dismutase (SOD), the scavenger of superoxide anions
	Inhibition of AGE formation improves endothelium-dependent relaxation and restores erectile function in diabetic rats.
	Impaired responses attributable to endothelium-derived hyperpolarizing factor (EDHF) in the vasculature of diabetic animals.
	Plasma concentration and vascular content of L-arginine are reduced in diabetic rats
	NO-dependent selective nitrergic nerve degeneration in diabetes
Diabetic rabbit	Production of cAMP in response to PGE_1 or forskolin is reduced after 6 months but not 3 months
	Increased glucose-induced production of PKC mediated by oxidative stress in rabbit corpus cavernosum smooth muscle cells
	Oxidative stress interferes with endothelial function in diabetic erectile tissue. This is supported by the potentiating effect of SOD or the natural antioxidant vitamin E on endothelium-dependent relaxation of corpus cavernosum from rabbits

AC, adenylyl cyclase; AGE, advanced glycation end product; cAMP, cyclic adenosine monophosphate; cGMP, cyclic guanosine monophosphate; ETA, endothelin receptor; PGE_1, prostaglandin E_1; PKC, protein kinase C.

increased with age, diabetes, and nonuse of ACE inhibitors. Many of the effects of persistent uremia can potentially contribute to the development of ED, including disturbance of the hypothalamic-pituitary-testis sex hormone axis, hyperprolactinemia, accelerated atheromatous disease, and psychologic factors (Ayub and Fletcher, 2000).

Studies of the L-arginine–NO pathway in erythrocytes suggest that uremia decreases NO bioavailability (Mendes Ribeiro et al, 2001). These findings have stimulated experiments to determine the effect of chronic uremia on cavernous smooth muscle in animal models. In in vitro experiments with cavernous strips from rabbit, Bagcivan and coworkers (2003) found that a chronic uremic state resulted in impaired neural and endothelium-mediated relaxation of cavernous smooth muscle, while relaxation induced by NO donors was preserved. These findings suggest either decreased production or reduced bioavailability of endogenous NO (Bagcivan et al, 2003). In a similar set of experiments from the same laboratory, the investigators found no change in the cavernous relaxant response to activation of the purinergic system (Kilicarslan et al, 2002). In a rat model, an earlier paper related low serum levels of testosterone to low intratesticular levels of zinc in uremic animals and suggested this as a factor in sexual dysfunction (Ribeiro et al, 1982). A more recent study with this model suggested that deficiency of functional NO may result from oxidative stress, leading to inactivation of NO by oxygen radicals. Interestingly this effect was reversed by treatment with vitamin E, an antioxidant (Vaziri et al, 2002). Evidence from animal models of chronic uremia therefore suggests that a decrease in functional NO may be responsible for vascular side effects, including ED. Several putative mechanisms may lead to such a deficiency, such as reduced bioavailability of the NO substrate L-arginine, reduced expression of NOS isoforms in the relevant organs, rapid quenching of NO by reactive oxygen species known to be increased in chronic renal failure, and the accumulation of uremic inhibitors of NOS (Vaziri, 2001).

Evidence of autonomic neuropathy as a factor contributing to ED in men with chronic renal failure comes from three studies that found a high rate of abnormality in vascular and bulbocavernous reflexes, suggesting nerve dysfunction (Campese et al, 1982; Vita et al, 1999). The putative role of hyperprolactinemia and zinc deficiency as factors reducing sexual and reproductive function in men and women receiving dialysis prompted researchers to determine a mechanism. The results were conflicting, with one controlled trial finding no benefit of treatment with either a prolactin inhibitor or zinc (Rodger et al, 1989), whereas others found that treatment with erythropoietin (to reduce prolactin) (Schaffer, 1989) or with zinc supplements (Mahajan et al, 1982) improved sexual and reproductive function in patients with uremia. The significance of nonspecific factors related to a chronic disease state, such as depression and fatigue, was suggested by a case-control study that found similar rates of ED in age-matched men receiving renal replacement therapy and in those with rheumatoid arthritis and normal renal function (Toorians et al, 1997). Investigation of cavernous vascular function in 20 men undergoing renal replacement therapy showed that 80% had both arterial insufficiency and veno-occlusive dysfunction (Kaufman et al, 1994). Current knowledge would suggest that

this combination represents failure of sinusoidal relaxation owing to functional or structural alterations of cavernous smooth muscle. A link with possible impairment of the NO-cGMP pathway relating to failure of cavernous relaxation is provided by the finding of increased serum levels of endogenous inhibitors of NO synthesis in uremic patients (Vallance et al, 1992).

Patients with severe pulmonary disease often fear worsening dyspnea during sexual intercourse. Patients with angina, heart failure, or myocardial infarction can become impotent because of anxiety, depression, or arterial insufficiency. Other systemic diseases such as cirrhosis of the liver, scleroderma, chronic debilitation, and cachexia are also known to cause ED.

Primary Erectile Dysfunction

Primary ED refers to a lifelong inability to initiate or maintain erections, or both, beginning with the first sexual encounter. Although most cases owe to psychologic factors, a small number of afflicted men have a physical cause resulting from maldevelopment of the penis or the blood and nerve supply. Primary psychologic dysfunction is usually related to anxiety about sexual performance stemming from adverse childhood events, traumatic early sexual experience, or misinformation. Endocrine abnormalities, particularly low testosterone levels, may also be implicated in primary ED, although lowered sex drive is likely to be the main symptom. Evidence to support these concepts is confined to observation studies with varying numbers of cases. The largest study described 67 patients, of whom 10 (15%) had a predominantly psychologic cause (Stief et al, 1989). Those with physical abnormalities had a variety of neurologic, arterial, and veno-occlusive dysfunction.

Micropenis. Symmetrical hypoplasia of the phallus, micropenis, is often related to urethral developmental abnormalities, such as hypospadias and epispadias (Reilly and Woodhouse, 1989), or endocrine deficiency. The erectile tissue in such cases often functions normally; sexual dysfunction usually relates to lack of penile length or the degree of chordee rather than to ED (Woodhouse, 1998).

Vascular Abnormalities. Primary ED in the presence of an externally normal phallus is unusual. Authors have described structural abnormalities of the cavernous tissue, such as absence (Teloken et al, 1993) or replacement by fibrous tissue (Aboseif et al, 1992). Others have found vascular abnormalities, including hypoplasia of the cavernous arteries (Montague et al, 1995) or veno-occlusive dysfunction owing to aberrant cavernous venous drainage (Lue, 1999). The underlying cause of these congenital abnormalities is unknown. Treatment in most cases has been vascular surgery or implantation of a penile prosthesis.

PERSPECTIVES

The past two decades have seen a continuing explosion of new information on the physiology of penile erection and the pathophysiology of ED. These new discoveries not only enhance our understanding of the disease process but also provide a solid basis for improving our diagnosis and treatment. We can expect that the application of new research tools and information in molecular biology, signal transduction, growth factors, microarrays, and stem cells will bring the investigation of erectile function and dysfunction to an even higher level in the near future.

SUGGESTED READINGS

Andersson K-E, Wagner G: Physiology of penile erection. Physiol Rev 1995;75:191-236.

Droupy S, Hessel A, Benoit G, et al: Assessment of the functional role of accessory pudendal arteries in erection by transrectal color Doppler ultrasound. J Urol 1999;162:1987-1991.

Feldman HA, Goldstein I, Hatzichristou DG, et al: Impotence and its medical and psychosocial correlates: Results of the Massachusetts Male Aging Study. J Urol 1994;151:54-61.

Lewis RW, Fugl-Meyer KS, Bosch R, et al: Epidemiology/risk factors of sexual dysfunction. J Sexual Med 2004;1:35-39.

Lin CS, Xin ZC, Lin G, Lue TF: Phosphodiesterases as therapeutic targets. Urology 2003;61:685-691.

Lizza EF, Rosen RC: Definition and classification of erectile dysfunction: Report of the Nomenclature Committee of the International Society of Impotence Research. Int J Impot Res 1999;11:141-143.

Lue TF: Erectile dysfunction. N Engl J Med 2000;342:1802-1813.

Mouras H, Stoleru S, Bittoun J, et al: Brain processing of visual sexual stimuli in healthy men: A functional magnetic resonance imaging study. Neuroimage 2003;20:855-869.

Saenz de Tejada I, Angulo J, Cellek S, et al: Physiology of erection and pathophysiology of erectile dysfunction. In Lue TF, Basson R, Rosen R, et al (eds): Sexual Medicine: Sexual Dysfunctions in Men and Women. Paris, Health Publications, 2004, pp 287-344.

Spektor M, Rodriguez R, Rosenbaum RS, et al: Potassium channels and human corporeal smooth muscle cell tone: Further evidence of the physiological relevance of the maxi-K channel subtype to the regulation of human corporeal smooth muscle tone in vitro. J Urol 2002;167:2628-2635.

KEY POINTS: PATHOPHYSIOLOGY

- The prevalence of ED increases with age and concomitant medical diseases. The incidence is about 25 to 30 cases per thousand person-years.
- ED is a symptom of many underlying conditions and diseases.
- Any condition that affects penile nerve, artery, endothelium, smooth muscle, or tunica albuginea can cause ED.
- Endothelial dysfunction seems to be a common final pathway to ED in patients with hyperlipidemia, diabetes mellitus, hypertension, and chronic renal failure.
- Drugs most commonly associated with ED include antiandrogens, antidepressants, and antihypertensives.

22 Evaluation and Nonsurgical Management of Erectile Dysfunction and Premature Ejaculation

TOM F. LUE, MD • GREGORY A. BRODERICK, MD

PATIENT-CENTERED EVALUATION

EVALUATION OF THE COMPLEX PATIENT

NONSURGICAL MANAGEMENT OF ERECTILE DYSFUNCTION

FUTURE RESEARCH

PREMATURE EJACULATION

PATIENT-CENTERED EVALUATION

The management of erectile dysfunction (ED) has changed in almost every decade since the 1970s (Table 22–1) thanks to the introduction of new diagnostic tests and the successful launch of less-invasive but highly effective therapies. As a result, the health care professional most frequently consulted has also changed from the psychologist to the urologist and, with the introduction of phosphodiesterase inhibitors, to primary care physicians.

In the era when the treatment of ED consisted of the penile prosthesis and psychotherapy, nocturnal penile tumescence monitoring in a sleep laboratory and the penile brachial pressure index were the available tests required for differential diagnosis so that a penile prosthesis would not be wrongly implanted in the patient with "psychogenic" ED. The era of penile injection brought about refined tests such as duplex ultrasonography and pharmacologic cavernosometry and cavernosography for penile vascular function. The RigiScan (Endocare, Inc., Irvine, CA), a computerized device for monitoring penile tumescence and rigidity, was developed for outpatient test. The widespread use and abuse of these tests led to the introduction of a **goal-directed approach,** devised to conserve health care dollars and minimize patient morbidity

from excessive testing (Lue, 1990). The goal-directed approach was introduced when urologists were the main health care providers for patients with ED. **Evaluation was based on a thorough medical and psychosexual history and a focused physical examination and on laboratory testing. It emphasized the role of patient education and dialogue and the need to consider the patient's goals and motivation in making diagnostic and treatment decisions.**

The first worldwide effort in ED evaluation and management was the First International Consultation on Erectile Dysfunction, convened in Paris in July of 1999, and co-sponsored by, among others, the World Health Organization, International Consultation on Urological Diseases, American Urological Association, and Société Internationale d'Urologie. Recommendations, the work of 18 focused committees, were peer reviewed through open presentation and commentary and published in 2000. ED was redefined as the consistent or recurrent inability to attain and/or maintain penile erection sufficient for sexual performance (Jardin et al, 2000). The evaluation and treatment algorithms were similar to those in the goal-directed approach; treatment options were also updated. The consultants emphasized that ED is a symptom of many underlying medical conditions and that treatment requires the direct involvement of a physician. The use of the Internet to prescribe therapy should be condemned because it fails to meet the requirement of physician-patient contact in all cases.

Four years later, the Second International Consultation on Sexual Medicine (ICSM) made additional recommendations. This approach to the management of ED is built on a **patient-centered and evidence-based principle** (Rosen et al, 2004a). **Traditionally, the dominant model in medicine has been the "disease-centered" approach, in which the patient maintains a passive role. In contrast, patient-centered care is "an approach that consciously adopts the patient's perspective" and respects his or her ideas, expectations, and values, as "the physician tries to enter the patient's world, to see the illness through the patient's eyes"** (Geirteis et al, 1993).

Table 22–1.	Evolution in the Diagnostic Workup for ED	
	Main Treatments	**Diagnostic Tests**
Before 1970	Psychosexual therapy	Psychosexual history
1970s	Penile prosthesis and psychosexual therapy	Medical and psychosexual history, sleep lab
1980s	Yohimbine, intracavernous or transurethral therapy, vacuum device	History, physical examination, testosterone, duplex ultrasound, DICC (goal-directed approach)
1990s–Present	Oral phosphodiesterase-5 inhibitors	Process-of-care model 1st ICUD algorithm 2nd ICUD algorithm (patient-centered approach)

DICC, dynamic infusion cavernosometry and cavernosography.
ICUD, International Consultation on Urological Diseases.

Patient-centered medicine assumes a holistic approach that takes into account not only the biologic dimension of disease but also its psychologic and social implications, in accordance with the definition of health of the World Health Organization (WHO Preamble, 1946).

Evidence-based evaluation implies that patients, as well as physicians, should be guided in their decision-making by the findings from controlled research. Because available treatments and diagnostic approaches for sexual dysfunction are evolving, the patient should be given every opportunity to choose among available options and to determine which best fits his individual needs. Patients vary also in their preference for information and involvement in the decision-making process, and for this reason the approach should be flexible and individualized.

In each case strong consideration should be given to the evidence basis for diagnostic evaluation. Costly or invasive procedures should not be recommended in the absence of supporting evidence of their specific applicability. The algorithms recommended by the ICSM for the diagnosis and treatment of ED are shown in Figures 22–1 and 22–2 (Lue et al, 2004).

Questionnaires and Sexual Function Symptom Scores

Many male sexual function profiles and ED questionnaires have been developed (Fineman and Rettinger, 1991; Geisser et al, 1993; Speckens et al, 1993; Corty et al, 1996). Formerly, the aim of these detailed questionnaires was to differentiate psychogenic from nonpsychogenic ED. More recently, a variety of self-report measures for assessing the levels of male sexual function or dysfunction have been described; self-administered questionnaires (SAQs) have seen their greatest use in clinical trials. SAQs provide quantifiable efficacy endpoints for new drug trials; they attempt to quantify sexual interest, performance, and satisfaction. **Those most commonly referenced include the International Index of Erectile Function (IIEF) by Rosen and associates** (1997), **the Brief Male Sexual Function Inventory (BMSFI) by O'Leary and colleagues** (1995), **and the Dysfunction Inventory for Treatment Satisfaction (EDITS) by Althof and associates** (1999). Other self-report measures include the Derogatis Sexual Function Inventory (245 items) (Derogatis and Melisaratos, 1979), the Center for Marital and Sexual Health Questionnaire (18 items) (Glick et al, 1997), and the recently added Male Sexual Function Scale (Rosen R, personal communication).

The BMSFI instrument covers sexual drive (2 items), erection (3 items), ejaculation (2 items), perceptions of problems in each area (3 items), and overall satisfaction (1 item). The EDITS questionnaire is very useful in drug studies; it supplies efficacy endpoints that permit companies to tabulate pre- and post-treatment responses in ways that, although subjectively based, provide quantifiable data for U.S. Food and Drug Administration (FDA) reviews. Ultimately, in the clinic,

ALGORITHM FOR DIAGNOSTIC EVALUATION OF ED

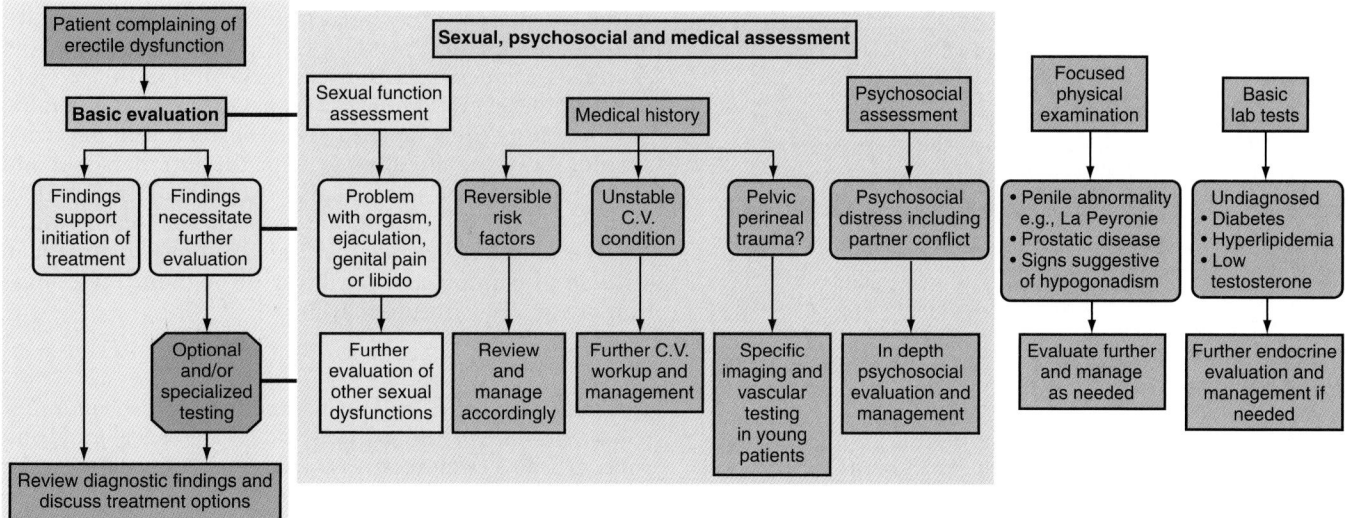

Figure 22–1. Diagnostic algorithm for ED recommended by the ICSM.

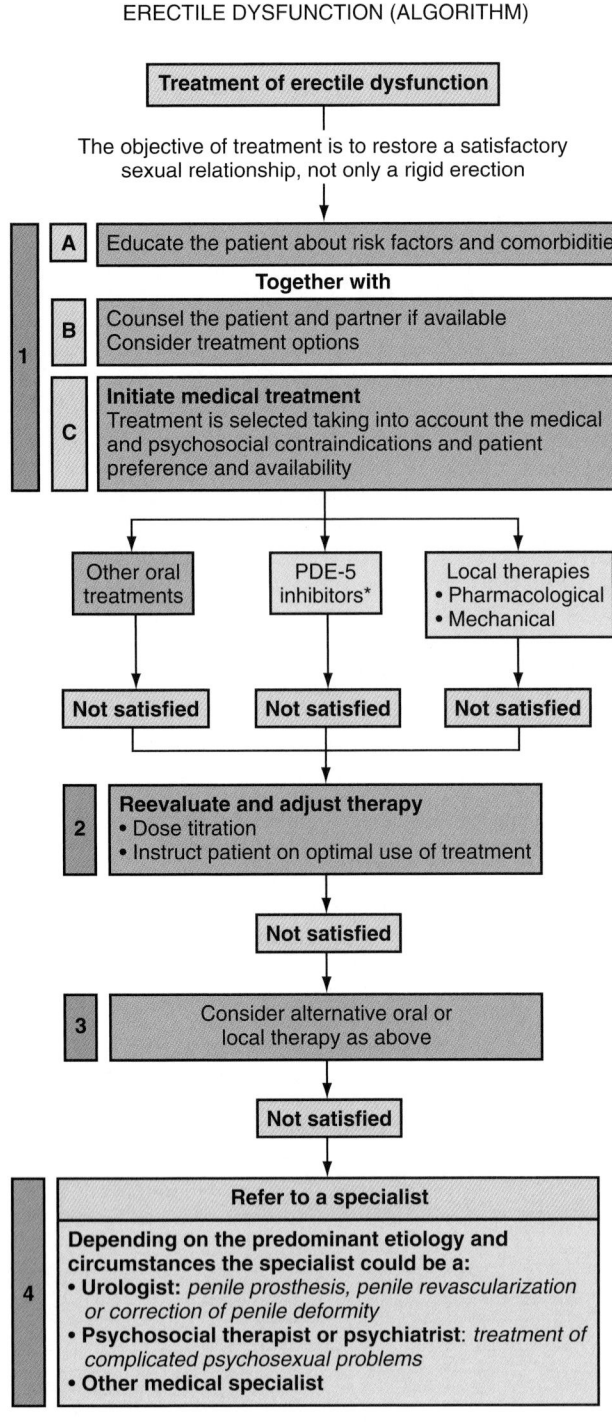

TREATMENT STRATEGY OF
ERECTILE DYSFUNCTION (ALGORITHM)

Treatment of erectile dysfunction

The objective of treatment is to restore a satisfactory
sexual relationship, not only a rigid erection

1

A Educate the patient about risk factors and comorbidities

Together with

B Counsel the patient and partner if available
Consider treatment options

C **Initiate medical treatment**
Treatment is selected taking into account the medical
and psychosocial contraindications and patient
preference and availability

| Other oral treatments | PDE-5 inhibitors* | Local therapies • Pharmacological • Mechanical |

Not satisfied · **Not satisfied** · **Not satisfied**

2 **Reevaluate and adjust therapy**
• Dose titration
• Instruct patient on optimal use of treatment

Not satisfied

3 Consider alternative oral or
local therapy as above

Not satisfied

4 **Refer to a specialist**
**Depending on the predominant etiology and
circumstances the specialist could be a:**
• **Urologist:** *penile prosthesis, penile revascularization
or correction of penile deformity*
• **Psychosocial therapist or psychiatrist:** *treatment of
complicated psychosexual problems*
• **Other medical specialist**

**PDE-5 inhibitors are the preferred treatment option in the large
majority of patients*

Figure 22–2. Treatment algorithm for ED recommended by the ICSM.

satisfaction rates are established by prescription refills, dropouts, and requests for further evaluation.

The IIEF is the most widely used SAQ, and it is statistically validated in many languages. Its 15 items address and quantify five domains: erectile function, orgasmic function, sexual desire, intercourse satisfaction, and overall satisfaction (Fig. 22–3) (Rosen et al, 1997).

In the hope of providing physicians with a "checklist" on erectile function that could be used in an office setting, an abridged 5-item version of the IIEF-15 has been developed (Rosen et al, 1999), in which 4 items are taken from the erectile function domain. The fifth item addresses sexual intercourse satisfaction; it was chosen to reflect the central element in the NIH Consensus Panel (1992) definition of ED, which ties erectile function to satisfaction: "maintain erection of sufficient rigidity and duration to permit satisfactory sexual performance." **Perhaps the most important difference between the IIEF-15 and the IIEF-5 is that the latter asks patients to self-assess erectile function and satisfaction over the past 6 months, a more clinically relevant and practical time frame than 4 weeks. ED severity is classified into five categories based on the IIEF-5: severe (5 to 7), moderate (8 to 11), mild to moderate (12 to 16), mild (17 to 21), and no ED (22 to 25).**

The Male Sexual Function Scale (Fig. 22–4) was developed in conjunction with the Second International Consultation on Sexual Dysfunction (Lue et al, 2004) and is based on qualitative research in normal and sexually dysfunctional men and assesses core components of male sexual function (desire, erection, ejaculation, satisfaction) in both clinical and research settings. The scale was designed by an independent advisory board of experts in male sexuality, without involvement or funding from industry. This new screening tool is suitable for use in both primary care and urology practice settings and may be valuable in screening patients for sexual dysfunction after pelvic surgery or with chronic illness or medications.

One major drawback of sexual inventories is their reliance on self-assessment. Blander and coworkers (1999) have demonstrated that SAQs do not differentiate among the various causes of ED (arterial, venous, or mixed vascular), and evidence-based assessments (diagnostic tests) are still necessary in patients with complex ED. **Therefore, in clinical evaluation, a good case history, preferably taken from both partners, physical examination, and proper laboratory studies still form the cornerstone in the evaluation of ED.**

Medical, Sexual, and Psychosocial History

Initial assessment of a sexual problem includes a detailed medical, sexual, and psychosocial history. Although brief checklists or questionnaires may be helpful in the recognition and initial evaluation of a sexual problem, they should not substitute for a detailed sexual history. The physician should always be attentive to both the intrapersonal and interpersonal aspects of sexual dysfunction. Careful attention should be paid to both the style and the content of the initial evaluation. Overall, the clinician should maintain an attitude of comfort and flexibility throughout the evaluation process (Rosen et al, 2004a).

Medical History

The examiner begins with a medical history, explaining the risk factors for ED, before directly addressing sexual problems; patients will feel more at ease talking about cardiovascular health and providing a list of medications.

The goals of medical history-taking are (1) to evaluate the potential role of underlying medical conditions (e.g.,

Patient Name: _____ MR#: _____ Date: _____

OVER THE PAST 4 WEEKS

1. How often were you able to get an erection during sexual activity?
   0 = No sexual activity
   1 = Almost never/never
   2 = A few times (much less than half the time)
   3 = Sometimes (about half the time)
   4 = Most times (much more than half the time)
   5 = Almost always/always

2. When you had erections with sexual stimulation, how often were your erections hard enough for penetration?
   0 = No sexual activity
   1 = Almost never/never
   2 = A few times (much less than half the time)
   3 = Sometimes (about half the time)
   4 = Most times (much more than half the time)
   5 = Almost always/always

3. When you attempted sexual intercourse, how often were you able to penetrate (enter)?
   0 = Did not attempt intercourse
   1 = Almost never/never
   2 = A few times (much less than half the time)
   3 = Sometimes (about half the time)
   4 = Most times (much more than half the time)
   5 = Almost always/always

4. During sexual intercourse, <u>how often</u> were you able to maintain your erection after you had penetrated (entered) you partner?
   0 = Did not attempt intercourse
   1 = Almost never/never
   2 = A few times (much less than half the time)
   3 = Sometimes (about half the time)
   4 = Most times (much more than half the time)
   5 = Almost always/always

5. During sexual intercourse, <u>how difficult</u> was it to maintain your erection to complete intercourse?
   0 = Did not attempt intercourse
   1 = Extremely difficult
   2 = Very difficult
   3 = Difficult
   4 = Slightly difficult
   5 = Not difficult

6. How many times have you attempted sexual intercourse?
   0 = No attempts
   1 = One to two attempts
   2 = Three to four attempts
   3 = Five to six attempts
   4 = Seven to ten attempts
   5 = Eleven or more attempts

7. When you attempted sexual intercourse, how often was it satisfactory to you?
   0 = Did not attempt intercourse
   1 = Almost never/never
   2 = A few times (much less than half the time)
   3 = Sometimes (about half the time)
   4 = Most times (much more than half the time)
   5 = Almost always/always

8. How much have you enjoyed sexual intercourse?
   0 = No intercourse
   1 = No enjoyment
   2 = Not very enjoyable
   3 = Fairly enjoyable
   4 = Highly enjoyable
   5 = Very highly enjoyable

9. When you had sexual stimulation or intercourse, how often did you ejaculate?
   0 = No sexual stimulation/intercourse
   1 = Almost never/never
   2 = A few times (much less than half the time)
   3 = Sometimes (about half the time)
   4 = Most times (much more than half the time)
   5 = Almost always/always

10. When you had sexual stimulation or intercourse, how often did you have the feeling of orgasm or climax?
    0 = No sexual stimulation/intercourse
    1 = Almost never/never
    2 = A few times (much less than half the time)
    3 = Sometimes (about half the time)
    4 = Most times (much more than half the time)
    5 = Almost always/always

11. How often have you felt sexual desire?
    1 = Almost never/never
    2 = A few times (much less than half the time)
    3 = Sometimes (about half the time)
    4 = Most times (much more than half the time)
    5 = Almost always/always

12. How would you rate your level of sexual desire?
    1 = Very low/none at all
    2 = Low
    3 = Moderate
    4 = High
    5 = Very high

13. How satisfied have you been with your overall <u>sex life</u>?
    1 = Very dissatisfied
    2 = Moderately dissatisfied
    3 = About equally satisfied and dissatisfied
    4 = Moderately satisfied
    5 = Very satisfied

14. How satisfied have you been with your <u>sexual relationship</u> with your partner?
    1 = Very dissatisfied
    2 = Moderately dissatisfied
    3 = About equally satisfied and dissatisfied
    4 = Moderately satisfied
    5 = Very satisfied

15. How do you rate your <u>confidence</u> that you could get and keep an erection?
    1 = Very low
    2 = Low
    3 = Moderate
    4 = High
    5 = Very high

Figure 22–3. International Index of Erectile Function Questionnaire.

Name: _____   Date: _____

Please answer the following questions about your sexual function in the <u>PAST 3 MONTHS</u>.

1a. Do you get erections? (please check one response)

yes, with normal stiffness	☐
yes, with reduced stiffness	☐
yes, with severely reduced stiffness	☐
no, erection not possible	☐

1b. How bothered or trouble are you by this? (please circle one response)
Please circle a number between 1 (not at all bothered) and 5 (extremely bothered)

1	2	3	4	5
not at all bothered		moderately bothered		extremely bothered

2a. Do you maintain your erection during sexual activity? (please check one response)

yes	☐
yes, but not every time	☐
yes, but only occasionally	☐
no, never able to maintain the erection	☐

2b. How bothered or troubled are you by this? (please circle one response)
Please circle a number between 1 (not at all bothered) and 5 (extremely bothered)

1	2	3	4	5
not at all bothered		moderately bothered		extremely bothered

Please answer the following questions about your ejaculations in the <u>PAST 3 MONTHS</u>.

3a. Are you able to <u>ejaculate</u> during sexual activity? (please check one response)

yes, every time	☐
yes, but not every time	☐
yes, but only occasionally	☐
no, ejaculation not possible	☐

3b. How bothered or troubled are you by this? (please circle one response)
Please circle a number between 1 (not at all bothered) and 5 (extremely bothered)

1	2	3	4	5
not at all bothered		moderately bothered		extremely bothered

4a. Does it take you longer than you wish to <u>ejaculate</u>? (please check one response)

no	☐
yes, but only occasionally	☐
yes, on most occasions	☐
yes, hardly ever able to ejaculate	☐
I do not ejaculate	☐

4b. How bothered or troubled are you by this? (please circle one response)
Please circle a number between 1 (not at all bothered) and 5 (extremely bothered)

1	2	3	4	5
not at all bothered		moderately bothered		extremely bothered

5a. Do you ejaculate too quickly? (please check one response)

no	☐
yes, but only occasionally	☐
yes, on most occasions	☐
yes, I always ejaculate too quickly	☐
I do not ejaculate	☐

5b. How bothered or troubled are you by this? (please circle one response)
Please circle a number between 1 (not at all bothered) and 5 (extremely bothered)

1	2	3	4	5
not at all bothered		moderately bothered		extremely bothered

Figure 22–4. Male sexual function scale.

Sexual desire is the wish or urge to engage in sexual activities.
Please answer the following questions about your sexual desire in the PAST 3 MONTHS.

6a. **How strong is your sexual desire? (please check one response)**

as strong as I would like ☐
less than I would like ☐
much less than I would like ☐
no desire at all ☐

6b. **How bothered or troubled are you by this? (please circle one response)**
Please circle a number between 1 (not at all bothered) and 5 (extremely bothered)

1	2	3	4	5
not at all bothered		moderately bothered		extremely bothered

7. **Overall, are you satisfied with your sexual activity? (please check one response)**

yes, very satisfied ☐
yes, moderately satisfied ☐
no, moderately dissatisfied ☐
no, very dissatisfied ☐

8. **Overall, how distressed by sexual problems or lack of sex have you been during the past 3 months? (please check one response)**

very much ☐
a moderate amount ☐
a slight amount ☐
very little ☐
not at all ☐

Figure 22–4, cont'd. Male sexual function scale.

atherosclerosis, diabetes) and comorbidities (e.g., depression); (2) to differentiate between potential organic and psychogenic causes (Table 22–2); and (3) to assess the potential role of medication (e.g., some may cause or contribute to the patient's sexual difficulties and some, such as nitrates, may be contraindications for specific treatments, such as phosphodiesterase inhibitors).

A patient's past surgical history may similarly yield insights. Radical pelvic surgery (e.g., prostatectomy, abdominoperineal resection) and pelvic trauma are well known to be associated with ED (Armenakas et al, 1993; Walsh et al, 1994).

Sexual History

A comprehensive sexual history is essential to confirm the diagnosis, as well as to evaluate the patient's overall sexual function. Ideally, the interview should be conducted face-to-face. Attention should be paid to the setting, in particular the need for privacy and confidentiality, and the clinician should make every effort to ensure patient trust, comfort, and openness.

The objective is to elicit the sexual history in a nonthreatening and permissive manner. The doctor and patient should have the opportunity to discuss matters privately, but interviewing the partner for corroboration of the history and assessment of mutual goals is no less important. If the patient presents with his partner, this goal is easily achieved; the physician may take the opportunity of the physical examination to inquire in private whether the patient has other specific concerns he was unwilling to share in the presence of his partner.

Sexual history-taking should be aimed at ascertaining the severity, onset, and duration of the problem, as well as the presence of concomitant medical or psychosocial factors. It

Table 22–2. Differentiation between Psychogenic and Organic ED

Characteristic	Organic	Psychogenic
Onset	Gradual	Acute
Circumstances	Global	Situational
Course	Constant	Varying
Noncoital erection	Poor	Rigid
Psychosexual problem	Secondary	Long history
Partner problem	Secondary	At onset
Anxiety and fear	Secondary	Primary

Modified from Hengeveld MW: Erectile disorder: A psychosexological review. In Jonas U, Thon WF, Stief CG (eds): Erectile Dysfunction. Berlin, Springer-Verlag, 1991.

is necessary to determine whether the presenting complaint (e.g., ED, premature ejaculation) is the primary sexual problem or if some other aspects of the sexual response cycle (desire, ejaculation, orgasm) are involved (Rosen et al, 2004a).

Psychosocial History

A detailed psychosocial assessment is essential. Given the interpersonal context of sexual problems, the physician should carefully assess the patient's past and present partner relationships. **Sexual dysfunction may affect the patient's self-esteem and coping ability, as well as social relationships and occupational performance.** The physician should not assume that every patient is involved in a monogamous, heterosexual relationship. In addition, questions should be asked about other relevant aspects of the patient's life, including interpersonal relationships, occupational status, financial security, family life, and social support.

In many cases, organic and psychogenic factors often coexist, particularly in individuals or couples with long-standing or chronic sexual dysfunction. Table 22–2 provides an overview of specific aspects of the patient's history that may be useful in differentiating organic from psychogenic ED (Hengeveld, 1991).

Physical Examination

The physical examination is an essential component of sexual dysfunction evaluation, although in most cases it may not identify the specific cause. It should include a general screening for medical risk factors or comorbidities, such as body habitus (secondary sexual characteristics), and an assessment of the cardiovascular, neurologic, and genital systems, with particular focus on the genitalia and secondary sex characteristics. Evaluation of sexual and genital development may occasionally reveal an obvious cause (e.g., micropenis, chordee, Peyronie's plaque). Patients with certain genetic syndromes, such as Kallmann's or Klinefelter's, may present with obvious physical signs of hypogonadism or a distinctive body habitus. Patients with degenerative neurologic disorders or diabetes may show evidence of peripheral neuropathy. Testing for genital and perineal sensation and the bulbocavernosus reflex (BCR) is also useful in assessing possible neurogenic impotence (Rosen et al, 2004a).

Laboratory Testing

Recommended laboratory tests for men with sexual problems typically include fasting glucose, lipids, and hormonal profiles. These tests are performed primarily to identify or confirm specific causes (e.g., hypogonadism) or to assess the role of medical comorbidities or concomitant illnesses (e.g., diabetes, hyperlipidemia).

The laboratory investigation may identify treatable conditions or previously undetected medical illnesses that may contribute directly to ED. Additional laboratory tests (e.g., thyroid function) may be performed at the discretion of the physician based on the medical history and clinician's judgment. Prostate-specific antigen (PSA) may be measured in patients over 50 or in those with a family history of prostate cancer. Furthermore, from the standpoint of ED management, a PSA should be obtained if hormonal replacement therapy is planned (Rosen et al, 2004a).

Review of Findings and Physician/Patient Dialogue

Results of the initial evaluation should be reviewed with the patient, and partner if available, before initiating therapy. This review should be used as an opportunity to educate patients on the anatomy and physiology of sexual function and to provide appropriate understanding of the pathophysiology. Potentially modifiable risk factors, such as stress, marital conflict, cigarette smoking, alcohol abuse, obesity, and bicycle riding, should be addressed. The potential role of prescription or nonprescription drugs, including psychotropic and cardiovascular agents, or other iatrogenic causes of sexual dysfunction should be discussed (Rosen et al, 2004a).

Shared Decision-Making and Treatment Planning

In accordance with the principle of patient-centered medicine, after the initial diagnostic evaluation patients (and partners where possible) should be given a detailed description of the available treatment options (Table 22–3). These should include both medical and nonmedical options, whenever indicated. Some patients may prefer no treatment or further consideration before selecting a specific option. Additionally, some patients may wish to consult with their partner or another health care provider. In each case, these options should be respected and encouraged, if appropriate. It is important for the clinician not to assume an authoritarian or patriarchal role in the selection (or rejection) of specific treatment options. Instead, the clinician should aim to educate the patient as fully as possible, making full use of evidence-based literature and guidelines regarding the risks and benefits of each treatment. The clinician should provide a supportive and empathic environment for shared decision-making (Rosen et al, 2004a).

Specialist Consultation and Referral

With the advent of effective oral treatment for ED, primary care practitioners currently manage the majority of cases of male sexual dysfunction. However, either the patient or primary care physician may wish to consult a specialist (e.g.,

Table 22–3. **Treatment Options for ED: Costs, Advantages, and Disadvantages**			
Treatment	*Cost ($)*	*Advantages*	*Disadvantages/Side Effects*
Counseling	500-2000	Noninvasive; resolves conflict	High recurrence rate of ED
Oral drugs (phosphodiesterase inhibitors)	10/pill	Noninvasive; 60%-70% efficacy	Systemic side effects; nitrate contraindications
Vacuum devices	200-550	Minimally invasive	Unnatural erection; absence of spontaneity; petechiae, pain; cold penis
Intracavernous injection	40-200/mo	90% efficacy	More invasive; priapism, fibrosis, pain
Prosthesis	20,000-30,000	High success rate	Requires surgery, anesthesia; infection, fibrosis
Vascular surgery	15,000-30,000	Restores natural erection	Low efficacy of venous surgery; arterial bypass limited to select patients; requires anesthesia and extensive workup

cardiologist, endocrinologist, psychologist, or urologist) for further diagnostic evaluation. In accordance with the principles of patient-centered medicine, patients (and partners where possible) should be included in the decision-making; they should be fully informed of the cost and potential risks of additional procedures, as well as the potential benefits and evidence basis supporting their use.

Follow-Up Strategy

Regardless of the treatment option chosen, follow-up is essential to ensure the best treatment outcome. Monitoring adverse events, assessing satisfaction or outcome associated with a given treatment, determining whether the partner may also suffer from a sexual dysfunction, and assessing overall health and psychosocial function are important aspects of follow-up. Consideration should also be given to whether an alteration in dose or treatment might be of value.

In patients who do not respond to so-called first-line treatments (e.g., oral therapy), second- and third-line options should always be considered, because most of these treatments have demonstrated reasonable response and satisfaction rates in controlled studies (Rosen et al, 2004a).

EVALUATION OF THE COMPLEX PATIENT

Advances in the understanding of erectile physiology and improvements in technology have greatly increased our ability to define the many types of impotence (neurogenic, psychogenic, and vasculogenic). The goal of specialized evaluation is to define the cause of ED. Generally in medicine a specific diagnosis is needed to formulate a treatment plan; in most cases of ED this can be done without extensive testing. However, in the absence of diagnostic testing, efficacy and satisfaction with treatment become a matter of chance. Generally accepted indications for specialized evaluation are failure of initial treatment, Peyronie's disease, primary ED, history of pelvic/perineal trauma, cases requiring vascular or neurosurgical intervention, complicated endocrinopathy, complicated psychiatric disorder, complex relationship problems, and medicolegal concerns. Table 22–4 summarizes the most frequently used evidence-based procedures for diagnostic evaluation of ED (Rosen et al, 2004a).

Vascular Evaluation

Vascular evaluation is aimed at diagnosis of arterial and veno-occlusive dysfunction. At least a decade of experience is available with several tests: combined intracavernous injection and stimulation (CIS), duplex ultrasound, dynamic infusion cavernosometry and cavernosography (DICC), and selective penile angiography. Specialized vascular testing is aimed at identifying and quantifying arterial and veno-occlusive erectile function.

First-Line Evaluation of Penile Blood Flow

Combined Intracavernous Injection and Stimulation. A CIS test consists of intracavernous injection of a vasodilator

Table 22–4. **Evidence-Based Tests for Organic ED and Recommendations**	
Test	Recommendation*
Vascular	
Dynamic infusion cavernosometry and cavernosography (DICC)	B
Intracavernous injection pharmacotesting (ICI)	B
ICI and color duplex ultrasound	B
Arteriography	C
CT angiography	D
MRI	D
Infrared spectrophotometry	D
Radioisotope penography	D
Audiovisual Sexual Stimulation (AVSS)	
Independent or jointly with vascular testing	C
With or without: pharmacologic stimulation (oral, ICI)	C
Neurophysiologic	
Nocturnal penile tumescence and rigidity (NPTR)	B
Erectiometer/rigidometer	D
Biothesiometry (vibratory thresholds)	C
Dorsal nerve conduction velocity	C
Bulbocavernosus reflex latency	B
Plethysmography/electrobioimpedance	D
Corpus cavernosum electromyography (CC-EMG)	C
MRI or PET scanning of brain (during AVSS)	D

*Grades of Recommendation
A: At least one meta-analysis, systematic review, or randomized controlled trial with a very low level of bias and directly applicable to the target population.
B: A body of evidence including high-quality systematic reviews of case-control or cohort studies directly applicable to the target population and demonstrating overall consistency of results.
C: A body of evidence including well-conducted case-control or cohort studies with a low risk of confounding, bias, or chance and a moderate probability that the relationship is causal, directly applicable to the target population, with overall consistency of results.
D: Nonanalytic studies (e.g., case reports, case series, and expert opinion).
Modified from Rosen RC, Hatzichristou D, Broderick G, et al: Clinical evaluation and symptom scales: Sexual dysfunction assessment in men. In Lue TF, Basson R, Rosen R, et al (eds): Sexual Medicine: Sexual Dysfunctions in Men and Women. Paris, Health Publications, 2004, pp 173-220; and Harbour R, Miller J: A new system for grading recommendations in evidence-based guidelines. BMJ 2001;323:334-336.

or a combination of two or three vasodilators, genital or audiovisual sexual stimulation, and assessment of the erection by an observer (Donatucci and Lue, 1992; Katlowitz et al, 1993). **This screening test is the most commonly performed diagnostic procedure for ED. It allows the clinician to bypass neurologic and hormonal influences and to evaluate the vascular status of the penis directly and objectively.**

Several vasodilators have been used, including alprostadil alone (Caverject or Edex, 10 to 20 μg), a combination of papaverine and phentolamine (Bimix, 0.3 mL), or a mixture of all three of these agents (Trimix, 0.3 mL). The technique involves injecting the medication through a $^5/_8$-inch needle (27 to 29 gauge) into the corpus cavernosum. The needle site is compressed manually for 5 minutes to prevent hematoma formation. The erectile response is periodically evaluated for both rigidity and duration. In our practice, 0.3 mL of Bimix solution is routinely used because the incidence of painful erections is lower than with alprostadil (a common complaint in patients after radical prostatectomy or cystectomy). A second injection of 0.3 mL of Trimix solution may be given if the erectile response is poor.

Comparison with other hemodynamic tests suggests a normal CIS response is associated with normal venous occlusion. However, results may be false negative in as many as 20% of patients with borderline arterial inflow (when normal is defined as >35 cm/s peak systolic flow on duplex ultrasound and borderline is defined as 25 to 35 cm/s) (Pescatori et al, 1994). False-positive findings occur most commonly because of patient anxiety, needle phobia, or inadequate dosage.

Before injection, the patient should be informed about the purpose, alternatives, risks, and benefits of the test. He should not leave the office until the penis becomes flaccid spontaneously or by injection of a diluted phenylephrine solution (500 µg/mL, given 1 mL every 3 to 5 minutes until detumescence). With this approach, only five patients in 20 years have developed priapism and needed to return to the clinic for further treatment.

Second-Line Evaluation of Penile Blood Flow

Duplex Ultrasonography (Gray Scale or Color-Coded). When further diagnostic testing is indicated in the evaluation of the complex patient, **the penile blood flow study, which consists of CIS and blood flow measurement by duplex ultrasound, is the most reliable and least invasive evidence-based assessment of ED.** In color-coded duplex ultrasound, the direction of the blood flow is designated with red (toward the probe) or blue (away from the probe), making the identification of the vessels and recording of blood flow easier (Broderick and Arger, 1993; Herbner et al, 1994; Landwehr, 1995). Duplex ultrasound consists of high-resolution (7 to 10 MHz) real-time ultrasonography and color pulsed Doppler, which enables the ultrasonographer to visualize the dorsal and cavernous arteries selectively and to perform dynamic blood flow analysis (Fig. 22–5). **It is also the best tool available for the diagnosis of high-flow priapism and localization of a ruptured artery** (Fig. 22–6).

Flow velocities should be measured 5 to 10 minutes after injection; a delayed response is typical in both the hypertensive and the anxious patient; a rapid response is typical in young neurogenic patients. Erectile quality should be rated each time a set of Doppler parameters is recorded. Each main cavernous artery (and dorsal artery, if desired) is individually assessed. Cavernous arterial diameters may be recorded. The presence of a communication between the paired cavernous arteries or between the dorsal and the cavernous arteries should be noted. Asymmetrical cavernous arterial flows greater than 10 cm/s or reversal of flow across a collateral may indicate a significant atherosclerotic lesion (Benson et al, 1993). In some patients, anxiety or fear of injection can lead to a poor erection; therefore, scanning should be repeated after stimulation and, if necessary, after redosing as described in the CIS test.

A portable Doppler unit has been introduced to evaluate penile blood flow in the urologist's office. The Midus pulsed Doppler unit records the Doppler waveform of the cavernous arteries without providing a real-time ultrasound image; it is based on a laptop computer design (UroMetrics, Anoka, MN). Cavernous arterial flow is studied in a fashion similar to that with duplex ultrasound. Two independent groups have vali-

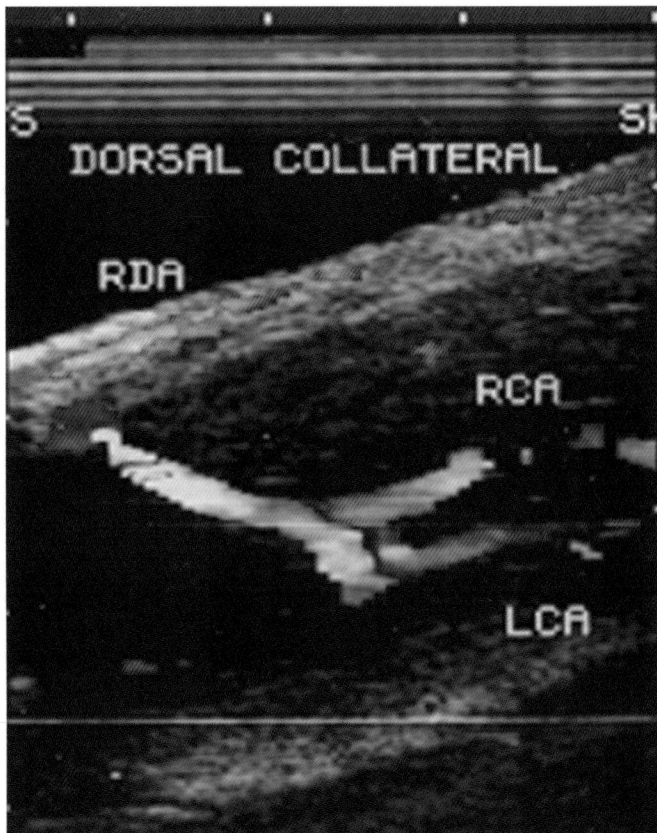

Figure 22–5. Collateral circulation connecting the right dorsal artery (RDA) to the right cavernous artery (RCA) and the left cavernous artery (LCA) is shown by color duplex ultrasound in a longitudinal view.

dated its reliability when compared with duplex ultrasound (Lee and Melman, 1999; Metro and Broderick, 1999).

Doppler Waveform Analysis. Schwartz and coworkers (1991) correlated changes in Doppler waveforms with hemodynamic changes in corporeal pressure during progression to full erection. In the filling phase when sinusoidal resistance is low (within 5 minutes after vasoactive injection), the waveform is characterized by high forward flow during both systole and diastole (Fig. 22–7). As intracavernous pressure increases, diastolic velocities decrease; with full erection, the systolic waveforms sharply peak and may be slightly less than during full tumescence; in rigid erection, diastolic flow may be zero or reversed when intracavernous pressure exceeds systemic diastolic blood pressure. With color duplex ultrasound, reversal of diastolic flow is associated with a dramatic color shift from red to blue in the cavernous artery. The absence of these expected Doppler spectral waveform changes allows the experienced sonographer to document penile hemodynamic pathology.

Peak Systolic Velocity (PSV) and Arterial Dilation. Total blood flow is a function of both arterial diameter and blood flow velocity. In patients with nonarteriogenic causes of ED (i.e., neurogenic, psychogenic), Lue and associates found that the PSV of the cavernous arteries consistently exceeds 25 cm/s within 5 minutes of intracavernous injection (Lue et al, 1985; Mueller and Lue, 1988). Additional studies from varying insti-

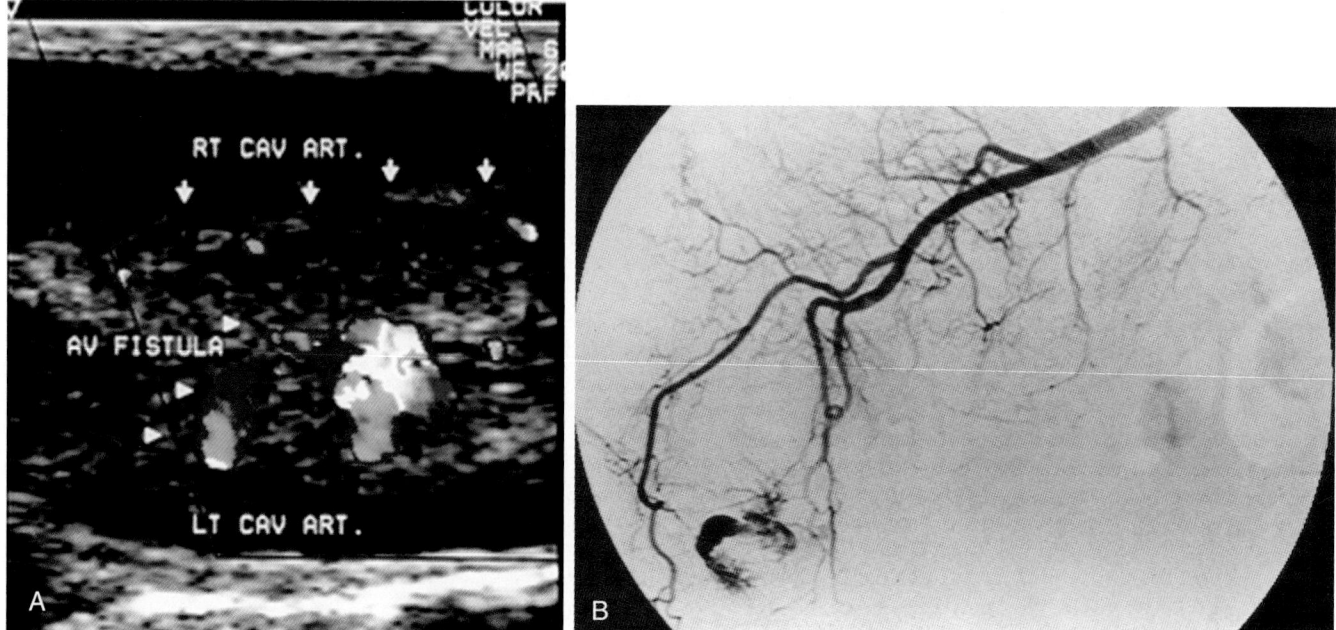

Figure 22–6. **A,** Color duplex ultrasonograph in a patient with high-flow priapism shows turbulent flow within the corpus cavernosum resulting from rupture of a branch of the left cavernous artery. **B,** On selective penile arteriography, a ruptured branch of the cavernous artery is seen filling the cavity.

tutions have reported the mean PSV in normal subjects as 34.8 cm/s (Broderick and Lue, 1991), 40 cm/s (Shabsigh et al, 1990), and 47 cm/s (Benson and Vickers, 1989). **In the Mayo Clinic series, PSV less than 25 cm/s had a sensitivity of 100% and a specificity of 95% in patients with abnormal pudendal arteriography** (Lewis and King, 1994). **Severe unilateral cavernous arterial insufficiency results in asymmetry of PSV greater than 10 cm/s.**

An increase in penile arterial blood flow velocity after injection is accompanied by an increase in cavernous arterial diameter. In patients with severe vascular ED, the diameter increase is usually less than 75% and post-injection luminal diameter rarely exceeds 0.7 mm (Lue and Tanagho, 1987; Mueller and Lue, 1988). Jarow and associates (1993) reported that, although PSV correlated well with findings on arteriography, the percentage of arterial vasodilation did not. Nevertheless, a forceful pulsation with an appreciable change of arterial diameter between the systolic and diastolic phases indicates normal

arterial compliance and function and is seen only in patients who develop full erection after intracavernous injection. The relationship of diameter and velocity changes to the phases of erection is shown in Figure 22–7.

Variation in Penile Arterial Anatomy. The variation in penile arterial anatomy can be a confounding factor. Jarow and associates (1993) found an excellent correlation between duplex sonography and pudendal arteriography in patients with classic penile arterial anatomy; however, the correlation was significantly lower in patients with variant anatomy. More significantly, both anatomic and radiographic studies show that a high percentage of patients have nonclassic penile arterial anatomy, which can potentially alter the interpretation of duplex sonography (Breza et al, 1989; Jarow et al, 1993). Significant variations include both the number and the location of the cavernous arteries. Early branching or the presence of multiple vessels, for example, may make it difficult for the

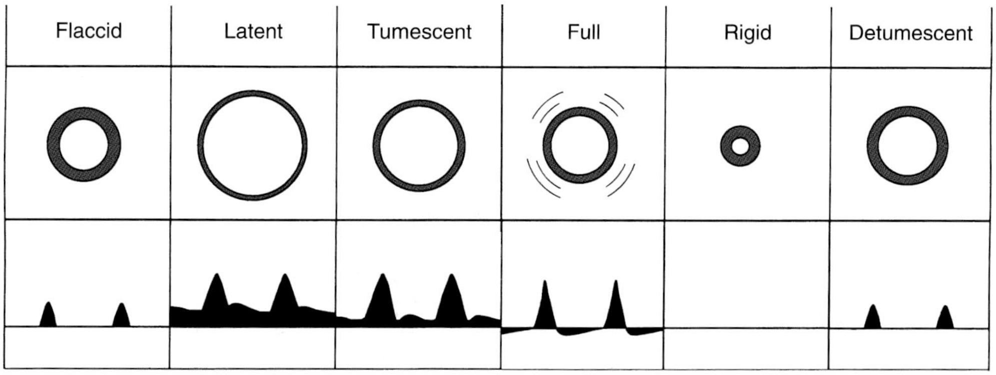

Figure 22–7. Artist's conception of the changes in diameter and flow waveform in the cavernous arteries induced by intracavernous injection of prostaglandin E$_1$ in a potent young man as demonstrated by duplex ultrasound. Forceful concentric pulsations are particularly noticeable during full erection.

Flaccid	Latent	Tumescent	Full	Rigid	Detumescent

clinician to evaluate blood flow velocity through the main cavernous artery. The presence of distal arterial perforators from the dorsal or spongiosal arteries, if undetected, may lead the clinician to underestimate the total arterial blood flow and wrongly assign a diagnosis of arteriogenic impotence. Fortunately, with color-coded duplex ultrasonography, an experienced sonographer can scan the entire penis from the crura to the tip and thus avoid underestimating penile blood flow.

Power Doppler. Some investigators have applied power Doppler to the study of penile "morphodynamics" (Sarteschi et al, 1998). They have visualized three orders of distal ramifications beyond the main cavernous artery. In power Doppler mode, the hue and brightness of the signal are functions not only of blood flow direction but also of the number of flowing red blood cells within the lumen; the dynamic range of imaging is increased, yielding resolution down to the level of arterioles.

Duplex Ultrasound Evaluation in Veno-occlusive Dysfunction. The trapping of blood within the corpora cavernosa, limiting venous outflow, is a necessary step to achieving and maintaining rigid erection. Cavernous veno-occlusive dysfunction is defined as the inability to achieve and maintain erection despite adequate arterial inflow. **When the Doppler spectral waveform continues to exhibit high systolic flow (>25 cm/s PSV) and persistent end-diastolic flow velocity (EDV) (>5 cm/s) accompanied by quick detumescence after self-stimulation, the patient is considered to have venogenic impotence.** Among patients with PSVs greater than 25 cm/s, venous leakage on cavernosometry was predicted with a sensitivity of 90% and specificity of 56% when EDV was greater than 5 cm/s (Quam et al, 1989; Lewis and King, 1994).

In 1974, Planiol and Pourcelot proposed a resistive index (RI) to describe vascular resistance from the Doppler spectrum. The formula follows: RI = PSV − EDV/PSV. As penile pressure equals or exceeds diastolic pressure, diastolic flow in the corpora will approach 0 and the value for RI approaches 1. During tumescence and until full rigidity, diastolic flow is antegrade (+); the value for RI remains less than 1.0. The RI correlates very well with visual ratings of erectile responses because both are reflections of intracavernous pressure. Both EDV and RI are useful parameters in predicting adequacy of veno-occlusion. **Naroda and associates (1994) found that an RI greater than 0.9 was associated with normal results during DICC in 90% of their series and an RI less than 0.75 was associated with venous leakage in 95%.** The conclusion reached from these investigations is that measurement of RI 20 minutes after injection and stimulation (or re-dosing) is a reliable, noninvasive method to diagnose cavernous venous leakage.

Third-Line Evaluation of Penile Blood Flow

Cavernous Arterial Occlusion Pressure. This variation of penile blood pressure determination was introduced by Padma-Nathan and associates in 1989. It involves intracavernous injection of a vasodilator (usually Trimix solution) followed by infusion of saline into the corpora cavernosa at a rate sufficient to raise the intracavernous pressure above the systolic blood pressure. A pencil Doppler transducer is then

ICSM RECOMMENDATIONS FOR DUPLEX ULTRASOUND

- When vascular evaluation is indicated, intracavernous injection with color duplex Doppler ultrasound is the most informative diagnostic test. This may be all that is needed to define and determine severity. Color duplex ultrasound should be used before other tests are considered because it is the least invasive technology for evaluating vascular ED, distinguishing high- from low-flow priapism, and assessing Peyronie's plaque. Recently, the combination of oral sildenafil citrate with visual erotic stimulation has been shown to be an effective noninvasive pharmacologic induction method for penile blood flow evaluation (Bacar et al, 2001; Speel et al, 2001; Park et al, 2002), but more studies are needed to confirm its validity.

  The parameters used to infer the integrity of the penile inflow tract are cavernous arterial diameters, peak systolic arterial velocity (PSV is the maximum of the systolic waveform), end-diastolic arterial velocity (EDV), systolic rise time (measured in msec from the start of systole to maximum value), cavernous artery acceleration time (AT; PSV ÷ systolic rise time), and index of vascular resistance (RI; PSV − EDV ÷ PSV). PSV less than 25 cm/s after intracavernous injection and sexual stimulation has a 100% sensitivity and 95% specificity in selecting patients with abnormal penile arteriography, because it reflects severe cavernous arterial insufficiency. A PSV consistently greater than 35 cm/s is associated with normal arteriography and defines normal cavernous arterial inflow. There is a negative relationship between age and PSV. Speel and associates (2003) have shown that AT has more power than PSV to diagnose atherosclerotic ED.

  Color duplex ultrasound accurately assesses venogenic ED and should be performed before cavernosometry and cavernosography.

applied to the side of the penile base. The saline infusion is stopped, and the intracavernous pressure is allowed to fall. **The pressure at which the cavernous arterial flow becomes detectable is defined as the cavernous artery systolic occlusion pressure (CASOP). A gradient between the cavernous and the brachial artery pressures of less than 35 mm Hg and an equal pressure between the right and the left cavernous arteries has been defined as normal** (Fig. 22–8). Results have been shown to correlate well with those of arteriography (Padma-Nathan et al, 1988) and PSV obtained by high-resolution duplex Doppler ultrasound (Rhee et al, 1995). However, despite these advantages, this is nonetheless a more invasive procedure prone to psychological inhibition and is not feasible if the intracavernous pressure cannot be raised above the systolic blood pressure (e.g., in patients with severe venous leakage).

Pharmacologic Arteriography. Arteriography is performed by intracavernous injection of a vasodilating agent

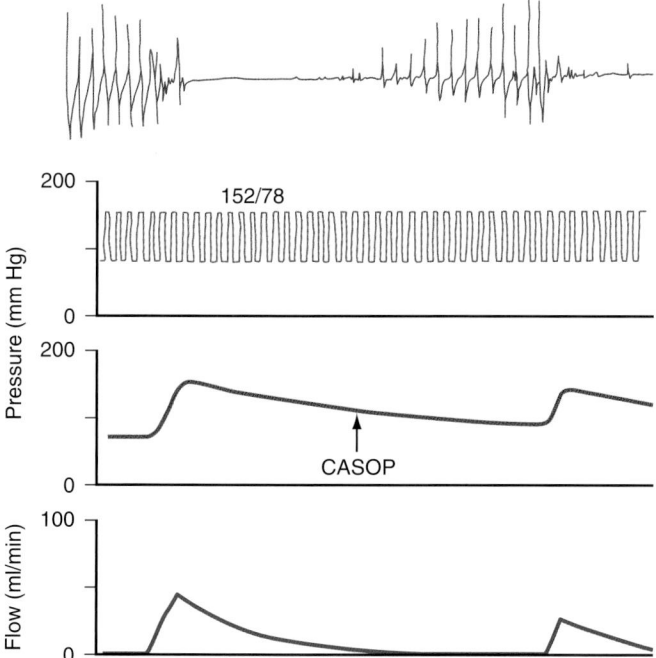

Figure 22–8. This tracing depicts four simultaneous variables obtained during the third phase of dynamic infusion cavernosometry and cavernosography. **Top to bottom,** Cavernosal artery flow recorded by using a continuous-wave Doppler ultrasound probe; systemic brachial systolic and diastolic arterial blood pressure (150/87 mm Hg); intracavernosal pressure, which varied from 70 to 160 mm Hg in this tracing; and intracavernosal heparinized saline inflow. The intracavernosal pressure at which the cavernosal artery pulsations returned, the effective cavernosal artery systolic occlusion pressure (CASOP), was 108 mm Hg. The gradient between the brachial and the cavernosal artery systolic occlusion pressures was 150 to 108, or 42 mm Hg, which is abnormal.

(papaverine, papaverine + phentolamine, or alprostadil) followed by selective cannulation of the internal pudendal artery and injection of radiographic contrast. The anatomy and radiographic appearance of the iliac, internal pudendal, and penile arteries are then evaluated according to established criteria (Fig. 22–9).

To image the cavernous arteries optimally, the contrast agent should be injected during the period of maximal vasodilation. Confounding interpretation of penile pharmacoarteriography is the fact that deviations from paired common penile arteries have been documented in 50% of normal potent volunteers (Bahren et al, 1988). Anatomic variation of intrapenile arterial anatomy appears to be the rule rather than the exception (Benson et al, 1993). For the angiographer, the problem is twofold: (1) how to differentiate congenital variations in penile arterial anatomy from acquired abnormalities and (2) how to correlate anatomic alternations.

Arteriography is most useful in providing anatomic rather than functional information. The inferior epigastric vessels also need to be studied because they are most commonly used for penile revascularization. Because of the high cost and invasive nature of the study, only a small percentage of patients with complex ED are appropriate candidates. Perhaps **the best indication is in the young patient with ED secondary to a traumatic arterial disruption or in a patient with a history of perineal compression injury. In these highly selected cases, a detailed "road map" of the arterial anatomy is essential to planning surgical reconstruction.**

Pharmacologic Cavernosometry and Cavernosography. Pharmacologic cavernosometry involves simultaneous saline infusion and intracavernous pressure monitoring to assess the penile outflow system after intracavernous injection of a strong vasodilating solution such as a high dose of alprostadil or Trimix. Veno-occlusive dysfunction is indicated by either the inability to increase intracavernous pressure to the level of the mean systolic blood pressure with saline

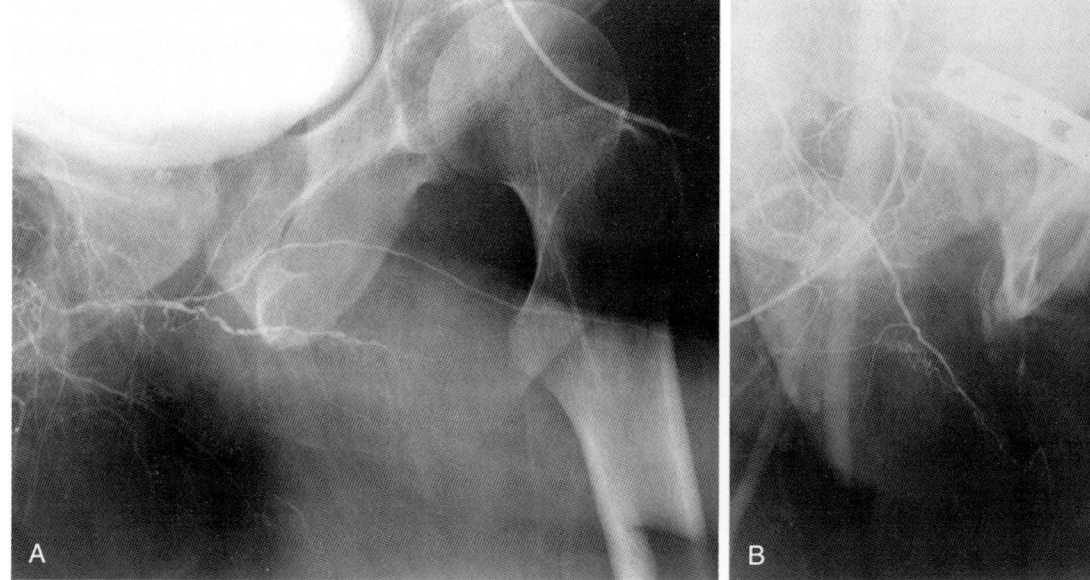

Figure 22–9. In this patient with a pelvic injury, pharmacologic penile arteriography (after intracavernous injection of 60 mg of papaverine) shows patent common penile, dorsal, and cavernous arteries (**A**) and nonvisualization of the common penile artery and its branches (**B**).

infusion or a rapid drop of intracavernous pressure after cessation of infusion (Puyau and Lewis, 1983; Rudnick et al, 1991; Shabsigh et al, 1991; Motiwala, 1993).

Pharmacologic cavernosography involves the infusion of radiographic contrast solution into the corpora cavernosa after a vasodilator-induced erection to visualize the site of venous leakage (Fig. 22–10). Leakage sites to the glans, corpus spongiosum, superficial dorsal veins, and cavernous and crural veins can then be detected. In the majority of patients, more than one site is visualized (Lue et al, 1986; Rajfer et al, 1988; Shabsigh et al, 1991).

Many technical factors may influence the findings. Dynamic infusion cavernosometry and cavernosography (DICC) is invasive, requiring that two needles remain in the penis for saline infusion and pressure recording. Saenz de Tejada and colleagues (1991) have suggested that, to avoid erroneous results, DICC should be performed under conditions of complete trabecular smooth muscle relaxation. Their data indicate this occurs in only 17% of patients after a single dose of vasoactive agent. Repeated dosages are required in the majority (Hatzichristou et al, 1995). To achieve complete smooth muscle relaxation, one to several intracavernous injections are given, followed by measurement of maintenance flow rate, pressure drop, and CASOP. **With complete smooth muscle relaxation, the flow rate required to maintain erection at an intracavernous pressure of more than 100 mm Hg is reported to be less than 3 to 5 mL/min, whereas the pressure decrease in 30 seconds from 150 mm Hg is less than 45 mm Hg.** Cavernosography is performed after cavernosometry and should reveal opacification of the corpora cavernosa but minimal or no visualization of venous structures or corpus spongiosum in men with normal veno-occlusive function. **DICC is reserved for young men who might be candidates for penile vascular operations, specifically those with a history of pelvic trauma or life-long ED (primary ED).**

Historical and Investigational Evaluations of Penile Blood Flow

Penile Brachial Pressure Index. The penile brachial pressure index (PBI) represents the penile systolic blood pressure divided by the brachial systolic blood pressure. The technique involves applying a small pediatric blood pressure cuff to the base of the flaccid penis and measuring the systolic blood pressure with a continuous-wave Doppler probe. A PBI of 0.7 or less has been used to indicate arteriogenic impotence (Metz and Bengtsson, 1981).

Attempts to correlate PBI with other more accurate techniques have been disappointing (Aitchison and associates, 1990; Mueller and associates, 1990), and the authors conclude that the PBI is inaccurate and poorly reproducible and suggest no justification for its continued use.

Penile Plethysmography (Penile Pulse Volume Recording). This test is performed by connecting a 2.5- or 3-cm cuff to an air plethysmograph. The cuff is applied to the base of the penis and inflated to a pressure above brachial systolic pressure, which is then decreased by 10-mm Hg increments, and tracings are obtained at each level. The pressure demonstrating the best waveform is recorded. The normal waveform is similar to a normal arterial waveform obtained from other part of body: a rapid upstroke, a sharp peak, a lower downstroke, and, occasionally, a dicrotic notch. In patients with vasculogenic ED, the waveform shows a slow upstroke, a low rounded peak, slow downstroke, and no dicrotic notch. Its height varies considerably; patients with vascular insufficiency usually have the lowest mean height (17.3 mm) (deWolfe, 1988). The proponents of this method argue that, because penile pulse volume recording measures the contributions of all the vessels at the root of the penis, it is more accurate than recording the pressure in an individual artery. However, this study is performed in the flaccid state and cannot distinguish dorsal or cavernous artery impairment.

Infrared Spectrophotometry. Burnett and coworkers (2000) described the use of a specialized near-infrared spectrophotometry instrument for continuous monitoring of the hemodynamics of erection. Near-infrared spectrophotometry is a safe, biomedical optics technique that provides quantitative measurements of the vascular physiology of penile erection. Further studies are needed before clinical application can be recommended.

Radioisotopic Penography. Radionuclide penography involves using ^{99m}Tc-labeled red blood cells to quantify

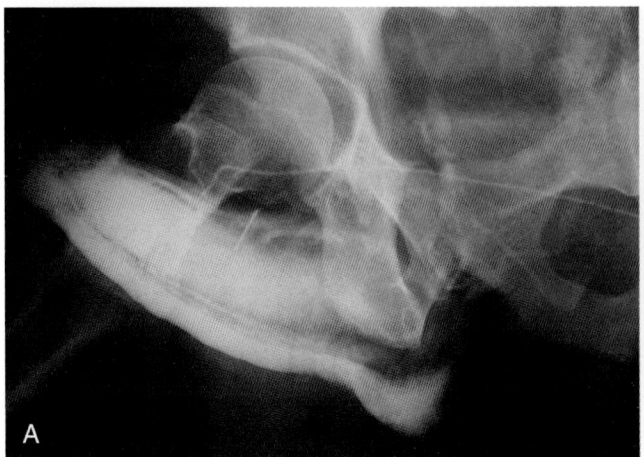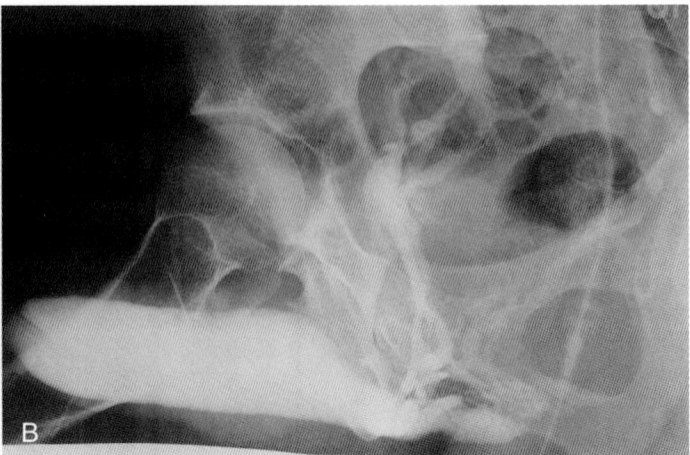

Figure 22–10. Pharmacologic cavernosography. **A,** In a patient 1 year after a penile fracture, a communication between the corpus cavernosum and the spongiosum is seen. **B,** In a 27-year-old man with primary impotence, venous leakage from the crura is seen.

changes in penile blood volume after injection of a vasoactive substance. Smith and colleagues (1998) noted that radioisotope penography measures penile blood flow, separating patients with extremely low flow (severe arteriogenic impotence) from those with a normal flow. Glass and associates (1996) evaluated 37 men with color duplex ultrasound and radionuclide penography but found little correlation between the two.

Magnetic Resonance Angiography (MRA). Several groups have evaluated the sensitivity and specificity of MRA of internal iliac and penile vessels. One group compared penile duplex ultrasound with digital subtraction MRA in patients being evaluated for arterial revascularization. Two studies with a total of 23 patients showed good correlation between MRA and duplex ultrasound; MRA localized the disease processes from the iliac arteries down to the internal pudendal arteries (Stehling et al, 1997; John et al, 1999). With further refinement, MRA may be useful in patients with a history of pelvic trauma who are candidates for vascular reconstruction (Munarriz et al, 1995).

Cavernous Smooth Muscle Content. Wespes and coworkers (1992) have advocated corporeal biopsies with light microscopy and computed morphometric analysis as an adjunctive technique in the diagnosis of vasculogenic impotence. When computed morphometry was used to compare young healthy men with penile curvature with elderly patients with ED, the corpora cavernosa in the young were composed of 40% to 52% smooth muscle; in the elderly with corporeal veno-occlusive dysfunction, the corpora cavernosa had 19% to 36% smooth muscle; and in the elderly with arterial impotence, corporeal smooth muscle was 10% to 25% (collagen was correspondingly increased) (Wespes et al, 1991). At present, cavernous biopsy for diagnosis of ED remains controversial and more studies are needed before its routine use can be recommended.

Psychophysiologic Evaluation

Nocturnal Penile Tumescence

Nocturnal penile tumescence (NPT) monitoring was first described by Halverson (1940), who documented nocturnal erections in infants. **Karacan and colleagues** (1966) **were the first to demonstrate that 80% of NPT occurs during rapid eye movement (REM) sleep.** Total tumescence time during sleep peaks at the age of puberty, when as much as 20% of total sleep time may be spent with an erection. In the second decade of life, the average duration of a nocturnal erection is 38 minutes; for adults, the average duration is 27 minutes (Karacan, 1970). Initially, NPT investigations were conducted by psychologists to study sleep and dreams; almost a decade later, NPT was applied to differentiate psychogenic from organic ED (Karacan, 1991).

NPT has been measured by a number of methods: stamp test (Barry et al, 1980); snap gauges (Diedrich et al, 1992); sleep laboratory nocturnal penile tumescence and rigidity (NPTR); RigiScan (Endocare, Inc., Irvine, CA); and, most recently, NPT electrobioimpedance (NEVA, American Medical Systems, Inc., Minnetonka, MN).

In its classic form, NPT consists of nocturnal monitoring devices that measure the number of episodes, tumescence

(circumference change by strain gauges), maximal penile rigidity, and duration of nocturnal erections (Kessler, 1988). Traditionally, NPT is recorded in conjunction with electroencephalography, electro-oculography, and electromyography (EMG), with nasal air flow, and with oxygen saturation to document REM sleep and the presence or absence of hypoxia (sleep apnea). Laboratories also monitor sleep movement patterns because periodic limb movement disorders are associated with abnormal NPT. The patient is awakened during maximal tumescence, and the erection is photographed and axial rigidity measured with a device applied to the tip of the penis. A buckling resistance of 500 g is considered the minimum for vaginal penetration; 1.5 kg is considered complete rigidity according to the original Karacan (1970) criteria. Because NPT occurs during REM sleep, tumescence monitoring may need to be repeated over two to three nights to overcome the so-called first-night effect. Formal NPT evaluations are costly, because they need to be conducted in specially equipped sleep centers with trained observers. Morales and coworkers (1994) were the first to use diurnal penile tumescence (monitoring during daytime napping) in the office.

In 1985, the RigiScan was introduced; it was the first device to provide automated, portable NPTR recording. The device combines the monitoring of radial rigidity, tumescence, number, and duration of erectile events with the convenience of a portable system that can be used at home (Bradley et al, 1985). It consists of a recording unit that can collect data for three separate nights for a maximum of 10 hours each night. The mechanics consist of two loops: one is placed at the base of the penis and the other at the coronal sulcus. By constricting the loops, the device records penile tumescence (circumference) and radial rigidity at the penile base and tip. Measurement (initialization) is first done in the office for 15 to 20 minutes with the patient awake to establish an individual baseline. At home, penile rigidity is registered every 3 minutes by constriction of the loops, applying a radial compression of 2.8 N. If the base detects a circumference increase of more than 10 mm, sampling is increased to every 30 seconds.

Radial rigidity above 70% represents a nonbuckling erection, and a rigidity of less than 40% represents a flaccid penis. The number of erections considered normal is three to six per 8-hour session, lasting an average of 10 to 15 minutes each (Levine and Lenting, 1995). **Cilurzo and colleagues** (1992) **recommend the following as normal NPTR criteria: four to five erectile episodes per night; mean duration longer than 30 minutes; an increase in circumference of more than 3 cm at the base and more than 2 cm at the tip; and maximal rigidity above 70% at both base and tip** (Fig. 22–11).

In 1994, Levine and Carroll studied 44 potent volunteers and noted considerable variation in individual responses over three night-time recordings. Furthermore, despite using normal subjects, they found no simple visual criteria for normal NPTR and thus developed a nomogram to allow rapid computerized comparison of NPTR. Data measurements consisted of cumulative distribution of time-intensity measures defined as tumescence activity units (TAU) and radial rigidity activity units (RAU). TAU and RAU are a refinement of the "area under the curve" measures suggested by Burris and

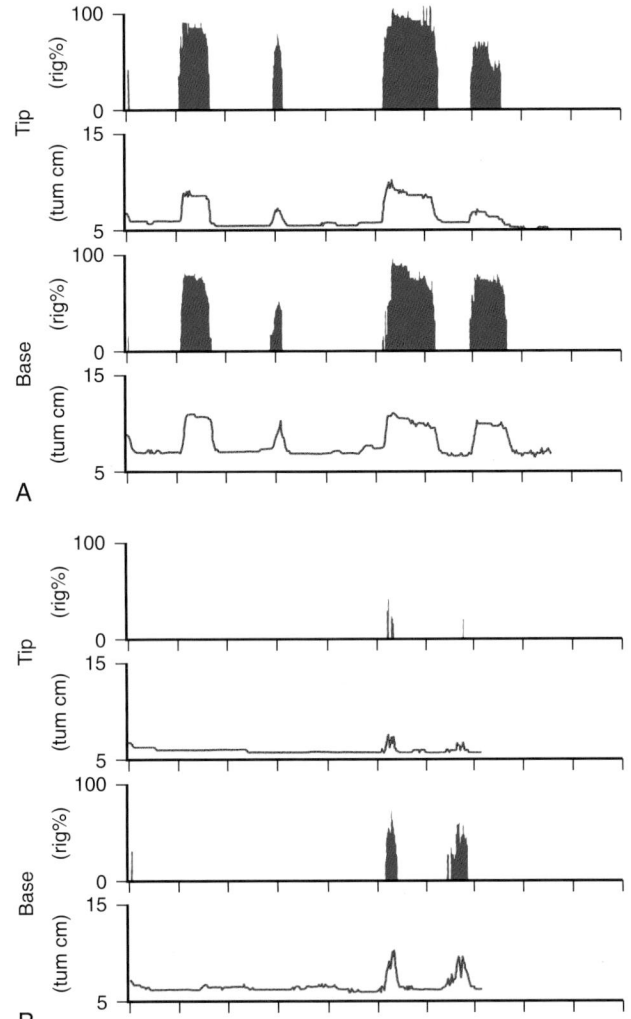

Figure 22–11. The RigiScan device has been designed to measure penile rigidity during home nocturnal monitoring. **A,** A study in a patient with at least two episodes of well-sustained, completely rigid nocturnal erections. **B,** A study with two episodes of poorly sustained, poorly rigid nocturnal erections. Such home studies fail to document sleep quality.

colleagues (1989). Levine and Carroll (1994) also demonstrated an overall tendency in normal men for tip rigidity to decrease with age.

There are few RigiScan studies done in aging normal men. Zimmern and colleagues (1999) evaluated a group of potent prostate cancer patients before surgery and concluded that RigiScan criteria developed in young volunteers are not applicable to the aging potent man, nor do RigiScan data correlate with patient self-assessment of potency.

One analysis comparing RigiScan radial rigidity, axial buckling rigidity, and intracavernous pressures has demonstrated that radial rigidity is not an accurate predictor of axial rigidity (Udelson et al, 1999). These investigators noted that, as intracavernous pressure increased during dynamic corporeal infusions, the RigiScan became increasingly insensitive to pressure, whereas axial buckling forces became more sensitive. In Europe, a home digital inflection rigidometer is available. Rossello (1996) has noted that two thirds of patients whose

radial rigidity was rated at 60% to 70% by RigiScan had insufficient axial rigidity measured by inflection rigidometry at home.

The newest addition to NPT testing is the NEVA device, which uses electrobioimpedance to assess volumetric changes in the penis during nocturnal erections. A small recording device is attached to the patient's thigh, and three small electrode pads are applied to the hip and the penile base and glans. An undetectable alternating current is sent from the glans electrode to the hip ground. The penile base electrode measures impedance and changes in penile length; as the cross-sectional area of the penis changes with nocturnal tumescence, impedance decreases (Knoll and Abrams, 1999a). Knoll and Abrams (1999b) have used this system to record the number and duration of erectile episodes and penile length and blood volume changes at night in controls and patients. The mean volume change in 10 controls was 213% (14.4 mL). The NEVA system can be used to document NPT, but the relationship to rigidity and volume change needs to be established.

In summary, **the main advantages of NPT testing are its relative freedom from psychologic influences and its ability to detect sleep-related abnormalities. The documented presence of a full erection indicates that the neurovascular axis is functionally intact and that the cause of the ED is most likely psychogenic. The disadvantages of NPT evaluation are that it is age dependent and costly, because it is ideally done with a RigiScan in a specially equipped sleep center. Because of problems associated with various NPTR tests, this is not recommended as a routine part of ED evaluation.** Nevertheless, NPT testing remains a valuable tool in certain conditions in which findings from other studies are inconclusive and additional objective data are needed to arrive at a final diagnosis. Heaton and Morales (1997) have suggested indications for NPTR as follows: (1) suspected sleep disorder; (2) obscure cause of ED; (3) nonresponse to therapy; (4) planned surgical treatment; (5) legally sensitive case; (6) measurement of drug effects in placebo-controlled drug trials; and (7) suspected psychogenic cause.

Audiovisual and Vibratory Stimulation

Audiovisual sexual stimulation (AVSS) appears to enhance penile responses to a variety of test stimuli: vibration, intracavernous injection, and topical and oral pharmacologic agents. Incrocci and coworkers (1996) documented their experience with over 400 patients: 34% exposed to AVSS alone achieved partial or full erection; 52% who underwent AVSS and vibratory stimulation were able to initiate erection, and 82% of patients shown AVSS in combination with intracavernous papaverine (15 to 60 mg) achieved erection.

Because nocturnal penile tumescence and rigidity declines in the aging male, the assumption is that awake penile tumescence and rigidity (PTR) with AVSS may have the same tendency. To the contrary, Incrocci and coworkers (1996) found AVSS responses from men younger than 40 years were distinctly different from those in men older than age 40, but when intracavernous agents were given in combination with AVSS and PTR monitoring (by Erectiometer), erectile responses in men between ages 40 and 60 years were not significantly different.

Psychological Evaluation

The contemporary definition of psychogenic ED, as elaborated by the nomenclature committee of the International Society of Impotence Research (Lizza et al, 1999), is the persistent inability to achieve or maintain erection satisfactory for sexual performance due predominantly or exclusively to psychological or interpersonal factors. If the medical and sexual histories suggest a combination of organic and psychological risk factors, these patients should be diagnosed as having mixed organic/psychogenic ED; successful treatment must address both components.

Contemporary population studies such as the Massachusetts Male Aging Study (MMAS) and National Health and Social Life Survey (NHSLS) document that ED is associated with anxiety, self-reported depressive symptoms, low degrees of self-esteem, negative outlook on life, self-reported emotional stress, and history of sexual coercion.

A skillful diagnostic interview is the mainstay of a good psychological evaluation. It should focus more on the current sexual problem and its immediate cause and less on general personality traits. Hartmann (1991) suggests that the interview should focus on (1) current sexual problem and its history; (2) deeper causes of sexual dysfunction; (3) the relationship; and (4) psychiatric symptoms. Immediate causes that should be brought out by the interviewer include fear of failure, performance anxiety (for widowers, this typically involves complex interactions of dating, new partners, and unresolved mourning/guilt), insufficient sexual stimulation, loss of attraction for partner, and relationship conflicts. Remote or "deeper" causes of psychogenic ED include unresolved parental attachments, sexual identity, sexual trauma, and cultural-religious taboos (Mohr and Beutler, 1990; Laumann et al, 1999).

In obtaining the current sexual history, the interviewer must keep in mind the clinical subtypes of psychogenic ED: (1) generalized versus situational and (2) lifelong (primary) versus acquired (secondary, including substance abuse or major psychiatric illness). The information should cover feelings during the course of sexual contact, the occurrence and timing of performance anxiety, or interfering thoughts. Masters and Johnson (1970) defined performance anxiety as "spectatoring," which they believed could be treated by a program of nongenital, nondemand pleasuring exercises that they named "sensate focus." The interviewer should also obtain information about noncoital erections (masturbatory, nocturnal, or morning). If the patient complains of decreased arousal, one should attempt to determine if this occurred before or after the development of ED.

The interviewer should determine whether the patient has an appropriate cognitive understanding of genital function and penile rigidity. Dysfunctional sexual beliefs and expectations for performance can be found not only in young and inexperienced men but also in older men who cannot accept age-related reductions in sexual functioning, such as the need for increased tactile stimulation and lessened responsiveness to psychological stimuli. Relationship conflicts may be the source of psychogenic ED or may aggravate organic ED. Couples issues include intimacy and trust, status and dominance, loss of sexual attraction, couples' ability to achieve sexual satisfaction without erection, and communication problems. In assessing a partner-related problem, the couple should be interviewed both together and apart.

Identifying the deeper intrapsychic causes of sexual dysfunction is an important aspect of the diagnostic interview but may be beyond the skill, comfort, and time constraints of the urologist. This portion of the interview solicits history related to traumatic experience, cultural or religious indoctrination, and neurotic processes. The interviewer should determine whether psychiatric comorbidities such as substance abuse, depressive symptoms, anxiety disorder, and personality disorders have a dynamic connection to the ED. One should remember that psychiatric illness can be the cause of sexual dysfunction or it can be secondary. Many psychiatric illnesses are associated with sexual problems, but it is equally true that many patients with severe psychiatric disorders are capable of having normal erectile responses. A psychiatric illness often affects sexual desire more than erectile function, and, unfortunately, many medications may affect both desire and erection (Hartmann, 1991).

Although psychological consultation is not indicated for most patients, it is very useful in evaluating and treating men with deep-seated psychological problems. Three groups of psychometric instruments are available for the evaluation of ED: (1) personality questionnaires; (2) depression inventories; and (3) questionnaires for sexual dysfunction and relationship factors. The Minnesota Multiphasic Personality Inventory (MMPI)-2 is a valuable tool for assessing the patient's personality and its relevance to sexual dysfunction (Arnau et al, 2005). The Beck Depression Inventory is a self-reported test for which a score above 18 is considered indicative of significant clinical depression (Trentini et al, 2005). For relationship assessment, the Short Marital Adjustment Test (for married couples) (Cramer, 2001) and the Dyadic Adjustment Inventory (for unmarried people) (Issac and Shah, 2004) can be used to determine overall relationship quality. Specific factors examined include fidelity and level of commitment as well as sexual relations, family finances, and relationships with friends. Although early reports of these tests claimed that they could differentiate psychogenic from physical causes, subsequent studies have been unable to substantiate these findings, and physiologic testing is often required in concert with the psychological assessment to diagnose and manage the patient with mixed or psychogenic ED.

Neurologic Evaluation

Physiologically, there are three types of erections: nocturnal, psychogenic, and reflexogenic. In a broader sense, neurologic testing should assess peripheral, spinal, and supraspinal centers and both somatic and autonomic pathways associated with all three types of erection and sexual arousal. However, the effect of a neurologic deficit on penile erection is a complicated phenomenon, and, with a few exceptions, neurologic testing will rarely change management. Moreover, there is no reliable test to assess neurotransmitter release, which leaves a major gap in the current assessment of overall neurologic function associated with penile erection. Therefore, neurologic testing is only recommended in specific research protocols or medicolegal investigations, including cases of trauma or surgical complications. Based on the available evidence, these tests lack adequate sensitivity and reliability for routine clinical diagnosis.

In the past 2 decades, tests have been developed to evaluate specific components of the neural network: somatic efferent (motor) pathways; afferent (sensory) pathways; and reflexes and autonomic responses. The somatic nerves are evaluated by testing nerve conduction velocities and evoked potentials, and these tests have well-known reproducibility and validity. Autonomic function tests are less reliable because they simultaneously measure a chain of events or reactions involving receptors, small fibers, and target organs. The complex interactions among central and peripheral sympathetic and parasympathetic nerve systems, as in the pelvic plexus, make autonomic testing difficult. Moreover, efferent autonomic function tests involve the evaluation of vasomotor and sudomotor fibers and target organs, which may not be equally affected by neuropathy. Current autonomic tests are not well standardized and lack reproducibility, validity, and comparability (Rosen et al, 2004a).

Somatic Nervous System

Biothesiometry. This test is designed to measure the sensory perception threshold to various amplitudes of vibratory stimulation produced by a hand-held electromagnetic device (biothesiometer) placed on the pulp of the index fingers, both sides of the penile shaft, and the glans penis. Goldstein and Krame (1992) have developed a nomogram and have advocated using biothesiometry to select patients for further comprehensive testing. In one study, Bemelmans and colleagues (1995) compared biothesiometry and neurourophysiologic investigations for the clinical evaluation of patients with ED and showed that penile glans biothesiometry yielded consistent results when measurements were repeated during one session. However, they found no relationship between results of penile glans biothesiometry and neurourophysiologic tests of the dorsal penile nerve, probably because vibration is not an adequate stimulus to the glanular skin, which contains only free nerve endings and hardly any vibration receptors. They argue that biothesiometric investigation of penile glans innervation is unsuited for the evaluation of penile innervation and cannot replace neurourophysiologic tests.

Sacral Evoked Response—Bulbocavernosus Reflex Latency. This test is performed by placing two stimulating ring electrodes around the penis, one near the corona and the other 3 cm proximal. Concentric needle electrodes are placed in the right and left bulbocavernous muscles to record the response. Square-wave impulses are delivered by means of a direct-current stimulator. The latency period for each stimulus response is measured from the beginning of the stimulus to the beginning of the response. An abnormal latency time, defined as a value more than 3 standard deviations above the mean (30 to 40 ms), denotes a high probability of neuropathology (Padma-Nathan, 1994). In a study of diabetic patients, Vodusek and coworkers (1993) showed a significant clinical/neurophysiologic correlation between the absence of the BCR on clinical examination and its prolonged latency on electrophysiologic measurement. However, the study also showed that the battery of electrophysiologic tests evaluating limb nerve function seems more sensitive in diagnosing

neuropathy than electrophysiologic assessment of pudendal nerve function alone.

Dorsal Nerve Conduction Velocity. In patients with adequate penile length, it is possible to use two BCR latency measurements, one from the glans and one from the base of the penis, to determine the conduction velocity of the dorsal nerve (i.e., by dividing the distance between the two stimulating electrodes by the difference in latency between the base and the glans). Gerstenberg and Bradley (1983) have determined an average conduction velocity of 23.5 m/s with a range of 21.4 to 29.1 m/s in normal subjects.

Genitocerebral Evoked Potential. This test involves electrical stimulation of the dorsal nerve of the penis as described for the BCR latency test. Instead of recording electromyographic responses, this study records the evoked potential waveforms overlying the sacral spinal cord and cerebral cortex. The cerebral response to peripheral nerve stimulation is one of potentials of extremely low amplitude, and complex electronic equipment is used to store and average data of thousands of waveforms recurring as often as every tenth of a millisecond. The first latency recorded is the time of stimulation to the first replicated spinal response—the peripheral conduction time. The second is from the time of stimulation to the first replicated cerebral response—the total conduction time. The difference between the two is the central conduction time (Padma-Nathan, 1994). Unlike BCR latency, this is a purely sensory evaluation. This study is not useful as a routine test, but it can provide an objective assessment of the presence, location, and nature of afferent penile sensory dysfunction in patients with subtle abnormalities on neurologic examination.

Autonomic Nervous System

Heart Rate Variability and Sympathetic Skin Response. The test of heart rate control (mainly parasympathetic) consists of measuring heart rate variations during quiet breathing, deep breathing, and in response to raising the feet. Normal parameters follow: (1) the heart rate variation coefficient of the mean respiratory rate (RR) variation during quiet breathing should be less than 1.88 in patients in the 41- to 60-year age group and 2.52 for adults younger than 40; (2) the maximal average difference between the minimal heart rate of inspiration and the maximal rate of expiration during three successive breathing cycles should be higher than 15 beats per minute in the younger group and 9 beats per minute in the older group; and (3) the ratio of the longest RR interval of the bradycardiac phase and the shortest RR interval of the tachycardiac phase should be greater than 1.11.

Sympathetic skin response (SSR) measures the skin potential evoked by electrical shock stimuli. For example, the electrical stimuli can be applied to the median or tibial nerve and the evoked potential recorded at the contralateral hand or foot or the penis. Zgur and associates (1993) studied 30 patients with moderate diabetic polyneuropathy and a control group of 30 normal subjects. In diabetics, two thirds reported autonomic symptoms and 60% reported ED. The SSR amplitudes were significantly lower (changed in 53%, absent in 20%) than in the control subjects. This abnormality correlated with some clinical and electroneurographic signs of neuropathy, suggesting similar impairment of sympathetic and somatic fibers.

The Valsalva index was abnormal in 37% of patients, showing no correlation with clinical, electroneurographic, or SSR changes. Especially if the SSR is recorded from the penis, this seems to be a useful method of testing penile autonomic innervation. However, basic questions regarding the technique are still unresolved and its clinical usefulness is limited.

Penile Thermal Sensory Testing. Thermal threshold measurements yield data on the conductance of small sensory nerve fibers, which can indirectly reflect autonomic disturbances, particularly in the context of a diffuse neuropathy such as diabetic polyneuropathy. Penile thermal sensory testing correlates strongly with the clinical evaluation of erectile function and is a new and promising tool for the diagnosis of neurogenic impotence (Lefaucheur et al, 2001; Bleustein et al, 2003).

Corpus Cavernosum Electromyography (CC-EMG) and Single Potential Analysis of Cavernous Electrical Activity. Direct recording of cavernous electrical activity with a needle electrode during flaccidity and with visual sexual stimulation was first reported by Wagner and coworkers (1989). They found the normal resting flaccid electrical activity from the corpora cavernosa to be a rhythmic slow wave with an intermittent burst of activity. These bursts virtually ceased during visual sexual stimulation or after intracavernous injection of a smooth muscle relaxant. The electrical activity returned during the detumescence phase. Patients with suspected autonomic neuropathy demonstrated a discordant pattern, with continuing electrical activity during visual sexual stimulation or after intracavernous injection.

Two international workshops on CC-EMG have been convened, and recording techniques have been standardized (Juenemann et al, 1993; Stief et al, 1994). It is now generally agreed that an analog recording of CC-EMG during flaccidity in normal subjects is reproducible. In patients, CC-EMG is characterized by reproducible waveforms (potentials) in the individual subject, mostly of comparable shape. The maximum peak-to-peak amplitude lies between 120 and 500 mV, and potentials have a mean duration of 12 seconds. Nevertheless, basic questions regarding the signal recorded, and how to interpret it, are still unresolved. Thus, despite some clinical use, this test must be regarded as experimental (Kellner et al, 2000; Jiang et al, 2003).

Hormonal Evaluation

Historically, hypogonadism as a cause of ED was thought to be rare, but **recent data support a significant increase of hypogonadism with age. The interrelationships among hypogonadism, depression, and ED are now recognized, underscoring the importance of the endocrine evaluation. In male sexual dysfunction most endocrinopathies center around testosterone.** The decrease or absence of hormonal secretion from the gonads in men is traditionally referred to as hypogonadism. More contemporary designations attempt to acknowledge aging as the primary cause of declining androgens: androgen deficiency of the aging male (ADAM), partial androgen deficiency of the aging male (PADAM), hypoandrogenism, symptomatic late-onset hypogonadism (SLOH), and andropause (see Chapter 27, "Androgen Deficiency in the Aging Male").

Testosterone is normally produced in men at a rate of 4 to 8 mg/day (~0.24 mol/day), occurring in a pulsatile manner (Schopohl et al, 1995). **The diurnal pattern has a peak level in the early morning and a nadir in the evening.** Testosterone can be converted to dihydrotestosterone (DHT) within androgen target cells (skin, liver, prostate, and other organs) that contain the enzyme 5α-reductase (Mooradian et al, 1987). Testosterone is also metabolized to estradiol by the aromatase enzyme complex in brain, fat, liver, and the testes (Mooradian et al, 1987). In normal men, 2% of testosterone is unbound (free testosterone) and 30% is bound to sex hormone–binding globulin (SHBG) (Basaria and Dobs, 2001; Freeman et al, 2001). The remainder is bound with lower affinity to albumin and other serum proteins. Free testosterone and albumin-bound portions make up the bioavailable testosterone fraction. The relative concentrations of these carrier proteins (SHBG and albumin) modulate androgen function. The synthesis of SHBG by the liver is downregulated by androgens and upregulated by estrogens. SHBG has a higher affinity for testosterone than for estradiol, and changes in SHBG concentration change or amplify the hormonal milieu. Elevated estrogens, thyroid hormone, and aging each variably increase serum SHBG levels and decrease bioavailable testosterone to some extent. On the other hand, exogenous androgens, growth hormone, and obesity depress SHBG levels and increase the free testosterone levels.

Serum Endocrine Evaluations: Choice of Assay. The most relevant measurement of testosterone bioavailability should be the unbound or free fraction, but commercial assays for free testosterone are inconsistent and have been considered invalid by some investigators. The best indicator of androgenicity is the calculated bioavailable testosterone (free testosterone and albumin-bound testosterone). A formula can be found on the website of the International Society for the Study for the Aging Male at http://www.issam.ch/. Once the values of total testosterone and SHBG are entered, the calculator automatically indicates the bioavailable testosterone. In men with serious liver disease or hypoalbuminemia, it may be appropriate to enter the serum albumin value for the calculation.

Serum Testosterone Range. The problem of identifying the normal cutoff level for testosterone beyond which therapy should be initiated remains unresolved. Wide individual variability in the threshold of serum testosterone below which impairment of androgen-dependent processes becomes evident makes both diagnosis and treatment difficult.

Although the range of normal values for serum testosterone varies among laboratories, **morning testosterone values below 350 ng/dL in a young man with chronically elevated gonadotropins make a clear diagnosis of hypogonadism. In an older man the diagnostic lines are not as clearly defined and additional information may be needed. Circadian rhythm of testosterone levels should be considered in measuring serum testosterone; blood should be drawn between 8:00 AM and 11:00 AM. For screening, a total testosterone determination is usually adequate. If the testosterone level is below or at the low limit of normal, it should be confirmed with a second determination together with assessment of luteinizing hormone (LH) and prolactin.** One or more of the following serum laboratory values may be required to diagnose hormone deficiencies: (1) total/free/bioavailable testosterone; (2) SHBG; (3) LH; and (4) follicle-stimulating hormone (FSH).

Hyperprolactinemia

Many believe that the very low prevalence of significant hyperprolactinemia can hardly justify the routine determination of prolactin in men with ED, considering the frequency of ED and the cost of the determination (Kropman et al, 1991; Johnson and Jarow, 1992). It has often been recommended to determine prolactin only in men with low serum testosterone or low sexual desire. **However, in a study by Buvat and Lemaire (1997), determining serum prolactin only in ED patients with low testosterone levels would have missed 50% of 12 marked hyperprolactinemias and three of seven pituitary tumors.** Likewise, in men with hyperprolactinemia, sexual desire may be normal or may be perceived as normal. In a study by Johri and coworkers (2001), determining serum prolactin only in ED patients with a score less than 3 in the Sexual Desire Domain of the IIEF would have missed 50% of the cases of hyperprolactinemia. **Buvat (1996) has reported that, by restricting the serum prolactin determination to men with low sexual desire, gynecomastia, or serum testosterone less than 4 ng/mL (low + low normal values), more than half of the laboratory determinations need not have been done in their ED patients;** 1 of 10 marked cases of hyperprolactinemia would have been missed, but none of the six pituitary tumors.

Precautions should be taken to avoid false diagnosis of hyperprolactinemia resulting from stress, meals, or the intake of certain types of drugs. Blood sampling ideally should be carried out fasting, after a 20-minute rest in a quiet place. Elevated serum prolactin levels should be confirmed. Finally, any man with a confirmed diagnosis of hyperprolactinemia (non–drug-induced) should undergo investigation of the hypothalamic-pituitary area (if possible with magnetic resonance imaging) to rule out the presence of a tumor responsible for the hyperprolactinemia.

Other Hormonal Abnormalities

Some men with gynecomastia or suspected androgen resistance (high serum testosterone and LH with undermasculinization) should undergo determination of serum estradiol and androgen receptors on the genital skin. Patients with a rapid loss of secondary sex characteristics may have both testicular and adrenal failure and should also be tested for adrenal function (McClure and Marshall, 1994). Other endocrine disorders such as hyperthyroidism and hypothyroidism and adrenocortical dysfunction or tumor may affect sexual function and should be investigated if suspected.

NONSURGICAL MANAGEMENT OF ERECTILE DYSFUNCTION

Although the penile prosthesis remains one of the most effective treatments for all types of ED, its dominance was replaced during the 1990s by nonsurgical management. **Both specific and nonspecific treatments are now available. The former includes lifestyle change, psychosexual therapy, replacement of offending medications, and hormonal therapy; the latter**

ICSM SUMMARY AND RECOMMENDATION ON DIAGNOSTIC EVALUATION OF ED

- The large majority of patients with ED do not require specialized evaluation. A physical examination, medical and sexual history, and basic laboratory tests are sufficient. Specialized consultation and evaluation may be indicated, however, for specific organic causes, for patients with specific preferences, or in medicolegal circumstances. Typical indications for specialized vascular, neurologic, or endocrine evaluation are failure of initial treatment, Peyronie's disease, primary ED, history of pelvic/perineal trauma, cases requiring vascular or neurosurgical intervention, complicated endocrinopathy, complicated neurologic or psychiatric disorders, and medicolegal concerns.

  Commonly used vascular evaluation procedures include combined injection and stimulation, color duplex ultrasound, and dynamic infusion cavernosometry and cavernosography (DICC). Less common procedures include arteriography, computed tomographic angiography, penile magnetic resonance imaging (MRI), infrared spectrophotometry, audiovisual sexual stimulation (AVSS), and radioisotope penography. These latter techniques except arteriography should be regarded as experimental and lacking evidence-based assessment.

  Specialized neurologic procedures include nocturnal penile tumescence and rigidity testing (NPTR), biothesiometry, dorsal nerve conduction studies, bulbocavernosus reflex latency, and corpus cavernosum electromyography (CC-EMG). These procedures may be helpful for evaluating specific neurologic deficits in individual cases but are not widely used or generally recommended at this time. Additional experimental procedures include MRI and positron emission tomographic (PET) scanning of the brain during VSS, but these are recommended only for research purposes.

  Patients with complicated endocrine or psychiatric disorders should be referred for specialized consultation and evaluation when possible. In accordance with the principle of a patient-based approach to sexual medicine, results of specialized testing and evaluation should be clearly communicated to the patient and taken into consideration in the mutual decision-making process.

includes oral phosphodiesterase type-5 (PDE-5) inhibitors, the vacuum constriction device, and intracavernous injection. Although nonspecific therapies appear to be more effective for most cases of ED, the patient should also be made aware of specific therapies so that an informed decision can be made.

Lifestyle Change

In a cohort study of a random sample of men age 40 to 70 years selected from street listings in Massachusetts, in-home interviews were completed by 1709 men at baseline in 1987 to 1989 and by 1156 men at follow-up in 1995 to 1997 (average follow-up 8.8 years). Analyses included 593 men without ED at baseline who were free of prostate cancer and had not been treated for heart disease or diabetes. The incidence of moderate to complete ED was determined by discriminant analysis of responses to a self-administered sexual function questionnaire.

Obesity was associated with ED ($P = .006$), with baseline obesity predicting a higher risk regardless of follow-up weight loss. Physical activity was also associated with ED ($P = .01$), with the highest risk among men who remained sedentary and the lowest among those who remained active or initiated activity. Although the probability of complete ED was not statistically different between smokers and non-smokers (11% vs. 9.3%), cigarette smoking significantly increased impotence associated with cardiovascular disease, hypertension, and medication use (Derby et al, 2000).

Shiri and associates (2004) reported similar findings in a 5-year study in Finland. The target population comprised men 50 to 70 years old. A questionnaire was mailed in 1994 and 1999, with the follow-up sample comprising 1442 men who responded to both baseline and follow-up questionnaires. The effect of sociodemographic and lifestyle factors on the incidence of ED among the 1130 men free of ED at baseline was assessed. The authors found no differences in incidence by level of education, marital status, urban/rural place of residence, and amount of alcohol and coffee consumed. Obesity (rate ratio [RR] = 1.7, 95% confidence interval [CI]: 1.1 to 2.5) and current smoking (RR = 1.5, 95% CI: 0.9 to 2.2) increased the incidence of ED. Current smokers free of comorbidity were also at higher risk of ED (RR = 1.3, 95% CI: 0.8 to 2.1), but no effect was observed among past smokers.

The beneficial effect of lifestyle change has been reported by Esposito and coworkers (2004), who conducted a randomized, single-blind trial of 110 obese men (body mass index ≥30) age 35 to 55 years, without diabetes, hypertension, or hyperlipidemia but with ED (a score of 21 or less on the IIEF). The 55 men randomly assigned to the intervention group received *detailed* advice on how to achieve a total body weight loss of 10% or more by reducing caloric intake and increasing physical activity. The 55 men in the control group were given *general* information about healthy food choices and exercise. **After 2 years, body mass index decreased more in the intervention group (from a mean [±SD] of 36.9 ± 2.5 to 31.2 ± 2.1) than in the control group (from 36.4 ± 2.3 to 35.7 ± 2.5) ($P < .001$), as did serum concentrations of interleukin-6 ($P = .03$), and C-reactive protein ($P = .02$). The mean (SD) level of physical activity increased more in the intervention group (from 48 ± 10 to 195 ± 36 min/wk; $P < .001$) than in the control group (from 51 ± 9 to 84 ± 28 min/wk; $P < .001$). The mean (SD) IIEF score improved in the intervention group (from 13.9 ± 4.0 to 17 ± 5; $P < .001$), but remained stable in the control group (from 13.5 ± 4.0 to 13.6 ± 4.1; $P = .89$); 17 men in the intervention group and 3 in the control group ($P = .001$) reported an IIEF score of 22 or higher. In multivariate analyses, changes in body mass index** ($P = .02$), physical activity ($P = .02$), and C-reactive protein ($P = .03$) were independently associated with changes in IIEF score.

The beneficial effect of using a statin drug to lower cholesterol in men in whom the only risk factor for ED is hypercholesterolemia was reported by Saltzman and coworkers (2004). Of 18 such patients, 9 agreed to participate in a study in which they were given atorvastatin with a goal decrease of total cholesterol to less than 200 mg/dL and low-density lipoprotein to less than 120 mg/dL. RigiScan measurements were compared before and after treatment. The authors reported that, after taking atorvastatin for a mean of 3.7 ± 2.1 months, 8 of the 9 men had improved erection adequate for penetration during sexual intercourse. Mean questionnaire scores improved from 14.2 to 20.7 ($P < .001$). Mean total and low-density lipoprotein cholesterol decreased significantly after treatment ($P < .001$). RigiScan measurements showed an increased average penile rigidity at the base ($P < .001$) and tip ($P < .005$).

Long-distance bicycling is another risk factor that should be discussed, because adherents of this sport have described genital numbness and ED. Schwarzer and associates (1999) surveyed amateur cyclists and swimmers who were members of Cologne, Germany, sports clubs and found the ED rate for cyclists to be 4% and that of age-matched swimmers 2% (age range, 18 to 75 years; mean, 43 years). Genital numbness and ED correlated with total time in the saddle weekly, with 83% of men riding 60 continuous minutes complaining of genital numbness. In one study, different saddles were used in an office setting: patients underwent pharmacologic testing and Doppler penile blood flow measurement standing and while sitting on different saddles (Broderick, 1999). Penile blood flow was significantly less when sitting, although not completely obstructed (deep dorsal vein, −53%; cavernous artery, −36%; dorsal artery, −29%). The reduction in cavernous arterial flow was minimized when a wide padded seat was used (−17%). Indeed, the detrimental effects of perineal compression on penile arteries may be lessened by changes in both seat design and riding practices. Nayal and colleagues (1999) found penile oxygenation, measured through transcutaneous glans PO_2, to be as follows: standing before biking, 61 mm Hg; sitting for 3 minutes on saddle, 18 mm Hg; after standing and cycling for 1 minute, 68 mm Hg. Changing the bicycle seat or pursuing another form of exercise may be necessary if penile vascular compromise is found.

Medication Change

When a patient complains of sexual dysfunction after a particular medication, it is important to determine whether the problem is related to loss of sexual drive, impaired erection, or rapid or delayed ejaculation. In many situations, changing to a different class of medication is a feasible first step. Antihypertensive agents therapeutically lower blood pressure, and this primary effect has long been thought the mechanism of their adverse action on erection. **Nonspecific α-adrenergic blockers clinically have the most severe effects on erectile function.** Older antihypertensive drugs, such as methyldopa and reserpine, have a high incidence of sexual dysfunction because of their central suppressive effect. Thiazide diuretics are commonly associated with ED, and spironolactone interferes with testosterone synthesis. Switching patients to newer agents, such as calcium-channel blockers and angiotensin-converting enzyme inhibitors, may reverse ED in some patients. Large-scale antihypertensive trials suggest that using α_1-adrenoceptor antagonists is protective of baseline erectile activity (Grimm et al, 1997). Doxazosin therapy has shown a reduced incidence of ED when compared with placebo (Guthrie and Siegel, 1997).

Male sexual dysfunction occurs in many patients experiencing major depression (Nurnberg et al, 2002; Nicolosi et al, 2004). Selective serotonin reuptake inhibitors (SSRIs) have replaced tricyclic antidepressants and monoamine oxidase inhibitors as primary therapy for depression because of equal or better efficacy and fewer adverse effects. Treatment-related arousal disorders (lubrication and anorgasmia in women, ED and retarded ejaculation in men) secondary to SSRIs have been reported to range as high as 70% (Montejo-Gonzalez et al, 1997). Rosen and colleagues (1999) noted that the incidence of ED with fluoxetine was 1.7%; with sertraline, 2.5%; and with paroxetine, 6.4%. Potential mechanisms of SSRI-induced ED are multiple and include central and peripheral effects. Treatment strategies include substitution (bupropion, nefazodone, buspirone, mirtazapine), drug holidays, SSRI dosage reduction, watchful waiting, and PDE-5 inhibitors (Rosen et al, 1999; Nurnberg et al, 2000).

Herbal Supplements

Various herbs and herbal preparations have been used for centuries in many parts of the world for the treatment of ED. The introduction of PDE-5 inhibitors has contributed to the promotion of numerous supplements. Whether these have merit is questionable: some may produce results opposite to those advertised; others may enjoy the benefits of the placebo effect (a 25% to 50% placebo response has been recorded in clinical trials with effective agents). Table 22–5 summarizes some popular ED supplements and general conclusions that can be drawn from clinical investigations.

Some dietary supplements may in fact have an active ingredient that benefits patients with certain types of ED. An exciting area for future research is the possibility of a synergistic effect with ED prescription drugs, especially oral agents, with the hope of improved response rates in men in whom approved therapy initially fails. Randomized clinical trials are the best method of determining which dietary supplements will become a part of conventional medicine. **The challenge for clinicians is to discuss the placebo response properly and the need for good research before any supplement or herbal preparation can be advocated for general use** (Moyad et al, 2004).

Pelvic Floor Muscle Exercises

In a randomized crossover trial of lifestyle change in 55 men with ED (median age, 59.2 years; range, 22 to 78 years), the intervention group of 28 engaged in pelvic floor exercises in addition to receiving biofeedback and suggestions for lifestyle change. The 27 control subjects were advised on lifestyle change solely (Dorey et al, 2004). Baseline, 3-, and 6-month assessments were made. After 3 months, the control group was transferred to the active arm. At 3 months, compared with

Table 22–5. Alternative Therapies and Commercially Available ED Supplements

Alternative/Supplement	Overall Evidence
Acupuncture	Psychogenic ED; needs a randomized trial.
Androstenedione/DHEA	Increases estradiol and testosterone levels in men with normal testosterone levels; lowers high-density lipoprotein by an average of 10%. May increase testosterone levels dramatically in hypogonadal men. May benefit men with nonorganic and other ED and suboptimal levels of these precursors.
Ginkgo biloba	May have a blood-thinning effect. Lacks benefit in a study with men with ED.
Korean red ginseng (Panax ginseng)	Three preliminary trials suggest a potential benefit for men with ED, but quality control is a serious issue and more randomized trials are needed.
L-Arginine	A precursor to nitric oxide. High doses may benefit men who secrete low levels of nitric oxide. May lower blood pressure. Needs more randomized trials.
Yohimbine	Supplements probably contain little to no yohimbine. Prescription form is best and may benefit some with psychogenic ED. Can cause serious side effects.
Zinc	May benefit those with a severe zinc deficiency. Otherwise, data are lacking and high dosages can be dangerous and immunosuppressive.
Other supplements	*Avena saliva* and other potential cholesterol and blood-pressure reducers and *Tribulus terrestris* (precursor to DHEA) need clinical trials. Recent study of a Chinese herbal combination demonstrated no impact on sexual function versus placebo.
Antioxidants in combination with orally approved FDA medications	Folic acid plus vitamin E may enhance the response to sildenafil in men who failed to respond initially. Other oral drugs plus other supplements (e.g., yohimbine and arginine) may enhance erection. Large placebo-controlled trials are needed.

controls, men in the intervention group showed significant mean increases in the erectile function domain of the IIEF (6.74 points, $P = .004$); anal pressure (44.16 cm H_2O, $P < .001$); and digital anal grades on anal manometry (1.5 grades, $P < .001$). All showed further improvement in these outcomes at 6 months, and benefits were similar in the control group after transfer to active treatment. A total of 22 (40.0%) participants attained normal function and 19 (34.5%) had improved function; 14 (25.5%) failed to improve.

Psychosexual Therapy

Masters and Johnson's groundbreaking volume *Human Sexual Inadequacy* (1970) described their innovative format of using a mixed-sex team of two therapists working with couples in a quasi-residential setting with daily individual and joint treatment sessions. Basic treatment elements included an emphasis on sensate focus exercises and the elimination of performance anxiety. Masters and Johnson recommended beginning with nonsexual touching and then, in a desensitization paradigm, moving on to more genitally focused caressing. By emphasizing the nondemand nature of the sensual exchange, they sought to eliminate performance pressure. Masters and Johnson's treatment method was impractical to reproduce, because it was therapist-intensive and expensive. Therefore, modifications were investigated to ascertain if similar results could be achieved with more conventional outpatient treatment models.

Clinicians examined the impact of single therapist versus dual teams, weekly versus daily sessions, and a group versus individual/couple format. The results indicated that couples did as well when seen on a weekly basis and by a single therapist (Crowe et al, 1981; Heiman and Lopiccolo, 1983; Hawton, 1995). Two studies examined whether matching the gender of the therapist with the gender of the symptom-bearer would result in improved outcome; no differences were found (Crowe et al, 1981; Lopiccolo et al, 1985). When researchers examined the efficacy of individual versus group treatment formats, the latter was found to be advantageous not only because it was less costly in terms of therapist time but also because it offered peer support and allowed patients to learn from the experiences of others. Additionally, competition within the group motivated patients to change behaviors and desensitized them to discussions of their sexual lives (Spence, 1991).

However, the use of groups in sex therapy has been limited because of organizing and scheduling difficulties as well as finding enough patients with the same disorder available for treatment at the same time. **More recent approaches to sex therapy have included cognitive-behavioral interventions focused on challenging or correcting maladaptive cognitions, behavioral techniques such as desensitization and assertiveness exercises, family-of-origin and psychodynamic explorations exploring the role of past developmental experiences on present behavior, and systemic and couples therapy.**

Psychosexual therapy is also effective in a number of men with "organic" ED, and medical and surgical treatments are sometimes choices for psychogenic ED (Hengeveld, 1991). In some cases, the highly effective therapies that are minimally invasive (or not at all) such as PDE-5 inhibitors, a vacuum constriction device, or intracavernous injection may be better than a prolonged course of psychosexual therapy. Nevertheless, **in some patients with mixed psychogenic and organic ED, psychosexual therapy may help relieve anxiety and remove unrealistic expectations associated with medical or surgical therapy.**

Hormonal Therapy

We refer patients with thyroid, adrenal, pituitary, or hypothalamic dysfunction to endocrinologists for further evaluation and treatment. This discussion is limited to the treatment of hypogonadism and hyperprolactinemia as they relate to ED. Our experience and that of others is that, although most patients report improved libido, far fewer note increased erectile ability (Nieschlag et al, 1998).

Testosterone Preparations (See Table 22–6 and also Chapter 27.)

Injectable. Injectable depot preparations of testosterone, such as testosterone cypionate and enanthate, are the least

Table 22-6. Testosterone Preparations

Preparation	Dose	Route	Schedule
Oral			
Methyltestosterone (Metandren)	10-30 mg	Sublingual	Daily
Testosterone undecanoate (Andriol)	120-160 mg	Oral	Daily
Fluoxymesterone (Halotestin)	5-20 mg	Oral	Daily
Methandrostenolone	5-10 mg	Oral	Daily
Buccal			
Striant	30 mg	Buccal	q 12 hr
Transdermal Patches			
Testoderm TTS	5 mg	Skin	Daily
Testoderm	4-6 mg	Scrotum	Daily
Androderm	2.5-5 mg	Skin	Daily
Transdermal Gel			
Androgel 1%	5 g	Skin	Daily
Testim 1%	5 g	Skin	Daily
Intramuscular			
Cypionate (Depo-testosterone)	150-300 mg	IM	q 2-4 wk
Enanthate (Delatestryl)	150-300 mg	IM	q 2-4 wk
Pellet			
Testopel	150-450 mg	SC	q 3-6 mo

Modified from Maas D, Jochen A, Lalande B: Age-related changes in male gonadal function. Drugs Aging 1997;11:45-50.

expensive form of androgen supplementation. They are administered through deep intramuscular injection (200 to 250 mg every 2 weeks) and result in supraphysiologic levels of testosterone for 72 hours with steady exponential decline to subphysiologic levels by 10 to 12 days. **These depot preparations do not replicate the normal circadian rhythm.** The initial supraphysiologic testosterone "rush" may be disconcerting to some patients, but others enjoy an improved sense of well-being, aggression, and libido. The subphysiologic phase is reported by many patients as unpleasant, with decreased energy and libido as well as depressed mood.

Transdermal. This means of delivery more closely simulates normal circadian levels of testosterone if patients apply the patch in the morning; higher initial absorption will mimic normal diurnal variations. Several FDA-approved preparations are available in the United States.

Patch. Testoderm was initially available only as a scrotal patch without adhesive (4 to 6 mg). With this system, physiologic blood levels could be achieved in 65% of patients. Scrotal skin patches required shaving and were difficult to keep in place; additionally, because of high levels of 5α-reductase activity in scrotal skin, significantly high levels of dihydrotestosterone (DHT) were produced.

Testoderm TTS is applied daily as a 5-mg patch to the arm, back, or upper buttocks, avoiding the inconveniences of scrotal therapy. Another product, Androderm, comes as a patch that delivers 2.5 or 5 mg testosterone per day. The most common adverse reactions to both are itching, chronic skin irritation, and allergic contact dermatitis. Patients should alternate application sites and avoid sun-exposed areas. Local application of cortisone cream may relieve irritated skin.

Gel. AndroGel 1% gel pack contains 50 mg, 75 mg, or 100 mg of testosterone; it is applied once daily in the morning to clean, dry skin over the shoulders, upper arms, or abdomen. After the skin begins to dry, patients may dress. **They should wash their hands thoroughly, because skin contact can transmit testosterone: in clinical studies, 15 minutes of direct skin contact resulted in doubling the female partner's basal testosterone levels.** Another product, Testim, is likewise a topical gel containing 1% testosterone. It provides continuous transdermal delivery of testosterone for 24 hours after a single application to intact, clean, dry skin of the shoulders and upper arms. One 5-g tube of Testim contains 50 mg of testosterone.

Pellet. Each Testopel pellet contains 75 mg of testosterone. The usual dosage is two to six pellets (150 to 450 mg testosterone) implanted subcutaneously every 3 to 6 months.

Buccal. Striant is a tablet-like, mucoadhesive buccal system that adheres to the gum tissue above the incisors and provides sustained release of testosterone through the buccal mucosa. Each system contains 30 mg of testosterone; it is to be used twice a day to provide continuous systemic delivery.

Oral. **When taken orally, testosterone preparations are largely rendered metabolically inactive during the "first-pass" circulation through the liver.** Metabolic inactivation requires oral dosing to exceed 200 mg/day to maintain normal serum levels. **Large dosages of testosterone are toxic to the liver and can lead to hepatitis, cholestatic jaundice, hepatomas, hemorrhagic liver cysts, and hepatocarcinoma** (Bagatell and Bremner, 1996). Chemical modification to 17α-methyltestosterone or fluoxymesterone reduces the amount of testosterone necessary to reach normal serum levels, but significant patient variability remains. The only orally active and safe form is testosterone undecanoate in oleic acid (TU), which, owing to its lipophilic side chain, is partly taken up by the lymph and partly escapes hepatic inactivation. TU should be administered two to three times daily, always with a meal to improve absorption (Bagehus et al, 2003). A dosage of 40 mg three times a day generally provides adequate androgen replacement, yielding testosterone levels within the (low) normal range, whereas DHT levels are moderately increased (2 to 4 nMol/L) (Davidson et al, 1987). TU is not available in the United States.

Dihydrotestosterone

In contrast to testosterone, DHT cannot be aromatized to estradiol and therefore acts as a pure androgen. In patients with certain clinical conditions, a pure androgen might have advantages over aromatizable testosterone, as in hypogonadal men with a propensity to gynecomastia or boys with constitutionally delayed puberty (estrogens are pivotal in closure of the epiphyses). The available studies in hypogonadal men show that DHT maintains sex characteristics, increases muscle mass, and improves sexual function without a significant increase in prostate size (Schaison and Couzinet, 1998). (The lack of aromatization of DHT to estradiol reduces the hypothesized synergism between androgens and estrogens on the prostate.) In a recent study of 6 months of DHT therapy, a reduction of plasma estradiol was noted without a change in prostate size or detrimental effects on lipid profiles

(Kunelius et al, 2002). On the basis of these findings, it may be a potentially useful androgen for the aging man. DHT gel is available at a dose of 125 to 250 mg/day, which yields plasma DHT levels comparable to physiologic testosterone levels; more recently it has been shown that, in healthy elderly men, a lower dose of 32 to 64 mg/day yields comparable levels.

Dehydroepiandrosterone

The effect of DHEA replacement therapy on sexual function is controversial (Barnhart et al, 1999; Flynn et al, 1999; Artl et al, 2001). The most comprehensive long-term study was reported by Beaulieu and associates (2000): 140 men and 140 women (70 aged 60 to 69 years and 70 aged 70 to 79 in each group) received either 50 mg DHEA or a placebo daily for 12 months in a double-blind design. No significant difference between groups was found in the men (sexual function, bone mineral density, cardiovascular system). Conversely, several significant differences were found in women: in the DHEA group, at any age, there was an increase in sebum production (an androgen-like effect) and skin hydration, as well as an increase in bone mineral density (an estrogen-like effect). Only in the subgroup 70 to 79 years old was an increase in sexual interest found, from the sixth month of supplementation, and in sexual arousal, sexual activity, and sexual satisfaction at 12 months. These different effects probably resulted from the increase in serum levels of testosterone and estradiol observed on DHEA supplementation. In men, serum estradiol, but not serum testosterone, significantly increased on DHEA. No effect on different measures of well-being was observed in any gender. No important deleterious clinical or biologic effects were observed during this study.

A consequence of the conversion of DHEA to androgens and estrogens is that the effects of DHEA administration are not necessarily harmless. They may influence hormone-sensitive diseases such as breast or prostate cancer. Well-designed human studies, with specific endpoints aimed at investigating the effects of adrenal androgen deficiency and replacement therapy, are required to clarify the long-term effect of DHEA therapy (Yaffe et al, 1998).

Human Chorionic Gonadotropin

Only one study has monitored the effects of 3 months' administration of human chorionic gonadotropin to aging men with plasma testosterone levels in the lower range of normal (Liu et al, 2002). Plasma levels of total and free testosterone and estradiol increased 50% above baseline. The effects were very similar to those of androgen administration to aging men: a decrease in fat mass, an increase in lean body mass, but no effect on muscle strength. No adverse effect on hemoglobin or prostate was noted.

Adequacy of Androgen Replacement and Clinical Endpoints

It is a common clinical practice to judge the adequacy of androgen replacement by the effects on general well-being, mood, sexual interest, and sexual activity. Bone mineral density, although determined by multiple factors, can be regarded as an indicator of adequacy of sex steroid replacement, but changes are slow and obtaining a measurement more than every 2 years is usually not informative. **A general principle in hormone replacement therapy is that plasma** levels to be achieved over the 24 hours of the day must come close to normal reference values and ideally follow the normal diurnal pattern. Thus, an impression of adequate levels might be gained by determining plasma testosterone before administration of the next dose of the androgen preparation. On the specific activity of androgens in ED, recent reports suggest a marginal synergistic effect when testosterone is added to PDE-5 inhibitors in hypogonadal men in whom the latter failed as a single therapy (Rosenthal et al, 2003; Shabsigh et al, 2003); this effect is apparently mediated by increased inflow in the cavernous arteries (Aversa et al, 2003). These studies are preliminary and involve only small groups of patients followed for limited periods. The results must be interpreted with much caution.

Potential Adverse Effects of Androgen Therapy

In a young hypogonadal man, testosterone replacement is clearly the treatment of choice. However, the risks may outweigh the benefits in some patients. Supraphysiologic levels of testosterone will suppress LH and FSH production and result in infertility; breast tenderness and/or gynecomastia is not uncommon with parenteral testosterone. Long-term androgen therapy requires a commitment from the patient and the specialist for follow-up. Testosterone and its metabolite DHT are growth factors. Erythrocytosis is the most common laboratory alteration noted with long-term therapy. Morley and coworkers (1993) noted that the mean hematocrit increased from 42% to 49% after 3 months of treatment. Androgens may induce or worsen sleep apnea (Schneider et al, 1986). Cardiovascular risks are increased in some patients by increases in red cell mass; additionally, in young patients, testosterone abuse moderately elevates low-density lipoprotein and decreases high-density lipoprotein (Gutai et al, 1981). Increases in thromboxane A_2 and platelet aggregation have also been attributed to testosterone therapy (Ajayi et al, 1995).

Regarding **prostate safety**, Morgantaler and associates (1996) raised concerns when their group found that 11 of 77 hypogonadal men on supplemental testosterone with normal findings on digital rectal examination and normal PSA levels had occult prostate cancer on biopsy. Morley and associates (1993) noted a mean increase in PSA from 1.7 to 2.5 ng/L after 3 months of testosterone therapy. Tenover (1992) has noted a similar mean increase in PSA levels of 0.6 ng/L after 3 months of androgen therapy. **A number of studies in the literature suggest that androgen replacement does not induce prostate cancer in men with normal prostates, and placebo-controlled studies show little difference in prostate volume, PSA, and obstructive symptoms** (Nomura et al, 1988; Behere, 1994; Cooper et al, 1998).

The fear of exacerbating an occult cancer of the prostate in men undergoing testosterone replacement remains a urologist's nightmare. Nevertheless, there are a number of older hypogonadal patients whose libido and erectile function can be restored by testosterone therapy and who should not be denied the option. When a patient desires this, the physician should perform a digital rectal examination and obtain a serum PSA level. When in doubt, ultrasound-guided biopsy should also be done before androgen therapy is given. The presence of prostate or breast cancer is an *absolute contraindication* to androgen supplementation. Patients are followed every 6 months with a rectal examination and serum PSA testing as long as they are on therapy. Laboratory surveillance should also include periodic hemoglobin/hematocrit levels, liver function tests, cholesterol, and lipid profile. The efficacy of testosterone supplementation is reasonably determined by clinical response rather than by repeating testosterone determinations.

In patients with *hyperprolactinemia* with or without hypogonadism, testosterone therapy does not improve sexual function. Treatment should first be aimed at eliminating the offending drugs, such as estrogens, morphine, sedatives, or neuroleptics. Bromocriptine is a dopamine agonist that lowers the prolactin level and restores testosterone to normal. It is used to reduce tumor size of a prolactin-secreting adenoma. Neurosurgery may occasionally be needed if the response is not satisfactory or if there are changes in the visual field secondary to optic nerve compression. In a study of 600 patients with ED, Netto Junior and Claro (1993) reported that moderate elevations of prolactin levels, without any associated disorder, occurred in 3.8% (23 of the 600). In patients with prolactin levels ranging from 20 to 40 ng/mL, bromocriptine brought the values down to normal in all, but only 1 patient achieved full erection. In patients with levels higher than 40 ng/mL, 9 of 11 achieved normal levels after treatment and 77.7% achieved full erection. These findings indicate that, in patients with a mild elevation of prolactin, other factors such as a vascular or neurologic deficit may be the underlying cause of ED. **If a pituitary adenoma is identified (usually in patients with marked [10-fold] prolactin elevation), the treatment of choice is bromocriptine or surgical ablation.**

Pharmacologic Therapy

Peripherally Acting Agents

Oral Therapy

Phosphodiesterase Type-5 Inhibitors. Sildenafil (Viagra), the first of this class, was approved by the FDA in 1998 and has since been joined by *vardenafil* (Levitra) and *tadalafil* (Cialis). Vardenafil has a similar structure to sildenafil's, but the structure of tadalafil is quite different (Fig. 22–12).

The normal pathway for penile erection is initiated by sexual arousal, which stimulates release of nitric oxide at nerve endings in the penis. Another source of nitric oxide is vascular endothelial cells. Nitric oxide diffuses into vascular and cavernous smooth muscle cells in the corpus cavernosum to cause stimulation of guanylyl cyclase and elevation of cyclic guanosine monophosphate (GMP) in these cells. This leads to hyperpolarization and lowering of cytoplasmic calcium, which in turn results in smooth muscle relaxation and penile erection. PDE-5 inhibitors do not increase the nitric oxide level, but they potentiate nitric oxide's effect to enhance erection. **Without sexual stimulation and resultant nitric oxide release, these inhibitors are ineffective.**

The biochemical selectivity of an inhibitor is a key factor in determining its side-effect profile (Corbin and Francis, 2002). For PDE-5 inhibitors, selectivity is usually expressed in terms of potency (IC50) to inhibit PDE-5 as opposed to inhibiting nontarget PDEs (or other proteins). The selectivity is computed by dividing the IC50s of the two compounds that are compared. The PDEs comprise families of enzymes that cat-

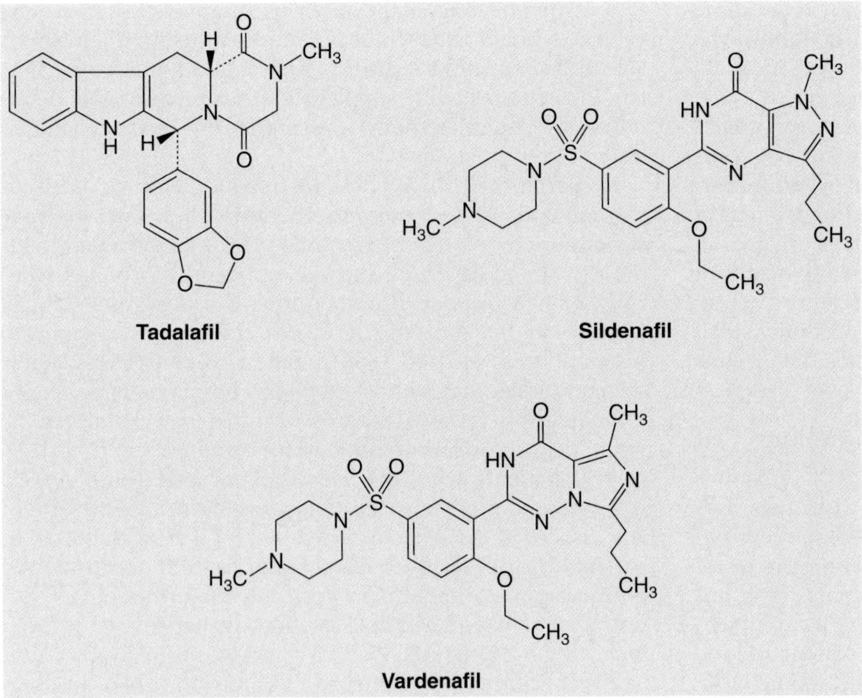

Figure 22–12. The structures of sildenafil, vardenafil, and tadalafil.

alyze the termination of second messenger activity in cells by breaking the phosphodiester bond of either cyclic adenosine monophosphate (AMP) or cyclic GMP. Eleven distinct families have been identified (PDE-1 to PDE-11) that are known to have or are implicated in a broad range of cellular functions. PDE-5 is present in high concentrations in the smooth muscle of the penile corpora cavernosa. **Sildenafil and vardenafil crossreact slightly with PDE-6, that is, their IC50s for PDE-5 are only 4- to 10-fold lower than those for PDE-6. This may explain the complaint of some patients that sildenafil causes visual disturbances. Tadalafil minimally crossreacts with PDE-11, but the consequences of this effect are unknown** (Weeks et al, 2005). None of the three PDE-5 inhibitors crossreacts to a large extent with PDEs other than PDE-6 and PDE-11. **Except for visual disturbances, the other reported side effects of PDE-5 inhibitors (e.g., headaches, flushing, slight lowering of blood pressure, dyspepsia) are** likely caused by **PDE-5 inhibition in vascular or gastrointestinal smooth muscle.**

Sildenafil, vardenafil, and tadalafil have broadly similar times required for attaining maximal plasma concentration (Tmax). The time required for elimination of one half of the medication from plasma of tadalafil is considerably longer than that of the other two PDE-5 inhibitors, which could be due to slower degradation of this drug by the liver or to other factors. The extended half-life of tadalafil might provide a longer therapeutic effect, which may be preferred for spontaneous sexual activity, but could subject the patient to greater drug exposure and prolonged adverse events. **Despite the lack of direct comparative studies, all three PDE-5 inhibitors appear to have equivalent efficacy in the treatment of ED. All appear to be generally well tolerated and have similar contraindications and warnings. However, vardenafil is the only PDE-5 inhibitor with a cardiac conduction precaution** (Table 22–7).

Table 22–7. Comparison of Three PDE-5 Inhibitors Currently Available in the United States

	Sildenafil	*Vardenafil*	*Tadalafil*
Cmax (ng/mL)	450	20.9	378
Tmax (hr)	0.8	0.7-0.9	2
Onset of action	15 min to 1 hr	15 min to 1 hr	15 min to 2 hr
Half-life	3-5 hr	4-5 hr	17.5 hr
Bioavailability	40%	15%	Not tested
Fatty food	Reduced absorption	Reduced absorption	No effect
Recommended dosage	25, 50, 100 mg	5, 10, 20 mg	5, 10, 20 mg
Side effects			
Headache, dyspepsia, facial flushing	Yes	Yes	Yes
Backache, myalgia	Rare	Rare	Yes
Blurred/blue vision	Yes	Rare	Rare
Precaution with antiarrhythmics	No	Yes	No
Contraindication with nitrates	Yes	Yes	Yes

Cmax, maximal plasma concentration; Tmax, time required to attain Cmax.

One particular concern is the development of nonarteritic anterior ischemic optic neuropathy (NAION), which has been reported in men using sildenafil, vardenafil, and tadalafil (n = 38, 1, and 4, respectively, from a total of 30 million users up to June 2005) (Pomeranz and Bhavsar, 2005). Although many of those affected had risk factors such as hypertension, diabetes, or hyperlipidemia, recurrence of NAION after rechallenge with PDE-5 inhibitors in several reports indicates a causal relationship in some men. PDE-5 inhibitors are also shown to be beneficial in patients with pulmonary hypertension (Chua et al, 2005). In June 2005, FDA approved the use of sildenafil 20 mg (under the brand name of Revatio) three times a day for pulmonary artery hypertension.

Effect of PDE-5 Inhibitors in the General ED Population. Sildenafil, vardenafil, and tadalafil are highly effective in enhancing erectile function across a wide range of outcome measures, causes of ED, patient subgroups, and regional populations (Jackson et al, 2005; Mirone et al, 2005; Montorsi et al, 2005). Because of differences in trial designs, comparisons among the three PDE-5 inhibitors across published studies are not feasible (Carson and Lue, 2005).

The effects of sildenafil, vardenafil, and tadalafil on nocturnal penile erections have been evaluated in several studies, and all three medications improved erections in men with ED (Klotz et al, 2001; Terradas et al, 2001). Many randomized controlled trials have also been conducted, and the three agents show similar efficacy and tolerability in men with ED of varying severity and cause. The pivotal studies are presented below (Carson and Lue, 2005).

In a 1998 report of a dose-escalation (50 to 100 mg) sildenafil phase 3 trial involving 329 men (mean age 59 years) who had had ED for 5 years (organic ED ≥ 55%), the mean score for the IIEF erectile function domain at the end of 12 weeks of treatment was 22.1 in the sildenafil group and 12.2 in the placebo group ($P < .001$). Scores on the orgasmic function, intercourse satisfaction, and overall satisfaction domains (but not the sexual desire domain) also significantly improved (Goldstein et al, 1998). It is to be noted that randomized controlled trials with each of the three PDE-5 inhibitors have shown no significant improvement in libido between patients receiving active treatment and those given placebo (Goldstein et al, 1998; Brock et al, 2002; Hellstrom et al, 2002).

The efficacy of vardenafil at differing doses was evaluated in 805 men (age 57 years) with a duration of ED ≥ 2.9 years (Hellstrom et al, 2002). At least 54% of men in each treatment group had organic ED. The mean IIEF erectile function score increased from 12.8 at baseline to 21 at week 12 of 20-mg treatment with vardenafil compared with an increase from 13.6 to only 15.0 in the placebo group (Hellstrom et al, 2002). In addition, 73% of patients randomized to vardenafil, 10 mg, and 81% of those randomized to the 20-mg dose reported that treatment improved their erections, in contrast to 39% of placebo-treated patients ($P < .001$ for each comparison vs. placebo). About 40% of patients with severe ED had an IIEF erectile function domain score ≥ 26 after 12 weeks of treatment with vardenafil 20 mg, as did half of those with moderate ED and 79% of those with mild ED at baseline. The vardenafil pivotal trials excluded sildenafil nonresponders (Hellstrom et al, 2002).

An integrated phase 3 tadalafil study (Brock et al, 2002) involving 1112 patients showed that the IIEF erectile function domain score at the end of 12 weeks of treatment was 24 in men receiving tadalafil 20 mg, compared with 15 in men receiving placebo ($P < .001$). Patients were 59 years old on average, 61% had organic ED, and 90% had ED of more than 1 year's duration. Treatment with tadalafil, 20 mg, also significantly enhanced the intercourse satisfaction and overall satisfaction domains of the IIEF. A total of 81% of responses to the GAQ indicated improved erections in the tadalafil, 20 mg, group, in contrast to 35% in the placebo group ($P < .001$). More than 70% of intercourse attempts were successfully completed with tadalafil, 20 mg, from more than 30 minutes to 36 hours after dosing (Brock et al, 2002).

Effect of PDE-5 Inhibitors in Difficult-to-Treat Patients. The Sildenafil Diabetes Study Group (Rendell et al, 1999) showed that 56% of men with ED and **diabetes mellitus** who underwent sildenafil (25 to 100 mg) treatment for 12 weeks reported improved erections, in contrast to 10% of patients receiving placebo ($P < .001$). In that study, 61% of men randomized to sildenafil reported at least one successful attempt at sexual intercourse, compared with 22% of controls ($P < .001$). Similarly, 452 diabetic men with ED treated with vardenafil for 12 weeks had significant increases in the erectile function domain score: 5.9 for vardenafil, 10 mg; 7.8 for vardenafil, 20 mg; 1.4 for placebo ($P < .001$ for each comparison) (Goldstein et al, 2003). Based on positive responses to the global assessment questions (GAQ) after 12 weeks of treatment, 54% and 72% of patients receiving vardenafil 10 mg and 20 mg, respectively, reported that their erections were improved, in contrast to 13% of placebo controls ($P < .001$ for each comparison vs. placebo) (Goldstein et al, 2003). At the endpoint, 54% of intercourse attempts were successful in men receiving vardenafil, 20 mg, and 49% in those receiving vardenafil, 10 mg, compared with 23% in placebo controls ($P < .001$ for each comparison vs. placebo). Among men with severe ED, the intercourse success rate was 40% in patients receiving vardenafil, 20 mg, compared with 11% in placebo controls ($P < .001$). In the study of diabetic men with ED reported by Saenz de Tejada and colleagues (2002), tadalafil, 10 mg or 20 mg, significantly improved the IIEF erectile function domain score by 6.4 and 7.3, respectively, compared with 0.1 for placebo ($P < .001$ for each comparison). The scores were similar to those reported in a retrospective analysis of 12 randomized controlled trials involving 637 men with ED and diabetes mellitus (Fonseca et al, 2004).

Sildenafil, vardenafil, and tadalafil have all been shown to be effective in diabetic men with ED, although longer-term studies are needed. In the longitudinal Exploratory Comprehensive Evaluation of Erectile Dysfunction study (Penson et al, 2003), men in an observational disease registry showed substantial improvements in the erectile function and intercourse satisfaction domains of the IIEF after 6 months of treatment but relapse to nearly pretreatment levels occurred at 12 months. A similar relapsing trend was seen in the Emotional Life domain of the Psychological Impact of Erectile Dysfunction scale.

In patients with prostate cancer, ED is a well-known side effect after either surgery or radiation. Among such patients, treatment with each of the PDE-5 inhibitors results in significant improvements. In a sildenafil open-label study involving 84 men (mean age 62 years) with ED 2.1 years after radical prostatectomy, 53% receiving sildenafil at 50 to 100 mg reported improved erections and 40% reported an enhanced ability to achieve and maintain erection (Lowentritt et al, 1999). **Erectile function was directly related to the degree of nerve-sparing, with men after bilateral nerve-sparing tending to respond better than those receiving unilateral or non–nerve-sparing surgery. A lower pathologic stage and younger age were also predictive of improved outcomes.** Daily sildenafil use in patients after radical prostatectomy has also been reported to be beneficial. A study with nightly administration of sildenafil or placebo for 36 weeks after a bilateral nerve-sparing prostatectomy revealed a sevenfold improvement in return of spontaneous, normal erectile function 2 months after drug discontinuation in sildenafil-treated group as compared with placebo-treated group (27% vs. 4%) (Padma-Nathan et al, 2004).

Therapy with vardenafil 10 and 20 mg for 12 weeks also significantly enhanced erectile function in 440 men with ED associated with either bilateral or unilateral nerve-sparing radical prostatectomy (Brock et al, 2003). Patients averaged 60 years of age and were a mean of 2 years post surgery at randomization. On the basis of responses to the GAQ, about 65% of patients who completed treatment with vardenafil, 20 mg, reported improved erections, in contrast to 13% of placebo controls ($P < .001$). The average intercourse success rate per patient receiving 20 mg vardenafil was 74% in men with mild to moderate ED and 28% in men with severe ED, compared with 49% and 4% for placebo, respectively.

A double-blind randomized controlled trial involving 303 men (mean age 60 years) with ED seen 12 to 48 months (mean 25 months) after bilateral nerve-sparing radical prostatectomy showed that treatment with tadalafil, 20 mg, for 12 weeks significantly enhanced erectile function (Montorsi et al, 2004). Among all tadalafil patients, 62% reported improved erections at the completion of the study, compared with 23% of controls ($P < .001$). About 54% of intercourse attempts resulted in successful penetration among men randomized to tadalafil, compared with 32% in controls ($P < .001$); 41% of intercourse attempts were successfully completed among patients on tadalafil compared with 19% among controls ($P < .001$) (Montorsi et al, 2004).

Onset of Action. The onset of activity, in reports with similar methods, is 14 minutes with sildenafil, 10 minutes with vardenafil, and 16 minutes with tadalafil (Padma-Nathan et al, 2003; Montorsi et al, 2004; Rosen et al, 2004b). **However, the success rates 20 minutes after medication are much less than those after 1 hour; therefore, if patients do not experience a rapid beneficial effect, they should be advised to delay sexual intercourse for 1 (sildenafil) or 2 hours (tadalafil) when serum concentrations have peaked.**

Patient Satisfaction. Two critical components of therapeutic effectiveness, patient and partner satisfaction, have also been well documented with sildenafil. In a meta-analysis of 14 randomized controlled trials, Montorsi and Althof (2004) reported that 74% of female partners of men aged younger than 65 years who were receiving sildenafil were satisfied with treatment (i.e., EDITS score 50), in contrast to 35% of partners of men receiving placebo ($P < .001$). Similar findings were reported among partners of elderly men. Correlations between patient and partner EDITS scores were significant ($P < .001$) in both placebo ($r = .80$) and sildenafil ($r = .86$) groups. In a review of sildenafil data (2002), Seftel reported that some

patients (14% to 47%) have suboptimal acceptance or lack of long-term adherence to therapy with sildenafil. These findings reflect the fact that drug adherence is a complex matter, with potential psychosocial and physiologic underpinnings. From the psychosocial perspective, restoration of erectile function can reveal other difficulties in a relationship, acting as a "therapeutic probe" for other sources of discord.

For men with low testosterone levels who did not respond to sildenafil, adjunctive testosterone "rescue" therapy (testosterone gel) has been used successfully. In a randomized controlled trial, 75 hypogonadal men with ED and testosterone levels of less than 4 mg/L who had not responded to sildenafil alone received placebo or a 1% testosterone gel (5 mg) daily together with 100 mg of sildenafil (Shabsigh et al, 2004). After 12 weeks, men receiving testosterone and sildenafil had greater improvements in the erectile function domain of the IIEF (4.4 units) than did those with placebo and sildenafil (2.1 units; $P = .029$). The adjunctive testosterone-sildenafil regimen also significantly improved overall satisfaction and orgasmic satisfaction domains, as well as other efficacy outcome measures, compared with sildenafil alone (Shabsigh et al, 2004). Patients should also be counseled to use a PDE-5 inhibitor several times before declaring it "ineffective"; for instance, the cumulative probability of success with sildenafil increases with the first 9 to 10 attempts, after which it stabilizes (McCullough et al, 2002).

Tadalafil therapy has a broader window of clinical responsiveness than either sildenafil or vardenafil because of its longer half-life (17.5 vs. 4 to 5 hours for sildenafil or vardenafil). Tadalafil enhances erectile function in men with ED for up to 36 hours and, thus, may mean less planning and pressure to have sexual intercourse to a schedule, which can result in greater patient and/or partner convenience.

Crossover trials evaluating preferences for one PDE-5 inhibitor over another among patients with ED receiving sildenafil or tadalafil have been conducted. In prospective randomized crossover studies involving about 600 men with ED, patients preferred tadalafil over sildenafil by statistically significant margins (von Keitz et al, 2002; Govier et al, 2003; Stroberg et al, 2003), which remained stable irrespective of comorbidity or previous sildenafil use (von Keitz et al, 2002) Despite patient preference for tadalafil over sildenafil in these prospective clinical trials, comparing the efficacy of either vardenafil or tadalafil against sildenafil cannot readily control for the relative novelty of the newer agents (Carson and Lue, 2005).

Tolerance. Most side effects associated with PDE-5 inhibitor therapy result from inhibition of PDE-5 in other tissue or organs. Untoward events observed with the three agents include headache, dyspepsia, flushing, myalgia/back pain, and rhinitis. In randomized controlled trials, flushing and visual side effects were more common in patients receiving sildenafil or vardenafil, and back pain/myalgia was more common in those receiving tadalafil. These events were mostly mild, abated with time, and prompted treatment discontinuation in only a small number of patients (Goldstein et al, 1998; Brock et al, 2003; Porst et al, 2003).

In the long-term study by Stief and associates (2004), the incidence of treatment-emergent adverse events was highest within the first few weeks of vardenafil treatment, then rapidly declined with further use up to 2 years. Similar findings were recorded in an analysis of 4348 patients (average age, 55 years) in 17 double-blind flexible-dose (25 to 100 mg) sildenafil randomized controlled trials ranging from 8 to 26 weeks in duration. Treatment-related adverse events, including headache, dizziness, dyspepsia, rhinitis, and abnormal vision, peaked at 15% during the first 2 weeks of treatment and declined to 4% at treatment weeks 6 to 8.

WARNINGS AND DRUG INTERACTIONS

The package inserts of all three PDE-5 inhibitors warn against the use in patients with severe cardiovascular diseases and left ventricular outflow obstruction and patients not studied in clinical trials (U.S. prescribing information of Viagra, Cialis and Levitra, July, 2005). These include patients with:

- Myocardial infarction within the previous 90 days

- Unstable angina or angina occurring during sexual intercourse

- New York Heart Association class II or greater heart failure in the previous 6 months

- Uncontrolled arrhythmias, hypotension (<90/50 mm Hg), or uncontrolled hypertension (>170/100 mm Hg)

- Stroke within the previous 6 months

- Known hereditary degenerative retinal disorders, including retinitis pigmentosa

- Tendency to develop priapism (e.g., sickle cell anemia, leukemia)

Certain drugs, such as ketoconazole and itraconazole, and protease inhibitors, such as ritonavir, can impair the metabolic breakdown of PDE-5 inhibitors by blocking the CYP3A4 pathway. Such agents may increase blood levels of inhibitors, requiring a PDE-5 dose reduction. On the other hand, agents such as rifampin may induce CYP3A4, enhancing the breakdown of inhibitors and requiring higher PDE-5 doses. Severe kidney or hepatic dysfunction may require dose adjustments or warnings.

The recommended starting doses are 50 mg for sildenafil and 10 mg for vardenafil and tadalafil taken by mouth. The dose may be increased to 100 mg (sildenafil) or 20 mg (vardenafil and tadalafil) or decreased to 25 mg or 5 mg, respectively, based on individual efficacy and tolerability. The maximal recommended dosing frequency is once per day in most patients.

PDE-5 Inhibitors and Cardiovascular Safety. Many men have both ED and cardiovascular disease, and thus the risks of an acute cardiovascular event during sexual activity and adverse drug interactions are major concerns. **A risk-stratification algorithm was developed by the first Princeton Consensus Panel to evaluate the degree of risk associated** with sexual activity for men with varying degrees of cardiovascular disease (DeBusk et al, 2000): **low risk, intermediate risk (including those requiring further evaluation), and high risk.** A Second Princeton Conference was convened in June, 2004 (Kostis et al, 2005), and the participants reaffirmed the applicability of the original stratification algorithm by which exercise tolerance ascertained by history guides the clinician. The ability to perform exercise of modest intensity without symptoms typically implies low risk. In this category are patients for whom sexual activity does not represent a significant cardiac risk, and no special cardiac testing or evaluation is indicated before the initiation or resumption of sexual activity or institution of a PDE-5 inhibitor. The three risk categories are shown in Tables 22-8 and 22-9, and the management algorithm is shown in Figure 22–13.

Most patients at low risk may safely engage in sexual activity or receive treatment for ED as needed. Patients at high risk should be stabilized by cardiologic treatment before resumption of sexual activity treatment of sexual

Table 22–8. Major Cardiovascular Risk Factors*

Age
Male gender
Hypertension
Diabetes mellitus
Cigarette smoking
Dyslipidemia
Sedentary lifestyle
Family history of premature coronary artery disease

*Emerging and less well validated risk factors such as obesity, the metabolic syndrome, inflammatory markers, ethnicity, psychological stress, and recreational drug use are not included. A history of atherosclerotic disease is a very strong risk factor for a future event.

Table 22–9. Stratification of Cardiovascular Risk in ED Patients

The Low-Risk Patient

Asymptomatic, less than three cardiovascular risk factors (see Table 22-10.)
Controlled hypertension
Mild, stable angina pectoris
Post revascularization
Past myocardial infarction (>6 to 8 wk)
Mild valvular disease
Left ventricular dysfunction (NYHA class I)
Other cardiovascular conditions (pericarditis, mitral valve prolapse, or atrial fibrillation with controlled ventricular response)

The High-Risk Patient

Unstable or refractory angina pectoris
Uncontrolled hypertension
Congestive heart failure (NYHA class III or IV)
Recent myocardial infarction (<2 wk)
High-risk arrhythmia
Obstructive hypertrophic cardiomyopathy
Moderate-to-severe valve disease, particularly aortic stenosis

The Intermediate- or Indeterminate-Risk Patient

Asymptomatic, three or more risk factors (excluding gender)
Moderate, stable angina pectoris
History of myocardial infarction (>2 wk, <6 wk)
Left ventricular dysfunction/congestive heart failure (NYHA class II)
Noncardiac sequelae of atherosclerotic disease

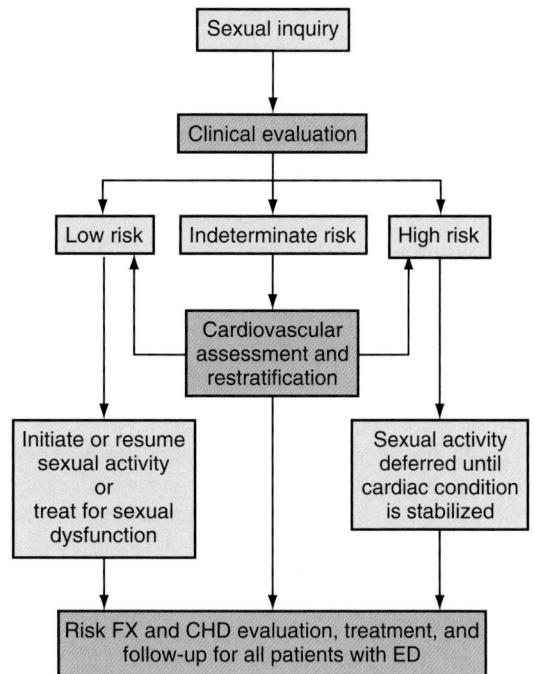

Figure 22–13. Algorithm for evaluation of the patient with cardiovascular disease recommended by the Second Princeton Panel.

dysfunction is considered. Specialized cardiovascular testing is recommended to reclassify patients at intermediate levels of risk into the low- or high-risk category. Patient follow-up and reassessment at regular intervals is recommended in all cases.

With regard to *overall cardiac safety,* controlled and post-marketing studies of the three FDA-approved PDE-5 inhibitors demonstrated no increase in myocardial infarction or death rates in either double-blind, placebo-controlled trials, or open-label studies when compared with expected rates in the study populations (Zussman et al, 1999; Shakir et al, 2001; Emmick et al, 2002; Kloner et al, 2002; Wysowski et al, 2002). Patients with known coronary artery disease or heart failure receiving PDE-5 inhibitors did not exhibit worsening ischemia, coronary vasoconstriction, or worsening hemodynamics on exercise testing or cardiac catheterization (Jackson, 1999; Hermann, 2000; Thadani et al, 2002; Kloner et al, 2003).

PDE-5 inhibitors have a minimal effect on QTc interval (Morganroth et al, 2004). However, **vardenafil is the only one not recommended in patients who take type-1A antiarrhythmics (e.g., quinidine or procainamide) or type-3 antiarrhythmics (e.g., sotalol or amiodarone) or in patients with congenital prolonged QT syndrome.**

The *vasodilator effects* of sildenafil, vardenafil, and tadalafil may be more marked in patients with hypertension or coronary artery disease. As with all vasodilators, caution is advised in certain conditions: aortic stenosis, left ventricular outflow obstruction, hypotension, and hypovolemia (Cheitlin et al, 1999).

Nitrates are *absolutely contraindicated* in patients taking PDE-5 inhibitors. These include organic nitrates, including sublingual nitroglycerin, isosorbide mononitrate, isosorbide dinitrate, and other nitrate preparations used to treat

angina, as well as amyl nitrite or amyl nitrate (so-called poppers, a recreational drug). Past use of nitrates, that is, more than 2 weeks before the use of PDE-5 inhibitors, is not considered a contraindication. Patients who develop angina during sexual activity with a PDE-5 inhibitor should be instructed to discontinue sexual activity, relax for 5 to 10 minutes, and, if the pain persists, seek emergency care and inform emergency medical personnel that a PDE-5 inhibitor was taken.

Patients who develop chest pain after taking a short-acting PDE-5 inhibitor (sildenafil, vardenafil) are advised against taking nitroglycerin for at least 24 hours, as suggested by the guidelines (Cheitlin et al, 1999). A period of 48 hours is recommended after tadalafil. Patients who have acute myocardial infarction after a PDE-5 inhibitor may be given the usual therapies (except for organic nitrates). Patients who develop hypotension after organic nitrates and PDE-5 inhibitors should be placed in the Trendelenburg position and given intravenous fluids, with α-adrenergic agonists (e.g., phenylephrine) as needed. In patients with refractory hypotension, intra-aortic balloon counterpulsation should be administered, as suggested by the American College of Cardiology/American Heart Association guidelines. At present, there is no pharmacologic antidote to the PDE-5 inhibitor/nitrate interaction (Cheitlin et al, 1999).

Caution is advised when an **α-adrenergic blocker** and a PDE-5 inhibitor are given together, because interaction can lead to excessive vasodilation and hypotension.

PDE-5 Inhibitor Combination Therapy. The FDA has not approved PDE-5 inhibitors in combination with other vasoactive penile pharmacotherapies; therefore, any combination treatments should be considered "off label" and undertaken with clinical precautions. Porst (1998) reported salvage of intracavernous injection failure with a combination of sildenafil and alprostadil, although the format was more case report than clinical trial. In a more comprehensive study of 93 men in whom home intracavernous injection therapy had failed (high-dosage alprostadil [20 μg] or Trimix [alprostadil, 20 μg/mL; papaverine, 24 mg/mL; phentolamine, 1.6 mg/mL] in trials of up to 2 mL), McMahon and coworkers (1991) found that 34% responded to sildenafil alone: 30 required 100 mg, and 2 required 50 mg. To a sildenafil-Trimix combination, responders were 31% of the group: all required 100 mg of sildenafil with 0.6 mL Trimix (mean dosage). These authors concluded that two thirds of intracavernous injection failures could be salvaged with sildenafil monotherapy or combination therapies. Adverse events were considerably different from those in previously reported sildenafil trials: dizziness was noted in 5% treated with tablets alone and in 20% of patients on combination therapy. Overall, 37% of patients taking tablets reported side effects: headache (30/34), facial flushing (25/34), dyspepsia (12/34), nasal congestion (9/34), dizziness (5/34), and visual disturbances (1/34). Of those on combination therapy, 49% reported side effects: penile pain (15/41), headache (15/41), facial flushing (12/41), dyspepsia (7/41), nasal congestion (3/41), dizziness (12/41), and syncope (1/41).

Adrenoceptor Antagonists. Oral phentolamine has been used in two pilot studies with some reported improvement in erectile function (Gwinup, 1988; Zorgniotti, 1994). Phentolamine is a nonspecific α-adrenergic antagonist with equal affinity for blocking both α_1 and α_2 adrenoreceptors. In long-term antihypertensive drug trials, a "protective" erectile effect of α-adrenergic blockers has been observed; these patients may have lesser degrees of ED than patients on other antihypertensive agents. In a U.S. multicenter, double-blind, placebo-controlled trial, oral phentolamine (Vasomax) demonstrated mild efficacy over placebo. The treatment effect was measured in a group of patients categorized as having "minimal to mild ED" by IIEF self-assessment. Improvement was noted in 37% of men on 40 mg (n = 152) and 45% of men on 80 mg (n = 159). Side effects were headache, facial flushing, and nasal congestion in fewer than 10% of patients. The study has been criticized for patient selection (minimal and mild ED) as well as for low placebo-response rates, which were typically 20% to 30% in the PDE-5 inhibitor trials (Goldstein et al, 2001).

Intracavernous Injection. One of the most dramatic changes in urology has been the introduction of intracavernous injection of vasoactive drugs for the diagnosis and treatment of ED. At the 1983 annual meeting of the American Urological Association, Brindley personally demonstrated erection after injection of phenoxybenzamine. Subsequently, Zorgniotti and Lefleur (1985) reported their experience instructing patients in the technique of autoinjection of a mixture of papaverine and phentolamine for home use. A list of drugs that have been used clinically is presented in Table 22–10. Several of the most common are discussed in more detail next.

Papaverine. **Papaverine, an alkaloid isolated from the opium poppy, exerts an inhibitory effect on PDE, leading to increased cyclic AMP and cyclic GMP in penile erectile tissue.** Papaverine also blocks voltage-dependent calcium channels, thus impairing calcium influx, and it may also impair calcium-activated potassium and chloride currents (Brading et al, 1983). All these actions relax cavernous smooth muscle and penile vessels. Papaverine is metabolized in the liver, and the plasma half-life is 1 to 2 hours.

Virag and colleagues (1984) originally used papaverine office injection followed by saline infusion to maintain a rigid erection for 15 minutes as a form of corporeal dilation therapy. However, the result was not as successful as expected. Home self-injection has since become popular. **The advantages are its low cost and stability at room temperature. The major disadvantages are the incidences of priapism (up to 35%) and corporeal fibrosis (1% to 33%), thought to be a result of low acidity** (pH, 3 to 4) (Barada and McKimmy, 1994), and occasional elevation of liver enzymes. Several recent reports indicate that papaverine may be toxic to endothelial cells, cavernous fibroblast, or smooth muscle cells (Pilatz et al, 2005), although these studies were performed in

primary cell culture with high concentrations of papaverine for 30 minutes. Whether the results are applicable to intracavernous injection therapy, where the effect is on three-dimensional erectile tissue rather than on a monolayer cell culture and is diluted by large arterial inflow, is uncertain. In our experience, fibrosis seems to be associated with poor technique, minimal compression time to the injection site, and more than 1-mL injection volume. Systemic side effects include dizziness, pallor, and cold sweats, which may be the result of vasovagal reflex. The clinical dosages of papaverine monotherapy range from 20 to 80 mg. Its general efficacy as monotherapy is less than 55%; although it was the very first agent for promoting erection, it has never been reviewed or approved by the FDA for that specific purpose.

α-Adrenergic Antagonists. **Phentolamine methylate (Regitine) is a competitive α-adrenoceptor antagonist with equal affinity for α_1- and α_2-adrenergic receptors. Systemic hypotension, reflex tachycardia, nasal congestion, and gastrointestinal upset are the most common systemic side effects.** It has a short plasma half-life (30 minutes). When injected intracavernously alone, it increases corporeal blood flow but does not result in a significant rise in intracavernous pressure. It is hypothesized that, by blocking prejunctional α_2 adrenoreceptors, phentolamine inadvertently increases intracavernous norepinephrine, preventing complete sinusoidal relaxation (Juenemann et al, 1986; Juenemann and Alken, 1989). *Moxisylyte (thymoxamine)* is a competitive blocker of α_1 adrenoceptors approved in several European countries but not in the United States. It has a short duration of action, 3 to 4 hours, and some antihistaminic properties. Buvat and colleagues (1993) compared results in 72 patients receiving moxisylyte with those in 34 patients treated with papaverine during the same time period. Complete and sustained erection was induced in 68% of patients treated with moxisylyte and 79% with papaverine. The rate of prolonged erection (1.3% vs. 8.8%) and corporeal fibrosis (1.3% vs. 32%) was significantly less with moxisylyte.

Alprostadil (Prostaglandin E₁). **Alprostadil is the synthetic form of a naturally occurring fatty acid (i.e., alprostadil refers to the exogenous form, PGE₁ to the endogenous compound). It causes smooth muscle relaxation, vasodilation, and inhibition of platelet aggregation through elevation of intracellular cyclic AMP.** Alprostadil is metabolized by the enzyme prostaglandin-15-hydroxydehydrogenase, which has been shown to be active in human corpus cavernosum (Roy et al, 1989). After intracavernous injection, 96% of alprostadil is locally metabolized within 60 minutes and no change in peripheral blood levels has been observed (van Ahlen et al, 1994). In patients with veno-occlusive dysfunction, alprostadil may rise to 10 times

Drug	Dose Range	Advantages	Disadvantages/Side Effects
Papaverine	7.5-60 mg	Low cost; Stable at room temp	Fibrosis, priapism; Elevation of liver enzymes
Papaverine + phentolamine	0.1-1 mL	More potent than papaverine alone	Fibrosis, priapism
Alprostadil	1-60 µg	Metabolized in penis; Priapism rare	Painful erection; Requires refrigeration; Relatively expensive
Moxisylyte	10-30 mg	Priapism rare	Less potent
Papaverine + phentolamine + alprostadil	0.1-1.0 mL	Most potent	Requires refrigeration

Table 22-10. Common Intracavernous Agents

baseline, but up to 90% is metabolized on the first pass through the lungs.

In a review of the published literature, Linet and Neff (1994) found that, in doses of 10 to 20 μg, alprostadil produced full erections in 70% to 80% of patients with ED. The most frequent side effects were pain at the injection site or during erection (in 16.8% of patients), hematoma/ecchymosis (1.5%), and prolonged erection/priapism (1.3%). Systemic side effects occurred rarely. In the 1996 worldwide clinical trials conducted by the Alprostadil Study group, efficacy of PGE1 was 87% in 683 subjects. Only 6% of subjects withdrew from the study because of penile pain, although 11% of individual injections were noted to cause pain. Prolonged erection was noted in 5% (4 to 6 hours) and priapism (>6 hours) in 1%; penile fibrotic lesions were found in 2% of all subjects regardless of history of normal or prolonged erections (Linet and Ogrinc, 1996).

In the United States, injectable alprostadil for ED therapy is available in two proprietary forms: Caverject (Pfizer) and Edex (Schwarz Pharma). The clinical dose ranges from 2 to 40 mcg. Its advantages are lower incidences of prolonged erection, systemic side effects, and fibrosis. The disadvantages include a higher incidence of painful erection and higher cost, and, once reconstituted into liquid from powder, it has a shortened half-life if not refrigerated.

Commonly Used Drug Combinations. **Zorgniotti and Lefleur** (1985) **first reported the use of a combination of papaverine (30 mg) and phentolamine (0.5 mg) for self-injection.** This was effective in 72% of 250 patients. Prolonged erection occurred in 1.6% during titration and in one patient on home therapy. Fibrosis developed in 4.1%. The combination has been used successfully in patients with different types of ED. In a study by Armstrong and associates (1993), a total of 160 men with erectile failure received treatment with 13,030 intracavernous papaverine and phentolamine injections. An erection sufficient for sexual intercourse was achieved in 115 (72%). The response rates were as follows: vasculogenic (48%), psychogenic (93%), neurogenic (92%), diabetic (68%), idiopathic (63%), traumatic (60%), alcohol-related (80%), and drug-related (75%). After a mean follow-up period of 14.1 months, 55 (48%) were still successfully using intracavernous therapy. A total of 22 episodes of priapism occurred in 16 patients and one patient developed corporeal fibrosis.

In 1991, **Bennett and coworkers introduced a three-drug mixture containing 2.5 mL papaverine (30 mg/mL), 0.5 mL phentolamine (5 mg/mL), and 0.05 mL alprostadil (500 μg/mL) for intracavernous injection;** 89% of the patients tested had adequate erection and went on to home injection therapy. Overall, 74% of the 78 patients were maintained at a dose of less than 0.25 mL per injection with a frequency averaging 3.1 uses per month. Two patients had prolonged erection that required treatment. In another report from the same group, Barada and Bennett (1991) contacted 110 patients with 12 to 28 months of follow-up: 65% were continuing injection therapy and of these, 89% were satisfied with the drug combination. Seven prolonged erections (5.6%) of more than 3 hours occurred. No patient developed fibrosis or nodules.

In another study (Goldstein et al, 1990), 32 patients in whom alprostadil alone or the dual combination of papaver-

ine/phentolamine had failed had adequate erection when the triple combination was used. Eight patients reported painful erection. No prolonged erections or systemic side effects were noted. In a randomized crossover study of 228 patients, McMahon (1991) likewise compared the triple-drug combination with papaverine/phentolamine and alprostadil alone. **In summary, the triple-drug combination has been shown to be as effective as alprostadil alone, or more so, and has a much lower incidence of painful erection. It is generally reserved for men in whom PGE₁ or papaverine/phentolamine therapy has failed or who have significant penile pain with PGE₁.**

Other Drug Combinations. Several other drug combinations have also been studied. Virag and associates (1991) first used a combination of six drugs (Ceritine [which contains atropine], dipyridamole, ifenprodil, papaverine, piribedil, and yohimbine) in treating ED. Floth and Schramek (1991) reported that the combination of papaverine (7.5 mg) and alprostadil (5 μg) is more effective than alprostadil alone (10 μg). Gerstenberg and coworkers (1992) reported a combination of vasoactive intestinal polypeptide (VIP) (30 μg) and phentolamine (0.5 to 2.0 mg) in 52 men with a total of 1380 self-injections. After sexual stimulation, all patients obtained adequate erection, and none developed priapism, fibrosis, or systemic side effects. Although intracavernous VIP alone produced disappointing responses, in combination with papaverine it potentiated the response to this drug. Kiely and colleagues (1989) reported that a combination of papaverine and VIP produced penile rigidity similar to that with papaverine and phentolamine. Truss and coworkers (1994) reported the results of testing a mixture of calcitonin gene–related peptide (CGRP) (5 μg) and alprostadil (10 μg) in 28 patients with ED and venous leakage. Erections sufficient for intercourse were noted in 19 of the 28 patients (68%). Mulhall and coworkers (1997) reported that approximately 20% of men in whom Trimix fails (papaverine, 30 mg/mL; phentolamine, 2 mg/mL; PGE₁, 20 μg/mL) can be salvaged by Quadmix, that is, the addition of forskolin (1000 μg/mL), which resulted in substantial improvements in 61% of 31 patients studied.

Facilitation of Erectile Function Recovery after Radical Prostatectomy. In a small study, 30 potent patients who had undergone nerve-sparing radical retropubic prostatectomy were randomized to alprostadil injections three times a week for 12 weeks (15 patients) or observation without any treatment (15 patients). Patients were assessed at the 6-month follow-up by sexual history, physical examination, color Doppler sonography of the cavernous arteries, and polysomnographic recording of nocturnal erections. In the alprostadil-treated group, 12 patients (80%) completed the entire treatment schedule and were evaluated at the follow-up. In this group 8 patients (67%) reported the recovery of spontaneous erection sufficient for satisfactory sexual intercourse, compared with 3 patients (20%) in the control group ($P <$ .01). In the injection group, all but one patient reporting normal postoperative erections also showed normal erections at nocturnal testing, whereas color Doppler sonography demonstrated normal penile hemodynamics in all. Failure in the injection group was the result of cavernous veno-occlusive dysfunction (2 patients, 17%) and cavernous nerve injury (2 patients, 17%). In the control group, patients with normal erections (n = 3) showed both normal nocturnal testing and penile hemodynamics, whereas failures were the result of cavernous veno-occlusive dysfunction (8 patients, 53%), cavernous arterial insufficiency (2 patients, 13%), and cavernous nerve injury (3 patients, 20%). Complications in patients treated with alprostadil injections comprised two cases of penile nodule and one case of prolonged penile erection. Complications were not seen in the control group. **The authors suggest that programmed vasoactive injections improve cavernous oxygenation, thereby limiting the development of hypoxia-induced tissue damage** (Montorsi et al, 1997).

Patient Acceptance and Dropout. In several studies, the percentage of patients accepting injection therapy when offered in the office ranges from 49% to 84% (Gerber and Levine, 1991; Chandeck Montesa et al, 1992). In long-term studies, 13% to 60% of patients drop out for a number of reasons. These include loss of interest, loss of partner, poor erectile response, penile pain, concomitant illness, recovery of spontaneous erection, and ultimate choice of other therapy. De la Taille and coworkers (1999) segregated dropouts into short- and long-term dropouts. They found that, of patients who were instructed in self-injection therapy and never initiated home treatment, dissatisfaction and unnaturalness of the process were most commonly cited. Among dropouts from home therapy (63%), the most common complaints were drug costs and insufficient erection for penetration.

Serious Adverse Effects. **Priapism and fibrosis are the two more serious side effects associated with intracavernous injection therapy.** Linet and Neff (1994) calculated that priapism occurred in 1.3% of 8090 patients in 48 studies with alprostadil, an incidence about five times lower than with papaverine or papaverine/phentolamine (1.5% vs. 10% vs. 7%). Fibrosis can occur as a nodule, diffuse scarring, plaque, or curvature. The incidence is about ten times lower with alprostadil than with papaverine or papaverine/phentolamine (1% vs. 12% vs. 9% of patients) (Pastorini et al, 1993), although one study reported a 12% incidence with alprostadil.

Dosage and Administration. Patients must have the first injection performed by medical personnel and receive appropriate training and education before home injection. For alprostadil, an initial dose of 2.5 µg is recommended. If the response is inadequate, increases in 2.5-µg increments can be given until a full erection is achieved or a maximum of 60 µg is reached. There is no manufacturer's recommendation for other drugs used in intracavernous injection.

As a general rule, one should start with a small dose (e.g., 7.5 mg of papaverine, 0.1 mL of combination drugs), especially in patients with nonvascular ED. The goal is to achieve an erection adequate for sexual intercourse but that lasts for less than 1 hour. In patients who use excessive amounts to maintain erection for more than 1 hour, increasing doses may be required to achieve and maintain the same erection and eventually may fail to achieve erection at all.

Contraindications. The use of intracavernous injection therapy is contraindicated in patients with sickle cell anemia, schizophrenia or other severe psychiatric disorders, or severe systemic disease. In patients taking an anticoagulant or aspirin, compressing the injection site for 7 to 10 minutes after injection is recommended. In patients with poor manual dexterity, the sexual partner can be instructed to perform the injection.

Intraurethral Therapy. Alprostadil, the synthetic formulation of PGE_1, is the only pharmacologic agent with FDA approval for ED management by both intracavernous and intraurethral routes. When inserted into the urethra, the drug is absorbed from the urethra by the corpus spongiosum and then transported to the corpus cavernosum through venous channels (through circumflex and emissary veins perforating the tunica albuginea). **The medicated urethral system for erection (MUSE; Vivus, Inc, Mountain View, CA) consists of a very small semisolid pellet (3 × 1 mm) administered into the distal urethra (3 cm) by a proprietary applicator (MUSE).** The alprostadil is rapidly absorbed by the urethral mucosa (residual urine in the urethra helps the pellet to dissolve); 20% of a 1000-µg dosage remains after 20 minutes (Vivus, Inc, Pharmacokinetic and Toxicological Data, FDA submission, 1996). Some female partners report vaginal discomfort (about 10%) after ejaculation by a man using MUSE. Dosages of 500 µg of MUSE have equivalent vasodilatory effects of 10 µg of injected alprostadil (as measured by duplex Doppler peak systolic velocity changes in cavernous arteries), but significantly inferior degrees of veno-occlusion are seen (Padma-Nathan et al, 1997). This translates into reduced penile rigidity.

Clinical trials involved 1511 men, who were first treated in the office with intraurethral pellets of varying dosages (125, 250, 500, 1000 µg). **To this in-office trial, 66% responded; of these, 65% had successful intercourse at least once at home with MUSE, for a rate of 43%. Only 50.4% of episodes of home administrations resulted in intercourse in those men who were office responders** (Hellstrom et al, 1996; Padma-Nathan et al, 1997). Penile rigidity can be enhanced by an elastic ring placed at the base of the penis (ACTIS; Vivus, Inc) to assist veno-occlusion mechanically.

Penile pain is a ubiquitous side effect of alprostadil-based therapies and is clearly dose related; in MUSE patients, the discomfort, a dull ache, can range from the penis to the scrotum and lower extremities. **The reported penile pain rate was up to 10.6% in Caverject trials and 33% in MUSE trials. In the latter, hypotension and syncope have been noted in 1% to 5.8%, mandating the office setting for initial administration.**

Transdermal Therapy. Two companies are currently conducting U.S. clinical trials of transglanular monotherapy (Macrochem Corporation and NexMed, Inc). Topiglan (Macrochem) is a mixture of a PGE_1 gel (0.5 to 2.5 mg) and a proprietary transdermal permeation enhancer (SEPA). In a recent single-blind, nonrandomized dosage study of Topiglan, 48 ED patients were screened by positive responses to injectable PGE_1 (an erection score of 4 or 5 on a 5-point scale). Topiglan responses were 3 or greater in up to 67% to 75% of patients, but, unlike injectable dosing, all men required audiovisual self-stimulation and/or tactile self-stimulation to achieve any erection. Nearly 20% of patients had penile discomfort, described as warmth to severe burning.

Alprox-TD is also an enhancer-driven alprostadil gel. In two multicenter, placebo-controlled, phase 2 studies, patients with mild-to-moderate (n = 161, study 1) or severe (n = 142, study 2) ED were randomized to receive placebo or Alprox-TD (0.05, 0.1, or 0.2 mg in study 1 and 0.1, 0.2, or 0.3 mg in study 2). The primary efficacy endpoint in both studies was the change in erectile function score from baseline to final visit: −0.8 ± 1.1,

1.8 ± 1.1, 0.7 ± 1.2, and 3.7 ± 1.2 ($P < .01$; study 1); and 2.7 ± 1.3, 6.29 ± 1.4, 6.49 ± 1.5, and 9.44 ± 1.5 ($P < .001$; study 2) for placebo and ascending dose groups in each study. Topical alprostadil was well tolerated, with the most common adverse event being urogenital pain (Padma-Nathan et al, 2003).

Centrally Acting Drugs

Yohimbine is an α_2-adrenergic antagonist obtained from the bark of the yohim tree. It acts centrally to promote sexual behavior by blocking presynaptic autoreceptors and increasing adrenergic receptor activity, which also alters serotonin and dopamine transmission. Documented experimental effects on the male sexual response from either systemically or intracranially administered yohimbine are behavioral. Although yohimbine has been highly effective in castrated rats, several clinical studies have shown only moderate success in men. **In a controlled randomized study of patients with organic ED receiving 6 mg of yohimbine orally three times a day for 10 weeks, no significant difference from those taking placebo was found** (Morales et al, 1987). However, in a study in patients with psychogenic ED, a positive response rate of 62% was noted, whereas the placebo group achieved only a 16% response rate (Reid et al, 1987). Despite these relatively poor results, yohimbine has been traditionally prescribed because of its mild side effects (anxiety, nervousness, slight increase of blood pressure) (Ernst and Pittler, 1998). As an initial treatment, 5.4 mg three times a day has been recommended; others have reported efficacy by doubling that dosage or using it on an as-needed basis (two tablets 1 to 2 hours before anticipated sexual activity). Side effects of yohimbine include gastrointestinal intolerance, palpitations, headache, agitation, anxiety, and increased blood pressure. The American Urological Association in its guidelines for the management of organic ED published in 1996 advised that there was no efficacy of yohimbine over placebo in patients with organic ED.

Trazodone is a commonly prescribed mild antidepressant with a rare incidence of priapism. Several small clinical trials have shown a positive effect on nocturnal penile erection (Saenz de Tejada et al, 1991) and sexually stimulated erection (Lal et al, 1987). However, in a double-blind study of 51 ED patients taking either 50 mg of trazodone or placebo at bedtime for 3 months, 19% of patients receiving trazodone had improved erections compared with 24% receiving placebo ($P < .50$). The authors concluded that, in patients with severe physiologic ED, trazodone is no more effective than placebo in improving erections and sexual function (Costabile et al, 1999). Side effects include drowsiness, nausea, emesis, blood pressure changes (both hypotension and hypertension), urinary retention, and priapism (especially at therapeutic antidepressant levels).

Apomorphine has a well-known positive effect on sexual arousal in the rat model: intrathecal or subcutaneous injection causes yawning and erection. Apomorphine is not an opiate and is chemically unrelated to morphine; it acts in the brain within the paraventricular nucleus, which functions as the sexual drive center in mammals. **Apomorphine is a dopaminergic agonist, activating D_1 and D_2 receptors. Dopaminergic stimulation is proerectile;** early reports of patients treated for Parkinson's disease showed increased spontaneous erections, without increased libido.

In 1995, Heaton and associates demonstrated that a new formulation permitting buccal absorption (oral ingestion, without swallowing) induced erection in 67% of psychogenically impotent patients. Clinical trials were conducted in "typical ED patients," men with risk factors such as hypertension, diabetes, and atherosclerotic coronary artery disease. At dosages of 2 and 4 mg, subjects reporting erections firm enough for intercourse were 45% and 55%, respectively, with placebo responses of 35% and 36%. Sexual attempts resulting in intercourse were 40% and 49%, respectively, on 2 and 4 mg; placebo resulted in intercourse in 30% of attempts. Self-assessment of success was 47% and 59.9% at 2- and 4-mg dosages (data on file, Uprima, TAP Holdings, Inc).

Sexual arousal is necessary to enhance the effect of apomorphine. Also, if the tablet is swallowed, the erectile efficacy is lost. The drug has a rapid onset of action, with mean time to erection of 12 minutes, but the pharmacology permits a window of sexual opportunity of approximately 2 hours from ingestion. Maximal plasma concentrations are reached in 50 minutes, and eating beforehand has no effect. Adverse events described in clinical trials were nausea, 16.9%; dizziness, 8.3%; sweating, 5%; somnolence, 5.8%; yawning, 7.9%; and emesis, 3.7%. At the highest recommended dosage, syncope occurred in 0.6% of patients and was accompanied by a clear prodrome suggestive of a vasovagal event: nausea, vomiting, sweating, dizziness, and light-headedness. The vasovagal events were without cardiac sequelae in clinical trials and notably not consistent among subjects who chose to rechallenge. The reported severity of nausea was lowered in those subjects who were titrated from lower to higher dosages. There were no documented food/drug interactions in clinical trials (with the exception of ethanol) and, specifically, no documented pharmacologic interactions for subjects using nitrate drugs. Sublingual apomorphine was approved by European authority in early 2001.

Melanocortin-Receptor Agonists. **Melanocortin-4 receptor (MC4R) has been implicated in controlling food intake and energy expenditure as well as modulating erectile function and sexual behavior.** Wessells and associates (2000) reported that, in the absence of sexual stimulation, subcutaneous melanotan II led to penile erection in 17 of 20 men. Increased sexual desire was reported after 13/19 (68%) doses of melanotan II versus 4/21 (19%) of placebo ($P < .01$). Nausea and yawning were frequently reported; at a dose of 0.025 mg/kg, 12.9% of subjects had severe nausea.

Another melanocortin analog, PT-141, was also evaluated after subcutaneous administration in healthy men and in ED patients with an inadequate response to sildenafil. Erectile responses were assessed by RigiScan in healthy subjects in the absence of visual sexual stimulation (VSS); doses ranging from 0.3 to 10 mg resulted in a statistically significant erectile response at doses over 1.0 mg. ED patients were treated with placebo or 4 or 6 mg PT-141 in a crossover design in the presence of VSS; the erectile response was statistically significant at both doses (Rosen et al, 2004c).

Intranasal administration of PT-141 in healthy male subjects and in sildenafil-responsive ED patients was also studied. Erectile response was assessed by RigiScan in healthy men without VSS and in sildenafil-responsive ED patients with VSS. Median Tmax was 0.50 hr and mean half-life ranged from 1.85 to 2.09 hours. In both studies, an erectile response induced by PT-141 was significantly greater than the placebo's at doses over 7 mg, with the onset of the first erection occurring in approximately 30 minutes. Flushing and nausea were the most common adverse events reported in both studies, and no clinically significant changes in vital signs, laboratory tests, electrocardiograms, or physical examination were observed (Diamond et al, 2004).

Vacuum Constriction Device

The vacuum constriction device consists of a plastic cylinder connected directly or by tubing to a vacuum-generating source (manual or battery-operated pump). After the penis is engorged by the negative pressure, a constricting ring is applied to the base to maintain the erection. To avoid injury, the ring should not be left in place for longer than 30 minutes.

The erection produced by a vacuum device is different from a physiologic erection or one produced by intracavernous injection. The blood oxygen level in the corpus cavernosum is less and the portion of the penis proximal to the ring is not rigid, which may produce a pivoting effect. The penile skin may be cold and dusky, and ejaculation may be trapped by the constricting ring. The ring can be uncomfortable or even painful. However, in many patients, the device can produce an erection that is close to normal and rigidity sufficient for coitus. The device also engorges the glans and is useful for patients with glanular insufficiency.

In patients with severe proximal venous leakage or arterial insufficiency, fibrosis secondary to priapism, or an infection from a prosthesis, the device may not produce adequate erection. **The device can be used successfully by men with a malfunctioning penile prosthesis in place** (Sidi et al, 1990; Korenman and Viosca, 1992) **and has been used after explantation to prevent shortening. In men with severe vascular insufficiency, combining intracavernous injection with the vacuum constriction device may enhance the erection** (Marmar et al, 1988).

The majority of men using the device report satisfaction with penile rigidity, length, and circumference; partner satisfaction is likewise good (Sidi and Lewis, 1992). Patients also report an improvement in self-esteem and sense of well-being. Complications include penile pain and numbness, difficult ejaculation, ecchymosis, and petechiae. **Patients taking aspirin or warfarin (Coumadin) should exercise caution when using these devices.**

The patient satisfaction rate has been reported to range from 68% to 83% (Cookson and Nadig, 1993). Derouet and coworkers (1999) performed a retrospective review of their patients and reported that 20% rejected the device primarily and another 30.9% after a period of up to 16 weeks. They cite a primary dropout rate of 50.9% and a secondary dropout rate of 7.3% after 10 months. Long-term users (41.8%) reported 98% satisfaction; partner satisfaction was 85%. Dutta and Eid (1999) describe an attrition rate of 65% at a mean of 4 months; in their experience, 35% of patients continued with the vacuum constriction device long term (mean, 37 months). The device is more acceptable to older men in a steady relationship than to young single men in search of a partner. It is safe when used properly and is one of the least costly treatment options available. Although it can be used by any patient with ED, it is recommend that a reasonable evaluation be conducted so that some easily correctable cause of the dysfunction will not be overlooked.

FUTURE RESEARCH

The American Urological Association Guidelines Panel on ED has made a number of recommendations (2005). To develop new and more effective agents for treatment, the panel recommends more research in the areas of pathophysiology, natural history, and epidemiology (e.g., the role of hypogonadism in ED, the epidemiology of bothersomeness in men and their partners before and after treatment, and the prevalence and severity of ED in men with hypertension, hyperlipidemia, diabetes, and smoking).

Improvement in clinically applicable instruments is needed to improve diagnosis and assess satisfaction. The panel identified two urgent needs: testing for both neurologic and venoocclusive function of the corpus cavernosum. Evidence-based criteria are also needed to classify arterial and venous origins.

A number of research priorities are recommended regarding treatment of ED.

RESEARCH PRIORITIES IN ED DIAGNOSIS AND TREATMENT

- Outcomes of oral PDE-5 inhibitors characterized/stratified based on testosterone levels
- Better characterization of the adverse events associated with ED therapies (e.g., duration of headache)
- Effect of lifestyle modification
- Identification of patients who should not be sexually active with or without PDE-5 inhibitors
- Effect of PDE-5 inhibitors that crossreact with PDE-11 in patients with abnormal spermatogenesis
- Applicability of PDE-5 inhibitors after radical prostatectomy
- Role of testosterone therapy in ED patients with low, borderline-normal, and normal testosterone levels
- Additional randomized controlled trials of various herbal therapies
- Efficacy and safety of combining pharmacotherapies and/or mechanical therapies, such as oral and intrapenile vasoconstrictive therapies, PDE-5 inhibitors and prostheses, or vacuum constriction and vasoconstriction devices
- Randomized controlled trial on the efficacy of drugs in veno-occlusive ED
- Cost-effectiveness analyses of the fixed and unfixed costs involved with the various ED treatments
- Standardized measure of patient-partner satisfaction beyond the IIEF

PREMATURE EJACULATION
Definition

The definition of premature ejaculation (PE) is still evolving. Those most often quoted are from the American Psychiatric Association's *Diagnostic and Statistical Manual of Mental Disorders* (4th edition, revised, 1994) (DSM-IV-R) and the World Health Organization's 1994 *International Classification of Diseases* (ICD-10). The former defines it as "persistent or recurrent ejaculation with minimal stimulation before, on, or shortly after penetration and before the person wishes it. The disturbance causes marked distress or interpersonal difficulty." The latter defines it as "an inability to delay ejaculation sufficiently to enjoy lovemaking, manifest as either of the following: occurrence of ejaculation before or very soon after the beginning of intercourse (if a time limit is required: before or within 15 seconds of the beginning of intercourse); occurrence of ejaculation in the absence of sufficient erection to make intercourse possible. The problem is not the result of prolonged absence from sexual activity."

The Triad of Premature Ejaculation

Both DSM-IV-R and ICD-10 definitions refer to three essential components for the diagnosis of PE: short ejaculatory latency; lack of control; and sexual dissatisfaction.

The short ejaculatory latency is typically measured by intravaginal ejaculatory latency time (IVELT), defined as the time between vaginal intromission and ejaculation, averaged over a number of sexual encounters. The DSM-IV-R definition indicates that latencies of 15 seconds or less are consistent with the diagnosis. Others suggest latencies of up to 1 or 2 minutes (Waldinger et al, 1998a; Rowland et al, 2000). **Latencies of 2 minutes or less show minimal overlap with those of men without PE, which typically range from 2 to 10 minutes. Accordingly, any latency less than 2 minutes** (Waldinger et al, 1998a; Rowland et al, 2000) **suggests a possible PE diagnosis.** Others suggest that the "number of penile thrusts" to ejaculation represents a more valid assessment of the amount of penile stimulation. However, IVELT is generally considered the more reliable measure and, within the larger population of men, correlates with the number of penile thrusts (Rowland et al, 1998). Whether IVELT should be precisely timed with a stopwatch or by estimation is yet undecided. Recent data indicate that estimations of IVELT tend to overestimate rather than underestimate ejaculatory latencies.

The second component—the patient's ability to control the dysfunctional response—distinguishes men who ejaculate rapidly because they have difficulty controlling ejaculation from those who do so intentionally. In recent research, self-ratings of "control over ejaculation" have been used successfully as a self-efficacy measure that differentiates affected men from sexually functional men (Rowland et al, 1997; Strassberg et al, 1999). Men with PE rate their ejaculatory control at around 2 to 4 (1 = not at all; 7 = complete control), whereas functional men typically rate their control at 4 or higher.

The third criterion—concern or distress about the condition—is usually satisfied by the mere fact that the man approaches the clinic seeking help for the sexual problem. In situations where participants are recruited into a clinical investigation, several questions might be included in a screening questionnaire addressing concern or distress (McMahon et al, 2004).

Exclusionary Factors

Both the American Psychiatric Association and the World Health Organization definitions describe conditions that exclude diagnosis: PE mediated by alcohol, substance use, or medication; a context that leads to very high levels of arousal because of novelty of partner or situation; and a low frequency of sexual activity.

Classification

Most clinicians and researchers distinguish between lifelong and acquired PE, and between PE that is limited to specific situations or partners and that which is global. Knowing that the patient has had a lifelong history of PE not specific to one partner may argue toward a biologic cause, and the need to address interpersonal issues may be less important in these men. In contrast, knowing that the PE developed recently in specific situations and in conjunction with erectile dysfunction may suggest the need to address relationship issues and attend less to a biologic cause.

Etiology

A number of theories have been proposed regarding the causes of PE (Table 22–11). However, because most of these are not evidence based and are speculative at best, only the two most likely are discussed below.

Penile Hypersensitivity

Multiple authors have proposed that men with PE have a hypersensitive penis and either reach the ejaculatory threshold more rapidly or have a lower threshold than men with normal control (Rowland et al, 1989; Strassberg et al, 1990). Xin and associates (1996, 1997b) reported that men with PE have lower biothesiometric vibration perception thresholds and significantly shorter mean somatosensory evoked poten-

Table 22–11. Proposed Causes of Premature Ejaculation

Psychogenic

Anxiety
Early sexual experience
Infrequent sexual intercourse
Poor ejaculatory control techniques
Evolutional
Psychodynamic

Biogenic

Penile hypersensitivity
Hyperexcitable ejaculatory reflex
Hyperarousability
Endocrinopathy
Genetic predisposition
5-HT-receptor dysfunction

tial latency times of the glans and penile shaft than controls. Paick and colleagues (1998) and Rowland and associates (1993), however, have reported no significant statistical differences between normal controls and patients with primary PE. Fanciullacci and coworkers (1988) found that, in response to penile electrostimulation, men with severe lifelong PE had cortical somatosensory evoked potentials of significantly higher amplitude than those in control subjects. They hypothesized that men with PE have a greater representation of the penile sensory nerve supply in the cerebral cortex than controls and suggested this as an indication of an organic basis for PE. Yang and Bradley (1998) also reported that the cortical distribution of the dorsal nerve of the penis is larger in men with lifelong PE.

5-Hydroxytryptamine (5-HT)-Receptor Sensitivity

Studies in male rats show the hypothalamic medial preoptic area (MPOA) and the medullary nucleus paragigantocellularis (nPGI) in the ventral medulla to have pivotal roles in the central control of ejaculation (Marson and McKenna, 1990; Yells et al, 1994). In the MPOA, electrostimulation or microinjection of dopamine agonists promotes ejaculation (MacLean, 1975). It has been suggested that descending serotonergic pathways from the nPGI to the lumbosacral motor nuclei tonically inhibit ejaculation and that disinhibition of the nPGI results in ejaculation (Yells et al, 1992).

Coolen and coworkers (1996, 1997, 1998) identified ejaculation-initiated neural activation in several brain regions, including the posterodorsal medial amygdala, the posteromedial bed nucleus of the stria terminalis, and the medial parvicellular subparafascicular nucleus of the thalamus. These areas are extensively and reciprocally interconnected and likely form the basis of an ejaculation "brain circuit" in response to afferent neurons ascending in the spinal cord (Coolen et al, 1998).

Multiple dopamine- and 5-HT-receptor types have been identified. Studies have described a pivotal role for 5-HT2C and 5-HT1A receptors in the central control of ejaculation, the former to delay and the latter to facilitate (Ahlenius et al, 1981; Waldinger et al, 1998a). Waldinger and colleagues (1998a) hypothesized that lifelong PE in humans may be explained by hyposensitivity of the 5-HT2C and/or hypersensitivity of the 5-HT1A receptor. Treatment with a serotonin reuptake inhibitor (SSRI) activates the 5-HT2C receptor, adjusts the ejaculatory threshold set point, and delays ejaculation. The extent of delay may vary widely in different men according to the dosage and frequency of SSRI administration and the genetically determined ejaculatory threshold set point. Cessation of treatment results in re-establishment of the previous set point within 5 to 7 days in men with lifelong PE.

Treatment

Psychological/Behavioral Treatment

Although the more expedient pharmacologic therapies are overshadowing the traditional psychological/behavioral methods, the latter approach remains an attractive option for several reasons. The treatment is specific to the problem, is neither harmful nor painful, produces few adverse side effects or none, and encourages open communication about sexuality in the couple, which is likely to lead to a more satisfying relationship (Wincze and Carey, 1991; Verhulst and Heiman, 1988). At the same time, the psychological/behavioral approach does have drawbacks: it is time consuming, often requiring a substantial commitment of both time and money; lacks immediacy; requires the partner's cooperation; and yields results that are mixed (and less well documented than those of pharmacologic treatment) (Heiman, 1997; Hawton, 1998).

Empirically Supported Psychological Approaches. Two psychological/behavioral strategies enjoy substantial popularity among sex therapists. The first is the stop-squeeze method, developed by Semans (1956) and later adopted by Masters and Johnson (1970). The second, advocated by Kaplan (1983), is the stop-pause method. Both suppress the urge to ejaculate by stopping sexual stimulation, but the latter substitutes a squeeze of the glans penis with a pause in stimulation at the point of impending ejaculation.

Although Masters and Johnson's initial report of only a 2% short-term and a 3% long-term failure rate for the stop-squeeze method revolutionized PE treatment, subsequent studies have reported much lower success rates, in the neighborhood of 50% to 60% (Grenier and Byers, 1995; Madakasira and St. Lawrence, 1997; Metz et al, 1997). Long-term success rates may be even lower.

The second behavioral approach simulates the natural behaviors required to prolong ejaculation latency during intercourse. Weekly outpatient therapy resulted in a high success rate (80% to 90%) in men with primary and generalized PE, although Kaplan's rates have also been challenged (Metz et al, 1997).

Pharmacologic Treatment

SSRIs. The introduction of SSRIs resulted in another revolutionary change. SSRIs that have been evaluated for the treatment of PE include citalopram, fluoxetine, fluvoxamine, paroxetine, and sertraline. In the past decade, these SSRIs and clomipramine have repeatedly been studied for their propensity to delay ejaculation (Althof et al, 1995; Kim et al, 1998; Waldinger et al, 1998c, 2001), and there is some evidence that fluvoxamine and citalopram are less effective than paroxetine, sertraline, and fluoxetine (Waldinger et al, 1998c, 2001).

Daily Treatment with Serotonergic Antidepressants. **Daily treatment can be undertaken with paroxetine (20 to 40 mg), clomipramine (10 to 50 mg), sertraline (50 to 100 mg), and fluoxetine (20 to 40 mg)** (Table 22–12). **Meta-analysis of drug treatment studies has demonstrated that paroxetine exerts the strongest ejaculation delay** (Waldinger et al, 2004b). Paroxetine, sertraline, and fluoxetine may give rise to side effects such as fatigue, yawning, mild nausea, loose stools, or perspiration. These often start in the first week and gradually disappear within 2 to 3 weeks. Ejaculation delay with daily treatment usually manifests itself at the end of the first or second week and sometimes even earlier. With the exception of fluoxetine, SSRIs should not be withdrawn acutely, but gradually within 3 to 4 weeks. Side effects of clomipramine may consist of nausea, dry mouth, and fatigue. Sometimes clomipramine and the SSRIs may give rise to reversible feelings of diminished libido or moderately decreased penile rigidity. Patients should be informed of all the aforementioned side effects when starting treatment.

On-Demand Treatment with Antidepressants. It has been reported that clomipramine (25 mg), but not paroxetine (20 mg), taken about 5 hours before intercourse can delay ejaculation in men with lifelong PE (Waldinger et al, 2004a). Another strategy is the daily use of paroxetine, sertraline, and fluoxetine in a low dose combined with higher doses as needed shortly before intercourse.

Based on the Level of Evidence rating of the studies reviewed, both the SSRIs and clomipramine received a grade A recommendation from an expert panel of the Second International Consultation on Sexual Medicine.

Topical Local Anesthetics. The use of topical local anesthetics such as lidocaine and/or prilocaine as a cream, gel, or spray is well established. They appear moderately effective in retarding ejaculation but do so at the price of possibly significant penile hypoanesthesia and possible transvaginal absorption, resulting in vaginal numbness, unless a condom is used (Berkovitch et al, 1995; Atikeler et al, 2002). The optimal time of application is reported to be 20 minutes before intromission (Atikeler et al, 2002). In 43 men with PE, Atan and colleagues (2000) studied the combined use of fluoxetine and topical lidocaine: 83.3% improved, compared with 72% of those treated with fluoxetine alone.

Xin and associates (1995, 1997) reported significantly improved ejaculatory control in 89.2% of patients treated with

SS-cream, a natural compound made with extracts from nine herbs, some of which have a local anesthetic property. One hour before coitus, it is applied to the glans penis and immediately washed off. Adverse effects were noted in 5.9% of patients, including mild local irritation and delayed ejaculation. Both the latency and amplitude of somatosensory evoked potentials measured at the glans penis were increased over baseline after application.

Based on the Level of Evidence rating of the studies reviewed, treatment of PE with topical anesthetics has a grade A recommendation.

PDE-5 Inhibitors

Several authors have reported their experience with sildenafil citrate as a treatment for PE. In a prospective randomized double-blind crossover study of 31 potent men with lifelong PE, Abdel-Hamid and associates (2001) compared the efficacy and safety of "on-demand" clomipramine, sertraline, paroxetine, sildenafil, and the pause/squeeze technique. Sildenafil was associated with a significantly higher IVELT and sexual satisfaction score than all other treatments. In an open label study of 80 potent men, Salonia and colleagues (2002) compared treatment with paroxetine alone (first chronic, then "on-demand") with a combination of paroxetine and sildenafil. Both treatments significantly improved the ejaculatory latency time and intercourse satisfaction domain of the IIEF. The combination's results were better, albeit associated with a mild increase in drug-related side effects.

Chen and coworkers (2003) treated 138 men with PE in a progressive manner, instituting a new regimen if results were unsatisfactory: first 5% lidocaine ointment, then paroxetine alone, and finally paroxetine with sildenafil. Psychological and behavioral therapy was also provided. The authors reported that sildenafil combined with paroxetine and psychological and behavioral counseling alleviated PE in patients in whom other treatments had failed.

One must note that none of the just discussed studies was placebo controlled and the results are difficult to interpret. Interestingly, in a placebo-controlled study with placebo, EMLA cream alone, sildenafil (50 mg) alone, and EMLA cream with sildenafil (50 mg), the authors reported that sildenafil alone was not more effective than placebo and that topical EMLA cream alone was as effective as EMLA plus sildenafil (Atan et al, 2006). Therefore, **it is unlikely that PDE-5 inhibitors have a significant role in the treatment of PE—with the exception of men with acquired PE secondary to ED.**

Based on the Level of Evidence rating of the studies reviewed, treatment of PE with PDE-5 inhibitors has a grade C recommendation.

Office Management

Men with PE should be evaluated with a detailed medical and sexual history, a physical examination, and appropriate investigations to establish the true presenting complaint, identify obvious biologic causes such as medication or recent pelvic surgery, and uncover sufficient detail to establish the optimal treatment plan. Relevant information to obtain from the patient is included in Table 22–13.

Table 22–12. Medical Therapy Options for the Treatment of Premature Ejaculation*

	Trade Names[†]	Recommended Dose[‡§]
Oral Therapies		
Nonselective Serotonin Reuptake Inhibitor		
Clomipramine	Anafranil	25 to 50 mg/day or 25 mg 4 to 24 hr before intercourse
Selective Serotonin Reuptake Inhibitors		
Fluoxetine	Prozac, Sarafem	5 to 20 mg/day
Paroxetine	Paxil	10, 20, 40 mg/day or 20 mg 3 to 4 hr before intercourse
Sertraline	Zoloft	25 to 200 mg/day or 50 mg 4 to 8 hr before intercourse
Topical Therapies		
Lidocaine/ prilocaine cream	EMLA Cream	Lidocaine 2.5% Prilocaine 2.5% 20 to 30 minutes before intercourse

*This list does not reflect order of choice or efficacy.
[†]Trade names listed may not be all-inclusive.
[‡]Peak plasma concentrations occur 2 to 8 hours post dose, and half-lives range from 1 to 3 days.
[§]Titrate dose from low to high based on response.

Table 22–13. Office Evaluation of the Patient Complaining of Premature Ejaculation

1. A basic medical history, including use of prescribed and recreational medications
2. The cultural context and developmental history of the disorder, including whether the problem is global or situational or lifelong or recent in its development
3. Measures of the quality of each of the three phases of the sexual response cycle (desire, arousal, and ejaculation), because the desire and arousal phases may impact the ejaculatory response
4. Details about the ejaculatory response, including the patient's subjective assessment of his intravaginal ejaculatory latency time (IVELT) and sense of ejaculatory control, the level of sexual dissatisfaction and distress, the frequency of sexual activity, etc.
5. The partner's assessment of the situation, including whether the partner suffers from female sexual dysfunction
6. Assessment of the sexual and overall relationship

KEY POINT: PREMATURE EJACULATION

■ Men with PE secondary to ED, other sexual dysfunction, or genitourinary infection should receive appropriate cause-specific treatment. Men with lifelong PE should be managed with pharmacotherapy. Men with significant contributing psychogenic or relationship factors may benefit from concomitant behavioral therapy. PE is highly likely to recur after withdrawal of treatment. Men with acquired PE can be treated with pharmacotherapy and/or behavioral therapy according to patient/partner preference. In men with acquired PE, ejaculatory control is likely to be restored after completion of treatment, but this is unlikely in men with lifelong PE. Behavioral therapy may augment pharmacotherapy and prevent relapse.

SUGGESTED READINGS

Broderick GA, Arger P: Duplex Doppler ultrasonography: Noninvasive assessment of penile anatomy and function. Semin Roentgenol 1993;28:43-56.

Carson CC, Lue TF: Great drug classes: Phosphodiesterase type 5 inhibitors for erectile dysfunction. BJU Int 2005;96:257-280.

Donatucci CF, Lue TF: The combined intracavernous injection and stimulation test: Diagnostic accuracy. J Urol 1992;148:61-62.

Esposito K, Giugliano F, Di Palo C, et al: Effect of lifestyle changes on erectile dysfunction in obese men: A randomized controlled trial. JAMA 2004;291:2978-2984.

Goldstein I, Lue TF, Padma-Nathan H, et al: Oral sildenafil in the treatment of erectile dysfunction. Sildenafil Study Group. N Engl J Med 1998; 338:1397-1404.

Hatzichristou DG, Saenz de Tejada I, Kupferman S, et al: In vivo assessment of trabecular smooth muscle tone, its application in pharmaco-cavernosometry and analysis of intracavernous pressure determinants. J Urol 1995;153:1126-1135.

Lue TF: Impotence: A patient's goal-directed approach to treatment. World J Urol 1990;8:67.

McMahon CG, Abdo C, Hull E, et al: Disorders of orgasm and ejaculation in men. In Lue TF, Basson R, Rosen R, et al (eds): Sexual Medicine: Sexual Dysfunctions in Men and Women. Paris, Health Publications, 2004, pp 241-286.

Morales A, Buvat J, Gooren LJ, et al: Endocrine aspects of men sexual dysfunction. In Lue TF, Basson R, Rosen R, et al (eds): Sexual Medicine: Sexual Dysfunctions in Men and Women. Paris, Health Publications, 2004, pp 345-382.

Morley JE, Charlton E, Patrick P, et al: Validation of a screening questionnaire for androgen deficiency in ageing males. Metabolism 2000;49:1239-1242.

Moyad MA, Barada JH, Lue TF, et al: Sexual Medicine Society Nutraceutical Committee: Prevention and treatment of erectile dysfunction using lifestyle changes and dietary supplements: What works and what is worthless: II. Urol Clin North Am 2004;31:259-273.

Rosen RC, Capelleri JC, Smith MD, et al: Development and evaluation of an abridged, 5-item version of the International Index of Erectile Function (IIEF-5) as a diagnostic tool for erectile function. Int J Impot Res 1999;11:319.

Rosen, RC, Hatzichristou D, Broderick G, et al: Clinical evaluation and symptom scales: Sexual dysfunction assessment in men. In Lue TF, Basson R, Rosen R, et al (eds): Sexual Medicine: Sexual Dysfunctions in Men and Women. Paris, Health Publications, 2004, pp 173-220.

Rosen RC, Riley A, Wagner G, et al: The international index of erectile function (IIEF): A multidimensional scale for assessment of erectile dysfunction. Urology 1997;49:822-830.

Schwartz AN, Lowe M, Berger RE, et al: Assessment of normal and abnormal erectile function: Color Doppler flow sonography versus conventional techniques. Radiology 1991;180:105-109.

Waldinger MD, Zwinderman AH, Schweitzer DH, Olivier B: Relevance of methodological design for the interpretation of efficacy of drug treatment of premature ejaculation: A systematic review and meta-analysis. Int J Impot Res 2004b;16:369-381.

Prosthetic Surgery for Erectile Dysfunction

DROGO K. MONTAGUE, MD

Three sentinel events define the history of the treatment of erectile dysfunction (ED). These are the introduction of the inflatable penile prosthesis in 1973 (Scott et al, 1973), intracavernous injection therapy in 1982 (Virag, 1982), and effective systemic therapy with sildenafil citrate in 1998 (Goldstein et al, 1998). Today, the treatment of ED can be likened to the treatment of osteoarthritis, another common disorder that also becomes more prevalent with age. In both, a progressive treatment model may be employed (Table 23–1). Most men with ED are initially offered systemic therapy with a phosphodiesterase type 5 (PDE-5) inhibitor. When that fails and the man wishes to continue treatment, second- and third-line therapies should be discussed. When these fail or are rejected, penile prosthesis implantation is usually appropriate.

TYPES OF PROSTHESES

The currently available penile prostheses in the United States are shown in Table 23–2. Malleable prostheses are semirigid devices with a central core that allows the penis to be bent down for dressing and bent upward for coitus. However, for most men this malleable core does not maintain these positions very well. Malleable devices have the advantage of very low mechanical failure rates and ease of use. Disadvantages include constant penile rigidity and an increased risk of erosion (Steidle and Mulcahy, 1989).

The postionable penile prosthesis (Dura II) is a semirigid device with a central series of articulating segments held together with a spring on each end. This device, compared with malleable prostheses, is better able to maintain its upward and downward positions.

The two-piece inflatable penile prosthesis (AMS Ambicor) consists of two cylinders connected to a small scrotal pump (Fig. 23–1). Squeezing this pump transfers a small volume of fluid from the rear tip reservoirs of the cylinders into a nondistensible central chamber, producing rigidity comparable to that of a malleable device. When the device is deflated, the central chamber partially collapses, providing better flaccidity than a malleable implant. The two-piece prosthesis has as its primary advantage ease of implantation because there is no third piece (abdominal fluid reservoir). A disadvantage compared with malleable devices is the increased risk of mechanical failure.

The ideal prosthesis would provide its recipient with a penis that provides as closely as possible normal penile flaccidity and erection. Only three-piece inflatable devices that transfer a large volume of fluid into the penile cylinders for erection and out of the cylinders for flaccidity approach this ideal. Three-piece prostheses have paired corporeal cylinders, a scrotal pump, and an abdominal fluid reservoir. An example of a three-piece inflatable prosthesis is the Mentor Titan (Fig. 23–2). All three-piece devices provide penile girth expansion and rigidity similar to that of a normal erection. One device, the AMS 700 Ultrex, also provides length expansion (Fig. 23–3).

PREOPERATIVE PATIENT-PARTNER COUNSELING

Discussions regarding the treatment of ED ideally should include the partner; however, this is not always possible. When a decision has been made that penile prosthesis implantation should be considered, it is important to inform the patient about alternative treatments and the advantages and disadvantages of each. By this time, the patient has either failed or is not a candidate for systemic treatment with PDE-5 inhibitors. He should be aware that in addition to penile prosthesis implantation, therapies with vacuum constriction devices, intraurethral prostaglandin, and intracavernous injection are available. **An option such as penile prosthesis implantation should not be considered to treat a man with ED that is situational, the result of a relationship conflict,**

Table 23-1. Progressive Treatment Model

	Osteoarthritis	*Erectile Dysfunction*
First-line therapy	NSAIDs	PDE-5 inhibitors
Second-line therapy	Joint injections	VCDs, IUD
Third-line therapy	Arthroscopic surgery	Intracavernous injections
Fourth-line therapy	Prosthetic joint replacement	Penile prosthesis implantation

IUD, intraurethral drug; NSAIDs, nonsteroidal anti-inflammatory drugs; PDE-5, type 5 phosphodiesterase; VCDs, vacuum constriction devices.

Table 23-2. Penile Prosthesis Types

Prosthesis Type	*American Medical Systems**	*Mentor Corporation†*
Semirigid rod	AMS Malleable 600	Acu-Form
	AMS Malleable 650	
Positionable	Dura II	
Two-piece inflatable	AMS Ambicor	
Three-piece inflatable	AMS 700 CX	Alpha I
	AMS 700 CXM	Titan
	AMS 700 CXR	Titan Narrow Base
	AMS 700 Ultrex	

*American Medical Systems (AMS), Minnetonka, MN.
†Mentor Corporation, Santa Barbara, CA.

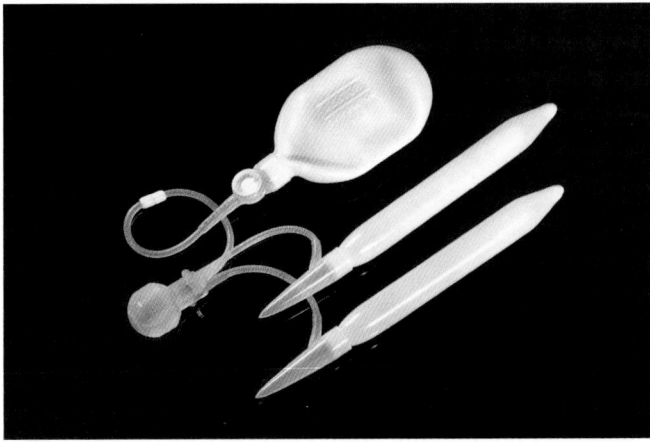

Figure 23-2. Mentor Titan three-piece inflatable penile prosthesis. (Courtesy of Mentor Corp, Santa Barbara, CA.)

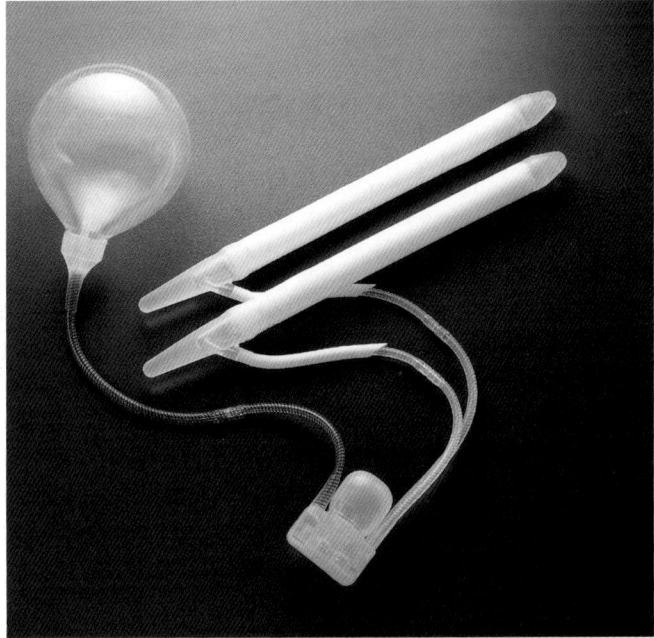

Figure 23-3. AMS 700 Ultrex® three-piece inflatable penile prosthesis. Courtesy of the American Medical Systems, Inc., Minnetonka, MN.

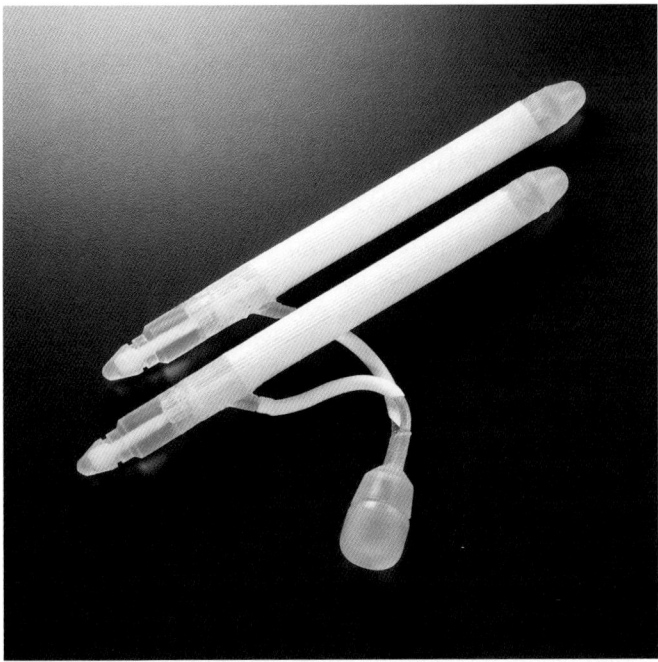

Figure 23-1. AMS Ambicor® two-piece inflatable penile prosthesis. Courtesy of the American Medical Systems, Inc., Minnetonka, MN.

or potentially reversible. For these men and their partners, psychological consultation and sex therapy are more appropriate.

The various types of penile prostheses along with their advantages and disadvantages (see earlier) should be explored. Most penile prosthesis implantation is done under spinal or general anesthesia on an outpatient basis with discharge on the same or the next day. The intensity and duration of post-operative pain are variable. Most men require oral narcotics for about 1 week. After that, pain can often be managed with a nonsteroidal anti-inflammatory agent. When an abdominal fluid reservoir has been placed, strenuous activity and heavy lifting are proscribed for 4 weeks. Patients can drive and return to nonstrenuous work when they are no longer taking narcotics. Coitus is usually possible in 4 to 6 weeks.

The patient should understand that penile prostheses produce an erection-like state. The following considerations refer to the three-piece inflatable devices. With the prosthesis deflated, most men feel comfortable in a locker room situation. With inflation, the erection-like state produces girth expansion and rigidity that for most men approach those of a normal erection. **The glans penis, however, is not included in the erection, and for most men the erection is shorter than their normal erection. We demonstrate to men their**

Table 23–3.   Comparison of Infrapubic and Penoscrotal Implant Approaches

	Infrapubic Approach	Penoscrotal Approach
Advantages	Reservoir placement under direct vision	Better corporeal exposure No dorsal nerve injury Pump fixation possible
Disadvantages	Limited corporeal exposure Possible dorsal nerve injury Inability to anchor pump	Blind reservoir placement

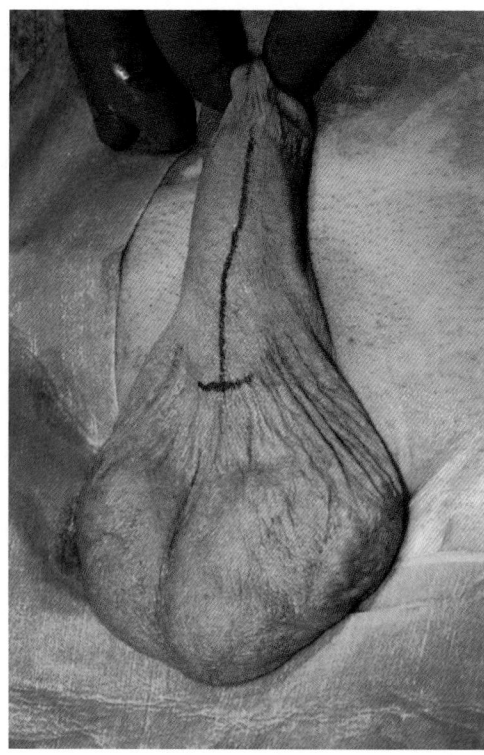

Figure 23–4. The transverse penoscrotal incision extended in an inverted-T fashion to provide nearly complete corporeal exposure.

stretched penile length and tell them that this will be the approximate length of their prosthetic erection. One device, the AMS 700 Ultrex, produces both girth and length expansion, with length expansion ranging from 1 to 4 cm (mean 1.9 cm) (Montague and Lakin, 1992).

Many men with ED have normal libido, and most have normal penile sensation and orgasm with ejaculation. Penile prosthesis implantation preserves orgasm and ejaculation if present but does not restore them if they are absent.

The patient should be informed that infection will probably require complete removal of the implant with resulting scarring of the corporeal smooth muscle. With prosthesis reimplantation after infection, the penis is frequently smaller and cylinder implantation is usually difficult and on rare occasions may not be possible. Erosion of the prosthesis through the skin or into the urethra also requires device removal. **The potential implant recipient should understand that mechanical failure is possible and correcting it requires device revision or replacement.**

SURGICAL APPROACHES

Surgical approaches for penile prosthesis implantation include subcoronal (used only for implantation of malleable or positionable devices), infrapubic, and penoscrotal. We prefer the penoscrotal approach for the reasons listed in Table 23–3. When corporeal fibrosis is present, the transverse version of the penoscrotal incision can be extended in an inverted-T fashion to expose almost the entire extent of both corpora cavernosa (Fig. 23–4). A potential disadvantage of the penoscrotal incision not listed in Table 23–3 is the presence of excess tubing in the scrotum or at the base of the penis. This is a problem when preconnected versions of the inflatable prostheses are used. We avoid this by implanting the cylinders and pump separately. We then route pump tubing through the back wall of the subdartos pouch. This requires making three connections rather than one. However, doing this helps anchor the pump in its pouch and results in minimal tubing that becomes buried in the upper scrotum under dartos fascia. Buried tubing under the fascia not only is advantageous from a cosmetic standpoint but also reduces the risk of device infection. If a superficial penoscrotal wound infection occurs and the fascia is intact, a deep infection in the space around the prosthesis that would require device removal is not likely to occur.

AMS 700 ULTREX INFLATABLE PENILE PROSTHESIS IMPLANTATION BY THE TRANSVERSE PENOSCROTAL APPROACH

We perform this procedure with the patient in the supine position under either spinal or general anesthesia. Shaving of the skin is done in the operating room to avoid bacterial colonization of small skin breaks that might occur if shaving were done before the surgery. A 10-minute skin preparation is performed. Paper drapes are used because cloth drapes do not provide a good bacterial barrier when they become wet. We do not place a urethral catheter at this point because it is easier to judge the quality of the erection when a catheter is not present.

A 4-cm transverse incision is made about 1 cm below the penoscrotal junction. After the skin incision is made, the transverse incision is carried down through dartos fascia. This transverse incision through the fascia should be directed toward the urethra and corporeal bodies rather than toward the scrotum. Allis clamps are placed on the lower margin of the fascia, and the underside of dartos fascia is dissected off the urethra and the proximal corpora (crura). We use a ring retractor that we have modified by placing slits in the ring so that exposure may be maintained by a combination of hook stays and retractor blades (Fig. 23–5).

Two-centimeter corporotomies are made, and two horizontal mattress sutures of 2-0 PDS II (polydioxanone, Ethicon, Somerville, NJ) are placed on each side of the corporotomy (Fig. 23–6). These sutures are used as guide sutures during corporeal dilation and measurement, and they are also

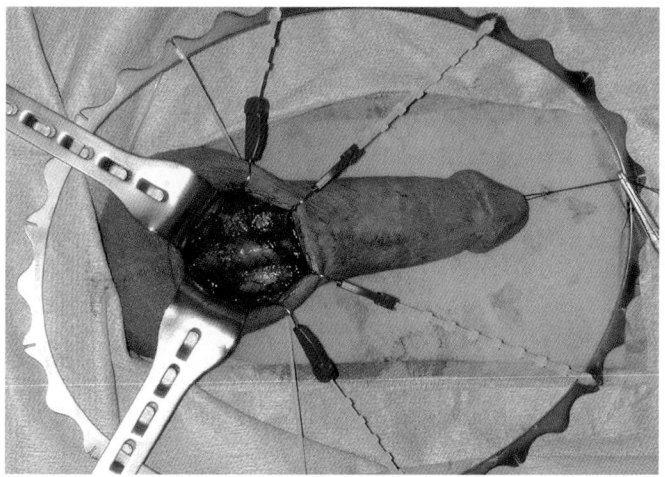

Figure 23–5. The standard transverse penoscrotal incision with exposure maintained by a ring retractor.

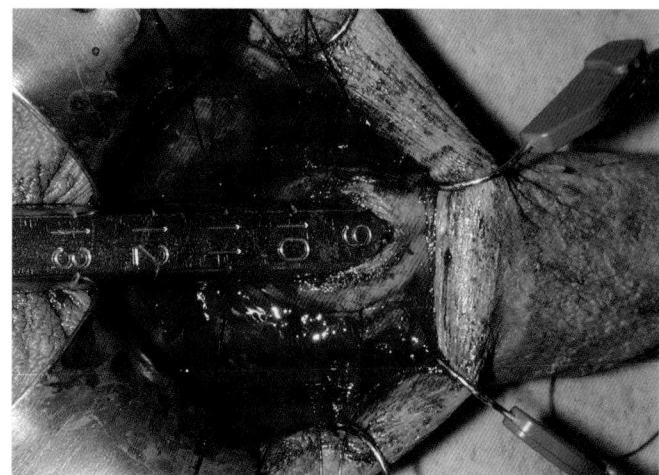

Figure 23–7. The distal measurement is 9 cm.

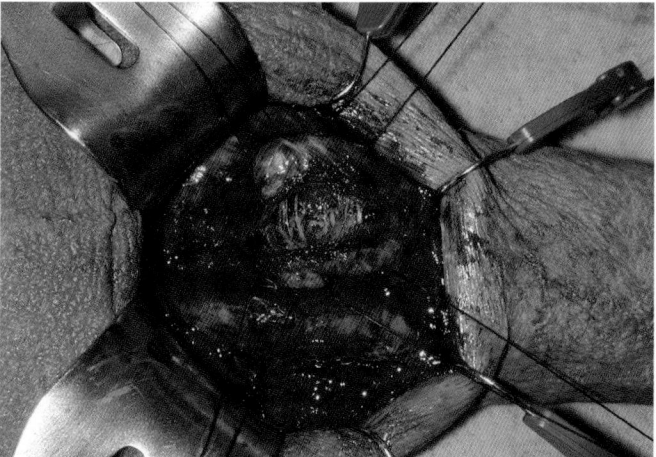

Figure 23–6. Four horizontal mattress sutures have been placed. These serve as traction sutures and are then used to close the corporotomy over the cylinder.

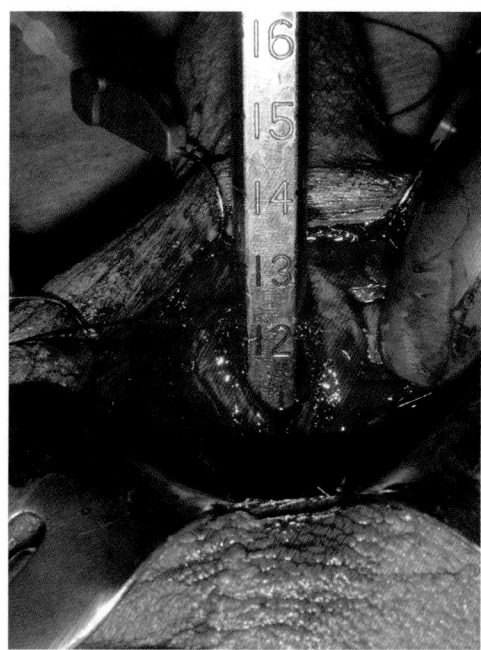

Figure 23–8. The proximal measurement is 11 cm.

used to close the corporotomy after the cylinders are placed (Montague, 1993). Dilation starts with an 8-mm Hegar dilator and proceeds to 16 mm proximally and to 14 mm distally. The greater proximal dilation is needed to accommodate both the cylinder and the cylinder tubing. If dilation to these diameters is not possible, the smaller diameter AMS 700 CXR or the Mentor Titan Narrow Base prosthesis should be used.

Using a sizing instrument, the distal measurement is taken from the distal end of the corporotomy (9 cm) (Fig. 23–7), and the proximal measurement is taken from the proximal end of the corporotomy (11 cm) (Fig. 23–8). **We do not include the 2-cm corporotomy in the measurement because we believe that surface sizing with a rigid measuring tool introduces a 2-cm measuring error** (Montague and Angermeier, 2003). With standard measuring techniques from a midcorporotomy reference point, the cylinder placed is about 2 cm too long. When the length-expanding Ultrex cylinder is used, this leads to the so-called S-shaped cylinder deformity (Wilson et al, 1996). Although there are no data to support this, we believe that with non–length-expanding cylinders, too

long a cylinder may cause premature failure (cylinder failures are most common in the area where the bend with a too long cylinder occurs).

After corporeal measurements are taken, the appropriate cylinder size is selected. Ultrex and CX cylinders come in the following lengths: 12, 15, 18, and 21 cm. Adjustments between these sizes are made by the addition of rear tip extenders (1, 2, or 3 cm). The cylinders are filled with normal saline, and we inject saline until the cylinders are full (rounded) but not inflated under pressure. Having the cylinders full rather than collapsed facilitates judging whether the cylinder fit after insertion is correct. The pump is filled by cycling the pump while the pump tubes are submersed in a basin of normal saline. The reservoir is filled with normal saline to displace air; the saline is then removed because the reservoir will be filled after it is implanted. In this case the total corporeal length was

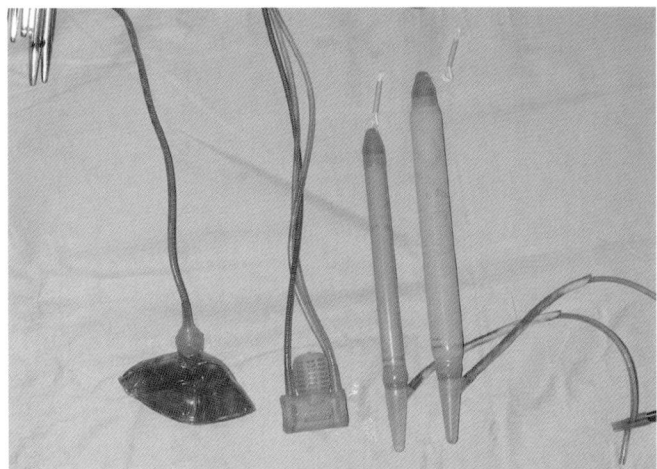

Figure 23–9. The prosthesis components prepared for implantation. One cylinder is inflated to demonstrate its girth- and length-expanding capabilities. It is deflated prior to implantation.

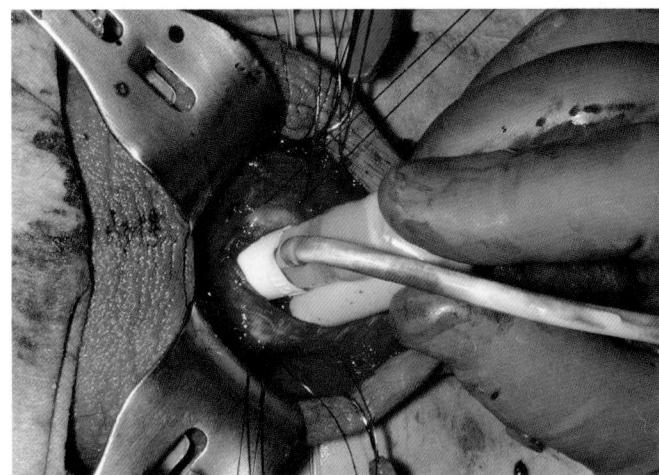

Figure 23–11. A 2-cm rear tip extender has been placed, and the proximal portion of the cylinder is being introduced into the crus.

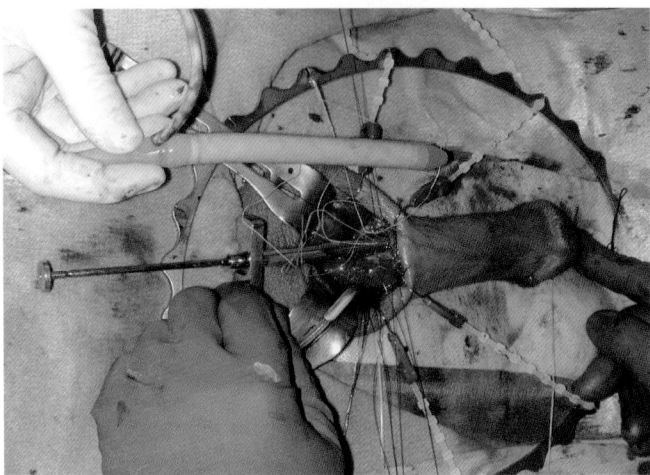

Figure 23–10. The Furlow cylinder inserter is in place.

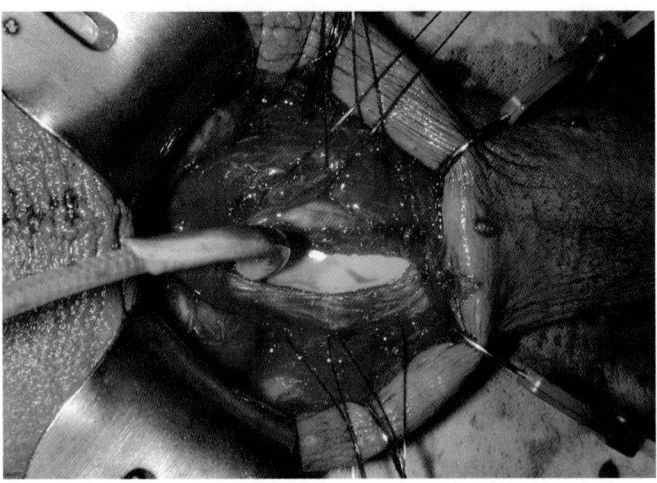

Figure 23–12. The cylinder, which has been correctly sized, lies flat within the corpus cavernosum.

20 cm (9 cm + 11 cm), and we elected to use 18-cm Ultrex cylinders with 2 cm of rear tip extension. Figure 23–9 shows the filled prosthesis components ready for implantation. For illustrative purposes, one cylinder is inflated to show both its girth and length expansion. It is deflated prior to implantation.

Distal cylinder insertion is aided by use of the Furlow cylinder inserter (American Medical Systems, Minnetonka, MN). The guide sutures in the tip of the cylinder are threaded through the needle provided in the accessory package, and this needle with its sutures is placed into the distal end of the inserter. The inserter is then placed to the distal end of the corpus cavernosum (Fig. 23–10). The plunger of the cylinder inserter is pushed in delivering the needle and guide sutures through the tip of the corpus cavernosum and out through the glans. The guide sutures are used to pull the distal cylinder into the distal corpus cavernosum. If rear tip extenders are needed they are added now, and the proximal portion of the cylinder is manually inserted (Fig. 23–11). If the cylinder fit is proper, the proximal portion is all the way down to the attach-

ment of the crus to the pelvic bone and the distal portion is in the distal corpus cavernosum under the midglans penis. When these conditions have been met, the rounded visible portion of the cylinder lies flatly in the open corporotomy (Fig. 23–12). If the cylinder is too long or too short, the proximal portion can be removed, and length can be adjusted by adding or removing rear tip extenders. Note that rear tip extenders can be stacked; for example, 1 cm and 3 cm can be used together if 4 cm of rear tip extension is needed. The corporotomies are closed (Fig. 23–13) by tying the proximal ends (dark glove) and then the distal ends (light glove) of the preplaced horizontal mattress sutures (Montague, 1993).

In preparation for pump placement, a second incision through dartos fascia is made in the scrotal septum. A deep septal pouch is developed with ring forceps (Fig. 23–14). The pump is placed in this pouch with the reservoir tube in front and the two cylinder tubes in back. A right angle clamp is used to route each pump tube through three separate stab incisions through the back wall of the pouch (Fig. 23–15). After this step is completed, all three tubes from the pump are

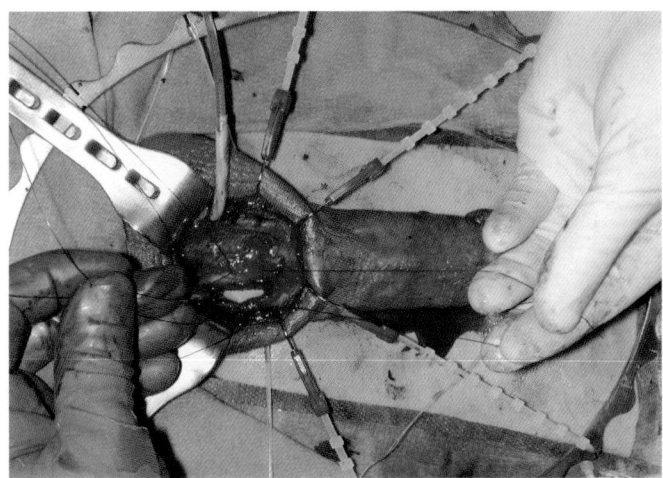

Figure 23–13. The two proximal suture strands from each side (dark gloves) are tied, and then the two distal sutures (light gloves) are tied.

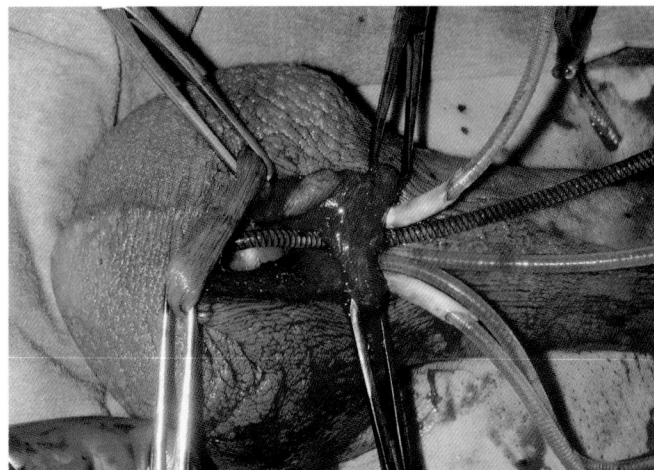

Figure 23–16. All three pump tubes have been transposed.

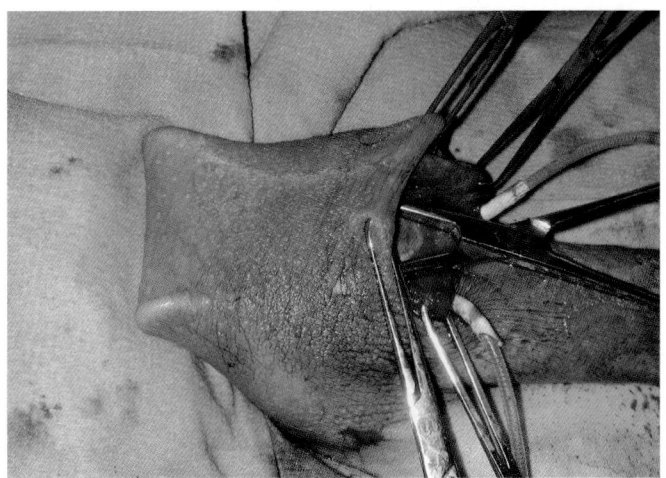

Figure 23–14. A deep septal subdartos pouch is developed for the pump.

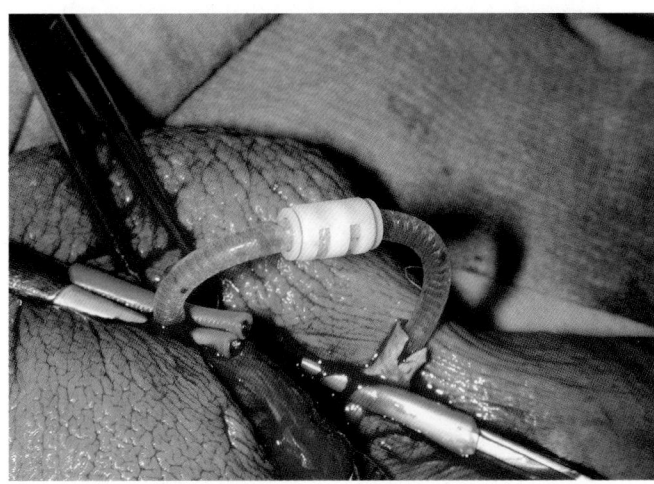

Figure 23–17. A connection between the pump and one of the cylinders has been completed.

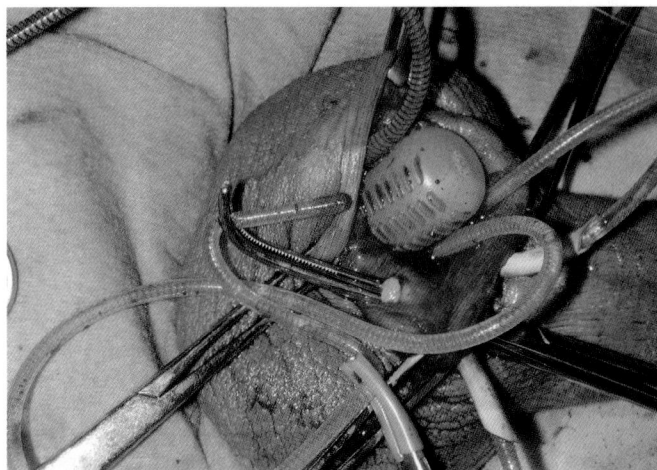

Figure 23–15. Each of the three pump tubes is routed through the back wall of the pouch.

transposed to the area exposed by the first transverse dartos incision (Fig. 23–16). After irrigation with antibiotic solution, the second dartos incision is closed with running 3-0 Dexon II (polyglycolic acid suture, United States Surgical, Tyco Healthcare Group, Norwalk, CT).

The tubing is cut just long enough to make connections with the sutureless connectors between the pump and each cylinder (Fig. 23–17). A 50-mL syringe filled with normal saline that serves as a temporary reservoir is then connected to the reservoir tube from the pump. The pubis to glans tip penile length measurement is made with the cylinders both deflated (12.5 cm) (Fig. 23–18) and inflated (15.5 cm) (Fig. 23–19).

Safe reservoir insertion into the retropubic space through the primary penoscrotal incision is possible only if the bladder is completely empty. We insert an 18 French urethral catheter attached to closed gravity drainage and apply suprapubic pressure over the bladder until it is empty. The surgeon introduces a finger into the incision and moves it up to the external inguinal ring on either side. If the external ring is not palpable, a point just above the pubic tubercle is chosen.

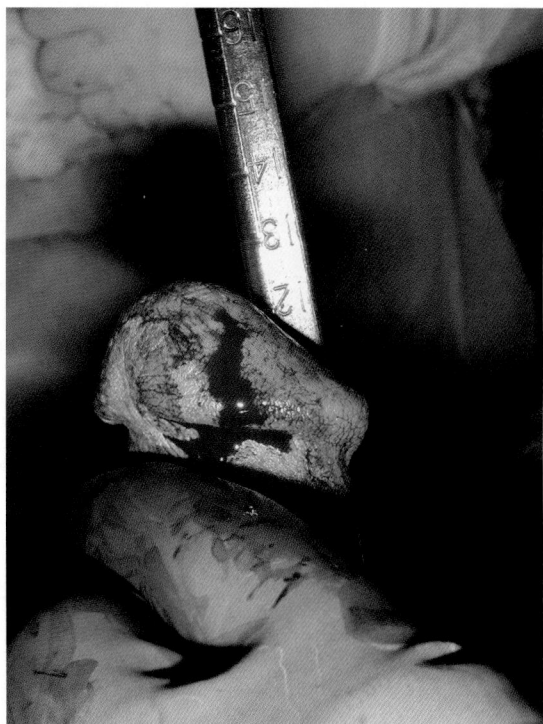

Figure 23–18. The pubis to glans tip measurement with the cylinders deflated is 12.5 cm.

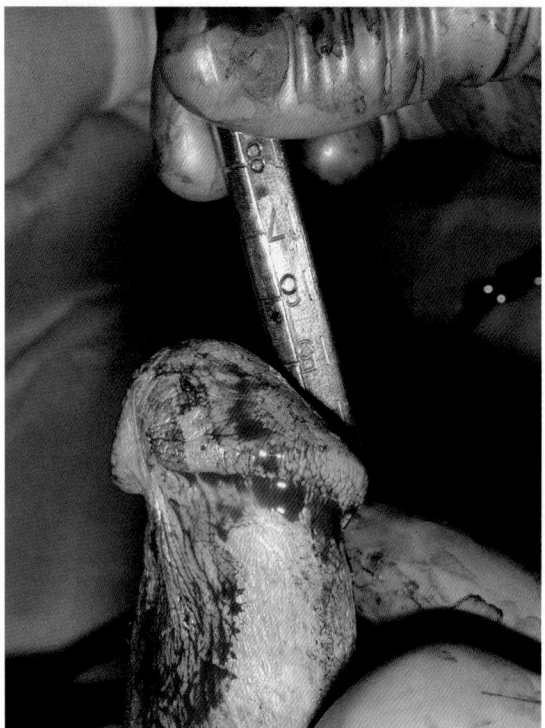

Figure 23–19. The pubis to glans tip measurement with the cylinders inflated is 15.5 cm.

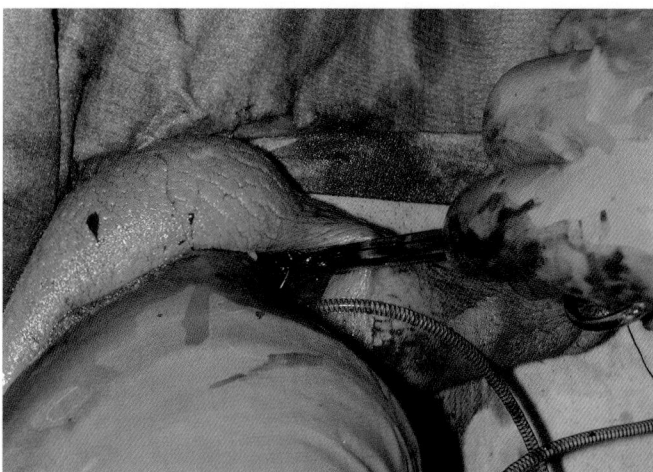

Figure 23–20. Metzenbaum scissors are used to perforate the fascia in the floor of the external inguinal ring to gain entry into the retropubic (prevesical) space.

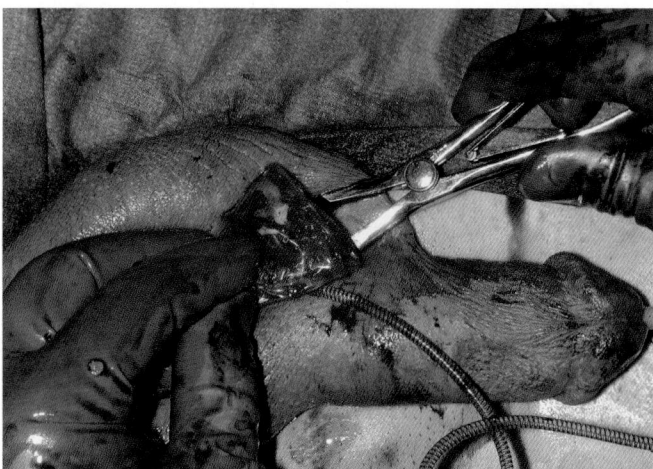

Figure 23–21. The empty reservoir is inserted into the prevesical space. A nasal speculum is maintaining the fascial opening.

Metzenbaum scissors or a Kelly clamp is used to perforate the transversalis fascia (Fig. 23–20). **If all layers of the fascia are perforated, the surgeon's index finger enters the retropubic space. Correct entry is confirmed if the back of the symphysis pubis and the balloon in the empty bladder are pal-** pated. A nasal speculum with long blades is substituted for the finger; this maintains the fascial opening. The empty reservoir is introduced into the retropubic space (Fig. 23–21); the hublike junction between the reservoir and the tube should be located in the fascial defect.

The AMS reservoirs are available in two sizes: 65 mL and 100 mL. The former is recommended for all cylinder sizes except for the 18- and 21-cm Ultrex cylinders, which require the 100 mL reservoir size. The reservoir is then filled with the requisite amount of normal saline, and the position of the reservoir is confirmed by palpation. The reservoir itself, which is below the fascia, should not be palpable. The tubing hub should be palpable as it protrudes through the fascia. **To avoid autoinflation, the fluid pressure in the reservoir should be zero even when pressure is applied to the suprapubic area.** To achieve zero pressure, a 50-mL syringe without a plunger is attached to the reservoir tubing and held at the bladder (reservoir) level. Manual suprapubic pressure is then applied, allowing fluid to escape from the reservoir (Fig. 23–22). This maneuver should leave 50 to 55 mL in a 65-mL reservoir and

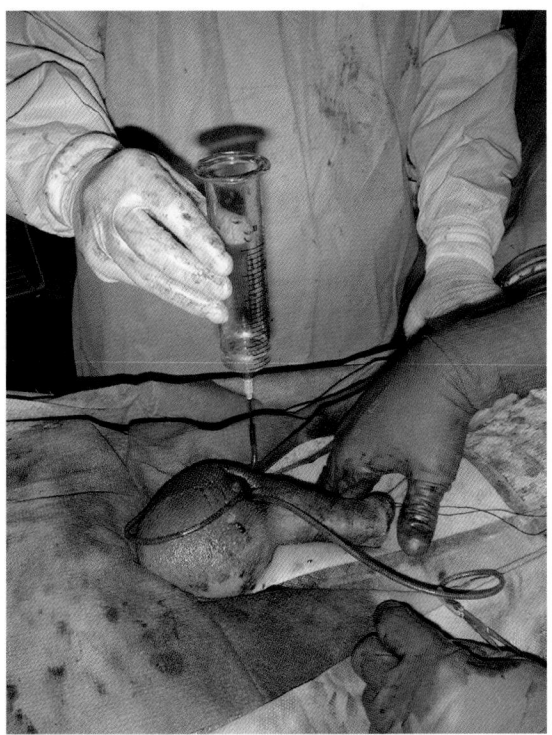

Figure 23-22. A back pressure test is performed with manual pressure being applied over the reservoir site.

80 to 85 mL in a 100-mL reservoir. If less fluid is in the reservoir after performing this maneuver, the reservoir is probably not in the retropubic space. The reservoir tubing is brought down into the incision in the upper scrotum where the third sutureless connection is made (all three connections are made with the straight connectors).

A long right angle clamp is introduced through the incision to the inguinal area on the side of the reservoir. A stab incision is made, and through this a closed suction type of drain is introduced. The drain is brought down to the base of the penis, where it lies on top of the tubes and connectors. Dartos fascia is then closed transversely with running 3-0 Dexon. The skin is closed with running subcuticular 4-0 Vicryl.

POSTOPERATIVE CARE

The urethral catheter and the closed suction drain are removed the next morning after an overnight stay in the ambulatory surgery center. We continue antibiotic treatment with an oral cephalosporin for 1 week. Most men require an oral narcotic for about 1 week. After that, a nonsteroidal anti-inflammatory agent usually suffices. If an abdominal fluid reservoir has been placed, lifting and other activities that might result in reservoir displacement from the retropubic space into the inguinal area are proscribed for 1 month. The patient is instructed to keep his penis up on the lower abdomen pointing to the umbilicus. If the penis is worn in a downward position as healing takes place, ventral curvature of the penis may result.

One month after surgery, most men are ready for instructions on cycling the device. We instruct the patient to inflate and deflate his device fully twice daily for 1 month. This serves a dual purpose: practice in cycling and activity that stretches the pseudocapsule that by now has formed around the cylinders. In the beginning pumping requires considerable force, but with time it becomes much easier.

The patient is given permission to begin coitus whenever inflation can be accomplished without discomfort. Because anxiety on the part of the partner may inhibit vaginal lubrication, the couple is advised to use a water-soluble lubricant at least initially. **Retarded ejaculation (failure to reach orgasm) may occur when men first use their prosthesis for coitus. To avoid this, the couple is counseled to have adequate foreplay so that both partners are sexually aroused before intromission.**

COMPLICATIONS
Infection

Infection in the periprosthetic space usually does not cause significant illness; however, to eradicate the infection, removal of all components of the prosthesis is almost always required. Therefore, infection is considered by many to be the most significant complication of genitourinary prosthetic surgery.

Penile prosthesis implantation should be delayed in patients with urinary tract infections or cutaneous infections in the operative area. Shaving of the operative area is done just before surgery to avoid bacterial colonization of small skin breaks, which might occur if shaving was done before the day of surgery. The operative area is prepared with a 10-minute skin preparation. Broad-spectrum prophylactic antibiotics are given 1 hour before the case begins so that adequate tissue levels are present when the incision is made. We use gentamicin and vancomycin for this purpose. Paper rather than cloth drapes are used because the latter are permeable to bacteria when wet. The prosthesis is kept in its sterile package until it is ready to be filled and implanted. It is then submersed in an antibiotic solution unless it has an antibiotic coating, in which case it is placed in a sterile basin and covered with a paper towel. Silicone has a positive charge and attracts airborne particles; therefore, as it is placed in the body it is irrigated with antibiotic solution, and it is irrigated again as tissues are closed over it. For our antibiotic solution we use 50,000 units of bacitracin in a liter of normal saline.

Infections occurring after penile prosthesis implantation are either early (in the first few weeks following implantation) or late (6 months to 1 or 2 years after implantation). The former are often associated with gram-negative bacteria, whereas the later are usually associated with gram-positive bacteria such as *Staphylococcus epidermidis* (Kabalin and Kessler, 1988; Licht et al, 1995). Infections with other organisms such as fungi (Peppas et al, 1988) and gonococci (Nelson and Gregory, 1988) have also been rarely reported. It was originally believed that all infections originated from the time of surgery. Carson showed that late prosthetic infections can occur by hematogenous spread from a distant source (Carson and Robertson, 1988). We have shown that late infection can also arise after a mechanical malfunction (fluid leak) from a prosthetic device (Milbank et al, 2004). Fluid leak probably disrupts the balance with a biofilm, favoring bacterial growth

(Silverstein and Donatucci, 2003). Alternatively, the fluid itself could be a bacterial reservoir.

Evidence is divided as to whether men with diabetes mellitus are at increased risk for infection after penile prosthesis implantation and whether the degree of diabetes control at the time of surgery is related to the risk of infection. In one study, four infections occurred in 13 diabetics with a glycosylated hemoglobin above 11.5%; whereas in 19 diabetics with a glycosylated hemoglobin under 11.5% only one infection occurred (Bishop et al, 1992). In another study of penile prosthesis recipients, infections occurred in 10 of 114 diabetics (8.7%) and in 11 of 275 nondiabetics (4.0%). However, there was no statistically significant increased infection rate with increased levels of glycosylated hemoglobin (Wilson et al, 1998). In a study of 556 prosthesis recipients, there was no significant difference in the incidence of infection in diabetic versus nondiabetic patients (Montague, 1987).

In a study investigating the surgical approach for penile prosthesis implantation, 4 of 139 devices implanted by the infrapubic approach became infected (2.9%), whereas 2 of 221 implanted by the penoscrotal approach became infected. This difference was not statistically significant (Garber and Marcus, 1998).

Early infections are likely to be evident by swelling, erythema, tenderness, possible purulent drainage, and occasionally fever. Late infections may be manifested only by persistent or recurrent long-term pain. With long-term infections the scrotal skin may be adherent to the pump. Infections are sometimes evident by erosion, particularly of the pump through the scrotum (Fig. 23–23). This should never be considered infection of the pump alone. All components of the device are connected by tubing, and the entire device is considered to be infected.

Treatment of a prosthetic infection with appropriate antibiotics usually results in clinical improvement; however, antibiotic treatment rarely permanently eradicates this type of infection. This is thought to be due to harboring of microorganisms within a biofilm that is adherent to the device (Abouassaly et al, 2004). **For this reason, when a prosthetic infection is present, all components of the prosthesis should be removed.**

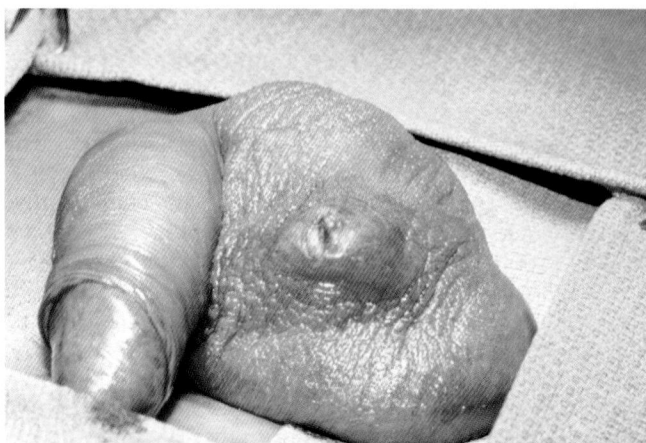

Figure 23–23. Impending scrotal pump erosion in a patient with an infected prosthesis.

Penile prosthesis reimplantation following infected device removal presents certain difficulties. Pump and reservoir reimplantation is seldom a problem. However, after infected device removal, the corporeal smooth muscle becomes replaced in varying degrees with scar. In the past, reimplantation was often delayed as long as a year. During this time the scar within the corpora would mature, resulting in contraction, a smaller penis size, and more difficulty with dilation prior to cylinder reimplantation. **To minimize loss of penile size and to facilitate corporeal dilation, we now perform prosthesis reimplantation as soon as possible after device removal for infection.** When all incisions have healed and postoperative edema has resolved (usually 2 to 3 months after device removal), reimplantation is advised because early fibrosis is easier to dilate and the scar contraction that leads to shortening has not yet occurred.

Mulcahy introduced the concept of prosthesis salvage for infection in 1996 (Brant et al, 1996) and updated his experience with this in 2000 (Mulcahy, 2000). His protocol involves removal of all prosthetic components and foreign bodies followed by irrigation with seven antibacterial solutions. A new device is implanted, and the patient is prescribed antibiotics. Of 55 patients available for follow-up, 45 (82%) were free of infection with follow-up ranging from 6 to 93 months. **When salvage procedures are successful, they maintain penile size and correct the problem with only one operation.**

Advances in prosthetic design have been made in attempts to reduce infection. A surface treatment combining rifampin and minocycline (InhibiZone) was introduced in 2001 by American Medical Systems for its three-piece inflatable penile prosthesis product line. In a report comparing 2261 rifampin-minocycline–coated devices with 1944 controls, the infection rate at 180 days was 0.68% in the treated group and 1.61% in the control group (Carson, 2004).

Mentor introduced a hydrophilic surface coating for their three-piece inflatable prosthesis in 2002 (Mentor Titan). This coating, polyvinylpyrrolidone (PVP), reduces bacterial adhesion and absorbs the antibiotics in which the prosthesis is submerged by the surgeon just before implantation. In a report comparing 2357 hydrophilic-coated devices with 482 controls, the infection rate was 1.06% in the treated group and 2.07% in the control group (Wolter and Hellstrom, 2004).

The incidence of infection during first-time penile prosthesis implantation ranges from 1% to 3%, whereas with revision surgery it is considerably higher (7% to 18%) (Kabalin and Kessler, 1988; Wilson and Delk, 1995; Jarow, 1996; Henry et al, 2005). In the early days of penile prosthesis surgery, mechanical failures were common and frequently occurred within the first few years after device implantation. Increased infection rates following prosthesis revision were reported when only the failed component of the prosthesis was replaced.

Mechanical failures today are less common and typically occur more than 5 years after implantation. **If the entire device is explanted and all prosthesis compartments are thoroughly irrigated before a new prosthesis is implanted, the infection rate is not significantly different from the rates seen with first-time prosthesis implantation** (Montague et al, 2001; Henry et al, 2005).

Perforation and Erosion

Perforation is an event that occurs intraoperatively; whereas erosion is an event that occurs or is recognized only post-operatively. When the surgeon is dilating the proximal corpora (crura), a sudden give of the dilator suggests that the crus has been perforated on its medial aspect near its attachment to the pelvic bone. The dilator, almost always a smaller size, travels out into the soft tissues of the perineum. Mulcahy (1987) suggested the "wind sock" correction for this, but it is rarely necessary if the perforation is recognized and larger diameter dilators are used to dilate the correct track. When the proximal portion of the cylinder is inserted, it stays within the crus and the small area of perforation heals over it.

With distal dilation, crossover to the opposite side may occur or the urethra may be perforated. **If urethral perforation occurs, the implant procedure should be abandoned and a urethral catheter should be left in for 7 to 10 days.** Prosthesis reimplantation may be done at a later date. To avoid urethral perforation, the surgeon should keep the tip of the dilator under the dorsolateral surface of the corpus cavernosum. This maneuver also helps to prevent crossover to the opposite side. After the first cylinder is implanted, the surgeon should resound the other side both proximally and distally to see whether crossover in either direction has occurred.

Erosion of the distal cylinder lateral to the distal corpus cavernosum is usually most effectively corrected by a technique described by Mulcahy (1999). With this approach, the distal cylinder is removed (folded back) and an incision through the back wall of the capsule of the cylinder compartment is made in an area proximal to the erosion site. This allows distal dilation within the true corpus cavernosum. Using the Furlow cylinder inserter, the distal cylinder is then reimplanted within the distal corpus cavernosum.

Erosion of the distal end of the prosthesis may occur into the urethra, in which case it is visible through the meatus. This occurs more commonly after semirigid rod implantation, presumably because of constant internal pressure from the rod device (Steidle and Mulcahy, 1989). It also occurs more commonly in men with spinal cord injury because of their lack of sensation. In the case of a semirigid rod device, only the eroded side needs to be removed, and this can usually be done in the office by grasping the distal end of the rod with a towel clip and pulling it out. In the case of urethral erosion, a urethral catheter is placed for 10 days to allow urethral healing. Many patients are able to have adequate coitus with only one rod in place; hence, a procedure to reimplant the second rod is usually not necessary.

In the case of erosion of one cylinder of an inflatable device into the meatus or through the glans, this cylinder should be removed as soon as possible to avoid spread of bacteria along the cylinder to its tubing and thus to the rest of the prosthesis. After the cylinder is removed, an implantable plug (supplied by the device manufacturer) is placed in the pump tubing that led to that cylinder. Again, many men are able to have coitus with only one inflatable cylinder; thus, a later procedure to reimplant the second cylinder is not always necessary.

Poor Glans Support

Poor support of the glans penis by cylinder or rod tips leads to a drooping appearance of the glans, which is commonly referred to as the SST deformity after the supersonic transport (Concorde) nose appearance on takeoff and landing. This deformity may result from inadequate distal dilation, too short cylinders, or, in the case of minor deformity, variations in anatomy.

Correction of this deformity can be done in one of two ways. The definitive correction involves removing both cylinders, perforating the distal capsule with Metzenbaum scissors, redilating the distal corpora, resizing, and then inserting longer cylinders or the same cylinders with longer rear tip extenders. Alternatively, dorsal plication of the glans back onto the shaft of the penis (Fig. 23–24) can be performed (Ball, 1980; Mulhall and Kim, 2001). The latter procedure is preferable when there are minor but otherwise bothersome degrees of SST deformity.

Oversized Cylinder or Rod

When a semirigid rod prosthesis that is too long is implanted, the patient may complain of pain that does not subside as healing takes place after device implantation. Alternatively, it may lead to erosion of the rod either into the meatus or through the glans. Reoperation with placement of smaller rods usually relieves the pain and avoids impending erosion.

As already discussed, cylinders that are too long may result in a sigmoid (S) penile deformity in the case of Ultrex cylinders. In the case of non–length-expanding cylinders, there is usually not a problem, although theoretically it might lead to premature cylinder failure.

Pump Complications

The technique for pump implantation discussed previously helps to avoid upward pump migration, which tends to take place during healing because of the action of the cremasteric muscles. If upward pump migration occurs, the pump may impinge on the base of the penis, making use of the pump difficult and also interfering with intromission. Revision is sometimes necessary, at which time the pump is relocated to its correct position.

The pump may also be difficult to use if a hematoma or seroma forms around it. These may reabsorb with time; if they do not, pump revision may be necessary.

Autoinflation

Autoinflation occurs when the inflatable penile prosthesis partially inflates with physical activity. It can be minimized by placing the reservoir in the prevesical (retropubic) space and by performing the back pressure test as described previously. The cylinders should also be kept deflated during healing after surgery and when the prosthesis is not being used.

Mentor has a reservoir with a lock-out valve available as an option. Initial experience with this device suggests that it reduces the incidence of this complication (Hollenbeck et al, 2002; Wilson et al, 2002).

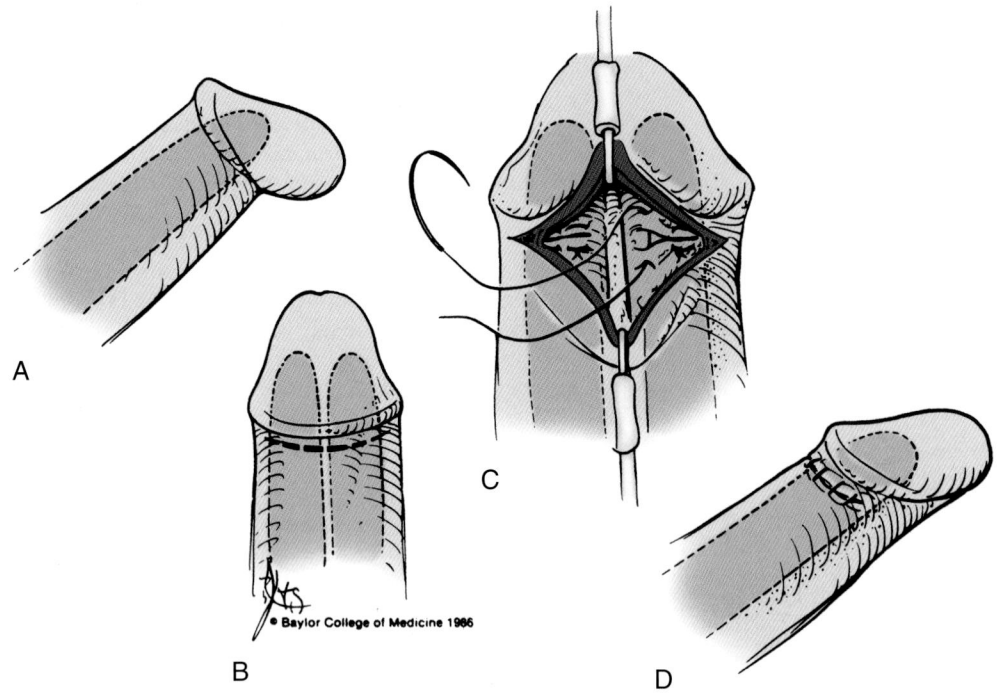

A

B

© Baylor College of Medicine 1986

C

D

Figure 23–24. Plication sutures pull the dorsal aspect of the glans back onto the corporeal bodies to correct an SST deformity.

PENILE PROSTHESIS IMPLANTATION IN SPECIAL CASES
Peyronie's Disease

Men who have acquired erectile deformity secondary to Peyronie's disease along with significant ED may be candidates for penile prosthesis implantation. When prosthesis implantation by itself does not produce satisfactory straightening of the penis, a corporoplasty may also be necessary (Mulcahy and Wilson, 2002). We showed that corporoplasty was frequently needed when girth- plus length-expanding Ultrex cylinders were used and not necessary when girth-only expanding CX cylinders were used (Montague et al, 1996). Wilson and colleagues (2001) showed that modeling or forcefully bending the penis with the cylinders inflated usually obviated the need for corporoplasty.

Multiple relaxing incisions to correct curvature and increase penile length have been used in men with Peyronie's disease undergoing penile prosthesis implantation (Rajpurkar et al, 1999; Montorsi et al, 2001). When a relaxing incision leaves a gap greater than 1 cm, covering the defect to prevent herniation of the cylinder is recommended. Materials used to cover the defect include human cadaveric dura mater (Fallon, 1990), polytetrafluoroethylene (Fig. 23–25) (Herschorn and Ordorica, 1995), human cadaveric pericardium (Palese and Burnett, 2001), and porcine small intestinal submucosa (Knoll, 2002).

Cavernosal Fibrosis

In contrast to Peyronie's disease, in which scarring is present in the tunica albuginea, scarring may occur in the cavernosal

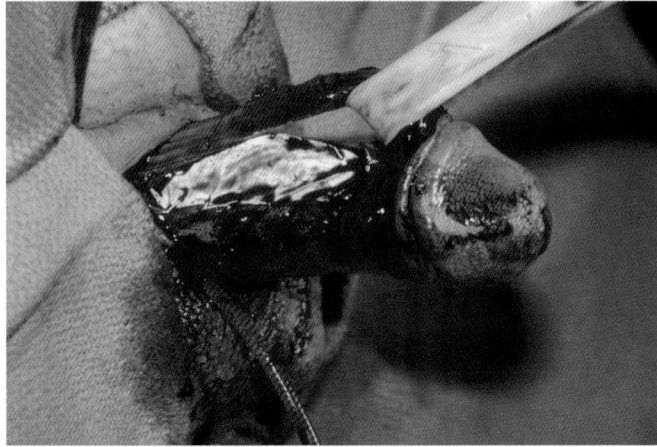

Figure 23–25. After inflatable penile prosthesis implantation, a large plaque required excision. The exposed cylinders are covered with a polytetrafluorethylene patch.

smooth muscle that forms much of the contents of the corporeal bodies. **Cavernosal fibrosis is most often seen after removal of an infected penile prosthesis; it also occurs in men with ED as a result of ischemic priapism. In both of these cases, the penis is often significantly smaller owing to decreased volume of the corpora cavernosa. Dilation of the corpora and placement of semirigid rods or cylinders are also frequently quite difficult.**

In preparing the corpora for cylinder implantation, we start with a 2-cm standard corporotomy. If the corpora cannot be dilated without force, we abandon the use of Hegar dilators and instead use Metzenbaum scissors with rounded tips.

Gently spreading the tips as the scissors are advanced is often effective. After the scissors tips reach the distal and proximal ends of the corpora, dilation with special cutting dilators is often helpful (Mooreville et al, 1999).

If these maneuvers are not successful, we extend the transverse penoscrotal incision in an inverted-T fashion (see Fig. 23–4). Extended corporotomies are made permitting either dilation with more control or resection of scar tissue by establishing a plane between the fibrotic core and the inner surface of the tunica albuginea (Figs. 23–26 and 23–27) (Montague and Angermeier, 2004). This results in the removal of the fibrotic contents of the corpus cavernosum (Fig. 23–28). Multiple horizontal mattress sutures of 2-0 PDS are then placed along the edges of the tunica albuginea (Fig. 23–29). The prosthetic cylinder can then be laid into the empty corporeal shell (Fig. 23–30), with primary closure of the tunica albuginea being possible (Fig. 23–31).

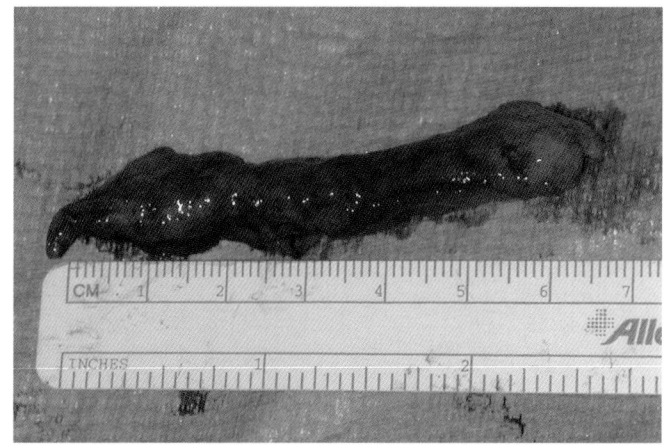

Figure 23–28. The excised core of fibrotic tissue.

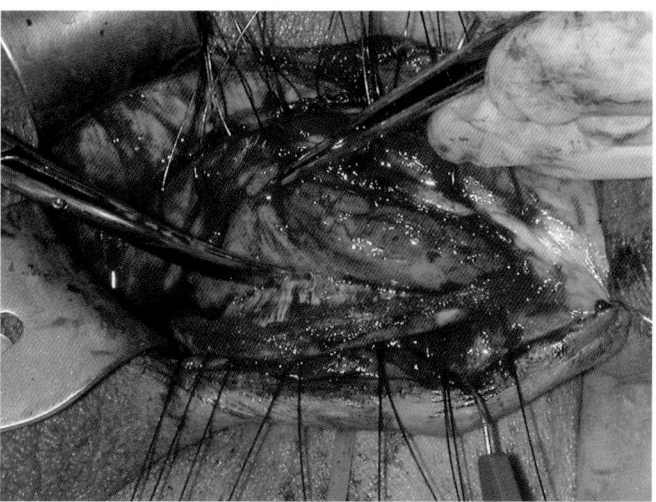

Figure 23–26. A plane of dissection is established between the fibrotic core and the inner surface of the tunica albuginea.

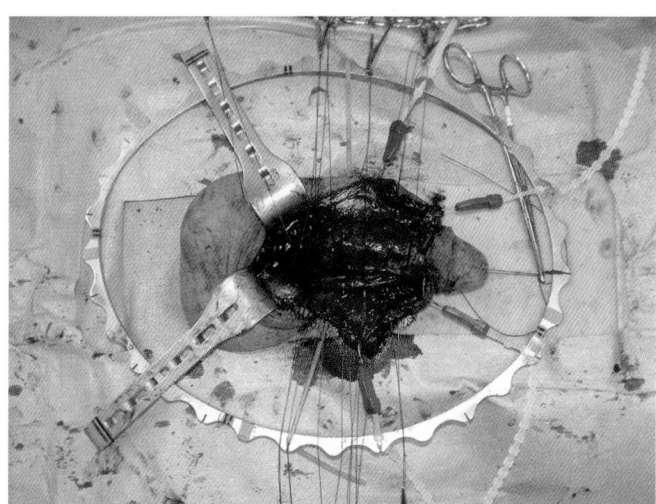

Figure 23–29. Multiple horizontal mattress sutures are placed along the cut edges of the tunica albuginea.

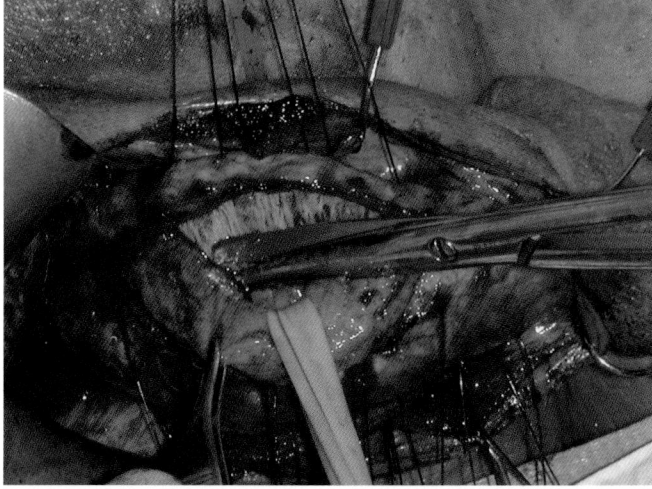

Figure 23–27. A Penrose drain is used to place traction on the fibrotic core, facilitating further dissection.

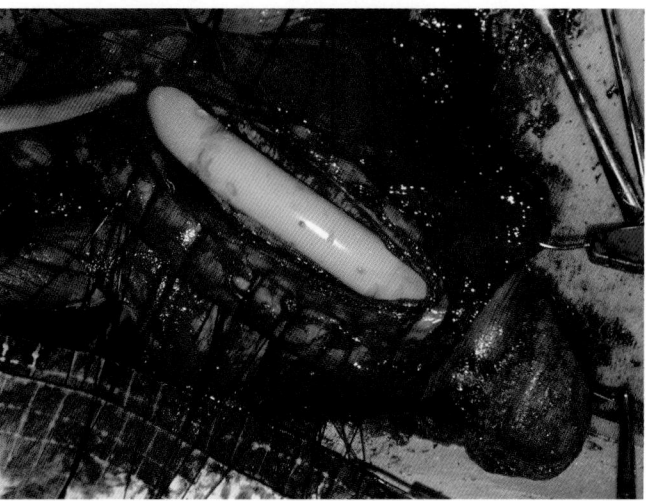

Figure 23–30. The cylinder can be laid into place.

Table 23–4. Inflatable Penile Prostheses: Survival Free of Mechanical Failure*

Reference	Number of Patients	Follow-Up Months Range (mean)	Data before or after Modification	% of Devices Free of Mechanical Failure[†]
AMS 700 CX/CXM (Not Modified)				
Deuk Choi et al, 2001	273	6-100 (49)	NA	90.4
Carson et al, 2000	372	38-134 (57)	NA	86.2
Montorsi et al, 2000	90	(60)	NA	93.1
Daitch et al, 1997	111	1-112 (47.2)	NA	90.8
Dubocq et al, 1998	103	(66 across three groups)	NA	83.9[‡]
AMS 700 Ultrex (Modified 1993)				
Montorsi et al, 2000	110	(58)	Both	79.4
Dubocq et al, 1998	103	(66 across three groups)	Both	84.2[‡]
Milbank et al, 2002	85	<1-136 (75)	Pre-1993	64.7
Milbank et al, 2002	52	<1-92 (46)	Post-1993	93.7
Mentor Alpha-1 (Modified 1992)				
Goldstein et al, 1997	434	<1-44 (22)	Both	85[§]
Dubocq et al, 1998	117	(66 across three groups)	Both	95.7[‡]
Wilson et al, 1999	410	Not specified	Pre-1992	75.3
Wilson et al, 1999	971	Not specified	Post-1992	92.6

*With permission from AUA Erectile Dysfunction Guidelines Update Panel.
[†]Kaplan-Meier survival estimates; 5-year estimates unless otherwise noted.
[‡]63-month estimate.
[§]Three-year estimate.
NA, not applicable.

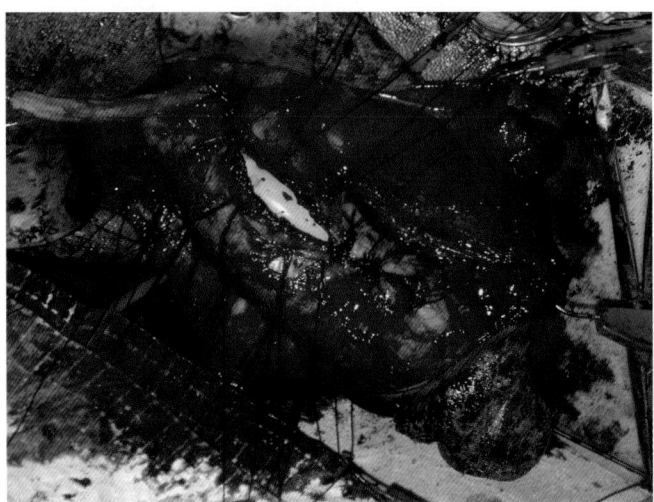

Figure 23–31. Partial closure over the cylinder.

RESULTS
Mechanical Failure Rates

Much of the early reporting of penile prosthesis results in terms of survival free of mechanical failure was limited because of data that usually gave only the range and mean follow-up for the entire series. It was not possible with this type of reporting to compare meaningfully different devices or the same device in different series because of failures to take into account differences in follow-up. **Contemporary reporting standards should require reporting device survival free of mechanical failure by using Kaplan-Meier projections** (Kaplan and Meier, 1958).

The results reported herein are limited to the three-piece inflatable penile prostheses available today (the AMS 700 CX/CXM, the AMS 700 Ultrex, and the Mentor Alpha-1) and include only studies that report Kaplan-Meier projections. Eight such studies were found (Table 23–4). The AMS 700 CX/CXM prosthesis was introduced in 1987; no significant design changes have been made with this device since its introduction. Five studies with a total of 949 implant recipients revealed that freedom from mechanical failure ranged from 83.9% (63 months) to 93.1% (5 years).

The AMS 700 Ultrex prosthesis was introduced in 1990, and the cylinders were modified in 1993. Results from two studies (Dubocq et al, 1998; Montorsi et al, 2000) with a total of 213 device recipients included both pre- and post-1993 Ultrex modified devices. Survival free of mechanical failure was reported as 79.4% (5 years) and 84.2% (63 months). One study compared 5-year device survival before the 1993 cylinder modification (64.7%, $N = 85$) and after the 1993 cylinder modification (93.7%, $N = 52$) (Milbank et al, 2002).

The Mentor Alpha-1 prosthesis introduced in 1989 underwent pump modification in November 1992. Two studies with a total of 551 implant recipients included devices both before and after pump modification. Survival free of mechanical failure was 85% at 3 years (Goldstein et al, 1997) and 95.7% at 63 months (Dubocq et al, 1998). One study compared 5-year device survival before pump modification (75.3%, $N = 410$) and after pump modification (92.6%, $N = 971$) (Wilson et al, 1999).

Patient (Partner) Satisfaction

Early satisfaction studies were retrospective and used non-standardized questionnaires. In one such study of the AMS 700 inflatable (pre-CX and pre-Ultrex) prosthesis, 387 recipients were mailed questionnaires and 272 returned them. This retrospective review showed that 83% of the men and 70% of their partners were satisfied with the use of this device (McLaren and Barrett, 1992). In another retrospective study of 145 AMS 700 Ultrex inflatable penile prosthesis recipients using a nonstandardized questionnaire, 85% of the men and 76% of their partners were satisfied (Holloway and Farah, 1997).

Prospective studies using structured questionnaires can provide more useful information regarding satisfaction of patients and partners after penile prosthesis implantation. In one such study, a psychosexual questionnaire containing 13 questions scored on a scale of 1 to 5 was administered to 35 recipients of inflatable penile prostheses preoperatively and again at 3, 6, and 12 months after surgery. This study demonstrated significant improvements in the psychosexual well-being of these prosthesis recipients with attainment of a high level of satisfaction of patients up to 1 year after surgery. This study permitted these results to be broken down into erectile ability, libido, frequency of sexual activity, satisfaction with sexual activity, and a decrease in feelings of sadness, depression, anxiety, anger, frustration, and embarrassment related to sexual activity (Tefilli et al, 1998).

In another prospective study of 96 inflatable penile prosthesis recipients, the International Index of Erectile Function (IIEF) (Rosen et al, 1997) and the Erectile Dysfunction Inventory of Treatment Satisfaction (EDITS) (Althof et al, 1999) were administered preoperatively and 3, 6, and 12 months postoperatively (IIEF) and 3, 6, and 12 months postoperatively (EDITS). All 12-month scores were significantly higher than baseline scores, and the 12-month scores were significantly higher than the 6-month scores for the IIEF satisfaction domain and for EDITS (Mulhall et al, 2003).

One study compared penile prosthesis implantation with penile injection therapy. In this retrospective study a structured telephone questionnaire was administered to 115 intracavernosal injection patients and 65 penile prosthesis recipients. Mean follow-up of all patients was 5.4 years. At the time of contact, 70% of the patients with prostheses were still sexually active whereas only 41% of the penile injection patients were sexually active (Sexton et al, 1998).

Another retrospective study compared erectile function status and satisfaction in patients receiving treatment with sildenafil citrate, intracavernous injection therapy, and inflatable penile prosthesis implantation. The patients were administered EDITS and the erectile function domain of the IIEF. There were 31 patients in the sildenafil citrate group, 22 in the penile injection therapy group, and 32 who had received a penile prosthesis. At a mean follow-up of 19.54 months, penile prosthesis recipients had significantly better erectile function and treatment satisfaction than patients in the other two groups (Rajpurkar and Dhabuwala, 2003).

SUGGESTED READINGS

Abouassaly R, Montague DK, Angermeier KW: Antibiotic-coated medical devices: With an emphasis on inflatable penile prosthesis. Asian J Androl 2004;6:249-257.

Milbank AJ, Montague DK, Angermeier KW, et al: Mechanical failure of the American Medical Systems Ultrex inflatable penile prosthesis: Before and after 1993 structural modification. J Urol 2002;167:2502-2506.

Mulcahy JJ: Long-term experience with salvage of infected penile implants. J Urol 2000;163:481-482.

Mulhall JP, Ahmed A, Branch J, et al: Serial assessment of efficacy and satisfaction profiles following penile prosthesis surgery. J Urol 2003;169: 1429-1433.

Tefilli MV, Dubocq F, Rajpurkar A, et al: Assessment of psychosexual adjustment after insertion of inflatable penile prosthesis. Urology 1998;52:1106-1112.

Wilson SK, Cleves MA, Delk JR 2nd: Comparison of mechanical reliability of original and enhanced Mentor Alpha I penile prosthesis. J Urol 1999;162:715-718.

24 Vascular Surgery for Erectile Dysfunction

RONALD W. LEWIS, MD • RICARDO MUNARRIZ, MD

A HISTORY AND REVIEW OF VASCULAR ERECTILE DYSFUNCTION SURGERY

Surgical interventions have consisted primarily of penile prosthesis insertion and vascular surgery. Venous leak surgery for corporal veno-occlusive dysfunction, popular among urologic surgeons in the mid-1980s to early 1990s, has been associated with poor long-term success rates, and this surgical procedure is no longer widely used. The American Urological Association Clinical Guidelines Panel on Erectile Dysfunction has recommended only one surgical treatment alternative as standard care for the patient with acquired organic erectile dysfunction, that is, the implantation of a penile prosthesis (Montague et al, 1996). These guidelines still consider vascular surgery experimental. Currently, penile revascularization is the only treatment modality with the capability of restoring fully natural penile erections for a long period without the necessity of external mechanical devices, chronic use of vasoactive medication, or surgical placement of internal penile prosthetic devices.

Historically, the first cases of penile arterial bypass surgery for erectile dysfunction were reported by Michal in the early 1970s with use of the inferior epigastric artery as the donor vessel (Michal et al, 1973, 1974; Michal, 1980). Subsequent modifications by Virag and others resulted in a multitude of procedures that used the deep dorsal vein as the recipient vessel (Virag et al, 1981; Virag ,1982; Hauri, 1986). Crespo and others presented procedures for revascularization of the cavernous artery directly by use of the inferior epigastric artery as a donor source (Crespo et al, 1982; Konnak and Ohl, 1989).

Lack of standardized techniques and selection criteria may have contributed to the current low popularity of arterial revascularization such that no one procedure has been universally accepted. On the other hand, a number of review and technique articles exist and are recommended for further details that are not presented in these pages (Metz, 1986; Lewis, 1990a, 1990b, 1993; Sohn et al, 1992; Hatzichristou and Goldstein, 1993; Goldstein et al, 1994; Sharlip, 1994; DePalma, 1997; Mulhall et al, 1999; Rao and Donatucci, 2001; Jarow, 2002; Licht and Lewis, 2002; Munarriz et al, 2004).

Vascular surgical procedures, in particular penile revascularization and penile venous surgery, are recommended only for a select group of patients. An example is the case of a young man who has significant vascular injury of vessels leading directly to the corpora cavernosa; revascularization surgery is often successful in such a case. The overall goal of penile revascularization surgery is to bypass obstructive arterial lesions in the hypogastric-cavernosal arterial bed. The specific objective of the surgery is to increase the cavernosal arterial perfusion pressure and blood inflow in patients with vasculogenic erectile dysfunction secondary to pure arterial insufficiency. Part of the failure of revascularization surgery may be that many of those patients in whom revascularization is used have significant end-organ disease already, such that revascularization is doomed to failure even though vascular lesions may be part of the pathologic process. In addition, in some arterialization surgery, there is a problem because of poor runoff after rearterialization for damaged arterial systems. The corpora cavernosa are areas of high resistance, and unless adequate runoff into the corpora tissue is present, vascular surgery may, again, be doomed to failure.

Penile venous surgery can still be indicated in patients who have congenital venous abnormalities of drainage of the corpora cavernosa tissue, but most of the venous surgery addressed to erectile dysfunction has occurred in patients who have significant intracorporeal tissue disease. Therefore, surgery directed at decreasing venous runoff beyond the corpora may provide only temporary relief.

There is a large mixture of organic and psychological properties to the disorder, and the high placebo effect in any type of treatment of erectile dysfunction must be constantly kept in mind by the surgeon. The history of erectile dysfunction surgery has been reviewed by several authors (Gee, 1975; Lewis, 1990b; Das, 1994). Some of these early procedures were amazingly similar to procedures that later became popular, such as the venous plication procedure and venous ligation surgery as proposed by Lowsley and Reuda (1953) in their presentation of a large group of patients that updated their previous report of the surgery in 1936. Ebbehoj and Wagner (1979) can be given credit for the first modern surgical approach to correction of abnormal drainage of the cavernous tissue based on diagnostic dynamic cavernosography techniques.

COUNSELING OF THE PATIENT FOR VASCULAR ERECTILE DYSFUNCTION SURGERY

It is imperative that alternative nonsurgical treatment modalities be fully explained to the potential patient. Decisions for management of impotence should be in the context of goal-directed therapy for the patient (and, when at all possible, the partner), as presented by Lue in Chapter 22, "Evaluation and Nonsurgical Management of Erectile Dysfunction and Premature Ejaculation." Patients for whom more conservative first treatment of their erectile problem has failed will tend to be more satisfied with a later choice of surgical intervention. There are individual patients, however, who will benefit from surgical intervention as a primary choice.

The choice of incision for erectile vascular surgery varies markedly, and this should also be explained to the patient in the preoperative counseling sessions. A semicircular incision on one side of the scrotal skin around the base of the penis, through which the entire penile shaft and access to the infrapubic region can be obtained, is the incision of choice for penile vein dissection and ligation surgery (Fig. 24–1). Although some authors believe that a paramedian incision is the best way to expose the inferior epigastric vessel complex in penile revascularization, others prefer a midline abdominal incision from umbilicus to base of penis, which will provide access to bilateral inferior epigastric vessel complexes, if this

becomes necessary, without having to make a second paramedian incision or a separate peripenile incision for recipient vessel exposure in penile arterial reconstruction.

PENILE ARTERIAL RECONSTRUCTION (PENILE REVASCULARIZATION)
Selection Criteria

It is a rare patient with erectile dysfunction who should be offered the choice of arterial vascular surgery (Table 24–1). Those patients with discrete focal arterial lesions found on selective pudendal arteriography, particularly younger patients who have a history of trauma (pelvic fracture or perineal blunt trauma), who do not have diabetes or neurologic disease and who are not currently users of tobacco, are the best candidates for penile revascularization procedures. They should not have systemic arteriosclerosis or major veno-occlusive dysfunction. These patients should have demonstrated functional arterial disease, based on findings on the second phase of the dynamic infusion cavernosometry and cavernosography of Goldstein (a gradient of more than 30 mm Hg between the penile occlusion pressure and the mean brachial pressure) or poor peak systolic velocities (<25 cm/sec) in the corporal penile arteries on color duplex Doppler sonographic studies (Quam et al, 1989), before pudendal arteriography is considered (Fig. 24–2).

A common iliac arteriogram and a selective internal pudendal arteriogram are necessary to demonstrate the adequacy of the proposed donor artery, such as the inferior epigastric artery, and the focal lesion in the artery or arteries supplying the corpora cavernosa. The selective internal pudendal study also is necessary for planning the exact nature of the surgery. It is preferable to connect the donor arterial vessel, usually the inferior epigastric artery (Fig. 24–3), to a branch of the dorsal penile artery in an end-to-end fashion, which allows the most

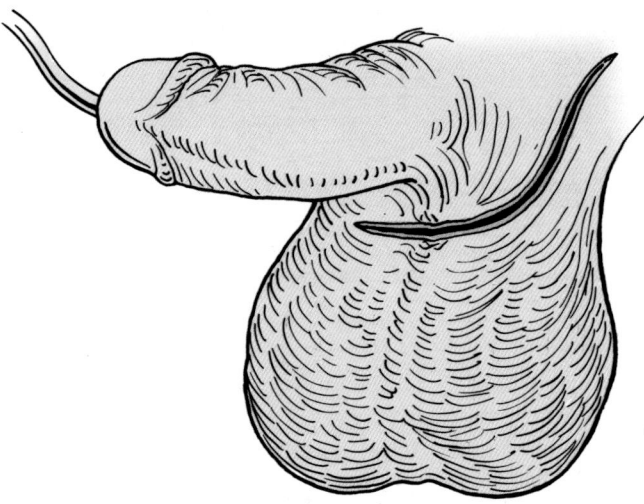

Figure 24–1. The peripenile inguinoscrotal incision that is used for both arterial revascularization and penile venous occlusive surgery. This incision affords excellent approach to the arterial and venous vessels of the penile shaft.

Table 24–1. Ideal Candidate for Microvascular Arterial Bypass Surgery

Young and psychologically stable
Without vascular risk factor exposure (diabetes mellitus, hypertension, coronary artery disease)
History of blunt perineal or pelvic trauma
  Obvious recollection of event
  Probable occurrence of event
Has considered conservative treatment options (all patients respond to low-dose injections with a sustained, relatively rigid erection)
Is highly motivated for natural, spontaneous, rigid sustained erections without need for chronic pharmacologic support, external mechanical devices, or internal mechanical devices
Symptoms
  Failure to fill erectile dysfunction pattern
    Reduced erectile rigidity
    Reduced erectile spontaneity
    Variable sustaining capability (normal or improved ability in AM)
  Normal libido, ejaculation and orgasm, and penile sensation
Physical examination
  Appropriate penile geometry (flaccid and erect penile diameter-to-length ratio)
  Normal penile extensibility during stretching
  No Peyronie's plaques, intracavernosal masses, or nodules
  No sensory neuropathy

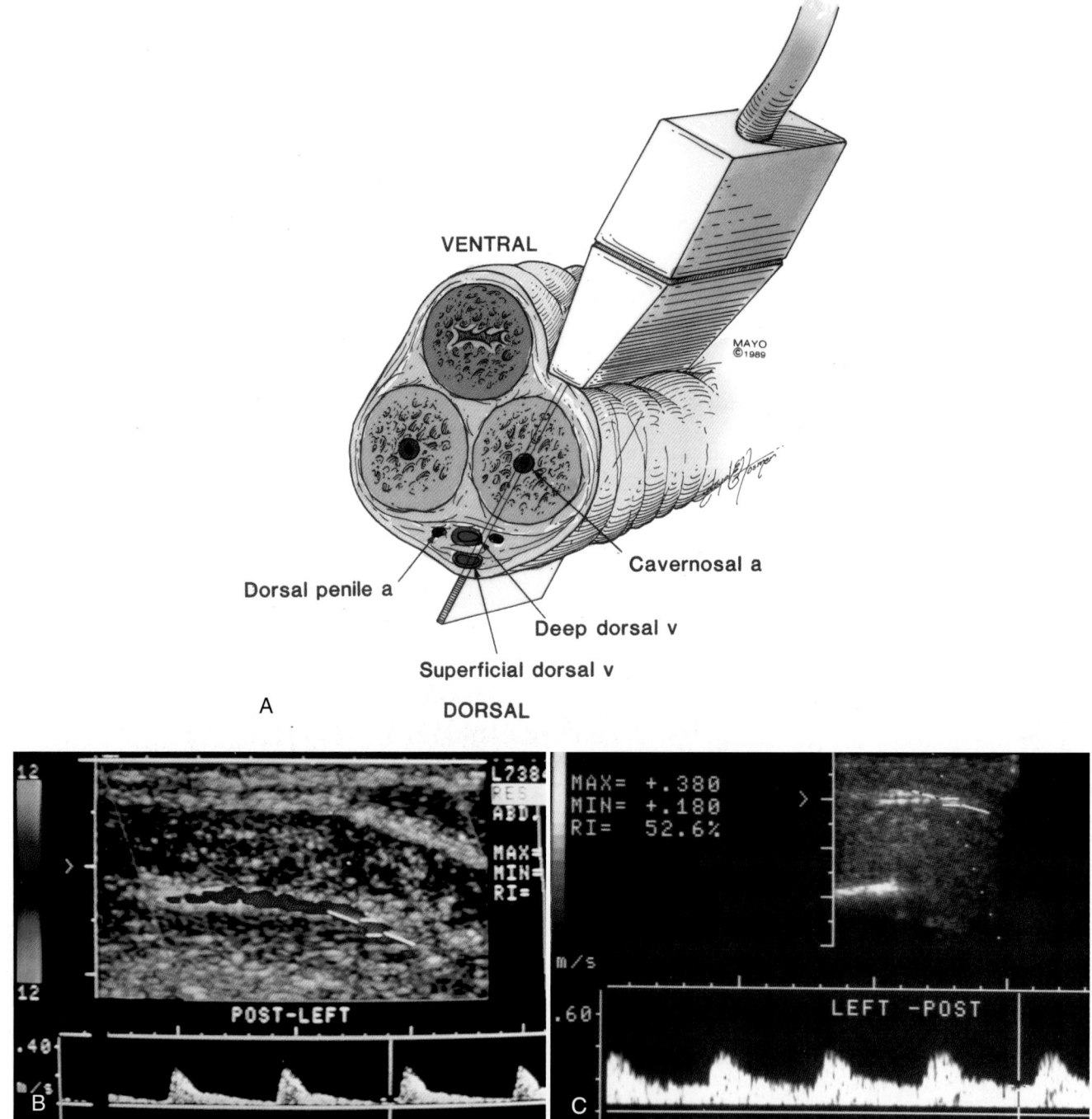

VENTRAL

MAYO
©1989

Dorsal penile a

Cavernosal a

Deep dorsal v

Superficial dorsal v

A

DORSAL

Figure 24–2. **A,** Use of a Doppler probe on the ventral surface of the penis to image the cavernosal artery of the penis. **B,** The typical color duplex Doppler image shows the cursors used to produce the most accurate measurement of arterial flow, which is demonstrated as a pulse image on the lower portion of the screen. **C,** Imaging of an arterial pulse in the cavernosal artery in a patient with veno-occlusive disorder. The patient has a peak systolic velocity of 38 cm per second and an end-diastolic velocity of 18 cm per second with a resistive index of 52.6%.

efficient runoff, or, when this is not possible, with an end-to-side anastomosis. This is possible if the dorsal artery has demonstrated good connections to the intracavernosal deep penile artery on the preoperative arteriogram. On occasion, in the absence of a suitable epigastric artery, a reversed saphenous vein connected to the superficial femoral artery may serve as the input arterial supply (Sohn et al, 1992; Jarow, 2002). When there is no suitable dorsal artery, revascularization of an isolated segment of deep dorsal vein with good communicators to the intracavernous tissue is the choice for recipient vessel. Another possibility is the use of a Y branch of the inferior epigastric artery or two inferior epigastric arteries

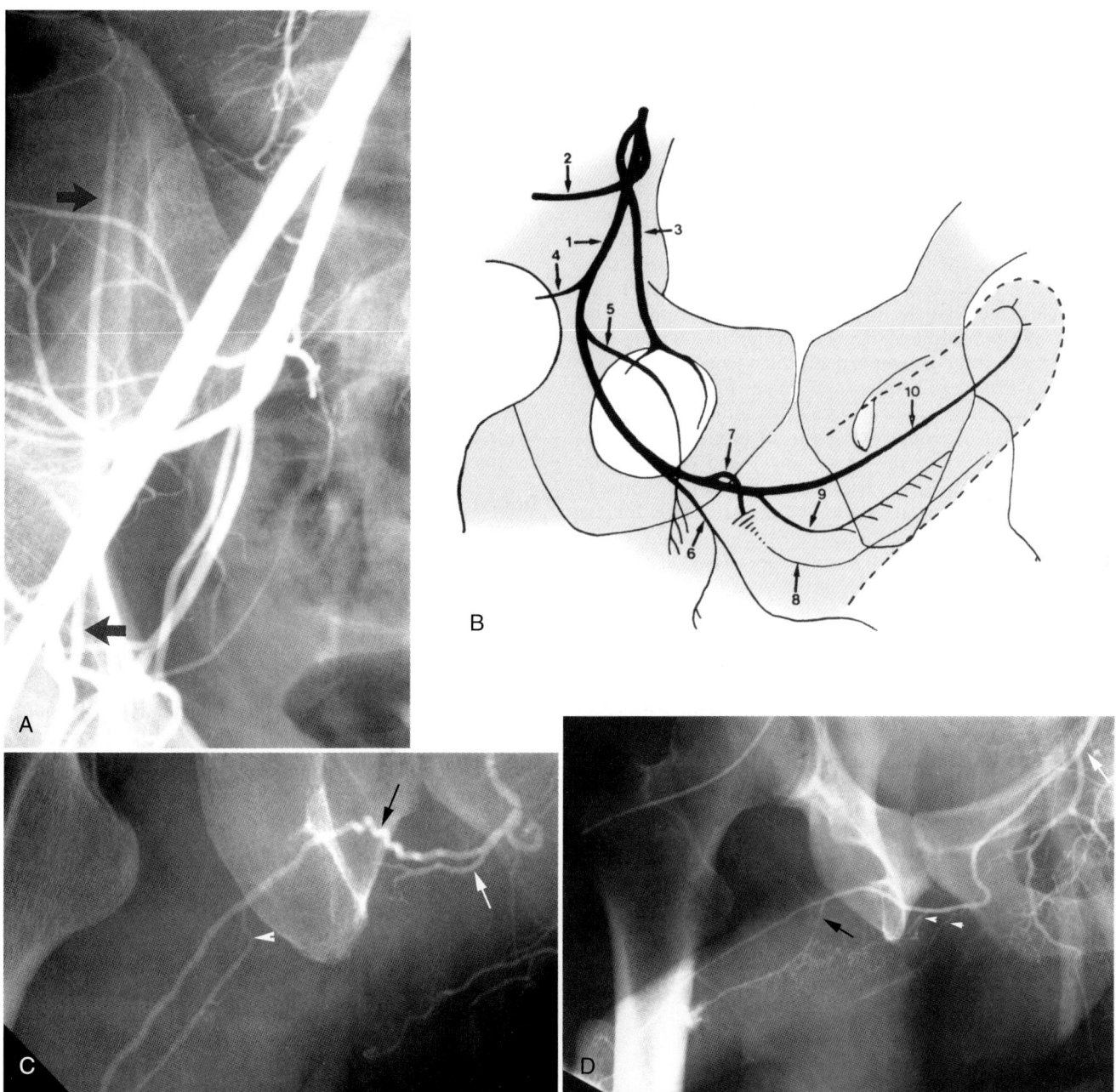

Figure 24–3. **A,** A flush pelvic arteriogram demonstrates an excellent donor artery of the inferior epigastric artery on the right side (*black arrows* indicate the potential donor artery). **B,** Diagram of the anterior division of the hypogastric artery: 1, internal pudendal artery, which is the artery that is cannulated for a detailed study of the vessels supplying the penis; 2, superior gluteal artery; 3, obturator artery; 4, inferior gluteal artery; 5, hemorrhoidal artery; 6, superficial perineal artery; 7, artery to the bulb; 8, continuation of the bulbar artery as the urethral artery; 9, cavernosal artery; 10, dorsal artery of the penis. **C,** A selective internal pudendal artery study at the base of the penis shows some tortuosity of the first portion of the dorsal artery of the penis (*black arrow*), a very short segment of the cavernosal artery (*white arrow*) with reentry of flow into the cavernous artery by a distal branch (*arrowhead*) off of the dorsal artery of the penis. **D,** Another selective internal pudendal artery study. In this particular study, the first branch vessel is the obturator vessel (*white arrow*) that comes off of the internal pudendal. One can then see proximal small arteries (*arrowheads*) supplying each of the cavernosal spaces and another vessel (*black arrow*) feeding the cavernosal space on the right from the dorsal artery of the penis.

for anastomosis to the dorsal artery and an isolated segment of deep dorsal vein. Hauri (1986, 1999) used the inferior epigastric artery anastomosed as the input source to a side-to-side recipient anastomosed dorsal artery to deep dorsal vein.

Patients with arterial disease or a combination of arterial and veno-occlusive disease should be offered an in-depth discussion of alternative therapeutic choices, such as vacuum devices and penile prostheses. Many patients with mild to moderate vascular disease will also respond to injection of a vasoactive agent or oral administration of sildenafil with improved erections that are suitable for vaginal intercourse.

Surgical Technique

Penile vascular surgery is performed with the patient under general intubated or spinal anesthesia. The patient is placed supine with the legs in a slightly abducted position. Since these are long operations (often exceeding 5 hours), extremity padding and placement to protect from transient nerve palsies is recommended. Securing arms next to the body and alternating the blood pressure cuff periodically through the procedure are examples of protection of neurovascular points. The patient's abdomen and genitalia are carefully shaved, prepared, and draped; this is then followed by placement of a 16 French Foley catheter with use of sterile technique. The patient is given one dose of preoperative antibiotics (cefazolin or vancomycin if the patient is penicillin allergic).

Some surgeons prefer the use of loupes for the early dissection in the arterial cases and for all of the venous surgery cases. A hand-held Doppler probe is an excellent accessory tool for monitoring of the dorsal artery and checking for runoff into revascularized arteries or arterialized veins. A lighted suction instrument is also useful, particularly for the arterial cases; it is also helpful for any venous dissection near the urethra. The choice of incision for the venous surgery and for preparation of the recipient dorsal artery for revascularization is the anterior scrotal peripenile incision, first introduced by Lue (1988). Use of a ring retractor with its elastic hooks maximizes operative exposure of the penis. The choice of incision for the senior author for arterial surgery is the lower abdominal midline because both inferior epigastric artery vessel bundles can be dissected from the lower surface of the rectus muscle, if necessary (Fig. 24–4). Others prefer a

Table 24–2. Current Major Penile Revascularization Procedures

Use of inferior epigastric artery or reversed saphenous vein bypass from superficial femoral vein as input source
Microvascular surgery (endothelium preserving)
Modification of Michal procedure: distal or proximal end-to-end to dorsal artery or end-to-side dorsal artery
Arterialization (modification of Virag procedure) of isolated segment of deep dorsal vein
Arterialization of dorsal vein–penile artery fistula (Hauri)

transverse semilunar abdominal incision or a paramedian incision for dissection of the inferior epigastric artery complex. The general nature of this type of vascular surgery is presented in Table 24–2. Certain points of technique are stressed in the next three sections. **There is no single type of revascularization surgery that fits every case** (Fig. 24–5).

Dorsal Artery Dissection

The junior author's group prefers this as the first step. The senior author exposes the donor artery first (see next section). A curvilinear peripenile incision is made, in general on the side opposite the planned abdominal incision for inferior epigastric artery harvesting (see Fig. 24–1). The incision is made two fingerbreadths from the base of the penis and is carried down through the dartos layer by use of cautery. The advantages of this incision are that it offers excellent proximal and distal exposure of the penile neurovascular bundle, preserves the fundiform and suspensory ligaments (thus preventing

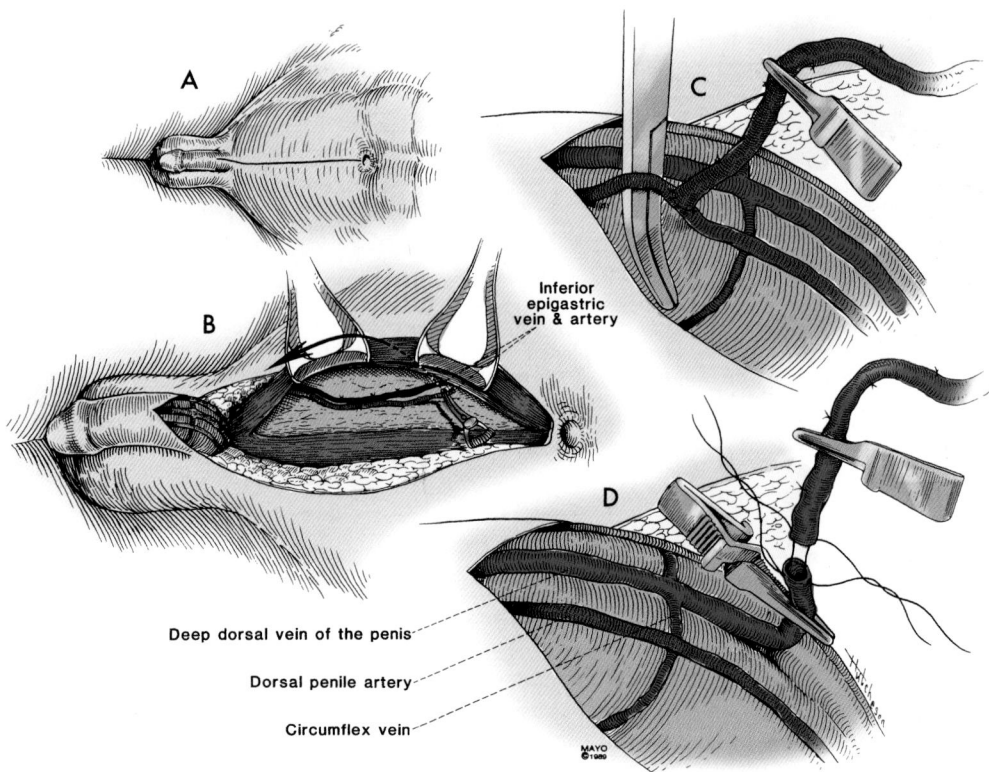

Figure 24–4. Steps in revascularization procedures of the penis with the inferior epigastric artery. **A,** Midline incision. **B,** Dissection of the inferior epigastric vessels from the lower surface of the rectus muscle. **C,** Anastomosis of the inferior epigastric artery in an end-to-side fashion to the left dorsal artery. **D,** Anastomosis of the inferior epigastric artery to the deep dorsal vein in an end-to-end configuration. Details are described in the text. (**A** to **D,** reproduced from the Mayo Clinic Foundation.)

Inferior epigastric vein & artery

Deep dorsal vein of the penis
Dorsal penile artery
Circumflex vein

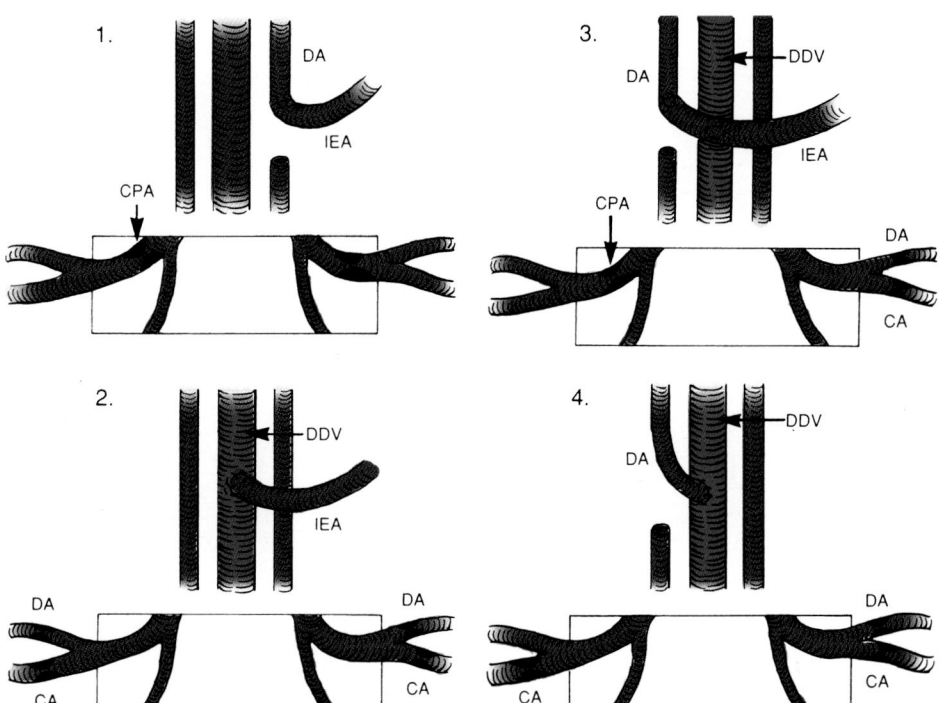

Figure 24–5. Types of arteriographic patterns and the associated types of bypass procedures. CA, cavernosal artery; CPA, common penile artery; DA, dorsal artery; DDV, deep dorsal vein; IEA, inferior epigastric artery. (From Hatzichristou D, Goldstein I: Penile microvascular arterial bypass surgery. Urol Clin North Am 1993;1:42.)

penile shortening), and avoids unsightly postoperative scars on the penile shaft or at the base of the penis.

With the penis stretched, blunt finger dissection along the tunica albuginea is performed in a distal direction deep and inferior to the spermatic cord structures along the lateral aspect of the penile shaft. Injury to the fundiform ligament is avoided. The penis is then inverted through the skin incision, with care taken to push the glans in fully toward the incision site (Fig. 24–6). If a partial erection or tumescence is present, intracavernosal α-adrenergic agonist (preferably 100 to 500 μg phenylephrine) should be administered. Blunt finger dissection around the distal penile shaft enables a plane to be established between Buck's fascia and Colles' fascia, and a Penrose drain can be secured in this plane.

Exposure of the neurovascular bundle and, in particular, the right and left dorsal penile arteries is now performed. The arteries are usually obvious, located on either side of the deep dorsal vein and surrounded predominantly laterally by the dorsal nerves. Isolation of the dorsal penile arteries for such arterial bypass surgery requires limited dissection at this stage of the procedure, thus limiting ischemic, mechanical, and thermal trauma to the dorsal penile arteries. The right and left dorsal penile arteries are identified first in the midpenile shaft. Their course is followed proximally underneath the fundiform ligament, with care being taken to leave the fundiform ligament intact. To avoid injurious vasospasm, topical papaverine hydrochloride irrigations may be applied frequently. In this way, preservation of endothelial and smooth muscle cell morphologic features during dorsal artery preparation is ensured. This step is critical as the room temperature of the operating room, the use of room-temperature irrigating solution, and even the skin incision can induce vasoconstriction, spasm, and possible endothelial cell damage.

A window is fashioned in the fundiform ligament proximally, usually near the junction of the fundiform and suspensory ligaments at a location where the pendulous penile shaft becomes fixed proximally. Blunt dissection is performed under the proximal aspect of the fundiform ligament above the pubic bone toward the external ring opposite to the peripenile incision. This dissection provides a path for the inferior epigastric artery to pass from its abdominal location to the appropriate location in the penis while simultaneously preserving the fundiform ligament. The penis is placed back in its normal anatomic position, and the inguinoscrotal incision is temporarily closed with staples.

For the deep dorsal vein arterialization procedure, the senior author prefers an end-to-end anastomosis to the deep dorsal vein and thus takes down the fundiform and suspensory ligaments of the penis to prepare the free vein for anastomosis. Reanastomosis of the base of the penis to the infrapubic periosteum after such vein preparation is accomplished with a silk suture. When anastomosis to the deep dorsal artery in either an end-to-side or an end-to-end fashion is performed, the two ligaments can be preserved as described before. Also for dorsal vein arterialization, the initial multiple branches of the deep dorsal vein near the glans are ligated with a nonpermanent suture, as well as large trunks of the deep dorsal vein that anastomose to the spongiosum laterally along the shaft of the penis. Valves in the deep dorsal vein are removed with a 2-mm LeMaitre valvulotome or a similarly sized Fogarty balloon catheter.

Harvesting of the Inferior Epigastric Artery

The senior author prefers a lower midline incision for this step for reasons mentioned before (see Fig. 24–4). A transverse semilunar abdominal incision following Langer's lines (Fig.

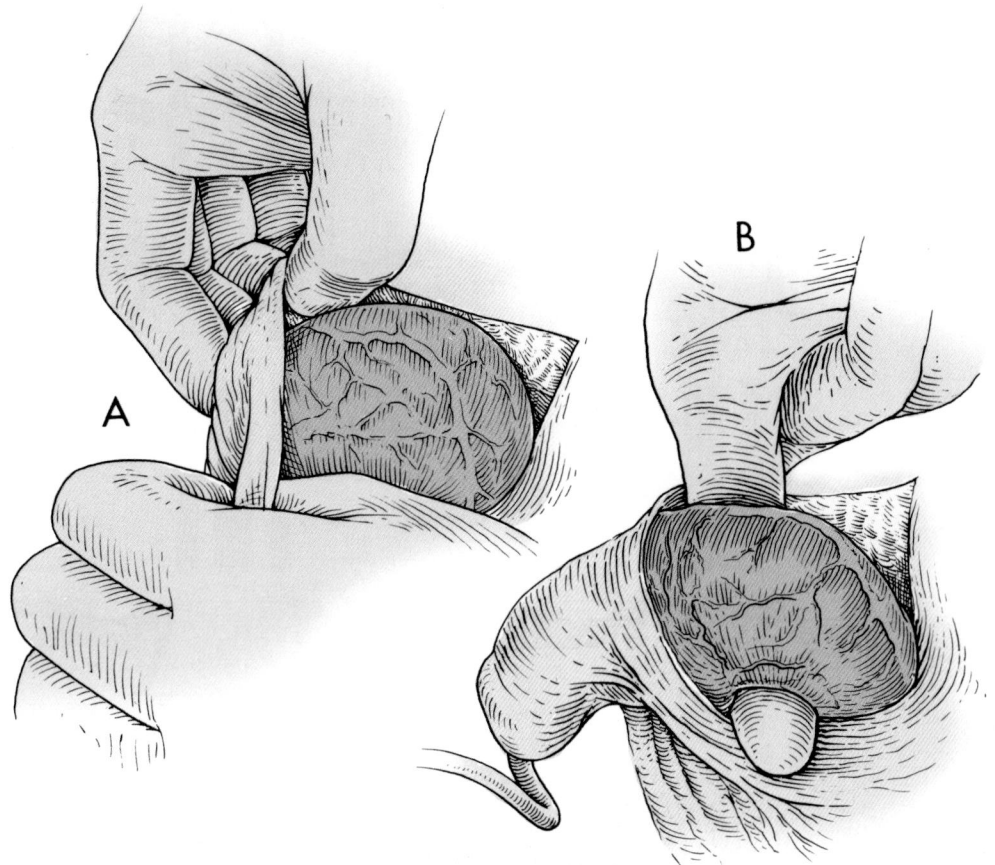

Figure 24–6. **A,** Eversion of the penile shaft through the peripenile incision by pushing into the glans of the penis. **B,** The skin and dartos layer have been stripped away from the shaft of the penis. A Penrose drain can be placed for retraction in the plane that is demonstrated by the index finger.

24–7) is the preferred incision for the junior author, although a paramedian incision can be used, especially if the desired inferior epigastric artery is short or has several branches or the patient's habitus precludes a standard transverse incision. The transverse incision provides excellent operative exposure of the inferior epigastric artery and heals with a more cosmetic scar compared with those observed with paramedian skin incisions. The starting point of the transverse incision is approximately $^{11}/_{16}$ of the total distance from the pubic bone to the umbilicus in the midline. It extends laterally along the skin lines for approximately 5 cm. The rectus fascia is incised vertically. The junction between the rectus muscle and underlying preperitoneal fat is identified, and the preperitoneal space is entered. The rectus muscle is reflected medially. The inferior epigastric artery and its accompanying veins are located beneath the rectus muscle in the preperitoneal plane.

A ring retractor is again used to optimize operative exposure. It is critical to harvest an inferior epigastric artery of sufficient length to prevent tension on the microvascular anastomosis. Topical papaverine is applied on the inferior epigastric artery throughout the dissection. Thermal injury is avoided by use of low-current microbipolar cautery set at the minimum level necessary for adequate coagulation. **The vasa vasorum are preserved by dissecting the artery en bloc with its surrounding veins and fat.** Usually, branches isolated during the dissection are both artery and vein, which can be commonly ligated or clipped with small vascular clips or cauterized with a bipolar cautery. Dissection of the inferior

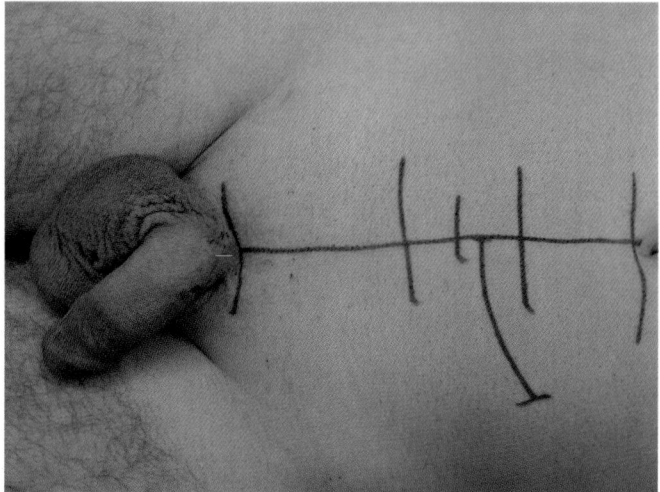

Figure 24–7. The transverse semilunar abdominal incision (to be placed on the patient's left 60% from the pubic bone) for harvesting of the inferior epigastric artery.

epigastric artery is required from its origin at the level of the external iliac artery to a point at the level of the umbilicus (see Fig. 24–4). It is at this point that the artery usually bifurcates. In the past, we made every effort to use the bifurcation where possible to allow anastomoses to both dorsal arteries, but we have not seen a significant improvement in erectile function in patients who underwent anastomosis of the inferior epigastric artery to both dorsal arteries compared with patients who had a single anastomosis. Thus, we are currently performing a single anastomosis, minimizing surgical time and preserving a dorsal artery in case a second penile revascularization is desired.

The transfer route of the neoarterial inflow source is prepared from the abdominal perspective before transection of the vessel distally (the penile transfer route has previously been dissected). The temporary scrotal staples are removed, and the penis is reinverted. The internal ring on the side of the harvested artery is identified medial to the origin of the inferior epigastric artery. By use of blunt finger dissection through the inguinal canal, a long fine vascular clamp is passed through the fenestration in the fundiform ligament and the external inguinal rings. A Penrose drain is placed to protect this transfer route.

The donor vascular bundle is transected at the level of the umbilicus between two Ligaclips and carefully inspected for any proximal bleeding points. A long fine vascular clamp is brought through the internal inguinal ring again, this time to grasp the end of the transected inferior epigastric artery. The inferior epigastric vascular bundle is transferred to the base of the penis. It should be briskly pulsating and of adequate length. The origin of the inferior epigastric artery should be inspected for kinking or twisting, eliminating this if it is found. Closure of the abdominal wound is performed in two layers after achievement of complete hemostasis. The rectus fascia is closed with a running 0 polyglycolic acid suture. The skin edges are apposed with skin staples or a subcuticular 4-0 polyglycolic acid suture.

Microvascular Anastomosis

A ring retractor and the associated elastic hooks are used once again on the inguinoscrotal incision and the fenestration of the fundiform ligament to gain exposure of the proximal dorsal neurovascular bundle. The pulsating inferior epigastric artery is placed against the recipient dorsal penile arteries, and a convenient location is selected for the vascular anastomosis. The anastomosis is based on the arteriographic and duplex Doppler ultrasound findings. An end-to-end anastomosis is best under conditions whereby dorsal penile artery communications exist to the cavernous artery. In addition, an end-to-end anastomosis transfers perfusion pressure more effectively than does an end-to-side anastomosis with less turbulence. This end-to-end anastomosis can be to the proximal dorsal artery, where good communication exists between this artery and the cavernous artery proximally (usually injuries to the common penile artery). Anastomosis to the distal dorsal artery must have distal communication to the cavernous artery (usually injuries to the deep artery are present at or near the bifurcation into the deep and dorsal penile artery). It has been our experience that ligation of both dorsal penile arteries to perform bilateral proximal end-to-end anastomoses has never caused ischemic injury to the glans penis since one or both donor inferior epigastric arteries provide excellent blood supply to the glans.

The appropriate dorsal penile artery segment is freed from its attachments to the tunica albuginea, with care being taken to avoid injury to any communicating branches to the cavernosal artery. Vascular hemostasis of this segment of the dorsal penile artery may be achieved with either gold-plated (low-pressure) aneurysm vascular clamps or vessel loops under minimal tension for the minimal operating time. The only location where the adventitia must be carefully removed is at the site of the vascular anastomosis, that is, the distal end of the inferior epigastric artery and the free end of the dorsal artery, to avoid causing subsequent thrombosis (Fig. 24-8). If segments of adventitia enter the anastomosis, patency of the anastomosis is in jeopardy as adventitia activates clotting factors from the extrinsic clotting system. The remaining adventitia should be preserved on the vessels since the vasa vasorum provide a nutritional and innervation role to the vessel wall.

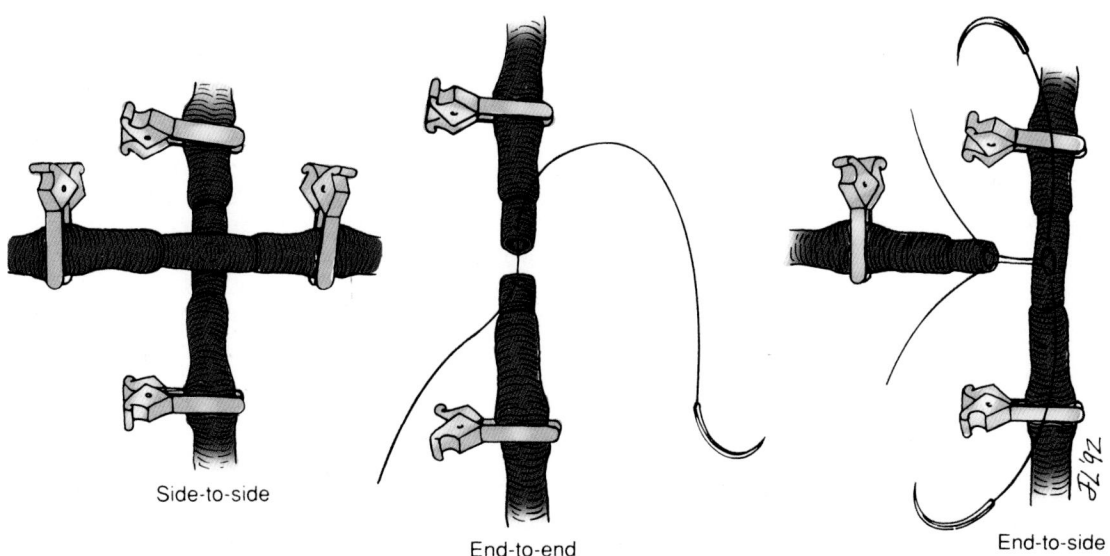

Side-to-side

End-to-end

End-to-side

Figure 24-8. The different types of microvascular anastomoses. Notice that the adventitial tissue is removed from the vessel only at the site of the anastomosis. (From Hatzichristou D, Goldstein I: Penile microvascular arterial bypass surgery. Urol Clin North Am 1993;1:42.)

We use a plastic colored background material to aid in vessel visualization under the microscope. An end-to-end anastomosis is performed between the inferior epigastric artery and the dorsal artery with interrupted 10-0 nylon sutures (single-armed, 100-μm, 149-degree curved needle) under 10× magnification. For intraluminal irrigation, we use a dilute papaverine, heparin, and electrolytic solution believed to be capable of inhibiting the early development of myointimal proliferative lesions during surgical preparation. After release of the temporary occluding vascular clamps (or vessel loops) on the dorsal penile artery, the anastomosed segment should reveal arterial pulsations along its length and retrograde into the inferior epigastric artery. Such an observation implies a patent anastomosis. At this time, the inferior epigastric artery gold-plated aneurysm clamp may be removed. The intensity of the arterial pulsations in the anastomosis usually increases. Good flow can be checked with a Doppler probe. On occasion, the application of a small amount of hemostatic material may be needed to aid in promoting hemostasis from suture needle holes in the vessel walls. After complete hemostasis has been achieved and correct instrument and sponge counts are ensured, closure of the inguinoscrotal incision may begin. The dartos layer is reapproximated with 3-0 polyglycolic acid sutures in a running fashion. The skin edges are closed with subcuticular running closure or with skin staples; no drains are used. The Foley catheter is left to closed-system gravity drainage overnight.

Modifications of this procedure may be used. The most common alternative arterial anastomosis is an end-to-side anastomosis between the inferior epigastric artery and dorsal penile artery. A 10-0 suture is placed along the longitudinal axis of the dorsal penile artery in a 1-mm segment in the region of the intended anastomosis. After tension is placed on the suture, an oval section of the artery wall is excised with a curved microscissors, resulting in a 1.2- to 1.5-mm horizontal arteriotomy (Fig. 24–9). A temporary 2 French Silastic stent is placed within the arteriotomy for clearer definition of the vessel lumen. The sutures are placed initially at each apex of the anastomosis, and then subsequently three to five interrupted sutures are placed into each sidewall. All sutures used to complete the anastomosis are inserted equidistant from each other to avoid an uneven anastomosis. One side of the anastomosis is completed before the other side is commenced. If a temporary vascular stent is used, it is removed after placement of all sutures. The use of a temporary vascular stent enables careful inspection of the vessel backwall.

Other modifications for recipient vessels include the original Hauri procedure in which the dorsal penile artery and dorsal penile vein are opened longitudinally for an extended length of approximately 1.5 to 2 cm and the adjacent sidewalls of each vessel are joined with 7-0 continuous suture, creating a common backwall. The donor inferior epigastric artery is then connected to these joined vessels in an end-to-side fashion. A modification of this procedure was described later by Löbelenz et al (1992), who divides the dorsal penile artery proximally and distally and performs an end-to-side anastomosis of each of these to the deep dorsal vein. The inferior epigastric artery is also brought down as an end-to-side anastomosis to the deep dorsal vein of the penis.

Another alternative donor vessel for the inferior epigastric artery is the reverse saphenous vein graft that can be attached

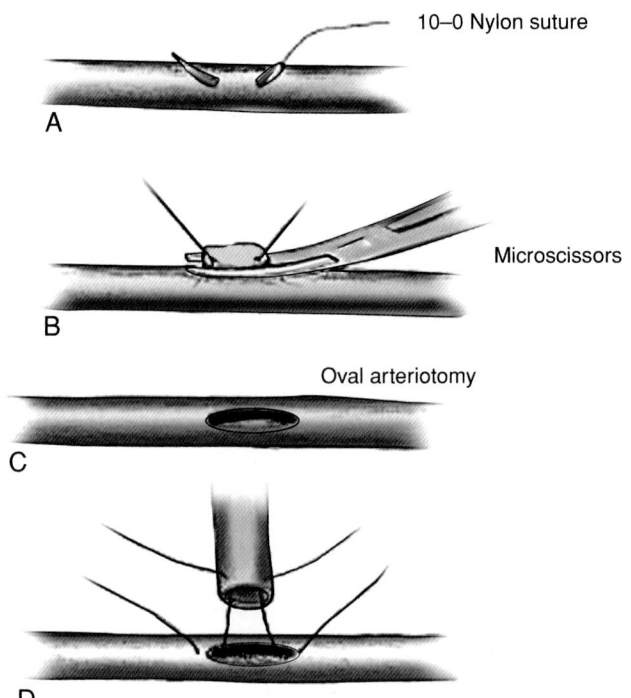

Figure 24–9. **A** to **C**, The technique of preparing the recipient vessel for an end-to-side anastomosis. **D**, The alignment of the donor vessel in an end fashion to the recipient vessel in a side fashion and fixed by two initial sutures.

to the superficial femoral artery. An end-to-side anastomosis is made between the reversed saphenous vein and the superficial femoral artery, and this vessel is subsequently anastomosed to the recipient vessel of the penis.

Complications

Penile edema is common after vascular surgery of the penis. A lightly applied elastic dressing of the penis for 24 hours after surgery greatly aids in controlling this postoperative minor complication, and any mild to moderate edema after the removal of the dressing usually resolves without sequelae 2 to 3 weeks after surgery. Superficial ecchymosis and bruising of the penile shaft and scrotum are not unusual or debilitating; serious wound hematomas can be avoided by use of the tubular fenestrated drain postoperatively for 24 to 48 hours.

Two significant complications of penile vascular surgery are penile numbness (or hypoesthesia) and penile shortening from scar entrapment, which is experienced in as many as 20% of patients. Preservation of the suspensory and fundiform ligaments has markedly diminished penile shortening. Penile sensation usually returns 12 to 18 months after surgery if no major penile sensory nerve has been significantly severed. On occasion, penile shortening from severe scar entrapment may require subsequent scar release surgery and the use of relaxing Z-plasty incisions or scrotal flap coverage.

Mechanical disruption of the microvascular anastomosis has been reported by Hatzichristou and Goldstein (1993). This disruption of the microvascular anastomosis and subsequent uncontrolled arterial hemorrhage may occur from blunt trauma in the first few postoperative weeks from coitus, masturbation, or accidents. Resumption of sexual activity should begin 6 weeks after this surgery. Another complication of deep dorsal penile vein arterialization is glans hyperemia, which occurs when a communicating vein from the revascularized deep dorsal vein to the glans in the distal dissection is missed. Surgical exploration and ligation of the arterialized communicator resolves the problem.

Results

Table 24–3 lists reported results of arterial surgery for erectile dysfunction. In summary, long-term success rates of 50% to 60% are less than optimal and have led some to question the possible benefits from this type of surgery (Barada and Gennett, 1990; Lewis, 1992; Sohn et al, 1992; Sharlip, 1994). The report of Sohn and associates (1992) of the lack of correlation of results (as reported by the patient) to preoperative and postoperative objective testing in the arterial surgical treatment of erectile dysfunction would suggest that much scientific understanding is lacking for this treatment modality. Of the 31 publications on penile revascularization surgery reviewed by the American Urological Association committee, only four reports for a total of 64 patients met the peer review criteria: age younger than 55 years; absence of major vascular risk factors (diabetes, tobacco); minimum follow-up of 1 year; classic findings by penile duplex Doppler ultrasound examination, dynamic infusion cavernosometry and cavernosography, and selective internal pudendal arteriography; and objective follow-up data. These reports document a success rate of 36% to 91% (Grasso et al, 1992; Jarow and DeFranzo, 1996; Ang and Lim, 1997; Kayigil et al, 2000). The article by Kayigil and associates (2000) dealt with 3-year results of deep

dorsal vein arterialization in 25 patients who had pure caverno-occlusive dysfunction. The article by Ang and Lim (1997) described results in six men who had pure arteriogenic (two patients) or mixed arteriogenic-venogenic (four patients) erectile dysfunction. This too was a deep dorsal vein arterialization revascularization, sometimes associated with venous channel dissection and ligation. At a mean follow-up of 19.8 months (range, 8 to 37 months), two patients had excellent surgical outcome and two had improved outcome, having ability to have intercourse with intracavernosal injection. Many of the reports that are included in Table 24–3 have tried to analyze the population of patients that has had success from the surgery compared with patent anastomoses measured objectively and have found discrepancy between patency and success and lack of patency and failure.

Munarriz and colleagues (2004) have reported on the objective postoperative hemodynamic status, including steady-state equilibrium intracavernosal pressures and veno-occlusive and arterial function testing parameters, in patients who experienced successful as well as unsuccessful clinical results after microvascular arterial bypass surgery for impotence. Of the 226 patients who underwent penile microvascular arterial bypass surgery from 1985 to 1992, 68 (30%) (mean age, 34 ± 10 years) underwent both preoperative and postoperative pharmacocavernosometry-pharmacocavernosography. The mean duration between the bypass procedure and follow-up postoperative testing was 8 ± 6 months. Surgical bypasses in these 68 patients included 65 inferior epigastric artery to dorsal penile artery, including 30 with dual dorsal arterial anastomosis. There were, in addition, nine artery to deep dorsal vein anastomoses, including six performed in conjunction with an arterial anastomosis. Twelve patients (21%)

Table 24–3. Success Rate of Arterial Surgery for Impotence

Study (yr)	Procedure	Patients (N)	Result
Virag (1982)	V4-V6	36	41.6% good, 33.3% fair
Michal et al (1986)	Michal	73	60% success
Balko et al (1986)	V6	11	73% significantly improved
U.S. Society for Study of Impotence (1988)*	V5 or modified V5	50	78% success
Lizza and Zorgniotti (1988)	V5 or modified V5	13	77% success
Sharlip (1990)	Mixed	30	20% success, 27% improved
Virag and Bennett (1991)	V5	100	38% good, 30% improved
Furlow et al (1990)	Modified V5	95	78%
Sohn (1992)	Mixed	65	31% success, 54% good or improved
Bock and Lewis (1992)	Mixed	36	53% success, 28% improved
Löbelenz et al (1992)	Mixed	19	58% success, 40% improved
Schramek et al (1992)	Hauri	35	60% success, 23% improved
			54% excellent postoperative Doppler
			23% good postoperative Doppler
Melman and Riccardi (1993)	Mixed	18	33% success
Janssen et al (1994)	Mixed	21	62% success, 5% improved
Lizza and Zorgniotti (1994)	Mixed	36 (1 yr)	53% success, 31% improved
		32 (2 yr)	41% success, 34% improved
		26 (3 yr)	54% success, 19% improved
Jarow and DeFranzo (1996)	Mixed	11	64% success, 27% improved
Benet et al (1997)	Mixed	36 (8 lost to follow-up)	46% success, 14% improved
Sarramon et al (1997)	Mixed	114	47.8% success, 14.6% improved
Manning et al (1998)	Mixed	62	34% success, 20% improved
Kayigil et al (2000)†	Furlow-Fisher modification of Virag	25 (1 yr)	80% subjective success
		16 (2 yr)	75% subjective success
		10 (3 yr)	70% subjective success

*Reported by Belker and Bennett (1988).
†Deep dorsal vein arterialization for pure veno-occlusive dysfunction.

with pure arteriogenic impotence had a postoperative mean increase in steady-state equilibrium intracavernosal pressure of 25 ± 12.3 mm Hg (range, 13 to 45 mm Hg). Of the remaining 56 patients, 49 had concomitant venous surgery. In this group, there was no significant change in mean steady-state equilibrium intracavernosal pressure, mean pressure decay in 30 seconds, or mean flow to maintain values. The remaining seven who did not have venous surgery had normal veno-occlusive function preoperatively and postoperatively; however, the postoperative intracavernosal pressure did not increase.

PENILE VENOUS SURGERY
Selection Criteria

Criteria for recommending surgery for a veno-occlusive disorder consist of the following:
1. complaint by a patient of short-duration erections or tumescence only with sexual stimulation;
2. failure to obtain or to maintain an erection from the use of oral sildenafil or intracavernous injection on multiple trials with different agents with sexual stimulation;
3. normal cavernous arteries on color duplex Doppler studies or the second phase of dynamic infusion cavernosometry and cavernosography (see Fig. 24–2C);
4. faulty veno-occlusive mechanism as determined by infusion pump or gravity pharmacocavernosometry that is amenable to surgery (no massive venous leakage);
5. location of the site of venous leakage from the corpora cavernosa on pharmacocavernosography (Fig. 24–10);
6. no medical contraindication to surgery;
7. complete elimination of tobacco use; and
8. selection on presentation of alternative therapeutic choices in the presence of a long-term success rate of 40% to 50%.

It is a rare patient who should be offered venous surgery for the treatment of erectile dysfunction. Wespes and coworkers (1994) have suggested that responders to surgery need to have a crucial percentage of smooth muscle (>29%) present in the cavernosal tissue. In fact, the same authors, in 1997, questioned the wisdom of venous surgery because sinus smooth muscle seems to play such a crucial role in the veno-occlusive mechanism (Wespes et al, 1997, 2003). However, when smooth muscle content is determined before surgery, as a criterion for selection, long-term results are not better, being 52% at more than 1 year (Sasso et al, 1999).

Surgical Technique

For venous dissection and ligation surgery, the entire penis can be inverted into the wound for access to all-important venous channels along the shaft of the penis by a combination of sharp and blunt dissection through the previously described peripenile incision. Some surgeons prefer a dorsal lithotomy position for venous dissection and ligation surgery; if crural banding or ligation is planned as a part of the procedure, this is also the position of choice. Figure 24–11 outlines the general steps of venous dissection surgery. Communicating veins between the deep and the superficial systems are ligated as exposed with absorbable suture because the patient will be able to palpate permanent ligatures, and these can often be a nuisance. After the penile shaft eversion is accomplished, a butterfly needle can be placed into one of the corpora cavernosa, fixing this in place with a purse-string ligature in the tunica albuginea, for introduction of indigo carmine for greater demarcation of draining cavernosal veins or intraoperative or postdissection pharmacocavernosometry.

As the penis is dissected more proximally and as the fundiform and suspensory ligaments are dissected and divided, communicating veins to the perineal sidewall and the pubic regions are usually isolated and divided so that exposure of the deeper venous drainage system is facilitated. The suspensory ligament must be taken down in its entirety for proper exposure to the more distal deep dorsal penile vein and the cavernosal veins, when present.

Once the penis is fully mobilized, an incision in Buck's fascia directly over the deep dorsal penile vein is made in the midshaft, the vein is divided between ligatures, and then distal or proximal dissection is begun; communicating tributaries encountered in this dissection of the deep dorsal vein or veins are ligated. Care is taken to stay in the midline over the deep dorsal vein to avoid injury to the slightly more laterally positioned dorsal penile arteries and penile sensory nerves. Distally along the penile shaft, the dissection of the deep dorsal vein is taken to 1 to 1.5 cm from the glandular sulcus, where the multitrunk origins of this vein are dissected and individually ligated.

Along the penile shaft, communicating circumflex veins near the corpora cavernosa and the spongiosum are identified, exposed under Buck's fascia, and ligated. Any use of electrocoagulation along the penile shaft should be performed with a bipolar unit to prevent transmission of possible coagulation to arteries or nerves of the penile shaft. The deep dorsal vein is dissected proximally to under the pubis, where it is ligated with a heavy permanent suture. It is in this area that the cavernosal veins can be found for dissection and ligation. Some expert surgeons also recommend crural plication sutures along the lateral surface of the tunica albuginea of each of the corpora cavernosa.

An attempt is made, after the venous dissection, to reapproximate the suspensory ligament attachment of the base of the penis with a permanent suture from the pubis to the midline tunica albuginea of the corpora in the midline sulcus, where the deep dorsal vein had been. A fenestrated tubular drain is placed in the infrapubic region and exited out a separate stab wound, where it is affixed to the skin. This remains usually for 24 to 48 hours and is removed at the time of minimal drainage. The skin closure is done carefully to match the various layers of depth and equal side-to-side approximation; failure to do so will result in dense fixation of this scrotal or infrapubic skin to the penile shaft. A loose elastic dressing is applied to the penile shaft, and the catheter is usually removed the following morning. This dressing is used to avoid glanular edema. Some authors recommend perineal plication procedures or spongiolysis, but these procedures are rarely indicated (Lewis, 1993; Licht and Lewis, 2002).

Some authors have proposed deep dorsal vein arterialization for veno-occlusive erectile dysfunction (Virag et al, 1981; Furlow et al, 1990; Kayigil et al, 2000; Sarramon et al, 2001). However, others have described poor outcome of such surgery for veno-occlusive disease (Anafarta et al, 1997). The article

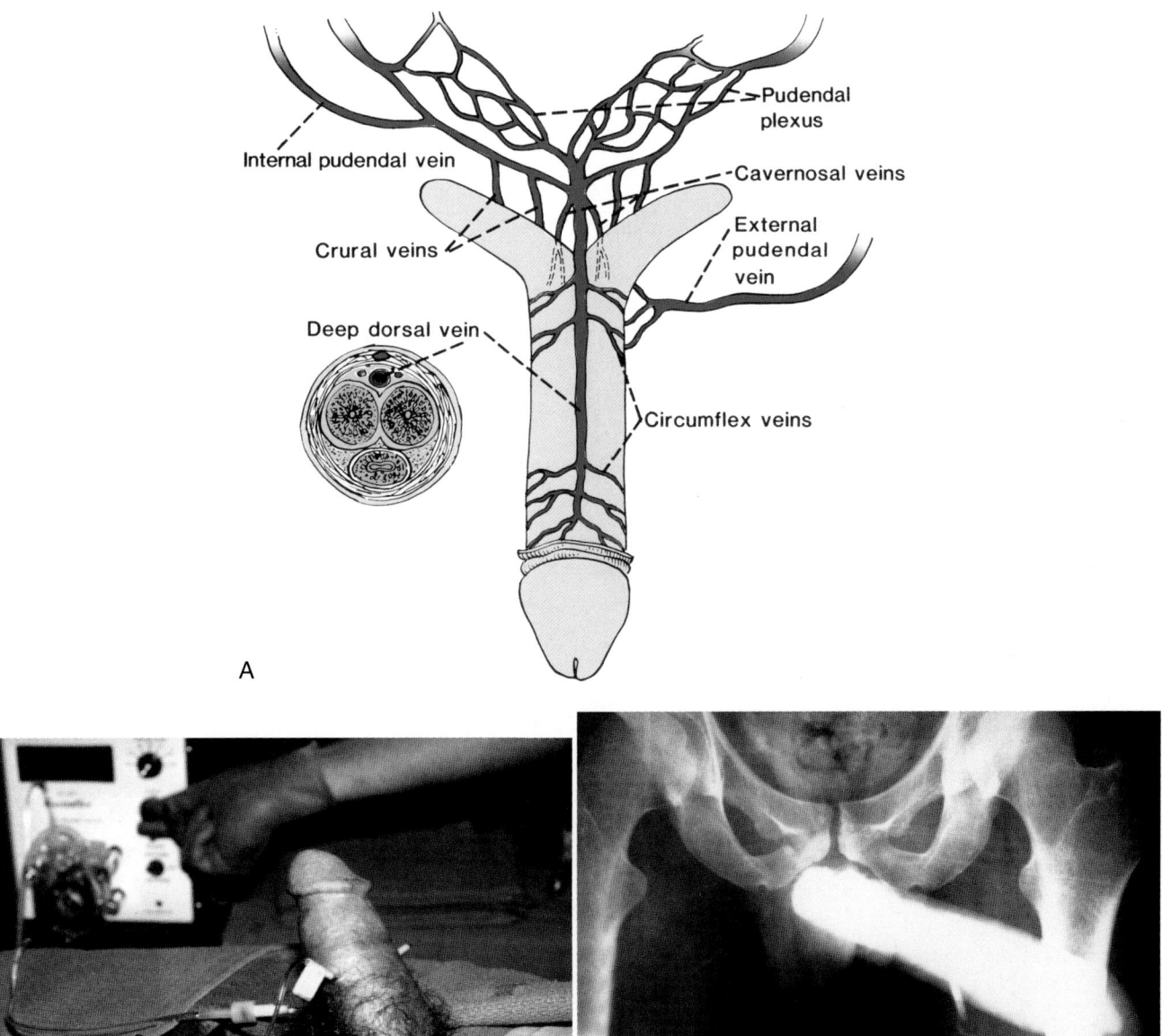

VENOUS DRAINAGE OF CORPORA CAVERNOSA

Figure 24–10. **A,** The venous drainage of the penis including the deep dorsal vein, circumflex veins, and superficial veins at the base of the penis that feed into the external pudendal vein and subsequently the saphenous vein. Veins are seen directly draining from the crural region of the penis (labeled crural veins) and cavernosal veins that are often found at the region where the corpora cavernosal crura diverge. The rest of the vessels drain in the pudendal plexus. On occasion, there can be connection to the internal pudendal vein. **B,** Infusion pump is used for cavernosometry and cavernosography. The other needle is connected to a pressure transducer. **C,** Normal veno-occlusive function as demonstrated by pharmacocavernosography. There is no venous drainage, and a rigid corpus cavernosum is filled completely with contrast material. *Continued*

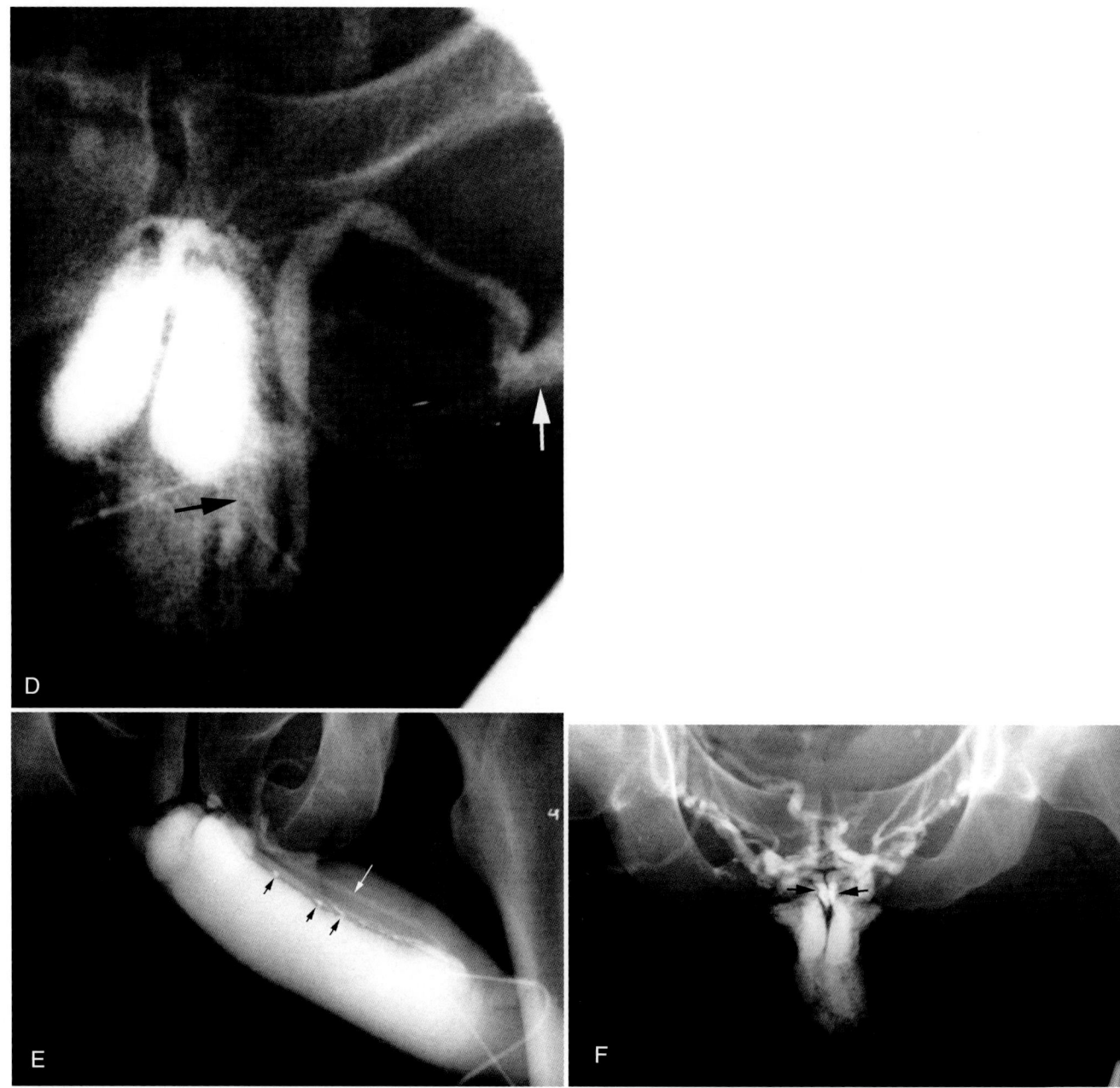

Figure 24–10, cont'd.   D, A congenital abnormality in which the distal tunica albuginea has a malformation at the level of the tunic *(black arrow)* that drains into a superficial penile vein and subsequently to the saphenous system *(white arrow).* The venous system was dissected out and the defect in the tunica closed with an excellent result for the patient, who was last observed at 3 years. **E,** Minimal drainage into the intermediate venous system. Direct vessels *(black arrows)* filling the deep dorsal vein of the penis are clearly shown as well as communication to the superficial dorsal vein of the penis *(white arrow).* **F,** Massive venous drainage. This also demonstrates two cavernosal veins *(black arrows)* at the base of the penis.

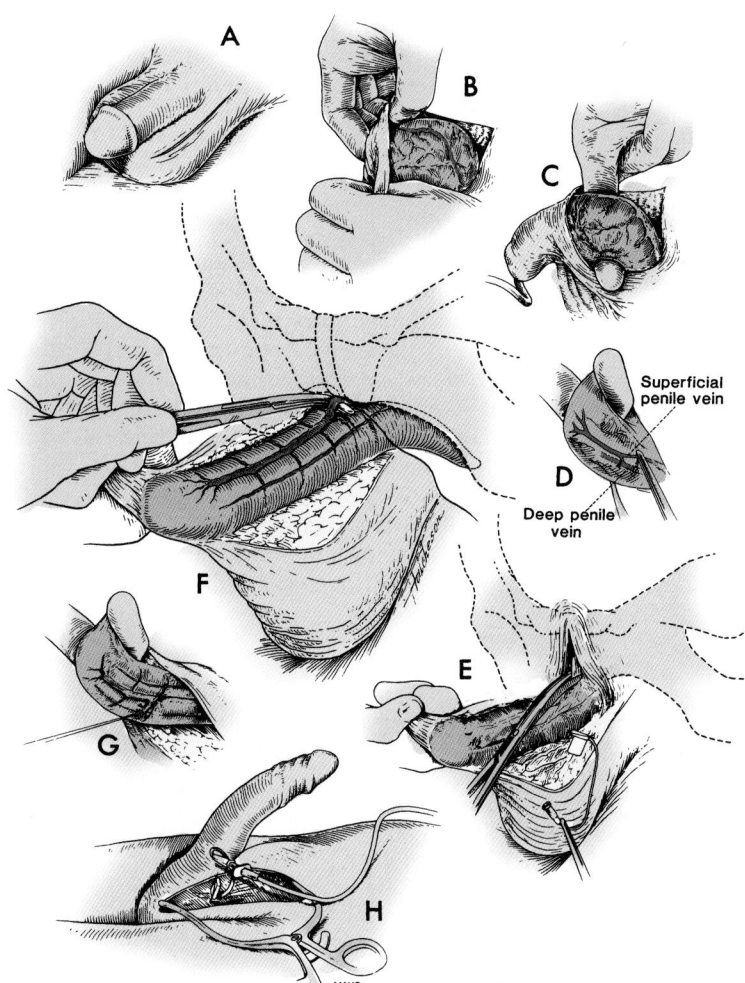

Figure 24–11. Steps in the performance of deep penile vein ligation and dissection surgery. **A,** The peripenile anterior scrotal incision. **B** and **C,** Eversion of the penile deep tissues through the wound. **D,** Ligation of communicators identified between the superficial and the deep penile venous systems. **E,** Release of the suspensory ligament in the infrapubic region. **F,** Ligation of the vein on the penile shaft. Once this ligation is accomplished, the vein is dissected proximally and distally. **G,** Distal dissection of the penile vein in the midpenile shaft. Direct communicators and communicators from the circumflex vessels are ligated and exposed. **H,** An operative cavernosometry to produce an erection and to show that adequate veno-occlusion has been obtained from the surgery. (**A** to **H,** reproduced from the Mayo Clinic Foundation.)

by Sarramon and colleagues was a report of deep dorsal vein arterialization of the penis for isolated veno-occlusive dysfunction and veno-occlusive dysfunction associated with decreased arterial inflow; this is mixed origin for the erectile dysfunction. At a later mail survey in which the International Index of Erectile Function (IIEF) questionnaire was used, those patients who had received the deep dorsal vein arterialization had a higher score on the IIEF for the erectile function domain compared with untreated patients with erectile dysfunction, but the score was below that obtained with a control group of patients who did not have erectile dysfunction but who were age matched. There was no IIEF evaluation performed in the patients in a preoperative manner.

Complications

Complications of penile venous surgery can be divided into two categories, immediate complications and long-term complications. Common immediate complications are penile and scrotal skin bruising, penile edema, and pain from nocturnal erections in the immediate time after surgery. Rare complica-

tions of an immediate nature are wound infection and hematoma. Hematoma formation has been drastically reduced by placement of a superficial drain that is left in for several days after the extensive vein dissection procedure. Common long-term complications are penile shortening and decreased penile sensation. The penile shortening occurs in approximately 20% to 30% of patients. The amount of loss of length, however, is rarely functionally or clinically significant. Hypoesthesia or numbness of the glans of the shaft of the penis is common after surgery, and on occasion it can impair the ability to achieve orgasm. Most often the penile sensation completely returns 7 to 9 months postoperatively. The decreased ability for orgasm is extremely rare.

A rare disfiguring later complication is wound scar contraction that leads to penile tethering. Revision of surgery with release of scar tissue and skin Z-plasty is necessary for treatment under some conditions. There has been a report by Austoni and colleagues (1989) of patients who have undergone venous ligation surgery who have developed priapism. One of the authors of this chapter has seen priapism in only one patient, in whom a vasoactive agent was injected after the surgery had been performed to test for significant improvement and leakage. Later in the recovery room, the patient was found to have priapism that rapidly responded to intracavernosal phenylephrine.

Results

Results of surgery for veno-occlusive sexual dysfunction are presented in Table 24–4. Early results during the first year have been much higher by almost double rates than the success after 12 months. As shown in Table 24–4, long-term results (for which most of these studies are reported for 12 months or more) show success of about 25%. Complete and detailed dissection surgery as opposed to simple ligation leads to better success. Some authors have stated, however, that most of the veno-occlusive dysfunction is due to faulty filling of the sinuses of the corpora and inadequate occlusion of the subtunical veins. Since this occurs beneath the tunica albuginea and does not involve the veins that are commonly dissected in venous surgery, some authors have been led to abandon venous surgery for erectile dysfunction. Other authors have proposed in the patient with good arterial inflow that venous surgery still be offered to the patient who may not wish to use more invasive therapy or move to the most invasive therapy of penile prostheses.

Other venous surgery, though, such as varicocele surgery, surgery for varicose veins of the lower extremities, and surgery directed at venous malformations such as hemangiomas, also are known to have recurrences. This reflects the rich anastomosis of venous drainage in the body, which later will produce the same abnormalities. There are rare cases of congenital defects in the tunica albuginea, such as shown in Figure 24–10D, that are usually associated with a primary erectile dysfunction that is consistent with a treatable veno-occlusive disorder. As mentioned earlier, some authors have proposed that there may be a crucial number of smooth muscles needed to be present in the underlying cavernosal space for the veno-occlusive mechanism to work or to be aided by more distal vein dissection procedures.

Table 24–4. Results of Surgery for Veno-occlusive Sexual Dysfunction

Study (years of study)	Patients (N)	Excellent	Improved	Immediate Success–Later Failure	Failures	Average Follow-up (mo)
Lewis-Tulane series (1981-1987)	49	12 (24%)	12 (24%)	8 (16%)	17 (35%)	15
Wespes et al (1982-1986)	67*	31 (46%)	16 (24%)	—	20 (30%)	24
Donatucci and Lue (1986-1988)	100	44 (44%)	24 (24%)	—	32 (32%)	(12-50)
Bondil et al (1981-1988)	60	25 (42%)[†]		—	35 (58%)	22
Lunglmayr et al (1984-1986)	29	9 (31%)		10 (34.5%)	10	to 22
Weidner et al (1985-1987)	51	28 (55%)	—	8 (16%)[‡]	15 (29%)[‡]	12
Weidner et al (1988-1989)	40	24 (60%)	—	11 (27.5%)[‡]	5 (12.5%)[‡]	12
Gilbert et al (1985-1990)	134	26 (19.4%)	47 (35.1%)	—	61 (45.5%)	12.9
Lewis-Mayo series (1987-1988)	28	7 (25%)	4 (14%)	8 (29%)	9 (32%)	48
Lewis-Mayo series (1988-1989)	32	9 (28%)	13 (41%)	5 (15.5%)	5 (15.5%)	24
Knoll et al (1987-1989)	41	19 (46%)	unknown	unknown	22 (54%)	28
Kropman et al (1987-1989)	20	6 (30%)	4 (20%)	8 (40%)	2 (10%)	15
Rossman et al (1985-1988)	16	2 (12.5%)	2 (12.5%)	10 (62.5%)	2 (12.5%)	unknown
Claes and Baert (1987-1989)	72	30 (41.7%)	23 (31.9%)	—	19 (26.4%)	>12
Montague et al (1988-1990)	18	11 (61%)	—	6 (33%)	1 (6%)	24
Freedman et al (1986-1991)	46	11 (24%)	8 (17%)	23 (50%)	4 (9%)	31-33
Popken et al (1987-1991)	122	17 (14%)	23 (19%)	(43%)	(24%)	70
Hassan et al (1988-1991)	32	10 (31%)	9 (28%)	7 (21%)	6 (20%)	36
Kim and McVary (1989-1992)	15	6 (40%)	3 (20%)	2 (13%)	4 (27%)	29
Stief et al (1989-1992)	77	31 (40.3%)[§]	8 (10.4%)	38 (49.4%)	6	
Berardinucci et al (1985-1993)	94	31%	11%	31%	27%	40
Vale et al (1995)	22	45%	18%	—	37%	12
Sasso et al (1984-1995)	15	4 (28.6%)	1 (7.1%)	4 (28.6%)	5 (35.7%)	35.2 ± 29.6 (3-96)
	29 (+corporopexy)	15 (51.7%)	3 (10.3%)	5 (19%)	6 (19%)	16.1 ± 9.3 (2-48)
Sasso et al (1999)	23 (+corporopexy)	12 (52%)	5 (22%)	3 (13%)	3 (13%)	17.2
Schultheiss et al (1987-1996)	126	14 (11%)	24 (19%)	56 (44%)	32 (25%)	33 ± 19.6

*Sixty-seven questionnaire responses to 105 letters sent.
[†]Series reported as excellent or improved as a group, not in each individual category.
[‡]Seventeen of 39 are now able to achieve erection with pharmacologic agent injection.
[§]Four of 31, when observed for an extended time (18.5 months), needed pharmacotherapy to obtain an erection.

KEY POINTS: VASCULAR SURGERY FOR ERECTILE DYSFUNCTION

■ Vascular surgical procedures are recommended only for a select group of patients.

■ The overall goal of penile revascularization surgery is the bypass of specific obstructive arterial lesions in the hypogastric-cavernosal arterial bed.

■ This surgery is not indicated in the patient with generalized arterial disease or diabetes mellitus.

■ It is imperative that alternative nonsurgical treatment modalities be fully explained to the potential surgical patient.

■ For penile revascularization, a common iliac arteriogram and a selective internal pudendal arteriogram are absolutely necessary.

■ The most common donor artery for penile revascularization is the inferior epigastric artery, usually connected to the dorsal artery of the penis by microvascular surgery. An end-to-end anastomosis from the arterial donor site to the recipient vessel is the most physiologic choice.

■ Penile veno-occlusive surgery, indicated in a select group of patients, should consist of a thorough complete penile vein dissection and ligation.

■ Early results of penile veno-occlusive surgery are much better than long-term results after 2 years.

■ Complications of penile vascular surgery are penile numbness and hypoesthesia and some minor penile shortening.

SUGGESTED READINGS

Goldstein I, Hatzichristou DG, Pescatori EG: Pelvic, perineal, and penile trauma–associated arteriogenic impotence: Pathophysiologic mechanisms and the role of microvascular arterial bypass surgery. In Bennett HA, ed: Impotence—Diagnosis and Management of Erectile Dysfunction. Philadelphia, WB Saunders, 1994:213-228.

Jarow JP: Penile revascularization for arterial occlusive disease. Atlas Urol Clin North Am 2002;10:127-140.

Licht MR, Lewis RW: Surgery for venous leak impotence. Atlas Urol Clin North Am 2002;10:141-151.

Munarriz R, Mulhall J, Goldstein I: Penile arterial reconstruction. In Graham SD, ed: Glenn's Urologic Surgery, 6th ed. Philadelphia, Lippincott Williams & Wilkins, 2004:573-587.

Sohn MH, Sikora RR, Bohndorf KK, et al: Objective follow-up after penile revascularization. Int J Impot Res 1992;4:73-84.

25 Peyronie's Disease

GERALD H. JORDAN, MD

Credit for the first description of Peyronie's disease is given to François Gigot de la Peyronie in 1743 (Peyronie, 1743). **Fallopius, however, first reported the entity in 1561.** Peyronie's disease is also known as induratio plastica of the penis. **In most patients, reassurance is sufficient and a necessity.** For others, medical therapy is useful. Fortunately, only a minority of patients will have deformity that precludes them from having intercourse. **Most of the patients with Peyronie's disease do not require surgery. Surgery, at best, can be viewed as palliation for the mechanical effects of Peyronie's disease and erectile dysfunction.**

The literature associates Peyronie's disease with many entities. Some have stood the test of time; in others, the association has not. In a study by Nyberg and colleagues (1982), **Peyronie's disease was associated with Dupuytren's contracture. Dupuytren's contracture has a familial pattern known to be transmitted in an autosomal dominant pattern.** Thirty percent to 40% of men with Peyronie's disease will also have Dupuytren's contracture (Ralph et al, 1997). Other associated fibrotic conditions are plantar fascial contracture (Ledderhose's disease) and tympanosclerosis. Peyronie's disease is also reported to occur in patients after external trauma to the penis (e.g., seat belt injuries). To the author's knowledge, no reported incidence rate appears in the literature for such patients. However, all urologists who see any volume of patients with Peyronie's disease will inevitably encounter one or two such patients a year who can attribute the onset of Peyronie's disease only to an incident of external trauma to the penis. The relationship of Peyronie's disease to diabetes mellitus likewise remains unclear. Certainly if one accepts the notion that erectile dysfunction can be an inciting event for the development of Peyronie's disease, the relationship with diabetes mellitus will follow. To date, however,

because the incidence of Peyronie's disease as associated with diabetes mellitus has not been defined, the relationship must be regarded as anecdotal. This follows also for the relationship noted with gout.

The relationship with Paget's disease of the bone, however, was noted in a nicely done study reported by Lyles (1997). In that study, patients with Paget's disease were noted to have Peyronie's disease at an incidence rate higher than that quoted for the population in general. Certain HLA subtypes have been incriminated as being causally related to the development of Peyronie's disease. However, for an HLA subtype to be positively linked to the development of Peyronie's disease, a study of many thousands of patients would be required. Nyberg in 1982, Leffell in 1997, and Ralph in 1997 suggested an association.

The use of β blockers has been causally incriminated with regard to the development of Peyronie's disease. However, the association was made when first-generation β blockers had just been released to the market. Like diabetes mellitus, those first-generation β blockers were also causally associated with erectile dysfunction. Thus, the comment made about diabetes mellitus could hold true for the relationship to β blockers. No further studies substantiating that relationship exist to the author's knowledge.

Urethral instrumentation has been implicated as a cause of Peyronie's disease. Any urologist who sees a large volume of patients with Peyronie's disease will encounter, on a one or two per year basis, patients who had straight erections before transurethral surgery but with the resumption of intercourse after surgery noted curvature. Most of these patients do not complain of ventral curvature. This association should not be confused with Kelami's syndrome, which is fibrosis of the corpus spongiosum so severe that it limits expansion of the ventral corpora cavernosa. Again, to the author's knowledge, no incidence figures exist for the relationship to urethral instrumentation (Carrieri et al, 1998).

A prime example of an association that has never stood the test of time is the association with phenytoin. In the post-marketing study for phenytoin, there were patients taking phenytoin who developed Peyronie's disease. Because phenytoin is associated with hyperplastic tissue growth phenomena (gingival hyperplasia), the association of Peyronie's disease with phenytoin was thought logical and published in the *Physicians' Desk Reference*. No other report of a causal relationship, and in fact no other report linking phenytoin use with Peyronie's disease, has been published.

The symptomatic incidence of Peyronie's disease has been estimated at 1%. In white men, the average age at onset of

Peyronie's disease is 53 years. The asymptomatic prevalence is estimated at 0.4% to 1.0%. In a study of 100 men without known Peyronie's disease, 22 of the 100, on autopsy, were found to have fibrotic lesions of the tunica albuginea compatible with Peyronie's disease (Smith, 1969; Gelbard et al, 1990; Lindsay et al, 1991; Carson et al, 1999). Clearly, many think that the clinical incidence of Peyronie's disease is increasing. The increase, however, may be associated with and seems to coincide with the increased use of erection-enhancing medications. The phosphodiesterase type 5 (PDE5) inhibitor medications and the approved intracavernosal injection agents are not indicated for Peyronie's patients. That does not mean that they are contraindicated; it means that during the final phase studies reviewed for drug approval, Peyronie's patients were excluded. **To the author's knowledge, there has never been any suggestion that PDE5 inhibitors are in any way directly causally related to the development of Peyronie's disease, nor is there suggestion that their use would worsen the course of Peyronie's disease.** Data are emerging to suggest that certain endothelial impairment may be reversed with the initiation of PDE5 inhibitor therapy. However, the concept of "endothelial rehabilitation" with PDE inhibitor therapy should be considered as suggested only (Rosano et al, 2005). Likewise, it is the author's belief that the scarring seen with intracavernosal injection therapy is related not to the medications necessarily but rather to the injection technique. There are certainly patients who can recall a given event in which they used their injection medication. The injection was accompanied by undue pain, a good erection was not achieved, and the patient then noticed an area of induration in the penis. After that, patients often notice deformity of the penis. Also, it could be theorized that the repetitive trauma of the needle may initiate a "Peyronie's process." The prolonged use of papaverine and phentolamine (Regitine) has been implicated as a cause of intracorporal fibrosis, which is different from the fibrotic process of the tunica albuginea that is recognized as Peyronie's disease.

KEY POINTS: EPIDEMIOLOGY

- Peyronie's disease presents with a variety of deformities of the penis. The symptomatic incidence has been estimated at 1%, but most think that the incidence is increasing and now can be conservatively estimated at around 4% to 5%. Fortunately, most patients do not require surgery. Most do require reassurance and education. Surgery for Peyronie's disease is considered palliation for the mechanical effects of the disease.

- Peyronie's disease has been related to a number of conditions. The strongest relation is to Dupuytren's contracture.

- Whereas the increased incidence of Peyronie's disease seems to correspond with the use of pharmacotherapy for the management of erectile dysfunction, to the author's knowledge there has never been any suggestion that PDE5 inhibitors are in any way directly causally related to the development of Peyronie's disease. Nor is there any evidence that intracavernosal injection therapy is directly implicated in the process of Peyronie's disease. The development of Peyronie's disease does seem to be related to the unique anatomy of the tunica albuginea and its relationship to the septal fibers.

ANATOMIC CONSIDERATIONS AND ETIOLOGIC FACTORS

In examining the etiology of Peyronie's disease, it is important to review some facts concerning the anatomy of the corpora cavernosa (Fig. 25–1). The tunica albuginea is bilaminar throughout most of its circumference. It is composed of an

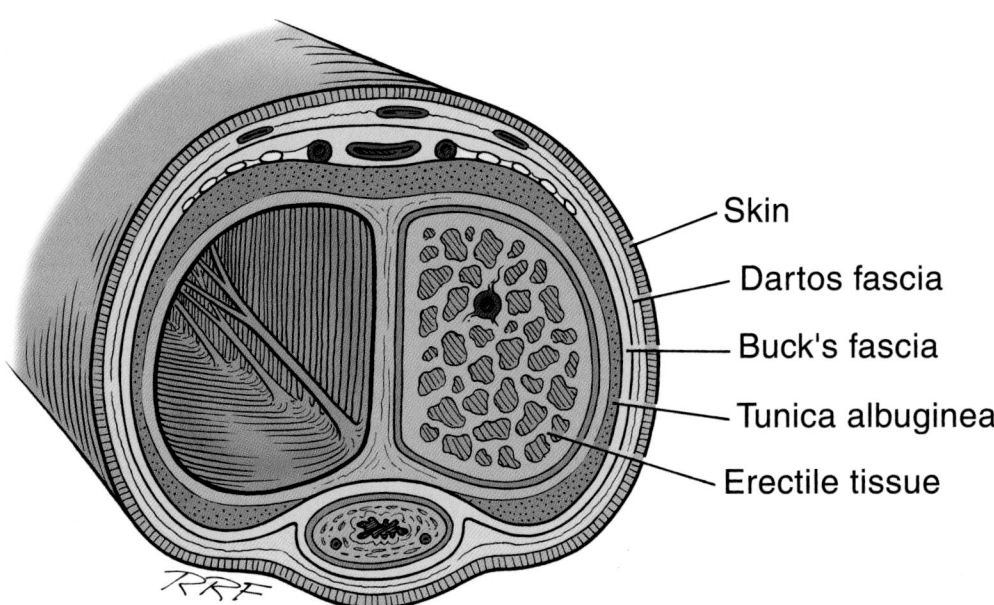

Figure 25–1. Diagram of the penis. The fibers of the septum are attached to the inner layer of the tunica albuginea of the corpora cavernosa along the dorsal and ventral midlines. Plaques of Peyronie's disease occur in the tunica albuginea at the site of attachment of the septal fibers.

Skin
Dartos fascia
Buck's fascia
Tunica albuginea
Erectile tissue

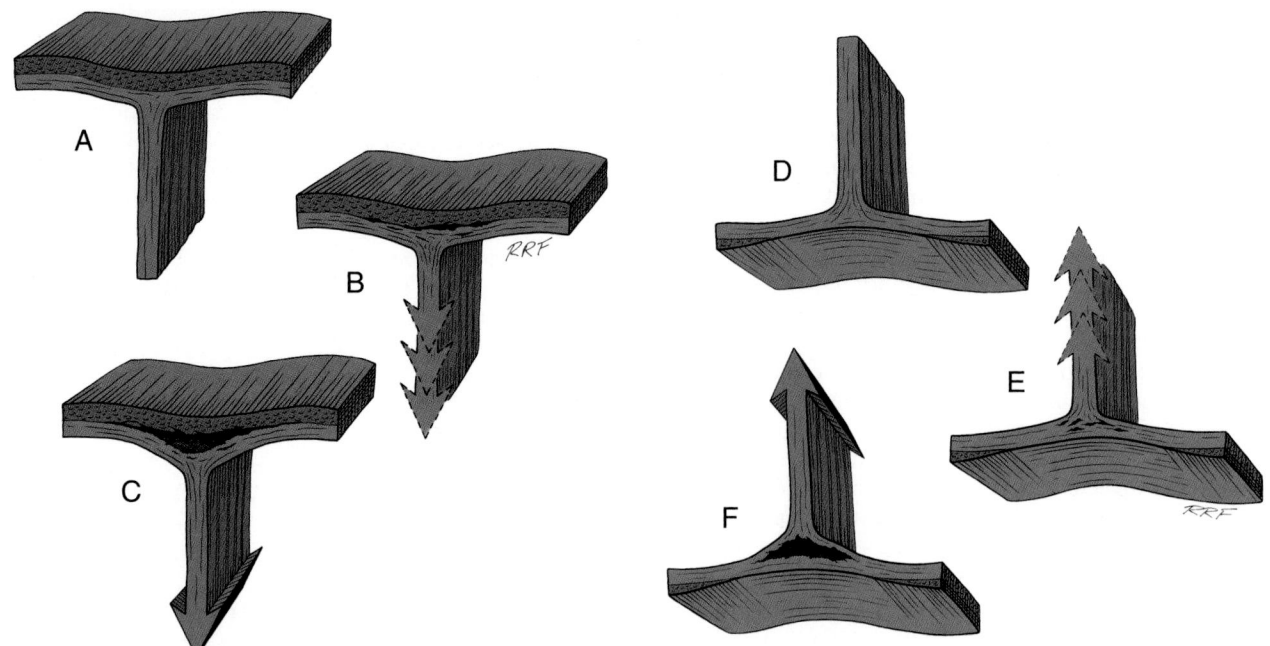

Figure 25–2. Demonstration of the mechanism of injury during buckling injuries to the penis. **A,** Fibers of the septal strands dorsally fan out and are interwoven with the inner circular lamina fibers of the tunica albuginea. The outer lamina consists of longitudinal fibers. **B,** In the chronic form of Peyronie's disease, less turgid erections allow flexion of the penis during intercourse, producing elastic tissue fatigue, further reducing elasticity of the tissue and leading to multiple smaller ruptures of the fibers of the tunica with smaller collections of blood, possibly producing multiple scars. **C,** In the acute form of Peyronie's disease bending the erect penis out of column produces tension on the strands of the septum, delaminating the layers of the tunica albuginea. Bleeding occurs, and the space fills with clot. The scar generated by the response of the tissue to this process becomes Peyronie's disease plaque. **D,** Illustration of the situation on the ventrum of the penis, where the bilaminar arrangement of the tunica albuginea becomes thinned, with the midline being monolaminar. The fibers of the septal strands fan out and are interwoven with the inner circular layer. There is no outer circular layer. **E,** In the chronic form of Peyronie's disease, less turgid erections allow buckling of the penis as in **B. F,** In the acute form of Peyronie's disease, buckling of the erect penis out of column produces tension on the strands of the septum, causing the septal fibers to tear.

outer longitudinal layer and an inner circular layer. The corpora are separated by an incompetent septum. In the pendulous portion of the penis, there are intracavernous supporting fibers that anchor the inner layer of the corpora cavernosa at the 2-o'clock and 6-o'clock positions. The tunica albuginea varies in thickness from 1.5 to 3 mm, depending on the position on the circumference. The outer longitudinal layer attenuates in the ventral midline, and thus the tunica is monolaminar at that point. The outer longitudinal layer is thickest on the ventrum adjacent to the corpus spongiosum and on the dorsum and thinnest on the lateral aspects. Most patients with Peyronie's disease demonstrate lesions dorsally. Because the tunica albuginea is bilaminar on the dorsum, it is possible that these layers might delaminate with buckling trauma. Also, on the ventrum, the longitudinal layer is absent, thus potentially allowing dorsal buckling more easily (Devine and Horton, 1988; Border and Ruoslahti, 1992; Brock et al, 1997; Devine et al, 1997; Jarow and Lowe, 1997).

Somers and Dawson (1997), in studies, have shown that Peyronie's disease most likely begins with buckling trauma that causes injury to the septal insertion of the tunica albuginea. Intravasation of blood occurs with activation of fibrinogen (Fig. 25–2). The body responds to the effects of trauma, and macrophages, as well as neutrophils and mast cells, migrate to the area. Platelets are present because of the intravasation of blood, and fibrin becomes incarcerated in the healing process. Platelets, neutrophils, and mast cells

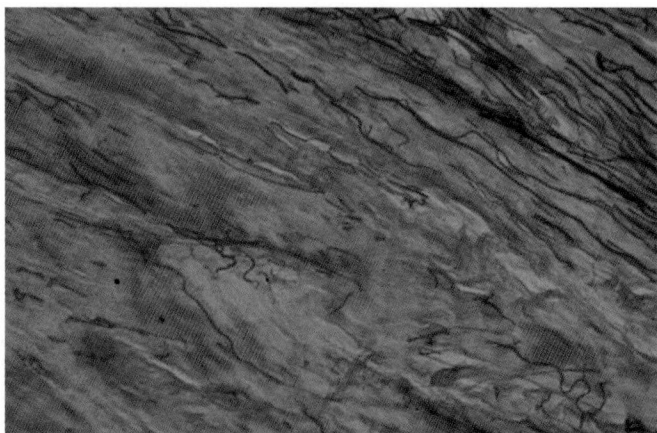

Figure 25–3. Photomicrograph of Peyronie's plaque demonstrating entrapped fibrin. The fibrin stains pink; the collagen fibers stain Prussian blue.

secrete cytokines, autacoids, and vasoactive factors, many of which become involved in fibrosis. Platelets release serotonin and platelet-derived growth factors as well as transforming growth factors. The formation of thrombus leads to the deposition of fibronectin, which binds a number of growth factors, keeping them localized to the area of injury. Fibrinogen leakage leads to the deposition and incarceration of fibrin (Fig. 25–3).

It has been proposed that the avascular nature of the tunica albuginea may impede clearance of many of these growth factors. The transforming growth factors, particularly transforming growth factor-β (TGF-β), are capable of autoinducement. Thus, the accumulation of TGF-β1 is capable of inducement of further accumulation. The presence of TGF-β stimulating further release of TGF-β1 could possibly lead to an ongoing, smoldering, inflammatory process ending with disordered healing. There is good reason to suspect TGF-β1 as possibly involved with the formation of Peyronie's plaque because it has been implicated in a number of soft tissue fibroses as well as with erectile dysfunction (Border and Ruoslahti, 1992; Border and Noble, 1994; Davis, 1997; Diegelmann, 1997; Van De Water, 1997; Moreland, 1998).

TGF-β1 is synthesized as a latent peptide by many cells; those pertinent to this discussion are platelets, macrophages, and fibroblasts. On activation, TGF-β1 binds to cell surface receptors and eventually results in synthesis of connective tissues with inhibition of collagenases (El-Sakka et al, 1997a, 1997b, 1998a). The net result of this trauma with disordered healing is the formation of plaques that appear as scars and impede expansion of the tunica albuginea during erection, which results in curvature, and/or indentation, and/or foreshortening (Fig. 25–4). On histologic examination, there is aberrant cicatrization with nonpolarization of collagen and diminished and erratic distribution of the elastin fibers (Fig. 25–5).

Recent work at the University of California–San Francisco has examined the role of matrix metalloproteinase in this

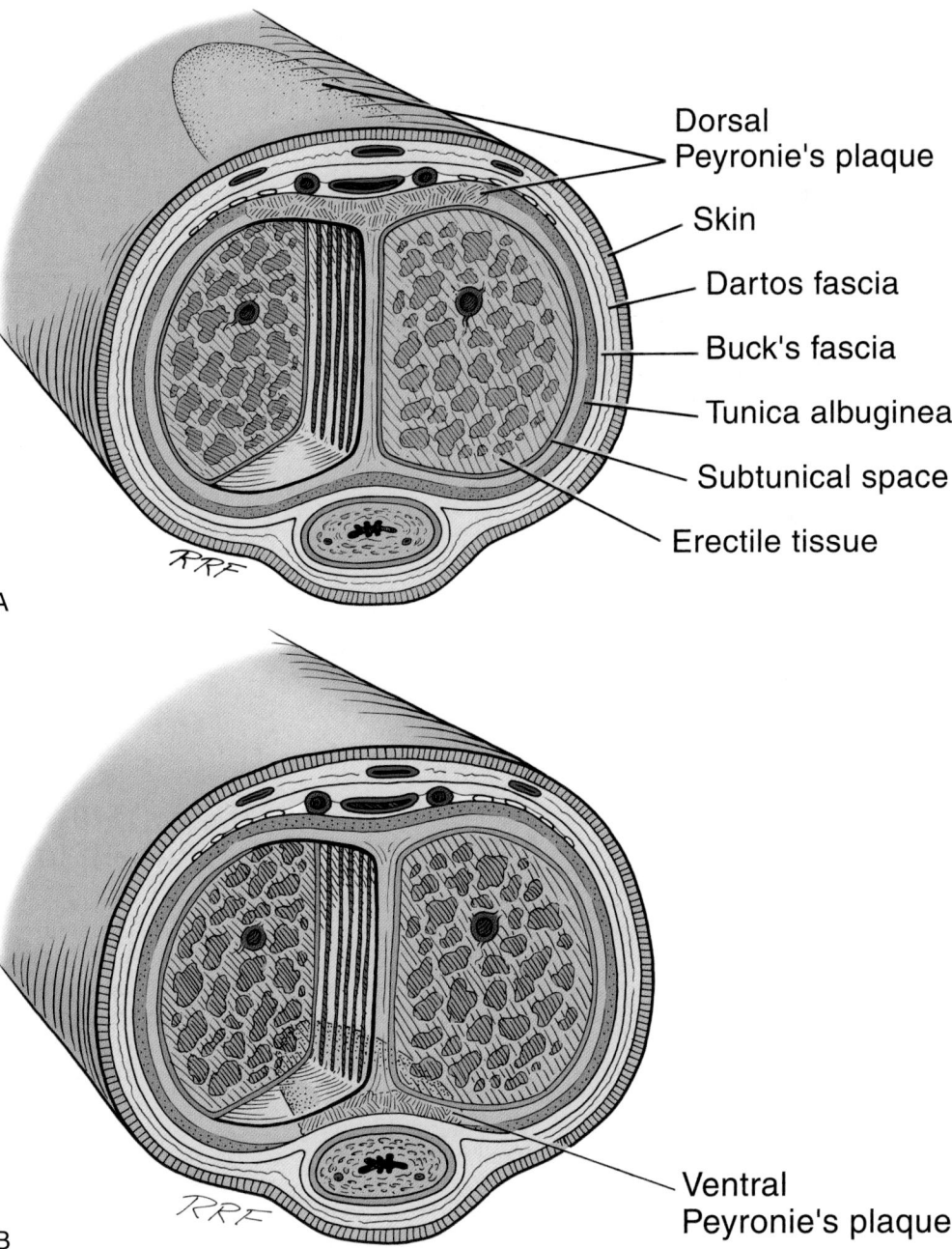

Figure 25–4. **A** and **B,** Under the influence of inflammation and cytokines, the disease progresses through an active or immature phase during which there appears to be disordered healing that eventually leads to a scar, which almost always is associated with the septal fibers.

Dorsal Peyronie's plaque

Skin

Dartos fascia

Buck's fascia

Tunica albuginea

Subtunical space

Erectile tissue

A

B

Ventral Peyronie's plaque

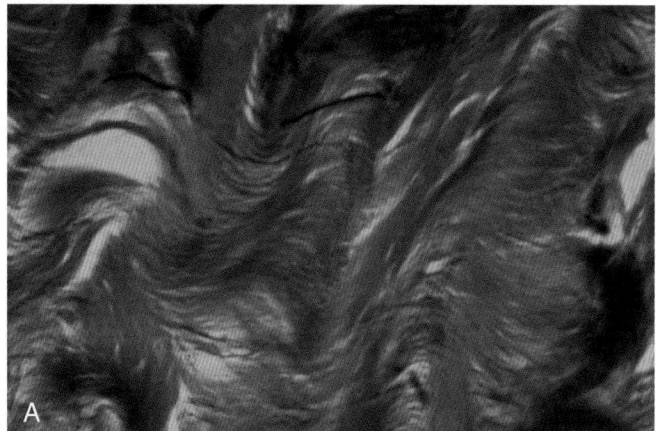
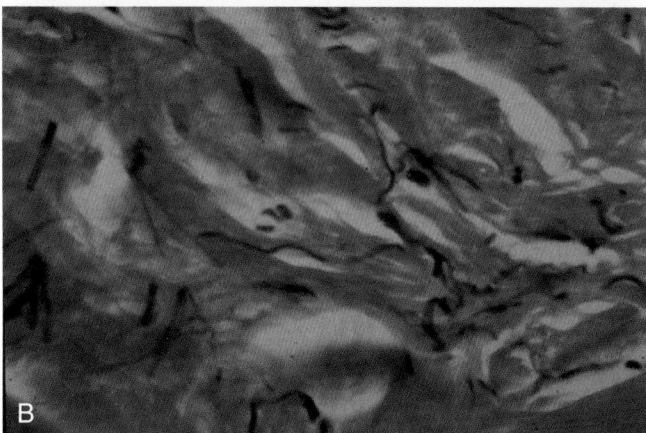

Figure 25–5. Photomicrographs of the tunica albuginea. **A,** Normal tunica albuginea demonstrating the polarized arrangement of collagen. **B,** Peyronie's plaque demonstrating the nonpolarized arrangement of collagen and the haphazard arrangement of elastin. Collagen stains green; the elastin stains black.

abnormal scarring process. Matrix metalloproteinases are enzymes that are involved in the remodeling of extracellular matrix proteins. These remodeling enzymes are regulated by tissue inhibitors of metalloproteinase. **Failure of downregulation of matrix metalloproteinase has been implicated in a number of disease processes. In the case of Peyronie's disease, if matrix metalloproteinases are not downregulated, they could function as a possible mechanism for the scarring process in Peyronie's disease.** In the studies, image analyses were used to examine the cavernosal tissues of Peyronie's disease patients compared with controlled patients having only prosthetic placement for other reasons. Those analyses showed a higher expression of the tissue inhibitors of metalloproteinase in all of the components of the Peyronie's plaques compared with the controls. Thus, inhibition of anti-scarring enzymes can perhaps represent another facet of the etiology of the lesion we recognize as Peyronie's plaque (Grazziotin et al, 2004).

In a similar vein, Hauck and coworkers (2004) examined the role of α_1-antitrypsin, which is a proteinase inhibitor, as a possible factor in the development of Peyronie's disease. Reduction in α_1-antitrypsin levels could result in a change in collagen metabolism. Previous work had suggested diminished levels, and such diminished levels could be associated with diminished tissue degradation (remodeling) and hence increased cicatrization. Hauck did find diminished α_1-antitrypsin levels in patients with Peyronie's disease; however, compared with age-matched controls, the levels were not diminished in Peyronie's disease with regard to the controls. Thus α_1-antitrypsin levels may vary with age, but the association with Peyronie's disease was not made.

Studies also demonstrate the role of oxidative stress in addition to cytokine release in the development of Peyronie's disease plaques. Acting as profibrotic factors, they interact with antifibrotic defense mechanisms, which, as already mentioned, may be inhibited. Oxidative stress intensifies in the fibroblasts of human Peyronie's disease plaques and rat-modeled fibrosis (Ferrini et al, 2002; Vernet et al, 2002; Valente et al, 2003). Reactive oxygen species trigger profibrotic processes in a number of disease processes (Becker et al, 2001; Intengan et al, 2001). There is interplay between a number of mechanisms as they relate to fibrosis. Possibly of particular importance is cyclic guanosine monophosphate (GMP), one of the mediators of penile erection. Cyclic GMP has been found to be antifibrotic in Peyronie's disease plaques. Long-term administration of PDE5 inhibitors prevents plaque formation in rat fibrosis models. PDE5 is expressed in tunical and Peyronie's disease fibroblasts (Valente et al, 2003). Thus, as earlier mentioned, the use of PDE5 inhibitors in patients with Peyronie's disease may be helpful on a number of fronts.

KEY POINTS: ETIOLOGIC FACTORS

■ Buckling trauma of the penis, usually occurring during intercourse, has been implicated in the development of Peyronie's disease. TGF-β has been found to be related to the disordered healing process that leads to the scarring of Peyronie's plaque. In addition, failure of downregulation of a number of "antifibrotic" factors has been implicated.

■ Basic science research into the etiology of Peyronie's disease is limited by the failure, to date, to develop a true animal model of Peyronie's disease. There are animal models and models of fibrosis, however, that have led to a number of interesting proposals, many of which eventually will be translational with therapeutic options.

PATHOPHYSIOLOGY AND NATURAL HISTORY

Basic science research into the etiology of Peyronie's disease is limited by the failure, to date, to develop a true reliable animal model of Peyronie's disease. A couple of animal models have examined the injection of cytomodulin, a TGF-β promoter, and the injection of blood. Clearly, in both models, fibrotic lesions were produced. Whether these represent true models of Peyronie's disease remains to be proved or disproved. These models of fibrosis, however, have led to interesting research regarding the pathogenesis of Peyronie's disease. In addition, a number of cell culture models have been proposed and have allowed significant enlightenment with regard to cell cycle regulators and gene expression. The obvious comment about these models is that, of course, these do enlighten us with regard to the essential cell aberrations; however, most probably fail to truly represent what would be the in vivo condition. They do allow, however, investigation with regard to agents that potentially can manipulate the behavior of the individual cell (El-Sakka et al, 1999; Perinchery et al, 2000; Bivalacqua et al, 2001; Mulhall et al, 2001a; Ferrini et al, 2002; Gonzalez-Cadavid et al, 2002; Lin et al, 2002; Magee et al, 2002; Hauck et al, 2003b; Kim et al, 2004).

Several studies have examined the natural history of Peyronie's disease. **In most cases of Peyronie's disease, there are two phases. The first is an active phase, which not uncommonly is associated with painful erections and changing deformity of the penis. It is followed by a quiescent secondary phase, which is characterized by stabilization of the deformity, with disappearance of painful erections, if they were present, and, in general, stability of the process. Up to a third of patients, however, present with what appears to be sudden development of painless deformity.** It is said that Peyronie's disease totally resolves in some patients. This is probably a misstatement. Clearly, there are some patients who traumatize their penises and then develop curvature secondary to the inflammatory process and its associated loss of compliance. In some, the inflammation resolves without seeming to enter into the phase of smoldering inflammation that ends in disordered healing and scar formation. Thus, the process is resolved. Semantically, however, these patients probably cannot be said to have resolved Peyronie's disease; rather, the trauma has resolved without the development of Peyronie's disease. In Mulhall's study of men diagnosed promptly after development of Peyronie's disease symptoms and findings who elected to avoid all therapy, few were found to show much improvement in curvature during a period of 12 months (O'Brien et al, 2004). Obviously this study could be faulted for not having observed the patients longer, but the point is made that "spontaneous resolution" of Peyronie's disease is an infrequent occurrence.

When the urologist is confronted with a patient with Peyronie's disease, it is imperative that he or she understand the mindset of that patient and indeed of the couple. It has been shown that couples in which the man has Peyronie's disease, compared with age-matched adult couples, seem to engage in more frequent and more vigorous intercourse and often use positions that are potentially traumatic to the penis. These couples seem to relate by intercourse. It could be said that **Peyronie's disease is a disease of aging tissue in a patient with a youthful libido** (Williams and Thomas, 1970; Gelbard et al, 1990; Carson et al, 1999).

The relationship of erectile dysfunction with Peyronie's disease is a difficult one to ascertain. Mention of erectile dysfunction after surgery begins with the first report of surgery for Peyronie's disease (Lowsley and Boyce, 1950) by excision and grafting. In that series, erectile dysfunction postoperatively was a major source of failure. Interestingly, in that series, patients with ventral curvature were singled out as particularly at risk for postoperative problems with erectile dysfunction. The poor prognosis for that group of patients seems to persist into current series. Returning to articles concerning the natural history (Williams and Thomas, 1970; Gelbard et al, 1990), erectile dysfunction again is prominently mentioned. In Gelbard and colleagues' manuscript (1990), a large number of patients discussed poor erections and erectile dysfunction.

In the author's experience, erectile dysfunction precedes the onset of Peyronie's disease in many patients. In our analysis in 1993 (Jordan and Angermeier, 1993), it was clear that erectile dysfunction is a significant factor in patients examined preoperatively. A review by Mulhall further clarifies the association of erectile dysfunction with Peyronie's disease (Palese et al, 2004). In that analysis, a large cohort of men were questioned with the International Index of Erectile Function, erectile function domain (IIEF/EF). The data showed that one third of men with Peyronie's disease presented with erectile dysfunction at the time that they presented with Peyronie's disease. Further, a significant percentage of them had erectile dysfunction that preceded their notice of the onset of Peyronie's disease and its diagnosis. The investigators also examined patients with dynamic infusion cavernosometry and cavernosography (DICC) and found that venous leak is seen more commonly in men who develop erectile dysfunction with Peyronie's disease; however, site-specific venous leak was not noted. There also was the confusing factor of those men with normal vascular parameters who by questionnaire had erectile dysfunction. This further emphasizes the strong psychological component seen in these patients.

In that analysis, almost 80% of the patients complained of "the psychological effects" of Peyronie's disease. Of note is that of those 80%, 70% complained that their psychological complaints did not improve despite the fact that their disease went into a quiescent phase. A major failure of the literature is that patients are not stratified with regard to functional issues versus organic issues as they relate to erectile dysfunction.

Since Brock and Lue's analysis (1993), there are now a number of reports that have attempted to stratify patients preoperatively with functional testing. In those articles, there is wide variance of opinion concerning the coexistence of erectile dysfunction with Peyronie's disease. Jordan and Angermeier (1993) showed erectile dysfunction in almost 100% of patients; Jarow and Lowe (1997) showed that 76 of 95 patients were impotent by testing; and Ralph and coworkers (1992) showed that of 20 patients with erectile dysfunction who were studied with duplex ultrasonography, 90% had complaints of erectile dysfunction because of functional, not organic, causes. In Mulhall's study cited earlier, by IIEF/EF criteria, 30% of that cohort had erectile dysfunction associated with Peyronie's disease (Palese et al, 2004). Hellstrom's analysis of more than 500 men, all evaluated with duplex ultrasonography, showed a significant relationship between the type of penile deformity and penile hemodynamics. The study showed that patients with hourglass deformity most commonly had arterial insufficiency. Veno-occlusive dysfunction was most prevalent in patients with ventral curvature. This fact makes Lowsley's final statement in his 1950 paper almost prophetic: "Patients with ventral curvature do not do well with graft operations." However, Hellstrom's study did not demonstrate any statistical relationship between the type of deformity and the frequency of erectile dysfunction. All patients were evaluated with the IIEF/EF questionnaire (Kendirci et al, 2005).

Thus, what is in the literature is not clear other than the fact that patients preoperatively complain in large numbers of the psychological impact of their Peyronie's disease, and those psychological aspects continue to plague good surgical results.

On the basis of a study still to be published, men with and without Peyronie's disease participated in a series of focus groups that were conducted in several cities. Most men indicated that the impact Peyronie's disease has had on their life has been severe. The emotions expressed by many of the men who were interviewed ranged from anger to frustration to hopelessness. Although many men—even those not in a steady relationship—were still having sex, most of those who were still having sex said that it was different from what it used to be, and many were concerned that their condition would worsen and that they would not be able to have sexual intercourse in the future. In every focus group, most men said they had become resigned to the fact that there was nothing that could be done. Additional work is under way to develop a questionnaire to measure the impact of Peyronie's disease on various aspects of a man's life (R. C. Rosen, data on file; personal communication, May 2005).

Jones (1997) deals best with the counseling issues of men with sexual dysfunction resulting from Peyronie's disease. His comments are based on interviews of more than 1500 men with Peyronie's disease. **He describes counseling a patient with Peyronie's disease as being much the same as counseling a person who has suffered a death and is grieving.** As with death, grieving is complicated by denial, ambivalence, anxiety, depression, shame, embarrassment, and, in the case of this particular group of patients, self-disgust. Most of these patients are not good talkers. Jones (1997) suggests that these patients tend not to like to talk about their problems with their spouses and initially spurn counseling in many instances.

A major point made by Jones (1997) in dealing with Peyronie's patients is that to avoid or to limit emotional factors, patients and their partners need to hear the suggestion that they must "keep sexual expression alive, be active to whatever degree possible at every stage of the progression or regression of their Peyronie's disease course." Patients' understanding of Peyronie's disease is made worse many times by the comments of urologists and primary care physicians who in general do not understand the disease. Many patients have been told that Peyronie's disease is probably the end of their sex life. Many of these couples have related by the belief that "sex is intercourse." Thus, when coitus is precluded, they avoid all sexual activity. Most men with Peyronie's disease have ignored, at one point, the plea of their partners who have asked for intimacy regardless of whether there was intercourse. As mentioned, the relationship of the functional aspects to the organic aspects remains elusive. To define these aspects, there must be uniformity in history taking; there must be uniformity in preoperative assessment with regard to erectile function; and, in failures, there must be uniformity in postoperative assessment with regard to erectile dysfunction.

SYMPTOMS

The presenting symptoms of Peyronie's disease include, in many patients, penile pain with erection; penile deformity, both flaccid and erect; shortening with and without an erection; plaque or indurated areas in the penis; and in many patients, erectile dysfunction. On physical examination, virtually all patients have either a well-defined plaque or an area of induration palpable. The plaque is usually on the dorsal surface of the penis, intimately associated with the

---

KEY POINTS: PATHOPHYSIOLOGY AND NATURAL HISTORY

- Studies that examine the natural history of Peyronie's disease show that Peyronie's disease presents usually with two phases. The first is an active phase; the second is a quiescent phase. Thus, studies to evaluate the efficacy of pharmacotherapy are difficult; when the disease process enters the quiescent phase, many things noted during the acute phase disappear or become less apparent.

- The relationship of Peyronie's disease to erectile dysfunction has been difficult to determine. Studies estimate the occurrence of simultaneous erectile dysfunction with Peyronie's disease to be in some cases as high as 100%. A study showed that one third of a cohort of patients with Peyronie's disease presented with erectile dysfunction at the time they presented with Peyronie's disease. A significant percentage of them noted that the erectile dysfunction preceded their notice of Peyronie's disease.

- Older articles fail to stratify patients with regard to their erectile function, and this has led to the variance of opinion concerning the relationship of erectile dysfunction with Peyronie's disease. It is clear that the issues of erectile dysfunction make the psychological effects of Peyronie's disease worse. Recent data suggest that one major concern of patients with Peyronie's disease is that the condition will worsen and eventually they will completely lose the ability to have sexual intercourse. Patients must be encouraged to keep their sexual expression alive.

---

insertion of the septal fibers. Patients not uncommonly can remain sexually active with significant dorsal curvature (up to 45 degrees). Patients with lateral components or ventral Peyronie's disease tolerate the deformity far less well. Mulhall's analysis of the natural history of Peyronie's disease in a group of men who avoided treatment but were observed carefully documents the frequent occurrence of penile shortening in this population (O'Brien et al, 2004).

Pain may be persistent in the inflammatory stage of the disease; it is usually not severe, but it can interfere with sexual function. Some patients also complain of being awakened in the morning or at night with pain during erection. **Spontaneous improvement in pain virtually always occurs as the inflammation resolves.** A small group of patients with extensive disease will have "circumferential plaques" and an unstable penis due to the resulting hinge effect. Most patients complain of distal flaccidity. In DICC studies, it was found, however, that the pressures were equal proximal and distal to the plaque (Jordan and Angermeier, 1993). There is variance of opinion with regard to the cause of distal tip flaccidity; one ultrasound study seemingly showed cavernosal fibrosis that ostensibly could interfere with distal perfusion of the corpus cavernosum (Ralph et al, 1992). However, in the author's experience, the fibrotic process is limited to the tunica albuginea, although the process can clearly involve the septal fibers and thicken them appreciably. Thus, to my knowledge, there is no corroboration of the finding of diffuse cavernosal fibrosis when these patients are taken to the operating room (Ralph et al, 1996).

EVALUATION OF THE PATIENT

When the urologist is confronted with the patient with Peyronie's disease, the medical history should include the mode of onset (sudden versus gradual) and time at onset. The course of disease is helpful with regard to determining the phase the patient is in. The history is obtained of prior penile surgery, urethral instrumentation or external trauma, medication or drug abuse, and fibromatosis including Dupuytren's contracture and Ledderhose's disease. Family history of the other fibromatoses is revealing. **Because most patients with Peyronie's disease have an element or at least the aura of erectile dysfunction, risk factors for erectile dysfunction should also be assessed.** The recent literature suggests that erectile dysfunction may be a sensitive hallmark of many vasculopathic conditions. Endothelial dysfunction is an important abnormality contributing to a decrease in penile vascular responses to sexual stimuli. Vascular disease has been shown to be the most common cause of erectile dysfunction. Cardiovascular disease and erectile dysfunction share a host of risk factors including age, smoking, hyperlipidemia, hypertension, and diabetes mellitus. Further, the severity of coronary artery disease has been shown to correlate with the severity of erectile dysfunction (Feldman et al, 1994; Greenstein et al, 1997; Lue, 2000; Martin-Morales et al, 2001; Roumeguere et al, 2003). Thus, in addition to trying to glean factors from the patient about smoking, hypertension, diabetes mellitus, and other suggestions of vascular disease, the inquiries must also extend to the patient's family with regard to those same issues. Likewise, since a few of these patients will require surgery, the surgeon must carefully assess the need for screening with regard to a patient's total vascular health.

A detailed psychosexual history is imperative. Photographs of the patient's erect penis are helpful in identifying the direction of curvature and degree of curvature, and they provide some information about the patient's erectile function.

The penis should be examined on stretch. This amplifies the plaque and often allows the examiner to feel plaques that are not obvious when the penis is examined flaccid. The location and size of the plaque as well as the consistency (e.g., tender, indurated) are better defined. Most of the recent clinical trials examining intralesional injection have included a diagram in the chart. The diagram illustrates the plaque or plaques both longitudinally and in cross section. Most of these protocols emphasize the need to measure total penile length (pubis to mid glans) as well as length of the plaque. It can certainly be argued that measuring the length of the plaque really does not offer much clinical information, as plaques that are indurated tend to feel much larger and more prominent than mature plaques. Thus, the actual diagram of the plaque may be more useful in tracking the course of the disease. The hands and feet must be examined; and in the rare patient, examination of the ears will identify tympanosclerosis. Although many patients will have thickening in the palmar area of the dominant hand,

except in manual laborers, callus formation in the palmar area of the nondominant hand is indicative of noncontractile Dupuytren's contracture. Contractile Dupuytren's contracture is obvious. Examination of the feet for Ledderhose's disease often will reveal nodules compatible with plantar fascial involvement. Whether Ledderhose's disease is just a manifestation of plantar fasciitis remains to be seen, and certainly the author's experience would suggest that in the current American population, an element of plantar fasciitis is almost a ubiquitous finding in well above half of the men older than 50 years.

Imaging of the plaque is important for one purpose only, that is, the demonstration of calcification. Imaging to record plaque size is probably as useful as measuring plaque size and recording it on a diagram. **Demonstration of calcification is easily accomplished with ultrasound examination.** The calcified plaque will be shown as shadowed areas (Fig. 25–6). The plaque itself will be prominently imaged (Altaffer and Jordan, 1981; Hauck et al, 2003a). **Plain radiography is also equally effective in demonstrating calcification within the plaque** (Fig. 25–7). We use a high-definition film (Kodak X-Omat ready-pack 8 × 10). This is accurate in imaging the calcification and allows minimal radiation exposure (20 mA at 49 kV). The testicles are shielded with a lead sheet. Zero radiography is an effective way of demonstrating the plaque; however, the technology is not readily available with the increase in other imaging modalities. **Computed tomographic scanning has no place in the examination of the penis.** However, magnetic resonance imaging (MRI), which does not effectively demonstrate plaque calcification, does image the plaque well. **There is not universal agreement about the use of MRI for imaging of the plaque** (Helweg et al, 1992; Vosshenrich et al, 1995;

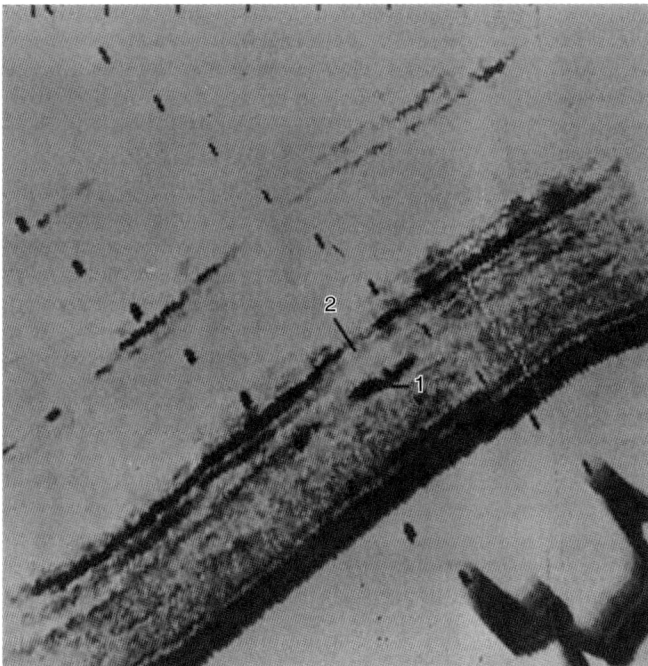

Figure 25–6. B-mode ultrasound examination of calcified Peyronie's plaque. The plaque is imaged as an echodense area (1); the area of calcification is accompanied by shadowing (2).

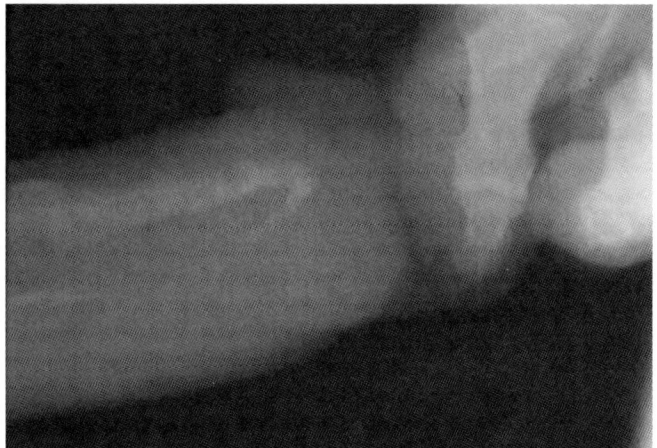

Figure 25–7. Radiograph of an extensively calcified dorsal plaque.

Andresen et al, 1998; Hauck et al, 2003a; Moncada, 2003; Perovic, 2003). In the author's opinion, at present, MRI evaluation is overkill. For the purposes of assessing the results of clinical trials, MRI may have a place.

The place of vascular testing is not clearly defined. Currently, the use of vascular testing is variable. Some centers perform duplex Doppler testing on all patients with Peyronie's disease; other centers do not perform vascular testing at all, despite that patients are routinely operated on for Peyronie's disease and, in some cases, receive prostheses as the primary treatment option (Kendirci et al, 2004, 2005; Pak et al, 2004). At our center, vascular testing is done on all patients who are prospective surgical candidates and who indicate motivation for the option of surgery. Initially, these patients are examined with color Doppler ultrasonography. If the peak systolic velocity, end-diastolic velocity, and resistive index are normal, the patients are not further tested. If the end-diastolic velocity and the resistive indices are not normal, our patients are tested with DICC. Our studies have reported that there is a linear association between preoperative erectile function and postoperative results (Jordan and Angermeier, 1993). We thus lean heavily on these results in discussing potential options for surgical management. One group of patients whose results are clear outliers are those with ventral Peyronie's disease. As mentioned, in our experience and the experience of many others, patients with ventral Peyronie's disease do not do well with surgery that involves grafting. In Hellstrom's analysis of the relationship of penile deformity to the vascular status of Peyronie's patients, patients with ventral curvature have the greatest likelihood of having cavernous veno-occlusive dysfunction (Lowsley and Boyce, 1950; Jordan and Angermeier, 1993; Kendirci et al, 2005).

There are a number of proposed treatment protocols or algorithms. The original classification system proposed by Kelami sought to include all categories of importance in evaluation of the patient with Peyronie's disease. Indeed, most of the important entities were included with the exception of erectile dysfunction (Kelami, 1983). In 1993, Gelbard, as part of the original collagenase intralesional injection protocol, used a modification of the Kelami classification. Several other treatment algorithms have been proposed (Gelbard, 1993; Novak et al, 2001; Levine and Greenfield, 2003; Bokarica et al,

2005; Viviano and Honig, 2005). It is imperative to understand that these algorithms serve only as guidelines. **Individualization with regard to patients' requirements and their findings and assessments is imperative.** This individualization will allow us to determine which patients require only reassurance, which need vigorous investigation, which are appropriately treated with medical management, and which few patients are appropriately treated with surgery. Shabsigh and colleagues (2003) published a Peyronie's disease index that is derived from a standardized patient questionnaire. That questionnaire seeks to specifically address issues most pertinent to the patient with Peyronie's disease. Issues such as duration of disease, recollection of injury, and presenting symptom or symptoms are addressed. Strategies to ideally assess degree and direction of curvature could include the use of visual analog scales. In association with future studies to examine intralesional injection protocols, a validated questionnaire is in the process of being developed. Interviews with Peyronie's patients have highlighted areas of concern, and the questions are in the process of being validated (Moncala-Iribarren et al, 2004; Fragas, 2004; R. C. Rosen/Auxilium Pharmaceuticals, personal communication, 2005).

KEY POINTS: EVALUATION OF THE PATIENT

- Patients with Peyronie's disease present with a variety of deformities of the penis. In addition, most have noted an indurated area in the penis that has been identified as the plaque. Many patients have noticed erectile dysfunction. It is important to understand that pain with erection, if it is present, inevitably disappears as patients progress to the quiescent stage. It is not unusual for the deformities to be migratory before stabilizing.

- All patients must be evaluated with a medical history as well as a detailed psychosexual history. Approximately one third of the patients will develop dystrophic calcification in the plaque that can be demonstrated by ultrasonography or plain radiography. The place for MRI in the evaluation of Peyronie's plaque has not been defined, nor has the place for vascular testing been clearly defined. However, most investigators now would agree that in patients who are to be operated on, vascular testing to stratify the vascular parameters of erectile function is a necessity. Once all of the data have been assembled, individualization with regard to the patient's requirements, findings, and assessment is imperative.

MANAGEMENT
Medical Management

Any section on the medical management of Peyronie's disease must begin with the disclaimer that few medical methods of management have been subjected to double-blind drug testing. The use of vitamin E was proposed by

Scardino and Scott (1949). Vitamin E, a tocopherol, is an antioxidant. In 1983, Pryor convened a randomly allocated placebo-controlled study. Men were randomized to vitamin E, 200 mg three times a day, versus placebo for a 3-month course. Basic disease status was assessed and in particular pain and deformity; in that study, no difference was found between vitamin E and placebo (Pryor and Farrell, 1983). In 1990, Gelbard also conducted a controlled study, and again that study failed to demonstrate any significant difference between vitamin E and placebo with regard to overall disease status and in particular pain and bend (Gelbard et al, 1990). That said, however, vitamin E is inexpensive and probably safe. Recent cautions have been raised about the use of high-dose vitamin E. It has long been recognized that vitamin E in high dose, in some individuals, can have a significant warfarin effect. **If one chooses to use vitamin E for Peyronie's disease, it should be used in divided doses of 800 to 1000 units a day. Treatment should be continued for no longer than 3 to 6 months, and patients must be cautioned about the possibility of anticoagulative side effects.** Should they notice these effects, the vitamin E should be stopped and the physician should be notified. In addition, some concerns have been raised about general cardiac health and vitamin E. It is still probably a reasonable treatment to initiate during the early phases of the disease.

Zarafonetis and Horrax (1959) published an article on the use of potassium aminobenzoate (Potaba). This drug has been looked at in a small blinded study that showed it to be efficacious (Hasche-Klunder, 1978). Two subsequent reports examining the use of potassium aminobenzoate for Peyronie's disease have been published. First, a multicenter study with random allocation between 12 g of p-aminobenzoate and matching placebo showed little benefit to treatment with the exception possibly of improving pain (Shah et al, 1983). A subsequent randomized placebo-controlled double-blind prospective multicenter trial showed no improvement with regard to pain but less worsening of other symptoms. A study by Weidner and colleagues (2005) enrolled 103 patients, with 75 completing follow-up. Many were excluded because of side effects (predominantly gastrointestinal side effects) or noncompliance for reasons not stated. Fifty-one patients were randomized against 52 patients receiving placebo control. Patients received potassium aminobenzoate or placebo at a dose of 3 g, four times a day. Endpoints studied were plaque regression and reduction of curvature. There was not a reduction in curvature noted; however, regression of plaque size was noted to be significantly better in the treatment group. Interestingly, progression of curvature or "deterioration of disease" was noted at a significantly increased rate in the placebo group. The dosage of potassium aminobenzoate is 12 g/day in four to six doses. The literature supports the fact that **potassium aminobenzoate is poorly tolerated by many patients because of gastrointestinal upset and is relatively costly.** The use of potassium aminobenzoate cannot be strongly advocated on the basis of the evidence to date.

Jordan (personal experience) has used terfenadine (Seldane) and now fexofenadine (Allegra). Its use is clearly anecdotal. It is used as a nonspecific antihistamine and has been used in patients who have had an unusually long, painful course. The medication is expensive; it is well tolerated and, if used, should be in a dosage of 60 mg twice a day.

Ralph and coworkers (1992) have suggested the use of oral tamoxifen. Tamoxifen, it is believed, facilitates the release of TGF-β from fibroblasts. **Teloken and coworkers (1999), in a small controlled report, used tamoxifen versus a placebo and did not demonstrate a therapeutic advantage.** Should one desire to prescribe tamoxifen, it is used at a dosage of 20 mg twice daily.

The use of colchicine was originally proposed by M. K. Gelbard (personal communication, 1995). There are no blinded or controlled studies that have examined the use of colchicine. Akkus and coworkers (1994), in an uncontrolled study of 24 patients, reported some efficaciousness for colchicine. The patients were in the early phase of disease and received colchicine at a dose of 0.6 mg three times a day. **In that study, diminished plaque size and improved penile curvature were reported in approximately 50% of the patients.** Four actions are attributed to colchicine. Colchicine binds tubulin and causes it to depolymerize; thus, it inhibits mobility and adhesion of leukocytes. It inhibits cell mitosis by disrupting spindle cell fibers and thus functions as a potent anti-inflammatory agent. It blocks the lipoxygenase pathway of arachidonic acid metabolism, furthering its anti-inflammatory effect. It interferes with the transcellular movement of protocollagen. Colchicine is reasonably well tolerated. Approximately one third of patients, however, will have diarrhea. It is inexpensive. If it is used, the dosage is 0.6 mg three times per day with meals.

Biagiotti and Cavallini (2001) convened a study of 48 patients with Peyronie's disease, approximately one third in the acute phase and two thirds in the chronic phase. The groups were randomized between tamoxifen, 20 mg twice daily for 3 months, and acetyl-L-carnitine, 1 g twice daily for 3 months. Oral carnitine is thought to have several mechanisms of action involving free radical metabolism. It has been useful in degenerative oxidative diseases and vasculitides. **The authors found that the carnitine was more effective in reducing pain and seemed to inhibit disease progression. Thus, they thought it was more effective and safer than tamoxifen in therapy for Peyronie's disease.** Propionyl-L-carnitine in the same dose can also be used for oral therapy. Nonsteroidal anti-inflammatory drugs and corticosteroids have been used anecdotally on the basis of the belief that inflammation is integral to the development of Peyronie's disease. No studies support an indication for the use of these drugs.

A number of intralesional injection protocols have been examined. Teasley (1954) reported the use of intralesional corticosteroids, as did other studies (Bodner et al, 1954). **It is the recommendation of the consensus committee on penile curvatures that the use of intralesional corticosteroids be eliminated or at least initiated with extreme caution because of the significant local side effects, the inconsistent pattern of improvement in well-established curvature, the lack of studies showing proven efficacy,** and the reports of patients who believed that their condition deteriorated after the injections (Jardin et al, 2000).

The calcium antagonist verapamil was first used as intralesional therapy by Levine and colleagues (1994). Verapamil is thought to have efficacy on the basis of its ability to inhibit the exocytosis of collagen, fibronectin, and glycosaminoglycans. This inhibition works at the basic metabolic step involved with the manufacture of collagen and hence is thought to inhibit the ultimate formation of scar. Since that report, several observational studies have been performed. **A single-blind controlled study comparing verapamil with saline showed a diminished plaque volume but no change in deformity** (Rehman et al, 1998). **In a prospective study of 156 patients, of those who completed the protocol, 60% had a decrease in curvature and 80% reported improvement in tip flaccidity** (Levine et al, 2002). A number of injection protocols have been discussed. A "full course" could consist of 12 injections (10 mg/10 mL) given once every 2 to 4 weeks. In many hands, up to that total dose, injections are discontinued when satisfactory improvement is noted. Patients must understand that improvement may not be noted immediately, and hence they must be prepared to proceed with the entire 12-injection series. **The use of intralesional verapamil for patients with acute disease is thought reasonable on the basis of the available data to date.**

The use of purified clostridial collagenase was first studied in vitro by Gelbard and associates (1982, 1983). Collagenase is a naturally occurring enzyme that has been found to be intimately involved with the process of scar remodeling. Simply stated, the use of collagenase as an intralesional agent is thought to create "chemical incisions," thus initiating areas of remodeling. **Collagenase has since been subjected to two double-blind studies and an additional small pilot study using intralesional collagenase combined with modeling** (Gelbard, 1993; Jordan, in preparation). **In that study, 10 patients were enrolled and 9 completed follow-up; improvement was noted in curvature in all 9 as judged by photographs submitted at intervals by the patients and questionnaire endpoints** (Jordan, data in analysis, April 2005). A double-blind, placebo-controlled, multicenter study is planned for enrollment in the fourth quarter of 2006. Intralesional collagenase is thus available only on study protocol.

The use of interferons as intralesional therapy for Peyronie's disease was reported in 1991 by Duncan and associates. Interferons are thought to have action based on their abilities to inhibit the synthesis of collagen, fibronectin, and glycosaminoglycans. Thus, the mechanism of action of interferon is thought to be similar to that proposed for verapamil. An observational study using interferon alfa enrolled 35 patients. Some of the patients received a 12-week course and some a 24-week course. **Seventy-five percent of the patients reported treatment satisfaction as judged by improvement in their ability to have intercourse.** The authors thought that treatment with interferon can be done safely and is reasonable to offer patients (Hakim et al, 2004).

A number of topical therapies have been reported, with delivery often combined with iontophoresis or electromotive therapy. Agents used are orgotein (recently withdrawn from all markets), steroids, verapamil, and β-aminopropionitrile, either singly or as "cocktails." No blinded studies have shown efficacy (Montorsi et al, 2000a). These are only single observational reports. Corticosteroids have been used in association with ultrasound (iontophoresis). Again, no blinded studies have shown efficacy.

Radiotherapy has been proposed as a treatment of Peyronie's disease. In recent years, radiotherapy was proposed for the treatment of pain that was thought to be "abnormally persistent." In 1975, a retrospective study examined the use of radiotherapy and found it to be no more effective than "no treatment." **It is the consensus of the World Health Organization committee that radiotherapy be avoided because of potential risk of malignant change and the potential for increasing the risk of erectile dysfunction in aging patients** (Lue et al, 2004).

Extracorporeal shockwave therapy has been proposed as a treatment of Peyronie's disease since 1989 (Lebret et al, 2002). There has been little standardization with regard to the treatment (varying dosages and machines) (Butz and Teichert, 1998; Colombo et al, 1999; Gianneo et al, 1999; Lebret et al, 2002; Manikandan et al, 2002; Sytenko, 2004). **There are no controlled trials, but one case-controlled trial** (Hauck et al, 2000) **reported favorable results.** No studies examining the efficacy of extracorporeal shockwave lithotripsy in the treatment of Peyronie's disease have been convened in the United States.

The vacuum erection device has been proposed as a treatment of Peyronie's disease. A report (Kirsch-Noir et al, 2004) examined six patients with Peyronie's disease treated with the vacuum erection device. The authors concluded that the vacuum device might limit penile fibrosis, but no comment was made concerning plaque volume or curvature. Verheyden is quoted as stating that in a series of patients treated with vacuum therapy for Peyronie's disease at the Andrology Unit, Department of Urology, Antwerp, Belgium, more than 50% stated that their plaques softened and they noted improvement in curvature (Augusta Medical Systems, product information, 2005). **Treatment of Peyronie's disease with the vacuum erection device has thus not been adequately studied.**

A number of studies have examined combined medical management. These include a study of intralesional injection and oral therapy with interferon alfa-2b plus vitamin E (Novak et al, 2001). Another study examined the use of oral vitamin E plus colchicine (Prieto Castro et al, 2003), and another series of studies of intralesional injection and oral therapy looked at the combination of verapamil with carnitine and verapamil with tamoxifen (Cavallini et al, 2002). These single observational studies represent the thrust of current work with regard to medical management. A study is currently being convened to examine the efficacy of the vacuum device both singly and in combination with intralesional therapy. Rajfer has proposed the use of PDE5 inhibitors. As briefly discussed earlier, there is an interplay between oxidative and nitrosative mechanisms in fibrosis that is not restricted to Peyronie's disease fibroblasts. Cyclic GMP, the mediator of penile erection, is produced by nitric oxide activation of guanylate cyclase, which is also antifibrotic in Peyronie's disease plaques. Long-term administration of sildenafil, a phosphodiesterase inhibitor that impedes GMP breakdown, prevented Peyronie's disease plaque formation in rat models (Gonzalez-Cadavid and Rajfer, 2005).

Surgical Management

For a patient to be a surgical candidate, he must have stable and mature disease. In review, the signs of disease stability (quiescence) include resolution of pain and stabilization of curvature or other deformity. Likewise, the experienced examiner will recognize the palpatory findings of a mature plaque.

KEY POINTS: MEDICAL MANAGEMENT

- The efficacy of medical management of Peyronie's disease is difficult to determine because, in the past, few studies were properly done. Vitamin E has been used historically. Potassium aminobenzoate, in a small study, was found to reduce plaque size, not curvature, and thus in that study was found "efficacious." However, the side effects make it difficult to tolerate. From an intellectual standpoint, the use of colchicine makes a great deal of sense in patients with Peyronie's disease who are in the acute phase. For the most part, colchicine is reasonably well tolerated. Tamoxifen, in a small controlled study, was not found to demonstrate any therapeutic advantage. The neutraceutical carnitine, in either its propionyl or acetyl ester, in preliminary studies was thought to be effective for certain disease parameters.

- A number of intralesional protocols have been proposed. The use of verapamil as an intralesional agent has been studied. A prospective study did show decrease in curvature in about 80% of the patients. The use of collagenase as an intralesional agent has been subjected to a number of double-blind placebo-controlled protocols, and in all, efficacy was suggested. However, collagenase is currently available only as part of clinical trials.

- Radiotherapy should be avoided.

- The vacuum erection device has not been adequately studied.

- The place of extracorporeal shockwave therapy has likewise not been adequately determined.

Most investigators arbitrarily impose a 12- to 18-month period from onset of disease. Most suggest a period of at least 6 months of disease stability (i.e., stable deformity). Indications for surgery include deformity that precludes intercourse and erectile dysfunction that precludes intercourse.

Surgical Correction of Peyronie's Disease

A number of surgical procedures have been used for the straightening of the deformity of Peyronie's disease. Pryor and Fitzpatrick (1979) described a procedure of excision and plicating closure of the aspect opposite the Peyronie lesion. This procedure counteracted the effects of the inelastic lesion by shortening the opposite, more compliant aspect of the corpora cavernosa.

Lue performs a correction in which he omits the excision of the tunica albuginea and merely plicates the opposite aspect of the corpora cavernosa (Akkus et al, 1997; Gholami and Lue, 2002). Although this technique historically did not yield durable results in patients with congenital curvature, in the patient with Peyronie's disease, in whom accumulated intracavernosal pressures are probably less, it possibly can be expected to be more effective. Lue emphasizes the use of permanent suture that is "loosely tied" to correct the deformity. Although the techniques of both Pryor and Fitzpatrick (1979) and Lue are valid in some patients, many patients are already

concerned by the shortening of their penis as a result of Peyronie's disease; thus, surgery that offers the suggestion of further shortening of the penis is unacceptable to them. The use of permanent suture as described by Lue is also not well accepted by some patients.

The procedure described by Yachia (1993), discussed in Chapter 33 "Surgery of the Penis and Urethra," under the correction of congenital curvatures, represents a corporoplasty technique that can be effectively used for curvatures associated with Peyronie's disease. Plication and corporoplasty techniques seem to be useful especially for patients with associated erectile dysfunction, in whom grafting procedures could be expected to cause further deterioration of erectile function. The author relies on this procedure for those patients with ventral curvature for reasons already discussed. The perceived shortening associated with these procedures in a number of studies, in properly selected patients, is not clinically significant (Klevmark et al, 1994; Nooter et al, 1994; Sulaiman and Gingell, 1994; Kummerling and Schubert, 1995; Poulson and Kikeby, 1995; Ralph et al, 1995; Porst, 1997; Savoca et al, 2000; Chahal et al, 2001; Gholami and Lue, 2002; Van Drift et al, 2002; Lucas et al, 2004; Seipp and Schukfeh, 2004).

Gelbard (1989) described a surgical technique that involved incising the plaque of Peyronie's disease. He reported a series of patients in whom incisions were made in the plaque and grafts of temporalis fascia were used to fill the defects. His technique was based on the theory that by making a number of incisions, thus expanding the scar, and then filling them with compliant material, a smoother correction of curvature would result. He has reported good results with this procedure.

Das and Amar (1982) described a procedure in which the plaque is excised and the corporotomy defect is grafted with tunica vaginalis. They believed that the tunica vaginalis is an easy donor site for the urologist and that it gives the same results as the dermal graft. Our experience has been that tunica vaginalis is a suitable substitute for dermis in select patients with well-defined, small lesions. In patients in whom the corporotomy defect is large, however, we have not been pleased with the use of tunica vaginalis. A report has described tunica vaginalis double folded to limit the problem with larger corporotomy defects. In an observational series, the authors reported acceptable results (Geavlete et al, 2004).

Lockhart has employed a procedure in which the plaque is excised and the corporotomy defect is closed with tunica vaginalis as an island based on a dartos fascial and cremasteric flap (J. L. Lockhart, personal communication, 1991). He found that his results were better with the improved vascularity of the tunica vaginalis transposed as a paddle on a flap.

Buncke (cited in Stefanovic et al, 1994) reported an experimental animal series in which the lesion is excised and the corporotomy defect is replaced with temporalis fascia transferred to the area of the penis as a microvascular free transfer flap. To date, this procedure has not been reported in humans.

Lue and El-Sakka (1998) have also described a procedure using incisions but patching the corporotomy defects with vein grafts. They initially believed that the excised deep dorsal vein provided an adequate donor site for the vein grafts. With time, however, it was found that the donor site offered inadequate amounts of donor tissue, and later the saphenous vein was harvested to design the vein graft patches. Lue believes

SECTION VI

that the intracorporal space represents a large vessel, and therefore a patch of vessel wall represents a physiologic procedure. He reports good results with this procedure. Montorsi and colleagues (2000b) reported a series of 50 men treated with plaque incision and vein grafting for Peyronie's disease. All patients were evaluated preoperatively with sexual history, examination, determination of penile length and degree of curvature, and dynamic color power Doppler sonography of the penile vessels and three nights of nocturnal RigiScan. All were evaluated postoperatively with the same variables including color duplex Doppler sonography and RigiScan. They reported either complete or adequate straightening in 94% of patients. Penile rigidity was equal to that preoperatively in 94% of patients. Power Doppler sonography showed vascular impairment in 10% of patients, and RigiScan revealed significant decrease in nightly erections in 10% of patients. They concluded, thus, that plaque incision with vein grafting achieved satisfactory results in the majority of patients with severe and stable Peyronie's disease who have intact penile rigidity preoperatively. Akkus and colleagues (2001) quoted a series of 58 patients. The patients in that study were similarly evaluated with history, counseling, and duplex Doppler ultrasound examination. They reported complete or adequate straightening in 95% of patients and preservation of preoperative erectile function in 93% of patients. They concluded that plaque incision with venous patch grafting is a satisfactory surgical method for the treatment of the curvature in Peyronie's disease.

Krishnamurti (1995) reported the use of de-epithelialized penile skin as a paddle carried on the dartos fascia. He cited increased dependability of flaps, not a fact that is totally validated in the literature. We have attempted to "de-epithelialize" penile skin with the dermabrader as described by Krishnamurti. However, histologic evaluation of these "de-epithelialized islands" actually shows many areas where the entire thickness of the skin has been removed. Thus, in our minds, the precise histologic composition of Krishnamurti's de-epithelialized islands is not clear.

Hellstrom (1994) has reported the use of a number of nonautologous grafts. Hellstrom and Reddy (2000) reported the use of cadaver pericardium in a small series. Chun and associates (2001) compared the results of plaque incision or excision and grafting with either dermal or cadaveric pericardial graft techniques, and they suggest that the minimal preoperative preparation and decreased patient morbidity with cadaveric pericardium makes it a more efficacious and appropriate graft compared with dermis. They do not report that the graft provides clinical results superior to those of dermis. Levine and Estrade in 2003 reported results of the use of human cadaveric pericardial graft for the surgical correction of Peyronie's disease. That was a retrospective evaluation of 40 men. Postoperatively, all patients reported sufficient rigid erection for coitus after the procedure; many required, however, intracorporal papaverine injection. Thus, a 98% success with penile straightening and a 95% success with intercourse as previously described were reported; 70% of the patients had unaided full erections, and 30% required pharmacologic assistance. Palese and Burnett (2001) reported the use of pericardial allograft in patients requiring complex penile prosthetic surgery. Hellstrom thought that the pericardial graft essentially serves as an inert collagen matrix or scaf-

fold for the adjoining tunica albuginea. As the graft is overgrown or ingrown and the new tissues are vascularized, the graft is enzymatically dissolved (Leungwattanakij et al, 2001). Arap and colleagues (Egydio et al, 2002) reported the results of their series using plaque incision with bovine pericardial graft; they described 33 patients. It is unclear in the report how the patients were stratified preoperatively with regard to erectile function. They reported a good correction of deformity in 88% of cases with adequate correction in the rest of their series. They stated that all recovered their ability to "penetrate with no difficulty." They thus think that the procedure is an effective one.

Knoll in 2001 reported the use of porcine small intestinal submucosal graft (SIS) in the surgical management of Peyronie's disease. His initial report was of 12 patients, the majority of whom had adequate straightening and adequate preservation of erectile function. He later described 97 patients with curvatures of 60 degrees or more secondary to Peyronie's disease. Some patients were preoperatively stratified with color Doppler ultrasonography; the majority were evaluated with examination by intracavernous injection. He reported successful correction of curvature in 90% of patients. Mean follow-up was 20 months. Preservation of erectile function is not clearly stated. The author thought that the technique offers an excellent alternative. Our experience is that foreign material "grafts" (e.g., Silastic, Gore-Tex, Dacron), in the absence of concomitant prosthetic implantation, inevitably yield poor results.

Devine and Horton (1974) described a procedure for correction of deformity of Peyronie's disease in which the plaque is excised and replaced with a dermal graft. This procedure continues to be used selectively in the author's center. The use of dermal graft for corporoplasty has been variously applied. Austoni and coworkers (1995) reported a large series of 418 men. In that series, 17% required further surgery for curvature and 20% had troublesome postoperative erectile dysfunction. However, what one must realize is that Austoni used an aggressive dissection of the penis, in many patients, disassembling the glans from the tip of the corporal bodies. Thus, the results may not be a fair representation of the procedure of excision of Peyronie's plaque with dermal graft in general. The World Health Organization consensus (Lue et al, 2004) reports that the operation of excision of Peyronie's plaque with dermal graft is regarded as outmoded. I disagree with that opinion. The procedure selectively still has use; however, I would agree that there are many suitable alternatives.

In addition, we now have a relatively large series of patients who have been treated by incisions through the plaque and patching of the corporotomy defects with dermis. With the exception of those patients with severely calcified plaques, we have preferentially used the technique of incision with dermal grafting and more recently with porcine intestinal submucosal grafting. Our early results indicate that the technique of plaque incision is at least as successful as the technique of plaque excision; however, it has not yet been determined whether there is a difference between the techniques with regard to preservation of erectile function or limitation of graft-induced veno-occlusive dysfunction. Likewise, our early analysis of the porcine intestinal submucosal graft has been promising. The advantage of an off-the-shelf graft cannot be overemphasized.

The initial skin incision is dependent on the location of the lesion or the location of the proposed intervention; ventral plaques or patients who will have corpora plication can be approached through a midline incision of the ventral aspect of the penis, and dorsal plaques are most effectively approached by a circumferential incision. In the patient who has been previously circumcised, the incision should be placed through the original circumcision incision (Fig. 25–8). In many patients, the circumcision scar may be displaced far down the shaft of the penis. We have not encountered any problems, however, with reapproaching the penis through the circumcising incision, even when this is the case.

The shaft of the penis is then degloved to its base. This maneuver gives good exposure for midshaft and distal lesions. For proximal plaques or in patients who have relatively redundant foreskin, a second peripenile periscrotal incision is made. After the shaft of the penis is degloved, it is delivered into the periscrotal incision; the shaft skin is laid aside and covered with a warm sponge. This protects the penile skin from trauma until the end of the procedure, when it is returned to the shaft. Optionally, a counterincision can be made at the penoscrotal junction in the scrotal raphe.

The dorsal neurovascular bundle is elevated in concert with Buck's fascia. This can be accomplished by several techniques. Incisions can be made just lateral to the corpus spongiosum, with Buck's fascia and the dorsal neurovascular bundle dissected off the lateral and dorsal aspects of the corpora caver-

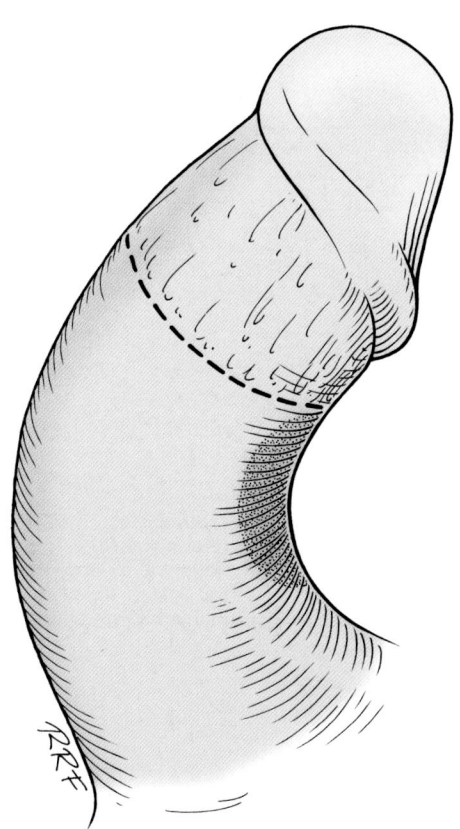

Figure 25–8. An erection demonstrates the dorsal curvature of the penis caused by the inelastic scar tissue in a dorsal plaque of Peyronie's disease. The incision to be made in the scar of the previous circumcision has been marked.

nosa. Alternatively, we currently approach dorsal plaques by dissecting sharply through the bed of the deep dorsal vein and perform a modified vein dissection (Figs. 25–9 to 25–12). We initially used this approach to investigate the potential effect of a modified vein dissection with regard to limitation of graft-induced veno-occlusive dysfunction. Although the beneficial effects of this are yet to be proved, approaching the dorsal plaque through the bed of the dorsal vein appears to be a superior approach technically.

In the past, if preoperative testing suggested veno-occlusive dysfunction, we proceeded with a formal vein dissection, ligation, and excision. More recent experience has shown, however, that vein dissection does not offer durable results in patients with Peyronie's disease, and it is currently believed that patients who demonstrate severe veno-occlusive dysfunction are better treated by a surgical approach or modeling to straighten the penis and prosthetic implantation for their erectile dysfunction (Wilson and Delk, 1994). Some patients might do well with a plication or corporoplasty technique and then postoperatively undergo management of the erectile dysfunction pharmaceutically.

After dorsal exposure of the tunica (see Fig. 25–12), the inelasticity of the plaque will be evident, and its extent can be delineated by feeling the surface of the tunica albuginea. An artificial erection accurately defines the curvature. Incisions are then planned either to incise or to excise the plaque. We place Prolene stay sutures in the midline, proximal and distal to the plaque, and mark the planned incisions. Depending on the technique selected, the plaque can be excised or incised. We do not favor the use of a tourniquet for either control of bleeding or induction of an artificial erection as tourniquets can conceal proximal curvatures.

Once the plaque has been excised or incisions have been made, we measure the defect, stretching the penis to ensure accurate coverage. The dermal graft, if that is what we used, is then outlined on the donor site. We prefer to use the skin of the abdomen just above the iliac crest, lateral to the hairline, as the donor site for the dermal graft. The donor site is closed per primam by subcuticular sutures, with use of either a pull-out or the newer absorbable long-acting monofilament suture.

In the case of dermal graft, we then carefully tailor the graft to measure approximately 30% larger in all dimensions than the corporotomy defect and place it into either the incisional or the excisional defect. The graft, when it is released from the inherent tissue tension at the donor site, "contracts" about 30%. This should not be confused with graft contraction during "take." After completing the graft inlay with polydioxanone suture, we perform another artificial erection to demonstrate that the penis is straight and the suture lines are watertight. If there are leaks, they are oversewn. If the penis is not straight during surgery, it will not be straight postoperatively. If curvature persists, therefore, further modification by means of incisions and grafting or "touch-up" plications is necessary.

After completion of the dermal graft inlays, we anatomically close the penis. Buck's fascia is reapposed with polydioxanone suture, and small suction drains are placed superficial to Buck's fascia but deep to the dartos layer. We then coapt the skin incisions with either chromic or small Vicryl sutures. If a ventral midline incision was made that crosses the penoscro-

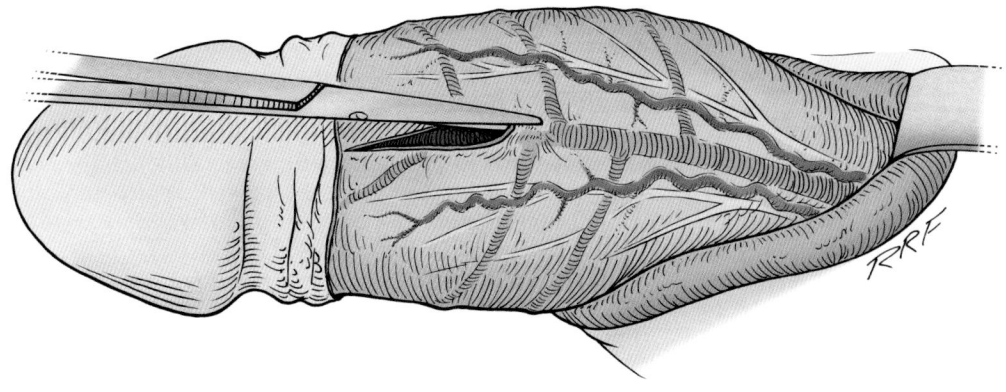

Figure 25–9. The skin has been degloved to the base of the penis by dissection in the layer immediately superficial to Buck's fascia. An incision in the dorsal midline of Buck's fascia exposes the deep dorsal vein. The coiled dorsal arteries and the circumflex veins are demonstrated.

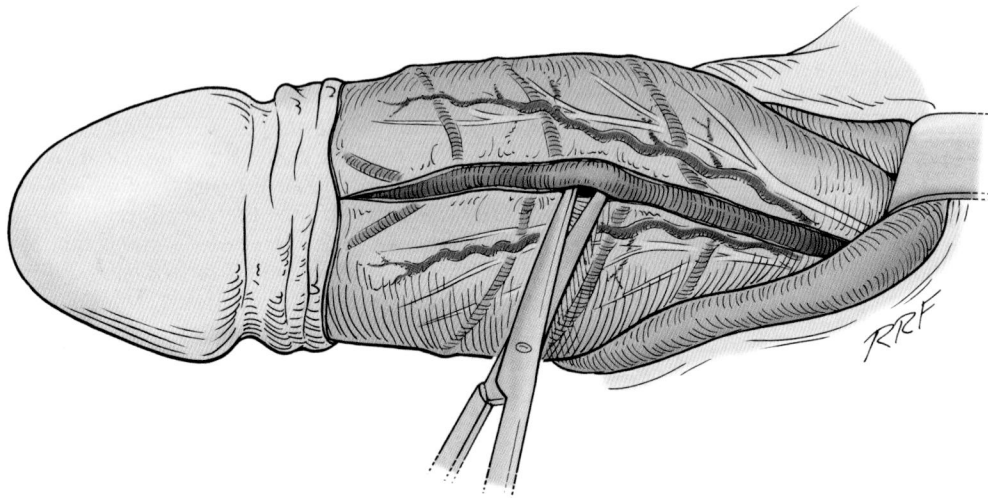

Figure 25–10. The deep dorsal vein is mobilized.

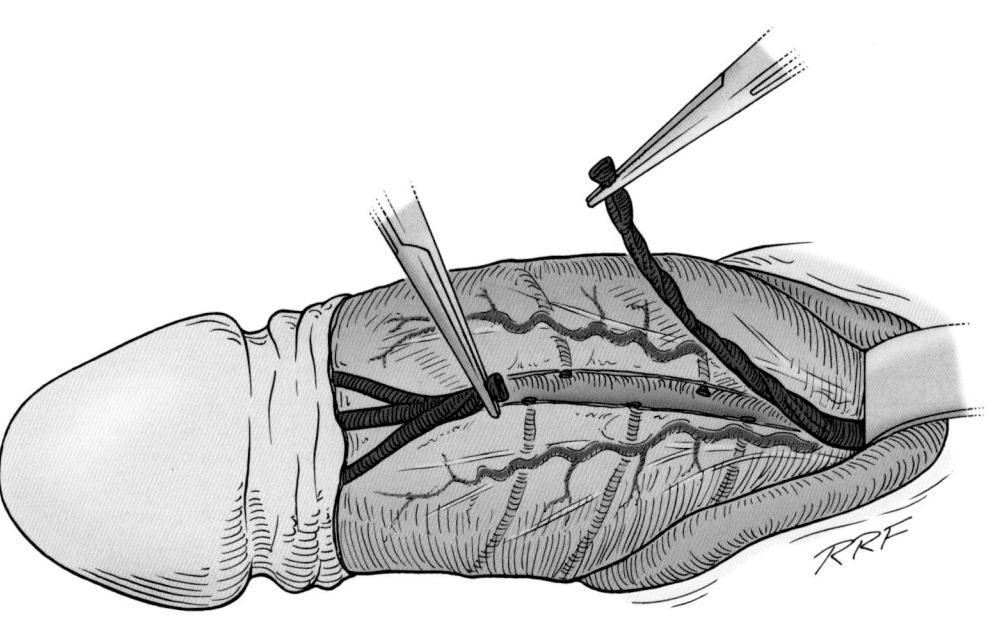

Figure 25–11. After the deep dorsal vein is divided, it is dissected proximally; the emissary veins are divided and ligated. The subcoronal veins and the dorsal vein proximally are suture ligated.

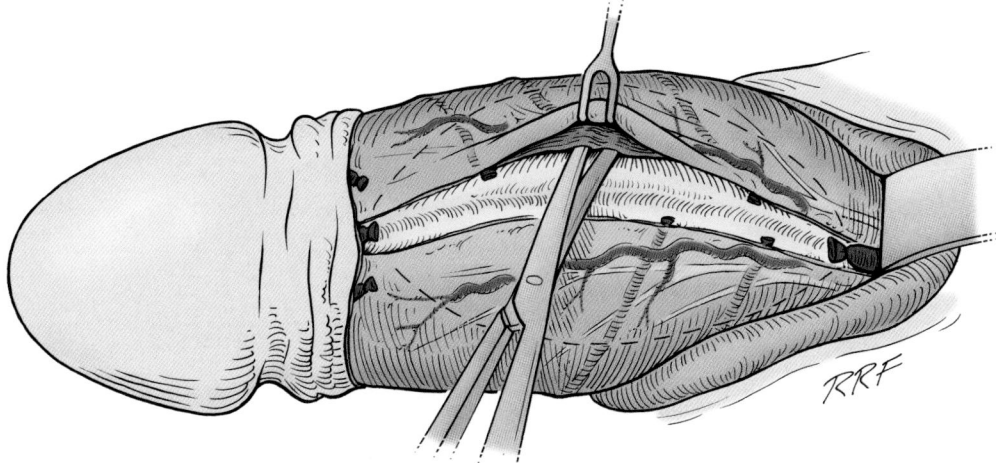

Figure 25–12. Buck's fascia is elevated from Peyronie's plaque. The area of dissection is outlined by the *dashed line,* continued far enough proximally, distally, and laterally to allow excision of the plaque without distraction or stretching of the nerves in Buck's fascia.

tal junction, a Z-plasty should be used to prevent penoscrotal tethering.

Beginning in 1998, in suitable patients, we further modified our technique of plaque incision. The technique of incision was described by Lue. In this technique, the plaque is exposed as already illustrated and discussed. Artificial erection is used to identify the curvature and the point of maximal curvature. At that point, an H-shaped incision is made; the flaps are elevated, allowed to slide (Figs. 25–13 to 25–16), and sutured, leaving an approximately square defect. Since 2001, the sliding H incision has been modified. At the point of maximal curvature, which can be accurately identified during artificial erection, a stitch is placed and a strip of tunica albuginea is excised. This indeed does make a larger corporotomy defect; however, the corporotomy defect remains approximately square, and the graft inlay can be placed without difficulty. After either H incision is made, the sliding flaps are sutured. If there is indentation, the flaps are darted, allowing expansion. A graft is then sutured into the defect, and preferentially since 2003 we have used the SIS graft; however, dermis or vein can also be used

(Fig. 25–17; see also Fig. 25–16). It is clear that the penis can be effectively straightened with this incision and graft technique alone in about 70% of patients. The addition of the small strip excision allows straightening in almost all patients. Only about 5% of patients will require touch-up plication, and generally that is for persistent tilt of the glans as mentioned. Beginning about 2 years ago, the modified sliding H technique (excision of a small strip across the midline) has been used. By doing this, we find that touch-up plications are usually not required (Figs. 25–18 to 25–20). It is also clear that the H technique limits graft size, whether it is dermis, vein, or SIS graft. It is not clear whether this technique is more reliable or effective with regard to preservation of erectile function. It is our distinct early impression that the SIS graft is clearly as efficacious as dermis or vein, and perhaps superior.

The penis is dressed with a Bioclusive dressing, loosely applied and extending from the base of the penis to the level of the midglans. A mildly compressing Kling dressing is wrapped over the Bioclusive dressing to limit edema and to

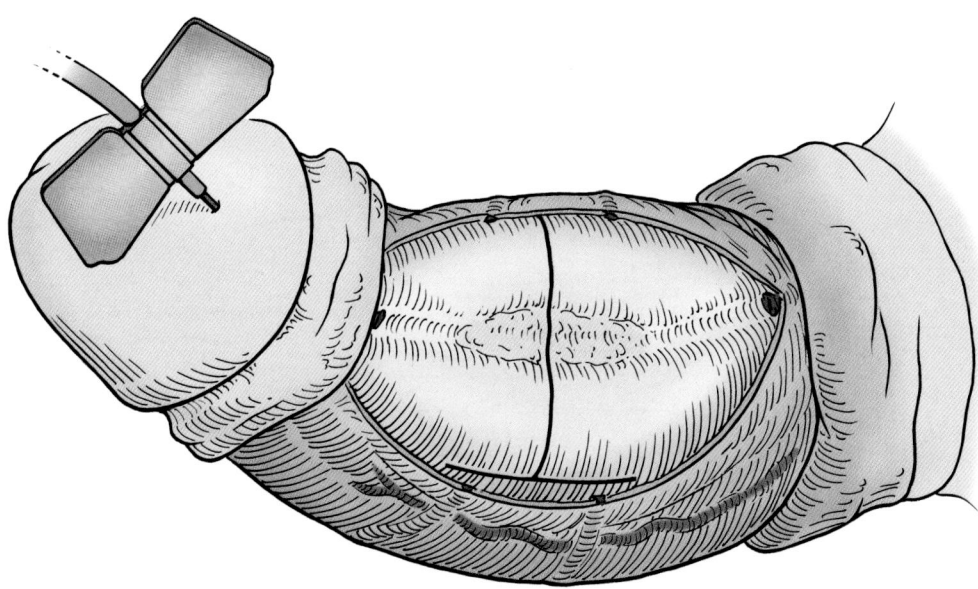

Figure 25–13. Illustration of "sliding H" technique of incision. The dorsal tunica and plaque are exposed as already described. An H-shaped incision is marked at the site of maximal curvature.

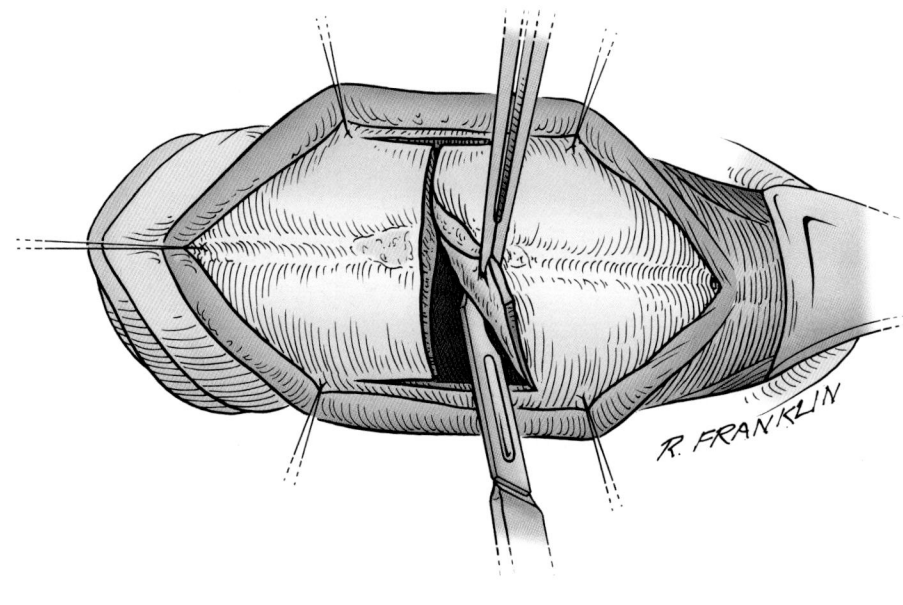

Figure 25–14. The flaps of the H are incised and elevated from the underlying erectile tissue. The septal fibers are divided. The septal fibers are detached back to the point of normal tunica albuginea both proximally and distally. This maneuver is extremely important in achieving straightening with this technique.

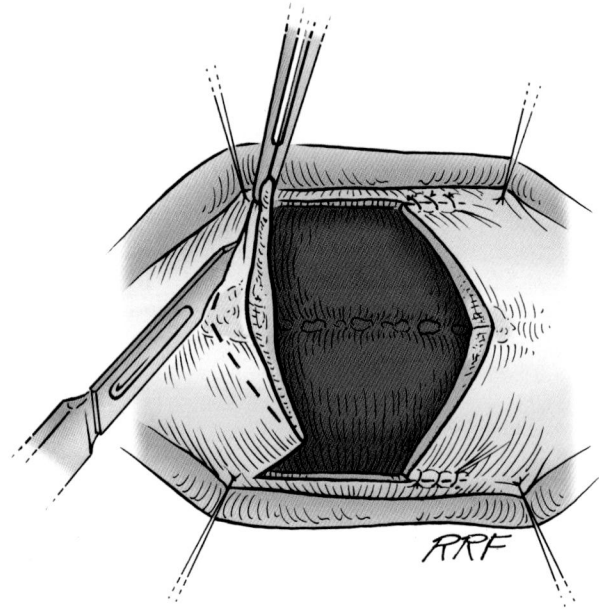

Figure 25–15. The flaps are elevated, and darting incisions are marked to allow some expansion of the defect circumferentially.

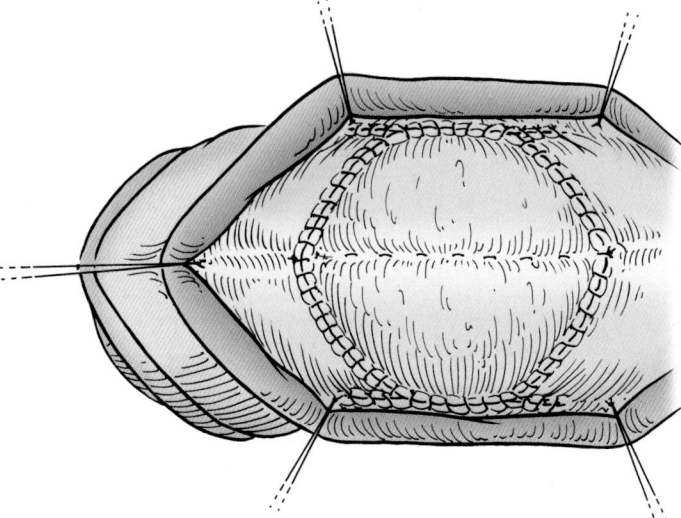

Figure 25–16. The flaps are sutured in place, creating a square corporotomy defect. Appearence with either dermis or SIS.

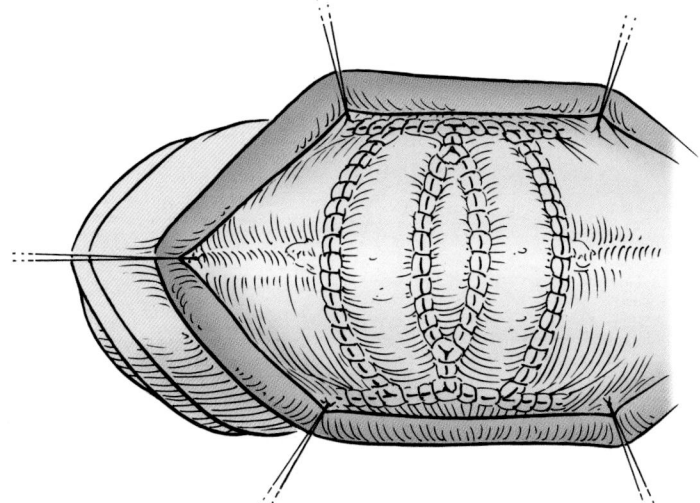

Figure 25–17. Alternatively, the corporotomy defect can be replaced with a vein graft. Notice that the vein graft is oriented so that the circumferential distensibility allows long axial lengthening.

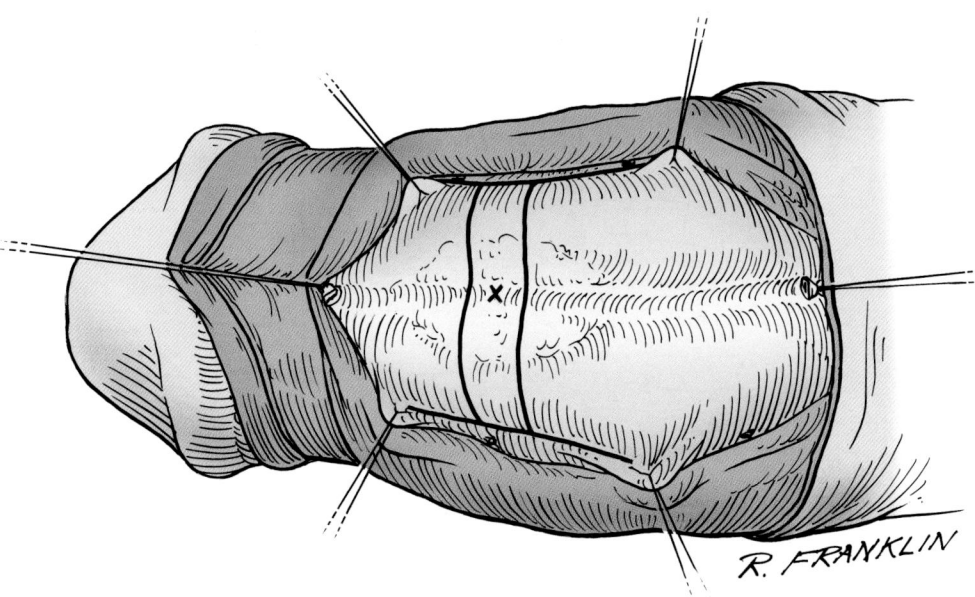

Figure 25–18. Modification of the sliding H technique, in which a small strip is excised at the point of maximal curvature. The stitch marks that point.

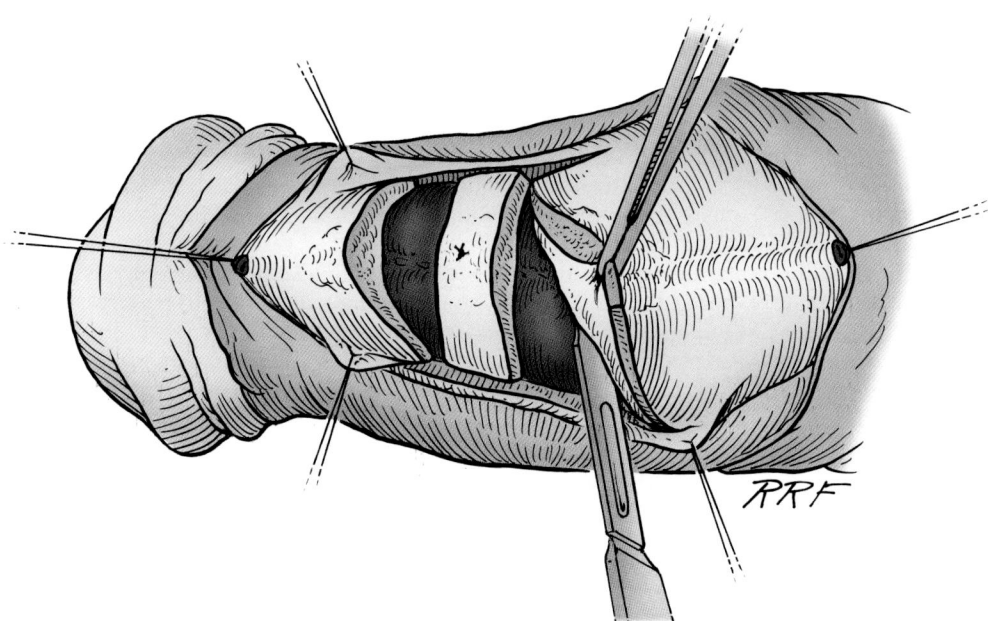

Figure 25–19. The incisions are made; the H flaps are elevated extensively as discussed in Figure 25–14. Note the expansion of the corporotomy defect.

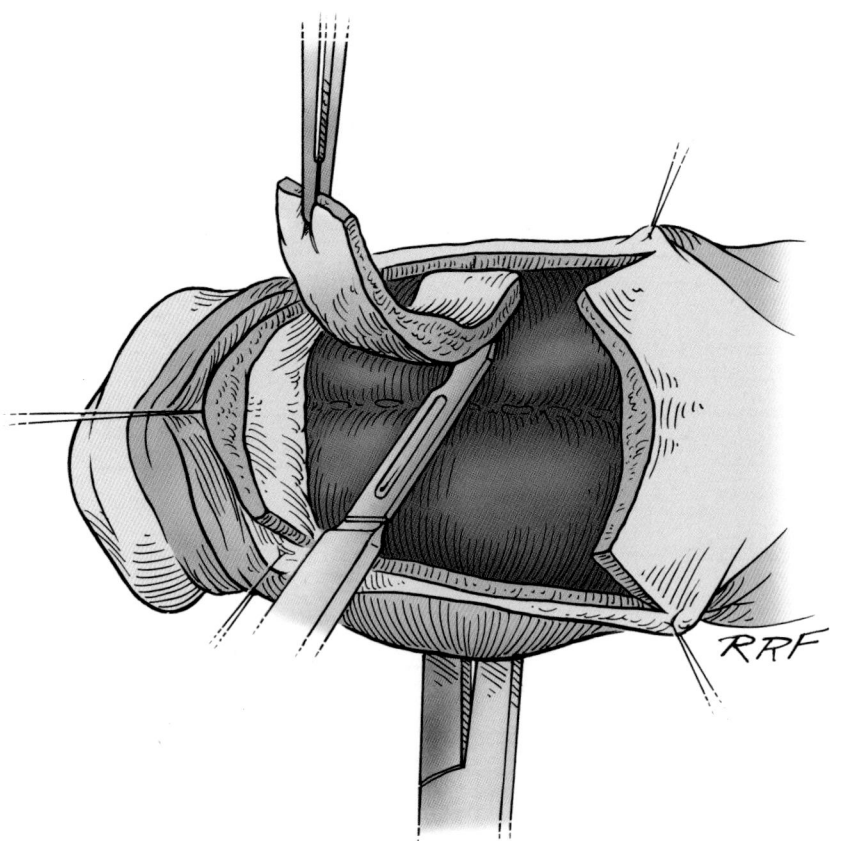

Figure 25–20. The transverse strip is excised; the H flaps are then sutured as discussed in Figure 25–15. The flap can be darted if lateral expansion is needed.

allow better collapse of the surgical spaces around the suction drains. The Kling dressing is left in place for 4 hours, during which the glans is checked every 30 minutes. A No. 14 French Foley catheter is left until the patient ambulates on the morning after surgery. The suction drains are removed on the first postoperative day, and usually the patient is discharged on that day. We suppress erections with diazepam and amyl nitrite.

Dermal grafts mature in the same manner as other grafts do: first nourished by imbibition of tissue fluids while inosculation occurs from adjacent blood vessels. Remodeling takes place during the late phase of maturation, with the graft tending first to contract and then to become compliant. In the first 3 months, the graft may contract enough to re-create some of the curvature, but as the graft softens, straightening occurs. This is seen less in patients who have had incisions as opposed to excisions. Patients should be forewarned of this sequence of events to avoid undue anxiety. With vein and also SIS grafts, this initial contraction can be seen, but seemingly less often and less severely.

After the first 2 weeks, we encourage patients to have erections but discourage them from intercourse. During this time, it is desirable for the penis to be manipulated so that the skin does not adhere to the deeper layers of the penis. In addition,

erections stretch the graft and aid in the maturation phases of graft take. In some patients, we encourage the use of the vacuum erection device without the constriction ring as a means of distending and stretching the graft.

Penile Prosthesis in Peyronie's Disease

It is the consensus of the committee on Peyronie's disease at the World Health Organization Second International Consultation on Sexual Dysfunctions that the penile prosthesis is a reliable option for the older man with vascular impairment, erectile dysfunction, and acquired deformity of the penis (Lue et al, 2004). It is hence not the only treatment for Peyronie's disease but rather a prudent treatment for the patient with significant erectile dysfunction in association with Peyronie's disease. In past years, semirigid devices have been preferred; however, with improvement in the three-piece hydraulic devices, they would appear to be preferable (Marzi et al, 1997; Ghanem, 1998). In 1993, Montorsi published a study that showed greater patient and partner dissatisfaction with semirigid devices when they were used for the treatment of erectile dysfunction combined with Peyronie's disease. Before 1994, correction of the curvature of Peyronie's disease, at the time of prosthesis placement, was accomplished by degloving of the penis and incision of the tunica albuginea in the area

■ For a patient to be a surgical candidate, he must have
stable and mature disease. Most investigators
consider curvature or erectile dysfunction that
precludes intercourse the indication for surgery.
The surgeon must consider all options of surgical
therapy. Plication and corporoplasty techniques can
be lumped under those operations that shorten the
less involved side, and the application of those
techniques is preferential in many patients.
Procedures that incise or excise the plaque require
the use of graft materials, and a number of graft
materials have been successfully employed.

■ Overall, plication or corporoplasty techniques seem
to preserve the patient's erectile function more
effectively; however, excellent results can be achieved
with incision and grafting techniques. The use of a
prosthesis for all Peyronie's patients is condemned.

of curvature. In 1994, however, Wilson and Delk advised the
modeling procedure. Since that report, the modeling procedure has proved to be an excellent means for straightening the
penis in the majority of patients. However, when the patient
is to be modeled, it is imperative to explain to the patient that
urethral injury at the time of modeling is possible. This can
occur with the extension of the modeling into the urethra at
the point of maximal curvature, or the tips of the prosthesis
can actually be forced through the tip of the corporal bodies
and into the urethra in some cases. If modeling does not work,
one can resort to what was previously applied, and that is incision with or without grafts as described earlier. In 1996,
Montague and associates published a comparative study of the
AMS CX cylinders versus the AMS Ultrex cylinders in
Peyronie's disease. In that study, it was found that the CX
cylinders were superior. The message is that a controlled
expansion cylinder provides better results; thus, the AMS
700CX or the Mentor Alpha I/Titan system would be preferable (Wilson and Delk, 1994; Montague et al, 1996). If incisions are required, I recommend closing the incisions with a
synthetic patch. Materials that I have used include Gore-Tex,
but I now prefer to use the SIS graft.

The recent publications showing superiority of the antibiotic-coated prostheses or the hydrophilic-coated prosthesis
with regard to infection rate suggest to me that in cases of
Peyronie's disease, the antibiotic-coated devices should be
used (Carson, 2004; Wolter and Hellstrom, 2004). Wilson
reported the use of the Ambicor prosthesis in Peyronie's
patients. A series of 77 consecutive patients were studied.
Thirty-two were primary implants; of these patients, 20 had
bothersome Peyronie's disease. The remaining 34 were
replacement devices for a malfunctioning AMS 700 prosthesis, and many of these patients had Peyronie's disease. All of
the Peyronie's patients had satisfactory straightening without
another adjunctive procedure. There were no infections

reported in the series. Thus, it was concluded that the Ambicor
two-piece inflatable prosthesis has good patient satisfaction
even when it is implanted for Peyronie's disease and in
patients who have had previous three-piece devices (Scarzella
and Wilson, 2004).

Peyronie's disease is not the "terminal–no hope" diagnosis
that many patients believe it is. Peyronie's patients and their
partners must be educated about what is happening and what
might happen. They must be told that in the majority of cases,
their sexual relationship can be adequately restored. They
must also understand that for most cases, all we have to offer
will, at best, make their sex lives adequate. There is not one
best operation or approach but rather a menu of options that
for a given individual will have benefits and disadvantages.
With counseling, they must match their "have to haves and
can't stand to haves" to those advantages and disadvantages.
This approach, in my experience, will lead to the best management for most.

■ The consensus committee on Peyronie's disease at
the World Health Organization Second International
Consultation on Sexual Dysfunctions stated that the
penile prosthesis is a reliable option for the older
man with vascular impairment, erectile dysfunction,
and acquired deformity of the penis.

■ It is not the only treatment of Peyronie's disease
but rather a prudent treatment for the patient with
significant erectile dysfunction in association
with Peyronie's disease. Hydraulic prostheses are
preferred, and those prostheses that have true
controlled expansion cylinders have been shown to
provide better results.

SUGGESTED READINGS

Akkus E, Carrier S, Baba K, et al: Structural alterations in the tunica albug-
inea of the penis: Impact of Peyronie's disease, ageing and impotence. Br J
Urol 1997;80:190.
Brock G, Hsu GL, Nunes L, et al: The anatomy of the tunica albuginea in the
normal penis and Peyronie's disease. J Urol 1997;157:276-281.
Carson CC, Jordan GH, Gelbard MK: Peyronie's disease: New concepts in eti-
ology, diagnosis and treatment. Contemp Urol 1999;11:44-64.
Davis CJ Jr: The microscopic pathology of Peyronie's disease. J Urol 1997;157:
282-284.
Gelbard MK, Dorey F, James K: The natural history of Peyronie's disease.
J Urol 1990;144:1376-1379.
Jardin A, Wagner G, Khoury S, et al: Erectile Dysfunction. First International
Consultation on Erectile Dysfunction. Co-sponsored by World Health
Organization, International Society for Impotence Research, and Société
Internationale d'Urologie, Paris, July 1-3, 1999.
Jones WJ: Counseling men with sexual dysfunction. AUA Update Series
1997;XVI(lesson 23):178-184.
Kelami A: Classification of congenital and acquired penile deviation. Urol Int
1983;38:229-233.
Kendirci M, Nowfar S, Gur S, et al: The relationship between the type of penile
deformity and penile vascular status in patients with Peyronie's disease. J
Urol 2005;174:632-635.

Lue TF, Basson R, Rosen R, et al, eds: Second International Consultation on Sexual Dysfunctions. Sexual Medicine: Sexual Dysfunctions in Men and Women. Paris, Health Publications, 2004.

Nyberg LM Jr, Bias WB, Hochbert MC, Walsh PC: Identification of an inherited form of Peyronie's disease with autosomal dominant inheritance and association with Dupuytren's contracture and histocompatibility B7 cross-reacting antigens. J Urol 1982;128:48-51.

O'Brien K, Parker M, Guhring P, et al: Analysis of the natural history of Peyronie's disease [abstract 69]. J Sex Med 2004;1(suppl 1):50.

Williams J, Thomas G: The natural history of Peyronie's disease. J Urol 1970;103:75.

26 Priapism

ARTHUR L. BURNETT, MD

Priapism refers to an obscure disorder of unwanted, persistent penile erection. Its obscurity pertains variously to its relative rarity, its often inconsistent clinical presentation, and its fairly unclear pathophysiologic mechanisms. Moreover, the disorder has paradoxical implications, invoking superior sexual prowess and virility while actually signifying a pathologic and nontrivial entity. Indeed, priapism is a significant medical problem associated with risks of structural damage of the penis and erectile dysfunction, which may adversely affect normal sexual health and well-being and cause psychological distress. Such significance supports its proper recognition and management.

DEFINITION

The origin of the term *priapism* is historically attributed to the ancient Greek and Roman mythologic figure Priapus, a deity of fertility and gardens (Papadopoulos and Kelami, 1988; Burnett, 2003). Consistent with perceptions of his male generative powers, Priapus was generally portrayed as ithyphallic (in reference to genital organs of disproportionately enlarged size with respect to the whole body). In various cultures over time, effigies of genitals displayed in ritualistic worship of Priapus or his personage have served therapeutic purposes. The first account in the medical literature of priapism as a medical problem appears to be the publication entitled

Gonorrhoea, Satyriasi et Priapisme by Petraens, recorded in 1616 (Hinman, 1914).

By conventional definition, priapism is a pathologic condition of penile erection characterized as prolonged and devoid of sexual stimulation or excitement (Berger et al, 2001; Montague et al, 2003). Correctly, it is distinguishable from normal sleep-related erections, which do not constitute pathologic phenomena. The penis is familiarly recognized as being the affected body organ, although priapism of the clitoris has also been described in the medical literature (Monllor et al, 1996). The corpora cavernosa are the anatomic structures typically sustaining penile rigidity, although the corpus spongiosum may similarly become tumescent (Hashmat et al, 1989; Sharpsteen et al, 1993). Its pathologic determinants include a host of disease states or circumstances secondarily affecting hemodynamics of the genital region. However, an inherent primary disorder of the erectile process that resists physiologic genital organ flaccidity is also understood. A time interval of 4 hours has frequently been cited as a qualifying criterion since on a practical basis, pathologic consequences are associated with priapism extending beyond this time limit (Montague et al, 2003). However, presentations of shorter durations and conversely those lasting days or months that may not overtly result in erectile tissue damage are identifiable as representing priapism. Pain is a common descriptor, perceived to be a consequence of genital tissue ischemia and increased pressure generated within the corporal bodies, although this feature is not a requirement for the designation of priapism. **In light of these multiple observations, the meaning of the term appropriately encompasses a multifactorial entity of genital organ tumescence or rigidity that develops and persists in a pathologically uncontrolled fashion for any duration without sexual purpose.** This chapter focuses on priapism of the penis and emphasizes clinical objectives to preserve male erectile function.

EPIDEMIOLOGY

Although priapism is presumed to be an infrequently occurring phenomenon, it does occur in the population to a measurable extent. Cases per 100,000 person-years (the number of patients with a first episode of priapism divided by the accumulated amount of person-time in the study population) were calculated to be 0.34 to 0.52 in Finland during the years 1975-1990 (Kulmala et al, 1995a), 1.5 in the Netherlands during the years 1995-1999 (Eland et al, 2001), and 0.84 in western Australia during the years 1985-2000 (Earle et al, 2003). Whereas estimates of priapism incidence from these population-based studies seem roughly comparable, an accurate sense of the frequency of the problem must account for the influence of intracavernous pharmacotherapy for erectile dysfunction, which has a known risk for priapism (Lomas and Jarow, 1992), introduced in the time frame of these studies. The overall incidence rate cited in the Finnish study excludes priapism related to this factor, although the incidence rate doubly increased to 1.1 cases per 100,000 person-years in the final 3 years of the study after the introduction of intracavernous pharmacotherapy (Kulmala et al, 1995a). The adjusted incidence rate in the Netherlands was found to be 0.9 case per 100,000 person-years after exclusion of cases associated with intracavernous vasoactive drug use (Eland et al, 2001). Interestingly, the incidence rate in western Australia declined to 0.43 case per 100,000 person-years after 1989 coincident with the change to intracavernously administered prostaglandin E_1 monotherapy for erectile dysfunction (Earle et al, 2003), a practice identified to have a lesser risk profile for priapism than previously used intracavernous pharmacotherapy regimens (Porst, 1996).

Additional factors may influence incidence estimates for priapism. The presentations of this disorder inventoried in these studies are only those that came to medical attention and consequently were likely to be the most prolonged or painful cases. Apparently, repeated episodes and cases that resolved with or without major clinical consequences were not registered and thus were excluded from the calculations. Furthermore, as recognized by some of the investigators of these studies, the results may have been limited by potential diagnosis misclassifications and inaccuracies associated with retrospectively collected registry data. Thus, these representative studies may yet have underestimated the frequency of the problem.

The estimation of incidence rates of priapism also depends on the population group under study. This matter applies particularly to populations in which sickle cell disease, a major risk category for priapism, is highly prevalent. **Cohort studies involving populations with sickle disease demonstrate lifetime probabilities for development of priapism to be between 29% and 42%** (Emond et al, 1980; Fowler et al, 1991; Mantadakis et al, 1999; Adeyoju et al, 2002). Furthermore, the actuarial probability of experiencing priapism by 20 years of age in this population is estimated to be 89% (Mantadakis et al, 1999). As such, sickle cell disease ranks as the most frequent basis for priapism in the pediatric age range (Fowler et al, 1991; Miller et al, 1995). The fact that certain population groups are highly affected by priapism emphasizes the public health significance of the problem and, moreover, a needful role for preventive efforts in addressing the problem particularly in these groups.

ETIOLOGY

Priapism has been linked with many different disease states and other situations that constitute risk associations for the condition. Several etiologic categories are presented here.

Hematologic Dyscrasias

Priapism is associated with hematologic disease, most notably sickle cell disease, although a relationship with sickle cell trait has also been described (Emond et al, 1980; Fowler et al, 1991). Priapism secondary to sickle cell disease is reported to account for approximately 23% of adult cases and as much as 63% of pediatric cases (Nelson and Winter, 1977). Other hemoglobinopathies, including hemoglobin Hb Olmsted and thrombophilia, have also been associated (Thuret et al, 1996; Quigley and Fawcett, 1999). Leukemia is recognized to have an association, particularly chronic granulocytic leukemia; priapism develops in as many as 50% of patients with this disease (Schreibman et al, 1974; Steinhardt and Steinhardt, 1981; Morano et al, 2000).

Thrombotic risk associations for priapism have also been identified. Asplenism is an apparent risk factor for priapism (Atala et al, 1992; Thuret et al, 1996). Erythropoietin use has also been linked with the disorder (Brown and Nehra, 1998). Priapism has followed hemodialysis with heparin administration as well as cessation of oral warfarin (Coumadin) therapy, both believed to constitute rebound hypercoagulable states (Fassbinder et al, 1976; Routledge et al, 1998). Intracavernous heparin administration intended as a priapism treatment has actually exacerbated the problem (Bschleipfer et al, 2001). Priapism has been related to total parenteral nutrition containing 20% fat emulsion (Klein et al, 1985; Hebuterne et al, 1992). It has also been associated with Fabry's disease, a genetically determined enzyme deficiency disorder of glycosphingolipid metabolism (Foda et al, 1996).

Neurologic Conditions

A variety of neurologic conditions may serve as risk conditions for priapism. Causative roles have been suggested for neurologic infections such as syphilis, brain tumors, epilepsy, intoxication, and brain and spinal cord injury (Hinman, 1914; Munro et al, 1948). Other associations include lumbar disk herniation (Ravindran, 1979), lumbar spinal cord stenosis (Hopkins et al, 1987; Ram et al, 1987), cauda equina compression from metastatic cancer (Greschner et al, 1998), and even cervical spinal cord trauma from legalized hanging (Gallagher, 1995).

Anesthesia, either general or regional (spinal or epidural) administration, has also been associated with priapism, with a heightened risk in the presence of genital manipulation as part of the surgical procedure (Wasmer et al, 1981; Chin and Sharpe, 1983; Van Arsdalen et al, 1983; Shantha et al, 1989; Dittrich et al, 1991).

Nonhematologic Malignant Neoplasms

Local primary or metastatic neoplastic processes are also known to carry priapism risks. Organs of cancer origin include penis, urethra, prostate, bladder, kidney, and rectosigmoid colon (Powell et al, 1985; Chan et al, 1998; Nezu et al, 1998; Morga Egea et al, 2000; Hettiarachchi et al, 2001).

Trauma

Priapism has been associated with direct penile and perineal trauma (Burt et al, 1960; Hinman, 1960) as well as traumatic needle insertion with intracavernosal pharmacotherapy (Witt et al, 1990). The onset may be delayed in many instances, occurring after a subsequent sexual or sleep-related erection generates intracorporal pressure increase that results in disruption of earlier damaged intracavernous arteries (Ricciardi et al, 1993).

Erectile Dysfunction Pharmacotherapy

After the introduction of intracavernously administered vasoactive agents for the treatment of erectile dysfunction, priapism resulting from the use of these agents was immediately recognized (Virag, 1985; Halsted et al, 1986; Lomas and Jarow, 1992). Lomas and Jarow (1992) defined the risk profile of priapism in this setting, finding that younger men with better baseline erectile function, patients with overt neurologic disease, and patients without significant cardiovascular disease were most susceptible. Other vasoactive therapies for erectile dysfunction have also been implicated, including intraurethral alprostadil (Bettochi et al, 1998; Lue, 1999) and oral sildenafil (Sur and Kane, 2000).

Pharmacologic Exposures

Medication use constitutes a risk factor for priapism. The earliest association was made with the antihypertensive agents hydralazine and guanethidine (Rubin, 1968) and later with α-adrenergic antagonists (Siegel et al, 1988; Vaidyanathan et al, 1998). Priapism has also been linked with the use of psychotropic and antidepressant medications such as phenothiazines, sedative-hypnotics, selective serotonin reuptake inhibitors, and trazodone (Abber et al, 1987; Carson and Mino, 1988; Segraves, 1989; Saenz de Tejada et al, 1991; Seftel et al, 1992; Kulmala et al, 1995b; Compton and Miller, 2001).

Heavy alcohol intake has been associated with the development of priapism (Pohl et al, 1986; Kulmala et al, 1995b). Topical and intranasal cocaine administration has been described to induce priapism (Fiorelli et al, 1990; Rodriguez-Blaquez et al, 1990; Altman et al, 1999). Other pharmacologic agents demonstrated to constitute risk associations for priapism include the immunosuppressant agent FK506 (tacrolimus) (Harmon et al, 1999), androgen supplements (Kachhi and Henderson, 2000; Zargooshi, 2000), and scorpion toxin (Teixeira et al, 2004).

Idiopathic

Priapism occurring without any discernible cause is considered to be idiopathic. Some investigators have estimated that this disorder accounts for as many as half of all documented cases (Larocque and Cosgrove, 1974; Pohl et al, 1986; Winter and McDowell, 1988).

NATURAL HISTORY

After its onset, the recognized outcome from priapism is either its permanent resolution or its progression to recurrent episodes with or without some degree of erectile impairment. Understandably, the administration of effective treatment would alter the natural course of the condition and predispose to its resolution with optimization of erectile function.

Resolution of a major episode of ischemic priapism is characterized by return of the penis to a flaccid, nonpainful state, although penile edema and enlargement sometimes persist, mimicking unresolved priapism. In the absence of effective treatment, it has long been recognized that even major episodes of ischemic priapism will eventually resolve in time, although permanent damage of the penis may be expected. Pryor (2004) reported that 90% of men with ischemic priapism lasting 24 hours fail to regain ability to perform sexual intercourse. An erectile dysfunction rate of 35% was determined by literature review of published cases of ischemic priapism treated systemically without apparent direct relief of penile ischemia (Montague et al, 2003). Among patients with sickle cell disease having priapism, a separate report found that 29% had erectile dysfunction, and 24% were unable to perform sexual intercourse to their satisfaction (Adeyoju et al, 2002). Whereas the age at onset of priapism and erectile dysfunction were not found to be statistically related, a trend was shown indicating that sexual ability was better preserved with a later age at onset (Adeyoju et al, 2002).

Nonischemic priapism, which is typically not painful, follows a natural course different from that of ischemic priapism. Whereas its spontaneous resolution is also characterized by a return to a completely flaccid state, this form, if untreated, may persist unresolved in some individuals for extended periods (Hakim et al, 1996). **It is perceived that individuals with nonischemic priapism generally preserve erectile ability.** However, cavernosometric descriptions of veno-occlusive abnormalities in patients with this entity suggest that erectile dysfunction may occur in some individuals (Brock et al, 1993).

Recurrent forms of ischemic priapism adhere to a clinical pattern distinct from a single major episode of priapism, in that they occur repeatedly with intervening periods of detumescence. Patients with idiopathic presentations and those with hematologic abnormalities such as sickle cell disease are most commonly represented. In the population of men with sickle cell disease, Emond and associates (1980) described "stuttering attacks" in reference to multiple, typically self-limited (characteristically less than 3 hours in duration) recurrences. These recurrent episodes have been commonly observed to begin soon after puberty and evolve in variable intervals of weeks, months, or even years, with some culminating in a major episode lasting 3 to 5 days and up to several weeks (Emond et al, 1980; Serjeant et al, 1985). Interestingly, these episodes do not appear to have any relationship to other vaso-occlusive crises characteristic of sickle cell disease (Serjeant et al, 1985; Tarry et al, 1987). Stuttering episodes have not been generally associated with a significant extent of erectile dysfunction, in contrast with acute or major episodes (Emond, 1980; Serjeant et al, 1985; Fowler et al, 1991). However, Adeyoju and associates (2002) documented a 25% erectile dysfunction rate among patients with sickle cell disease who reported a prior history of only stuttering priapism.

PATHOLOGY

Priapism is associated with pathologic changes of the penis that may occur on morphologic, biochemical, and functional grounds. Grossly obvious is the distended and deformed, megalophallic penis that frequently occurs in patients with recurrent priapism of sickle cell disease (Datta, 1977). **Penile** tissue necrosis and progressive fibrosis are the end-stage manifestations of ischemic priapism, hampering the physical reactivity of the erectile tissue and its elasticity needed for physiologic blood engorgement (Hinman, 1960).

Hinman (1960) early described the histopathologic features of the ischemic penis as edematous changes in the trabecular structure of the cavernous tissue, which accounts for penile turgidity even after early priapism resolution. Sequential ultrastructural changes of the corpora cavernosa can also be identified as penile ischemia progresses. Spycher and Hauri (1986) found that after 12 hours, trabecular interstitial edema develops; after 24 hours, the sinusoidal endothelium is denuded and thrombocytes adhere to the exposed basement membrane; and after 48 hours, thrombi form in the sinusoidal spaces and smooth muscle cells undergo necrosis or become transformed to fibroblast-like cells. Such changes were not observed in the priapic penis that is not ischemic. However, a unique feature of intracorporal blood stasis during prolonged penile erection is the lack of thrombus formation because of heightened fibrinolytic activity in the penis relative to the systemic circulation (Rolle et al, 1991). In correlation with the fibrotic progression of priapism, the fibrosis factor transforming growth factor-β1 becomes elevated (Ul-Hasan et al, 1998).

Biochemical changes occurring in the course of ischemic priapism have been investigated and found to correlate with cavernosal tissue damage. Juenemann and associates (1986), using blood gas measurement of penile aspirates in men with ischemic priapism, documented the presence of hypoxia and the accumulation of metabolic acid products as soon as 4 hours after priapism onset. Broderick and Harkaway (1994) observed increasingly altered metabolic changes (i.e., deoxygenation, acidosis, and hypercapnia) in penile aspirates from men developing prolonged erections up to 6 hours while using intracavernous pharmacotherapy for erectile dysfunction. Conditions of anoxia (Broderick et al, 1994; Kim et al, 1996), acidosis (Saenz de Tejada et al, 1997; Moon et al, 1999), and glucopenia (Liu et al, 1999) have been shown to independently impair corpus cavernosal smooth muscle tone and contractile responses to physiologic and pharmacologic stimuli in both in vitro and in vivo experimental animal models of priapism. Muneer and associates (2005) further demonstrated the relationship of ischemic metabolic changes and irreversible cavernosal smooth muscle contractile dysfunction applying an in vitro experimental model. **These investigators established that the irreversible effects resulted most consistently from the combination of hypoxia, acidosis, and glucopenia at a time interval of 4 hours. It is apparent that the 4-hour duration of ischemic priapism is relevant as an interval after which definite erectile tissue functional damage occurs.**

Pathologic changes also occur in the penis when ischemic priapism is relieved. In this event, as a result of reperfusion injury, the cavernosal tissue sustains damage from oxidative stress. Penile tissue reoxygenation after ischemia interferes with prostacyclin (prostaglandin I_2) production, hence diminishing the roles of this prostanoid as an inhibitor of platelet aggregation and white cell adhesion (Daley et al, 1996). Further studies have confirmed lipid peroxidation as an indicator of tissue injury involving reactive oxygen metabolites in experimental animal models of reperfused ischemic priapism (Evliyaoglu et al, 1997; Munarriz et al, 2003).

PATHOPHYSIOLOGY

In evaluating the origins of idiopathic priapism, Hinman (1960) proposed that vascular stasis in the penis and decreased venous outflow from the organ were the primary circumstances that mechanically or physically interfered with detumescence. This contention stemmed mainly from the invariable finding of dark, viscous blood in the corpora cavernosa when priapic penes were incised or aspirated. Additional support for the venous congestion hypothesis was provided by clinical examples of priapism in which mechanical factors were presumably responsible for impeding blood drainage, most notably veno-occlusive erythrocytes in patients with sickle cell disease (Hinman, 1960). Hinman (1960) further reasoned that deoxygenated blood (decreased oxygen tension or increased carbon dioxide tension) associated with ischemia combined with venous congestion to enhance blood viscosity in all idiopathic presentations and contributed to the deformity of erythrocytes locally in the penis, particularly in patients with sickle cell disease.

Whereas this classic paradigm of veno-occlusion has been applied to the mechanism of priapism associated with sickle cell disease, it has also been generally accepted as a pathophysiologic basis for priapism associated with a host of other circumstances. Such deranged veno-occlusive mechanisms conceivably pertain to penile intravascular viscosity changes and increased blood coagulability associated with parenteral hyperalimentation, particularly in combination with fat emulsion (Klein et al, 1985; Hebuterne et al, 1992); hemoconcentration and hypovolemia leading to intracavernous blood viscosity associated with hemodialysis (Fassbinder et al, 1976); increased blood coagulability related to heparin-induced platelet aggregation (Bschleipfer et al, 2001); venous outflow obstruction of the corporal bodies based on the invasion or infiltration of local primary or metastatic neoplastic processes (Chan et al, 1998; Morano et al, 2000; Morga Egea et al, 2000; Hettiarachchi et al, 2001); and venous outflow obstruction of the corporal bodies and increased intracavernous blood viscosity associated with hematologic dyscrasias (Pond, 1969; Larocque and Cosgrove, 1974; Winter and McDowell, 1988; Brown and Nehra, 1998).

Early theories regarding the pathophysiologic process of traumatically induced priapism have centered on a mechanism of excessive arterial inflow (Burt et al, 1960; Hauri et al, 1983). Burt and associates (1960) observed bright red blood at initial incision and irrigation of one of the engorged corpus cavernosal bodies in a man whose priapism followed traumatic coitus, and they resolved the priapism only after staged reoperation involving ipsilateral internal pudendal artery ligation. Others have further supported vascular injury from blunt trauma to the perineum or genitalia as having an etiologic relationship (Winter, 1978; Llado et al, 1980; Ricciardi et al, 1993). A similar pathophysiologic process is attributed to direct vascular laceration resulting from needle passage within the corpora cavernosa in association with intracavernous pharmacotherapy (Witt et al, 1990). **In all of these settings, the traumatic disruption of the penile vasculature results in unregulated blood entry and filling within the corpora cavernosa. Fistula formation between the cavernous artery and lacunar spaces of the cavernous tissue, which allows blood to bypass the normal helicine arteriolar bed, then accounts** for this form of priapism (Hauri et al, 1983; Brock et al, 1993; Hakim et al, 1996). Penile arterial revascularization surgery for arteriogenic erectile dysfunction is an iatrogenic manifestation of this effect (Michal et al, 1980; Jarow and DeFranzo, 1992).

Observations about the clinical features of priapism have also suggested that predisposing conditions or susceptibility factors play roles in its pathogenesis. Hinman (1960) associated idiopathic priapism (including priapism associated with sickle cell disease) with sporadic previous priapism episodes and suggested that sexual activity was a commonly preceding circumstance. Others also correlated priapism recurrences with sexual activity and particularly with erections sustained for prolonged durations of sexual activity (Larocque and Cosgrove, 1974; Lue et al, 1986; Pohl et al, 1986; Winter and McDowell, 1988; Levine et al, 1991). Sleep-related erections are also identified to precede priapism (Hinman, 1914; Lue et al, 1986; Fowler et al, 1991; Levine et al, 1991). **Thus, in predisposed individuals, heightened erection stimulatory conditions apparently provoke priapism.**

Several investigators have conjectured that upsetting or resetting the control level of corporal smooth muscle tone may account for some forms of priapism (Lue et al, 1986; Levine et al, 1991; Melman and Serels, 2000; Burnett, 2003). **A dysregulatory hypothesis for priapism suggests that either common determinants of corporal smooth muscle responses somehow operate in a dysfunctional manner or, alternatively, specific pathophysiologic mechanisms are responsible.** The dysregulation may in theory occur at the penile tissue level or at central or peripheral levels of the neurologic system controlling penile erection. Among currently known molecular mechanisms controlling the erectile tissue response, recent support has gone to aberrations in the nitric oxide signaling pathway, the main erection mediatory system in the penis. Lin and associates (2003) showed that phosphodiesterase-5, which hydrolyzes the pathway's second-messenger molecule cyclic guanosine monophosphate, is downregulated in ischemic corpus cavernosal smooth muscle cells in vitro. On this basis, the investigators proposed that ischemic priapism yields pathologic conditions for priapism recurrences (Lin et al, 2003). In another study, Champion and associates (2005) found decreased phosphodiesterase-5 expression and activity in penes of genetically altered mouse models lacking endothelial nitric oxide synthase and transgenic sickle cell mice, both having priapism phenotypes. The investigators viewed this finding to offer a molecular explanation for idiopathic, stuttering, and other primary forms of priapism.

CLASSIFICATION

A classification system is commonly used to differentiate clinical presentations of priapism. To a large extent, the main divisions of ischemic and nonischemic priapism convey conventional belief that presentations are generally discernible by both their local rheologic differences and their related pathologic consequences (Hinman, 1960). The division also has practical ramifications with respect to overall clinical management. **Presentations classified as ischemic priapism are frequently associated with irreversible cavernosal tissue damage and subsequent erectile function loss, whereas** those classified as nonischemic priapism presumably do not incur such consequences. The extension of this understanding is that ischemic priapism warrants emergency management, whereas nonischemic priapism does not demand such intervention.

Ischemic Priapism

Ischemic priapism, also termed veno-occlusive or low-flow priapism, features little or absent intracorporal blood flow. It represents a true compartment syndrome involving the penis, having characteristic metabolic changes and excessive pressure increases localized to the corpora cavernosa. Hinman (1914) should be acknowledged for initial descriptions of this predominant form of priapism, which he purported resulted from "mechanical" disturbances of blood flow in the penis causing "thrombosis of the veins of the corpora." Many local and systemic clinical conditions have been etiologically associated with this form of priapism. The corpora cavernosa are standardly rigid and tender to palpation. Pain is typically reported. Cavernous blood gas values are consistent with hypoxia, hypercapnia, and acidosis.

Nonischemic Priapism

Nonischemic priapism, also termed arterial or high-flow priapism, features elevated vascular flow through the corpora cavernosa. Initial descriptions of this less common form of priapism identified arteriogenic unregulation as its pathogenic basis (Burt et al, 1960; Hauri et al, 1983). Penile or perineal trauma is most frequently associated. However, other clinical conditions that are evidently atraumatic also fit criteria for this form of priapism. The corpora cavernosa are not usually fully rigid or painful (Das and Leidinger, 1992). Cavernous blood gas values do not reveal hypoxia or acidosis.

Priapism Variants

A review of priapism presentations described in the medical literature reveals the existence of anomalous priapic phenomena that do not conveniently fit classic hemodynamic models of the disorder. **These so-termed priapism variants plausibly involve primary pathophysiologic mechanisms that differ from those invoked with classic descriptions of the disorder. Their distinction carries potential importance for devising effective categorical approaches to clinical management.**

Recurrent (Stuttering) Priapism

Hinman (1914) first recognized that some recurrent forms of priapism are endured in limited durations compared with an isolated, long-lasting episode, which he termed acute transitory attacks. The more familiar term *stuttering priapism* was coined by Emond and associates (1980), in reference to the frequently recurrent episodes of priapism observed in sickle cell patients. Such priapism that progresses in severity may be considered to represent ischemic priapism (Montague et al, 2003).

Refractory Priapism

The immediately recurrent nonischemic erectile state that follows aspiration or incision of the corpora cavernosa for apparently ischemic priapism represents a priapism variant. Hinman (1960) first speculated that this entity resulted from rapid arterial blood refilling of the penis after surgical treatment rather than further venous congestion. Other investigators using blood gas determinations of penile aspirates and penile color duplex ultrasonography have documented the conversion of veno-occlusive ischemic priapism after initial treatment to a high-flow nonischemic form despite the absence of a traumatic insult or evidence of arteriocavernous fistulas (Lue et al, 1986; Ramos et al, 1995; Hakim et al, 1996; Seftel et al, 1998). High-flow arterial characteristics are also evident in surgically refractory priapism related to medical diseases including sickle cell disease (Ramos et al, 1995) and Fabry's disease (Foda et al, 1996).

Neurogenic Priapism

Given the recognized relationship between neurologic disorders and priapism, a neurologic basis for priapism is well postulated. Hinman's early characterization of priapism distinguished a minority of clinical presentations as "nervous," having associations with known or suspected neurologic disorders affecting "erectile centers of the nervous system" (Hinman, 1914). Others have also contended that disturbances in the neuroregulation of penile erection at central or peripheral nervous system levels remain a probable basis for priapism (Melman and Serels, 2000). Examples of this category fit characteristics of both ischemic and nonischemic priapism.

Idiopathic Priapism

Priapism lacking a recognizable clinical association establishes this category. Although the pathophysiologic mechanism of this form of priapism remains unclear, prolonged or painful presentations tend to fit an ischemic priapism model.

Drug-Induced Priapism

Although priapism associated with medication use does not represent spontaneously occurring priapism, it is recognized as being a major distinct form of the entity. Examples of this category fit characteristics of both ischemic and nonischemic priapism.

DIAGNOSIS

Because of the physical conspicuousness of priapism, the diagnosis of the disorder is generally straightforward (Fig. 26–1). **A key principle in the evaluation is to determine whether the clinical presentation is consistent with an ischemic pathologic process since emergent treatment is required in this situation. Thus, differentiating features between ischemic and nonischemic priapism should be borne in mind while proceeding with the evaluation.** Decisions to initiate treatment may be made on completion of the initial portion of the evaluation even if laboratory results are awaited and certain radiologic studies are postponed.

History and Physical Examination

Clinical history and physical examination, as for any clinical disorder presentation, are appropriately done (Berger et al, 2001; Montague et al, 2003). The clinical history should produce information such as the presence of pain, duration of priapism, role of antecedent factors, prior priapism episodes, use and success of relieving maneuvers or prior clinical treatments, existence of etiologic conditions, and erectile function status before the priapism episode. Inspection and palpation of the penis may indicate the extent of tumescence or rigidity, corporal body involvement (i.e., whether rigidity involves only the corpora cavernosa with a soft glans penis and corpus spongiosum or all three corporal bodies), and presence and extent of tenderness. Abdominal, perineal, and rectal examinations may reveal signs of trauma or malignant disease.

Laboratory Testing

Several laboratory tests are recommended in the routine evaluation of the patient with priapism (Berger et al, 2001; Montague et al, 2003). These include complete blood count,

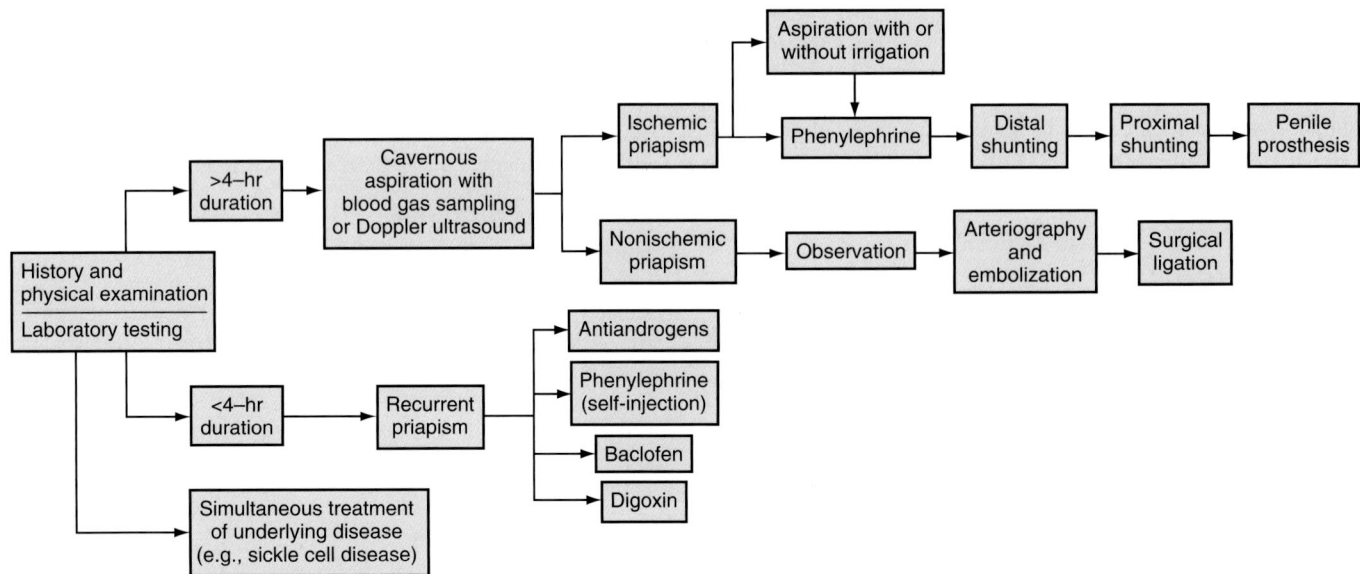

Figure 26–1. Priapism treatment algorithm.

white blood cell differential, and platelet count, which may reveal the presence of acute infections or hematologic abnormalities. Reticulocyte count and hemoglobin electrophoresis can be used to identify the presence of sickle cell disease or trait as well as other hemoglobinopathies and should be considered in all men unless another cause of priapism is obvious. The recommendation is based on the fact that hemoglobinopathies are not restricted to black men and may occur in nonobviously affected ethnic groups, including white men of Mediterranean descent (e.g., thalassemia). Screening for psychoactive drugs and urine toxicology to identify overdoses of legal and illegal drugs may also be performed.

Penile Diagnostics

Direct evaluation of the aspirated blood from the corpus cavernosum is a critical element of the diagnostic assessment (Berger et al, 2001; Montague et al, 2003). Aspirates should be visually inspected and submitted for blood gas testing. In patients with ischemic priapism, the blood is standardly hypoxic and therefore dark, whereas that of patients with nonischemic priapism is normally oxygenated and therefore bright red. The early observations that blood gas determinations and intracavernous pressure recordings differ between ischemic and nonischemic priapism suggested the immediate value of these tools (Lue et al, 1986), although the former has had practical clinical use. **Cavernous blood gas determinations in patients with ischemic priapism typically show a PO_2 of less than 30 mm Hg, PCO_2 of greater than 60 mm Hg, and pH below 7.25; whereas cavernous blood gas determinations in patients with nonischemic priapism commonly show a PO_2 of greater than 90 mm Hg, PCO_2 of less than 40 mm Hg, and pH of 7.40 consistent with normal arterial blood at room air** (Montague et al, 2003). **Normal flaccid penis cavernous blood gas levels are approximately equal to those of normal mixed venous blood at room air (PO_2 of 40 mm Hg, PCO_2 of 50 mm Hg, and pH of 7.35)** (Montague et al, 2003).

Radiologic Evaluation

Color duplex ultrasonography offers another reliable diagnostic method for distinguishing ischemic from nonischemic priapism (Berger et al, 2001; Montague et al, 2003). It can be done alternatively to cavernous blood gas testing as long as significant delay in ischemic priapism treatment is not incurred. **Patients with ischemic priapism have minimal or absent blood flow in the cavernosal arteries as well as within the corpora cavernosa; patients with nonischemic priapism have normal to high blood flow velocities in the cavernosal arteries and evidence of blood flow in the corpora cavernosa** (Feldstein, 1993; Hakim et al, 1996). Ultrasonography may also reveal anatomic abnormalities, such as a cavernous arterial fistula or pseudoaneurysm, which would help confirm the diagnosis of nonischemic priapism. An important technical aspect is that color duplex ultrasonography should be done in the lithotomy or frogleg position, scanning the perineum first and then the entire penile shaft. This recommendation follows the observation that intracavernous abnormalities indicative of nonischemic priapism often result from straddle injury or direct scrotal trauma and therefore commonly are identified

sonographically in the perineal portions of the corpora cavernosa.

Penile arteriography has use as an adjunctive study to identify the presence and site of a cavernous artery fistula (ruptured helicine artery) in the patient with nonischemic priapism. **At this time, arteriography is not routinely used for diagnosis and is otherwise usually performed as part of an embolization procedure.**

Other radiographic studies, such as penile scintigraphy (Hashmat et al, 1989) and cavernosography (Bruhlmann et al, 1983), have also been described as having properties to differentiate between ischemic and nonischemic priapism.

TREATMENT

Treatment decisions are based extensively on diagnostic findings. Interventions differ for ischemic, nonischemic, and recurrent priapism. **However, a stepwise treatment approach is essentially applied across all priapism forms on the basis of reversibility and invasiveness of specific therapies** (Berger et al, 2001). Treatment offerings of mainly historical interest include medical (e.g., warm baths, hot or cold packs, enemas, leeches, sedatives) and surgical (e.g., dorsal artery ligation, perineal nerve transection, penile amputation) therapies.

Ischemic Priapism

The management of a major episode of ischemic priapism is immediate. In general, since ischemic priapism of more than 4 hours in duration irrespective of etiology implies a compartment syndrome, decompression of the corpora cavernosa is recommended for counteracting the ischemic effects including pain sensations (Berger et al, 2001; Montague et al, 2003). Thus, therapeutic aspiration may be performed simultaneously with cavernous blood gas sampling after insertion of a scalp vein needle (19- or 21-gauge) directly into the corpus cavernosum. **Definitive first-line treatment consists of evacuation of blood and irrigation of the corpora cavernosa along with intracavernous injection of an α-adrenergic sympathomimetic agent** (Montague et al, 2003). A dorsal nerve block or local penile shaft block as a preceding penile anesthetic maneuver is usually done (Berger et al, 2001). This technique may best involve transglanular intracorporal needle insertion with an angiocatheter (16- or 18-gauge) in the manner of the Winter shunt (see later) since it apparently lessens penile hematoma formation from that associated with a laterally placed intracorporal needle; it may also facilitate blood drainage into the corpus spongiosum after the angiocatheter is removed. Alternatively, placement of needles into the corpora cavernosa distally and proximally at the penile crura with the patient in the lithotomy position offers an approach for maximally irrigating the corporal bodies (Chung et al, 2003). Priapism resolution employing aspiration with or without irrigation is approximately 30% (Montague et al, 2003).

Sympathomimetic agents can be expected to exert contractile effects on the cavernous tissue and thus facilitate detumescence (Lee et al, 1995). **Among these, phenylephrine as an α_1-selective adrenergic agonist is the preferred drug for this application since it minimizes the risk of cardiovascular side effects compared with other sympathomimetic agents**

Table 26-1. Pharmacologic Therapies for Priapism

Drug	Class/Mechanism	Dosage	Administration	Adverse Effects	Special Considerations
Sympathomimetics (α-adrenergic agents)					
Phenylephrine	α_1 agonist	100-200 µg every 5-10 min until detumescence (maximum 1000 µg)	Intracavernous injection	Hypertension, tachycardia, palpitations, headache, arrhythmia, sweating	Preferred agent based on selectivity
Epinephrine	α, $\beta_{1/2}$ agonist	10-20 µg every 5-10 min until detumescence	Intracavernous injection	Hypertension, tachycardia, palpitations, headache, arrhythmia, sweating	Potential for cardiac stimulation based on β-adrenergic receptor activity
Antiandrogens					
Leuprolide	Gonadotropin-releasing hormone agonist	7.5 mg once a month	Intramuscular injection	Hot flashes, gynecomastia, loss of sexually induced erections, asthenia	Not applicable for children
Bicalutamide	Androgen receptor antagonist	50 mg once a day	Oral tablets	Hot flashes, gynecomastia, diarrhea, asthenia, loss of libido	Precaution if moderate to severe hepatic impairment
Flutamide	Androgen receptor antagonist	250 mg every 8 hours	Oral capsules	Hot flashes, gynecomastia, diarrhea, loss of libido, edema, rash	Monitor for liver dysfunction
Miscellaneous					
Baclofen	γ-Aminobutyric acid agonist	20-40 mg once a day (bedtime)	Oral tablets	Drowsiness, confusion, dizziness, weakness, fatigue, headache, hypotension, nausea	Possible role for "neurogenic" priapism
Digoxin	Cardiac glycoside	0.5 mg every day	Oral tablets	Anorexia, nausea, vomiting, confusion, blurred vision, headache, gynecomastia, rash, arrhythmia	Monitor digoxin levels, electrolytes, renal function

having β-adrenergic activity (Table 26-1). Monitoring for potential side effects from the medication that may occur through its entry to the systemic circulation is recommended. These side effects encompass subjective symptoms and objective findings, including acute hypertension, headache, reflex bradycardia, tachycardia, palpitations, and cardiac arrhythmia. Blood pressure and electrocardiogram monitoring is recommended in patients with high cardiovascular risk (Montague et al, 2003). Evacuation of stagnant intracorporal blood may be required for the medication to be most effective. On the other hand, ischemic priapism of relatively short durations may not necessitate blood evacuation.

Repeated aspirations or irrigations and sympathomimetic injections during several hours may be necessary and should be performed before initiation of surgical intervention. Whereas clinical judgment based on interval physical examination findings is primarily employed to evaluate for resolution, repeated diagnostic studies including color duplex ultrasonography may assist in this regard. Review of the literature has revealed significantly higher resolution of ischemic priapism after sympathomimetic injection with or without irrigation (43% to 81%) than aspiration with or without irrigation alone (24% to 36%) (Montague et al, 2003). Because of the lack of consistent literature support for the use of oral sympathomimetic treatment (e.g., terbutaline and pseudoephedrine) for ischemic priapism, these medications are not recommended for such presentations (Montague et al, 2003).

In patients with an underlying etiologic disorder, intracavernous treatment of ischemic priapism should be provided concurrent with appropriate systemic treatment.

This recommendation applies to priapism associated with sickle cell disease as well as that associated with other hematologic diseases, metastatic neoplasia, or other causes having standard treatments. Support for this recommendation is provided by literature review showing that ischemic priapism resolved in 37% or less of patients with sickle cell disease managed with systemic medical treatments, whereas much better resolution rates were achieved with therapies directed at the penis (Montague et al, 2003). Thus, for priapism related to sickle cell disease, conventionally recommended medical therapies such as analgesia, hydration, oxygenation, alkalinization, and even transfusion may be performed, but these interventions should not lead to delays in intracavernous treatment if prolonged periods of ischemia have occurred (Mantadakis et al, 2000). Clearly, nonischemic priapism associated with sickle cell disease or other hematologic disorders, if confirmed diagnostically, should ideally be managed conservatively consistent with recommendations for this form of priapism.

As a matter of clinical discretion, the surgeon may proceed with surgical intervention once it is apparent that intracavernous treatment has failed. **It is recognized that ischemic priapism of particularly extended durations, such as 48 to 72 hours, is unlikely to resolve with intracavernous treatment, and surgical shunting may be rapidly instituted in this instance** (Montague et al, 2003). A surgical shunt has the objective of facilitating blood drainage from the corpora cavernosa, bypassing the veno-occlusive mechanism of these structures. A variety of shunt procedures may be performed (Fig. 26-2). **A distal cavernoglanular (corporoglanular)**

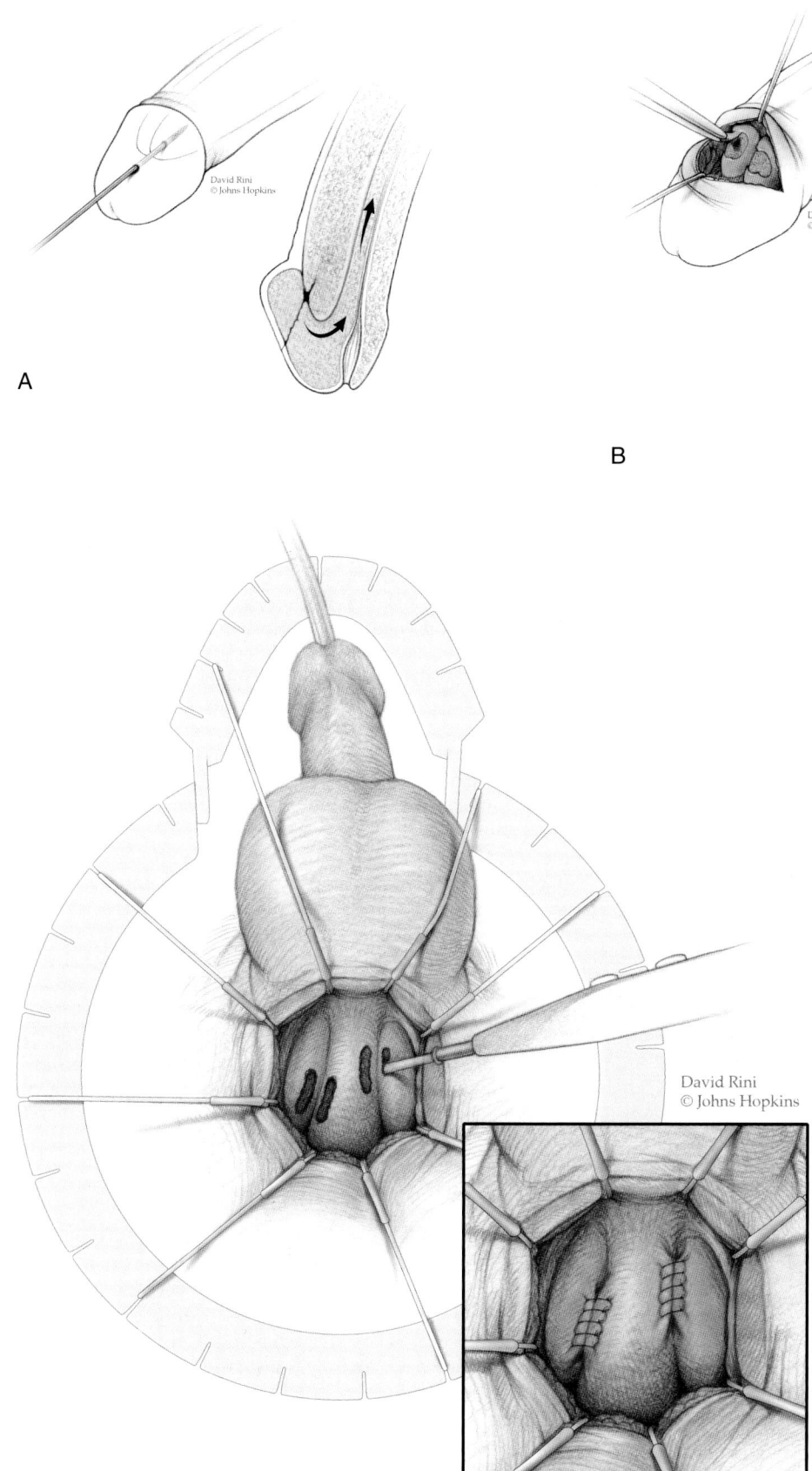

A

B

C

Figure 26–2. Surgical shunts for the treatment of priapism. **A,** Winter shunt, a distal cavernoglanular (corporoglanular) shunt procedure, is depicted by the transglanular placement of a needle or angiocatheter (16- or 18-gauge) into the distal aspect of the corpus cavernosum for blood drainage. **B,** El-Ghorab shunt, a distal cavernoglanular (corporoglanular) shunt procedure; an incision is made dorsally into the glans penis, and portions of the distal corpus cavernosum are excised as a vent for blood drainage. **C,** Quackels or Sacher shunt, a proximal cavernospongiosal (corporospongiosal) shunt procedure; openings are placed in a staggered fashion connecting the cavernosum and spongiosum bilaterally for blood drainage.
Continued

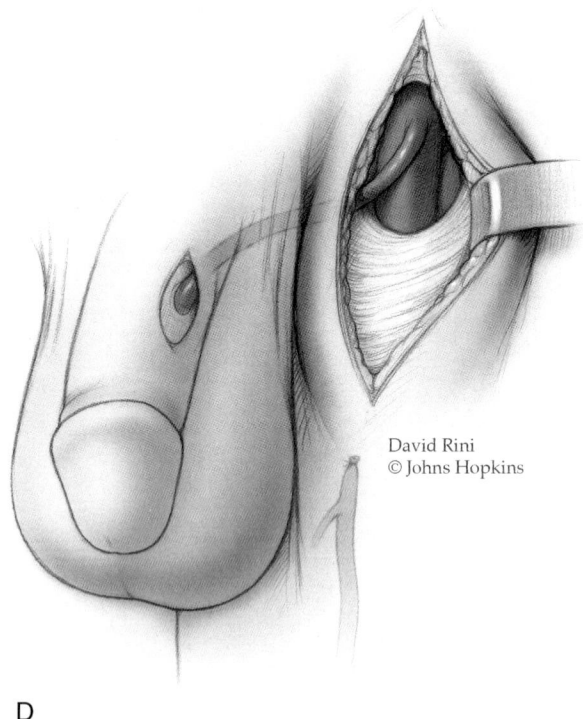

David Rini
© Johns Hopkins

D

Figure 26–2, cont'd. D, Grayhack shunt, also a proximal shunt procedure; the saphenous vein is anastomosed to the corpus cavernosum for blood drainage. (Copyright Johns Hopkins, Baltimore, Md.)

shunt should be the first choice given its ease of performance and association with few complications (Montague et al, 2003). Such shunting procedures include placement of a large biopsy needle (Winter shunt) (Winter, 1976) or a scalpel (Ebbehoj shunt) (Ebbehoj, 1974) percutaneously through the glans or excision of the tunica albuginea at the tip of the corpus cavernosum (El-Ghorab shunt) (Ercole et al, 1981). The El-Ghorab procedure is regarded as the most effective distal shunt, although it is more invasive and thus commonly performed secondarily (Montague et al, 2003; Nixon et al, 2003). **Proximal shunting by creation of a window between the corpus cavernosum and corpus spongiosum (Quackels or Sacher shunt)** (Quackels, 1964; Sacher et al, 1972) **or by anastomosis of the saphenous vein to one of the corpora cavernosa (Grayhack shunt)** (Grayhack et al, 1964) **may be warranted if distal shunting fails.** Serious complications, such as urethral fistulas and purulent cavernositis, have been reported after the various shunt procedures (Ochoa Urdangarain and Hermida Perez, 1998; De Stefani et al, 2001); pulmonary embolism has been reported after the Grayhack procedure (Kandel et al, 1968).

Since most shunts appear to close in time, it is believed that shunting does not produce permanent erectile dysfunction. However, persistence of a shunt has been described to be a cause for erectile dysfunction (Kulmala et al, 1995c), and shunt closure has succeeded in erectile function recovery (Stein et al, 2005). Erectile dysfunction in patients after shunting procedures may be a direct result of the prolonged priapism itself (Nixon et al, 2003).

Ischemic priapism presenting in a significantly delayed fashion may predictably fail to resolve with intracavernous treatment as well as surgical shunting and suggests that erectile dysfunction will be the inevitable outcome. In these cases, some investigators have advocated immediate placement of a penile prosthesis (Monga et al, 1996; Rees et al, 2002). The recommendation is based in part on the knowledge that performance of the surgery at a later time after significant fibrosis has evolved is extremely difficult and fraught with higher complication rates. Also, it has been observed that patients at this clinical juncture commonly do not respond satisfactorily to lesser invasive therapies for erectile dysfunction (Pryor et al, 2004).

Nonischemic Priapism

The initial management of nonischemic priapism should be observation (Berger et al, 2001; Montague et al, 2003). The recommendation is based on the finding that spontaneous resolution is the outcome of untreated nonischemic priapism in up to 62% of reported cases (Montague et al, 2003). Whereas immediate invasive interventions such as embolization and surgery can be performed at the request of the patient, the patient should be thoroughly counseled about the chances for spontaneous resolution, complication risks after treatment, and lack of significant adverse consequences resulting from delayed intervention (Montague et al, 2003). The duration of the priapism even in the time frame of years is not believed to have any impact on subsequent outcome.

Selective arterial embolization offers the next step for the patient desirous of an immediate resolution. **Whereas both nonpermanent (i.e., autologous clot, absorbable gels) and permanent (i.e., coils, ethanol, polyvinyl alcohol particles, and acrylic glue) embolization materials similarly achieve an approximate 75% resolution rate, the nonpermanent materials are preferred as producing a lesser erectile dysfunction rate (5% versus 39% with permanent substances)** (Montague et al, 2003). A complication of perineal abscess after embolization has been reported (Sandock et al, 1996). As an option of last resort, penile exploration and direct surgical ligation of sinusoidal fistulas or pseudoaneurysms may be performed with the assistance of intraoperative color duplex ultrasonography (Montague et al, 2003). Efficacy rates are noted in up to 63% of cases, although erectile dysfunction may occur in up to 50% of cases (Montague et al, 2003).

Recurrent (Stuttering) Priapism

In principle, all episodes of recurrent priapism should be readily treated according to recommendations for ischemic priapism (Montague et al, 2003). **However, the recurrent nature of this form of priapism has prompted the implementation of preventive strategies to offset future episodes.** Such strategies have included systemic therapies, intracavernous self-injection of sympathomimetic agents, and penile prosthesis surgery. Whereas several systemic therapies including hormonal agents (Serjeant et al, 1985; Levine and Guss, 1993; Steinberg and Eyre, 1995; Dahm et al, 2002; Gbadoe et al, 2002), baclofen (Rourke et al, 2002), digoxin (Gupta et al, 1998), and terbutaline (Ahmed and Shaikh, 1997) have been proposed, the most consistently successful treatment has been hormonal treatment, such that this therapy is supported as a primary recommendation (Montague et al, 2003; Levine et al, 2004). Accordingly, a trial of gonadotropin-releasing hormone agonist or androgen receptor antagonist therapy may be used (see Table 26–1). However, hormonal agents should not be used in patients who have not achieved full sexual maturation and adult stature since the therapy may have a contraceptive effect and interfere with the timing of the closure of the epiphyseal plates, respectively. Intracavernous self-injection of phenylephrine may alternatively be explored (Van Driel et al, 1990; Steinberg and Eyre, 1995; Virag et al, 1996; Gbadoe et al, 2001), with proper instruction given to patients in regard to injection site, dosing, potential local and systemic side effects, and duration of erection prompting treatment (Montague et al, 2003).

Miscellaneous Medical Therapies

A host of medical therapies have been reported to produce successful outcomes in the management of priapism. These include hydroxyurea in the treatment of sickle cell–associated priapism (Al Jam'a and Al Dabbous, 1998), methylene blue for high-flow priapism (Steers and Selby, 1991), and thrombolytics such as streptokinase (Gibel et al, 1985) and tissue plasminogen activator (Rutchik et al, 2001) for ischemic priapism. However, limited outcomes data for these treatments preclude strong recommendations for their support at this time.

SUMMARY

Although priapism is an uncommon medical disorder, it deserves proper clinical attention in light of its major potential complications. Significant strides have been made in recent years with regard to its diagnosis and treatment. However, improved treatments remain necessary to avoid adverse consequences, which are still all too prevalent. Innovative potential treatments directed toward reducing pathologic changes (e.g., antioxidant therapy) or impeding pathophysiologic mechanisms (e.g., phosphodiesterase-5 regulators) associated with the disorder carry enormous interest.

Whereas management guidelines have been produced for priapism (Berger et al, 2001; Montague et al, 2003), these are mostly consensus based. Future recommendations will be assisted by continued scientific progress and controlled clinical trial outcomes in the field.

KEY POINTS: PRIAPISM MANAGEMENT

- Ischemic priapism of more than 4 hours in duration irrespective of etiology implies a compartment syndrome and requires decompression of the corpora cavernosa.

- Blood gas testing and color duplex ultrasonography are highly reliable diagnostic methods to distinguish between ischemic and nonischemic priapism.

- Arteriography is not routinely used for diagnosis and is otherwise usually performed as part of an embolization procedure for nonischemic priapism.

- For ischemic priapism, definitive first-line treatment consists of blood aspiration and irrigation of the corpora cavernosa along with intracavernous injection of an α-adrenergic sympathomimetic agent. Secondarily, surgical intervention is applied.

- For nonischemic priapism, initial management consists of observation and only careful secondary application of selective arterial embolization.

SUGGESTED READINGS

Berger R, Billups K, Brock G, et al: Report of the American Foundation for Urologic Disease (AFUD) Thought Leader Panel for evaluation and treatment of priapism. Int J Impot Res 2001;13(suppl 5):S39-S43.
Hinman F: Priapism. Ann Surg 1914;60:689-716.
Montague DK, Jarow J, Broderick GA, et al, members of the Erectile Dysfunction Guideline Update Panel: American Urological Association guideline on the management of priapism. J Urol 2003;170:1318-1324.

27 Androgen Deficiency in the Aging Male

ALVARO MORALES, MD, FRCSC, FACS • JOHN MORLEY, MB, BCH • JEREMY P. W. HEATON, MD, FRCSC, FACS

KEY POINT: SYMPTOMATIC LATE-ONSET HYPOGONADISM

- Symptomatic late-onset hypogonadism (SLOH) is a clinical and biochemical syndrome frequently associated with advancing age and characterized by a deficiency in serum androgen levels with or without changes in receptor sensitivity to androgens. It may affect the function of multiple organ systems and result in a significant detriment in the quality of life.

DEFINITION

Gonadal function diminishes as part of normal aging (Kaufman, 1999). In men this process is not universal, and when it occurs it is usually subtle in its clinical manifestations. Also, there is significant interindividual variability in the age of onset and speed and depth of the androgen decline associated with age, but no factors have emerged that predict the characteristics or effects of the age-related hypotestosteronemia. The syndrome is variously known as androgen decline in the aging male (ADAM), late-onset hypogonadism (LOH), or, less accurately, andropause. When symptomatic (SLOH), it is characterized by multiple clinical manifestations (Table 27–1) (Liu et al, 2004). Urologists often see the same presentation more acutely and dramatically in men subjected to castration for advanced prostate cancer (Nishiyama et al, 2005).

HISTORICAL PERSPECTIVE
Aging and Hormones: From Antiquity to the 21st Century

The importance of the gonads in the maintenance of homeostasis has been recognized since antiquity (Plinius Secundum, 2004). The association of aging with a decline in gonadal function, although a more recent medical observation, has been widely acknowledged since the end of the 19th century

with the report in the scientific literature by Brown-Séquard on his observations about the improvement in his own physical strength and intellectual capacity after administration of a *liquid testiculaire* prepared by him from animal gonads. These reports gave origin to a series of medical claims—reaching its apogee in the 1920s—that exploited testicular extracts and testicular transplants as effective treatments for the infirmities of aging, particularly sexual dysfunction. These techniques of extract administration and heterologous transplantation were eventually exposed as hoaxes (Current Comment, 1927).

Concurrently with the pseudoscience at the turn of the last century, serious investigators were exploring the effects of substances produced and secreted by the testicles. Animal models were employed to demonstrate the activity of autologous testicular transplants, eventually resulting in the isolation of androsterone and testosterone by Laqueur and colleagues (David et al, 1935). By 1935, almost simultaneously and independently, three research teams led by Adolf Butenandt, Kàroly Gyula, and Leopold Ruzicka, who were individually sponsored by three different corporations (Schering, Organon, and Ciba, respectively), synthesized the more powerful testicular hormone, ultimately named testosterone (T). **For this work, Butenandt and Ruzicka received the Nobel Prize for Chemistry in 1939.** After synthesis of the hormone, injectable preparations for human use were developed, and shortly before the onset of World War II clinical trials on T were under way. Interest grew in the use of T for a variety of ailments ranging from sexual difficulties to the prevention of benign prostatic hypertrophy (Cuneo and Jomain, 1938). By the end of World War II, the clinical picture of a syndrome

Table 27–1. **Clinical Manifestations of Late-Onset Hypogonadism and Their Anticipated Response to Treatment**

System/Function	Aging	Response to Testosterone
Erectile function	↓	↑
Sexual desire	↓	↑
Mood/cognition	→/↓	⟡
Tiredness/lack of motivation	↓	↑
Sleep disturbances	→/↑	→
Spatial cognition	↓	⟡
Vasomotor (hot flushes)	↑	↓
Quality of life	↓	↑
Hematocrit	↓	↑
Leptin production	↑	↓
LDL and HDL cholesterol	→	↓
Fat mass	↑	↓
Muscle mass	↓	↑
Bone mass	↓	↑
Hair and skin changes	↓	→

↑, increases/improves; ↓, decreases/deteriorates; →, no change; ⟡, suspected/not proved.
HDL, high-density lipoprotein; LDL, low-density lipoprotein.

named "male climacteric" associated with low T levels was fully recognized (Werner, 1946). T substitution became so widely used that warnings about the indiscriminate use and abuse of the hormone were already being sounded in medical journals by the 1940s (Thompson, 1946).

EPIDEMIOLOGY OF HYPOGONADISM IN AGING

The mean life span in Imperial Rome was about 20 years. Data from United Nations estimates and projections of world population trends over a 75-year period (United Nations Department for Economical and Social Information and Policy Analysis, 1995) tell the full story: In the last decade of the 20th century the number of humans increased by 1 billion, and it will become close to 2 billion over the next 25 years (United Nations Secretariat, 1998). In addition, life expectancy over this period will increase by more than 30 years (United Nations Secretariat, 2004). It follows that the prevalence of hormonal alterations in general and hypogonadism in particular is bound to rise significantly in the first half of this century.

The prevalence of LOH is not accurately known, but it can be inferred from population projections that it is on the rise. **In an attempt to alleviate the scarcity of descriptive epidemiology of androgen deficiency, the Massachusetts Male Aging Study (MMAS) reported a crude incidence rate of 12.3 per 1000 person-years, leading to a prevalence of 481,000 new cases of LOH per year in American men 40 to 69 years old** (Araujo et al, 2004).

PHYSIOLOGIC PRINCIPLES
Regulation of Testosterone Production—Central Mechanisms

Luteinizing hormone (LH) modulates T biosynthesis by Leydig cells and also controls their population (Habert et al,

2001). An example exists in aged animals, in which "hibernation" of Leydig cells develops after prolonged LH suppression (Chen and Zirkin, 1999). **In rodents, aging of the hypothalamus results in an apoptotic process leading to decreased production of gonadotropins** (Morales and Heaton, 2003). **Although not proved in humans, this process may explain a fundamental cause of LOH.** In the testicle the local cellular environment has the potential for impact on regulation and function in a paracrine fashion, mostly in the form of T acting in seminiferous tubules (Fig. 27–1). But Sertoli cells do not appear to have a major impact as long as LH control is active (Young et al, 2000). **Neural influences on Leydig cells have been demonstrated, independent of the pituitary, in the paraventricular nucleus of the hypothalamus** (Selvage and Rivier, 2003), and the peptide gherelin actively regulates Leydig cell activity (Barreiro et al, 2004). These findings have implications for T production independent of central endocrine mechanisms.

Androgen Production in Aging—Peripheral Mechanisms

T and dihydrotestosterone (DHT) are the two main androgens that play the key regulatory roles in determining and later supporting the male phenotype. Androgen effects require the delivery of androgens to the site of action, penetration into the cells, metabolic conversion where necessary, and action with the androgen receptor (AR) on the genome. T is the predominant circulating androgen; the adrenal cortex secretes 19-carbon steroids with weak androgenic activity that serve as precursors for estrogens and active androgens such as T. Very small amounts of steroids are produced in brain cells, but local production may be functionally important (King et al, 2002) and not be represented in serum-based measurements. Leydig cells decrease in numbers in the testes of older men and these men have less T secreted per burst and a decline in secretory bursts in response to LH, suggesting partial desensitization of Leydig cells to LH with aging. Taken together, these studies demonstrate that a component of the decline in T with aging in men is due to testicular failure.

The Transport and Metabolism of Testosterone

T is exchanged readily through cellular membranes with the extracellular environment. The passive transfer of T through membranes means that serum concentrations reflect general tissue androgen levels except where local sources of production or conversion exist. T is 98% bound to proteins (sex hormone–binding globulin [SHBG] and albumin; see Fig. 27–1) in the circulation, in which form it is relatively spared hepatic metabolism. The binding to SHBG and that to albumin have different affinities, providing the concept of bioavailable T: T bound to albumin is more readily unbound for use.

Metabolism. T levels are determined by the relative rates of production and metabolism. T can be aromatized to 17β-estradiol or reduced to 5α-DHT. Aromatization by cytochrome P450$_{arom}$ and the supply of T substrate determine estrogen availability in estrogen-dependent cells such as those in the testis, fat, liver, hair follicles, and brain (de Ronde et al, 2003). There are two isoforms of 5α-reductase, and the cellular availability of 5α-DHT depends on T reduction and the

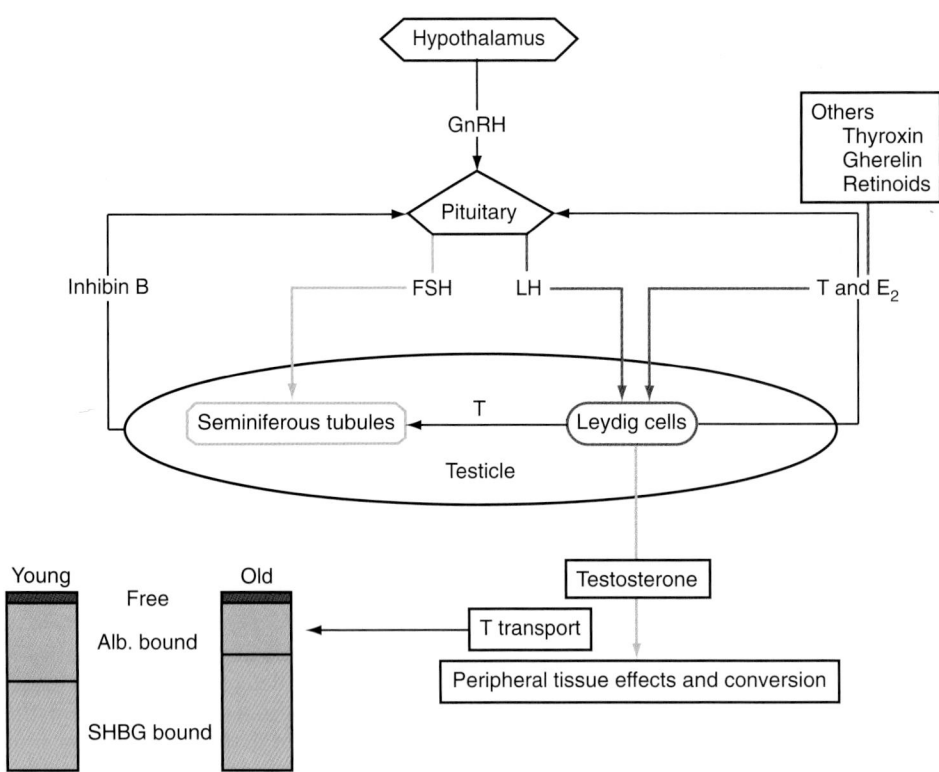

Figure 27–1. Effect of aging on the production, transport, and metabolism of testosterone (T). Luteinizing hormone (LH) is the major but not the only regulator of T production. Aging of the hypothalamus and the pituitary results in decreased production of gonadotropin-releasing hormone (GnRH) and LH, respectively. T circulates free (2%) or bound to albumin or sex hormone–binding globulin (SHBG). Binding of T to SHBG renders it unavailable to most tissues. SHBG increases with aging. Bioavailable T (free and albumin-bound fractions) is metabolically active and can be converted to other hormones (dihydrotestosterone, dehydroepiandrosterone, estradiol [E_2]). FSH, follicle-stimulating hormone.

rate of DHT metabolism. **The balance between T and DHT metabolic enzyme activity is more critical to the cells in which it is occurring than to the overall rate of T metabolism.** With aging, changes occur in enzyme functions that can potentially skew cellular activities in a way that is hidden from any systemic measures of androgen status. T catabolism takes place mostly in the liver, prostate, and skin, and catabolic products are largely excreted in the urine.

The Androgen Receptor

T and DHT act through the androgen receptor (AR), which is a ligand-inducible transcription factor. The AR structure includes a COOH-terminal ligand binding domain, a DNA binding domain, a hinge region, a variable-length CAG repeat region, and an NH_2-terminal transactivation domain (Glass et al, 1997). Most of the transactivational activity is associated with the NH_2 terminus. The CAG repeat stretch is maximal in man (about 22 triplets) and decreases with evolutionary distance from man (Choong and Wilson, 1998). The hinge region is responsible for nuclear function after hormone binding. The ligand binding domain acts with the help of molecular chaperones, which increase the affinity for the hormone of the unbound AR (Fang et al, 1996).

T is transported through the cellular membrane, binds to the inactive AR complex, and is translocated to the nucleus. The binding of T to DNA activates the basal transcription machinery, so regulating the transcription of target genes. Although the time frame for this genomic activity is of the order of 30 to 60 minutes, there are nongenomic actions that take place too rapidly to follow this pathway. These rapid actions may be due to activation or possibly binding to undetermined membrane-bound receptors. **The AR may be activated without the presence of ligand, for example, by protein kinase C, a factor that has great importance in the androgen interaction with prostate cancer cells** (Culig, 2004).

CAG Repeat Polymorphism and Aging

The CAG repeat lengths of the AR vary from 6 to 39, depending on race (Valdehuis et al, 2005). In general, increased androgenic effect is seen at any level of T in men with shorter CAG repeat length. In older men, lower T is associated with fewer CAG repeats. The association of polymorphic AR with LOH symptoms showed that older men with more than 23 CAG repeats had less elevated LH, normal T, and less decreased potency but more depression, more anxiety, more deterioration of general well-being, and decreased beard growth (Harkonen et al, 2003). Changes in the AR can play a major role in the symptomatic response to T, potentially explaining some of the variability in clinical presentation in men with similar serum T.

Androgen Actions

T actions on sexual function, spermatogenesis, and the prostate are dealt with in other chapters. Action of T in other systems (i.e., musculoskeletal) are included later in the chapter. The remainder are outlined in the following.

Testosterone and Glucose Metabolism

The metabolic syndrome (MS) is a complex association of several interrelated abnormalities that increase the risk for cardiovascular disease and progression to diabetes mellitus. Insulin resistance is the key factor for the clustering of risk factors. Hypogonadism is seen frequently in association with the MS (Dhindsa et al, 2004), and several studies show that the fundamental cardiovascular risk parameters can be improved by the administration of T to these men. Hypogonadal men have increased leptin, obesity, and insulin that become normal with exogenous T treatment, which also reduces abdominal fat mass and improves insulin action (Zitzmann and Nieschlag, 2003). T administration to older men is associated with decreased visceral fat and glucose concentrations and increased insulin sensitivity (Bhasin, 2003). Hypogonadism correlates with high serum glucose, high triglycerides, high body mass, high waist-to-hip ratio, high total body fat mass, and high fasting insulin resistance index. Treatment with T improves the MS, especially in overweight older men (Schroeder et al, 2004).

Androgens and the Brain

A relationship between hypogonadism and depression has not been conclusively established. However, there are studies showing improvements in measures of well-being in aging men with hypogonadism (Azad et al, 2003) and in hypogonadal men with human immunodeficiency virus (Grinspoon et al, 2000). Depression scores are higher and T levels lower in men with shorter CAG repeats, and these men are more susceptible to the depressive effects of low T (Seidman et al, 2001). There are well-researched gender differences in selected areas of cognition such as verbal skills and spatial tests that point to the developmental influence of T (Halpern et al, 1998). Studies of hypogonadal men suggest that some cognitive skills can be improved with replacement therapy (O'Connor et al, 2001), but this is not invariably seen as there are clearly many potential causes of impaired cognition.

DIAGNOSIS
Clinical Diagnosis

Clinical diagnosis of LOH is problematic because neither a low serum T nor symptoms are truly diagnostic of the condition. The presence of symptoms, however, is a sine qua non for diagnosis and should be coupled with a low or borderline low objective biochemical measure of T status. In practice, this ideal is not always achievable. Thus, it has been suggested (Black et al, 2004) that in the presence of symptoms but without strong biochemical support, a therapeutic trial would be an acceptable diagnostic approach; it should be noted that a sustained placebo response can be observed for up to a year (Haren et al, 2005).

KEY POINT: LOH DEFINITION

■ A dichotomy exists in the definition of LOH: the statistical approach defines LOH purely on the basis of biochemical parameters and selects percentile cutoff values from young healthy males to determine prevalence. The clinical approach relies primarily on clinical findings. Neither in isolation is sufficient. The combination of both approaches together with adequate clinical judgment is of paramount importance in the management of this condition.

The clinical picture has been recognized for many years (see Table 27–1). Among the most prominent symptoms are tiredness, hypoactive sexual desire, and dysphoria. These manifestations need not all be present to identify the syndrome. In addition, the severity of one or more of them does not necessarily match the severity of the others, nor do we yet understand the uneven appearance of these manifestations. **LOH symptoms recur after discontinuation of therapy at highly reproducible intraindividual T levels, but the trigger level differs widely among individuals** (Table 27–2) (Kelleher et al, 2004).

The **physical examination** suffers the same shortcomings as the history, mainly lack of specificity. Testicular atrophy may be present together with a decrease in pubic and facial hair. Sarcopenia and increase in visceral fat can also be part of the findings. The sequelae of osteoporosis become evident in long-standing cases. None of these are, alone or in combination, sufficient to make a definitive diagnosis, although the composite of history and findings on examination provides a strong case for a presumptive diagnosis of LOH.

Screening Questionnaires for Late-Onset Hypogonadism

Three questionnaires have been developed to detect hypogonadism in adult men: (1) St. Louis University's ADAM, (2) the Aging Male Survey (AMS), and (3) the MMAS. The first two are symptom questionnaires, and the last one represents a mixture of symptoms and epidemiologic findings. The ADAM questionnaire (Table 27–3) in the original validation had a sensitivity and specificity of 88% and 60%, respectively, against serum bioavailable T (BT) levels (Morley et al, 2000). In a follow-up study, BT and calculated free T (cFT) were lower in ADAM positive than in ADAM negative men. The effectiveness of the ADAM questionnaire as a screening tool has been confirmed by most independent investigators (Tancredi et al, 2004). The AMS (Fig. 27–2) (Moore et al, 2004), in our hands, has sensitivity (83%) and specificity (39%) similar to those of the ADAM, but in a European study none of the three AMS domains correlated significantly with serum levels of total, bioavailable, or free T in men older than 70 (T'Sjoen

Table 27-2. Spectrum and Severity of Late-Onset Hypogonadism Symptoms*

Symptom (N = 52)	Minimally to Mildly Problematic	Moderately Problematic	Very Problematic
Loss of energy	10 (19%)	17 (33%)	19 (36%)
Diminished libido	14 (27%)	10 (20%)	8 (15%)
Lack of motivation	9 (18%)	12 (23%)	8 (15%)
Irritability	4 (8%)	10 (20%)	11 (20%)
Sleepiness after meal	6 (12%)	5 (10%)	12 (23%)
Inability to concentrate	14 (26%)	4 (8%)	4 (8%)
Hot flashes	10 (20%)	2 (4%)	2 (4%)
Muscular aches	2 (4%)	0	6 (12%)

*Symptoms appearing after discontinuation of treatment with depot subdermal administration of testosterone (see text for details).
Adapted from Kelleher S, Conway AJ, Handelsman DJ: Blood testosterone threshold for androgen deficiency symptoms. J Clin Endocrinol Metab 2004;89:3813–3817.

AMS Questionnaire

Which of the following symptoms apply to you at this time? Please mark the appropriate box for each symptom. For symptoms that do not apply, please mark "none."

Symptoms Score =	None 1	Mild 2	Moderate 3	Severe 4	Extremely severe 5
1. **Decline in your feeling of general well-being** (general state of health, subjective feeling)	☐	☐	☐	☐	☐
2. **Joint pain and muscular ache** (lower back pain, joint pain, pain in a limb, general back ache)	☐	☐	☐	☐	☐
3. **Excessive sweating** (unexpected/sudden episodes of sweating, hot flushes independent of strain)	☐	☐	☐	☐	☐
4. **Sleep problems** (difficulty in falling asleep, difficulty in sleeping through, waking up early and feeling tired, poor sleep, sleeplessness)	☐	☐	☐	☐	☐
5. **Increased need for sleep, often feeling tired**	☐	☐	☐	☐	☐
6. **Irritability** (feeling aggressive, easily upset about little things, moody)	☐	☐	☐	☐	☐
7. **Nervousness** (inner tension, restlessness, feeling fidgety)	☐	☐	☐	☐	☐
8. **Anxiety** (feeling panicky)	☐	☐	☐	☐	☐
9. **Physical exhaustion/lacking vitality** (general decrease in performance, reduced activity, lacking interest in leisure activities, feeling of getting less done, of achieving less, of having to force oneself to undertake activities)	☐	☐	☐	☐	☐
10. **Decrease in muscular strength** (feeling of weakness)	☐	☐	☐	☐	☐
11. **Depressive mood** (feeling down, sad, on the verge of tears, lack of drive, mood swings, feeling nothing is of any use)	☐	☐	☐	☐	☐
12. **Feeling that you have passed your peak**	☐	☐	☐	☐	☐
13. **Feeling burnt out, having hit rock-bottom**	☐	☐	☐	☐	☐
14. **Decrease in beard growth**	☐	☐	☐	☐	☐
15. **Decrease in ability/frequency to perform sexually**	☐	☐	☐	☐	☐
16. **Decrease in the number of morning erections**	☐	☐	☐	☐	☐
17. **Decrease in sexual desire/libido** (lacking pleasure in sex, lacking desire for sexual intercourse)	☐	☐	☐	☐	☐

Have you got any other major symptoms?   Yes.......☐   No.....☐
If Yes, please describe: _____

Thank you very much for your cooperation

Figure 27–2. The Aging Male Survey (AMS). This questionnaire has three domains: Psychological (questions 6, 7, 8, 11, 13), Somatovegetative (questions 1, 2, 3, 4, 5, 9, 10), and Sexual (questions 12, 14, 15, 16, 17). The minimum and maximum scores are 5 and 25, respectively, for the Psychological and Sexual domains and 7 and 35 for the Somatovegetative domain. The higher the score, the more severe the symptoms.

Table 27–3. The Androgen Deficiency in Aging Male (ADAM) Questionnaire

A positive answer represents yes to 1 or 7 or any 3 other questions. (Circle one)

Yes No	1.	Do you have a decrease in libido (sex drive)?
Yes No	2.	Do you have a lack of energy?
Yes No	3.	Do you have a decrease in strength and/or endurance?
Yes No	4.	Have you lost height?
Yes No	5.	Have you noticed a decreased enjoyment of life?
Yes No	6.	Are you sad and/or grumpy?
Yes No	7.	Are your erections less strong?
Yes No	8.	Have you noticed a recent deterioration in your ability to play sports?
Yes No	9.	Are you falling asleep after dinner?
Yes No	10.	Has there been a recent deterioration in your work performance?

et al, 2004). In contrast, the MMAS showed a sensitivity of 60% and a specificity of 59%. **These questionnaires are useful as a screening tools but fall short of expectation for diagnostic purposes.** Their value as outcome measures after T treatment remains undetermined.

Biochemical Diagnosis

T values decline while SHBG levels increase with aging. In young men, about 60% of circulating T is bound to SHBG, 38% is bound to albumin, and 1% to 2% is free (see Fig. 27–1). The T that is free and bound to albumin is considered to be capable of entering tissues and to be responsible for the actions of T. SHBG-bound T is inaccessible to tissues and not active. **It should be recognized that in some tissues, such as** the prostate, T bound to SHBG can activate SHBG receptors and produce effects within the cell (Rosner et al, 1999). The active component (free plus albumin bound) is called bioavailable or bioeffective T (BT). Epidemiologic studies suggest that BT correlates better with symptoms associated with T deficiency than total T.

Assays for Testosterone

Establishing the presence of hypogonadism on a purely clinical basis is difficult. Only the most severe cases bring up clinical suspicion. The support of the biochemical evaluation is, therefore, fundamental in the diagnosis of the condition.

KEY POINT: BIOCHEMISTRY

■ In patients at risk for or suspected of having hypogonadism, the following investigations should be done: (1) T determination from blood taken between 8:00 and 11:00 AM. For screening purposes total T determination is usually sufficient. (2) If T levels are below or at the lower limit of the accepted normal values, it is prudent to confirm the results with a second determination together with assessment of gonadotropins (LH) and prolactin. (3) In the younger male, low levels of T (<12 nmol/L or <350 ng/dL) with chronically elevated gonadotropins make a clear diagnosis of primary hypogonadism. (4) In an older man the diagnostic lines are not as clearly defined and additional information may be needed (see Fig. 27–3).

The urologist should become familiar with the range and quality of the T assays offered by the local laboratory as well as the intra- and interindividual variations in serum T levels. Assay techniques have improved greatly, but many laboratories have paid scant attention to the accuracy or the normal range of their assays. Three assays for measurement of total T are commonly used: (1) radioimmunoassay, (2) nonradioactive immunoassay kits, and (3) automated platform assays that use chemiluminescent detection. There is significant interassay variability: a value of 297 ng/dL (10.3 nmol) showed a variation from 160 to 508 ng/dL (5.5 to 17.6 nmol). In addition, the coefficients of variation ranged from 5.1% to 22.7%. Fortunately, most of the assay techniques had regression slopes close to 1 and correlation coefficients of 0.92 to 0.97 compared with liquid chromatography–tandem mass spectroscopy (Wang et al, 2004a).

In young men, but not in older men, there is a substantial circadian rhythm with higher values being obtained in the morning. In addition, in both young and old persons there is substantial variability (+20%) from week to week (Morley et al, 2002). Thus, two samples obtained a week or two apart, ideally in the morning, would seem to be a minimal criterion. The assays that more closely reflect tissue available T are (1) free T only if measured by ultracentrifugal ultrafiltration or dialysis techniques, (2) BT, generally measured by an ammonium sulfate precipitation technique, and (3) calculated free T or BT that can be obtained by measuring T and SHBG with or without an albumin level (see later).

Assays for BT and free T are cumbersome, costly, and not readily available. Vermeulen and colleagues (1999) provided a solution for situations in which the more reliable BT or free T determinations are not accessible: a calculation can be made from the values obtained for total T and the determination of SHBG. It has become known as calculated free T or simply cFT. This method provides a good correlation with the values of nonbound T. The formula is available at http://www.issam.ch. Although this approach, in general, works well, there are pitfalls: (1) different SHBG levels varying up to twofold with different assays and (2) altered binding characteristics (either SHBG or serum) related to aging or illness. The relative advantages, drawbacks, and usefulness of the various assays are given in Table 27–4.

KEY POINT: INAPPROPRIATE ASSAY

■ The assay that should not be used is commonly available and frequently ordered: direct radioimmunoassay of free T using a labeled T analog with low affinity for SHBG and albumin that binds to an immobilized antibody that is specific for T. This assay has poor accuracy and precision. It is most closely related to the measurement of total T. Clinicians are thus misled to believe that true "free T" is being measured.

Table 27–4. **Assays for Testosterone and Their Attributes**

Assay	Utility	Comments
Total testosterone	Low/intermediate	Variable normal ranges; below 200 ng/dL very likely to be hypogonadal; above 600 ng/dL unlikely to be
Free testosterone		
Dialysis	High	Difficult to do; requires ³H-T
Ultrafiltration	High	
Analog	Poor	Commonly available in N/A
Calculated free	Intermediate	Requires SHBG and T measurements
Bioavailable testosterone		
Ammonium sulfate	High	Easier to do than free T; excellent precipitation assay; good correlation with symptoms
Calculated bioavailable	Intermediate	Requires SHBG and T measurements
Free androgen index		
Testosterone/SHBG	Poor	Requires SHBG and T measurements
Salivary testosterone	Undetermined	Uncertain value

SHBG, sex hormone–binding globulin; T, testosterone.

DIAGNOSTIC ALGORITHM FOR SLOH

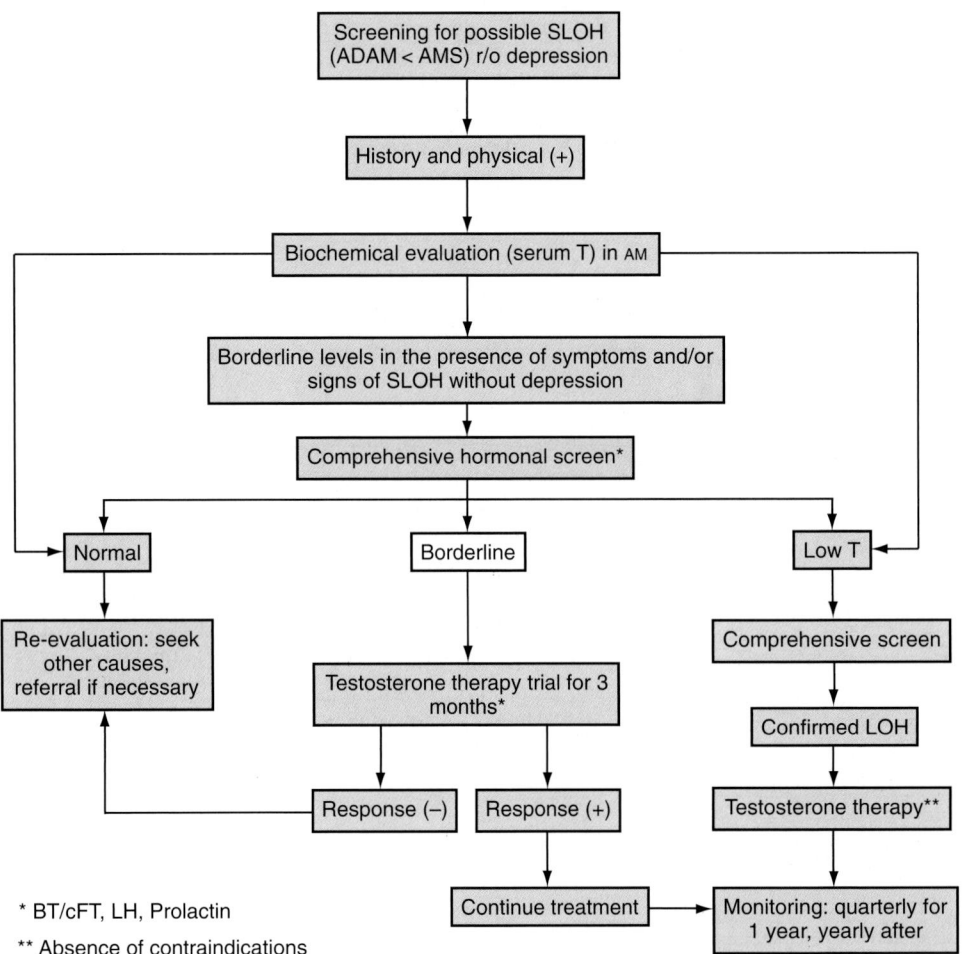

Figure 27–3. Diagnostic algorithm for symptomatic late-onset hypogonadism (SLOH). Screening questionnaires are appropriate for initial assessment. A comprehensive hormonal screen includes either a repeated measurement of total testosterone (T) or bioavailable or calculated free T (BT/cFT) to assess the non–sex hormone–binding globulin fraction. A basic evaluation of the pituitary (prolactin, luteinizing hormone [LH]) is indicated in the presence of low T levels. Other hormones (dihydrotestosterone, dehydroepiandrosterone, growth hormone, melatonin) are not generally necessary. ADAM, Androgen Deficiency in Aging Male; AMS, Aging Male Survey; r/o, rule out.

Because of the controversial nature of the biochemical assessment, **when the biochemistry does not support a strong clinical picture, other causes have been ruled out, and no contraindications exist, a 90-day therapeutic/diagnostic trial of T administration is justified** (Black et al, 2000) (Fig. 27–3).

Other Hormones

It is important to dispel the concept that endocrinopathies resulting from the normal process of aging in men are narrowly focused on sex steroids. Although hypotestosteronemia is most widely recognized, the production of several other hormones is also profoundly affected by age (Table 27–5).

Dehydroepiandrosterone

Production of dehydroepiandrosterone (DHEA) reaches a peak in the second to third decade of life and decreases steadily afterward, to very low values (<30% of those in the young) by the age of 70 (Vermeulen, 1995). The finding of a putative specific DHEA receptor on the plasma membrane of bovine aortic endothelial cells (Liu and Dillon, 2002) is radically changing our understanding of the role of DHEA in many functions, particularly in the vascular system. Kawano and colleagues (2003) and Simoncini and associates (2003) have

Table 27–5. Hormones, besides Testosterone, Most Commonly Affected by the Aging Process*		
Hormone	*Production*	*Function and Real/Putative Effects*
DHEA	⇩	Neurosteroid. Regulation of vascular endothelium
Growth hormone	⇩	Somatic growth. Anabolic effects mediated by IGF-I (protein synthesis and cell proliferation)
Melatonin	⇩	Regulation of biorhythms and sleep patterns. Prevention of oxidative stress
Thyroxin	⇩	
Leptin	⇧	Regulation of appetite and fat distribution. Receptor expressed in prostate gland

*For most, their functions are not fully understood in most cases. It is known, however, that there is a great deal of cross talk among them in their production, function, and activity.
DHEA, dehydroepiandrosterone; IGF, insulin-like growth factor.

documented an improvement in vascular endothelial function in middle-aged men with a variety of vascular problems. These findings may have direct and significant implications for the mechanisms of sexual function. DHEA may have a dual role in sexual function: an indirect endocrinologic and a direct vascular role.

Growth Hormone

The production of growth hormone (GH) also decreases with age, about 14% per decade (Veldhuis, 1997). This reduction is associated with changes in lean muscle mass, bone density, hair distribution, and the pattern of obesity described also in hypogonadal states (Molitch, 2002). **Administration of GH reverses these alterations** (Murray and Shalet, 2002) **and does it more efficiently in eugonadal men than in their hypogonadal counterparts** (Lesse et al, 1998). Although the body of evidence favors the use of androgens in the treatment of some of the manifestations of ADAM, more recent studies clearly indicate that elderly patients respond to GH administration alone (Gola et al, 2005). Some of the concerns about androgen supplementation in elderly men (e.g., prostate health) may be shared by GH administration. Although no changes in prostate-specific antigen (PSA) were found in adults receiving injectable GH (Colao et al, 2003), the simultaneous administration of GH and T may lead to significant increases in prostate size (Vance, 2003).

Melatonin

Melatonin is secreted in response to hypoglycemia and darkness. Its production by the pineal gland also decreases with age regardless of these stimuli (Liu et al, 1999). The physiologic role of the pineal gland is not completely understood, but it is involved in gonadal function and regulation of biorhythms. However, the popular enthusiasm about the hormone has a precarious scientific basis. It is likely that administration of melatonin may improve sleep disorders, frequently seen in elderly persons, but profound hypogonadism is associated with alterations in melatonin production, making it difficult to attribute some symptoms exclusively to deficits of one or the other hormone. Evidence is emerging of a wide range of direct and indirect activities of melatonin on many human organ systems (Reiter and Tan, 2004), although its role in sleep disturbances in the aging population has been challenged (Tozawa et al, 2003).

Thyroxin

Changes occur with aging in the hypothalamic-pituitary-thyroid axis resulting in the development of hypothyroidism, which may reach an incidence of close to 20% in the elderly population (Leitolf et al, 2002). The production of prolactin, corticosteroids, and estradiol (E_2) in males remains fairly constant throughout life. On the contrary, leptin is altered in hypotestosteronemia, which explains, in part, some of the changes in fat distribution observed in these men (Bray and York, 1997). Levels of leptin can be brought down by androgen supplementation (Luukkaa et al, 1998), which usually results in an improvement in obesity (Behere et al, 1997). **The linkage between obesity and prostate cancer is of interest. Obesity contributes to a higher risk for prostate cancer incidence and mortality as well as its aggressiveness and recurrence** (Ribeiro et al, 2004). It appears that the relationship is not simply due to the excess fats. The leptin receptor is expressed in prostatic tissue, leptin promotes prostate growth during puberty, and it might stimulate cancer development by a direct effect on the gland (Stattin et al, 2001). It has been shown that there exists an inverse correlation between plasma leptin and T levels in men with advanced prostate cancer. Equally relevant is the finding that leptin is capable of inducing proliferation of androgen-independent prostate cancer cells. The role of leptin in prostate cancer remains to be fully explored.

TREATMENT OF SYMPTOMATIC LATE-ONSET HYPOGONADISM

The clinical picture of SLOH is not specific, and some manifestations can be effectively treated with methods other than sex hormone administration. Changes in lifestyle (smoking and alcohol abuse cessation) should be advised to all patients. Diet and exercise do decrease visceral obesity and improve muscle strength and sensation of well-being. Biphosphonates are effective drugs for osteoporosis, and antidepressants and counseling work well for dysphoria. However, programs of lifestyle changes are characterized by a high dropout rate or only intermittent adherence. In most cases, in the presence of confirmed hypogonadism, the administration of T alone results in significant improvement in many of the signs and symptoms of the condition. That better results are achieved with lifestyle changes and additional nonhormonal medications is not debatable.

In clinical practice there are few valid and specific reasons to withhold T treatment in men with SLOH. The case for treatment is compelling. Hypogonadism in itself did not appear to influence life expectancy, as reported in a historical analysis of castrati ($n = 50$) (Nieschlag and Behre, 2004). A retrospective study (Tomlinson et al, 2001) suggests a more credible view: standardized mortality ratio is significantly higher in men with untreated gonadotropin deficiency compared with those treated with sex steroids and healthy control subjects.

Options for Treatment with Testosterone

There is an ever increasing selection of T delivery formulations available, of which the vast majority are safe and effective. Currently obtainable preparations of T are listed in Table 27–6.

Intramuscular Injections

Intramuscular injections of T are long acting and reach a maximum concentration at about 72 hours. They do not provide normal circadian patterns of serum T. Levels of DHT are usually normal, but E_2 levels may become excessive in some men. In the first few days after injection, supraphysiologic serum T levels occur. These injections are commonly administered every 10 to 21 days to maintain normal average T levels; baseline values are reached at approximately 21 days. These T preparations are cost efficient and proven effective (Amory et al, 2004). T undecanoate (TU, Nebido) for injection (1000 mg per dose) has been introduced. After a loading dose, administration of 1000 mg every 12 weeks resulted in stable serum levels within the normal range (Schubert et al, 2004). This product is not yet available in North America.

Oral Preparations

Oral agents available in the United States include the alkylated (to prevent rapid hepatic metabolism) androgen preparations, which are generally associated with erratic androgenic effects,

Table 27–6. Most Frequently Used Testosterone Preparations

	Generic Name	Trade Name	Dose	Comments
Injectable	Testosterone cypionate	Depo-Testosterone cypionate	200-400 mg every 3-4 weeks	Supraphysiologic levels. Roller-coaster effect
	Testosterone enanthate	Delatestryl	200-400 mg every 4 weeks	Same as cypionate
	Testosterone undecanoate*	Nebido	1000 mg every 12-14 weeks*	Stable levels. Short experience
Oral/buccal	Buccal tabs	Striant	30 mg twice daily	Inconvenient
	Methyltestosterone[†]	Metandren	10-30 mg daily	Liver toxicity
	Testosterone undecanoate	Andriol Testocaps	120-160 mg daily	Not available in United States
Transdermal	Testosterone patch	Androderm	5 mg daily	Skin reactions Visible
		Testoderm	10-15 mg/day	Skin reactions
	Testosterone gel	Androgel/Testim	5-10 g/day	Good tolerability. Reproduces circadian rhythm

*Requires a loading 3 × 1000 mg every 6 weeks for naïve patients or 2 × 1000 mg every 8 weeks for those switching from a different testosterone formulation.
[†]As 17α alkylated testosterone products, both fluoxymesterone and methyltestosterone are associated with potential for serious liver toxicity.

significant changes in lipid profile, and a risk of liver toxicity. They are rarely used. Although not available in the United States, oral TU (Andriol) is commonly used throughout the world. It is free of liver toxicity but may result in supraphysiologic levels of DHT (Gooren, 1994). It is taken with meals in two divided doses.

Buccal

This mucoadhesive delivery system (Striant) is placed against the gum above the incisor tooth twice a day (30 mg). To diminish the incidence of local irritation (about 9%), the site of application should be alternated. It is somewhat inconvenient.

Transdermal Testosterone Therapy

Transdermal T therapy is available in patches and gels. Both result in normal serum T levels and reproduce the diurnal physiologic variations with normal E_2 and DHT levels. Drawbacks of the patches include their visibility and skin reactions (Jordan and Atkinson, 1998). Transdermal T gel preparations are better tolerated (minimal skin irritation). The experience with one of these formulations (Androgel) is now beyond 3 years. They result in improved sexual function and mood and increased lean body mass and muscle strength associated with a decrease in fat mass (Wang et al, 2004b). The studies, however, are limited in the size of the sample, the age range of the participants, and the length of follow-up.

Dihydrotestosterone

The use of DHT as an alternative to T appears occasionally in the literature (Kunelius et al, 2002). **The main argument for the use of DHT is that it is not aromatizable and, as such, may prevent prostate enlargement (believed to require both androgens and estrogens).** The transdermal DHT preparation is easy to use, but long-term studies are still lacking and its use outside proper trials is not recommended (Wang and Swerdloff, 2002).

7α-Methyl-19-Nortestosterone

Much interest exists in the use of androgens that spare the most prominent adverse effects of T supplementation. Among the drugs better recognized and most promising, although not yet commercially available, is 7α-methyl-19-nortestosterone

(MENT). It has high biopotency per molecule (about 10 times more than T), does not undergo 5α reduction, but retains its capacity to be aromatized to E_2. It has antigonadotropic properties and anabolic effects on muscles. It maintains sexual function in hypogonadotropic men, and its effects on the prostate are less pronounced than those of T (Kumar et al, 1999).

Selective Androgen Receptor Modulators

The therapeutic potential of selective estrogen receptor modulators (SERMs) in women has set the stage for the development of selective androgen receptor modulators (SARMs). The availability of these molecules with their diversity of ligands provides the opportunity to explore the utility and activities of SARMs (Negro-Vilar, 1999). Various SARMs are under active investigation but not available for the foreseeable future.

KEY POINT: CHOICE OF PREPARATION

- The choice among T preparations depends on **a**vailability, **s**afety, **t**olerability, **e**fficacy, and **p**reference (by patient and physician): ASTEP.

Objective Effects of Testosterone

Administration of T to hypogonadal men results in a variety of positive effects (Table 27–1) including the following.

Body Composition and Strength

Studies consistently report changes in body composition with T therapy (Snyder et al, 1999). The magnitude of the fat mass changes in older men appeared similar to that seen with T replacement in young hypogonadal men, whereas the lean body mass changes produced were usually less dramatic. In terms of strength changes, the effects are more limited in older men. Most studies noted an increase in grip strength with T treatment (Vermeulen, 2002) but **the effects are significant even when T is administered with finasteride, indicating** that DHT is not necessary for these positive actions (Page et al, 2005).

Bone

A number of studies have evaluated the effects of T therapy on bone mineral density or biochemical parameters of bone turnover in older men. These studies have lasted from 3 to 36 months, with the shorter-term trials evaluating only bone turnover parameters. T therapy was reported to slow the rate of bone degradation and significantly increase bone mineral density, especially in the lumbar spine (Szule et al, 2003). No study has yet evaluated the effect of T therapy on the occurrence of osteoporotic fractures.

Cardiovascular System

Most epidemiologic studies have shown that higher serum T levels correlate with lower, rather than higher, cardiovascular disease risk in men (Zamuda et al, 1997). Cardiovascular disease risk factors that might be affected by sex steroids include serum lipoprotein profiles, vascular tone, platelet and red blood cell clotting parameters, and the direct process of atherogenesis (Muller et al, 2003). The effects on serum lipoprotein levels in older men are the one area in which T therapy has been more extensively evaluated (Jockenhovel et al, 1999). In general, **T therapy in older men leads to a decrease in total and low-density lipoprotein cholesterol levels with no change or a small decrease in high-density lipoprotein cholesterol** levels. These lipoprotein changes are modest, and the ultimate impact on cardiovascular disease is unknown.

Sexual Function

The efficacy of T administration to men with sexual dysfunction needs to be discussed in two different areas: sexual desire and erectile function.

Sexual Desire. Hypogonadal men frequently experience hypoactive sexual desire disorder (HSDD). The threshold of serum androgen levels for adequate libido, however, exhibits large interindividual variability and is largely dependent on a number of intrapsychical and environmental factors (Morley, 2003). As monotherapy, T administration is successful in a majority of patients, but it is difficult to assess outcomes of sexual interest and there is a need for large controlled studies in this area. It is, however, widely recognized that HSDD and low serum T levels are a clear indication for therapy.

Erectile Dysfunction. An adequate amount of T is essential for the cascading of mechanisms driving the penile erectile response: production of nitric oxide synthase, release of nitric oxide, and augmentation of the synthesis of cyclic guanine monophosphate leading to arteriolar dilatation and relaxation of the corporeal smooth muscle. **When a critical low-androgen milieu is reached, this complex process is blunted or fails altogether.** The critical androgen level for adequate maintenance of the process remains to be determined, but, undoubtedly, it exhibits large interindividual (and possibly some intraindividual) inconsistency. For this reason, in the presence of a combination of erectile insufficiency and hypotestosteronemia, a trial of supplemental androgen is justified. If no success is evident, other causes need to be explored.

Synergism of Testosterone with Phosphodiesterase 5 Inhibitors

In cases of recalcitrant erectile dysfunction (ED), a multi-pronged pharmacologic approach may be more effective than the single-agent management. Specifically in cases of ED and hypogonadism, the available evidence is encouraging. Aversa and coauthors (2003) showed in a small, controlled, randomized study that hypogonadal patients in whom sildenafil failed could be rescued by the administration of T. The proposed mechanism of action in the study was vascular because increased arterial dilatation was documented by Doppler ultrasonography. These findings have been supported by the report of Shabsigh and coworkers (2004) showing a significantly better response in the erectile function domains for the combination of T plus sildenafil compared with sildenafil alone in hypogonadal men. Kalinchenko and colleagues (2003) treated a group of type 2 diabetics with sildenafil. In the group of hypogonadal patients who had initially failed a trial of sildenafil alone, 70% responded to the combination of sildenafil and oral TU. Further exploration of class agents (i.e., phosphodiesterase 5 inhibitors, dopaminergic agonists) in combination with androgens needs to be pursued vigorously.

Adverse Effects of Testosterone Treatment

The presence of prostate or breast carcinoma is an absolute contraindication for T treatment. However, T administration can result in adverse effects that are particularly significant in elderly persons. These include the following.

Fluid retention is rarely seen. In the chronically ill or more frail older man, fluid retention might pose a concern.

Liver toxicity is not a problem with modern T preparations.

Sleep apnea has been reported to be exacerbated by T therapy. A 36-month trial of T in older men found no effect on apneic or hypoapneic episodes (Liu et al, 2003).

Gynecomastia occurs rarely because of the relatively greater increase in serum E_2 levels. Often this side effect can be overcome with a downward adjustment of the T dose.

Prostate

Both benign prostatic hyperplasia (BPH) and prostate cancer are diseases common in older men and both are promoted by androgens. Androgen deprivation therapy has been used for the treatment of both of these processes, but whether T therapy for an older man places him at increased risk for developing clinically significant prostate disease from a preexisting but subclinical condition is unknown. There have been at least 22 T replacement trials, involving a total of 583 men aged 45 to 89 years, in which serum PSA levels were measured. Sixteen of the 22 studies showed no increase in prostate-specific antigen (PSA) with T therapy. In the six studies showing a PSA rise with T, the average PSA change was 0.48 ng/mL and the average PSA velocity was 0.52 ng/mL/year. Seven T replacement trials in older men have evaluated prostate size, maximum urine flow rates, and International Prostate Symptom Scores. None of them showed any change in these parameters with treatment (Morales, 2002). The data suggest that, in the short term (up to 3 years), T therapy in the older man has little effect on the prostate. **However, because both prostate cancer and BPH are diseases with long natural histories and the observation time to date with T therapy in older men is limited to less than 900 man-years, it is possible that T therapy might have long-term effects on the prostates of older men.**

Polycythemia

T therapy in older men can often result in a significant increase in red blood cell mass and hemoglobin levels. This may lead to termination of therapy, a decrease of dose, or a switch to a different formulation of T. The method of T replacement may affect the magnitude of the change in red blood cell mass.

RECOMMENDATIONS AND GUIDELINES

Despite the long time since the synthesis and initial use of T in clinical practice, there is a scarcity of credible, well-designed trials to document its safety and efficacy. The completion of large studies on hormone replacement in postmenopausal women brought into sharp focus the inadequacy of limited trials (Writing Group for the Women's Health Initiative Investigators, 2002). **It is, however, unhelpful and misleading to assume that the results of the Women's Health Initiative on hormone replacement therapy (HRT: estrogen ± progesterone) in postmenopausal women apply equally to the men's situation; such an assumption does not take into consideration the large differences in the molecular structures and actions of the hormones themselves and the gender responses to them** (Goderie-Plomp et al, 2004). Although it is tempting to equate the possible effects of HRT in the development of breast cancer to androgen replacement therapy (ART) in prostate cancer, the biologic behavior and clinical management of the two tumors are markedly dissimilar. It is estimated (Bhasin et al, 2003) that some 5000 hypogonadal men receiving T supplementation for a period of 5 years are needed to have a study of the magnitude of the Women's Health Initiative.

The Institute of Medicine Report

In an extensive and comprehensive publication, a committee of the Institute of Medicine (IOM) analyzed the current status of androgen therapy in men. The report (available electronically at http://www.iom.edu or in hard copy) (Liverman and Blazer, 2004) contains several recommendations (Table 27–7). The gist of the report is that initially the efficacy of T treat-

Table 27–7. Summary of the Institute of Medicine Recommendations

Clinical trials are needed.
Focus on populations most likely to benefit.
Use for treatment not for prevention.
Focus on clinical outcomes with preliminary evidence of benefit.
Begin with short-term efficacy trials.
Conduct longer-term studies if short-term efficacy is established.
Ensure safety of research participants.

ment should be assessed in a limited trial. Only if a positive response is found should the investigations proceed to the large studies designed to evaluate safety. **Although no one would question the need for and importance of these studies, it is also clear that reliable answers will not be available for at least 10 to 15 years after the completion of the efficacy studies and the subsequent safety trials.** For the practicing physician, it is not logical to wait that long until all conclusive evidence is complete. When indicated, action needs to be taken on the basis of the most reliable information at hand regarding the advantages and drawbacks of T treatment and guidelines and recommendations available from professional societies.

Sexual Medicine Society of North America

The position statement of the Sexual Medicine Society of North America preceded the IOM report but expresses its essence superbly: **T supplementation is indicated for men who have signs and symptoms of hypogonadism accompanied by subnormal serum T measurements. T supplementation can provide important health benefits to these hypogonadal men. T supplementation requires medical surveillance in order to identify early signs of possible adverse effects. Although the benefits and risks of long-term T supplementation have not yet been definitively established, the weight of current evidence does not suggest an increased risk of heart disease or prostate cancer with long-term use of T. T is not medically indicated in men who do not have hypogonadism.** An expert panel of urologists and endocrinologists produced a set of recommendations with succinctness, wide appeal, and practicality (Liu et al, 2004; Morales et al, 2004). Because of their impact in urologic practice, they are included (with some modifications) here. The grading refers to the degree of evidence available supporting each recommendation (Morales et al, 2004).

Recommendations

Definition (Grade B)

Adult-onset hypogonadism is a clinical **and** biochemical syndrome frequently associated with advancing age and characterized by a deficiency in serum androgen levels, with or without changes in receptor sensitivity to androgens. It **may** affect the function of multiple organ systems and result in a significant detriment in the quality of life, including major alterations in sexual function

Clinical Diagnosis (Grade A)

The clinical manifestations of adult hypogonadism are not specific. Sexual dysfunction is prominent and often the presenting symptom. Depression, irritability, changes in cognition and sleep patterns, and diminished strength and endurance may also be present. The physical examination is frequently unhelpful, but alterations in testicular size and consistency, hair distribution, muscle mass, and body shape and sequelae of osteoporosis can be detected. **Not all the manifestations need to be evident simultaneously, and their intensity shows marked interindividual variability.**

Biochemical Diagnosis (Grade A)

In patients at risk for or suspected of having hypogonadism, the following biochemical investigations are recommended: a blood sample for T determination between 8:00 and 11:00 AM. The most accessible and reliable assays to establish the presence of hypogonadism are measurements of bioavailable T or the cFT. Assays for total T, particularly in elderly men, may not reflect the true androgenic status. If T levels are below or at the lower limit of the accepted normal values, it is prudent to confirm the results with a second determination together with assessment of LH, follicle-stimulating hormone, and prolactin.

Other Hormonal Alterations besides Sex Hormones (Grade C)

It is recognized that alterations in other endocrine systems occur in association with aging, but the significance of these changes is not well understood. In general terms, determinations of E_2, DHEA, melatonin, GH, and insulin-like growth factor 1 are not indicated in the uncomplicated evaluation of hypogonadism. Under special circumstances or for well-defined clinical research, assessment of these and other hormones may be warranted.

Indications for Therapy (Grade A)

A clear indication (a clinical picture together with biochemical evidence of hypogonadism) should exist prior to initiation of androgen therapy.

Age (Grade C)

In the absence of defined contraindications, age is not a limiting factor to initiate ART in aged men with hypoandrogenism.

Sexual Function (Grade A)

Hypogonadal men with specific sexual dysfunctions (e.g., ED or diminished interest, or both) are candidates for androgen therapy. Absence of an adequate response after appropriate T treatment calls for further investigation to rule out associated comorbidities.

Combined Treatment for Erectile Dysfunction (Grade C)

Evidence is emerging suggesting therapeutic synergism with combined use of T and phosphodiesterase 5 inhibitors **in hypogonadal or borderline eugonadal** men. These observations are preliminary and require additional study. However, the combination treatment can be considered in patients who do not respond to adequate treatment with phosphodiesterase inhibitors alone. No credible evidence for or against exists with other drugs in combination with androgens.

Testosterone Commercial Formulations (Grade B)

Currently commercially available preparations of T (**with the exception of the alkylated ones**) are safe and effective. The treating physician should have sufficient knowledge and adequate understanding of the advantages and drawbacks of each preparation. The patient should be given the opportunity to participate actively in the choice of androgen formulation.

Serum Levels (Grade B)

The purpose of ART is to bring and maintain serum T levels within the physiologic range. Supraphysiologic levels are to be avoided. Although it may appear desirable, **no evidence exists for or against the need to maintain a circadian rhythm of serum T levels.**

Other Androgens (Grade B)

The use of DHEA and DHT has not been proved to be effective specifically in male sexual dysfunction. Current evidence concerning DHT efficacy is also insufficient. There is a need for additional studies aimed expressly at investigating the effects of these hormones on aging men.

Monitoring—Liver (Grade A)

Currently available T preparations are largely free of hepatic toxicity (methylated forms are an exception). Liver function studies are advisable before the onset of therapy. Despite the lack of evidence, commercial manufacturers (for regulatory purposes) include warnings about hepatic risks in their product inserts.

Monitoring—Lipids (Grade A)

A fasting lipid profile before initiation of treatment, if not obtained as part of the initial evaluation, and reassessment at 3 or 6 months after onset of T administration are also recommended.

Monitoring—Prostate (Grade A)

In men older than 40 years, digital rectal examination and determination of serum PSA are mandatory as baseline measurements of prostate health before therapy with androgens, every 3 to 6 months for the first 12 months, and yearly thereafter. **Transrectal ultrasound-guided biopsies of the prostate are indicated only if the digital rectal examination or the PSA is abnormal.**

Prostate and Breast Safety—I (Grade A)

Androgen administration is absolutely contraindicated in men suspected of harboring carcinoma of the prostate or breast.

Prostate Safety—II (Grade D)

Men successfully treated for prostate cancer and suffering from symptomatic hypogonadism may become candidates for androgen therapy, **after a prudent interval,** if there is no evidence of residual cancer. The risk and benefits must be clearly understood by the patient and the follow-up must be particularly careful. No reliable evidence exists in favor of or against this recommendation. The clinician must exercise good clinical judgment together with adequate knowledge of the advantages and drawbacks of androgen therapy in this situation.

Prostate Safety—III (Grade A)

Androgen supplementation is contraindicated in men with severe bladder outlet obstruction related to an enlarged, clinically benign prostate. Moderate obstruction represents a partial contraindication to ART. After successful treatment of the obstruction, the contraindication can be lifted.

Monitoring—Mood (Grade B)

ART normally results in improvements in mood and well-being. The development of negative behavioral patterns (aggressiveness, hypersexuality) during treatment calls for dose modifications or discontinuation of therapy.

Monitoring—Hematology (Grade A)

Polycythemia may develop during ART. Periodic hematologic assessment is indicated. Dose adjustments, change of preparation, periodic phlebotomies, or discontinuation of treatment may be necessary.

Monitoring—Sleep Apnea (Grade C)

Exacerbation of sleep apnea may occur during T supplementation therapy. Proper assessment and treatment of the sleep apnea are indicated during T supplementation. Careful consideration should be given to the need for T treatment if the sleep disturbances deteriorate.

Physician's Responsibilities

ART is normally for life. This demands a lifelong commitment for follow-up. The treating physician must be familiar with the diagnostic, therapeutic, and monitoring aspects of androgen therapy. Good clinical judgment is equally important. Inadequate therapeutic response or the appearance of significant adverse effects calls for reassessment of treatment indications.

SUGGESTED READINGS

Bhasin S, Singh AB, Mac RP, et al: Managing the risks of prostate disease during testosterone replacement therapy of older men: Recommendations for a standardized monitoring plan. J Androl 2003;24:299-306.

Liverman CT, Blazer DG (eds): Testosterone and Aging. Clinical Research Directions. Institute of Medicine of the National Academies. Washington, DC, Washington, DC, The National Academies Press, 2004. http://www.iom.edu.

Morales A, Buvat J, Gooren LJ, et al: Endocrine aspects of sexual dysfunction in man. J Sex Med 2004;1:69-81.

Morley JE, Patrick P, Perry HM III: Evaluation of assays available to measure free testosterone. Metabolism 2002;51:554-559.

28 Urologic Management of Women with Sexual Health Concerns

IRWIN GOLDSTEIN, MD

<table>
<tr><td>CLASSIFICATION AND EPIDEMIOLOGY</td></tr>
<tr><td>DIAGNOSIS</td></tr>
<tr><td>TREATMENT</td></tr>
<tr><td>SUMMARY</td></tr>
</table>

At the present time there are limited urologic specialists who offer comprehensive sexual health care for women. This is likely only a temporary situation. **Multiple population-based studies reveal a high prevalence of sexual health concerns in women of all ages** (Rosen et al, 1993; Laumann et al, 1999, 2001; Nusbaum et al, 2000; Simons and Carey, 2001; Kadri et al, 2002; Danielsson et al, 2003; Lewis RW et al, 2004; Salonia et al, 2004; Basson, 2005; Hayes, 2005; Nappi et al, 2005; Öberg, 2005, Weijmar Schultz, 2005). Historically, the urologist has contributed significantly to the basic science knowledge and contemporary management strategies of men's sexual health care (Fisher et al, 2004; Hatzichristou et al, 2004; Hirsch et al, 2004; Lue et al, 2004; Rowland et al, 2004). Furthermore, urologists provide urologic health care to women. They are in a unique position to understand the specialized female pelvic floor anatomy and physiology, especially in terms of muscular support, and the effects of pharmacology and surgical treatments on bladder and urethra and to know that female peripheral sexual organs are an essential component of the pelvic floor (Glazer and MacConkey, 1996; Glazer et al, 1999; Bergeron et al, 2001a, 2002; Shafik and El-Sibai, 2002). At the end of the decade, it would be probable that many academic urology departments will have trained faculty members to provide safe and effective, evidence-based sexual health care for women.

To provide state-of-the-art care to afflicted women and couples, sexual medicine centers devoted to the study, diagnosis, and treatment of men and women with sexual disorders are being launched in this decade. Many of these facilities are composed of multidisciplinary groups. Women in these centers are typically managed by a team of allied health care professionals, mental health care professionals, and physical therapists, under the direction of sexual medicine physicians who may be board certified in urology (Goldstein, 2005; Kang and Ducharme, 2005).

Women's (and men's) sexual health concerns are, in general, secondary to mind, body, and relationship issues that are interrelated in unique and individual ways, molded with distinct couple dynamics, to cause the particular sexual problem. Psychological factors include previous sexual trauma and abuse, sexual neuroses, sexual inhibitions or idiosyncrasies, and/or interpersonal relationship issues. Biologic factors may involve such pertinent factors as aging; exposure to vascular risk factors; urologic conditions such as interstitial cystitis, post-radical cystectomy, and recurrent urinary tract infections; and gynecologic conditions such as endometriosis, post-hysterectomy, childbirth, infertility issues, genital tissue sexually transmitted infections, inflammation, abnormal immunologic conditions, abnormal hormonal states, tumors, mechanical compartment syndromes, blunt or penetrating traumatic injury, tissue weakness with organ prolapse, and others (Bergeron et al, 2001a; Basson et al, 2004a; Heiman et al, 2004; Salonia et al, 2004; Basson, 2005, Öberg, 2005; Nappi et al, 2005).

While recognizing the need for multiple trained specialists in the overall management of women with sexual health issues, **the aim of this chapter is to selectively provide the urologist with relevant evidence-based clinical information to help identify and treat specific biologic-based pathophysiologic processes.** Even though urologists (and all health care professionals) need to be holistic in managing women (and men) with sexual dysfunction, the goal is to educate the urologic biologic-focused clinician how to identify the biologic pathology or pathologic processes associated with the sexual health concern and to provide evidence-based safe and effective management strategies.

There have been limited clinical and basic science research investigations in the area of women's sexual health concerns.

Sexual health problems are associated with multiple theories and anecdotes with little evidence-based medicine documentation. Unfortunately, randomized, multi-institutional, multicultural controlled treatment outcome studies in the management of women with sexual dysfunctions are limited. In this chapter existing evidence-based data are reviewed concerning epidemiology, diagnosis, and treatments (medical and surgical) of women's sexual health problems. Because of space constraints, there is limited discussion concerning contemporary advances in the basic science (animal model) understanding of the physiology of female sexual function and the pathophysiology of female sexual dysfunction (Sjoberg, 1968; MacLean et al, 1990; McKenna et al, 1991; Kaleczyc, 1994; Hodgins et al, 1998; Park et al, 2001a; Yoon et al, 2001; Min et al, 2002; Traish et al, 2002, 2003; Giraldi et al, 2004; Kim NN et al, 2004; Kim SW et al, 2004; Ting et al, 2004; Nappi et al, 2005). For the most part, relevant basic science research data are embedded within the clinically oriented diagnosis and treatment sections. In the future, as basic science research and clinical management data expand, it is hoped that the section on women's sexual health will include a separate physiology and pathophysiology contribution.

CLASSIFICATION AND EPIDEMIOLOGY

There are limited population-based epidemiologic studies in women with sexual health concerns (Laumann et al, 1999, 2001; Lewis et al, 2004; Nappi et al, 2005). Measurements of women's sexual problems have varied, including how the sexual problem is defined and classified and which instruments are utilized. Experts are still discussing the appropriateness of presently utilized women's sexual health definitions at recent international consensus meetings (Basson et al, 2000, 2003, 2004b). The type of definitions selected in any study will obviously affect the epidemiologic prevalence estimates of women's sexual problems. Based on current published information, the following is the most contemporary international classification system (Basson et al, 2004b):

Women's Sexual Interest/Desire Disorder: Absent or diminished feelings of sexual interest or desire, absent sexual thoughts or fantasies, and a lack of responsive desire. Motivations (here defined as reasons/incentives) for attempting to become sexually aroused are scarce or absent. The lack of interest is considered to be beyond a normative lessening with life cycle and relationship duration.

Subjective Sexual Arousal Disorder: Absence of or markedly diminished feelings of sexual arousal (sexual excitement and sexual pleasure) from any type of sexual stimulation. Vaginal lubrication or other signs of physical response still occur.

Genital Sexual Arousal Disorder: Complaints of absent or impaired genital sexual arousal. Self-reports may include minimal vulvar swelling or vaginal lubrication from any type of sexual stimulation and reduced sexual sensations from caressing genitalia. Subjective sexual excitement still occurs from nongenital sexual stimuli.

Combined Genital and Subjective Arousal Disorder: Absence of, or markedly diminished feelings of, sexual arousal (sexual excitement and sexual pleasure) from any type of sexual stimulation as well as complaints of absent or impaired genital sexual arousal (vulvar swelling, lubrication).

Persistent Sexual Arousal Disorder: Spontaneous, intrusive, and unwanted genital arousal (e.g., tingling, throbbing, pulsating) in the absence of sexual interest and desire. Any awareness of subjective arousal is typically but not invariably unpleasant. The arousal is unrelieved by one or more orgasms, and the feelings of arousal persist for hours or days.

Women's Orgasmic Disorder: Despite the self-report of high sexual arousal/excitement, there is either lack of orgasm, markedly diminished intensity of orgasmic sensations, or marked delay of orgasm from any kind of stimulation.

Dyspareunia: Persistent or recurrent pain with attempted or complete vaginal entry and/or penile vaginal intercourse.

Vaginismus: Persistent difficulties to allow vaginal entry of a penis, a finger, and/or any object, despite the woman's expressed wish to do so. There is variable involuntary pelvic muscle contraction (phobic) avoidance and anticipation/fear/experience of pain. Structural or other physical abnormalities must be ruled out/addressed.

Sexual Aversion Disorder: Extreme anxiety and/or disgust at the anticipation of/or attempt to have any sexual activity.

The following represent contemporary international prevalence data concerning women's sexual health problems. **For problems with sexual desire or sexual interest,** the reported estimates range from 7% current (sexual health concerns that exist in the woman at the time of study) to 31% lifetime (sexual health concerns that have ever occurred in the woman) prevalence. For problems with excitement or pleasure, estimates for a 1-year (sexual health concerns that may have existed in the woman over the past year) prevalence are 23%. **For lubrication difficulties or vaginal dryness,** prevalence estimates are 20% for a 1-year prevalence and range from 19% to 23% for lifetime prevalence. **For infrequent orgasm or difficulties in reaching orgasm,** lifetime prevalence estimates range from 4% to 41%. **For an inability to experience orgasm** for several months, one population-based study estimated the lifetime prevalence to be 16% of women, whereas another reported that 18% had problems with orgasm for 2 months or more and 25% had trouble reaching orgasm more than 50% of the time. **For pain during or after sex,** prevalence estimates range from 3% to 48%, lifetime estimates from population-based studies range from 17% to 19%, whereas clinic-based studies report prevalence estimates of 10% to 20%. **For women experiencing a problem with desire, arousal, orgasm, or pain,** two population-based surveys, using similar instruments, estimate a lifetime prevalence of 33% and 35%. **For women experiencing a current sexual problem,** one national study estimated a 1-month prevalence of 45% (Rosen et al, 1993; Laumann et al, 1999, 2001; Nusbaum et al, 2000; Simons and Carey, 2001; Kadri et al, 2002; Danielsson et al, 2003; Lewis et al, 2004; Salonia et al, 2004; Basson, 2005; Hayes, 2005; Nappi et al, 2005; Öberg, 2005; Weijmar Schultz, 2005).

DIAGNOSIS
History

There are limited management paradigms for the diagnosis of women with sexual health complaints (Basson et al, 2004a; Hatzichristou et al, 2004; Basson, 2005). **The cornerstone of the physical-based diagnosis of women with sexual dysfunction is a detailed history and physical examination performed by the biologic-focused health care professional.** Specifically, history taking is crucial because it establishes the diagnostic impressions and forms the basis of search on physical examination. It is customary that the history includes sexual, medical, and psychosocial aspects, so that the many physical and psychological factors that often contribute to the sexual health difficulty can be characterized. **It is advised that women with sexual health concerns undergo a separate and concomitant psychological interview by a psychologic-focused health care professional** to broaden the psychosocial information derived during the interview process (Basson et al, 2000, 2003, 2004a).

The sexual history should begin with the patient describing the sexual problem (Masters and Johnson, 1970; Kaplan, 1974; Gagnon et al, 1982; Basson, 2000, 2005; Basson et al, 2000, 2003, 2004a, 2004b; Warnock, 2001; Rosen, 2002; Lewis et al, 2004; Hatzichristou et al, 2004; Heiman et al, 2004; Nappi et al, 2005; Weijmar Schultz, 2005). The following questions may be utilized to help obtain maximal descriptive information. What is the sexual problem? When did the sexual problem manifest? How long have you had the sexual problem? Does the sexual problem happen all the time? Does the sexual problem occur during partner-related sexual activity? Does the sexual problem occur during self-stimulation? In which situations is the sexual problem minimized? In which situations is the sexual problem maximized? Did you ever experience full capabilities for sexual interest, sexual arousal, and sexual orgasm? How many years were you at peak sexual function? What is your current sexual functioning in terms of interest, arousal, and orgasm compared with when you were at peak sexual function? Is the sexual problem associated with any degree of discomfort, tenderness, soreness, or pain? If so, can you localize the site of the pain on a schematic diagram of a woman's genitalia? What tests have you already had in the evaluation of your sexual health concern? What treatments have you already received, and what are the outcome of the various treatments? How does the sexual problem affect you? How is your partner affected by the sexual problem? Does the sexual problem cause you to withdraw from partner-related sexual activity, from self-stimulated sexual activity, or from the relationship? How would you feel if the sexual problem were cured? It is relevant to inquire of the sexual health of the partner. For women with men, there may exist male sexual dysfunctions such as erectile dysfunction, early ejaculation, or an anatomic concern, such as Peyronie's disease.

The use of validated, reliable, standardized self-rated questionnaires are a very useful clinical starting point to assist the identification of the presence or absence of a sexual problem, and which of the disorders of desire, arousal, orgasm, and sexual pain subtypes of women's sexual dysfunction are involved. Such self-report measures are valuable screening tools that are easy to administer and score and have normative values for populations of women with and without sexual dysfunction. Common self-rated questionnaires include the Female Sexual Function and the Sexual Function Questionnaire (Rosen et al, 2000; Quirk et al, 2002; Meston, 2003; Wiegel et al, 2005). As in all areas of clinical medicine, the use of screening tools for clinical diagnosis has recognized limitations. The determination of particular psychological contributors or confounds, contextual conditions, and other features and characteristics that cause individual women their unique sexual concerns requires more traditional assessment through structured history and physical examination.

The medical history should include focused questions on any accompanying medical/surgical illnesses and/or the use of medications (Masters and Johnson, 1970; Kaplan, 1974; Gagnon et al, 1982; Basson, 2000, 2005; Warnock, 2001; Rosen, 2002; Basson et al, 2003, 2004a, 2004b; Hatzichristou et al, 2004; Heiman et al, 2004; Nappi et al, 2005; Weijmar Schultz, 2005). Topics of importance in the medical history may include (1) chronic/medical illnesses such as diabetes, anemia, or renal failure; (2) neurologic illnesses such as spinal cord injury, multiple sclerosis, or lumbosacral disc disease; (3) endocrinologic illnesses such as hypogonadism, hyperprolactinemia, or thyroid disorders; (4) atherosclerotic vascular risk factor exposure such as hypercholesterolemia, hypertension, diabetes, smoking, or family history; (5) nonhormonal medication/recreational drug use such as antihypertensive agents, selective serotonin reuptake inhibitors, over-the-counter drugs, street drugs, alcohol, or cocaine; (6) hormonal medication use such as combined oral contraceptives, infertility drugs, and leuprolide acetate; (7) pelvic/perineal/genital trauma such as pelvic fracture or bicycling injury; (8) gynecologic history such as childbirth, abortions, episiotomy, abnormal Papanicolaou smears, sexually transmitted diseases, pelvic inflammatory disorder, endometriosis, fibroids, hysterectomy with or without oophorectomy, and menopause; (9) urologic history such as incontinence, frequent urinary tract infections, interstitial cystitis, and pelvic surgeries; (10) surgical history such as laminectomy, colon/anal surgery, vascular bypass surgery; and (11) psychiatric history such as depression, panic, or anxiety.

Because sex **steroid hormones are critical for genital structure and function** (McKenna et al, 1991; Park et al, 2001a; Yoon et al, 2001; Min et al, 2002; Traish et al, 2003; Giraldi et al, 2004; Kim NN et al, 2004; Kim SW et al, 2004), the medical history should routinely probe and evaluate for symptoms of estrogen deficiency such as vaginal dryness, vaginal bleeding with minimal sexual contact, pain and soreness after sexual activity, hot flashes, and night sweats. Symptoms of androgen insufficiency include fatigue, lack of energy, diminished skeletal muscle strength, depressed mood, falling asleep after meals, decreased athletic performance, or lack of interest in sexual activity.

The psychosocial history should assess such issues as social factors, past sexual beliefs, past sexual abuse and trauma, emotional concerns, and interpersonal relationship matters (Masters and Johnson, 1970; Kaplan, 1974; Gagnon et al, 1982; Basson 2000; Warnock, 2001; Rosen, 2002; Basson et al, 2003, 2004a, 2004b). Any past history of mood or psychiatric disorders should be identified.

There are multiple caveats to history taking in women with sexual health concerns. One is that the health care professional should consider history taking as having more significance than the first diagnostic step toward resolution of the sexual problem. **The fact is that history taking may be viewed as actually the beginning of treatment for the women with sexual health concerns.** Women are often empowered after the detailed discussion about their sexual health, because they have now taken the first step in overcoming their past failures to take action in this area. It is not uncommon for the discussion with the health care provider to become a model of what is possible about sexual health conversation. Many patients will thereafter initiate a sexual health conversation with their partner, close friend, or family member.

The second is that the health care professional should be cognizant that, **whereas the women may have a specific complaint, such as lack of interest, there may be additional and more complex mind, body, and relationship issues in the overall pathophysiology** (Nappi et al, 2005). For example, a woman may experience sexual pain during intercourse. She may be quite psychologically distracted by the discomfort, throbbing, stinging, aching, soreness, burning, and/or tenderness that physiologic desire, arousal, and orgasm responses during sexual stimulation are not able to manifest. It is possible that this woman may present with a primary sexual complaint such as lack of interest or orgasm, whereas more detailed history and physical examination may yield the concomitant long-standing genital sexual pain problem.

Physical Examination

The physical examination for a woman with sexual health concerns should be tailored to the sexual medicine complaint obtained on history taking. For example, if during history taking genital itching is a major sexual health problem, a careful assessment would follow for the presence of a genital dermatitis condition. If a woman with sexual health problems is younger than the age of 50 and has sexual pain, a careful physical examination would evaluate for the presence or absence of vulvar vestibulitis syndrome/vestibular adenitis. Similar complaints of sexual pain in a woman older than age 50 years of age would assess for the presence of vaginal atrophy with dryness, loss of rugae, mucosal thinning, pale hue, and lack of shiny vaginal secretions. The physical examination should be performed ideally without menses and without intercourse or douching for 24 hours before the examination. If dysfunction occurs at a specific time, such as midcycle dyspareunia, the physical examination should be scheduled at the time of the sexual problem. Such scheduling may require two visits: one for history taking and one for the physical examination.

The genital-focused examination should be considered routine in the diagnosis of women's sexual health problem, but its personal character demands that a rational explanation exist for its inclusion in the diagnostic process. A focused peripheral genital examination is recommended in women with sexual dysfunction for complaints of dyspareunia, vaginismus, genital arousal disorder, and combined arousal disorder, orgasmic disorder, pelvic trauma history, and any disease affecting genital health such as herpes or lichen sclerosus

(Basson et al, 2004a). For women with suspected neurologic disorders, the examiner may also assess for anal and vaginal tone, voluntary tightening of anus, and bulbocavernosal reflexes.

It is particularly important that the patient with sexual dysfunction has full communication with the health care provider and final authority during the physical examination to terminate at any time, to ask questions, to have control over who is in attendance, and to understand the extent of the assessment. It is vital that the patient is aware of the purpose. Inclusion of the sexual partner, with permission of the patient, is advantageous and provides needed patient support. Allowing the patient (and the partner) to observe any pathology via mirrors or digital photography is often therapeutic, allowing, for the first time in many cases, an illustration and connection of a detected physical abnormality with the sexual health problem. If there exists a genital sexual pain history, the patient should point with her finger to the locations of the discomfort during the physical examination.

Independent of the gender of the examining health care provider, it is strongly recommended that a female chaperone health care provider be present in the examination room. The following equipment should be available: examination table, hospital gown, bed sheet, disposable absorbing chucks, patient covering sheet, surgical loupes or magnifying glass, examination light source, examination gloves, gauze, lubricant, cotton-tipped swabs, speculum, pH paper, glass slide, saline, and microscope. The patient should wear a hospital gown and a sheet should cover her lower torso. The patient should be placed in the lithotomy position and the examining health care provider, using magnified vision and a carefully focused light source, should be sitting comfortably.

The first part of the examination involves inspection. If appropriate, lubricant should be placed on the vulva. Gauze can be grasped between thumb and index finger and used to retract the labia majora for a full inspection of the vestibular contents. Two gloved fingers are placed on either side of the clitoral shaft and, using an upward force in the cephalic direction, the prepuce is retracted to gain full exposure of the glans clitoris, corona, and right and left frenulum emanating at the 5 and 7 o'clock positions from the posterior portion of the glans clitoris (Fig. 28–1). After using gauze to retract the labia minora, the labial-hymenal junction is identified. A cotton swab test is performed by gently applying pressure on the minor vestibular glands, documenting the quality of the discomfort or pain (Fig. 28–2). The cotton swab may also be placed at multiple locations in the vulva and vestibule. **Palpation is next performed using a single-digit examination** (Fig. 28–3). This procedure occurs before speculum insertion or bimanual searches for vaginismus. Single-digit palpation is achieved by gently placing a finger into the vaginal opening and depressing the bulbocavernosus muscle. The test is positive if there is hypertonicity and pain (Basson et al, 2004c; Goldstein, 2005).

The goals of the physical examination for a woman with sexual health concerns are to confirm normal architecture, detect any existing pathology or abnormalities, educate the woman about normal anatomy and physiology, and, if pain is a feature, to reproduce and localize the pain to potential tender areas of the vulva, vagina, or pelvis or hypertonicity of the pelvic floor (Basson et al, 2004a; Hatzichristou et al,

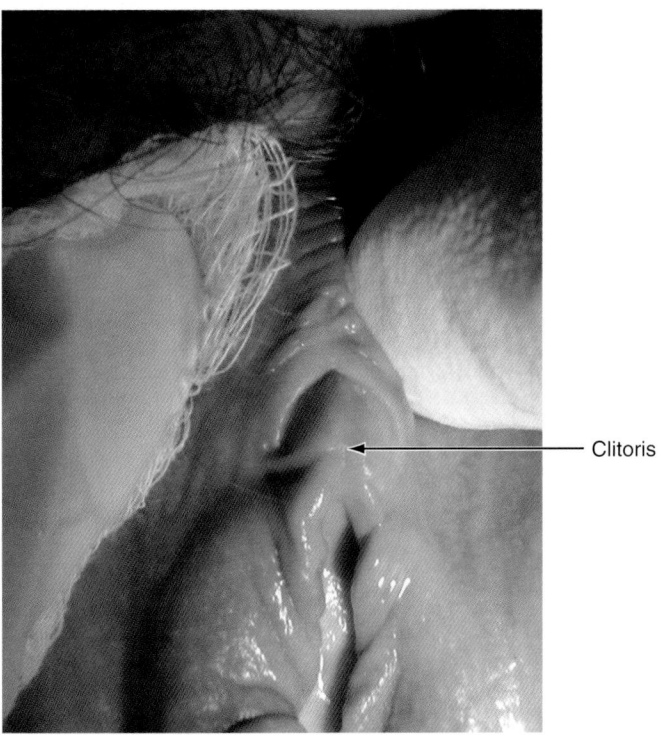

Figure 28–1. Physical examination of the clitoris is performed by carefully and gently elevating the prepuce on either side of the clitoral shaft and inspecting the glans, corona, and frenular regions.

2004; Heiman et al, 2004; Basson, 2005; Nappi et al, 2005) (Figs. 28–4 to 28–10).

A bimanual examination and evaluation of the pelvic floor may be subsequently performed if indicated. Two fingers are placed against the lateral walls, and the levators and underlying obturator are assessed for tenderness or taut bands. In addition, a bimanual examination can evaluate the integrity of the fornices, bladder and urethral bases, and pelvic organs. A rectovaginal examination and speculum examination can be performed if indicated. For the speculum examination, a warm, lubricated speculum is used. The vaginal wall is examined for estrogen milieu integrity, inflammation of the walls, and any vaginal lesions (Basson et al, 2004c; Goldstein, 2005).

The astute urologist should also perform a complete physical examination, such as examining for a thyroid goiter, to rule out other comorbid conditions that might be causing sexual dysfunction. A general physical examination is highly recommended in women with chronic illnesses and as part of good medical care, such as simple evaluation of blood pressure, pulse, and a detailed breast exam. The general physical examination would inspect the oral cavity for gingival erosions from lichen planus or cold sores from herpes simplex. The skin should be inspected for psoriasis on extremities that may also be seen on the vestibule. Pigment changes may signify Addison's disease and the potential for altered orgasm. Spider veins and palmar erythema may signify alcoholism and a substance abuse reason for sexual problems. Breast examinations may reveal evidence of previous lumpectomy or

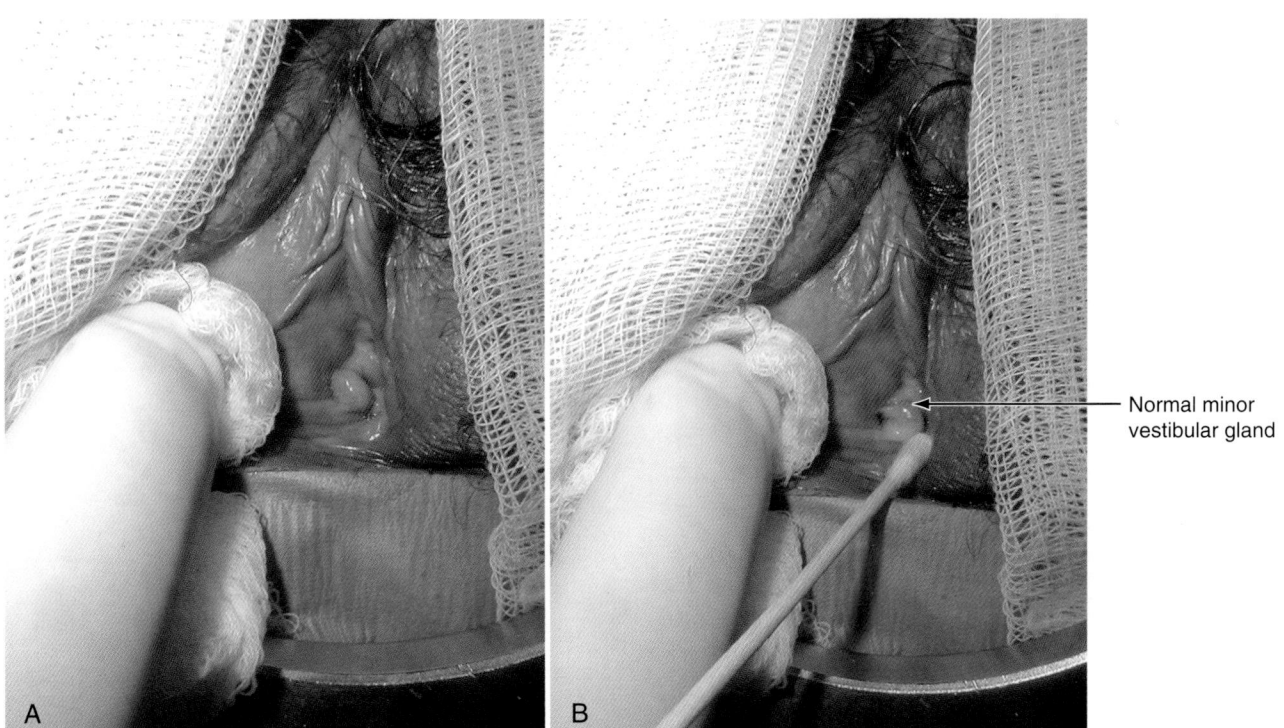

Figure 28–2. **A** and **B,** Physical examination of the minor vestibular glands (embryologically related to the glands of Littre) is performed by carefully and gently stretching the labia minora laterally and using a cotton-tipped swab to reflect the hymenal tissue medially. The minor vestibular glands are located at the labial-hymenal junction in the vestibule.

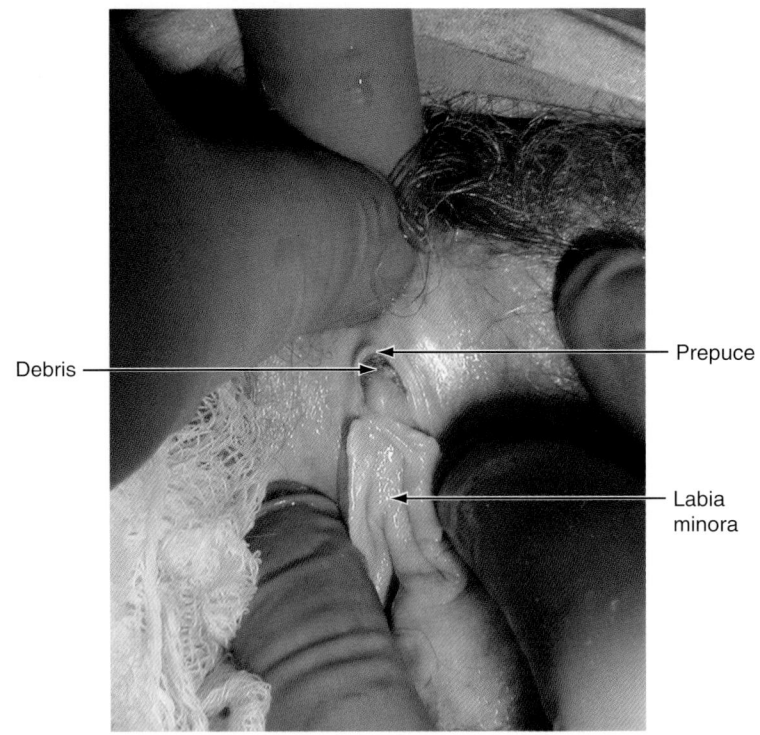

Debris

Prepuce

Labia
minora

Figure 28–3. A 53-year-old woman presented with a 5-year history of unrelenting clitoral pain. Physical examination revealed clitoral phimosis and abundant dark-colored smegma-like debris.

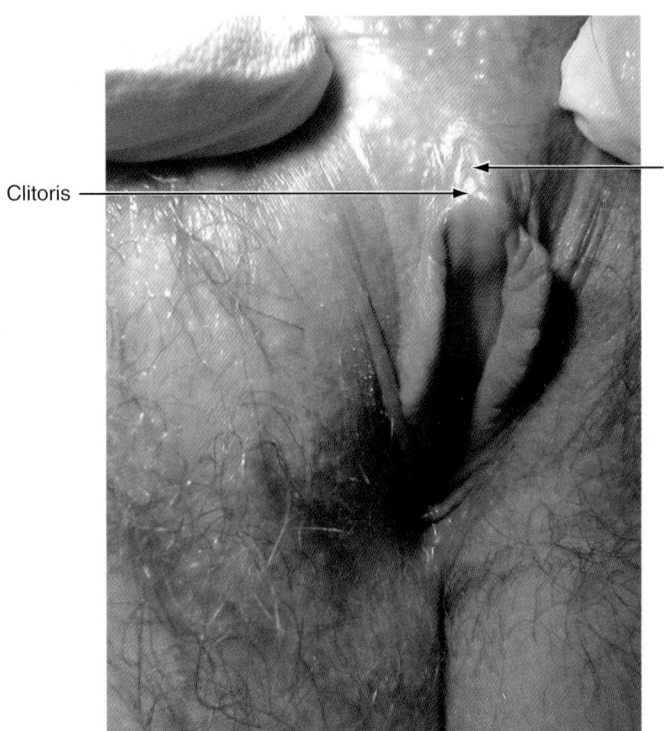

Clitoris

Prepuce

Figure 28–4. A 42-year-old woman presented with a 2-year history of recurrent clitoral itching postcoitally. Physical examination revealed complete clitoral phimosis.

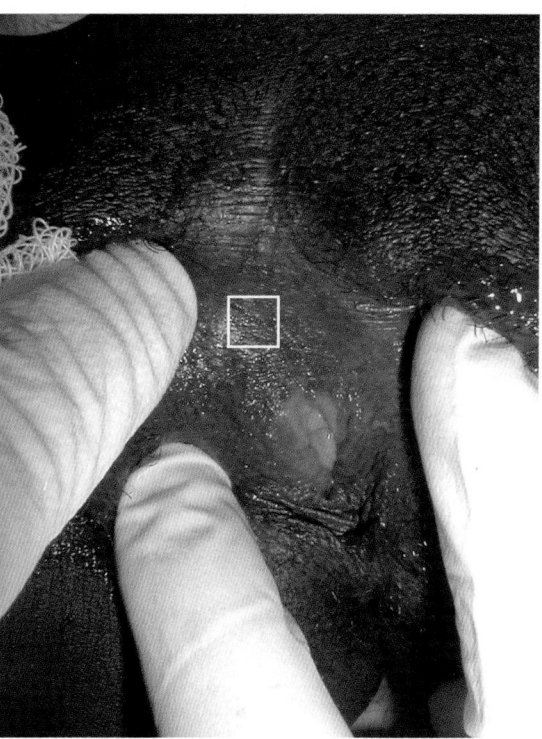

Figure 28–5. A 33-year-old African woman presented with lifetime anorgasmia revealing absent clitoris glans and prepuce secondary to ritualistic "genital mutilation" performed when she was a young child. The *box* indicates the normal location of the clitoris.

Figure 28–6. Physical examination of a 29-year-old woman with lifetime anorgasmia revealing clitoral phimosis and a preputial cyst measuring 2.5 cm in diameter.

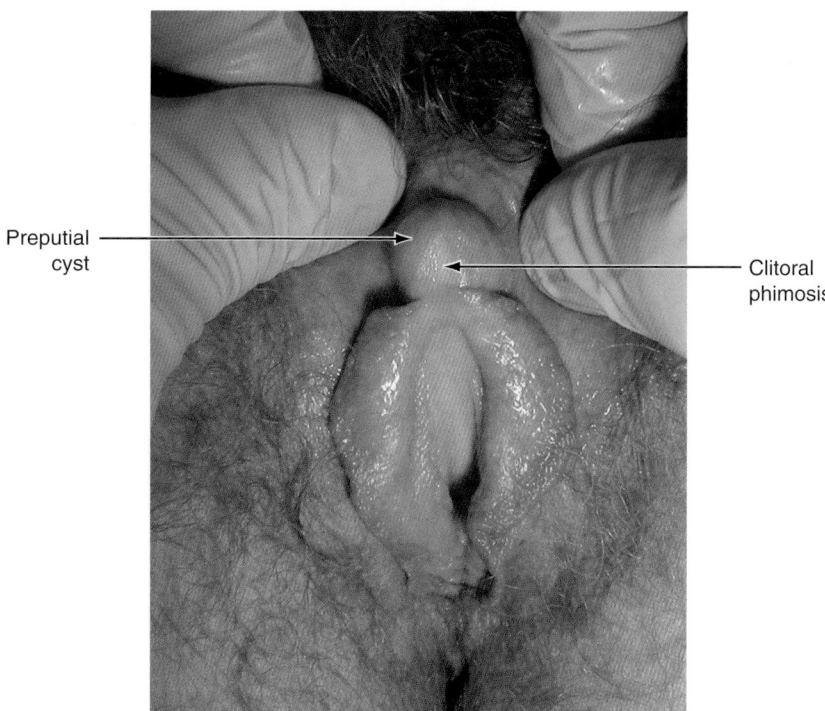

Preputial cyst

Clitoral phimosis

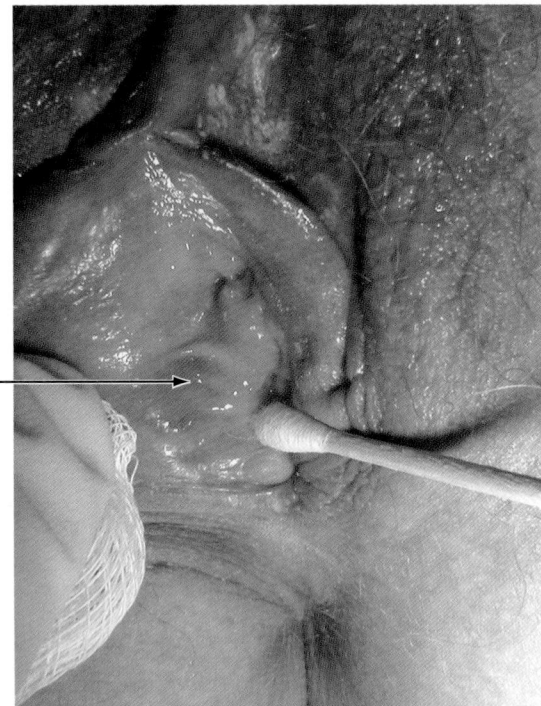

Abnormal
minor
vestibular
glands

Figure 28–7. Physical examination of a 30-year-old woman complaining of dyspareunia for 3 years revealed vestibular adenitis and positive cotton-tipped swab testing of abnormal minor vestibular glands at the 9 o'clock position.

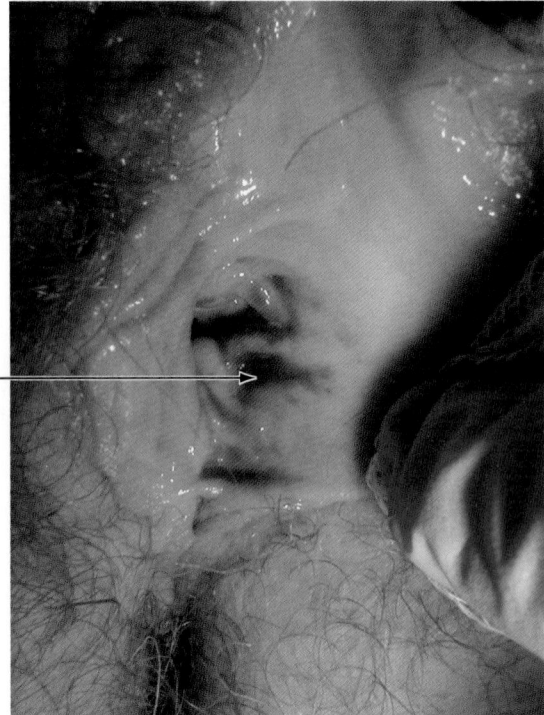

Abnormal and
erythematous
minor vestibular
glands

Figure 28–8. Physical examination of a 34-year-old woman complaining of severe dyspareunia for 7 years revealed erythema and vestibular adenitis with positive cotton-tipped swab testing of multiple minor vestibular glands from the 1 o'clock to 6 o'clock positions.

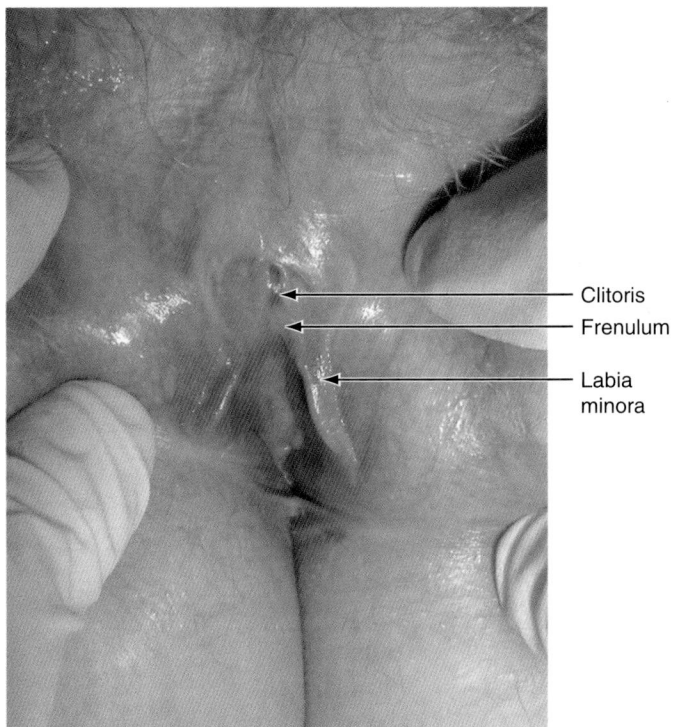

Clitoris

Frenulum

Labia minora

Figure 28–9. A 28-year-old woman on oral contraceptive pills for 12 years presented with hypoactive sexual desire. Physical examination revealed genital atrophy with clitoral, preputial, and labia minor atrophy.

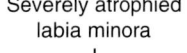

Severely atrophied labia minora

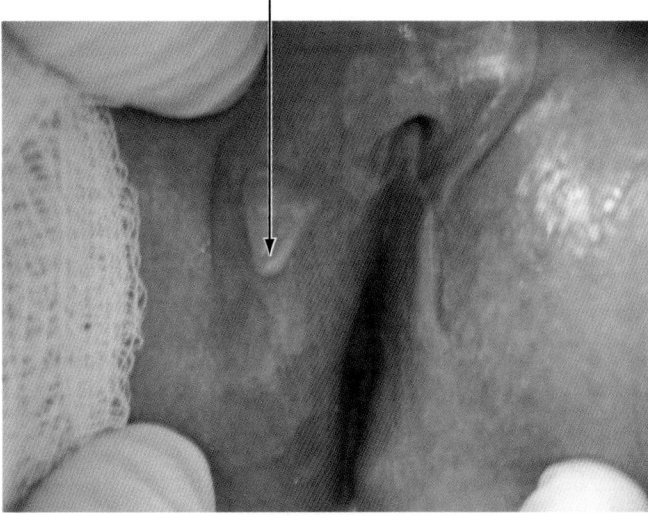

Figure 28–10. Physical examination of a 58-year-old woman who was 7 years postmenopausal with hypoactive sexual desire disorder and sexual arousal and orgasmic disorder revealed genital atrophy with clitoral and preputial atrophy and severe labial atrophy with only fragments of labia remaining at the 2 and 10 o'clock positions.

mastectomy with potential for altered body image. Galactorrhea may indicate a prolactinoma that may also be associated with low sexual desire. Neurologic symptoms such as paraplegia or a cerebrovascular accident may herald mechanical difficulties with intercourse.

Laboratory Testing

Vaginal pH

Vaginal pH testing can be performed as indicated in a woman with a sexual health concern, especially if the physical examination identifies vaginal discharge, vaginal odor, or vaginal atrophy. The vaginal pH in a healthy vaginal milieu is 3.5 to 4.5 (Stewart, 2002). An acid pH rules out a bacterial vaginitis other than candidiasis. For vaginal pH values more than 4.5, several conditions need to be considered, including vaginitis, vaginosis, and/or atrophic vaginitis.

Wet Mount Testing

During the speculum examination, an evaluation should be performed for discharge. Samples should be collected for wet mount and culture (Haefner, 1999; Anderson et al, 2004). Normal vaginal secretions are odorless and are not associated with the clinical complaint of itching or irritation. On wet mount, one should note a heterogeneous suspension of desquamated vaginal epithelial cells with lactobacilli as the predominant microorganism. The wet prep has four important elements: background flora, vaginal epithelial cells, pathogens, and white blood cells.

Concerning background flora, lactobacilli dominate in the healthy vagina. If lactobacilli are seen to dominate the background flora and the vaginal pH is acidic, it likely does not matter what vaginal culture grows. There is likely no bacterial infection, independent of any vaginal culture reports. If, however, there are absent lactobacilli in the background flora, there are several causes, including bacterial vaginosis, desquamative vaginitis, vaginal lichen planus, and the recent use of antibiotics. **Concerning vaginal epithelial cells, the frequency of noting parabasal cells on the wet mount can help the urologist assess the woman's estrogen status and/or presence or absence of inflammation.** In normally estrogenized vaginal epithelium, the wet mount should reveal very few parabasal epithelial cells. If there is an ongoing inflammatory process in the vagina, the inflamed epithelium will shed, thereby increasing the occurrence of parabasal epithelial cells. In addition, the presence of so-called clue cells may be a sign for the existence of the condition of bacterial vaginosis. Concerning vaginal pathogens, these may include *Trichomonas* and *Candida*. These organisms may be identified on wet mount in approximately 60% of cases. Vaginal cultures that show *Escherichia coli*, enterococcus, and/or group B *Streptococcus* are normal vaginal organisms. *Gardnerella* may be seen in the vaginal cultures of 50% to 70% of normal women. Concerning white blood cells on the wet mount, the observation of an increased white blood cell count is considered to be more than 1 white blood cell per epithelial cell. The observation of an increased white blood cell count on a wet mount may occur under the following conditions: vaginitis secondary to *Trichomonas*, yeast, and/or atrophy; cervicitis secondary to gonorrhea, chlamydia, and/or herpes; and upper genital/reproductive tract disease such as endometritis and/or pelvic inflammatory disease (Haefner, 1999; Anderson et al, 2004).

BIOSYNTHESIS OF ANDROGENS

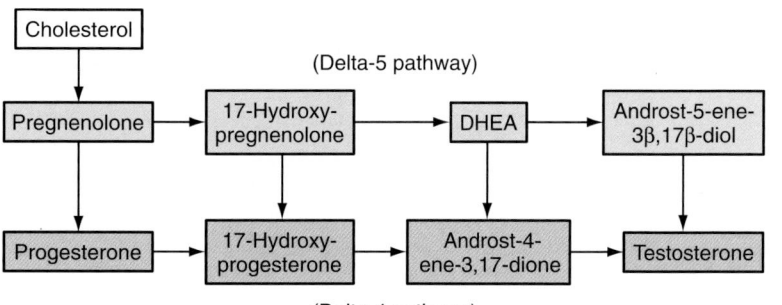

Figure 28–11. A schematic revealing the intermediate androgen sex steroids in the synthesis of testosterone and dihydrotestosterone.

Blood Testing

There are no recommended routine laboratory tests for women's sexual health concern (Bachmann et al, 2002; Guay and Davis, 2002; Basson et al, 2004a, 2004c; Davis et al, 2004; Guay et al, 2004a, 2004b). There are 10 sex steroids, including 7 androgens and 3 estrogens. Measurement of multiple sex steroids may be of clinical relevance to gain a better understanding of the hormonal integrity in a woman with sexual health concerns. **Blood testing should be dictated by the clinical suspicion of medical disease. If appropriate, the urologist may assess various androgen values,** such as dehydroepiandrosterone sulfate (DHEAS), androstenedione, total testosterone, free testosterone, sex hormone–binding globulin (SHBG), and dihydrotestosterone (Fig. 28–11). For example, assessment of the DHEAS and androstenedione values may provide insight as to the function of the zona reticularis of the adrenal gland. The SHBG value would be of great interest if the woman was taking exogenous estrogen steroids (e.g., oral contraceptive pill). The blood test for dihydrotestosterone may be of interest if the woman has acne or alopecia side effects after treatment with a topical testosterone gel. If the results are elevated, a 5α-reductase inhibitor may be considered. **If appropriate, the urologist may assess estrogen values** such as estradiol and estrone (Fig. 28–12). Estradiol is the most biologically active form of estrogen. The blood levels of estradiol may not be representative of the exogenous estrogen administration in women on exogenous conjugated equine estrogens, because the latter estrogens are not bioidentical. Pituitary function may be measured by obtaining luteinizing hormone, follicle-stimulating hormone, and prolactin. Thyroid-stimulating hormone should be measured to exclude subclinical thyroid disease.

There are multiple concerns and caveats to the determination of serum hormone levels in women with sexual health concerns (Sodergard et al, 1982; Zumoff et al, 1995; Baulieu, 1996; Mushayandebyu et al, 1996; Labrie et al, 1997a; Vierhapper et al, 1997; Arlt et al, 1999; Barnhart et al, 1999; Vermeulen et al, 1999; Baulieu et al, 2000; Shifren et al, 2000; Bachmann et al, 2002; Davis et al, 2002; Guay and Davis, 2002; Goldstat et al, 2003; Basson et al, 2004a, 2004c; Davis et al, 2004; Guay et al, 2004a, 2004b; Simon et al, 2004). **For example, testosterone assays are not uniformly found to be sensitive or reliable enough to accurately measure testosterone at the low serum concentrations typically found in women** (Davis et al, 2004). **The normal ranges of testos-**

BIOSYNTHESIS OF ESTROGENS

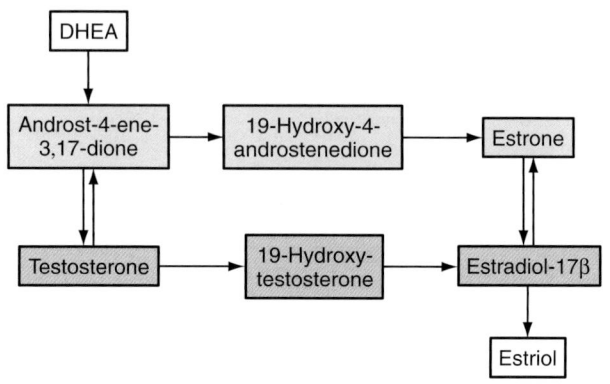

Figure 28–12. A schematic revealing the intermediate androgen and estrogen sex steroids in the synthesis of estradiol.

terone concentration values for women of different age groups are also not well defined (Zumoff et al, 1995; Vierhapper et al, 1997; Davis et al, 2002; Guay and Davis, 2002; Guay et al, 2004b). **Free testosterone is more important than total testosterone in sexual function because most testosterone is bound to SHBG and only a very small amount of total testosterone is biologically available** (Guay and Davis, 2002; Davis et al, 2004). Equilibrium dialysis is a highly sensitive assay for free testosterone, but this method is labor intensive and expensive and not feasible for clinical practice. Measurement of free testosterone by analog assay is unreliable and should not be used in clinical practice (Guay and Davis, 2002; Davis et al, 2004). Free androgen may also be estimated using the free androgen index, which is defined as the total testosterone concentration (in nmol/L; multiply testosterone units in ng/dL × 3.47 = nmol/L) divided by the concentration of SHBG (in nmol/L). The free androgen index is unreliable when SHBG levels are low. A calculated free testosterone value may also be determined, which takes into account total testosterone, SHBG, and albumin (Sodergard et al, 1982; Vermeulen et al, 1999). A calculator for this value is available online at http://www.issam.ch/freetesto.htm. The measurement of SHBG is not controversial and is relatively simple to perform with good reproducibility. Timing of measurement to prevent misdiagnosis of low testosterone may be of importance. If possible, blood should be drawn between 8 and 10 AM owing to the diurnal variation of testosterone, which results in higher levels at this time (Vierhapper et al, 1997). Testosterone levels reach a nadir during the early follicular phase, with small but less significant variation across the rest of the cycle. Thus, blood should be drawn after day 8 of the cycle and preferably before day 20. The gold standard methodology for measurement of free testosterone is considered by many investigators to be equilibrium dialysis.

Dehydroepiandrosterone (DHEA) is usually measured in the sulfated form, DHEAS, because the half-life is much longer, resulting in more stable levels. The immunoassay for DHEAS is relatively robust and simple to perform. DHEAS does not vary in concentration within the various phases of the menstrual cycle and is not bound significantly to DHEA. It also does not seem to be affected by estrogen therapy at standard doses. A number of authors (Zumoff et al, 1995; Baulieu, 1996; Mushayandebyu et al, 1996; Labrie et al, 1997a; Vierhapper et al, 1997; Baulieu et al, 2000; Davis et al, 2002; Guay and Davis, 2002; Guay et al, 2004a, 2004b) have shown consistent, age-related decline curves for DHEAS. If low levels are found, a morning cortisol level should be drawn to rule out adrenal insufficiency.

In summary, **although clinical consensus is lacking as to the value, specificity, and sensitivity of individual hormone blood tests, there are evidence-based, placebo-controlled, double-blind data supporting the efficacy of exogenous sex steroid hormone treatment in women with sexual health concerns** (Arlt et al, 1999; Barnhart et al, 1999; Shifren et al, 2000; Goldstat et al, 2003; Simon et al, 2004). As such, the prudent physician may wish to discuss with the patient the strategy of serial blood test surveillance testing to enhance safety concerns during such treatment.

A most common and controversial question concerns what is the "normal range" for sex steroid blood test values in women with sexual health problems. It is well recognized that the circulating testosterone concentration decreases with age in women. Zumoff and colleagues (1995) examined the 24-hour mean plasma concentration of free testosterone in 33 "healthy women" with regular menstrual cycles. A significant inverse correlation was noted between age and testosterone concentration (r = −0.54; P < .003). The testosterone concentration of women age 40 to 49 years was less than half the testosterone concentration in women age 20 to 29 years. Because the women in the study by Zumoff and colleagues were not screened for sexual dysfunction, it is likely, by virtue of the high prevalence of female sexual dysfunction, that some women with sexual dysfunction were included. If so, then the resulting data would be biased downward and may have underestimated the normal range of testosterone values in premenopausal women with normal sexual functioning, because some women with sexual dysfunction have low androgen levels. Guay and coworkers (2004a, 2004b) examined androgen values in women "without sexual dysfunction" as determined by a validated Female Sexual Questionnaire (Quirk et al, 2002). Androgen concentrations were highest in the women age 20 to 29 years, decreased at approximately age 30, and remained relatively constant thereafter. The free androgen index in women "without sexual dysfunction" was approximately 3.7 for women age 20 to 29 years and 2.0 for women between the ages of 30 and 39.

One final caveat concerning the clinical measurement of circulating sex steroid hormone levels concerns the fact that

determination of serum levels can only measure deficiency or excess. **Sex steroid hormone actions are quite complex and involve critical enzymes and critical hormone receptors that also determine tissue exposure, tissue sensitivity, and tissue responsiveness.** For example, in individuals, there are variations in the amount and activity of critical enzymes such as 5α-reductase and aromatase. In addition, individuals have variations in individual sex steroid hormone receptor sequencing. For example, the number of repeat sequences of cytosine, adenine, and guanine nucleotides, CAG repeats, in the DNA molecule coding for the sex steroid hormone receptor may vary widely in individuals. Thus, independent of the values of sex steroid hormones, the unique individual variations in critical enzymes and sex steroid hormone receptors result in individual differences in tissue exposure, tissue sensitivity, and tissue responsiveness. As can be seen, more research is needed in the blood testing of sex steroid hormones in women with sexual health concerns (Basson, 2005).

Specialized Testing

Vascular Testing

The biologic evaluation of women with sexual health problems involves an assessment of the integrity of multiple systems contributing to physiologic sexual function, including vascular factors when indicated (Basson et al, 2004a; Lewis et al, 2004; Nappi et al, 2005). During sexual arousal, the increased pelvic blood flow through the ilio-hypogastric-pudendal arterial bed leading to increased perfusion of the peripheral sexual organs results in an increased engorgement of the clitoral, labial, and vaginal erectile tissues, increased diameter of the clitoral corpora cavernosa and the labial corpora spongiosa (vestibular bulb erectile tissue), and increased diameter and length of the vagina (Giraldi et al, 2004). **The clinical relevance of diagnostic hemodynamic investigations in women with sexual dysfunction has not yet been established** (Basson et al, 2004a). It is likely, however, that there are sexual arousal problems and tissue integrity changes in women that are associated with ilio-hypogastric-pudendal arterial occlusive disease (Park et al, 1997, 2000; Tarcan et al, 1999; Lewis et al, 2004; Nappi et al, 2005). Vascular assessment by duplex Doppler ultrasound may be performed in the evaluation of women with sexual health concerns (Khalife et al, 2000; Bechara et al, 2003; Munarriz et al, 2003). Likely indications include women who are menopausal with sexual arousal disorders, women who have exposure to multiple vascular risk factors, women who have suffered pelvic fractures, or women with sexual arousal disorders unresponsive to other treatments.

It has been particularly difficult to observe and to quantify the blood flow changes that occur in women during arousal in a nonintrusive manner. Some of the physiologic measures for the assessment of genital blood flow during arousal have included vaginal photoplethysmography and oxygen-temperature measuring system; such tests have been used for psychophysiologic research in women since the 1970s (Levin and Wagner, 1977; Levin, 1997; Laan et al, 1995). Newer strategies include duplex Doppler ultrasonography (Akkus et al, 1995; Khalife et al, 2000; Becher et al, 2001; Bechara et al, 2003, Munarriz et al, 2003) and magnetic resonance imaging (MRI)

(Park et al, 2001b; Deliganis et al, 2002; Maravilla et al, 2003a, 2003b, 2005; Suh et al, 2003, 2004; Komisaruk et al, 2004).

In particular, urologists are familiar with **duplex Doppler ultrasonography** equipment to record hemodynamic integrity. This procedure **can be adapted for measuring vaginal, clitoral, and labial blood flow during arousal** (Fig. 28–13). There have been limited publications concerning duplex ultrasonographic findings in women with sexual dysfunction (Akkus et al, 1995; Khalife et al, 2000; Becher et al, 2001; Bechara et al, 2003; Munarriz et al, 2003). A high-frequency (12.5-MHz) external probe can be used to provide continuous, real-time imaging of arterial and erectile tissue components recorded at baseline and after sexual stimulation with an audiovisual sexual stimulation on a surround sound headset and a vibrator. Only visual stimulation is maintained during the actual ultrasound examination. Duplex Doppler ultrasonography can assess the changes in peak systolic velocity in centimeters per second that occur in the clitoral cavernosal and labial artery during sexual arousal. Genital tumescence is visually demonstrated on ultrasound, anatomically by increased venous pooling, and physiologically by increased end-diastolic velocities in the genital arteries. Duplex Doppler ultrasonography can also be used to assess the changes in clitoral and labial diameter associated with sexual stimulation. A transvaginal probe may be used to measure vaginal arterial peak systolic velocity changes. There is a paucity of "control" duplex Doppler ultrasound values in women without sexual dysfunction (Akkus et al, 1995; Khalife et al, 2000; Becher et al, 2001; Bechara et al, 2003; Munarriz et al, 2003).

MRI has been applied in recent years as a new method to evaluate changes in tissue signal intensity in the pelvic genital area and in the brain associated with sexual arousal in women. MRI is exquisitely sensitive to subtle changes in tissue composition, is noninvasive, and utilizes no ionizing radiation. MRI is capable of providing dynamic assessment of tissue changes over time and can also provide quantitative physiologic information such as information about three-dimensional anatomic volumes of specific structures, regional blood flow changes, and information about regional metabolite composition. **MRI can be utilized to define the normal anatomic relationships of the female genital structures in vivo** (Deliganis et al, 2002; Maravilla et al, 2003a, 2003b, 2005; Suh et al, 2003, 2004). This provides a more accurate picture and a better understanding of the functional anatomy of women compared with cadaver dissection studies. For example, just deep to the glans clitoris is the body of the clitoris not visible on direct visual examination of the introitus. The clitoral body is seen as a paired structure that gives rise to the two crura of the clitoris, which are also hidden from direct visual examination. The vestibular bulbs, oblong-shaped structures on either side of the vaginal opening in the midline, track alongside the clitoral crura and form an inverted V-shaped configuration. During arousal MR images show characteristic changes with engorgement that are most evident in the clitoris, especially in the crura and body of the clitoris. The vaginal mucosa does not show any increase in size and signal intensity because it is only a few cell layers thick, below the limit of resolution of the MRI technique, and is not resolvable separate from the muscular wall of the vagina itself (Suh et al, 2003).

Functional brain imaging or functional MRI represents the ability to observe anatomic sites of brain activation in response to a specific task performed by a subject using rapid dynamic MRI. This technique is an experimental tool for exploring brain function associated with emotional attraction, feelings of pleasure, and even sites of activation associated with sexual arousal. There have been a number of studies applying functional MRI techniques to the evaluation of sexual arousal or emotional response in women. Brain regions that activated with sexual arousal were related with visual association areas (posterior temporal-occipital cortices, paralimbic areas, anterior cingulate cortex) (Park et al, 2001b; Komisaruk et al, 2004).

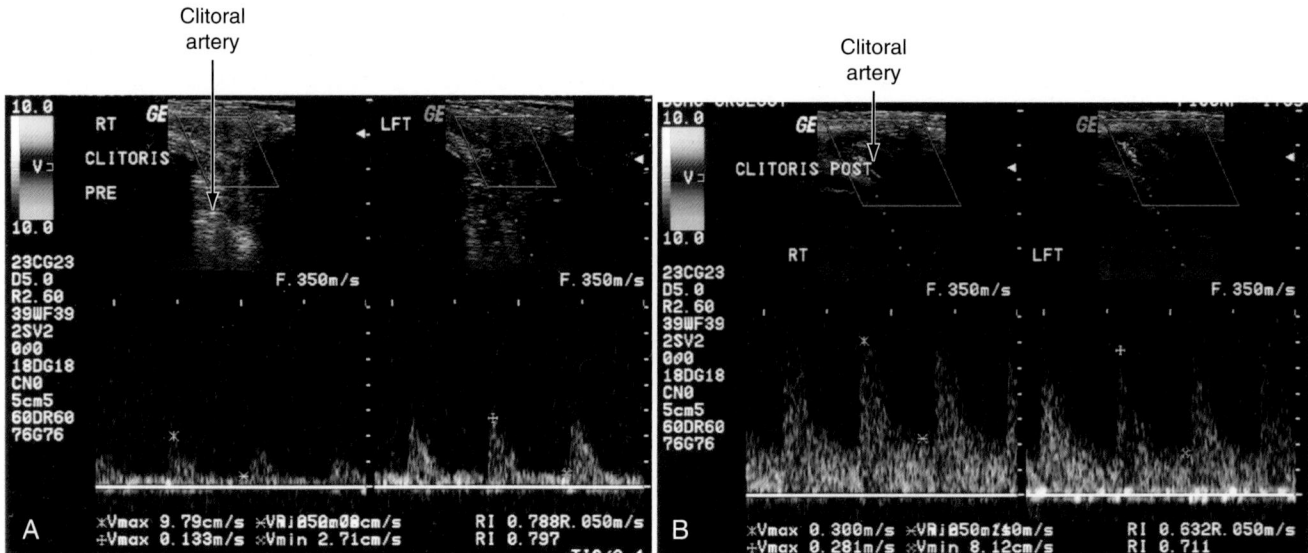

Figure 28–13. Duplex Doppler ultrasound of the right and left clitoral arteries before (**A**) and after (**B**) audiovisual mechanical sexual stimulation. After sexual arousal there are marked increases in both peak systolic and end-diastolic velocity values.

Neurologic Testing

There is only limited knowledge concerning central and peripheral nervous system physiologic regulation of a woman's sexual response (McKenna et al, 1991; Giraldi et al, 2004). Neurologic pathology adversely influencing the integrity of genital sensory and/or motor innervation may result in women's sexual dysfunction.

Neurologic testing of the integrity of the motor and sensory innervation of a woman's external genitalia is indicated in cases in which the history suggests neurologic pathophysiology of the sexual health concern (Basson et al, 2004a; Hatzichristou et al, 2004). For example, if the history is consistent with spinal cord injury, peripheral neuropathy, toxic neuropathy, uremic neuropathy, lumbar radiculopathy, and/or multiple sclerosis, there is a need for the urologist to quantitatively measure the neurologic function of the female genitalia. In such cases, neurophysiologic testing becomes an expansion of the genital physical examination.

In suspected neurologic disorders, in-office–based vibratory or thermal stimuli can be administered in a controlled manner via Quantitative Sensory Testing (QST) (Zaslansky and Yarnitsky, 1998; Vardi et al, 2000; Lowenstein et al, 2004). The subject determines the sensation threshold either verbally or by electronic means. Collected data are compared with a normal set of age-corrected threshold values to determine if sensory hypersensitivity or hyposensitivity is present. Specially designed probes exist for the quantitative measurement of sensation for the vaginal and clitoral region. The thermal probe has a working temperature range of 0°C to 50°C at both thermal surfaces. The vibration probe has a fixed vibration frequency at 100 Hz, with an amplitude range of 0 to 130 Hz. Like any other sensory measuring test, the Quantitative Sensory Testing is not fully objective, because it is dependent on the patients' subjective feeling and individual reaction time until pressing the button. It can be used as a valid initial clinical tool to evaluate the sensory state of the genital area in the woman (Zaslansky and Yarnitsky, 1998; Vardi et al, 2000; Lowenstein et al, 2004).

More sophisticated neurophysiologic testing of the motor and sensory nerve integrity of the woman's genitalia involves the performance of electrodiagnostic testing. Electrodiagnostic studies include nerve conduction studies, somatosensory evoked potential testing, bulbocavernosus reflex testing, and electromyography (Vodusek, 1990; Yang et al, 2000; Yilmaz et al, 2002; Yang and Kromm, 2004). Such tests should be referred to clinical and research settings where such specialized expertise exists.

TREATMENT

Hormonal Therapy: Premenopausal Women

As long as the premenopausal woman continues to regularly ovulate, estrogen and progesterone levels are maintained until the time of menopause. In premenopausal women, therefore, throughout their reproductive years, the primary source of estradiol is cyclical production by the ovaries (Simpson et al, 2000; Davis et al, 2004; Giraldi et al, 2004). The ovarian synthesis of estradiol in premenopause remains under the control

of the pituitary via follicle-stimulating hormone and inhibin. Estrogen synthesis throughout reproductive life also occurs, outside of the ovary, via adrenal and ovarian androgen precursors. In premenopausal women with regular menstrual cycles there is a rise in estradiol in the late follicular phase of the menstrual cycle and in the luteal phase. The luteal phase is characterized by a rise in progesterone, another sex steroid whose primary source of synthesis is the ovary. Estradiol and progesterone levels fall abruptly at the time of menopause when ovulation ceases (Simpson et al, 2000; Davis et al, 2004; Giraldi et al, 2004).

Estradiol and progesterone actions on central and peripheral target tissues are extensive. Estradiol is present centrally, with the highest concentrations of estradiol measured in the hypothalamus and the preoptic area (Bixo et al, 1995). In these central regions, there is high aromatase activity. **It is scientifically possible that estradiol is aromatized from testosterone conversion, resulting in high local estradiol concentrations in critical brain regions, resulting in modification of sexual behavior** (Roselli and Resko, 1993). Estrogen exhibits widespread actions throughout the brain (McEwen, 2002). Via estrogen receptors, estradiol is involved in a genomic process that utilizes transcription to induce protein synthesis and tissue structure and function. Estradiol also acts in a nongenomic fashion with direct interactions with numerous neurotransmitter systems, including catecholaminergic, serotoninergic, cholinergic, and γ-aminobutyric acidergic systems. Progesterone, like estrogen, has genomic activity via progesterone receptors that modulates gene expression and thus regulates neuronal networks that control sexual behavior. Estradiol increases the expression of progesterone receptor, which in turn functions as a critical coordinator of the sexual response. In summary, **there are much animal data to support that estradiol and progesterone as well as estrogen and progesterone receptors are crucial for genomic and nongenomic regulation of sexual behavior** (Roselli and Resko, 1993; Bixo et al, 1995; McEwen, 2002).

Evidence-Based Basic Science/Clinical Research Data—Estrogen and Progesterone

There is no evidence that premenopausal women who have sexual dysfunction and who have regular menstrual cycles with ovulation require exogenous estrogen and/or estrogen and progesterone therapy to improve their sexual function. On the other hand, premenopausal women with sexual dysfunction who do not have regular, normal menstrual cycles and are otherwise amenorrheic, or dysmenorrheic or menorrhagic, should have the underlying pathophysiology managed and, if indicated, receive estrogen and progestin hormonal therapy. During the premenopausal years there are other medical issues that interfere with cyclical estrogen and progesterone production. Clinical examples include rapid weight loss and anorexia nervosa, in which it has been well documented that estrogen and progesterone levels in such conditions may fall (Basson et al, 2004a; Davis et al, 2004; Lewis et al, 2004; Basson, 2005).

Should there be the need for exogenous estrogen and progesterone treatment, there are many choices of estrogen and progesterone for women, including bioidentical and synthetic forms of estradiol and progesterone as well as multiple delivery systems for administration, including oral, transdermal, transvaginal, or parenteral routes (Davis et al, 2004). The choice of estrogen and progesterone utilized (synthetic or nonsynthetic) may have important implications on the woman's sex steroid hormonal milieu, especially the SHBG and androgen values (Dunn et al, 1981). Thus **the choice of estrogen and/or progesterone may adversely influence sexual function** (Davis et al, 2004).

For example, premenopausal women who are otherwise healthy, have no sexual health issues, and have normal menstrual cycles may elect to use exogenous potent synthetic estrogen, such as ethinyl estradiol, in combination with various synthetic progestogens for reversible pharmacologic birth control. These oral contraceptives diminish FSH and LH levels and reduce metabolic activity of the ovary, including suppression of ovulation. **Circulating levels of androgens, recognized sex steroids that are major modulators of sexual function in women, are decreased by oral contraceptives by two separate mechanisms:** (1) direct inhibition of androgen production in the ovaries and (2) marked increase in the hepatic synthesis of SHBG. **The combination of these two mechanisms may lead to very low circulating levels of free and bioavailable testosterone. Several studies have already reported negative effects of oral contraceptives on sexual function,** including diminished sexual interest and arousal, suppression of female-initiated sexual activity, and decreased frequency of sexual intercourse and sexual enjoyment (Basson et al, 2004a; Davis et al, 2004; Nappi et al, 2005).

KEY POINT: HORMONAL THERAPY: PREMENOPAUSAL WOMEN: ESTROGEN AND PROGESTERONE

■ There are limited studies in premenopausal women concerning the risks and benefits of the various exogenous synthetic and nonsynthetic estrogens and progestins on their sexual function. In summary, should a premenopausal woman require exogenous estrogen and/or progesterone treatment to manage amenorrhea, dysmenorrhea, or menorrhagia, the choice of hormones may have an adverse impact on SHBG and androgen levels and the quality of her sexual function. Should exogenous estrogens and progestins be utilized in a woman for elective pharmacologic birth control or for management of menstrual disorders, use of surveillance blood tests at regular intervals to assess SHBG and androgen levels may be useful should sexual dysfunction result. Alternative nonestrogen/progesterone treatments may be considered should hormonal-based sexual problems be linked to the use of estrogen/progestin treatment (Davis et al, 2004).

Evidence-Based Basic Science/Clinical Research Data—Androgens

Dehydroepiandrosterone. DHEA is an adrenal precursor sex steroid hormone that is converted to other androgens, such as Δ-5-androstenediol, Δ-4-androstenedione, and testos-

terone via the enzymes 3β and 17β hydroxysteroid dehydrogenase, and ultimately to estradiol via aromatase or to dihydrotestosterone via 5α-reductase (Baulieu, 1996; Barnhart et al, 1999; Baulieu et al, 2000). New research shows that DHEA has its own receptors, primarily on endothelial cells, and that DHEA is involved in the process of vascular smooth muscle relaxation. Additional research notes that Δ-5-androstenediol acts on its own receptors on the vaginal mucosa and is involved in the mucin content of vaginal lubrication (Traish et al, 2004). It is thus important to note that **any positive effects of DHEA on sexual function must take into account all the actions of DHEA, that is DHEA alone and as a precursor of multiple androgens** (such as Δ-5-androstenediol and Δ-4-androstenedione and estrogens), especially testosterone and estradiol (Labrie et al, 1997a, 1997b; Baulieu, 1996; Baulieu et al, 2000; Davis et al, 2004).

There are limited studies evaluating the effects of oral DHEA on the sexual function of women. One placebo-controlled randomized clinical trial involved a 4-month crossover design of 24 women with adrenal insufficiency (Arlt et al, 1999). Compared with those subjects who received 50 mg/day of DHEA versus placebo, the active drug increased serum testosterone from below normal to the normal range and significantly increased sexual thoughts, interest, and mental and physical satisfaction. Two other studies of women with Addison's disease involved the use of 50 mg/day dose of DHEA and, in both, significant improvements were noted in self-esteem, mood, and fatigue (Hunt et al, 2000; Lovas et al, 2003). A retrospective open-label study of DHEA treatment (50 mg/day) in 113 healthy women with sexual dysfunction secondary to diminished desire, arousal, and orgasmic capacity noted increases in desire, arousal, lubrication, orgasm, and satisfaction compared with baseline function ($P < .05$) (Munarriz et al, 2002a).

The androgen precursors DHEA and androstenedione are both available without prescription as dietary supplements. As such there is wide disparity in the purity and formulation of these products, making it difficult to compare among the various safety and efficacy studies. **Administration of DHEA to women has also been shown to increase testosterone levels appreciably** (Labrie et al, 1997b). In one study, 100 mg of androstenedione administered orally to women raised testosterone levels by approximately 100 ng/dL. **Safety issues for any androgen therapy, including DHEA and androstenedione, include the development of acne and hirsutism** (Labrie et al, 1997b; Arlt et al, 1999; Barnhart et al, 1999; Hunt et al, 2000; Munarriz et al, 2002a; Kicman et al, 2003; Lovas et al, 2003). **To prevent other safety issues, routine blood test surveillance testing is indicated. Markedly supraphysiologic testosterone levels could result in possible hepatotoxicity, reduction in high-density lipoprotein cholesterol, and elevation of estradiol and estrone levels.** Further research is needed to better understand the role of androgen precursors in women with sexual dysfunction.

Testosterone. In premenopausal women with regular menstrual cycles throughout their reproductive years there is a rise in testosterone and androstenedione in the late follicular phase of the menstrual cycle and in the luteal phase (Vierhapper et al, 1997). **In premenopausal women, there is also a diurnal variation in testosterone, with the peak in the**

morning (Vierhapper et al, 1997). Whereas in men nearly all testosterone synthesis occurs in the testis, **in women testosterone synthesis occurs from approximately 50% directly by the ovaries and the adrenal glands and the remaining 50% from testosterone precursors such as androstenedione and DHEA processed in the peripheral tissues** (Simpson et al, 2000).

Aging, in premenopausal women, adversely affects serum testosterone levels in a slow and progressive decline (Zumoff et al, 1995; Baulieu, 1996; Mushayandebyu et al, 1996; Vierhapper et al, 1997; Baulieu et al, 2000; Bachmann et al, 2002; Davis, 2002; Guay and Davis, 2002; Guay et al, 2004a, 2004b; Davis et al, 2004). This is in sharp contrast to estrogen and progesterone levels, which fall abruptly with menopause. Total and free testosterone levels fall from the 20s to the 40s such that women in their 40s have about half the circulating levels of testosterone and free testosterone as do women in their 20s (Zumoff et al, 1995; Guay et al, 2004a, 2004b). **In addition, in the late reproductive years the mid-cycle rise in free testosterone, a hallmark of the menstrual cycle in young ovulating women, begins to diminish** (Mushayandebyu et al, 1996). Another factor is the level of adrenal precursors that serve as a prehormone for about half of ovarian testosterone production; serum levels of DHEAS and DHEA also fall with increasing age (Baulieu, 1996; Baulieu et al, 2000).

Other than aging, there are several clinical conditions in premenopausal women that are associated with low testosterone levels (Bachmann et al, 2002; Guay and Davis, 2002; Davis et al, 2004; Guay et al, 2004a, 2004b). For example, **hyperprolactinemia** may occur either secondary to a prolactinoma or secondary to medications. Hyperprolactinemia results in hypogonadotropic hypogonadism and loss of libido. Another example is **adrenal insufficiency.** In such conditions there are associated reductions in DHEAS and total testosterone. Similarly, Cushing's disease or endogenous or exogenous glucocorticosteroid excess leads to adrenal suppression and androgen insufficiency and thus may indirectly inhibit sexual function. As discussed earlier, **the oral contraceptive pill suppresses both ovarian testosterone production and increases SHBG, thus reducing free testosterone** (Bachmann et al, 2002; Guay and Davis, 2002; Davis et al, 2004, Guay et al, 2004a, 2004b).

A multinational expert panel developed a consensus statement on the role of androgen insufficiency in female sexual dysfunction (Bachmann et al, 2002; Nappi et al, 2005). **Androgen insufficiency was defined as a pattern of characteristic clinical symptoms in the presence of decreased bioavailable or free testosterone.** These symptoms include diminished sense of well-being or dysphoric mood; persistent unexplained fatigue; changes in sexual function, including decreased libido, sexual receptivity, and pleasure; and vasomotor instability or decreased vaginal lubrication, even with adequate estrogen treatment. Bone loss, decreased muscle strength, and changes in memory or cognitive function are also possible as a result of diminished androgen production.

There are limited basic science studies relating testosterone to sexual behavior in the woman. Animal studies reveal that androgen receptor messenger RNA-containing neurons are widely distributed in the central brain regions thought to play a key role in mediating the hormonal control of sexual behavior, such as the hypothalamus, and in locations, including the telencephalon, that provide strong input to the medial preoptic and ventromedial nuclei (Simerley et al, 1990). Furthermore, in the animal brain, high densities of the enzyme aromatase are observed co-localized with high densities of androgen receptor mRNA-containing neurons in numerous regions of the brain integral to central control of sexual behavior. At least in animal models, testosterone, in conjunction with estrogen, appears to be associated with sexual behavior (Simerley et al, 1990).

Androgens may also play a role in peripheral genital structure and function. Whereas a lack of estrogen is the common cause of dyspareunia in postmenopausal women, there have been reports of associations between androstenedione and testosterone levels and vaginal physiologic function (Giraldi et al, 2004; Traish et al, 2002, 2004). Androgen receptors have been reported in the vagina, and these may play a role in vaginal health (Traish et al, 2004).

There are limited clinical studies in premenopausal women examining the relationships between serum testosterone levels and sexual activity (Bachmann et al, 2002; Guay and Davis, 2002; Davis et al, 2004; Guay et al, 2004a, 2004b; Nappi et al, 2005). Low sexual desire has been associated with lower testosterone and DHEAS levels in some studies. In 45 premenopausal women presenting with low libido, one randomized crossover clinical trial of transdermal testosterone therapy versus placebo has been reported. Those who received the active drug significantly improved sexual motivation, fantasy, frequency of sexual activity, pleasure, orgasm, and satisfaction. Testosterone also significantly improved the total score and all subscale scores of the Personal General Well-Being Index in the premenopausal women (Goldstat et al, 2003).

Testosterone may one day prove to be an efficacious therapy for premenopausal women with sexual health concerns; currently there are limited data on long-term safety (Bachmann et al, 2002; Guay and Davis, 2002; Goldstat et al, 2003; Davis et al, 2004; Guay et al, 2004a, 2004b). In premenopausal women, adverse effects of testosterone therapy include hirsutism and acne. Other side effects may include balding, voice deepening, clitoromegaly, and polycythemia. Although oral testosterone therapy as methyltestosterone results in lowering of high-density lipoprotein cholesterol, there is no evidence that parenteral testosterone therapy has adverse cardiovascular effects. High doses of orally administered androgens such as methyltestosterone and, to a lesser extent, testosterone undecanoate may be associated with hepatotoxicity (peliosis hepatis, hepatic neoplasms, and cholestatic jaundice), but this has not been a problem for lower-dose therapy (Bachmann et al, 2002; Guay and Davis, 2002; Goldstat et al, 2003; Davis et al, 2004; Guay et al, 2004a, 2004b). There is no evidence that exogenous testosterone increases the risk of endometrial cancer or endometriosis (Goldstat et al, 2003).

A major concern for premenopausal reproductive-aged women is the potential for harm to either the mother or fetus should pregnancy occur during the administration of testosterone. Virilization of the fetus does not commonly occur, and high levels of testosterone are required for maternal virilization to occur, consistent with the fact that normal pregnancy is a hyperandrogenic state (Ben-Chetrit and Greenblatt, 1995). Testosterone levels begin to rise in the first trimester, with free testosterone peaking in the third trimester of normal pregnancy. It is believed that high circulating SHBG and progesterone (which binds the androgen receptor) may protect the mother and fetus from virilization unless androgens are massively elevated. Wolf and coworkers (2002) studied the effects of a range of doses of testosterone propionate administered subcutaneously to pregnant Sprague-Dawley rats. Androgenic effects were seen at a dose of 0.5 mg that elevated maternal levels of testosterone 10-fold but had no effect on fetal levels. Viability of the offspring was unaffected at any dose. Adverse fetal effects included increased anogenital distance, reduced number of areolas and nipples, cleft phallus, small vaginal orifice, and presence of prostatic tissue. The 0.1-mg dose, which would be estimated to have increased female serum levels about 2-fold, did not cause any adverse effects.

Any premenopausal woman treated with androgen therapy needs to be thoroughly counseled regarding risks and benefits and the need for routine follow-up and blood test surveillance testing (Bachmann et al, 2002; Guay and Davis, 2002; Davis et al, 2004; Guay et al, 2004a, 2004b). Ongoing monitoring should include assessment for signs of androgen excess (acne and hirsutism), the presence of abnormal vaginal bleeding, regular breast and pelvic examinations, every 3-month monitoring of serum androgen levels, yearly monitoring of liver function tests, and lipid profiles. In the presence of a family history of diabetes or significant obesity, fasting insulin and glucose levels should be considered. Contraception and the risk of adverse effects on a fetus should be discussed (Bachmann et al, 2002; Guay and Davis, 2002; Davis et al, 2004; Guay et al, 2004a, 2004b).

KEY POINT: HORMONAL THERAPY: PREMENOPAUSAL WOMEN: ANDROGENS

■ Sex steroid hormones have a critical role in the maintenance of structure and function of women's genital organs and tissues and an essential role in the central regulation of sexual behavior. Androgen levels fall for various medical reasons and as a result of aging. Currently, there are limited human safety and efficacy data in the management of premenopausal women with sexual heath concerns. Although initial studies may support preliminary evidence for effectiveness of testosterone for increasing libido, arousal, and orgasm in premenopausal women, more long-term safety data in premenopausal women with sexual health concerns are needed (Bachmann et al, 2002; Guay and Davis, 2002; Davis et al, 2004; Guay et al, 2004a, 2004b).

Hormonal Therapy: Perimenopausal and Postmenopausal Women

Women will experience the natural evolution from prepuberty, to puberty (reproductive capabilities), to perimenopause (transition leading up to the final menstrual period), and to menopause (cessation of estradiol production by the ovaries) (Bachmann and Leiblum, 2004). The mean age at the onset of menopause is approximately 51 years of age (Reynolds and Obermeyer, 2005). **Due to expanded life expectancy until their mid-80s, women will live approximately one third of their lives in menopause,** an average of 30 or more years beyond the onset of the menopause. In this perimenopausal and postmenopausal era, women frequently encounter a range of new medical issues, such as hypertension, hyperlipidemia, obesity, diabetes mellitus, coronary heart disease, osteopenia, osteoporosis, depression, and breast cancer. As it concerns this chapter, women in the perimenopause and postmenopause period frequently encounter sexual health concerns. Although quality of life may not be negatively impacted as the result of sexual dysfunction in all women, for some, sexual problems can be associated with significant personal distress and may result in diminution of their ego, self-worth, and self-esteem, as well as a significant reduction in life satisfaction and quality of the couple's relationship (Freedman, 2002; Bachmann and Leiblum, 2004; Kovalvsky, 2004; Reynolds and Obermeyer, 2005).

In postmenopausal women, sexual problems are less likely to be reversible or situational than in younger, premenopausal women. For example, premenopausal women often experience temporary sexual problems during couple infertility concerns, during pregnancy, during breast-feeding post partum, during the time her young child has a short-term illness, or during a period of fatigue or relationship discord. During perimenopause and postmenopause, however, sexual dysfunctions occur more frequently, are more often irreversible, and are more likely to be progressive, particularly if the pathophysiology of the dysfunction is related to vaginal atrophy secondary to estrogen deficiency. The consequences of hormonal insufficiency may not be reversible unless local or systemic estrogen treatment is initiated, and hormonal insufficiency is not a condition that decreases in intensity over time (Freedman, 2002; Bachmann and Leiblum, 2004; Kovalevsky, 2004; Nappi et al, 2005).

Because the prevalence of sexual dysfunction is so high in women during menopause, it is important for health care professionals who treat women with general health concerns to initiate direct discussion of their patient's sexual function and any subsequent consequences. Health care providers who are interested in providing the medical care but feel uncomfortable owing to lack of training should consider receiving postgraduate education on evidence-based management principles for woman's sexual health concerns (available from the International Society for the Study of Women's Sexual Health [www.isswsh.org]). Armed with such knowledge, health care professionals may be more amenable to discuss basic and initial management principles with their postmenopausal patients who have sexual health concerns. It should be emphasized that a woman's sexual response is a complex interactive process involving a unique set of mind, body, and partner issues. All contributors to woman's sexual health should be evaluated when considering therapeutic approach (Basson et al, 2004a).

Evidence-Based Basic Science/Clinical Research Data—Estrogen and Progesterone

All women in the menopause will have cessation of ovarian estradiol production. Estrogen continues to be synthesized in the periphery (e.g., skin, adipose tissue, bone, muscle) in post-menopausal women through conversion of androstenedione to estrone and testosterone to estradiol, but the amount of estradiol synthesized depends, in part, on the enzymatic activity of aromatase (Simpson et al, 2000).

The important principle is that estrogens are required for genital tissue structure and function (McKenna et al, 1991; Haefner, 1999; Park et al, 2001a; Yoon et al, 2001; Min et al, 2002; Stewart, 2002; Traish et al, 2002, 2003; Anderson et al, 2004; Basson et al, 2004c; Davis et al, 2004; Giraldi et al, 2004; Kim NN et al, 2004; Kim SW et al, 2004). Estrogens act on estrogen receptors that exist in high levels in the genital tissues, including epithelial/endothelial cells and smooth muscle cells of the vagina, vulva, vestibule, labia, and urethra, suggesting that these genital tissues require estrogen for structure and function. **Diminished estrogen production in the menopause renders these genital tissues highly susceptible to atrophy.** Following weeks to months of exposure to low estrogen, atrophic changes can be identified. The host of genital tissue structural changes and cellular dysfunctions that occur in the genital tissues as a result of estrogen deficiency are as follows. Specifically in the vagina, estrogen deficiency leads to vaginal atrophy (Fig. 28–14). One consequence of the atrophic vagina secondary to estrogen deficiency is an alteration of the normally acidic vaginal pH that usually discourages growth of pathogenic bacteria. In an estrogen-rich environment, glycogen from sloughed epithelial cells is hydrolyzed into glucose and then metabolized to lactic acid by normal vaginal flora. In the postmenopausal women, epithelial thinning reduces the available glycogen. The change to an alkaline pH value leads to a shift in the vaginal flora, resulting in the likelihood of vaginal yeast infections, discharge, and odor (McKenna et al, 1991; Haefner, 1999; Park et al, 2001a; Yoon et al, 2001; Freedman, 2002; Min et al, 2002; Stewart, 2002; Traish et al, 2002, 2003; Anderson et al, 2004; Bachmann and Leiblum, 2004; Basson et al, 2004c; Davis et al, 2004; Giraldi et al, 2004; Kim NN et al, 2004; Kim SW et al, 2004; Kovalevsky, 2004; Nappi et al, 2005).

Other consequences of chronic estrogen deficiency in the vagina are that the epithelium and vascular, muscular, and connective tissues of the vagina atrophy. This leads to the vaginal vault becoming pale or colorless, with loss of multiple folds or rugae normally present in the estrogenized vagina. The atrophy of the lamina propria blood vessels leads to diminished blood flow to the tissues, decreased lubrication, and vaginal dryness. Estrogen deficiency may lead also to adverse changes in vestibular sensation, with diminished perception to vibratory sensation and hot and cold sensation. Reduction of vestibular sensation may be a cause for diminution and muffling of the orgasmic intensity. Thinning of the vaginal epithelial layer leads to increased friability and lowered elasticity of vaginal tissues. When coital activity is attempted in the presence of estrogen deficiency, the marked shortening and narrowing of the vaginal vault may make sexual activity painful, unpleasant, and unsatisfactory (Haefner, 1999; Freedman, 2002; Stewart, 2002; Anderson et al, 2004; Bachmann and Leiblum, 2004; Kovalevsky, 2004; Basson et al, 2004c; Davis et al, 2004; Nappi et al, 2005).

Estrogen deficiency also adversely affects other genital tissues. The clitoral hood may become phimotic, and the glans clitoris may atrophy and become fibrosed with persistent estrogen deficiency and diminished genital blood flow. There is thinning of the hair of the mons, and shrinkage of the labia minora. The labia majora atrophy because there is decreased subcutaneous fat and skin elasticity. It is common for women to experience itching as tissues undergo atrophy. The endocervical glandular tissue produces less mucin, further contributing to vaginal dryness. Estrogen deficiency can also decrease vibratory sensation of the clitoris and labia. Estrogen deficiency also adversely affects the bladder, and women frequently note dysuria, urinary frequency, urgency, incontinence, and postcoital urinary tract infections. In summary,

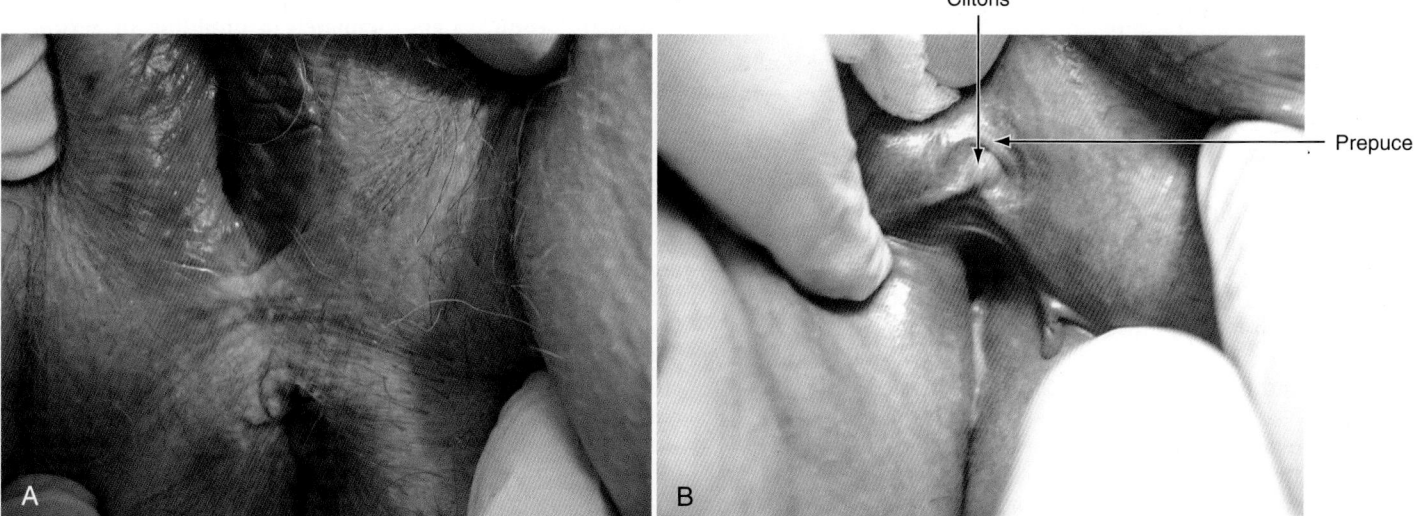

Figure 28–14. **A** and **B,** Abnormal physical examination of a postmenopausal 64-year-old woman. The patient has multidimensional sexual dysfunction involving problems with desire, arousal, vaginal dryness, orgasm, and pain. This woman has various degrees of clitoral and preputial atrophy, labial atrophy, pale color of the vaginal vault, and loss of rugae in the vaginal wall. She was found to have diminished clitoral blood flow and diminished vestibular sensation with diminished perception to vibratory sensation. The important principle is that estrogens are required for genital tissue structure and function.

the routine clinical symptoms of estrogen deficiency include vaginal atrophy, vaginal dryness, diminished vaginal sensation, painful intercourse, and vaginal bleeding after minimal trauma. Other common symptoms of low estrogen include hot flushes, night sweats, and nocturnal awakening (Haefner, 1999; Freedman, 2002; Stewart, 2002; Anderson et al, 2004; Bachmann and Leiblum, 2004; Basson et al, 2004c; Davis et al, 2004; Kovalevsky, 2004; Nappi et al, 2005).

The use of systemic and/or localized estrogen and/or progesterone must be individualized to each patient's desires, wishes, requirements, and expectations. Systemic estrogen therapy can successfully improve hot flushes, night sweats, and sleep disturbances that can otherwise markedly diminish afflicted women's body image, mood, and sexual desire. Local estrogen therapy can successfully improve vaginal lubrication, vaginal dryness, and dyspareunia. Alleviation of such symptoms by systemic and/or localized estrogen can increase quality of life, desire, arousal, and orgasmic function (Freedman, 2002; Bachmann and Leiblum, 2004; Kovalevsky, 2004).

Systemic Estrogen/Progesterone Therapy and Vaginal Atrophy. Several clinical trials have shown that the distressing symptoms of vaginal atrophy associated with low estrogen states are ameliorated after estrogen therapy. Low doses of systemic conjugated equine estrogen with and without medroxyprogesterone acetate reduced vaginal atrophy compared with placebo in several thousand healthy menopausal women (Utian et al, 2001). One placebo-controlled trial was conducted in postmenopausal ovariectomized women with sexual dysfunction receiving estrogen therapy. A significant improvement in vaginal symptoms, and also mood, sexual desire, enjoyment, and orgasmic frequency, was reported in the women receiving ethinyl estradiol (50 μg) compared with levonorgestrel (250 μg/day), a combination of these two substances, or placebo (Dennerstein et al, 1980).

Local Estrogen Therapy and Vaginal Atrophy. Local estrogen therapy can within weeks to months effectively restore vaginal epithelium and relieve atrophy. There are a variety of local vaginal estrogen therapies such as creams consisting of conjugated equine estrogen, estradiol, and estriol. Other forms of local estrogen delivery systems include rings and tablets. A 2-mg estradiol ring, placed in the vagina for 3 months, slowly releases the estradiol locally. A 17β-estradiol tablet in a 25-μg single vaginal dose applicator is administered daily for the first 2 weeks of treatment, then decreased to 1 vaginal tablet twice weekly as maintenance therapy (Barentsen et al, 1997). Several studies have shown restoration of vaginal cytology and improvement of vaginal atrophy and dryness (Buckler and Al-Azzawi, 2003; Bachmann and Leiblum, 2004; Davis et al, 2004; Kovalevsky, 2004). A randomized clinical trial found that among postmenopausal women with vaginal atrophy, a continuous low-dose estradiol-releasing vaginal ring provided relief and was more acceptable compared with conjugated equine estrogen vaginal cream (Ayton et al, 1996). Another comparative study of menopausal women found that local 25-hydroxy-17β-estradiol vaginal tablets and conjugated equine estrogen vaginal cream were equally efficacious in relieving vaginal atrophy but the vaginal tablets produced less endometrial proliferation and were more favorable than the

cream (Rioux et al, 2000). Higher estrogen dosages of vaginal creams can result in increased systemic estrogen concentrations owing to the bolus absorption of the product.

Evidence-Based Basic Science/Clinical Research Data—Androgens

In menopausal women, androgens are also critical in maintaining genital tissue structure and function (McKenna et al, 1991; Traish et al, 2002; Basson et al, 2004c; Giraldi et al, 2004; Nappi et al, 2005). **Androgens, like estrogens, contribute to other sexual and nonsexual physiologic functions,** including desire and orgasm responses, bone and skeletal muscle metabolism, cognition, energy, and feelings of well-being. The synthesis of the seven androgens, from the ovaries and zona reticularis of the adrenal gland from cholesterol, and in the periphery from DHEA, decline with aging in premenopausal women and continue to decrease with advancing age in the menopause. After menopause, androgen insufficiency occurs, in part, due to contributions from reduced synthetic function in both the adrenals and the ovaries. Furthermore, SHBG, which has a high affinity for binding testosterone, increases in postmenopausal women, especially those treated with oral estrogen therapy. The net effect of a diminished androgen synthesis and an increase in SHBG is a reduced amount of free testosterone. **Classic complaints of low androgen levels include decreased libido and impaired sexual functioning, but also muscle wasting, osteoporosis, loss of energy, changes in mood, and depression** (Nappi et al, 2005).

Androgen treatments have been evaluated for postmenopausal women with sexual dysfunction for many years, and there are evidence-based data regarding the safety and efficacy (Davis et al, 2004).

Dehydroepiandrosterone. There are limited clinical trials that have examined the effects of DHEA therapy on sexual function in postmenopausal women, in part owing to a lack of pharmaceutical-grade DHEA consistent in preparation and free from contaminants. Baulieu and colleagues (2000) administered DHEA (50 mg) or placebo to 140 women between the ages of 60 and 79 years for 12 months. **DHEA treatment produced approximately a doubling of serum total testosterone concentration and also significantly increased skin hydration and bone density.** Libidinal interest was increased after 6 months of treatment, and sexual activity and sexual satisfaction were increased after 12 months.

Testosterone. Although there were a number of clinical trials using testosterone-like products (e.g., methyltestosterone with or without synthetic estrogens) in the past, contemporary data are reported from multi-institutional, placebo-controlled trials utilizing transdermal testosterone in postmenopausal women (Shifren et al, 2000; Simon et al, 2004).

One such trial (Shifren et al, 2000) examined the safety and efficacy of 12-week treatment with transdermal testosterone patches (150 μg/day, 300 μg/day vs. placebo patches) in 75 women between the ages of 31 and 56 with sexual health concerns who had undergone hysterectomy and oophorectomy and received replacement conjugated equine estrogens. Those women who received the 150-μg dose patch increased total testosterone to approximately the upper limit of the normal range. Those who received the 300-μg dose patch increased testosterone to well above the upper limit of the normal range.

There were significant increases in free testosterone, bioavailable testosterone, and dihydrotestosterone from the lower limit of the normal range to higher values within the normal range. The SHBG concentration was very high in all treatment groups as a result of the exogenous estrogen administration. Of note, DHEA levels did not change significantly with testosterone treatment. **For measures of the frequency of sexual activity and pleasure and orgasm, those who utilized the testosterone patch observed significantly greater improvements than placebo.** No significant adverse effects were noted from baseline on measures of blood lipids, including total cholesterol, high-density lipoprotein cholesterol, low-density lipoprotein cholesterol, or triglycerides. The incidence of hirsutism and acne were unchanged from baseline with the 150-µg/day or the 300-µg/day testosterone dose. Patients reported an increase in depilation of facial hair by an average of one time per month more with the 300-µg/day testosterone dose.

Other studies (Simon et al, 2004) reported on the use of 24 weeks of double-blind treatment with placebo or testosterone transdermal patch (300 µg/day) in women (mean age 49 years; in their current relationship for an average of 18 to 19 years) with surgically induced menopause (mean 8 to 9 years earlier) and hypoactive sexual desire disorder on oral or transdermal estrogen. The primary efficacy outcome parameter was total satisfying sexual activity, which significantly increased with testosterone administration in both studies. Treatment produced an increase from baseline of approximately one episode of sexual activity per 4 weeks in the placebo group to two episodes per 4 weeks in the testosterone group ($P = .0003$ for study 1; $P = .001$ for study 2). Scores on a sexual desire rating scale increased by 56% from baseline with the testosterone patch versus 29% from baseline with placebo ($P = .0006$) in one study and by 49% with the testosterone patch versus 18% from baseline with placebo ($P = .0006$) in the other study. **Testosterone treatment was also associated with significant improvement in a number of secondary sexual function outcome measures, including arousal, orgasm, pleasure, and body image.** Women assigned to testosterone also reported decreased concern or distress about sexual functioning. The most common adverse events were application site reactions and hirsutism. No differences were observed in the prevalence of adverse events or in clinical laboratory value changes between the testosterone groups versus placebo.

Nonhormonal Medical Therapy

Dopamine Agonist Administration

Sexual motivation is encouraged, sustained, and ended by a number of central nervous system neurotransmitter and receptor changes induced, in part, by the action of sex steroids, androgens, estrogens, progestins, and the central neurotransmitter dopamine. The activation of dopamine receptors may be a key intermediary in the stimulation of incentive sexual motivation and sexual reward. These neurotransmitter and receptor changes, in turn, activate central sexual arousal and desire (Pfaus 1999; Giuliano and Allard, 2001; Pfaus et al, 2003; Giraldi et al, 2004).

Androgens may be accommodating in this by allowing more estradiol to be distributed to central nervous system

target tissues via aromatase (Pfaus 1999; Giuliano and Allard, 2001; Pfaus et al, 2003, 2004). Progestins appear to play a role in females, with small amounts activating progestin receptors in important central hypothalamic and limbic structures to increase sexual motivation. Contemporary animal research reveals that dopamine neurotransmitter systems may play a critical intermediary role in the central regulation of sexual arousal and excitation, mood, and incentive-related sexual behavior, in particular, in the motivational responses to conditioned external stimuli. In summary, the complex central neurochemical actions of steroid hormones stimulate sensory awareness, central sexual arousal, mood, and reward and relate them to the relevant individual's sexual experiences involving a partner, a place, and an action (Pfaus, 1999; Giuliano and Allard, 2001; Pfaus et al, 2003, 2004).

A clinical effect was noted with the dopamine receptor agonist apomorphine, stimulating sexual solicitation in ovariectomized rats treated with estradiol (Beharry et al, 2003). Evidence exists for the participation of the dopaminergic system and D_1/D_2 dopamine receptor agonists in the control of women's sexual function. A placebo-controlled study (Caruso et al, 2004) was performed to verify whether a D_1/D_2 dopamine receptor agonist was effective in premenopausal women affected by arousal disorder and hypoactive sexual desire disorder. Women were randomly allocated to treatment in one of six possible sequences of three 2-week double-blind, crossover study periods with the D_1/D_2 dopamine receptor agonist apomorphine, 2 mg or 3 mg, washout, and placebo. The daily intake of the drug was effective with both the 2-mg and 3-mg dosages compared with placebo for arousal and desire. The effects of 3 mg of apomorphine were better than those obtained with 2 mg. **The orgasm, enjoyment, and satisfaction with frequency scores improved during treatment with daily D_1/D_2 dopamine receptor agonist compared with baseline and placebo.** Adverse events were mild or moderate, occurring both during the "as required" part and during daily usage, and were mainly nausea, vomiting, dizziness, or headache. However, during the placebo period, two women had adverse events, mainly headache (Caruso et al, 2004).

A randomized, double-blind, placebo-controlled study (Bechara et al, 2004) was performed to evaluate changes in female sexual response in premenopausal women with orgasmic sexual dysfunction treated with 3 mg of sublingual apomorphine. Sexual response was evaluated objectively by Doppler sonography and subjectively by self-reported questionnaire, following vibrator stimulation with the addition of apomorphine or placebo. Clitoral hemodynamic changes were higher with the D_1/D_2 dopamine receptor agonist than placebo, even when there were no differences between D_1/D_2 dopamine receptor agonist and placebo in regard to orgasm, probably due to confounding factors such as study situation, lack of intimacy, and a single apomorphine dose (Bechara et al, 2004).

A number of studies have examined the effects of pharmacologic agents for treating antidepressant-induced sexual dysfunction (Clayton et al, 2004). Some such drugs include dopaminergic agents such as amantadine (Balon, 1996) and mianserin (Aizenberg et al, 1999). Bupropion may have a beneficial effect on premenopausal women with hypoactive sexual desire disorder (Segraves et al, 2004). In a placebo-controlled trial, bupropion produced an increase in desire and frequency of sexual activity compared with placebo. However, frequency was correlated to total testosterone level at baseline and during treatment (Segraves et al, 2004).

Vasodilator Administration

There are limited basic science studies investigating the physiology of sexual function utilizing female animal models (Giraldi et al, 2004). Those studies that have been performed to support the role of nitric oxide/cyclic guanosine monophosphate/phosphodiesterase type 5 pathways in the peripheral arousal physiology of the clitoral corpus cavernosum, corpus spongiosum, vaginal epithelium, and vaginal lamina propria (Burnett et al, 1997; Park et al, 1998; Giraldi et al, 2004).

There have been several clinical studies on selective phosphodiesterase type 5 inhibitors over the past few years (Caruso et al, 2001, 2003; Basson et al, 2003; Berman et al, 2003), conducted with either premenopausal or postmenopausal women with sexual health concerns as well as healthy women without sexual dysfunction. Many studies did not take into account the hormonal milieu of the subjects in the inclusion and exclusion criteria (Giraldi et al, 2004). **An important point in treating women with sexual health concerns is that an adequate sex steroid (androgen and estrogens) hormonal milieu is critical for benefits from selective phosphodiesterase type 5 inhibitor treatment.** The following studies did assess safety and efficacy of selective phosphodiesterase type 5 inhibitors in subjects with a normal hormonal milieu (Caruso et al, 2001, 2003; Berman et al, 2003).

A double-blind, crossover, placebo-controlled safety and efficacy study (Caruso et al, 2001) with a selective phosphodiesterase type 5 inhibitor was performed in premenopausal women with normal ovulatory cycles and normal levels of steroid hormones who were affected by female sexual arousal disorder without hypoactive sexual desire disorder. Subjects were observed to benefit from treatment with the active selective phosphodiesterase type 5 inhibitor showing improvement in sexual arousal, orgasm, frequency, and enjoyment of sexual intercourse versus placebo (Caruso et al, 2001).

A double-blind, placebo-controlled safety and efficacy study with a selective phosphodiesterase type 5 inhibitor was performed in postmenopausal women with female sexual arousal disorder who had adequate serum estradiol and free testosterone values (Berman et al, 2003). Women with female sexual arousal disorder without hypoactive sexual desire disorder assigned the active drug had a significantly greater improvement in sexual arousal, orgasm, intercourse, and overall satisfaction with sexual life compared with placebo. No efficacy was shown for women with concomitant hypoactive sexual desire disorder.

A randomized, double-blind, crossover, placebo-controlled safety and efficacy study with a selective phosphodiesterase type 5 inhibitor was performed in premenopausal women asymptomatic for sexual disorders, with normal ovulatory cycles and with normal levels of steroid hormones (Caruso et al, 2003). The selective phosphodiesterase type 5 inhibitor improved general sexual behavior, including sexual arousal, orgasm, and enjoyment versus placebo. Adverse events associated with the use of selective phosphodiesterase type 5 inhibitors were related to vasodilatation, such as headache, or to gastrointestinal events with nausea, or to visual effects. **The study suggested that selective phosphodiesterase type 5 inhibitors act on different sexual pathways in healthy women, improving their sexual experience, including multiple orgasms** (Caruso et al, et al, 2003).

Selective phosphodiesterase type 5 inhibitor use has been studied as an antidote to psychotropic-induced sexual dysfunction in women. In one study (Salerian et al, 2000), women reported significant improvements in all domains of sexual function, with improvement in overall sexual satisfaction, after selective phosphodiesterase type 5 inhibitor treatment.

Significant improvements were reported regardless of psychotropic medication type. Patients taking selective serotonin reuptake inhibitors reported less improvement in arousal, libido, and overall sexual satisfaction than did other patients, whereas patients taking benzodiazepines reported significantly more improvement in libido and overall sexual satisfaction (Salerian et al, 2000).

Another study was performed utilizing selective phosphodiesterase type 5 inhibitors in women with psychotropic-induced sexual dysfunction (Nurnberg et al, 1999). Women who had normal premorbid sexual function and who had developed sexual dysfunction, particularly anorgasmia with or without other sexual disturbances (i.e., loss of libido, lubrication difficulties, uncomfortable or painful intercourse), were treated with a selective phosphodiesterase type 5 inhibitor. The subjects showed improvement of the presenting condition, usually depression, anxiety, or both, and experienced sexual side effects continuously for more than 4 weeks. Patients took selective phosphodiesterase type 5 inhibitors and reported a complete or very significant reversal of their sexual dysfunction. This included return of effective duration and intensity of adequate arousal, lubrication, and orgasmic function (Nurnberg et al, 1999).

Other vasodilators, oral and topical, that have been studied in women with sexual health concerns include L-arginine, yohimbine, phentolamine, and prostaglandin E_1. Data from most of these agents are preliminary (Basson et al, 2004a, 2004c).

In conclusion, **selective phosphodiesterase type 5 inhibitors seem to be effective in highly selected populations of premenopausal and menopausal women with sexual arousal disorder** (Caruso et al, 2001, 2003; Berman et al, 2003). Selection criteria best associated with success included having normal sex steroid hormonal milieu and no hypoactive sexual desire disorder. Selective phosphodiesterase type 5 inhibitors may have a role as an antidote to psychotropic-induced sexual dysfunction (Nurnberg et al, 1999).

Medical Therapy for Genital Sexual Pain Disorders

Biologic pathophysiologic processes resulting in women's sexual health problems associated with sexual pain may occur in the clitoris, urethra, bladder, vulva, vestibule, vagina, and pelvic floor muscles.

Clitoris, Prepuce and Frenulae

Phimosis/Balanitis. In women with focused clitoral pain, clitoral itching, or clitoral burning, careful inspection of the glans clitoris should be performed. Failure to visualize the whole glans clitoris with the corona is consistent with some degree (mild, moderate, or severe) of preputial phimosis, based on the elasticity of the prepuce and its ability to retract on examination (Haefner, 1999; Munarriz et al, 2002b; Anderson et al, 2004). Because phimosis may create a closed compartment, phimosis is often the underlying pathology in clitoral glans balanitis associated with recurrent fungal infections. Initial treatment may be conservative with topical estrogen (Crandall, 2002) and/or testosterone creams to see if the prepuce can be made more elastic and retractile. Topical anti-

fungal agents such as nystatin or oral antifungal agents such as fluconazole (Sobel et al, 2001) may be considered. Infections can also be related to herpesvirus, with appropriate treatment administered such as acyclovir. If a chronic genital dermatitis condition such as lichen sclerosus involves the prepuce, phimosis and fusion of the prepuce is a likely sequela (Bracco et al, 1993). An uncommon chronic genital dermatitis condition, lichen planus, may lead to hypertrophic, white scarring of the glans clitoris, prepuce, and frenulae. A useful treatment consideration for lichen sclerosus or lichen planus of the peri-glans clitoral tissue is clobetasol cream (Bracco et al, 1993). If conservative treatment fails due to the phimotic prepuce, surgical management by dorsal slit procedure should be considered.

Preputial Infections. Severe swelling, pain, tenderness, fever, or purulent drainage may emanate from the prepuce. The most likely diagnosis is an infected sebaceous cyst with extension from surrounding vulvar or pubic skin into the prepuce. Conservative treatments include antibiotics, soaking, and sitz baths. Often the situation is only resolved with incision and drainage.

Traumatic Neuropathy. In some cases, women with genital sexual pain claim that symptoms started after traumatic injuries to regional or local nerves associated with childbirth, especially associated with forceps delivery or regional anesthetic procedures or postoperative injuries to the iliohypogastric or ilioinguinal nerves, especially with wide lower abdominal Pfannenstiel incisions. Some women provide a history of sudden-onset pain in the clitoris after a sharp blow to the perineum. This may result from bicycle riding injuries, especially after a fall onto the nose of the saddle or the bar of the bicycle frame, or from other blunt perineal or pelvic trauma such as a fall onto a tree branch, horn of a horse saddle, or after a pelvic fracture as a result of a motor vehicle accident. Psychotropic agents such as amitriptyline or gabapentin have become the mainstay of conservative therapy (McKay, 1993; Rowbotham et al, 1998).

Urethral Meatus, Urethra/Bladder Neck, Skene's Glands

Gentle retraction of the labia minora should provide full view of the urethral meatus. This orifice is 1 to 2 cm posterior in the midline from the glans and frenula and should be flush to the vestibule.

Urethral Prolapse. Prolapse of the urethral mucosa out the urethral lumen is highly associated with estrogen deficiency states such as after bilateral oophorectomy, natural menopause, or after chemotherapy for malignancy (Haefner, 1999; Harlow et al, 2001; Stewart, 2002; Anderson et al, 2004). Clinical symptoms include urgency, frequency, and discomfort on urination; and also spotting of blood may be observed on the toilet paper after wiping after voiding. The abnormal voiding history is often accompanied by a unique sexual history. Women with urethral prolapse often have the ability to have full sexual pleasure and satisfaction during self-stimulation of the clitoris; however, during sexual activity with the partner or with a mechanical device, she experiences pain and/or urgency to urinate and/or inability to have orgasm secondary to distracting pain. Conservative treatment options include topical or systemic estrogens, although the risks and benefits of estrogen treatment need to be fully discussed (Haefner, 1999; Harlow et al, 2001; Stewart, 2002; Anderson et al, 2004).

Skene's Gland Adenitis. Skene's glands drain to the side of the meatus at various locations. The pathophysiology of Skene's gland adenitis is not known but there appears to be a relation to abnormal immunologic and/or sex steroid deficiency states. The diagnosis is made by a history of significant localized urethral meatal discomfort and/or dysuria during penetrative sexual activity. Women who are able to have self-stimulation sexual activity that avoids contact with the urethral meatus are able to have excellent sexual satisfaction. The classic physical finding of Skene's gland adenitis is a swollen, edematous, protruding urethral meatus without mucosal prolapse. Conservative treatment is by topical and systemic estrogen administration. Risks and benefits of estrogen treatment need to be fully discussed (Haefner, 1999, Harlow et al, 2001; Stewart, 2002, Anderson et al, 2004).

Urethritis/Recurrent Urinary Tract Infections/Interstitial Cystitis. It is very common for women, especially during transition and in the menopause, to complain of irritative voiding symptoms, especially burning, frequency, urgency, and nocturia, which significantly interfere with sexual activity (Haefner, 1999; Harlow et al, 2001; Stewart, 2002; Anderson et al, 2004). In such women the vulvovaginal and urinary irritative and burning symptoms are often poorly defined. The patient and physician confusion in this area occurs because **the differential diagnosis of irritation and burning in the perineum, especially after coitus, involves multiple different urologic and gynecologic conditions.** Urologic conditions that do not involve the urethral meatus include, for example, recurrent urethritis, recurrent urinary tract infections, urethral diverticula, irritable bladder, cystocele, ureteral stones, and endometriosis of the ureter and/or bladder. Irritative symptoms during voiding, especially after coitus, may also be associated with inflammatory gynecologic conditions. In such situations, the contact of voided urine against the inflamed vestibular, vulvar, and/or vaginal tissues can result in significant perineal burning and stinging. Vaginal yeast infections, vulvar dermatitis conditions, and uterine prolapse with or without rectocele are common gynecologic pathophysiologic processes. In many cases, expert urologic and gynecologic consultations are required to confirm the various diagnoses involved in the individual patient so that varied specific focused treatments may be initiated (Haefner, 1999; Harlow et al, 2001; Stewart, 2002, Anderson et al, 2004).

One rare genital sexual pain condition that is confusing and ill-defined is termed *painful bladder syndrome* or *interstitial cystitis* and is associated with severe urogenital and pelvic pain, urgency, frequency, nocturia, and dyspareunia (Stewart and Berger, 1997; Lukban and Whitmore, 2000). The pathophysiology of interstitial cystitis is unknown at this time but appears unrelated to any recognized bacterial pathophysiology. Interstitial cystitis symptoms, including the dyspareunia, often increase with menses, increase during bladder filling, and decrease with bladder emptying. There is no definitive diagnostic test for interstitial cystitis. Treatment of interstitial cystitis is fully discussed in Chapter 10, "Painful Bladder Syndrome/Interstitial Cystitis and Related Disorders" (Stewart and Berger, 1997; Lukban and Whitmore, 2000).

Vulva

Genital sexual pain in the vulva may be related to varied specific disorders.

Lichen Sclerosus/Lichen Planus. Lichen sclerosus (Bracco et al, 1993; Wakelin et al, 1997) **is a chronic genital dermatitis condition that is associated with varying intensity of symptoms including vulvar itch and/or burning and various degrees of vulvar scarring leading to narrowing of the introitus and dyspareunia** (Haefner, 1999; Harlow et al, 2001; Stewart, 2002; Anderson et al, 2004). There is a wide variation in presenting symptoms. In some women, especially those not sexually active, there can be minimal symptoms and the patient may be unaware of the condition of lichen sclerosus for years. Alternatively, the burning and itching symptoms can be so intense as to severely interfere with sexual activity, day-to-day activities, and even sleep. If the scarring of lichen sclerosus involves the perianal area, the patient may also complain of perianal fissuring and painful defecation. The diagnosis of lichen sclerosus is suspected by physical examination showing white genital, vulvar, and vestibular tissue, with paleness, loss of pigmentation, and a characteristic "cigarette paper" wrinkling. Classically, the genital tissue changes do not involve the inside of the vagina and if they involve the perianal area there is a traditional "figure of eight" extension. The lichen sclerosus condition commonly involves the vestibule, with associated labia minora atrophy, and the vaginal introitus, with loss of elasticity and narrowing. The treatment of choice for lichen sclerosus is the ultrapotent fluorinated steroid clobetasol (Bracco et al, 1993). Safety and efficacy (especially for control of itching) studies for clobetasol treatment of vulvar lichen sclerosus have been reported for more than a decade.

Lichen planus (Lewis et al, 1996) is another chronic genital dermatitis condition likely pathophysiologically related to varied altered immunologic disorders. The presenting symptoms vary widely in different patients, likely owing to the varied pathophysiologic processes. Lichen planus may occur secondary to drugs, such as antihypertensive agents, diuretics, oral hypoglycemic agents, and nonsteroidal anti-inflammatory agents, which may rarely induce a lichen planus–like eruption. One type of lichen planus is primarily associated with itching and does not result in scarring. Another type of lichen planus is erosive and destructive. Overall patient complaints may include severe vulvar itching, pain, burning, and irritation. Dyspareunia (Haefner, 1999; Harlow et al, 2001; Stewart, 2002; Anderson et al, 2004) occurs in sexually active women secondary to vaginal introital scarring. Some types of lichen planus, unlike lichen sclerosus, may involve the vaginal mucosa. If there is vaginal involvement, a purulent malodorous discharge may be noted. Findings on physical examination of women with lichen planus vary widely. The pruritic type of lichen planus is associated with a purple color and multiple papules and plaques on the vulva and vestibule. The erosive type is associated with vestibular ulcers, scarring, and atrophy of the clitoris and labia minora, and occasionally destruction of the vagina has been reported. A biopsy and dermatopathologic review may be needed to establish the diagnosis of lichen planus. Treatment of lichen planus involves use of ultrapotent topical steroids such as clobetasol, topically and vaginally as indicated (Bracco et al, 1993; Lewis et al, 1996).

Vestibule

Generalized Vulvodynia. Generalized vulvodynia (Bergeron et al, 2001a, 2002; Harlow and Stewart, 2003) refers to a diffuse, constant, burning pain anywhere on the vulva, from mons to anus, which is hyperpathic and greatly out of proportion to the stimulus. Afflicted patients have a constant or sporadic awareness of the vulva with widespread "everything hurts," vulvar soreness, rawness, constant irritation, various paresthesias, aching, and/or stinging. Generalized vulvodynia may be considered primary if it occurs with the first penetrative sexual encounter or with a tampon or speculum examination. Generalized vulvodynia may be considered as secondary if it occurs after previous nonpainful vaginal penetrations.

The diagnosis of generalized vulvodynia (Stewart and Berger, 1997; Haefner, 1999; Bergeron et al, 2001a, 2002; Harlow et al, 2001; Stewart, 2002; Harlow and Stewart, 2003) is made by ruling out, on physical examination and laboratory testing, such diagnoses as *Candida* vaginitis and chronic genital dermatitis conditions. Testing with a cotton-tipped swab shows all vulvar areas positive for pain and/or tenderness. **The treatment of any genital sexual pain disorder involves the multidisciplinary team approach, and this is especially true for the disabling condition of generalized vulvodynia.** Patient management includes education and support, especially regarding avoidance of contacts and practice of healthy vulvar hygiene, pelvic floor physical therapy treatment, management of concomitant depression, and management of any associated neurologic, dermatologic, gynecologic, orthopedic, or urologic conditions. Medical management includes amitriptyline and/or gabapentin (McKay, 1993; Rowbotham et al, 1998).

Vulvar Vestibulitis Syndrome/Vestibular Adenitis. Friedrich's criteria (1987) for a woman to have vulvar vestibulitis syndrome include the following. On history, there is severe pain on vestibular touch or attempted vaginal entry. On physical examination, there is erythema of various degrees within the vestibule. During cotton-tipped swab testing, there is tenderness to pressure "localized" within the vulvar vestibule. Often the tender localized region is along the labial hymen junction associated with the presence of minor vestibular glands.

Vulvar vestibulitis syndrome (Friedrich, 1987; Stewart and Berger, 1997; Bergeron et al, 2001a, 2001b, 2002; Harlow et al, 2001; Harlow and Stewart, 2003) **is one of the most likely causes of dyspareunia, especially in women younger than 50 years old.** Afflicted patients with vulvar vestibulitis syndrome will complain of severe pain during sexual activity often described as raw, red burning, feeling like sandpaper or burnt tissue being rubbed. Most women experience the pain in the vulvar region with initial penetration. There is another group of women who do not experience pain during initial penetration but experience severe pain on deep penetration when the man's perineum comes into contact with the woman's perineum, resulting in the genital sexual pain. In this latter group of women, physicians are misguided to the cervix when the site of the pain trigger is really within the vulvar region. With vulvar vestibulitis syndrome, genital sexual pain may also be experienced with the use of tampons, during speculum examination, wearing tight pants, or straddling while cycling or horseback riding. Although there is no known pathophysiology, there are several possible pathophysiologic factors, including exposure to human papillomavirus or the irritant oxalate, abnormal immunologic conditions, psychopathology, and an abnormal sex steroid hormonal milieu. The treatment of vulvar vestibulitis syndrome involves conservative measures, including education, support, counseling, physical therapy, and/or biofeedback. Elimination of the pain trigger should be performed. Topical estrogen and topical lidocaine creams and/or ointments should be considered. Systemic medications include tricyclic antidepressants or gabapentin. Correction of the sex steroid hormonal milieu should be considered. Unlike generalized vulvodynia, in women with vulvar vestibulitis syndrome, if medical management fails, surgery such as vestibulectomy can be considered (Friedrich, 1987; Stewart and Berger, 1997, Bergeron et al, 2001a, 2001b, 2002; Harlow et al, 2001; Harlow and Stewart, 2003).

Vagina

Atrophic Vaginitis. The symptoms of atrophic vaginitis (Dennerstein et al, 1980; Ayton et al, 1996; Barentsen et al, 1997; Haefner, 1999; Rioux et al, 2000; Utian et al, 2001; Freeman, 2002; Stewart, 2002; Buckler and Al-Azzawi, 2003; Anderson et al, 2004; Basson et al, 2004a; Kovalevsky, 2004; Lewis et al, 2004; Nappi et al, 2005) include vaginal dryness, dyspareunia, stinging, bleeding, and dysuria. **On physical examination, women with atrophic vaginitis reveal vaginal mucosal changes.** The classic healthy-appearing vagina has a pink hue with vaginal folds and rugae that, when touched with a cotton-tipped swab, reveal a shiny lubricating substance and, when rubbed with the swab, do not bleed. In atrophic vaginitis, the vagina transforms to an unhealthy pale complexion, with a lack of vaginal folds and rugae, a lack of lubricating substance on the surface, and tissue that bleeds with minimal contact. On wet mount, the microscopic examination reveals parabasal cells, increased white blood cells, and absent background flora of lactobacilli. The vaginal pH is elevated to 6.0 to 7.0 (Dennerstein et al, 1980; Ayton et al, 1996; Barentsen et al, 1997; Haefner, 1999; Rioux et al, 2000; Utian et al, 2001; Freeman, 2002; Stewart, 2002; Buckler and Al-Azzawi, 2003; Anderson et al, 2004; Kovalevsky, 2004).

The conservative treatment involves the use of local topical vestibular and/or intravaginal estrogen. There are multiple products on the market, including intravaginal rings, suppositories, and creams. In some rare patients, plasma estradiol levels may increase to values similar to systemic estrogen administration so monitoring is required as indicated by the physician. Also, there are some patients who are allergic to the various additives in the topical estradiol product. For example, some women react negatively to the propylene glycol in several topical estrogen products. There are also multiple estrogen alternatives, such as soy, although there are limited double-blind, placebo-controlled safety and efficacy trials with these products (Dennerstein et al, 1980; Ayton et al, 1996; Barentsen et al, 1997; Haefner, 1999; Rioux et al, 2000; Utian et al, 2001; Freeman, 2002; Stewart, 2002; Buckler and Al-Azzawi, 2003; Anderson et al, 2004; Kovalevsky, 2004).

Pelvic Floor Disorders

Urologists are familiar with the diagnosis and treatment of women with disorders of the female pelvic floor, especially bladder/urethra and sexual dysfunction (Glazer and Mac-Conkey, 1996; Glazer et al, 1999; Lukban and Whitmore, 2000; Weber et al, 2000; Bergeron et al, 2001a, 2002; Glazener et al, 2001; Shafik and El-Sibai, 2002; Fitzgerald and Kotarinos, 2003; Reissing et al, 2004; Goldstein, 2005). Normal function of the pelvic floor musculature is essential in maintaining appropriate sexual function. Both "low-tone pelvic floor dysfunction "or "high-tone pelvic floor muscle dysfunction" can be closely associated with women's sexual health concerns. Hypotonus of the pelvic floor muscles, secondary to childbirth, trauma, and/or aging, is related to urinary incontinence during orgasm, vaginal laxity, and/or thrusting dyspareunia secondary to pelvic organ prolapse. Hypertonus of the pelvic floor secondary to childbirth, postural stressors, microtrauma, infection, adhesions, and surgical trauma can contribute to symptoms of urinary retention, reduced force of stream, dysuria, urgency, penetrative dyspareunia, and/or vaginismus (Glazer and MacConkey, 1996; Glazer et al, 1999; Lukban and Whitmore, 2000; Weber et al, 2000; Bergeron et al, 2001a, 2002; Glazener et al, 2001; Shafik and El-Sibai, 2002; Fitzgerald and Kotarinos, 2003; Reissing et al, 2004; Goldstein, 2005).

The assessment of tone in the pelvic floor is determined by the woman's ability to isolate, contract, and relax the pelvic floor muscles. During a pelvic examination, a digital exam, by exerting light pressure on the lateral walls of the vagina, should assess whether the woman is able to squeeze on the examining finger and to elevate the pelvic floor, without simultaneously contracting the abdominal, gluteal, or adductor muscle groups. If the patient is not able to produce sufficient muscle strength to compress the finger or is not able to sustain that pressure for several seconds, she may be exhibiting a low-tone pelvic floor dysfunction pattern. If, conversely, the woman experiences muscle tenderness or pain when pressure is applied to the lateral vaginal wall or during an attempted squeeze against resistance, she may be exhibiting a high-tone pelvic floor dysfunction pattern. A perineometer or an electromyography probe, designed to measure muscle activity, can verify these physical examination findings (Glazer and MacConkey, 1996; Glazer et al, 1999; Lukban and Whitmore, 2000; Weber et al, 2000; Bergeron et al, 2001a, 2002; Glazener et al, 2001; Shafik and El-Sibai, 2002; Fitzgerald and Kotarinos, 2003; Reissing et al, 2004; Goldstein, 2005). Hypersensitivity disorders involving the genitourinary tract represent a spectrum of symptoms and conditions that include chronic bacterial cystitis, urgency and frequency syndrome, sensory urgency, urethral syndrome, interstitial cystitis, vulvar pain, vaginal pain, and perineal and pelvic pain. Hypersensitivity disorders, associated with hypertonus of the pelvic floor musculature, account for some of the concerns of female patients who present for evaluation of sexual health concerns. **Sexuality is adversely affected for the majority of women with hypersensitivity disorders of the bladder, bowel, and vulva and high-tone pelvic floor dysfunction.** Those who are able to tolerate coitus often suffer a flare of their symptoms for days as a result of sexual activity, which then becomes negative reinforcement for future sexual activity. Conservative therapy for pelvic floor dysfunction is aimed at muscle reeducation. A pelvic floor rehabilitation program aimed at facilitating sexual comfort and pleasure for patients can be designed. Massage of the pelvic floor can be performed to elongate shortened muscles and decrease high-tone spasm in

such patients (Glazer and MacConkey, 1996; Glazer et al, 1999; Lukban and Whitmore, 2000; Weber et al, 2000; Bergeron et al, 2001a, 2002; Glazener et al, 2001; Shafik and El-Sibai, 2002; Fitzgerald and Kotarinos, 2003; Reissing et al, 2004; Goldstein, 2005).

Weakness and laxity of the pelvic floor muscles represent a spectrum of symptoms and conditions that include women with pelvic organ prolapse with or without urinary or fecal incontinence. Risk factors include age, heredity, vaginal birth trauma, previous pelvic/vaginal surgery, history of radiation therapy, menopausal status, lifestyle factors such as strenuous lifting, and chronic medical conditions, including obstructive pulmonary disease, obesity, and constipation. Stress incontinence that occurs with increased intra-abdominal pressure and maneuvers such as sneezing, coughing, and straining is related to abnormalities in urethral closure and poor pelvic muscle support. Sexuality is often adversely affected for women with severe low-tone pelvic floor dysfunction, especially those with severe incontinence and prolapse when symptoms are a source of anxiety and interfere with the overall sense of sexual satisfaction. Women who experience incontinence during intercourse express concern about feeling undesirable, fearing embarrassment, and possibly infecting themselves or their partner. Conservative therapy for low-tone pelvic floor dysfunction is also aimed at muscle reeducation. Pelvic floor muscle strengthening exercises, augmented with biofeedback and/or electrical stimulation to the pelvic floor, can be initiated. If this and other conservative treatment options fail, surgical procedures, including sling and tension-free vaginal tape placement, provide cure rates as high as 95% when performed in appropriate candidates (Glazer and MacConkey, 1996; Glazer et al, 1999; Lukban and Whitmore, 2000; Weber et al, 2000; Bergeron et al, 2001a, 2002; Glazener et al, 2001; Shafik and El-Sibai, 2002; Fitzgerald and Kotarinos, 2003; Reissing et al, 2004; Goldstein, 2005).

KEY POINT: NONHORMONAL MEDICAL THERAPY

- A woman's sense of well-being is closely tied to the quality of her relationships, including her intimate physical relationships. Unfortunately, genital sexual pain problems are common and often disabling, interfering with relationships and intimacy. Genital sexual pain disorders are multifactorial syndromes of pain, sexual dysfunction, and psychological disability. Ideal patient management involves a multimodal approach including psychological support, sexual therapy, physical therapy, and medical management of the pain. There are multiple physiologic causes for genital sexual pain and, similar to other medical issues, accurate diagnosis is essential to appropriate treatment. The basis for diagnosis is a careful history and physical examination with appropriate laboratory testing. By taking the time to assess and address patients' sexual concerns, the urologist can assist women with chronic genital sexual pain to reclaim a sense of themselves as individuals capable of intimacy. Additional research is needed in this very important aspect of women's sexual health.

Surgical Therapy for Genital Sexual Pain Disorders

Surgical Treatment of Vulvar Vestibulitis Syndrome

Surgical intervention for management of women with vulvar vestibulitis syndrome is offered to those who have failed initial conservative medical, psychological, and/or physical therapy focused treatment (Glazer and MacConkey, 1996; Glazer et al, 1999; Shafik et al, 2002; Basson et al, 2004a; Bergeron et al, 2001a, 2002; Goldstein, 2005). **Surgery is based on the hypothesis that the pathophysiology of vulvar vestibulitis syndrome is associated with inflamed, irritated, and hypersensitive vestibular glandular tissue and related increased nerve density in the vestibular mucosa** (Bergeron et al, 2001a). Surgical success is therefore based on excision of this abnormal glandular and nerve tissue in the vestibule. Vestibular tissue is embryologically distinct from vaginal tissue; thus there is low symptom recurrence after surgical resection of the vestibule tissue with vaginal advancement.

With regard to women with vulvar vestibulitis syndrome, the first surgical excision and reconstructive procedure was described by Woodruff and colleagues (1981) approximately 25 years ago. In the original report, excision consisted of a semicircular segment of perineal skin, the mucosa of the posterior vulvar vestibule, and the posterior hymenal ring. The reconstruction consisted of undermining 3 cm of the vaginal mucosa and approximating this directly to the perineum.

Subsequently, variations and modifications have evolved (Woodruff et al, 1981; Kehoe and Luesley, 1999; Bergeron et al, 2001a; Edwards, 2003; Gaunt et al, 2003). Specifically, in contemporary "vulvar vestibulectomy" the posterior incision extends only to the posterior fourchette and does not include excisions of perineal skin. A "complete vulvar vestibulectomy" includes excision of the vestibular mucosa adjacent to the urethral meatus/Skene's glands region anteriorly, excision of vestibular mucosa laterally and posteriorly, with reconstruction including the posterior vaginal flap advancement. A "modified vulvar vestibulectomy" limits the excision of vestibular mucosa to the posterior vestibule (Fig. 28–15). Both procedures are usually performed under general or regional anesthesia. During vestibulectomy, the vaginal advancement may cover the ostia of Bartholin's glands, but the risk of postoperative Bartholin's gland cysts is only 1%.

A "vestibuloplasty" or "excision of vestibular adenitis" consists only of excision of localized painful areas of vestibular mucosa without vaginal advancement and can be performed with local anesthesia (Fig. 28–16). Before the procedure, a cotton swab is used to delineate painful areas of the vestibule. These areas are outlined with a marking pen and then injected with lidocaine 1%. A scalpel is then used to excise the tender vestibular mucosa, including the tissue at the base of the hymen. The defects are then closed with interrupted sutures of 4-0 Vicryl (Woodruff et al, 1981; Kehoe and Luesley, 1999; Bergeron et al, 2001a; Edwards, 2003; Gaunt et al, 2003).

Most surgeons choose the procedure based on the individual needs and symptoms of the patient. For example, if a patient has an area of tenderness confined to a small portion of the vestibule, consideration of "excision of vestibular adenitis" would be the most appropriate procedure. If a woman has pain and tenderness throughout the majority of the vestibule, then complete vulvar vestibulectomy would be the most

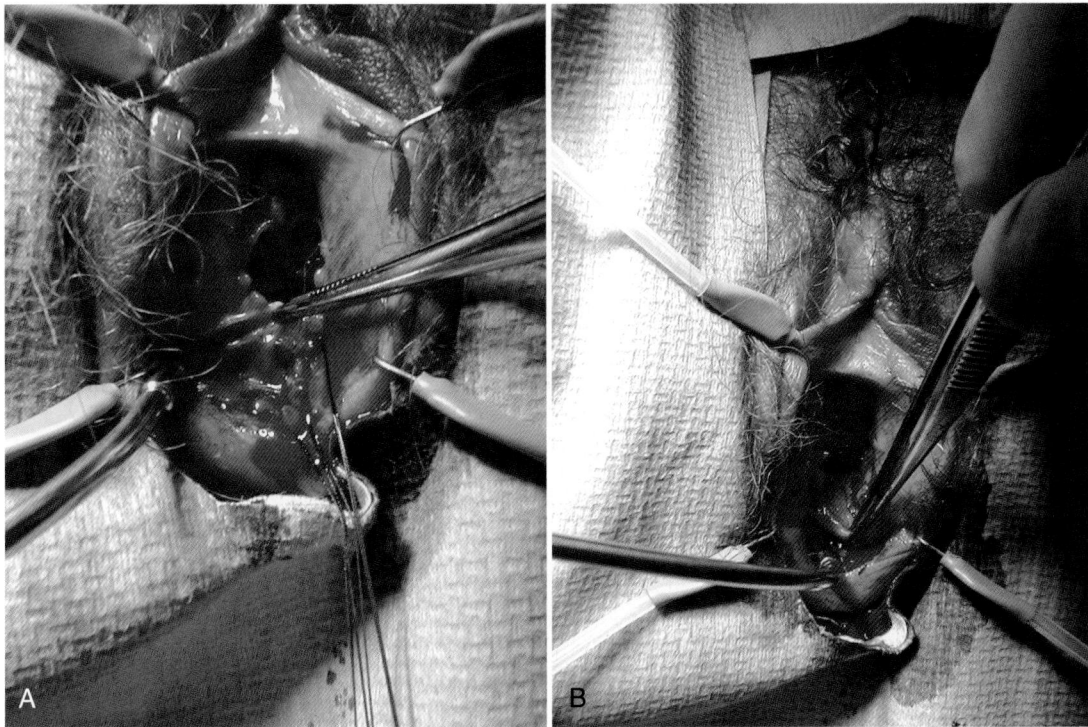

Figure 28–15. Intraoperative photographs of a 36-year-old woman with severe dyspareunia for 3 years who failed all conservative treatment options and opted for a surgical solution to the vulvar vestibulitis syndrome. **A,** Vestibular adenitis is present in the region of the posterior fourchette at the 6 and 7 o'clock positions. A "modified vulvar vestibulectomy" limited the excision of vestibular mucosa to the posterior vestibule. **B,** The posterior reconstruction included a posterior vaginal flap advancement.

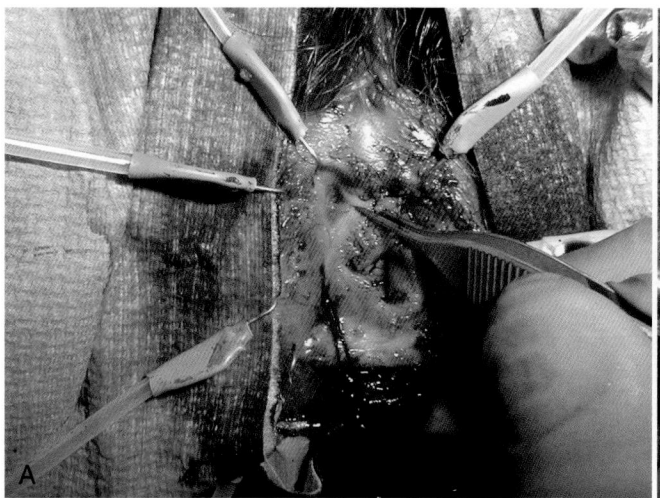

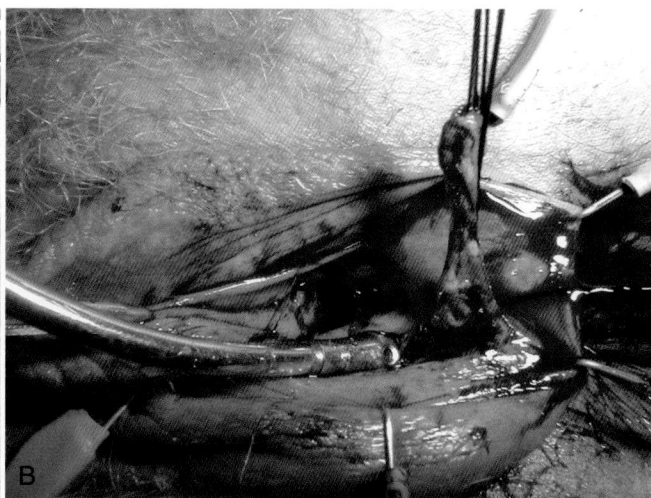

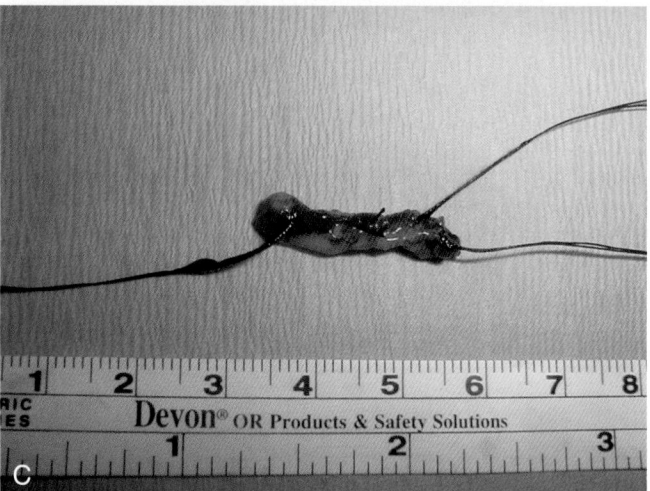

Figure 28–16. Intraoperative photographs from a 25-year-old woman with severe dyspareunia for 4 years who failed conservative treatments and elected to undergo surgical intervention. She did not wish to undergo any surgery that involved destruction of the vestibule. **A,** Minor vestibular glands localized to the 11 o'clock position. **B,** Excision of localized painful areas of vestibular mucosa without vaginal advancement. **C,** Specimen that is 2 cm long, 0.5 cm deep, and 1 cm wide. Histologic examination *(not shown)* with hematoxylin and eosin staining revealed a chronic inflammatory infiltrate surrounding the vestibular glands and replacement of columnar epithelium by squamous metaplasia.

appropriate procedure (Woodruff et al, 1981; Kehoe and Luesley, 1999; Bergeron et al, 2001a; Edwards, 2003; Gaunt et al, 2003).

Appropriate postoperative care is important. Nothing enters the vagina postoperatively unless permission is granted by the patient. In the immediate postoperative period, liberal use of ice packs prevents swelling and helps with pain. Sitz baths starting 3 days after the surgery can help with postoperative pain and may help prevent infection. Physical activity should be limited for the first 4 to 6 weeks while the surgical site heals. Close communication and frequent visits to a certified woman's physical therapist specializing in pelvic floor disorders are encouraged beginning at 4 weeks postoperatively. Under physical therapist and biofeedback pelvic floor electromyography monitoring, vaginal dilators can be used beginning at 4 weeks postoperatively after the surgical site has healed to help the postoperative patient resume normal sexual functioning (Woodruff et al, 1981; Kehoe and Luesley, 1999; Bergeron et al, 2001a; Edwards, 2003; Gaunt et al, 2003).

The complications of surgery (Woodruff et al, 1981; Kehoe and Luesley, 1999; Edwards, 2003; Gaunt et al, 2003) for vulvar vestibulitis syndrome increase with the invasiveness of the procedure performed. Specifically, complications include

bleeding, infection, increased pain, hematoma, wound dehiscence, vaginal stenosis, scar tissue formation, and Bartholin's duct cyst formation. As always with surgery, the risk of these complications can be reduced with appropriate surgical techniques. Various closure techniques have been described to minimize the risks of postoperative complications. Specifically, the vaginal advancement flap should be anchored by multiple subcutaneous mattress sutures of 3-0 Vicryl placed in an anteroposterior direction and should be approximated to the perineum with interrupted stitches of 4-0 Vicryl.

At the present time, outcome data from surgical management of women with vulvar vestibulitis syndrome involving more than 1000 patients from multiple case series have been reported in the literature (Woodruff et al, 1981; Kehoe and Luesley, 1999; Bergeron et al, 2001a; Edwards, 2003; Gaunt et al, 2003). The overall surgical success rate is difficult to assess because of conflicting use of (1) terminology describing the severity and extent of vestibulitis preoperatively, (2) preoperative patient selection criteria, (3) surgical techniques, (4) postoperative surgical outcome criteria, and (5) postoperative follow-up period. Based on the existing data, the surgical treatment of vulvar vestibulitis syndrome resulted in a high degree of patient satisfaction, in significant resolution of dyspareunia in more than half of the patients operated, and in a clinically meaningful reduction in dyspareunia in approximately one third of the remaining patients (Woodruff et al, 1981; Kehoe and Luesley, 1999; Bergeron et al, 2001a; Edwards, 2003; Gaunt et al, 2003).

Surgery for Other Sexual Pain Disorders within the Vestibule

Distressing and disabling clitoral pain may occur secondary to phimosis of the clitoral prepuce and recurrent fungal balanitis of the clitoral glans or frenulae (Haefner, 1999; Munarriz et al, 2002b; Anderson et al, 2004). If conservative treatment fails, a dorsal slit procedure of the prepuce may be indicated to relieve the woman of the closed compartment perpetuating the recurrent fungal clitoral glans infection.

Distressing and disabling clitoral pain may occur secondary to a clitoral or frenular tumor. A common such tumor is a vestibular fibroepithelioma (Val-Bernal et al, 2002). Local excision with careful preservation of underlying clitoral, frenular, and vestibular tissues may be indicated.

Distressing and disabling clitoral pain and swelling may occur secondary to an infected expanding sebaceous cyst/abscess (Guelinckx and Sinsel, 2002) dissecting subcutaneous tissues to involve the prepuce. If conservative treatment fails, incision and drainage of the abscess may be indicated.

Distressing and disabling vulvar/vestibular pain with destruction of the vulvar architecture and scarring of the posterior fourchette and perineum may occur secondary to dermatologic conditions of the vulva/vestibule, such as lichen sclerosus (Wakelin and Marren, 1997). If conservative treatment fails, a complete vulvar vestibulectomy with vaginal flap advancement may be indicated. Rouzier and colleagues (2002) described a series of 62 women with introital stenosis caused by lichen sclerosus who underwent excision and reconstructive vestibular surgery with many realizing significant improvement in their sexual function after surgery.

Distressing and disabling vulvar/vestibular pain may occur secondary to recurrent idiopathic fissuring at the posterior fourchette. If conservative treatment fails, simple excision of recurrent fissures may be indicated. This excision-only procedure may fail, however, because the introitus may be narrowed postoperatively. Even though a "modified vulvar vestibulectomy" is a more invasive procedure, this may be indicated because in this procedure, excision of vestibular mucosa is limited to the posterior vestibule and the vaginal flap advancement widens the introitus (Woodruff et al, 1981; Kehoe and Luesley, 1999; Edwards, 2003; Gaunt et al, 2003).

Distressing and disabling vestibular pain, urinary urgency and frequency, and genital sexual pain may occur secondary to urethral prolapse (Glazener et al, 2001). If conservative treatments fail, surgical excision of the prolapsed urethral mucosa may be indicated.

Distressing vulvar/vestibular discomfort may occur secondary to Bartholin's cyst (Omole et al, 2003). If conservative treatments fail, marsupialization of the cyst may be indicated to enable drainage of the highly viscous and mucinous cyst fluid.

Distressing vulvar/vestibular discomfort may occur secondary to redundant labia minora greater than 4 to 8 cm. In several cases, the redundant labia minora (Fliegner, 1997; Alter, 1998; Choi and Kim, 2000) have been the source of dyspareunia as the tissue gets dragged into the vaginal introitus during penetrative coitus. Redundant labia minora have also been the source of disabling clitoral pain secondary to an unrelenting clitoral glans and frenular fungal infection. The pathophysiology is similar to the closed compartment of the phimotic prepuce. The coated redundant labia minora create a similar closed compartment preventing adequate treatment of the fungal infection. If conservative treatments fail, surgical reduction of the labia minora to approximately 1 cm width may be indicated. Labial varicosities within the redundant labia may be another indication for surgical reduction (Fliegner, 1997).

SUMMARY

The basic premise of urologic biologic-focused management of women with sexual health concerns is that physiologic processes can be altered by pathology. How specific medical conditions modulate female sexual health requires much investment in basic science investigation. From the perspective of the biologic-focused clinician, the essential principle guiding his/her medical decision making is identification of the underlying pathophysiology of the sexual dysfunction. If the biologic basis of the dysfunction can be diagnosed, management outcome may be successfully directed to the source pathophysiology.

The continuing message throughout the chapter is that the comprehension of epidemiology, basic physiology, pathophysiology, diagnosis, and treatment of female sexual health issues remains limited. Despite the limited knowledge, there are many women with sexual health concerns who have become empowered to seek help from health care professionals. One of many dilemmas faced by the health care profession in general and the urologist in particular is to face the challenge of safely and effectively diagnosing the increasing number of women who present with sexual dysfunctions and offer them the best, evidence-based available treatment options. The goal of this chapter is to provide the urologist with evidence-based, state-of-the-art, inclusive data concerning contemporary biologic-focused management strategies for women with sexual health concerns. The management strategies discussed in the chapter will continue to evolve. We look forward to the future when the biologic-focused urologist has more robust high levels of evidence supporting additional safe and effective treatment options for women with sexual health problems.

SUGGESTED READINGS

Bancroft JH: Human Sexuality and Its Problems. New York, Churchill Livingstone, 1983.
Goldstein I, Meston CM, Davis S, Traish AM (eds): Women's Sexual Function and Dysfunction. London, Taylor and Francis, 2005.
Kaplan HS: The New Sex Therapy. New York, Brunner/Mazel, 1974.
Kaplan HS: Disorders of Sexual Desire. New York, Brunner/Mazel, 1979.
Kinsey AC, Pomeroy WB, Martin CE: Sexual Behavior in the Human Male. Philadelphia, WB Saunders, 1948.
Kinsey AC, Pomeroy WB, Martin CE, et al: Sexual Behavior in the Human Female. Philadelphia, WB Saunders, 1953.
Lue TF, Basson R, Rosen R (eds): Sexual Medicine: Sexual Dysfunction in Men and Women. Paris, Editions 21, 2004.
Masters WH, Johnson VE: Human Sexual Response. Boston, Little, Brown, 1966.
Masters WH, Johnson VE: Human Sexual Inadequacy. Boston, Little, Brown, 1970.

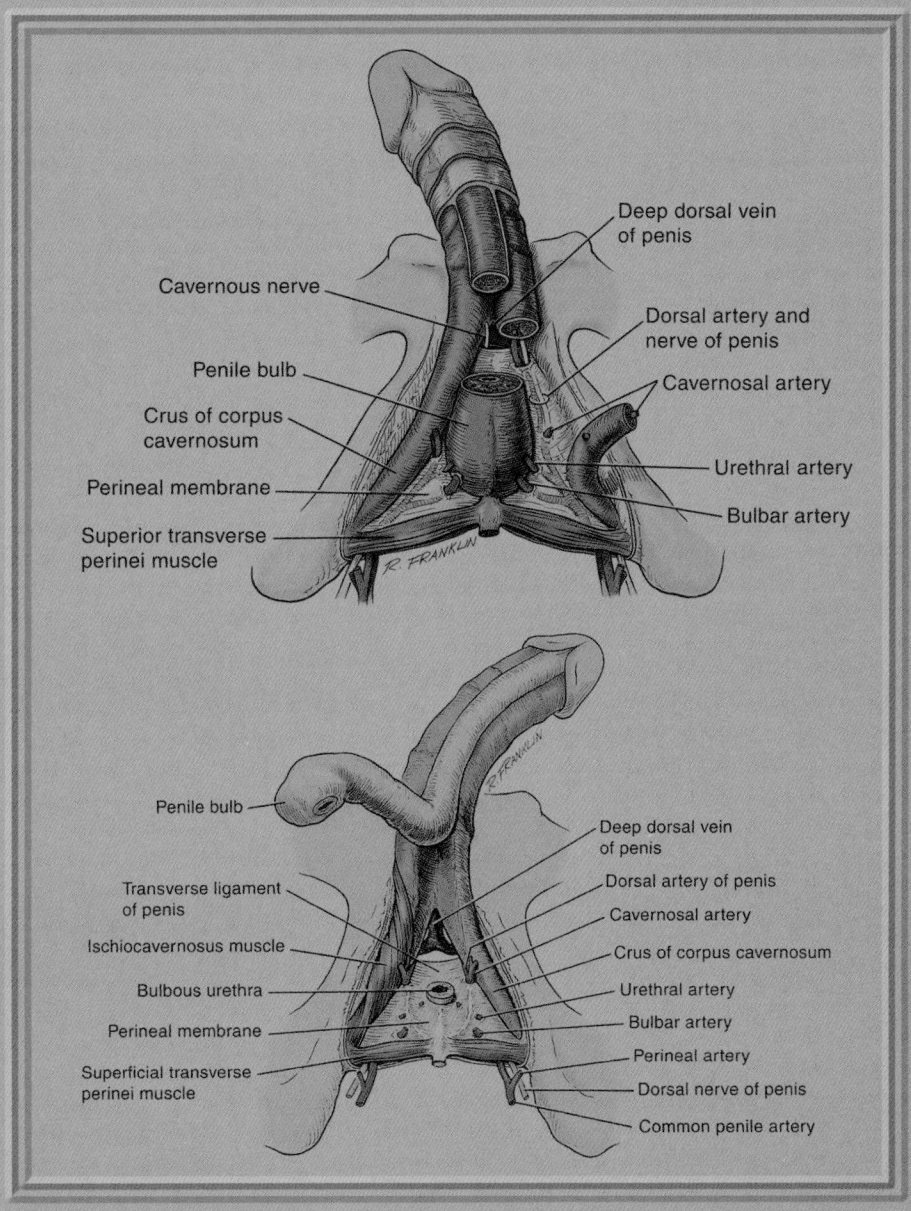

Deep dorsal vein of penis

Cavernous nerve

Dorsal artery and nerve of penis

Penile bulb

Cavernosal artery

Crus of corpus cavernosum

Perineal membrane

Urethral artery

Superior transverse perinei muscle

Bulbar artery

R. FRANKLIN

Penile bulb

Deep dorsal vein of penis

Transverse ligament of penis

Dorsal artery of penis

Cavernosal artery

Ischiocavernosus muscle

Crus of corpus cavernosum

Bulbous urethra

Urethral artery

Perineal membrane

Bulbar artery

Perineal artery

Superficial transverse perinei muscle

Dorsal nerve of penis

Common penile artery

MALE GENITALIA

29 Neoplasms of the Testis

JEROME P. RICHIE, MD · GRAEME S. STEELE, MD

GERM CELL TUMORS

CLINICAL STAGING

EXTRAGONADAL GERM CELL TUMORS

OTHER TESTICULAR NEOPLASMS

TUMORS OF TESTICULAR ADNEXA

Testicular cancer, although relatively rare, is the most common malignancy in men in the 15- to 35-year age group and evokes widespread interest for several reasons. Testicular cancer has become one of the most curable solid neoplasms and serves as a paradigm for the multimodal treatment of malignancies. The dramatic improvement in survival resulting from the combination of effective diagnostic techniques, improved tumor markers, effective multidrug chemotherapeutic regimens, and modifications of surgical technique has led to a decrease in patient mortality from more than 50% before 1970 to less than 5% in 1997 (Bosl and Motzer, 1997). With the availability of effective treatment, even for patients with advanced disease, attention has been turned to reduction of morbidity by altering therapeutic protocols in selected subsets of patients. These changes in treatment philosophy are based on knowledge of the effective backup methods available should alternative methods of treatment fail.

Testicular cancer is one of the few neoplasms associated with accurate serum markers: β-human chorionic gonadotropin (β-hCG) and α-fetoprotein (AFP). These accurate tumor markers allow careful follow-up, with intervention earlier in the course of disease. Additional characteristics of testicular tumors that favor successful therapeutic manipulation include origin in germ cells, which are generally sensitive to both radiation therapy and a wide variety of chemotherapeutic agents; capacity for differentiation into histologically more benign counterparts; rapid rate of growth; predictable, systematic pattern of spread; and occurrence in young individuals without comorbid disease who may tolerate multimodal treatment. Nonetheless, in patients whose tumors arise outside the testis (extragonadal germ cell tumors [EGCTs]), the prognosis with similar treatment is approximately half that which can be expected in patients with tumors of primary germ cell origin (GCTs).

The burgeoning field of molecular biology holds promise for identification of intracellular changes that alter the kinet-ics of growth of normal testicular cells. Whereas in the 1980s cell surface antigens and morphologic characteristics could be evaluated, the potential for better understanding and possible elucidation of the etiology of testicular cancer may well be achieved in the not too distant future.

GERM CELL TUMORS
Histologic Classification of GCTs

Histologic classifications, grading systems, and staging evaluations have traditionally provided a major clinical basis for therapeutic decisions. Morphologic descriptions provide standardized means of identifying a given tumor and, in conjunction with past clinical experience, of estimating its potential for local growth, distant metastases, or both. Clinical and surgical staging indicates the extent to which a given tumor's potential has been realized at the time of evaluation. Although histologic and staging systems play important roles in treatment selection, grading schema have not been uniformly employed.

There have been at least six major attempts since 1940 to classify germinal tumors. **The World Health Organization (WHO) standardized pathologic criteria for diagnosis of testis cancer, has gone a long way toward eradicating confusion associated with various histologic staging systems** (Table 29–1) (Mostofi et al, 1998). GCTs are composed of five basic cell types: seminoma, embryonal cell carcinoma, yolk sac tumor, teratoma, and choriocarcinoma. More than half of GCTs contain more than one cell type and are therefore known as mixed GCTs. In that GCTs arise from pluripotential cells, a variety of elements may inhabit a given primary tumor or its secondary metastatic sites. Ray and coworkers (1974) noted that in the majority of patients (71 of 75, or 95%), a primary tumor containing embryonal carcinoma and seminoma either metastasized as pure embryonal carcinoma or combined with other elements but rarely metastasized as pure seminoma (2 of 75, or 3%). Heterogeneity among germ cell neoplasms is an expected consequence of their pluripotential origin. Biochemical marker "probes" can provide a means of delineating tumor heterogeneity, which may be useful in treatment selection.

Classification of germ cell neoplasms according to morphologic appearance is invaluable in treatment selection. The broad distinction between seminomas and nonseminomas has been particularly important in determining management strategies for retroperitoneal lymph node metastasis.

893

Table 29–1. World Health Organization Classification of Testicular Tumors

Germ Cell Tumors

Precursor lesions—intratubular malignant germ cells (carcinoma in situ)
Tumors of one histologic type (pure forms)
  Seminoma
    Variant—seminoma with syncytiotrophoblastic cells
  Spermatocytic seminoma
    Variant—spermatocytic seminoma with sarcoma
  Embryonal carcinoma
  Yolk sac tumor
  Polyembryoma
  Trophoblastic tumors
    Choriocarcinoma
    Choriocarcinoma with other cell types
    Placental site trophoblastic tumor
  Teratoma
    Mature teratoma
    Dermoid cyst
    Immature teratoma
    Teratoma with malignant areas
Tumors of more than one histologic type (mixed forms)—specify types and estimate percentage

Sex Cord/Gonadal Stromal Tumors

Pure forms
  Leydig's cell tumor
  Sertoli's cell tumor
    Large-cell calcifying Sertoli's cell tumor
    Lipid-rich Sertoli's cell tumor
  Granulosa cell tumor
    Adult-type granulosa cell tumor
    Juvenile-type granulosa cell tumor
  Tumors of thecoma/fibroma group
  Incompletely differentiated sex cord/gonadal stromal tumors
  Mixed forms

Unclassified Forms

Tumors Containing Both Germ Cell and Sex Cord/Gonadal Stromal Elements

Gonadoblastoma
Mixed germ cell-sex cord/gonadal stromal tumors, unclassified

Miscellaneous Tumors

Carcinoid tumor
Tumors of ovarian epithelial types

Lymphoid and Hematopoietic Tumors

Lymphoma
Plasmacytoma
Leukemia

Tumors of Collecting Ducts and Rete

Adenoma
Carcinoma

Tumors of the Tunica, Epididymis, Spermatic Cord, Supporting Structures, and Appendices

Adenomatoid tumor
Mesothelioma
  Benign
  Malignant
Adenoma
Carcinoma
Melanotic neuroectodermal
Desmoplastic small round cell tumor

Soft Tissue Tumors

Unclassified Tumors

Secondary Tumors

Tumor-like Lesions

Nodules of immature tubules
Testicular lesions of adrenogenital syndrome
Testicular lesions of androgen-insensitivity syndrome
Nodular precocious maturation
Specific orchitis
Nonspecific orchitis
Granulomatous orchitis
Malakoplakia
Adrenal cortical rest
Fibromatous peritonitis
Funiculitis
Residue of meconium peritonitis
Sperm granuloma
Vasitis nodosa
Sclerosing lipogranuloma
Gonadal splenic fusion
Mesonephric remnants
Endometriosis
Epidermal cyst
Cystic dysplasia
Mesolithial cyst
Others

Data from Vogelzang NJ, Scardino PT, Shipley WU, Coffey DS (eds): Genitourinary Oncology. Philadelphia, Lippincott, Williams & Wilkins, 1999.

Seminoma

Three subtypes of pure seminomas have been described: classic, anaplastic, and spermatocytic. The histologic and biochemical properties, natural history, and response to therapy of these subtypes have been characterized.

Several histopathologic characteristics of the primary tumor have been evaluated with regard to prognostic features as well as predictive value for likelihood of metastatic involvement (Hoeltl et al, 1987). In the past, most patients with low-stage disease were treated with radiation, and therefore prognostic factors for seminoma were largely ignored. More recently, however, surveillance as an option for low-stage disease has increased interest in prognostic factors for seminoma, as outlined subsequently.

Typical Seminoma. Typical, or classic, seminoma accounts for 82% to 85% of all seminomas and occurs most commonly in men in their thirties but not uncommonly in men in their forties or fifties. Seminoma rarely, if ever, occurs in the adolescent or infant population, but it may occur in patients older than age 60 years. Histologically, it is composed of islands or sheets of relatively large cells with clear cytoplasm and densely staining nuclei. **Syncytiotrophoblastic elements occur in 10% to 15%, and lymphocytic infiltration occurs in approximately 20%. The incidence of syncytiotrophoblastic**

elements corresponds to the frequency of β-hCG production. The slower growth rate of seminomas may be inferred from the observation that treatment failures may become evident 2 to 10 years after apparently adequate irradiation of metastatic sites.

Anaplastic Seminoma. Anaplastic seminoma accounts for 5% to 10% of all seminomas and has an age distribution similar to that of the typical subtype. Despite its rarity, discrimination of anaplastic seminoma is noteworthy because up to 30% of patients dying with seminoma have an anaplastic morphology. **A number of features suggest that anaplastic seminoma is a more aggressive and potentially more lethal variant of typical seminoma. These characteristics include (1) greater mitotic activity, (2) higher rate of local invasion, (3) increased rate of metastatic spread, and (4) higher rate of tumor marker (β-hCG) production.**

Histologically, anaplastic seminoma is typified by increased mitotic activity (three or more mitoses per high-power field), nuclear pleomorphism, and cellular anaplasia (Mostofi and Price, 1973). Morphologically, histiocytic lymphoma and embryonal carcinoma may closely resemble anaplastic seminoma. Relative to the rate of metastasis, Percarpio and associates (1979) noted in a series of 77 patients with anaplastic seminoma that 19 (25%) had clinical evidence of stage II disease. Shulman and coworkers (1983) reported a similar incidence of metastatic disease (29%), a relatively high rate of extragonadal extension (46%), and an unexpectedly high rate of elevated β-hCG (36%) in 14 patients with anaplastic seminoma.

The less favorable results of treatment for patients with anaplastic seminoma may merely reflect greater metastatic potential; there is no difference from classic seminoma when patients are treated appropriately and compared stage for stage. Analyses of treatment results indicate that inguinal orchiectomy plus radiation therapy is equally effective in controlling both anaplastic and classic seminoma.

Spermatocytic Seminoma. This lesion is composed of cells that vary in size and have deeply pigmented cytoplasm and rounded nuclei containing characteristic filamentous chromatin. The cells closely resemble different phases of maturing spermatogonia. Spermatocytic seminoma accounts for 2% to 12% of all seminomas, and nearly half occur in men older than age 50 years. Bilateral tumors have been reported, but no cases have occurred in conjunction with cryptorchidism. The association of spermatocytic seminoma with other nonseminomatous tumors is rare.

The metastatic potential of spermatocytic seminoma is extremely low, and prognosis is accordingly favorable. Reviews by Thackray and Crane (1976) and Weitzner (1979) documented no cases of metastatic disease. When histologic and staging evaluations have confirmed the diagnosis and the fact that disease is limited to the testis, treatment beyond inguinal orchiectomy appears unwarranted.

Nonseminomatous Germ Cell Tumors (NSGCTs)

Embryonal carcinoma is generally discovered as a small, rounded, but irregular mass invading the tunica vaginalis testis and not infrequently involving contiguous cord structures. The cut surface reveals a variegated, grayish white, fleshy tumor, often with areas of necrosis or hemorrhage and a poorly defined capsule. The typical histologic appearance is that of distinctly malignant epithelioid cells arranged in glands or tubules. The cell borders are usually indistinct, the cytoplasm pale or vacuolated, and the nuclei rounded with coarse chromatin and one or more large nucleoli. Pleomorphism, mitotic figures, and giant cells are features common to these highly malignant tumors.

Choriocarcinoma may occur as a palpable nodule; the size depends on the extent of local hemorrhage. Patients with pure choriocarcinoma may present with evidence of advanced distant metastasis and what seems to be a paradoxically small intratesticular lesion that may not distort the normal testicular size or shape. Central hemorrhage with viable, grayish white tumor at the periphery may be seen on the cut surface if the lesion can be demonstrated grossly. Microscopically, two distinct and appropriately oriented cell types must be demonstrated to satisfy the histologic diagnosis of choriocarcinoma: syncytiotrophoblasts and cytotrophoblasts. The syncytiotrophoblasts may be large, multinucleated cells containing abundant, often vacuolated, eosinophilic cytoplasm and large, hyperchromatic, irregular nuclei. Less commonly, the syncytial elements may be spindle shaped and contain one large, dark-staining nucleus. The cytotrophoblasts are closely packed, intermediate-sized, uniform cells with a distinct cell border, clear cytoplasm, and a single vesicular nucleus.

Teratoma contains more than one germ cell layer in various stages of maturation and differentiation. Mature elements resemble benign structures derived from normal ectoderm, entoderm, and mesoderm. Immature teratoma consists of undifferentiated primitive tissues from each of the three germ cell layers. Grossly, the tumors are usually large, lobulated, and nonhomogeneous in consistency. The cut surface may reveal variably sized cysts containing gelatinous, mucinous, or hyalinized material interspersed with islands of solid tissue often containing cartilage or bone. Histologically, the cysts may be lined by squamous, cuboidal, columnar, or transitional epithelium, and the solid component may contain any combination of cartilage; bone; intestinal, pancreatic, or liver tissue; smooth or skeletal muscle; and neural or connective tissue elements. On rare occasions, malignant changes may be recognized in such differentiated tissues, justifying the designation *malignant teratoma.*

Yolk sac tumor is the most common testis tumor of infants and children. In adults, it occurs most frequently in combination with other histologic types and is presumably responsible for the production of AFP. The terms *endodermal sinus tumor, adenocarcinoma of the infantile testis, juvenile embryonal carcinoma,* and *orchioblastoma* are all used synonymously. In its pure form, the lesion has a homogeneous, yellowish, mucinous appearance. Microscopically, the tumor is composed of epithelioid cells that form glandular and ductal structures arranged in columns, papillary projections, or solid islands within a primitive mesenchymal stroma. The individual epithelial tumor cells may be columnar, cuboidal, or flat, with poorly defined cell borders and vacuolated cytoplasm containing glycogen and fat. The large, irregularly shaped nuclei contain one or more prominent nucleoli and variable amounts of chromatin. Embryoid bodies, a common finding in yolk sac tumors, resemble 1- to 2-week-old embryos. These

Table 29–2. Presentation, Pathology, and Treatment of Yolk Sac Tumor (Embryonal Cell Carcinoma of Infants and Children)

Presentation	Pathology	Treatment
Most common testis tumor in prepubertal boys. Slow-growing scrotal mass in a young boy Hydrocele present in 25% of cases α-Fetoprotein elevated in >90%	Gross appearance similar to that of embryonal cell carcinoma. Yolk sac elements are found in one third of mixed adult germ cell tumors. Three most common microscopic patterns: Microcystic—honeycomb appearance, with hyaline globules Endodermal sinus—perivascular formations known as Schiller-Duval bodies Solid—small polygonal cells, clear cytoplasm, frequent mitoses The pattern of metastatic disease of yolk sac tumors in childhood differs from the pattern in adult germ cell tumors, owing to a higher incidence of hematogenous spread.	Over 80% of yolk sac tumors are confined to the testis at the time of diagnosis and are cured by radical inguinal orchiectomy. Radiographic evidence of low-volume retroperitoneal lymph node involvement is best treated by retroperitoneal lymph node dissection. Advanced disease: chemotherapy Radiotherapy can be used for residual disease that has failed to respond to chemotherapy. Overall prognosis is good; mean survival is 87% for all stages of disease.

ovoid structures, commonly measuring less than 1 mm in diameter, consist of a cavity surrounded by loose mesenchyma containing syncytiotrophoblasts and cytotrophoblasts (Table 29–2).

Mixed Tumors

In classifying more than 6000 testis tumors, Mostofi (1973) found that in roughly 60% more than one histologic pattern was identified. The most frequent combination is embryonal carcinoma, yolk sac tumor, teratoma, and syncytiotrophoblasts.

Metastatic deposits associated with teratomas usually contain embryonal carcinoma (80%) and, less frequently, teratoma or choriocarcinoma. The bisected tumor exhibits cysts, typical of teratoma, within the solid, sometimes hemorrhagic, stroma that contains embryonal elements.

The pluripotential nature of GCTs and, in particular, nonseminomatous tumors is evident from the varied histologic patterns of metastasis, more than half of which display different morphologies in primary versus metastatic sites, although pure choriocarcinoma invariably spreads unaltered. Whereas postmortem studies indicate that 30% to 45% of patients dying with seminoma harbor nonseminomatous metastases, the converse is rarely documented (Ray et al, 1974). Although the clinical incidence of nonseminomatous metastasis from an apparently pure seminoma is less than 10%, 30% to 45% of patients dying of apparently pure seminoma harbor nonseminomatous metastases (Bredael et al, 1982) (Table 29–3).

Intratubular Germ Cell Neoplasia: Carcinoma in Situ of the Testis

The early detection of preneoplastic change could improve survival for patients with many types of tumors, including testicular cancer. **Testicular carcinoma in situ (CIS) is widely regarded as the preinvasive precursor of all testicular GCTs except spermatocytic seminoma** (Skakkebaek et al, 1987). Controversy exists, however, regarding clinical significance, need for detection, and management of testicular CIS.

Skakkebaek (1972) described the occurrence of atypical intratubular germ cells seen on testicular biopsy of infertile men. **Early studies in infertile men and in patients with testicular GCTs showed that 50% of men in whom CIS was found on biopsy developed "invasive" disease within 5 years if left untreated** (Berthelsen et al, 1982; Skakkebaek et al, 1982). In one series, four of six patients with intratubular germ cell neoplasia developed "invasive tumor" between 1 and 5 years after initial biopsy (Skakkebaek, 1978). However, *invasive* disease was defined as invasion through the basement membrane, a distinctly different scenario from the frankly malignant GCT seen in patients with a palpable testicular mass.

To investigate the preinvasive phase of adult GCTs detected in childhood, Parkinson and associates (1994) evaluated 70 testicular biopsy specimens taken at orchidopexy with follow-up data available. CIS was seen in only 1 of the 70 specimens, and it preceded the appearance of a teratoma by 4 years. CIS was not seen in biopsy specimens 11 and 22 years before tumor diagnosis, raising questions regarding the role of testicular biopsy at the time of orchiopexy. **Nevertheless, the incidence of CIS in the male population is 0.8%, which correlates well with the lifetime risk for the development of testis cancer in Danish men. Furthermore, in patients with testicular cancer, the cumulative risk of developing a GCT in the contralateral testis was found to be 5.2%, which is similar to the prevalence of CIS in the contralateral testis** (von der Maase et al, 1986b; Giwercan et al, 1993).

Testicular CIS develops from fetal gonocytes and is characterized histologically by seminiferous tubules containing only Sertoli's cells and malignant germ cells located in a single row along the tubular membrane, characterized by nuclear pleomorphism. Several cell surface glycoprotein antigens have been identified that distinguish CIS cells from those of normal germ cells in the postpubertal testis. These proteins have also been shown to be highly expressed by primordial germ cells, as well as by testicular fetal germ cells, between the 8th and 12th weeks of development (Jorgensen et al, 1995). It is therefore postulated that malignant initiation of germ cells takes place in utero and is possibly influenced by external factors as well, such as exposure to high levels of estrogens (Sharpe et al, 1993).

Although the prevalence of testicular CIS in the general male population is low, a number of men fall into a

Table 29–3. Germ Cell Tumors: Incidence, Pathology, Tumor Markers, Presentation

Type	Incidence (%)	Pathology	Serum Tumor Markers	Presentation
Seminoma: Classic Spermatocytic	35–70	Classic seminoma: predominantly solitary homogeneous tumor comprising uniform cells with clear cytoplasm and well-defined borders. Cells are arranged in nests, surrounded by fibrous septa infiltrated with lymphocytes. Nuclei are spherical and hyperchromatic with 1-2 enlarged nucleoli. Mitoses are variable and associated with intratubular germ cell neoplasia (ITGCN) but have no prognostic significance. The separate pathologic classification of anaplastic seminoma is no longer used. Immunohistochemistry can be used to distinguish seminoma from embryonal carcinoma (EC); most seminomas express PLAP and do not stain with antibodies to keratin. The reverse applies to embryonal tumors. In addition, most seminomas express CD117 (c-*kit* proto-oncogene protein) and not CD30 (transmembrane glycoprotein), whereas most embryonal cell carcinomas are CD30 positive and CD117 negative.	PLAP: 90% hCG: <10% (produced by syncytiotrophoblasts found in small numbers of seminomas)	Typically enlarged painless testis (can be 10× normal). Testis is normal or decreased in size in 15%. Age range: 35-55 years for classic seminomas and >60 years for spermatocytic seminomas. Extragonadal sites include mediastinum, pituitary and pineal gland. Spermatocytic seminoma: comprises 9% of seminomas, occurs most frequently in men > 40 years of age. In men > 65 years this tumor is the most common germ cell tumor. It generally behaves in a benign fashion and very rarely may be associated with a sarcoma, which may metastasize.
Embryonal carcinoma (EC)	3–6	EC cells are undifferentiated malignant cells resembling developmentally pluripotential cells from early stages of embryogenesis. Glycogen-containing pleomorphic cells have less distinct cell membranes and increased numbers of mitoses. The cytoplasm is scant, and thus cells appear to be overlapping. Cells may be arranged in sheets or may be papillary or tubular structures. Necrosis and vascular invasion may be evident. Approximately 40% of GCT contain embryonal elements. EC is the smallest of the germ cell tumors: 40% are <2 cm in diameter and often in close proximity to the rete testis. Vascular and lymphatic invasion may be noted and represent a risk factor for metastatic disease. Presence of more than 40% EC in mixed GCT (more than one histologic entity) represents a risk factor for metastatic disease. Syncytiotrophoblastic cells are commonly found adjacent to EC cells. Immunohistochemistry: EC cells are positive for CD 30, keratin, and occasionally PLAP. Syncytiotrophoblastic cells are positive for hCG.	Elevation of hCG not due to EC cells but rather to syncytiotrophoblastic cells that may be present in the stroma. Elevation of hCG does not occur in pure EC, which does not contain syncytiotrophoblastic cells. α-Fetoprotein elevation rare in pure embryonal carcinoma and when it occurs is usually due to yolk sac elements.	Hard irregular testis, often of normal size. Age range: 25-35 years.

Continued

high-risk group, characterized by significantly higher rates of CIS. Risk factors for the development of testicular CIS include a history of testicular carcinoma (5% to 6%), EGCT (40%), cryptorchidism (3%), contralateral testis with unilateral testicular cancer (5% to 6%), atrophic contralateral testis with unilateral testicular cancer (30%), somatosexual ambiguity (25% to 100%), and infertility (0.4% to 1.1%) (Harland et al, 1998).

CIS is usually evenly distributed throughout the testis; therefore, open surgical biopsy (3 mm³) is generally positive in cases where CIS exists (Giwercan et al, 1993). Although needle biopsy of the testis has been shown to result in fewer seminiferous tubules than open biopsy, the prevalence of CIS in one study was shown to be the same for open versus needle biopsy. **Presently, there is no established tumor marker for CIS, and testicular ultrasound has been shown to be unreliable with respect to diagnosing CIS. Therefore, testicular biopsy remains the "gold standard" for diagnosing CIS.** In the future, seminal analysis, fine-needle aspiration, or serum markers may become available for screening patients at high risk for CIS.

Management of testicular CIS depends on a variety of factors, such as patient age, whether the patient has bilateral or unilateral CIS, associated testicular atrophy, and the philosophy of the treating physician. In GCT, CIS of the contralateral testis is present in 5% of patients and, with time,

Table 29–3. Germ Cell Tumors: Incidence, Pathology, Tumor Markers, Presentation—cont'd

Type	Incidence (%)	Pathology	Serum Tumor Markers	Presentation
Teratoma: Mature Immature With malignant transformation Simple epidermoid cysts	3% in adults; 38% in children	By definition this tumor is composed of two or more embryonic germ cell layers that may be both mature and immature. Endoderm: mucus-secreting glands (may degenerate into adenocarcinoma) Mesoderm: cartilage, bone, muscle, or lymphoid tissue Ectoderm: stratified squamous epithelium and neural tissue. Tumor is very heterogeneous with both solid and cystic components. Divided into three subsets: Mature: well-differentiated ectodermal, mesodermal, or endodermal tissues Immature: incompletely differentiated tissues Teratoma with areas of malignant transformation: sarcoma, squamous carcinoma, adenocarcinoma Simple epidermoid cysts: keratinizing, stratified squamous cell–lined cysts supported by fibrous tissue are therefore not strictly teratomas because only one germ cell layer is present. Mature teratoma is considered to be a fully differentiated form of mixed NSGCT in which all EC cells have differentiated into somatic tissue. Thus teratomas are potentially malignant, and it is generally recommended that these tumors are managed in similar fashion to other NSGCTs.	α-Fetoprotein in 20%-25%; associated with mucinous glands and areas of hepatoid differentiation.	Age range: first, second, and third decades. Mature and immature forms have metastatic potential in adults but in children are uniformly benign. Although these tumors do not contain EC cells, they may produce metastatic disease composed of somatic tissue or even EC cells. The latter are probably accounted for by unrecognized EC cells in the primary tumor. The primary tumor generally presents as an enlarged testis with both solid and cystic components. Epidermoid cysts have a uniformly benign course. The teratoma component of metastatic GCT is resistant to chemotherapy and radiotherapy.
Choriocarcinoma	1-2	Occurs as either pure choriocarcinoma or in tumors with more than one histologic type (mixed GCT) Pure choriocarcinoma: hemorrhagic mass with viable tumor at the periphery. Choriocarcinoma cells tend to destroy tissue and invade blood vessels, causing necrosis and hemorrhage. These tumors are associated with two other cells types: Syncytiotrophoblasts: large multinucleated giant cells with multiple irregular nuclei Cytotrophoblasts: medium-sized closely packed cells with single uniform nucleus	hCG > 99%; levels may be extremely high PLAP	Age range: second and third decades Testis usually not enlarged Patient may present with manifestations of metastatic disease such as pulmonary insufficiency or features of brain secondary tumors.
Mixed tumors (tumors of more than one histologic type)	60	Mixed tumors occurs in various combinations Most frequent mixed tumor is one of EC, seminoma, yolk sac tumor, teratoma, and syncytiotrophoblasts Tumor cell types and their relative contributions to tumor volume should be documented.	Depends on the cell types; usually α-fetoprotein due to yolk sac elements and hCG due to syncytiotrophoblasts	Age range: second and third decades. Despite the presence of seminoma, these tumors are managed as NSGCTs. A subset of patients present with symptoms of advanced disease, including chronic cough, abdominal or back discomfort and occasionally central nervous system manifestations. Delay in diagnosis due to delay in seeking medical evaluation and/or incorrect diagnosis averages 6 weeks to 3 months.

Table 29–4.   Presentation, Pathology, and Treatment of Intratubular Germ Cell Neoplasia (ITGCN)

Presentation	Pathology	Treatment

Risk factors:
  Contralateral gonad in men with unilateral testis cancer; incidence ranges from 2%-38%
  Cryptorchidism
  Infertility: infertile men have an incidence of 0.4%-1%
  Extragonadal GCT: 35%-50% incidence of ITGCN in one or both testes
  Intersex individuals with Y chromosome karyotype
Testis may be atrophic but is usually normal to palpation.
Testis biopsy reliably diagnoses ITGCN because the ITGCN is almost always found throughout the testis
Progression of ITGCN to invasive disease may take 15 years.
	ITGCN cells are located on the basement membrane of the seminiferous tubule and possess morphologic features of malignancy: large irregular nucleus, coarse chromatin, and abundant cytoplasm.
	Typically only one layer of ITGCN cells is seen, but occasionally the whole tubule is filled with ITGCN cells, which may represent an early stage in progression to GCT
		Theoretically with long enough follow-up, ITGCN will progress to invasive disease.
		Treatment options:
		  Observation
		  Orchiectomy
		  Radiation
		Although observation may be complicated by delayed diagnosis of GCT, it is unlikely that observation affects ultimate prognosis.
		Low-dose radiation is widely used in some European centers.
		Chemotherapy so far appears to be ineffective against ITGCN.

probably evolves into invasive cancer in the majority of these patients. Although CIS can easily be cured by radiation, this therapy may have undesirable side effects on both fertility and androgen production. Furthermore, the incidence of CIS in the general population is low and screening programs are therefore not generally recommended (von der Maase et al, 1987; Herr et al, 1997). On the other hand, screening of high-risk groups is recommended by some physicians, especially for patients with extragonadal tumors and patients with intersex disorders; both types of patients are at very high risk for CIS.

Treatment options for CIS include observation, radiation therapy, chemotherapy, and orchiectomy (Table 29–4). Radiation therapy was introduced by Skakkebaek in 1985 for patients with CIS in the remaining testis after contralateral orchiectomy for GCT (von der Maase et al, 1986a). Initially, patients received 20 Gy of radiation therapy, but experience with reduced doses of 14 Gy revealed that a pattern of only Sertoli's cells, similar to that found in patients treated with higher doses of radiation therapy, was noted on follow-up testis biopsy. All men who receive radiation therapy for CIS of a solitary testis are rendered infertile. These concerns, however, must be tempered by the fact that fertility in patients with testis cancer may be significantly compromised before any adjuvant therapy is administered (Fordham et al, 1990). Cisplatin-based chemotherapy has been shown to eradicate CIS; however, the response is somewhat unpredictable. Persistence of CIS and development of second GCTs have been described after cisplatin-based chemotherapy (Christensen et al, 1998). In a survey of 33 patients with CIS in the contralateral testis treated with chemotherapy, CIS was not reported on follow-up biopsy in 30 of the patients. CIS was subsequently detected in six patients, and the estimated cumulative risk of developing CIS 5 and 10 years after chemotherapy was 21% and 42%, respectively. Therefore, chemotherapy is not recommended in patients with contralateral testis CIS unless it is planned as adjuvant therapy for the primary tumor.

In summary, we do not advocate biopsy of the contralateral testis in patients with GCT, owing to the protracted course of CIS, the side effects of therapy, and the realization that second primary GCTs respond well to treatment.

Despite the argument that early diagnosis and therapy for CIS allows preservation of the testis, whereas development of a second GCT usually results in anorchia, we nevertheless believe that a conservative approach is warranted in view of the low risks involved. High-risk patients (those with infertility, cryptorchidism, atrophic testis, EGCTs, and intersex conditions) require close observation, and some may elect to undergo biopsy and CIS therapy after having clearly understood all the risks and benefits involved.

Epidemiology of Germ Cell Tumors

Incidence

Approximately 6900 new cases related to testicular cancer are reported in the United States annually (Greenlee et al, 2000). Estimates indicate that for American white males, the lifetime probability of developing testicular cancer is approximately 0.2%, or 1 in 500 (Zdeb, 1977). **The average annual age-adjusted incidence rate for American men from 1969 to 1971 was 3.7 per 100,000—nearly twice the rate of 2 per 100,000 from 1937 to 1939.** The average rate among American black males is 0.9 per 100,000, unchanged since the 1960s.

Similar trends have been noted in Denmark, where the age-adjusted incidence rose from 3.4 to 6.4 per 100,000 between 1945 and 1970 (Clemmesen, 1974). Data compiled by Muir and Nectoux (1979) indicated considerable variability in the worldwide incidence of adult GCTs. The average annual age-adjusted rate is highest in Scandinavia (Denmark and Norway), Switzerland, Germany, and New Zealand; it is intermediate in the United States and Great Britain and low in Africa and Asia. In data collected by Clemmesen (1974), the age-adjusted rate rose from 3.2 to 6.7 per 100,000 in Copenhagen between 1943 and 1967. Prevalence rates in Copenhagen were double those in rural Denmark during the same period.

Age

Peak incidences of testicular tumors occur in late adolescence to early adulthood (20 to 40 years), in late adulthood (older than 60 years), and in infancy (0 to 10 years). **Overall, the highest incidence is noted in young adult males, making these neoplasms the most common solid tumors of men age 20 to 34 years and the second most common of men age 35 to 40 years in the United States and Great Britain. Seminoma is rare before age 10 years and after age 60 years, but it is the most common histologic type overall, with a peak incidence between 35 and 39 years.** Spermatocytic seminoma (approximately 10% of all seminomas) occurs most often in patients older than 50 years. Embryonal carcinoma and teratocarcinoma occur predominantly between 25 and 35 years. Choriocarcinoma (1% to 2% of all GCTs) occurs more often in the 20- to 30-year age group. Yolk sac tumors are the predominant lesions of infancy and childhood but are frequently found in combination with other germ cell elements in young adults. Histologically benign, pure teratoma occurs most often in children but frequently appears in combination with other elements in adulthood. Malignant testicular lymphomas are predominantly tumors of men older than age 50 years.

Racial Factors

Variable incidence rates are noted among different ethnic groups within a given region. The incidence of testicular tumors in American blacks is approximately one third that in American whites but 10 times that in African blacks. In Israel, Jewish people have at least an eightfold higher incidence of testis tumors in comparison with non-Jewish people. In Hawaii, the incidence in the Filipino and Japanese sectors is approximately one tenth that in the Chinese, white, and native Hawaiian populations.

Graham and Gibson (1972) presented data indicating a higher incidence among professional men. Mack and Henderson (1980) noted higher incidence rates in the upper and middle socioeconomic classes of whites in Los Angeles County, California. Although similar trends have been noted in American blacks (Ross et al, 1979), the rate is still less than one third that of whites of comparable social status.

Genetic Factors

Although a relatively higher incidence of testicular tumors has been reported in twins, brothers, and family members, the evidence for a predominantly genetic influence is not overwhelming (Johnson, 1976). In nearly 7000 sets of twins from the Danish Twin Registry, Harvald and Hauge (1963) found no higher incidence of cancer in twins than was expected in the general population. Nicholson and Harland (1995) reported that one third of all testicular cancer patients are genetically predisposed to disease, likely a homozygous (recessive) inheritance of a single predisposing gene. The 2% to 3% incidence of bilateral tumors may suggest the potential importance of genetic (or congenital) factors.

Laterality and Bilaterality

Testicular neoplasms appear to be slightly more common in the right testis than in the left, similar to the slightly greater incidence of right-sided cryptorchidism. **Two to 3 percent of testicular tumors are bilateral, occurring either simultaneously or successively.** If secondary testicular tumors are excluded, the incidence of bilateral tumors is between 1% and 2.8% of all cases of germinal neoplasms (Sokal et al, 1980). Similar, rather than different, histology in the two testes

predominates with bilateral tumors. Bach and coworkers (1983) tabulated the histology in 337 cases of bilateral testicular tumors. Bilateral seminoma was the most common histologic type (48%); bilateral similar nonseminomas were found in 15%; germinal tumors with different histology were present in 15%; and nongerminal tumors with similar histology occurred in 22%. A history of cryptorchidism (unilateral or bilateral) in nearly half these men is consistent with observations that bilateral dysgenesis occurs frequently in unilateral maldescent (Sohval, 1956). Long-term surveillance of patients with a history of cryptorchidism or previous orchiectomy for GCT is mandatory.

Frequency of Histologic Types

Germinal tumors constitute between 90% and 95% of all primary testicular malignancies. Variability in the reported frequency of histologic types may reflect true differences in the incidence of such tumors. Such variations, however, may instead reflect demographic differences, variance of histologic interpretations, or other unquantified selection factors. **The overall incidence rates vary and have been tabulated as follows: seminoma, 30% to 60%; embryonal carcinoma in its pure form, 3% to 4%, although it is present in 40% of NSGCTs; teratoma, 5% to 10%; and pure choriocarcinoma, 1%. Tumors of more than one histologic type are considered a separate entity and are also known as mixed GCTs; they make up approximately 60% of all GCTs** (Mostofi, 1973).

Etiology

Experimental and clinical evidence supports the importance of congenital factors in the etiology of GCTs. During development, the primordial germ cell may be altered by environmental factors, resulting in disturbed differentiation. The germ cell is conceivably detained from normal development by cryptorchidism, gonadal dysgenesis, or hereditary predisposition or by chemical carcinogens, trauma, or orchitis. The teratocarcinoma tumor model (Stevens, 1968) suggests the crucial influence of temporal relationships on normal versus abnormal differentiation.

Congenital Causes

Cryptorchidism. LeComete (1851) is credited with the initial observation that testicular maldescent and tumor formation are interrelated (Grove, 1954). Pooled data from several large series indicate that 7% to 10% of patients with testicular tumors have a prior history of cryptorchidism (Whitaker, 1970). Mostofi (1973) listed five possible, but unquantified, factors that may play a causative role in the cryptorchid/malignant testis: abnormal germ cell morphology, elevated temperature, interference with blood supply, endocrine dysfunction, and gonadal dysgenesis.

The exact incidence of cryptorchidism is unknown because much of the relevant information on testicular maldescent includes data on patients with retractile testes. From accumulated series, Scorer and Farrington (1971) estimated that approximately 4.3% of neonates, 0.8% of infants and children, and 0.7% of adults older than 18 years (military inductees) harbor a truly cryptorchid testis. In reviewing more than 7000 cases of testicular tumor, Gilbert and Hamilton (1940) found a history of cryptorchidism in 840 men (12%). Based on the observed incidence of cryptorchidism in military inductees (0.23%, roughly 1 in 500), they calculated the estimated risk of tumorigenesis in a man with a history of maldescent to be 48 times that of a man with normally descended testes. **More recent epidemiologic studies have reported the relative risk of testicular cancer in patients with cryptorchidism to be much lower: 3 to 14 times the normal expected incidence** (Henderson et al, 1979; Schottenfeld et al, 1980; Farrer et al, 1985).

Between 5% and 10% of patients with a history of cryptorchidism develop malignancy in the contralateral, normally descended gonad. This observation is consistent with the findings of Berthelsen and colleagues (1982). They provided biopsy data in 250 patients with testis cancer relative to the contralateral testis. CIS was found in 13 (5.2%), representing one third of patients with atrophy of the remaining testis and one fifth of patients with a history of cryptorchidism. Two of the patients (10%) with contralateral CIS subsequently developed a second testis cancer. Campbell (1942) noted that roughly 25% of patients with bilateral cryptorchidism and a history of testis cancer were subject to the risk of a second GCT.

Ultrastructural abnormalities of spermatogonia and Sertoli's cells are readily apparent in cryptorchid testis by age 3 years. Cellular degeneration is followed by progressive fibrosis, destruction of the basement membrane, and deposition of myelin and lipids (Mengel et al, 1982). Consideration of these histologic changes and other social factors has favored the practice of early orchiopexy. Such a philosophy, however, has not completely prevented tumor formation in the testis (Martin, 1979; Batata et al, 1982). **It is, therefore, generally believed that orchiopexy does not prevent carcinogenesis but rather allows clinical surveillance of patients with a previously impalpable gonad.**

Acquired Causes

Trauma. Although trauma is considered a contributing factor in zinc-induced or copper-induced fowl teratomas, there is little to suggest a cause-and-effect relationship in humans (Carleton et al, 1953). Most investigators conclude that trauma to the enlarged testis is an event that prompts medical evaluation rather than a causative factor.

Hormones. Sex hormone fluctuations may contribute to the development of testicular tumors in experimental animals and humans. The administration of estrogen to pregnant mice may cause maldescent and dysgenesis of the testis in the offspring (Nomura and Kanzak, 1977). Similar findings have been noted in the sons of women exposed to diethylstilbestrol (Cosgrove et al, 1977) or oral contraceptives (Rothman and Louik, 1978). Exogenous estrogen administration has also been linked to the induction of Leydig's cell tumors. Epidemiologic studies found relative risk rates ranging from 2.8% to 5.3% for testicular tumor in the sons of diethylstilbestrol-treated mothers (Schottenfeld et al, 1980; Henderson et al, 1983).

Atrophy. Nonspecific or mumps-associated atrophy of the testis has been suggested as a potential causative factor in testicular cancer. Gilbert (1944) found 80 cases of testicular tumors occurring in patients with a history of nonspecific atrophy and 24 additional cases related to a previous history of mumps-associated orchitis among 5500 cases of testicular tumor. Although a causative role for atrophy remains speculative, it is tempting to invoke local hormonal imbalance as a possible cause of malignant transformation.

Pathogenesis and Natural History of Germ Cell Tumors

Local growth characteristics and patterns of spread have been well defined by the clinical observation of patients with germinal testicular tumors. After malignant transformation, intratubular CIS extends beyond the basement membrane and may eventually replace most of the testicular parenchyma. Local involvement of the epididymis or spermatic cord is hindered by the tunica albuginea, and, seemingly as a consequence, lymphatic or hematogenous spread may occur first. Approximately half of patients with nonseminomatous tumors present with disseminated disease (Bosl et al, 1981). **Involvement of the epididymis or cord may lead to pelvic and inguinal lymph node metastasis, whereas tumors confined to the testis proper usually spread to retroperitoneal nodes.** Hematogenous spread to lung, bone, or liver occurs by direct vascular invasion or indirectly from previously established lymphatic metastasis, by way of the thoracic duct and subclavian veins, or through other lymphaticovenous communications. The natural history of germinal testis tumors has been the subject of numerous treatises and appears sufficiently well defined to permit the following generalizations (Whitmore, 1968):

- Complete spontaneous regressions are rare.
- All germinal testis tumors in adults should be regarded as malignant. Although infantile teratoma may be regarded as benign, teratoma of the adult testis may be associated with vascular invasion microscopically and with a definite mortality risk in patients treated with orchiectomy alone (as high as 29%, according to Mostofi and Price [1973]). Clinical experience has shown that retroperitoneal teratoma in the adult, whether resulting from maturation of embryonal carcinoma or from regression of the embryonal carcinoma component of a teratocarcinoma (spontaneous or induced), may be accompanied by unrelenting local growth and ultimate fatality (Hong et al, 1977).
- The tunica albuginea is a natural barrier to expansile local growth. Extension through this dense membrane occurs at the testicular mediastinum, where the blood vessels, lymphatics, nerves, and efferent tubules exit the testis proper. Local involvement of the epididymis or spermatic cord occurs in 10% to 15% of cases and increases the risks of lymphatic or bloodborne metastasis.
- Lymphatic metastasis is common to all forms of germinal testis tumors, although pure choriocarcinoma almost uniformly disseminates by means of vascular invasion as well.

Patterns of Spread of Germ Cell Tumors

The principles that underlie the modern surgical treatment of GCT of the testis are based on the fact that testicular cancer spreads in a predictable and stepwise fashion (as described), with the notable exception of choriocarcinoma.

Anatomic studies at the turn of the century by Most (1898) and Cuneo (1901), as well as later work by Jamieson and Dobson (1910) and Rouviere (1938), demonstrated the lymphatic drainage of the testis, with the primary echelon of drainage for right-sided tumors to be interaortocaval and for left-sided tumors to be left para-aortic and preaortic nodes. There exists some crossover, especially from right to left. These anatomic studies provided the basis for regional control after establishing local control by orchiectomy.

The spermatic cord contains four to eight lymphatic channels that traverse the inguinal canal and retroperitoneal space. As the spermatic vessels cross ventral to the ureter, these lymphatics fan out medially and drain into the retroperitoneal lymph node chain. **The primary drainage of the right testis is usually located within the group of lymph nodes in the interaortocaval region at the level of the second vertebral body; the first echelon of nodes draining the left testis is located in the para-aortic region in the compartment bounded by the left ureter, the left renal vein, the aorta, and the origin of the inferior mesenteric artery. Lymphatic drainage has been shown to cross over from right to left, and, therefore, cross-metastases occur more commonly in patients with right-sided tumors. In a review of 104 consecutive cases of stage II NSGCT, the Indiana group made a number of important observations confirming the predictability of lymphatic spread in testicular cancer** (Donohue et al, 1982). They reported that suprahilar lymph node spread was rare in stage N1 disease; on the other hand, suprahilar spread was not uncommon in stage N2 disease. In low-stage disease, the absence of contralateral node involvement was noted. Cross-metastases were reported to occur more commonly in patients with right-sided tumors because of lymphatic drainage from right to left. These observations obviously have important implications for the surgical management of testicular cancer.

Subsequent cephalad drainage is to the cisterna chyli, thoracic duct, and supraclavicular nodes (usually left), but retrograde spread may occur to common, external, and inguinal lymph nodes. Although the thoracic duct–subclavian vein juncture is the major site of communication, other lymphaticovenous communications may be occasioned by massive retroperitoneal lymph node deposits. Furthermore, it has been demonstrated by spermatic lymphangiography that testicular lymphatics can, rarely, communicate directly with the thoracic duct, bypassing the retroperitoneal nodes. **Lymphatics of the epididymis drain into the external iliac chain, affording locally extensive testicular tumors access to pelvic lymph nodes. Inguinal node metastasis may result from scrotal involvement by the primary tumor, prior inguinal or scrotal surgery, or retrograde lymphatic spread secondary to massive retroperitoneal lymph node deposits.**

Extranodal distant metastasis results from either direct vascular invasion or tumor emboli from lymphatic metastasis via major thoracoabdominal channels or minor lymphaticovenous communications. Most, but not all, bloodborne metastases occur after lymph node involvement. This is of obvious practical importance in treatment and prognosis. **Despite surgical excision of negative retroperitoneal lymph nodes, the distant failure rate is approximately 5%** (Whitmore, 1973). This is probably because testicular lymphatics may very occasionally bypass retroperitoneal

lymph nodes altogether and communicate directly with the thoracic duct.

In patients undergoing surveillance alone after inguinal orchiectomy for clinical stage A nonseminoma, approximately 30% fail, most with retroperitoneal lymph node metastasis (80% of failures) and the remainder with extralymphatic distant metastasis (20% of failures) independent of retroperitoneal deposits (Duchesne et al, 1990).

With the exception of seminoma, the growth rate among GCTs tends to be high. **Doubling times calculated on the basis of serial chest radiographs usually range from 10 to 30 days.** Alterations in the production of tumor marker substances (β-hCG, AFP, lactic acid dehydrogenase [LDH]) are in keeping with rapid metabolic activity and growth. The anticipated rapid demise of patients failing treatment has been confirmed by clinical observation; 85% of patients dying of GCTs do so within 2 years and the majority of the remainder within 3 years. Because of a sometimes indolent course, seminoma may recur from 2 to 10 years after apparently successful initial management.

Because of the short natural history of germinal tumors, it has become customary to regard 2-year survival as an endpoint for judging the effectiveness of therapy. With the evolution of multimodal therapy, surviving patients may not be actually cured of their neoplasm, and a disease-free interval of 5 years may be a more appropriate yardstick for assessing curability. Longer follow-up after chemotherapy is mandatory, however, because relapse has been noted up to 10 years after treatment.

In summary, with the notable exception of choriocarcinoma, testicular cancer generally spreads in a predictable pattern. This has led to the development of new surgical techniques, which provide accurate pathologic staging while at the same time providing therapeutic benefit. These techniques are also associated with reduced morbidity when compared with the classic full retroperitoneal lymph node dissection (RPLND).

Clinical Manifestations

In general, survival in patients with GCT is related to the stage at presentation and therefore to the amount of tumor burden as well as to the effectiveness of subsequent treatment. Patients who present with advanced disease (stage III) generally have a much poorer prognosis than do those with disease confined to the testis or those with regional nodal involvement only. Delay in diagnosis of 1 to 2 months or more is not uncommon in these patients and seems to be related directly to patient factors such as ignorance, denial, and fear as well as physician factors such as misdiagnosis. Almost half of patients present with metastatic disease (Bosl et al, 1981). The need clearly exists for patient education through programs such as those advocating testicular self-examination. Only through widespread public health techniques will the knowledge of testicular tumors be promulgated so that diagnosis can occur earlier. Physician-related causes still remain major factors in delay of treatment, which emphasizes the need for continuing education. It is of interest that denial is such a strong force in patients with testicular tumor. Some of these patients present with masses as large as a grapefruit in the scrotal contents.

Signs and Symptoms

The usual presentation of a testicular tumor is a nodule or painless swelling of one gonad. This may be noted incidentally by the patient or by his sexual partner. The classic description is that of a lump, swelling, or hardness of the testis. Thirty to 40 percent of patients may complain of a dull ache or a heavy sensation in the lower abdomen, anal area, or scrotum. In approximately 10% of patients, acute pain is the presenting symptom. Occasionally, patients with a previously small atrophic testis note enlargement. On rare occasions, infertility may be the presenting complaint (Skakkebaek, 1972). Acute onset of pain is rare unless there is associated epididymitis or bleeding within the tumor.

In approximately 10% of patients, the presenting manifestations may be due to metastases and include a neck mass (supraclavicular lymph node metastasis); respiratory symptoms, such as cough or dyspnea (pulmonary metastasis); gastrointestinal disturbances, such as anorexia, nausea, vomiting, or hemorrhage (retroduodenal metastasis); lumbar back pain (bulky retroperitoneal disease involving the psoas muscle or nerve roots); bone pain (skeletal metastasis); central and peripheral nervous system manifestations (cerebral, spinal cord, or peripheral root involvement); or unilateral or bilateral lower-extremity swelling (iliac or caval venous obstruction or thrombosis).

Gynecomastia, seen in about 5% of patients with testicular GCTs, may be regarded as a systemic endocrine manifestation of these neoplasms. Gynecomastia may or may not be associated with elevated levels of hCG, human chorionic somatomammotropin, prolactin, estrogens, or androgens. Relationships among gynecomastia, morphologic characteristics of the primary tumor, and endocrine abnormalities remain incompletely defined.

Physical Examination

Physical examination of the testis is performed by bimanual examination of the scrotal contents, beginning with the normal contralateral testis. This provides a baseline and allows the examiner to note the relative size, contour, and consistency of the normal testis as well as the suspected gonad. Physical examination of the testis is performed by careful palpation of the testis between the thumb and the first two fingers of the examining hand. The normal testis is homogeneous in consistency, freely movable, and separable from the epididymis. Any firm, hard, or fixed area within the substance of the tunica albuginea should be considered suspicious until proved otherwise. Further examination of the suspected tumor should be directed toward possible involvement of the cord, scrotal investments, or skin. In general, seminoma tends to expand within the testis as a painless, rubbery enlargement. Embryonal carcinoma or teratocarcinoma may produce an irregular, rather than discrete, mass, although this distinction is not always easily appreciated.

Testicular tumors tend to remain ovoid, being limited by the tough investing tunica albuginea. In 10% to 15% of patients, spread to the epididymis or cord may occur. A hydrocele may be present and increase the difficulty of appreciation of a testicular neoplasm. **Ultrasonography of the scrotum is a rapid, reliable technique to exclude hydrocele or** epididymitis and should be used if there is any suspicion of testicular tumor.

Physical examination should also include palpation of the abdomen for evidence of nodal disease or visceral involvement. Routine assessment of the supraclavicular lymph nodes may reveal adenopathy in patients with advanced disease. Examination of the chest may disclose gynecomastia or the presence of respiratory tract involvement.

Differential Diagnosis

The differential diagnosis of a testicular mass includes testicular torsion, epididymitis, or epididymo-orchitis. Less common problems include hydrocele, hernia, hematoma, spermatocele, or syphilitic gumma. **In any patient with a solid, firm, intratesticular mass, testicular cancer must be the considered diagnosis until proved otherwise.** In patients in whom the diagnosis is unclear or in whom a hydrocele precludes adequate examination, imaging studies should be used as an important second step.

Scrotal Ultrasonography

Ultrasonography of the scrotum is basically an extension of the physical examination. Any hypoechoic area within the tunica albuginea is markedly suspicious for testicular cancer. With the advent of scrotal ultrasonography and its general availability throughout the United States, the delay in diagnosis from confusion with epididymitis should be markedly reduced (Friedrich et al, 1981; Richie et al, 1982). Intrascrotal fluid collection is no barrier to examination of the underlying testicular parenchyma by ultrasonography. In patients with palpably normal genitalia and evidence of extragonadal germ cell malignancy, sonography has been reported to be successful in identifying occult testicular neoplasms (Glazer et al, 1982).

Rarely, patients present with advanced disease without a recognizable primary tumor in the testis. Some of these may be EGCTs, with an inherently worse prognosis, whereas others may represent a small primary testicular tumor with large extragonadal metastases. In this latter subset of patients, scrotal ultrasonography is important to establish the testis as the organ of GCT origin. Furthermore, in patients with a diagnosis of EGCT, ultrasound of the testis is mandatory to be certain that one is not dealing with a primary GCT. Nonpalpable intratesticular masses are more frequently detected now than in the past owing to the increased use of scrotal ultrasound. Horstman and colleagues (1994) reported that 78% of nonpalpable lesions were benign Leydig's and Sertoli's cell tumors. Another study, however, reported that of 15 impalpable masses detected among 3019 scrotal ultrasound studies performed over a 10-year period, 73% were malignant. Intraoperative ultrasound can be useful in these patients to locate the tumor, allowing performance of testis-sparing surgery.

CLINICAL STAGING

Findings noted at orchiectomy—predominantly histologic findings in the primary tumor, radiologic procedures, and laboratory studies—are essential in assessing clinical stage

of disease. The importance of clinical staging cannot be overemphasized because it leads to orderly decision making with respect to appropriate treatment and it provides important prognostic data. With the advent of alternative treatment protocols for patients with clinical low-stage testicular cancer, the impact of staging and its accuracy are even more critical. The accuracy of clinical assessment is imperative if the physician is to be able to make a logical decision about therapy.

It is important to appreciate that, in general, clinical staging systems are based on pathologic analysis of the primary tumor and imaging studies of the chest and retroperitoneum. Modern staging techniques have reduced false-negative staging errors in clinical stage T1-T3 N0 M0 disease to approximately 20%. In patients with clinical stage I disease subjected to RPLND, 10% to 15% harbor undetected nodal metastasis, and another 5% to 10% relapse after surgery, almost always in extranodal sites. These figures underscore the need for patients on surveillance protocols to adhere diligently to the protocol.

A convenient division for staging systems is those patients with seminomas and those with nonseminomatous tumors. Patients with pure seminoma are usually staged by clinical means, whereas staging in patients with NSGCTs sometimes employs surgical techniques such as RPLND as well.

The extent of staging is determined in part by decisions for therapy; for example, if surveillance protocols are to be considered, every effort should be made to exclude patients with any evidence of retroperitoneal disease. If retroperitoneal lymphadenectomy is likely to be elected as the primary treatment for low-stage, nonseminomatous tumors, efforts should be directed toward delineation of regional and nodal versus distant metastases.

Staging Systems

The predictable mode of metastasis in patients with GCTs, along with technologic advances in imaging and biochemical marker assays, has improved the accuracy of initial clinical evaluations, although they are far from perfect. A variety of clinical staging systems have been advocated since the 1960s.

The numerous staging systems for seminoma and NSGCT, however, led to confusion because of differences among clinical and pathologic staging systems and subsequently resulted in difficulty comparing interinstitutional data.

In 1997, an internationally agreed-on consensus classification applicable to both seminoma and nonseminoma was published. The American Joint Committee on Cancer (AJCC) staging for GCTs is unique because, for the first time, a serum tumor marker category (S) is used to supplement the prognostic stages defined by anatomy alone. This tumor, nodes, and metastasis staging (TNMS) system should replace all prior staging systems and should, it is hoped, standardize patient reporting (Table 29–5).

The AJCC TNMS system subdivides stage I disease into stages Ia and Ib depending on the T stage, as well as into stage Is according to serum tumor marker levels; stage II is subdivided into stages IIa, IIb, and IIc depending on volume of retroperitoneal lymph node involvement; and stage III is subdivided into stages IIIa, IIIb, and IIIc according to the degree of metastatic involvement and serum tumor marker levels (Table 29–6).

Table 29–5. Testicular Cancer Staging System of the American Joint Committee on Cancer and the International Union Against Cancer

Definition of TNM

Primary Tumor (T)

pTX	Primary tumor cannot be assessed (if no radical orchiectomy has been performed, TX is used)
pT0	No evidence of primary tumor (e.g., histologic scar in testis)
pTis	Intratubular germ cell neoplasia (carcinoma in situ)
pT1	Tumor limited to the testis and epididymis and no vascular/lymphatic invasion
pT2	Tumor limited to the testis and epididymis with vascular/lymphatic invasion or tumor extending through the tunica albuginea with involvement of tunica vaginalis
pT3	Tumor invades the spermatic cord with or without vascular/lymphatic invasion
pT4	Tumor invades the scrotum with or without vascular/lymphatic invasion

Regional Lymph Nodes (N)

Clinical

NX	Regional lymph nodes cannot be assessed
N0	No regional lymph node metastasis
N1	Lymph node mass 2 cm or less in greatest dimension or multiple lymph node masses, none more than 2 cm in greatest dimension
N2	Lymph node mass, more than 2 cm but not more than 5 cm in greatest dimension, or multiple lymph node masses, any one mass greater than 2 cm but not more than 5 cm in greatest dimension
N3	Lymph node mass more than 5 cm in greatest dimension

Pathologic

pN0	No evidence of tumor in lymph nodes
pN1	Lymph node mass, 2 cm or less in greatest dimension and ≤6 nodes positive, none >2 cm in greatest dimension
pN2	Lymph node mass, more than 2 cm but not more than 5 cm in greatest dimension; more than 5 nodes positive, none >5 cm; evidence of extranodal extension of tumor
pN3	Lymph node mass more than 5 cm in greatest dimension

Distant Metastases (M)

M0	No evidence of distant metastases
M1	Nonregional nodal or pulmonary metastases
M2	Nonpulmonary visceral masses

Serum Tumor Markers (S)

	LDH	hCG (mIU/mL)	AFP (ng/mL)
S0	≤N	≤N	≤N
S1	<1.5 × N	<5,000	<1,000
S2	1.5–10 × N	5,000–50,000	1,000–10,000
S3	>10 × N	>50,000	>10,000

AFP, α-fetoprotein, hCG, human chorionic gonadotropin; LDH, lactate dehydrogenase; N, upper limit of normal for the LDH assay.
Data from Vogelzang NJ, Scardino PT, Shipley WU, Coffey DS (eds): Genitourinary Oncology. Philadelphia, Lippincott, Williams & Wilkins, 1999.

Findings at Orchiectomy

Removal of the testis via an inguinal approach, the so-called radical orchiectomy, remains the definitive procedure for pathologic diagnosis as well as for local treatment of testicular neoplasms. Morbidity is minimal, and mortality should be virtually zero while allowing 100% local control. Transscrotal biopsy is to be condemned. The inguinal approach permits early control of the vascular and lymphatic supply as well as en-bloc removal of the testis with all its tunicae.

Table 29–6. Stage Grouping for Testicular Cancer According to the AJCC Staging System

Stage Grouping	T	N	M	S
Stage 0	pTis	N0	M0	S0
Stage I	T1-T4	N0	M0	SX
Ia	T1	N0	M0	S0
Ib	T2	N0	M0	S0
	T3	N0	M0	S0
	T4	N0	M0	S0
Is	Any T	N0	M0	S1-S3
Stage II	Any T	Any N	M0	SX
IIa	Any T	N1	M0	S0
	Any T	N1	M0	S1
IIb	Any T	N2	M0	S0
	Any T	N2	M0	S1
IIc	Any T	N3	M0	S0
	Any T	N3	M0	S1
Stage III	Any T	Any N	M1	SX
IIIa	Any T	Any N	M1	S0
	Any T	Any N	M1	S1
IIIb	Any T	Any N	M0	S2
	Any T	Any N	M1	S2
IIIc	Any T	Any N	M0	S3
	Any T	Any N	M1a	S3
	Any T	Any N	M1b	Any S

AJCC, American Joint Committee on Cancer; TNM, tumor, nodes, metastasis.
Data from Vogelzang NJ, Scardino PT, Shipley WU, Coffey DS (eds): Genitourinary Oncology. Philadelphia, Lippincott, Williams & Wilkins, 1999.

The decision to proceed to radical inguinal orchiectomy is made after careful consideration of all available data, including clinical findings, imaging studies, and tumor markers, samples of which should always be drawn before orchiectomy.

We do not delay radical orchiectomy in patients with clinically advanced disease, because the testis has been shown to be a privileged site with respect to its ability to harbor viable tumor despite chemotherapy.

Radical or inguinal orchiectomy, with early clamping of the spermatic cord at the deep inguinal ring, effectively removes a primary tumor and allows staging in patients with testicular cancer. The orchiectomy specimen should be processed carefully to ensure that all elements within the tumor are recognized and that the histologic diagnosis is reasonably accurate. Of equal importance is determination of the local extent of tumor. **In addition to the histologic nature and percentage of tumor subtypes, the pathologist should record the T stage of the primary tumor and should also determine whether lymphatic or vascular invasion is seen within the tumor mass.**

Imaging Studies

Chest Radiography

Posteroanterior and lateral chest radiographs should be the initial radiographic procedures performed. These x-ray films provide the minimal assessment of the lung parenchyma and mediastinal structures. Whole-lung tomography is not obtained routinely at Brigham and Women's Hospital and the Dana Farber Cancer Institute. In a study of 120 whole-lung tomographic scans performed, whole-lung tomography altered the therapeutic decision in only 4 of 120 patients (Jochelson et al, 1984).

Chest computed tomography (CT) provides more sensitive evaluations of the thorax and may increase the detection of pulmonary metastases. Chest CT, however, delineates lesions as small as 2 mm in size. Approximately 70% of these small lesions turn out to be benign processes. Thus, if CT is used, a critical high index of suspicion should be present, with recognition that small lesions may, in fact, be benign and not related to the primary testicular cancer. See and Hoxie (1993) evaluated the added benefit of chest CT. They found in patients with negative abdominal CT that chest CT failed to increase diagnostic sensitivity above chest radiography alone. In patients with abnormal abdominal CT scans, however, chest CT identified abnormalities missed on routine, standard chest radiography alone.

Computed Tomography

Abdominal CT has been touted as being the most effective means to identify retroperitoneal lymph node involvement. CT has replaced intravenous urography and pedal lymphangiography as the procedure of choice for evaluation of the retroperitoneum. Pedal lymphangiography has an error rate of roughly 25% false-negative and 10% false-positive results. Given its overall inaccuracy coupled with its invasive nature, lymphangiography is no longer used for staging purposes (Bussar-Maatz and Weissbach, 1993). CT has largely supplanted intravenous pyelography for visualization of the kidneys and the course of the ureters and is much more sensitive in the detection of extensive retroperitoneal disease. Abdominal CT, especially with third-generation and fourth-generation scanners, can identify small lymph node deposits less than 2 cm in diameter in the upper para-aortic regions. CT provides a generally accurate three-dimensional estimate of tumor size and involvement of soft tissue structures and regional viscera. In addition, CT provides a view of the retrocrural space in the para-aortic region above the crus of the diaphragm, an important site of metastasis. CT, however, is not sufficiently accurate to distinguish fibrosis, teratoma, or malignancy by size criteria alone (Stomper et al, 1985).

Magnetic Resonance Imaging

In magnetic resonance imaging (MRI), the normal testis is homogeneous in signal by both T1-weighted and T2-weighted imaging. Relative to the normal testicular parenchyma, tumors are usually hypointense on T2-weighted images and show brisk and early enhancement after intravenous administration of gadolinium. In general, differentiation of tumor types with MRI is unreliable. Furthermore, MRI offers no advantage over CT for imaging and staging of the retroperitoneum in patients with testicular cancer.

Positron Emission Tomography

The use of positron emission tomography (PET) in the evaluation of retroperitoneal lymph nodes and radiographic abnormalities after chemotherapy in patients with testis cancer has been reported. No apparent advantage over CT has been demonstrated, mainly because neither PET nor CT has the ability to detect microscopic nodal disease (Cremerius et al, 1999; Ganjoo et al, 1999).

Tumor Markers

Germinal testicular tumors are among a select group of neoplasms identified as producing so-called marker proteins that are relatively specific and readily measurable in minute quantities using highly sensitive radioimmunoassay technology. Applied to the study of body fluids and tissue sections, these biochemical markers theoretically may be capable of detecting small tumor burdens (10^5 cells) that are not detectable by currently available imaging techniques (Bagshawe and Searle, 1977). The study of biochemical marker substances, particularly AFP and β-hCG, is clinically useful in the diagnosis, staging, and monitoring of treatment response in patients with germ cell neoplasms and may be useful as a prognostic index. GCT markers belong to two main classes: (1) oncofetal substances associated with embryonic development (AFP and β-hCG) and (2) certain cellular enzymes, such as LDH and placental alkaline phosphatase (PLAP).

The production by GCTs of oncofetal substances provides evidence that oncogenesis and ontogenesis are closely related. AFP is a dominant serum protein of the early embryo, and hCG is a secretory product of the placenta. During normal maturation of the fetus, both products fall to barely detectable levels soon after birth. **The production of AFP and hCG by trophoblastic and syncytiotrophoblastic cells, respectively, within germ cell neoplasms implies the re-expression of repressed genes (presumably lost during differentiation) or the malignant transformation of a pluripotential cell that has retained the ability to differentiate into cells capable of producing oncofetal proteins** (Abelev, 1974; Uriel, 1979).

α-Fetoprotein

AFP is a single-chain glycoprotein (molecular weight: ~70,000 daltons) first demonstrated by Bergstrand and Czar (1954) in normal human fetal serum. In the fetus, AFP is a major serum binding protein produced by the fetal yolk sac, liver, and gastrointestinal tract. **The highest concentrations noted during the 12th to 14th weeks of gestation gradually decline so that at 1 year after birth AFP is detectable only at low levels (<40 ng/mL).** In 1963, Abelev and colleagues detected AFP in mouse embryos and in the sera of mice with chemically induced liver tumors. Further investigation led to the discovery of elevated levels in humans with hepatomas and testicular tumors. The metabolic half-life of AFP in humans is between 5 and 7 days, a fact useful in evaluating treatment response.

After the first 6 weeks of postnatal life, elevated AFP may be detected in association with a number of malignancies (testis, liver, pancreas, stomach, lung), normal pregnancy, benign liver disease, ataxia-telangiectasia, and tyrosinemia. In endodermal sinus (or yolk sac) tumors, immunofluorescent methods indicate that the epithelial lining of the cysts and tubules is the site of synthesis of AFP (Teilum et al, 1975). **AFP may be produced by pure embryonal carcinoma, teratocarcinoma, yolk sac tumor, or combined tumors but not by pure choriocarcinoma or pure seminoma** (Javadpour, 1980a, 1980b). Taken together, these observations indicate that yolk sac elements are not always recognizable by conventional light microscopy in individuals with elevated serum AFP owing to GCTs. Binding studies with lectins have shown that AFP produced in the fetal liver has a molecular structure different from that produced in yolk sac tumors, a characteristic that may discriminate benign from malignant liver disease (Ruoslahti et al, 1978).

Human Chorionic Gonadotropin

This glycoprotein (molecular weight: 38,000 daltons) is composed of α and β polypeptide chains and is normally produced by trophoblastic tissue. Pituitary hormones (luteinizing hormone, follicle-stimulating hormone, thyroid-stimulating hormone) possess α subunits closely resembling that of hCG. The β subunit of hCG is structurally and antigenically distinct from that of the pituitary hormones and allows the production of specific antibodies against the purified β-hCG subunit used in radioimmunoassay techniques (Vaitukaitis, 1979).

During pregnancy, hCG is secreted by the placenta for the maintenance of the corpus luteum. Zondek (1930) was the first to demonstrate that hCG is detectable in the sera of some patients with GCTs. Elevated hCG levels may also be demonstrated in patients with various other malignancies (liver, pancreas, stomach, lung, breast, kidney, bladder) and, perhaps, in marijuana smokers. **In GCTs, syncytiotrophoblastic cells have been found responsible for the production of hCG. Some of the radioimmunoassay techniques for hCG variously cross react with luteinizing hormone, and, accordingly, caution should be exercised with patients whose luteinizing hormone may be physiologically elevated (e.g., after castration).**

The serum half-life of hCG is between 24 and 36 hours, but the individual subunits are cleared much more rapidly (20 minutes for the α subunit and 45 minutes for the β subunit). All patients with choriocarcinoma and 40% to 60% of patients with embryonal carcinoma are expected to have elevated serum levels of hCG. Five to 10 percent of patients with pure seminoma have detectable levels of hCG (usually below the level of 500 ng/mL), apparently produced by the syncytiotrophoblast-like giant cells occurring in some seminomas.

Lactic Acid Dehydrogenase

LDH is a ubiquitous cellular enzyme (molecular weight: 134,000 daltons), with particularly high levels detectable in smooth, cardiac, and skeletal muscles; liver; kidney; and brain. Elevation of serum LDH or one of its isoenzymes (LDH I to IV) has been reported as a useful finding in monitoring the treatment of GCTs. **Because of its low specificity (high false-positive rate), serum LDH levels must be correlated with other clinical findings in making therapeutic decisions.**

In evaluating experience with serum LDH as a tumor marker for NSGCTs, **Boyle and Samuels (1977) reported a direct relationship between tumor burden and LDH levels.** Increased LDH values were noted in 7 of 92 (8%) patients with stage I disease, 15 of 42 (32%) with stage II disease, and 57 of 70 (81%) with stage III disease. Recurrence rates in patients with stage I and II disease were higher—15 of 22 (77%) if pretreatment LDH values were elevated—than those in patients with normal levels—42 of 112 (40%). The first fraction (LDH I), as determined by agar gel electrophoresis, was responsible for LDH elevation in 25 of 29 patients studied. Skinner and Scardino (1980) found that an elevated LDH value may be the sole biochemical abnormality in as many as 10% of patients with persistent or recurrent nonseminomatous tumors. Serum LDH may be even more useful as a marker substance in the surveillance of patients with advanced seminoma. In reviewing their experience in patients with advanced, pure seminoma, Stanton and associates (1983) found elevation of LDH levels in 21 of 26 patients (81%). LDH seems to be most useful as a marker for "bulk" tissue.

Placental Alkaline Phosphatase and Gamma-Glutamyl-Transpeptidase

PLAP is a fetal isoenzyme structurally different from adult alkaline phosphatase. **Small studies using enzyme-linked immunosorbent assays indicate that as many as 40% of patients with advanced disease have elevated levels of PLAP** (Javadpour, 1983). Gamma-glutamyl-transpeptidase (GGTP) is a hepatocellular enzyme frequently elevated in benign or neoplastic diseases of the liver. Its presence has been documented in humans in the early placenta, normal testis, and seminal fluid and in sacrococcygeal teratocarcinoma and testicular seminoma (Krishnaswamy et al, 1977). Javadpour (1983) found that one third of patients with active seminomas had elevated levels of GGTP. Although the individual sensitivities of PLAP and GGTP are low, simultaneous determinations revealed elevation of one or both in 25 of 30 patients (80%) considered to have active disease. CD30 antigen has been evaluated as a possible marker for embryonal carcinoma, with detection of soluble CD30 molecule noted in a high percentage of patients with embryonal carcinoma but not in patients with other testicular GCTs (Latza et al, 1995).

Clinical Applications of Tumor Markers

Among patients with nonseminomatous testis tumors, 50% to 70% have elevated levels of AFP and 40% to 60% have elevated levels of hCG when sensitive radioimmunoassay techniques are used. If both markers are measured simultaneously, approximately 90% of patients have elevations of one or both marker substances (Barzell and Whitmore, 1979; Fraley et al, 1979; Javadpour, 1980b). These values are derived from patient populations with clinical stage I, II, and III tumors. In patients with clinical stage I tumors only, the incidence of positive markers is significantly lower.

The overall sensitivity of any test or marker varies with the amount of tumor burden. Determinations of AFP and hCG, in concert with other staging modalities, have helped reduce the understaging error in GCTs to a level of 10% to 15%. **Expressed another way, 10% to 15% of patients with NSGCTs can be expected to have normal marker levels even at advanced stages of disease.** Although large numbers of patients with clinical stage I nonseminoma have not had markers evaluated before orchiectomy, data from the University of Minnesota suggest that roughly two thirds have elevated levels of AFP or hCG or both (Lange and Raghavan, 1983). Up to 90% of such patients are expected to produce marker substances in the presence of advanced disease.

Tumor marker levels should be evaluated before orchiectomy especially when one is considering a surveillance protocol. Persistent serum tumor marker elevations after radical inguinal orchiectomy must be interpreted with caution to avoid unnecessary adjuvant treatment. Elevation of serum levels of AFP in patients with GCTs can be produced by liver dysfunction, and serum elevations of hCG can occur in hypogonadotropic patients. However, in general, persistently elevated tumor markers after orchiectomy reflect systemic metastases rather than tumor confined to retroperitoneal nodes, and for this reason chemotherapy is recommended for this subset of patients.

Monitoring Therapeutic Response

The rate of tumor marker decline relative to expected marker half-life after treatment has been proposed as a prognostic index. Patients whose values decline according to negative half-lives after treatment appear more likely to be disease free than those whose marker decline is slower or whose markers never return to normal levels (Lange and Raghavan, 1983). Serial determinations of AFP and hCG closely reflect the effectiveness of therapy in patients with testicular tumors. The rate of marker decline after treatment (surgery, irradiation, chemotherapy) is proportional to the decrease in tumor burden and viability. After apparently successful treatment, serologic relapse may precede clinical detection by an appreciable but unquantified interval. Alternative therapy may be initiated when minimal tumor burden is thereby perceived.

After treatment of metastatic disease with irradiation, systemic drugs, or surgery, persistent marker elevation indicates an incomplete response. Because of a therapeutic lag after irradiation or chemotherapy, definition of the "expected" rate of decline and subsequent normalization of markers remains somewhat uncertain; no clear endpoint of tumor destruction can be identified. Such an endpoint has been precisely defined for surgery, in that serum markers should fall immediately, according to half-life, if such a procedure eradicates the tumor. Nevertheless, marker determinations do act as guidelines after primary chemotherapy or irradiation. Clinical experience has shown that if a patient with advanced disease fails to achieve normalization of tumor markers after aggressive combination chemotherapy, attempts at surgical excision invariably fail.

Normalization of marker levels after treatment cannot be equated with the absence of residual disease. Between 10% and 20% of patients receiving combined systemic chemotherapy for bulky metastatic disease and subsequently subjected to RPLND have viable tumor confirmed histologically despite normal preoperative tumor marker levels. Similarly, failure to achieve normal levels of AFP and β-hCG after definitive irradiation indicates persistent tumor. However, there are nonmalignant causes of persistently elevated levels of both AFP and hCG. Liver damage secondary to drugs (chemotherapy, anesthetics, or antiepileptics), viral hepatitis, and alcohol abuse may all lead to an elevated AFP level. Furthermore, nonmalignant causes of persistent hCG elevations include hypogonadism and marijuana use. Clearly, every effort should be made to exclude all false-positive causes of tumor marker elevation before subjecting patients to adjuvant therapy.

Predicting Histologic Subtype

Relative to seminoma, the detection of elevated AFP strongly suggests the presence of a nonseminomatous element. Step sections of the primary tumor may further define the source of the marker abnormality. Metastatic disease accompanied by elevated serum AFP from a pure seminoma indicates a nonseminomatous element, and treatment plans should be restructured accordingly. Parenthetically, 30% to 45% of patients dying with seminoma are found to have elements of nonseminomatous histology at autopsy. It is generally accepted that between 5% and 10% of patients with pure seminoma have mild elevation of hCG because of the presence of syncytiotrophoblastic giant cell forms. If step sections of the primary tumor fail to disclose nonseminomatous elements, conventional therapy is justified. If the hCG value normalizes after orchiectomy, patients should be treated as having pure seminoma. Current clinical evidence has indicated that hCG levels as high as 500 ng/mL may be found in association with pure seminoma, although such an occurrence is rare.

Prognostic Value of Tumor Markers

The degree of AFP or hCG elevation does appear to be directly proportional to the amount of tumor burden (stage and number of metastatic sites). The importance attached to the elevation of one tumor marker or another is not readily appreciated unless all potential variables are subjected to multivariate analysis. In studying interrelationships among tumor histology, tumor markers, tumor burden, and number of metastatic sites, **Bosl and colleagues** (1983) **identified elevation of hCG, LDH, or both and number of metastatic sites as the most important prognostic factors for determining survival in patients with GCTs.** Elevation of tumor markers and multiple sites of metastasis, as well as bulk of disease, are generally recognized as the major determinants of prognosis. For this reason, tumor markers have been included in the AJCC classification of testis tumors. In addition, tumor marker levels are used in combination with the presence of metastatic disease to categorize disease as good risk or poor risk.

Germ Cell Tumors: Principles of Treatment

Principal treatment strategies for patients with GCTs have evolved from conceptions of tumor natural history, clinical staging (assessment of the extent of disease), and effectiveness of treatment (alteration of natural history). Analysis of tumor histology and of frequency and pattern of spread indicates some predictable features of germ cell neoplasms. Pathologic stage is a function of disease progression, and clinical staging is an application of the methods available for assessment of pathologic stage. Selection of treatment alternatives depends on the relative advantages and disadvantages of different regimens. **Multimodal therapy has been largely credited with treatment success, but the accuracy of clinical staging, the ability to recognize failure early, and the high probability of successful treatment of such failures have prompted investigations aimed at reducing the therapeutic burden.**

Each of the major treatment alternatives—surgery, irradiation, and chemotherapy—has a particular but imperfectly defined role in the management of testicular tumors. **As a means of establishing local control, inguinal or "radical" orchiectomy is clearly preferred. Such a procedure provides histologic diagnosis and local staging information (P category); controls the neoplasm locally with virtually 100% effectiveness, the rare exception usually being attributable**

to iatrogenic influence; results in cure of patients with tumor confined to the testis; and is accomplished with minimal morbidity and virtually no mortality. Surgical excision of a retained spermatic cord remnant or of the "contaminated" scrotum is recommended after scrotal violation or tumor spillage, although additional irradiation of groin and ipsilateral hemiscrotum suffices when pure seminoma is diagnosed. Because more than half of patients with testicular tumors present with metastatic disease, further treatment after orchiectomy is usual.

Clinical staging in addition to treatment of the retroperitoneal lymph nodes is a logical next step if no evidence of disease is detected in supradiaphragmatic or extralymphatic sites. It is now generally acknowledged that most patients with large retroperitoneal metastatic deposits are best managed by chemotherapy initially.

Histologic diagnosis is a major factor in the natural history of testicular neoplasms. Between 65% and 85% of all seminomas are clinically confined to the testis, whereas 60% to 70% of nonseminomas present as recognizable metastatic disease. Both the relatively low rate of spread and the radiosensitivity of seminomas have made radiation therapy the most widely accepted form of treatment after inguinal orchiectomy. Radiation therapy, principally used in Europe, and surgical excision, used in North America, have been employed in the management of regional lymph node metastasis from nonseminomas.

Organ-Preserving Surgery for Testicular Neoplasms

Tumor enucleation was first reported by Richie in 1984. He performed a partial orchiectomy in a patient with bilateral seminoma. Heidenreich and associates (2001) described organ-preserving surgery in patients with testicular GCT.

Shukla and colleagues (2004) reported that partial orchiectomy could safely be performed in patients younger than the age of 18 years with a cystic polar mass. Of 16 patients with testicular teratomas, 13 were treated with partial orchiectomy and at a mean 7-year follow-up not a single recurrence was reported. Furthermore, postoperative physical examination and scrotal ultrasound were obtained in 9 patients at a median follow-up of 10.2 months, at which time there was no evidence of testicular atrophy or persistent discomfort.

The German Testicular Cancer Study Group performed organ-sparing surgery in 73 patients treated at eight centers between January, 1994, and December, 2000. Seventeen tumors (23.3%) were synchronous, 52 (71.2%) were metachronous, and 4 (5.5%) occurred in a solitary testis. All patients presenting with synchronous and metachronous bilateral testicular GCTs or tumors in a solitary testis were considered to be appropriate candidates for testis-sparing surgery if the testicular tumor did not involve more than 75% of the testicular volume (Heidenreich et al, 2001).

The standard surgical technique involves inguinal exploration of the testis, gentle occlusion of the spermatic cord vessels, and tumor identification by palpation or intraoperative ultrasonography. Incision of the tunica albuginea is performed above the tumor, which is enucleated with a small margin of the adjacent parenchyma. The tumor and additional biopsies from the tumor bed are sent for frozen section analysis to exclude tumor infiltration. In this study,

the majority of tumor enucleation procedures were performed under cold ischemia with the testis being placed in crushed ice while the frozen section was analyzed (Heidenreich et al, 2001).

Of the 73 patients who underwent tumor excision, 72 (98.6%) survived without evidence of disease. Local recurrence occurred in 4 patients, detected by transscrotal ultrasound; these patients were all managed by completion orchiectomy. Eighty-five percent of the patients had normal endogenous serum testosterone levels and did not need exogenous androgen replacement. Hypogonadism developed in 15% of the patients who needed testosterone substitution. Half of the patients who wanted to father a child did so successfully due to the organ-sparing approach. Interestingly, associated intratubular germ cell neoplasia (ITGCN) was diagnosed in 82% of patients, who were subsequently treated with 18 Gy of local radiation. It is well known that ITGCN is exquisitely sensitive to radiation therapy. Patients, however, should be informed of the potential benefits of seminal cryopreservation preoperatively.

Despite the established relationship between Leydig cell impairment and radiation exposure, investigators report encouraging results with respect to serum testosterone levels in those patients who underwent organ-sparing surgery for testicular cancer; in all of these patients associated ITGCN was treated with adjuvant radiation therapy. Weissbach (1995) found normal postoperative levels of testosterone in 11 of 14 patients treated by sparing of the testis. However, Willemse and associates point out that the long-term endocrinologic benefit of partial orchiectomy to the patient remains debatable and correctly recommend that patients with pre-existing androgen deficiency should probably be excluded from testis-sparing surgery (Willemse et al, 1983).

In our experience, in adult patients, testis-sparing surgery can be considered for small, suspicious nonpalpable lesions detected by scrotal ultrasound commonly performed for infertility or scrotal symptoms. In addition, those patients with a GCT in a solitary testis can also be considered candidates for testis-sparing surgery, as well as those patients with the rare occurrence of bilateral testicular tumors.

We have had experience with all categories of patients. Our approach for GCTs in a solitary testis is to consider testis-sparing surgery for organ-confined tumors less than 2 cm in size, especially polar tumors. Intraoperative scrotal ultrasound can be invaluable for impalpable lesions, and frozen section analysis of tumor margins is imperative. We have not opted for testicular cooling during partial orchiectomy and in addition do not advocate low-dose radiation therapy for ITGCN.

In summary, testis-sparing surgery is an option in patients with organ-confined tumors less than 2 cm in diameter occurring in a solitary testis or associated with a contralateral tumor. Surgical technique mandates careful frozen section analysis of both tumor margins and tumor bed. Cryopreservation of semen preoperatively is recommended, and for those patients with impaired endocrinologic function this technique is not an appropriate option.

Seminoma: Therapeutic Principles

Seminomas make up 30% to 60% of all GCTs of the testis, depending on the hospital population from which the statistics are being reported (Steele et al, 1999). Approximately 75% of seminomas are confined to the testis at the time of clinical presentation (Whitmore, 1968). Between 10% and 15% harbor metastatic disease in regional retroperitoneal lymph nodes, and no more than 5% to 10% have advanced to juxtaregional lymph nodes or visceral metastases, which represents a smaller percentage than that among patients with NSGCTs, in whom the incidence of occult metastatic retroperitoneal disease is significantly higher.

The established treatment of low-stage seminoma is inguinal orchiectomy followed by therapeutic or adjuvant radiation therapy (Fig. 29–1). This treatment is a highly effective method of treating low-stage disease with minimal morbidity; with the advent of multidrug chemotherapy for cure of patients with more disseminated disease, the overall cure rate for all stages exceeds 90%.

The optimal treatment of patients who present with distant metastases or bulky retroperitoneal disease is initially chemotherapy. The role of salvage chemotherapy, surgical removal, or radiation therapy for persistent radiographic masses remains controversial. Controversy exists about the treatment of bulk stage II disease as well.

Autopsy studies in patients who died with seminoma reveal that liver and lung involvement is common, occurring in approximately 75% of patients. Bone and brain metastases are found in 50% and 25% of patients, respectively. Of major importance is the fact that roughly one third of patients with histologically pure seminoma of the testes who ultimately die of the disease are found to harbor nonseminomatous elements in metastatic sites (Bredael et al, 1982).

Because seminoma occurs in a young population, and because surgical extirpation, radiation therapy, and multidrug chemotherapy all have salient benefits, treatment should be aimed not only at consideration of cure but also at attempted maintenance of fertility and avoidance of potentially harmful long-term sequelae.

Stage I Seminoma

In patients with clinically localized disease, treatment options after orchiectomy include adjuvant radiation therapy to retroperitoneal lymph nodes and single-agent therapeutic and chemotherapeutic surveillance. Currently, adjuvant radiation therapy remains the treatment of choice; however, the success of surveillance protocols for low-stage NSGCT has encouraged the use of surveillance protocols in stage I seminoma (T1-T3 N0 M0 S0) patients as well. Although acute morbidity from low-dose adjuvant radiation therapy is minimal, reports of long-term side effects, such as infertility, gastrointestinal complications, and possible induction of second malignancies, have prompted a review of the standard approach, which subjects all stage I seminoma patients to adjuvant radiation therapy. When discussing seminoma that is clinically confined to the testis, it must be borne in mind that staging error may be 15% to 25%; therefore, any adjuvant therapy (or lack of it) should produce a cure in 75% of patients or more.

Primary Radiation Therapy. The natural history and radiosensitivity of seminoma favor megavoltage irradiation in relatively modest amounts as the treatment of choice in the vast majority of patients after inguinal orchiectomy. In the

SECTION VII

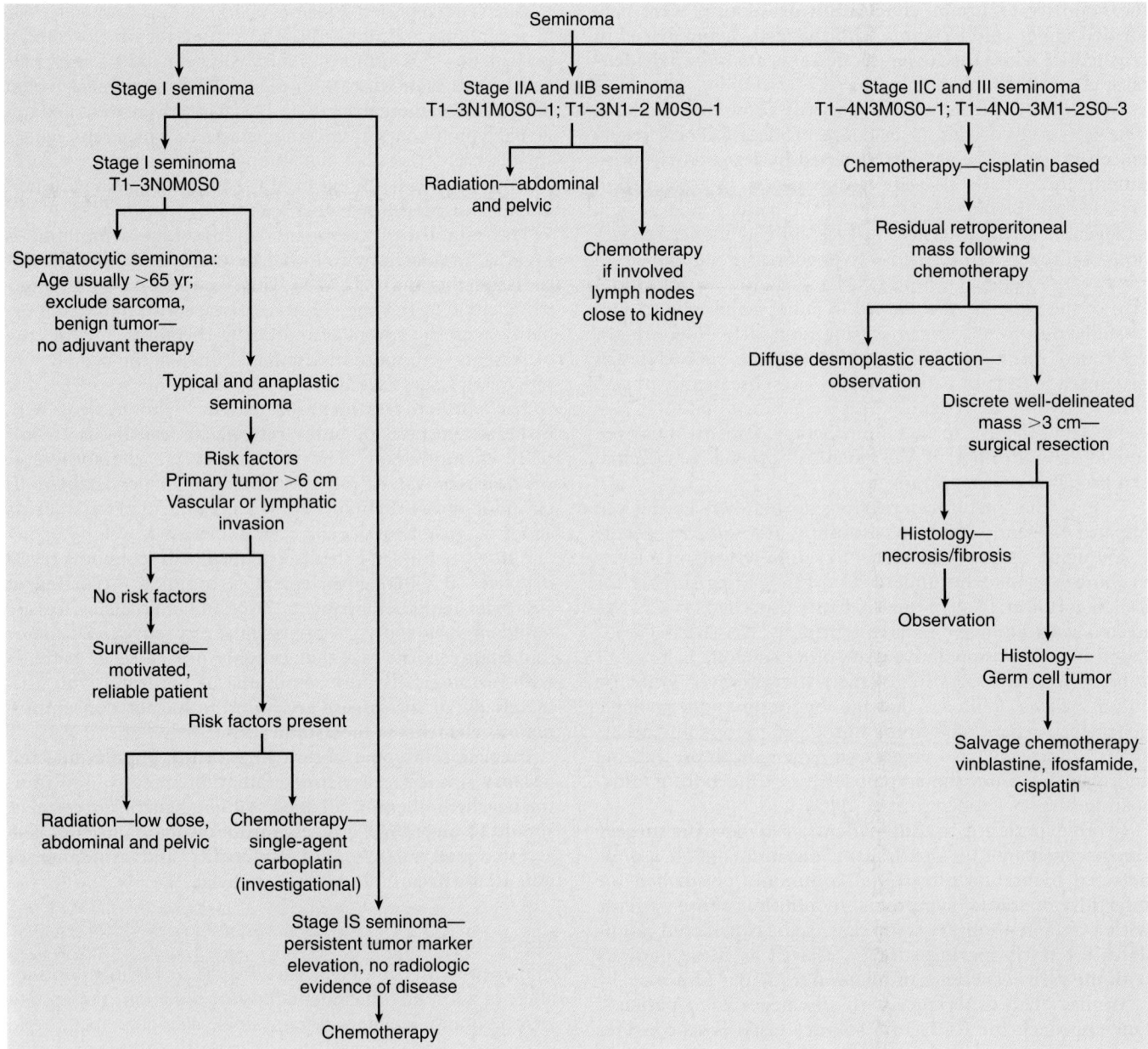

Figure 29-1. Treatment algorithm for patients with low- and high-stage seminoma.

past, 35 Gy was administered to both para-aortic and ipsilateral iliac lymph nodes and, in many institutions, prophylactic mediastinal irradiation was administered as well. However, mediastinal irradiation that could potentially compromise the patient's ability to receive effective therapy has generally been discontinued for low-stage seminoma (Loehrer et al, 1987). Today, most centers administer 25 Gy to para-aortic nodes only, which has been shown to be associated with reduced hematologic, gastrointestinal, and gonadal toxicity (Thomas et al, 1982; Fiveash et al, 1998).

The overall effectiveness of radiation therapy for stage I seminoma (T1-T3) has been confirmed by numerous studies reporting 5-year survival rates in excess of 95% (Table 29–7). The Medical Research Council (MRC) Testicular Tumor

Working Group reported 3-year survival rates approximating 100% (Fossa et al, 1999). Five-year disease-free survival rates roughly equate with cure, in that late relapses with death are exceedingly rare beyond that time frame. Results for disease-free survival in patients with postorchiectomy radiation therapy in clinical stages I and II seminoma are presented in Table 29–7. Routine survival rates above 95% are to be expected in patients with clinical stage I seminoma.

Primary Chemotherapy. The success of chemotherapy for high-stage seminoma has led investigators to examine its use in low-stage disease. Single-agent carboplatin for stage I seminoma has been evaluated by several nonrandomized trials (Krege et al, 1997). The efficacy of this approach has been

Table 29-7. Radiation Therapy in Clinical Stages I and II Seminoma (Disease-Free Survival)

	Stage I		Stage II		
Author	**No. Patients**	**Survival (%)**	**No. Patients**	**Survival (%)**	**Years Follow-Up (A/C)**
Maier and Sulak (1973)	284	97	34	91	5 (A)
Earle et al (1973)	71	100	27	85	5 (A)
Peckham and McElwain (1974)	78	98	27	93	4 (A)
Doornbos et al (1975)	79	94	48	77	3 (C)
Blandy (1976)	98	93	35	71	5 (A)
van der WerfMessing (1976)	91	100	67	85	5 (A)
Batata et al (1979)	227	88	53	62	5 (C)
Dosoretz et al (1981)	135	97	18	92	5 (A)
Thomas et al (1982)	338	94	86	74	5 (A)

A, actuarial survival; C, crude survival.

Table 29-8. Surveillance Studies in Clinical Stage I Seminoma

Author	Year	No.	Nodal Relapse (%)	Relapses (%)	Follow-up, Months	Time to Relapse, Months	RT/Chemotherapy at Relapse	4-5 Year % Relapse-Free Survival	Overall Survival, %
Horwich et al	1992	103	16 (15)	17 (16)	62 (14-41)	15 (6-56)	Carboplatin	82	97
von der Maase et al	1992	261	48 (18)	49 (19)	48 (6-67)	14 (2-37)	PVB/BEP	80	98
Warde et al	1995	172	27 (16)	27 (16)	50 (7-20)	16 (3-108)	Etoposide and cisplatin	82	98
Allhof et al	1991	33	3	3 (3)					
TOTAL		536	90 (17)	93 (17)	53 (6-141)	15 (2-108)			98

BEP, bleomycin, etoposide, cisplatin; PVB, cisplatin, vinblastine, bleomycin; RT, radiation therapy.
Data from Sternberg CN: The management of stage I testis cancer. Urol Clin North Am 1998;25:435-449.

found to compare favorably with adjuvant radiation therapy for low-stage disease. A retrospective comparison of patient quality of life after adjuvant radiation therapy versus adjuvant chemotherapy revealed only minor differences. Dieckmann and colleagues (2000) showed that although a single adjuvant course of carboplatin was associated with low myelotoxicity and gonadal toxicity, the recurrence rate was almost 9%. However, two courses of carboplatin were associated with no relapses and a favorable toxicity profile.

Before this approach can be generally adopted, however, further study is necessary. In this regard, the MRC is presently conducting a phase III trial comparing carboplatin with standard retroperitoneal irradiation in stage I seminoma.

Surveillance. Available data from surveillance and adjuvant radiation therapy series suggest that almost 100% of patients with stage I seminoma are cured whichever approach is selected after orchiectomy. Long-term late clinical effects of irradiation have previously been reported to be minimal. In the United States, the morbidity of radiation therapy is generally considered to be low; for this reason, surveillance has rarely been offered to patients with clinical stage I seminoma. In a study of 104 patients observed for more than 10 years, there were no serious acute toxic effects or late complications. Six patients developed second malignancies at a mean of 10 years after treatment, none of which was considered to be radiation induced (van Rooy and Sagerman, 1994). More recently, however, convincing data from long-term studies indicate that patients with seminoma treated with radiation therapy have an increased risk of developing a second malignancy (Travis et al, 1997). This factor is

now an important reason for recommending surveillance in some patients with stage I seminoma.

Surveillance protocols mandate careful, long-term follow-up, and seminoma patients are disadvantaged by the fact that a reliable serum tumor marker does not exist for this disease. Furthermore, the optimal postorchiectomy surveillance regimen for seminoma is unknown, and therefore its economic impact is also unclear. Despite these difficulties, only four deaths have been reported among 826 patients in surveillance studies with stage I seminoma (Warde et al, 1998).

There are relatively few clinical trials evaluating the role of surveillance for low-stage seminoma. However, published data report that without radiation therapy, 17% of patients experience relapse at a median time of 15 months (2 to 108 months). The overall survival is reported to be 98%, which is similar to that of patients who undergo routine primary radiation therapy (Table 29-8).

The surveillance series with the most data on recurrence after surgery is a nationwide Danish study involving 261 patients (von der Maase et al, 1993). Univariate analysis showed tumor size, histologic subtype, presence of necrosis, and invasion of rete testis to be predictive of recurrence, but only tumor size was a statistically significant predictor on multivariate analysis. The 4-year recurrence rate was 6% for tumors less than 3 cm, 18% for tumors 3 to 6 cm, and 36% for tumors larger than 6 cm. **In this study, tumors larger than 6 cm represented approximately 25% of the study population. Other studies have reported that vascular invasion increases the risk for failure in stage I seminoma patients.**

Therefore, although reliable prognostic factors for seminoma have not been developed, it seems appropriate for patients with tumors smaller than 6 cm in diameter, absence of vascular invasion, and normal β-hCG levels to be given the option of surveillance.

Stage IIA and IIb Seminoma

Seminoma patients with bulky retroperitoneal disease have traditionally received adjuvant irradiation. More recently, however, adjuvant chemotherapy has been preferred to retroperitoneal irradiation for retroperitoneal disease larger than 5 cm in diameter. At Brigham and Women's Hospital and the Dana Farber Cancer Institute, this policy is adhered to, with N1 disease receiving 30 Gy and N2 disease receiving 35 Gy.

Radiation Therapy. The retroperitoneal lymph node groups included in radiation treatment fields for stage II seminoma are the ipsilateral external iliac, the bilateral common iliac, the paracaval, and the para-aortic nodes superiorly, including coverage of the cisterna chyli. CT is useful in planning and simulation of treatment fields. The exact field depends on characteristics of the individual patient and the tumor as well as the equipment used. The para-aortic field is bounded superiorly by the origin of the thoracic duct and includes the anterior surface of the 10th or 11th thoracic vertebra anterior to the internal inguinal ring and inguinal excision laterally to include the ipsilateral renal hilum—more generously on the left side than on the right. The contralateral para-aortic nodes are treated on an individual basis. Irradiation of the kidney is avoided owing to the sensitivity of renal parenchyma to radiation. Therefore, in those patients with retroperitoneal disease in close relation to the kidney, chemotherapy is usually preferred to avoid exposing the kidney to radiation. The pelvic segment stretches from the fourth lumbar vertebra to the inguinal ligament and includes the orchiectomy scar. In patients with retained spermatic cord remnant or contaminated scrotum, the field may be widened considerably. Fields are treated with conventional fractionation of 150 cGy/day, 5 days per week, including both anterior and posterior fields treated on a daily basis.

In patients with a history of herniorrhaphy or prior orchiopexy, with potential alteration in lymphatic drainage, the inferior portion of the field should include the contralateral inguinal region as well. The contralateral testis should be shielded.

Patients with clinical stage II seminoma treated with postorchiectomy radiation therapy enjoy 5-year survival rates of approximately 80%, with a range of 70% to 92% (see Table 29–7). The management of patients with stage II seminoma has created controversy in the past, with respect to the use of radiation therapy alone in the subset of patients with bulky retroperitoneal disease (N3). Furthermore, when analyzing stage II seminoma treatment results, it is important to take note that treatment results are reported depending on the staging system used. For example, some centers have designated stage IIA as less than 10 cm in diameter and stage IIB as greater than 10 cm in diameter. Standardization of staging will avoid confusion in this regard.

In a study from the Royal Marsden Hospital, 10% of patients with stage II (N1) disease experienced relapse; 18% of patients with stage II (N2) disease experienced relapse; and 38% of patients with nodes greater than 5 cm (N3 disease) experienced relapse (Peckham et al, 1981). Therefore, patients with retroperitoneal disease less than 5 cm in diameter (N2) enjoy a reasonably good 5-year survival with radiation therapy alone. **In fact, patients with stage II (N1) disease have enjoyed survival rates above 90%, which statistically do not differ from those of patients with stage I disease. For patients with stage II (N3) disease treated by radiation therapy alone, approximately half of patients develop metastatic disease outside the treated fields.** Warde and coworkers (1998) reported 11% and 56% relapse rates when comparing patients with N1-N2 and N3 disease, respectively, who received adjuvant irradiation in a nonrandomized trial.

In summary, stage II (N1-N2) disease generally responds well to radiation therapy alone, whereas those patients with stage II (N3) disease are appropriate candidates for cisplatin-based chemotherapy, as outlined subsequently.

Stage IIc and Stage III Disease: Advanced Seminoma

Radiation therapy was the treatment of choice for patients with advanced seminoma before the advent of platinum-based combination chemotherapy. Patients experienced relapse with equal frequency in the abdomen or in distant sites regardless of whether prophylactic mediastinal or supraclavicular irradiation was used. In patients who experience relapse salvage might be achieved with radiation therapy, although the response rate is poor.

Cisplatin-based chemotherapy has been found to be highly effective against disseminated testicular seminoma as well as nonseminomatous tumors. More than 90% of patients who present with stage III (T1-T4 N0-N3 M1-M2 S0-S3) disease achieve a complete response to chemotherapy alone, and approximately 90% of the responders remain disease free during follow-up evaluation to 4 years (Table 29–9). Horwich and associates (1996) randomized patients with advanced seminoma to treatment with either carboplatin or etoposide and cisplatin. Two-year progression-free rates were improved with combination therapy. Similarly, Bosl and colleagues (1988) performed a randomized trial comparing etoposide and cisplatin to vinblastine, bleomycin, cisplatin, cyclophosphamide, and dactinomycin and found the former combination preferable.

Response rates seem to be somewhat better when cisplatin-based chemotherapy is given as the primary treatment with no prior radiation, but reasonable results can be obtained for relapse after initial irradiation. Extensive prior irradiation can have an impact on the amount of chemotherapy received as well as the response rate. Thus, response rates seem to be higher in patients treated with chemotherapy than in those treated with primary radiation therapy alone.

Management of Postchemotherapy Residual Mass. One difficulty in patients with advanced seminoma treated with cisplatin combination chemotherapy is the lack of complete resolution of radiographic masses on CT. Controversy exists about the need for further treatment as opposed to observation. **Attempts to remove bulk residual disease after chemotherapy for seminoma are fraught with difficulty.**

Table 29–9. Primary Chemotherapy for Advanced Seminoma

Author	Regimen	Patients	Prior Irradiation No. (%)	Follow-Up CR + PR	NED (%)	Months
Einhorn and Williams (1980)	PVB (A)	19	13 (68)	12 + 7	11 (58)	19
Vugrin et al (1981)*	DDP + Cy	9	6 (67)	5 + 4	7 (78)	19
Morse et al (1983)*	VAB VI	22	8 (38)	9 + 10	17 (77)	17
Wajsman et al (1983)	DDP + VBP/VP16	12	4 (33)	12 + 00	12 (100)	—
Crawford et al (1983)†	VAC	16	1 (7)	15 + 00	15 (94)	48
Mencel et al (1994)	VAB-V6/EP	140	N/A	105 + 25	120 (86)	43
Fossa et al (1995)	VIP	42	N/A	26 + 11	36 (90)	36

*Series contains patients with extragonadal primary tumors and patients who received additional surgery with or without radiation therapy.
†15 of 16 patients received radiation therapy following chemotherapy.
CR + PR, complete response plus partial response; DDP, cisplatin; EP, etoposide and cisplatin; NED, no evidence of disease; PVB, cisplatin, vinblastine, and bleomycin; VAB, vinblastine, actinomycin D, and bleomycin; VAB-6, VAB plus cyclophosphamide and cisplatin; VAC, vincristine, doxorubicin, and cyclophosphamide; VBP, vinblastine, bleomycin, and cisplatin; VIP, vinblastine, ifosfamide, and cisplatin.

Because seminoma involves the retroperitoneum as a fibrotic process similar to retroperitoneal fibrosis, clean retroperitoneal dissection is rarely achieved. In most patients explored after chemotherapy, only residual necrosis or fibrosis is found. A Memorial Sloan-Kettering review of patients with advanced seminoma reported viable tumor in approximately 30% of patients in whom the residual mass after chemotherapy was 3 cm or greater (Herr et al, 1997). Experience at Brigham and Women's Hospital and the Dana Farber Cancer Institute, however, has revealed a much lower incidence of viable tumor in residual retroperitoneal masses after chemotherapy.

Fortunately, the occurrence of a residual mass after chemotherapy for pure seminoma is rare. Clinical experience has shown that there are generally two presentations with respect to residual masses in seminoma patients after chemotherapy (Herr et al, 1997). First, residual disease may have the appearance of a sheet of tissue around the great vessels obliterating radiographic planes. This form of residual disease merges with the great vessels, the psoas muscles, and other retroperitoneal structures; it usually represents fibrosis and is often unresectable. Second, residual disease may be well delineated and distinct from surrounding structures and thus usually resectable. According to the Memorial Sloan-Kettering group, surgery is justifiable in this setting because these masses often represent residual seminoma (Herr et al, 1997). Their current recommendations are that well-delineated, post-chemotherapy, retroperitoneal masses (detected by CT) in seminoma patients should be resected if the diameter is larger than 3 cm. On the other hand, the Indiana group follows up such patients with repeat abdominal CT every 3 months for the first year, then every 4 months for the second year, and then once or twice a year for the next 3 years (Schultz et al, 1989). Moreover, in a study from the Royal Marsden Hospital, Horwich and associates (1997) showed that residual masses persisted after cisplatin-based combination chemotherapy for seminoma in 73% of cases; however, they reported that recurrence was rare and that there was no evidence that it was influenced by either the size of the residual mass or the use of adjuvant therapy.

In summary, both irradiation and chemotherapy are highly effective against pure seminoma. The natural history of seminoma generally favors a minimal therapeutic burden, which justifies either surveillance or radiation therapy after orchiectomy in the majority of patients (see Fig. 29–1). Although surveillance can be justifiably considered in patients after orchiectomy for stage I seminoma, it must be remembered that excellent results with minimal morbidity and toxicity from low-dose retroperitoneal irradiation make this the treatment of choice in many centers, despite reports of radiation-induced malignancies.

In patients with advanced disease, however, initial treatment should be cisplatin-based chemotherapy, with surgery or radiation therapy reserved for treatment failures. Patients with advanced seminoma generally have chemosensitive tumors and potential cure with chemotherapy that is comparable to that seen with patients with NSGCTs. More than 85% of patients have achieved continuous, disease-free status with cisplatin combination chemotherapy. Therefore, multidrug, cisplatin-based chemotherapy should be used initially in patients with advanced seminoma, and no further treatment should be used in patients with radiographic complete responses. With residual mass, close, careful observation is favored, as opposed to consolidation with radiation therapy or surgical excision (Fossa et al, 1987), unless the mass is well defined, larger than 3 cm in diameter, and surgically amenable to resection.

Nonseminomatous Germ Cell Tumor: Therapeutic Principles

In general, patients presenting with NSGCT are subdivided into low- and high- or advanced-stage disease. Patients with low-stage NSGCT may be candidates for surveillance, chemotherapy, or RPLND, depending on a variety of factors, such as the clinical staging, serum tumor markers, and tumor histologic findings. On the other hand, patients with advanced disease are further subcategorized into good- and poor-risk categories and are then subjected to primary chemotherapy depending on the nature of their disease (Fig. 29–2). For those patients predicted to have a more favorable outcome (i.e., good risk), the goals have been to maintain high cure rates while reducing treatment-related toxicity. However, the goal of treating poor-risk patients has been to improve the proportion of patients achieving a complete response while at the same time achieving tolerable treatment side effects.

Stage I and Stage IIa Disease: Low-Stage Nonseminomatous Germ Cell Tumors

Principles of Retroperitoneal Lymph Node Dissection. RPLND was established as a primary therapy for NSGCTs by

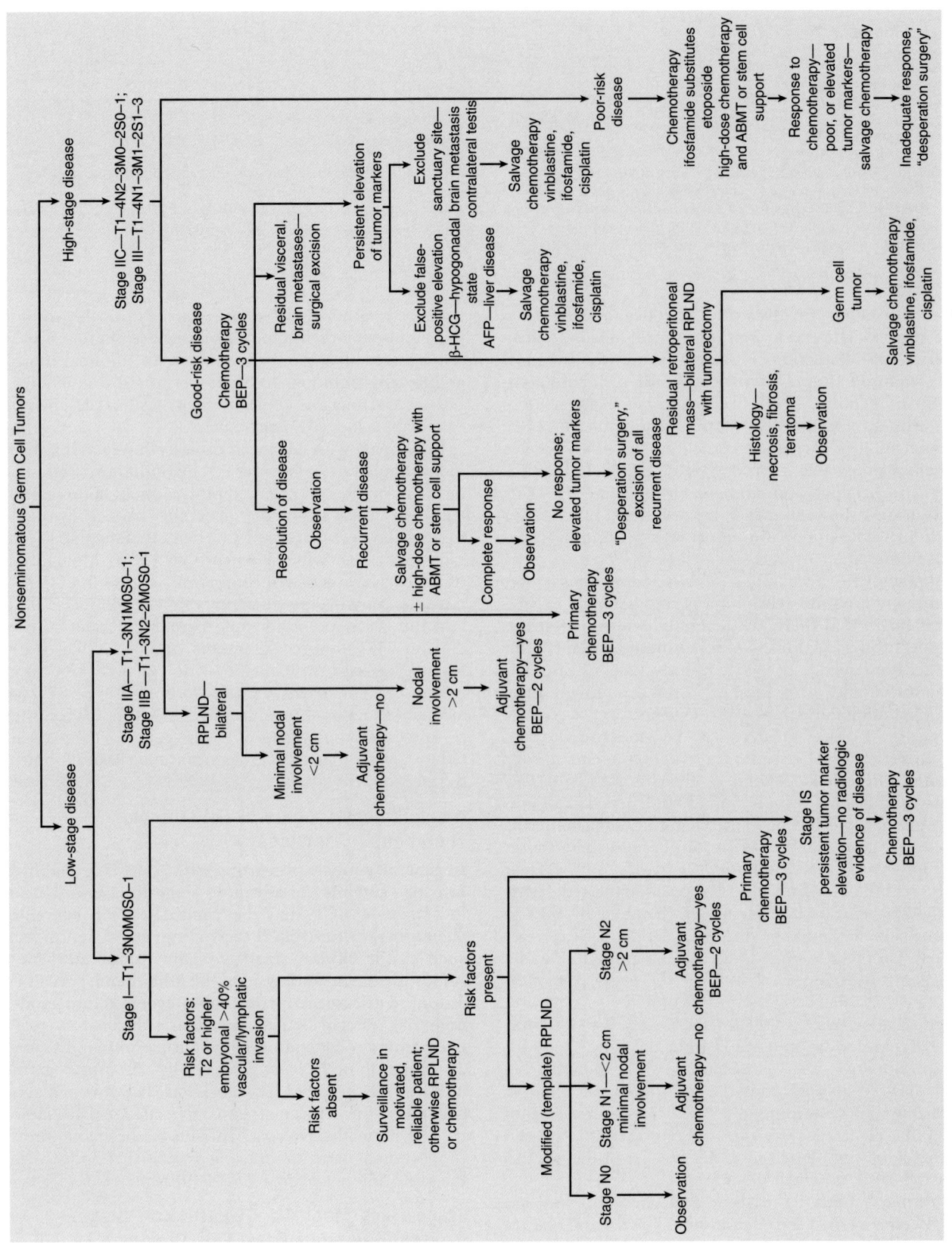

Figure 29–2. Treatment algorithm for patients with low- and high-stage nonseminomatous germ cell tumor.

Lewis in 1948. Kimbrough and Cook (1953) fostered inguinal orchiectomy plus retroperitoneal lymphadenectomy as the preferred locoregional treatment for patients with testis tumors. In Europe, conversely, radiation therapy was used as a primary means of sterilizing nodal deposits. Lewis reported a 46% 5-year survival among 28 patients treated with lymphadenectomy, radiation therapy, or both after orchiectomy.

The potential advantages of RPLND in the treatment of testicular cancer stem from the fact that retroperitoneal deposits are usually the first and frequently the sole evidence of extragonadal spread. Such therapy is capable of eradicating resectable disease in the majority of patients with stage N1-N2 tumors. Thorough excision of the retroperitoneal lymph nodes, therefore, remains the "gold standard" of staging. Although noninvasive staging techniques are somewhat accurate, 20% to 25% of patients with clinical stage T1-T3 N0 M0 disease are understaged by all available modalities of nonsurgical staging. The cure rate for patients with pathologically confirmed stage I disease is roughly 95% with surgery alone. The 5% to 10% of patients who may experience relapse after negative RPLND for low-stage disease have a high cure rate with chemotherapy.

RPLND, via a transabdominal approach, is a generally well-tolerated, 2- to 3-hour procedure with negligible mortality and minimal morbidity. The mortality rate is less than 1%. Morbidity ranges from 5% to 25% and is usually related to atelectasis, pneumonitis, ileus, lymphocele, or pancreatitis.

Modified (template) RPLND has significant advantages. By using this technique, a complete dissection can be performed in the area most likely to be involved with retroperitoneal nodal disease, yet modification in a less likely area can spare some of the ejaculatory consequences (Figs. 29-3 and 29-4). Jewett and Torbey (1988) and Donohue and associates (1990) reported excellent return of ejaculation with nerve-sparing RPLND. These techniques involve removal of node-bearing tissue from around the postganglionic fibers, are somewhat more time consuming, and may require a steeper learning curve as well. Nonetheless, ejaculation can be preserved in 100% of patients and fertility noted in 75% of patients undergoing this procedure (Foster et al, 1994).

Primary Radiation Therapy. Megavoltage irradiation has been available since the 1950s and has been in common use since the 1960s, by which time RPLND had already become established, especially in the United States. Radiation therapy of the retroperitoneum in patients with clinical stage I (T1-T3 N0 M0 S1) NSGCTs remains accepted practice in many treatment centers outside North America.

The efficacy of lymph node irradiation, however, remains in question, although one randomized study that has reached maturity now exists. Between 1980 and 1984, 153 patients with clinical stage T1-T3 N0 M0 nonseminoma were randomized after orchiectomy to either prophylactic irradiation or observation. With a minimal follow-up of 5 years, 23 of 85 (27%) of the patients who were observed experienced relapse; in 14 of the 23 (61%) relapse occurred primarily in the retroperitoneum. Only 11 of 68 (16%) patients treated with irradiation experienced relapse, with none of the relapses occurring in the retroperitoneum. All patients in both groups who experienced relapse had chemotherapy for salvage with

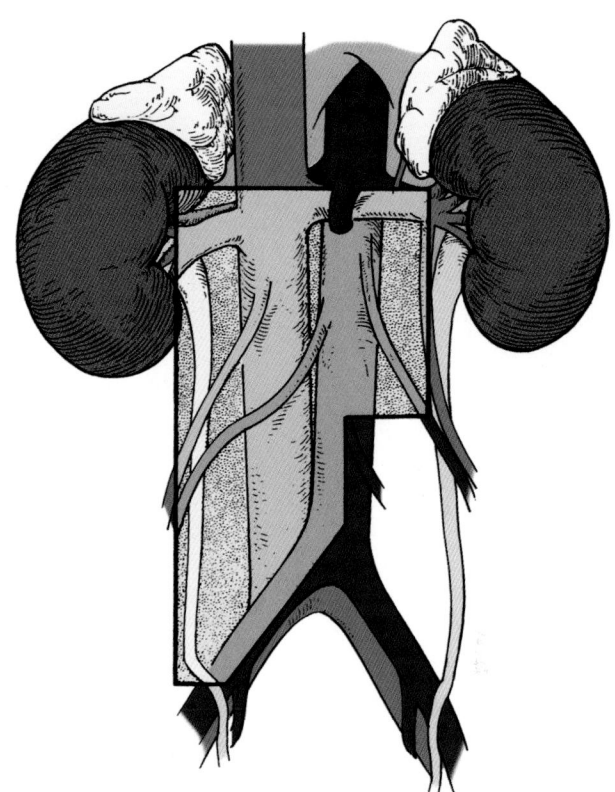

Figure 29–3. Template for modified, right-sided retroperitoneal lymph node dissection.

the exception of 1 patient in the irradiation-treated group. These data suggest that irradiation can be an effective modality for low-stage nonseminoma, and the failure to demonstrate its efficacy previously may be due to a high proportion of understaged patients in historical controls not evaluated by CT.

The main objections to the use of retroperitoneal lymph node irradiation have been the inaccuracy of clinical staging of the retroperitoneal lymph nodes; the resultant lack of survival data that could be reasonably compared with surgical data; and the concern that, in the event of postirradiation relapse, the prior irradiation might preclude adequate chemotherapy or surgical excision.

The tumoricidal dose for NSGCTs ranges between 4000 and 5000 cGy, far in excess of that required to sterilize seminoma. A dose of 4000 to 4500 cGy delivered in 4 to 5 weeks to the para-aortic and ipsilateral pelvic lymph nodes is the recommended radiation standard in clinical stage I nonseminoma. The long-term complications of para-aortic irradiation include radiation enteritis, bowel obstruction, and bone marrow suppression, with a reported frequency between 5% and 10%. **Travis and associates (1997) described the risk of second malignant neoplasms among long-term survivors of testicular cancer. More than 28,000 patients with testicular cancer were evaluated; overall, 1406 second cancers, excluding contralateral testis, were described. The actuarial risk of developing a second malignancy increased over time and was 18% at 25 years. Secondary malignancy was linked with radiation therapy and chemotherapy, whereas an excess of**

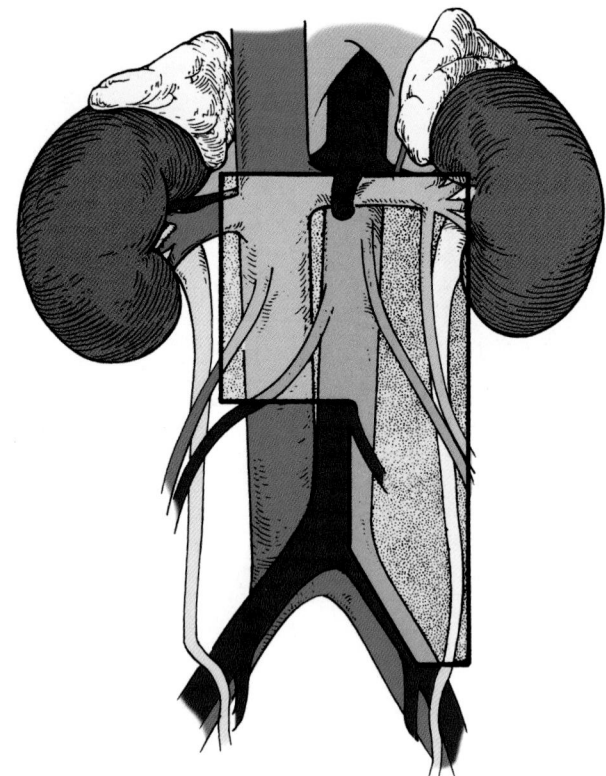

Figure 29–4. Template for modified, left-sided retroperitoneal lymph node dissection.

Table 29–10. **Survival after Orchiectomy and Radiotherapy for Clinical Stages I and II Nonseminomatous Germ Cell Tumors (2-5 Years)**

Author	Stage I (%)	Stage II (%)	Total (%)
Battermann et al (1973)	24/30 (80)	6/19 (32)	30/49 (61)
Tyrell and Peckham (1976)	73/88 (84)	14/29 (48)	87/117 (74)
van der WerfMessing (1976)*	26/29 (90)	16/35 (46)	42/64 (66)
Maier and Mittemeyer (1977)	25/29 (86)	9/11 (82)	34/40 (85)
Peckham et al (1981)†	37/39 (95)	17/21 (81)	54/60 (90)
Blandy et al (1983)	125/162 (77)	—	125/162 (77)
Total	310/377 (82)	62/115 (54)	372/492 (76)

*Extrapolated from actuarial tables.
†Includes patients treated successfully for relapse and patients in stage II treated primarily with preirradiation chemotherapy.

stomach, bladder, and possibly pancreas tumors was associated with prior radiation therapy.

The overall success rate of radiation therapy in the treatment of clinical stage T1-T3 N0 M0 NSGCT in terms of 5-year survival is between 80% and 95% when chemotherapy is used to treat relapses. Relapse rates after radiation therapy for clinical stage I NSGCT are as high as 24% (14 of 59), 3% within the irradiated volume and 21% outside (Raghavan et al, 1982) (Table 29–10).

Surveillance. If staging modalities were sufficiently accurate to identify patients whose disease is truly confined to the testis, orchiectomy alone would yield survival results equal to therapeutic strategies that incorporate treatment of the regional lymph nodes. With the inaccuracies of staging, however, RPLND remains the only modality that can accurately delineate pathologic stage I from pathologic stage II testicular cancer. Clinical understaging is approximately 25% even in the best of series. Nonetheless, approximately 70% of patients who undergo RPLND are found to have pathologic stage T1-T3 N0 M0 disease and, therefore, receive no therapeutic benefit from the operation. Additionally, 5% to 10% of patients relapse outside the field of the RPLND. Thus, careful follow-up is necessary for the first 2 years, generally with chest radiographs and evaluation of tumor markers every 2 months for the first year and every 4 months for the second year. Because relapse beyond 2 years is rare, these patients can be observed annually for the next several years. Patients who experience relapse generally do so in the lungs, suggesting hematogenous spread that preceded lymphatic dissemination.

Recurrences in the retroperitoneum have been recognized rarely in patients who previously had a negative RPLND.

With the advent of effective chemotherapy, concerns about the need for RPLND in all patients with clinical stage T1-T3 N0 M0 testicular cancer, and concerns about the complications of loss of ejaculation and infertility, postorchiectomy observation or surveillance has gained certain appeal. Peckham and colleagues (1982) introduced this concept in 1979. **Several large surveillance programs were subsequently undertaken throughout the world.** In the largest series, detailed in Table 29–11, the relapse rate was approximately 28%, of which just over half (54%) were in the retroperitoneum. Unfortunately the death rate in those patients who experienced relapse was 7%, or 1.8% of the entire series. Even with monitoring, 80% of relapses are noted at more advanced stages compared with patients who undergo RPLND, who tend to have relapse with pulmonary metastases at a lower stage of advanced disease (Rowland et al, 1982). Considering that the majority of these patients have favorable factors to enter a surveillance protocol, death rates should be exceedingly rare in this subset of patients.

A valid concern with respect to surveillance strategies for testicular cancer is patient compliance with the protocol. Hao and associates (1998) defined noncompliance as missing more than one CT scan or two consecutive clinic visits, marker evaluation studies, or radiographs. Among 76 patients with clinical stage T1-T3 N0 M0 disease on surveillance protocols, they reported that compliance was 61% in the first year but only 35% in the second year. Compliance was especially poor with respect to CT scans (Table 29–12).

Several series have evaluated prognostic factors for clinical stage T1-T3 N0 M0 disease that predict positive nodes after orchiectomy and relapse after orchiectomy and RPLND (Freedman et al, 1987; Dunphy et al, 1988; Fung et al, 1988; Moul et al, 1994; Albers et al, 1995). Six factors have been analyzed in many of these studies, including stage of the primary tumor (pT ≥ 2), vascular (including lymphatic) invasion, presence of embryonal carcinoma, absence of yolk sac elements, and elevated preorchiectomy markers. In an MRC series, Freedman and associates (1987) found that four

Table 29–11. Surveillance Trials in Clinical Stage I Nonseminomatous Germ Cell Tumor

Author	Year	No.	Relapses (%)	RPLN Relapses (%)	Months to Relapse	Median Follow-Up in Months (Range)	Overall Survival (%)
Freedman et al	1987	259	70 (27)	27 (10)	12 (3-48)	54	99
Pizzocaro et al	1987	85	23 (27)	14 (17)	10 (4-36)	42 (24-64)	99
Dewar et al	1987	28	9 (32)	3 (11)	7 (1-16)	36 (9-72)	96
Raghavan et al	1988	46	13 (28)	2 (4)	4 (1-36)	40 (6-88)	96
Crawford et al	1988	46	16 (35)	4 (9)	4 (16)	36	100
Thompson et al	1988	36	12 (33)	4 (11)	7 (2-28)	36 (9-72)	97
Freiha and Torti	1989	23	3 (13)	2 (9)	6 (3-8)	44 (24-66)	100
Sogani	1991	105	27 (26)	17 (16)	5 (3-24)	82 (36-132)	97
Rorth et al	1991	77	23 (30)	14 (18)	4 (2-62)	64 (33-103)	100
Sturgeon et al	1992	105	37 (35)	24 (24)	6 (2-21)	60 (12-121)	99
Read et al	1992	373	100 (27)	48 (13)	6 (0-42)	60 (4-60)	98
Colls et al	1992	115	34 (30)	—	6 (6-28)	36 (3-119)	98
Swanson	1993	99	27 (27)	—	—	81	98
Ondrus and Hornak	1994	80	29 (36)	22 (28)	13* (3-58)	83* (61-110)	95
Gels et al†	1995	154	42 (27)	38 (25)	4 (2-24)	84 (24-144)	98
Sogani et al	1998	105	27 (26)	17 (63)	5 (2-24)	136 (49-202)	99
Sharir et al	1999	170	48 (28)	—	7 (2-21)	76 (1-173)	99
Colls et al	1999	248	70 (28)	—	—	5 (31-85)	98
Hendry et al	2000	357	89 (25)	45 (18)	—	103 (12-244)	99
Napier and Rustin	2000	185	26 (14)	13 (7)	4 (1-4)	98 (2-180)	100
Francis et al	2000	183	52 (23)	24 (46)	6 (1-22)	70 (1-260)	99
Alexandre et al	2001	88	24 (27)	14 (16)	—	—	96
Spermon et al	2002	90	23 (26)	18 (20)	12 (3-44)	92 (12-179)	99
Germa-Lluch et al	2002	262	58 (22)	—	—	33	—
Daugaard et al	2003	301	86 (29)	—	5 (1-171)	60 (1-226)	99
Atsu et al	2003	132	32 (24)	18 (14)	5 (2-23)	38 (6-265)	99
Amato et al	2004	23	2 (9)	—	—	38 (9-69)	100
Oliver et al	2004	234	71 (30)	—	—	84 (2-219)	97
Total		4009	1073 (27)	348 (9)			99

*Mean follow-up.
†Not strictly a surveillance protocol because 33 patients had palpitation of retroperitoneal lymph nodes at exploratory laparotomy.
RPLN, retroperitoneal lymph node.
Data from Sternberg CN: The management of stage I testis cancer. Urol Clin North Am 1998;25:435-449.

Table 29–12. Protocol for Surveillance in Stage I Seminoma and Nonseminomatous Germ Cell Tumor

	Baseline	Years 1 and 2		Years 3 and 4		Year 5	
		2 monthly	4 monthly	4 monthly	6 monthly	6 monthly	Yearly
History and physical examination	√	√		√		√	
Serum tumor markers	√	√		√		√	
Metabolic panel							
Liver function tests and complete blood cell count	√	√		√		√	
Chest radiography	√	√					
Computed tomography	√		√		√		√

Data from Vogelzang NJ, Scardino PT, Shipley WU, Coffey DS (eds): Genitourinary Oncology. Philadelphia, Lippincott, Williams & Wilkins, 1999.

features were independently predictive of relapse: invasion of testicular veins, invasion of lymphatics, absence of yolk sac elements, and presence of embryonal cell carcinoma. Of the 259 patients in this series, 55 patients had three or four factors and a relapse rate of 58%, 89 patients had two factors and a relapse rate of 24%, 81 patients had one factor and a relapse rate of 10%, and 8 patients had no factors and thus a relapse rate of 0%.

Based on the work of Folkman and a description of angiogenesis as a predictor of prognosis, Olivarez and coworkers (1994) conducted a blinded review in 65 clinical stage A testicular cancer patients to evaluate usefulness of angiogenesis. They found that angiogenesis measured by quantization of microvessel counts using factor VIII staining was significantly predictive of occult nodal metastatic disease by a univariate analysis. This study needs prospective evaluation for confirmation.

In general, patients with a significant percentage (>40%) of embryonal carcinoma in the primary tumor are believed to be at high risk of relapse. The local T stage or extent of disease is also an important prognostic factor. Patients with invasion of the epididymis or tunica albuginea (stage T2 or greater) have a higher rate of relapse. Finally, and most importantly, the presence of vascular or lymphatic invasion is significantly associated with relapse.

Treatment decisions can, therefore, be individualized based on these risk factors; in other words, patients with low risk of metastatic disease may undergo surveillance, whereas patients with significant risk of occult metastatic disease may be given the option of undergoing either chemotherapy or RPLND.

However, despite the prognostic criteria, it is still not possible to establish highly accurate distinctions between high- and low-risk patients with clinical stage I NSGCT. Moreover, patients with high-risk stage I disease constitute less than 25% of patients with testicular cancer and account for less than half of relapses. Therefore, investigators are actively searching for more accurate ways of predicting the presence of occult metastatic disease. In this regard, the Indiana University group reported that the percentage of embryonal carcinoma and the S-phase fraction in aneuploid cells were predictive of occult metastases. In addition, this group proposed a model that used embryonal cell volume, percentage of cells that stain with MIB-1 monoclonal antibody against Ki-67, and retroperitoneal lymph node diameters on CT (Studer et al, 2000). Specificity and overall accuracy of the model were 61% and 70%, respectively. The advantages of a highly accurate predictive model are self-evident, and it is hoped that this goal will be achieved in the future.

Surveillance is, therefore, appropriate only in patients with clinical stage T1-T3 N0 M0 disease, without any risk factors for relapse, who are motivated to rigidly adhere to a surveillance protocol and who fully understand the risks of failure to comply with the follow-up schedule. These patients require meticulous evaluation before entering a well-designed and well-managed surveillance protocol. Tumor staging should be carried out compulsively in this selected group of patients with no evidence of suspicious nodes or pulmonary masses.

An additional concern about surveillance is the extraordinary period of time necessary to observe patients. At least two reports have documented relapses at 6 and 9 years for patients with NSGCT on surveillance protocols (Hurley and Libertino, 1995; McCrystal et al, 1995). In addition to potential problems with inadequate follow-up, imaging study difficulties, and higher mortality with relapse, one must consider costs and labor for longer surveillance periods. **Lashley and Lowe (1998) compared economic implications of surveillance therapy, modified RPLND, and chemotherapy for stage T1-T3 N0 M0 disease. Costs involved were found to be not substantially different, and there was, therefore, no** significant economic advantage to any of the three treatment options.

Surveillance therapy should be considered an active form of treatment, with careful follow-up being mandatory. **Physical examination, chest radiographs, and tumor marker studies are performed monthly for the first year, every 2 months for the second year, and every 3 to 6 months thereafter. Because of the difficulty of assessment of the retroperitoneum, CT should be performed every 2 to 3 months for the first 2 years and at least every 6 months thereafter. Finally, surveillance is necessary for a minimum of 5 years, possibly 10 years, after orchiectomy.**

Primary Chemotherapy. The rationale for primary chemotherapy in patients with stage T1-T3 N0 M0 disease is that although chemotherapy is less invasive than RPLND, it is just as effective and simultaneously eliminates the uncertainties of a surveillance protocol. A number of published reports have indicated that survival in patients who receive two cycles of bleomycin, etoposide, and cisplatin for stage T1-T3 N0 M0 NSGCT is between 95% and 100% (Table 29-13). Primary chemotherapy has the added advantage of treating metastatic disease outside the retroperitoneum, which RPLND clearly fails to do and which accounts for the 5% to 10% relapse rate after RPLND. The studies that evaluated the role of primary chemotherapy in stage I NSGCT, however, were not randomized against RPLND, and selection criteria were not standardized in terms of prognostic risk factors (T stage, vascular invasion, and embryonal carcinoma volume). Nevertheless, survival appears to be comparable to that of RPLND, and some patients may choose adjuvant chemotherapy over RPLND, especially in those centers where the necessary expertise required to perform RPLND is unavailable. However, the long-term effects in young adults who receive chemotherapy are unclear and remain a real concern. Proponents of adjuvant chemotherapy for T1-T3 N0 M0 disease point out that although two cycles of adjuvant bleomycin, etoposide, and cisplatin represent overtreatment for some patients, low relapse rates and less intensive follow-up are clear benefits. Furthermore, adjuvant chemotherapy prevents relapses that would require a higher total dose of chemotherapy (Studer et al, 2000).

Table 29-13.	Primary Chemotherapy in Stage I Nonseminomatous Germ Cell Tumor						
Author	**Year**	**No.**	**Patient Characteristics**	**Chemo/ Surveillance**	**Relapses (%)**	**Median Follow-Up, Mo**	**Overall Survival**
Madej and Pawinski	1991	30	Vascular/lymphatic invasion pT ≥ 2 (≥1 of 3)	PVB surveillance	0	31 (12-60)	100
		42	Low risk		1 (2)	31 (12-60)	100
Oliver et al	1992	22	MRC intermediate/high risk	EBCi3 surveillance	1 (5)	43	95
		19	MRC low risk		3 (16)	44	100
Kratzik et al	1996	87	Vascular invasion	PEB surveillance	4 (5)	62	98
		114	No vascular invasion		16 (14)	62	97
Cullen et al	1996	114	MRC (≥3 of 4)	BEP	2 (2)	48 (7-48)	98
Böhlen et al	1997	59	Embryonal carcinoma Vascular invasion pT ≥ 2	BEP/PVB	1 (2)	65	100
Chevreau et al	1997	38	Embryonal carcinoma Vascular invasion	BEP/PVB	0	36 (2-114)	100

EBCi, etoposide, bleomycin, cisplatin (3 days); MRC, Medical Research Council; PEB/BEP, bleomycin, etoposide, cisplatin; PVB, cisplatin, vinblastine, bleomycin.
Data from Sternberg CN: The management of stage I testis cancer. Urol Clin North Am 1998;25:435-449.

Stage IIb Nonseminomatous Germ Cell Tumors: Principles of Treatment

Surgical Management. Clinical experience has shown that surgical exploration alone is more than 90% accurate in assessing the presence or absence of lymph node metastasis. When suspicious lymph nodes are encountered at laparotomy, a complete bilateral lymphadenectomy is recommended, although nerve-sparing techniques can be used in selected cases. Suprarenal nodal metastasis occurs infrequently in the absence of advanced infrarenal disease. Routine suprahilar lymph node dissection in the absence of palpable metastasis in this region has not demonstrably improved local control rates. Several nonrandomized studies of stage II NSGCT treated with bilateral RPLND followed by surveillance have confirmed the efficacy of this approach (Table 29–14). Although Williams and colleagues (1987) could find no significant associations among recurrence, histopathologic features, and volume of disease, other series reported significantly lower relapse rates with low-volume disease (Richie et al, 1982; Hartlapp et al, 1987).

Adjuvant Chemotherapy after RPLND. Surgical excision has been the standard treatment for patients with clinical stage IIa (T1-T3 N0-N1 M0 S0-S1) NSGCT. **At issue is whether adjuvant chemotherapy is necessary in patients with disease in the retroperitoneum that has been resected completely.** In patients with pathologic stage IIa and IIb (T1-T3 N2 M0 S0-S1) NSGCT, controversy exists concerning the role of adjunctive chemotherapy. Two-year disease-free survival rate for such patients is 60% to 80%, indicating that 20% to 40% of these patients experience recurrence, usually in the lungs. These patients can be salvaged with three or four cycles of combination chemotherapy.

A national intergroup study published by Williams and associates (1987) reported a 48% relapse rate for patients with any positive nodes who were observed after retroperitoneal lymphadenectomy. This relapse rate was compared with a 2% relapse rate in patients who received two postoperative cycles of adjuvant chemotherapy, either vinblastine, dactinomycin, bleomycin, cyclophosphamide, and cisplatin or cisplatin, vinblastine, and bleomycin. This study included all patients with positive retroperitoneal lymph nodes dissected, from stage N1 to N3. There was no significant difference in relapse rate among patients with different nodal stages: 40% for N1, 53% for N2, and 60% for N3.

In a review of 39 patients who underwent RPLND at Brigham and Women's Hospital for pathologic stage T1-T3 N1-N2 M0 disease, with fewer than six positive nodes and no node greater than 2 cm, only 3 of 39 patients experienced relapse, with a median follow-up of 3.5 years (Richie and Kantoff, 1991). Thus, for patients with minimal retroperitoneal disease, who had complete resection, careful follow-up is recommended. For patients with more extensive disease, two cycles of adjuvant chemotherapy can be initiated relatively soon after RPLND and almost always prevents relapse. The disadvantage of adjuvant chemotherapy for all patients with positive nodal disease is that 50% of patients (those cured by bilateral RPLND alone) receive unnecessary treatment, with associated short- and long-term complications. The other alternative is careful follow-up, with three or four cycles of chemotherapy to be used at the time of relapse. The disadvantage of this approach is that it requires patients to adhere to stringent surveillance protocols with attendant anxiety and the ever-present possibility of noncompliance.

Primary Chemotherapy. The high relapse and unresectability rates in patients with bulky stage N3 retroperitoneal disease, coupled with the demonstrated effectiveness of multidrug regimens in treating disseminated cancer, prompted the use of chemotherapy as initial therapy for those with advanced nodal or pulmonary metastases during the mid 1970s. Almost simultaneously, advances in clinical staging identified patients who might benefit from such a strategy. **Because chemotherapy was so effective in treating disseminated disease, it appeared prudent to redefine the role of surgery after primary chemotherapy** (Table 29–15).

In many centers in the United States, primary bilateral RPLND remains the standard of treatment for clinical stage IIa and stage IIb disease. However, several series support the use of primary chemotherapy for this subset of patients (Peckham et al, 1981; Vugrin et al, 1981; Logothetis et al, 1982;

Table 29–14. Observation after RPLND for Stage II NSGCT Patients

Author	Extent of Nodal Disease	No. Patients	Relapse (%)
Richie, 1991	Nodes ≤2 cm, <6 nodes, no extranodal extension	39	3 (8)
Hartlapp et al, 1987	Solitary node <2 cm, no extranodal extension	49	1 (2)
Williams et al, 1987	Microscopically positive nodes	30	12 (40)
	Nodes <2 cm, no extranodal extension	17	9 (53)
	Nodes >2 cm, no extranodal extension	43	26 (60)
	Extranodal extension	5	1 (20)
Fraley et al, 1985	Stage IIa (not defined by authors)	12	5 (42)
	Stage IIb, "small retroperitoneal metastases"	14	13 (93)
	Stage IIc, "large but resectable metastases"	3	3 (100)
Pizzocaro et al, 1984	Nodes ≤2 cm, ≤5 nodes, no extranodal extension	2	0 (0)
	Nodes ≤5 cm or >5 nodes or microscopic extranodal extension	7	2 (28)
	Nodes >5 cm or macroscopic extranodal extension or retroperitoneal vein invasion	7	6 (86)
Pizzocaro et al, 1984	Nodes ≤2 cm, ≤5 nodes	6	4 (36)
	Nodes 2-5 cm or >5 nodes, microscopic extranodal extension	5	5 (33)
Vogelzang et al, 1983	Microscopic metastases in <5 nodes	6	2 (33)
	Nodes <2 cm or >5 nodes microscopically involved	5	3 (60)
Total		265	95 (36)

NSGCT, nonseminomatous germ cell tumor; RPLND, retroperitoneal lymph node disection.

Table 29–15. **Standard Chemotherapy for Nonseminomatous Germ Cell Tumors**

Chemotherapy	Dose	Days	Toxicity
BEP (per cycle)			
Bleomycin	30 units	2, 9, 16	Pulmonary fibrosis
Etoposide	100 mg/m²	1–5	Myelosuppression
			Alopecia
			Renal insufficiency (mild)
			Secondary leukemia
Cisplatin	20 mg/m²	1–5	Renal insufficiency
			Nausea, vomiting
			Neuropathy
VIP (per cycle)			
Etoposide	75 mg/m²	1–5	Myelosuppression
			Alopecia
			Renal insufficiency (mild)
			Secondary leukemia
Ifosfamide	1.2 g/m²	1–5	Hemorrhagic cystitis
Cisplatin	20 mg/m²	1–5	Renal insufficiency
			Nausea, vomiting
			Neuropathy
Mesna	240 mg/m² every 4 hr		

Horwich et al, 1997). In a series by Horwich and colleagues (1994) 17% of patients with stage IIa disease and 39% of patients with stage IIb disease required RPLND after chemotherapy for radiologic evidence of residual disease. Therefore, although this approach avoids bilateral RPLND in the majority of patients and therefore avoids ejaculatory failure as well, primary chemotherapy is associated with complications of its own. Azoospermia is seen in a significant subset of patients after chemotherapy, and the risk of second malignancies is well described (Wanderas et al, 1997).

Controversy, therefore, persists regarding the role of retroperitoneal lymphadenectomy versus primary chemotherapy in patients with clinical stage T1-T3 N1-N2 M0 testicular cancer. Although it is apparent that both RPLND and chemotherapy are similarly effective for clinical low-volume stage T1-T3 N1-N2 M0 NSGCT, at Brigham and Women's Hospital and the Dana Farber Cancer Center, chemotherapy is favored as primary treatment for patients with nodes larger than 3 cm in diameter. In a review by Donohue and associates (1995), 174 patients considered to have clinical stage T1-T3 N1-N2 M0 disease underwent RPLND. Twenty-three percent actually had pathologic stage T1-T3 N0 M0 disease. Sixty-five percent of the pathologic stage T1-T3 N1-N2 M0 cancer patients were cured by RPLND alone, indicating that surgery has diagnostic and therapeutic importance. Patients who had relapses were uniformly salvaged with chemotherapy. From a cost analysis using the Indiana University experience, overall direct costs for 100 patients undergoing primary RPLND were compared with direct costs for 100 patients receiving primary chemotherapy for low-volume stage II disease (Baniel et al, 1995b). The overall 5-year costs of RPLND were significantly less than the costs of primary chemotherapy, although the two options did not differ in terms of survival or quality of life.

Radiation Therapy. An alternative approach to patients with clinical stage T1-T3 N1-N2 M0 NSGCT is lymph node irradiation, which was fairly routine outside the United States before the development of effective chemotherapy and routine abdominal CT. However, this approach has largely fallen into disuse with the development of effective chemotherapy.

Similar to RPLND, prophylactic irradiation likely eradicates disease in the retroperitoneum; however, in many patients with clinical stage T1-T3 N3 M0 tumors, disease coexists outside the retroperitoneum. In contrast to RPLND, irradiation gives no information regarding the need for adjuvant chemotherapy and for those patients who experience relapse there is potentially a greater likelihood of morbid consequences from chemotherapy.

The evolution of effective multidrug regimens has changed the attitudes of both radiation and surgical oncologists. Many radiotherapists now recommend the use of chemotherapy as initial treatment for clinical stage T1-T3 N2-N3 M1-M2 disease. Supplementary irradiation may then be delivered to initially large nodal deposits, with surgical excision being reserved for selected patients with residual masses (Peckham et al, 1981).

Finally, it must be pointed out that if relapse does occur after radiation therapy for small-volume disease or after an integrated scheme, the effectiveness of chemotherapy may be undermined by cumulative myelosuppression. Furthermore, surgical treatment of focally persistent disease may be complicated by prior irradiation.

Stage IIc and Stage III Nonseminomatous Germ Cell Tumors: Principles of Treatment

Good-Risk Versus Poor-Risk Disease. While chemotherapeutic trials were being conducted, it became clear that prognosis varied and that patients should therefore be divided into low-risk (good-risk) and high-risk (poor-risk) categories. Several schemes were developed, which made comparison across various trials difficult (Einhorn et al, 1989). In 1997, an international conference was convened to address the multiplicity of prognostic systems. As a result of this meeting, a new prognostic classification was published: the International Germ Cell Consensus Classification (Table 29–16). This validated model facilitates collaboration of clinical trials and provides a means of comparison of clinical results across studies. This collaboration provided agreement on the use of pretreatment serum tumor marker levels (AFP, β-hCG, and LDH) and on the poor-risk prognostic factors of metastases to organs other than the lung. The classification contains three subclassifications of good-, intermediate-, and poor-prognosis disease, but for clinical purposes patients are classified as having either good-risk (good or intermediate prognosis) disease or poor-risk (poor prognosis) disease.

Chemotherapy is tailored according to this classification. For those patients predicted to have a more favorable outcome (i.e., good risk), the goals have been to maintain high cure rates while reducing treatment-related toxicity. Patients with minimal or moderate disease do well with standard chemotherapy, with response rates in the 91% to 95% category (Birch et al, 1986). Patients with advanced disease, however, have only a 53% therapeutic response. Therefore, more aggressive chemotherapy should be used in patients with advanced disease according to this category.

Einhorn and associates (1989) showed that three versus four cycles of bleomycin, etoposide, and cisplatin resulted in

Table 29–16. International Germ Cell Consensus Prognostic Classification System for Testicular Cancer

Good Prognosis

Nonseminoma

Testis or retroperitoneal primary
No nonpulmonary visceral metastases
AFP < 1000 ng/mL, hCG < 5000 IU/L, and LDH < 1.5 times upper limit or normal

Seminoma

Any primary site
No nonpulmonary visceral metastases
Normal AFP; any hCG or LDH

Intermediate Prognosis

Nonseminoma

Testis or retroperitoneal primary
No nonpulmonary visceral metastases
Any of: AFP 1000-10,000 ng/mL; hCG 5000-50,000 IU/L; or LDH 1.5-10 times upper limit of normal

Seminoma

Testis or retroperitoneal primary site
Normal AFP; any hCG or LDH
Nonpulmonary visceral metastases

Poor Prognosis

Nonseminoma only

Any of the following criteria:
   Mediastinal primary
   Nonpulmonary visceral metastases
   AFP > 10,000 ng/mL; hCG > 50,000 IU/L, or LDH > 10 times upper limit of normal

AFP, α-fetoprotein; hCG, human chorionic gonadotropin; LDH, lactate dehydrogenase.

the same complete response rates (97%) and disease-free states (92%). Thus, for good-risk patients with disseminated disease, three cycles of bleomycin, etoposide, and cisplatin have become the standard of care. The Memorial Sloan-Kettering group compared the vinblastine, dactinomycin, bleomycin, cyclophosphamide, and cisplatin regimen with four cycles of etoposide and cisplatin and demonstrated therapeutic equivalence. However, inferior results were obtained when carboplatin was substituted for cisplatin or bleomycin was deleted. An Eastern Cooperative Oncology Group study demonstrated an inferior outcome with only three cycles of etoposide and cisplatin compared with three cycles of bleomycin, etoposide, and cisplatin (Loehrer et al, 1995). **More recently, a study comparing four cycles of etoposide and cisplatin to three cycles of bleomycin, etoposide, and cisplatin has shown equivalent results and toxicity** (Culine et al, 1999).

On the other hand, the goal of treating poor-risk patients has been to improve the proportion of patients achieving a complete response while at the same time achieving tolerable treatment side effects. These patients are often unwell at the time of diagnosis owing to factors such as bulky abdominal disease, vena caval compression, and malnutrition.

Because poor-prognosis disease can progress rapidly, we advocate beginning chemotherapy as soon as possible. Standard management of poor-risk disease has traditionally been four cycles of bleomycin, etoposide, and cisplatin,

resulting in cure rates of less than 60% to 70%. Based on its success in salvage therapy, ifosfamide was substituted for etoposide, and a regimen of vinblastine, ifosfamide, and cisplatin has been compared with one of bleomycin, etoposide, and cisplatin in two studies (de Wit et al, 1998; Nichols et al, 1998). At 2 years, overall survival was not significantly different between the two groups; however, the regimen of vinblastine, ifosfamide, and cisplatin proved to be far more toxic.

Studies are being performed to compare four cycles of bleomycin, etoposide, and cisplatin with two cycles followed by two cycles of high-dose chemotherapy. However, Nichols and associates (1991) previously showed that high-dose cisplatin is markedly toxic when comparing standard-dose bleomycin, etoposide, and cisplatin to bleomycin, etoposide, and cisplatin given with high-dose cisplatin. Furthermore, no survival advantage was shown by this study. Other chemotherapy regimens for poor-risk disease include cyclic alternating chemotherapy, which exposes the tumor to a variety of chemotherapeutic agents in an attempt to anticipate and avoid drug resistance (Bower et al, 1997). Randomized trials, however, have not validated single-center studies using cyclic chemotherapy regimens.

High-dose chemotherapy and autologous bone marrow transplantation can be used in patients with poor-prognosis tumors, resulting in a complete response rate of 35% to 45% and long-term survival in about 25% (Barnett et al, 1993; Lotz et al, 1995). **Although the majority of patients with poor-risk GCTs achieve durable complete remission with standard first-line therapy, 20% to 30% of them either experience relapse or fail to achieve an initial complete response and eventually die. For this reason, the strategy of using high-dose chemotherapy with autologous stem cell support has been investigated as first-line therapy in patients with poor-risk GCTs. This application of high-dose chemotherapy with autologous bone marrow transplantation has yielded some promising results.** The Memorial Sloan-Kettering group published results regarding high-dose chemotherapy and autologous bone marrow transplantation in patients with poor-risk, previously untreated GCTs (Motzer et al, 1997). Patients in this latter study received four cycles of bleomycin, etoposide, and cisplatin and then two additional cycles of etoposide and carboplatin with autologous bone marrow transplantation. Almost 50% of patients were disease free at a median follow-up of 31 months. For poor-risk GCT, the survival of a cohort of 58 patients treated with high-dose chemotherapy was compared with that of patients treated with conventional-dose cisplatin chemotherapy alone. Patients treated with marker-dependent, early-intervention, high-dose chemotherapy were found to experience longer survival.

In addition, peripheral blood stem cell support in combination with high-dose chemotherapy has been used with promising results in patients with poor-risk disease.

In summary, there is no regimen based on conventional chemotherapy that has been shown to significantly improve survival of patients with poor-risk GCT. Results of current trials involving two cycles of bleomycin, etoposide, and cisplatin followed by two cycles of high-dose chemotherapy with stem cell or autologous bone marrow transplantation rescue are eagerly awaited (Schmoll et al, 1996).

Management of Postchemotherapy Residual Masses in Advanced Germ Cell Tumors. Despite the well-described hazards of residual viable GCT in the retroperitoneum after chemotherapy, the indications for RPLND in patients with residual disease after chemotherapy are controversial, and there are no clear guidelines. The presence of elevated levels of tumor markers, however, remains the only generally accepted contraindication to adjunctive surgery in patients after chemotherapy.

The management of patients whose tumor markers have normalized after chemotherapy ranges from observation, irrespective of the results of imaging studies, to surgery for all patients. A residual mass is usually detected by CT after chemotherapy; however, the definition of a normal CT differs from one institution to another. Definitions include no visible mass, lymph nodes no larger than 1 cm, and lymph nodes less than 1.5 to 2 cm in diameter (Fossa et al, 1989).

In view of the well-described complications of RPLND in patients with residual disease, patient selection plays an important role in excluding those patients who are unlikely to have viable disease. In earlier series, roughly one third of patients with advanced NSGCT who had normal serum tumor markers after preoperative cytoreductive chemotherapy had a malignant component within the excised residual tissues (Einhorn et al, 1981; Vugrin et al, 1981). In 1995, approximately 10% of patients had residual malignancy. Although pathologic techniques vary, it is unlikely that step sectioning is routine in the assessment of all resected material, which implies that a malignant element may be missed by sampling error.

Debono and colleagues (1997) found that in cases where no teratomatous elements were detected in the primary tumor and a greater than 90% decrease was seen in the volume of retroperitoneal disease by sequential CT scans after chemotherapy, viable GCT or teratoma was not seen in the resected specimen. Other reports, however, have indicated that predicting presence or absence of residual viable GCT or teratoma with any degree of accuracy is not possible with currently available technology (Toner et al, 1990). Moreover, RPLND after chemotherapy in patients with advanced GCT provides essential information for future patient management: it evaluates the response to chemotherapy, removes viable GCT, and therefore improves chances for cure and directs the need for further therapy.

Early retrospective studies revealed that RPLND defines three subsets of patients based on histopathologic analysis of the resected specimen: 40%, necrosis/fibrosis; 40%, adult teratoma; and 20%, residual NSGCT (Einhorn et al, 1981). Therefore, approximately 60% of patients with evidence of a residual mass on postchemotherapy imaging studies either have viable cancer or teratoma. More recently, however, the Memorial Sloan-Kettering group reported that the likelihood of malignancy in postchemotherapy resected tumor was 13%, with the remainder of tumor specimens containing teratoma or necrosis. In addition, the Indiana group reported that of 417 patients who underwent postchemotherapy RPLND for residual disease, only 10% were found to have viable GCT in their pathology specimens (Fox et al, 1993).

The finding of only necrotic/fibrotic tissue implies that no further treatment is required, whereas patients with viable GCT require additional chemotherapy. Herr and colleagues

(1997) showed that if frozen-section analysis shows only necrosis at the time of RPLND, then surgical resection of residual masses followed by only limited RPLND is safe, as opposed to residual mass resection and complete RPLND, which is considered the standard of care. In addition, histologic findings of necrosis/fibrosis were shown to be strongly predictive of necrosis/fibrosis in patients with concomitant pulmonary disease. This information can be used to avoid thoracic exploration in some patients. However, other studies confirmed that all sites of residual disease require resection despite the results of RPLND (Sheinfeld and Bajorin, 1993). In this case, resections of thoracic, neck, and retroperitoneal disease can be contemplated as either simultaneous or staged procedures, depending on the patient's performance status (Tiffany et al, 1986). At our institution, we frequently combine RPLND with resection of pulmonary or mediastinal disease, at which time special attention is paid to avoiding excessive intravascular fluid infusion because of the dangers of hypoxemia owing to bleomycin toxicity. Surgeons should be aware of potential bleomycin-related complications, especially pulmonary fibrosis. Barneveld and colleagues (1987) reported on 8 of 93 patients with evidence of bleomycin pneumonitis, one of whom died of bleomycin toxicity. Bleomycin toxicity can be minimized by careful monitoring intraoperatively and postoperatively, reduction in the forced inspiratory oxygen (<0.25), and restriction of free water intraoperatively and immediately postoperatively.

The recognition of teratoma within surgically excised residual masses after combination chemotherapy for advanced disease is a relatively recent phenomenon (Merrin et al, 1975; Hong et al, 1977; Logothetis et al, 1982). **The rationale to resect residual teratoma is multifactorial. Indolent teratoma growth, known as growing teratoma syndrome, may compromise vital organ function. Malignant transformation of mature teratoma to sarcoma and adenocarcinoma, which is resistant to chemotherapy, has been well described. Chemotherapy and radiation therapy are relatively ineffective against benign or malignant teratoma, and expansion of benign solid and cystic teratomatous elements may compromise vital organ function.**

RPLND after chemotherapy involves both resection of residual disease and full bilateral node dissection. In the best of hands, this procedure is associated with an 18% complication rate owing to the technically demanding nature of the surgery as well as other factors such as reduced pulmonary reserve resulting from bleomycin therapy (Baniel et al, 1995a; Steyerberg et al, 1997).

Summary: Indications for Resection of Residual Masses

- Complete remission after chemotherapy for NSGCT can be defined as the presence of normal serum levels of tumor markers in association with complete absence of an identifiable residual mass on imaging studies. In this group of patients postchemotherapy RPLND can safely be omitted.
- Postchemotherapy RPLND, on the other hand, should be considered for the following subsets of patients:
  - Residual mass and normal serum tumor markers after primary chemotherapy. Within this subset of patients,

RPLND can be excluded in those patients with greater than 90% chemotherapy-induced reduction in tumor volume, and the absence of teratoma in the primary tumor (Debono et al, 1997).

- Residual mass irrespective of serum tumor markers after salvage chemotherapy.
- Recurrent resectable mass after salvage chemotherapy.
- Resectable chemorefractory NSGCT with or without elevated serum tumor markers.

Salvage Chemotherapy. Cisplatin combination chemotherapy effects cure in approximately 70% of patients with disseminated GCTs. In patients in whom serum markers have normalized after three cycles of chemotherapy, residual masses should be resected surgically.

For patients with residual cancer that has been resected after chemotherapy or, more commonly, for patients who do not respond to the traditional courses of induction therapy, salvage therapy with different agents is available and should be considered (see Fig. 29-2). In patients who show evidence of progression during cisplatin combination chemotherapy, salvage chemotherapy with cisplatin should not be used. In patients whose disease progresses after cisplatin therapy, cisplatin may still be useful and should be considered in salvage regimens.

Ifosfamide is an active agent in patients with testicular cancer, with a 22% single-agent response rate (Wheeler et al, 1986). **Ifosfamide in combination with vinblastine and cisplatin has achieved approximately 30% disease-free status in patients who failed initial chemotherapy regimens** (see Table 29-15). In patients who receive ifosfamide, mesna should be used before starting ifosfamide to prevent the complication of hemorrhagic cystitis. In patients who have initially received vinblastine, etoposide should be used in the vinblastine, ifosfamide, and cisplatin regimen. In patients who receive etoposide, vinblastine should be used.

Third-line chemotherapy for patients who have not responded to first-line and second-line therapy includes autologous bone marrow transplantation or stem-cell support with high-dose chemotherapy regimens. Carboplatin, an agent with activity similar to that of cisplatin, has myelosuppression as its dose-limiting toxicity. Therefore, carboplatin can be used in lieu of cisplatin in patients who are undergoing autologous bone marrow transplantation. Early salvage therapy using autologous bone marrow support, including carboplatin, has resulted in complete response in 9 and partial response in 6 of 18 patients in a relatively small series of first relapse (Broun et al, 1994).

Finally, it should be noted that distribution of histologic findings after salvage chemotherapy is quite different, with viable GCT noted in approximately 50% of specimens, teratoma in 40% of specimens, and necrosis in only 10% of specimens. The Indiana group analyzed patients who underwent RPLND after salvage chemotherapy. This study showed that the importance of complete and adequate surgical excision at initial RPLND after chemotherapy cannot be overemphasized (Donohue et al, 1998).

Toxicity of Chemotherapy. Toxicity related to chemotherapy for GCTs is well recognized. Bohlen and associates (1999) reviewed toxicity related to chemotherapy for NSGCT. With two cycles of chemotherapy for stage I NSGCT, myelosup-

pression, nausea, vomiting, and hair loss were the most common acute toxicities.

Late toxicity, defined as morbidity occurring at least 1 year after chemotherapy has been completed, includes second malignancies and pulmonary, vascular, and renal toxicity. This entity is now recognized as an increasingly important issue.

Second Malignancy. **The most serious long-term side effects of chemotherapy are the development of second malignancies. Travis and colleagues (1997) reviewed the Surveillance, Epidemiology and End Results (SEER) database to evaluate long-term testicular cancer survivors treated with chemotherapy or radiation therapy. The study cohort consisted of 28,843 men identified within 16 population-based tumor registries in North America and Europe; more than 3300 men had survived more than 20 years. This study revealed a greater than expected occurrence of second malignancies. For the entire group, the observed to expected malignancies rate (O/E ratio) was 1.43 (95% confidence interval [CI], 1.36-1.51) with a statistically significant cancer excess for acute lymphoblastic leukemia, acute nonlymphocytic leukemia, melanoma, non-Hodgkin's lymphoma, and cancers of the colon, stomach, kidney, prostate, bladder, thyroid, rectum, pancreas, and connective soft tissue.** Wanderas and associates (1997) described a high incidence of second malignancy in the setting of radiation therapy used in combination with chemotherapy. This study group consisted of 2006 male patients treated for germ cell cancer at the Norwegian Radium Hospital from 1952 to 1990 with a mean follow-up of 12.5 years. A total number of 153 subsequent non–germ cell cancers were diagnosed after a mean interval of 15.9 years. The relative risk was 1.65 (95% CI), and the mean cumulative risk after 15 years, 7.8% (95% CI). Significantly, elevated relative risks were found for gastrointestinal cancer; cancer of the stomach, liver and biliary system, lung, and bladder; melanoma; and sarcoma. Patients given both radiation therapy and chemotherapy experienced the highest risk.

The relationship between etoposide and the development of leukemia has been well described in patients treated for germ cell neoplasms. This effect is thought to be dose dependent. In one review, leukemia occurred in 5 of 82 patients treated with greater than 2000 mg/m^2 as opposed to no cases of leukemia in 130 patients who received less than 20,000 mg/m^2 (Aass et al, 1990).

A Danish report described the use of high-dose etoposide (more than 2000 mg/m^2) treatment for testicular cancer was associated with a cumulative risk of 11.3% of myelodysplasia and of acute leukemia (Pedersen-Bjergaard et al, 1991).

Hartmann and associates (2000a) reported that the overall risk of developing second malignancies in EGCT patients appear to be comparable to that in patients with primary testicular carcinoma. In a study involving 635 consecutive patients with EGCT, 17 patients with hematologic disorders were identified, All cases occurred in patients with nonseminomatous histology and with primary mediastinal localization of the GCT. This association represents a known biologic syndrome. Furthermore, an increased incidence of skin malignancies in patients treated with chemotherapy was reported.

The relative risks of a second malignancy need to be reviewed with patients considering primary chemotherapy for

GCTs and in our experience has persuaded some patients to opt for primary RPLND.

Pulmonary Toxicity. Bleomycin is a well-known cause of pulmonary toxicity, with associated mortality rates of 1%. Histopathologic changes include destruction of types I and II pneumocytes and alveolar wall and capillary damage. These histologic changes can progress to irreversible pulmonary fibrosis with demonstrable long-term changes in pulmonary function in a small proportion of patients (Donat and Levy, 1998).

O'Sullivan and associates (2003) reviewed 835 patients treated at the Royal Marsden NHS Trust (Sutton, UK) with bleomycin-containing regimens for germ-cell tumors between January 1982 and December 1999, to identify those with bleomycin pulmonary toxicity (BPT). Fifty-seven (6.8%) patients had BPT, ranging from chest radiography and CT changes to dyspnea. There were eight deaths (1% of patients treated) directly attributed to BPT. The median time from the start of bleomycin administration to documented lung toxicity was 4.2 months (range: 1.2 to 8.2 months).

On multivariate analysis, the factors independently predicting for increased risk of BPT were glomerular filtration rate less than 80 mL/min, age older than 40 years, advanced disease at presentation, and cumulative dose of bleomycin. This study concluded that in those patients with risk factors for BPT, alternative drug regimens or dose restriction should be considered.

Donat and Levy (1998) reviewed predictive factors for pulmonary morbidity in patients who received combination chemotherapy with bleomycin and who subsequently underwent surgical resection of residual disease. A total of 77 patients with high-volume stage II to IV NSGCT underwent 97 major surgical procedures a mean of 6.4 months after combination chemotherapy, including bleomycin, between 1988 and 1995. The importance of preoperative pulmonary status, anesthesia time, fraction of inspired oxygen, fluid balance, bleomycin dose, number of acute toxicity episodes, oxygen saturation problems, and pulmonary symptoms was examined. These researchers concluded that perioperative oxygen restriction in patients treated with bleomycin is not necessary. Intravenous fluid management, including transfusion, was the most significant factor affecting postoperative pulmonary morbidity.

Vascular Toxicity. Meinardi and coworkers (2000) reported on vascular complications after chemotherapy for germ cell neoplasms. They compared 87 patients who underwent cisplatin-based chemotherapy with age-matched controls and reported an increased incidence of both central and peripheral vascular disease. An O/E ratio for coronary artery disease of 7.1 was calculated (95% CI, 1.9-18.3). At a mean follow-up of 10 years, 25% of the chemotherapy group still experienced Raynaud's phenomenon. Aass and associates (1990) also reported a high incidence of Raynaud's phenomenon, which occurred in 46% of patients who received three to four cycles of cisplatin-based chemotherapy. Endothelial cell damage caused by bleomycin-induced activation of the coagulation cascade is one hypothesis used to explain vascular toxicity (Doll et al, 1986).

Raghavan and colleagues (1992) prospectively studied cholesterol measurements before and after chemotherapy for GCTs and reported absolute increases in fasting cholesterol in 80% of patients.

Nephrotoxicity. Cisplatin-induced nephrotoxicity may range from mild biochemical changes to acute and chronic renal insufficiency. Histologic changes associated with cisplatin administration include focal cortical necrosis and the formation of casts. Despite attempts to prevent nephrotoxicity by administration of copious volumes of intravenous fluids and diuresis, persistent reduction in glomerular filtration rate is observed in 20% to 30% of patients long term (Fjeldborg et al, 1986).

In addition to a reduction in glomerular filtration rate, cisplatin has also been shown to cause hypomagnesemia, which may result in tremors, tetany, and convulsions.

High-dose carboplatin used in salvage regimens for disease relapse has been shown to possess similar nephrotoxicity to standard cisplatin doses (Hartmann et al, 1999). Furthermore, patients receiving primary and salvage chemotherapy are also at risk for receiving other nephrotoxic drugs, such as aminoglycosides, which can contribute to overall nephrotoxicity (Kollmannsberger et al, 1999).

Neurotoxicity and Ototoxicity. Cisplatin is also associated with both neurotoxicity and ototoxicity. Long-term sensory peripheral neuropathy is most common, but motor and autonomic dysfunction is also reported. Long-term ototoxicity is reported in 30% to 40% of patients (Kollmannsberger et al, 1999).

Surgery in Patients with Positive Serum Tumor Markers. The standard treatment for patients with marker-positive disease is chemotherapy. However, the Indiana group confirmed long-term survival in marker-positive patients with chemorefractory disease who underwent salvage surgical resection. Of 48 marker-positive patients who underwent surgery, 79% were rendered grossly disease free, whereas 60% normalized their markers (Murphy et al, 1993).

EXTRAGONADAL GERM CELL TUMORS

Primary tumors of extragonadal origin are rare, with fewer than 1000 cases described in the literature. Distinction between primary EGCT and metastatic disease from an undetected testis primary tumor may be difficult but has obviously important clinical implications. Surgical and autopsy series have confirmed the absence of a "burned out" testicular primary lesion in a number of cases, laying to rest some of the skepticism surrounding past diagnosis of EGCT (Luna and Valenzuela-Tamariz, 1976). More recently, testicular ultrasonography has emerged as a sensitive technique for the detection of tiny neoplasms a few millimeters in size within the clinically normal testis. Although the exact incidence of EGCTs is unknown, clinical data suggest that 3% to 5% of all GCTs are of extragonadal origin.

The most common sites of origin are, in decreasing order of frequency, mediastinum, retroperitoneum, sacrococcygeal region, and pineal gland, although many unusual sites have also been reported. Two schools of thought exist as to the origin of these neoplasms: (1) displacement of primitive germ cells during early embryonic migration from the yolk sac entoderm and (2) persistence of pluripotential cells in sequestered primitive rests during early somatic development. The theory of misplaced germ cells holds that during ontogeny, migration through the retroperitoneum is misdirected cephalad to the mediastinum and pineal gland or caudad to the sacrococcygeal region, rather than to the genital ridges. The alternative hypothesis maintains that primitive pluripotential cells may be dislocated during early embryogenesis (blastema or morula phase). A germ cell at rest in the third brachial cleft, for example, could result in a mediastinal tumor, which, interestingly, often resembles a thymoma histologically.

Males are predominantly affected, although a female predominance has been noted with sacrococcygeal lesions. With the exception of sacrococcygeal tumors in the newborn, these tumors generally lack encapsulation, in contrast to their testicular counterparts, and tend to invade or envelope contiguous structures. **The majority of adults with EGCT present with advanced local disease and distant metastases.** These tumors most commonly spread to regional lymph nodes, lung, liver, and bone. Histologically, all germ cell types are represented, with pure seminoma accounting for roughly half the tumors in the mediastinum and retroperitoneum. In general, sacrococcygeal tumors of newborns and young adults are functionally and histologically benign, whereas tumors discovered during infancy prove malignant in about half of cases.

EGCTs may reach a large size with no or relatively few symptoms. Diagnosis of mediastinal EGCT is most commonly established in patients during their twenties, with or without signs and symptoms of chest pain, cough, or dyspnea. Patients with primary retroperitoneal tumors may present with abdominal or back pain, a palpable mass, vascular obstruction, or other vague constitutional symptoms. Sacrococcygeal tumors are most often diagnosed in the neonate (1 in 40,000 births) and are less frequently diagnosed during infancy or adulthood, with findings of a palpable mass, skin discoloration or hairy nevus, or bowel or urinary obstruction. Tumors of the pineal gland occur in children and young adults, producing symptoms of increased intracranial pressure (headache, visual impairment), oculomotor dysfunction (diplopia, ptosis), hearing loss, hypopituitarism (abnormal menses), and hypothalamic disturbances (diabetes insipidus).

Complete local excision of mediastinal or retroperitoneal tumors is rarely feasible because of frequent local extension and high rates of metastatic disease. In reviewing 30 cases of primary mediastinal tumors, Martini and associates (1974) found that only 4 of the 30 patients presented with no metastasis. Three of these 4 had pure seminoma. In the 10 total patients with pure seminoma, only 4 were long-term survivors after surgery or radiation therapy. Of 20 patients with elements of embryonal carcinoma, only 1 was alive at 20 months after surgery, radiation therapy, and chemotherapy. Sterchi and Cordell (1975) reviewed 108 patients with mediastinal seminoma, finding a 5-year survival rate of 58% after primary radiation therapy or surgery. The Memorial Sloan-Kettering experience with 21 cases of extragonadal seminoma was reviewed with primary cisplatin-based chemotherapy; only 1 patient died of metastatic disease, with the remainder disease free at more than 19 to 46 months of follow-up. Patients with primary retroperitoneal seminoma appear equally responsive to intensive chemotherapy regimens (Stanton et al, 1983). In contrast, patients with nonseminomatous EGCT do poorly despite surgery, radiation therapy, and chemotherapy (Recondo and Libshitz, 1978; Reynolds et al, 1979). Disappointingly, only 2 of 18 patients treated at Memorial Sloan-Kettering with successive vinblastine, dactinomycin, and

bleomycin protocols achieved complete remission. Although Garnick and colleagues (1983) reported similar results, those of Hainsworth and coworkers (1982), using the vinblastine, bleomycin, and cisplatin regimen, were superior. The reason for this apparent discrepancy remains unclear.

Wide local excision is the treatment of choice for sacrococcygeal tumors because most are benign. Limited experience renders uncertain the advisability of adjunctive irradiation or chemotherapy for malignant tumors. Radical excisions for pineal tumors have been disappointing from the standpoints of local control and operative morbidity. Such procedures have been largely abandoned in favor of primary radiation therapy, although a cerebrospinal fluid shunt may be required (Cole, 1971).

OTHER TESTICULAR NEOPLASMS

The designation "other testicular neoplasms" includes a heterogeneous group of tumors of relatively infrequent occurrence. Together, they constitute between 5% and 10% of all testicular tumors (Table 29–17).

Sex Cord–Mesenchyma Tumors

Both semantic and histogenetic uncertainties have contributed to the continuing difficulties in the classification of such lesions. Distinguishing between hyperplasia and benign and malignant tumors has added to the problems of classification. Teilum (1946, 1971) was principally responsible for calling attention to this group of tumors and for emphasizing the comparative pathology of the analogous ovarian and testicular neoplasms. **The cell type, architecture, and degree of differentiation of these tumors may closely duplicate the supporting tissues in the gonads of either sex. The microscopic appearance of the testis may show undifferentiated gonadal stroma, Sertoli's cell tumor in germ cell-free seminiferous tubules, or Leydig's cell tumor. More rarely, tumors that are apparently composed of granulosa cells or theca cells occur.**

Interstitial Cell Lesions (Leydig's Cell Tumors)

Varying degrees of apparent focal or diffuse interstitial cell hyperplasia may be noted with a variety of conditions associated with seminiferous tubule atrophy. To what extent these represent absolute or relative increases in interstitial cells may be difficult to assess. **Interstitial cell tumors, the most common of the sex cord–mesenchyma lesions, make up between 1% and 3% of all testis tumors.** Although most have been recognized in men between the ages of 20 and 60 years, approximately one fourth have been reported in prepubertal patients.

The etiology of Leydig's cell tumors is unknown. In contrast to GCTs, there appears to be no association with cryptorchidism. The experimental production of Leydig's cell tumors in mice after chronic estrogen administration or after intrasplenic testicular autografting is consistent with a hormonal basis.

The lesions are generally small, yellow to brown, and well circumscribed and rarely exhibit hemorrhage or necrosis. Microscopically, the tumors consist of relatively uniform, polyhedral, closely packed cells with round, slightly eccen-

Table 29-17. Non-GCT Type: Presentation, Pathology, Treatment

Type	Presentation	Pathology	Treatment
Sex Cord and Stromal Tumors			
Leydig cell tumor (1%-3% of testis tumors)	In adults, clinical features of both excessive androgen or estrogen production may be present. Gynecomastia may be present before a testicular mass is palpable. All children with Leydig's cell tumors manifest signs and symptoms of excessive androgen production.	Homogeneous well-circumscribed tumor, characterized by hexagonal cells with pathognomonic cigar-shaped crystals in the cytoplasm (Reinke's crystals) found in 40% of tumors. Ten percent are malignant; necrosis, mitoses, pleomorphism, and vascular invasion should raise this suspicion. Most malignant tumors are 6 to 10 cm.	Radical inguinal orchiectomy is the initial treatment of choice. If there are histopathologic features of malignancy then retroperitoneal lymph node dissection is an option. Virilizing and feminizing features may take a while to resolve, and thus initial persistence is not an indication of metastatic disease.
Sertoli's cell tumor (less than 1% of testis tumors)	Most often in patients < age 40 years. Vary in size from 1 to 20 cm. Metastases to both retroperitoneal lymph nodes and viscera occur.	Homogeneous tumor, medium-sized bland and uniform cells, with round and oval nuclei. Essential diagnostic feature: epithelioid cells representing Sertoli's cells and varying amounts of stroma between tubules, cords, or nests of cells. Ten to 20% are malignant and are characterized by vascular invasion, necrosis, and increased size.	Radical inguinal orchiectomy is the initial treatment of choice and cures 80% to 90% of patients. If there are histopathologic features of malignancy, then retroperitoneal lymph node dissection may have therapeutic benefit.
Mixed Germ Cell and Stromal Tumor			
Gonadoblastoma (less than 0.5% of testis tumors)	Associated with dysgenetic gonads: either a streak gonad or testis. 80% of patients are phenotypic females and usually present with primary amenorrhea and sometimes with a lower abdominal mass. High incidence occurs of bilaterality.	Mixed tumor containing large germ cells similar to seminoma and small immature Sertoli's cells. Leydig's cells may also be present.	Treatment is radical inguinal orchiectomy and contralateral orchiectomy when gonadal dysgenesis is present on that side.

tric nuclei and eosinophilic granular cytoplasm with lipoid vacuoles, brownish pigmentation, and occasional characteristic inclusions known as Reinke's crystals. Pleomorphism with large and bizarre cell forms may occur, and mitotic figures may or may not be identified. None of these features appears to be consistently related to malignant potential. Furthermore, limited observations suggest that ultrastructural features do not categorically distinguish between normal and neoplastic Leydig's cells, whether benign or malignant.

Approximately 10% of interstitial cell tumors are malignant, but there are no consistently reliable histologic criteria for making this judgment. Large size, extensive necrosis, gross or microscopic evidence of infiltration, invasion of blood vessels, and excessive mitotic activity are all features that suggest the possibility of malignancy, but metastasis is generally regarded as the only reliable criterion of malignancy. Similar to other testis tumors, malignant lesions may involve retroperitoneal lymph nodes, lung, and bone. Of importance is the observation that malignancy is nonexistent in the prepubertal age group.

Clinical Presentation. In prepubertal cases (average age, 5 years), presenting manifestations are usually those of isosexual precocity with prominent external genitalia, mature masculine voice, and pubic hair growth. Hormonal assays in such patients have been few and generally incomplete or have been carried out by antiquated techniques. Increased testosterone production is usually demonstrable, and urinary 17-keto-

steroid output may or may not be elevated. Virilizing types of congenital adrenocortical hyperplasia may also produce the endocrine signs and symptoms of interstitial cell tumors, so differential tests must be carried out to clarify the diagnosis. Such tests include estimation of urinary 17-hydroxysteroid and 17-ketosteroid levels as well as plasma cortisol before and after adrenocorticotropic hormone stimulation and dexamethasone suppression. Because interstitial cell carcinomas have been shown to possess 21-hydroxylase activity and to be capable of forming cortisol and hydroxylating steroids at the 11β position, it is clear that interstitial cell tumors may possess some of the same functional activities as adrenocortical tissue. The similar embryologic origin of interstitial cells and adrenocortical cells and the occurrence of adrenal rests in the testis complicate interpretation. The paradox of the tumor's arising in the interstitial cells of a prepubertal testis and behaving metabolically similar to its adult counterpart, in conjunction with cells in the normal prepubertal testis containing enzymes capable of producing testosterone, explains the occurrence of spermatogenesis in the seminiferous tubules more remote from the tumor.

In adults, the majority of reported cases have shown manifestations of endocrine imbalance, although some have not. The endocrinologic manifestations may precede the palpable testis mass, which is the most common presenting feature. In the remaining adult cases, symptoms of a feminizing nature, such as impotence and gynecomastia, may occur, along with decreased libido. **The slow progression of these neoplasms is suggested by the long duration of gynecomastia, which may precede recognition of the testicular mass.** In contrast to the situation of adult GCTs, the duration of gynecomastia with adult interstitial cell tumors has ranged from 6 months to 10 years and averages more than 3 years. Elevation of urinary and plasma estrogens in association with this tumor is relatively common. Lockhart and colleagues (1976) reported a nonfunctioning interstitial cell tumor in the testis of a malignant type in which there were neither clinical nor chemical manifestations of endocrinopathy. Hormonal disturbance, therefore, is not an essential feature. In cases in which a testicular swelling was not clinically apparent, Gabrilove and associates (1975) performed selective venous catheterization and measurement of the testicular venous effluent to assess gynecomastia of obscure etiology. Measurement of AFP and β-hCG may be helpful in differential diagnosis. Occasionally, MRI detects a small, nonpalpable Leydig's cell tumor not seen by ultrasonography (Kaufman et al, 1990). Other considerations in the differential diagnosis include feminizing adrenocortical disorders, Klinefelter's syndrome, and other feminizing testicular disorders.

Treatment. Radical inguinal orchiectomy is the initial procedure of choice. With documentation of Leydig's cell tumor, endocrinologic studies and further clinical staging evaluations are indicated. In the event of histopathologic suspicion of malignancy, CT of the retroperitoneum is indicated to seek retroperitoneal adenopathy. As with GCTs of the adult testis, spread to the lung, liver, or supradiaphragmatic lymph nodes is possible. The potential production of hormones by metastatic tumor invites exploration of these substances as markers for metastatic disease, but data are lacking. Urinary estrogens, androgens, corticoids, and pregnanediol have each demonstrated abnormalities based on the metabolic activity of different interstitial cell tumors. RPLND has been recommended as routine in patients whose interstitial cell tumors appear histologically or biochemically malignant. Total experience with any form of therapy, however, is limited by the small number of patients who have been treated, although the existing data suggest the relative radioresistance of this tumor. Ortho-para-DDD has been used with evidence of benefit in some patients (Azer and Braumstein, 1981). Various chemotherapeutic agents, including cisplatin, vinblastine, bleomycin, cyclophosphamide, doxorubicin, and vincristine, have been used in a variety of combination regimens without convincing benefit, but experience is limited. Experimental evidence of estrogen receptors in various mouse Leydig's cell tumor lines provided an experimental basis for trials of endocrine therapy (Sato et al, 1978). In addition, inhibition of mitochondrial protein synthesis with concomitant arrest of in-vivo growth of solid Leydig's cell tumors in rats by oxytetracycline has been reported (van der Bogert et al, 1983).

The prognosis for Leydig's cell tumors is good because of their generally benign nature. The persistence of virilizing and feminizing features after orchiectomy is not necessarily an indication of malignancy because these changes are to some extent irreversible. As might be anticipated from the characterization of malignancy (i.e., metastasis), the average survival time from surgery for patients with a malignant Leydig's cell tumor is approximately 3 years.

Sertoli's Cell Tumors: Androblastoma, Gonadal Stromal Tumor, Sertoli's Cell–Mesenchyma Tumor

Nodules of immature seminiferous tubules with lumens lined by undifferentiated cells are found not infrequently in cryptorchid testes and in roughly one fourth of patients with testicular feminization. Such lesions were formerly considered tubular adenomas, but it seems probable that they are not neoplastic, and malignant change appears not to have been reported.

True Sertoli's cell–mesenchyma tumors constitute less than 1% of all testicular tumors and may occur in any age group, including infancy. Although rare in humans, they are the most common testicular tumor in dogs. The majority of Sertoli's cell tumors are benign, but approximately 10% have proved malignant based on the currently accepted criterion of malignancy—the demonstration of metastasis. As with Leydig's cell tumors, definitive histologic criteria of malignancy remain to be established.

The etiology of these tumors has not been determined. The majority have arisen in apparently normal intrascrotal testes, although occurrence in maldescended or cryptorchid testes has been reported.

Grossly, these tumors vary in size from 1 cm to more than 20 cm. The cut surface is usually gray white to creamy yellow, with a uniform consistency interrupted by cystic change that becomes increasingly evident with increasing tumor size. The benign lesions are usually well circumscribed, whereas the malignant lesions tend to be larger and less well demarcated. Invasion of paratesticular structures may occur and is suggestive of malignancy.

The precise origin of these tumors remains somewhat uncertain, although derivation from the primitive gonadal mesenchyma is suspected. A diversity of microscopic appearances is evident not only between tumors but also between different areas within the same tumor. **Essential diagnostic features include epithelial elements resembling Sertoli's cells and varying amounts of stroma. The amount and organization of these two components have led to various attempts to subclassify the tumors.** The epithelial elements, on the one hand, may be arranged in tubules with or without lumens and lined by radially arranged cells in one or multiple layers; the epithelial cells, on the other hand, may form columns or sheets of trabeculae growing between stromal elements. The stromal elements may be scant, or the tumor may be largely composed of stroma resembling a fibroma but containing strands of epithelial cells. Secretory materials forming Call-Exner–like bodies are occasionally seen within tubules, the morphologic appearance resembling that of granulosa cell tumors. Furthermore, the stromal elements may be sufficiently well differentiated to be recognizable as Leydig's cells. The enormous potential for variation in both stromal and epithelial components and in degrees of differentiation accounts for the wide range of morphologic appearances described for these lesions and contributes to the difficulty in their classification.

Although large size, poor tumor demarcation, invasion of adjacent structures, blood vessel and lymphatic invasion, and increased mitotic activity are all suggestive of malignant potential, as with Leydig's cell tumors, the designation of malignancy can be made with certainty only in the presence of metastasis.

Clinical Presentation. The presenting signs and symptoms are those of testicular mass with or without pain and with or without gynecomastia. Although the lesions have been reported in all age groups, approximately one third of the recorded patients have been 12 years or younger. About one third of the patients have had gynecomastia. Gynecomastia in the presence of a testicular tumor in the prepubertal age group is an important finding in differential diagnosis because feminization in boys with Leydig's cell tumors is always superimposed on virilism.

Studies of the endocrinologic activity of these tumors have been uncommon. Gynecomastia is presumably a consequence of estrogen production, but whether the Sertoli's cells or the stromal elements are responsible for estrogen production remains to some extent uncertain. Gabrilove and colleagues (1975) reported an elevated plasma testosterone value in association with some virilizing features in a young patient with Sertoli's cell tumor.

Treatment. Radical orchiectomy is the initial procedure of choice and is, of course, curative in the 90% of cases that are benign. In the small proportion of patients in whom malignancy has been demonstrated by the presence of metastasis, retroperitoneal lymph node involvement has been common, and RPLND has been performed with apparent therapeutic success (Rosvoll and Woodard, 1968). The course of the disease, even in patients with metastasis, may be protracted compared with that of patients with metastatic GCTs. Lung and bone metastasis may occur and warrants the inclusion of chest films and bone scans in the staging evaluation. The value of radiation therapy and chemotherapy in the management of patients with this disease is uncertain. Although hormone production is a potential marker for follow-up in patients with apparently malignant tumors, clinical evidence on this point is lacking.

Gonadoblastoma

These rare tumors, occurring almost exclusively in patients with some form of gonadal dysgenesis, constitute approximately 0.5% of all testis neoplasms and occur in all age groups from infancy to beyond 70 years, although the majority occur in individuals younger than 30 years.

Grossly, the lesions may be unilateral or bilateral and may vary in size from microscopic to larger than 20 cm in diameter. Aggressive growth may replace and obscure the nature of the gonad from which the tumor arose, and lesions weighing more than 1000 g have been reported. The tumors generally are round, with a smooth, slightly lobulated surface, and vary from soft and fleshy to firm or hard in consistency. Calcified areas are frequent and probably reflect the extensive spontaneous retrogressive changes common with these lesions. The cut surface is grayish white to yellow but may vary considerably, depending on the histologic makeup of the tumor.

Although gonadoblastomas are regarded as neoplasms, the possibility that they represent hamartomas or nodular hyperplasia in response to pituitary gonadotropins has been suggested. **First clearly described by Scully (1953), the tumors consist of three elements: Sertoli's cells, interstitial tissue, and germ cells, the proportions of which show considerable variation.** In about half of such tumors, germ cell overgrowth, with the evolution of what is readily recognized as seminoma, or germ cell elements with histologic features of embryonal carcinoma, teratoma, choriocarcinoma, or yolk sac tumor may occur. Throughout the tubules, characteristic Call-Exner bodies may be identified, consisting of periodic acid-Schiff–positive material similar to that seen in the basement membrane of the tubules.

Clinical Presentation

The clinical manifestations of patients with this tumor are the consequence of three factors: (1) the usual concurrence of gonadal dysgenesis with resultant abnormalities in the external genitalia and gonads, (2) the presence of germ cells with malignant potential, and (3) the endocrine function of the gonadal stromal components of the tumor, usually with the production of androgen. Although interstitial cells may not be evident by light microscopy, a steroidogenic potential of the tumor may exist. Furthermore, demonstration of Leydig's cells in the tumor does not necessarily dictate virilism, either because the resultant steroids may be biologically inactive or because the end organs may be defective. The usual appearance is that of solid tubules of varying size containing germ cells in close association with Sertoli's cells and of mature interstitial cells evident between the tubules.

The germ cells of gonadoblastoma are similar to those of seminoma, and if germ cell proliferation occurs, it may progress from the in-situ stage to invasive germinoma (or seminoma), referred to as gonadoblastoma with germinoma.

Approximately four fifths of patients with gonadoblastoma are phenotypic females, usually presenting with primary amenorrhea and sometimes with a lower abdominal mass. The remainder are phenotypic males, almost always presenting with cryptorchidism, hypospadias, and some female internal genitalia. Gonadoblastoma, however, has been described in an anatomically normal male (Talerman, 1972). In phenotypic females, the breasts are small, the internal genitalia hypoplastic, and the gonads usually of the streak type. Sex chromatin is negative, and the chromosome analysis usually shows XY or XO or XO/XY patterns. Virilization in the phenotypic female usually manifests as hypertrophy of the clitoris. In the phenotypic male, gynecomastia may occasionally be present, and there is usually hypospadias, some female internal genitalia, and dysgenetic testes usually located in the abdomen or inguinal region; sex chromatin is negative, and the chromosome pattern is XY or XO/XY.

In general, 90% of patients with gonadal dysgenesis and gonadoblastoma are chromatin negative, and more than half have an XY karyotype, with the remainder demonstrating mosaicism. The external sex organs of patients with gonadoblastoma show a wide range of appearances ranging from normal to completely ambiguous. The secondary sex organs usually consist of a hypoplastic uterus and two normal or slightly hypoplastic fallopian tubes. Male internal sex organs, such as epididymis, vas deferens, and prostate, are found sometimes in phenotypic virilized females and always in phenotypic male pseudohermaphrodites.

Treatment

Radical orchiectomy is the first step in therapy, and the high incidence of bilaterality (50%) argues for contralateral gonadectomy when gonadal dysgenesis is present. The prognosis is excellent for patients with gonadoblastoma or gonadoblastoma with germinoma. In the presence of seminoma or other germ cell types, clinical staging employing the techniques used for the staging of GCTs of the adult testis may be indicated, although experience is too limited to justify categorical recommendations. As with GCTs of the adult testis, therapy may logically be based on tumor histology and the results of clinical staging.

Neoplasms of Mesenchymal Origin

A variety of neoplasms derived from mesenchymal elements may arise on the tunica albuginea or, more rarely, within the testis. Included are benign fibroma, angioma, neurofibroma, and leiomyoma. Occurring as painless masses, they are of concern chiefly because of the possibility of a malignant tumor. Differential diagnosis includes abnormalities of the testicular appendages, fibrous pseudotumors, adenomatoid tumors, and non-neoplastic cystic lesions. Varying from minute, "shotlike" lesions on the surface of the testis to masses of several centimeters, the reported lesions have been variously treated by local excision or orchiectomy.

Malignant mesothelioma may arise from any site on the mesothelial membrane—pleura, peritoneum, pericardium, or tunica vaginalis. Fewer than 20 cases involving the tunica vaginalis have been reported. The lesion occurs in patients from 21 to 78 years old, and the usual presentation is with a hydrocele. Radical orchiectomy is indicated for local control, but local recurrence and abdominal and pulmonary metastases may ensue. Limited experience suggests that surgery and irradiation may be of some value in controlling intra-abdominal metastasis. The value of chemotherapy remains to be defined, although doxorubicin appears active.

Miscellaneous Primary Non–Germ Cell Tumors

The testis may be the primary site of a number of tumors of unrelated histogenesis and varied pathologic type.

Epidermoid Cyst

Representing an estimated 1% of testis tumors (Shah et al, 1981), approximately half of epidermoid cysts occur in patients in their twenties, and most of the remainder occur in patients between their teens and thirties. Grossly, these lesions present as round, sharply circumscribed, firm, encapsulated intratesticular nodules; the cut surface reveals a grayish white to yellowish, cheesy, amorphous mass. Microscopically, the wall is composed of dense fibrous tissue lined by stratified squamous keratinized epithelium, desquamations from which, with degeneration and microcalcification, make up the amorphous interior.

Although the histogenesis remains uncertain, a common thesis is that the tumor represents a monolayer teratoma. This thesis is circumstantially supported by the age and racial incidences of such tumors and by the occasional association with cryptorchidism. This histogenesis, in turn, supports the use of radical orchiectomy as the usual treatment because the possibility of other germ cell elements in association with such lesions can be excluded only by careful microscopic examination. Nevertheless, the clinical behavior of these tumors has been consistently benign; apparently, no instance of associated, clinically unrecognized but microscopically confirmed GCT has been reported. Rare instances of bilaterality have been reported (as with GCTs) (Forrest and Whitmore, 1984). Testicular ultrasonography may demonstrate a well-circumscribed lesion with a solid central core and may aid in the distinction from a GCT. Although most have been managed by radical orchiectomy, local excision in a small number of patients appears to have been equally successful. The weakness in the latter approach stems from uncertainty in clinical diagnosis and the potential risks of spillage of a GCT.

Adenocarcinoma of the Rete Testis

These rare but highly malignant tumors occur uniformly in adults over a wide age range (20 to 80 years). Jacobellis and coworkers (1981) reported on only the 19th case. The usual presentation is a painless scrotal mass, commonly with an associated hydrocele. Pathologic evaluation reveals a multicystic papillary adenocarcinoma composed of small cuboidal cells with elongated nuclei and scanty cytoplasm, presumably arising from the rete tubules of the testicular mediastinum. Despite radical orchiectomy, half the patients die within 1 year of diagnosis. Metastasis occurs in inguinal and retroperitoneal lymph nodes, lungs, bone, and liver. The observation that retroperitoneal deposits may represent the sole site of metastasis supports the rationale of retroperitoneal lymphadenectomy in the absence of distant metastasis. Irradiation and chemotherapy with methotrexate, fluorouracil, dactinomycin, or cyclophosphamide in the treatment of metastasis have been of limited, if any, benefit.

Adrenal Rest Tumors

The association of bilateral testis tumors with congenital adrenal hyperplasia and the remission of both endocrine manifestations and tumors after appropriate corticoid treatment call attention to these unusual lesions. Whether they represent neoplasms or hyperplasia and whether they derive from "normal" adrenal rests or from abnormal interstitial cells remain uncertain in some cases. Kirkland and associates (1977) suggested that luteinizing hormones may contribute to the growth of these tumors because high serum luteinizing hormone levels may be seen in association with incomplete suppression of adrenal steroid secretion and there is evidence of gonadotropin secretion with testicular tumors in some patients with congenital adrenal hyperplasia. Nevertheless, these tumors are primarily dependent on adrenocorticotropic hormone for growth and steroid secretion; the most likely circumstance is that they arise from the adrenocortical rests that may occur normally in the testis but that are abnormally stimulated in the syndrome of congenital adrenal hyperplasia. Recognition of congenital adrenal hyperplasia and appropriate medical treatment may obviate surgical treatment of these testicular "tumors."

Adenomatoid Tumors

These lesions are characteristically small, benign tumors peculiar to the genital tracts of males and females. They consist of a fibrous stroma in which disoriented spaces of epithelial cells occur, resembling endothelium, epithelium, or mesothelium. Histogenesis remains debatable; although the lesion occurs primarily in the epididymis in the male, occasional instances of tumor confined to the testis have been reported.

Carcinoid

Carcinoid is uncommon outside the gastrointestinal tract. Nearly 150 cases of carcinoid in the ovary have been recorded, as well as 23 in the testis, 17 of which were primary and 6 metastatic (Talerman et al, 1978). On gross pathologic examination, the tumors have been circumscribed and limited to the testis, with diameters up to 8 cm. Microscopically, the tumors are composed of islands, nests, or discrete masses of round, oval, or polygonal cells separated by fibrous strands and exhibiting a solid acinar structure. Although most of the reported cases have been pure carcinoids, a few have arisen in association with teratoma. In primary ovarian carcinoids, the majority have arisen in association with teratoma. The histogenesis of these tumors remains uncertain, but one-sided development of a teratoma and origin from argentaffin or enterochromaffin cells within the gonad are the alternatives. A slow, progressive, painless testicular enlargement is the most frequent presentation. Although minimal symptoms suggestive of carcinoid syndrome were noted in one patient, estimations of serum serotonin and 5-hydroxyindoleacetic acid have not been performed preoperatively. Treatment has been inguinal orchiectomy, which has apparently been curative in patients with primary testicular carcinoid. In contrast, patients with metastatic carcinoid to the testis have a poor prognosis.

Secondary Tumors of the Testis

Lymphoma

Testicular involvement by lymphoma may be (1) a manifestation of primary extranodal disease, (2) the initial manifestation of clinically occult nodal disease, or (3) a later manifestation of disseminated nodal lymphoma. **Accounting for about 5% of all testis tumors, these lesions constitute the most common secondary neoplasms of the testis and the most frequent of all testicular tumors in patients older than 50 years. The median age of occurrence is approximately 60 years.** Primary lymphoma of the testis may occur in children; eight cases in patients ranging from 2 to 12 years old were reviewed by Weitzner and Gropp (1976).

Grossly, the testis is diffusely enlarged, usually to a diameter of 4 to 5 cm or more, bulging with a granular gray to light tan to pink solid tumor. Foci of hemorrhage and necrosis may be evident, and there may be gross extension to the epididymis or cord. Microscopically, all varieties of reticuloendothelial neoplasms, including Hodgkin's disease, have been described in the testis. The vast majority, however, are diffuse; of these, most are histiocytic (74%), according to the Rappaport classification, or large and noncleaved (70%), according to the Lukes and Collins classification. Diffuse replacement of the normal architecture is the rule, with focal sparing of the seminiferous tubules.

Malignant lymphoma confined to the testis at the time of clinical onset of disease is rare compared with the frequency with which the gonadal mass represents the initial clinical manifestation of occult or apparent nodal disease. When lymph node disease is limited to the regional nodes, however, it is possible that the neoplasm arose in the gonad and metastasized to the regional nodes. The pattern of dissemination of testicular lymphomas is similar to that of testicular GCTs. In autopsy cases, a pattern of pulmonary nodules not contiguous to the mediastinum or hilum strongly suggests a propensity of testicular lymphomas to spread by the hematogenous route, consistent with the observation of vascular invasion seen not infrequently in patients with testicular lymphoma.

A poor prognosis may be anticipated when there is evidence of generalized disease within a year after diagnosis. **As with lymphomas elsewhere, patients with poorly differentiated lymphocytic types tend to survive longer than those with histiocytic types.** Disease-free survivals of 60 months or longer in patients with testicular lymphoma treated by orchiectomy alone provide strong circumstantial evidence that a true primary testicular lymphoma occurs occasionally. Even patients whose disease seems to be limited to the gonads after clinical and surgical staging, however, may still have a short survival time. Patients who have no clinical evidence of systemic spread 1 year after therapy have a high probability of cure. Whether the long-term survival after orchiectomy alone is a reflection of a cured primary testicular tumor or of a spontaneous regression or prolonged remission of a generalized disease remains debatable.

A common clinical presentation is a painless enlargement of the testis, although about one fourth of patients present with generalized constitutional symptoms, including weight loss, weakness, and anorexia. Bilateral tumors occur in almost half of patients—simultaneously in roughly 10% and metachronously in the remainder.

Investigation may include complete blood cell count, peripheral smears, bone marrow studies, chest radiography, bone scan, CT or intravenous pyelogram, lymphogram, and liver and spleen scans. **There appears to be a high probability of generalized disease if para-aortic nodes are involved, indicating the importance of retroperitoneal staging.** Although radical orchiectomy provides the diagnosis and initial treatment, once the diagnosis of lymphoma has been established, referral to a medical oncologist is advisable for staging evaluation and decisions about further treatment.

Survival is poor with bilateral disease and poor in patients presenting with lymphoma at other sites and later experiencing a testicular relapse; but among patients with disease apparently confined to the testis, Turner and colleagues (1981) reported 8 of 14 to be alive and well for 7 to 87 months (mean: 2.5 years).

Leukemic Infiltration of the Testis

The testis appears to be a prime initial site of relapse in boys with acute lymphocytic leukemia. Stoffel and colleagues (1975) reported an 8% incidence of extramedullary involvement of the testis in children with acute leukemia, the

majority of patients being in complete remission at the time of testicular enlargement. The interval from testicular involvement to death ranges from 5 to 27 months, with a median of 9 months. Kuo and associates (1976) reported on seven children who developed testicular swelling during bone marrow remission in whom needle biopsy was used to confirm leukemic infiltration.

Leukemic infiltration occurs mainly in interstitial spaces, with destruction of the tubules by infiltration in advanced cases. Enlargement is bilateral in 50% of cases and is commonly associated with scrotal discoloration. Testicular irradiation with doses of 1200 cGy over 6 to 8 days is clinically successful in local control. Because of the frequency of bilateral involvement microscopically, bilateral irradiation seems advisable even with apparent unilateral involvement. Almost all patients can be expected to develop subsequent marrow relapse, despite control of testicular involvement by irradiation, unless effective systemic chemotherapy is given.

Biopsy is essential to diagnosis, orchiectomy is probably unwarranted, and the treatment of choice is testicular irradiation with 2000 cGy in 10 fractions plus reinstitution of adjunctive chemotherapy or re-induction therapy for children who relapse in the testis while on chemotherapy. The prognosis of boys who undergo such a bout of testicular infiltration is guarded.

Metastatic Tumors

Approximately 200 cases of metastatic carcinoma to the testis have been reported. In the vast majority, it is discovered incidentally at autopsy in patients dying of widespread metastatic disease. In rare circumstances, a metastatic focus in the testis may be the presenting feature of an occult neoplasm or the first evidence of a recurrent, previously diagnosed and treated neoplasm.

The usual pathologic feature of secondary testicular cancers is the microscopic demonstration of neoplastic cells in the interstitium, with relative sparing of the tubules. The route of dissemination to the testis may be hematogenous, lymphatic, or by direct invasion from contiguous masses. Renal adenocarcinoma may involve the testis via the spermatic vessels; rarely, dropped metastasis from a diffuse intra-abdominal malignancy can involve the cord and testis via a patent processus vaginalis. Retrograde extension through the vas deferens presumably may be a source as well. The common primary sources, in decreasing order of frequency, are prostate, lung, gastrointestinal tract, melanoma, and kidney. A relatively high incidence of prostatic lesions reflects, in part, the frequency with which carcinoma of the prostate occurs and the use of orchiectomy in its treatment. Metastatic tumors to the testis occur later in life, usually in the fifties or sixties, in contrast to primary testicular tumors. Metastasis has been bilateral in a small proportion of cases. Approximately 2.5% of lymphomas are found in the testis in metastatic fashion (Table 29–18).

TUMORS OF TESTICULAR ADNEXA
Epithelial Tumors

Epithelial tumors of the testicular adnexal structures are rare, even though the epididymis and paratesticular tissues may be involved by extensions from primary germinal cell testicular tumors. With the exception of cystadenomas of the epididymis, most tumors involving the testicular adnexal structures are of mesenchymal origin.

Adenomatoid Tumors

Adenomatoid tumors are the most common tumors of the paratesticular tissues, accounting for approximately 30% of all paratesticular tumors. In the male, they are located in a restricted anatomic distribution of the epididymis, testicular tunicae, and, rarely, the spermatic cord; in the female, they have been described in the uterus and fallopian tubes and, rarely, in the ovary. In the male, most of these tumors arise in or adjacent to the lower or upper pole of the epididymis, with a slightly higher incidence in the lower pole.

Most of these tumors occur in individuals in their twenties or thirties, but tumors have been seen in patients ranging from 20 to 80 years old. Clinically, adenomatoid tumors present as small, solid, asymptomatic masses generally found on routine examination. These rounded, discrete masses lie anywhere in the epididymis and may be embedded in the testicular tunicae. An occasional patient presents with mild pain or discomfort in association with the nodule. Most of these tumors have been present for several years without obvious change in size. These tumors uniformly behave in a benign fashion.

On gross examination, the tumors are small, ranging from 0.5 to 5 cm in diameter. The tumors are usually attached to the testicular tunicae. On sectioning, the tumors appear uniformly white, yellow, or tan with a fibrous appearance.

On microscopic examination, there are two different elements: epithelium-like cells and fibrous stroma. The epithelium-like cells are usually arranged in a framework of poorly delineated spaces, sometimes with flattened or cuboidal cells.

A fairly common feature of adenomatoid tumors is the presence of vacuoles within the epithelial cells (Mostofi and Price, 1973). The vacuoles may range in size from minute to large and may, in fact, replace most of the cytoplasm of the cell. The nuclei show marked uniformity in size and chromatin distribution. Nuclei are generally round or oval and centrally placed with a single nucleolus. The cytoplasm is acidophilic and finely granular. The stroma ranges from loose tissue to dense collagenized tissue with occasional hyalinization. Variations in the amount of stroma are common.

The origin of this tumor is unknown. Some pathologists have considered it to be a reaction to injury or inflammation. Jackson (1958), as well as other authors, has suggested that adenomatoid tumor may be of mesothelial origin, predominantly on the basis of histology. Occasional misclassification of adenomatoid tumors has been reported as mesothelioma. Others have suggested that adenomatoid tumors are of endothelial origin and may represent a specialized hemangioma or lymphangioma. Ultrastructural findings by Marcus and Lynn (1970) failed to confirm any similarities to hemangioma. These authors found morphologic similarity to pleural mesotheliomas.

These tumors behave in a benign fashion, and there has never been a documented case of metastasis. Cellular atypia and local invasion have been observed occasionally. Nonethe-

Table 29–18. **Testicular Lymphoma, Testicular Secondary Tumors, Adnexal Tumors: Presentation, Pathology, Treatment**

Type	Presentation	Pathology	Treatment
Hematopoietic Tumor			
Lymphoma	Most common testis tumor in men > age 50 years. Most common secondary neoplasm of the testis. Tumors may be primary (cured by radical orchiectomy alone) or secondary and may be unilateral or bilateral.	Large homogeneous tumor with marked intertubular and interstitial infiltration with lymphoma cells.	Orchiectomy for primary disease. Chemotherapy for secondary lymphoma.
Secondary Tumors			
Malignant melanoma, lung, skin, gastrointestinal, thyroid, prostate (most common)	Depends on stage and site of primary tumor	Depends on the primary tumor	Depends on stage and site of primary tumor
Tumors of Testicular Adnexa			
Adenomatoid tumor (most common paratesticular tumor)	Epididymis is most frequent location. Within the epididymis the globus minor is the most frequent site. Well circumscribed 0.5- to 4-cm mass, usually asymptomatic. These tumors behave in a benign fashion; metastases have never been reported.	Benign tumor, consisting of mesothelial cells which may resemble endothelium. Tumor cells are characterized by vacuoles. Smooth muscle may be present.	Surgical excision
Primary malignant tumors of epididymis	Scrotal mass that may be large and fixed.	Primary adenocarcinoma of the epididymis is described but is exceedingly rare and mandates a workup for the possibility of adenocarcinoma metastatic to the epididymis. A variety of primary sarcomas including fibrosarcoma, leiomyosarcoma, and rhabdomyosarcoma are described.	Wide surgical excision with intraoperative frozen section to determine margin status.
Tumors of spermatic cord structures	Tumors are usually distal (i.e., close to the epididymis and testis) and can therefore be difficult to distinguish from primary testicular or epididymal tumors.	Majority are sarcomas; rhabdomyosarcoma accounts for 40% of all paratesticular tumors.	Combination of surgery, radiotherapy, and chemotherapy, depending on stage of disease
Rete testis tumor	Scrotal mass or scrotal pain. Tumor may be concealed by hydrocele.	Adenocarcinoma	Surgical excision

less, the long history of these tumors and the absence of distant metastases suggest a benign nature. Treatment, therefore, is surgical excision (Söderström and Leidberg, 1966).

Mesothelioma

Paratesticular mesothelioma is more common in older individuals but may be encountered in any age group, including children. Usually, the tumor presents as a firm, painless scrotal mass in association with a hydrocele. Gradual enlargement of the hydrocele or sometimes the mass itself is seen in approximately 50% of patients. Most of these tumors are treated by orchiectomy.

On gross examination there is a poorly demarcated lesion that is whitish or yellowish with intermittent firm, shaggy, and friable areas. Microscopically, there is a background of papillary and solid structures against densely fibrous fibroconnective tissue. The complex structure has papillary processes combined with solid sheets of cells. Tumor cells tend to have a generous amount of cytoplasm and poorly defined cytoplasmic borders. Nuclei are often vesicular with a single small nucleolus. Mitotic activity is usually absent. Calcifications

may be seen scattered throughout these neoplastic structures. Solid mesotheliomas may have small or rather extensive areas of spindle-shaped cells resembling sarcomas. This feature, although devoid of clinical significance, may lead to an erroneous diagnosis of soft tissue sarcoma. Psammoma bodies are sometimes found within papillary areas in the tumor.

Approximately 15% of testicular mesotheliomas have been documented to result in metastatic involvement of inguinal lymph nodes or abdominal structures (Kasdon, 1969). The pure papillary tumors nearly always prove benign. Those of a more complex structure, however, may recur and may develop multiple recurrences or even metastases.

Clinical management should consist of adequate surgical excision with follow-up examination and local biopsy if a metastatic focus is suspected (Hollands et al, 1982). Antman and associates (1984) reported on a patient in whom conservative management failed. Limited experience with chemotherapy and radiation therapy in these rare tumors has not produced any conclusions. Staging includes CT of the chest and abdomen and, rarely, laparotomy if there is clinical suspicion of recurrent disease.

Cystadenoma

Cystadenoma of the epididymis corresponds to benign epithelial hyperplasia. Sherrick described the first case in 1956, and about 20 cases have been the subjects of subsequent reports. **Approximately one third of the cases are bilateral and may be seen as part of von Hippel-Lindau disease.** The tumor occurs most often in young adults and produces either minimal local discomfort or no symptoms. When seen in elderly patients, it is frequently an incidental finding at orchiectomy.

On gross examination, the lesion is partially cystic, ranging from 1.5 to 5 cm in diameter. The cut section may be multicystic, well-encapsulated, or circumscribed. The wall is studded with one or several nodules of epithelial cells arranged in small glands and papillary structures. Many of the glands are lined by columnar and ciliated cells, many of which display a vacuolated or clear cytoplasm. Staining shows abundant glycogen as well as stainable lipids in the clear cells. This pattern is similar to that of renal cell carcinoma, and distinction from metastases of renal cell carcinoma may be difficult.

Paratesticular Tumors

There are occasional reports of purely testicular mesenchymal tumors (one-sided teratomas) (Davis, 1962), but, for the most part, the overwhelming majority of mesenchymal tumors in this area arise from paratesticular structures, although it may sometimes be difficult to determine whether the primary origin is the spermatic cord, the epididymis, or the tunica vaginalis.

Most series agree that rhabdomyosarcoma in its juvenile form probably accounts for approximately 40% of all paratesticular tumors, benign and malignant. Leiomyosarcoma appears to be the second most common lesion in this area, followed by occasional occurrences of fibrosarcoma, liposarcoma, and undifferentiated mesenchymal tumors, which complete the spectrum of this group. Cooperative study groups have described some of their results with these tumors as well. One is dependent on this sort of accrual because the rarity of the tumor makes certain conclusions about therapy still tentative. In one report (Kingston et al, 1983), four boys with primary paratesticular tumors were seen. There are now late relapses, defined as recurrence or tumor persistence 2 years after diagnosis and treatment. This should be kept in mind for follow-up evaluation of such tumors.

Rhabdomyosarcoma

Paratesticular rhabdomyosarcoma occurs predominantly in children and adolescents and, with some exceptions, is most commonly seen during the first 2 decades of life. Clinically, this tumor usually presents as a large interscrotal mass that compresses the testis and the epididymis, sometimes reaching the external inguinal ring; the location varies somewhat, depending on the exact point of origin. On gross inspection, it can appear circumscribed, but on microscopic examination, it often extends well beyond the margin seen by the naked eye. The cut surface is solid, grayish white, and firm and is rarely hemorrhagic. Some patches of necrosis can be noted, especially around the central portion of the lesion.

The microscopic features of paratesticular rhabdomyosarcoma are largely characterized by pronounced variation from case to case and even within the same tumor. Most of them show more than one pattern of the spectrum, ranging from totally undifferentiated mesenchymal elements to distinctive features of skeletal muscle fibers. It is characteristic to find a combination of various patterns containing an admixture of cellular elements, as accurately described by Patton and Horn (1962).

Some paratesticular rhabdomyosarcomas are partially or predominantly arranged in an "alveolar" fashion identical with the distinctive pattern frequently seen in other locations that was first termed *alveolar rhabdomyosarcoma* by Riopelle and Thériault (1956) and is currently accepted as a variant of embryonal rhabdomyosarcoma.

Riehle and Venkatachalam (1982) made the point that has often been made about other sarcomas—that electron microscopic diagnosis has frequently assisted in sorting out aberrations, variance, and, particularly, identification of the sarcoma in question. Electron microscopy has been successfully used to identify the cytoplasmic myofilaments and Z bands in a paratesticular rhabdomyosarcoma. This, of course, applies to paratesticular tumors as well.

Testicular and Paratesticular Tumor Management

The primary testicular or paratesticular tumor should be removed by inguinal orchiectomy with high ligation of the cord. The primary lymphatic drainage of the testis and the cord courses through lymphatics parallel to the testicular vessels; these intercommunicate with para-aortic nodes at the level of the renal vessels. The lower para-aortic and iliac nodes serve as a route of lymphatic spread when the primary spermatic lymphatics have become occluded by fibrosis or tumor. Several papers discussing these tumors have recommended routine RPLND (Ghavimi et al, 1973; Johnson, 1975). The fact that rhabdomyosarcoma is the most common malignant spermatic cord tumor has been reaffirmed. A 5-year survival rate of 75%, using multimodal treatment, remains the current goal. Current adjuvant therapy is as follows.

Radiation Therapy. Cobalt-60 teletherapy can be delivered in a total tumor dose of 4000 to 6000 cGy over a period of 5 to 8 weeks through ports extending well beyond the known confines of the tumor. Dose and port size are determined by the primary site and extent of the tumor and by the age of the patient. Radiation therapy can be used for local tumors even when the tumor is generalized.

Chemotherapy. Chemotherapy with vincristine (1.5 mg/m^2), cyclophosphamide (300 mg/m^2), and dactinomycin (0.4 mg/m^2) is used. A report by Ghavimi and coworkers (1973) described 29 children younger than 15 years with embryonal rhabdomyosarcoma who were treated according to a multidisciplinary protocol that consisted of surgical removal of the tumor, if possible, followed by chemotherapy and by radiation therapy in patients with gross or microscopic residual disease. Radiation therapy was given in a dose of 4500 to 7000 cGy. Additional new trials of chemotherapy consisted of cycles of sequential administration of dactinomycin, doxorubicin, vincristine, and cyclophosphamide, with obligatory periods of rest. The drug therapy was continued for 2 years. In addition, early phase II trials are also employing a method of intravenous administration of semustine that appears promising.

Tumor stage and site are now considered important prognostic indicators. Grosfeld and colleagues (1983) **stated that chemotherapy improves survival in stage I (91%) and stage II (86%) tumors and may shrink bulky stage III tumors, allowing less radical procedures in certain selective sites, particularly the urinary tract.** It is still true, however, that survival is poor in stage III, with 35% survival, and dismal in stage IV, with 5.2% survival, despite combined therapy. Relapses are generally fatal despite attempts at second-look resection, altered chemotherapy, and radiation therapy.

Leiomyosarcoma

Smooth muscle tumors of the spermatic cord and epididymis are rare, and their exact incidence is difficult to determine: first, because the clinical and histologic differences between benign smooth muscle tumors and malignant ones are slight and, second, because some adenomatoid tumors are erroneously classified as leiomyomas, especially those that exhibit a significant component of smooth muscle (Wilson, 1949). Most benign and malignant smooth muscle tumors described in the literature are in patients ranging in age from their forties to their seventies. Ninety percent of extratesticular tumors occurring within the scrotum are found in the spermatic cord. Of the latter, 30% are malignant and 70% are benign. Of the malignant variety, the majority are mesenchymal sarcomas (i.e., fibrosarcoma, myxosarcoma, liposarcoma, rhabdomyosarcoma, and leiomyosarcoma). More than 25 cases of leiomyosarcoma of the spermatic cord have been reported. Local invasion of the adjacent tissues was found in 5 of the 13 cases in which this detail was described. The first recurrence was usually local, in the scrotum or at the distal spermatic stump. This feature was described in six cases.

Distant spread has been hematogenous in a large number of cases (i.e., in tumors of humerus, liver, ileum, and lung). Autopsies were not done in many cases, however, and the clinical finding of abdominally palpable masses probably represented metastatic disease in the para-aortic lymph nodes. The ratio of cases with known hematogenous spread to cases with known lymphatic spread is 6:2. These facts, at least, support the opinion of Strong (1942) and of others who believe that spread is as frequently hematogenous as lymphatic. The importance of electron microscopy in the documentation of these particular tumors, as contrasted to light microscopy, has been emphasized (Gaffney et al, 1984).

The philosophy and planning of treatment have been greatly affected by the mode of spread. It is agreed that all cases of tumor of the spermatic cord should be explored and that the growth should be removed. If it is benign, simple excision is all that is necessary. The standard therapy for leiomyosarcoma has been radical orchiectomy in which a high ligation of the cord is carried out. Because of the high incidence of hematogenous spread, the surgeon should carry out early clamping of the cord to prevent escape of tumor cells.

Electron microscopy is extremely helpful in the differentiation of the type of testicular sarcoma. Although, at present, management may not be radically changed, depending on the histologic description, there are differences as to the extent of dissection of the nodes. In children and adolescents, the complications of node dissection have been minimal, although these obviously have to be considered, as well as in adults (Waters et al, 1982). Particularly important for children and adolescents is a discussion with their parents concerning obvious difficulties with fertility in the future. This aspect has been addressed, but chiefly in adult patients (Lipshultz, 1982). The additional use of tumor markers must be further explored in these entities, and experience is limited in contrast to experience with what might be called adult testicular tumors (Vugrin et al, 1982).

Miscellaneous Mesenchymal Tumors of the Spermatic Cord

Isolated cases of other mesenchymal tumors of the spermatic cord, including liposarcoma, lipoma, fibrosarcoma, and myxochondrosarcoma, have been recorded. **Liposarcoma is probably the most significant of this group because of its greater frequency.** Samellas (1964), in a review of 112 tumors of the spermatic cord, added one case to three cases already reported, and Gowing and Morgan (1964) found two cases in their review of paratesticular tumors of connective tissue.

On histologic examination, liposarcomas of the spermatic cord and of the scrotal area show essentially the same features as those described in other soft tissue sites, although most of the recorded cases mentioned previously were predominantly characterized as well differentiated. The Armed Forces Institute of Pathology collected 14 paratesticular liposarcomas that also appeared to show this tendency to be well differentiated. In most cases, they appeared as a discrete nodular mass, sometimes attaining a large size and frequently located near the spermatic cord, entirely separate from the testis.

On histologic examination, mesenchymal tumors of the spermatic cord are characterized by the presence of a rather uniform pattern of interwoven bundles of long, spindle-shaped cells with blunt-ended nuclei and with cytoplasmic myofibrils extending along their longitudinal axis. Leiomyoma is distinguished from leiomyosarcoma based on occasional or absent mitotic figures and uniform cellular arrangement. Approximately 70% of tumors considered malignant on initial histologic examination either recur or metastasize (or both), regardless of their location.

Malignant neoplasms arising within the spermatic cord are uncommon, with 161 cases reported in the literature (Arlen et al, 1969). Sporadic cases have continued to appear, but the cumulative number remains relatively small. Although Banowsky and Shultz (1970) have described 19 histologic types of sarcoma originating from the spermatic cord and the tunicae, none was classified as neurofibrosarcoma. Johnson and associates (1975) have described such a case.

KEY POINTS: FERTILITY IN TESTICULAR CANCER PATIENTS

■ Testicular cancer affects young adult men; therefore, fertility becomes an important issue.

■ Approximately 25% of patients have defects in spermatogenesis at the time of presentation.

■ Higher concentrations of anti-sperm antibodies are present in serum of patients with testicular cancer than in the normal population.

■ Approximately 50% of patients are at least temporarily hypofertile after orchiectomy before any adjuvant therapy. This may be due to a variety of factors, such as stress, hormone production by the tumor, and surgical trauma to one testis that may have an effect on the contralateral testis.

■ Fertility can be further impaired by adjuvant therapy (RPLND, radiation therapy, and chemotherapy).

■ Fifty percent of patients who receive chemotherapy experience return of normal sperm counts by 2 years, whereas 25% continue to remain azoospermic after chemotherapy.

■ The best measurement of fertility is pregnancy. One study reported that only 35% of patients achieved paternity after chemotherapy. On the other hand, the Indiana group reported a 76% paternity rate after RPLND for clinical stage I NSGCT.

■ Cryopreservation of semen is therefore applicable to patients who undergo chemotherapy. Recent developments such as intracytoplasmic sperm injection, however, may make sperm banking less relevant in the future.

SUGGESTED READINGS

Bosl GJ, Motzer RJ: Testicular germ-cell cancer. N Engl J Med 1997;337:242-253.

Donohue JP, Thornhill JA, Foster RS: The role of retroperitoneal lymphadenectomy in clinical stage B testis cancer: The Indiana University experience (1965-1989). J Urol 1995;153:85.

Donohue JP, Zachary JM, Maynard BR: Distribution of nodal metastases in nonseminomatous testis cancer. J Urol 1982;128:315.

Foster RS, McNulty A, Rubin LR: The fertility of patients with clinical stage I testis cancer managed by nerve sparing retroperitoneal lymph node dissection. J Urol 1994;152:1139.

Freedman LS, Jones WG, Peckham MJ, et al: Histopathology in the prediction of relapse of patients with stage I testicular teratoma treated by orchidectomy alone. Lancet 1987;2:294.

Group International Germ Cell Consensus Classification: A prognostic factor based staging system for metastatic germ cell cancers. J Clin Oncol 1997;15:594-603.

Hao D, Seidel J, Brant R, et al: Compliance of clinical stage I nonseminomatous germ cell tumor patients with surveillance. J Urol 1998;160:768-771.

Heidenreich A, Weibach L, Höltl W, et al, for the German Testicular Cancer Study Group: Organ sparing surgery for malignant germ cell tumor of the testis. J Urol 2001;166:2161-2165.

Read G, Stenning SP, Cullen MH, et al: Medical Research Council prospective study of surveillance for stage I testicular teratoma. Medical Research Council Testicular Tumors Working Party. J Clin Oncol 1992;10:1762-1768.

Richie JP, Kantoff P: Is adjuvant chemotherapy necessary for patients with stage B$_1$ testicular cancer? J Clin Oncol 1991;9:1393-1396.

Sheinfeld J, Bajorin D: Management of the postchemotherapy residual mass. Urol Clin North Am 1993;20:133-143.

30 Surgery of Testicular Tumors

JOEL SHEINFELD, MD • GEORG BARTSCH, MD • GEORGE J. BOSL, MD

Each year, approximately 8000 new cases and almost 400 deaths due to testicular cancer are expected (Jemal et al, 2005). The incidence of germ cell tumors (GCTs), the most common solid tumor in men between the ages of 20 and 35 years, is rising both in the United States and Europe (Bergstrom et al, 1996; McKiernan et al, 1999).

Given the dramatic improvements in survival rates from 60% to 65% in the 1960s to more than 90% in the 1990s, the management of testicular cancer has come to represent a model in the successful multidisciplinary approach to solid tumors (Einhorn et al, 1981). Although testicular cancer is highly curable, it requires appropriate management at all stages (Bosl et al, 2000). Both the cure rate and the morbidity are highly sensitive to nuances of management. The clinician and, more importantly, the patient, pay a high price for inappropriate management. Surgery remains an integral part of the management of patients with GCTs; however, the advent of effective chemotherapy and improvements in clinical staging, including sophisticated imaging modalities and reliable serum tumor markers, have altered its role over the past 25 years (Sheinfeld and Herr, 1998).

In this chapter we summarize the principal indications and controversies of surgery in the management of testicular neoplasms, describe common surgical techniques and their associated complications, and discuss established and investigational alternatives to surgery in both low- and high-stage GCTs.

MANAGEMENT OF THE PRIMARY TUMOR
Diagnosis

Unfortunately, delays in the timely and accurate diagnosis of testicular cancer continue to be a significant problem. Moul noted a mean duration of symptoms of 26 weeks before diagnosis in a review of 4948 testicular cancer patients (Moul et al, 1994). Both patient and physician factors contribute to this delay in diagnosis. Bosl and colleagues (1981) reported that the median interval of delay for patients with clinical stage I disease was 75 days compared to 101 and 134 days for patients with clinical stages II and III disease, respectively. Painless scrotal masses are often ignored, whereas testicular cancers presenting as scrotal pain are treated as epididymitis up to 18% to 30% of the time (Bosl et al, 1981; Prout et al, 1984). Almost 20% of patients present with signs or symptoms of metastatic disease such as back or abdominal pain, weight loss, neck mass, gynecomastia, or breast tenderness (Bosl et al, 1981, 2000; Thornhill et al, 1978). Patients have undergone unnecessary mastectomy or laparotomy or prolonged therapy for back pain without considering the diagnosis of testicular cancer (Post et al, 1980; Moul et al, 1992, 2000). Stephenson and coworkers (2004) reported on 40 patients with a midline retroperitoneal mass who underwent unnecessary laparotomy. At the time of laparotomy all patients had an abnormality on testicular examination or sonography or an elevated serum tumor marker to suggest the diagnosis of GCT. The laparotomy contributed to therapeutic delay in a substantial number of patients and complicated their therapy (Stephenson et al, 2004).

A careful history and physical examination, as well as serum β-human chorionic gonadotropin (β-hCG), α-fetoprotein (AFP), and lactate dehydrogenase (LDH) levels, are helpful in establishing a correct diagnosis. Scrotal sonography is extremely accurate in identifying solid intratesticular lesions, with greater than 95% sensitivity and specificity.

Radical Orchiectomy

A radical orchiectomy with high ligation of the spermatic cord at the level of the internal ring is the first step in the treatment of patients suspected of harboring a testicular neoplasm. This procedure provides histopathologic diagnosis and T categorization, is associated with minimal morbidity

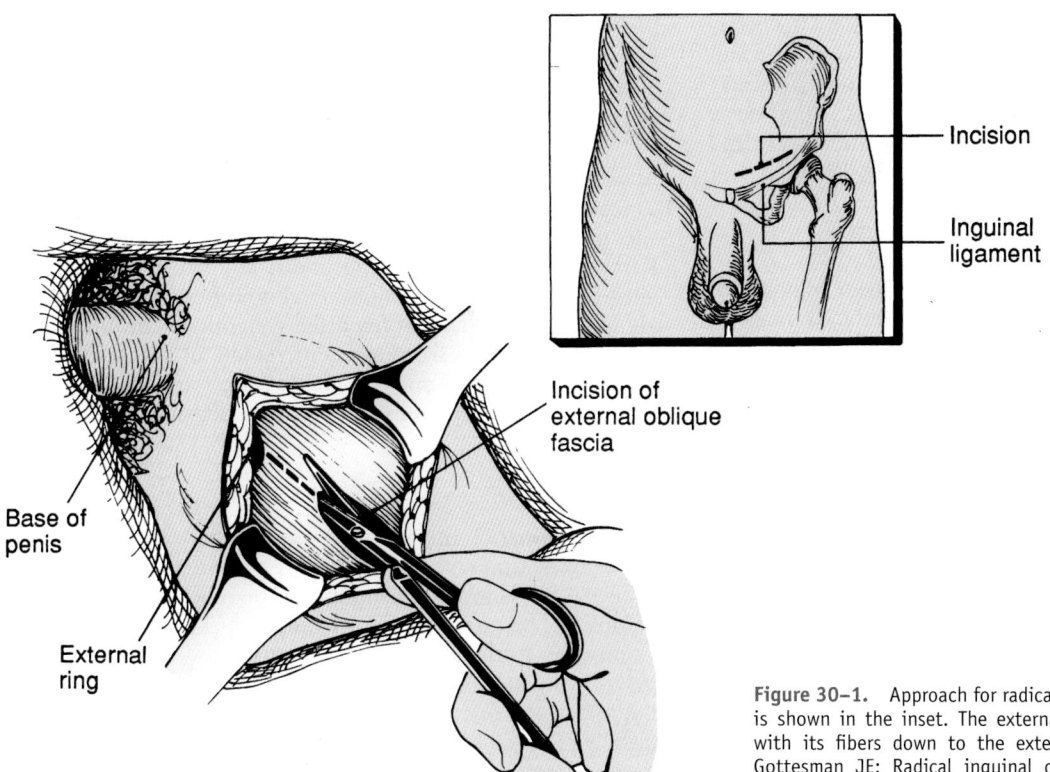

Incision

Inguinal ligament

Incision of external oblique fascia

Base of penis

External ring

Figure 30–1. Approach for radical inguinal orchiectomy. The incision is shown in the inset. The external oblique fascia is divided in line with its fibers down to the external inguinal ring. (Adapted from Gottesman JE: Radical inguinal orchiectomy. In Crawford ED [ed]: Current Genitourinary Cancer Surgery. Philadelphia, Lea & Febiger, 1990, p 319.)

and no mortality, and provides local control of the tumor in the vast majority of patients. The rare exceptions are usually due to tumor spillage, suboptimal orchiectomy, or transscrotal surgery (Whitmore et al, 1982).

The procedure is performed under general, spinal, or local anesthesia on an outpatient basis. The patient is placed in the supine position with the scrotum prepped in the sterile field. A 5- to 7-cm oblique incision is made in the inguinal area along Langerhans' skin lines approximately 2 cm above the pubic tubercle. This incision can be extended onto the upper scrotum to facilitate removal of large tumors. Camper's and Scarpa's fascia are incised to the level of the external oblique aponeurosis, which is then incised in the direction of its fibers to the level of the internal ring (Fig. 30–1). The ilioinguinal nerve is identified, dissected free of the cord, and preserved. The spermatic cord is isolated and either occluded with a noncrushing clamp or a 0.5-inch Penrose tourniquet at the level of the internal ring. The testis and its investing tunics are delivered into a carefully draped off field as gubernacular attachments are divided. If a diagnostic biopsy or subtotal orchiectomy is planned, meticulous draping off is necessary before opening the tunica vaginalis and incising testicular parenchyma. Radical orchiectomy is completed by mobilizing the cord 1 to 2 cm inside the internal ring and individually ligating the vas deferens and the cord vessels between separate clamps (Fig. 30–2). The cord vessels are secured with silk ligatures, which can then be used to identify the stump if a retroperitoneal lymph node dissection (RPLND) is performed. The wound and scrotum are thoroughly irrigated, and hemostasis is secured. A testicular prosthesis can be placed at this time. The external oblique aponeurosis is closed

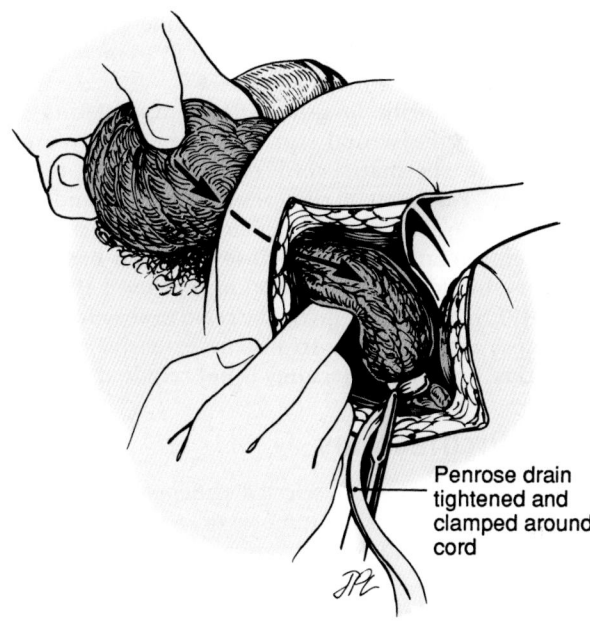

Penrose drain tightened and clamped around cord

Figure 30–2. After the cord has been controlled with a tightened Penrose drain or rubber-shod clamp, the testis is mobilized out of the scrotum using blunt dissection. (Adapted from Gottesman JE: Radical inguinal orchiectomy. In Crawford ED [ed]: Current Genitourinary Cancer Surgery. Philadelphia, Lea & Febiger, 1990, p 319.)

with a running 2-0 Prolene suture. Scarpa's fascia is closed with absorbable sutures and the skin with either skin staples or a subcuticular suture. Compressive fluff dressings with a scrotal support minimize postoperative edema.

The most common complication of radical orchiectomy remains postoperative bleeding, which may occasionally result in either a scrotal or a retroperitoneal hematoma. Furthermore, significant retroperitoneal hematomas may delay further therapy or be misinterpreted as metastatic disease and result in unnecessary treatment (Bochner et al, 1995).

Scrotal Violation

Sayegh and associates (1966) reported that prior inguinal or scrotal surgery could alter the normal lymphatic drainage of the testis; consequently, many patients with scrotal violation have undergone extensive local surgery and/or adjuvant therapy to prevent an adverse outcome.

Suboptimal approaches to testicular neoplasms, including scrotal orchiectomy, transscrotal biopsy, or fine-needle aspiration are reported from 4% to 17% of the time (Capelouto et al, 1995; Leibovitch et al, 1995a).

A recent meta-analysis of 206 cases of scrotal violation reported a local recurrence rate of 2.9% compared with 0.4% of patients treated by inguinal orchiectomy but, no difference in systemic relapse or survival rates. There did not appear to be any advantage to adjuvant therapy (Capelouto et al, 1995). Others have reported an increased local recurrence rate in patients with scrotal contamination (Giguere et al, 1988) and an 11% presence of tumor in hemiscrotectomy specimens of patients with scrotal violation. Therefore, the following recommendations for patients with scrotal violation seem prudent:

1. **In patients with low-stage seminoma, the radiation portals should be extended to include the ipsilateral groin and scrotum.** This may result in an increased risk of azoospermia (Amelar et al, 1971).
2. **In patients with low-stage nonseminomatous GCT (NSGCT), the scrotal scar should be widely excised with the spermatic cord remnant at the time of RPLND.** Patients with clinical stage I NSGCT and scrotal violation are not good candidates for surveillance.
3. **Patients treated with full-dose platinum-based regimens should have the cord stump removed at the time of RPLND; however, given the relative absence of local relapse after systemic treatment, extensive groin dissection or hemiscrotectomy is not required.**

Partial Orchiectomy

A small subset of carefully selected patients with a solitary testis or bilateral testicular tumors, or a suspected benign lesion, may be candidates for "testis-sparing" surgery. The German Testicular Cancer Intergroup reported on 63 patients with median follow-up of 74 months and found only four local recurrences, all in patients with untreated intratubular germ cell neoplasia (ITGCN) (van der Schyff et al, 2000). Almost 90% of patients maintained normal testosterone levels. **Favorable selection criteria include organ-confined disease with a mass less than 20 mm, negative postresection biopsies of the tumor bed, and absence of intratubular germ cell neoplasia in the remaining testicular parenchyma. The procedure is performed under conditions of cold ischemia with great care to avoid tumor spillage or contamination.** Patient compliance for rigorous follow-up must be assured,

particularly because most patients with GCT have associated ITGCN.

Delayed Orchiectomy

A subset of patients with documented advanced germ cell cancer that includes histologic verification from a metastatic site undergo systemic chemotherapy without orchiectomy. Rarely, postoperative complications following orchiectomy have resulted in delays initiating chemotherapy. **The rationale for delayed orchiectomy after systemic chemotherapy is supported by data from a recent review of 160 patients in which 40 (25%) patients had viable cancer and 50 (31%) had teratoma in the resected testis** (Simmonds et al, 1995).

STAGING

Staging evaluation must include a thorough history and physical examination with particular attention to the contralateral testis. Serum tumor markers should be repeated immediately before RPLND and should include β-hCG, LDH, and AFP. Computed tomography (CT) of the chest, abdomen, and pelvis is the most efficient and cost-effective means of detecting metastatic disease. Magnetic resonance imaging (MRI) is usually reserved for the setting of major vascular involvement to assess patency of the inferior vena cava (IVC) and renal vessels (Bosl et al, 2000).

In 1997 the American Joint Committee on Cancer and Union Internationale Contre le Cancer (UICC) adopted a comprehensive staging system that now includes serum tumor markers (TNMS). Stage I refers to disease confined to the testis, stage II implies retroperitoneal metastases, and stage III disease indicates supradiaphragmatic or visceral metastases. In the TNMS system, vascular or lymphatic invasion in the primary tumor is classified in the T2 category and serum tumor markers are included because of their independent prognostic significance (AJCC, 1998).

THE RETROPERITONEUM AND GERM CELL TUMORS
Natural History, Patterns of Metastasis, Anatomic Considerations

The natural history of testicular cancer provides the basis for its evaluation and management, and, in turn, is favorably influenced by effective treatment (Whitmore et al, 1982). GCTs share several features that have contributed significantly to their successful management. **These include (1) a germ cell origin, which is associated with responsiveness to irradiation (seminoma) and a number of chemotherapeutic agents and with a potential for differentiation to histologically benign teratoma; (2) a rapid growth rate; (3) frequent production of specific tumor markers such as AFP and β-hCG; (4) usual occurrence in otherwise healthy young adults who can tolerate the necessary therapy; and (5) a very predictable and systematic pattern of metastatic spread from the primary site to the retroperitoneal lymph nodes and, subsequently, to the lung and posterior mediastinum** (Richie et al, 1992; Whitmore et al, 1982; Sheinfeld, 1994).

Lymphatic spread is common to all forms of GCTs, although in the case of choriocarcinoma, vascular dissemination is often a more common clinical feature. In 1899, Most and colleagues were the first to accurately describe the lymphatic drainage of the testis (Most et al, 1899; Skinner et al, 1971). Other anatomic studies in the early 20th century confirmed these findings and noted that the primary lymphatic drainage of the testis was to the area of its embryologic origin, that is, the retroperitoneal lymph nodes adjacent to the great vessels (Cuneo et al, 1901; Jamieson and Dobsin, 1910; Skinner et al, 1971). *Right-sided testicular drainage included the interaortocaval lymph nodes, followed by the precaval and paracaval nodes, whereas left-sided drainage included the left para-aortic and preaortic lymph nodes* (Weinstein et al, 1999).

Further anatomic studies and detailed mapping studies of RPLNDs have increased our understanding of the testicular lymphatic drainage and sharpened the focus of clinical staging and treatment by identifying the most likely sites of metastatic disease (Busch and Sayegh, 1963; Chiappa et al, 1966; Sheinfeld, 1994). There are four to eight lymphatic vessels that accompany the spermatic vessels through the internal ring into the retroperitoneum. Although the majority of lymphatic channels continue to accompany the spermatic vessels to the point where those vessels cross the ureter and to their origin, some may drain directly into a lymph node on the anterior surface of the proximal third of the external iliac artery. At the point where the spermatic vessels cross ventral to the ureter, lymph channels fan out medially in relation to the aorta and IVC and drain into the retroperitoneal lymph node chain extending from approximately L5 to T11 (Weinstein et al, 1999). Contralateral lymphatic flow is often seen, particularly for right-sided lymphatics (Weinstein et al, 1999).

Surgical mapping studies by Donohue and colleagues (1982), Weissbach and Boedefeld (1987), and Ray and associates (1974) have divided the retroperitoneum into specific anatomic regions: right and left suprahilar, right paracaval, precaval, interaortocaval, preaortic, left para-aortic, right and left iliac, interiliac, and gonadal vessels (right or left) (Weinstein et al, 1999) (Fig. 30–3).

The first echelon of lymph nodes draining the right testis is located in the interaortocaval area, followed by the precaval and preaortic nodes. The primary "landing zone" for left-sided tumors includes the para-aortic and preaortic lymph nodes, followed by the interoartocaval nodes (Donohue et al, 1982). More caudal deposits of metastatic disease usually reflect retrograde spread secondary to large-volume disease and, rarely, aberrant drainage. **Contralateral spread is more common with right-sided tumors, rare with left-sided tumors, and usually associated with large-volume disease** (Sogani, 1991; Richie et al, 1992).

Testicular tumors have the capacity to spread by direct extension and involve the epididymis and/or scrotum. The lymphatic drainage of the epididymis is to the external iliac chain, whereas that of the scrotum is to the inguinal lymph nodes (Osler et al, 1907; Weinstein et al, 1999).

The rationale for treatment of the retroperitoneal lymph nodes in patients with testicular cancer is based on several factors. First, there is evidence that retroperitoneal lymph node spread is usually the first and often the only site of metastatic disease (Whitmore et al, 1979). This is supported

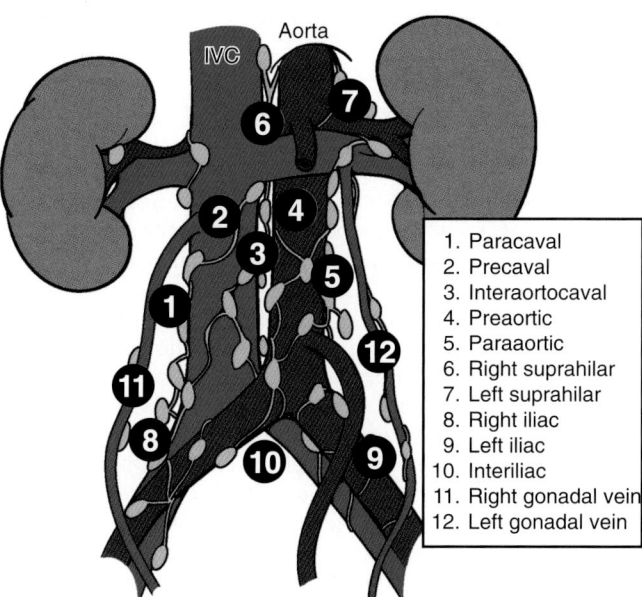

Figure 30–3. Anatomic regions of the retroperitoneum.

1. Paracaval
2. Precaval
3. Interaortocaval
4. Preaortic
5. Paraaortic
6. Right suprahilar
7. Left suprahilar
8. Right iliac
9. Left iliac
10. Interiliac
11. Right gonadal vein
12. Left gonadal vein

by several clinical observations: (1) the survival rates in patients with retroperitoneal lymph node metastases treated by RPLND alone (Richie et al, 1991; Sheinfeld et al, 1999a) and (2) patients whose regional lymph nodes are found to be pathologically negative after adequate RPLND; these patients are usually cured by orchiectomy, and the rare treatment failures are usually a result of pulmonary metastases and/or elevated serum levels of tumor markers. Relapse rates average approximately 10%, and disease-free survival rates range from 96% to 100% (Staubitz et al, 1973; Whitmore et al, 1979; Bredael et al, 1983).

Second, although clinical staging continues to improve through refinements of radiologic imaging such as CT (Hilton et al, 1997), **15% to 40% of patients are clinically understaged, particularly in the retroperitoneum.** This is supported by the 20% to 30% incidence of pathologic stage II disease in clinical stage I patients, the approximately 25% relapse rate in the retroperitoneum on surveillance protocols (Lashley and Lowe, 1998), and the 20% incidence of teratoma and/or viable carcinoma in resected masses of patients with radiographically normal CT scans after chemotherapy (Fossa et al, 1989c; Toner, 1990; Sheinfeld et al, 1993).

Third, untreated retroperitoneal lymph node metastases are usually fatal (Whitmore et al, 1979). **Autopsy studies of patients dying with GCTs of the testis indicate that brain, liver, and bone metastases were late occurrences in the course of the disease and that most patients had concomitant and usually bulky retroperitoneal metastases** (Johnson et al, 1976; Bredael et al, 1982). Interestingly, autopsy data did not reveal any significant differences in the site or frequency of metastasis between those treated before and after introduction of cisplatin-based chemotherapy (Bredael et al, 1982). **Furthermore, the most common site of late recurrence of both teratoma and viable GCT is the retroperitoneum** (Baniel et al, 1995b). **Late recurrences are usually chemorefractory, and survival rates are poor** (Borge et al, 1988; Baniel et al, 1995b; George et al, 2003; Carver et al, 2005).

RETROPERITONEAL LYMPH NODE DISSECTION
Evolution of Surgical Templates and Techniques

Although RPLND has been well established in the management of NSGCT since 1948, both its role and the surgical template itself have undergone considerable change over the past 30 years.

Either a transabdominal or thoracoabdominal approach to the retroperitoneum for lymph node dissection may be used (Whitmore et al, 1962; Skinner and Leadbetter, 1971; Donohue, 1977). Initially, RPLND included bilateral suprahilar dissections, as well as all the nodal tissue between both ureters down to the bifurcation of the common iliac arteries.

Given the significant limitations in clinical staging at the time, and the absence of other effective therapeutic modalities, emphasis was necessarily placed on extensive dissection of all lymph nodes. Although its therapeutic efficacy was confirmed (Skinner, 1976; Donohue, 1977; Donohue et al, 1993), extensive suprahilar dissection can result in increased pancreatic and renovascular complications. Several studies have confirmed that suprahilar metastases are rare in low-stage NSGCT, and, currently, suprahilar dissections are usually performed for residual hilar or suprahilar masses after cytoreductive chemotherapy for advanced stage NSGCT (Ray et al, 1974; Donohue et al, 1982). In this setting, the most common site of suprahilar disease is in the retrocrural space (Schmeller et al, 1981).

In an effort to reduce surgical perioperative morbidity, bilateral infrahilar RPLND replaced the original suprahilar dissections (see Fig. 30–2) (Donohue et al, 1982, 1993). The procedure was associated with minimal morbidity and a mortality rate less than 1% (Baniel et al, 1994).

The most consistent long-term morbidity of a standard bilateral RPLND has been the loss of antegrade ejaculation and, consequently, potential infertility, owing to damage of sympathetic nerve fibers (Lange et al, 1983, 1984; Jewett et al, 1988). Therefore, patients are advised to complete sperm banking before surgery. The incidence of this complication is related to the extent of the retroperitoneal dissection (Lange et al, 1984; Jewett et al, 1988).

Antegrade ejaculation requires the coordination of three separate events: (1) closure of the bladder neck, (2) seminal emission, and (3) ejaculation. The sympathetic fibers that mediate seminal emission originate primarily from the T12 to L3 thoracolumbar spinal cord. In the midretroperitoneum after leaving the sympathetic trunk, the fibers converge toward the midline and form the hypogastric plexus near the takeoff of the inferior mesenteric artery (IMA) just above the aortic bifurcation. From the hypogastric plexus, the sympathetic fibers travel via the pelvic plexus to innervate the seminal vesicles, vas deferens, prostate, and bladder neck (Fig. 30–4). Ejaculation is mediated by nerves originating at the sacral and lumbar spinal cord levels. Sympathetic fibers tighten the bladder neck, while pudendal somatic innervation from S2 to S4 causes relaxation of the external urethral sphincter and rhythmic contractions of the bulbourethral and perineal muscles (Lange et al, 1983, 1984; Sogani et al, 1991; Sheinfeld, 1994).

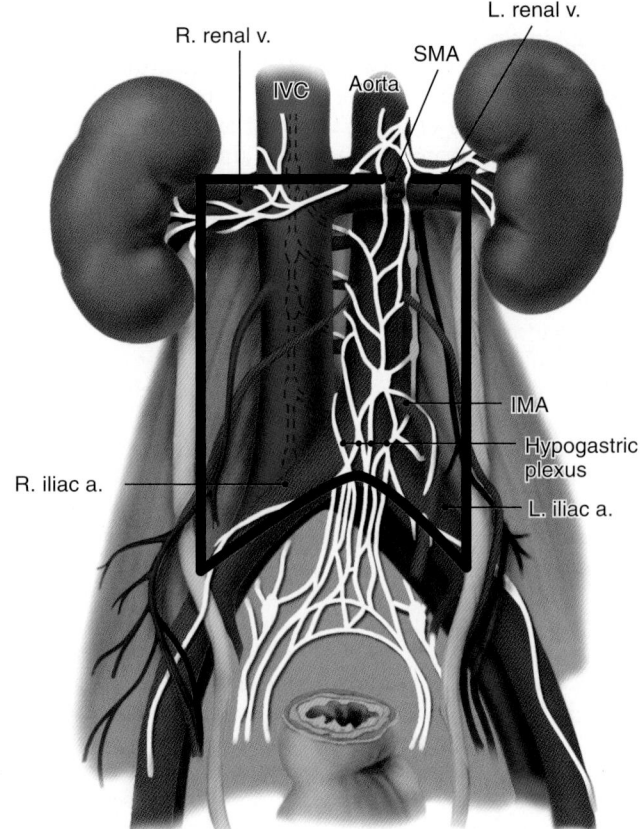

Figure 30–4. Surgical template for bilateral RPLND. IVC, inferior vena cava; SMA, superior mesenteric artery; IMA, inferior mesenteric artery.

An improved understanding of the neuroanatomy of seminal emission and ejaculation, anatomic studies of the distribution of retroperitoneal metastasis for right- and left-sided tumors, and surgical mapping studies (Ray et al, 1974; Donohue et al, 1982; Weissbach et al, 1987) have resulted in further modifications of surgical templates and techniques in an effort to reduce the incidence of ejaculatory dysfunction (Bosl and Motzer, 1997).

As noted, the paravertebral sympathetic ganglia, postganglionic sympathetic fibers T2-L4, and their convergence at the hypogastric plexus are most crucial in the preservation of antegrade ejaculation. Minimizing damage to these structures has resulted in higher rates of ejaculation (Lange et al, 1984; Sheinfeld et al, 1998). Two general approaches have been utilized to protect theses structures: modified template RPLND and, more recently, "nerve-sparing" dissections.

Narayan and coworkers (1982) first reported that modification of surgical boundaries resulted in spontaneous return of ejaculation, with 25 of 55 patients recovering ejaculation at 3 years. Subsequently, a number of investigators have proposed a variety of modified RPLND templates for both right- and left-sided primary tumors with rates of return of ejaculation ranging from 51% to 88% (Fossa et al, 1984; Pizzocaro et al, 1985; Donohue et al, 1990; Richie et al, 1990). Successful preservation of ejaculation is higher for right-sided dissections compared with left-sided ones. In an effort to avoid disrupting the sympathetic nerves and the hypogastric plexus, all modified templates share several goals: (1) to thoroughly resect all interaortocaval and ipsilateral lymph nodes between the level of the renal vessels and the bifurcation of the common iliac artery and (2) to minimize contralateral dissection, particularly below the level of the IMA (Sheinfeld et al, 1998) (Figs. 30–5 and 30–6).

The highest rates of preserved ejaculation are reported with "nerve-sparing" RPLND, in which the sympathetic chains, the postganglionic sympathetic fibers, and the hypogastric plexus are prospectively identified, meticulously dissected, and preserved (Jewett et al, 1988; Donohue et al, 1990). "Nerve-sparing" techniques can be utilized either in the primary or post-chemotherapy setting and within standard bilateral or modified templates, depending on clinical and surgical circumstances; however, **margins of resection should never be compromised in an attempt to maintain ejaculatory function** (Bosl et al, 2000).

Surgical Technique

Strict adherence to basic surgical principles is critical to perform an RPLND safely. First, it is imperative that the surgeon have an in-depth understanding of retroperitoneal anatomy and be able to recognize common variations and their potential implications. Second, excellent exposure of the

retroperitoneum must be ensured to properly set up the RPLND; finally, a thorough lymphadenectomy using meticulous "split and roll" technique should be carried out.

Exposing the Retroperitoneum

Adequate exposure of the retroperitoneum can be accomplished with either a transabdominal or a thoracoabdominal approach.

Thoracoabdominal Approach

The extraperitoneal thoracoabdominal approach to RPLND was originally described by Cooper and colleagues (1950) and later refined and popularized by Skinner and associates (1982). The main advantages of this approach are to allow easier visualization and dissection of the suprahilar lymphatic tissues and less risk of postoperative small bowel obstruction. In addition, simultaneous thoracic procedures can be performed through the same incision.

The patient is placed in the torqued position with the lower extremities and pelvis supine and the chest and upper extremities rotated medially. The operating table is hyperextended to allow exposure and retraction of the rib cage. The incision starts obliquely over the eighth or ninth rib and curves downward as a paramedian toward the pubic ramus. A subperiosteal rib resection is performed, and the ipsilateral rectus muscle is divided. The peritoneum and contents are mobilized

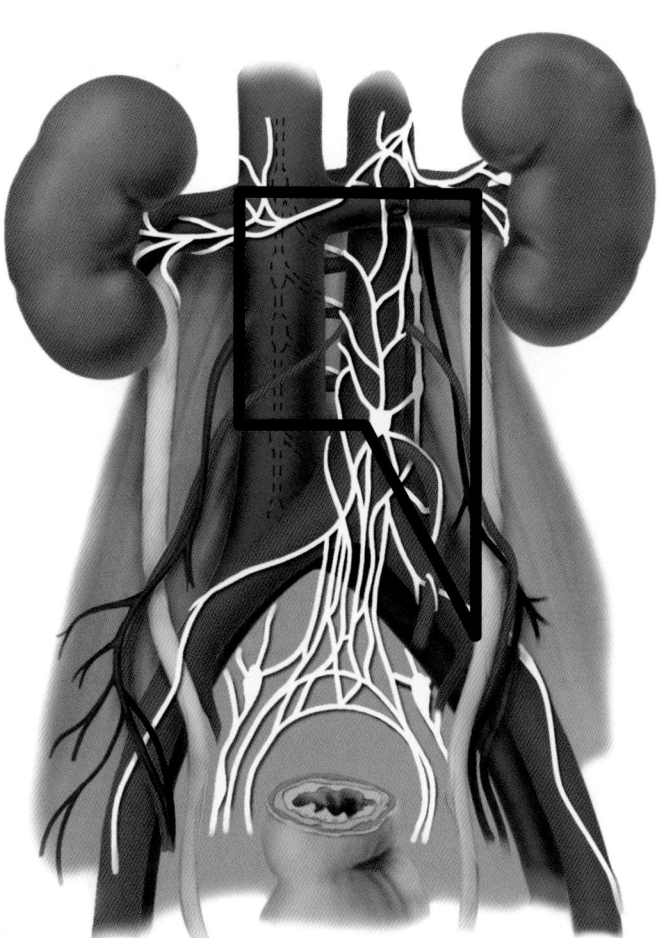

Figure 30–5. Surgical template for modified left-sided RPLND.

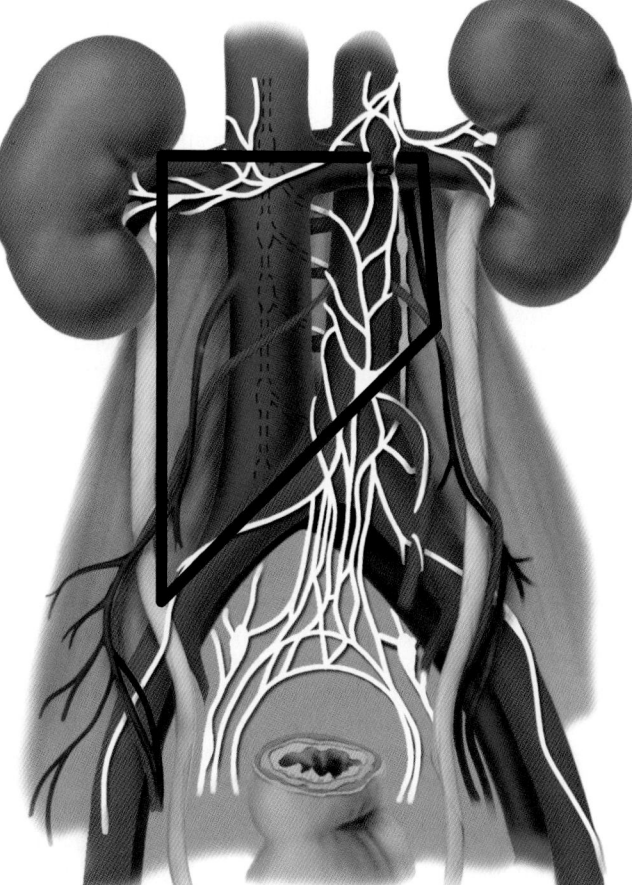

Figure 30–6. Surgical template for modified right-sided RPLND.

from the undersurface of the rectus sheath, and the diaphragm is divided and the pleura is entered. The chest can be inspected and pulmonary or mediastinal procedures performed through the same incision. The retroperitoneum is exposed to the level of the contralateral ureter. Full bilateral RPLND can be carried out as described for the transabdominal approach. In primary RPLND, routine suprahilar dissection is not warranted, because the incidence of suprahilar or retrocrural disease is extremely low. In advanced disease, suprahilar dissection is directed by preoperative imaging studies and intraoperative palpation. The most common site of residual suprahilar disease is in the retrocrural space (Schmeller et al, 1981).

The wound is closed by reapproximation of the diaphragm with silk sutures and of the costal cartilage with Prolene. Chest tube drainage is established, and the flank is closed.

Complications specific to the thoracoabdominal approach are pulmonary in nature, including atelectasis, prolonged chest tube drainage, and increased need for postoperative analgesia. In 1982, Skinner and colleagues described their complications with this technique in 149 patients both before and after chemotherapy. Overall operative mortality was 1.3% with both deaths due to hepatic failure. The overall complication rate was 13%, and major complications included small bowel obstruction, lymphocele, and wound dehiscence (Skinner et al, 1982).

Transabdominal Approach

After successful induction of general endotracheal anesthesia with the patient in the supine position, the skin of the chest wall, abdomen, pubis, genitalia, and upper thighs is prepared. A Foley catheter is placed and connected to closed drainage. A nasogastric tube is placed and connected to intermittent suction.

A midline incision is made from the xipho-costal junction to a point 2 cm above the symphysis pubis. It is carried down through the subcutaneous tissues, and the linea alba and peritoneum are opened. The falciform ligament is either divided between silk ligatures or excised en bloc with the preperitoneal fat. This prevents hepatic capsular tears and allows upward displacement of the liver as the wound edges are spread by two self-retaining Balfour retractors. Careful inspection of the abdomen, retroperitoneum, and pelvis is then carried out to assess resectability and the presence of metastatic disease. The greater omentum and the transverse colon are then displaced superiorly onto the chest between warm moist packs.

The small bowel is reflected to the right, and an incision is made in the posterior peritoneum medial to the inferior mesenteric vein (Fig. 30–7). This incision is continued cephalad to the ligament of Treitz and is extended superiorly and medially to the duodenojejunal flexure, allowing for superior mobilization of the fourth portion of the duodenum and pancreas. The left leaf of the incised posterior peritoneum is further developed, with the colonic mesentery located anteriorly and the para-aortic retroperitoneal space posteriorly (Fig. 30–8). The proper plane of dissection is the avascular plane between the inferior mesenteric vein and the left gonadal vein. This maneuver further defines a thick condensation of fibrovascular tissue (ligament of Treitz) and several large lymphatic trunks, which should be divided between silk sutures, further mobilizing the tail of the pancreas.

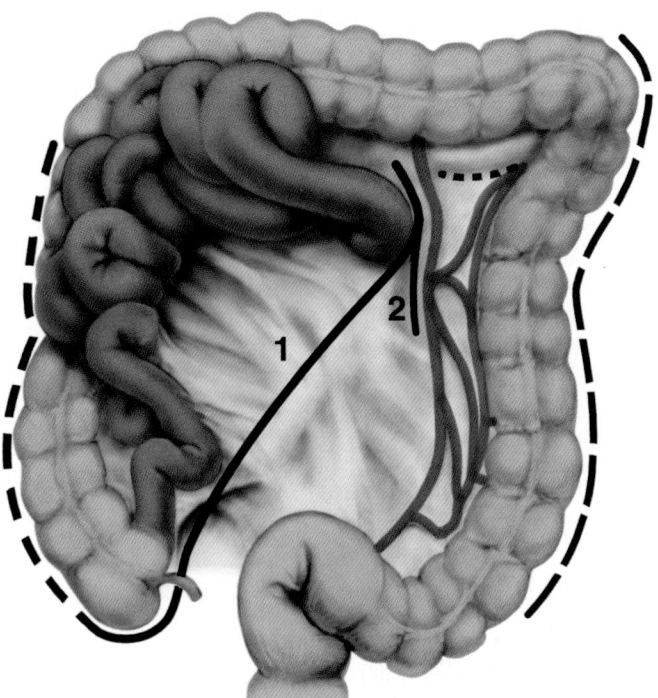

Figure 30–7. Incision of the posterior parietal peritoneum. The incision extends from the ligament of Treitz along the left side of the root of the small bowel mesentery to the ileocecal region (1). It may be extended superiorly and medially to the duodenojejunal flexure and inferolaterally around the cecum and ascending colon. The left leaf of the incised posterior peritoneum is defined (2).

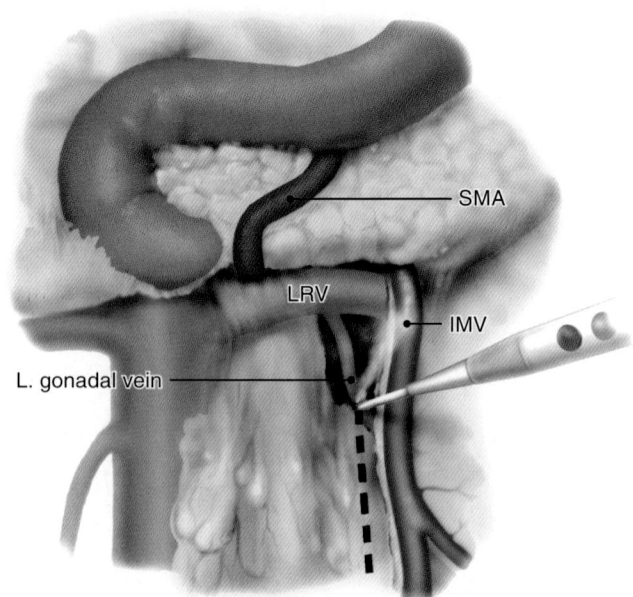

Figure 30–8. Development of the left leaf of the incised posterior peritoneum in the avascular plane between the inferior mesenteric vein (IMV) and the left gonadal vein. The colonic mesentery lies anteriorly and the para-aortic space and Gerota's fascia lie posteriorly. LRV, left renal vein; SMA, superior mesenteric artery.

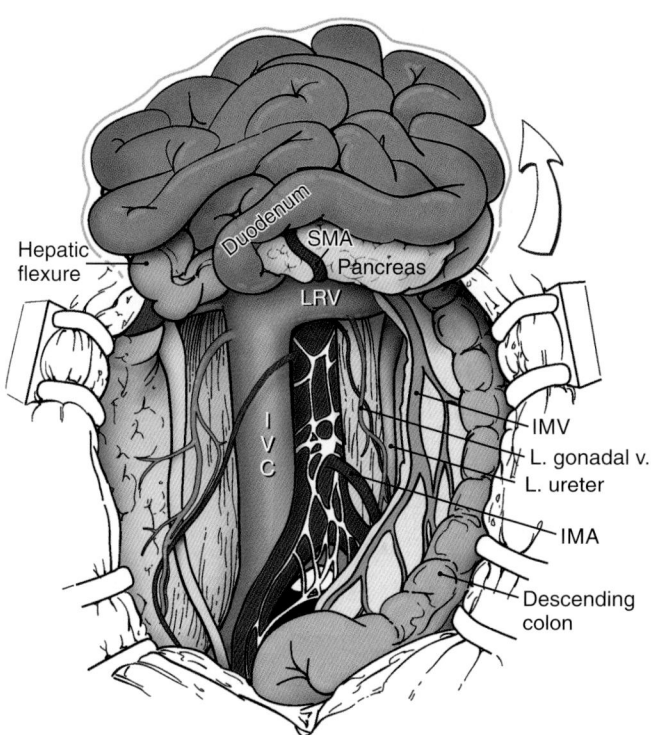

Figure 30–9. The retroperitoneal space has been exposed. The duodenum has been kocherized; its second, third, and fourth portions have been reflected superiorly along with the pancreas and superior mesenteric artery (SMA). The entire right colon has been mobilized and exteriorized. LRV, left renal vein; IMV, inferior mesenteric vein; IVC, inferior vena cava; IMA, inferior mesenteric artery.

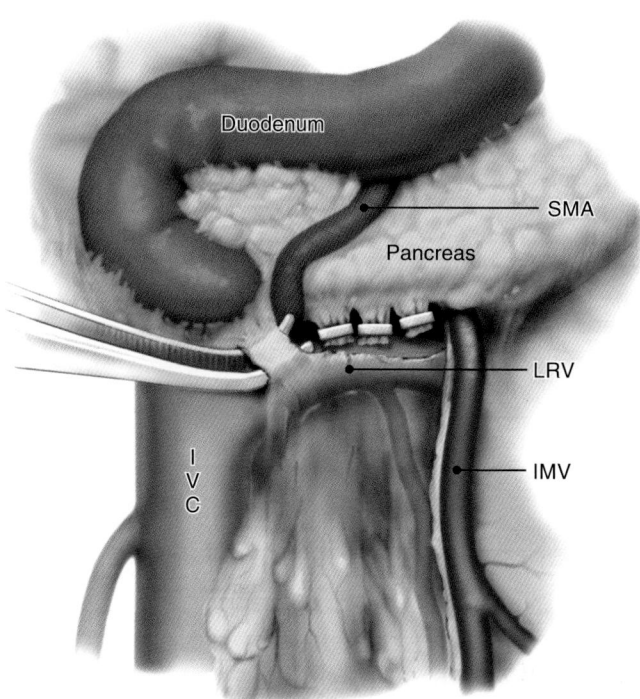

Figure 30–10. Division of attachments between the undersurface of the duodenum and pancreas and the anterior surface of the left renal vein (LRV). It is important to clip or ligate the numerous lymphatic channels in this area. Prominent lacteals in the vicinity of superior mesenteric artery (SMA) are often seen. IMV, inferior mesenteric artery; IVC, inferior vena cava.

Alternatively, to gain adequate exposure in the area of the left renal hilum, particularly with large postchemotherapy masses, the inferior mesenteric vein can be doubly ligated and divided.

The incision in the posterior parietal peritoneum is continued inferiorly along the medial aspect of the small bowel mesentery, lateral to the right gonadal vein and its branches, and extended around the cecum and up the right paracolic gutter to the foramen of Winslow. The duodenum is then kocherized, allowing cephalad reflection and exteriorization of the small bowel, cecum, and right colon onto the chest wall, where they can be either placed in a Lahey bag or protected by moist laparotomy pads (Fig. 30–9). To facilitate retraction of the exteriorized viscera and minimize traction when self-retaining Gallagher and large Deaver retractors are placed, careful and thorough division of attachments between the undersurface of the duodenum and pancreas and the anterior surface of the left renal vein is necessary (Fig. 30–10). It is also important to ligate or clip the numerous lymphatic vessels in this area to minimize postoperative lymphatic complications. In placing self-retaining retractors, great care must be taken in identifying the superior mesenteric artery (SMA) to avoid vascular compromise of the small bowel. Periodic inspection of small bowel color or SMA pulsation is prudent. These maneuvers allow for excellent exposure of the retroperitoneal space from the level of the right and left suprahilar areas distally to the bifurcation of the right common iliac artery. Additional exposure of the distal left para-aortic and left parailiac space can be accomplished by further extending the incision in the left leaf of the parietal peritoneum inferiorly and, if nec-

essary, sacrificing the IMA. Alternatively, the left colon can be reflected medially by incising the left white line of Toldt and developing the plane between the colonic mesentery and the anterior surface of Gerota's fascia.

Setting Up the RPLND

Injury to important structures can be avoided by being aware of the following structures: the SMA and IMA, the pancreas, the renal vessels, and the ureters. Up to 20% of patients will have accessory renal arteries, and approximately 2% to 3% of patients will have a retroaortic left renal vein. It is particularly important to recognize a retroaortic left renal vein because it may be inadvertently mistaken for a lumbar vein and ligated or, as the surgeon extends the cephalad dissection in search of the left renal vein, the pancreas and SMA may be injured. In the absence of a normally positioned left renal vein, the attachments of the undersurface of the pancreas and duodenum may lie directly on the aorta.

Soft vessel loops are placed around the ureters as they are retracted laterally, and their medial aspect defines the lateral margins of resection. The ipsilateral gonadal vein is mobilized from its insertion in the IVC (right) or left renal vein (left) to the internal ring. It is important to encompass all the branches as well as the fibroalveolar and lymphatic tissue surrounding the gonadal vessels to avoid late paracolic recurrences from incomplete excision of the spermatic cord (Chang et al, 2002c).

Lymphadenectomy

Attention is initially directed to the left renal vein, and the renal perivascular lymphatic tissue is mobilized inferiorly. The anterior surface of the aorta is thus exposed. Then adrenal, spermatic, and lumbar branches are tied with 3-0 silk and divided. The dissection along the anterior surface of the left renal vein continues to the right until the anterior surface of the IVC is encountered, and the first anterior "split" is then performed. The split and roll technique is illustrated in Figure 30–11. The right gonadal vein is ligated at the vena cava. Lymphatic tissue can then be rolled off the IVC laterally and medially as the dissection proceeds inferiorly. Lumbar veins are dissected, doubly ligated with 3-0 silk, and divided. At this point, nerve-sparing techniques can be performed if clinically indicated (see later).

Having secured control of the postganglionic sympathetic fibers with soft vessel loops as they course medially under the IVC to the anterior surface of the aorta, they are then retracted laterally. The anterior split on the surface of the aorta should then be carried inferiorly to the bifurcation of the common iliac arteries. The origin of the IMA is identified. If necessary, this artery can be sacrificed without detrimental effects, provided the marginal colonic artery is intact. The gonadal arteries should be ligated early to prevent the subadventitial hematoma that may result if they are avulsed. Following the anterior aortic split, lymphatic tissue is retracted medially and laterally and lumbar arteries are dissected, doubly ligated with 3-0 silk, and divided. At this point, the aorta and IVC have been separated from the retroperitoneal lymphatic tissue, which is attached to the posterior body wall and the renal arteries. The right and left renal arteries are skeletonized, and the lymphatic tissue is separated from the psoas fascia and anterior spinous ligament, which are the posterior limits of dissection. Great care should be taken to control lumbar vessels as they pass into the posterior body wall near the sympathetic chains to avoid possible injury to sympathetic innervation in attempting to control problematic bleeding.

Throughout the procedure it is important to ligate or clip the cut ends of lymphatic vessels, particularly in the region of the right renal artery, where large tributaries to the cisternae chyli are located.

Modified templates using these techniques may be used if clinically indicated; however, surgical margins should never be compromised in an effort to preserve ejaculation. Furthermore, in the face of documented or suspected metastatic disease in a primary RPLND, a full bilateral dissection remains the standard.

At the completion of a bilateral dissection, the aorta, IVC, and renal vessels should be skeletonized and the anterior spinous ligament visible, as are the stumps of the right and left gonadal vessels and IMA.

The area of dissection is thoroughly irrigated with warm water, and lymphostasis and hemostasis must be ensured. The bowel and mesentery are inspected for injury, as are the kidneys and ureters. Indigo carmine may be instilled to rule out a urinary leak if ureteral integrity is in doubt. The posterior parietal peritoneum is loosely approximated with interrupted 3-0 silk sutures to minimize the risk of small bowel obstruction and prevent direct adherence of bowel to the anterior surface of a great vessel. The fascia is closed in a single layer with interrupted 1-0 PDS sutures.

Most postoperative patients can usually be extubated immediately after surgery and are managed with nasogastric tube drainage until ileus resolves. **Postoperative tachycardia is common due to sympathetic discharge.** Fluid requirements are monitored closely, and third space volume losses replaced as indicated. Diet is resumed when bowel activity returns, and volume status is monitored by pulmonary examination, net fluid balance, and daily weights. The remainder of the postoperative care is routine, with average hospital stays of 5 to 7 days.

Prospective Nerve-Sparing Techniques

Appropriate candidates for nerve-sparing techniques include patients with clinical stage I and low-volume stage II NSGCT undergoing primary RPLND, as well as a carefully selected subset of patients undergoing post-chemotherapy lymphadenectomy.

The most important aspect in performing nerve-sparing RPLND is the prospective identification and preservation of relevant sympathetic nerves, specifically (1) the sympathetic chains bilaterally; (2) the postganglionic sympathetic nerves arising from the sympathetic chains; and (3) the hypogastric

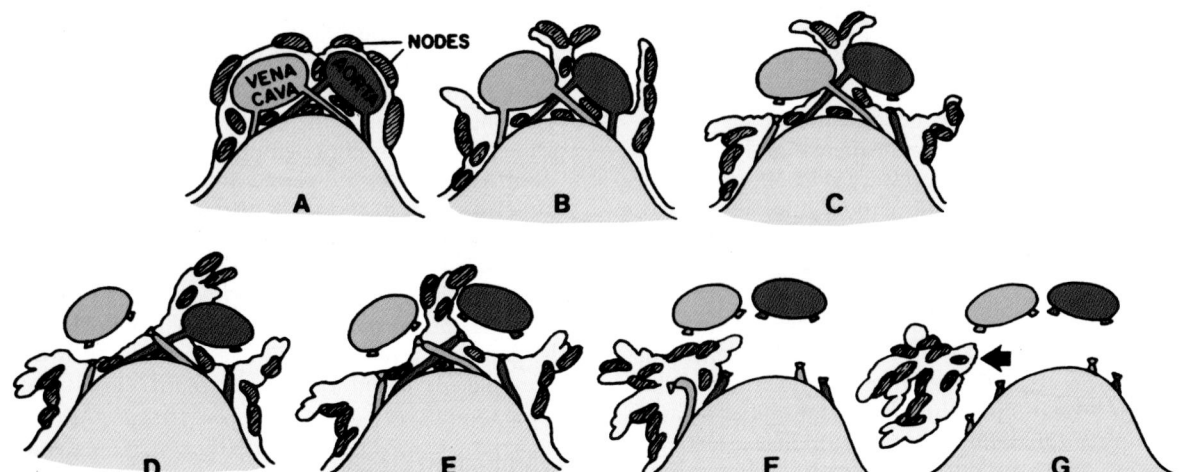

Figure 30–11. **A** to **G,** Sequentially, this diagram shows the "split and roll" technique that allows for en bloc removal of the nodal package. The lumbar vessels must be divided twice, first at the wall of the great vessels and again as they enter the foramina alongside the vertebral bodies.

plexus, which is the anastomosing network of nerve fibers anterior to the lower aorta (Fig. 30–12).

The sympathetic chains run parallel to the great vessels on either side of the spine. On the left side, the sympathetic chain is lateral and posterior to the lateral border of the aorta (see Fig. 30–10) and postganglionic fibers leave at an oblique angle transversing lymphatic tissue posterolateral to the aorta as they join the hypogastric plexus (Klein et al, 1995). On the right side the sympathetic chain lies posterior to the IVC and the postganglionic fibers emerge from the medial edge of the vena cava and course at an oblique angle anterior to the aorta to join the hypogastric plexus. **Therefore, it is important to note that an anterior "split" maneuver over the IVC does not damage these fibers; however, dissection along the aorta before isolating and preserving these nerves individually results in their disruption** (Klein et al, 1995).

It appears that the most important nerves to preserve antegrade ejaculation are those arising from the L3 and L4 ganglia. It is often possible to preserve three or four separate nerve trunks. Nerve fibers often exit in close proximity to lumbar vessels, and great care must be taken in ligating them to avoid injury to these delicate fibers.

These nerves are dissected free of surrounding fibrofatty and lymphatic tissue, encircled with soft vessel loops, and gently retracted out of harm's way. The lymphadenectomy then proceeds as just described within the appropriate template. Again, when performing nerve-sparing RPLND, dissection on the aorta should be done only after the nerve fibers have been isolated and protected. Proper nerve-sparing techniques result in greater than 95% rates of antegrade ejaculation.

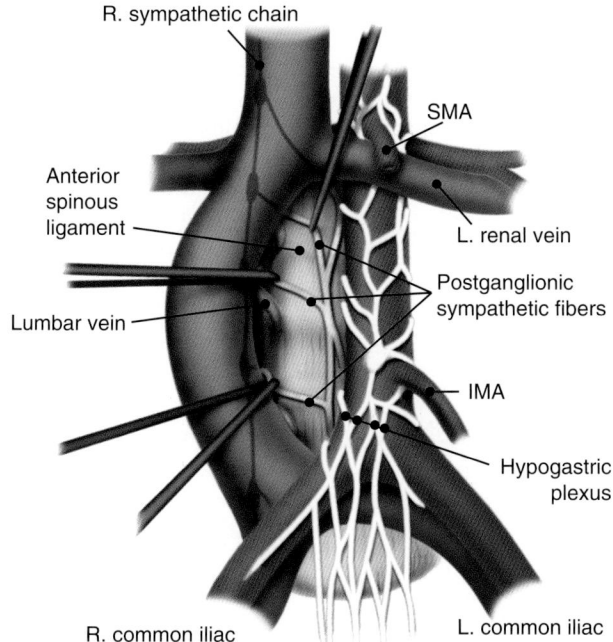

Figure 30–12. Nerve-sparing technique with soft vascular tapes around the right postganglionic branches of the sympathetic chains as they course in an oblique fashion toward the hypogastric plexus. Their relationship to the great vessels, lumbar veins, and root of the inferior mesenteric artery (IMA) is shown. SMA, superior mesenteric artery.

Intraoperative Neurostimulation

Several investigators have reported the use of intraoperative electrical stimulation of individual postganglionic sympathetic fibers to identify the most important nerves for antegrade emission (Recker and Tscholl, 1993; Kell and Jewett, 1999). Bladder neck closure and seminal emission can be documented endoscopically.

Laparoscopic RPLND (L-RPLND)

In an effort to reduce the perioperative morbidity, improve cosmesis, and shorten convalescence, minimally invasive techniques have been utilized to perform retroperitoneal surgery since the early 1990s. This has been possible because of dramatic improvement in camera, video, and imaging technologies, as well as the introduction of automated suturing devices, microstaples, and tissue adhesives such as fibrin glue.

L-RPLND is a technically demanding procedure that should be undertaken only by very experienced laparoscopic surgeons who are also comfortable and adept with advanced vascular techniques in the event of an open conversion. The indications for L-RPLND in low-stage NSCGT are the same as those for open primary RPLND, namely, clinical stage I or IIA, negative serum tumor, and the absence of comorbidities that would preclude safe surgery, such as a bleeding diathesis. After chemotherapy, L-RPLND has been limited to unifocal small-volume residual masses.

Preoperative Patient Preparation

All patients considered candidates for L-RPLND must be fully informed of all treatment options, including open RPLND and surveillance. All potential complications, including bleeding requiring blood transfusion, injury to adjacent organs (liver, bowel, kidney, pancreas), and orthopedic, neurologic, or pulmonary complications, as well as conversion to open surgery due to complications or incomplete resection, should be discussed (Winfield et al, 2000). Patients are encouraged to undergo preoperative sperm banking. To reduce the risk of chylous ascites, patients are started on a low-fat diet 2 weeks before surgery. Patients undergo a mechanical bowel preparation the afternoon before surgery and take only clear liquids until midnight. Broad-spectrum antibiotics are administered before starting the operation, and sequential antiembolic pneumatic boots are placed on the lower extremities.

Patient Positioning

General anesthesia is obtained, and a nasogastric tube and a Foley catheter are placed. The patient is placed in a modified lateral position (60 degrees) with elevation of the ipsilateral side. This position allows the surgeon to change between the flank and supine position by just rotating the table. The patient is secured to the table, and all pressure points are adequately padded. Preparing and draping the patient includes the entire middle from the xiphoid to the symphysis pubis. An open laparotomy tray with vascular instruments should be available in the room in the event of an open conversion. The use of a robot for the camera allows the assistant to be positioned behind the patient, thus giving the primary surgeon more working space. The video equipment is placed behind the patient, and the second screen for the assistant is behind the primary surgeon.

Transperitoneal Approach

Although some laparoscopic surgeons use an extraperitoneal approach (Le Blanc et al, 2001), most favor the transperitoneal route. Access into the peritoneal cavity is accomplished either by Veress needle or open Hasson technique. Once the pneumoperitoneum is established, the camera trocar is placed in the umbilicus. Three 10-mm trocars are then placed under vision: two pararectally above and below the umbilicus and the third one more laterally. Alternatively, all trocars may be placed in the midline equally spaced, beginning 2 cm below the xiphoid and extending 3 cm above the pubic symphysis.

The surgical template for the procedure is dictated by laterality and intraoperative findings. Surgical margins should not be compromised to minimize morbidity, preserve ejaculation or due to technical constraints.

Right-Sided L-RPLND

After placement of the ports, the operating table is rotated and the patient is brought almost to the flank position with the right side elevated. The ascending colon is mobilized medially by incising along the white line of Toldt from the pelvis around the hepatic flexure to Winslow's foramen. The second portion of the duodenum is then kocherized, providing wide exposure of the entire IVC as well as the renal veins and aorta below the level of the SMA.

Dissection of the Gonadal Vessels. The lymphatic tissue overlying the IVC is split medially from the level of the renal veins until the crossing of the right ureter. Great care should be taken during this maneuver to identify potential accessory renal arteries anterior to the IVC. During the ventral split, the insertion of the right spermatic vein into the IVC is identified, immediately clipped, and transected before significant manipulation, thereby minimizing the potential of a pseudoaneurysm. The spermatic artery is clipped and transected. The dissection then follows the spermatic vein, encompassing all the surrounding nodal and fibroadipose tissue down to the spermatic cord stump in the internal inguinal ring. The ureter should be identified to prevent injury as the gonadal vessels cross anteriorly. The vas deferens is clipped medial to the external iliac vessels. The specimen is retrieved in an entrapment bag (Endocatch, U.S. Surgical Inc., Norwalk, CT).

Lymphadenectomy. Lymph node dissection includes the right iliac, paracaval, interaortocaval, and preaortic nodes. Extension of the template to the para-aortic nodes is possible. As a first step the left border of the dissection is defined. The area from the crossing of the ureter with the iliac vessels in the lymphatic tissue along the common iliac artery is divided, and the incision is carried out on the anterior surface of the aorta up to the renal vein. If the dissection is limited to the preaortic nodes, the incision above the IMA is carried on the left side of the aorta.

The lymphatic tissue is rolled from the aorta medially until the level of the lumbar arteries is reached. If the para-aortic nodes are going to be removed, the lumbar arteries are clipped and transected and the dorsal lymphatic tissue split, the longitudinal incision behind the aorta is then made. Then the lymphatic tissue cranial to the IMA is rolled laterally until the lumbar vessels are reached again.

Lower pole arteries are present in approximately 20% of cases, and care is needed to identify and preserve them. The para-aortic lymphatic tissue can now be rolled laterally until it is fixed to the sympathic chain only by postganglionic fibers and by lumbar vessels that pass into the posterior body wall. These vessels are clipped carefully, and then the specimen is entrapped in an organ bag and either immediately delivered or stored inside and delivered at the end of the operation.

It is important to do most of the left-sided dissection early in the procedure to prevent problems with exposure secondary to bowel distention. Before the interaortocaval nodes can be removed, the right renal artery must be dissected from its origin as far as possible behind the IVC. The ventral split on the IVC has already been done and tissue from the IVC is rolled medially down to the level of the lumbar veins. Clipping and dividing of the lumbar vessels allows dissection of the retrocaval lymphatic tissue. Without clipping the lumbar veins the posterior split behind the cava is more difficult.

After the posterior split has been performed, the tissue is released from its attachments to the spine. On the most cranial borders of the dissection care has to be taken to achieve lymphostasis with clips or ligature device to minimize the risks of lymphatic complications. The interaortocaval tissue can now be removed. Again, the specimen is placed in an organ bag and removed either immediately or at the end of the operation.

Before the paracaval nodes can be removed, the ureter as the lateral border is followed in its full length, from the crossing with the common iliac artery up to the renal pelvis. The renal hilum is defined, and the lymphatic tissue is rolled laterally from the cava until the region of the dorsal split is reached and the vena caval resection can be completed. At this point the lymphatic tissue is fixed to the sympathetic chain. After dissection of the postganglionic fibers the specimen can be entrapped and all specimens are retrieved.

After control of the operating field the bowel contents are brought back to their anatomic position. The table is rotated, bringing the patient to the supine position. The right colonic flexure is fixed with one interrupted suture. The trocar sites are closed with fascial sutures. Drains are not used.

Left-Sided L-RPLND

Exposure of the Retroperitoneum. The peritoneum is incised lateral to the descending colon along the colonic flexure. The splenocolic ligament is incised, and the mesocolon is swept medially from the anterior aspect of Gerota's fascia using blunt dissection. The tail of the pancreas is carefully dissected and swept medially, and the retroperitoneum is exposed. Wide exposure is mandatory to achieve a complete and safe lymph node dissection.

Excision of the Gonadal Vein. The first step is the dissection of the left renal vein, thus marking the cranial border of dissection. The spermatic vein is clipped and transected at its insertion into the renal vein. The gonadal vein is dissected caudally together with the surrounding lymphatic tissue. The spermatic artery is either clipped or coagulated and transected. Special care when using cautery has to be taken at the level of the spermatic vessels and the ureter to prevent thermal injury of the ureter. The spermatic vessels are followed caudally to the inguinal ring, and the ligature of the previous orchiectomy is reached. The specimen is entrapped in an organ bag and removed.

Lymphadenectomy. The lymph node dissection includes the left iliac, the preaortic, and the para-aortic lymph nodes. Extension of the template with excision of the interaortocaval nodes is possible.

The renal vein has already been dissected. The lymphatic tissue overlying the aorta is clipped and divided beneath the renal vein and then split in a caudal direction along the right side of the aorta down to the IMA. At this point the dissection moves to the anterior side of the aorta and along the iliac artery down to the level of the ureter. This anterior split defines the right border of dissection. Following the ureter upward until the kidney is reached again defines the left border of dissection.

The preaortic lymphatic tissue is rolled laterally down to the lumbar arteries. Again, special care has to be taken to preserve lower pole renal vessels. The renal artery, the upper border of dissection, is completely freed from the surrounding tissue. Usually, the descending lumbar vein draining posteriorly into the renal vein has to be transected to achieve good exposure of the renal artery. Once the lumbar vessels are reached they should be either transected or completely freed from the surrounding lymphatic tissue, allowing the dorsal split behind the aorta to be completed. The lymphatic tissue is rolled laterally, and special care should be taken when approaching the sympathetic chain, as the lumbar vessels extend into the posterior body wall. After transection of the postganglionic fibers, the specimen is removed within an organ bag, regardless of tumor volume (Nelson et al, 1999; Bianchi et al, 1999).

Prospective Nerve-Sparing Techniques

As in open RPLND, the nerve-sparing technique involves prospectively identifying, dissecting, and preserving the sympathetic chains, hypogastric plexus, and the postganglionic sympathetic fibers before any split along the aorta. On the right side, the postganglionic sympathetic fibers are most easily identified behind the IVC as they cross anterior to the aorta to insert in the hypogastric plexus. Their takeoff from the sympathetic chains is always near lumbar veins, so great care should be taken in clipping lumbar vessels. On the left side, it is easiest to identify the postganglionic sympathetic nerves at the ganglia, as they leave the sympathetic chain, and then dissect them prospectively as they course anterior to the aorta before joining the hypogastric plexus. Care should be taken to avoid cautery when dissecting nerve fibers (Peschel et al, 2002).

Bilateral L-RPLND

The indications for bilateral templates are the same as for open RPLND, with repositioning and additional trocar placement as necessary. Prospective nerve-sparing techniques are possible using the principles described earlier.

Complications

Meticulous lymphostasis and a low-fat diet perioperatively have reduced the incidence of chylous ascites, which initially approached 20%. Retrograde ejaculation is reported in 2% to 5% of cases. Most cases of intraoperative bleeding can be controlled laparoscopically by experienced surgeons, and open conversion rates range from 2% to 5%. Fibrin glue is reported to be effective in controlling venous bleeding. The incidence of injury to adjacent viscera, particularly bowel, is approximately 1% to 2%.

The morbidity and open conversion rate of L-RPLND after chemotherapy is significantly higher. The major complication rate reported in the Johns Hopkins experience was 57%, including transection of the external iliac artery requiring grafting, duodenal perforation, and two renal artery injuries requiring either nephrectomy or grafting (Palese et al, 1999). Rassweiler and associates (1996) converted seven (78%) of nine post-chemotherapy stage II patients; however, more recently, Steiner and colleagues (2003) reported no open conversions in 57 post-chemotherapy L-RPLND cases.

Results and Current Status

At the present time, L-RPLND is a diagnostic procedure; however, its role as a therapeutic operation for low-stage NSGCT is very controversial. On the positive side, after a lengthy and steep learning curve, in the hands of dedicated experts (Bosl et al, 2005), are quicker convalescence and more favorable cosmetic results, less postoperative pain and morbidity, and reduced operative blood loss and length of hospital stay. **Unfortunately, the therapeutic efficacy remains difficult to assess for several reasons. First of all, virtually all patients with positive nodes (pathologic stage II) received postoperative chemotherapy following L-RPLND, regardless of tumor volume** (Nelson et al, 1999, Bianchi et al, 1999). In the combined experience of four of the largest published series in the English literature comprising 144 patients, only three patients with positive retroperitoneal lymph nodes did *not* receive postoperative chemotherapy; and one of these three relapsed in the retroperitoneum outside the limits of a modified template (Janetschek et al, 2000; Nelson et al, 1999; Carver, 2004).

Secondly, it is unclear whether L-RPLND has been performed with therapeutic intent (Sheinfeld, 2004). One report noted that "the dissection was limited if grossly positive nodes were encountered," and the total number of nodes resected was significantly different if the nodes were positive or negative (14 ± 2 and 25 ± 3, respectively) (Nelson et al, 1999). A second group reports that "laparoscopic RPLND is used for diagnostic purposes only and patients with positive nodes are definitively treated with adjuvant chemotherapy" (Janetschek et al, 1999).

Thirdly, the suggested boundaries of resection in most series appear too restrictive, particularly in the presence of positive nodes. Omitting the pre- and para-aortic lymph nodes in a right modified template and the interaortocaval nodes in a left modified template is not prudent and has resulted in the necessity for reoperative surgery and late relapse when done in the open setting for pathologic state II NSGCT. **Despite their inherent limitations, all mapping studies demonstrate increased multifocality and contralat-**

eral disease in the presence of positive retroperitoneal nodes (Ray et al, 1973; Donohue et al, 1982; Weissbach et al, 1987). **The liberal use of chemotherapy will not necessarily prevent relapses and compensate for incomplete resection.** The recommendation to delete the dissection behind the great vessels and posterior to lumbar vessels is based on the absence of relapse in chemotherapy-treated patients in whom it is impossible to assess the presence of disease prior to therapy (Höltl et al, 2002; Carver, 2004). One of us (GB) continues to resect all tissue behind the great vessels. A valid comparison of open versus L-RPLND would require comparable templates.

Finally, the absence of retroperitoneal relapse in patients with pathologic stage I (pN0) does not prove "oncologic efficacy," since these patients were cured at the time of the radical orchiectomy (Carver et al, 2004). A less complete dissection might be expected to be associated with a higher rate of local recurrence. Larger number of patients with comparable clinical and pathologic findings, identical templates for RPLND and indications for chemotherapy will be necessary to explore this issue.

In the postchemotherapy setting, the conversion rates to open surgery in some initial reports were high and the postoperative morbidity was significant (Rasweiler et al, 1996; Palese et al, 2002). More recently Steiner and associates (2003) reported no open conversions and minimal morbidity in a series of 57 carefully selected patients with low-volume residual masses. Following chemotherapy, RPLND should be undertaken in a formal study by surgeons highly experienced in laparoscopic techniques who apply the same criteria regarding patient selection, surgical templates, and perioperative management.

Treatment Options for Low-Stage GCTs

Clinical Stage I NSGCT

RPLND. In the United States and parts of Europe the conventional approach to patients with clinical stage I NSGCT has been bilateral RPLND, and it remains the standard against which all diagnostic and therapeutic alternatives must be judged (Whitmore, 1983; Hesketh et al, 1990; Chang and Sheinfeld, 2000). **As noted earlier, RPLND (1) provides the most accurate N categorization of the retroperitoneal lymph nodes that are the first site of metastatic spread in approximately 90% of GCT and (2) is curative in the majority of patients with pathologic stage I (pN0) and low-volume retroperitoneal disease (pN1) and avoids the persistence of chemorefractory teratoma in the retroperitoneum** (Sheinfeld et al, 2003a). **Relapses in the retroperitoneum are rare in the hands of experienced surgeons, after properly performed RPLND. Primary RPLND is associated with negligible mortality and minimal morbidity rates** (Baniel et al, 1994).

Nerve-sparing techniques should be considered the operation of choice and surgical templates determined by clinical and intraoperative findings. Surgical margins should not be compromised in an attempt to preserve ejaculation, and if positive nodes are noted at the time of RPLND, a bilateral dissection is warranted, particularly for right-sided primary tumors, because contralateral crossover is more common than for left-sided primaries.

Surveillance. The strategy of surveillance after orchiectomy was first reported by Peckham in 1979. The rationale for surveillance protocols rests with the improved accuracy of clinical staging, the ability of cisplatin-based chemotherapy to cure early relapses, the probability of surgical cure after radical orchiectomy alone, and the possible infertility resulting from RPLND due to retrograde ejaculation (Sheinfeld, 1994; Bosl et al, 2000, 2005).

Approximately 25% of patients with T1N0M0 disease and normal serum tumor markers experience relapse while on surveillance protocols (Hoskin et al, 1986; Swanson et al, 1993; Lashley and Lowe, 1998; Sogani et al, 1998). **The retroperitoneum is the most common site of relapse; the lungs or markers alone occur less frequently, and other visceral metastases are rare.** Survival rates after therapy for surveillance failures range from 96% to 100% (Hoskin et al, 1986; Swanson et al, 1993; Lashley and Lowe, 1998; Sogani et al, 1998).

A number of factors predictive for retroperitoneal and/or systemic failure have been identified. The presence of lymphovascular invasion within the primary tumor (now included as T2), higher T stage (T2 to T4) (i.e., tumor involvement of the cord, capsule, or scrotum), and a high percentage of embryonal carcinoma are associated with a higher likelihood of relapse (Read et al, 1992; Gels et al, 1995; Nicolai et al, 1995; Heidenreich et al, 1998; Sogani et al, 1998). Approximately 50% of patients with T2 to T4 tumors experience relapse, compared with 15% of patients with T1 tumors. A study from Memorial Sloan-Kettering Cancer Center (MSKCC) noted that almost 80% of patients with clinical stage I and pure embryonal carcinoma who underwent RPLND had pathologic stage II disease (Pohar et al, 2003).

Patient compliance cannot be overemphasized, and strict adherence to periodic follow-up evaluations is critical. Most relapses occur within the first 2 years and are rare after 5 years (Bosl et al, 2005).

Chemotherapy. In an attempt to avoid the potential morbidity of an RPLND, several European groups have studied the role of two cycles of cisplatin-based adjuvant chemotherapy in high-risk clinical stage I NSGCT (Oliver et al, 1992; Cullen et al, 1995; Studer et al, 2000). Although less than 5% of these patients experience relapse, they are exposed to both the short- and long-term toxicities of chemotherapy, such as myelosuppression, neuropathy, Raynaud's phenomenon, ototoxicity, nephrotoxicity, and the risk of acute leukemia. Furthermore, given the paucity of long-term follow-up, the risk of late relapse secondary to unresected chemoresistant teratoma remains unknown.

Investigators at MSKCC reported a 21% incidence of teratoma in patients with pathologic stage II disease, including 6 of 64 (9%) with clinical stage I (Sheinfeld et al, 2003a). Although teratomatous elements in the orchiectomy specimen predict for teratoma in retroperitoneal metastasis, its absence in the primary tumor does not preclude its presence in the retroperitoneum (Toner et al, 1990; Foster et al, 1998; Beck et al, 2002; Sheinfeld et al, 2003a).

Clinical Stage IS ("Marker Only" Disease)

Patients with persistently elevated serum tumor markers after radical orchiectomy but negative CT scans of the chest, abdomen, and pelvis should undergo primary cisplatin-

based chemotherapy because systemic disease is usually present. Davis and coworkers (1994) reported that all 11 patients with "marker only" disease who underwent primary RPLND had persistently elevated markers postoperatively. Saxman and associates (1996) also reported a high rate of systemic failures in patients with "serologic disease" only after initial surgery. An RPLND should be performed if there is radiographic evidence of retroperitoneal disease after chemotherapy.

Clinical Stage II NSGCT

The decision to treat patients with clinical stage II NSGCT initially with either RPLND or cisplatin-based chemotherapy depends primarily on (1) extent of disease, (2) serum tumor marker status, and (3) presence or absence of tumor-related back pain (Bosl and Motzer, 1997).

RPLND. Patients best suited for RPLND are those with clinical stage IIA and some IIB tumors with ipsilateral disease restricted to the primary landing zone and normal serum tumor markers (Bosl and Motzer, 1997; Bosl et al, 2005). **The presence of suprahilar, retrocrural, pelvic, or inguinal lymphadenopathy, contralateral or multifocal disease, or back pain implies either unresectable disease or metastases beyond the locoregional lymph nodes, and these patients should receive initial cisplatin-based chemotherapy** (Bosl et al, 2005).

Patients with clinical IIA or IIB tumors and elevated serum levels of tumor markers should be considered for primary cisplatin-based chemotherapy, because this usually reflects systemic disease (Sheinfeld et al, 2004). Investigators at MSKCC reported that the finding of elevated serum levels of tumor markers before RPLND was the most predictive factor for (1) systemic relapse in patients with low-volume (pN1) retroperitoneal disease treated without adjuvant chemotherapy and (2) for persistent NSGCT (usually persistent marker elevation) despite complete resection of high-volume (pN2, pN3) retroperitoneal disease (Rabbani et al, 1999a,b; Sheinfeld et al, 1999a,b; Bosl et al, 2000; Stephenson et al, 2005).

A study of 453 patients who underwent primary RPLND at MSKCC showed that by excluding patients whose markers fail to normalize or who were clinical stage IIB after 1999, the proportion of pathologic stage II patients with low-volume (pN1) retroperitoneal disease increased significantly (40% before vs. 64% after 1999, $P = .01$) without significantly affecting the rate of retroperitoneal teratoma (21% vs. 22%, $P = .89$) or pathologic stage I (56% vs. 67%, $P = .06$). For patients who did *not* receive chemotherapy, the 4-year progression-free probability improved significantly from 83% before 1999 to 96% after 1999. Consequently, for patients with normal serum tumor markers and clinical stage I-IIA tumors, the low rate of systemic progression and the 22% incidence of retroperitoneal teratoma support the therapeutic role of RPLND (Stephenson et al, 2005).

Adjuvant Chemotherapy

After RPLND, a meticulous pathologic assessment of the retroperitoneal lymph nodes is essential to assess prognosis and direct further therapy (Motzer and Bosl, 1993). With the exception of the Testicular Cancer Intergroup Study, most

investigators have reported that the risk of relapse is related to the size and/or number of involved lymph nodes (Motzer and Bosl, 1993; Sheinfeld et al, 1994). Careful observation is preferred in compliant patients with fully resected low-volume (pN1) disease, that is, fewer than five positive nodes *and* all nodes less than 2 cm with no evidence of extranodal extension, because these patients have a low risk of relapse (Pizzocaro et al, 1985; Richie et al, 1991; Rabbani et al, 2001). Three cycles of cisplatin, etoposide, and bleomycin (PEB) or four cycles of etoposide and cisplatin (EP) will be necessary in the event of relapse.

Conversely, patients with high-volume nodal disease have a relapse rate of 50% to 90% (Fraley et al, 1985; Williams et al, 1987; Donohue et al, 1995); therefore, patients with at least 6 positive nodes, any node greater than 2 cm, or any extranodal extension should be considered for two cycles of adjuvant cisplatin-based chemotherapy.

The randomized Testicular Cancer Intergroup Study showed that in patients with pathologic stage II NSGCT, observation with standard treatment at relapse and two cycles of adjuvant chemotherapy had equivalent survival rates (Williams et al, 1987). A number of cisplatin-based regimens have proven efficacy in preventing relapse after RPLND (Williams et al, 1987; Weissbach et al, 1991). The PEB regimen is favored by the Indiana Group, but Kondagunta and coworkers (2005) showed that treatment with etoposide and cisplatin was adequate in preventing relapse in patients with resected high-volume disease.

It is important to note that only patients who are completely resected and are clinically free of disease after RPLND are candidates for two cycles of cisplatin-based chemotherapy to prevent relapse. The management of patients with incompletely resected adenopathy or with any clinical evidence of disease (elevated β-hCG and/or AFP, lung nodule, retrocrural adenopathy) is the same as that for patients with systemic metastasis: three or four cycles of cisplatin-based chemotherapy (Motzer et al, 1993).

Fertility in Low-Stage Germ Cell Tumors

Up to 60% of patients diagnosed with testicular cancer have subnormal pretreatment semen analysis (Nijman et al, 1988). When compared with healthy controls or males with lymphoma, testicular cancer patients were found to have lower total sperm counts and higher serum follicle-stimulating hormone (FSH) levels. Similar findings have also been reported in patients with carcinoma in situ (Petersen et al, 1999). These abnormal parameters before treatment suggest a primary germ cell defect in testicular cancer patients. After orchiectomy, improvement in sperm parameters is seen, implying a reversible defect in fertility that may be due to circulating β-hCG or psychological stress. Despite this high incidence of oligospermia at the time of diagnosis, 65% of men are able to impregnate their partner after orchiectomy while on surveillance (Herr et al, 1998).

Antegrade ejaculation can be preserved in 95% to 98% of clinical stage I patients undergoing nerve-sparing RPLND. Paternity rates as high as 76% have been reported after RPLND for stage I disease (Foster et al, 1994). In this subfertile population, primary nerve-sparing RPLND does not significantly affect fertility.

KEY POINTS: LOW-STAGE NSGCT

- Patients whose tumor markers fail to normalize after radical orchiectomy should receive cisplatin-based induction chemotherapy, regardless of radiographic findings.

- Bilateral RPLND is the standard template for patients with pathologic stage II NSGCT.

- Nerve-sparing techniques involve preservation of both sympathetic chains, the postganglionic sympathetic fibers, and the hypogastric plexus.

- Incidence of teratoma in the retroperitoneum after primary RPLND in patients with pathologic stage II NSGCT is approximately 20% to 30%.

- Incompletely resected patients with pathologic stage II NSGCT, or those with any clinical evidence of disease (elevated β-hCG and/or AFP, lung nodules, retrocrural adenopathy) after primary RPLND, require cisplatin-based *induction* chemotherapy.

- The therapeutic impact of L-RPLND remains unknown.

Surgery for High-Stage Germ Cell Tumors

The initial treatment of patients with advanced GCT is cisplatin-based combination chemotherapy (Sheinfeld et al, 1994; Bosl et al, 2000), and a number of effective regimens have been used over the past 25 years (Einhorn et al, 1977; Vugrin et al, 1981; Bosl et al, 1988).

Preoperative Preparation and Timing of Surgery

The post-chemotherapy patient mandates thorough reevaluation to assess response to therapy before surgical intervention. This must include repeat determination of serum tumor markers, complete blood cell count, and blood chemistries with attention directed to platelet, neutrophil, and white blood cell count. Operative blood chemistries are checked with particular attention to serum creatinine after cisplatin-based therapy. Repeat CT of the retroperitoneum and repeat imaging of any other site of pre-chemotherapy disease should be done. Surgical intervention should be delayed until recovery of white blood cell ($>3.5/mm^3$) and platelet ($>100,000/mm^3$) counts into the normal range, which usually occurs 3 to 4 weeks after the final cycle of chemotherapy.

Preoperative evaluation should include pulmonary function testing in all patients treated with bleomycin. A restrictive pulmonary fibrosis due to alveolar edema and increased collagen deposition after bleomycin treatment can occur (Hay et al, 1991). This pulmonary fibrosis is believed to increase susceptibility to alveolar edema when patients are exposed to high levels of inspired oxygen concentration and fluid overload (Goldiner et al, 1978; Zwikler et al, 1994). Donat and Levy (1998) reviewed perioperative pulmonary complications of 77 patients treated with RPLND after bleomycin chemotherapy and found a 57% rate of pulmonary complications. Preoperative symptoms, pulmonary function testing,

and history of acute bleomycin were not predictive of postoperative pulmonary complications. The strongest risk factors for postoperative complications were overall fluid requirements and blood transfusions (Donat and Levy, 1998). **Meticulous management of intravenous fluid in the perioperative period is imperative in patients treated with bleomycin-containing chemotherapy regimens** (Donat and Levy, 1998).

NONSEMINOMATOUS GERM CELL TUMORS
Histologic Findings and Management Controversies

Post-chemotherapy surgery has evolved into an integral part of the management of patients with advanced GCTs; however, its role has undergone continued refinement over the past 2 decades (Sheinfeld et al, 1997). Before the development of cisplatin-based chemotherapy, surgical cytoreduction or "debulking" was followed by postoperative chemotherapy, resulting in high relapse rates, significant morbidity, and poor survival rates (Merrin et al, 1976; Donohue et al, 1980).

Improvements in staging techniques, such as CT and MRI, the reliability of serum tumor markers AFP and β-hCG, and the advent of effective cisplatin-based chemotherapy have led to the integration of surgery as an adjunct after cytoreductive chemotherapy (Donohue et al, 1982; Sheinfeld and Bajorin, 1993; Donohue et al, 1998). This multidisciplinary approach has resulted in survival rates of 70% to 80% of patients with advanced GCT (Einhorn et al, 1981; Bosl et al, 1986, 2000).

Increased serum concentrations of AFP and β-hCG after primary cisplatin-based chemotherapy are often characterized by unresectable, viable GCT; and second-line "salvage" chemotherapy is usually recommended for these nonresponders (Sheinfeld and Bajorin, 1993; Bosl et al, 2000). On the other hand, the recommendations for adjunctive surgery for patients who have undergone chemotherapy with appropriate normalization of serum tumor markers are variable and occasionally contradictory (Bajorin et al, 1992). **Whereas most clinicians agree that surgical exploration is indicated for patients with normal tumor markers and residual radiographic abnormalities, at the present time there are no standard guidelines for observation rather than adjunctive surgery** (Bajorin et al, 1992; Sheinfeld et al, 1997). Reported variables for patients in whom surgery can be safely omitted include residual masses less than 1.5 cm (Stomper et al, 1985; Carter et al, 1987), "normal" post-chemotherapy CT and absence of teratomatous elements in the primary tumor (Gelderman et al, 1988) and more than 90% volume reduction of the pre-chemotherapy mass, a residual mass less than 1.5 cm, and no teratoma in the primary tumor (Donohue et al, 1987).

Earlier published reports demonstrated that the pathologic findings at RPLND after cisplatin-based chemotherapy and normalization of serum tumor markers were necrosis/fibrosis, teratoma, or persistent viable carcinoma, each in approximately one third of cases (Donohue et al, 1980). More recently, investigators have reported a decrease in the proportion of patients with viable GCT (Table 30–1). This is com-

Table 30-1. Post-chemotherapy Pathologic Findings in Patients with High-Stage Germ Cell Tumors

Study	No. of Patients	Necrosis	Teratoma	Carcinoma
Donohue et al (1982)	51	16 (31%)	16 (31%)	19 (38%)
Bracken et al (1983)	23	9 (40%)	7 (30%)	7 (30%)
Tait et al (1984)	73	25 (34%)	32 (44%)	16 (22%)
Freiha et al (1984)	40	21 (53%)	18 (45%)	1 (2%)
Pizzocaro et al (1985)	36	16 (44%)	10 (28%)	10 (28%)
Donohue et al (1987)	80	35 (44%)	33 (41%)	12 (15%)
Gelderman et al (1988)	24	17 (71%)	7 (29%)	—
Harding et al (1989)	42	19 (45%)	14 (33%)	9 (22%)
Toner et al (1990)	122	57 (47%)	48 (39%)	17 (14%)
Mulder et al (1990)	55	31 (56%)	12 (22%)	12 (22%)
Aass et al (1991)	173	85 (49%)	50 (29%)	38 (22%)
Fossa et al (1992)	78	51 (65%)	22 (28%)	5 (7%)
Sonneveld et al (1998)*	110	49 (45%)	51 (46%)	10 (9%)
Stenning et al (1998)	153	45 (29%)	85 (56%)	23 (15%)
Donohue et al (1998)	870	221 (26%)	452 (52%)	197 (22%)
Steyerberg et al (1998)	172	77 (45%)	72 (42%)	23 (13%)

*Three additional patients underwent exploratory laparotomy but no specimen was resected.

monly attributed to stage migration and more effective chemotherapy regimens (Bosl et al, 1988).

Current investigators note that in the retroperitoneum, necrosis/fibrosis comprises 40% to 45% of pathologic findings after primary chemotherapy; teratoma, another 40%; and viable GCT, the remaining 15% to 20%, although variations in the various series probably reflect patient selection (see Table 30–1). After second-line or "salvage" chemotherapy, the distribution of histologic findings is markedly different, with viable GCT noted in approximately 50% of resected specimens, teratoma in 40%, and necrosis/fibrosis in only 10% of cases (Fox et al, 1993).

The patient's prognosis is related to serum marker level at the time of RPLND, prior treatment burden, and the pathologic findings of the resected specimen and completeness of resection (Donohue et al, 1998). The relapse rate of patients with necrosis/fibrosis or mature or immature teratoma is 5% to 10% after complete resection (Toner et al, 1990; Fossa et al, 1992; Donohue et al, 1994, 1998); therefore, additional chemotherapy is not required. **However, if viable GCT is present at any site but all disease is completely resected, two additional cycles provide survival benefit in this subset of patients** (Fox et al, 1993). **Fox and associates (1993) reported that 19 of 27 (70%) patients with completely resected viable GCT after primary chemotherapy followed by two cycles of postoperative chemotherapy remained disease free, compared with none of 7 patients without additional chemotherapy. Similarly, Logothetis and coworkers (1984) and Geller and colleagues (1989) reported survival rates of 53% and 66%, respectively, in patients undergoing complete resection of viable GCT and additional postoperative chemotherapy. Fizazi and associates (2001) challenged the therapeutic benefit of additional chemotherapy in completely resected GCT after induction chemotherapy in a multicenter, retrospective analysis of 146 patients. Three independent prognostic variables for survival were identified: (1) complete resection; (2) good risk IGCCGT classification; and (3) less than 10% viable malignant cells. Additional chemotherapy appeared to benefit only those with one risk factor but not those without risk factors or with two or more risk factors** (Fizazi et al, 2001). **Fox and

associates (1993) reported that two additional cycles of chemotherapy did not have any therapeutic benefit after** *salvage* **chemotherapy.**

Teratoma

Despite the histologically benign nature of teratoma, there are significant advantages in complete resection. First, teratomas may grow, obstruct, or invade adjacent structures and become unresectable (Logothetis et al, 1982; Logothetis and Samuels, 1984; Morgentaler et al, 1988; Sheinfeld and Bajorin, 1993).

Second, there is the risk of malignant transformation, that is, the development of non–germ cell malignant elements such as sarcoma or carcinoma (Little et al, 1994; Comiter et al, 1998; Motzer et al, 1998). The overall incidence is approximately 6% to 8%, and the most common histologic subtypes include sarcoma, particularly rhabdomyosarcoma and carcinomas (Little et al, 1994; Motzer et al, 1998). Toner and colleagues (1990) reported that 3 of 48 (6%) patients with resected teratoma had non–germ cell elements, whereas Little and coworkers (1994) noted that 45 of 557 (8%) patients undergoing post-chemotherapy RPLND (PC-RPLND) had malignant transformation of resected teratoma. Thirteen of the 19 patients with sarcomatous elements and 10 of 18 with nonsarcomatous tumors remain free of disease after surgery (Little et al, 1994). Complete surgical resection is the treatment of choice for this group of chemoresistant tumors and offers patients the best chance for survival (Little et al, 1994; Comiter et al, 1998; Motzer et al, 1998).

Motzer and colleagues performed conventional cytogenetic or molecular genetic techniques on 12 patients diagnosed with teratoma with malignant transformation. The isochromosome 12p was identified in 11 patients, confirming GCT clonality. Additionally, chromosomal abnormalities associated with the transformed histology were noted (Motzer et al, 1998).

Third, teratoma is associated with late recurrence (Loehrer et al, 1986; Borge et al, 1988; Gelderman et al, 1988; Gels et al, 1995). Loehrer and associates (1986) noted that 10 of 51 (19%) patients with teratoma developed late recurrence, with similar rates for mature teratoma (17%) and immature teratoma (23%). Borge and coworkers (1988) noted that 6 of 9 patients with NSGCT and late relapse had teratoma in the orchiectomy specimen. Roth and colleagues (1988) reported that all 7 patients with relapse after 24 months of achieving clinical remission had teratoma in the primary and/or retroperitoneal specimen. Furthermore, most recurrences developed locally, implying incomplete resection and foci of residual disease (Gelderman et al, 1988; Gerl et al, 1995).

Predicting Necrosis

Although the finding of necrosis/fibrosis alone in the resected retroperitoneal specimen is usually associated with a good long-term prognosis, the surgery offers no therapeutic advantage as it does in patients with viable GCT or teratoma (Foster and Donohue, 1998; Sheinfeld et al, 1997). Because almost 50% of resected residual retroperitoneal specimens have only necrosis/fibrosis, a number of investigators have attempted to reliably predict its presence and thus spare this subset of patients the associated morbidity of post-chemotherapy surgery (Steyerberg et al, 1996; Foster et al, 1998; Bosl et al, 2000).

Donohue and associates (1987) reported on 80 patients with sequential CT scans before and after chemotherapy at Indiana University. Among 15 of these patients without teratoma in the primary tumor and at least a 90% decrease in the retroperitoneal tumor volume determined by the formula $v = 0.52d^2$, none had viable GCT or teratoma. However, in a subsequent analysis from the same institution, Debono and coworkers (1997) found that only 74% of patients with these same criteria who were observed were continuously free of disease.

Observation has been recommended in patients whose tumor markers have normalized and in whom post-chemotherapy CT is "normal" (Debono et al, 1997; Foster et al, 1998). The definition of normal post-chemotherapy CT is variable and includes lymph node diameters of 10 mm or less (Fossa et al, 1989c) and 20 mm or less (Mead et al, 1992). A significant number of resected specimens will contain teratoma and/or viable GCT despite strict normal CT criteria (Sheinfeld et al, 1997). Fossa and colleagues (1989c) reported that 12 of 37 (30%) patients with normal post-chemotherapy serum tumor markers and CT (≤10 mm) had teratoma, and 1 patient had viable GCT. Toner and coworkers (1990) reported that 8 of 39 (21%) patients with residual masses less than 1.5 cm had residual teratoma or viable GCT. Oldenburg and associates (2003) reported that one third of retroperitoneal post-chemotherapy masses less than 2 cm harbored either teratoma or viable GCT, including 20% in masses less than 5 mm. Debono and colleagues (1997) reported 5 (6%) patients with recurrence in a group of 78 patients with normal post-chemotherapy CT who were observed.

CT criteria other than size, such as attenuation values, have been studied in an attempt to distinguish necrosis/fibrosis from residual teratoma or viable GCT (Soo et al, 1981; Husband et al, 1982; Stomper et al, 1985). Husband and associates (1982) noted that post-chemotherapy masses with low attenuation values were more likely to represent necrosis; however, Stomper and colleagues (1985) and Donohue and coworkers (1987) failed to confirm this finding. CT

criteria alone are not sufficiently reliable to distinguish viable tumor or teratoma from necrosis (Sheinfeld et al, 1997; Bosl et al, 2000).

Positron emission tomography (PET) has been studied in the evaluation of both seminoma and NSGCT post-chemotherapy residual masses (Stephens et al, 1996; Ganjoo et al, 1999). In NSGCT, the major limitation is the inability to distinguish teratoma from necrosis (Stephens et al, 1996). In the seminoma setting, viable GCT was not reliably predicted in an initial study (Ganjoo et al, 1999); however, more recently De Santis and associates (2003) reported that 50 of 52 PET scans correctly predicted clinical outcome.

Although teratoma in the primary tumor predicts the presence of teratoma and viable GCT in the post-chemotherapy resection despite volume reduction of the original mass (Donohue et al, 1987; Toner et al, 1990; Fossa et al, 1992; Debono et al, 1997; Beck et al, 2002), **teratoma may be found in the retroperitoneum despite its absence in the orchiectomy specimen** (Toner et al, 1990, Beck et al, 2002). Toner and colleagues (1990) reported that of 75 patients without teratoma in the orchiectomy specimen, 25 had resected teratoma after chemotherapy. Furthermore, of 17 patients with a residual mass less than 1.5 cm, 90% or greater shrinkage of the retroperitoneal mass, and no evidence of teratoma in the primary specimen, 3 (18%) patients had teratoma and 2 (12%) patients had viable GCT in the resected specimen (Toner et al, 1990). Beck and associates (2002) noted that 48% of patients with teratoma in the retroperitoneal specimen after chemotherapy did not have teratomatous elements in the primary tumor.

Several logistic regression models have been developed to calculate the probability of necrosis (Toner et al, 1990; Steyerberg et al, 1995). In the Steyerberg model, predictors of necrosis included the absence of teratoma in the primary tumor, normal pre-chemotherapy β-hCG and AFP, a small pre- or post-chemotherapy mass, and a large volume reduction in the retroperitoneal mass (Steyerberg et al, 1995).

Multiple studies show that approximately 20% of patients predicted to have necrosis/fibrosis will harbor either teratoma or viable GCT (Toner et al, 1990; Steyerberg et al, 1995). **No single criterion or combination of criteria predict a negative pathology with sufficient accuracy to eliminate the risk of residual teratoma or viable GCT and thus obviate PC-RPLND** (Bosl et al, 2000; Sheinfeld et al, 1997). **Therefore, the decision to recommend post-chemotherapy surgery depends on the frequency of viable GCT, the biologic potential of teratoma, and the morbidity of the RPLND** (Bosl et al, 2000). **If viable GCT is present, it is partially drug resistant and will progress if left unresected. The cure rate of recurrent GCT to ifosfamide-based salvage regimens is approximately 25%** (Motzer et al, 1992; Loehrer et al, 1988). **Conversely, if viable GCT is completely resected, and two additional cycles of cisplatin-based chemotherapy are given, cure rates between 50% and 70% are possible** (Toner, 1990; Fox, 1993). **As noted earlier, unresected teratoma may grow rapidly ("growing teratoma syndrome"), invade local structures, become unresectable, or undergo malignant transformation** (Logothetis et al, 1984; Sheinfeld and Bajorin, 1993; Little et al, 1994; Motzer et al, 1998).

The data suggest that undertreatment of patients with advanced GCT after chemotherapy may result in inferior clinical outcomes compared with those who have immediate surgery. Prompt recognition and appropriate treatment of disease progression or relapse after chemotherapy do not appear to compare favorably with immediate post-chemotherapy surgery.

In a nonrandomized study comparing 330 patients who underwent salvage surgery after relapse, Hendry and colleagues (2002) reported lower rates of complete resection (72% vs. 87%), relapse-free survival (62% vs. 83%), and overall survival (56% vs. 89%) and higher rates of viable GCT (49% vs. 8%) and teratoma with malignant transformation (6% vs. 1%) in the salvage group. Debono and colleagues (1997) reported that 4 of 78 patients with a complete clinical response who were observed after chemotherapy subsequently died of disease and that only 78% of 27 patients with a teratoma-negative primary tumor, normal serum markers, and a 90% or greater radiographic response who were initially treated expectantly were free of disease. Conversely, of 140 patients with less favorable clinical parameters (less than 90% radiographic response with or without teratoma in primary tumor) who underwent immediate post-chemotherapy surgery, 4 were dead of disease and 94% were free of disease.

Furthermore, the data suggest that an uncontrolled retroperitoneum is a predisposing factor for late relapse (see later) (Baniel et al, 1995a,b; George et al, 2003; Carver et al, 2005).

Late Relapse

Late recurrence of GCT of the testis is defined as relapse after a disease-free interval of at least 2 years in the absence of a second primary testicular tumor. The reported incidence of late relapse of GCT is 2% to 4% and appears to be increasing (George et al, 2003; Carver et al, 2005). Almost 60% of late relapses occur beyond 10 years, emphasizing the need for prolonged follow-up. Approximately 50% of patients with late relapses will be symptomatic, and approximately 60% will have an elevated AFP (Baniel et al, 1995b; Carver et al, 2005; Dieckmann et al, 2005; George et al, 2005).

Although late relapses of GCT have been reported in the chest, neck, liver, brain, and pelvis, the most common site is the retroperitoneum, regardless of initial stage, clinical presentation, or prior treatment. Approximately 50% to 80% of late relapses occur in the retroperitoneum, which further underscores the need for initial complete surgical resection. Postoperative, cisplatin-based chemotherapy did not prevent late local recurrence in the retroperitoneum after suboptimal RPLND for initial low-stage disease (Baniel et al, 1995a; Carver et al, 2005). More than 50% of patients with late relapse referred to MSKCC after induction chemotherapy for advanced disease had unresected retroperitoneal masses (Carver et al, 2005). Similarly, only 22 of 37 (59%) patients had undergone PC-RPLND in the Indiana series (Baniel et al, 1995b). Late relapse is more common when teratoma is present in a metastatic site (Loehrer et al, 1986; Sonneveld et al, 1998).

Late relapses of GCT are usually refractory to chemotherapy, although Motzer and colleagues (2000) reported encouraging results with paclitaxel, cisplatin, and ifosfamide. Survival rates range from 26% to 46% and are rare without complete resection (Baniel et al, 1995b; Carver et al, 2005; Dieckmann et al, 2005; George et al, 2003).

High-Risk Post-Chemotherapy NSGCT Patients

In a review of 801 patients who underwent PC-RPLND at Indiana University between 1974 and 1994 after cisplatin-based chemotherapy, Donohue and associates (1998) identified several unfavorable subsets of patients characterized by higher relapse and lower survival rates. The overall relapse rate for all PC-RPLND (n = 801) was 27.8%. Whereas the favorable group of PC-RPLND patients (n = 414) had a relapse rate of 11.8%, 174 of 387 (45%) patients with one or more unfavorable risk factors relapsed and 29% died of GCT (Donohue et al, 1998).

The first high-risk group are patients undergoing PC-RPLND after salvage chemotherapy, that is, patients with advanced GCT who experience relapse or fail to achieve a complete response to standard cisplatin-based chemotherapy and receive either conventional-dose salvage therapy or high-dose chemotherapy regimens with bone marrow or stem cell support (Donohue et al, 1998). Surgery in this setting is characterized by lower rates of complete resection and a higher proportion of viable cancer (approximately 50%) (Fox et al, 1993). Additional standard-dose chemotherapy does not appear to benefit patients in this setting, compared with a clear benefit in the setting of complete resection of viable GCT after *primary* chemotherapy (Fox et al, 1993).

Second, "desperation" PC-RPLND is done in patients with an elevated serum tumor marker (AFP or β-hCG) at the time of surgery. Historically, surgery has been avoided in patients with persistently elevated serum tumor markers, because most were believed to have unresectable or incurable disease (Nijman et al, 1988). Recent studies have identified highly selected patients in this setting in whom surgery has curative potential (Wood et al, 1992; Murphy et al, 1993; Eastham et al, 1994). Murphy and colleagues (1993) reported that 38 of 48 (79%) such patients were rendered free of disease, 29 (60%) normalized their markers, and 10 (21%) remain disease free with a median follow-up of 46 months. Eastham and associates (1994) noted that 6 of 16 (31%) patients undergoing desperation PC-RPLND were cured, whereas Wood and coworkers (1992) reported 7 of 15 (47%) patients were rendered free of disease.

Patients deemed to have unresectable disease do very poorly, with 17 of 19 (90%) patients experiencing relapse and only 4 (21%) survivors in the study of Donohue and colleagues (1998).

The fourth high-risk group is the "redo" PC-RPLND, that is, patients who have undergone a prior attempt at PC-RPLND who present with recurrence in the surgical field (Donohue et al, 1998; Foster et al, 1998). **The importance of complete initial post-chemotherapy surgery cannot be overemphasized. The data from Indiana University clearly demonstrate that patients who require repeat RPLND are severely disadvantaged,** *regardless of other risk factors* (Donohue et al, 1998). The relapse rates for primary versus redo PC-RPLND are 20.6% and 51.6%, respectively, and the survival rates are 55.3% for the redo group compared with 84.1% in the primary PC-RPLND group (Donohue et al, 1998).

To ensure complete surgical resection of residual retroperitoneal masses, adjunctive procedures are sometimes necessary. En bloc nephrectomy is the most common adjunctive procedure, with almost a 20% rate in the Indiana post-chemotherapy experience (Nash et al, 1998). These are predominantly left-sided primary tumors with large-volume residual disease densely adherent to the left renal vessels and/or hilum.

Multiple investigators have reported en bloc resection of a great vessel to achieve complete resection of densely adherent, bulky retroperitoneal masses (Donohue et al, 1991; Kelly et al, 1995; Spitz et al, 1997; Beck et al, 1999). Long-term survivors are reported with both IVC and aortic resections (Kelly et al, 1995; Spitz et al, 1997). Of 65 patients who had a portion of the infrarenal IVC resected without reconstruction, Beck and coworkers (1999) reported no long-term sequelae in 75% with 7-year follow-up. However, significant morbidity with venous congestion of the lower extremities and persistent lymphatic drainage into the retroperitoneal space is possible (Waters et al, 2000). If necessary, venous reconstruction can be accomplished with synthetic graft material (Mullen et al, 1996; Spitz et al, 1997). Similarly, aortic resection is occasionally necessary to achieve a complete resection and, again, vascular continuity can be achieved with synthetic grafts (Kelly et al, 1995).

This aggressive surgical approach in a subset of appropriately selected patients is justified by the high proportion of teratoma or viable cancer in the resected specimen, the high survival rates in completely resected patients, and acceptable morbidity when performed by experienced surgeons in tertiary centers (Donohue et al, 1991; Kelly et al, 1995; Spitz et al, 1997).

Post-Chemotherapy RPLND

While many of the techniques previously described for primary RPLND are applicable in performing post-chemotherapy lymphadenectomy, several important points should be emphasized. Large retroperitoneal tumors and severe desmoplastic reaction make PC-RPLND one of the most difficult and dangerous operations undertaken by urologists (Skinner and Skinner, 1992). Therefore, this operation should be performed by experienced surgeons in referral centers.

The choice of incision is based on tumor location and size. Large masses, located high in the retroperitoneum, may require a thoracoabdominal approach or costal extension of a midline incision. For large left-sided tumors, particularly those that cause lateral displacement of the left kidney with stretching of the renal vessels, massive suprahilar infradiaphragmatic extension is often seen. In this setting, a "visceral roll" provides good exposure of the para-aortic area above the left renal artery. By incising (1) the peritoneum of the left lumbar gutter along the white line of Toldt, (2) the splenophrenic ligament, and (3) the parietal peritoneal attachments of the stomach, the descending colon, spleen, stomach, and tail of the pancreas can be reflected medially, exposing the

aorta to the level of the diaphragmatic hiatus (Whitmore and Morse, 1986).

The "split and roll" technique is used to perform the lymphadenectomy. While separating the fibrous wall of the tumor mass and lymph nodes from the great vessels, great care must be taken to avoid subadventitial dissection along the aorta. Aortic wall stripped of adventitia is not amenable to conventional suture repair and may result in delayed rupture. Direct invasion of the aorta or vena cava may require resection with graft interposition. Adjunctive procedures such as nephrectomy may be necessary to achieve complete resection, particularly for left-sided tumors. Extensive violation of bowel serosa or enterotomies predispose patients to possible life-threatening fistulas, and omental interposition is advisable.

Tumor involvement of the SMA, celiac axis, or porta hepatis often precludes resection (Whitmore and Morse, 1986).

The standard bilateral RPLND should be performed. A significant number of patients will have residual teratoma or viable cancer outside the limits of a modified RPLND (Wood et al, 1992). **Modified templates, originally developed for patients with low-stage disease in an effort to preserve ejaculation, are not acceptable alternatives for patients with advanced disease who are at higher risk for disease in sites outside the limits of reduced surgical templates. Similarly, resection of a residual mass without RPLND is inappropriate.**

Approximately 20% of patients, particularly those with low-volume residual disease, are candidates for nerve-sparing PC-RPLND (Coogan et al, 1996). Again, the oncologic aspects of the procedure should not be compromised to preserve antegrade ejaculation.

Reoperative Retroperitoneal Surgery

Completeness of resection is an independent and consistent predictive variable of relapse-free survival for patients with NSGCT, and those who are incompletely resected and require reoperative surgery after either primary RPLND or PC-RPLND are compromised (Donohue et al, 1998; Sheinfeld, 2002a; McKiernan et al, 2003). As noted earlier, Donohue and coworkers (1998) noted that patients undergoing "redo" PC-RPLND were significantly disadvantaged in terms of survival (55% vs. 84%) compared with those who did not require reoperation, despite controlling for marker status, histologic findings, and prior need for salvage chemotherapy. Similarly, McKiernan and colleagues (2003) reported the MSKCC reoperative experience and noted a 56% 5-year disease-specific survival rate in patients requiring reoperation after PC-RPLND compared with 86% in those without reoperation.

Investigators at MSKCC also showed that inadequate initial surgery in low-stage NSGCT cannot be reliably remedied by postoperative chemotherapy. Twenty (90%) of 22 patients who underwent reoperative retroperitoneal surgery after primary RPLND had received postoperative cisplatin-based chemotherapy, including 19 patients who received full induction regimens (McKiernan et al, 2003). Survival in this group of patients was also compromised (86% vs. 99.3% in patients not requiring reoperation).

In the MSKCC series, 10 of 22 (45%) patients undergoing primary RPLND and 20 of 34 (59%) undergoing PC-RPLND had teratomatous elements present at initial surgery before local recurrence, underscoring the need for complete and meticulous resection of teratoma (McKiernan et al, 2003).

The left para-aortic region is the most common site of local recurrence prompting reoperation. This is due to the increased technical demands of obtaining adequate exposure in this area, including pancreatic mobilization and dissection of the renal vessels; and the fact that, unfortunately, surgeons often exclude the preaortic and para-aortic lymph nodes in modified templates for right-sided primary tumors (McKiernan et al, 2003). Data from MSKCC and Indiana have shown that a significant subset of patients with right-sided primary NSGCT and pathologic stage II disease will have involved lymph nodes in the para-aortic area (Leibovitch et al, 1995a; Koppie et al, 2004). Reoperative retroperitoneal surgery can be performed with acceptable morbidity in dedicated tertiary centers with experienced surgeons (Donohue et al, 1998; McKiernan et al, 2003; Sexton et al, 2003).

Lung, Mediastinal, and Neck Resections

The indications and timing for post-chemotherapy resection of residual masses in the chest are less controversial. Early investigators reported discordant histologic findings ranging from 29% to 46% between the retroperitoneum and the chest (Mandelbaum et al, 1983; Tiffany et al, 1986; Qvist et al, 1991).

Toner and coworkers (1990) reported on 39 patients who underwent 57 procedures for pulmonary nodules. Six of 14 patients with nodules not larger than 1 cm had either teratoma (5 patients) or viable cancer (1 patient), whereas 3 of 8 patients who underwent bilateral thoracotomies had different histologic findings in each lung.

Logistic regression analysis of multiple clinical parameters to estimate the probability of necrosis at thoracotomy found that necrosis in the retroperitoneum was most often the predictive variable (Steyerberg et al, 1997). Other predictors included primary tumor histology, pre-chemotherapy tumor markers, change in size after chemotherapy, and the presence of a single mass (Steyerberg et al, 1997).

More recently, Tognini and colleagues (1998) reported that although retroperitoneal histology was most predictive of thoracic histology, only 31 of 40 (78%) patients with necrosis in the abdomen had necrosis in the chest. Further categorization of the RPLND as standard or complicated increased the predictive accuracy to 86%.

Finally, the recent MSKCC experience of 93 patients who had RPLND and thoracotomy revealed histologic discordance between RPLND and thoracotomy in 27 of 93 (29%) patients; 7 of 59 (14%) patients with fibrosis in the retroperitoneum had teratoma or viable cancer in the chest (McGuire et al, 1999).

Post-chemotherapy thoracotomy yields important prognostic information and is therapeutic in most patients with resected teratoma and a subset of patients with viable cancer. Criteria predictive of necrosis are not sufficiently accurate to omit resection of post-chemotherapy residual thoracic masses; therefore, all sites of disease should be resected regardless of size (McGuire et al, 2003). Furthermore, investigators have demonstrated the feasibility of simultaneous RPLND and thoracic resection in experienced tertiary centers (Brenner et al, 1996; Tognini et al, 1998; McGuire et al, 2003).

Mohseni and associates (2002) reported on 16 patients with a residual neck mass who underwent resection of 61 residual masses in multiple sites. Histologic discordance in different sites was seen in 7 of 16 (44%) patients, and 13 of 16 patients had teratoma (10 patients) or viable GCT (3 patients) in the neck. All 10 patients with teratoma in the residual neck mass and 1 of 3 with viable GCT have no evidence of disease after complete resection. There were no perioperative deaths, and no patient suffered relapse in the neck.

KEY POINTS: HIGH-STAGE GERM CELL TUMORS

- The initial treatment for patients with advanced GCT is cisplatin-based combination chemotherapy.

- Post-chemotherapy pathologic findings in patients with advanced NSGCT after *induction* therapy are approximately as follows: necrosis, 50%; teratoma, 40%; viable carcinoma, 10%.

- Post-chemotherapy pathologic findings in patients with advanced NSGCT following *salvage* therapy are approximately as follows: necrosis, 10%; teratoma, 40%; viable carcinoma, 50%.

- Variables and statistical models to predict necrosis in the retroperitoneum after induction therapy have approximately a 30% error.

- Teratomatous elements may be found in the retroperitoneum despite their absence in the orchiectomy specimen.

- Teratoma may grow and obstruct or invade local structures, undergo malignant transformation, and may result in late relapse.

- Bilateral RPLND is the standard template in the post-chemotherapy NSGCT setting; resection of residual mass *alone* is an *unacceptable* alternative.

- Histologic discordance between different sites (e.g., retroperitoneum, thorax, neck) after post-chemotherapy resection is found in approximately 30% of cases.

Complications

The rate of complications for post-chemotherapy surgery is higher than for primary RPLND. Baniel and associates (1995c) reported 38 (8%) major complications in 478 patients who underwent primary RPLND compared with 106 (18%) in 603 patients after PC-RPLND. Furthermore, there were 5 deaths in the post-chemotherapy group and none in the primary group (Baniel et al, 1995c). Large-volume residual disease, post-chemotherapy desmoplastic reaction, prior exposure to bleomycin, and more extensive retroperitoneal resection increase the technical and perioperative demands of the procedure and result in higher morbidity rates. Fortunately, the morbidity appears to be decreasing with time. Mosharafa and associates (2004) reported that the rate of perioperative complications and length of hospital stay decreased from July 2000 to July 2002 compared with patients who underwent PC-RPLND from July 1990 to 1992. Careful monitoring of perioperative oxygen concentrations, meticulous fluid management with strict replacement criteria, and an emphasis on colloid rather than crystalloid have reduced pulmonary toxicity. Knowledge of the retroperitoneal anatomy, careful technique, and improved perioperative management have resulted in lower morbidity when PC-RPLND is performed by experienced surgeons. Data from a retrospective analysis suggested a beneficial impact of clinical care pathways on the reduction of perioperative morbidity (Chang et al, 2002c).

Lymphatic Complications. The incidence of chylous ascites is 2% to 3%, and predisposing factors included resection of the vena cava, suprahilar dissection, or simultaneous hepatic resection. Familiarity with retroperitoneal lymphovascular anatomy and meticulous lymphostasis with clips or ligatures will minimize this complication.

Patients with chylous ascites may present with abdominal distention, prolonged ileus, an abdominal fluid wave, a pleural effusion, or chylous leakage from the incision. Ultrasound or CT with paracentesis is diagnostic and may provide symptomatic relief. Chylous fluid has a characteristic milky or turbid appearance with a fat content of 4 to 40 g/L and a total protein content greater than 30 g/L. Initial management is with diuretics and dietary manipulation (low-fat diet with medium-chain triglycerides) and/or total parenteral nutrition. Persistent drainage of chyle refractory to conservative measures may require peritoneovenous shunting (Baniel et al, 1995a). Reoperation to repair lymphatic leakage is associated with a high failure rate and should be avoided.

Asymptomatic lymphoceles require no treatment; however, percutaneous drainage for infection, hydronephrosis, or bowel obstruction is necessary in 1% to 2% of cases. Persistent drainage may require treatment with a sclerosing agent.

Pulmonary Complications. Pulmonary complications include (1) atelectasis, which is treated by vigorous pulmonary physiotherapy; (2) pneumonia, which requires appropriate antibiotic therapy; and (3) acute respiratory distress syndrome, which often requires prolonged mechanical ventilation and corticosteroids and may be fatal. The signs and symptoms of acute respiratory distress syndrome include a dry nonproductive cough, dyspnea, rales, fever, and interstitial pneumonitis on chest radiography. **It is our practice to judiciously monitor the perioperative fluid administered to bleomycin-treated patients and to avoid unnecessary exposure to high concentrations of inspired oxygen.**

Infectious Complications. Superficial wound infections comprise the majority of infectious problems, whereas urinary tract infections account for less than 1%. *Clostridium difficile* infections require appropriate antibiotic therapy with metronidazole (Flagyl) or vancomycin. Incidental appendectomy increases the risk of infection and is contraindicated (Leibovitch et al, 1995b).

Vascular Complications. Renovascular injury is seen in 2% to 3% of cases and can result in renovascular hypertension or require nephrectomy at the time of RPLND. Minor injury of the great vessels during dissection can be managed with 5-0 vascular sutures. Major vascular injury requiring unplanned grafting or prolonged cross clamping is uncommon in experienced centers.

Neurologic Complications. Peripheral nerve injury due to neural compression secondary to positioning is rare and accounts for less than 1% of all complications, particularly with the transabdominal approach. Femoral and brachial neurapraxias have been reported (Baniel et al, 1995c). The more serious complication of spinal cord ischemia with aortic mobilization is encountered in less than 1% of all cases and has been associated with older age, simultaneous mediastinal and retroperitoneal dissections, previous radiation therapy, and intraoperative hypotension (Leibovitch et al, 1996). This complication can be minimized by selective preservation of lumbar arterial branches in suprahilar and thoracic dissections.

Gastrointestinal Complications. Prolonged paralytic ileus may be associated with mechanical obstruction or, less commonly, with retroperitoneal hematoma, pancreatitis, urinary extravasation, mesenteric hematoma, and bowel infarction (Whitmore and Morse, 1986). Small bowel obstruction is seen in 2% to 3% of all patients and can be managed conservatively, with exploration being reserved for signs of toxicity or failure to respond to prolonged nasogastric tube decompression. Pancreatitis usually presents as prolonged ileus and hyperamylasemia and can be avoided by minimizing traction on the pancreas during RPLND. Therapy is usually conservative with nasogastric tube decompression and occasional need for hyperalimentation. Isolated hyperamylasemia may be seen in up to 40% of asymptomatic patients and is self-limiting (Baniel et al, 1995d). Gastrointestinal bleeding is rare and can be minimized by the use of perioperative histamine-2 antagonists. Sacrifice of the IMA is common and is rarely associated with any lower gastrointestinal complication. Duodenal hematomas and laceration have been reported and are seen in the setting of high-volume disease behind the duodenum, making dissection in this area particularly demanding. In the past, routine appendectomy at the time of RPLND was performed, but it has been found to be associated with an increased risk of infectious complications and therefore is no longer recommended (Leibovitch et al, 1995b).

SEMINOMA

The approach to the patient with pure seminoma and a residual mass after chemotherapy is controversial. **There are two important differences between seminoma and NSGCT in this setting. First, teratoma in the residual mass is very rare. Second, a complete RPLND is often not technically possible owing to obliteration of tissue planes secondary to the severe desmoplastic reaction of these tumors after chemotherapy** (Horwich et al, 1997; Sheinfeld and Herr, 1998; Bosl et al, 2000). **Consequently, perioperative morbidity is higher than for NSGCT** (Fossa et al, 1987; Ellison et al, 1988).

Several studies have evaluated the role of surgery for residual masses in seminoma patients (Fossa et al, 1987; Loehrer et al, 1987; Puc et al, 1996; Herr et al, 1997; Horwich et al, 1997). Loehrer and associates (1987) reported on 62 patients with advanced-stage seminoma who received cisplatin-based chemotherapy. Of the 13 patients who underwent attempted surgical resection, 3 (23%) had residual malignancy, and the size of the residual mass was not predictive of histologic findings. Fossa and colleagues (1987) reported 39 patients with advanced seminoma, 15 of whom had received prior radiation therapy. Three (25%) of 12 patients who underwent surgical exploration had viable seminoma, and one postoperative death secondary to pulmonary toxicity was reported. Both groups concluded that observation was preferable in these patients given the significant surgical morbidity and the fact that the majority of post-chemotherapy seminoma patients with residual radiographic abnormalities do not have persistent malignant disease (Fossa et al, 1987; Loeher et al, 1987). Investigators at the Royal Marsden Hospital report only a 12% relapse rate in post-chemotherapy seminoma patients with observation alone despite radiographic abnormalities in over 80% of patients (Peckham et al, 1985).

In a group of 104 post-chemotherapy seminoma patients, investigators at MSKCC reported that 8 of 30 (27%) patients with a residual mass of ≥3 cm experienced relapse or had residual seminoma, whereas only 2 of 74 (3%) patients with tumors less than 3 cm in diameter relapsed at the site of residual disease. Of the 55 patients who underwent surgery, 32 (58%) had masses resected, whereas 23 (42%) underwent multiple biopsies. There were no postoperative deaths (Puc et al, 1996; Herr et al, 1997).

Although there is general agreement that residual masses less than 3 cm should be managed with observation, management of the minority of patients with residual masses larger than 3 cm remains controversial. Investigators at MSKCC believe that resection or biopsy of residual masses greater than 3 cm was preferable to observation because it can identify residual disease and direct immediate therapy (Puc et al, 1996; Bosl et al, 2000). If viable seminoma is identified, additional chemotherapy is necessary (Puc et al, 1996). Alternatively, radiation therapy is possible; however, approximately 75% of patients will receive it unnecessarily and it did not appear to reduce the risk of relapse (Horwich et al, 1997; Bosl et al, 2000). Observation is a third option; however, ifosfamide-based salvage chemotherapy for patients who relapsed had a low cure rate (Bosl et al, 2000).

Recently, a 2-^{18}fluoro-deoxy-D-glucose PET scan in 52 patients with residual masses after chemotherapy for bulky seminoma reported that all 8 positive scans and 42 of 44 negative scans correlated with clinical outcome (DeSantis et al, 2004).

In summary, patients with residual masses smaller than 3 cm after chemotherapy may be observed. An FDT PET scan should be done for masses 3 cm or larger. A negative PET scan usually implies freedom from disease, whereas a positive PET scan is often associated with residual viable seminoma and additional therapy should be considered. If surgical resection appears feasible, it should be done at centers with experienced surgeons (Bosl et al, 2005).

FERTILITY IN ADVANCED GERM CELL TUMORS

Subnormal pretreatment semen parameters in conjunction with cytotoxic chemotherapy and more extensive surgical

RPLND make fertility less common in the post-chemotherapy setting. Cytotoxic chemotherapy has been shown to have long-term deleterious effects on Leydig cell function (Brennemann et al, 1997; Howell et al, 1999). Platinum-based chemotherapy regimens cause both Leydig and Sertoli cell dysfunction. After two or four cycles of platinum-based chemotherapy, a nadir in spermatogenesis is reached in 10 to 14 months. The majority of patients with normal pretreatment spermatogenesis will return to baseline function by 3 years (Brennemann et al, 1997). Overall fertility rates after chemotherapy are directly related to the total dose of platinum delivered during treatment (Pont and Albrecht, 1997). Patient age and pretreatment FSH levels are also predictive of long-term fertility after chemotherapy (Brennemann et al, 1997). Cryopreservation of sperm is now widely available and is recommended before chemotherapy for testicular cancer. However, many patients will recover adequate spermatogenesis and not require the use of cryopreserved sperm (Fossa et al, 1989a). Despite defects in spermatogenesis and exposure to cytotoxic therapy, the incidence of birth defects is not increased in children conceived after treatment for testicular cancer (Byrne et al, 1990; Hartmann et al, 1999).

Acknowledgment

The authors are grateful for the expert and invaluable assistance of Mary Jane Harris in the preparation of this manuscript.

SELECTED READINGS

Baniel J, Foster RS, Gonin R, et al: Late relapse of testicular cancer. J Clin Oncol 1995b;13:1170-1176.

Beck SD, Foster R, Bihrle R, et al: Teratoma in the orchiectomy specimen and volume of metastasis are predictors of retroperitoneal teratoma in postchemotherapy nonseminomatous testis cancer. J Urol 2002;168:1402-1404.

Bosl GJ, Vogelzang NJ, Goldman A, et al: Impact of delay in diagnosis on clinical stage of testicular cancer. Lancet 1981;2:970-973.

Debono DJ, Heilman DK, Einhorn LH, Donohue JP: Decision analysis for avoiding postchemotherapy surgery in patients with disseminated nonseminomatous germ cell tumors. J Clin Oncol 1997;15:1455-1464.

Donohue JP, Zachary JM, Maynard BR: Distribution of nodal metastases in nonseminomatous testis cancer. J Urol 1982;128:315-320.

Donohue JP, Thornhill JA, Foster RS, et al: Retroperitoneal lymphadenectomy for clinical stage A testis cancer (1965 to 1989): Modifications of technique and impact on ejaculation. J Urol 1993;149:237-243.

Donohue JP, Leviovitch I, Foster RS, et al: Integration of surgery and systemic therapy: Results and principles of integration. Semin Urol Oncol 1998;16:65-71.

Fox EP, Weathers TD, Williams SD, et al: Outcome analysis for patients with persistent nonteratomatous germ cell tumor in postchemotherapy retroperitoneal lymph node dissections. J Clin Oncol 1993;11:1294-1299.

George DW, Foster RS, Hromas RA, et al: Update on late relapse of germ cell tumors: A clinical and molecular analysis. J Clin Oncol 2003; 21:113-122.

Jewett MA, Kong YS, Goldberg SD, et al: Retroperitoneal lymphadenectomy for testis tumor with nerve sparing for ejaculation. J Urol 1988;139:1220-1224.

Klein EA: Nerve-sparing retroperitoneal lymphadenectomy. Atlas Urol Clin 1995;3:63-79.

Kondagunta GV, Sheinfeld J, Mazumdar M, et al: Relapse-free and overall survival in patients with pathologic stage II nonseminomatous germ cell cancer treated with etoposide and cisplatin adjuvant chemotherapy. J Clin Oncol 2004;22:464-467.

McKiernan JM, Motzer RJ, Bajorin DF, et al: Reoperative RPLND for germ cell tumor; clinical presentation, patterns of recurrence, and outcome. Urology 2003;62:732-736.

Meinardi MT, Gietema JA, van der Graaf WTA, et al: Cardiovascular morbidity in long-term survivors of metastatic testicular cancer. J Clin Urol 2000;18:1725-1732.

Motzer RJ, Amsterdam A, Prieto V, et al: Teratoma with malignant transformation: Diverse malignant histologies arising in men with germ cell tumors. J Urol 1998;159:133-138.

Oldenburg J, Alfsen GC, Lien HH, et al: Postchemotherapy retroperitoneal surgery remains necessary in patients with nonseminomatous testicular cancer and minimal residual tumor masses. J Clin Oncol 2003;21:3310-3317.

Pohar KS, Rabbani F, Bosl GJ, et al: Results of retroperitoneal lymph node dissection for clinical stage I and II pure embryonal carcinoma of the testis. J Urol 2003;170:1155-1158.

Rabbani F, Sheinfeld J, Farivar-Mohseni H, et al: Low-volume nodal metastasis detected at retroperitoneal lymphadenectomy for testicular cancer: Pattern and prognostic factors for relapse. J Clin Oncol 1999a;19:2020-2025.

Richie JP, Kantoff PW: Is adjuvant chemotherapy necessary for patients with stage B1 testicular cancer? J Clin Oncol 1991;9:1393-1396.

Sheinfeld J: Adjuvant postchemotherapy surgery for nonseminomatous germ cell tumors: Current concepts and controversies. Semin Urol Oncol 2002a;20:262-271.

Sheinfeld J, Motzer RJ, Rabbani F, et al: Incidence and clinical outcome of patients with teratoma in the retroperitoneum following primary RPLND for clinical stages I and IIA NSGCT. J Urol 2003a;170:1159-1162.

Sheinfeld J, Pohar K, Rabbani F, et al: Results of retroperitoneal lymph node dissection for clinical stage I and II pure embryonal carcinoma of the testis. J Urol 2003b;170:1155-1158.

Sheinfeld J, Rabbani F, Mohsein H, et al: Elevated serum tumor markers (STM) prior to 1° RPLND predicts clinical outcome and requirements for systemic chemotherapy in patients with pN1, N2, and N3 nonseminomatous germ cell tumor (NSGCT) [Abstract]. Proc ASCO 1999a;18:308A.

Sogani PC, Perrotti M, Herr HW, et al: Clinical stage I testis cancer: Long-term outcome of patients on surveillance. J Urol 1998;159:855-858.

Stephenson AJ, Sheinfeld J: The role of retroperitoneal lymph node dissection in the management of testicular cancer. Urol Oncol 2004;22:225-235.

Stephenson AJ, Bosl GJ, Motzer RJ, et al: Impact of trends in patient selection on clinical outcome after retroperitoneal lymph node dissection for nonseminomatous germ cell testicular cancer. J Clinical Oncol 2005;23:2781-2788.

Steyerberg EW, Keizer HJ, Fossa SD, et al: Prediction of residual retroperitoneal mass histology after chemotherapy for metastatic nonseminomatous germ cell tumor: Multivariate analysis of individual patient data from six study groups. J Clin Oncol 1995;13:1177-1187.

Studer U, Burkhard F, Sountag R: Risk adapted management with adjuvant chemotherapy in patients with high risk clinical stage I nonseminomatous germ cell tumor. J Urol 2000;163:1785-1787.

Toner GC, Panicek DM, Heelan RT, et al: Adjunctive surgery after chemotherapy for nonseminomatous germ cell tumors: Recommendations for patient selection. J Clin Oncol 1990;8:1683-1694.

Weissbach L, Boedefeld EA: Localization of solitary and multiple metastases in stage II nonseminomatous testis tumor as basis for a modified staging lymph node dissection in stage I. J Urol 1987;138:77-82.

Williams SD, Stablein DM, Einhorn LH, et al: Immediate adjuvant chemotherapy versus observation with treatment at relapse in pathological stage II testicular cancer. N Engl J Med 1987;317:1433-1438.

31 Tumors of the Penis

CURTIS A. PETTAWAY, MD • DONALD F. LYNCH, JR., MD • JOHN W. DAVIS, MD

Cancers of the penis are uncommon tumors that are often devastating for the patient and frequently diagnostically and therapeutically challenging for the urologist. Although rare in North America and Europe, penile malignant neoplasms constitute a substantial health concern in many African, South American, and Asian countries.

Any discussion of penile cancers must begin by addressing both benign and malignant tumors of the penis. **Some penile lesions are strictly benign, whereas others have the potential to evolve into malignant neoplasms.** A description of these lesions serves to establish their anatomic, etiologic, and histologic relationship to squamous cell carcinoma, which is the most common malignant tumor of the penis, as well as to other malignant neoplasms that involve the penis. Developments in the etiology of various benign, premalignant, and malignant penile tumors are reviewed in this chapter.

A detailed discussion of surgical management of penile cancer is undertaken in Chapter 32. Here we review the epidemiology, etiology, and natural history of squamous carcinoma and its contemporary management. **Reports have confirmed the importance of pathologic stage and histologic features of the primary tumor as well as the presence and extent of lymph node metastasis in determining prognosis and treatment planning of penile squamous carcinoma** (Ravi, 1993b; McDougal, 1995; Theodorescu, 1996; Pizzocaro et al, 1997; Slaton et al, 2001). In addition, developments in staging of the disease, including novel imaging modalities and the use of lymphatic mapping, and modified surgical approaches to improve staging accuracy and reduce potential morbidities are presented. The selection of patients for organ-preserving surgical strategies is discussed.

The role of radiation therapy as both a primary treatment and a palliative measure is reviewed. Contemporary developments in chemotherapy as well as in combination therapy with multiple therapeutic modalities are also discussed. A contemporary scheme for the management of the inguinal region, based on histologic and clinical features, is presented.

Finally, the various nonsquamous malignant neoplasms that may involve the penis are reviewed and discussed.

BENIGN LESIONS
Noncutaneous Lesions

Benign tumors of the penile shaft skin include congenital and acquired inclusion cysts, retention cysts, syringomas, and neurilemomas. Congenital inclusion cysts have occurred in the penoscrotal raphe (Cole and Helwig, 1976). Acquired inclusion cysts from circumcision or trauma are more common. Retention cysts arise from the sebaceous glands located on the mucosal surface of the prepuce and on the skin of the penile shaft. Retention cysts may arise in the parameatal area as a result of obstruction of the urethral glands (Shiraki, 1975). Syringomas, benign tumors of the sweat glands, may become large and symptomatic (Lipshutz et al, 1991; Sola Casas et al, 1993). Neurilemomas have been reported in the frenulum and prepuce (Chan et al, 1990; Hamilton et al, 1996).

Benign tumors of the supporting structures include angiomas, fibromas, neuromas, lipomas, and myomas. Angiomas are usually superficial and appear most frequently as punctate reddish papules or macules on the corona. They resemble the small angiokeratomas found on the scrotum. Neuromas present as firm, whitish papules at the corona or frenulum (Montgomery et al, 1990). Fibroepithelial polyps may occasionally arise from the glans (Yildrim et al, 2004).

Penile masses and deformities, or pseudotumors, may develop after self-administered injections or implantation of foreign bodies (Nitidandhaprabhas, 1975). Testosterone in oil (Zalar et al, 1969) and other common oils (Engleman et al,

SECTION VII

1974) have been applied to or injected into the penis, producing a destructive lipogranulomatous process that may grossly mimic carcinoma. Pyogenic granuloma may arise at the site of self-injection in impotence therapy (Summers, 1990). Early or atypical Peyronie's plaques may present as masses within the shaft and base of the penis.

On occasion, phlebitis, lymphangitis, and angiitis may produce subcutaneous cords or nodules in the penis (Grossman et al, 1965; Ball and Pickett, 1975).

When a diagnosis is in question, all benign lesions are best treated with local excision and thorough histologic evaluation to rule out malignant transformation.

Cutaneous Lesions

Pearly penile papules, hirsute papillomas, and coronal papillae are normal and commonly encountered lesions of the glans penis. They occur in about 15% of postpubertal men and are more common in uncircumcised men (Neinstein and Goldenring, 1984). These lesions present as linear, curved, or irregular rows of conical or globular excrescences, varying from white to yellow to red, arranged along the coronal sulcus. They are considered acral angiofibromas. When larger than usual, they may be mistaken for condylomata acuminata (Evans and Patten, 1990). Treatment is usually unnecessary, but when it is indicated, lesions have responded to fulguration with the carbon dioxide laser (Magid and Garden, 1989; Lane et al, 2002). These lesions have not been associated with malignant transformation (Tannenbaum and Becker, 1965; Ferenczy et al, 1990).

Zoon's balanitis is characterized by a shiny, erythematous plaque or erosion that on biopsy demonstrates normal cell layers but a dense plasma cell infiltrate. It most commonly involves the glans but may involve the prepuce. Treatment is by circumcision, although there are reports of successful management with the carbon dioxide laser (Baldwin and Geronemus, 1989).

The full range of rashes and ulceration due to irritation, allergy, or infection must be considered in the differential diagnosis of the cutaneous lesion (Schneede et al, 2003).

PREMALIGNANT CUTANEOUS LESIONS

Some histologically benign penile lesions have been recognized as having malignant potential or close association with the development of squamous carcinoma. In one large series, 42% of patients with squamous cell cancer had a history of preexisting penile lesions (Bouchot et al, 1989). Although the incidence of progression of these lesions to squamous cell carcinoma is not known, all have been associated with the disease.

Cutaneous Horn

The penile cutaneous horn is a rare lesion. It usually develops over a preexisting skin lesion (wart, nevus, traumatic abrasion, or malignant neoplasm) and is characterized by overgrowth and cornification of the epithelium, which forms a solid protuberance. On microscopic examination, extreme hyperkeratosis, dyskeratosis, and acanthosis are noted. It is associated with human papillomavirus (HPV) type 16. Treatment

consists of surgical excision with a margin of normal tissue about the base of the horn. These lesions may recur and may demonstrate malignant change on subsequent biopsy, even when initial histologic appearance is benign (Fields et al, 1987). **Because this tumor may evolve into a carcinoma or may develop as a result of an underlying carcinoma, careful histologic evaluation of the base and close follow-up of the excision site are essential** (Pressman et al, 1962; Hassan et al, 1967; Solivan et al, 1990).

Pseudoepitheliomatous Micaceous and Keratotic Balanitis

These unusual lesions present as hyperkeratotic, micaceous growths on the glans and may have some of the microscopic features of verrucous carcinoma. They tend to recur and may represent an early form of that tumor (Jenkins and Jakubovic, 1988; Gray and Ansell, 1990). Treatment includes excision, laser ablation, and cryotherapy. These lesions require aggressive treatment and close follow-up. Fibrosarcoma of the glans after treatment of a pseudoepitheliomatous micaceous and keratotic balanitis lesion with cryotherapy has been reported (Irvine et al, 1987).

Balanitis Xerotica Obliterans (Lichen Sclerosus)

This genital variation of lichen sclerosus et atrophicus presents as a whitish patch on the prepuce or glans, often involving the meatus and sometimes extending into the fossa navicularis. The lesions may be multiple and may assume a mosaic appearance. The meatus may appear white, indurated, and edematous. Glanular erosions, fissures, and meatal stenosis may occur. The disorder is most common in uncircumcised men and occurs most commonly in middle-aged men, but it does occur in boys (McKay et al, 1975). Symptoms include pain, local penile discomfort, pruritus, painful erections, and urinary obstruction (Bainbridge et al, 1971).

On histologic examination, these lesions show atrophic epidermis with loss of the rete pegs and homogenization of collagen on the upper third of the dermis combined with a zone of lymphocytic and histiocytic infiltration. They resemble the lesions of lichen sclerosus et atrophicus found elsewhere (Laymon and Freeman, 1944). **There are reports documenting the association of balanitis xerotica obliterans with squamous cell carcinoma as well as with the development of carcinoma long after a lesion of balanitis xerotica obliterans has been treated** (Laymon and Freeman, 1944; Bart and Kopf, 1978; Jamieson et al, 1986; Dore et al, 1990; Simonart et al, 1998; Velazquez and Cubilla, 2003; Kumaran and Kanwar, 2004). A report describes a well-differentiated nonverruciform variant of squamous cell carcinoma associated with lichen sclerosus et atrophicus that preferentially involves the prepuce (Cubilla et al, 2004).

Treatment consists of topical steroid cream, injectable steroids, and surgical excision. Meatal stenosis is a common problem often requiring repeated dilations, steroid injection, or even formal meatoplasty (Poynter and Levy, 1967). Close follow-up is essential, with biopsy if a change in appearance or behavior occurs.

Leukoplakia

These lesions present as solitary or multiple whitish plaques that often involve the meatus. On histologic examination, there is hyperkeratosis, parakeratosis, and hypertrophy of the rete pegs with dermal edema and lymphocytic infiltration. Careful microscopic examination is necessary to determine malignant change.

Treatment involves elimination of chronic irritation, and circumcision may be indicated. Surgical excision and radiation have been used in the treatment of leukoplakia. **This disorder has been associated with both in situ squamous cell cancer and verrucous cancer of the penis** (Hanash et al, 1970; Reece and Koontz, 1975; Bain and Geronemus, 1989). Because of this close relationship with carcinoma, meticulous follow-up of the excision site with periodic biopsy of incompletely excised lesions is necessary to detect early malignant change.

KEY POINTS: BENIGN AND PREMALIGNANT CUTANEOUS LESIONS

- When in doubt, biopsy of penile lesions should be considered to establish a diagnosis.

- Lesions associated with the development of penile carcinoma that require treatment or close follow-up include cutaneous horn, balanitis xerotica obliterans, pseudoepitheliomatous micaceous and keratotic balanitis, and leukoplakia.

VIRUS-RELATED DERMATOLOGIC LESIONS

There is increasing evidence to suggest that a number of penile lesions share viral etiologies. **Condyloma acuminatum and bowenoid papulosis appear to be related to infection with human papillomavirus. Human herpesvirus 8, also known as Kaposi's sarcoma–associated herpesvirus, is strongly suspected of being the etiologic agent of epidemic (AIDS-related) Kaposi's sarcoma** (Miller et al, 1996; Simpson et al, 1996; Jaffe and Pellett, 1999; Dianzani et al, 2004).

Human Papillomavirus in Malignant Transformation

Condylomata acuminata are soft, papillomatous growths generally considered to be benign. Also known as genital warts or venereal warts, they have a predilection for the moist, glabrous areas of the body and the mucocutaneous surfaces of the perineal and genital areas. The lesions are soft and friable and may occur singly on a pedicle or in a moruloid cluster on a broad base. These lesions are rare before puberty (Redman and Meacham, 1973; Copulsky et al, 1975) and when encountered may suggest sexual abuse (Handly et al, 1993).

In the male, condylomata occur most commonly on the glans, the penile shaft, and the prepuce. The meatus should also be carefully inspected. Lesions recur frequently, both in new and in previously treated sites. Approximately 5% of patients will demonstrate urethral involvement, which may extend to the prostatic urethra (Culp et al, 1944). Rarely, extreme involvement of the urethra may require urethroplasty (Feneley et al, 1992). Bladder involvement, although rare, is extremely difficult to treat effectively (Bissada et al, 1974).

On microscopic examination, condylomata acuminata demonstrate an outer layer of keratinized tissue covering papillary fronds, which are supported by connective tissue stroma. The epithelial layer consists of well-ordered rows of squamous cells. A dermal lymphocytic infiltrate is usually present. **Treatment of these lesions with podophyllin may induce histologic changes suggestive of carcinoma** (King and Sullivan, 1947). **Consequently, preliminary biopsy of large lesions that appear to be condylomata acuminata should precede any treatment with topical podophyllin.**

Interest in genital condylomata has increased dramatically, stimulated by an increased understanding of the relationship between HPV infection and certain human cancers. The terms *genital condyloma, venereal warts, genital warts,* and *genital HPV infection* all refer to a sexually transmitted disease caused by HPV. Although HPV is not a reportable sexually transmitted disease, a current estimate puts the number of new infections at 500,000 to 1 million annually. Prevalence figures are unknown (Stone, 1989). **HPV is recognized as the principal etiologic agent in cervical dysplasia and cervical cancer** (Lancaster et al, 1986; Alani and Munger, 1998; Gross and Pfister, 2004). Significant numbers of male partners of women with cervical condylomata will have lesions not identified by simple inspection and may not be aware that they are infected or have the potential to infect others (Sedlacek et al, 1986).

On histologic examination, the koilocyte—a cell characterized by an empty cavity surrounding an atypical nucleus—is pathognomonic for HPV infection (Schneider, 1989). DNA hybridization techniques have been used to identify and classify HPV infections, and some 40 subtypes of HPV virus have been identified (Lowhagen et al, 1993). **Virus types 6, 11, and 42 to 44 are associated with gross condylomata and low-grade dysplasia. Types 16, 18, 31, 33, 35, and 39 have a higher association with malignant disease** (Smotkin, 1989). **More recently, reports have suggested that tumor virus transforming proteins from HPV types 16 and 18, particularly the E6 and E7 proteins, may target tumor suppressor gene products pRB and p53 and may be the causative agents in a subset of penile cancers** (Levi et al, 1998; Griffiths and Mellon, 1999). E6 appears to bind to cellular tumor suppressor protein p53, leading to its rapid degradation, resulting in chromosome instability, DNA mutations, and aneuploidy. E7 binds to and phosphorylates the pRB retinoblastoma protein, leading to the release of transcription factor E2F that activates mitosis (zur Hausen, 1996). Human immunodeficiency virus (HIV) infection may predispose affected patients to rapid development of squamous carcinoma from preexisting condyloma infection (Sanders, 1997). Whereas subtyping of HPV has been largely a research tool, it is being developed as a means of identifying potentially aggressive lesions to assist in treatment planning (Carpiniello et al, 1990; Noel et al, 1992).

Subclinical disease may be detected by the application of 5% acetic acid solution to the penis, followed by inspection with a magnifying glass. Lesions will turn white, and flat lesions often invisible on regular inspection may be detected.

These "aceto-white" lesions are not always due to HPV, and biopsy must be performed to confirm the diagnosis (Krebs, 1987). Careful inspection of the base of the shaft, the scrotum, and the inguinal folds is essential. The meatus should be examined, and if lesions are present, urethroscopy should be performed (Culp et al, 1944; Barrasso et al, 1987).

Topical podophyllin (Condylox 0.5%) or trichloroacetic acid has been a well-established and often successful treatment for small condyloma lesions (Culp et al, 1944; Kinghorn et al, 1993). **More recently, however, imiquimod cream (5%) has become the topical treatment of choice for condyloma. Imiquimod is an immune modulator that enhances natural killer cell activity and is the only topical treatment having the potential to eliminate HPV** (Buechner, 2002; Sanchez-Ortiz and Pettaway, 2003).

Circumcision will remove preputial lesions, gain exposure for treatment, and allow post-treatment monitoring. Fulguration and excision may be advisable to avoid large areas of maceration, ulceration, and secondary infection.

Surgical laser therapy has been used extensively in the management of condylomata and is covered in Chapter 32. Surgical therapy with use of a pediatric resectoscope may be helpful in debulking large intraurethral lesions. The lowest power required to resect the lesions should be used, and electrocautery should be minimized to avoid the development of urethral stricture.

Intraurethral lesions may be extremely difficult to treat. 5-Fluorouracil cream applied weekly for 3 weeks has been successful in eliminating urethral lesions (Bissada et al, 1974; Boxer and Skinner, 1977; Dretler and Klein, 1975). Care must be taken to work the cream down the urethra and to avoid exposure of the scrotal skin. Use of a scrotal support or zinc oxide cream may be helpful. The addition of 5-fluorouracil cream to laser therapy did not improve the success rate (Carpiniello et al, 1987).

Various interferons have been used in condyloma treatment (Geffen et al, 1984). A randomized study has shown that short-term intralesional interferon alfa-2b has activity against condyloma (Eron et al, 1986). The outcome of studies using other interferons has been less clear (Zouboulis et al, 1991). Interferon therapy continues to be reserved for extensive and recalcitrant lesions (Krebs, 1989a, 1989b; Ferenczy, 1990).

HPV infection is common and, as noted earlier, potentially carcinogenic. Condylomata have been associated with squamous cell carcinoma of the penis (Beggs and Spratt, 1964; Dawson et al, 1965; Rhatigan et al, 1972). Malignant transformation of condyloma to squamous cell carcinoma has been reported (Boxer and Skinner, 1977; Coetzee, 1977; Malek et al, 1993). Condylomata acuminata located in the perianal, scrotal, and oral areas have also demonstrated malignant degeneration (Siegel, 1962; Burmer et al, 1993). An increased incidence of penile intraepithelial neoplasia has been found in the male partners of women with cervical intraepithelial neoplasia (Barrasso et al, 1987; Iversen et al, 1997). The role of HPV in the transformation of condylomatous lesions to malignant neoplasms continues to undergo careful study.

Bowenoid Papulosis

Carcinoma in situ of the penis has been well recognized since its first description by Queyrat in 1911. Kopf and Bart described bowenoid papulosis, a condition having a histologic appearance similar to that of carcinoma in situ but a benign course, in 1977.

Bowenoid papulosis presents as multiple papules on the penile skin or female vulva, usually during the second or third decade of life. The lesions are usually pigmented and range from 0.2 to 3.0 cm in diameter, and smaller lesions may coalesce into larger ones (Patterson et al, 1986). Pigmented lesions present on the penile skin, whereas glanular lesions tend to be flat papules (Gross et al, 1985). Diagnosis is confirmed by biopsy (Peters and Perry, 1981). These lesions meet all the histologic criteria of carcinoma in situ but display differing growth patterns relative to flat, endophytic, or exophytic clinical appearance (Wade et al, 1978; Peters and Perry, 1981; Gross et al, 1985; Patterson et al, 1986; Bhojwani et al, 1997). DNA sequences suggestive of HPV-16 have been found in specimens of bowenoid papulosis, and a causative role for HPV is suspected (Gross et al, 1985; Endo et al, 2003). **Whereas histologically this condition is a carcinoma in situ, the clinical course of bowenoid papulosis is invariably benign** (Su and Shipley, 1997).

Treatment has included electrodesiccation, cryotherapy, laser fulguration, topical 5-fluorouracil cream, and excision with skin grafting.

Kaposi's Sarcoma

Kaposi's sarcoma, first described in 1972, is a tumor of the reticuloendothelial system (Kaposi, 1982). It presents as a cutaneous neovascular lesion, a raised, painful, bleeding papule or ulcer with bluish discoloration. On histologic examination, the tumor is vasoformative with endothelial proliferation and spindle cell formation.

Initially, Kaposi's sarcoma occurred rarely in Europe and North America. It was characterized by a slowly progressive tumor affecting the lower extremities of older men, usually of eastern European Jewish or Italian descent. Kaposi's sarcoma was also found in young black African men and patients receiving immunosuppressive therapy. The disease is now closely linked with patients having acquired immunodeficiency syndrome (AIDS) and takes a much more aggressive clinical course in this group.

Kaposi's sarcoma is now subcategorized as follows: (1) classic Kaposi's sarcoma, which occurs in patients without known immunodeficiency and has an indolent and rarely fatal course; (2) immunosuppressive treatment–related Kaposi's sarcoma, which occurs in a patient receiving immunosuppressive therapy for organ transplantation or other indications and is often reversed with dosage modification of the immunosuppressive agents; (3) African Kaposi's sarcoma, which occurs in young men and may be indolent or aggressive in course; and (4) epidemic or HIV-related Kaposi's sarcoma, which occurs in the patient with AIDS.

The classic and immunosuppressive forms of the disease are considered nonepidemic. Nonepidemic Kaposi's sarcoma limited to penile involvement should be aggressively treated because it is rarely associated with diffuse organ involvement. Localized surgical excision or small-field external beam or electron beam radiation has been effective (Lands et al, 1992). With wider areas of involvement, partial penectomy is indicated. In the immunosuppressed patient, Kaposi's sarcoma will often regress with the discontinuation of immunosuppressive therapy. If regression does not occur, local excision or radiation should be considered. Systemic management for multisystem involvement has employed interferon and cytotoxic therapy (National Cancer Institute Position Statement, 1990).

In the patient with AIDS, the underlying immune deficiency predisposes the host to Kaposi's sarcoma by a factor of 7000 (Miles, 1994). The first case of HIV-related epidemic Kaposi's sarcoma was reported in 1981 (Friedman, 1981) and the first with penile involvement in 1986 (Seftel et al, 1986). Subsequently, Kaposi's sarcoma of the penis has become a relatively common lesion in the patient with AIDS. Penile involvement is more common in the homosexual man than in others with AIDS. In the first 1000 cases of AIDS reported by the Centers for Disease Control and Prevention, incidence of penile Kaposi's sarcoma was 44% in homosexual and bisexual patients compared with only 16% in intravenous drug abusers with AIDS and 0% of hemophiliac patients with AIDS (Jaffe et al, 1983; Bayne and Wise, 1988). Some studies have found epidemic Kaposi's sarcoma in patients who are HIV negative, which suggests that certain sexual practices and a separate sexually transmitted agent may be responsible for this form of the disease (Miles, 1994; Chitale et al, 2002). **Several reports suggest a strong relationship between infection with human herpesvirus 8, also known as Kaposi's sarcoma–related herpesvirus, and the development of Kaposi's sarcoma lesions in patients with HIV infection** (Jaffe and Pellett, 1999; Sitas et al, 1999). **Largely because of the explosion of AIDS in the past decade, Kaposi's sarcoma of the penis is now probably the second most common malignant neoplasm of the penis after squamous cell carcinoma.**

Whereas Kaposi's sarcoma may be the presenting sign of the disease in many patients with AIDS, early involvement of the penis is rare in this group (Grunwald et al, 1994). Treatment is directed toward palliation (Lowe et al, 1989). Glans penis or corpus spongiosum involvement may produce urethral obstruction, necessitating proximal urethrostomy. This will usually allow voiding in the upright position. With large lesions involving the penis, partial or total penectomy may be necessary. Radiation therapy and use of the neodymium:yttrium-aluminum-garnet (Nd:YAG) laser to alleviate distal urethral obstruction have also been reported (Wishnow and Johnson, 1988; Ruszczak et al, 1996).

BUSCHKE-LÖWENSTEIN TUMOR (VERRUCOUS CARCINOMA, GIANT CONDYLOMA ACUMINATUM)

The Buschke-Löwenstein tumor was initially described by Buschke and Löwenstein in 1925 and later by Löwenstein in 1939 in the United States. Ackerman (1948) described a histologically similar tumor presenting in the oral cavity. Verrucous carcinomas of the larynx, vulva, and penis were described by Goethals and colleagues (1963). **Whereas some verrucous carcinomas of nonpenile sites do metastasize, metastasis from the Buschke-Löwenstein tumor does not appear to occur.** Rather, the Buschke-Löwenstein tumor invades locally, compressing and destroying adjacent tissues to produce

urethral erosion and fistulization. This aggressive local growth, combined with bleeding, discharge, and odor, prompts the patient to seek medical evaluation and treatment.

The true incidence of the Buschke-Löwenstein tumor is unknown, but it is probably higher than reported because many cases have been labeled low-grade squamous carcinoma of the penis. Retrospective analyses of several reports have revealed a number of cases of verrucous cancer or giant condylomata under the category of low-grade squamous cell carcinomas (Davies, 1965; Hanash et al, 1970; Grussendorf-Conen, 1997).

The Buschke-Löwenstein tumor differs from condyloma acuminatum in that condylomata, regardless of size, always remain superficial and never invade adjacent tissue. Buschke-Löwenstein tumor displaces, invades, and destroys adjacent structures by compression. Aside from this unrestrained local growth, it demonstrates no signs of malignant change on histologic examination and does not metastasize. On microscopic examination, the tumor forms a luxuriant mass composed of broad rounded rete pegs, often extending far into underlying tissue. The pegs are composed of well-differentiated squamous cells that show no cellular anaplasia. These epithelial pegs are characteristically surrounded by a dense band of acute and chronic inflammatory cells. As with condyloma acuminatum, the etiology may be viral (Dawson et al, 1965; Ubben et al, 1979; Antony et al, 2003). DNA from HPV types 6 and 11 has been identified in these tumors (Boshart and zur Hausen, 1986).

Lymph node metastases are rare with verrucous carcinoma (Ackerman, 1948; Davies, 1965; Seixas, 1994), **and their presence probably reflects malignant degeneration in the primary lesion.** Such changes are known to occur in verrucous carcinoma of nonpenile sites (Davies, 1965; Dawson et al, 1965). Anecdotal cases of malignant degeneration in association with penile carcinoma have been reported (Youngberg et al, 1983).

Either excisional biopsy or multiple deep biopsies are required to distinguish the lesion from true penile carcinoma. Treatment consists of excision, sparing as much of the penis as possible. Large lesions may necessitate total penectomy.

Recurrence is common, and close follow-up is essential. Topical therapy with either podophyllin or 5-fluorouracil has been unsuccessful, probably because the characteristic thickened stratum corneum is impervious to the medication (Bruns et al, 1975).

Radiation therapy is ineffective and has been associated with subsequent rapid malignant changes of verrucous carcinomas in other locations (Lepor and Leffler, 1960; Kraus and Perez-Mesa, 1966; Proffitt et al, 1970). Bleomycin has been used in both a primary and an adjunctive mode for verrucous carcinoma (Mishima and Matunaka, 1972). Successful treatment of a Buschke-Löwenstein tumor with systemic interferon therapy combined with Nd:YAG laser therapy has been reported (Gilbert and Beckert, 1990). Cryosurgery has also been employed with success (Michelman et al, 2002).

KEY POINTS: VERRUCOUS CARCINOMA

- Verrucous penile carcinoma exhibits progressive local growth but does not metastasize.

- It often requires surgical excision for definitive treatment.

- Treatment with radiation therapy has been associated with malignant degeneration of these lesions in other sites.

SQUAMOUS CELL CARCINOMA
Carcinoma In Situ

Carcinoma in situ (Tis) of the penis is called erythroplasia of Queyrat by urologists and dermatologists if it involves the glans penis, prepuce, or penile shaft and Bowen's disease if it involves the remainder of the genitalia or perineal region. This nomenclature has served to separate carcinoma in situ from the mainstream of thinking and reporting of penile carcinoma. However, the epidemiology and natural history of this lesion parallel those of early carcinoma of the penis, and carcinoma in situ can progress to invasive carcinoma.

The erythroplasia originally described by Queyrat in 1911 consists of a red, velvety, well-marginated lesion of the glans penis or, less frequently, the prepuce of the uncircumcised man (Aragona et al, 1985). It may ulcerate and may be associated with discharge and pain. On histologic examination, the normal mucosa is replaced by atypical hyperplastic cells characterized by disorientation, vacuolation, multiple hyperchromatic nuclei, and mitotic figures at all levels. The epithelial rete extends into the submucosa and appears elongated, broadened, and bulbous. The submucosa shows capillary proliferation and ectasia with a surrounding inflammatory infiltrate, usually rich in plasma cells. These microscopic features distinguish erythroplasia of Queyrat from chronic localized balanitis. HPV has been identified in penile carcinoma in situ (Pfister and Haneke, 1984).

In 1912, Bowen described an intraepithelial neoplasm of the skin associated with a high occurrence of subsequent internal malignant disease as a distinct entity. Bowen's disease and erythroplasia of Queyrat are histologically similar (Graham and Helwig, 1973). Both tumors are characterized by the noninvasive changes of carcinoma in situ. **Visceral malignant disease is not associated with erythroplasia of Queyrat, and subsequent case-control studies have shown no association of Bowen's disease with internal malignant tumors** (Anderson et al, 1973). Thus, penile carcinoma in situ does not in itself warrant a specific search for internal malignant tumors. **Graham and Helwig noted that 10% of cases of carcinoma in situ were associated with invasive cancer. Thus, progression to invasion can occur. Metastasis is extremely rare but has been reported** (Eng et al, 1995).

Treatment is based on proper histopathologic confirmation of malignancy with multiple biopsies of adequate depth to rule out invasion. When lesions are located on the foreskin, circumcision or excision with a 5-mm margin is adequate for local control (Bissada, 1992). In this regard, lesions on the glans penis are difficult to treat by excisional strategies while maintaining normal penile anatomy. Alternative strategies include topical 5-fluorouracil cream (Lewis and Bendl, 1971; Graham and Helwig, 1973; Goette, 1974) and laser ablation with Nd:YAG (Landthaler et al, 1986; Frimberger et al, 2002a), potassium titanyl phosphate (KTP) 532-nm, or carbon dioxide lasers (Rosemberg and Fuller, 1980; Tietjen and Malek, 1998; van Bezooijen et al, 2001). Such strategies have been shown to produce excellent cosmetic and functional results. Radiotherapy can be used to treat tumors that are resistant to topical treatment, especially among patients who are not surgical candidates (Kelley et al, 1974; Grabstald and Kelley, 1980).

KEY POINTS: CARCINOMA IN SITU (Tis) IS AN INTRAEPITHELIAL MALIGNANT PROCESS

- Tis may progress to invasive carcinoma in about 10% of cases.

- Metastasis has rarely occurred.

- Cancer eradication with organ-preserving strategies is the goal of therapy.

Invasive Carcinoma

Penile carcinoma accounts for 0.4% to 0.6% of all malignant neoplasms among men in the United States and Europe; it may represent up to 10% of malignant neoplasms in men in some Asian, African, and South American countries (Gloeckler-Ries et al, 1990; Vatanasapt et al, 1995). **However, reports suggest that the incidence of penile cancer is decreasing in many countries, including Finland, the United States, India, and other Asian countries** (Maiche et al, 1991; Frisch et al, 1995; Vatanasapt et al, 1995; Yeole and Jussawalla, 1997). The reasons are unclear but may be related in part to increased attention to personal hygiene.

Penile cancer is a disease of older men, with an abrupt increase in incidence in the sixth decade of life and a peak around 80 years of age (Persky, 1977). In two studies, the mean age was 58 years (Gursel et al, 1973) and 55 years (Derrick et al, 1973). The tumor is not unusual in younger men; in one large series, 22% of patients were younger than 40 years and 7% were younger than 30 years (Dean, 1935); the disease has also been reported in children (Kini, 1944; Narasimharao et al, 1985). The Surveillance, Epidemiology, and End Results (SEER) database reveals no racial difference in incidence of penile cancer between black and white men in the United States (incidence for white men, 0.8 of 100,000; for black men, 0.7 of 100,000) (Vatanasapt et al, 1995).

However, a study using SEER data suggested that race is associated with outcome. Rippentrop and colleagues (2004) noted there were 1605 patients diagnosed with penile cancer from 1973 to 1998, with 22.4% (360) dying of the disease. They found factors independently predictive of worsened survival to be higher stage at diagnosis, age older than 65 years, African American ethnicity, and disease within lymph nodes. They demonstrated a statistically significant disease-specific risk of death that was 2.2-fold higher in African American patients than in white patients. Although the reason for this disparity is likely to be multifactorial, possibilities include differences in cancer biology, in health care access, or in treatment. These provocative findings clearly deserve further study.

Etiology

The incidence of carcinoma of the penis varies according to circumcision practice, hygienic standard, phimosis, number of sexual partners, HPV infection, exposure to tobacco products, and other factors (Barrasso et al, 1987; Maiche, 1992; Maden et al, 1993; Misra et al, 2004).

Neonatal circumcision has been well established as a prophylactic measure that virtually eliminates the occurrence of penile carcinoma because it eliminates the closed preputial environment where penile carcinoma develops. The chronic irritative effects of smegma, a byproduct of bacterial action on desquamated cells that are within the preputial sac, have been proposed as an etiologic agent. Although definitive evidence that human smegma itself is a carcinogen has not been established (Reddy and Baruah, 1963), its relationship to the development of penile carcinoma has been widely observed. Improper hygiene can lead to buildup of smegma beneath the preputial foreskin, with resulting inflammation. Healing by fibrosis leads to phimosis of the preputial skin, which tends to perpetuate the cycle. Phimosis is found in 25% to 75% of patients described in most large series. Reddy and associates (1984) studied the foreskins of 26 men undergoing circumcision because of phimosis and found epithelial atypia in one third of the specimens.

Carcinoma of the penis is rare among the Jewish population, for whom neonatal circumcision is a universal practice (Licklider, 1961). Similarly, in the United States, where neonatal circumcision is widely practiced, penile cancer represents less than 1% of male malignant neoplasms. Among uncircumcised tribes of Africa and within uncircumcised Asian cultures, penile cancer may amount to 10% to 20% of all male malignant neoplasms (Dodge, 1965; Narayana et al, 1982). Data from most large series show that penile cancer is rare among neonatally circumcised individuals but more frequent when circumcision is delayed until puberty (Frew et al, 1967; Gursel et al, 1973; Johnson et al, 1973). Adult circumcision

appears to offer little or no protection from subsequent development of the disease (Maden et al, 1993). **These data suggest that the critical period of exposure to certain etiologic agents may have already occurred at puberty and certainly by adulthood, rendering later circumcision relatively ineffective as a prophylactic tool for penile cancer.**

Recent population-based data reveal that whereas neonatal circumcision is highly protective for invasive penile cancer, it does not afford the same level of protection for carcinoma in situ. Schoen and colleagues (2000) evaluated the incidence of invasive penile cancer or carcinoma in situ during a 10-year period and found only 2 cases of 89 (2.3%) occurring among neonatally circumcised men, whereas of 118 men with carcinoma in situ, 16 cases were noted in men circumcised at birth (15.7%). Considering that the protective effects of circumcision on invasive penile cancer are likely to be mediated by avoidance of phimosis, it is noteworthy that another study associated phimosis with the development of invasive penile cancer but not carcinoma in situ (Hung-fu et al, 2001).

Male circumcision has also been shown to be effective against HIV-1 infection. This effect was shown to be specific by Reynolds and colleagues (2004). There was no protective effect of circumcision for other sexually transmitted diseases, such as herpes simplex virus type 2 infection, syphilis, or gonorrhea.

HPV infection and exposure to tobacco products appear to be associated with development of penile cancer. Epidemiologic data provided the first clues to a relationship between a sexually transmitted agent and cancer by demonstrating that the wives or ex-wives of men with penile cancer had a threefold higher risk of cervical carcinoma (Graham et al, 1979). Further investigation revealed that the male partners of women with cervical intraepithelial neoplasia had a significantly higher incidence of penile intraepithelial neoplasia (Barrasso et al, 1987). These same male patients were also found to have a greater incidence of HPV infection.

Advanced molecular biologic techniques such as polymerase chain reaction and in situ hybridization have provided increased evidence for an etiologic role of HPV by identifying specific DNA sequences from different HPV types in primary penile lesions (malignant and benign) but not in normal foreskins (Varma et al, 1991; Iwasawa et al, 1993). More than 25 types of HPV infect genital sites. HPV types 6 and 11 are most commonly associated with nondysplastic lesions such as genital warts, but these are also noted in nonmetastatic verrucous carcinomas. In contrast, HPV types 16, 18, 31, and 33 are associated with in situ and invasive carcinomas (Wiener and Walther, 1995). **HPV-16 appears to be the most frequently detected type in primary carcinomas and has also been detected in metastatic lesions** (Varma et al, 1991; Iwasawa et al, 1993; Wiener and Walther, 1995). As noted previously, the HPV genome encodes oncoprotein E6, which complexes with the tumor suppressor protein p53, and oncoprotein E7, which binds the retinoblastoma protein, thus affecting cell cycle regulation (Munger et al, 1989; zur Hausen, 1996; Levi et al, 1998; Griffiths and Mellon, 1999). **Maden and colleagues (1993) found that the incidence of HPV infection directly correlated with the number of lifetime sexual partners, which was also related to risk of penile cancer.** Further, Castellsague and colleagues (1997) noted a direct correlation between the number of sexual partners, HPV-infected men, and incidence of cervical neoplasia among their female partners. Thus, for both cervical and penile cancer, HPV infection represents a preventable etiology.

Poblet and coworkers (1999) reported on two cases of coexisting HIV-1 and HPV infection and postulated that HIV-1 could synergize with HPV to increase the progression of HPV penile lesions into penile carcinoma. Whereas there is evidence supporting this effect in cervical and anal neoplasia, definitive proof for penile cancer awaits further study (Northfelt, 1994).

Although HPV infection is probably an important factor in the development of penile cancer, its presence is not invariable (31% to 63% of patients with penile carcinoma test positive) (Wiener and Walther, 1995), **indicating that additional factors may be involved in the development of the disease or its subtypes.** Additional evidence for Rubin and associates (2001), who performed a sensitive polymerase chain reaction assay, provided this hypothesis-based essay on penile cancer specimens from the United States and Paraguay. Overall, 42% of penile carcinomas were HPV positive. However, only 34.9% and 33.3% of keratinizing and verrucous carcinomas, respectively, were positive, whereas 80% and 100% of basaloid and warty tumor subtypes, respectively, exhibited HPV DNA.

Four studies have shown a significant association between exposure to cigarette smoke and development of penile cancer (Hellberg et al, 1987; Daling et al, 1992; Maden et al, 1993; Harish and Ravi, 1995). Hellberg and colleagues (1987) studied the smoking history of 244 men with penile cancer and matched controls. They found a significantly increased odds ratio for penile cancer based on whether an individual had smoked, and the risk increased with the number of cigarettes smoked. This observation held even when the presence of phimosis was controlled. **Harish and Ravi (1995) extended these observations by showing that all forms of tobacco products, including cigarettes, chewing tobacco, and snuff, were significantly and independently related to the incidence of penile cancer subsequent to multivariate regression analysis.** It has been hypothesized that tobacco products can act in the presence of HPV infection or bacteria associated with chronic inflammation to promote malignant transformation. These same risk factors are also common to other anogenital carcinomas (Daling et al, 1992; Maden et al, 1993).

Penile trauma may be another risk factor for penile cancer. The development of carcinoma in the scarred penile shaft after mutilating circumcision has been reported as a distinct entity (Bissada et al, 1986). Further, Maden and colleagues (1993) found a greater than threefold risk of penile cancer in men with penile tears and rashes. A case-control study also revealed an odds ratio of 18:1 for the development of penile cancer for those men reporting a penile injury 2 years before the onset of the disease (Hung-fu et al, 2001).

Genital ultraviolet radiation, alone and combined with 8-methoxypsoralen, increases the risk of squamous carcinoma at genital sites. A 12-year follow-up study reported that the risk of penile and scrotal cancer was increased 286 times that of the general population for those exposed to ultraviolet A photochemotherapy and 8-methoxysoralen (PUVA) (Stern et al, 1990). The risk was dose related. For those treated with ultraviolet B exposure, the risk was 4.6-fold enhanced. Another long-term follow-up study of PUVA-associated malignant neoplasia from Sweden revealed a 30-fold increased risk for skin cancer (but not for penile cancer) among males. In this study, PUVA was also associated with respiratory and pancreatic cancers (Lindelof et al, 1991). Lichen sclerosus (also known as balanitis xerotica obliterans), as previously discussed, is a risk factor for the development of penile cancer. **Studies have shown the incidence of subsequent cancer with long-term follow-up to be between 3% and 9% of men with lichen sclerosus** (Depasquale et al, 2000; Micali et al, 2001). Velasquez and Cubilla (2003) studied lichen sclerosus occurring in association with penile cancer and noted its presence distinctly among the subset of penile carcinomas that were not associated with HPV.

Larger studies performed in areas where the disease is endemic, incorporating the many risk factors for penile cancer into a multivariate analysis, are clearly needed to define which factors independently confer risk. Thus far, no convincing evidence has been found linking penile cancer to other factors such as occupation, other venereal diseases (gonorrhea, syphilis, herpes), marijuana use, or alcohol intake (Maden et al, 1993).

Prevention

The role of routine neonatal circumcision as a preventive strategy for penile cancer has been, to say the least, a controversial topic. The position of the American Academy of Pediatrics has changed from one of denial of any medical benefits (Schoen et al, 1989) to the more moderate recent position stating, **"There are potential medical benefits of newborn circumcision; however, these data are not sufficient to recommend routine neonatal circumcision. In such situations where the procedure is not essential to the child's well being, parents should determine what is in the best interest of the child subsequent to being presented unbiased information"** (Shapiro, 1999).

Any argument against circumcision must consider that penile carcinoma represents the only neoplasm for which there exists a predictable and simple means of prophylaxis to spare the organ at risk (Dagher et al, 1973). Although circumcision can obviate the disease, especially where facilities for daily hygiene may be lacking, it may not be as important in countries where good hygiene is practiced. Frisch and colleagues (1995) reported a falling incidence of penile cancer (from 1.15 of 100,000 men to 0.82 of 100,000 men) in the Danish population, which has a circumcision rate of only 1.6%. They attributed this trend to improved hygiene because the incidence of dwellings having a bath facility increased from 35% in the 1940s to 90% in the 1990s. Thus, considering the benefits of circumcision (including the prevention of infections, HIV infection and its transmission, and penile and cervical cancer), enhanced education about the potential benefits of circumcision, especially in developing countries, seems rational (Schoen et al, 1989; Reynolds et al, 2004; Kinkade et al, 2005).

Although neonatal circumcision and good hygiene to prevent the occurrence of phimosis represent important prevention strategies, additional efforts to prevent malignant transformation include avoidance of HPV infection, ultraviolet light exposure, and tobacco products. Thus, modifiable behaviors can potentially prevent penile cancer (Munger et al, 1989; Maden et al, 1993; Harish and Ravi, 1995; Levi et al, 1998; Griffiths and Mellon, 1999).

Natural History

Carcinoma of the penis usually begins with a small lesion that gradually extends to involve the entire glans, shaft, and corpora. The lesion may be papillary and exophytic or flat and ulcerative; if it is untreated, penile autoamputation may occur as a late result. The rates of growth of the papillary and ulcerative lesions are similar, but the flat, ulcerative tumor has a tendency toward earlier nodal metastasis and is associated with poorer 5-year survival rates (Dean, 1935; Marcial et al, 1962; Ornellas et al, 1994). Lesions larger than 5 cm (Beggs and Spratt, 1964) and those extending over 75% of the shaft (Staubitz et al, 1955) are also associated with an increased incidence of metastases and a decreased survival rate. However, others have not found a consistent relationship between lesion sizes, presence of metastases, and decreased survival (Ekstrom and Edsmyr, 1958; Puras et al, 1978).

Buck's fascia acts as a temporary natural barrier to local extension of the tumor, protecting the corporal bodies from invasion. Penetration of Buck's fascia and the tunica albuginea permits invasion of the vascular corpora and establishes the potential for vascular dissemination. Urethral and bladder involvement are rare (Riveros and Gorostiaga, 1962; Thomas and Small, 1968).

The earliest route of dissemination from penile carcinoma is metastasis to the regional femoral and iliac nodes. A detailed description of lymphatic drainage of the penis is found elsewhere in this text and is well documented in the literature (Dewire and Lepor, 1992). Briefly, the lymphatics of the prepuce form a connecting network that joins with the lymphatics from the skin of the shaft. These tributaries drain into the superficial inguinal nodes (the nodes external to the fascia lata). The lymphatics of the glans join the lymphatics draining the corporal bodies, and they form a collar of connecting channels at the base of the penis that drain by way of the superficial nodes. The superficial nodes drain to the deep inguinal nodes (those deep to the fascia lata). From there, drainage is to the pelvic nodes (external iliac, internal iliac, and obturator). Penile lymphangiographic studies demonstrate a consistent pattern of drainage that proceeds from superficial inguinal to deep inguinal to pelvic node sites without evidence of "skip" drainage (Cabanas, 1977, 1992). Multiple cross-connections exist at all levels of drainage, so that penile lymphatic drainage is bilateral to both inguinal areas.

Metastatic enlargement of the regional nodes eventually leads to skin necrosis, chronic infection, and death from inanition, sepsis, or hemorrhage secondary to erosion into the femoral vessels. Clinically detectable distant metastatic lesions to the lung, liver, bone, or brain are uncommon and are reported to occur in 1% to 10% of cases in most large series (Staubitz et al, 1955; Riveros and Gorostiaga, 1962; Beggs and Spratt, 1964; Derrick et al, 1973; Johnson et al, 1973; Kossow et al, 1973; Puras et al, 1978). Such metastases usually occur late in the course of the disease after the local lesion has been treated. Distant metastases in the absence of regional node metastases are unusual.

Carcinoma of the penis is characterized by a relentless progressive course, causing death for the majority of untreated patients within 2 years (Beggs and Spratt, 1964; Skinner et al, 1972; Derrick et al, 1973). Rarely, long-term survival occurs, even with advanced local disease and regional node metastases (Furlong and Uhle, 1953; Beggs and Spratt, 1964). No report of spontaneous remission of carcinoma of the penis is known. About 5% to 15% of patients have been reported to develop a second primary neoplasm (Buddington et al, 1963; Beggs and Spratt, 1964; Gursel et al, 1973), and one series reported secondary carcinoma in 17% of patients (Hubbell et al, 1988).

Modes of Presentation
Signs

It is the penile lesion itself that usually alerts the patient to the presence of penile cancer. The presentation ranges from a relatively subtle induration or small excrescence to a small papule, pustule, warty growth, or more luxuriant exophytic lesion. It may appear as a shallow erosion or as a deeply excavated ulcer with elevated or rolled-in edges. Phimosis may obscure a lesion and allow a tumor to progress silently. Eventually, erosion through the prepuce, foul preputial odor, and discharge with or without bleeding call attention to the disease.

Penile tumors may present anywhere on the penis but occur most commonly on the glans (48%) and prepuce (21%). Other tumors involve the glans and prepuce (9%), the coronal sulcus (6%), or the shaft (<2%) (Sufrin and Huben, 1991). This distribution of lesions may be due to constant exposure of the glans, coronal sulcus, and interior prepuce to irritants (e.g., smegma, HPV infection) within the preputial sac, whereas the shaft is relatively spared.

Rarely, a mass, ulceration, suppuration, or hemorrhage in the inguinal area may be due to nodal metastases from a lesion concealed within a phimotic foreskin. Urinary retention or urethral fistula due to local corporal involvement is a rare presenting sign.

Symptoms

Pain does not develop in proportion to the extent of the local destructive process and usually is not a presenting complaint.

Weakness, weight loss, fatigue, and systemic malaise occur secondary to chronic suppuration. On occasion, significant blood loss from the penile lesion, the nodal lesion, or both may occur. Because local disease and regional disease are usually far advanced by the time distant metastases occur, presenting symptoms referable to such metastases are rare.

Diagnosis

Delay

Patients with cancer of the penis, more than patients with other types of cancer, seem to delay seeking medical attention (Lynch and Krush, 1969). In large series, 15% to 50% of patients delayed medical care for more than a year (Dean, 1935; Buddington et al, 1963; Hardner et al, 1972; Gursel et al, 1973). Explanations include embarrassment, guilt, fear, ignorance, and personal neglect. This level of denial is substantial, given that the penis is observed and handled on a daily basis.

Delay on the part of the physician in initiating both diagnosis and treatment may also be considerable. In some instances, patients have been given prolonged courses of antibiotics or topical antifungal preparations before being referred for biopsy. Although some studies show that the difference in survival rates between patients who present early and those who present later is negligible (Ekstrom and Edsmyr, 1958; Johnson et al, 1973), other series show decreased survival with longer delay (Hardner et al, 1972). It appears logical that earlier diagnosis and treatment should improve outcome.

Examination

At presentation, most lesions are confined to the penis (Skinner et al, 1972; Derrick et al, 1973; Johnson et al, 1973). The penile lesion is assessed with regard to size, location, fixation, and involvement of the corporal bodies. Inspection of the base of the penis and scrotum is necessary to rule out extension into these areas. Rectal and bimanual examination provides information about perineal body involvement and presence of a pelvic mass. Careful bilateral palpation of the inguinal area for adenopathy is extremely important.

KEY POINTS: NATURAL HISTORY AND PRESENTATION

- Penile cancer often begins on the surface of the glans penis or in the preputial area, where it progressively enlarges.

- Delay in seeking medical attention and then subsequent definitive biopsy is common.

- Examination of both the penile primary tumor and inguinal region is critical to treatment planning.

- Metastasis occurs by embolization of tumor deposits from the penile tumor through penile lymphatics to the inguinal lymph nodes.

- Distant metastases occur late in the history of the disease.

Biopsy

Confirmation of the diagnosis of carcinoma of the penis and assessment of the depth of invasion, the presence of vascular invasion, and the histologic grade of the lesion by microscopic examination of a biopsy specimen are mandatory before the initiation of any therapy. This provides insight into the therapeutic options for treatment of the primary lesion as well as the likelihood of nodal metastases in patients with no palpable adenopathy (McDougal, 1995; Lopes et al, 1996; Theodorescu et al, 1996).

Biopsy may be a separate procedure from definitive surgical treatment. A dorsal slit is frequently necessary to gain adequate exposure of the lesion for satisfactory biopsy. An alternative approach to treatment is biopsy with frozen-section confirmation followed by partial or total penectomy. Full informed consent must be obtained before the procedure. Velazquez and colleagues (2004) demonstrated the shortcomings of superficial diagnostic biopsies in a study evaluating specimens from 57 patients. There was difficulty in delineating the extent of depth in 91% of patients, discordance with the histologic grade in 30% of patients (specifically with verrucous and mixed histologic patterns), and failure to detect any cancer in 3.5% of patients with well-differentiated cancers. The importance of obtaining an adequate biopsy specimen cannot be overemphasized.

Histologic Features

Most tumors of the penis are squamous cell carcinomas demonstrating keratinization, epithelial pearl formation, and various degrees of mitotic activity. The normal rete pegs are disrupted. Invasive lesions penetrate the basement membrane and the surrounding structures. Cubilla and associates (1993) originally divided penile cancers into superficially spreading squamous carcinoma, vertical growth carcinoma, verrucous carcinoma, and multicentric carcinoma. The superficially spreading carcinoma occurred most frequently, and inguinal lymph node metastases were found in 42% of patients. However, lymph node metastases were noted in 82% of patients with a vertical growth pattern, in none of those with a verrucous pattern, and in 33% of those with multicentric carcinomas. Subsequent to review of 61 cases from Memorial Sloan-Kettering Cancer Center, Cubilla and colleagues (2001) classified the cases as follows: usual type, 59% of cases; papillary, 15%; basaloid, 10%; warty (condylomatous), 10%; verrucous, 3%; and sarcomatoid, 3%. Of note, both the basaloid and sarcomatous types were associated with aggressive behavior; five of seven patients with these histologic patterns exhibited metastasis, and five of eight (63%) died. In contrast, the verruciform histologic patterns were more favorable (one patient with metastasis and no deaths). The typical squamous histologic type was intermediate in biologic potential; 14 of 26 exhibited metastases, and 13 of 36 (36%) died.

The basaloid variant, in addition to its aggressive behavior as noted previously, is associated with HPV expression in approximately 80% of cases (Gregoire et al, 1995; Cubilla et al, 1998, 2001; Rubin et al, 2001).

From a histologic standpoint, squamous cell carcinomas are graded by Broders' classification to define the level of differentiation on the basis of keratinization, nuclear pleomorphism, number of mitoses, and several other features

(Broders, 1921; Lucia and Miller, 1992). This grading system was originally designed for squamous carcinoma of the skin and has been adapted by pathologists for penile squamous carcinoma. Four grades were originally described, but it is common for authors to modify this to a three-grade system by combining grades (Maiche et al, 1991). Low-grade lesions (grade 1 and grade 2) constitute 70% to 80% of the reported cases at diagnosis, whether a three- or four-grade system is used (Maiche et al, 1991). These well-differentiated lesions show cords of atypical squamous cells projecting downward from a hyperkeratotic epidermis. The lower grade carcinomas typically demonstrate keratin, prominent intercellular bridges, and keratin pearls, characteristics that are absent in high-grade tumors. Almost half the tumors originating in the shaft are poorly differentiated (grade 3 and grade 4, depending on scale), whereas only 10% of tumors located in the prepuce are high-grade tumors (Maiche et al, 1991). Thus, grade and stage are often correlated.

Lack of correlation between grade and survival has been noted by a number of investigators (Staubitz et al, 1955; Beggs and Spratt, 1964; Edwards and Sawyers, 1968; Kuruvilla et al, 1971; Hardner et al, 1972; Johnson et al, 1973). Other series report reduced survival among patients with anaplastic tumors (Ekstrom and Edsmyr, 1958; Marcial et al, 1962; Frew et al, 1967; Hanash et al, 1970; Puras et al, 1978). Several studies have also emphasized the association of high-grade disease with regional nodal metastases (Fraley et al, 1989; Ravi, 1993b; McDougal, 1995; Theodorescu et al, 1996; Heyns et al, 1997). Overall, there is a significant body of agreement as to the histologic features that characterize high tumor grade (grade 3 and grade 4) and its correlation with nodal metastasis. However, as noted previously, most tumors are of lower grades. Histologic features that would better stratify the prognosis for patients with invasive, low- to intermediate-grade penile cancers would also be of value for management of patients.

Slaton and colleagues (2001) found that describing the percentage of poorly differentiated cancer in the primary penile tumor specimen correlated with lymph node metastasis. In this study, a semiquantitative system that estimated the amount of high-grade cancer (i.e., 50% or less versus more than 50%) was significantly associated with nodal metastases and was more predictive than the Broders' three-grade system in stratifying those with or without nodal metastasis.

Vascular invasion by tumor cells has significant prognostic importance but may not be specifically mentioned in pathology reports. When vascular invasion is present, it provides valuable information. Four studies have assessed its presence or absence, and it was an important predictor of nodal metastasis in all the reports (Fraley et al, 1989; Lopes et al, 1996; Heyns et al, 1997; Slaton et al, 2001). **Thus, the pathologist should specifically comment on the presence or absence of vascular invasion in the surgical specimen.**

Laboratory Studies

The results of laboratory tests in patients with penile cancer are often normal. Anemia, leukocytosis, and hypoalbuminemia may be present in patients with chronic illness, malnutrition, and extensive suppuration at the area of the primary and inguinal metastatic sites. Azotemia may develop secondary to urethral or ureteral obstruction.

KEY POINTS: BIOPSY AND HISTOLOGIC FEATURES

- Adequate tumor biopsy is essential to diagnosis and treatment planning.

- Squamous carcinoma subtypes include usual type, papillary, basaloid, warty, verrucous, and sarcomatoid.

- Basaloid histologic pattern is associated with aggressive behavior and HPV expression.

- Pathologic description of anatomic structures invaded (i.e., stage), grade, and status of vascular invasion provide important information to assess the risk of metastasis.

Hypercalcemia without detectable osseous metastases has been associated with penile cancer (Anderson and Glenn, 1965; Rudd et al, 1972). In a review from Memorial Sloan-Kettering Cancer Center (Sklaroff and Yagoda, 1982), 17 of 81 patients (20.9%) were hypercalcemic. Hypercalcemia seems to be largely a function of the bulk of the disease. It is often associated with inguinal metastases and may resolve after excision of involved inguinal nodes (Block et al, 1973). **Parathyroid hormone and related substances may be produced by both tumor and metastases that activate osteoclastic bone resorption** (Malakoff and Schmidt, 1975). Medical treatment of hypercalcemia includes aggressive saline hydration to restore the extracellular fluid volume and to promote both sodium and calcium excretion. The administration of diuretics is performed if volume overload is suspected. Bisphosphonates (e.g., pamidronate, etidronate) have become first-line therapy because they possess demonstrated efficacy as antiresorptive agents and are relatively safer than mithramycin, an older agent (Videtic et al, 1997; Morton and Lipton, 2000). For severe hypercalcemia associated with neurologic manifestations, the antiresorptive bisphosphonates can be combined with an agent that produces calciuria, such as calcitonin, to rapidly lower serum calcium levels.

Radiologic Studies

Penile Tumor Imaging. In patients with penile cancer, both the primary tumor and the inguinal lymph nodes are readily assessed by palpation. However, Horenblas and associates (1991) found that physical examination incorrectly established the actual pathologic stage in 26% of cases, with understaging in 10% and overstaging in 16%. It is clear that more accurate means of staging for penile tumors are needed.

Penile ultrasonography was performed on 16 patients referred for primary therapy by Horenblas and colleagues (1994). With use of a 7.5-MHz linear array small parts transducer, they found that the ultrasound appearance of cancer was invariably hypoechoic. However, ultrasound examination often underestimated the thickness of tumors and could not delineate invasion into the subepithelial connective tissue of the glans penis from corpus spongiosum involvement (i.e., glanular stage T1 versus glanular stage T2). However, the tunica albuginea separating the corpus cavernosum from the glans was easily identified in all patients, and the sensitivity for detecting corpus cavernosum invasion was 100%. This study confirmed the value of ultrasonography in assessing the primary tumor, as reported by others (Yamashita and Ogawa, 1989; Dorak et al, 1992).

Several studies have assessed the role of magnetic resonance imaging (MRI) in evaluating both the normal penis and its involvement by cancer. Vapnek and associates (1992) described the MRI appearance of the normal corpus cavernosum, corpus spongiosum, tunica albuginea, and Buck's fascia. Of six patients with urethral cancer, the disease was accurately staged in five (83%). de Kerviler and colleagues (1995) used gadolinium contrast–enhanced MRI to compare both clinical and MRI findings with tumor pathologic stage. Clinical examination correctly staged six of nine tumors; MRI was correct in seven of nine cases. MRI was not useful for clinical T1 lesions. Compared with MRI and ultrasonography, computed tomography (CT) scan has poor soft tissue resolution and has not been useful for imaging the extent of the primary tumor (Vapnek et al, 1992).

Lont and associates (2003) directly compared physical examination with ultrasonography and MRI to assess their ability to determine the tumor stage. They evaluated 33 patients with penile squamous cell carcinoma, all of whom underwent ultrasound examination, MRI, and physical examination of the primary tumor. Findings were correlated with histologic evaluation of the specimens obtained at surgery with a focus on determining the invasion of the corpus cavernosum. The respective positive predictive value, sensitivity, and specificity for the study were as follows—physical examination: 100%, 86%, 100%; ultrasound examination: 67%, 57%, 91%; and MRI: 75%, 100%, 91%. This comparative study concluded that physical examination is reliable in determining corporal invasion and that additional tests are mainly of value when physical examination cannot be properly performed.

The technique of artificial erection (by intracorporal injection of prostaglandin E_1) may augment the use of contrast-enhanced MRI in staging of the primary tumor. A study by the European Institute of Oncology evaluated nine patients to compare clinical, pathologic, and MRI staging (Scardino et al, 2004). MRI aided by artificial erection and contrast enhancement was shown to be of value as it correlated with pathologic stage in eight of nine cases, whereas physical examination correlated with only five of nine cases. These data suggest that this novel MRI approach could be beneficial in staging of glanular tumors, specifically when physical examination findings are equivocal. **Thus, for small-volume glanular lesions, imaging studies add virtually no additional information to palpation in most cases. However, for lesions thought to invade the corpus cavernosum, contrast-enhanced MRI (perhaps augmented with artificial erection) may provide unique information, especially when physical examination findings are equivocal and organ-sparing techniques are being considered.**

The ability to noninvasively determine the presence or absence of inguinal and pelvic metastases in patients with penile cancer remains problematic because physical examination exhibits varying reliability based on the grade and stage of the primary tumor. Historically, lymphangiography was used as an adjunct to physical examination in the identification of microscopic inguinal and pelvic nodal metastases and to direct needle biopsy (Vapnek et al, 1992). The technical difficulty of the procedure, combined with the availability of CT scanning and MRI, has made lymphangiography obsolete in staging of this disease. Both CT and MRI scanning techniques depend solely on lymph node enlargement for detection of metastases but are unable to define the internal architecture of normal-sized nodes. Because CT and MRI have similar accuracy in determining lymphadenopathy in other cancers, CT has often been the imaging modality chosen in penile cancer to examine the inguinal and pelvic areas as well as to rule out more distant metastases.

Horenblas and associates (1991) compared the ability of physical examination, CT scan, and lymphangiography to assess the inguinal region in patients who were surgically staged or had prolonged follow-up. In 102 patients with a 39% prevalence of positive nodes, the sensitivity and specificity of physical examination were 82% and 79%, respectively. Of note, both CT and lymphangiography were performed in patients who were thought to have metastases. The sensitivity of lymphangiography was only 31%, but there were no false positives. Similarly, the sensitivity and specificity of CT scanning were 36% and 100%, respectively. The combination of CT and lymphangiography performed simultaneously demonstrated equally poor sensitivity. Only one fifth of patients had positive nodes detected with either test. **On the basis of these data, the authors concluded that CT scan and lymphangiography offer no useful additional information over physical examination, especially in patients with no palpable adenopathy.** An important caveat is that CT scanning may have a role in examination of the inguinal region in obese patients or in those who have had prior inguinal surgery, for whom the physical examination may be unreliable. In addition, in patients with known inguinal metastases, CT-guided biopsy of enlarged pelvic nodes may provide important information for consideration of neoadjuvant chemotherapeutic strategies.

Recent insights in the field of nanoparticle technology are being applied to imaging of genitourinary malignant neoplasms to enhance detection of microscopic metastases. Ferumoxtran-10 particles (size = 35 nm), administered at a dose of 2.6 mg of iron per kilogram of body weight intravenously, are now capable of imaging microscopic metastasis in lymph nodes that are by size criteria normal (<1 cm). Deserno and coworkers (2004) used this technology in 58 patients with bladder cancer who underwent lymph node dissection to compare imaging characteristics before and after ferumoxtran-10 administration with pathologically proven nodal metastases. At post-contrast imaging, metastases (4 to 9 mm) were prospectively found in 10 of 12 normal-sized (<1 cm) lymph nodes. Application of this novel technology in penile cancer awaits further study.

In general, distant metastases occur late in the course of the disease, usually in patients with recognized significant inguinal and pelvic adenopathy. The most common metastatic sites are the lung, bone, and liver. In addition to an abdominal and pelvic CT scan, a radionuclide bone scan and chest radiograph may be indicated to stage the extent of disease in patients thought to have widespread metastases (Vapnek et al, 1992).

KEY POINTS: RADIOLOGIC STUDIES

■ Soft tissue detail of penile tumors is best imaged by ultrasonography or MRI.

■ Physical examination provides the most reliable staging information for small distal lesions.

■ MRI may provide unique staging information when physical examination findings are equivocal.

■ Physical examination of the inguinal region remains the clinical gold standard for evaluating the presence of metastasis.

■ CT or MRI studies can be useful in evaluating the inguinal region of obese patients and in those having prior inguinal surgery.

Staging

No universally accepted staging system for carcinoma of the penis exists. However, the older Union Internationale Contre le Cancer (UICC) tumor, nodes, metastasis (TNM) system and the more recent unified UICC and American Joint Committee on Cancer (AJCC) TNM system are most commonly used in contemporary series (Table 31–1) (Harmer, 1978; Union Internationale Contre le Cancer, 1989; Fleming et al, 1997).

The strengths of the TNM systems are that they stage both the primary tumor and the regional lymph nodes by the extent of disease. In the 1978 TNM version, the primary tumor was characterized by size, with rather vague terms (extension, deep extension) for invasive lesions. Inguinal staging was clinical and based on palpation, with important distinctions made for unilateral, bilateral, and fixed adenopathy. The 1978 TNM version did not provide a designation for pelvic nodal status, a known indicator of poor prognosis (Harmer, 1978). Horenblas and associates (1994) favored this system, emphasizing that clinical stage can be assigned before definitive therapy and that such staging has prognostic significance.

Some of the weaknesses of the earlier TNM system were addressed in the 1989 revision (Union Internationale Contre le Cancer, 1989). In that system, and in the current AJCC-UICC TNM system (1997), the primary tumor is staged according to histologic features and the precise anatomic structure invaded (Fig. 31–1 and Table 31–1). Experience documented in contemporary literature supports this system. Considering those patients with no palpable adenopathy, it is clear that patients with Tis and Ta lesions have a prognosis different from that of patients exhibiting T1 and T2 lesions (Johnson et al, 1985; Solsona et al, 1992; Gerber, 1994; Villavicencio et al, 1997). Because these histologic features are directly related to the risk of lymph node metastasis, such a staging arrangement is practical and informative with respect to surgical decision-making and prognosis.

The current TNM version also recognizes the importance of the extent of nodal involvement as a prognostic factor in survival, in that separate categories are used for patients with a single positive node (N1) versus those with bilateral nodes (N2) and deep inguinal or pelvic involvement (i.e., Cloquet's node or iliac nodes). The problem with this system, as pointed

Table 31–1. American Joint Committee on Cancer Staging for Penile Cancer

Primary tumor (T)

TX	Primary tumor cannot be assessed
T0	No evidence of primary tumor
Tis	Carcinoma in situ
Ta	Noninvasive verrucous carcinoma
T1	Tumor invades subepithelial connective tissue
T2	Tumor invades corpus spongiosum or cavernosum
T3	Tumor invades urethra or prostate
T4	Tumor invades other adjacent structures

Lymph nodes (N)

NX	Regional nodes cannot be assessed
N0	No regional lymph node metastases
N1	Metastasis in a single regional lymph node
	Metastases in multiple or bilateral superficial inguinal lymph nodes
	Metastases in deep inguinal or pelvic lymph nodes; unilateral or bilateral

Distant metastasis (M)

MX	Distant metastasis cannot be assessed
M0	No distant metastasis
M1	Distant metastasis

Stage grouping

Stage 0	Tis	N0	M0
	Ta	N0	M0
Stage I	T1	N0	M0
Stage II	T1	N1	M0
	T2	N0	M0
	T2	N1	M0
Stage III	T1	N2	M0
	T2	N2	M0
	T3	N0	M0
	T3	N1	M0
	T3	N2	M0
Stage IV	T4	Any N	M0
	Any T	N3	M0
	Any T	Any N	M1

Data from Greene FL, Page DL, Fleming ID, et al (eds): AJCC Cancer Staging Manual. New York, Springer-Verlag, 2002.

out by Horenblas and colleagues (1994), is that it is difficult to assign nodal status before definitive therapy. Thus, the current TNM staging system represents a pathologic staging system in which nodal histology must be assessed (i.e., aspiration, biopsy, lymphadenectomy). However, even if one considers the current version a pathologic staging system, important nodal prognostic factors for survival are not adequately considered. The 5-year survival for patients exhibiting bilateral versus unilateral positive nodes is inferior (Srinivas et al, 1987; Ravi, 1993b). Thus, consideration should be given to separation of these categories in future versions. In addition, the 5-year survival for patients exhibiting extranodal extension of cancer is dismal (5% to 6%) (Srinivas et al, 1987; Ravi, 1993b), yet this factor is not considered. Considering that the pathologic status of inguinal nodes is the driving factor determining survival, future stage groupings (i.e., stage 0 to stage IV) should consider using the extent of nodal involvement with consideration of these prognostic factors. Thus, the strength of the unified AJCC-UICC 1997 TNM system is that it provides an accurate assessment of the primary tumor based on clinical staging (examination, biopsy) but requires more invasive procedures to assess nodal status. This is reasonable considering the inaccuracy of assigning nodal stage with current noninvasive techniques or simple clinical examination.

In the 1997 AJCC-UICC TNM staging system, the primary tumor stage is assigned by biopsy, and additional prognostic factors within the primary tumor not included in the TNM system (i.e., tumor grade and the presence of vascular

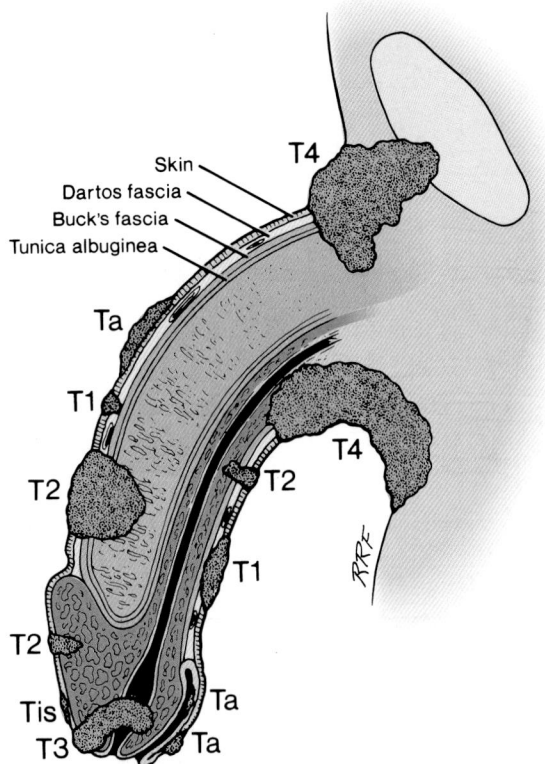

Figure 31–1. Because treatment decisions for inguinal node dissections are based on the characteristics of the primary lesion (see section on treatment of inguinal nodes), a careful assessment of the depth of invasion of the primary tumor is required. This diagram illustrates the importance of depth of invasion in assigning tumor (T) stage.

Table 31–2. Minimal Diagnostic Criteria for Carcinoma of the Penis

Primary tumor (T)

Clinical examination
Incisional-excisional biopsy of lesion and histologic examination
For grade, anatomic structure invaded and presence of vascular invasion

Regional and juxtaregional lymph nodes (N)

Clinical examination
Computed tomographic scan, if inguinal adenopathy is palpable*
Superficial inguinal node dissection (as indicated for high grade, vascular invasion, or invasive histologic pattern)
Aspiration cytology (as indicated)

Distant metastases (M)

Clinical examination
Chest radiograph
Biochemical determinations (liver functions, calcium)
Magnetic resonance imaging, bone scan (as indicated)

*Computed tomography should also be performed in obese patients and those having prior inguinal surgery, whose physical examination findings may be unreliable.

invasion) are also assessed. In most cases, the presence of palpable adenopathy, along with the histologic features of the primary tumor, determines the need for additional imaging studies. Positive fine-needle aspiration of palpably enlarged inguinal nodes or fine-needle biopsy of pelvic adenopathy identified by CT scan can assist in assigning nodal stage before therapy. In those patients requiring surgical staging (palpable lymph nodes or those with adverse primary tumor histologic features), pathologic nodal status assigned according to TNM stage provides valuable prognostic information. The suggested diagnostic criteria for TNM staging are listed in Table 31–2.

KEY POINTS: STAGING

- The current unified TNM staging system is a pathologic system and reflects the importance of the histologic features of the primary tumor and the penile structure invaded in determining outcome.

- Pathologic assessment of nodal status requires invasive procedures to accurately determine prognosis.

- Extranodal extension of cancer in inguinal metastases should be included in subsequent staging systems as a prognostic factor for survival.

Differential Diagnosis

A number of penile lesions must be considered in the differential diagnosis of penile carcinoma. They include some of the lesions previously discussed (condyloma acuminatum, Buschke-Löwenstein tumor, balanitis xerotica obliterans) as well as a number of infectious lesions (chancre, chancroid, herpes, lymphopathia venereum, granuloma inguinale, and tuberculosis). These diseases can be identified by appropriate skin tests, tissue studies, serologic examinations, cultures, or specialized staining techniques.

SURGICAL MANAGEMENT OF THE PRIMARY TUMOR
Organ Preservation

Surgical amputation of the primary tumor remains the oncologic "gold standard" for rapid definitive treatment of the penile primary tumor; local recurrence rates range from 0% to 8% (de Kernion et al, 1973; McDougal et al, 1986; Horenblas et al, 1992). Whereas amputation is often necessary for bulky stage T2-T4 tumors, it has been shown to decrease sexual quality of life (Opjordsmoen and Fossa, 1994). This is relevant because approximately 55% of penile cancer patients are 60 years of age or younger, and 30% are 55 years of age or younger (Narayana et al, 1982).

It is generally accepted that patients with penile primary tumors exhibiting favorable histologic features (stages Tis, Ta, T1; grade 1 and grade 2 tumors) are at a low risk for metastases. These patients are also best suited for organ-sparing or glans-sparing procedures (Solsona et al, 2004). The goal of treatment is to preserve glans sensation where possible or at least to maximize penile shaft length. Such approaches include topical treatments (5-fluorouracil or imiquimod cream for Tis only), radiotherapy, Mohs surgery, limited excision strategies, and laser ablation (Sanchez-Ortiz and Pettaway, 2003; Solsona et al, 2004). This section focuses on novel insights into surgical strategies to achieve organ preservation. Radiation-based strategies are discussed in the section "Radiation Therapy for the Primary Lesion."

Circumcision and Limited Excision Strategies

Circumcision, limited excisions of the glans, and glans removal with sparing of the penile shaft represent surgical strategies to maintain function and penile length. Historically, data on circumcision and limited excision of glanular lesions have been associated with recurrence rates in the range of 11% to 50% (Hanash et al, 1970; Skinner et al, 1972; McDougal et al, 1986). However, the grade, size, and exact location of the lesion and the status of surgical margins were often unavailable in such reports.

Recent reports have suggested that conservative surgery may be performed safely in well-selected patients with discrete tumors by intraoperative frozen-section analysis (Davis et al, 1999; Bissada et al, 2003). **In addition, two studies have challenged the dictum establishing that a 2-cm surgical margin is required for all patients undergoing partial penectomy** (Hoffman et al, 1999; Agrawal et al, 2000). After performing a prospective histologic analysis of 64 penectomy specimens, Agrawal and associates concluded that tumor grade highly correlated with microscopic tumor spread. The maximum proximal histologic extent was 5 mm for grade 1 and grade 2 tumors and 10 mm for grade 3 tumors. Furthermore, "skip" lesions were not encountered. After performing a retrospective pathologic review of 12 penectomy specimens, Hoffman and colleagues also found seven patients with disease of pathologic stage T1 or greater with microscopic margins measuring less than 10 mm. None of these patients had disease recurrence at a mean follow-up of 32.4 months. Pietrzak and colleagues (2004) documented the use of various techniques in a series of 39 patients to excise the tumor and to reconstruct or graft the glans and distal penis. With a mean follow-up of 16 months, only one patient (2.5%) who underwent a partial glans resection had a local recurrence. There were two early complications with grafts and two late complications with graft overgrowth intruding on the urethral meatus. Limitations of this approach include proximal lesions, deeply invasive tumors, and poor health status of patients who would not be candidates for salvage procedures if they experienced recurrence. Although these results seem to suggest that a 2-cm margin may not be necessary for small tumors of lower grade in the presence of a negative frozen section, these findings should be interpreted with caution. Patients managed with limited excision techniques should be considered to be at a higher risk for local recurrence until the surgical margin issue is addressed prospectively.

Mohs Micrographic Surgery

Mohs microsurgery has had a positive impact on the management of penile carcinoma in situ and small superficially invasive tumors. As originally described by Mohs and colleagues (1985), it involves layer-by-layer complete excision of the penile lesion in multiple sessions (fixed tissue technique), with microscopic examination of the undersurface of each

layer. Its sequential microscopic guidance offers improved precision and control of the negative margin while maximizing organ preservation. In a series of 29 consecutive cases of penile squamous cell carcinoma, the primary tumor was eradicated in 23 (92%) of 25 patients available for follow-up. Local recurrences were highly associated with tumor size (>3 cm), advanced stage, and failure of previous definitive therapy (Mohs et al, 1992). These excellent results have yet to be reproduced in a contemporary series, in which frozen-section analysis of margins has replaced the older fixed tissue technique. **Whereas results of Mohs microsurgery are likely to be equivalent to those of partial amputation for carcinoma in situ or for small, distal, superficially invasive tumors, the use of this technique in higher stage tumors (corpus cavernosum or urethral involvement) or in those larger than 3 cm should be discouraged** (Donat et al, 2002).

Laser Ablation

The four most widely used laser energy sources are the carbon dioxide, argon, Nd:YAG, and KTP lasers (Carpiniello et al, 1987; Malloy et al, 1988; von Eschenbach et al, 1991). Although the carbon dioxide laser has been widely used previously, the superficial depth of penetration (limited to 0.1 mm) makes it less than optimal for the treatment of penile carcinoma in situ or small T1 tumors. When the carbon dioxide laser is used, local recurrence rates have been shown to be as high as 50% (Bandieramonte et al, 1988; van Bezooijen et al, 2001). Conversely, the Nd:YAG laser results in protein denaturation at a depth of up to 6 mm by emitting at a wavelength of 1060 nm. Whereas overall recurrence rates after laser ablation have been reported at 7.7% for penile carcinoma in situ and have ranged from 10% to 25% for T1 lesions (Malloy et al, 1988; Windahl et al, 1995; Tietjen and Malek, 1998), results from more contemporary series using the Nd:YAG laser exclusively have been more encouraging. **Frimberger and colleagues (2002a) treated 29 men with carcinoma in situ and stage T1 tumors, combining Nd:YAG laser ablation with tumor base biopsies to ensure negative surgical margins. Only two recurrences (6.9%) were reported at a mean follow-up of 46.7 months, which is comparable to recurrence rates after partial penectomy.** In an effort to reduce the incidence of positive surgical margins, Frimberger and associates (2002b) have proposed the use of autofluorescence and 5-aminolevulinic acid–induced fluorescence for targeting of frozen-section biopsy specimens.

Laser ablation is feasible and may achieve results equivalent to those of extirpative surgery, especially when it is performed in well-selected patients in conjunction with frozen-section biopsies. However, until additional long-term studies become available, laser ablation should be performed with the understanding that local recurrences may develop and that close surveillance and patient self-examination are necessary for early detection. Although well-selected patients who develop small recurrent lesions may be candidates for repeated laser ablation, recurrences are best treated with wide local excision or partial amputation.

Contemporary Penile Amputation

Penile amputation remains the standard therapy for patients with invasive carcinoma. **Partial or total penectomy should** be considered in patients exhibiting adverse features for cure by organ preservation strategies. These are consistently associated with tumors of size 4 cm or more, grade 3 lesions, and those invading deeply into the glans urethra or corpora cavernosa (Mohs et al, 1992; Gotsadze et al, 2000; Kiltie et al, 2000). Because recurrence rates are higher with organ-preserving strategies, compliance with follow-up is also a consideration in recommending organ preservation versus amputation. On the basis of contemporary results, organ preservation strategies should be discussed with patients exhibiting optimal tumor characteristics (stages Tis, Ta, T1; grade 1 and grade 2 tumors) to assist them in making an informed decision about therapy.

KEY POINTS: SURGICAL TREATMENT OF THE PRIMARY TUMOR

- Patients with small lesions of low grade and stage (Tis, Ta, T1; grade 1 and grade 2) are the optimal candidates for organ preservation.

- The goals of organ preservation are to maintain glanular tissue for sensory purposes when possible and to maintain penile length.

- Surgical modalities include limited excision strategies, Mohs surgery, and laser ablation.

- Local recurrence rates after organ preservation are higher than with traditional amputation, and long-term follow-up is required.

- Amputation remains the standard for large or deeply invasive lesions to gain rapid tumor control.

TREATMENT OF THE INGUINAL NODES

The presence and the extent of metastasis to the inguinal region are the most important prognostic factors for survival in patients with squamous penile cancer. These findings affect the prognosis of the disease more than do tumor grade, gross appearance, and morphologic or microscopic patterns of the primary tumor.

Unlike with many other genitourinary tumors, which mandate systemic therapeutic strategies once metastasis has occurred, lymphadenectomy alone can be curative and should be performed. The biology of squamous penile cancer is such that it exhibits a prolonged locoregional phase before distant dissemination, providing a rationale for the therapeutic value of lymphadenectomy.

Still, there are several controversial issues in the treatment of regional lymph nodes. The first and major question remains, should lymphadenectomy be performed on a prophylactic or adjunctive basis in a patient with clinically negative inguinal nodes? Second, should lymphadenectomy be performed bilaterally if only unilateral nodes are palpable, or should node dissections be limited to the side of palpable abnormality? Third, should lymphadenectomy be extended to the pelvic lymph nodes, unilaterally or bilaterally, or should it be restricted to the inguinal lymph node area?

In this rare disease, prospective randomized trials have not been performed to answer many of these questions. However, with use of retrospective data from the literature as well as histopathologic insights, these questions are addressed, and treatment recommendations are presented.

Contemporary Indications for Inguinal Lymphadenectomy

Prognostic Significance of the Presence and Extent of Metastatic Disease. Table 31–3 reveals data collected from 24 surgical series during a 37-year period. Patients proved to have no evidence of inguinal metastases on the basis of histologic examination of the inguinal nodes or repeated normal examination findings over time; the average 5-year survival rate was 73% (46% to 100%). In patients with resected inguinal metastases, the 5-year survival averaged 60% (0% to 86%), but this varied widely and was directly attributable to the extent of nodal metastasis (Table 31–4). This point is illustrated in several series shown in Tables 31–3 and 31–4. Patients with minimal nodal metastases (generally fewer than two) exhibited an average 5-year survival of 77% (89 of 115 patients), compared with only a 25% survival (26 of 102 patients) when a greater degree of nodal involvement was present.

The extent of cancer in a lymph node was also of prognostic significance. Ravi (1993b) noted extranodal extension of cancer in lymph nodes 4 cm in size, and only 1 of 17 patients (6%) undergoing lymphadenectomy survived 5 years. Finally, pelvic lymph node involvement has been a particularly ominous finding with respect to long-term survival; the combined results of several small series reveal an average 5-year survival of 15% when pelvic nodal metastases are present (Table 31–5). **Taken together, these data suggest that the pathologic criteria associated with long-term survival after attempted curative surgical resection of inguinal metastases (i.e., 80% 5-year survival) include minimal nodal disease (up to two involved nodes in most series), unilateral involvement, no evidence of extranodal extension of cancer, and absence of pelvic nodal metastases.**

The Presence of Palpable Adenopathy as a Selection Factor for Inguinal Dissection. One can conclude from these data that it is advantageous to find and to treat nodal metastasis at the earliest possible opportunity. Data in Table 31–3 suggest that the presence of palpable adenopathy is associated with proven nodal metastasis in about 50% of cases. In the remainder, lymph node enlargement is secondary to inflammation. **Persistent adenopathy after treatment of the primary lesion and 4 to 6 weeks of antibiotic therapy is most often the consequence of metastatic disease.** Similarly, the development of new adenopathy during follow-up is much more likely to be due to tumor than inflammatory response. According to Srinivas and associates (1987), 66 of 76 patients (86%) with palpable adenopathy after 6 weeks of antibiotic therapy had pathologically positive nodes. A study by Ornellas and colleagues (1994) confirmed a 70% incidence of metastases in patients with clinically positive nodes after antibiotic treatment. **Thus, patients with palpable inguinal lymph nodes after an appropriate course of antibiotics should undergo inguinal lymphadenectomy.** An alternative approach for such

Table 31–3. Carcinoma of the Penis: Prognostic Indicators for Survival

Series	No. of Patients	Clinical and Pathologic Characteristics of Inguinal Adenopathy			5-Year Survival Rates (%)	
		Percentage with Palpable Nodes	Percentage Clinically False Positive (nodes palpable, histologic findings normal)	Percentage Clinically False Negative (nodes palpable, histologic findings abnormal)	Inguinal Nodes Negative*	Inguinal Nodes Resected and Positive†
Ekstrom and Edsmyer, 1958	229	33	48	—	80[a]	42
Beggs and Spratt, 1964	88	35	36	20	72.5	45
Thomas and Small, 1968	190	—	64	20	—	26
Edwards and Sawyers, 1968	77	—	—	0	68	25
Hanash et al, 1970	169	—	58[b]	2[b]	77[c]	—
Kuruvilla et al, 1971	153	39	63	10	69	33
Hardner et al, 1972	100	42	41[b]	16[b]	—	—
Gursel et al, 1973	64	53	60[b]	—	58	—
Skinner et al, 1972	34	29	40	—	75	20
					87[d]	50[d]
de Kernion et al, 1973	48	54	38[b]	—	84[e]	55[e]
Derrick et al, 1973	87	29	52	—	53	22
					76[d]	55[d]
Johnson et al, 1973	153	—	—	—	64.4	21.8
Kossow et al, 1973	100	51	49	25	—	—[f]
Puras et al, 1978	576	82	47	38[b]	89	67[g]
						29[h]
Cabanas, 1977	80	96	65	100	90	70[i]
						50[j]
						20[k]
Fossa et al, 1987	79	—	—	13	90	80[l]
						20[m]
Srinivas et al, 1987	199	63	14[n]	18	74	82[o]
						54[p]
						40[q]
						12[r]
McDougal et al, 1986	65	—	—	66	100	83[s]
						66[t]
						38[u]
Young et al, 1991	34	24	27	42	77	0
Horenblas et al, 1993	110	36	26	40	100	38
Ravi, 1993b	201	53	8	16	95	81[v]
						50[w]
						86[x]
						60[y]
Ornellas et al, 1994	414	50	51[y]	39	87	29
Theodorescu et al, 1996	40	70	35	—	46	45
Puras-Baez et al, 1995	272	—	—	—	89	38

*On histologic or repeated physical examination.

†On histologic examination of adenectomy specimen.

[a]Majority of patients received prophylactic or preoperative radiotherapy to inguinal area.

[b]Histologic classification based on node biopsy, not node dissection.

[c]Corrected 5-year survival (i.e., patients dying before 5 years without evidence of disease are excluded).

[d]Patients dying free of cancer before 5 years are considered surgical cures.

[e]Three-year survival.

[f]Omitted.

[g]Positive findings in inguinofemoral nodes.

[h]Positive findings in inguinofemoral and pelvic nodes.

[i]Single inguinal node with positive findings.

[j]More than one inguinal node with positive findings.

[k]Three-year survival with positive findings in inguinal and pelvic nodes.

[l]N1-2.

[m]N3.

[n]After antibiotic therapy.

[o]One node positive.

[p]One to six nodes positive.

[q]More than six nodes positive.

[r]Bilateral nodes positive.

[s]Adjunctive adenectomy.

[t]Immediate therapeutic adenectomy.

[u]Delayed therapeutic adenectomy.

[v]One to three positive nodes.

[w]More than three positive nodes.

[x]Unilateral.

[y]Some lymph node dissection done without antibiotic pretreatment.

Table 31–4. **Five-Year Survival Related to Extent of Nodal Metastasis**

| Series | No. of Patients | No. of Positive Nodes | |
		≤2	>2
Fraley et al, 1989	31	15/17 (88%)	1/14 (7%)
Johnson and Lo, 1984a	22	6/7 (85%)*	2/15 (13%)
Srinivas et al, 1987	119	5/6 (82%)	7/34 (20%)
			9/16 (54%)[†]
Fossa et al, 1987	18	11/12 (88%)[‡]	2/6 (33%)[§]
Ravi, 1993b	21	47/58 (81%)[‖]	5/10 (50%)[¶]
Horenblas et al, 1994	110	5/15 (67%)	9/23 (39%)

*Approximate.
[†]A subset with one to six positive nodes.
[‡]N1-2.
[§]N3.
[‖]One to three positive nodes.
[¶]More than three positive nodes.

Table 31–5. **Five-Year Survival Related to Pelvic Node Metastases**

Author	No. of Patients with Positive Nodes	5-Year Survival No. (%)
de Kernion et al, 1973	2	1 (50)
Horneblas et al, 1993	2	0 (0)
Srinivas et al, 1987	11	0 (0)
Pow-Sang et al, 1990	3	2 (66)
Kamat et al, 1993	6	2 (33)
Ravi, 1993b	30	0 (0)
Lopes et al, 2000	13	5 (38)
Total	67	10 (15)

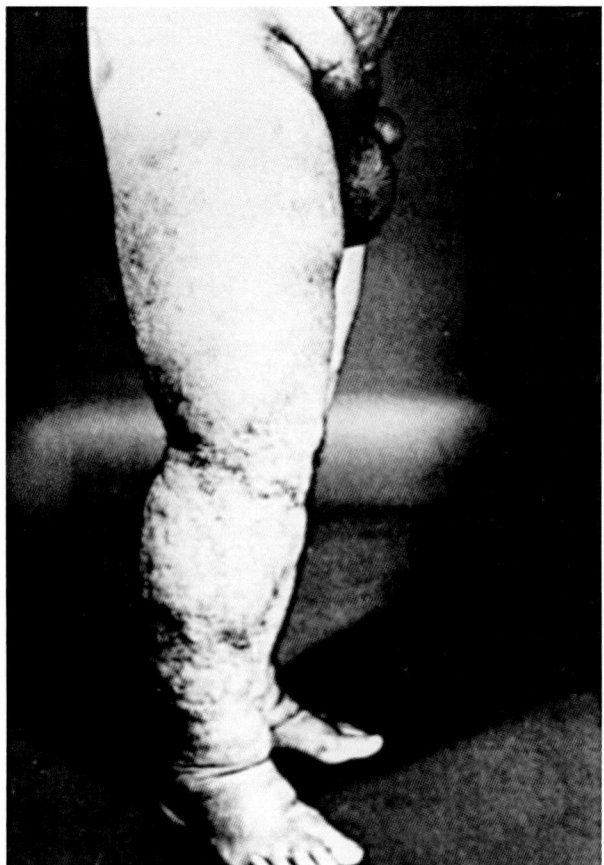

Figure 31–2. Extensive lymphedema and cutaneous changes secondary to recurrent lymphangitis and thrombophlebitis 2 years after a classic groin dissection.

patients is to perform fine-needle aspiration cytology of palpable nodes either at the time of or immediately after treatment of the primary tumor. In the case of a positive result, definite therapy can be planned without a 4- to 6-week delay. Should the result be negative, however, continued close observation and subsequent lymphadenectomy are required when adenopathy does not resolve because the false-negative rate of fine-needle aspiration cytology was 20% to 30% in two series (Scappini et al, 1986; Horenblas et al, 1991).

Evolving Indications for Lymphadenectomy in Patients without Palpable Adenopathy

The Dilemmas

Immediate Versus Delayed Surgery. Considering the value of early detection and treatment of metastasis, **should inguinal lymphadenectomy be routinely performed in patients with clinically normal groin examination findings at the time of presentation of the primary lesion?** This has been the most controversial issue in the management of patients with squamous penile cancer; however, the pendulum has moved toward earlier lymphadenectomy in "selected" patients with penile cancer. As noted, the cure rate with inguinal lymphadenectomy when nodes are positive for malignancy may be as high as 80%. A cure rate of this

magnitude with surgery in the face of regional nodal metastases parallels the urologist's experience with testicular cancer, in which retroperitoneal lymphadenectomy provides cure in many patients with minimal nodal metastasis. In contrast, for other common genitourinary malignant neoplasms—bladder, prostate, and kidney—surgical cure in the face of regional nodal metastases is rare. Given that node dissection can cure metastatic penile cancer, why is there debate about whether the procedure should be performed, especially given that regional node dissections are often advocated in other malignant neoplasms when evidence of their efficacy is marginal at best?

Morbidity Versus Benefit. The reluctance to advocate "automatic" ilioinguinal lymphadenectomy in all patients with penile cancer stems from the substantial morbidity the procedure can produce, as opposed to the relatively limited postoperative morbidity of pelvic or retroperitoneal lymphadenectomies. Early complications of phlebitis, pulmonary embolism, wound infection, flap necrosis, and permanent and disabling lymphedema of the scrotum and lower limbs were frequent after both inguinal and ilioinguinal node dissections (Fig. 31–2) (Skinner et al, 1972; Johnson and Lo, 1984b; McDougal et al, 1986; Fraley et al, 1989). **Postoperative complications have been reduced by improved preoperative and postoperative care; advances in surgical technique; plastic surgical consultation for myocutaneous flap**

coverage; and preservation of the dermis, Scarpa's fascia, and saphenous vein as well as modification of the extent of the dissection (Catalona, 1988; Colberg et al, 1997; Bevan-Thomas et al, 2002; Coblentz and Theodorescu, 2002; Nelson et al, 2004) (Fig. 31–3). In The University of Texas M. D. Anderson Cancer Center experience, both the incidence and severity of lymphedema and skin edge necrosis were significantly decreased (Table 31–6) (Bevan-Thomas et al, 2002).

Furthermore, experience has suggested that lymphadenectomy in the setting of microscopic disease may be less likely to produce complications than node dissection in the presence

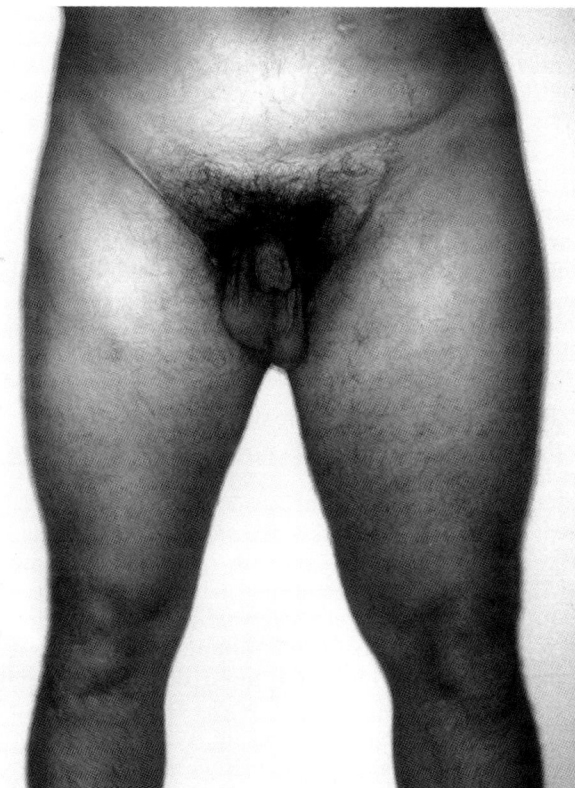

Figure 31–3. Postoperative appearance after contemporary lymphadenectomy. The patient's status is post left ilioinguinal lymphadenectomy and right superficial inguinal dissection for stage T2, N1, M0 squamous penile cancer. The patient has trace edema visible on the left 18 months after surgery.

of bulky nodal metastases (Fraley et al, 1989; Ornellas et al, 1994; Coblentz and Theodorescu, 2002). This is presumably due to the reduced amount of lymphatic tissue removed, preservation of venous drainage, and blood supply compromised. Together, these factors affect the viability of skin flaps and lymphatic flow.

Mortality after inguinal lymphadenectomy has been reported in association with surgery performed concomitantly with penectomy and after palliative inguinal dissection. In both scenarios, it was related to sepsis (Bevan-Thomas et al, 2002). An operative mortality of 3.3% was reported in earlier series (Beggs and Spratt, 1964). However, Johnson and Lo (1984b) and others (Ravi, 1993a; Ornellas et al, 1994; Coblentz and Theodorescu, 2002; Nelson et al, 2004) have reported no mortality in more recent series. Appropriate selection of patients along with routine preoperative antibiotic therapy and wound care to avoid septic complications has minimized this event.

Clearly, lymphadenectomy is not a trivial concern even though morbidity appears to be decreasing. If a policy of routine lymphadenectomy were adopted in all patients with clinically negative lymph nodes, the average risk of a false-negative examination (metastasis is actually present) would be approximately 29%, with wide-ranging variation (see Table 31–3). Stated another way, an average of 70% of patients could be subjected to the morbidity of inguinal lymphadenectomy with no benefit. Potential reasons for false-negative examinations include obesity, preexisting edema, and changes from prior therapy (radiation, inguinal surgery).

One alternative to immediate lymphadenectomy for all patients has been to "observe" patients with normal findings on inguinal examination. Lymphadenectomy is subsequently reserved for those patients who develop palpable lymph nodes. **The relevant question then becomes, can a delayed therapeutic dissection effectively salvage patients who have inguinal recurrence?**

Several studies have analyzed the survival of men undergoing early versus delayed lymphadenectomy according to pathologic evaluation of nodal status. McDougal and coworkers (1986) reported a series of 23 patients with invasive primary lesions and nonpalpable nodes; 9 patients were treated with immediate adjunctive lymph node dissection (6 were positive), and 14 were treated with surveillance and delayed lymph node dissection. The 5-year survival in the node-positive immediate adjunctive lymphadenectomy group

Table 31–6.	**Lymphadenectomy Complications in Four Surgical Series**			
	Johnson and Lo (1984a)	*Ravi (1993a)*	*Ornellas et al (1994)*	*Bevan-Thomas et al (2002)*
Number of dissections	101	405	200	106
Period	1948-1983	1962-1990	1972-1987	1989-1998
Complications (%)				
Skin edge necrosis	50	62	45	8*
Lymphedema	50	27	23	23†
Wound infection	14	17	15‡	10
Seroma formation	16	7	6	10
Death	0	1.3	Not stated	1.8

*Significantly lower than in the three other reported series (all *P* < .0001).
†Significantly lower than in the series of Johnson and Lo (*P* < .0001).
‡Incidence among 85 lymphadenectomies performed by Gibson-type incision.
From Bevan-Thomas R, Slaton JW, Pettaway CA: Contemporary morbidity from lymphadenectomy for penile squamous cell carcinoma: The M. D. Anderson Cancer Center experience. J Urol 2002;167:1638-1642.

was 83% (5 of 6 patients), whereas in the surveillance group, the 5-year survival was 36% (5 of 14 patients). However, only one patient in the surveillance group had a node dissection. Presumably, the other nine patients had progressed to inoperable local tumor or distant disease before presentation, emphasizing the role of careful, frequent follow-up and the difficulty of enforcing it. A third subset in this series had palpable nodes at presentation and had immediate therapeutic lymph node dissection, with 10 of 15 patients (66%) surviving 5 years (McDougal et al, 1986). The best results were from immediate adjunctive lymph node dissection (83%), with the next best from immediate therapeutic lymphadenectomy (66%). The worst results were from the surveillance and delayed lymphadenectomy group (36%), in whom dissection was delayed until palpable nodes developed. The interval of opportunity for cure in this third group appears to have been lost.

Similarly, Fraley reported that immediate adjunctive lymphadenectomy resulted in a 5-year disease-free survival in 6 of 8 node-positive patients (75%) compared with 1 of 12 patients (8%) who had been followed up and then treated by delayed lymphadenectomy when nodal enlargement occurred (Fraley et al, 1989). Six other patients in that series also presented with unresectable adenopathy after initial surveillance, and all died of disease. Although only two of six immediate lymphadenectomy patients had more than two positive nodes, all the patients treated by delayed lymph node dissection had three or more positive nodes.

Three other series suggest that early lymphadenectomy for varying degrees of "suspicious" or clinically positive nodes improves survival compared with the "surveillance" or delayed intervention approach in patients presenting with clinically negative nodes (Johnson and Lo, 1984a; Ornellas et al, 1994; Kroon et al, 2005a). A series from The University of Texas M. D. Anderson Cancer Center compared 5-year disease-free survival of 14 patients undergoing early lymphadenectomy for clinically suspicious and histologically node-positive disease with that of 8 patients who were followed up and later underwent lymphadenectomy when clinical nodal enlargement was undisputed (Johnson and Lo, 1984a). The primary tumors were of similar stage. The 5-year disease-free survival was 57% for early lymphadenectomy compared with 13% for delayed node dissection. Of note, the number of involved nodes in the immediate lymphadenectomy group (median, 2) was half that of the delayed lymphadenectomy group (median, 4), and no patient with more than two positive nodes survived more than 5 years.

Kroon and associates (2005a) from The Netherlands Cancer Institute compared survival of 20 patients found to have positive lymph nodes subsequent to prophylactic dynamic sentinel node biopsy with that of 20 patients who underwent delayed inguinal dissection after proven nodal metastasis. The 3-year survival for those patients detected during close surveillance was only 35% compared with 84% ($P = .0017$) for those undergoing early dissection. Pathologic evaluation of involved lymph nodes revealed extranodal extension of cancer among 19 of 20 patients in the delayed group versus only 4 of 20 patients ($P < .001$) in the early group. Thus, despite careful follow-up, survival was adversely affected by the extent of cancer in involved lymph nodes.

A single large study from India disputes the magnitude of the value of early prophylactic dissection. Ravi (1993a)

performed early prophylactic dissection in 113 patients with invasive penile cancer and compared the 5-year survival with that of 258 similarly staged patients who were initially observed. In the "early" group, 20 patients (18%) were found to have metastases, and all patients survived 5 years. The recurrence rate in the observed group was only 8% (21 patients). However, the 5-year survival in the patients who experienced recurrence was only 76% (compared with 100% in the early lymphadenectomy group). The enhanced survival of patients undergoing surveillance in India compared with other countries is probably attributable to patient selection factors, strict adherence to follow-up schedules, and aggressive treatment approach for recurrent disease (a combination of radiation and surgical resection) (Ravi, 1993b).

Thus, six series reveal an improvement in survival for patients undergoing early therapeutic versus delayed therapeutic dissection. Further, five of the six series show that delayed therapeutic dissection can rarely salvage patients who experience recurrence. Taken together, these data suggest that a policy of immediate adjunctive or early lymphadenectomy gives greater assurance that surgical intervention will occur when tumor volume is small (see Table 31–6) (Johnson and Lo, 1984b; Fossa et al, 1987; Srinivas et al, 1987; Fraley et al, 1989; Ravi, 1993a; Kroon et al, 2005a).

Impact of Primary Tumor Histology, Stage, Grade, and Vascular Invasion on Predicting Occult Nodal Metastasis

Although early lymphadenectomy improves survival in patients with inguinal metastases, the challenge remains to identify those patients who are truly lymph node negative to avoid the morbidity of traditional lymphadenectomy. **Data gained from analysis of a variety of histopathologic variables within the primary penile tumor allow the classification of patients into high- and low-risk groups for lymph node metastasis** (McDougal, 1995; Lopes et al, 1996; Theodorescu et al, 1996; Solsona et al, 1992).

Patients with primary tumors exhibiting carcinoma in situ or verrucous carcinoma have little or no risk for metastasis. Only two cases of metastasis in association with carcinoma in situ have been reported, and none of 47 cases of penile verrucous carcinoma has been shown to metastasize (Avrach and Christensen, 1976; Johnson et al, 1985; Seixas et al, 1994; Eng et al, 1995).

In contrast, patients with corporal invasion (TNM stage pT2) in the penile tumor exhibit a high risk for metastasis. The average risk for inguinal metastasis among 225 patients in seven different series was 59% (Table 31–7). **As noted in Table 31–7, the risk for metastasis among patients exhibiting corporal invasion was similar irrespective of whether palpable adenopathy was present.**

Stage T1 penile cancers exhibit involvement of the subepithelial connective tissue only and lack involvement of the corpus spongiosum, corpora cavernosa, or urethra (Fleming et al, 1997). Similarly staged tumors have been associated with a 4% to 14% incidence of nodal metastasis (Solsona et al, 1992; Villavicencio et al, 1997; Hall et al, 1998). Theodorescu and colleagues (1996) noted one exception to this relatively low rate of metastatic disease; 58% of patients (14 of 24) with pT1 primary tumors and initially negative nodes on clinical

Table 31-7. Penile Carcinoma: Corporal Invasion and Incidence of Lymph Node Metastasis

Author	Positive Nodes (%)	No. of Patients (%)	Clinical N Stage
McDougal et al, 1986	23	11 (48)	N0
Fraley et al, 1989	29	26 (90)	N0
Theodorescu et al, 1996	18	12 (67)	N0
Villavicencio et al, 1997	37	14 (38)	N0
Lopes et al, 1996	44	28 (64)	NS
Heyns et al, 1997	32	15 (47)	NS
Solsona et al, 1992	42	27 (64)	NS

N, node.

assessment subsequently developed inguinal nodal metastases. These data suggest that other variables present within the penile cancers of the cohort of patients studied (i.e., tumor grade and presence of vascular invasion) may have modified the effect of tumor stage on metastasis.

Tumor grade can also provide predictive information about the likelihood of nodal metastasis (Fraley et al, 1989; Horenblas et al, 1993). Fraley's study of tumor grade and its relationship to nodal metastases showed a higher correlation than most series show. One of 19 patients with well-differentiated tumor, 5 of 19 patients with moderately differentiated tumor, and all 16 patients with poorly differentiated tumor developed nodal metastases. Horenblas and associates (1993) also showed a close correlation between tumor differentiation and nodal metastases; 9 of 11 patients with grade 3 tumors (82%) and 13 of 28 patients with grade 2 tumors (46%) showed nodal metastases, whereas 17 of 59 (29%) of those with grade 1 lesions had nodal involvement. Subsequently, several authors have evaluated the risk of nodal metastasis for TNM stage T1 lesions according to tumor grade (Table 31–8). Among 64 patients with T1, grade 1 or grade 2 primary tumors, metastasis occurred in only 5 patients (8%). Thus, grade and stage can be used to identify a truly low-risk subset of patients. This concept was confirmed by two independent groups that analyzed the incidence of lymph node metastasis by risk groups generated by combining stage and grade information (Solsona et al, 2001, 2004; Ficarra et al, 2005).

The presence of vascular invasion as a prognostic indicator of inguinal lymph node metastasis in squamous penile cancer is now evident (Fraley et al, 1989; Lopes et al, 1996;

Heyns et al, 1997; Slaton et al, 2001; Ficarra et al, 2005). Lopes and colleagues studied the prognostic value of lymphatic invasion in 146 patients with penile cancer. In a univariate analysis, clinical nodal stage, tumor thickness, lymphatic and venous embolization, and urethral infiltration were all associated with lymph node metastasis. However, subsequent to multivariate analysis, only venous and lymphatic invasion remained significant predictors for positive lymph nodes. Data from the University of Texas M. D. Anderson Cancer Center revealed that vascular invasion was absent in all patients with T1 tumors (Slaton et al, 2001). These patients were also lymph node negative at surgery. In contrast, patients with stage pT2 primary tumors exhibited nodal metastasis in 75% of cases (15 of 20) when vascular invasion was present but in only 25% of cases (3 of 12) when it was absent.

Ficarra and colleagues (2005) described prognostic factors for lymph node metastasis in 175 patients undergoing surgery for penile cancer in a multicenter study from the Northeast Uro-Oncological Group from Italy. Subsequent to multivariate statistical analysis, the presence of venous or lymphatic invasion and pathologic invasion of the corpus spongiosum or urethra were the only independent risk factors for lymph node metastasis among patients who were clinically lymph node negative.

Analysis of gene expression was shown to be valuable in penile cancer. Nuclear accumulation of p53 (presumably mutated) was shown in a multivariate analysis to be an independent predictor of lymph node metastasis. Lopes and colleagues (2002) from Brazil analyzed the expression of p53 by immunohistochemical techniques among 82 patients undergoing amputation and bilateral lymphadenectomy. Thirty-four of 82 penile specimens (41.5%) exhibited staining. The risk of metastasis was enhanced 4.8 times among patients whose tumors were p53 positive. Further, those patients with tumors exhibiting both p53 and HPV staining exhibited the poorest 5- and 10-year survival. Among the same cohort of patients, lymphatic invasion was the only other factor providing independent prognostic information.

DNA flow cytometry has been studied in relatively small numbers of patients. Thus far, it has not been of value for the prediction of nodal metastasis (Hall et al, 1998). Data from these studies reveal that primary tumor pathologic and molecular factors provide important information with respect to predicting nodal metastasis. Prospective multi-institutional studies analyzing these variables among countries where the disease is endemic are needed to further validate which pathologic and molecular variables best stratify a patient's risk for metastasis.

Contemporary Indications for Expectant Management

Data reviewed in the preceding paragraphs demonstrate that patients with primary tumors exhibiting carcinoma in situ (Tis), verrucous carcinoma (Ta), and stage T1, grade 1 or grade 2 tumors exhibit less than a 10% incidence of positive lymph nodes and are optimal candidates for "watchful waiting" strategies. Table 31–9 provides guidelines for the follow-up of such patients.

Alternatively, patients with stage pT2 tumors or grade 3 tumors and those exhibiting vascular invasion have a greater

Table 31-8. Penile Carcinoma: Incidence of Nodal Metastasis for Stage T1, Grade 1 and Grade 2 Primary Tumors

Author	Stage and Grade	No. of Patients	No. of Patients with Metastasis (%)
Theodorescu et al, 1996	T1, G1	8	2 (25)
Solsona et al, 1992	T1, G1	19	0 (0)
	T1, G2	4	1 (25)
McDougal, 1995	T1, G1-2	24	1 (4)
Heyns et al, 1997	T1, G1-2	9	1 (11)
Total		64	5 (8)

Table 31-9. Penile Carcinoma: Suggested Follow-up for Patients with No Evidence of Inguinal Adenopathy Who Do Not Undergo Initial Lymphadenectomy

Year	Interval	
	Low-Risk Group*	High-Risk Group[†]
1-2	3 months	2 months
3	4 months	3 months
4	6 months	6 months
5+	Annually	Annually

*Tis; Ta; T1, grade 1 and grade 2; no vascular invasion.
[†]T2-T3, grade 3; vascular invasion.

than 50% incidence of metastasis, so prophylactic lymphadenectomy appears warranted. Noncompliant patients should be in the high-risk category. Table 31–9 provides a guideline for more intensive follow-up of high-risk patients, especially within the first 2 years. **It is imperative for both the patient and the physician to adhere to such follow-up "agreements" and be willing to intervene immediately if initial inguinal parameters change.**

Indications for Modified and Traditional Inguinal Procedures

Modified Procedures

In patients with no evidence of palpable adenopathy who are selected to undergo inguinal procedures by virtue of adverse prognostic factors within the primary tumor, the goal is to define if metastases exist with minimal morbidity for the patient. A variety of treatment options for this purpose have been reported and include fine-needle aspiration cytology, node biopsy, sentinel lymph node biopsy, extended sentinel lymph node dissection, intraoperative lymphatic mapping, superficial dissection, and modified complete dissection. The technical aspects of many of these procedures are discussed in Chapter 32.

Fine-Needle Aspiration Cytology. Experience with fine-needle aspiration cytology is limited, and most information is derived from a single series (Scappini et al, 1986). The procedure requires pedal or penile lymphangiography for nodal localization, followed by aspiration under fluoroscopic or CT scan guidance. Multiple nodes must be sampled (e.g., 170 node chains in 29 patients in this series). Of 20 patients who had lymphadenectomy for histologic confirmation, there was complete agreement between aspiration cytology and histologic results. However, two of nine patients whose cytologic analysis was negative subsequently died of metastatic disease, a presumptive 20% false-negative result. A series from Horenblas and colleagues (1991) also found that the sensitivity of fine-needle aspiration cytology was approximately 71% in 18 patients with clinically negative lymph nodes. This finding and the technical difficulty with lymphangiography make aspiration less practical as a staging technique for patients with no palpable lymph nodes. Kroon et al (2005c) described fine-needle aspiration cytology guided by ultrasonography as a preliminary study to surgical staging with dynamic sentinel lymph node biopsy. Thirty-four groins in 27 patients with clinically negative groins were found to have suspicious nodes by ultrasound examination and were aspirated. However, the sensitivity of the technique was only 39% subsequent to surgical staging. Thus, at present, fine-needle aspiration cytology of clinically negative groins does not exhibit the sensitivity for it to be relied on as a staging modality. However, direct aspiration of palpable inguinal nodes is easily performed, and if the result is positive, immediate information with which to advise patients about further treatment is provided.

Sentinel Lymph Node Biopsy, Extended Sentinel Lymph Node Dissection, and Node Biopsy. The concept of sentinel lymph node biopsy as described by Cabanas (1977) is predicated on detailed penile lymphangiographic studies that have demonstrated consistent drainage of the penile lymphatics into a sentinel node or group of nodes located superomedial to the junction of the saphenous and femoral veins in the area of the superficial epigastric vein. In this series, when this sentinel node was negative for tumor, metastases to other ilioinguinal lymph nodes did not occur. Metastases to this node indicated the need for a complete superficial and deep inguinal dissection.

The accuracy of the sentinel node histology to identify inguinal node metastases has been questioned by a number of reports (Perinetti et al, 1980; Fowler, 1984; Wespes et al, 1986). Because nodal metastases became palpable within 1 year of sentinel node biopsy with normal findings in some patients in these series, a false-negative biopsy result must be presumed. In one large series, 5 of 41 patients (12%) with normal findings on sentinel node biopsy subsequently developed inguinal node metastases (Fossa et al, 1987). In Cabanas' series, 3 of 31 patients with negative sentinel nodes died of disease, suggesting a false-negative rate for identifying metastases of 10% (Cabanas, 1992). McDougal and associates (1986) reported a 50% false-negative rate with inguinal node biopsy. A report by Pettaway and colleagues (1995), in which additional nodes around the sentinel node area were also removed, revealed that even this extended dissection was associated with a false-negative rate of 25%. The authors hypothesized that false-negative inguinal node biopsies were the result of anatomic variation in the position of the sentinel node within the inguinal field. **Thus, biopsies directed to a specific anatomic area can be unreliable in identifying microscopic metastasis and are no longer recommended.**

Intraoperative Lymphatic Mapping. Intraoperative lymphatic mapping offers the potential for precise localization of the sentinel node with the lowest morbidity of any surgical staging technique (Kroon et al, 2005b). The goal of lymphatic mapping is to define where in the inguinal lymph node field the sentinel lymph node resides by either visual (vital blue dyes) or gamma emission (hand-held gamma probe) techniques at the time of surgery.

The technique has been studied in patients with malignant melanoma and breast and vulvar carcinomas who required evaluation of the regional lymph nodes (Morton et al, 1992; Levenback et al, 1994; Albertini et al, 1996; Gershenwald et al, 1999). The technique involves intradermal injection of a vital blue dye (isosulfan blue or patent blue dyes) or technetium-labeled colloid adjacent to the lesion. The dye (or radioactive tracer) is transported by the afferent lymphatics to a specific node in the regional nodal basin. This node is designated the sentinel lymph node. In Morton's series of 237 patients with melanoma, the sentinel lymph node was identified in 194 patients. These patients then underwent full regional lymphadenectomy, with a false-negative sentinel node in only 1% of cases.

Few studies evaluating the results of intraoperative lymphatic mapping as a staging tool in penile cancer are available. In initial reports from the University of Texas M. D. Anderson Cancer Center (Pettaway et al, 1999) and The Netherlands Cancer Institute (Horenblas et al, 2000), both a vital blue dye and technetium-labeled colloid were used to identify the draining nodes. In the initial report from The Netherlands Cancer Institute, a false-negative rate of approximately 7% was noted among the initial 55 patients undergoing the procedure. Likewise, in the University of Texas M. D. Anderson Cancer Center experience, there were no false-negative findings among the initial 20 patients. Kroon and associates (2004) updated The Netherlands Cancer Institute experience, describing their experience using the combination of preoperative lymphoscintigraphy and intraoperative intradermally injected blue dye in 123 patients with penile cancer. They identified a sentinel node in 98% of patients for a sensitivity rate of 82% and a false-negative rate of 18% (six patients). Four of the six patients subsequently died of disease progression. This group has subsequently instituted several changes, including routine serial sectioning of the involved lymph nodes along with cytokeratin immunohistochemistry to increase the sensitivity of pathologic detection. In addition, routine exploration of groins with low or no signal subsequent to preoperative or intraoperative studies is now used in specific patients. The authors thought that direct palpation of the inguinal field or visualized blue dye could lead to the detection of positive lymph nodes that were not detected by gamma emission because of obstruction of lymphatics by cancer. Finally, the authors recommend the use of inguinal ultrasonography with fine-needle aspiration to detect subtle architectural changes (nonpalpable) in positive lymph nodes that could result in the redistribution of lymphatic flow (Kroon et al, 2005c).

Collectively, these data illustrate that intraoperative lymph node mapping in penile cancer is technically feasible but that the optimal technique to enhance the detection of microscopic metastases (i.e., sensitivity > 90%) remains to be defined. As noted, with many surgical techniques, the learning curve can initially be challenging, especially given the fact that the disease is rare. It was estimated that a surgeon technically capable of correctly identifying sentinel nodes (i.e., 5% false-negative rate) would have a 13% chance that the rate of nonidentification would be higher (i.e., ≥10%) if only 25 cases were performed (Tanis et al, 2002). **Thus, the number of cases for most urologists in developed countries, where the incidence is the lowest, is an impediment to the accurate performance of intraoperative lymph node mapping. At present, the technical aspects of intraoperative lymph node mapping and the associated learning curve limit its potential widespread application compared with other standard dissection techniques.**

Superficial and Modified Complete Inguinal Dissection. Both superficial inguinal and modified complete dis-

sections have been proposed as staging tools for the patient without palpable inguinal lymphadenopathy. Superficial node dissection involves removal of those nodes superficial to the fascia lata. A complete ilioinguinal lymphadenectomy (removal of those nodes deep to the fascia lata contained within the femoral triangle as well as the pelvic nodes) is then performed if the superficial nodes are positive at surgery by frozen-section analysis. The rationale for superficial dissection is that two series have shown no positive nodes deep to the fascia lata unless superficial nodes were also positive (Pompeo et al, 1995; Puras-Baez et al, 1995). A complete modified inguinal dissection was originally proposed by Catalona (1988) and involves smaller skin incision, limited field of inguinal dissection, preservation of the saphenous vein, and thicker skin flaps. This technique also avoids having to transpose the sartorius muscle to cover exposed femoral vessels. Unlike in superficial dissection, deep nodes within the fossa ovalis are also removed. Two reports involving 21 patients have confirmed the value of this technique, when it is properly performed, for identifying microscopic metastases with minimal morbidity (Parra, 1996; Colberg et al, 1997).

Of most importance, there has been no evidence of direct pelvic node drainage (i.e., bypassing inguinal nodes) by penile lymphangiography (Riveros et al, 1967). Thus, either superficial or complete modified inguinal dissection should adequately identify microscopic metastases in patients with clinically normal inguinal examination findings, without the need for a pelvic dissection if the inguinal nodes are negative. **These limited dissections have the following advantages: more information is provided than by biopsy of a single node or group of nodes; the possibility of not identifying the sentinel node is limited by removal of "all" potential first-echelon nodes; morbidity is minimal compared with standard lymphadenectomy; and the dissection is readily performed by any surgeon experienced in inguinal surgery.**

Traditional Inguinal and Ilioinguinal Lymphadenectomy

In patients with resectable metastatic adenopathy, the potential therapeutic value of lymphadenectomy justifies the morbidity of treatment. The goals are to eradicate all obvious cancer, to provide coverage for exposed vasculature, and to provide rapid wound healing (primary closure or myocutaneous flap coverage). Several issues remain with respect to surgical decision-making.

Should inguinal lymphadenectomy be bilateral rather than unilateral for patients presenting with unilateral adenopathy at initial presentation of the primary tumor? The answer to this question is yes. The anatomic crossover of penile lymphatics is well established, and bilateral drainage is the rule. In 43 of 54 patients (79%) undergoing intraoperative lymph node mapping at The Netherlands Cancer Institute, lymphatic drainage from the penis was bilateral (Horenblas et al, 2000). The contralateral node dissection may be limited to the area superficial to the fascia lata if no histologic evidence of positive superficial nodes is found at surgery by frozen-section analysis. Clinical support for a bilateral procedure is based on the finding of contralateral metastases in more than 50% of patients so treated, even if the contralateral nodal region was normal to palpation (Ekstrom and Edsmyr, 1958).

Should bilateral inguinal lymphadenectomy be performed in patients who present with unilateral lymphadenopathy some time after the initial presentation and treatment of the primary tumor? It is generally believed that bilateral node dissection in this setting is not necessary. The recommendation of unilateral rather than bilateral node dissection with delayed presentation of unilateral lymphadenopathy is supported by the elapsed disease-free interval of observation on the normal side. If one assumes that nodal metastases will enlarge at the same rate, the clinical palpation of nodal metastases, if present in both groins, should appear at approximately the same time. The absence of clinical adenopathy on one side despite prolonged observation suggests freedom from disease on that side (Ekstrom and Edsmyr, 1958). However, this concept may not apply to all patients with delayed recurrence. Horenblas and colleagues (2000) noted that in patients with two or more unilateral metastases, those contralateral occult metastases were noted in 30% of cases. Thus, in patients with a bulky unilateral recurrence, a contralateral inguinal staging procedure should be considered. Considering the current treatment recommendations for bilateral inguinal staging procedures in men at high risk for metastasis and the definition of low-risk groups for metastasis by use of available prognostic markers, this scenario should rarely occur.

Should pelvic lymphadenectomy be performed in patients with inguinal metastases? Patients with inguinal nodal metastases are at increased risk for spread to the pelvic nodes. Ravi (1993a) found no pelvic nodal metastases when inguinal nodes were negative but found positive pelvic nodes in 17 of 75 patients (22%) with one to three positive inguinal nodes and in 13 of 23 patients (57%) with more than three positive inguinal nodes. Srinivas and associates (1987) also found a similar correlation. Horenblas and colleagues (1993) showed that among patients with a single inguinal lymph node involved without extracapsular extension, the incidence of pelvic metastases was rare and recommended avoiding pelvic dissection among such patients. However, additional studies evaluating prognostic factors for pelvic metastasis in patients with positive inguinal lymph nodes are needed to determine which patients with positive inguinal node could avoid a pelvic dissection.

Unfortunately, the average 5-year survival for patients with positive pelvic nodes averages around 15% (see Table 31–5). However, data from some of the smaller series (see Table 31–5) suggest that in selected instances, 5-year survival can occur in patients treated with surgery alone. In the series reported by Ravi (1993a), however, even patients with a single positive pelvic node failed to survive 5 years (0 of 8 patients). The difficulty in determining the potential independent value of pelvic lymphadenectomy as a therapeutic procedure is related to the small numbers of patients reported, the coexisting extensive inguinal adenopathy in patients with resectable pelvic nodes, and the failure to specify sites of relapse in patients undergoing ilioinguinal lymphadenectomy (i.e., inguinal versus pelvic versus distant site). Although unproved, it is conceivable that patients with minimal inguinal disease who exhibit focal involvement of a pelvic node could benefit from pelvic dissection. The series reported from Lopes and coworkers (2000) provides support for this concept. Among 13 patients with pathologically proven lymph nodes, 5 of 13

(38%) were alive without disease with follow-up for more than 90 months in 4 of 5 survivors. This series is unique in that 4 of 5 survivors exhibited only a single iliac nodal metastasis and one inguinal lymph node metastasis; in fact, one patient with iliac metastases had no inguinal disease. This series is clearly the exception but reveals that selected patients with minimal inguinal and pelvic disease may be cured with surgery alone.

Until more information is available, a definitive statement about the advisability of pelvic node dissection among all patients with inguinal metastases is not possible. However, in patients undergoing inguinal lymphadenectomy for curative intent (in whom preoperative studies reveal no pelvic adenopathy), pelvic lymphadenectomy should be considered because it can serve as an effective staging tool for identifying those patients who should receive adjuvant combination chemotherapy. It also adds to local-regional control and provides little additional morbidity to the simultaneous inguinal procedure being performed. Alternatively, if pelvic nodal metastases are proven before lymphadenectomy, consideration should be given to neoadjuvant chemotherapeutic strategies followed by surgery in those patients who respond (Pizzocaro et al, 1997; Corral et al, 1998).

KEY POINTS: TREATMENT OF THE INGUINAL NODES

- The presence and extent of inguinal metastases determine survival in penile cancer.

- Patients with persistent palpable inguinal adenopathy should undergo an inguinal staging procedure.

- On the basis of the histologic features of the primary tumor, risk of lymph node metastases can be assessed in patients with no palpable adenopathy, and lymphadenectomy or close follow-up can be recommended.

- Factors associated with cure in surgically treated patients include no more than two inguinal metastases, unilateral involvement, no extranodal extension of cancer, and absence of pelvic metastases.

- Morbidity of lymphadenectomy is decreasing in contemporary series.

- Superficial and modified inguinal dissections remain the standard dissection techniques to reliably determine the presence of microscopic inguinal metastases.

- Intraoperative lymphatic mapping techniques to determine microscopic inguinal disease exhibit low morbidity, are in evolution, and remain investigational.

- Multi-institutional clinical trials integrating surgery, chemotherapy, and perhaps radiotherapy are needed to improve outcome among patients with bulky inguinal metastases.

Risk-Based Management of the Inguinal Region

A contemporary schema for management of the inguinal region is presented in Figure 31-4. Assumptions for these guidelines are that the primary tumor has been adequately controlled, that the pathologic stage of the primary tumor is available, and that an inguinal examination has been performed. CT of the abdomen and pelvis as well as chest radiography or other imaging studies should also be performed as clinically indicated.

Low-Risk Patients (Fig. 31–4A). Because the incidence of inguinal metastasis is anecdotal at best for patients with stage Tis or Ta primary tumors, observation is reasonable for those patients with normal inguinal examination findings. For patients with palpable adenopathy, a course of antibiotics should reveal those whose adenopathy is related to infection versus metastasis. A persistently palpable node should

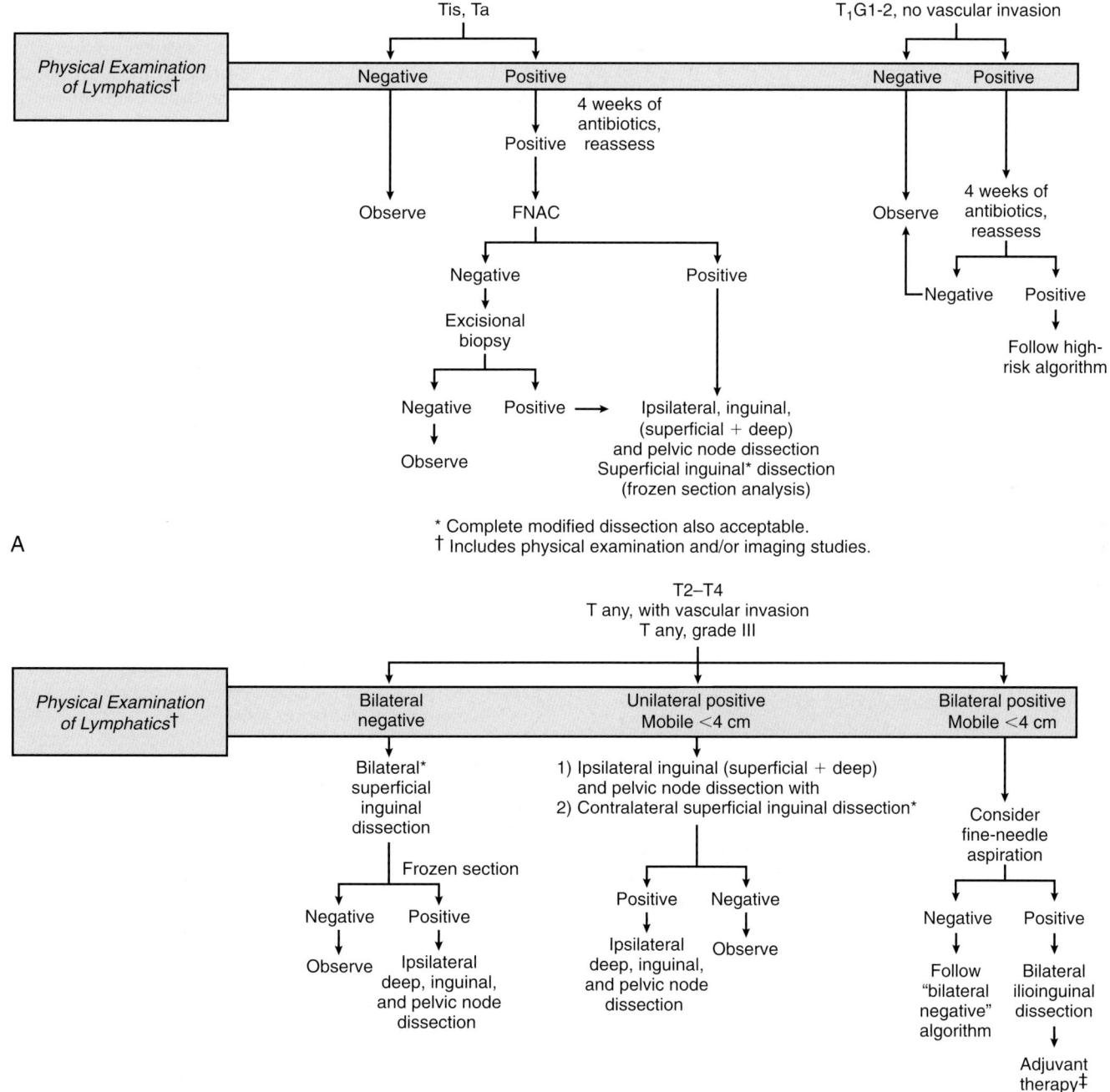

Figure 31–4. Management of regional disease. **A,** Low-risk patients. **B,** High-risk patients.   *Continued*

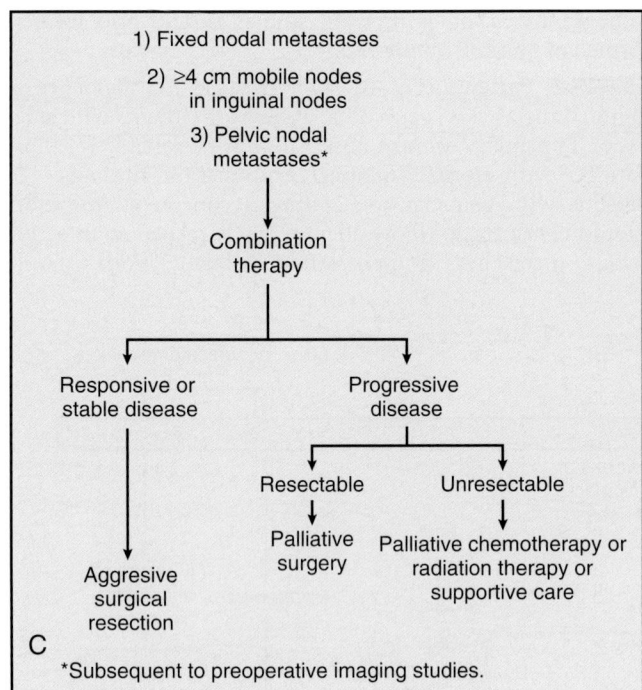

1) Fixed nodal metastases

2) ≥4 cm mobile nodes in inguinal nodes

3) Pelvic nodal metastases*

↓

Combination therapy

Responsive or stable disease

Progressive disease

Resectable

Unresectable

Palliative surgery

Palliative chemotherapy or radiation therapy or supportive care

Aggresive surgical resection

C

*Subsequent to preoperative imaging studies.

Figure 31–4, cont'd. C, Metastatic disease.

undergo fine-needle aspiration cytology; if the result is negative, an excisional biopsy is recommended. If the biopsy finding is abnormal, ipsilateral ilioinguinal dissection with contralateral superficial or modified complete dissection is performed.

On average, patients with stage T1, grade 1 and grade 2 tumors exhibit less than a 10% incidence of inguinal metastasis. Because vascular invasion is also another important predictor of metastasis, its absence in stage T1 tumors is thought to be important. Patients with low-grade stage T1 lesions that lack vascular invasion should also be treated with antibiotics for 4 to 6 weeks if they are noted to have palpable nodes on initial presentation. If adenopathy does not resolve, lymphadenectomy is recommended. Close follow-up is indicated for patients whose nodes resolve after antibiotic therapy, although the overall risk in this group remains low.

High-Risk Patients (Fig. 31–4B). For the high-risk cohort, the incidence of inguinal metastasis ranges from approximately 50% to 70%. The surgical approach is designed to maximize detection and treatment for those with proven nodal metastasis while limiting the morbidity of those with negative lymph nodes at surgery. Thus, surgical staging is indicated even in those patients with clinically normal inguinal examination findings. **In this setting, antibiotic use minimizes the risk of inguinal wound infections or septic complications after control of an infected primary tumor, rather than influencing the decision for surgical staging.**

Patients with normal inguinal examination findings are offered either bilateral superficial dissection or complete modified dissection. If frozen-section results reveal no metastasis, the procedure is concluded. If either side is positive, an ipsilateral ilioinguinal dissection is performed. Patients with

unilateral resectable adenopathy that is strongly suggestive of metastasis should undergo an ipsilateral ilioinguinal dissection and a contralateral superficial or complete modified dissection. Frozen-section analysis then determines if deep inguinal or pelvic nodes should be excised. Palpable adenopathy of less than 4 cm was arbitrarily selected as a cutoff point for surgery as monotherapy because nodal metastases larger than 4 cm are associated with extranodal extension of cancer (Ravi, 1993b).

For patients who present with bilateral palpable nodes that are strongly suggestive of metastasis, preoperative fine-needle aspiration cytology can be helpful for counseling of the patient as to the likelihood of the extent of surgery. For patients with negative results of fine-needle aspiration cytology, a staged surgical approach starting with superficial dissection is performed. Subsequent procedures in this setting depend on the results of frozen-section analysis. For patients requiring ilioinguinal lymphadenectomy because of metastases, adjuvant chemotherapy should be considered for those exhibiting more than two positive lymph nodes, extranodal extension of cancer, or pelvic nodal metastasis.

Bulky Adenopathy and Fixed Nodal Metastasis (Fig. 31–4C). **Survival in this cohort of patients is related to complete eradication of extensive disease. This task is difficult to achieve with surgery, chemotherapy, or radiotherapy alone. The combination of surgery and chemotherapy has shown some benefit in advanced penile carcinoma** (Pizzocaro et al, 1997; Corral et al, 1998). The optimal integration and timing of such therapy are unknown. A reasonable approach in this cohort of patients is to use neoadjuvant chemotherapy followed by an aggressive surgical resection for patients demonstrating either response to therapy or stable disease. This potentially improves surgical resectability and avoids long delays in the administration of chemotherapy resulting from delays in postoperative healing. **In patients exhibiting progression while they are receiving chemotherapy, the prognosis is poor.** Palliative groin dissection, if all gross disease can be resected, is a consideration for otherwise healthy patients. This often requires extensive surgery. Hemipelvectomy in patients without distant metastases has been reported. Palliative chemotherapy, radiation therapy, and other supportive care are provided to patients with unresectable disease or those with poor performance status.

RADIATION THERAPY
Radiation Therapy for the Primary Lesion

External Beam Radiotherapy

Primary radiation therapy may permit the preservation of penile structure and function in carefully selected patients. In reality, the number of patients for whom this treatment is appropriate is small. For most patients, advances in surgical therapy—laser therapy, Mohs micrographic surgery, and reconstructive surgery—can provide excellent surgical treatment while minimizing functional loss and avoiding the considerable complications associated with radiation therapy. In addition, among elderly patients, preservation of an aesthetic anatomic structure and sexual function are often of secondary importance. On occasion, concomitant medical problems may preclude major surgery, making radiation the preferred treatment.

Radiation therapy may be considered in a select group of patients: (1) young individuals presenting with small (2 to 4 cm), superficial, exophytic, noninvasive lesions on the glans or coronal sulcus; (2) patients refusing surgery as an initial form of treatment; and (3) patients with inoperable tumor or distant metastases who require local therapy for the primary tumor but who express a desire to retain the penis. Radiation may be considered after a course of topical 5-fluorouracil cream has failed in the treatment of carcinoma in situ. Before radiation therapy, circumcision is necessary to expose the lesion, to allow resolution of any surface infection, and to prevent maceration and preputial edema.

The success of radiation therapy in the treatment of penile cancers is difficult to assess because of the relative rarity of these tumors, the variability of treatment within single series, and the variations between different series. Treatment schedules, total radiation dosages, and modality—external beam (Jackson, 1966), electron beam (Kelley et al, 1974), radium mold (Jackson, 1966), silicon mold (Akimoto et al, 1997), and interstitial therapy (Pierquin et al, 1971; Delannes et al, 1992; Gerbaulet and Lambin, 1992; McLean et al, 1993; Rozan et al, 1995)—vary considerably.

Radiation therapy to select, small, superficial lesions is successful. A 90% rate of control of the primary tumor among 20 patients treated with megavoltage radiation has been reported (Duncan and Jackson, 1972). However, the dosages employed—5000 to 5700 rad during 3 weeks—produced significant complications: penile necrosis in 10% of patients and urethral stricture in 30%. Sensory loss and erectile dysfunction have also been reported.

The most successful series employing radiation therapy is that reported by Memorial Sloan-Kettering Cancer Center (Kelley et al, 1974). With electron beam therapy, a 100% success rate in controlling lesions in 10 carefully selected patients was achieved clinically and confirmed histologically by means of normal post-treatment biopsy findings. Nine patients retained sexual function. The most common complication was urethral stricture in four patients (Grabstald and Kelley, 1980). In one patient, squamous carcinoma developed at another penile site, suggesting a new primary tumor, a complication also reported by others (Ravi, 1995). A series from the University of Texas M. D. Anderson Cancer Center reported good control of smaller lesions without significant morbidity (Haile and Delclos, 1980), and similar success with well-selected cases has been reported by other centers (Raynal et al, 1977; Salaverria et al, 1979; Daly et al, 1982; Mazeron et al, 1984; McLean et al, 1993).

There are significant disadvantages to radiation therapy. Squamous cell carcinoma is characteristically radioresistant, and the dosage required to sterilize the tumor (i.e., 6000 rad) may cause urethral fistula, stricture, or stenosis, with or without penile necrosis, pain, and edema (Kelley et al, 1974). **In some instances, secondary penectomy may be required** (Duncan and Jackson, 1972).

Infection is frequently associated with newly diagnosed penile cancer. This markedly decreases the therapeutic effect of radiation while increasing the risk of damage to the radiosensitive penile tissue (Murrell and Williams, 1965).

In addition, radiation therapy is usually administered for a period of 3 to 6 weeks and is followed by several months of morbidity. This may pose a formidable burden in elderly patients. By contrast, partial penectomy offers a prompt and effective treatment, with relatively few side effects limiting activity in the postoperative period.

Finally, it must be accepted that should radiation therapy fail, prompt penectomy must be done to avoid jeopardizing survival. Careful long-term follow-up is essential to detect recurrence promptly, and it must be recognized that recurrence may develop relatively late. In one series, 7 of 11 recurrences were detected after 2 years (63%) and 2 (18%) after 5 years (Mazeron et al, 1984). Close follow-up may be difficult in a group of patients whose reliability is often poor and who have often neglected a markedly symptomatic primary lesion for an extended time before seeking treatment. Furthermore, distinguishing postirradiation ulcer, scar, and fibrosis from possible recurrent carcinoma is often impossible, and repeated biopsies of the lesions may be required.

Brachytherapy

As an alternative to external beam radiotherapy, interstitial brachytherapy with a variety of radioisotopes (radium 226, iridium 192, cesium 137) may be used. Gerbaulet and Lambin (1992), using percutaneously placed interstitial iridium 192 implants, reported successful local control in 82% of 109 patients, with long-term survivals of 75% to 80% in patients with tumor-free regional lymph nodes. Rozan and associates (1995) reviewed 259 patients from multiple centers, with 5- and 10-year disease-free survival rates of 78% and 67%, respectively. Twenty-two percent of patients also had surgery ranging from circumcision to total penectomy. Late side effects occurred in 53% of the group. Alternatively, iridium 192 wires are placed in a plastic mold worn in close apposition to the penile shaft for 12 hours or so daily for a period of 7 to 10 days for a total tumor dose of 60 Gy (El-Demiry et al, 1984; Akimoto et al, 1997).

Crook and associates (2002) reported a more recent cohort (1989-2000) of 30 men with cT1-cT3 squamous cell carcinoma treated with iridium 192 delivered by 17- to 19.5-gauge steel needles held in a three-dimensional array by predrilled acrylic plastic templates. With a median six needles, dosages of 55 to 65 Gy were delivered during an average of 93 hours. With a median 34 months of follow-up, there were four local failures and four regional failures, and one patient required partial penectomy for radionecrosis. The 2-year actuarial local failure-free rate was 85%, and successful penile conservation was 83%. Obviously, tumors could only be clinically staged, and the authors stated that clinical distinction between cT1 and cT2 is subjective. Failure related to tumor grade, but not tumor size. Kiltie and associates (2000), however, found local failures in 60% of tumors larger than 4 cm compared with 14% of tumors smaller than 4 cm. Mazeron and colleagues (1984) and Soria and coworkers (1997) both demonstrated more local failure as the tumor invaded the corpora and with tumor size larger than 4 cm. In the Crook series, prophylactic lymph node dissections were not routinely performed, and as one would expect, 50% of moderately or poorly differentiated tumors recurred regionally or distally. Therefore, selection of patients for prophylactic lymph node dissection should be the same as selection of patients having surgical removal of the primary tumor.

Conclusion: Radiation Therapy and Brachytherapy

When radiation therapy is employed as the initial treatment of penile carcinoma, control of the primary lesions occurs with much less frequency than when surgery is primarily employed (Table 31–10). A patient's prognosis is not altered if surgery is promptly performed when radiation fails to control the carcinoma (Murrell and Williams, 1965). Jackson (1966), however, did show that nodal metastases develop more frequently during or after a course of radiation therapy than after surgery; this suggests the potential for metastases to occur during or after a course of unsuccessful radiation therapy (see Table 31–10).

In summary, small, superficial tumors will respond well to radiotherapy, and with careful planning, complications can be minimized. Brachytherapy for tumors smaller than 4 cm may offer acceptable local control rates with faster dose delivery. The treatment of larger, invasive malignant neoplasms is less successful, may be associated with severe local complications, and theoretically may provide an interval during which metastatic dissemination may occur. Other untoward effects of radiation include testicular damage and secondary neoplasia (Lederman, 1953; Prescott and Mainwaring, 1990; Fukunaga et al, 1994; Ravi, 1995). In the case of a sexually active young patient with a deeply invasive or large tumor (i.e., ≥4 cm), the risks and benefits of all options should be discussed. However, surgical amputation remains the gold standard. Penile reconstruction should be considered when total penectomy is required (see Chapter 33).

Radiation Therapy of the Inguinal Areas

Assessment of the treatment of the inguinal area by primary radiation therapy is hampered by the uncertainty arising from the inaccuracy of clinical staging and the frequent lack of histologic confirmation of nodal metastases. Other objections to the treatment of inguinal node metastases are that the inguinal areas tolerate radiation poorly and are subject to skin maceration and ulceration. Infectious lymphadenopathy will reduce the effectiveness of radiation therapy and exacerbate complications. Information concerning the use of radiation therapy as a primary mode for the treatment of penile carcinoma comes primarily from European countries and India.

The adjunctive or therapeutic use of radiation in treatment is controversial. Even if metastases are documented by node biopsy, the efficacy of subsequent radiation is impossible to judge because all tumor may have been removed by the biopsy. In one series, 70% of nodal metastases involved a single node, and survival in this group was 70% (Cabanas, 1977). Radiotherapy for inguinal metastases documented by histologic examination has been compared with surgery for the node-positive groin. A 50% 5-year survival rate was observed among the surgically treated group, and a 25% 5-year survival rate was observed among the irradiated group (Staubitz et al, 1955). Other series report that radiation to the inguinal areas has not proved therapeutically effective (Murrell and Williams, 1965; Jensen, 1977).

Several Scandinavian centers have delivered radiation therapy to inguinal nodes as well as to the primary tumor in all cases of penile carcinoma. Surgical lymphadenectomy followed if palpable nodes persisted or appeared subsequently (Engelstad, 1948; Ekstrom and Edsmyr, 1958).

Ravi (1993b) reported on 201 patients, of whom 106 had clinically metastatic inguinal lymphadenopathy. Patients with inguinal nodes larger than 4 cm received 4000 cGY radiation before undergoing node dissection. Perinodal infiltration, thought to have an adverse impact on survival, was found in 14 of 43 nonirradiated groins (33%) but in only 3 of 34 irradiated groins (9%).

In a series of 130 patients initially having clinically impalpable nodes but treated with adjuvant radiation therapy, 18 subsequently developed palpable nodal disease requiring

Table 31-10.	Surgery Required after Radiation Therapy for Carcinoma of the Penis			
Series	No. of Patients	Amputation for Persistent or Recurrent Disease or Both (%)	Other Surgery (%)*	Total (%)
Engelstad, 1948	64	45[†]	8[‡]	53
Lederman, 1953	48	35	—	35
Murrell and Williams, 1965	92	48	—	48
Jackson, 1966	58	51	—	51
Knudsen and Brennhovd, 1967	145	62	6[‡]	68
Almgard and Edsmyr, 1973	33	52	18[§]	70
Raynal et al, 1977	45	22	8[‡]	30
Salverria et al, 1979	13	23	—	23
Haile and Delclos, 1980	20	10	10[‡]	20
Daly et al, 1982	22	5	10[‡]	15
Sagerman al, 1984	15	40	—	40
Mazeron et al, 1984	50	20	10	30
Fossa et al, 1987	11	33	—	33
Suchaud et al, 1989	53	42	—	42
McLean et al, 1993	26	19	12[‡]	31
Rozan et al, 1995	259	12	21	33
Zouhair et al, 2001	23	57	4	61

*Difference from 100% indicates cure by radiation alone.
[†]Includes seven failures of radiation therapy not having further surgery.
[‡]Penectomy for radiation complications.
[§]Local excision or electrocoagulation of recurrent neoplasm.

lymphadenectomy, and another 11 patients had metastases but no surgery. Therefore, 29 of 130 men (22%) who received prophylactic groin irradiation subsequently developed inguinal metastases (Ekstrom and Edsmyr, 1958).

Murrell and Williams (1965) found that 3 of 11 patients (25%) who received radiation therapy to the inguinal area without initially palpable nodes subsequently developed inguinal metastases. These percentages closely approximate the incidence of subclinical metastases that are encountered if node dissection is performed when the clinical examination is normal (see Table 31–3), and they suggest that radiation therapy did not alter the course of the disease. Furthermore, because of tissue changes that follow radiation to the groin, clinical evaluation of the groin is difficult, and the complications encountered with groin dissection after irradiation can be significant.

Last, the 5-year survival rate for patients with prophylactically irradiated groins followed as necessary by lymphadenectomy differs little from that for patients having surgery alone. Although a large, randomized, controlled study might definitely answer the question of efficacy of radiation therapy for inguinal metastases, both microscopic and macroscopic, it is unlikely that such a study could be realized. Present information supports surgical therapy for inguinal metastasis as superior to radiation therapy.

Radiation therapy may be considered in patients presenting with inoperable fixed and ulcerative inguinal lymph nodes. On occasion, radiation to these areas is well tolerated, may result in significant palliation, and may postpone local complications for prolonged periods (Furlong and Uhle, 1953; Staubitz et al, 1955; Vaeth et al, 1970).

An alternative use of radiation would be as adjuvant therapy for surgically treated, pN+ patients. In a small retrospective study from Taiwan, Chen and colleagues (2004) reported regional failure rates after positive inguinal lymph node dissections in 11% (1 of 9) versus 60% (3 of 5) with and without adjuvant inguinal radiotherapy.

In summary, radiation therapy to the inguinal area is not as effective therapeutically as lymph node dissection, but it may be useful for palliation in the situation of inoperable nodes.

KEY POINTS: RADIATION THERAPY

■ Primary radiation therapy for the penis may be successfully applied to select patients with T1 and T2 squamous cell carcinomas smaller than 4 cm with either external beam or brachytherapy techniques.

■ Salvage penectomy may be required after external beam radiation or brachytherapy for persistent or recurrent disease or radiation necrosis. Careful follow-up is required.

■ For patients selected for radiation therapy for the primary, surgical management of inguinal lymph nodes should be recommended by the same criteria as for patients selected for surgical management of the primary. Radiation to the inguinal area is not as effective as surgery, but it is useful for palliation of inoperable nodes.

CHEMOTHERAPY
Active Single Agents and Combination Strategies

Because of the relative rarity of penile carcinomas, experience with their chemotherapeutic management is limited. The use of topical 5-fluorouracil in superficial and precancerous lesions has already been discussed. 5-Fluorouracil has been administered as a continuous intravenous infusion in combination with DDCP (cisplatin) in a limited number of patients. Only three other drugs have been employed to any extent: cisplatin, bleomycin, and methotrexate. Experience with combination chemotherapy remains limited.

Because single-agent DDCP had demonstrated response in squamous carcinomas of the head and neck and elsewhere, it was used in two separate trials in advanced penile cancer. In a study from Memorial Sloan-Kettering Cancer Center, 13 patients with extensive disease and either prior radiotherapy or chemotherapy were treated with 70 to 120 mg/m² every 21 days. Three patients (23%) demonstrated partial responses (Ahmed et al, 1984). Gagliano and associates (1989) from the Southwest Oncology Group treated 26 patients, 12 of whom had had prior radiation with low-dose (50 mg/m²) DDCP, and observed a 15% response rate of limited duration.

Initial favorable reports from Japan suggested that bleomycin appeared to be effective in the treatment of penile and scrotal cancer. Ichikawa and associates (1969, 1977) reported a 50% response in 24 previously untreated patients with squamous carcinoma of the penis. A similar report from Uganda documented partial or complete tumor regression in 45% of treated patients (Kyalwazi et al, 1974). A review of 90 patients from the world literature demonstrated similar responses (Eisenberger, 1992).

Methotrexate produced partial responses in 8 of 13 patients (61%) treated at Memorial Sloan-Kettering Cancer Center (Ahmed et al, 1984). Five patients were treated with high-dose therapy with folinic acid rescue, and eight were treated with low-dose intravenous therapy (30 to 40 mg/m²/week). Methotrexate has been shown to be effective in other reports (Mills, 1972; Garnick et al, 1979).

Hussein and associates (1990) used a combination of 5-fluorouracil and DDCP in six patients, five with penile and one with urethral squamous cell carcinoma. The five patients with penile cancer had partial responses, whereas the patient with urethral cancer had complete disappearance of his tumor.

Combination vincristine, bleomycin, and methotrexate therapy was administered in 12 weekly courses to 17 patients as either a neoadjuvant (5 patients) or postoperative (12 patients) treatment program at the Milan National Tumor Institute (Table 31–11). The patients treated with adjuvant therapy were at high risk; nine showed extranodal tumor growth, five had pelvic nodal involvement, and five had bilateral metastases. At follow-up ranging between 18 and 102 months, only one relapse had occurred (Pizzocaro and Piva, 1988). Later reports from this center further confirmed the value of adjuvant chemotherapy. Of 56 node-positive patients, 82% of the 25 patients receiving adjuvant vincristine, bleomycin, and methotrexate therapy survived 5 years, compared with 37% of 31 patients treated with surgery alone (Pizzocaro et al, 1995, 1997). In the neoadjuvant treatment group, partial responses were noted in three of five patients

Table 31–11. Combination Chemotherapy for Penile Cancer

VBM (8-12 weekly courses)		
Vincristine	1 mg	IV day 1
Bleomycin	15 mg	IM 6 and 24 hours after vincristine
Methotrexate	30 mg	PO day 3
Principal toxicities		
Vincristine: alopecia, neurotoxicity		
Bleomycin: mucositis, pneumonitis		
Methotrexate: myelosuppression (nadir, 7-14 days), mucositis, nausea and vomiting		
PF (4 courses at intervals of 3 weeks)		
Cisplatin	100 mg/m^2	IV day 1
5-Fluorouracil	1.0 g/m^2	IV day 1, CI
Principal toxicities		
Cisplatin: myelosuppression (nadir, 18-23 days), nephrotoxicity, neurotoxicity, ototoxicity, severe nausea and vomiting		
5-Fluorouracil: myelosuppression (nadir, 7-14 days), mucositis, dermatitis		
MPB (every 28 days for 2-4 cycles)		
Methotrexate	200 mg/m^2	IV days 1, 15, 22
Leucovorin	25 mg	PO every 6 hours for 12 doses beginning day 2
Cisplatin	20 mg/m^2	IV days 2-6 (total = 100 mg/m^2)
Bleomycin	10 mg/m^2	IV days 2-6 CI (total = 50 mg/m^2)
Principal toxicities as noted above		
PMB (every 21 days for 4-6 cycles)		
Cisplatin	100 mg/m^2	IV day 1
Methotrexate	25 mg/m^2	IV bolus days 1 and 8
Bleomycin	10 mg/m^2	IV bolus days 1 and 8
Principal toxicities as noted above		

CI, continuous infusion; MPB, methotrexate, cisplatin, bleomycin; PF, cisplatin, 5-fluorouracil; PMB, cisplatin, methotrexate, bleomycin; VBM, vincristine, bleomycin, methotrexate.

with extremely large (6 to 11 cm) nodal metastases. These three patients subsequently were completely resected and were free of tumor at intervals ranging from 20 to 72 months.

In another neoadjuvant study, four patients with stage III tumors were treated with a regimen of DDCP and 5-fluorouracil and resected. Two patients showed no residual tumor in the lymphadenectomy specimen, and disease had not recurred in any patient 6 to 40 months after surgery (Fisher et al, 1990).

In a study from the University of Texas M. D. Anderson Cancer Center, combination chemotherapy with methotrexate, bleomycin, and cisplatin was administered to 14 men with inoperable or metastatic squamous cell carcinoma of the genital tract (Dexeus et al, 1991). In 12 patients, the primary tumor site was the penis. Several patients were given bleomycin and cisplatin intra-arterially. The overall response rate was 72% (14% complete responses, 57% partial responses), although the mean duration was only 6 months. **Corral and associates (1998) reported additional experience with this regimen in a phase II study** (see Table 31–11). **Of 21 evaluable patients with squamous cell carcinoma of the penis, 12 (57%) exhibited an objective response.** As noted previously, the response duration was brief. The overall median survival was 11 months, with survival of responders over nonresponders approaching statistical significance. More important, however, **in patients rendered disease free with chemotherapy alone or with chemotherapy followed by surgical resection or radiation therapy (one case), the median survival was 34 months. Thus, an aggressive multimodal approach to achieve disease-free status may be important in advanced penile cancer.**

The Southwest Oncology Group reported data with use of a modified regimen that reduced the total dose of all three agents; Haas and associates (1999) employed combination cisplatin, methotrexate, and bleomycin in 45 patients with locally advanced or metastatic penile cancer accrued from 31 different institutions (see Table 31–11). There were five complete and eight partial responses among 40 evaluable patients (32.5% response rate). Toxicity, including five treatment-related deaths, was high. Although this regimen can be associated with significant responses, toxicity can be significant, especially with administration outside of specialized settings.

Newer potentially effective strategies reported in a handful of patients include combination paclitaxel and carboplatin (Joerger et al, 2004) and paclitaxel, cisplatin, and ifosfamide (Bermejo et al, 2003).

Combined modality programs of chemotherapy plus surgery or radiotherapy have been employed with encouraging results in treatment of squamous cell carcinomas of both the larynx and the anus (Eisenberger, 1992; Pedrick et al, 1993). Similar strategies may be helpful in minimizing the disfigurement and functional loss associated with penile amputative surgery in selected cases. A report of successful treatment of localized invasive penile squamous carcinomas in two patients with combined modality therapy with laser hyperthermia, radiation therapy, and chemotherapy with intravenous peplomycin suggests that further evaluation of laser techniques in combination with other treatments is warranted (Shirahama et al, 1998).

A preliminary study of interferon-α in combination with a retinoid, etretinate, in a group of patients with squamous carcinomas of different sites including penile cancers showed moderate activity against the tumors. This suggests that combination therapies including retinoids may have a role in the treatment of metastatic penile tumors (Roth et al, 1999).

Combined modality approaches have been employed with some success in patients presenting with unresectable disease to convert the tumor to a potentially resectable lesion (Abratt et al, 1989; Germiyanoglu et al, 1993). Again, the low incidence of these tumors will necessitate evaluation of treatment protocols by means of multi-institutional cooperative studies with international scope.

In summary, chemotherapy can induce responses in metastatic penile cancer. These responses are generally partial in character and short in duration. Thus, disease consolidation with surgery and potentially radiotherapy is required in most cases to achieve disease-free status. The rarity of penile carcinoma in the United States is an obstacle to conducting successful phase II and phase III chemotherapy trials. This information will need to come from trials conducted in South America, Africa, or Asia. Studies must be designed to determine which agents will be most useful as (1) neoadjuvant therapy in stage III disease, (2) adjuvant therapy when pathologic evaluation of the nodes reveals extensive inguinal metastases or pelvic metastases that predict diminished survival (Johnson and Lo, 1984a; Srinivas et al, 1987; Fraley et al, 1989; Eisenberger, 1992; Lynch, 1997), and (3) palliative chemotherapy in patients with locally inoperable tumor or distant metastases.

KEY POINTS: CHEMOTHERAPY

- For advanced penile cancer, multiagent chemotherapy regimens such as cisplatin, methotrexate, and bleomycin demonstrate more than 50% response rates with a mean duration of only 6 months and median survival of less than 1 year. Toxicity can be significant.

- For locally advanced penile cancer, chemotherapy plus surgery or radiation therapy may improve results over single-modality therapy, but randomized trials are needed.

NONSQUAMOUS MALIGNANT NEOPLASMS
Basal Cell Carcinoma

Whereas basal cell carcinoma is frequently encountered on other cutaneous surfaces, it is rare on the penis. Fewer than 15 cases have been well documented (Goldminz et al, 1989; Ladocsi et al, 1998). **Treatment is by local excision, which is virtually always curative** (Hall et al, 1968; Goldminz et al, 1989). No instances of metastasis or local recurrence after local excision have been reported.

A benign variant of basal cell carcinoma, the premalignant fibroepithelioma of Pinkus, has been reported to occur on the penile shaft (Heymann et al, 1983). Diagnosis is made at excisional biopsy. Excision has been uniformly curative.

Melanoma and basal cell carcinoma rarely occur on the penis, presumably because the organ's skin is protected from exposure to the sun. Malignant neoplasms arising from the supporting structures of the penis are also rare and include any combination of tumors of smooth or striated muscle or of fibrous, fatty, or vascular tissue. Information about appropriate treatment of these malignant neoplasms is derived from the review of single case reports and small series (Belville and Cohen, 1992).

Melanoma

More than 150 cases of melanoma of the penis have been reported. Of 1200 melanomas treated at Memorial Sloan-Kettering Cancer Center, only two were of penile origin (Das Gupta and Grabstald, 1965). At the University of Texas M. D. Anderson Cancer Center, less than 1% of all primary penile cancers were malignant melanomas (Johnson and Ayala, 1973; de Bree et al, 1997).

Melanoma presents as a blue-black or reddish brown pigmented papule, plaque, or ulceration on the glans penis. It occurs on the prepuce less frequently. Diagnosis is made by histologic examination of biopsy specimens, which demonstrate atypical junctional cell activity with displacement of pigmented cells into the dermis.

Prognostic characteristics that have been found significant for melanoma in other sites, such as depth of invasion (Clark staging) and thickness of the tumor (Breslow classification), have not been prospectively applied to penile lesions as experience with these lesions is limited. Sanchez-Ortiz and colleagues (2005) used the AJCC system for classifying cutaneous melanomas (Fleming et al, 1997) in the largest report to date on melanoma of the penis. This system incorporates elements of the Clark and Breslow staging systems. When this information is favorable, local excision is feasible. Distant metastatic spread has been found in 60% of patients studied (Abeshouse, 1958; Johnson et al, 1973; de Bree et al, 1997) in older series. However, Sanchez-Ortiz found that patients with early stage melanomas had excellent outcomes if primary tumors were low stage and regional lymph nodes were negative. Hematogenous metastases occur by means of the vascular structures of the corporal bodies; lymphatic spread to the regional lymphatic ilioinguinal nodes occurs by lymphatic permeation.

Surgery is the primary mode of treatment; radiotherapy and chemotherapy are of only adjunctive or palliative benefit. For stage I melanoma (localized lesion without metastases) and stage II melanoma (metastases confined to one regional area), adequate excision of the primary tumor by partial or total penile amputation together with en bloc bilateral ilioinguinal node dissection offers the greatest prospect for cure (Johnson et al, 1973; Bracken and Diokno, 1974; Manivel and Fraley, 1988). In reviewing the University of Texas M. D. Anderson Cancer Center experience plus the literature to date, Sanchez-Ortiz and colleagues (2005) proposed a treatment algorithm for management of the primary tumor and inguinal lymph nodes. For tumors of the foreskin, circumcision may be adequate. For glans tumors, a partial penectomy can be performed; and for glans-shaft tumors, a partial or total penectomy can be performed. The prognosis for patients with penile melanoma is clearly dependent on stage of the primary tumor and the presence or absence of inguinal metastases. Contemporary staging and prognostic factors are reviewed by Sanchez-Ortiz and coworkers (2005).

Sarcomas

Primary mesenchymal tumors of the penis are rare. A thorough review of 46 such tumors from the Armed Forces Institute of Pathology revealed an equal number of benign and malignant lesions (Dehner and Smith, 1970). The patients ranged in age from newborn to the eighth decade of life. The presenting signs and symptoms of subcutaneous mass, penile pain and enlargement, priapism, and urinary obstruction were the same for both benign and malignant lesions. A sarcoma has been reported to "masquerade" as Peyronie's plaque (Moore et al, 1975).

Malignant lesions were found more frequently on the proximal shaft; benign lesions were more often located distally. The most common malignant lesions were those of vascular origin (hemangioepithelioma), followed in frequency by those of neural, myogenic, and fibrous origin (Ashley and Edwards, 1957). Single case reports of sarcomatous lesions have been published, for example, malignant fibrous histiocytoma (Parsons and Fox, 1988), angiosarcoma (Rasbridge and Parry, 1989), leiomyosarcoma (Planz et al, 1998), epithelioid sarcoma (Leviav et al, 1988), and osteosarcoma (Sacker et al, 1994).

Sarcomas have been classified as superficial when they arise from the integumentary supporting structures and as deep when they develop from the corporal body supporting structures (Pratt and Ross, 1969). Wide local surface excision and partial penile amputation for the superficial tumors have been suggested and used successfully in isolated case reports (Pak et al, 1986; Dalkin and Zaontz, 1989). Total penile amputation has been reserved for tumors of deep corporal origin. **However, local recurrences are characteristic of sarcomas** (Dehner and Smith, 1970). To avoid local recurrences, a total amputation, even for superficial malignant neoplasms of any cell type, should be considered.

Regional metastases are rare. Unless adenopathy is palpable, node dissections are not recommended (Hutcheson et al, 1969). Distant metastases have also been unusual (Dehner and Smith, 1970). This supports aggressive local treatment in anticipation of cure. Radiation therapy and chemotherapy have not been used extensively enough for comment on their efficacy.

Kaposi's sarcoma, usually a cutaneous manifestation of a generalized lymphoreticular disorder, may produce genital lesions but is now most frequently associated with HIV infection (see earlier).

Paget's Disease

Paget's disease of the penis is extremely rare. Fewer than 30 cases have been reported (Mitsudo et al, 1981; Macedo et al, 1997). It appears grossly as an erythematous, eczematoid, well-demarcated area that cannot be clinically distinguished from erythroplasia of Queyrat, Bowen's disease, or carcinoma in situ of the penis. Clinical presentation includes local discomfort, pruritus, and occasionally a serosanguineous discharge. On microscopic examination, identification is clearly made by the presence of large, round or oval, clear-staining hydropic cells with hypochromatic nuclei (i.e., "Paget cells").

Paget's disease may often herald a deeply seated carcinoma with Paget cells moving through ducts or lymphatics to the epidermal surface. In the penis, a sweat gland carcinoma (Mitsudo et al, 1981) or periurethral gland adenocarcinoma (Jenkins, 1989) may be the primary neoplasm. Paget's disease of the penis has developed after radiation therapy given for transitional cell carcinoma of the bladder (Hayes et al, 1997). Complete local surgical excision of the skin and subcutaneous tissue is the recommended form of therapy. If inguinal adenopathy is present, radical node dissection is advised (Hagan et al, 1975). Careful observation for recurrence at the margins is necessary.

Adenosquamous Carcinoma

This is a rare tumor characterized by both glandular and squamous histologic elements, which are independent of the urethral glands. In gross appearance, this tumor presents as a large (5 to 9 cm), firm, grayish white granular exophytic mass involving the distal shaft or glans. On microscopic examination, the glands contain mucin and are positive for carcinoembryonic antigen. In one reported case, tumor was metastatic to a single inguinal node. This patient was managed with local excision of the primary and a limited inguinal node dissection and lived 9 years after treatment. Other tumors were managed with local excision and surveillance (Cubilla et al, 1996).

Lymphoreticular Malignant Neoplasm

Primary lymphoreticular malignant neoplasm rarely occurs on the penis (Dehner and Smith, 1970). **Leukemia may infiltrate the corpora, resulting in priapism** (Pochedly et al, 1974). **When lymphomatous infiltration of the penis is diagnosed, a thorough search for systemic disease is necessary.** If the penile lesion is indeed a primary tumor, systemic chemotherapy may be administered. It is the most effective therapy for local disease, for potential occult deposits that may exist elsewhere, and for preservation of form and function (Marks et al, 1988). Local low-dose irradiation has also been reported to be successful (Stewart et al, 1985).

Metastases

Metastatic lesions to the penis are unusual. Approximately 200 cases have been reported in the literature. Their infrequency is somewhat puzzling when one considers the rich blood and lymphatic supply to the organ and its proximity to the bladder, prostate, and rectum—areas frequently involved with neoplasm. It is from these three organs that the majority of metastatic penile lesions originate (Abeshouse, 1958). Renal and respiratory neoplasms have also metastasized to the penis. The most likely routes of spread are by direct extension, retrograde venous and lymphatic transport, and arterial embolism.

The most frequent sign of penile metastasis is priapism; penile swelling, nodularity, and ulceration have also been reported (McCrea and Tobias, 1958; Abeshouse and Abeshouse, 1961; Weitzner, 1971). Urinary obstruction and hematuria may occur. The most common histologic feature of penile invasion by metastatic lesions is the replacement of one or both corpora cavernosa, which explains the frequent occurrence of priapism. Solitary cutaneous, preputial, and glanular deposits are less common.

The differential diagnosis includes idiopathic priapism; venereal or other infectious ulcerations; tuberculosis; Peyronie's plaque; and primary, benign, or malignant tumors.

Penile metastases represent an advanced form of virulent disease and usually appear rather rapidly after recognition and treatment of the primary lesion (Abeshouse and Abeshouse, 1961; Hayes and Young, 1967; Mukamel et al, 1987). On rare occasions, a long period may elapse between the treatment of the primary lesion and the appearance of penile metastases (Abeshouse and Abeshouse, 1961), or the penile lesion may occur as the initial and only site of metastasis.

Because of the association of a penile metastatic lesion with advanced disease, survival after its presentation is limited, and the majority of patients die within 1 year (Robey and Schellhammer, 1984; Mukamel et al, 1987; Fischer and Patrick, 1999). Successful treatment may occasionally be possible in the case of solitary nodules or localized distal penile involvement if complete excision by partial amputation succeeds in removing the entire area of malignant infiltration (Spaulding and Whitmore, 1978). The prospect for surgical cure is minimal if proximal corporal invasion is present. Penectomy is occasionally indicated after failure of other modalities to palliate intractable pain (Mukamel et al, 1987). Pain can also be managed by dorsal nerve section (Hill and Khalid, 1988). Radiation therapy has generally been unsuccessful, and chemotherapy has not been employed in a sufficient number of cases to warrant definitive recommendations.

KEY POINTS: NONSQUAMOUS MALIGNANT NEOPLASMS

- Rarely, nonsquamous cell skin or soft tissue cancers will occur on the penis and require prompt biopsy and control of the local tumor.

- Sarcomas are prone to local recurrence; regional and distant metastases are rare.

- Melanoma can be cured if diagnosed at an early stage.

- Melanoma has a propensity for early metastases and new systemic therapy is needed.

SUGGESTED READINGS

Agrawal A, Pai D, Ananthakrishnan N, et al: The histological extent of the local spread of carcinoma of the penis and its therapeutic implications. BJU Int 2000;85:299-301.

Alani RM, Munger K: Human papillomaviruses and associated malignancies. J Clin Oncol 1998;16:330-337.

Aragona F, Serretta V, Marconi A, et al: Queyrat's erythroplasia of the prepuce: A case-report. Acta Chir Belg 1985;85:303-304.

Bain L, Geronemus R: The association of lichen planus of the penis with squamous cell carcinoma in situ and with verrucous squamous carcinoma. J Dermatol Surg Oncol 1989;15:413-417.

Bevan-Thomas R, Slaton JW, Pettaway CA: Contemporary morbidity from lymphadenectomy for penile squamous cell carcinoma: The M. D. Anderson Cancer Center experience. J Urol 2002;167:1638-1642.

Bhojwani A, Biyani CS, Nicol A, Powell CS: Bowenoid papulosis of the penis. Br J Urol 1997;80:508.

Cabanas RM: Anatomy and biopsy of the sentinel lymph nodes. Urol Clin North Am 1992;19:267-276.

Castellsague X, Ghaffari A, Daniel RW, et al: Prevalence of penile human papillomavirus DNA in husbands of women with and without cervical neoplasia: A study in Spain and Colombia. J Infect Dis 1997;176:353-361.

Chen MF, Chen WC, Wu CT, Chuang CK: Contemporary management of penile cancer including surgery and adjuvant radiotherapy: An experience in Taiwan. World J Urol 2004;22:60-66.

Coblentz TR, Theodorescu D: Morbidity of modified prophylactic inguinal lymphadenectomy for squamous cell carcinoma of the penis. J Urol 2002;168(pt 1):1386-1389.

Colberg JW, Andriole GL, Catalona WJ: Long-term follow-up of men undergoing modified inguinal lymphadenectomy for carcinoma of the penis. Br J Urol 1997;79:54-57.

Corral DA, Sella A, Pettaway CA, et al: Combination chemotherapy for metastatic or locally advanced genitourinary squamous cell carcinoma: A phase II study of methotrexate, cisplatin and bleomycin. J Urol 1998;160:1770-1774.

Crook J, Grimard L, Tsihlias J, et al: Interstitial brachytherapy for penile cancer: An alternative to amputation. J Urol 2002;167:506-511.

Cubilla A, Reuter V, Gregoire L, et al: Basaloid squamous cell carcinoma: A distinctive human papilloma virus–related penile neoplasm: A report of 20 cases. Am J Surg Pathol 1998;22:755-761.

Cubilla AL, Reuter V, Velazquez E, et al: Histologic classification of penile carcinoma and its relation to outcome in 61 patients with primary resection. Int J Surg Pathol 2001;9:111-120.

Culkin DJ, Beer TM: Advanced penile carcinoma. J Urol 2003;170:359-365.

Danielson AG, Sand C, Weisman K: Treatment of Bowen's disease of the penis with 5% imiquimod cream. Clin Exp Dermatol 2003;28(suppl 1):7-9.

Davis JW, Schellhammer PF, Schlossberg SM: Conservative surgical therapy for penile and urethral carcinoma. Urology 1999;53:386-392.

Deserno WM, Harisinghani MG, Taupitz M, et al: Urinary bladder cancer: Preoperative nodal staging with ferumoxtran-10-enhanced MR imaging. Radiology 2004;233:449-456.

Dianzani C, Calvieri S, Pierangeli A, Degener AM: Identification of human papilloma viruses in male dysplastic genital lesions. New Microbiol 2004;27:65-69.

Eng TY, Petersen JP, Stack RS, Judson PH: Lymph node metastasis from carcinoma in situ of the penis: A case report. J Urol 1995;153:432-434.

Ficarra V, Zattoni F, Cunico SC, et al: Lymphatic and vascular embolizations are independent predictive variables of inguinal lymph node involvement in patients with squamous cell carcinoma of the penis. Gruppo Uro-Oncologico del Nord Est (Northeast Uro-Oncological Group) Penile Cancer data base. Cancer 2005;103:2507-2516.

Fleming ID, Cooper JS, Henson DE, et al: Penis. AJCC Cancer Staging Manual/American Joint Committee on Cancer, 5th ed. Philadelphia, Lippincott-Raven, 1997:215-217.

Frimberger D, Hungerhuber E, Zaak D, et al: Penile carcinoma. Is Nd:YAG laser therapy radical enough? J Urol 2002;168:2418-2421;discussion 2421.

Frimberger D, Schneede P, Hungerhuber E, et al: Autofluorescence and 5-aminolevulinic acid induced fluorescence diagnosis of penile carcinoma—new techniques to monitor Nd:YAG laser therapy. Urol Res 2002;30:295-300.

Frisch M, Friis S, Kjaer SK, Melbye KM: Falling incidence of penis cancer in an uncircumcised population (Denmark 1943-90). BMJ 1995;311:1471.

Graham JH, Helwig EB: Erythroplasia of Queyrat [review]. Cancer 1973;32:1396-1414.

Gross G, Pfister H: Role of human papillomavirus in penile cancer, penile intraepithelial squamous cell neoplasias and in genital warts. Med Microbiol Immunol (Berl) 2004;193:35-44.

Grussendorf-Conen EI: Anogenital premalignant and malignant tumors (including Buschke-Löwenstein tumors). Clin Dermatol 1997;15:377-388.

Haas GP, Blumenstein BA, Gagliano RG, et al: Cisplatin, methotrexate, and bleomycin for the treatment of carcinoma of the penis: A Southwest Oncology Group Study. J Urol 1999;161:1823-1825.

Harish K, Ravi R: The role of tobacco in penile carcinoma. Br J Urol 1995;75:375-377.

Harmer MH: Penis (ICD-0187). TNM Classification of Malignant Tumours, 3rd ed. Geneva, International Union Against Cancer, 1978:126-128.

Heyns CF, Van Vollenhoven P, Steenkamp JW, et al: Carcinoma of the penis—appraisal of a modified tumor-staging system. Br J Urol 1997;80:307-312.

Horenblas S, van Tinteren H: Squamous cell carcinoma of the penis. IV. Prognostic factors of survival: Analysis of tumor, nodes and metastasis classification system. J Urol 1994;151:1239-1243.

SECTION VII

Horenblas S, van Tinteren H, Delemarre JF, et al: Squamous cell carcinoma of the penis: Accuracy of tumor, nodes and metastases classification system and role of lymphangiography, computerized tomography scan, and fine needle aspiration cytology. J Urol 1991;146:1279-1283.

Horenblas S, van Tinteren H, Delemarre JF, et al: Squamous cell carcinoma of the penis. III. Treatment of regional lymph nodes. J Urol 1993;149:492-497.

Horenblas S, Jansen L, Meinhardt W, et al: Detection of occult metastasis in squamous cell carcinoma of the penis using a dynamic sentinel node procedure. J Urol 2000;163:100-104.

Hung-fu T, Morganstern H, Mack T, Peters RK: Risk factors for penile cancer: Results of a population-based case-control study in Los Angeles County. Cancer Causes Control 2001;12:267-277.

Johnson DE, Lo RK: Management of regional lymph nodes in penile carcinoma. Five-year results following therapeutic groin dissections. Urology 1984;24:308-311.

Kinkade S, Meadows S, Garcia-Trujillo J: Clinical inquiries. Does neonatal circumcision decrease morbidity? J Fam Pract 2005;54:81-82.

Kroon BK, Horenblas S, Estourgie SH, et al: How to avoid false-negative dynamic sentinel node procedures in penile carcinoma. J Urol 2004;171 (pt 1):2191-2194.

Kroon BK, Horenblas S, Deurloo EE, et al: Ultrasonography-guided fine-needle aspiration cytology before sentinel node biopsy in patients with penile carcinoma. BJU Int 2005;95:517-521.

Kroon BK, Horenblas S, Lont AP, et al: Patients with penile carcinoma benefit from immediate resection of clinically occult lymph node metastases. J Urol 2005;173:816-819.

Kroon BK, Lont AP, Valdes Olmos RA, et al: Morbidity of dynamic sentinel node biopsy in penile carcinoma [see comment]. J Urol 2005;173:813-815.

Lont AP, Besnard AP, Gallee MP, et al: A comparison of physical examination and imaging in determining the extent of primary penile carcinoma. BJU Int 2003;91:493-495.

Lopes A, Hidalgo GS, Kowalski LP, et al: Prognostic factors in carcinoma of the penis: Multivariate analysis of 145 patients treated with amputation and lymphadenectomy. J Urol 1996;156:1637-1642.

Lopes A, Bezerra AL, Serrano SV, Hidalgo GS: Iliac nodal metastases from carcinoma of the penis treated surgically. BJU Int 2000;86:690-693.

Lopes A, Bezerra AL, Pinto CA, et al: p53 as a new prognostic factor for lymph node metastasis in penile carcinoma: Analysis of 82 patients treated with amputation and bilateral lymphadenectomy. J Urol 2002;168:81-86.

Lowhagen GB, Bolmstedt A, Ryd W, Voog E: The prevalence of "high-risk" HPV types in penile condyloma-like lesions: Correlation between HPV type and morphology. Genitourin Med 1993;69:87-90.

Lucia MS, Miller GJ: Histopathology of malignant lesions of the penis. Urol Clin North Am 1992;19:227-246.

Maden C, Sherman KJ, Beckman AM, et al: History of circumcision, medical conditions, and sexual activity and risk of penile cancer. J Natl Cancer Inst 1993;85:19-24.

Malek RS: Laser treatment of premalignant and malignant squamous cell lesions of the penis. Lasers Surg Med 1992;12:246-253.

McDougal WS: Carcinoma of the penis: Improved survival by early regional lymphadenectomy based on the histological grade and depth of invasion of the primary lesion. J Urol 1995;154:1364-1366.

Micali G, Nasca MR, Innocenzi D: Lichen sclerosus of the glans is significantly associated with penile carcinoma. Sex Transm Infect 2001;77:226.

Micali G, Nasca MR, Tedeschi A: Topical treatment of intraepithelial penile carcinoma with imiquimod. Clin Exp Dermatol 2003;28(suppl 1):4-6.

Misra S, Chaturvedi A, Misra NC: Penile carcinoma: A challenge for the developing world. Lancet Oncol 2004;5:240-247.

Mohs FE, Snow SN, Larson PO: Mohs micrographic surgery for penile tumors. Urol Clin North Am 1992;19:291-304.

Nelson BA, Cookson MS, Smith JA Jr, Chang SS: Complications of inguinal and pelvic lymphadenectomy for squamous cell carcinoma of the penis: A contemporary series. J Urol 2004;172:494-497.

Opjordsmoen S, Fossa SD: Quality of life in patients treated for penile cancer. A follow-up study. Br J Urol 1994;74:652-657.

Pettaway CA, Pisters LL, Dinney CP, et al: Sentinel lymph node biopsy for penile squamous carcinoma: The M. D. Anderson Cancer Center Experience. J Urol 1995;154:1999-2003.

Pietrzak P, Corbishley C, Watkin N: Organ-sparing surgery for invasive penile cancer: Early follow-up data. BJU Int 2004;94:1253-1257.

Pizzocaro G, Piva L, Bandieramonte G, Tana S: Up-to-date management of carcinoma of the penis. Eur Urol 1997;32:5-15.

Poblet E, Alfaro L, Fernander-Segoviano P, et al: Human papillomavirus–associated penile squamous cell carcinoma in HIV positive patients. Am J Surg Pathol 1999;23:1119-1126.

Ravi R: Correlation between the extent of nodal involvement and survival following groin dissection for carcinoma of the penis. Br J Urol 1993;72:817-819.

Reynolds SJ, Shepherd ME, Risbud AR, et al: The highly protective effect of newborn circumcision against invasive penile cancer. Pediatrics 2000;105:E36.

Rippentrop JM, Joslyn SA, Konety BR: Squamous cell carcinoma of the penis: Evaluation of data from the Surveillance, Epidemiology, and End Results Program. Cancer 2004;101:1357-1363.

Rubin MA, Kleter B, Zhou M, et al: Detection and typing of human papillomavirus DNA in penile carcinoma. Am J Pathol 2001;159:1211-1218.

Sanchez-Ortiz R, Huang SF, Tamboli P, et al: Melanoma of the penis, scrotum and male urethra: A 40-year single institution experience. J Urol 2005;173:1958-1965.

Scappini P, Piscioli F, Pusiol T, et al: Penile cancer. Aspiration biopsy cytology for staging. Cancer 1986;58:1526-1533.

Scardino E, Villa G, Bonomo G, et al: Magnetic resonance imaging combined with artificial erection for local staging of penile cancer. Urology 2004; 63:1158-1162.

Seixas ALC, Ornellas AA, Marota A, et al: Verrucous carcinoma of the penis: Retrospective analysis of 32 cases. J Urol 1994;152:1476-1479.

Shapiro E: American Academy of Pediatrics policy statements on circumcision and urinary tract infection. Rev Urol 1999;1:154-156.

Slaton JW, Morgenstern N, Levy DA, et al: Tumor stage, vascular invasion and the percentage of poorly differentiated cancer: Independent prognosticators for inguinal lymph node metastasis in penile squamous cancer. J Urol 2001;165:1138-1142.

Solsona E, Iborra I, Ricos JV, et al: Corpus cavernosum invasion and tumor grade in the prediction of lymph node condition in penile carcinoma. Eur Urol 1992;22:115-118.

Solsona E, Algaba F, Horenblas S, et al: EAU guidelines on penile cancer. Eur Urol 2004;46:1-8.

Srinivas V, Morse MJ, Herr HW, et al: Penile cancer: Relation of extent of nodal metastasis to survival. J Urol 1987;137:880-882.

Su CK, Shipley WU: Bowenoid papulosis: A benign lesion of the shaft of the penis misdiagnosed as squamous carcinoma. J Urol 1997;157:1361-1362.

Tanis PJ, Lont AP, Meinhardt W, et al: Dynamic sentinel node biopsy for penile cancer: Reliability of a staging technique. J Urol 2002;168:76-80.

Theodorescu D, Russo P, Zhang ZF, et al: Outcomes of initial surveillance of invasive squamous cell carcinoma of the penis and negative nodes. J Urol 1996;155:1626-1631.

Tietjen DN, Malek RS: Laser therapy of squamous cell dysplasia and carcinoma of the penis. Urology 1998;52:559-565.

Vatanasapt V, Martin N, Sriplung MH, et al: Cancer incidence in Thailand, 1988-1991. Cancer Epidemiol Biomarkers Prev 1995;4:475-483.

Velazquez EF, Cubilla A: Lichen sclerosus in 68 patients with squamous cell carcinoma of the penis: Frequent atypias and correlation with special carcinoma variants suggests a precancerous role. Am J Surg Pathol 2003;27:1448-1453.

Velazquez EF, Barreto JE, Rodriguez I, et al: Limitations in the interpretation of biopsies in patients with penile squamous cell carcinoma. Int J Surg Pathol 2004;12:139-146.

Wiener JS, Walther PJ: The association of oncogenic human papillomaviruses with urologic malignancy. Surg Oncol Clin North Am 1995;4:257-276.

Zouhair A, Coucke PA, Jeanneret W, et al: Radiation therapy alone or combined surgery and radiation therapy in squamous-cell carcinoma of the penis? Eur J Cancer 2001;37:198-203.

32 Surgery of Penile and Urethral Carcinoma

DAVID S. SHARP, MD • KENNETH W. ANGERMEIER, MD

PENILE CANCER

MALE URETHRAL CANCER

FEMALE URETHRAL CANCER

PENILE CANCER

Despite ongoing clinical experience, the treatment of squamous cell carcinoma of the penis remains primarily surgical. Early meticulous surgical management with close follow-up generally provides the best opportunity for cure. A thorough understanding of the various operative procedures for treatment of the primary tumor and regional lymph nodes is therefore critical in the successful management of this condition.

Primary Tumor

Penile Biopsy

The majority of penile squamous cell carcinomas initially involve the glans penis, coronal sulcus, or inner preputial skin (Ekstrom and Edsmyr, 1958; Burgers et al, 1992). **When a suspicious lesion is identified, a biopsy is required to provide histologic confirmation of the diagnosis. It is important to include some adjacent normal tissue with the specimen to allow optimal evaluation of the depth of invasion of the cancer.** Biopsy may take the form of a punch biopsy, excisional biopsy of a relatively small tumor of the glans or foreskin, or incisional biopsy of a larger lesion that cannot be completely excised. A dorsal slit may be required to gain adequate exposure of the preputial cavity. If a lesion involves the urethral meatus, urethroscopy is indicated to evaluate the urethra, and directed biopsies are performed if any suspicious areas are noted.

Laser Therapy

Laser therapy has been extensively evaluated as a form of conservative treatment of penile squamous cell carcinoma. It is attractive in that it has the potential advantage of eliminating the primary tumor with preservation of surrounding tissues and penile function. The lasers most commonly reported for this purpose are the carbon dioxide (CO_2), neodymium:yttrium-aluminum-garnet (Nd:YAG), and potassium titanyl phosphate (KTP). Circumcision is generally recommended at the time of laser therapy if it has not already been done.

The CO_2 laser has a wavelength of 10,600 nm. The laser energy is absorbed by intracellular water, resulting in vaporization to a skin depth of 0.01 mm. Blood vessels up to 0.5 mm in size can be coagulated. For these reasons, it has been most often used as monotherapy for treatment of dysplastic lesions and squamous cell carcinoma in situ (Greenbaum et al, 1989; Tietjen and Malek, 1998; van Bezooijen et al, 2001). It remains unclear as to whether the CO_2 laser represents optimal therapy for carcinoma in situ, however, as a local recurrence rate of up to 33% has been reported (van Bezooijen et al, 2001).

Because of its cutting properties, the CO_2 laser has been shown to be technically capable of excising small superficial lesions of the penis (Bandieramonte et al, 1987). In this study, surgical specimens were adequate for pathologic examination in 87% of cases, and three patients underwent a repeated laser procedure for a positive margin. The mean distance between the resected lesion and the incision borders was 0.6 mm. A similar technique was used to completely resect the entire surface of the glans penis in a series of patients with diffuse glanular disease, 3 with carcinoma in situ and 11 with superficially invasive squamous cell carcinoma (Bandieramonte et al, 1988). Healing time varied from 5 to 8 weeks, and one patient had significant arterial hemorrhage controlled by cautery. Cosmetic appearance was good in all cases, and no meatal stenosis was noted. Only one patient had a recurrence with follow-up of 2 to 48 months.

The laser most commonly reported in the treatment of squamous cell carcinoma has been the Nd:YAG laser (Rothenberger, 1986; Boon, 1988; Malloy et al, 1988; von Eschenbach et al, 1991; Horenblas et al, 1992; Frimberger et al, 2002a; Windahl and Andersson, 2003). It has a depth of penetration of 3 to 6 mm and therefore is considered to potentially be more appropriate for treating small superficial penile lesions. The application of iced saline to the treatment area during laser coagulation may prevent carbonization of the surface and promote deeper penetration of the laser energy when desired. The local recurrence rate when the Nd:YAG laser is used alone for carcinoma in situ and T1 squamous cell carcinoma has been approximately 20% (Malloy et al, 1988; von Eschenbach et al, 1991). The Nd:YAG laser has also been used in combination with surgical excision, with the hope of improving treatment efficacy. The tumor is excised initially, followed by laser coagulation of the base and margins of the defect (Rothenberger, 1986; Boon, 1988; Horenblas et al, 1992; Windahl and Andersson, 2003). With this technique, the local recurrence has been reported to be 18% to 20%.

The KTP (532-nm wavelength) laser has also been used successfully in the treatment of superficial penile carcinoma (Tietjen and Malek, 1998). It has an intermediate depth of penetration relative to the CO_2 and Nd:YAG lasers and better hemostasis than the CO_2 laser.

Most reports of laser therapy for penile cancer have described treatment of the lesion with a margin of 3 to 5 mm, which may underestimate the extent of the lesion in some cases. In an attempt to decrease the recurrence rate, preparation of the genital skin with 5% acetic acid has been proposed along with the use of mapping biopsies and surgical excision during the procedure (Tietjen and Malek, 1998; Frimberger et al, 2002a). The acetic acid is applied for approximately 20 minutes before the procedure, and human papillomavirus–induced areas then appear whitened. In one study, the aceto-white staining was most prominent in the periphery of the grossly visible lesions (Tietjen and Malek, 1998). Laser therapy was then carried out with elimination of all abnormal areas, with a local recurrence rate of 7% to 11%. A more recent technique intended to decrease recurrences has been described by photodynamic diagnosis with 5-amino-levulinic acid and autofluorescence to visually direct frozen-section biopsies for assessment of margin status at the time of Nd:YAG tumor ablation (Frimberger et al, 2002b).

In general, laser therapy seems to be reasonable for patients with Tis and small T1 squamous cell carcinoma of the penis and for patients with manageable T2 tumors who refuse more aggressive surgical treatment. Disadvantages include difficulty in determining the exact depth of laser coagulation; inability to treat larger lesions; and potentially difficult healing in patients who are obese, immunocompromised, or receiving anticoagulation therapy (Tietjen and Malek, 1998). Postoperative healing generally requires 8 to 12 weeks for the Nd:YAG and KTP lasers, but overall cosmetic results are generally good. Erectile function after combined CO_2 and Nd:YAG laser treatment of penile squamous cell carcinoma was unaltered in 72% of patients in one study (Windahl et al, 2004). As with any form of conservative treatment, careful long-term surveillance is essential because of the remaining tissues of the preputial cavity that are at risk for carcinogenesis (Horenblas and Newling, 1993).

Mohs Micrographic Surgery

Mohs micrographic surgery is a technique allowing removal of penile cancer by excision of tissue in thin layers (Mohs et al, 1985). This was originally described as a fixed tissue technique, but a fresh tissue technique has increasingly been used as a result of treating smaller lesions and its shorter procedural time (Brown et al, 1988; Cottel et al, 1988; Mohs et al, 1992). Color coding of the excised layers with tissue dyes allows accurate orientation of the specimen and the creation of a tissue map. Frozen sections to evaluate the surgical margin are cut horizontally from the undersurface of the tissue specimens rather than vertically, allowing microscopic examination of the entire deep and peripheral margin. Any remaining tumor is marked on the tumor map. This is continued until the lesion is completely excised. Mohs micrographic surgery allows excellent local control rates while maximizing organ preservation. Mohs reported a cure rate of 81% for tumors on the glans or prepuce. For all tumor stages, 5-year cure rates were 100% for lesions smaller than 1 cm, 83% for lesions 1 to 2 cm, 75% for lesions 2 to 3 cm, and 50% for lesions larger than 3 cm (Mohs et al, 1985). With extended follow-up, the local control rate was 94% (Mohs et al, 1992), and this has been duplicated by others (Mikhail, 1976; Brown et al, 1988). In addition to tumor size, local recurrence has been associated with advanced stage and failure of previous definitive therapy.

Mohs micrographic surgery would seem to be best suited for patients with carcinoma in situ or small superficially invasive tumors, with cure rates comparable to partial penectomy. However, these results may be variable and dependent on the technique used and the experience of the surgeon (Cottel et al, 1988; Mohs et al, 1992). It should not be used in patients with higher stage or large lesions. Complications of Mohs micrographic surgery may include meatal stenosis and glans disfigurement.

Conservative Surgical Excision

Conservative surgical excision is another form of tissue-sparing therapy for low-stage penile cancer. **It may be attractive in some instances when there is inexperience on the part of the surgeon with regard to lasers or Mohs micrographic surgery or when these modalities are unavailable. In addition, compared with laser therapy, excision has the advantage of providing tissue for tumor grading and assessment of margins, and it does not require the technical support necessary for Mohs micrographic surgery.** Support for a conservative approach in selected patients has been provided by studies suggesting that the traditional 2-cm surgical margin may not always be necessary for cure. Pathologic analysis of 14 patients undergoing partial or total penectomy for squamous cell carcinoma revealed a mean surgical margin of approximately 14.5 mm; seven patients had a margin of 10 mm or less. No patient in this series had a local recurrence (Hoffman et al, 1999). Microscopic extent of penile carcinoma has also been shown to be dependent on tumor grade; grade 1 and grade 2 tumors demonstrated a maximum histologic extent of 5 mm in an analysis of 64 penectomy specimens (Agrawal et al, 2000). In addition, these authors were unable to identify any tumors with a pattern of discontinuous spread. The simplest form of conservative surgical excision is circumcision. Distal preputial tumors may be effectively treated in this fashion when a surgical margin of 2 cm can be achieved (Skinner et al, 1972; McDougal et al, 1986). If the cancer is more proximal and close to the coronal sulcus, however, recurrence rates may be as high as 50% (Narayana et al, 1982), and therefore excision of additional adjacent tissue is needed to ensure an adequate surgical margin.

Local excision of glanular tumors is more difficult because of the requirement of a surgical margin that may not preserve enough tissue to allow an adequate remaining glans penis. This is most often done in the form of excisional biopsy of a lesion with negative surgical margins. In some cases, the surgical defect is small and can be closed primarily. If the defect is larger and primary closure is not possible, the area can be covered with an outer preputial skin flap (Ubrig et al, 2001) (Fig. 32–1). Alternatively, a full-thickness graft of penile skin

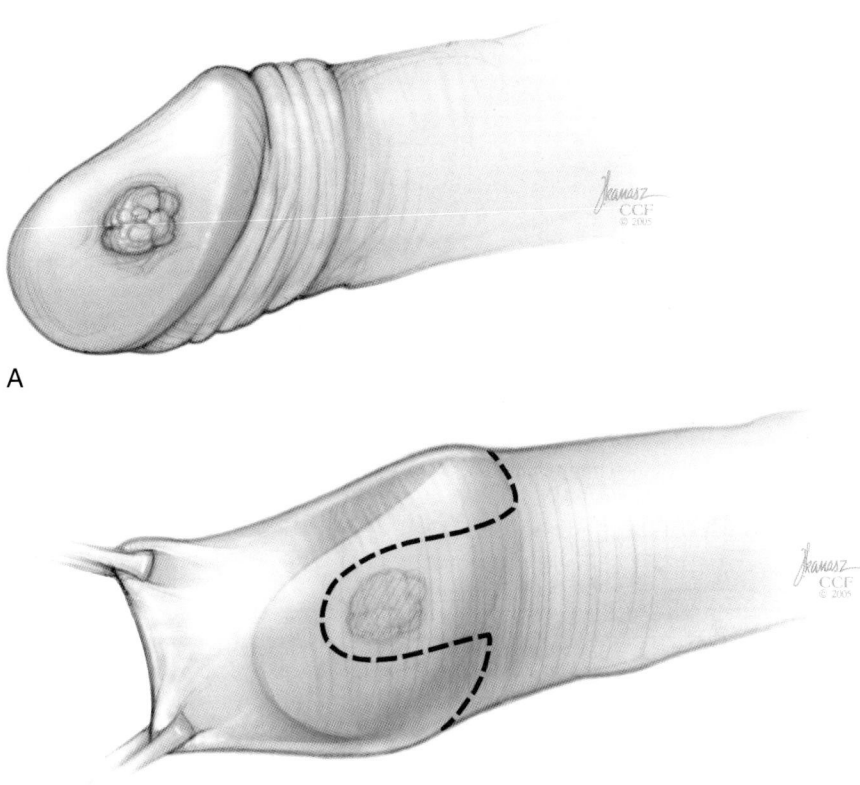

Figure 32–1. Surgical glans defect covered with outer preputial flap as described by Ubrig and colleagues (2001). **A**, Superficial glans tumor. **B**, Outer preputial flap outlined. **C**, Tumor excised and circumcision performed. **D**, Glans defect filled with outer preputial flap.

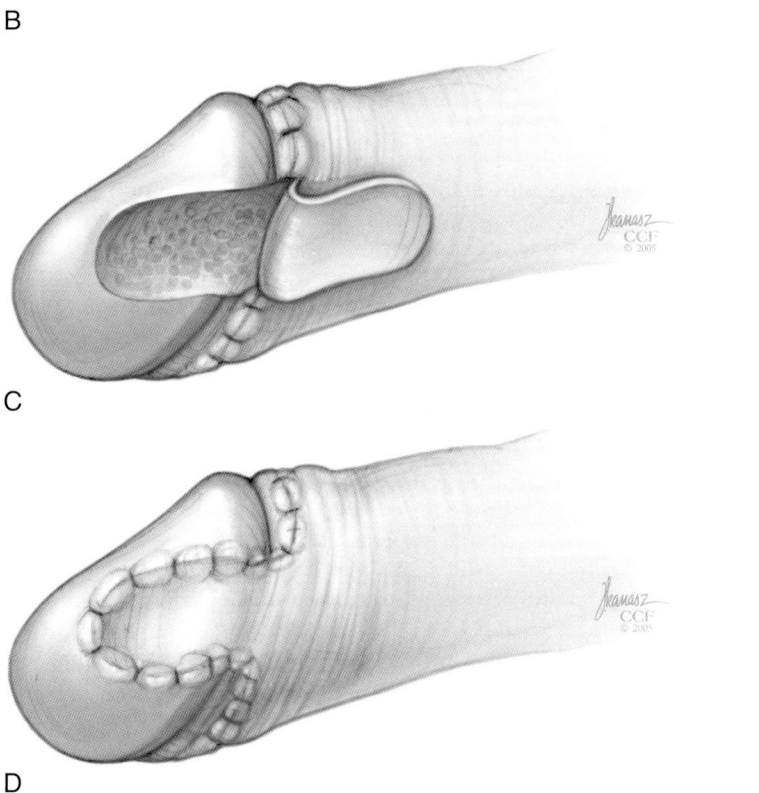

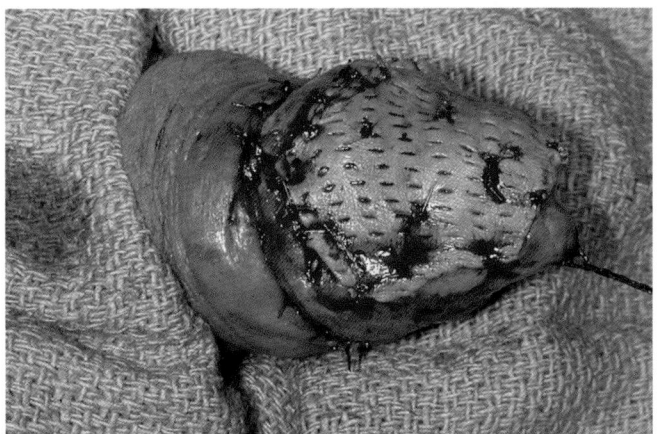

Figure 32–2. Finely meshed extragenital split-thickness skin graft quilted to glans defect after superficial tumor excision.

or extragenital split-thickness skin graft may be used to reconstruct the area (Pietrzak et al, 2004) (Fig. 32–2). Local recurrence rates after conservative penile surgery have varied. Two early publications reported recurrence in 32% and 40% of patients (Hanash et al, 1970; McDougal et al, 1986). In 1999, Ficarra and coworkers noted local recurrence after conservative penile surgery in three of eight patients with Tis and T1 disease. More recent data have been a bit more favorable, with reported local recurrence rates of 8% to 11% (Banon Perez et al, 2000; Bissada et al, 2003; Pietrzak et al, 2004).

Total glansectomy for penile malignant lesions was initially described in 1996 (Austoni et al, 1996). Since that time, excellent local tumor eradication has been described in a small number of patients with verrucous carcinoma and nonsquamous penile malignant neoplasms. Adequate voiding and erectile function was preserved in the majority of cases (Davis et al, 1999; Hatzichristou et al, 2001). In comparison, standard partial penectomy may be associated with significant impairment of sexual function (Opjordsmoen et al, 1994) and in our experience often results in the inability to void in a standing position with long-term follow-up. On the basis of this experience, a subsequent report described six patients with superficial, well to moderately differentiated squamous cell carcinoma limited to the glans penis who underwent glansectomy as primary therapy. With follow-up of 6 to 18 months, there were no local recurrences, and all patients maintained adequate sexual function (da Fonseca et al, 2003). The procedure begins with a distal circumferential skin incision to the level of Buck's fascia. The plane under Buck's fascia is developed proximal to the corona of the glans. Laterally, there are usually only a few small vessels within Buck's fascia that may be controlled with electrocautery. Dorsally, the neurovascular structures are divided between surgical ties. Ventrally, a plane is developed under the urethra, but it is not yet divided. Dorsal dissection is commenced in the plane between the glans penis and the tunica albuginea of the corpora cavernosa, and this is continued until the glans is attached by the urethra alone. The urethra is then divided, completing the excision. Frozen-section biopsy specimens are obtained from the tips of the corpora or any other suspicious area. Reconstruction is accomplished by fixing the remaining neurovascular bundle

to the tunica albuginea dorsally and the urethra ventrally if needed. The urethra is spatulated, and the penile skin is then approximated in the midline and around the neomeatus. A urethral catheter is left indwelling for 3 to 7 days.

Pietrzak and associates (2004) have reported the results of glansectomy or glansectomy and distal corporectomy in 29 men with primarily stage T1 and T2 squamous cell carcinoma of the glans, prepuce, and coronal sulcus. Patients undergoing glansectomy had circumcision and glans excision as described before, followed by mobilization of the urethra to allow formation of a urethrostomy near the tip of the penis. Frozen-section biopsy specimens are taken from the distal tunica albuginea and the urethral margin. The shaft skin is sutured in place approximately 2 cm from the end of the penis, leaving the corporal tips exposed. A split-thickness skin graft is harvested and quilted to the corpora, and a urethral catheter is placed. The patient is maintained at bed rest for 5 days. If the findings on frozen-section biopsy are abnormal, distal corporectomy is performed until the margins are negative, and the corpora are reconstructed as in partial penectomy. A distal split-thickness skin graft is then used to cover the corpora and to form the neoglans. Early results have been encouraging; there were no local recurrences in this group of patients at a mean follow-up of 16 months.

Partial Penectomy

Partial penectomy remains the most common surgical procedure for treatment of the primary tumor in patients with invasive squamous cell carcinoma. Successful local control is accomplished in the majority of patients by amputation of the penis at least 2 cm proximal to the tumor. Additional goals of the procedure are to preserve the ability to void in a standing position and possibly to allow sexual function. The lesion is initially excluded from the surgical field by a small towel or surgical glove (Fig. 32–3). Some authors have recommended the use of a tourniquet at the base of the penis, but we have not found this to be necessary. The skin and underlying dartos fascia at the proposed line of amputation are incised circumferentially to the level of Buck's fascia. Buck's fascia is incised laterally, and a plane is dissected between the tunica albuginea and the neurovascular structures dorsally. The dorsal penile vessels are sequentially ligated and divided. The corpora cavernosa are sharply divided, leaving the specimen attached only by the urethra. The urethra is dissected for a distance of 1 to 1.5 cm distal to the proximal corpora and then transected. The corpora are closed transversely with interrupted horizontal mattress sutures of 2-0 polydioxanone. The penile skin is closed in the midline over the corporal ends with interrupted 3-0 or 4-0 chromic suture material. A ventral urethrostomy is constructed by approximating the urethra to the adjacent penile skin with interrupted 4-0 chromic sutures (Fig. 32–4). An indwelling urethral catheter is left in place for 3 to 5 days. If additional stump length is needed to increase the probability of adequate voiding function, the suspensory ligament of the penis may be divided. The proximal corpora may subsequently be dissected off of the pubic arch for a short distance as well. Scrotal flaps are used to help with skin coverage as needed, and the skin is attached to the pubic arch to preserve the dissected penile length. Division of the penoscrotal fold with a Z-plasty at the penoscrotal junction ventrally may contribute to better

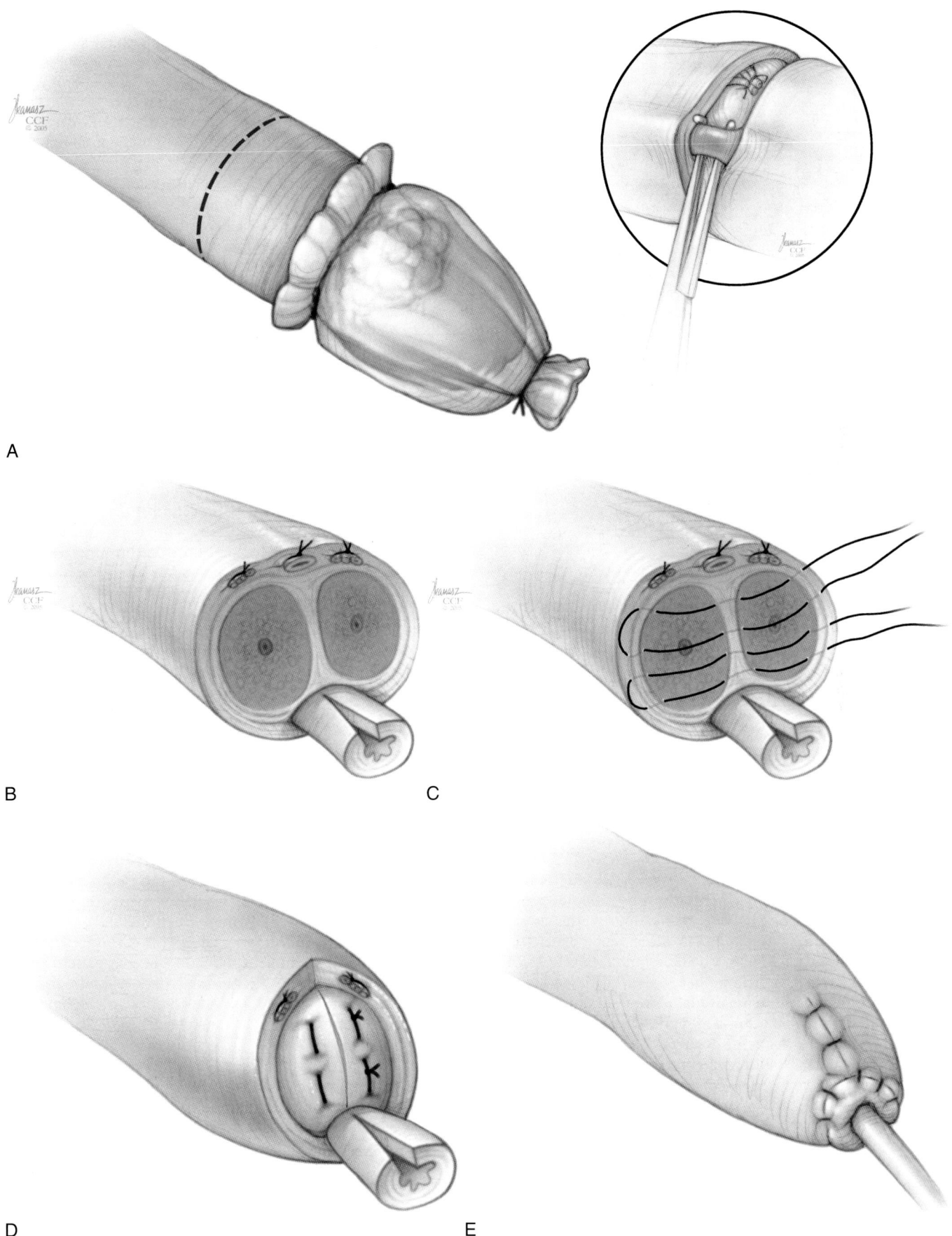

Figure 32–3. Partial penectomy. **A,** Incision with ligation and division of dorsal penile vessels within Buck's fascia *(inset)*. **B,** Corpora transected and urethra spatulated. **C** and **D,** Closure of corpora cavernosa. **E,** Final closure with construction of urethrostomy.

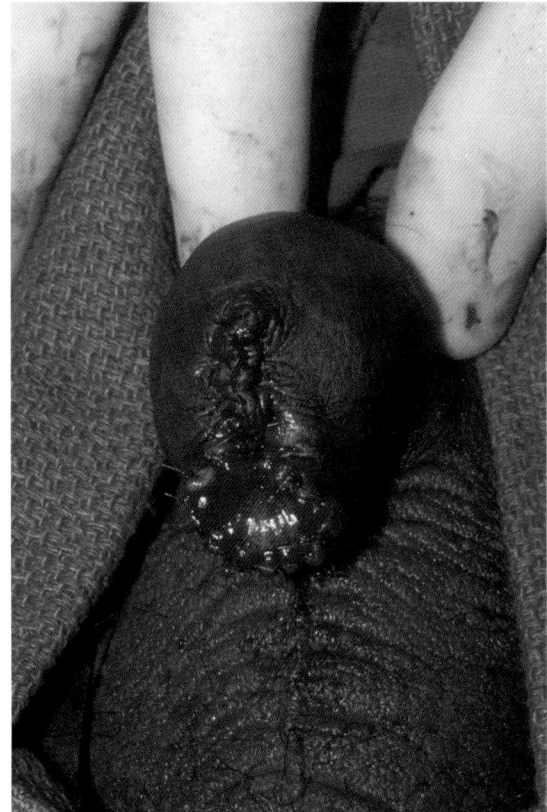

Figure 32–4. Penile stump after partial penectomy.

definition of the remaining penile stump (Parkash et al, 1986). In selected patients, glans reconstruction may be considered by covering the distal corpora with a split-thickness skin graft (de Souza, 1976) or a two-stage pedicled flap of scrotal skin (Mazza and Cheliz, 2001).

The reported local recurrence rate after partial or total penectomy has ranged from 0% to 8% (Hardner et al, 1972; de Kernion et al, 1973; McDougal et al, 1986; Horenblas et al, 1992). Two studies have suggested that recurrence rates are dependent on tumor stage, reporting a recurrence rate of 0% for patients with T1 tumors and 18% to 21% for T2 lesions (Lindegaard et al, 1996; Brkovic et al, 1997). Although one of the accepted goals of partial penectomy is to allow upright voiding, the percentage of patients able to do this after surgery has not been well documented. A 6% incidence of urethral meatal stenosis has been reported (Horenblas et al, 1992). In our experience, a significant number of men sit to void in the long term because of spraying of the urinary stream. In terms of sexual function, most published reports have indicated that approximately 20% of patients describe adequate sexual function postoperatively (Opjordsmoen et al, 1994; Ficarra et al, 1999; Mazza and Cheliz, 2001).

Total Penectomy

Total penectomy is a bit of a misnomer, as the penis is amputated at or near the level of the suspensory ligament of the penis without removal of the corpora cavernosa more proximally. **It is indicated for penile tumors whose size or location would not allow excision with an adequate surgical margin and preservation of a remnant sufficient for upright voiding.** The primary tumor is draped and an elliptical incision made around the base of the penis (Fig. 32–5). Dissection is commenced in the plane between the tunica albuginea and Buck's fascia dorsolaterally, and the dorsal vessels are ligated and divided. The corporal bodies are sharply transected, and the urethra is divided at the same level. The corpora are then closed with interrupted horizontal mattress sutures of 2-0 polydioxanone.

A perineal urethrostomy is then constructed by one of two techniques. The most commonly described method is to mobilize the urethra from the surrounding bulbospongiosus muscle and dorsally from the corporal bodies to near the departure of the urethra from the bulb (Fig. 32–6). A small U-shaped incision is made in the perineum. The mobilized urethra is transposed through the perineal opening without angulation. The urethra is spatulated dorsally, and the skin is sutured to the full-thickness urethra with 3-0 polyglactin sutures. Alternatively, a flap inlay urethrostomy may be constructed without mobilization of the urethra. A modified lambda incision is made in the perineum with a short vertical limb (Fig. 32–7). The soft tissues overlying the urethra are incised, and the bulbospongiosus muscle is divided in the midline to expose the corpus spongiosum of the bulbous urethra. A 3- to 4-cm ventral urethrotomy incision is made and carried proximally to a point just distal to the bulbomembranous junction (Fig. 32–8). The lateral aspects of the corpus spongiosum in the region of the urethrotomy are fixed to the adjacent corporal bodies with a few interrupted sutures of 4-0 polydioxanone to splay the opened urethra. The perineal skin flap is sutured to the full-thickness urethra with 3-0 polyglactin starting in the midline and working laterally as far as the flap will easily reach (Fig. 32–9). The urethrostomy is completed by approximation of the scrotal skin to the urethra dorsolaterally, and the resulting short lateral skin incisions are closed in standard fashion (Fig. 32–10).

After completion of the perineal urethrostomy, the primary skin incision is closed transversely and a small Penrose or suction drain is placed. A urethral catheter is left indwelling for 7 to 10 days.

Radical Penectomy

Although it is not commonly done, radical penectomy with excision of the corporal bodies in their entirety may on occasion be necessary. We have had experience with this procedure in three patients, one with epithelioid sarcoma of the penis involving multiple sites within the corpora cavernosa (Ormsby et al, 2000) and for palliation in two patients with extensive metastatic disease within the corporal bodies related to transitional cell carcinoma of the bladder and adenocarcinoma of the rectum.

The patient is placed into lithotomy position with adjustable stirrups so the level of the legs can be altered during the case as needed. The procedure begins with a peripenile incision as for total penectomy, and the corpora are mobilized off of the ischiopubic rami proximally to the point at which the dorsal vein may be seen coursing under the pubis, where it is ligated and divided (Fig. 32–11). A modified lambda incision is then made in the perineum, and the penis is maneuvered through this incision (Fig. 32–12). Dissection of the corporal bodies continues to the tips of the crura, which are

Text continued on p. 1002.

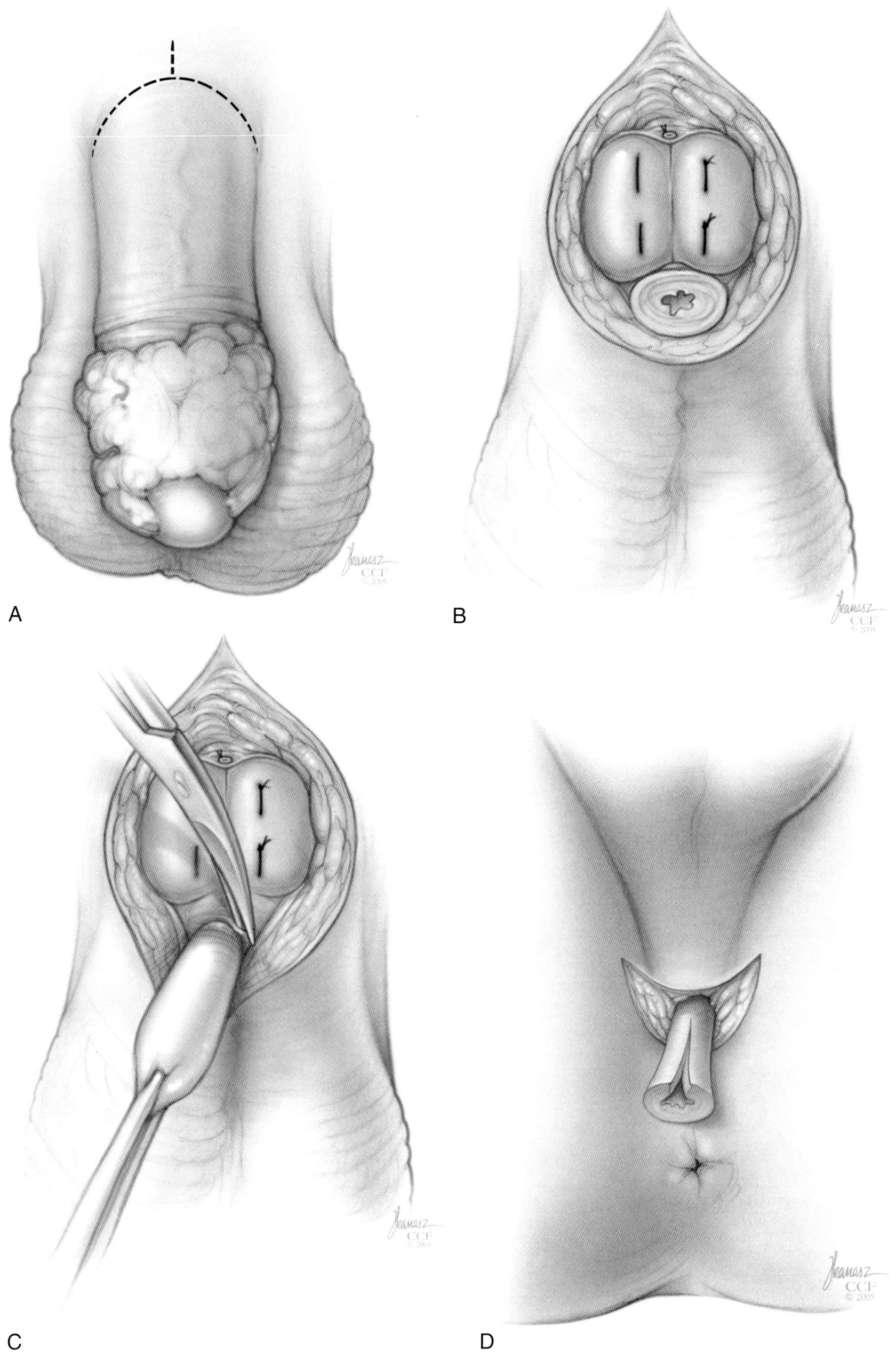

Figure 32–5.   Total penectomy. **A,** Incision. **B,** Transection of the corpora near the level of the pubis. **C,** Mobilization of the remaining urethra off of the proximal corporal bodies. **D,** Transposition of the urethra through a curvilinear perineal incision.   *Continued*

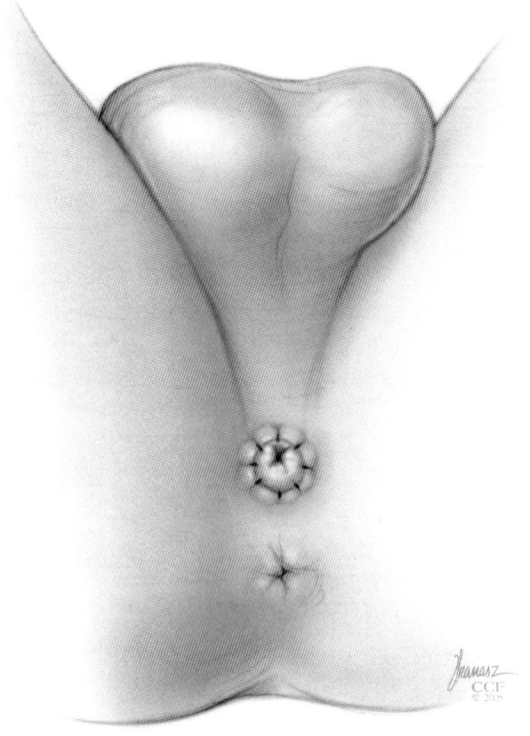

E

Figure 32-5, cont'd. **E,** Completion of perineal urethrostomy.

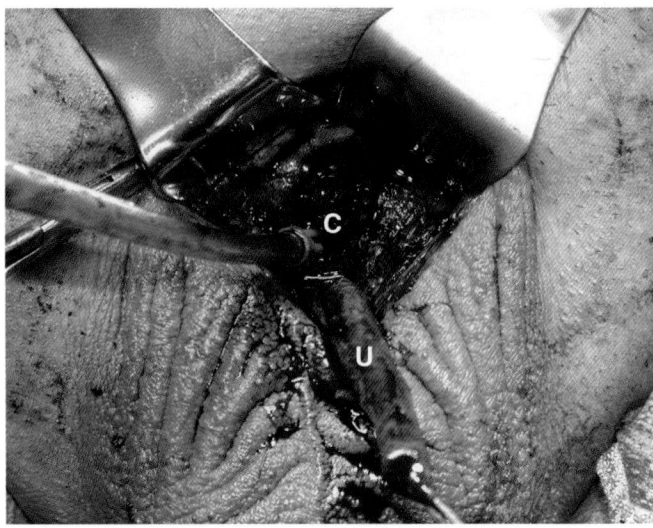

Figure 32-6. Intraoperative photograph demonstrating the bulbous urethra mobilized dorsally off of the corporal bodies before transposition. C, proximal corporal bodies; U, urethra.

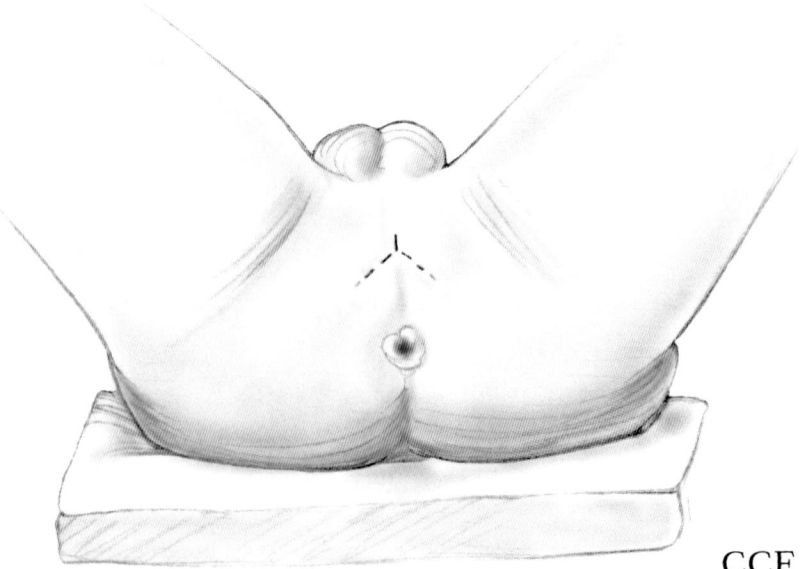

Figure 32-7. Incision for flap perineal urethrostomy.

CCF
© 2005

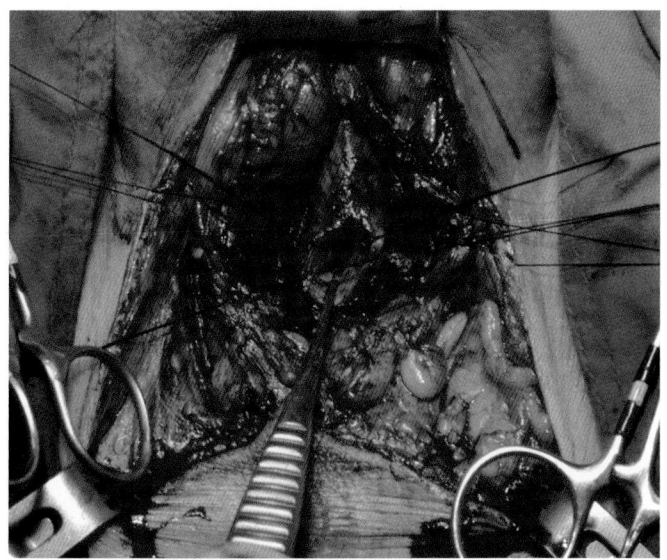

Figure 32–8. Ventral urethrotomy incision in the mid to proximal bulbous urethra.

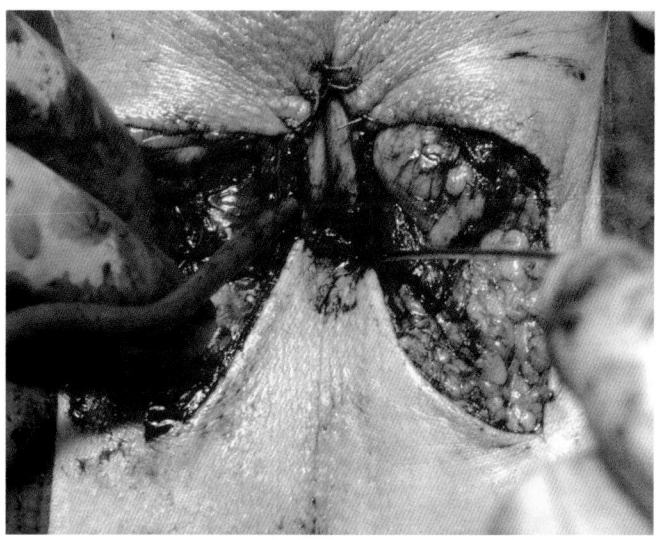

Figure 32–9. Perineal flap being sutured into place.

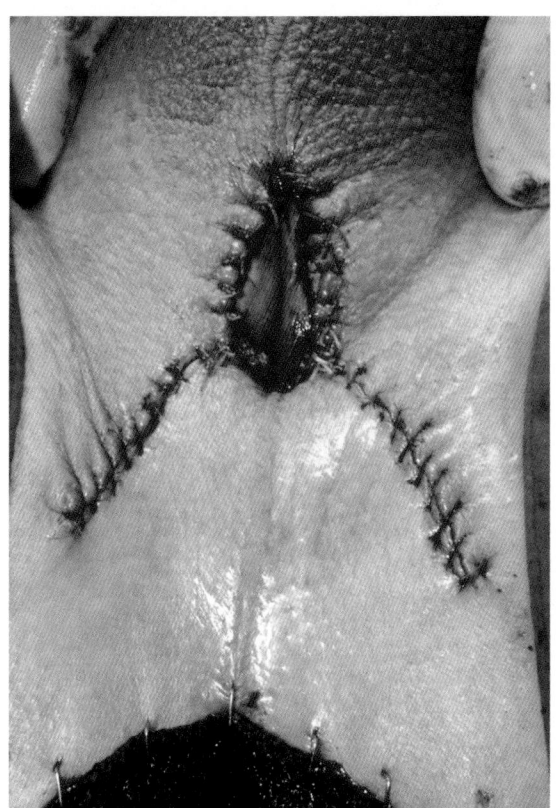

Figure 32–10. Completed perineal urethrostomy.

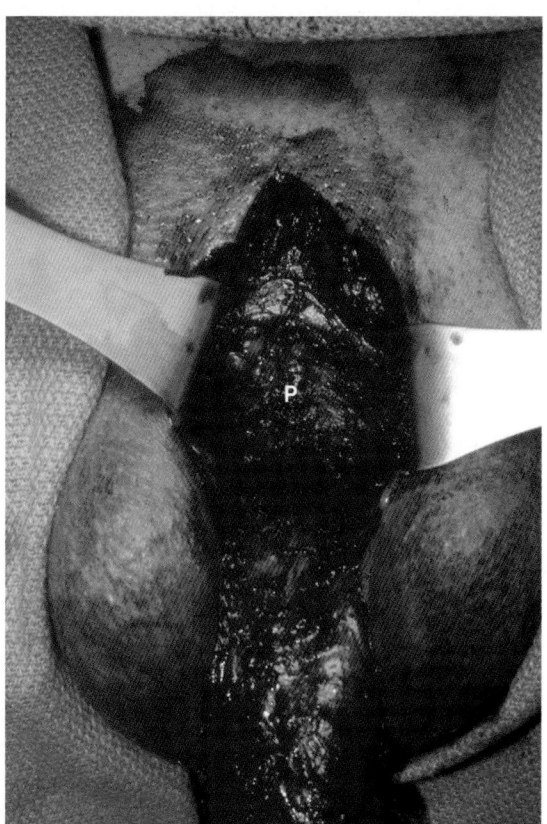

Figure 32–11. Penis retracted downward after mobilization off of the pubis (P).

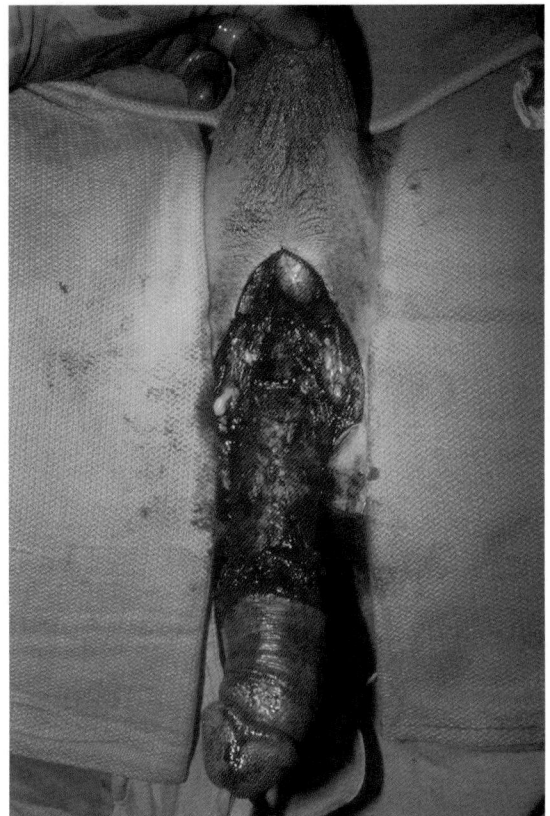

Figure 32–12.   Penis transposed through the perineal incision.

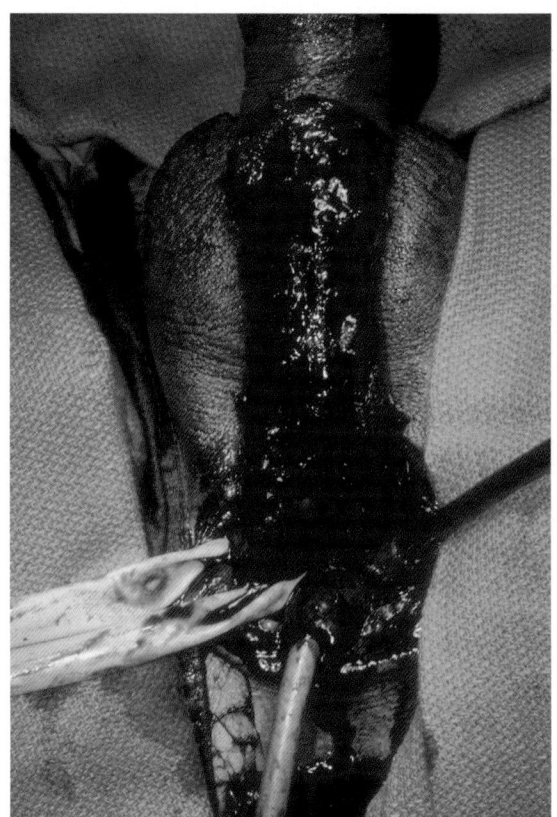

Figure 32–13.   Penrose drain around right crus of the corporal body after dissection of the urethra (with catheter indwelling).

completely excised. Suture ligatures are used to control the dorsal penile and cavernosal vasculature near the dorsal aspect of the crura and in the penile hilum. A plane is developed between the proximal urethra and the corpora, and the urethra is then transected, leaving 2 to 3 cm of urethra to form a perineal urethrostomy (Fig. 32–13). A standard flap perineal urethrostomy is then constructed as described previously and managed as described previously. A small suction drain is placed, and the peripenile incision is closed transversely.

Regional Lymph Nodes

Squamous cell carcinoma of the penis spreads initially to regional lymph nodes before the occurrence of distant metastatic disease. Lymphatic spread occurs in a systematic fashion along the normal route of penile lymphatic drainage. Lymphatic vessels draining the prepuce and skin of the penile shaft converge dorsally and then divide at the base of the penis to drain into the right and left superficial inguinal nodes. Drainage from the glans penis is toward the frenulum, where large trunks are formed and encircle the corona to unite with those from the other side on the dorsum. They traverse the penis to the base within Buck's fascia, draining through presymphyseal lymphatics into the superficial inguinal nodes and the deep inguinal nodes of the femoral triangle. It is not uncommon for the tumor to metastasize to the contralateral inguinal nodes. Drainage proceeds from the inguinal nodes to the ipsilateral pelvic lymph nodes. Although some anatomic

texts have stated that penile lymphatics may drain directly to the external iliac nodes, we are not aware of any patients or reports in the literature in which this has occurred clinically. **Although penile carcinoma metastatic to the inguinal lymph nodes confers a poorer prognosis overall, aggressive lymphadenectomy is associated with improved long-term survival and potential cure in 30% to 60% of patients** (McDougal et al, 1986; Horenblas and van Tinteren, 1994). If the tumor has spread to the pelvic nodes, long-term survival is less than 10%.

Inguinal Anatomy

The inguinal lymph nodes are divided into superficial and deep groups, which are anatomically separated by the fascia lata of the thigh. The superficial group is composed of 4 to 25 lymph nodes that are situated in the deep membranous layer of the superficial fascia of the thigh (Camper's fascia). The superficial inguinal nodes have been divided into five anatomic groups (Daseler et al, 1948): (1) central nodes around the saphenofemoral junction, (2) superolateral nodes around the superficial circumflex vein, (3) inferolateral nodes around the lateral femoral cutaneous and superficial circumflex veins, (4) superomedial nodes around the superficial external pudendal and superficial epigastric veins, and (5) inferomedial nodes around the greater saphenous vein (Fig. 32–14). The deep inguinal nodes are fewer and lie primarily medial to the femoral vein in the femoral canal. The node of Cloquet is the most cephalad of this deep group and is

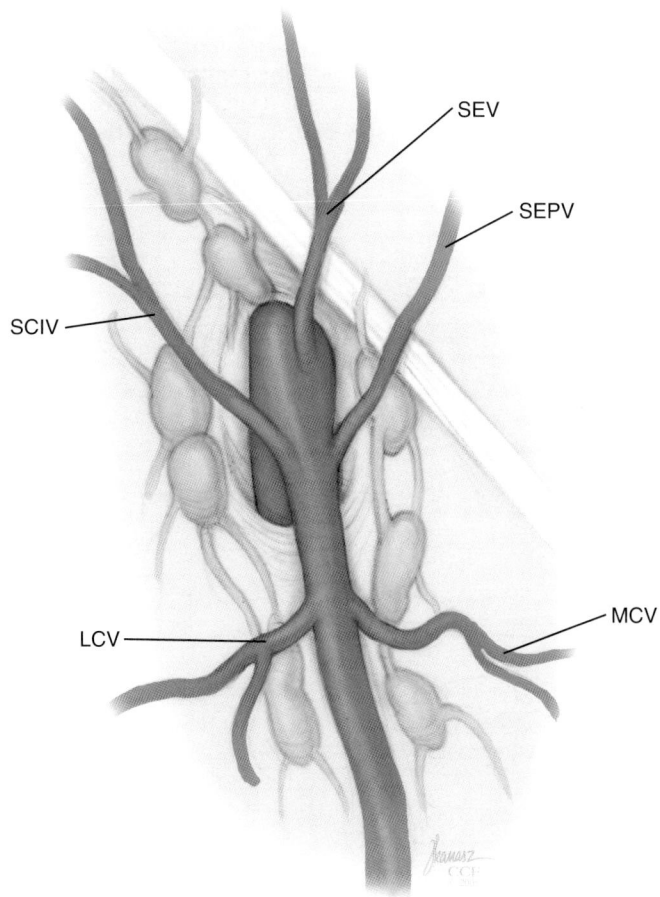

Figure 32–14. Superficial inguinal lymph nodes and the branches of the saphenous vein. SEV, superficial epigastric; SEPV, superficial external pudendal; MCV, medial cutaneous; LCV, lateral cutaneous; SCIV, superficial circumflex iliac.

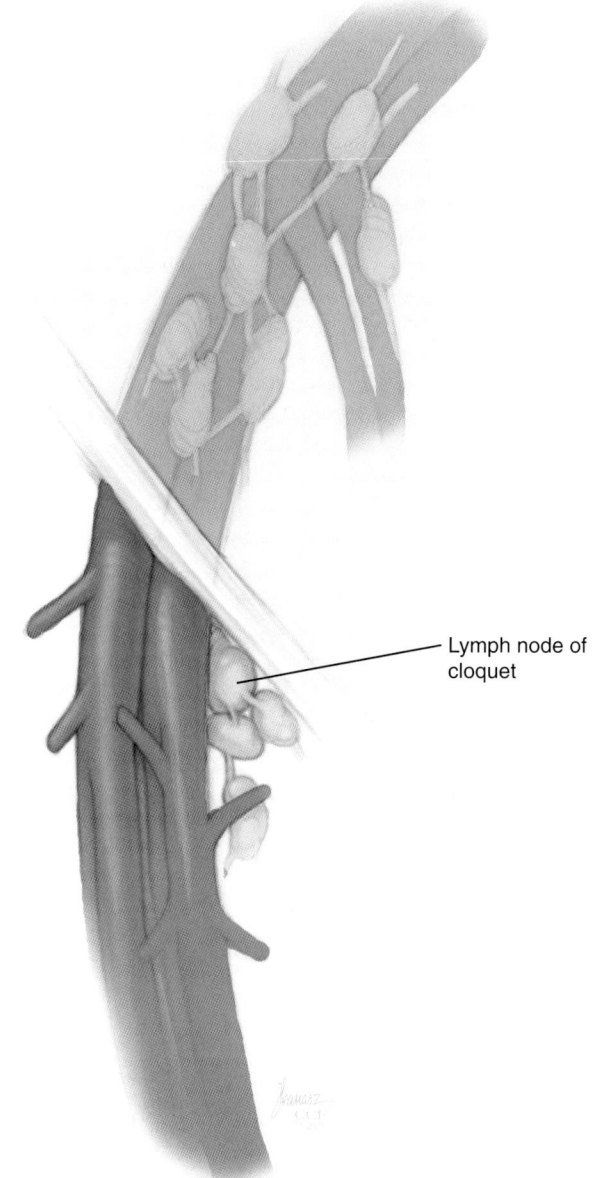

Figure 32–15. Deep inguinal lymph nodes.

situated between the femoral vein and the lacunar ligament (Fig. 32–15). The external iliac lymph nodes receive drainage from the deep inguinal, obturator, and hypogastric groups. In turn, drainage progresses to the common iliac and para-aortic nodes.

The blood supply to the skin of the inguinal region derives from branches of the common femoral artery—the superficial external pudendal, superficial circumflex iliac, and superficial epigastric arteries. Complete inguinal dissection necessitates ligation of these branches. Viability of the skin flaps raised during the dissection depends on anastomotic vessels in the superficial fatty layer of Camper's fascia that course lateral to medial along the natural skin lines. Because lymphatic drainage of the penis to the groin runs beneath Camper's fascia, this layer can be preserved and left attached to the overlying skin when the superior and inferior skin flaps are fashioned. On the basis of this anatomy, a transverse skin incision least compromises this blood supply. In this fashion, serious skin slough is prevented in the majority of cases. The femoral nerve lies deep to the iliacus fascia and supplies motor function to the pectineus, quadriceps femoris, and sartorius muscles. In addition, this nerve provides cutaneous sensation to the anterior thigh and should be preserved. Some of the

sensory branches, however, are commonly sacrificed in the regional node dissection.

The femoral triangle is bounded by the inguinal ligament superiorly, the sartorius muscle laterally, and the adductor longus medially. The floor of the triangle is composed of the pectineus muscle medially and the iliopsoas laterally. The location of the saphenofemoral junction is estimated to be at a point two fingerbreadths lateral and two fingerbreadths inferior to the pubic tubercle.

Sentinel Node Biopsy

The concept of sentinel node biopsy in patients with invasive squamous cell carcinoma of the penis and clinically negative inguinal regions was proposed by Cabanas (1977) after extensive study of lymphangiograms and anatomic dissections. The impetus for a conservative approach to evaluate this group of patients arose from the realization that surgical treatment of inguinal metastases is desirable and because of the significant morbidity associated with conventional inguinofemoral lymphadenectomy. A 5-cm incision is made parallel to the inguinal crease and centered two fingerbreadths lateral and inferior to the pubic tubercle. By insertion of the finger under the upper flap toward the pubic tubercle, the sentinel lymph node is encountered and excised (Fig. 32–16). **Although Cabanas reported 90% survival in patients with normal**

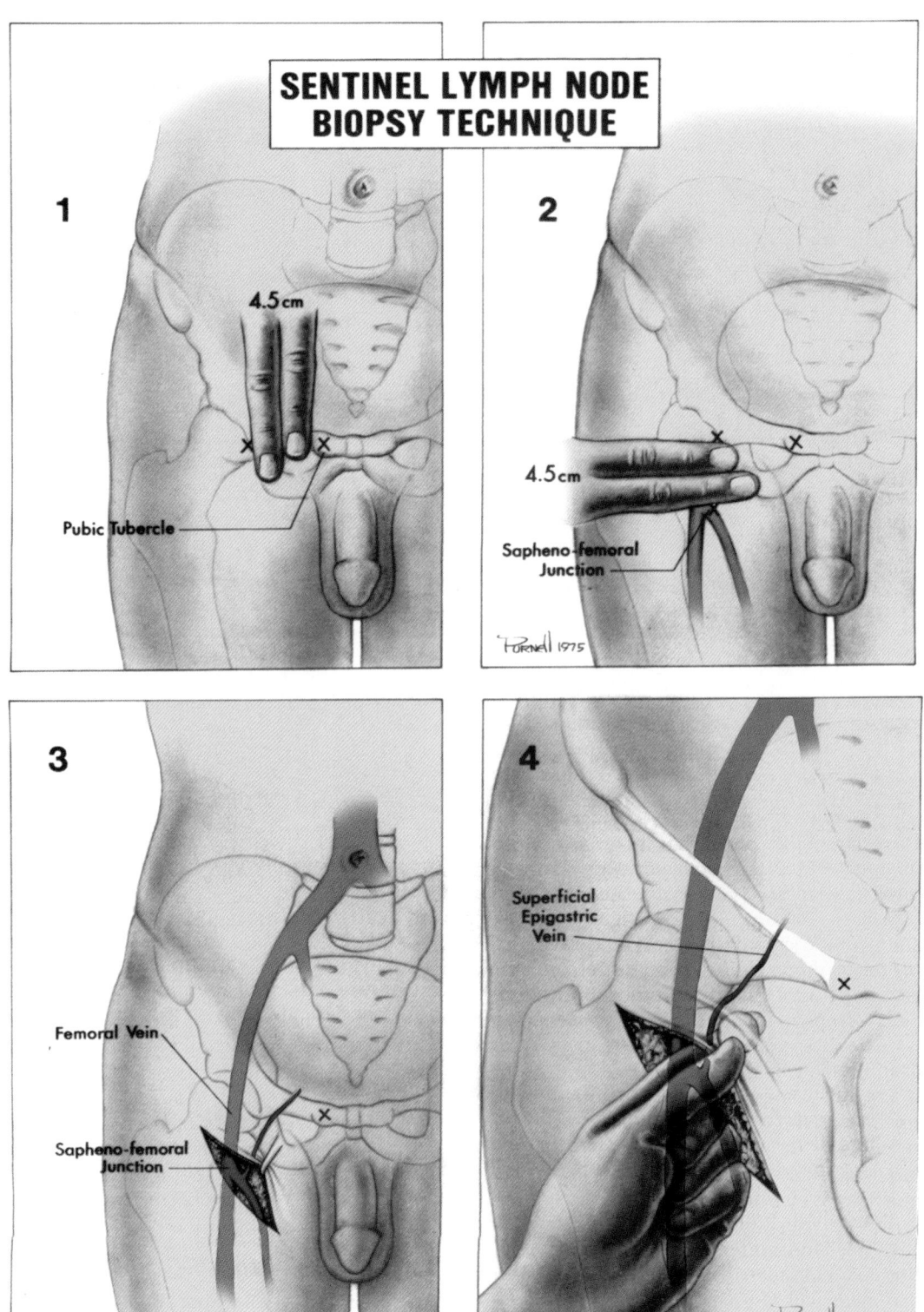

SENTINEL LYMPH NODE BIOPSY TECHNIQUE

Figure 32–16. Sentinel lymph node biopsy technique as described by Cabanas. (From Cabanas RM: An approach for the treatment of penile carcinoma. Cancer 1977;39:456-466.)

findings on sentinel node biopsy, subsequent authors found the results to be less satisfactory, with reports of development of extensive regional metastases after a biopsy with normal findings (Perinetti et al, 1980; Wespes et al, 1986). As an alternative, Pettaway and colleagues (1995) evaluated extended sentinel node biopsy, during which all of the lymph nodes between the inguinal ligament and the superficial external pudendal vein were removed. This approach has also been abandoned because it resulted in a false-negative rate of 15% to 25% (Ravi, 1993; Pettaway et al, 1995).

Efforts have been made to improve the accuracy of sentinel node biopsy. Dynamic sentinel node biopsy with lymphoscintigraphic imaging has been described on the basis of experience in other tumors (Horenblas et al, 2000). The technique starts the day before surgery with the intradermal injection of technetium Tc 99m nanocolloid at three or four sites around the primary tumor. Dynamic anterior lymphoscintigraphy is subsequently performed at defined intervals. The location of the sentinel node is marked on the skin. Shortly before surgery, 1 mL of patent blue dye is injected around the tumor in similar fashion. The sentinel node is harvested after dissection of blue lymphatic vessels and intraoperative detection of radioactivity by use of a gamma ray detection probe. Detection of positive nodes has also been aided by preoperative inguinal ultrasonography with fine-needle aspiration of any abnormal-appearing lymph nodes. A false-negative rate of 18% has been reported with this approach (Kroon et al, 2004). The authors recommended routine inguinal exploration in the absence of radiotracer visualization, intraoperative palpation of the wound for abnormal nodes, and extended pathologic analysis of excised nodes as means of decreasing the number of false-negative biopsy results.

Modified Inguinal Lymphadenectomy

In 1988, Catalona proposed a technique of modified inguinofemoral lymphadenectomy designed to provide staging information and therapeutic benefit similar to standard extended lymphadenectomy with less morbidity (Fig. 32–17). **Key aspects of the procedure are (1) shorter skin incision, (2) limitation of the dissection by excluding the area lateral to the femoral artery and caudal to the fossa ovalis, (3) preservation of the saphenous vein, and (4) elimination of the need to transpose the sartorius muscle.** All of the superficial lymph nodes within the described area are removed, as are the deep inguinal nodes that are located primarily medial to the femoral vein to the level of the inguinal ligament.

The procedure begins by placing the patient into a frog-legged position. A 10-cm skin incision is made approximately 1.5 to 2 cm below the inguinal crease. Skin flaps are developed in the plane just beneath Scarpa's fascia for a distance of 8 cm superiorly and 6 cm inferiorly. The superior dissection is carried to the level of the external oblique fascia with exposure of the spermatic cord. A funiculus of lymphofatty tissue extending from the base of the penis to the superomedial portion of the lymph node packet is ligated and divided. Dissection commences in a caudad direction with removal of the superficial and deep inguinal nodes with the boundaries consisting of the adductor longus muscle medially and the femoral artery laterally. The saphenous vein is identified and preserved, although a number of branches draining into it will need to be sacrificed. The nodal packet is dissected

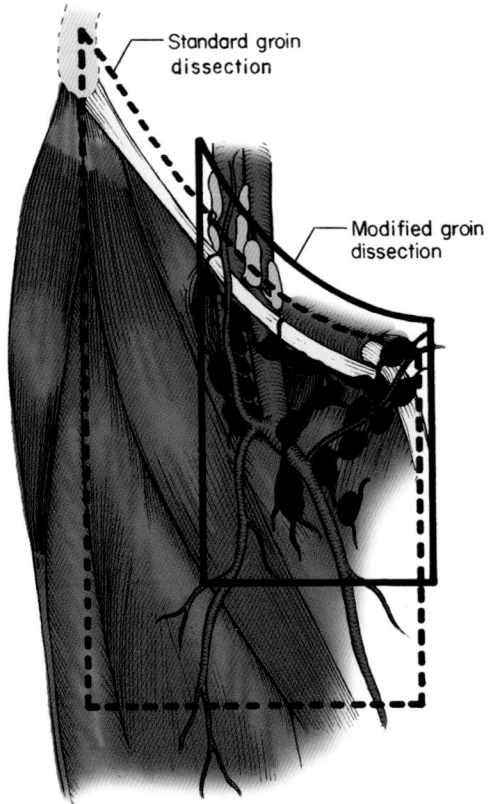

Figure 32–17. Limits of standard and modified groin dissection. (From Colberg JW, Andriole GL, Catalona WJ: Long-term follow-up of men undergoing modified inguinal lymphadenectomy for carcinoma of the penis. Br J Urol 1997;79:54-57.)

caudad to the level of the skin flap dissection (Fig. 32–18), at which point the lymphatics are carefully ligated and the specimen is delivered from the operative field (Fig. 32–19). A closed-suction drain is placed, and the incision is closed in standard fashion.

Morbidity after modified inguinal lymphadenectomy consists primarily of minor complications including seroma (25% to 27%), lymphorrhea (9% to 10%), and wound infection or skin necrosis (0% to 9%). These have been self-limited in the majority of cases (Parra, 1996; Coblentz and Theodorescu, 2002; Jacobellis, 2003; Bouchot et al, 2004; d'Ancona et al, 2004). Temporary lower extremity edema has been reported in approximately 20% of patients, and persistent edema is uncommon. Major complications are rare.

Although it is not universally accepted, the literature suggests that the primary use of modified inguinal lymphadenectomy currently is in patients with a primary tumor that places them at increased risk for inguinal metastasis and clinically negative groins on examination. If nodal metastasis is detected on frozen-section examination of the specimen, the procedure is converted to a standard extended lymphadenectomy. The false-negative rate for this procedure in terms of detecting inguinal metastatic disease ranges from 0% to 5.5% in the majority of published reports (Parra, 1996; Colberg et al, 1997; Coblentz and Theodorescu, 2002; Bouchot et al, 2004; d'Ancona et al, 2004).

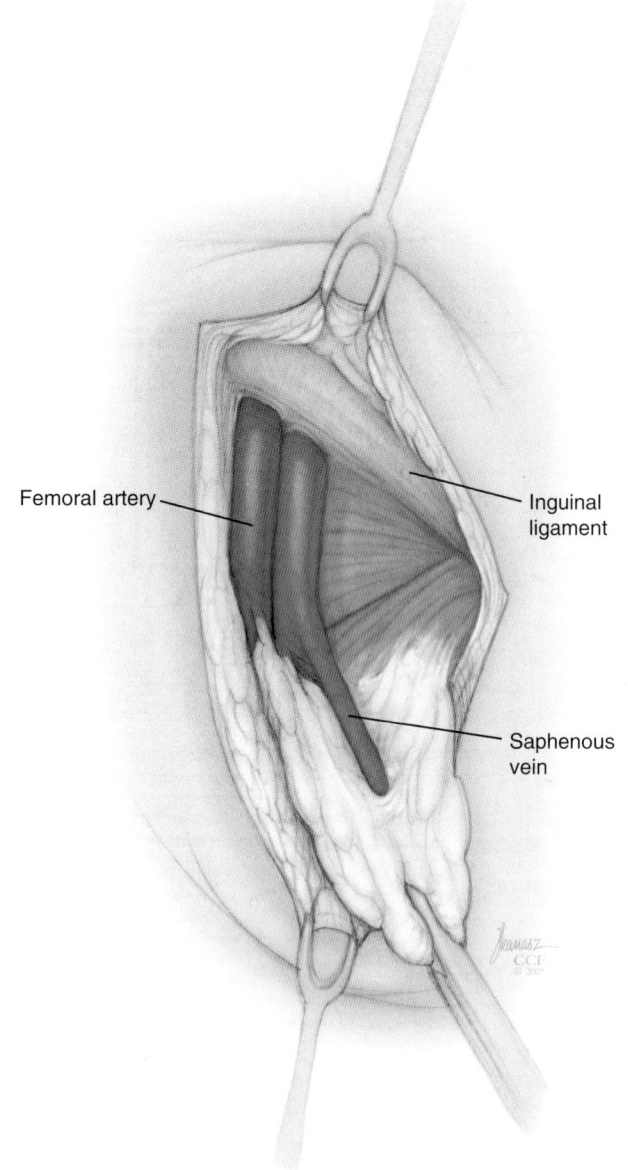

Figure 32–18.   Modified inguinal lymphadenectomy. Lymph node packet is medial to the femoral artery and includes superficial and deep inguinal nodes.

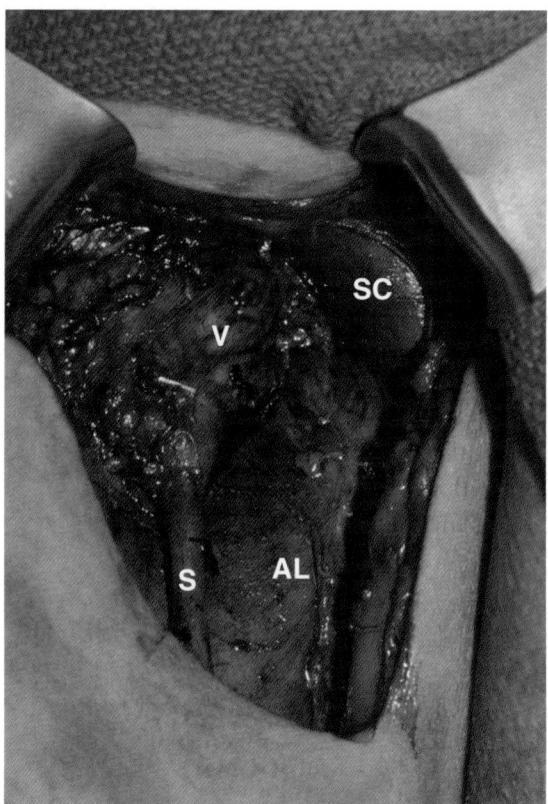

Figure 32–19.   Intraoperative photograph of right inguinal region after modified lymphadenectomy. SC, spermatic cord; V, femoral vein; S, saphenous vein; AL, adductor longus.

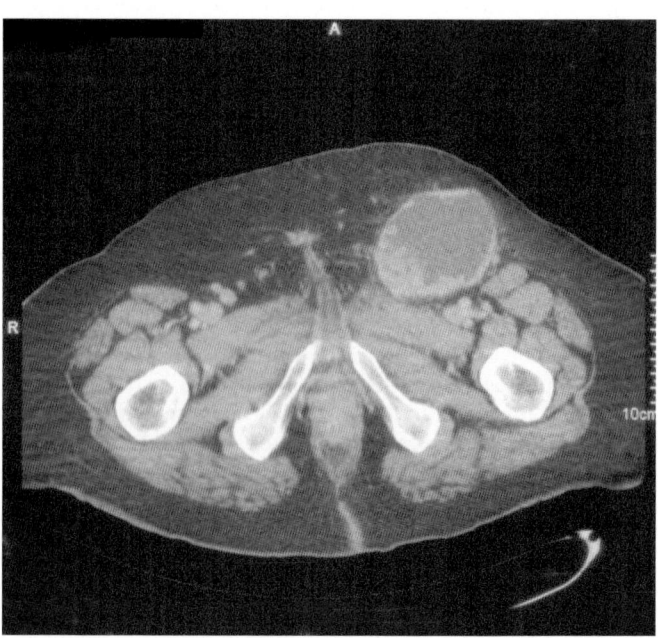

Figure 32–20.   Pelvic computed tomographic scan of patient with penile carcinoma demonstrating large left inguinal metastasis overlying the femoral vessels.

Radical Ilioinguinal Lymphadenectomy

Radical ilioinguinal lymphadenectomy is indicated in patients with resectable metastatic adenopathy and may be curative when the disease is limited to the inguinal nodes. We have also favored its use as a palliative procedure in patients with documented inguinal metastasis who are fit for surgery. If left unchecked, cancer-bearing inguinal nodes may lead to significant complications, such as infection or abscess with chronic foul-smelling drainage or life-threatening femoral hemorrhage (Fig. 32–20). The procedure is carried out 4 to 6 weeks after surgical treatment of the primary tumor. Antibiotics are administered during this time to reduce the inflammatory component of the regional adenopathy. The patient is positioned with the involved thigh slightly abducted and externally rotated with cushioned support under the flexed knee.

The inguinofemoral dissection is designed to cover an area outlined superiorly by a line drawn from the superior margin of the external ring to the anterior superior iliac spine, laterally by a line drawn from the anterior superior iliac spine extending 20 cm inferiorly, and medially by a line drawn from the pubic tubercle 15 cm down the medial thigh. In most situations, the procedure is carried out through an oblique inci-

sion approximately 3 cm below and parallel to the inguinal ligament and extending from the lateral to the medial limit of the dissection (Fig. 32–21). If an area of the skin overlying the cancer-bearing nodes is invaded or adherent and requires excision, an elliptical incision is made around the involved skin and then extended medially and laterally. In this setting, the incision may alternatively be extended superiorly from the lateral border of the ellipse and inferiorly from the medial border to make a single S-shaped incision for the iliac and inguinofemoral dissections (Fig. 32–22).

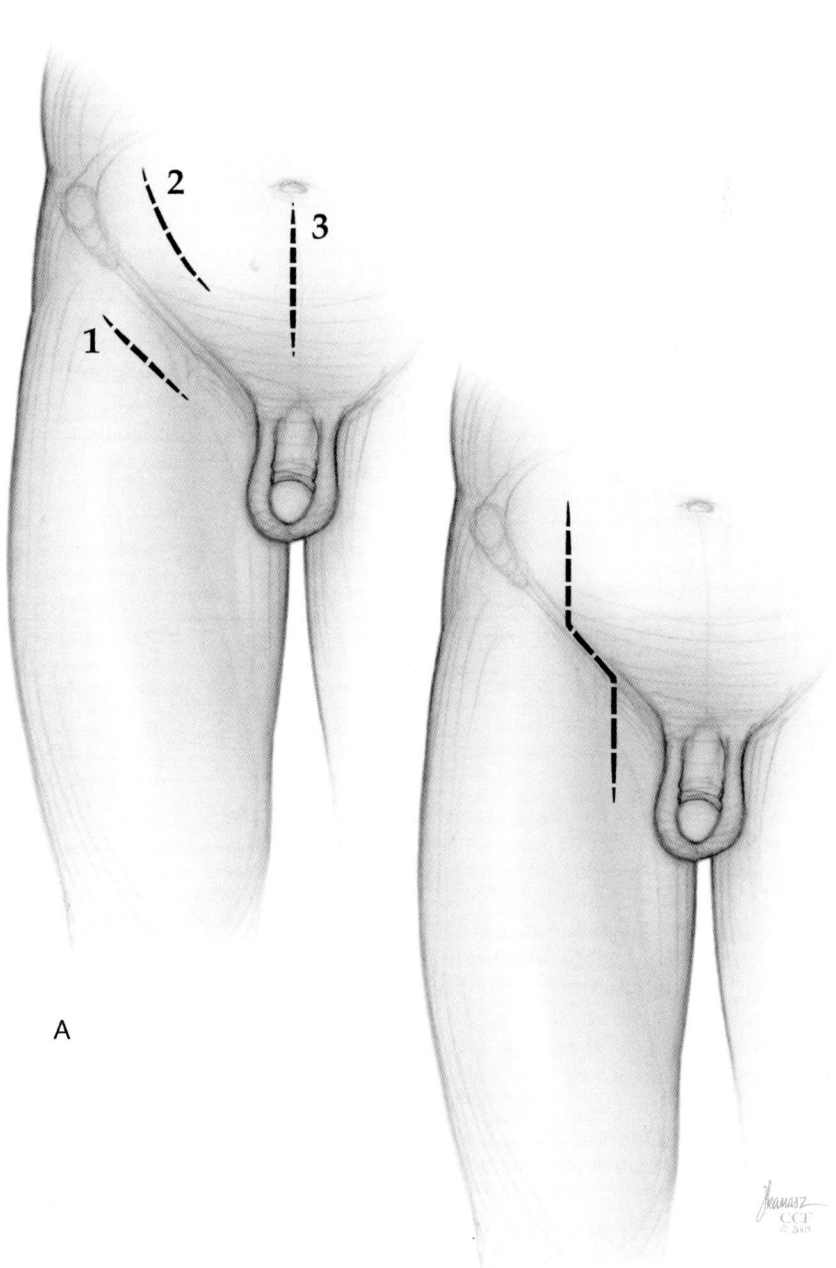

Figure 32–21. Ilioinguinal lymph node dissection. **A**, Incisions for inguinofemoral lymph node dissection (1), unilateral pelvic lymph node dissection (2), and bilateral pelvic lymph node dissection (3). **B**, Single incision approach for ilioinguinal lymph node dissection.

A

B

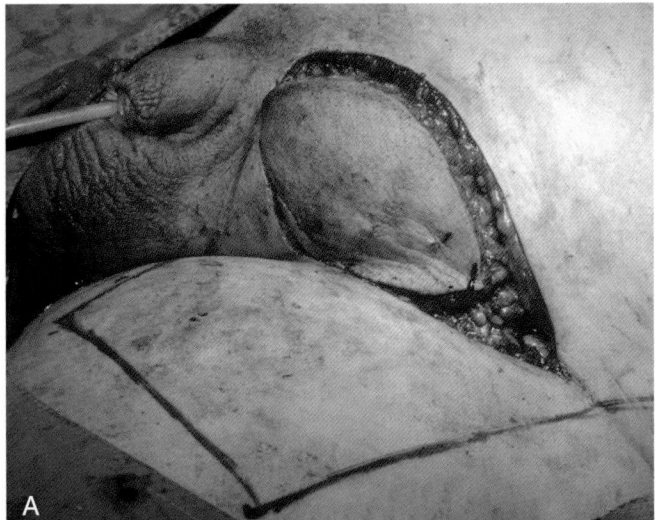

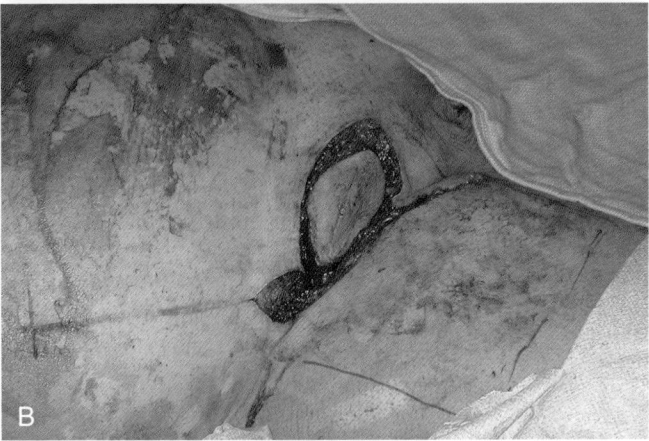

Figure 32–22. A, Incision and area of dissection for left inguinofemoral lymph node dissection with excision of adherent skin overlying nodal mass. **B,** Single incision approach and area of dissection for right ilioinguinal lymph node dissection with excision of overlying skin.

Superior and inferior skin flaps are developed in the plane just below Scarpa's fascia. The superior flap is elevated cephalad to a point 4 cm above the inguinal ligament and the inferior flap to the limit of the dissection. The fat and areolar tissues are dissected from the external oblique aponeurosis and the spermatic cord to the inferior border of the inguinal ligament, forming the superior boundary of the lymph node packet (Fig. 32–23). The inferior angle of the inguinofemoral exposure is at the apex of the femoral triangle, where the long saphenous vein is identified and divided. In patients with minimal metastatic disease, it may be feasible and beneficial to spare the saphenous vein, and this should be considered (Fig. 32–24). Dissection is deepened through the fascia lata overlying the sartorius muscle laterally and the thinner fascia covering the adductor longus muscle medially. At the apex of the femoral triangle, the femoral artery and vein are identified, and dissection is continued superiorly along the femoral vessels. Superficial cutaneous perforating arteries are ligated as they are encountered on the surface of the femoral artery.

The saphenous vein is divided at the saphenofemoral junction, and the dissection is continued superiorly to include the deep inguinal nodes medial and lateral to the femoral vein until continuity with the pelvic dissection is attained at the femoral canal (Fig. 32–25). The anterior aspects of the femoral vessels are dissected, but the femoral vessels are not skeletonized and the lateral surface of the femoral artery is not exposed. This avoids injury to the femoral nerve and the profunda femoris artery, and the femoral nerve is usually not visible as it runs beneath the iliacus fascia.

After the femoral triangle is dissected (Fig. 32–26), the sartorius muscle is mobilized from its origin at the anterior superior iliac spine and either transposed or rolled 180 degrees medially to cover the femoral vessels. The muscle is sutured to the inguinal ligament superiorly, and its margins are sutured to the muscles of the thigh immediately adjacent to the femoral vessels (Fig. 32–27). The femoral canal is closed if necessary by suturing the shelving edge of Poupart's ligament to Cooper's ligament, being careful not to compromise the lumen of the external iliac vein or to injure the inferior epigastric vessels in the process. Primary closure of the inguinofemoral dissection is usually possible with minimal or no further mobilization of the excision margins. When circumstances demand a large area of inguinal soft tissue sacrifice, primary closure may be obtained by scrotal skin rotation flaps (Skinner, 1974), an abdominal wall advancement flap (Tabatabaei and McDougal, 2003), or a myocutaneous flap based on the rectus abdominis or tensor fascia lata (Airhart et al, 1982) for more extensive defects.

Bilateral pelvic lymphadenectomy is best accomplished by an extraperitoneal approach through a lower midline incision. If a unilateral dissection is indicated, we favor a modified Gibson incision or an S-shaped ilioinguinal incision (see Figs. 32–21 and 32–22). **Pelvic lymphadenectomy should include the distal common iliac, external iliac, and obturator nodes. No further benefit is gained from proximal iliac or paraaortic dissection.**

Closed-suction drains are placed under the subcutaneous tissue and brought out inferiorly. During closure, the skin flaps are sutured to the surface of the exposed musculature to decrease dead space. The skin is closed with absorbable subcutaneous sutures and staples. The patient is maintained at bed rest for 2 or 3 days, and pneumatic compression stockings are used. The drains are removed after 5 to 7 days when drainage is less than 30 to 40 mL/day. Compression stockings are recommended postoperatively. We maintain the patient on a suppressive dose of a cephalosporin for 2 months to decrease the incidence of erythema and cellulitis, and this seems to improve overall wound healing.

In the past, complications related to radical ilioinguinal lymphadenectomy have been significant. In contemporary series, early minor complications have been reported in 40% to 54% of dissections (Bevan-Thomas et al, 2002; Bouchot et al, 2004; Nelson et al, 2004). These consist primarily of lymphocele, wound infection or necrosis, and lymphedema. Major complications, such as debilitating lymphedema, flap necrosis, and lymphocele requiring intervention, occur in 5% to 21% of cases (Bevan-Thomas et al, 2002; Nelson et al, 2004). Efforts to minimize lower extremity lymphedema include the use of elastic stockings and sequential compression devices. The trend seems to be toward earlier ambulation,

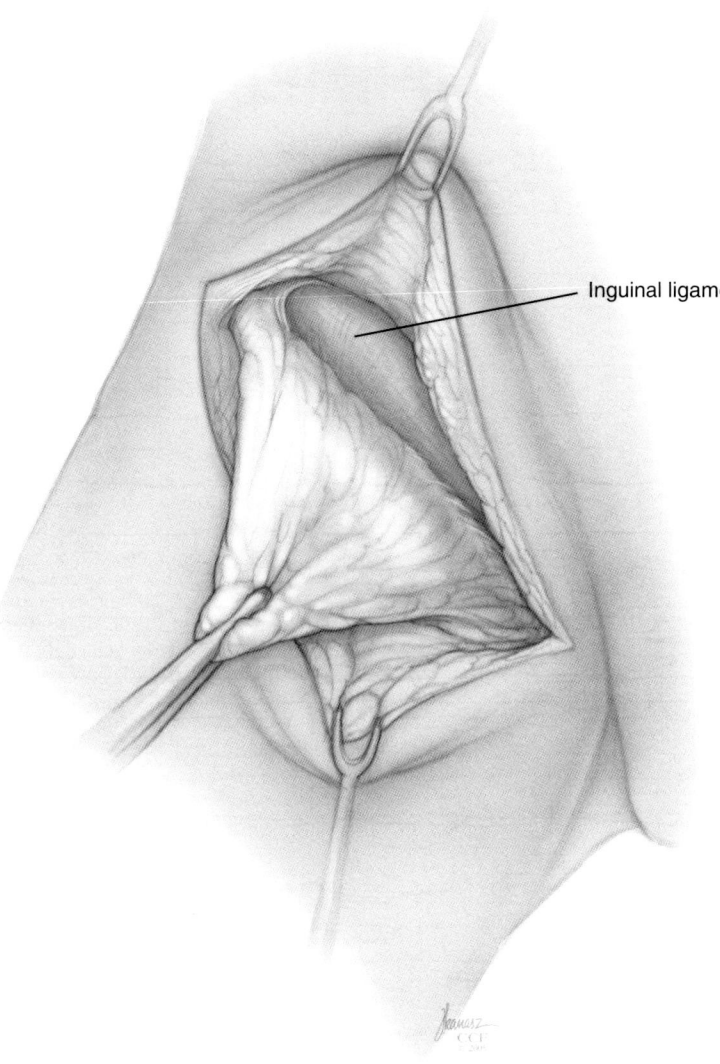

Inguinal ligament

Figure 32–23. Initial dissection for radical inguinofemoral lymph node dissection with exposure of superior border defined by the external oblique fascia.

Figure 32–24. Intraoperative photograph after saphenous-sparing radical left inguinofemoral lymph node dissection. A, femoral artery; S, sartorius muscle; SV, saphenous vein.

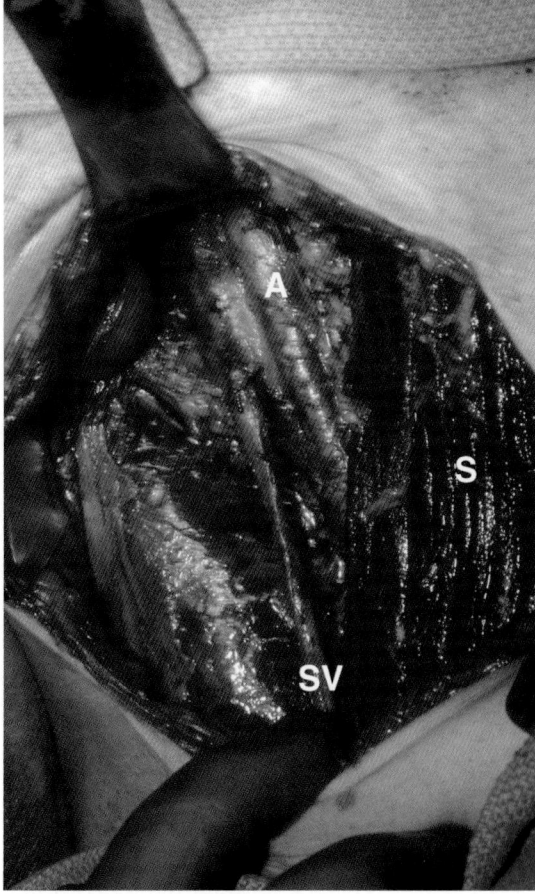

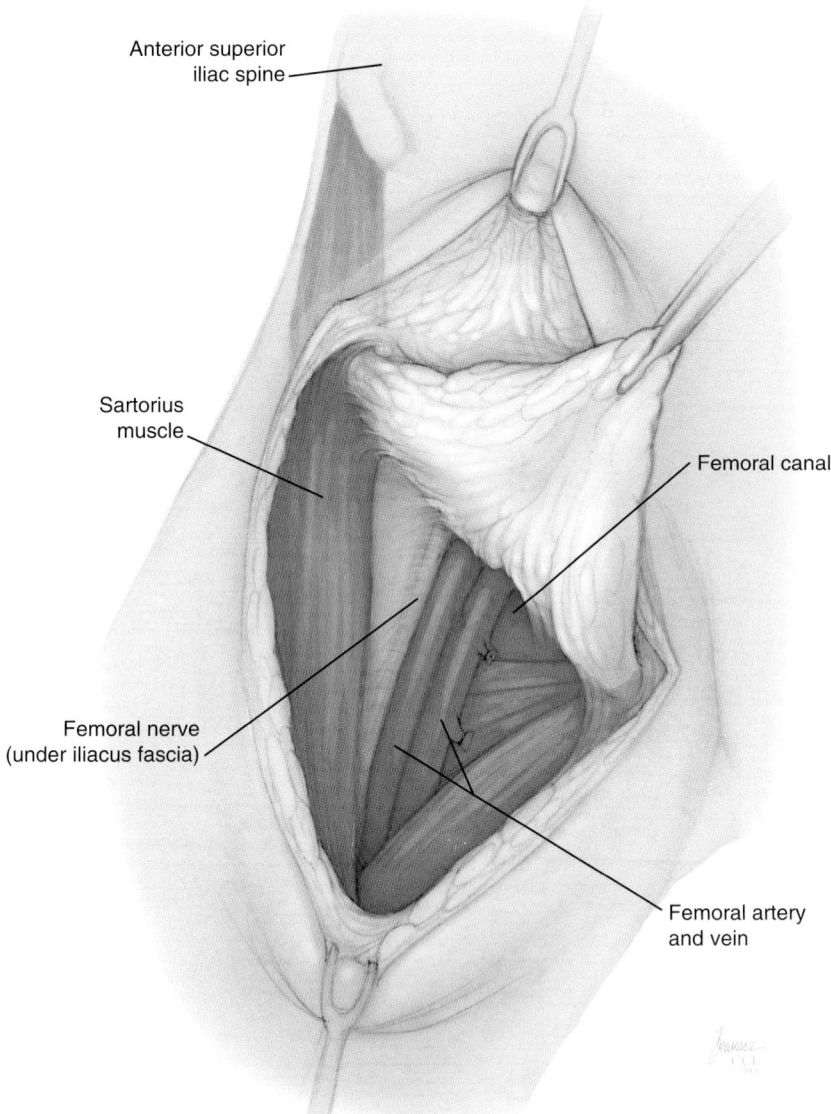

Anterior superior
iliac spine

Sartorius
muscle

Femoral canal

Femoral nerve
(under iliacus fascia)

Femoral artery
and vein

Figure 32–25. Inferior dissection during radical inguinofemoral lymph node dissection with removal of lymph node packet from the inferior border of the femoral triangle. After further lateral and medial dissection, the packet will remain in continuity with the pelvic dissection in the area of the femoral canal.

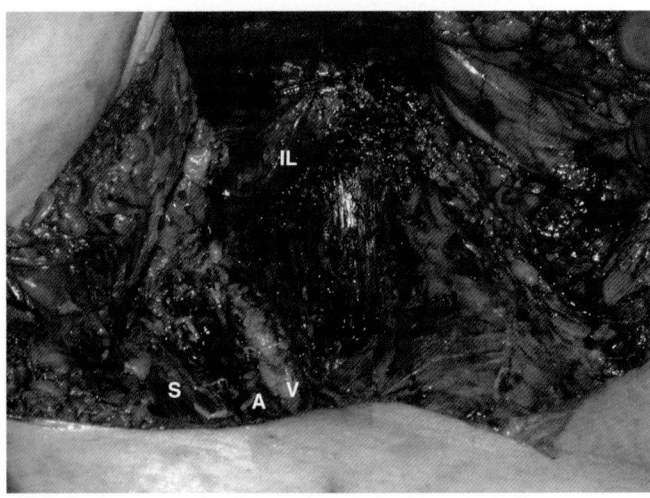

Figure 32–26. Intraoperative photograph after right radical inguinofemoral lymph node dissection in an obese patient. S, sartorius muscle; A, femoral artery; V, femoral vein; IL, inguinal ligament.

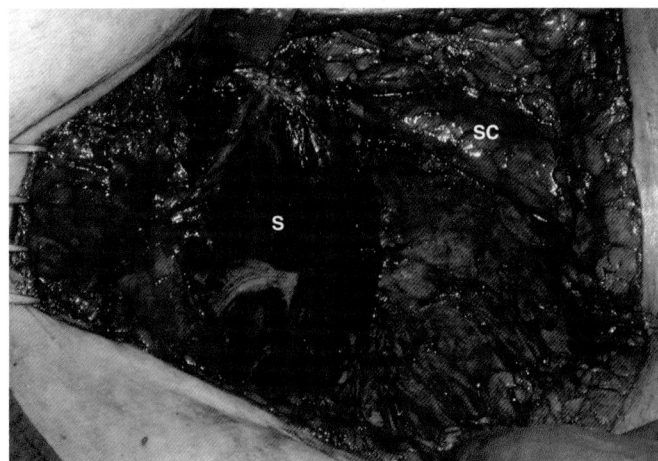

Figure 32–27. Sartorius muscle after detachment from the anterior superior iliac spine and 180-degree rotation medially, with suture fixation to the fascia of the inguinal ligament and the adductor longus. S, sartorius muscle; SC, spermatic cord.

Male Urethra

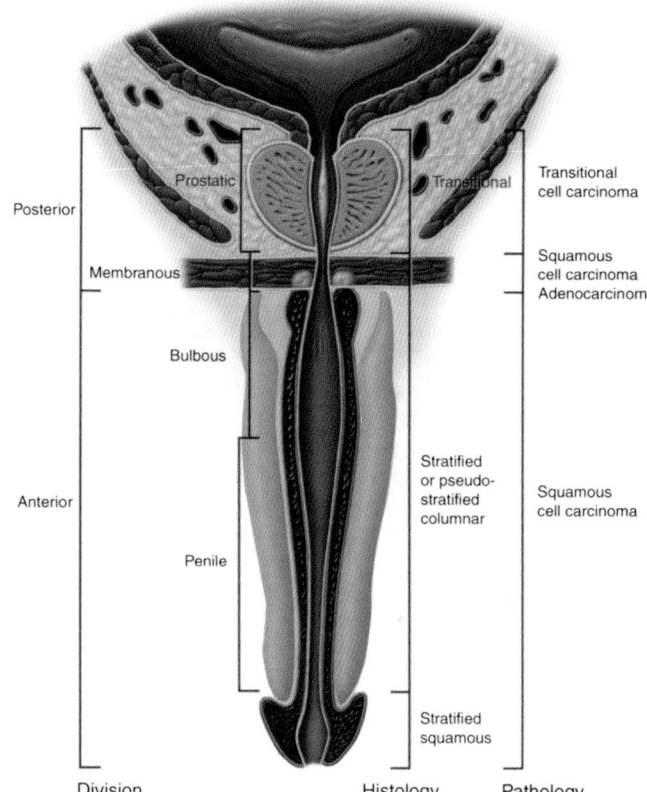

Figure 32–28. Anatomic regions of the male urethra and corresponding histology and histopathology.

with the avoidance of prophylactic low-dose heparin therapy because of the possibility of an increased risk of lymphocele formation (Tomic et al, 1994).

MALE URETHRAL CANCER
General Considerations

Carcinoma of the male urethra is rare and usually presents in the fifth decade of life (Dalbagni et al, 1999). **Etiologic factors include chronic inflammation due to a history of frequent sexually transmitted diseases, urethritis, and urethral stricture, and there is likely to be a causal role for human papillomavirus 16 in squamous cell carcinoma of the urethra** (Weiner et al, 1992; Cupp et al, 1996). The onset of malignant change in a patient with chronic urethral stricture disease may be insidious, and a high index of clinical suspicion is required to diagnose these tumors expediently. More than half of patients have a history of urethral stricture disease, almost one fourth have a history of sexually transmitted disease, and 96% are symptomatic at presentation (Dalbagni et al, 1999). The most common presenting symptoms are urethral bleeding, a palpable urethral mass, and obstructive voiding symptoms.

Pathology

Tumors of the male urethra are categorized according to location and histologic features of the cells lining the urethra (Mostofi et al, 1992) (Fig. 32–28). The bulbomembranous urethra is involved most frequently, accounting for 60% of tumors, followed by the penile urethra (30%) and the prostatic urethra (10%). Overall, 80% of male urethral cancers are squamous cell carcinoma; 15% are transitional cell carcinoma; and 5% are adenocarcinoma, melanoma, lymphoma, paraganglioma, sarcoma, or undifferentiated tumor. The histologic subtype of urethral cancer also varies by anatomic location. Carcinomas of the prostatic urethra are of transitional cell origin in 90% and of squamous cell origin in 10%; carcinomas of the penile urethra are of squamous cell origin in 90% and of transitional cell origin in 10%; and carcinomas of the bulbomembranous urethra are of squamous cell origin in 80%, of transitional cell origin in 10%, and adenocarcinoma or undifferentiated in 10% (Grigsby and Herr, 2000).

Male urethral carcinoma can spread by direct extension to adjacent structures, usually involving the vascular spaces of the corpus spongiosum and the periurethral tissues, or it can metastasize through lymphatic embolization to regional lymph nodes. The lymphatics from the anterior urethra drain into the superficial and deep inguinal lymph nodes and occasionally into the external iliac lymph nodes. Tumors of the posterior urethra most commonly spread to the pelvic lymph nodes. Palpable inguinal lymph nodes occur in about 20% of cases and almost always represent metastatic disease, in contrast to penile cancer, in which a large percentage of palpable nodes may be inflammatory. Hematogenous dissemination is uncommon except in advanced disease.

Evaluation and Staging

The tumor, nodes, metastasis (TNM) staging classification is based on depth of invasion of the primary tumor and presence or absence of regional lymph node involvement and distant metastasis (Table 32–1). Examination under anesthesia consisting of cystoscopy and bimanual palpation of the external genitalia, urethra, rectum, and perineum aids in evaluating the extent of local involvement by tumor. Transurethral or needle biopsy of the lesion is also performed. Cytologic studies of voided urine do not seem to be a reliable method for diagnosis of primary urethral carcinoma. In one study, sensitivity was greatest in men with transitional cell carcinoma (80%) and in those with tumors involving the pendulous urethra (73%) (Touijer and Dalbagni, 2004). If rectal involvement is suspected on bimanual examination or by the patient's symptoms, an evaluation of the lower colon by barium enema study and flexible sigmoidoscopy is recommended to assist with surgical planning. Local soft tissue involvement, lymph

node involvement, and bone extension are best evaluated by a computed tomographic scan of the abdomen and pelvis or by magnetic resonance imaging. Magnetic resonance imaging may be helpful for detecting invasion of the corpora cavernosa and is a useful staging modality (Vapnek et al, 1992).

Treatment

As in penile carcinoma, the primary form of treatment for men with urethral carcinoma is surgical excision. **In general, anterior urethral carcinoma is more amenable to surgical control, and the prognosis is better than that of posterior urethral carcinoma, which is often associated with extensive local invasion and distant metastasis** (Zeidman et al, 1992). A large series reported overall survival rates of 83% for low-stage tumors, 36% for high-stage tumors, 69% for anterior tumors, and 26% for those in the posterior urethra (Dalbagni et al, 1999).

Carcinoma of the Penile Urethra

Transurethral resection, local excision, or distal urethrectomy and perineal urethrostomy may be acceptable treatment in selected patients with superficial, papillary, or low-grade tumors. Long-term disease-free survival has been reported in this setting (Mandler and Pool, 1966; Konnak, 1980; Gheiler et al, 1998; Hakenberg et al, 2001). Squamous cell carcinoma in situ of the perimeatal glans may extend into the distal urethra (Fig. 32–29) and has been successfully treated with partial glansectomy and distal urethrectomy with simultaneous urethral reconstruction (Nash et al, 1996) or penile urethrostomy (Fig. 32–30). **Partial penectomy with a 2-cm negative margin is the treatment of choice for tumors infiltrating the corpus spongiosum and localized to the distal half of the penis. Excellent local control after this procedure has been documented** (Kaplan et al, 1967; Ray et al, 1977; Anderson and McAninch, 1984; Hopkins et al, 1984; Dinney et al, 1994; Gheiler et al, 1998). If invasive disease extends to or involves the proximal penile urethra, total penectomy is required to obtain an adequate margin of excision (Fig.

Table 32–1. Urethral Cancer TNM Staging System	
Primary tumor (T) (male and female)	
TX	Primary tumor cannot be assessed
T0	No evidence of primary tumor
Ta	Noninvasive papillary, polypoid, or verrucous carcinoma
Tis	Carcinoma in situ
T1	Tumor invades subepithelial connective tissue
T2	Tumor invades any of the following: corpus spongiosum, prostate, periurethral muscle
T3	Tumor invades any of the following: corpus cavernosum, beyond prostatic capsule, anterior vagina, bladder neck
T4	Tumor invades other adjacent organs
Transitional cell carcinoma of the prostate	
Tis-pu	Carcinoma in situ, involvement of the prostatic urethra
Tis-pd	Carcinoma in situ, involvement of the prostatic ducts
T1	Tumor invades subepithelial connective tissue
T2	Tumor invades any of the following: prostatic stroma, corpus spongiosum, periurethral muscle
T3	Tumor invades any of the following: corpus cavernosum, beyond prostatic capsule, bladder neck (extraprostatic extension)
T4	Tumor invades other adjacent organs (invasion of the bladder)
Regional lymph nodes (N)	
NX	Regional lymph nodes cannot be assessed
N0	No regional lymph node metastasis
N1	Metastasis in a single lymph node, 2 cm or less in greatest dimension
N2	Metastasis in a single lymph node, more than 2 cm but less than 5 cm in greatest dimension; or in multiple nodes, none greater than 5 cm
N3	Metastasis in a lymph node greater than 5 cm in greatest dimension
Distant metastasis (M)	
MX	Presence of distant metastasis cannot be assessed
M0	No distant metastasis
M1	Distant metastasis

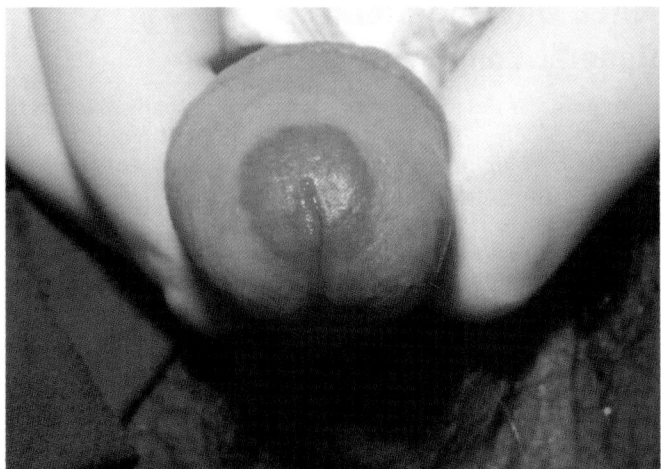

Figure 32–29. Squamous cell carcinoma in situ (erythroplasia of Queyrat) of the glans penis surrounding the urethral meatus. The patient also had significant extension of disease into the distal urethra.

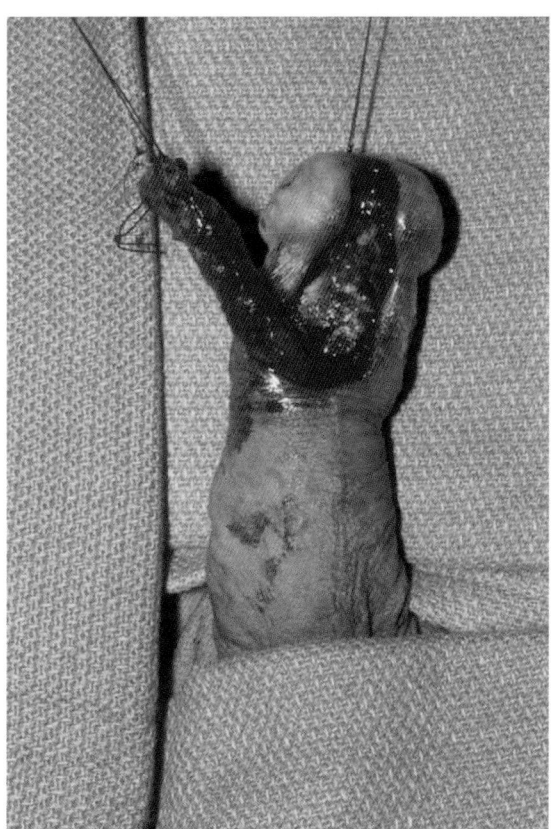

Figure 32–30. Partial glansectomy and distal urethrectomy (same patient as in Figure 32–29). After negative margins were ensured, penile urethrostomy completed the procedure.

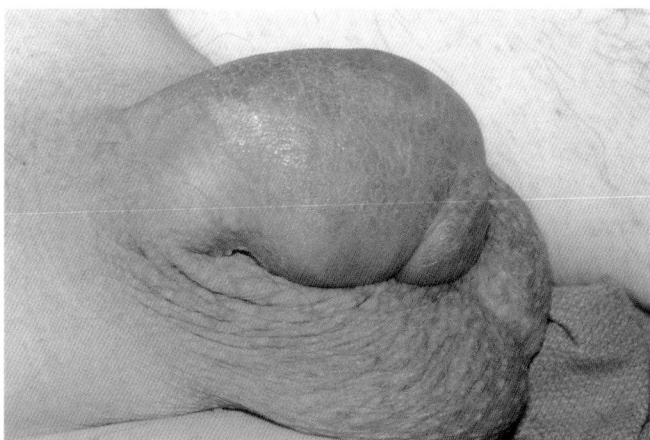

Figure 32–31. Large penile mass in a patient with transitional cell carcinoma of the penile urethra.

32–31). In the largest series to date, a local recurrence rate of 13% was reported after this procedure (Kaplan et al, 1967).

Accurate staging is important to avoid underestimation of the proximal extent of the tumor. Review of previous data would suggest that radical penectomy is an insufficient operation for bulbous urethral tumors (Zeidman et al, 1992). There have been limited reports of urethrectomy alone with perineal urethrostomy for infiltrating tumors confined to the corpus spongiosum (Hakenberg et al, 2001). The benefits of this more conservative approach need to be weighed against the probability of local relapse or dissemination of disease. **Ilioinguinal lymphadenectomy is indicated in the presence of palpable inguinal lymph nodes without evidence of metastatic disease. Benefit from prophylactic inguinal lymph node dissection has not been demonstrated in urethral cancer.**

Carcinoma of the Bulbomembranous Urethra

Early lesions of the bulbomembranous urethra have been treated successfully by transurethral resection or by segmental excision of the involved urethral segment with an end-to-end anastomosis. Unfortunately, cases appropriate for limited resection are rare. **Poor survival figures have been recorded for all forms of treatment, but it appears that radical excision offers the best opportunity for long-term disease control and the lowest incidence of local recurrence.** Radical cystoprostatectomy, pelvic lymphadenectomy, and total penectomy are usually required. Extending the operation to include in-continuity resection of the pubic rami and the adjacent urogenital diaphragm may improve the margin of resection and local control (Mackenzie and Whitmore, 1968; Shuttleworth and Lloyd-Davies, 1969; Bracken, 1982; Klein et al, 1983; Dinney et al, 1994).

With the patient in low lithotomy position to allow perineal access, the standard abdominal mobilization of the bladder is completed, except for preservation of the endopelvic fascia and the anterior pubic attachments. A modified lambda or inverted U-shaped perineal incision is performed, based just medial to the ischial tuberosities, with the apex in the mid-perineum. The ischiorectal fossae are developed as in perineal prostatectomy, and a tunnel is bluntly dissected just anterior to the rectum, extending from one fossa to the other. The inferior skin flap is mobilized by sharply dividing the intervening subcutaneous tissue and rectourethral muscle. The superior flap is mobilized by sharply incising the subcutaneous tissue to the superficial Colles' fascia and then continuing bilaterally to the adductor musculature at the inferior pubic rami. Circumferential incision of the skin and dartos fascia at the penoscrotal junction is performed, and the corporal bodies are mobilized for a short distance proximally off of the superior aspect of the symphysis pubis to allow subsequent inferior pubectomy. Care must be taken not to carry this dissection too far proximally to avoid breaching the anterior aspect of a locally advanced tumor. The penis is passed downward through the perineal incision. Wider exposure may be gained by dividing the scrotum in the midline if necessary. The scrotum can usually be preserved; however, bulky tumors may necessitate sacrifice of portions of the scrotum or perineal skin. In this setting, the testicles may be preserved in thigh pouches.

To complete the pubic arch resection, the adductor musculature is sharply divided bilaterally from the length of the inferior pubic ramus along the medial margin of the obturator foramen. A Gigli saw is passed along the inferior ramus just posterior to the origins of the transverse perineal musculature. An inferiorly beveled transection is made bilaterally to simplify perineal delivery of the specimen. Alternatively, an osteotome may be used for this purpose. The entire

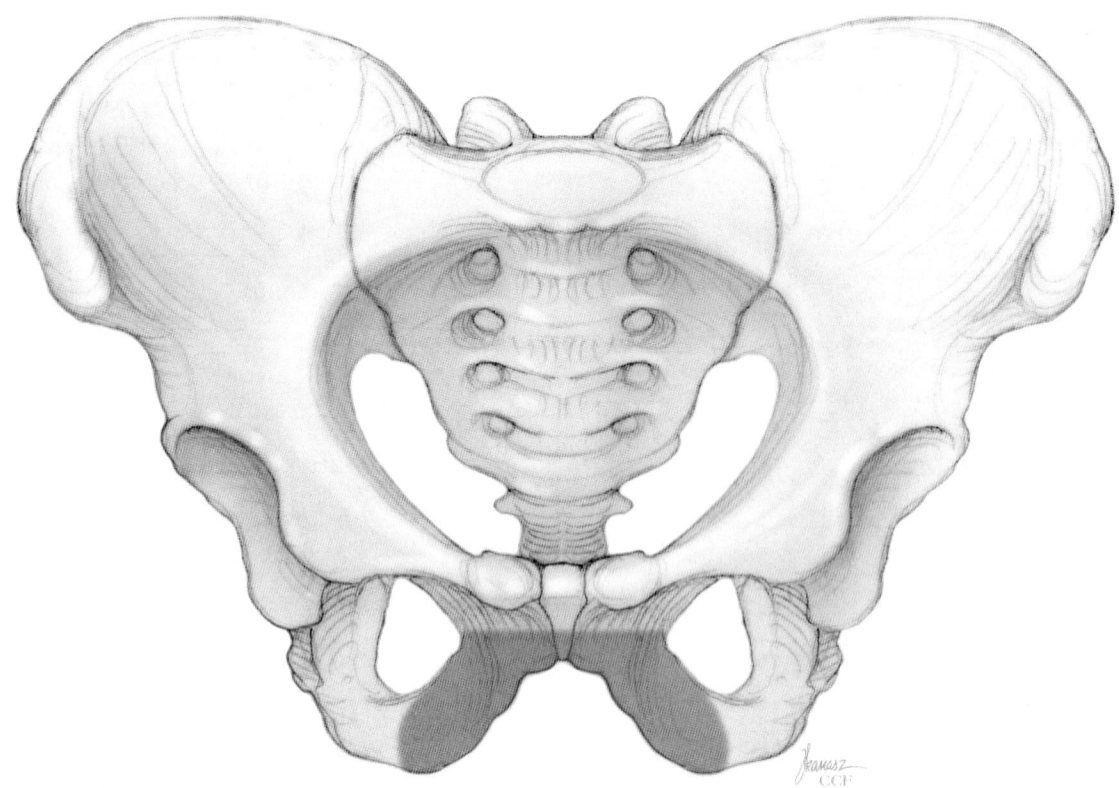

Figure 32–32. Shaded area outlines the portions of the ischiopubic rami excised at the time of inferior pubectomy during radical excision of bulbomembranous urethral cancer.

symphysis may be resected for bulky urethral lesions involving the presymphyseal tissues. This is accomplished by division of the superior rami at their junction with the symphysis. For most lesions, however, the bulk of the symphysis can be preserved with resection of the subsymphyseal arch. This procedure is preferred, when possible, to preserve stability of the pelvic girdle and results in a much smaller pelvic floor defect. A Gigli saw passed through the obturator foramina or an osteotome is used to incise the symphysis transversely, joining the foramina (Fig. 32–32). The specimen is delivered en bloc (Fig. 32–33). After hemostasis is secure, the omentum is mobilized to cover the bowel. Large pelvic floor defects such as after total pubectomy may be managed with a rectus abdominis muscle flap placed as a pelvic sling. Myocutaneous flaps can be fashioned to close large full-thickness perineal defects (Larson and Bracken, 1982).

Radiation Therapy and Chemotherapy

Although some instances of tumor control by irradiation have been reported, in general, radiation therapy has been reserved for patients with early-stage lesions of the anterior urethra who refuse surgery. The most commonly used technique consists of parallel opposed fields with the penis suspended vertically by a urethral catheter (Heysek et al, 1985). Radiation therapy has the advantage of preserving the penis, but it may result in skin ulceration or necrosis, urethral stricture, or chronic edema, and it does not prevent new tumor occur-

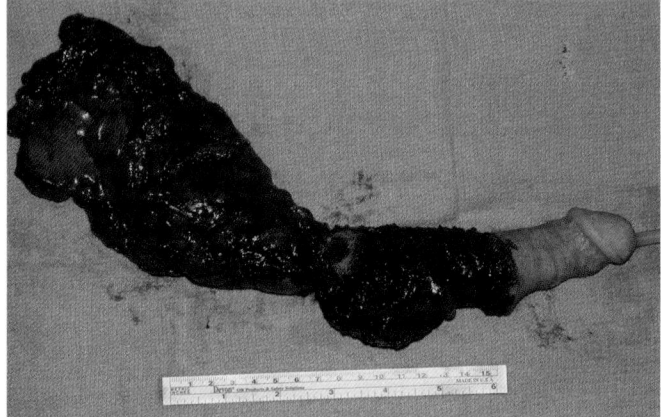

Figure 32–33. Surgical specimen after radical cystoprostatectomy, urethrectomy, penectomy, and inferior pubectomy for a large bulbomembranous squamous cell carcinoma.

rence. The long-term results of radiotherapy are difficult to evaluate because few reports are available of patients treated with this modality (Raghavaiah, 1978; Forman and Lichter, 1992).

A small number of studies have reported the results of neoadjuvant and adjuvant combination chemotherapy in patients with advanced stage or metastatic disease. A regimen including methotrexate, vinblastine, doxorubicin, and cis-platin (M-VAC) has been noted to have activity against transitional cell carcinoma but was ineffective against other tumor histologic types (Scher et al, 1988). Dinney and colleagues (1994) reported long-term survival in four of eight patients who presented with metastatic urethral carcinoma and were treated with cisplatin-based chemotherapy and surgical excision. On the basis of this experience, their favored regimen was noted to consist of cisplatin, bleomycin, and methotrexate for squamous cell carcinoma and M-VAC for transitional cell carcinoma.

The combination of chemotherapy and radiation therapy has shown some success in a small number of patients with localized and metastatic urethral cancer (Licht et al, 1995; Oberfield et al, 1996). More commonly, these forms of treatment are combined with surgery in a multimodal approach in patients with advanced stage or metastatic disease (Johnson et al, 1989; Gheiler et al, 1998; Grigsby and Herr, 2000).

Management of the Urethra after Cystectomy

General Considerations

Contemporary series have demonstrated the incidence of urethral cancer recurrence that follows cystoprostatectomy to range from 2.1% to 11.1% after cutaneous diversion (Freeman et al, 1996; Hassan et al, 2004; Nieder et al, 2004) and 0.5% to 4% after construction of an orthotopic neobladder (Freeman et al, 1996; Hassan et al, 2004; Nieder et al, 2004; Varol et al, 2004). Early studies indicated that transitional cell carcinoma involving the prostatic urethra, particularly with stromal invasion, significantly increased the probability of postoperative urethral recurrence (Hardeman and Soloway, 1990; Freeman et al, 1996). **However, the low incidence of urethral recurrence after orthotopic bladder replacement has led most authors to feel comfortable proceeding with this form of diversion as long as the findings on frozen-section biopsy of the distal prostatic urethral margin are normal at the time of cystoprostatectomy** (Freeman et al, 1996; Hassan et al, 2004; Nieder et al, 2004).

Approximately 40% of urethral recurrences are diagnosed within 1 year after cystoprostatectomy, with a median time to diagnosis of 18 months (Clark et al, 2004). However, a number of cases of late urethral recurrence have been reported, indicating the need for prolonged surveillance in these patients (Schellhammer and Whitmore, 1976; Freeman et al, 1996). Urethral wash cytology has traditionally been recommended for urethral monitoring after cutaneous diversion and leads to earlier diagnosis of urethral recurrence than when evaluation is delayed until symptoms occur. However, the presumed survival benefit afforded by surveillance with urethral wash cytology over symptomatic presentation has been called into question (Lin et al, 2003). Voided urine cytology is part of standard surveillance in patients who have undergone orthotopic diversion. Patients with positive results of urine or urethral wash cytology or symptoms of urethral bleeding, discharge, or palpable mass are evaluated with cystoscopy and biopsy. Pelvic computed tomography or magnetic resonance imaging may be necessary to aid in assessment of the

local extent of larger invasive tumors and to assess for metastatic disease. Patients who develop urethral carcinoma in situ after orthotopic diversion may respond to urethral perfusion with bacillus Calmette-Guérin, but this treatment is ineffective for those with papillary or invasive disease (Varol et al, 2004).

Total Urethrectomy after Cutaneous Diversion

The high or exaggerated lithotomy position provides optimal exposure for total urethrectomy, with the hips and knees gently flexed and the lower limbs abducted in boot-type stirrups. A modified lambda or midline perineal incision (Fig. 32–34) is made, and the subcutaneous tissue and bulbospongiosus muscle are then divided in the midline and retracted to expose the corpus spongiosum. The corpus spongiosum is mobilized circumferentially near the level of the mid bulbous urethra, and traction is applied to facilitate sharp dissection of the urethra distally, thus separating the corpus spongiosum from the adjacent corpora cavernosa. As dissection proceeds distally, the penis becomes inverted, the corpora cavernosa become bowed, and the glans recedes into the phallus. The penis is essentially turned inside out onto the perineum, and the dissection is completed to the base of the glans. To excise the meatus and glandular urethra, the penis is replaced in its anatomic position, and an incision is made around the meatus and extended on each side down the ventral aspect of the glans. The distal urethra is then freed from its investments within the glans, and the isolated pendulous urethra is delivered onto the perineum. The deep spongiosum of the glans penis is reapproximated with 4-0 polydioxanone sutures in a horizontal mattress fashion; the surface layer is closed with interrupted 4-0 chromic.

Proximal sharp dissection of the urethral bulb is carried out posteriorly and laterally, staying close to the bulb but avoiding entry if possible as bothersome bleeding will result. The urethra is detached from the corporal bodies anteriorly to the level of the departure of the urethra from the bulb, leaving the specimen attached only by the membranous urethra itself. The bulbar arteries are usually identified at the 4-o'clock and 8-o'clock positions just inferior to the perineal membrane after they are transected during the posterior bulb dissection. They are controlled with electrocautery or suture ligature, or they can be ligated if they are identified before transection. **Care must be exercised in completing the proximal dissection, in view of the possible postcystectomy adherence of intestine to the superior surface of the urogenital diaphragm.** This should be done under direct vision, and exposure can be aided by separating the crura of the corporal bodies in the midline to open the intracrural space. All that remains of the membranous urethra proximally is an ill-defined fibrotic band, and it should be completely excised. Frozen-section analysis of this region adds some assurance that a negative proximal margin has been attained. A small suction drain is placed in the urethral bed and brought out through the perineum. Closure of the bulbospongiosus muscle, subcutaneous tissue, and skin with interrupted absorbable sutures completes the procedure, and a light pressure dressing is applied. Superficial hematoma, edema along the penile shaft, and infection are uncommon complications.

SECTION VII

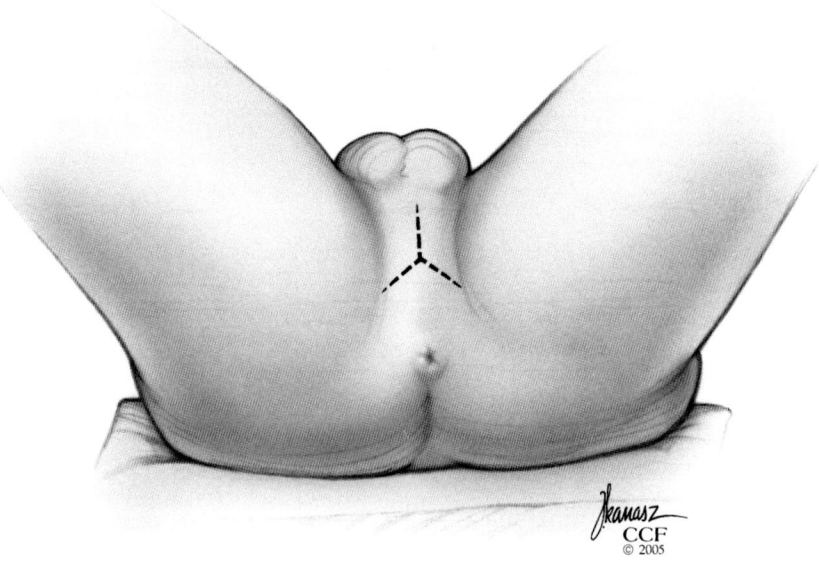

A

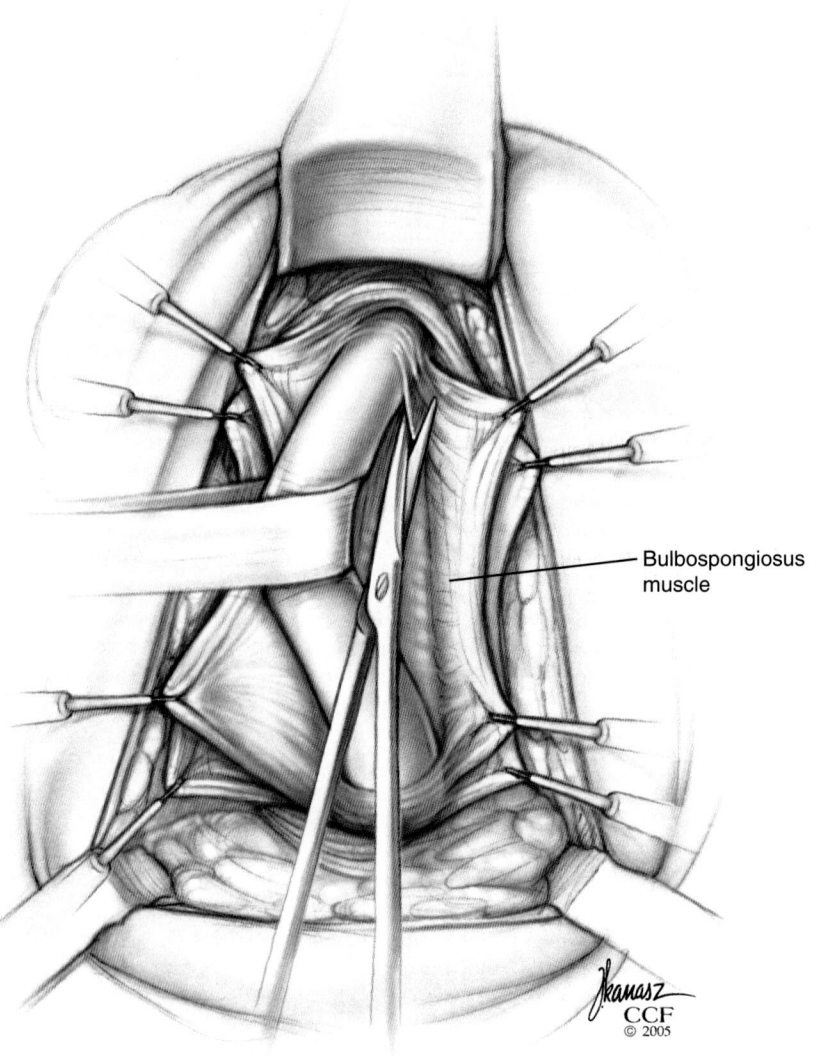

Figure 32–34. Secondary urethrectomy after previous cystoprostatectomy. **A,** Perineal incision. **B,** Division of bulbospongiosus muscle to expose the bulb of the corpus spongiosum and initial dissection of the urethra off of the corporal bodies.

Continued

Bulbospongiosus muscle

B

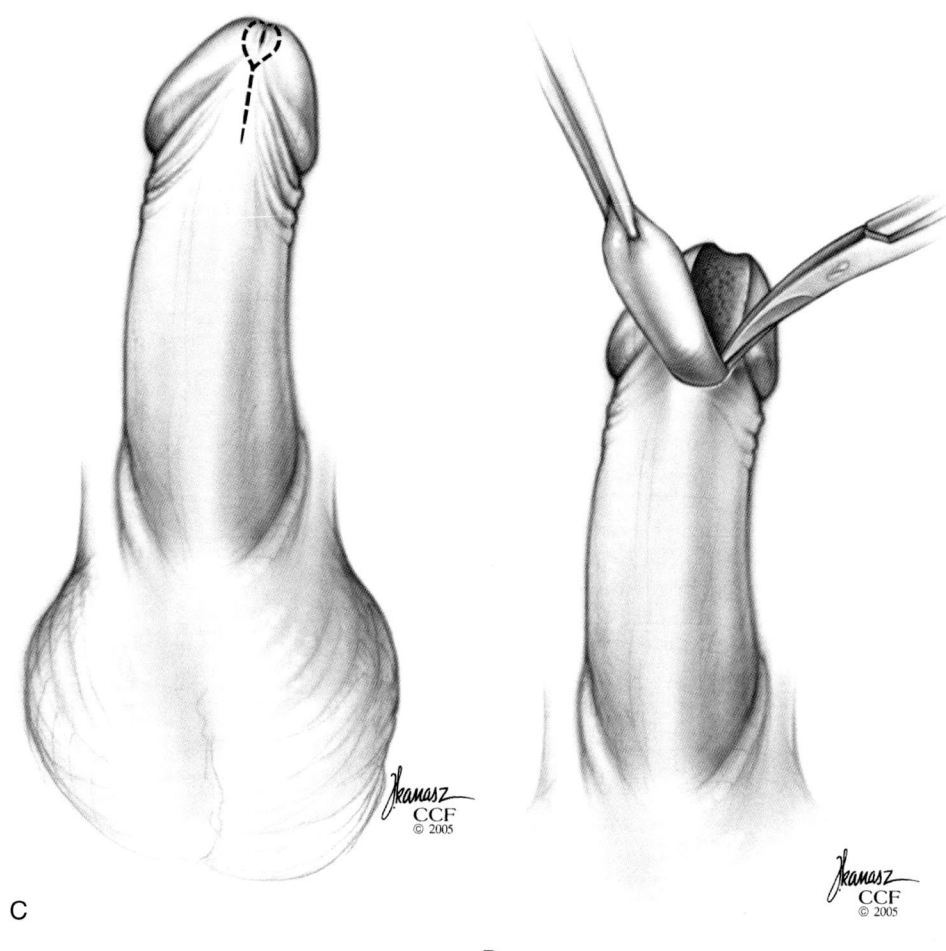

C

D

Figure 32–34, cont'd.   **C,** Distal incision circumscribing the urethral meatus. **D,** Distal urethral dissection, which then connects to the proximal dissection at the level of the distal shaft. **E,** Sagittal view demonstrating posterior bulb dissection and location of the bulbar artery.

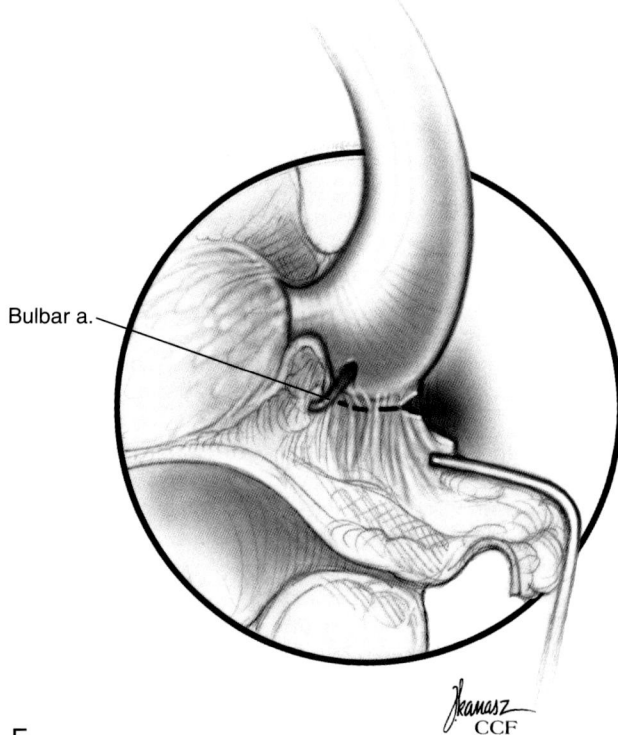

Bulbar a.

E

Total Urethrectomy after Orthotopic Diversion

Total urethrectomy after orthotopic urinary diversion is performed through an abdominoperineal approach. The patient is placed in lithotomy position with boot-type stirrups that can be adjusted during the case. Urethrectomy is carried out to the level of the membranous urethra as described previously. Abdominal exploration with lysis of adhesions and mobilization of the orthotopic neobladder is done to the level of the urethral anastomosis. Working with careful palpation from above and below, the area of the membranous urethra and the anastomosis are dissected free in their entirety. A circular area of the pouch adjacent to the anastomosis is excised to ensure an adequate surgical margin, and the specimen is delivered through the perineum. Bleeding from the musculature within the tunnel developed during excision of the membranous urethra can be bothersome and is best controlled with suture ligatures.

In most situations, urinary diversion is accomplished with an ileal conduit. **This can often be carried out with use of bowel from the orthotopic neobladder, which may be reconfigured when necessary, with care taken to incise the bowel along visible lines of previous closure with preservation of the mesenteric blood supply.** The remaining portions of the pouch are excised. If the existing diversion has an afferent limb (Studer pouch, for example), this segment can be used to construct the conduit without the need for manipulation of the ureters (Bissada et al, 2004). Conversion to a continent cutaneous diversion may also be possible in selected patients, depending on intra-abdominal anatomy and the motivation of the patient (Bartoletti et al, 1999).

FEMALE URETHRAL CANCER
Epidemiology, Etiology, and Clinical Presentation

Although the female urethra is much shorter than its male counterpart, primary urethral carcinoma is much more common in women than in men. The ratio of female to male predominance is reported as 4:1, and female urethral carcinoma is the only urologic malignant neoplasm that is more common in women than in men (Narayan and Konety, 1992). Female urethral carcinoma is rare, accounting for approximately 0.02% of all female cancers (Fagan and Hertig, 1955) and less than 1% of cancers in the female genitourinary tract (Srinivas and Khan, 1987). More than 1200 cases are reported in the literature, most diagnosed in the fifth and sixth decades of life (Srinivas and Khan, 1987). About 85% of urethral carcinoma cases occur in white women (Terry et al, 1997).

Although the cause of urethral carcinoma in women has not been identified, several factors have been implicated. **Etiologic factors associated with the development of urethral carcinoma include leukoplakia, chronic irritation, caruncles, polyps, parturition, and human papillomavirus infection or other viral infections** (Mevorach et al, 1990; Grigsby and Herr, 2000). Female urethral diverticula may also predispose the patient to malignant change, with perhaps 5% of female urethral carcinomas arising within a diverticulum (Rajan et al, 1993).

KEY POINTS: MALE URETHRAL CANCER

- Eighty percent of male urethral cancers are squamous cell carcinoma, and the region most commonly involved is the bulbomembranous urethra.

- In general, anterior urethral carcinoma is more amenable to surgical control, and the prognosis is better than that of posterior urethral carcinoma, which is often associated with extensive local invasion and distant metastasis.

- As opposed to penile carcinoma, benefit from prophylactic inguinal lymph node dissection has not been demonstrated in urethral cancer.

- The low incidence of urethral recurrence after orthotopic bladder replacement has led most authors to feel comfortable proceeding with this form of diversion as long as the findings on frozen-section biopsy of the distal prostatic urethral margin are normal at the time of cystoprostatectomy.

- In converting a patient to cutaneous conduit urinary diversion, bowel from the existing orthotopic neobladder can often be reconfigured with its blood supply intact and used for this purpose.

Ninety-five percent to 98% of patients are symptomatic at presentation. Many patients will present with obstructive symptoms, dysuria, urethral bleeding, urinary frequency, and often a palpable urethral mass or induration. A suspicion of a urethral tumor should be raised in any otherwise healthy middle-aged woman without prior urologic history who presents in urinary retention. Patients may also present with a small lesion prolapsing through the urethral meatus or with a small submucosal lesion on the anterior wall off the vagina. Tumors spread typically by local extension and may ulcerate as the tumor progresses to the skin and vulvar region. Proximal lesions may extend posteriorly into the vagina or proximally into the bladder. Lymphatic spread is uncommon at early stages, but clinically palpable nodes may be present in up to one third of patients at presentation and half of patients with advanced and proximal tumors (Grabstald et al, 1966). Hematogenous spread may occur to the lung, liver, bone, and brain, in order of frequency (Forman and Lichter, 1992).

Anatomy and Pathology

Knowledge of urethral anatomy is essential for surgical excision and reconstruction. The female urethra has been divided into an anterior segment (distal third) and a posterior segment (proximal two thirds). **The distal third may be excised while urinary continence is maintained.** The proximal third of the urethra is lined by typical transitional urothelium and the distal two thirds by stratified squamous epithelium (Fig. 32–35). Along its length are submucosal glands composed of columnar epithelium. Lymphatic drainage differs along the course of the female urethra, as in men. Although crossover and communications are possible, lymphatics from the posterior urethra drain to the external and internal iliac and obturator lymph node chains. The anterior urethra and labia drain to the superficial and then to the deep inguinal lymph nodes (Carroll and Dixon, 1992).

The histology of the malignant neoplasm depends primarily on the site of origin within the urethra (see Fig. 32–35). **Squamous cell carcinoma is the most common histologic type, accounting for 50% to 70% of all cases.** Transitional cell carcinoma and adenocarcinomas are the next most common cell types (10% to 25% each). Other rarer cell types include lymphoma, neuroendocrine carcinoma, sarcomas, paragangliomas, melanoma, and metastasis (Grabstald et al, 1966; Johnson and O'Connell, 1983; Foens et al, 1991; Forman and Lichter, 1992; Grigsby and Herr, 2000). Within urethral diverticula, an increased incidence of adenocarcinomas seems to exist, substantiating the theory that urethral diverticula in women may arise from a glandular origin (Rajan et al, 1993; Gheiler et al, 1998).

Diagnosis and Staging

The evaluation of women with suspected urethral carcinoma includes cystourethroscopy, examination under anesthesia, computed tomography of the abdomen and pelvis, and chest radiography. Magnetic resonance imaging has been used to evaluate pelvic lesions and may help determine local extension. TNM staging for female urethral cancer is identical to that for male urethral cancer (see Table 32–1). Clinically palpable inguinal nodes are found in 30% of patients overall, and these are confirmed to be malignant in approximately 90% of cases. Up to 50% of patients with proximal or advanced urethral cancers may have palpable nodes. Pelvic nodal metastases are also not uncommon, affecting 20% of cases. Metastasis outside of the pelvis at presentation is rare,

however. During follow-up, another 15% of patients will develop metastatic nodal disease (Grigsby and Herr, 2000).

Treatment and Prognosis

Because of the rarity of this tumor and heterogeneity of disease, insufficient experience at any single institution within a reasonable period has precluded attempts to effectively define the natural history of the disease, recommendations for therapy, and follow-up of these patients (Grigsby and Herr, 2000). **Although it is conceivable that different histologic subtypes may affect prognosis and the propensity for route of disease spread, most studies have failed to detect any differences in survival based on histologic subtype** (Foens et al, 1991; Dimarco et al, 2004). Consequently, lesions of varying histologic type are often treated in a similar fashion.

Treatment recommendations are primarily dependent on tumor location and clinical stage. Local excision, which should lead to excellent functional results, may be sufficient for the relatively uncommon small, superficial, distal urethral tumors. For more proximal and advanced urethral tumors, a more aggressive approach is warranted. **Compared with proximal urethral cancers, distal lesions are associated with improved survival.** Five-year disease-specific survival is reported at 71% for distal lesions, 48% for proximal lesions, and 24% for lesions that involve the majority of the urethra (Dalbagni et al, 1998). Surgical and radiotherapy series reflect overall 5-year survival rates of 30% to 40%. Unfortunately, little improvement has been made in treatment of this disease, and survival rates have remained statistically unchanged for the last 50 years (Bracken et al, 1976; Prempree et al, 1984; Foens et al, 1991; Dalbagni et al, 1998; Dimarco et al, 2004). Options for treatment of female urethral carcinoma include surgery, radiation therapy, and chemotherapy, alone or in combination. Treatment has trended toward a multimodality approach in recent years because of outcomes outlined in the following. Although representative of a heterogeneous group of studies with varying treatment technique and follow-up, reported

Figure 32–35. Anatomic regions of the female urethra and corresponding histology and histopathology.

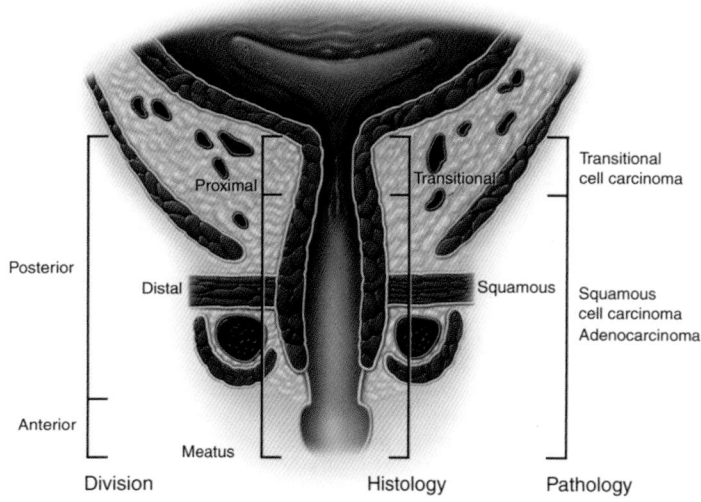

Female Urethra

results in series with more than two patients, based on primary treatment modalities, are summarized in Tables 32-2 and 32-3 for early and advanced disease, respectively.

Distal Female Urethral Carcinoma

Small, exophytic, superficial tumors arising from the urethral meatus or distal third of the urethra may be surgically treated with circumferential excision of the distal urethra and inclusion of a portion of the anterior vaginal wall. Frozen-section specimens of the proximal urethra should be obtained to ensure an adequate margin (Narayan and Konety, 1992). Laser coagulation of small distal tumors has been described (Staehler et al, 1985; Dann et al, 1989). In select patients with T2 or T3 cancer, bladder-sparing strategies have also been employed if the tumor is more anterior while an attempt is made to maintain a thorough resection. Dimarco and colleagues describe radical urethrectomy in the female patient, including excision up to the level of the bladder neck with wide resection of periurethral tissues and anterior vaginal wall. Urinary diversion is then accomplished with a catheterizable stoma (ileovesicostomy or appendicovesicostomy) to the native bladder. **Tumors in the distal urethra tend to be low stage, and cure rates of 70% to 90% have been achieved with local excision alone.** However, in a study by Dimarco and colleagues (2004), 21% of patients with stage T2 tumors or less treated with partial urethrectomy had local recurrence. Other studies of partial urethrectomy with or without radiation therapy for lower stage lesions have recurrence rates of 0% to 50% (Hahn et al, 1991; Gheiler et al, 1998). Meatal stenosis is a common complication, and incidence may be decreased by spatulation of the urethra. Approximation of the anterior vaginal wall and labia may help prevent urinary incontinence, although a sling procedure or

other procedure to treat urinary incontinence may need to be subsequently performed. Many authors report minimal complications and rare incontinence from partial urethrectomy, but one series noted de novo or worsening stress urinary incontinence in 42% of patients (Dimarco et al, 2004).

Radiation therapy, as well as surgery, has proved effective for the treatment of low-stage distal urethral carcinomas. An overall 5-year actuarial survival rate of 41% was reported in a series of 84 patients by Garden and colleagues (1993). This was subdivided into 5-year survival of 74% if only part of the urethra was involved and 55% if the entire urethra was involved. Survival appeared to be associated with clinical stage of the tumor (Garden et al, 1993). Radiation may be delivered as external beam, brachytherapy, or combined. In a series of 42 patients treated at the University of Iowa, radiotherapy delivered with combined interstitial and external beam radiation provided fewer local failures (14%) than all radiation–treated patients (36%) or those treated by surgery alone (60%). However, 5-year survival rates for irradiated and surgically treated groups are similar (Foens et al, 1991). Although doses may vary widely, a dose of between 55 and 70 Gy is reported in most series. Complication rates, now decreasing, have ranged from 20% to 40%, including urinary incontinence, urethral strictures, necrosis, fistula formation, cystitis, vulvar abscess, and cellulitis (Forman and Lichter, 1992).

Significant morbidity has been noted with ilioinguinal lymphadenectomy. In addition, female urethral carcinoma often

Table 32–2. Results of Various Treatment Modalities for Early Urethral Carcinoma in Women

Treatment	Study	No. of Patients	Survival* No. (%)
Radiotherapy	Weghaupt et al	42	30 (71)
	Pointon and Poole-Wilson	26	20 (77)[1]
	Taggart et al	15	8 (53)[2]
	Grabstald et al	11	3 (27)
	Delclos et al	11	6 (55)
	Chu	11	7 (64)
	Antoniades	8	8 (100)[3]
	Prempree et al	6	6 (100)
	Johnson and O'Connell	5	3 (60)[4]
	Klein et al	3	2 (66)[5]
	Total	138	93 (67)
Surgery	Grabstald et al	14	10 (71)
	Bracken et al	3	1 (33)
	Eng et al	4	4 (100)
	Total	21	15 (71)
Radiotherapy plus surgery	Grabstald et al	3	2 (67)
	Total	3	2 (67)

*Five- to 6-year survival unless otherwise noted.
[1]Three-year survival.
[2]Two-year survival with no evidence of disease.
[3]One patient dead of disease at 64 months.
[4]Patients had no evidence of disease at 4 years.
[5]Patients alive at 27 and 37 months.

Table 32–3. Results of Various Treatment Modalities for Advanced-Stage Urethral Carcinoma in Women

Treatment	Study	No. of Patients	Survival* No. (%)
Radiotherapy	Pointon and Poole-Wilson	52	21 (40)[1]
	Delclos et al	25	7 (28)
	Weghaupt et al	20	10 (50)
	Grabstald et al	19	1 (5)
	Antoniades	11	4 (36)[2]
	Prempree et al	7	4 (57)
	Hahn et al	8	3 (38)
	Chu	8	0 (0)
	Johnson and O'Connell	7	4 (57)[3]
	Total	157	54 (34)
Surgery	Grabstald et al	13	2 (15)
	Bracken et al	7	3 (43)[4]
	Moinuddin Ali et al	3	0 (0)
	Total	23	5 (22)
Radiotherapy plus surgery	Grabstald et al	20	5 (25)
	Johnson and O'Connell	7	3 (43)
	Hahn et al	3	9 (0)
	Moinuddin Ali et al	4	2 (50)[5]
	Total	34	19 (55)
Radiotherapy + chemotherapy ± surgery	Gheiler et al	6	3 (50)[6]
	Dalbagni et al	4	2 (50)[7]
	Total	10	5 (50)

*Five- to 6-year survival unless otherwise noted.
[1]Three-year survival.
[2]Two patients dead of disease at 8 and 21 years.
[3]No evidence of disease at 1, 1, 3, and 6 years.
[4]No evidence of disease at 2 months and 3, 8, and 12 years.
[5]Alive at 48 months.
[6]No evidence of disease at 0.5, 2, and 2 years.
[7]No evidence of disease at 1.5 and 4 years.

spreads systemically without regional lymph node involvement. Although studies are small, there has been no evidence for improved survival after pelvic or inguinal lymphadenectomy (Grabstald et al, 1966; Levine, 1980; Dimarco et al, 2004). These findings, as well as the inability to prognosticate likelihood for micrometastatic lymph node involvement, have led to the recommendation against prophylactic or diagnostic lymphadenectomy. **Acknowledging the fact that few objective data exist for definitive decisions to be made, recommendations have been made for groin dissection to be performed only on patients who present with positive inguinal or pelvic lymphadenopathy without distant metastasis or patients who develop regional adenopathy during surveillance.** Late inguinal lymph node recurrences up to 7 years have been noted. The technique of ilioinguinal lymphadenectomy is identical to the dissection performed in men for penile cancer (Narayan and Konety, 1992; Grigsby and Herr, 2000).

In patients with recurrence or radioresistant tumors, neoadjuvant irradiation followed by local excision has resulted in a survival advantage over radiotherapy alone (Grabstald et al, 1966; Peterson et al, 1973; Allen and Nelson, 1978). Despite early and aggressive therapy for anterior lesions, local recurrence rates and mortality remain high. Further studies are necessary to evaluate the potential role of multimodality therapy in these patients.

Proximal Female Urethral Carcinoma

Proximal female urethral carcinomas are more likely to be high stage and may extend into the bladder and vagina. Results with anterior exenteration alone resulted in a 10% to 17% 5-year survival rate and a local recurrence rate of 67% (Bracken et al, 1976; Klein et al, 1983). The poor disease-specific survival and high local recurrence rates observed with single-modality treatment of advanced female urethral carcinoma have led to the recommendation of combination therapy (Dalbagni et al, 1998, 2001; Gheiler et al, 1998). Advanced female urethral carcinoma includes tumors in a proximal location, a lesion that encompasses the entire urethra, or a locally invasive lesion that involves external genitalia, vagina, or bladder. Anterior exenteration (cystourethrectomy), pelvic lymph node dissection, and wide vaginal or complete vaginal excision are often required to obtain negative surgical margins. If the lesion extends into the external genitalia, partial vulvectomy or labial excision may be necessary. Anterior exenteration is performed as for bladder cancer in a female patient with a more extensive perineal portion of the procedure to provide wide margins around the urethra. The margins of the lymphadenectomy should include Cloquet's node distally and otherwise retain limits identical to the dissection encouraged for lymphadenectomy in bladder cancer. Anterior exenteration includes the en bloc removal of the entire urethra and bladder, the uterus and adnexa, and the anterior and lateral vaginal walls. On occasion, the entire vagina may need to be resected. The perineal portion is initiated by completing an inverted U-shaped incision to encircle widely around the urethral meatus. It has been suggested that this incision be extended onto the posterior vaginal wall to the labia minora and continued anteriorly to beyond and including the clitoris (Narayan and Konety, 1992). En bloc resection of the pubic symphysis and inferior pubic rami may be nec-

essary if the lesion encroaches anteriorly at the pubis, although the necessity of bone resection has been questioned in ensuring durable local control when intraoperative irradiation is added in suspect cases (Dalbagni et al, 2001).

Radiotherapy alone for proximal invasive urethral carcinoma has yielded poor local control, and 5-year survival rates of 0% to 57% are reported (Grabstald et al, 1966; Johnson and O'Connell, 1983; Prempree et al, 1984; Narayan and Konety, 1992). An improved mean survival rate of 54% at 5 years has resulted from the combination of radiation therapy and surgery for high-stage disease (Moinuddin Ali et al, 1988; Terry et al, 1997).

A combination of chemotherapy, radiation therapy, and surgery has been recommended for optimal local and distant disease control in advanced female urethral cancer. Patients whose treatment fails are thought likely to harbor micrometastatic disease at the time of primary treatment. For patients with squamous cell carcinoma, in part because of its effectiveness against anal cancers, 5-fluorouracil plus mitomycin C has been the most common empirically chosen regimen (Kalra et al, 1985). For transitional cell cancers, either M-VAC (methotrexate, vinblastine, doxorubicin, and cisplatin) or a gemcitabine regimen is recommended (Grigsby and Herr, 2000). Chemotherapy given concomitantly with radiation therapy has been shown to interfere with cell repair and thus act as a radiosensitizer. It is hoped that this rationale may serve to decrease local recurrence and improve survival by eliminating micrometastatic disease and preventing progression of local failures to systemic failures. The group at Memorial Sloan-Kettering has shown early results based on six patients with advanced proximal urethral tumors treated with a multimodality approach. The authors suggest that anterior exenteration with high-dose intraoperative brachytherapy followed by external beam radiation seems to improve local control. Studies must evaluate whether combined modality therapy proves to decrease distant metastasis and improve survival (Dalbagni et al, 1998, 2001).

Urethral Recurrence after Cystectomy in Women

Orthotopic neobladder construction in women is now an established form of urinary diversion after radical cystectomy for transitional cell carcinoma. **The incidence of carcinoma involving the urethra in female patients undergoing cystectomy for bladder cancer ranges from 1% to 13%** (Coloby et al, 1994; Stein et al, 1995, 1998; Stenzl et al, 1995). There is still debate whether involvement of the bladder neck is a contraindication to orthotopic diversion; a prospective study has revealed that although all patients with urethral transitional cell carcinoma on final pathologic analysis of the cystectomy specimen had involvement of the bladder neck, more than 60% of women with bladder neck involvement had no evidence of urethral transitional cell carcinoma (Stein et al, 1998). Intraoperative frozen-section analysis of the urethral stump has been subsequently espoused by some authors to determine the feasibility of urethra-sparing cystectomy and orthotopic diversion (Stein et al, 1998).

Despite the reported incidence of urethral involvement in cystectomy patients and the increased use of orthotopic

diversion in women, there are few reported cases of subsequent urethral malignant neoplasms in patients who have undergone this procedure. A review of 1054 patients undergoing radical cystectomy at a single center with a median follow-up of 10 years included 211 women, 44 of whom had an orthotopic urinary diversion. None of the 44 women developed a urethral recurrence (Clark et al, 2004). In a study by Ali-el-Dein and coworkers (2004), 145 women underwent orthotopic urinary diversion, 61% for squamous cell carcinoma and 21% for transitional cell carcinoma. At a median follow-up of 56 months, two patients (1.4%) developed an isolated urethral recurrence. One patient was reportedly not a surgical candidate, and the other patient underwent urethrectomy and conversion to a continent cutaneous reservoir but died 8 months later (Ali-el-Dein et al, 2004). One additional report described urethral transitional cell carcinoma in a woman after orthotopic diversion. This patient had a high-grade lesion of the bladder base with evidence of nodal metastasis. The patient was treated initially with chemotherapy, followed by urethral resection and conversion to a continent cutaneous diversion. The patient died 5 months later with visceral metastases (Jones et al, 2000). Limited experience to date precludes the ability to make definitive treatment recommendations for women with urethral cancer recurrence after orthotopic diversion. Urethrectomy and surgical resection of the area of the urethra-pouch anastomosis with conversion to a continent cutaneous urinary diversion seem feasible and reasonable in the absence of metastatic disease. Conversion to a cutaneous urinary conduit with use of reconfigured bowel from the existing orthotopic diversion is another option (Bissada et al, 2004).

SUGGESTED READINGS

Bissada NK, Yakout HH, Fahmy WE, et al: Multi-institutional long-term experience with conservative surgery for invasive penile carcinoma. J Urol 2003;169:500-502.

Catalona WJ: Modified inguinal lymphadenectomy for carcinoma of the penis with preservation of saphenous veins: Technique and preliminary results. J Urol 1988;140:306-310.

Clark PE, Stein JP, Groshen SG, et al: The management of urethral transitional cell carcinoma after radical cystectomy for invasive bladder cancer. J Urol 2004;172:1342-1347.

Dalbagni G, Zhang ZF, Lacombe L, et al: Male urethral carcinoma: Analysis of treatment outcome. Urology 1999;53:1126-1132.

KEY POINTS: FEMALE URETHRAL CANCER

- Squamous cell carcinoma is the most common histologic type of urethral cancer in women, accounting for 50% to 70% of all cases.

- Most studies have failed to detect any differences in survival based on histologic subtype.

- Compared with proximal urethral cancers, distal lesions are associated with improved survival.

- Tumors in the distal urethra tend to be low stage, and cure rates of 70% to 90% have been achieved with local excision alone.

- Proximal female urethral carcinomas are more likely to be high stage and may extend into the bladder and vagina.

- A combination of chemotherapy, radiation therapy, and surgery has been recommended for optimal local and distant disease control in advanced female urethral cancer.

- On the basis of results to date, it appears that in appropriately selected women undergoing orthotopic diversion, recurrence of cancer in the retained urethra is a rare event.

Dalbagni G, Donat SM, Eschwege P, et al: Results of high dose rate brachytherapy, anterior pelvic exenteration and external beam radiotherapy for carcinoma of the female urethra. J Urol 2001;166:1759-1761.

Dimarco DS, Dimarco CS, Zincke H, et al: Surgical treatment for local control of female urethral carcinoma. Urol Oncol 2004;22:404-409.

Horenblas S, van Tinteren H, Delemarre JF, et al: Squamous cell carcinoma of the penis. II. Treatment of the primary tumor. J Urol 1992;147:1533-1538.

McDougal WS, Kirchner FK, Edwards RH, et al: Treatment of carcinoma of the penis: The case for primary lymphadenectomy. J Urol 1986;136:38-41.

Tietjen DN, Malek RS: Laser therapy of squamous cell dysplasia and carcinoma of the penis. Urology 1998;52:559-565.

Zeidman EJ, Desmond P, Thompson I: Surgical treatment of carcinoma of the male urethra. Urol Clin North Am 1992;19:359-372.

33 Surgery of the Penis and Urethra

GERALD H. JORDAN, MD • STEVEN M. SCHLOSSBERG, MD

Improvements in microsurgery, tissue transfer techniques, and tissue handling have expanded the repertoire of the urologic surgeon and the genitourinary reconstructive surgeon in particular. Urologists are now able to reconstruct congenital and acquired genitourinary abnormalities with greater facility. Microvascular and microneurosurgical techniques have made it possible to construct a phallus that allows a patient to stand to void and to enjoy erotic sensibility; and because the phallus has both erotic sensibility and a protective function, the patient can eventually have a prosthetic implantation that allows an acceptable sexual life. This chapter discusses the general principles of male genital reconstructive surgery; specifics include male urethral surgery, surgery for congenital and traumatic penile lesions, and complex fistula and obliterative issues associated with the posterior urethra.

PRINCIPLES OF RECONSTRUCTIVE SURGERY

Many techniques in reconstructive surgery require the transfer of tissue. Skin is one of those tissues, and **its properties vary from individual to individual and from place to place on the same individual.** Variable characteristics such as color, texture, thickness, extensibility, innate skin tension, and blood supply can be useful in various situations.

The term *tissue transfer* implies the movement of tissue for purposes of reconstruction. Unlike extirpative surgery, the transfer of tissue for reconstruction requires an intimate knowledge of the anatomy of both the donor and the recipient sites as well as of the principles that will allow that tissue to survive once it is transferred.

The skin can be used as a model. The superficial layer of the skin is termed the epidermis (thickness, 0.8 to 1 mm). The deep layer of the skin is termed the dermis. The dermis has two layers, a superficial layer, the adventitial dermis (also called the papillary or periadnexal dermis, depending on the anatomy), and a deep layer, the reticular dermis. For genitourinary reconstruction, skin without adnexal structures is often used; thus, the papillary dermis is synonymous with the adventitial dermis. Other tissues commonly transferred for genitourinary reconstruction include bladder and buccal mucosa. The bladder epithelium is the superficial layer of the bladder; the deep layer of the bladder is termed the lamina propria, with superficial and deep layers. The buccal mucosa is the superficial layer of much of the oral cavity, which also has a deeper layer termed the lamina propria, again with superficial and deep layers.

All tissue has physical characteristics: extensibility, inherent tension, and the viscoelastic properties of stress relaxation and creep. The physical characteristics of a transferred unit are primarily a function of the helical arrangement of collagen along with the elastin cross-linkages. The collagen-elastin structure is suspended in a mucopolysaccharide matrix that influences the viscoelastic properties.

Tissue can be transferred as a graft (Fig. 33–1). **The term *graft* implies that tissue has been excised and transferred to a graft host bed, where a new blood supply develops by a process termed take. Take requires approximately 96 hours and occurs in two phases. The initial phase, imbibition, takes about 48 hours.** During that phase, the graft survives by "drinking" nutrients from the adjacent graft host bed, and the temperature of the graft is less than the core body temperature. **The second phase, inosculation, also requires about 48 hours and is the phase in which true microcirculation is reestablished in the graft.** During that phase, the temperature of the graft rises to core body temperature. The process of take is influenced by both the nature of the grafted tissue and the conditions of the graft host bed. Processes that interfere

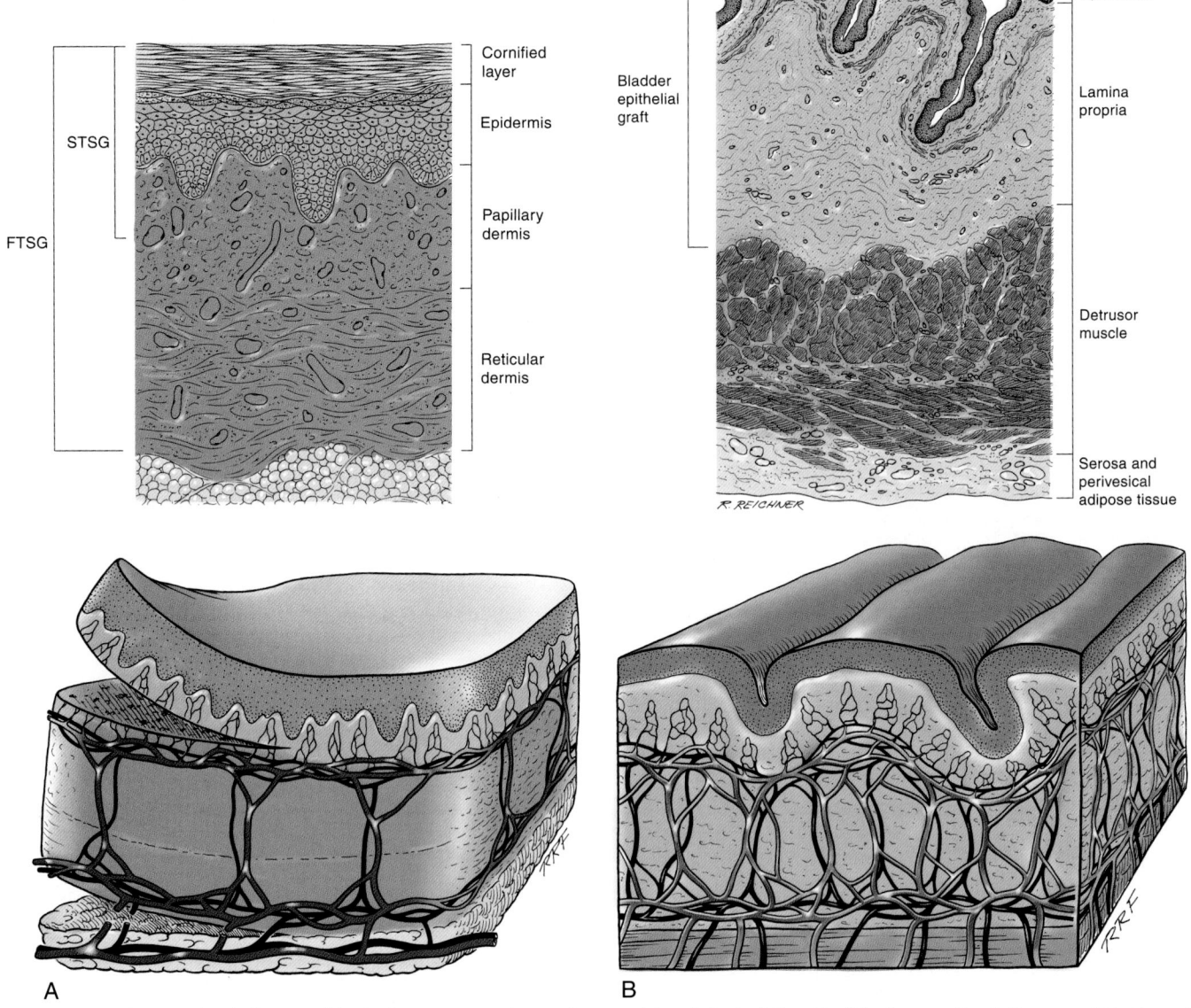

Figure 33–1. Cross-sectional diagrams (histologic appearance above, microvasculature below) of the skin (**A**). Cross-sectional diagrams of bladder wall (**B**). FTSG, full-thickness skin graft; STSG, split-thickness skin graft. (**A** to **C**, from Jordan GH, Schlossberg SM: Using tissue transfer for urethral reconstruction. Contemp Urol 1993;13:23.).

Continued

with the vascularity of the graft host bed thus interfere with graft take.

The epidermal or epithelial layer is a covering, the barrier to the "outside," and is adjacent to the superficial dermis or superficial lamina. At approximately that interface is the superficial plexus. In the case of skin, the plexus is the intradermal plexus. There are some lymphatics in the superficial dermal or tunica layer. On the undersurface of the deep dermal layer or deep lamina is the deep plexus. In the case of skin, this is the subdermal plexus. The deep dermis contains most of the lymphatics and greater collagen content than in the superficial dermal layer. The deep or reticular dermis is generally thought to account for the physical characteristics of the tissue.

Thus, **if a graft is a split-thickness unit, that graft carries the epidermis or the covering. That graft also exposes the superficial dermal (intradermal or intralaminar) plexus.** In most grafts, that superficial plexus is composed of small but numerous vessels. **This thus conveys favorable vascular characteristics to a split-thickness unit.** The unit has few lymphatics, and **the physical characteristics are not carried, which accounts for the tendency of split-thickness units to be brittle and less durable.** The reticular dermis is not carried with the split-thickness unit.

The mesh graft is usually an application of the split-thickness graft. After the harvest of a sheet graft, the sheet is placed on a carrier that cuts systematically placed slits in the graft. These slits can expand the graft by various ratios (i.e.,

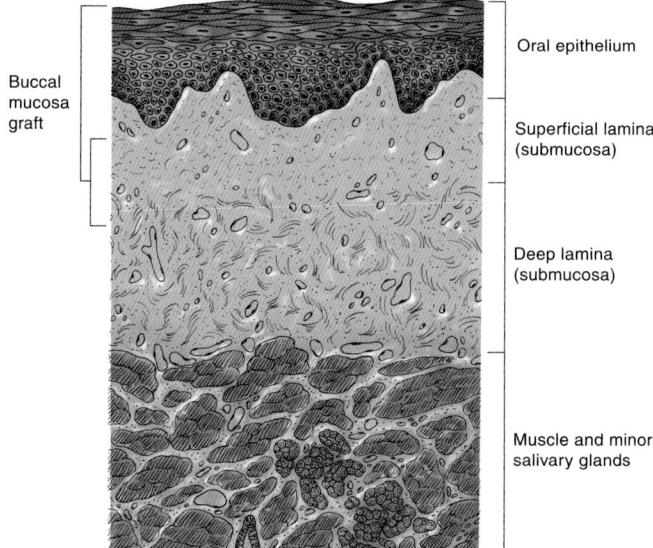

Buccal mucosa graft

Oral epithelium

Superficial lamina (submucosa)

Deep lamina (submucosa)

Muscle and minor salivary glands

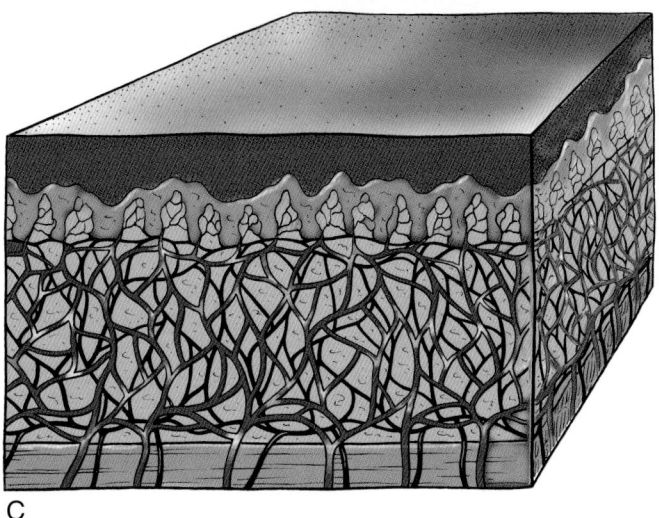

C

Figure 33–1, cont'd. Cross-sectional diagrams of buccal mucosa (**C**).

1.5:1, 2:1, 3:1). For most genital reconstructive surgery, the slits are not for expansion but rather to allow subgraft collections to escape; in some cases, the slits allow the graft to conform better to irregular graft host beds (e.g., the testes in split-thickness skin graft scrotal construction). It has also been proposed that mesh grafts take readily because of increased levels of growth factors, possibly as a function of the slits. In general, full-thickness skin grafts are not meshed.

If a graft is a full-thickness unit, it carries the covering and the superficial dermis or lamina with all the characteristics attributable to that layer. It also, however, carries the deep dermis or deep lamina. In skin, the subdermal plexus is exposed. In most cases, **that plexus is composed of larger vessels that are more sparsely distributed. The graft is thus fastidious in its vascular characteristics.** A full-thickness unit carries most of the lymphatics, and the physical characteristics are likewise carried with the transferred tissue.

If we examine the grafts that are most commonly used in genitourinary reconstructive surgery, **the split-thickness skin graft has favorable vascular characteristics but tends to contract** and be brittle when mature. **The full-thickness skin graft tends to have more fastidious vascular characteristics, but it does not contract as much and is more durable when mature** (Fig. 33–1A). There is a difference between genital full-thickness skin (penile and preputial skin grafts) and extragenital full-thickness skin. This is probably a reflection of the increased mass of the graft in extragenital skin grafts. This increased mass makes the graft more fastidious, and the poor results reported with urethral reconstruction with extragenital full-thickness skin grafts are probably due to poor or ischemic take. The posterior auricular graft (Wolff graft) is an exception to the rule concerning extragenital skin. The postauricular skin is thin and overlies the temporalis fascia and is thought to be carried on numerous perforators. The subdermal plexus of this graft thus mimics the characteristics of the intradermal plexus, and the total mass of the graft is more like that of the split-thickness unit. In the bladder epithelial graft (Fig. 33–1B), there is a superficial and a deep plexus; however, the plexuses are connected by many more perforators. Thus, **bladder epithelial grafts tend to have more favorable vascular characteristics.** In the case of the **buccal mucosal graft, there is a panlaminar plexus.** Thus, **the buccal mucosal graft can be thinned somewhat, provided a sufficient amount of deep lamina is carried to preserve the physical characteristics** (Fig. 33–1C). **The buccal mucosal graft is thought to have optimal vascular characteristics.** The thinned graft diminishes the total graft mass while preserving the physical characteristics and not adversely affecting the vascular characteristics. The enthusiasm for the buccal mucosal graft thus seems well founded. The fact that the graft has a "wet epithelial" surface is likewise thought to be a favorable characteristic for many cases of urethral reconstructive surgery.

A series reporting the use of buccal mucosal onlay grafts with mid- and long-term results seems to suggest durability for these grafts. In that series (Fichtner et al, 2004), 67 patients were described, all with follow-up exceeding 5 years and some with 10 years of follow-up. All failures occurred within 12 months of the original procedure.

The dermal graft has been used for years to augment the tunica albuginea of the corpora cavernosa. When it is harvested, the graft exposes both the intradermal plexus and the deep dermal plexus. The dermal graft thus takes readily (is not fastidious) and has the physical characteristics normal to skin. When it is properly prepared, the tunica vaginalis graft is essentially peritoneum. The tendency of peritoneum to take readily is well documented both in the literature that examines adhesion formation and in the urology literature concerning the application of peritoneal grafts for reconstruction of the urinary tract. With regard to physical characteristics, the literature fails to accurately define what the surgeon can expect. Tunica vaginalis grafts have been shown to be useful for small defects of the tunica albuginea of the corpora cavernosa, but there is a tendency to aneurysmal dilation when they are used for larger defects. Tunica vaginalis grafts have been tried for urethral reconstruction with uniformly poor results.

As described in the urologic literature, vein grafts are perhaps not true grafts according to the terminology used in this chapter. Vein patches are widely used in vascular surgery. The premise is that the vein survives by endothelial direct perfusion and re-establishment of vein wall blood flow by perfusion of the vasa vasorum. The vascular literature is at odds with this concept. The intima is the endothelial layer; it is thin and easily injured during the process of vein harvest and preparation, with areas of endothelial sloughing noted. Inflammatory cells and fibrin adhere to the exposed basement membrane. However, the endothelium does regenerate in the first 6 weeks. The media is a combination of smooth muscle and interlaced collagen. After graft harvest, smooth muscle injury is prominently noted and is thought to be related to warm ischemia. In more mature grafts, much of the smooth muscle is replaced by a process of fibrous transformation with collagen deposition. The adventitia is a loose collagenous network interspersed with vasa vasorum. Mature vein grafts show evidence of take to the vasa vasorum. However, the adventitia becomes incorporated by periadventitial connective tissues. Thrombosis in the vasa vasorum, early in the process of take, is not an unusual phenomenon. When vein grafts are exposed to arterial pressure and shear stress forces, the process colloquially described as "arterialization" occurs and is associated with changes of the vessel wall elastic properties, and the graft becomes rigid with low compliance. Once these changes are noted, at least when veins are used for vessel replacement, the graft remains noncompliant throughout the remaining life of the graft. Vein "grafts" are currently being widely used for replacement of defects of the tunica albuginea of the corpora cavernosa. The pertinent points with regard to the transfer of vein patches to the corpora cavernosa and their long-term behavior, however, have been inferred from the current vascular literature. Dermal grafts have been tried for urethral reconstruction, also with poor results in general. **Rectal mucosal grafts have been proposed for urethral reconstruction. In general, the vascularity of the bowel mucosa is based on the vascularity of the underlying muscle, with the mucosa carried on perforators. Little is found in the literature regarding the process of take of these grafts.**

Tissue can be transferred as a flap. **The term *flap* implies that the tissue is excised and transferred with the blood supply either preserved or surgically re-established at the recipient site.** There is some confusion with regard to the terminology of tissue transfer. Many use the term *graft* to refer to any tissue that is transferred. This confusion probably emanates from the use of the term *graft* to describe the donor

source. For example, the terms *allograft, xenograft, autograft,* and the like are used to define the genetic relationship of transferred tissue to the recipient. However, when one refers to terms of tissue transfer, the term *graft* implies a specific unit of transfer, and thus terms such as *pedicle graft* or *free graft* are confusing. It is best to avoid these terms in discussing tissue transfer.

Flaps can be classified by a number of criteria. We can classify flaps on the basis of their vascularity and thus characterize flaps as either random flaps (Fig. 33–2) **or axial flaps** (Fig. 33–3). **A *random flap* is a flap without a defined cuticular vascular territory.** The flap is carried on the dermal or laminar plexuses; the dimensions of random flaps can vary widely from individual to individual and from body site to body site. **The term *axial flap* means that there is a defined vessel in the base of the flap. There are three types of axial flaps. The direct cuticular axial flap is a flap based on a vessel superficial to the superficial layer of the deep body wall fascia** (Fig. 33–3A). The classic example of a direct cuticular flap is the groin flap. **A musculocutaneous flap** (Fig. 33–4A), **on the other hand, is based on the vascularity to the muscle. The overlying skin paddle is carried on perforators.** If the muscle alone is carried as a flap, the overlying skin survives as a random unit. **The fasciocutaneous system of vascularity** (Fig. 33–4B) **is similar to the musculocutaneous system.** However, the deep blood supply is carried on the fascia (both deep and superficial layers), and the overlying skin paddle is based again on perforators. Thus, one can transfer a fascial flap based on the deep blood supply associated with the flap; the overlying skin, if it is not carried with the flap, remains as a random unit. It has been argued that fascia is relatively avascular and hence cannot serve as "the blood supply" to the fasciocutaneous unit. Indeed, the fascial layer, in reality, acts as a trellis—thus the vessels are carried much like the limbs of a vine.

A flap can also be classified by the elevation technique. A peninsular flap is a flap in which the vascular continuity and the cutaneous continuity of the flap base are left intact (see Figs. 33–2 and 33–3A). **An island flap** (Fig. 33–3B) **is a flap in which the vascular continuity is maintained; however, the cuticular continuity is divided. Thus, a true island flap is elevated on dangling vessels. The microvascular free transfer flap (free flap)** (Fig. 33–3C) **has both the vascular continuity and the cuticular continuity interrupted. The vascular continuity is then re-established at the recipient site.**

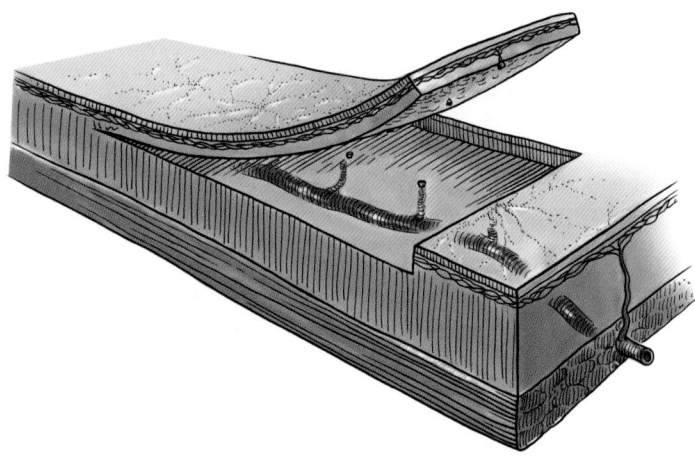

Figure 33–2. Random flap. The arterial perforators have been interrupted, and flap survival depends on the intradermal and subdermal plexuses.

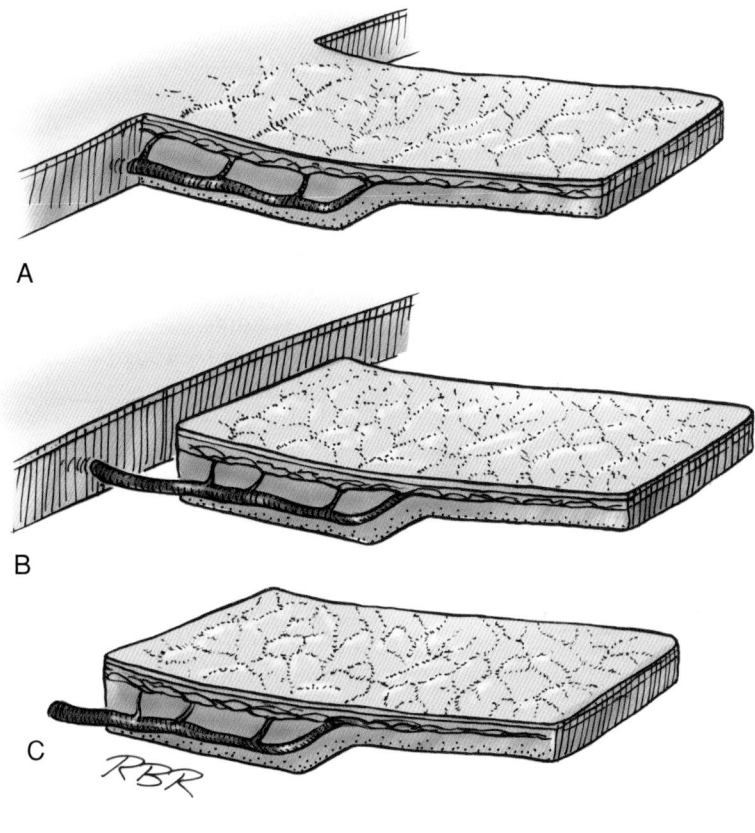

Figure 33–3. Axial flaps. Large vessels enter the base of the flaps. Survival depends on these vessels and on the random distal vascularity. **A,** Peninsula flap. The vascular continuity and the cutaneous continuity in the flap base are intact. **B,** Island flap. The vascular pedicle is intact; the cuticular continuity has been divided. These axial vessels are unsupported (dangling). **C,** Microvascular "free" transfer flap. The free flap cuticular and vascular connections are interrupted at the base of the flap. Vascular continuity is reconstituted in the recipient area by a microsurgical anastomosis. (**A** to **C,** from Jordan GH, et al: Tissue transfer techniques for genitourinary reconstructive surgery. AUA Update Series 1988;7:lesson 10.)

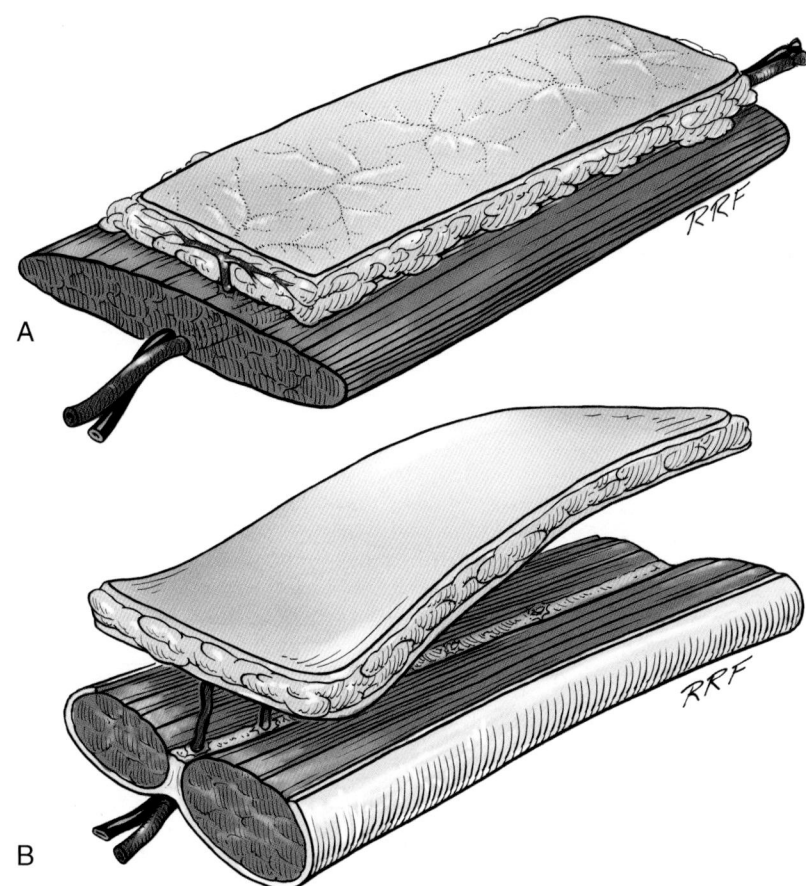

Figure 33–4. **A,** Musculocutaneous flap. Musculocutaneous perforators from the artery to a muscle vascularize the skin and overlying subcutaneous fat. They may be transferred as free flaps but are usually transferred locally, left attached to the vascular pedicle. **B,** Fasciocutaneous flap. Perforating blood vessels from rich plexuses on the superficial and deep aspects of the fascia connect to perforator vessels that communicate with the microvasculature of the overlying paddle. In genital reconstruction, these flaps are based on the dartos fascia of the penis or are free flaps from the forearm. (**A** and **B,** from Jordan GH, et al: Tissue transfer techniques for genitourinary reconstructive surgery. AUA Update Series 1988;7:lesson 10.)

Again, there is confusion in terminology. In genitourinary reconstructive surgical procedures, we tend to use the term *island flap*. As already mentioned, a true island flap is elevated on dangling vessels. The usual case, however, is that a skin island or paddle is elevated either on the muscle, as in the gracilis musculocutaneous flap, or on the fascia, as in local genital skin flaps. The term *island flap* is not synonymous with the terms *skin island* and *skin paddle*. The usefulness of these flaps and grafts is illustrated in the discussion of the surgical techniques in this chapter. There is continued interest in the use of tissue-cultured grafts or "manufactured" grafts. The likelihood of someday, soon, being able to successfully use off-the-shelf grafts or sheets of cultured material is right around the corner (Chen et al, 1999; Atala, 2002; Rotariu et al, 2002; El-Kassaby et al, 2003; Bhargava et al, 2004).

KEY POINTS: PRINCIPLES OF RECONSTRUCTIVE SURGERY

■ Many of the techniques in reconstructive surgery require the transfer of tissue. Tissue transfer implies the movement of tissue for purposes of reconstruction. All tissue has extensibility, inherent tension, and the viscoelastic properties of stress relaxation and creep. These physical characteristics are important in predicting the behavior of transferred tissue.

■ A graft is tissue that has been excised and transferred to a graft host bed, where a new blood supply develops by a process termed take. A flap is tissue that has been excised and transferred with the blood supply preserved or surgically re-established at the recipient site. The grafts that have been successfully used for primary urethral reconstruction are the full-thickness skin graft, the bladder epithelial graft, the buccal mucosal graft, and the rectal mucosal graft. Little is known about the characteristics of the rectal mucosal graft. The bladder epithelial graft and the buccal mucosal graft have a number of properties from the standpoint of vascularity that make them desirable for urethral reconstruction. The issue of desiccation and hypertrophic growth in the case of the bladder epithelial graft has limited its use in the distal urethra.

■ Full-thickness skin and split-thickness skin have been used for penile reconstruction. The results with split-thickness skin are so good that full-thickness grafts are rarely used for coverage of the penis. In complex cases, microvascular free transfer technology has become a mainstay. For urethral reconstruction, skin islands based on the dartos fascia or tunica dartos have been effectively used. The dermal graft has been used for years to augment the tunica albuginea of the corpora cavernosa.

■ The behavior of almost all forms of transfer can be predicted by examination of the histologic features and recognizing what layers provide what characteristics to the tissue.

Anatomy of the Penis and Male Perineum

An understanding of anatomy is of utmost importance to the surgeon performing reconstructive surgery. The anatomic relationships of the male genitourinary structures in the penis and male perineum must precede the discussion of specific reconstructive surgical techniques.

The penile shaft (Fig. 33–5) **comprises three erectile bodies, the two corpora cavernosa and the corpus spongiosum containing the urethra, along with their enveloping fascial layers, nerves, and vessels, all covered by skin.** All these structures continue into the perineum. **The corpora cavernosa make up the bulk of the penis.** They contain erectile tissue within a dense elastic sheath of connective tissue called the tunica albuginea. The corpora cavernosa are not separate structures but constitute a single space with free communication through an incompetent midline septum, composed of multiple strands of elastic tissue similar to that making up the tunica albuginea. The septum becomes more complete toward the base of the penis; the corpora cavernosa become truly independent only as they split to form the crura, which are attached to the inferior ramus of the pubis and ischium.

The erectile tissue containing arteries, nerves, muscle fibers, and venous sinuses lined with flat endothelial cells fills the space of the corpora cavernosa, making its cut surface look like that of a sponge. This tissue is separated from the tunica albuginea by a thin layer of areolar connective tissue. The paired cavernosal arteries run near the center of the corpora cavernosa. Blood is carried by these arteries and returns through the erectile space that connects through numerous anastomotic channels to the corpus spongiosum and venous drainage.

The third erectile body, the corpus spongiosum, lies in the ventral groove between the two corpora cavernosa. The tunica albuginea (adventitia) of the corpus spongiosum is thinner than the tunica albuginea of the corpora cavernosa, and the corpus spongiosum contains less erectile tissue than the corpora cavernosa. The urethra traverses the length of the penis within the corpus spongiosum. At its distal end, the corpus spongiosum expands to form the glans penis, a broad cap of erectile tissue covering the tips of the corpora cavernosa. The urethral meatus is slitlike, lying slightly on the ventral aspect of the tip of the glans, with its long axis oriented vertically. The edge of the glans overhangs the penile shaft, forming a rim called the corona or coronal margin, with the sulcus just proximal. A fold of skin, the frenulum, is attached at the most ventral point, just proximal to the meatus, where the corona forms a distally pointing triangle.

At its base, the penis is supported by two ligaments, composed primarily of elastic fibers that are continuous with the fascia of the penis. Posterior to this attachment, the right and left corpora cavernosa diverge, and the corpus spongiosum broadens between the two crura to form the bulbospongiosus (bulb).

Figure 33–5 also illustrates the relationship of the erectile bodies and the urethra to the structures in the perineum. For the discussion of trauma and reconstruction, it is the **consensus opinion of a World Health Organization conference**

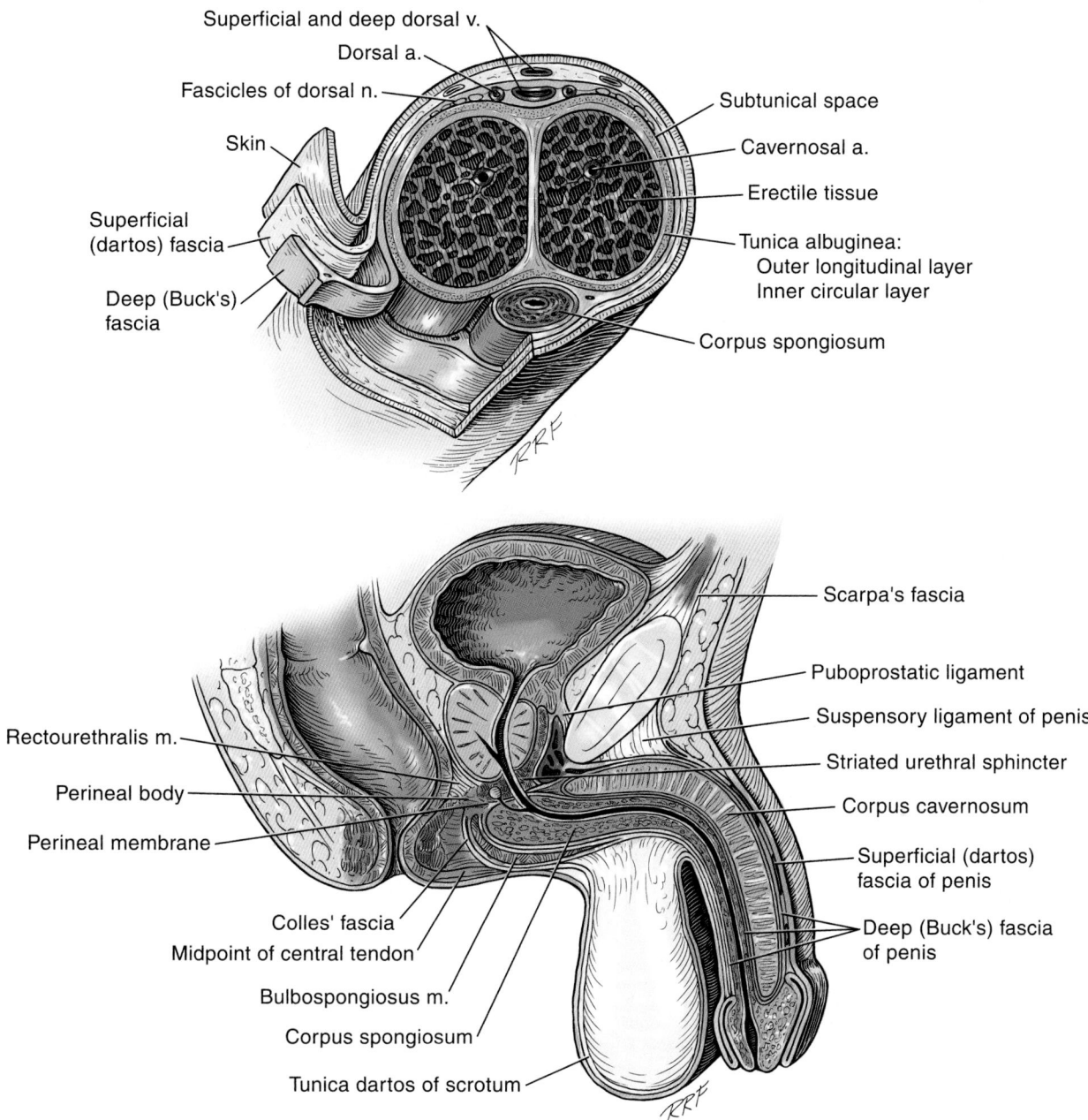

Figure 33–5. *Above,* Cross section of the penis at the junction of its middle and distal thirds. The septum is correctly illustrated as strands that interweave with the tunica albuginea both ventrally and dorsally. *Below,* Diagram of a sagittal section of the penis and perineum illustrating the fascial layers.

convened in Stockholm in 2002 that the common use of the terms *anterior urethra* and *posterior urethra* be departed from and that the urethra be subdivided into six separate areas. These portions of the urethra are numbered in Figure 33–6.

1. The **fossa navicularis** is contained within the spongy erectile tissue of the glans penis and terminates at the junction of the urethral epithelium with the skin of the glans. This portion of the urethra is lined with stratified squamous epithelium.
2. The **penile or pendulous urethra** lies distal to the investment of the ischiocavernosus musculature but is invested by the corpus spongiosum and maintains a con-

stant lumen size roughly centered in the corpus spongiosum. The pendulous urethra is lined with simple squamous epithelium.
3. The **bulbous urethra** is covered by the midline fusion of the ischiocavernosus musculature and is invested by the bulbospongiosus of the corpus spongiosum. It becomes larger and lies closer to the dorsal aspect of the corpus spongiosum, exiting from its dorsal surface before the posterior attachment of the bulbospongiosus to the perineal body. The bulbous urethra is lined distally with squamous epithelium that gradually changes to the transitional epithelium found in the membranous urethra as it swings upward (Devine PC and Horton, 1977).

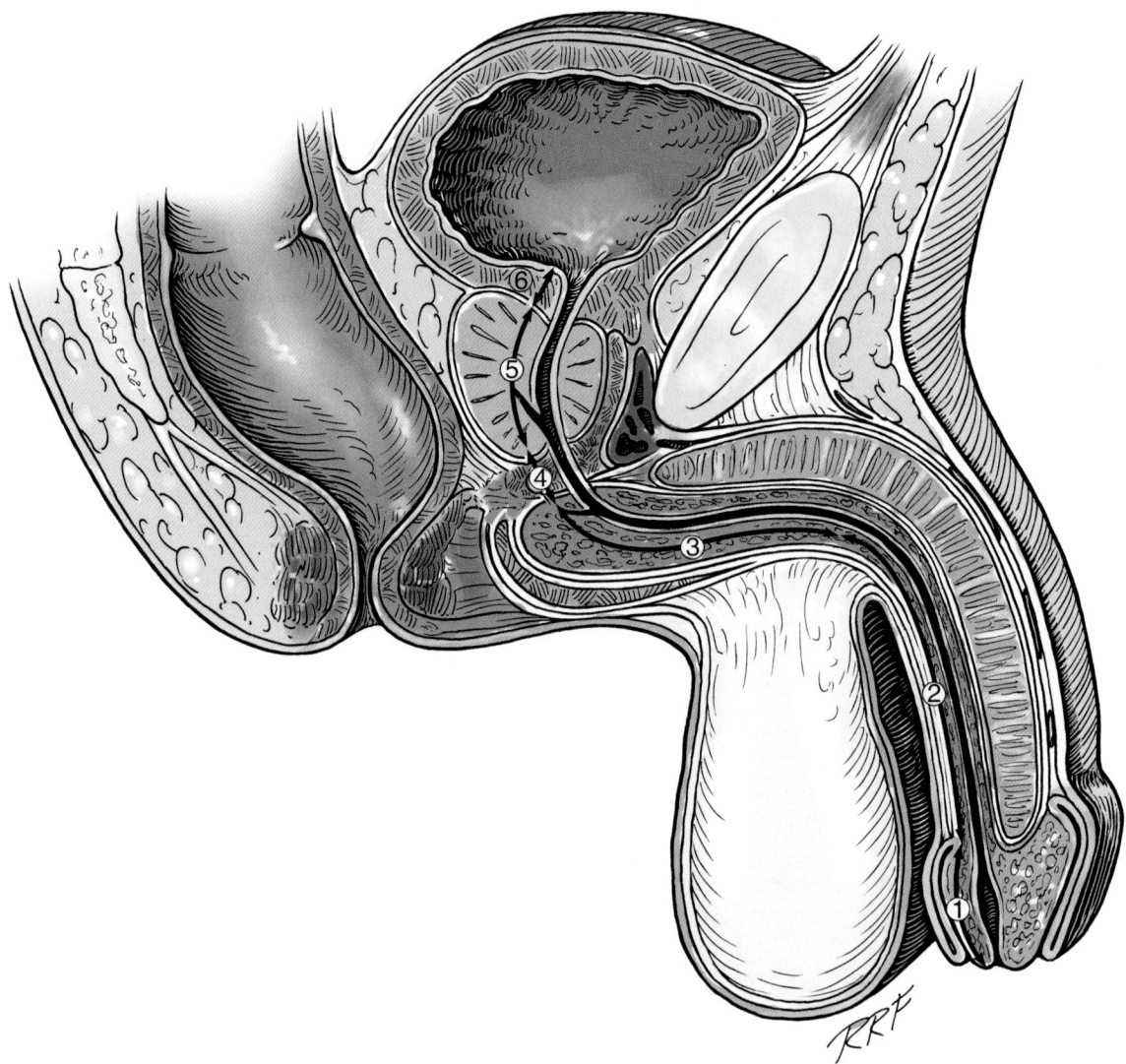

Figure 33–6. Sagittal section of the pelvis. The urethra is subdivided into the following sections: 1, fossa navicularis; 2, pendulous or penile urethra; 3, bulbous urethra; 4, membranous urethra; 5, prostatic urethra; 6, bladder neck. By common usage, the divisions of the fossa navicularis, pendulous urethra, and bulbous urethra compose the anterior urethra; and the divisions of the membranous urethra, prostatic urethra, and bladder neck compose the posterior urethra. (Modified from Devine CJ Jr, Angermeier KW: Anatomy of the penis and male perineum. AUA Update Series 1994;8:11.)

4. The **membranous urethra** is the portion that traverses the perineal pouch and is surrounded by the external urethral sphincter. This segment of the urethra is un-attached to fixed structures, has the distinction of being the only portion of the male urethra that is not invested by another structure, and is lined with a delicate transitional epithelium.

5. The **prostatic urethra,** in common use, is the portion of the urethra that is proximal to the membranous urethra and is mostly surrounded by the prostatic stromal and glandular tissue. Its epithelium is continuous with that of the trigone and bladder.

6. The **bladder neck** is the location of the bladder neck musculature, variably surrounded by intravesical protrusion of the prostate. Its epithelium is contiguous with that of the trigone and bladder.

A submucosal layer is noted throughout the length of the urethra. Five "sphincters" are recognized (Fig. 33–7).

1. If one begins proximally, first there is the bladder neck.
2. The prostate itself is composed of a muscular stroma.
3. The prostate muscle continues into the membranous urethra as the external smooth muscle sphincter.
4. The external rhabdosphincter is often referred to as the external sphincter.
5. In the area of the membranous urethra are the muscles of recruitment, which are not true sphincters but do provide aid with volitional continence.

Numerous glands of Littre open into the urethra along its dorsal surface and are distributed more numerously distally and less proximally. At times, these form small diverticula called lacunae of Morgagni. There is often a larger lacuna magna in the dorsal wall of the fossa navicularis. The ducts of Cowper's glands open into the urethra in the bulb and travel to the glands located in the urogenital membrane adjacent to the membranous urethra.

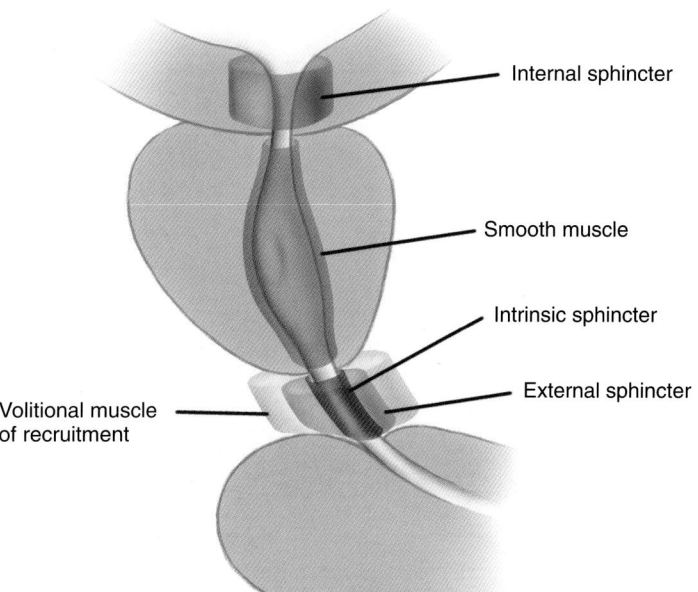

Figure 33–7. Diagrammatic representation of the sphincters surrounding the male posterior urethra.

In the penis, the erectile bodies are surrounded by Buck's fascia, dartos fascia, and skin. Buck's fascia is the tough, elastic layer immediately adjacent to the tunica albuginea (see Fig. 33–5). On the superior aspect of the corpora cavernosa, the deep dorsal vein, paired dorsal arteries, and multiple branches of the dorsal nerves are contained within the envelope of Buck's fascia. In the midline groove on the underside of the corpora cavernosa, Buck's fascia splits to surround the corpus spongiosum. Consolidation of the fascial layers (Fig. 33–8A), lateral to the corpus spongiosum, attaches it to the tunica albuginea of the corpora cavernosa. Attached distally to the undersurface of the glans penis at the corona, Buck's fascia extends into the perineum, enclosing each crus of the corpora cavernosa and the bulb of the corpus spongiosum and firmly fixing these structures to the pubis, ischium, and inferior fascia of the perineal membrane (urogenital diaphragm) (Fig. 33–8C).

Distally, the skin of the penis is confluent with the glabrous skin covering the glans. At the corona, it is folded on itself to form the foreskin (prepuce) that overlies the glans. The dartos fascia, a layer of areolar tissue remarkable for its lack of fat, separates these two layers of skin and continues into the perineum (Fig. 33–8B), where it fuses with the layers of the superficial perineal (Colles') fascia. In the penis, the dartos fascia is loosely attached to the skin and the deeper layer of Buck's fascia and contains the superficial arteries, veins, and nerves of the penis.

Blood is supplied to the skin of the penis by the left and right superficial external pudendal vessels (Fig. 33–9A) that arise from the first portion of the femoral artery, cross the upper medial portion of the femoral triangle, and divide into two main branches, running dorsolaterally and ventrolaterally in the shaft of the penis with collateralization across the midline. At intervals, they give off fine branches to the skin, forming a rich subdermal vascular plexus that can sustain the skin after its underlying dartos fascia has been mobilized. The arteries are accompanied by venous tributaries that are more prominent and easily seen than the arteries. Because of its remarkable thinness and mobility and the character of its vascular supply, the skin covering the penis is an ideal substitute, in some cases, for urethral reconstruction. A flap of skin can be elevated and the fascia containing its blood supply can be mobilized to construct a subcutaneous pedicle, allowing distal islands of preputial or penile skin to be transferred to virtually any part of the urethra. **The blood supply to the scrotal wall and ventral penile skin is based on the posterior scrotal artery, a superficial vessel from the deep internal pudendal artery (Fig. 33–9B).** As with the superficial external pudendal tributaries, the posterior scrotal system provides a series of tributaries carried within the tunica dartos.

Venous Drainage

The penis is drained by three venous systems: superficial, intermediate, and deep (Fig. 33–10) (Aboseif et al, 1989). The superficial veins contained in the dartos fascia on the dorsolateral aspects of the penis unite at its base to form a single superficial dorsal vein. The superficial dorsal vein usually drains into the left saphenous vein, rarely into the right, and occasionally forms two trunks that drain into both. Veins from more superficial tissue may drain into the external superficial pudendal veins.

The intermediate system contains the deep dorsal and circumflex veins, lying within and beneath Buck's fascia. Emissary veins begin within the erectile space of the corpora cavernosa and, following a perpendicular or oblique course through the tunica albuginea, emerge from the lateral and dorsal surfaces of the corpora cavernosa to empty into the circumflex veins or the deep dorsal vein. The circumflex veins are channels, usually more prominently present in the distal two thirds of the penile shaft. They arise from the corpus spongiosum, on the ventrum of the penis, and often receive the emissary veins as they travel around the lateral aspect of the corpora cavernosa, passing beneath the dorsal arteries and

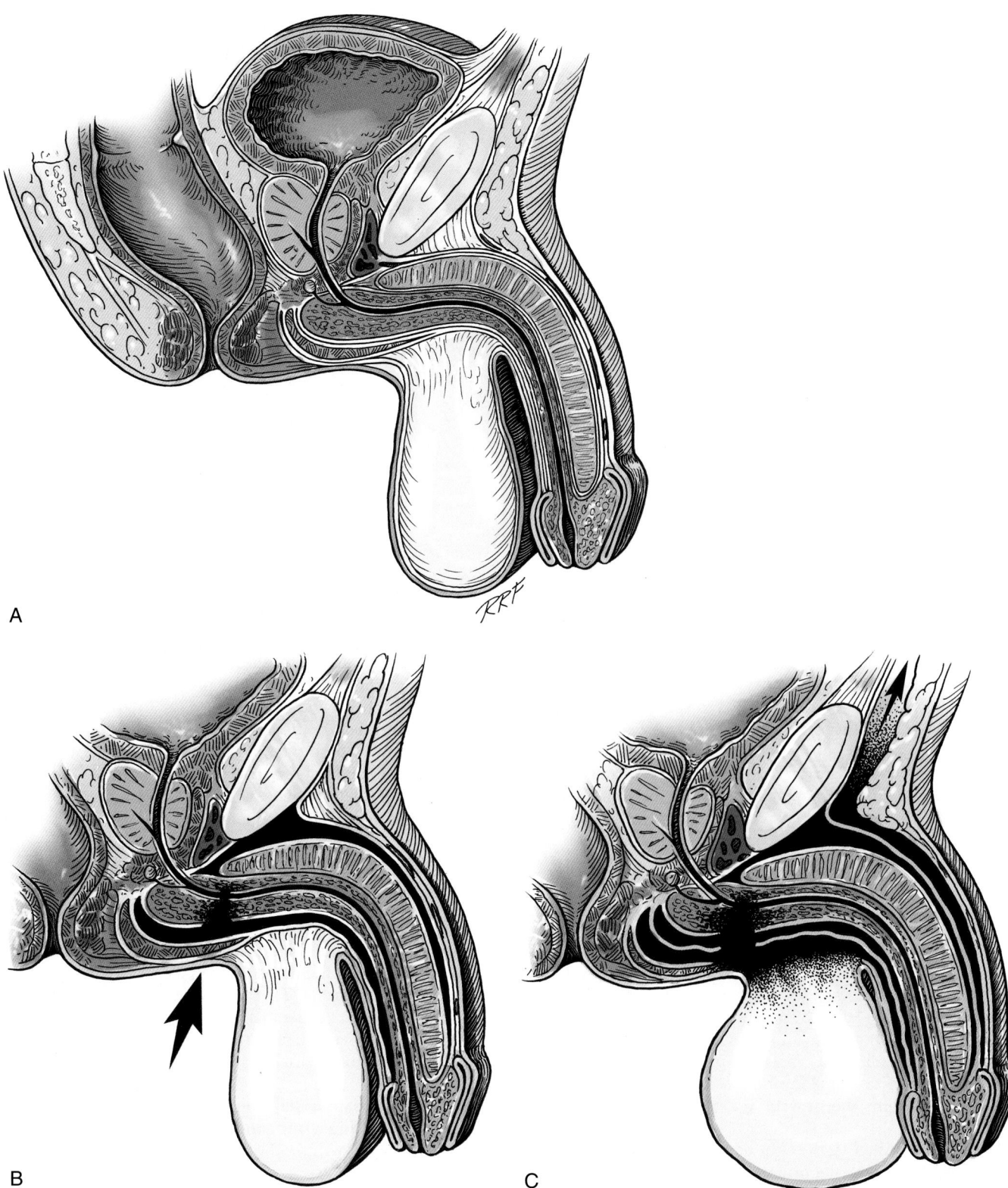

A

B

C

Figure 33–8. Cross sections of the pelvis. **A** illustrates the normal attachment of the fasciae enveloping the penile structures. The dartos fascia is contiguous with Scarpa's fascia onto the abdomen, with the tunica dartos of the scrotum, with Colles' fascia on the perineum, and over the thigh eventually to insert at the fascia lata. **B,** With trauma to the pelvis or perineum, the corpus spongiosum is injured; the hematoma, however, is confined by the attachment of Buck's fascia. **C,** With trauma to the perineum or pelvis, the corpus spongiosum is injured and Buck's fascia is violated; the hematoma thus can spread throughout the confines of the extended dartos fascia–tunica dartos system.

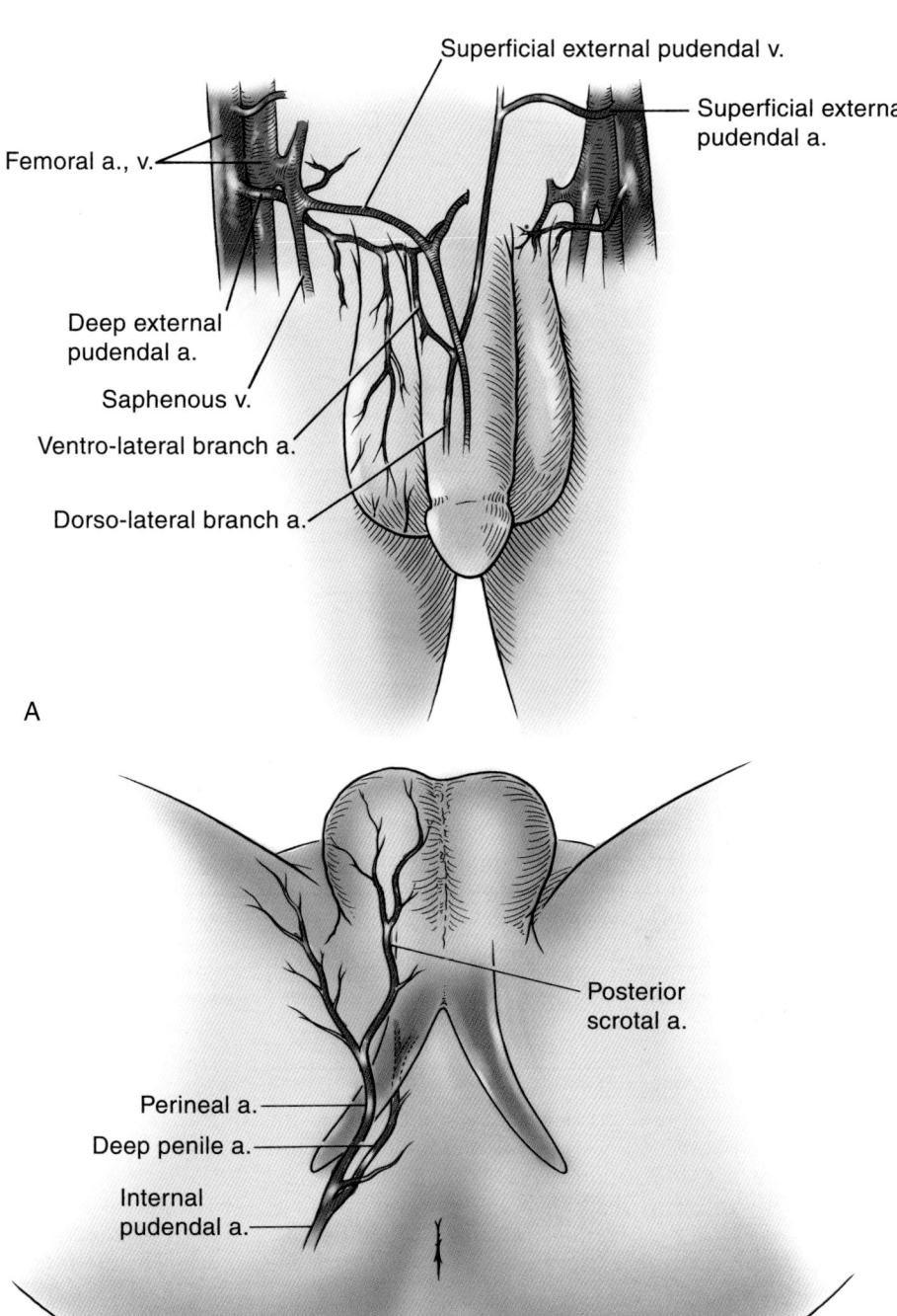

Figure 33–9.   Illustration of the vasculature to the genital skin. **A,** The superficial external pudendal vessels arborize to become the fascial blood supply contained in the dartos fascia of the penis. **B,** The scrotal artery is a terminal branch of the deep internal pudendal artery. This artery is thought to arborize in the tunica dartos of the scrotum and Colles' fascia of the perineum. The perineal artery continues lateral to the groin crease onto the thigh and extends toward the groin.

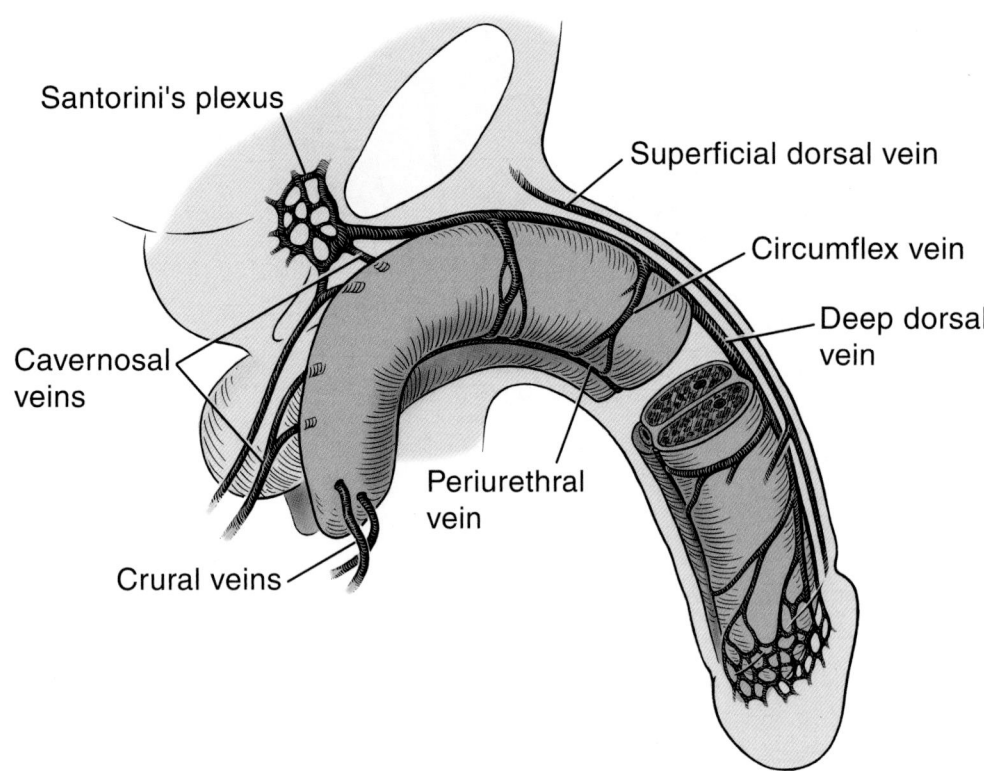

Santorini's plexus

Superficial dorsal vein

Circumflex vein

Deep dorsal vein

Cavernosal veins

Periurethral vein

Crural veins

Figure 33–10. Diagram illustrates the venous drainage of the deep structures of the penis. (From Horton CE, Stecker JF, Jordan GH: Management of erectile dysfunction, genital reconstruction following trauma and transsexualism. In McCarthy JG, ed: Plastic Surgery, vol 6. Philadelphia, WB Saunders, 1990:4213-4245.)

nerves to empty into the deep dorsal vein. They communicate with one another and those of the opposite side to form 3 to 12 common venous channels, usually accompanied by branches of the dorsal nerve and artery. The circumflex veins can also become confluent ventrally, forming periurethral veins on each side. These may become important in the treatment of impotence caused by veno-occlusive incompetence.

The deep dorsal vein is formed by five to eight small veins emerging from the glans penis to form the retrocoronal plexus, which drains into the deep dorsal vein lying in the midline groove between the corporal bodies. In a number of patients, there is a connection between the superficial and deep dorsal veins. In the shaft of the penis, the deep dorsal vein often consists of two and sometimes three tributaries that anastomose with each other. The vein gathers blood from the emissary and circumflex veins, and passing beneath the pubis at the level of the suspensory ligament, it leaves the shaft of the penis at the crus and drains into the periprostatic plexus.

The deep drainage system consists of the crural and cavernosal veins. The crural veins arise in the midline, in the space between the crura. Normally, they are small and almost indiscernible, joining the deep dorsal vein or the periprostatic plexus. If the deep dorsal vein has been ligated or obliterated after trauma, striking development of these veins can be noted as the intracrural space is entered during the perineal dissection for urethral repair. Emissary veins in the proximal third of the crura, near their attachment to the ischial tuberosities, join to form several thin-walled trunks on the dorsomedial surface of each corpus cavernosum. Some pass medially, joining the dorsal or crural veins, or extend proximally, entering the periprostatic plexus. Most consolidate into one or two cavernosal veins on each side. Running in the penile hilum, deep and medial to the cavernosal arteries and nerves, they join

to form a large venous channel that drains into the internal pudendal vein. Three or four small cavernosal veins emerge from the dorsolateral surface of each crus and course laterally between the bulbospongiosus and the crus of the penis for 2 to 3 cm before draining into the internal pudendal veins. These usually insignificant vessels become larger, and can be noted more readily, in patients with veno-occlusive erectile dysfunction. The internal pudendal veins (usually two) run together with the internal pudendal artery and nerve in Alcock's canal to empty into the internal iliac vein.

Arterial System

The blood supply to the deep structures of the penis is derived from the common penile artery, which is a continuation of the internal pudendal artery after it gives off its perineal branch (Fig. 33–11). **From that point, the artery is termed the common penile artery** and travels along the medial margin of the inferior pubic ramus. As it nears the urethral bulb, the artery divides into its three terminal branches, as follows:

The bulbourethral artery is a short artery or arteries of relatively large caliber that pierce Buck's fascia to enter the bulbospongiosus. These arteries are oriented almost parallel to the path of the membranous urethra.

The dorsal artery generally travels along the dorsum of the penis between the deep dorsal vein medially and the dorsal nerves laterally, with a coiled rather than a straight configuration. The artery uncoils as the penis elongates with erection, allowing flow to be maintained. Along its course, it gives off 3 to 10 circumflex branches (the circumflex cavernosal arteries) that accompany the circumflex veins around the lateral surface of the corpora cavernosa and that provide vascularity to the corpus

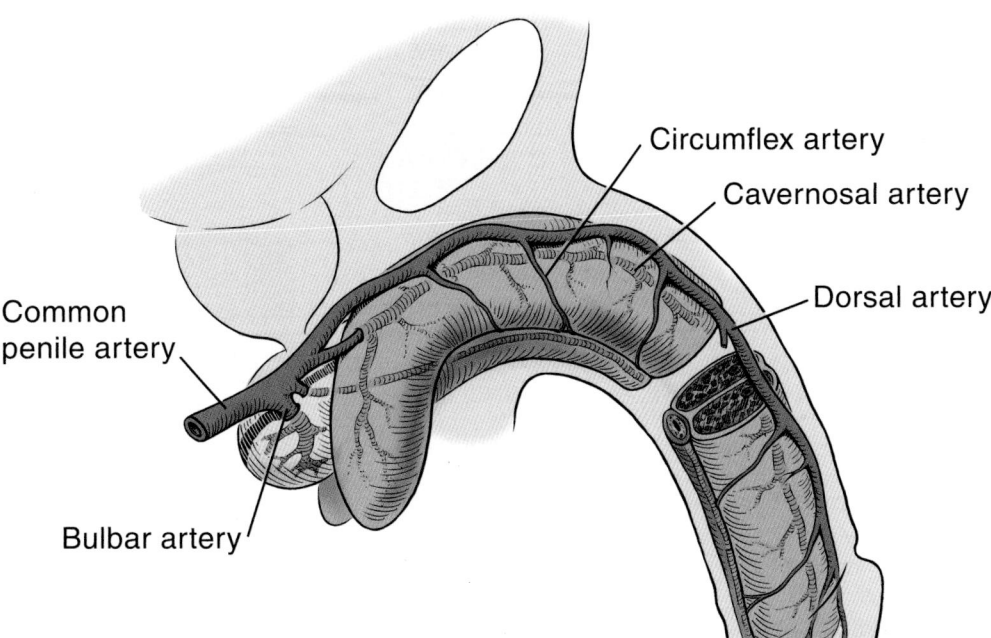

Circumflex artery

Cavernosal artery

Dorsal artery

Common penile artery

Bulbar artery

Figure 33–11. Diagram illustrates the arterial supply to the deep structures of the penis. (From Horton CE, Stecker JF, Jordan GH: Management of erectile dysfunction, genital reconstruction following trauma and transsexualism. In McCarthy JG, ed: Plastic Surgery, vol 6. Philadelphia, WB Saunders, 1990:4213-4245.)

spongiosum. Its terminal branches arborize in the glans penis. In many patients, branches penetrate the tunica and connect to the cavernosal arteries. The functional significance of these perforators varies from individual to individual.

The cavernosal artery, usually a single artery, arises on each side as the terminal branch of the penile artery. It enters the corpus cavernosum at the hilum and runs the length of the penile shaft, giving off the many helicine arteries that constitute the arterial portion of the erectile apparatus. The arteries frequently branch before entering the corporal body. Sometimes a branch enters the opposite corpus cavernosum, and occasionally a single artery branches in the penile shaft to supply both sides.

Lymphatics

Lymph drainage from the glans penis collects in large trunks in the area of the frenulum. The lymph vessels circle to the dorsal aspect of the corona, where they unite with those from the other side. The vessels traverse the penis beneath Buck's fascia, terminating mostly in the deep inguinal lymph nodes of the femoral triangle. Some drainage is to the presymphyseal lymph nodes and by way of these to the lateral lymph nodes of the external iliac group.

Nerve Supply

The nerves of the penis are derived from the pudendal and cavernosal nerves. The pudendal nerves supply somatic motor and sensory innervation to the penis. The cavernosal nerves are a combination of the parasympathetic and visceral afferent fibers and constitute the autonomic nerves of the penis. These provide the nerve supply to the erectile apparatus.

The pudendal nerves enter the perineum with the internal pudendal vessels through the lesser sciatic notch at the posterior border of the ischiorectal fossa. They run in the fibrofascial pudendal canal of Alcock to the edge of the urogenital diaphragm. Each dorsal nerve of the penis arises in Alcock's canal as the first branch of the pudendal nerve. Traveling ventral to the main pudendal trunk above the internal obturator and under the levator ani, the dorsal nerves perforate the transverse perinei muscles to attain the dorsum of the penis and continue distally along the respective dorsolateral penile surface lateral to the dorsal artery. On the shaft, their fascicles fan out to supply proprioceptive and sensory nerve terminals in the tunica of the corpora cavernosa and sensory terminals in the skin. These nerves terminate in the glans penis.

The autonomic innervation of the pelvic organs and external genitalia arises from the pelvic plexus. The plexus is formed by preganglionic parasympathetic visceral efferent and afferent fibers arising from the sacral center (S2-4) and sympathetic preganglionic afferent and visceral afferent fibers arising from the thoracolumbar center (T11-L2). Beyond the prostate, the parasympathetic nerves, the cavernosal nerves, run adjacent to and through the wall of the membranous urethra. As they pierce the perineal membrane, these nerves pass close to and supply Cowper's gland before entering the corpora cavernosa, where they are readily identified in the hilum of the penis, dorsomedial to the cavernosal arteries.

Perineum

The perineum is the diamond-shaped outlet bounded anteriorly by the pubic arch and the arcuate ligaments of the pubis, posteriorly by the tip of the coccyx, and laterally by the inferior rami of the pubis and ischium. A transverse line between the ischial tuberosities divides the perineum into

an anterior triangle containing the external urogenital organs and a posterior anal triangle (Fig. 33–12*A* and *B*).

Colles' Fascia. In the anterior triangle, Colles' fascia (Fig. 33–12*A*) attaches at its posterior margin to the perineal body at the posteroinferior margin of the urogenital diaphragm. The fascia curves below the superficial transverse perinei muscles and projects forward as two layers attached laterally to the ischium and the inferior ramus of the pelvis. The loose superficial layer is fatty and is continuous with the more substantial dartos fascia (tuncia dartos) of the scrotum. In the scrotum, the dartos fascial layer contains muscle fibers that cause the rugous appearance of the scrotum. The fascia also projects (but without muscle fibers) into the midline, to form the septum between the halves of the scrotum. The median raphe in the skin delineates the separation of the halves of the scrotum and is continued anteriorly as a darkly colored streak in the ventral midline of the penis and posteriorly as the median raphe of the perineum terminating at the anus.

The deep membranous layer of Colles' fascia is a more substantial layer that forms a roof over the scrotal cavity, separating it from the superficial perineal pouch. At the anterior aspect of the scrotum, Colles' fascia joins with the dartos fascia (tunica dartos) of the scrotum, and a fold of this fascia projects backward beneath the fibers of the bulbospongiosus muscle. At the base of the penis, it is continuous with the dartos fascia of the penis. Thickenings of the fascia at this level form the two suspensory ligaments of the penis. First, the outer fundiform ligament, which is continuous with the lower end of the linea alba, splits into laminae that surround the body of the penis and unite beneath it. Second, the inner triangle-shaped suspensory ligament is attached to the anterior aspect of the symphysis pubis and blends with the dartos fascia of the penis below it.

Anteriorly, Colles' fascia fuses and becomes continuous with the membranous layer of the subcutaneous connective tissue of the anterior abdominal wall (Scarpa's fascia). Laterally, Colles' fascia fuses to the pubic arch and with the fascia lata. Posteriorly, Colles' fascia sweeps beneath the transverse perinei muscles, fusing with the posterior aspect of the perineal membrane. The space beneath the continuous plane formed by these fascial attachments is the superficial perineal pouch, in which infections or extravasation of urine and collections of blood after trauma to the urethra may be confined (see Fig. 33–8*B* and *C*).

Superficial Perineal Space. In males, the superficial perineal space contains the continuation of the corpora cavernosa, the proximal part of the corpus spongiosum and urethra, the muscles associated with them, and the branches of the internal pudendal vessels and pudendal nerves (Fig. 33–12*B*).

The ischiocavernous muscles cover the crura of the corpora cavernosa. They attach to the inner surfaces of the ischium and ischial tuberosities on each side and insert at the midline into Buck's fascia, surrounding the crura at their junction below the arcuate ligament of the penis. The midline fusion of the ischiocavernosus muscles–bulbospongiosus muscles is in the midline of the perineum. They are attached to the perineal body posteriorly and to each other in the midline, as they encompass the bulbospongiosus and crura of the corpora cavernosa at the base of the penis. These muscles are confluent with the ischiocavernous muscles laterally and

at their insertion into Buck's fascia, covering the dorsal vessels and nerves at the base of the penis.

Central Perineal Tendon (Perineal Body). Lying just anterior to the anus, as a part of the plane separating the anterior and posterior perineal triangles, the **perineal body is formed**

KEY POINTS: ANATOMY OF THE PENIS AND MALE PERINEUM

■ An understanding of the anatomy is of utmost importance to the surgeon. The penile shaft is composed of three erectile bodies, the paired corpora cavernosa and the corpus spongiosum. The corpus spongiosum invests the anterior urethra.

■ By consensus, the urethra has been subdivided into six separate areas: the fossa navicularis, the penile or pendulous urethra, the bulbous urethra, the membranous urethra, the prostatic urethra, and the bladder neck.

■ In the male, five urethral "sphincters" are recognized. If one begins proximally, there is the bladder neck. The prostate itself is composed of a muscular stroma. The prostatic muscle continues into the membranous urethra as the external smooth muscle sphincter. The external rhabdosphincter is often referred to as the external sphincter, and in the area of the membranous urethra are the muscles of recruitment that are not true sphincters.

■ Buck's fascia is devoted to the deep structures of the penis. The more areolar and superficial fascia, the dartos fascia, is much more related to the skin and its vasculature.

■ The blood supply to the deep structures of the penis is based on the common penile artery, which is the extension of the deep internal pudendal artery. The blood supply to the skin of the genitalia is based on the perineal branch–scrotal branch of the deep internal pudendal artery as well as the superficial external pudendal vessels, branches of the femoral arteries. The penis is drained by three systems: the superficial, intermediate, and deep venous systems.

■ The nerves to the penis are derived from the pudendal and the cavernosal nerves. The pudendal nerve supplies somatic motor and sensory innervation to the penis. The cavernosal nerves are a combination of the parasympathetic and the visceral afferent fibers and constitute the autonomic nerves to the penis.

■ The perineum is a diamond-shaped outlet bounded anteriorly by the pubic arch and the circuate ligaments of the pubis, posteriorly by the tip of the coccyx, and laterally by the inferior rami of the pubis and ischium. A transverse line between the ischial tuberosities divides the perineum into an anterior triangle containing the external urogenital organs and a posterior anal triangle.

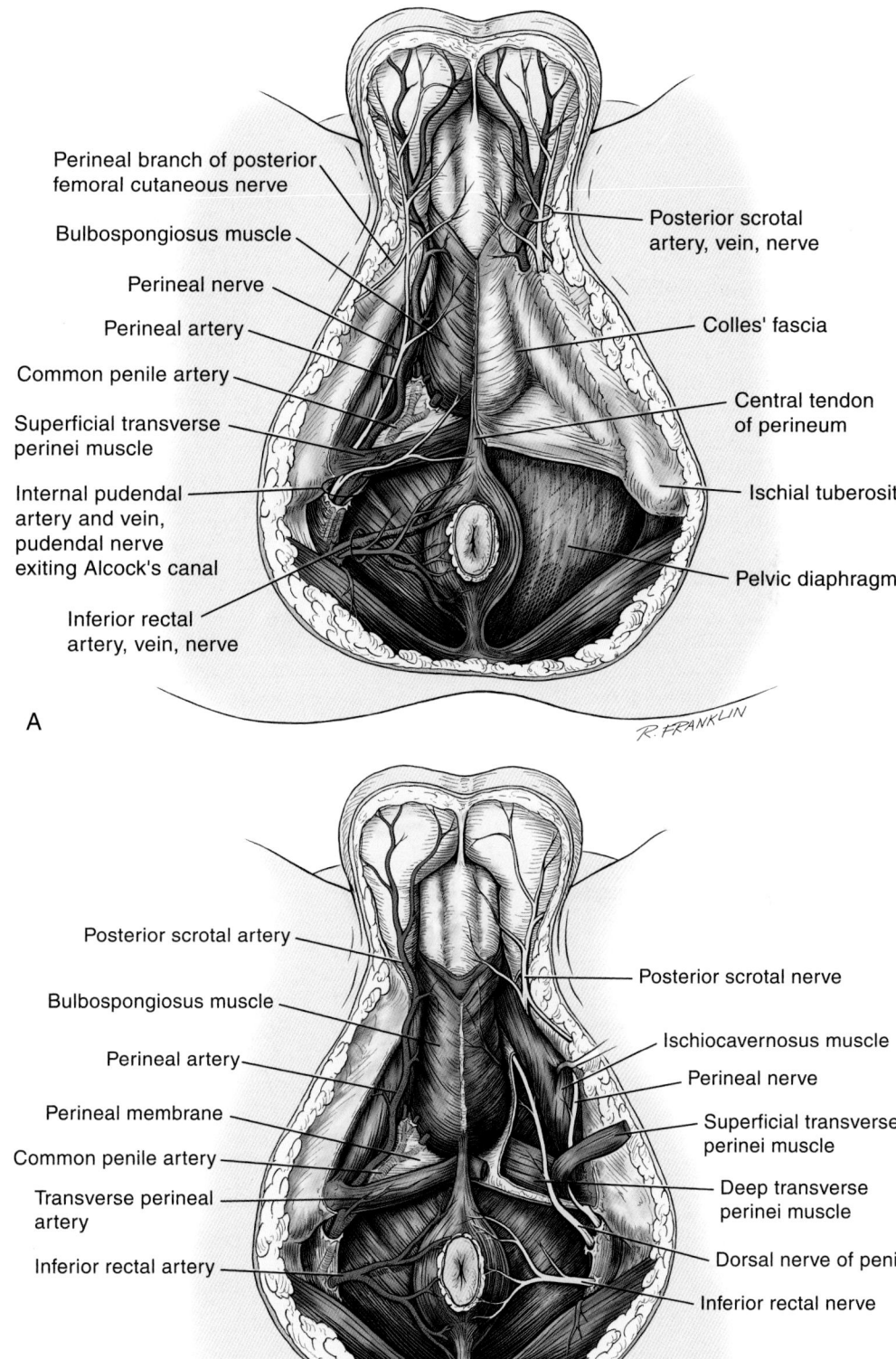

Perineal branch of posterior femoral cutaneous nerve

Bulbospongiosus muscle

Perineal nerve

Perineal artery

Common penile artery

Superficial transverse perinei muscle

Internal pudendal artery and vein, pudendal nerve exiting Alcock's canal

Inferior rectal artery, vein, nerve

Posterior scrotal artery, vein, nerve

Colles' fascia

Central tendon of perineum

Ischial tuberosity

Pelvic diaphragm

A

R. FRANKLIN

Figure 33–12. "Peel-away" diagrams of the anatomy of the perineum. **A,** The skin and subcuticular tissues have been removed. **B,** In the anterior perineal triangle, Colles' fascia has been removed. In the posterior anal triangle, the pelvic diaphragm has been removed. Note the division of the superficial transverse perinei muscle, exposing the deep transverse perinei muscle.

Continued

Posterior scrotal artery

Bulbospongiosus muscle

Perineal artery

Perineal membrane

Common penile artery

Transverse perineal artery

Inferior rectal artery

Posterior scrotal nerve

Ischiocavernosus muscle

Perineal nerve

Superficial transverse perinei muscle

Deep transverse perinei muscle

Dorsal nerve of penis

Inferior rectal nerve

B

R. FRANKLIN

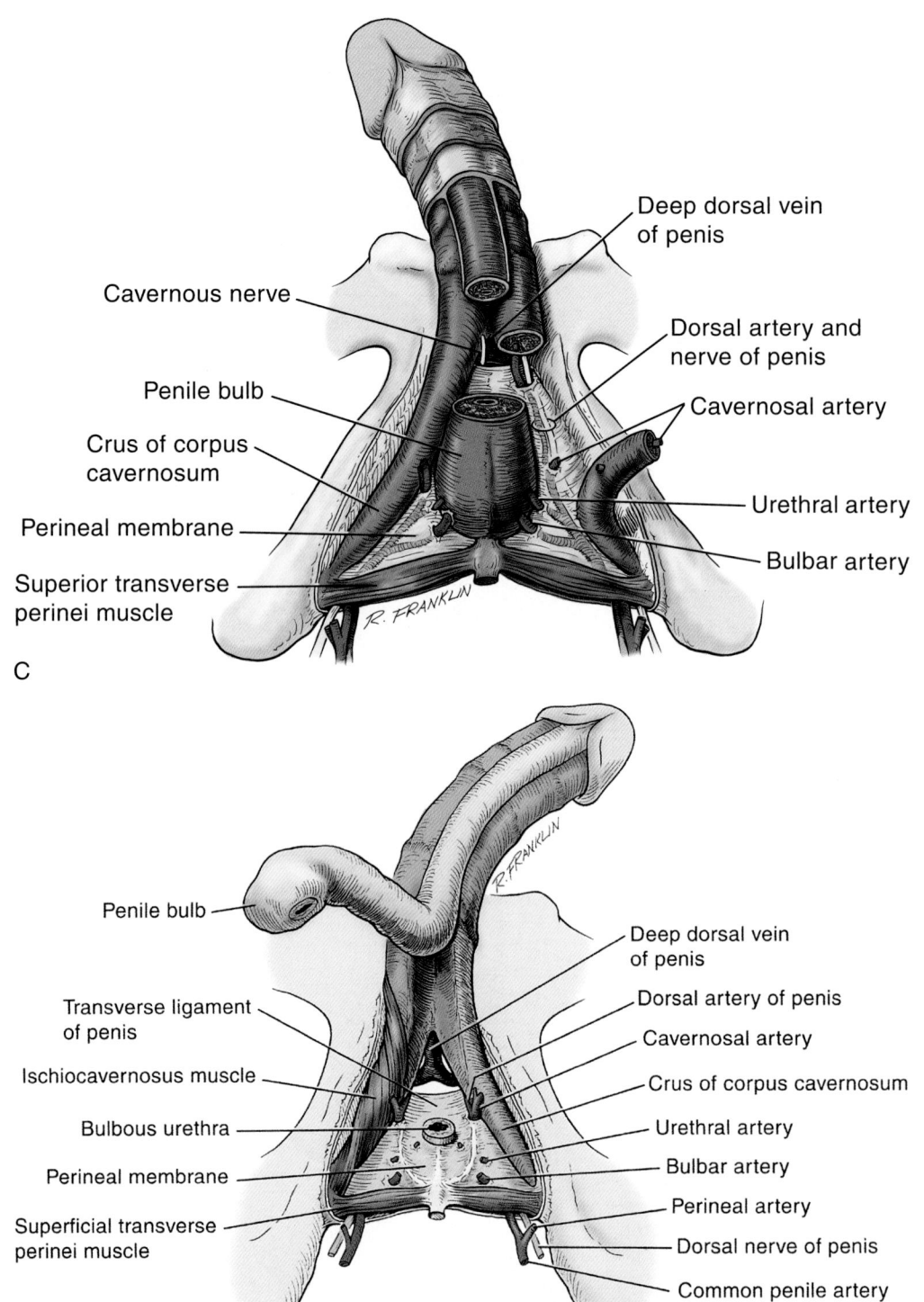

Deep dorsal vein of penis

Cavernous nerve

Dorsal artery and nerve of penis

Penile bulb

Cavernosal artery

Crus of corpus cavernosum

Urethral artery

Perineal membrane

Bulbar artery

Superior transverse perinei muscle

R. FRANKLIN

C

Penile bulb

Deep dorsal vein of penis

Dorsal artery of penis

Cavernosal artery

Transverse ligament of penis

Crus of corpus cavernosum

Ischiocavernosus muscle

Urethral artery

Bulbous urethra

Bulbar artery

Perineal membrane

Perineal artery

Superficial transverse perinei muscle

Dorsal nerve of penis

Common penile artery

R. FRANKLIN

D

Figure 33–12, cont'd. C, The anterior perineal triangle has been dissected to expose the erectile bodies. **D,** The corpus spongiosum has been divided at the departure of the urethra from the penile bulb. The intracrural space is exposed. (**A** to **D,** from Devine CJ Jr, Angermeier KW: Anatomy of the pelvis and male perineum. AUA Update Series 1994; 13:1015.)

by the interconnection of eight muscles of the perineum (Fig. 33–12A and B). **The perineal body receives fibers from the anterior portion of the anal sphincter and is the central point of insertion of the superficial transverse perinei muscles that arise at the ischial tuberosities.** The bulbospongiosus muscle (midline fusion of the ischiocavernosus muscle) is fixed to the perineal body by its most posterior fibers. The deep transverse perinei muscles and fibers from the anterior portions of the levator ani muscles attach to the deep aspect of the perineal body.

Deep Perineal Space. The urogenital diaphragm constitutes the deep perineal space (Fig. 33–12C and D). It is contained within two layers of fascia and incompletely covers the outlet of the pelvis anterior to the deep layer of the perineal body. The deep layer of fascia is an indistinct structure—the continuation of the endopelvic obturator fascia. The superficial fascia attaches laterally to the ischial rami and the inferior ramus of the pubis. This fascia blends with the deep layer behind the perineal body and anteriorly, where it terminates with a thickened edge, the transverse perineal ligament. A space between this ligament and the arcuate ligament of the pubis accommodates the deep dorsal vein of the penis.

The deep perineal pouch (Fig. 33–13; see also Fig. 33–12D) contains the deep transverse perinei muscles, the external sphincter of the urethra, the bulbourethral (Cowper's) glands, and the blood vessels and nerves associated with the structures within it. The sphincter urethral muscle fibers arise from the medial surface of the inferior pubic rami and pass medially toward the urethra, where they meet the fibers from the opposite side. In males, the muscle encircles the membranous urethra to function as the somatic sphincter of the urethra.

Generalities of Reconstructive Surgical Techniques

With any surgical procedure, there are basic rules and surgeons' biases as to the best way to perform a certain operation.

Certainly, this is true for reconstructive procedures of the external genitalia. In this section, the differences are highlighted.

Reconstructive surgery is performed with all efforts aimed at minimizing tissue injury and promoting healing. Adequate visualization is essential. Surgical loupes are used by almost all surgeons performing both adult and pediatric reconstructive genital surgery. A headlight or suction with attached light often adds to visualization, especially in deep perineal surgery. Both monopolar and bipolar cauteries are appropriate, depending on the procedure. In penile cases such as reconstruction of the fossa navicularis or correction of penile curvature, bipolar cautery is used exclusively. With cautery, the electric charge is grounded either to a pad (monopolar) or to the opposite tong of the forceps (bipolar). It is easy to see that in most instances, the field effects of the electricity are more confined with bipolar cautery. Because electricity is dissipated by conductors (in the case of human tissue, vessels and nerves), there is a possibility of damage to these delicate structures. In other cases, monopolar cautery can be used in the superficial structures, but bipolar cautery is better during dissection around the corpus spongiosum, elevation of penile and scrotal flaps, division of the perineal intracorporal space, and dissection of the dorsal neurovascular structures.

In general, the typical instruments that are used for open urologic surgery are inadequate for genital reconstructive surgery. Appropriate instruments can be found in a plastic surgery tray or on the peripheral vascular tray in the typical operating room. Some examples are fine tenotomy scissors, fine forceps, a variety of skin hooks, and delicate needle holders. Sharp scissors that cut with minimal collateral trauma are essential. These instruments minimize tissue injury from manipulation and permit more precise dissection. For urethral surgery, a set of bougie à boule sizers is essential to check the caliber of the urethral lumen. McCrea urethral sounds are a nice addition to the typical van Buren sounds available in the usual operating room. For calibration, sounds do not replace the need for bougie à boule calibrators. For

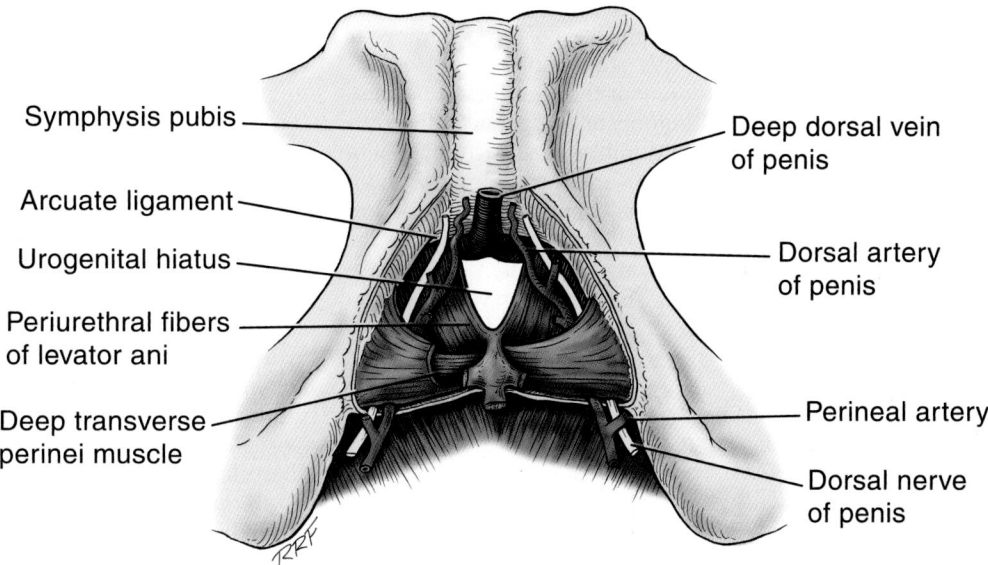

Figure 33–13. Illustration of the infrapubic space. The urethra has been dissected, as has the perineal diaphragm. (From Devine CJ Jr, Angermeier KW: Anatomy of the penis and male perineum. AUA Update Series 1994;8:11.)

Symphysis pubis

Arcuate ligament

Urogenital hiatus

Periurethral fibers of levator ani

Deep transverse perinei muscle

Deep dorsal vein of penis

Dorsal artery of penis

Perineal artery

Dorsal nerve of penis

posterior urethral reconstruction, a sound to pass through the cystostomy tract and prostate to find the proximal end for the reconstruction is often helpful. We find that a Haygrove staff serves this role nicely. Some centers use the cystoscope for this purpose, and often it suffices well, whereas at other times it is not as effective as the Haygrove-style sound. The Gelman sound* is essentially a Haygrove staff with a lumen that allows a true 16 French flexible scope to pass through it, offering the advantages of endoscopy with the convenient "round sound" shape.

The choice of suture material clearly evolves on the basis of the surgeon's experience and bias. However, there are some common principles with which most surgeons would agree. First, in urethral surgery, absorbable suture is the rule. Typical choices for most surgeons are braided absorbable sutures or the family of monofilament absorbable sutures. Chromic suture is rarely used now as the choices of other absorbable sutures seem superior in virtually all cases. Thus, in the case of tension-free closures, very small sutures can be used. In some cases, tying the suture can be awkward, and thus a larger suture may be warranted, even though the anastomosis is tension free. The caliber of suture should be the smallest possible to line up the tissue, which is typically not under tension. There is no reason to use suture that is stronger than the tissues that are being sutured. Fine suture such as 5-0 and 6-0 chromic or polyglactin can be used to suture the epithelium to the adventitia of the corpus spongiosum to control bleeding. For a flap or graft repair, 4-0 to 6-0 suture is usually adequate. For primary anastomosis of the corpus spongiosum or for a posterior urethral reconstruction, 3-0 suture may be appropriate because of tying concerns. The needle should be tapered if possible except when, as in urethroplasty, for example, severe spongiofibrosis or scarring is present. Some of the typical choices are taper needles, such as RB-1, TF, and SH-1, and cutting needles, such as P-3 and PC-3. The UR-6 half-circle taper needle that is often used in radical prostatectomy can be helpful for deep perineal anastomosis of the urethra.

Surgical position and retraction are critical to attaining good results. If possible, procedures are done with the patient supine or prone. Many procedures that previously were done with the patient in the lithotomy position can be done with the patient in the frog-leg or split-leg position. For penile surgery, a Scott retractor with stay hooks,[†] the Jordan-Bookwalter perineal retractor set,[‡] or the Omni-Tract perineal retractor[§] is often helpful. Lithotomy or exaggerated lithotomy positions are used only for the minimal time necessary. With appropriate padding for the foot and positioning without pressure on the back of the leg, the complications in the low lithotomy position are minimal. When the patient is in the supine, split-leg, and low lithotomy positions, venous compression stockings can be used. The controversy in positioning revolves around the use of the exaggerated lithotomy

position. It is our preference to use this position for all bulbar and posterior urethral reconstructions. Other surgeons use a lower lithotomy position. We find the more exaggerated position to be safe and believe that it provides unequaled access to the deep perineal structures (Angermeier and Jordan, 1994). Details of positioning as we do it are covered later. To minimize the patient's time in the exaggerated position, all graft harvesting or flap elevation is done with the patient in the flat supine position.

In addition to proper diagnosis and planning, the surgical technique is important for the overall success of reconstructive surgery. Unlike the results of extirpative surgery, the results of reconstructive surgery depend on methods that minimize tissue damage and maximize wound healing. The key ingredients are adequate visualization, appropriate choice of suture, delicate tissue handling, appropriate positioning, and adequate retraction.

KEY POINTS: RECONSTRUCTIVE SURGICAL TECHNIQUES

- Reconstructive surgery is performed with all efforts aimed at minimizing tissue injury and promoting healing. Loupe magnification is used by almost all surgeons performing adult and pediatric reconstructive surgery. For deep exposure, a headlight or lighted suction is advantageous. Instruments must be delicate because reconstructive surgery uses small sutures and small needles.

- The choice of suture material clearly evolves on the basis of the surgeon's experience. However, the caliber of sutures should be the smallest possible to align the tissue, which is not typically under tension. There is no reason to use suture that is stronger than the tissues being sutured.

- The choice of surgical positioning is clearly left to the surgeon's preference.

- Proper diagnosis and planning of the surgical technique are important for the success of reconstructive surgery.

SELECTED PROCESSES
Urethral Hemangioma

Although **urethral hemangioma is a rare condition, it is usually persistent** and offers a challenge to the surgeon when excision is deemed necessary. Patients typically present with hematuria or a bloody urethral discharge and occasionally with obstructive symptoms. The lesions may be either single or multiple, and the urethral meatus is a common location. Although diagnosis is often made at cystoscopy, which readily visualizes the dilated blood vessels, the lesion often extends beyond the point at which it is seen with cystoscopy.

Because all reported cases of urethral hemangioma have been benign, management depends on the size and location of the lesion. Asymptomatic lesions do not require treatment

---

*C. S. Surgical, 662 Whitney Drive, Slidell, LA 70461; 985-781-8292.
[†]Lone Star Industries; 800-331-7427.
[‡]J. Hugh Knight Instrument Company, 226 S. Villere St., New Orleans, LA 70112; 800-535-5645.
[§]Omni-Tract Surgical, Division of Minnesota Scientific Inc., 4849 White Bear Parkway, St. Paul, MN 55110; 800-367-8657.

and should be observed because hemangiomas can regress spontaneously. Symptomatic lesions that require treatment must be completely excised to prevent recurrence.

Although electrofulguration has been reported as a possible treatment of urethral hemangioma, it should be used only to control an acute episode. For smaller lesions, laser treatment has been successful and produces less scarring. Lasers that are used for this purpose include argon, potassium titanyl phosphate (KTP) 532-nm, and neodymium:yttrium-aluminum-garnet (Nd:YAG). The preferred treatment of larger lesions is open excision and urethral reconstruction. This in some cases means tubed reconstruction. It is clear that tubed graft reconstruction should be avoided; tubed flap reconstruction or tubed construction with mixed tissue transfer could be considered, although staged reconstruction may be preferable. In addition, good initial success has been reported with polidocanol as a sclerosing agent for extensive urethral hemangiomas.

Reiter's Syndrome

Reiter's syndrome is characterized by a classic triad of arthritis, conjunctivitis, and urethritis. In addition, **some patients have had an episode of diarrhea that preceded the development of arthritis.** In most cases, however, the classic triad is not present, and patients present with only arthritis affecting the knees, ankles, and feet in an asymmetrical distribution. The history of urethritis is obtained on detailed questioning.

Urethral involvement is usually mild, self-limited, and a minor portion of the disease. In approximately 10% to 20% of patients, a glanular lesion is present. Referred to as circinate balanitis, this lesion is diagnostic of Reiter's syndrome and typically appears as a shallow, painless ulcer with gray borders. On occasion, the lesion appears as small, red macules, 1 to 2 mm in diameter. When the urethritis is mild and self-limited, no treatment is necessary.

In rare cases, urethritis causes severe inflammation with necrosis of the mucosa, producing uncompromising stricture disease. We have not been successful in excision and replacement of the urethra in these cases. Alternatively, we perform a perineal urethrostomy and excise the entire distal urethra. This approach may decrease the rheumatic manifestations associated with Reiter's syndrome.

Lichen Sclerosus (Balanitis Xerotica Obliterans)

Lichen sclerosus is the preferred term for what was previously known as balanitis xerotica obliterans. On histologic examination, it is characterized by hyperkeratosis, homogenization of the collagen in the papillary dermis in association with stromal edema, and a lymphocytic infiltrate. The most common cause of meatal stenosis, lichen sclerosus appears as a whitish plaque that may involve the prepuce, glans penis, urethral meatus, and fossa navicularis. In the authors' experience, lichen sclerosus usually begins as a meatal or parameatal process in the circumcised patient, but it may involve other areas of the preputial space in the uncircumcised

patient. In severe, long-standing cases, the inflammation often involves the skin of the penile shaft. In uncircumcised men, the prepuce becomes edematous and thickened and often may be adherent to the glans (Bainbridge et al, 1971). **Diagnosis is made through biopsy.** Several reports have suggested the association with chronic infection by a spirochete, *Borrelia burgdorferi* (Shelley et al, 1999).

Although previously thought to be rare, lichen sclerosus is commonly found at the time of circumcision performed beyond the neonatal period (Rickwood et al, 1980; Ledwig and Weigland, 1989; Meuli et al, 1994). If only the foreskin is involved, circumcision may be curative. As stated before, more commonly the glans and meatus are also involved. A combination of topical steroids and antibiotics may help stabilize the inflammatory process. Conservative therapy may be warranted in patients whose meatus can easily be maintained at 14 to 16 French. In these cases, intermittent catheterization with lubrication of the catheter or meatal dilator with 0.05% clotrimazole may be adequate treatment. Long-term antibiotic therapy may also be helpful to improve the inflammation, as secondary infection of the inflamed tissue may occur. We have typically used tetracycline, but a trial of long-term penicillin (or advanced-generation erythromycin) therapy may be warranted (Shelley et al, 1999). This nonsurgical approach to treatment is used in older patients who are not good surgical candidates for other medical reasons, or in all older patients, and in younger patients who have demonstrated stable disease.

In young patients with severe meatal stenosis, surgery is indicated. Because patients with long-standing lichen sclerosus and meatal stenosis often have severe proximal urethral stricture disease, retrograde urethrography should be performed before the initiation of therapy. The etiology of stricture disease associated with lichen sclerosus is unclear. Possible causes include iatrogenic stricture resulting from repeated instrumentation and pressure voiding associated with meatal stenosis causing secondary intravasation of urine into the glands of Littre (Fig. 33-14). In cases of early lichen sclerosus, with only meatal involvement resulting in stenosis of the fossa navicularis, prompt reconstruction has been successful in the long term and seems to avoid the sequelae of panurethral stricture disease. Some surgeons believe that because lichen sclerosus is a disease of genital skin, a better tissue for reconstruction is buccal mucosa, and techniques are discussed later (Mundy, 1994). Long-standing cases with long lengths of urethral stricture are amenable to techniques of reconstruction but can be challenging. **It is becoming clear that except in the case of urethral disease confined only to the meatus and fossa navicularis, staged buccal graft reconstruction, at least in the short to mid term, seems to provide superior durable results.** If urethral disease is confined only to the meatus and fossa navicularis, after a course of topical steroid and oral antibiotics, the authors have found a 50% recurrence of stricture rate with the skin flaps.

We have also seen patients present with a buried penis. This occurs when the skin of the penile shaft has been lost because of severe inflammation, and the penis is trapped in the penopubic and scrotal skin. These patients are often profoundly overweight, and many are diabetic; they have often had prior surgical procedures. Their management is complex and

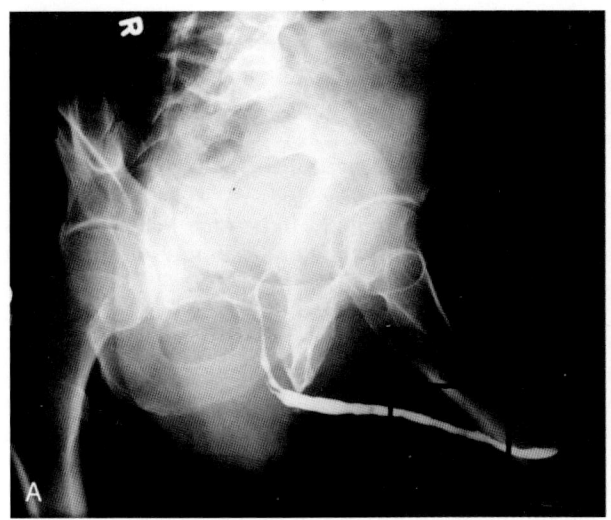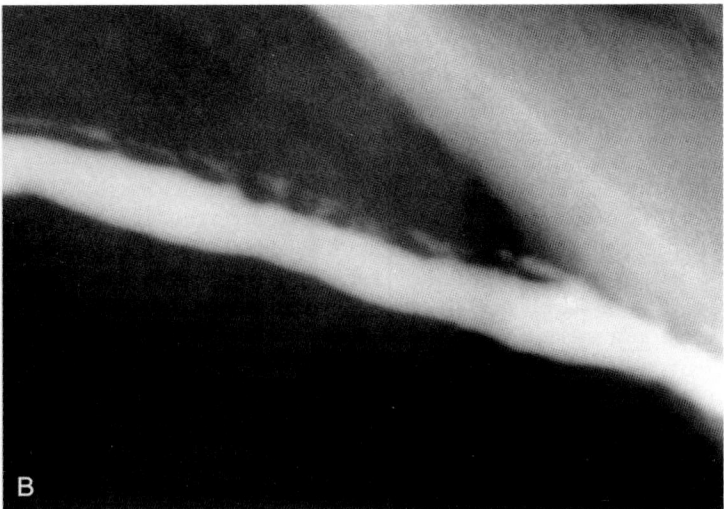

Figure 33–14. Urethrogram in a patient with urethral stricture disease associated with lichen sclerosus–balanitis xerotica obliterans. It illustrates the intravasation of contrast material into the dilated glands of Littre during voiding. (From Jordan GH: Management of membranous urethral strictures via the perineal approach. In McAninch J, Carroll P, Jordan GH, eds: Traumatic and Reconstructive Urology. Philadelphia, WB Saunders, 1996.)

ultimately determined by their desire and need for functional reconstruction. In some patients with severe urethral stricture disease, we have completely reconstructed the urethra; in others, we have simply performed a perineal urethrostomy. Perineal urethrostomy is usually technically straightforward, as the rule in most patients with lichen sclerosus is to spare the proximal anterior urethra. We have proposed that in many cases, the sparing of the proximal anterior urethra demonstrates the distribution of the glands of Littre for a given patient. Younger patients have requested mobilization and release of the penis with placement of a split-thickness skin graft. However, because the inflammation involves the glans penis (which is not removed), the secondary inflammation may also involve the skin graft. Therefore, lifelong monitoring of these patients for the secondary effects of inflammation is necessary.

Several reports have suggested the development of squamous cell carcinoma in patients with a long history of lichen sclerosus (Doré et al, 1990; Pride et al, 1993).

Amyloidosis

Although a rare disease, amyloidosis of the urethra should be considered in the evaluation of any patient with a urethral mass. Patients may present with hematuria, dysuria, or urethral obstruction. Since the differential diagnosis includes urethral neoplasm, cystoscopy with transurethral biopsy is indicated. Once the diagnosis is made, treatment should be based only on symptoms. Most patients can be observed expectantly and not require aggressive treatment. Some will require treatment for urethral stricture. Progression and recurrence are rare (Walzer et al, 1983; Dounis et al, 1985; Crook et al, 2002).

Urethrocutaneous Fistula

A urethrocutaneous fistula is a track lined with epithelium that leads from the urethra to the skin. The size of a fistula can vary from pinpoint to large. **Urethral fistulas may be a complication of urethral surgery or develop secondary to periurethral infection associated with inflammatory strictures or treatment of a urethral growth** (condyloma or papillary tumor). **Treatment of a urethral fistula must be directed not only to the defect but also to the underlying process that led to its development.** Treatment therefore varies according to the cause of the fistula. In cases of urethral reconstruction, especially reconstruction for hypospadias, fistula often occurs or recurs because of distal obstruction and high-pressure voiding.

After urethral surgery, fistulas can develop immediately or as delayed complications. An early fistula is the result of poor local healing, possibly secondary to hematoma, infection, or tension with closure. In addition, a mere breakdown of the urethral or overlying skin closure, or both, could occur. Very occasionally, with aggressive local care and continued urinary diversion, the fistula closes spontaneously.

If a fistula is noted after the removal of a urethral stent for a voiding trial, urinary diversion should be reinstituted in some cases. Before reinsertion of a urethral stenting catheter in the management of such an acute fistula, cystoscopy may help determine whether other complicating factors are present. If these measures fail, repair of the fistula should be delayed a minimum of 6 months to allow complete resolution of the inflammation associated with the healing process attendant to surgery.

Several techniques are used for fistula closure. Endoscopic and radiographic evaluation of the urethra must be performed before the repair in all cases. If the fistula is small and closure of the hole will not decrease the lumen of the urethra, a button of skin is removed from around the fistula and its edges are cut flush with the urethral wall (Fig. 33–15). The urethra is closed with small (6-0 or 7-0) absorbable suture, inverting the epithelial edge, and the repair is tested to ensure that it is watertight. The authors prefer either polyglycolic acid (Vicryl) or polydioxanone suture. Subsequent layers are designed and closed to avoid superimposed suture lines. Without question,

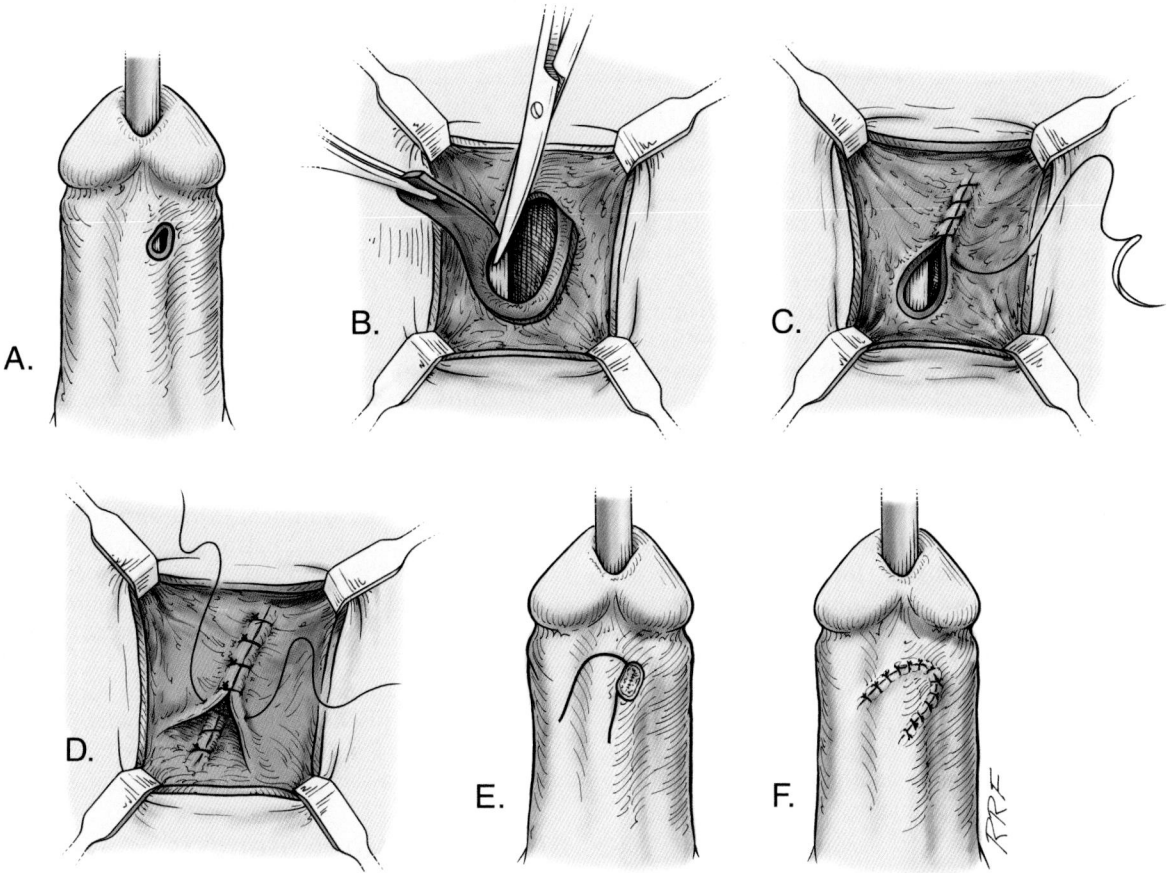

Figure 33–15. Example of fistula closure. **A,** An incision is marked surrounding the fistula, the closure of which will not compromise the lumen of the urethra. **B,** The skin is dissected peripherally, and the fistula track is excised. **C,** A running extraepithelial 6-0 polydioxanone suture secures a watertight closure. **D,** A second layer of sutures buries the urethral closure. **E,** A skin flap is designed to cover the repair to avoid overlapping suture lines. **F,** The closure is complete. (**A** to **F,** from Jordan GH, et al: AUA Update Series 1988;7.)

the safest diversion is a suprapubic catheter. However, in many cases, a silicone stent that reduces pressure during voiding for 7 to 14 days suffices. The operating microscope can be useful for the closure of small fistulas, allowing the use of 8-0 polyglycolic acid suture and limiting the size of the associated skin incision.

If the fistula is so large that simple closure will compromise the lumen of the urethra, a trap-door flap ("flip flap") of penile skin is left attached to one edge of the fistula, and the other edges are incised even with the urethral epithelium. The flap is trimmed to fit exactly and sewn in place with interrupted small absorbable sutures to invert the epithelium. These flaps are random flaps and must be carefully handled. For larger fistulas, a suprapubic tube for diversion is probably prudent. Large fistulas may require more extended tissue transfer that for the most part is just a urethral reconstruction. The mobilization of flaps such as the tunica dartos flap may be necessary to secure adequate tissue interposition.

Fistulas associated with inflammatory strictures occur as periurethral tracks and develop secondary to high-pressure voiding of infected urine. As multiple tracks develop, this problem becomes what is known as a "watering pot perineum." Repair requires suprapubic drainage, and treatment of the infection requires incision and drainage of any abscesses present. We widely excise the fistula tracks and associated

inflammatory tissue and wait 4 to 6 months before repairing the underlying stricture. When tissue is available, in these cases, a flap urethral reconstruction is our first choice. However, a staged graft procedure (discussed later) is also an excellent choice. One must be cautious in the patient with urethral fistulas but without a chronic history of obstructive voiding symptoms. In many cases, fistula or periurethral abscess may be the hallmark symptom of urethral carcinoma.

Treatment of a fistula occurring after electrocautery or laser destruction of a urethral lesion follows the principles outlined previously. If the original lesion was a papillary tumor or condyloma, however, it is imperative to determine whether there has been any seeding of the track that must be excised at the time of repair.

Urethral Diverticulum

A congenital diverticulum is a transitional cell epithelium–lined pouch that is the result of either a distention of a segment of the urethra or the attachment of a structure to the urethra by a narrow neck (i.e., a müllerian remnant). In males, a congenital anterior urethral diverticulum may result from incomplete development of the urethra, with a defect in only the ventral wall and subsequent distention of this segment by the hydraulic force of the voiding stream

(Valdivia et al, 1986; Bedos and Cibert, 1989; Ozgok et al, 1994). Furthermore, the downstream lip of the defect may serve as a valvular obstruction, increasing the pressure in the lumen and the rate at which the diverticulum enlarges. **Another possible etiology is injury of the urethra that may cause an intraspongiosal hematoma.** This could create a paraurethral space and subsequent diverticulum or defects (fistula or diverticulum). These can also be associated with urethral strictures (Bryden and Gough, 1999). It has also been suggested that congenital diverticula may represent giant cystic dilation of Cowper's ducts (Gil-Vernet, 1977; Jiminez Cruz and Rioja Sanz, 1993). The authors do not favor this proposed suggested etiology as the diverticula seem to be slightly more distal than the expected location of Cowper's ducts, and in our experience with reconstruction of a considerable number of these, no proximal limb of the ducts seems to exist in these diverticula.

A congenital diverticulum in the prostatic urethra may be a large remnant of the müllerian duct associated with defects of diminished virilization. However, it often occurs in proximal hypospadias and represents an enlarged utricle (Devine CJ et al, 1980). **These diverticula may not be demonstrated with voiding urethrography but are demonstrated with cystoscopy or retrograde urethrography.** The tip of a urethral catheter tends to catch in this opening, necessitating the use of something to direct the catheter tip toward the true lumen. Other than necessitating caution during evaluation, they do not usually cause problems or require treatment unless they are very large.

Large utricles can accumulate urine with voiding and then decompress after voiding. If they are large enough, the stasis of urine can be associated with recurrent urinary tract infection or difficult-to-manage "incontinence." A surgical approach to small lesions can be through a suprapubic incision, possibly opening the bladder to go through the center of the trigone. However, large diverticula can be approached transsacrally (Peña and Devries, 1982). Although this is a complex procedure, it seems to be associated with much less morbidity than an abdominal or a perineal approach and provides superior exposure. We excise the diverticulum after exposing and dissecting its communication with the urethra. After ensuring that there is no distal obstruction to interfere with healing, we close the urethra.

Diverticula of the female urethra are covered elsewhere in this text.

Paraphimosis, Balanitis, and Phimosis

Paraphimosis, or painful swelling of the foreskin distal to a phimotic ring, occurs if the foreskin remains retracted for a prolonged time. Swelling is sufficient to make reduction of the foreskin over the glans difficult. **In the very young child, paraphimosis is often seen after the foreskin has been traumatically reduced during an examination or sometimes by overzealous parental attempts at hygiene.** It serves to say that traumatic, sudden reduction of a tight foreskin should be avoided in all ages and circumstances. To reduce a paraphimosis, gentle steady pressure must be applied to the foreskin to decrease the swelling. Especially with a child, this is best accomplished in a quiet room by a parent squeezing it in the hand. Elastic wrap may be helpful in some cases. Putting an

ice pack on the area for a short time before gentle compression helps, not with the swelling but as an analgesic. When the swelling has been reduced, the surgeon can push against the glans with the thumbs, pulling on the foreskin with the fingers. Because paraphimosis tends to recur, a dorsal slit at a minimum or a circumcision should be carried out as an elective procedure at a later date. An occasional patient presents with acute paraphimosis that has been present for many hours to days. This is typically seen in an adolescent who is reluctant to reveal the problem to his parents. In these cases, reduction may be impossible and should be dealt with by emergency dorsal slit or circumcision. Considerable postoperative edema is the rule in these cases.

Balanitis, or inflammation of the glans, can occur as a result of poor hygiene, from failure to retract and clean under the foreskin. The subsequent swelling makes cleaning more difficult, but the inflammation usually responds to local care and antibiotic ointment. Oral antibiotic therapy may occasionally be necessary. Balanoposthitis is a severe balanitis and occurs when the phimotic band is tight enough to retain inflammatory secretions, creating what amounts to a preputial cavity abscess. On occasion, an emergent dorsal slit is required.

Phimosis, or the inability to retract the foreskin, can result from repeated episodes of balanitis. In older patients, balanitis may be a presenting sign of diabetes. In these cases, circumcision may be warranted.

Urethral Meatal Stenosis

A small urethral meatus in the newborn will probably not be called to a urologist's attention unless the stenosis is associated with other congenital deformities (e.g., hypospadias) or causes voiding difficulties or urinary tract infection (Allen and Summers, 1974). If the urethral meatus of a boy appears exceptionally narrow and there are associated symptoms, a meatotomy should be considered. For this decision to be made, voiding should be observed to note that the meatus opens as a full, forceful stream is passed. If the stream is narrow and excessively forceful, stenosis is probably present. The occluding skin is generally a thin layer that can sometimes be seen to pouch out, with the meatus opening at the dorsal lip as the child voids. **Meatal stenosis in a boy appears to be a consequence of circumcision that then allows subsequent ammoniacal meatitis.** If the child is seen with ammoniacal meatitis, we usually start meatal dilation with 0.05% clotrimazole cream. Within a week, the process seems to settle down. Anecdotally, the fusion of the ventral-meatal skin that causes meatal stenosis can be avoided. Parents must be counseled about the cause, that is, a wet diaper pressing for prolonged periods against the tip of the glans.

A ventral urethral meatotomy can at times be accomplished with the use of local anesthesia (Fig. 33–16). In the young child, general anesthesia is the preferred approach, avoiding trauma to the child, the parents, and the urologist. It is important to insert the anesthetic needle into the skin fold from the underside, so that the tip of the needle can be observed and controlled. If insertion is done from the outside, the needle will pass through both layers of the fold, and a wheal cannot be raised because of leakage of the anesthetic solution. After the meatotomy, the edges of the cut will seal together unless be necessary to perform a dorsal rather than a ventral meatotomy. This can be accomplished as a Y-V-plasty after the excision of any scarred ridge of neourethra. Dorsal meatotomy, although effective in opening the meatus, often creates a cosmetically less than optimal shape of the meatus. In the adult, it is unusual for the meatal stenosis to be an isolated finding. The stricture process usually involves the fossa navicularis to some extent as well.

Circumcision

Controversy continues about whether neonatal circumcision should or should not be performed (Poland, 1990; Schoen, 1990). Much attention has been focused on this issue, but despite this, many little boys in the United States are circumcised. Ritual circumcision will continue; however, in ritual circumcision, it is not necessary to remove the skin but only to draw blood. **It is important not to circumcise any boy with a penile abnormality (e.g., hypospadias, chordee) that may require the foreskin during repair. An indication for circumcision in the young boy presents when the child has had recurrent urinary tract infections thought to be associated with the redundant preputial skin.**

Most circumcisions performed just after birth are done with the Gomco clamp or one of the plastic disposable devices made for this purpose. Care should be taken to free the foreskin from the glans completely and to apply appropriate tension when the foreskin is pulled into the clamp. To prevent either a too generous or an inadequate circumcision, we find it useful to carefully mark the foreskin so that the correct level is ascertained. At this center, we do neonatal circumcision with a penile block for anesthesia.

The most common complication is bleeding due to inadequate control with vascular compression. Application of an epinephrine-soaked sponge may help in controlling a minimal ooze. Infection can also occur and responds to local care. Any resulting skin separation should be repaired after the inflammation resolves. Sometimes, too much skin is removed, or the urethra is included in the clamp, resulting in a fistula. In many if not most cases in which excess skin is removed, closure can still be accomplished with aggressive frenuloplasty along with remaining skin closure by transposition of the remaining skin. If the entire penis is "scalped," it may be best managed with a split-thickness skin graft or with reapplication of the excised foreskin, after it is prepared properly as a graft. In complicated cases, burying the penis in the scrotum and repairing it at a later date may be prudent. Monopolar electrocautery should be avoided in a neonatal circumcision as penile loss from the field distribution of the current can occur. The use of monopolar cautery with a Gomco or similar clamping device must be avoided because devastating loss of tissue can occur.

At present, whether a newborn who has lost his penis as a result of such a mishap should be gender reassigned is under review by the North American Task Force on Intersexuality (Oesterling et al, 1987; Gearhart and Rock, 1989). Our experience with phallic construction now includes a number of children and youths who had been converted to female after a circumcision accident. As they passed through puberty, they realized that this sexual assignment was wrong. We believe that with the present knowledge of reconstructive techniques, the matter is not clear, one way or the other. However, most

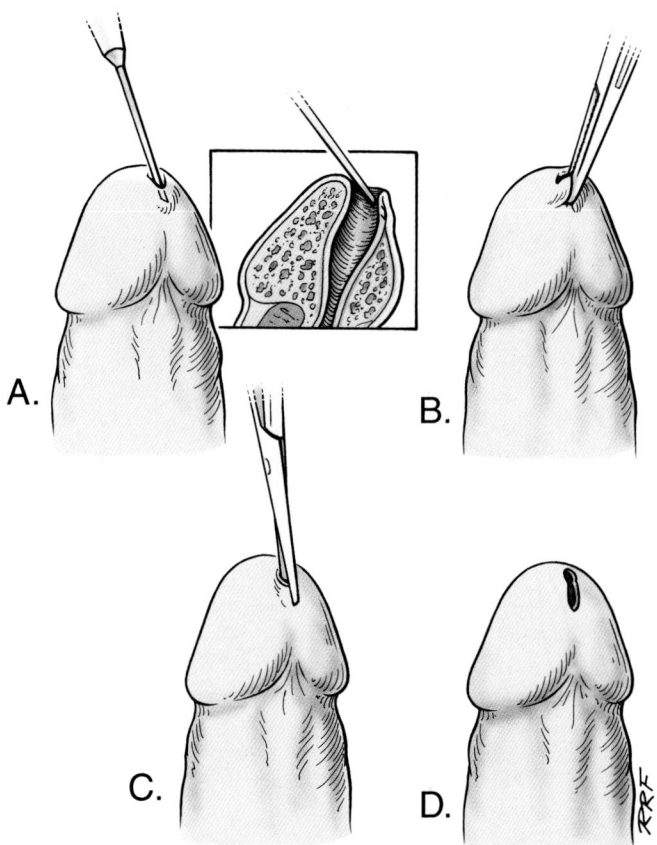

Figure 33–16. Illustration of ventral meatotomy. This procedure is useful for children with meatal stenosis secondary to ammoniacal meatitis. **A,** If it is performed under local anesthesia, a needle can be introduced into the obstructing diaphragm tissue from the inside. **B,** The ventral diaphragm is crushed with a small hemostat. **C,** The crushed tissue is incised. **D,** The appearance of the meatus after ventral meatotomy. The child's parent is instructed to use a meatal dilator, thus separating the crushed edges during healing.

they are kept open. The tip of a meatal dilator is the best instrument for this purpose. The child's parents are instructed to gently separate the edges with the tip of the dilator three times a day for 7 to 10 days. The surgeon should observe the parents carry out this procedure. Pediatric meatal dilators (see the later product reference) are available; however, the tip of an ophthalmic antibiotic tube also works well, and the antibiotic ointment can be used as the lubricant.

Meatal stenosis occurs in adults after inflammation, specific or nonspecific urethral infection, and trauma (especially in association with indwelling catheters, urethral instrumentation, or radical prostatectomy in some cases). It may also be the result of the failure of a previous hypospadias repair. To perform a ventral meatotomy in a normally developed penis in adolescents and adults, it is often necessary to place sutures to approximate the urethral mucosal edge to control bleeding. This step usually requires three sutures: one at the apex and one on either side. We have found a dilator made by Cook* to be helpful in keeping the meatus open. In some cases, it may

*Cook Urological, PO Box 227, Spencer, IN 47460; 800-457-4448. Catalog No. 073406, adult 6 to 34 French; No. 073403, pediatric 6 to 10 French.

of these boys could undergo reconstruction in such a manner as to preserve reproductive function.

In adults, circumcision can be done with local anesthesia, by blocking the dorsal nerves at the base of the penis and circumferentially infiltrating the superficial layers of the penile base. In men and older boys, we favor a sleeve circumcision. With the foreskin in its retracted position, a marking pen outlines an incision, leaving a small preputial cuff. This mark should go straight across the base of the frenulum. This incision is made and carried through the dartos fascia to the superficial lamina of Buck's fascia. The foreskin is reduced, and a second incision is marked, following the outlines of the coronal margin and the V of the frenulum on the ventral side. The frenulum usually retracts into a V. In some cases, the frenulum can be lengthened by closing the edges of the V in a longitudinal orientation for a short length (frenuloplasty). If frenuloplasty is done, the proximal incision does not need to follow the V of the retracted frenulum because the ventral skin is straight. We make the skin incision and fulgurate bleeding vessels with bipolar cautery as the incision is deepened and the skin edge mobilized. In older boys and adults, the vessels are more substantial and not easily sealed by compression, no matter how vigorous. Thus, circumcision clamps can be ineffective and are not recommended even though larger sizes are available. After the sleeve of preputial skin has been removed, hemostasis is obtained and the skin edges are reapproximated.

In smaller boys, some may consider this sleeve procedure to be tedious and difficult. If this is the case, after the skin is marked, a dorsal slit is made through both layers of the prepuce back to the level of the corona (Fig. 33–17). Following the marks, the two layers of the preputial skin are incised. Bleeders are controlled, and the skin edges are reapproximated.

Complications should be uncommon. Most patients develop some hyperesthesia of the glans, which resolves. A hematoma is probably the most common immediate complication. Some patients notice minor cosmetic imperfections that are functionally insignificant. One of the most distressing problems we see, however, is a patient who complains that the surgeon has removed too much skin. To avoid this unfortunate occurrence, a circumcision should be done precisely, and, whatever the procedure to be carried out, the incisions should first be marked with the skin lying undistorted on the shaft. Adults requesting circumcision must be carefully evaluated from a psychosexual standpoint because many of these patients, who are the most persistent in requesting circumcision, become the most dissatisfied after the surgery.

Failed Hypospadias Repair

In treating a patient in whom hypospadias repair has failed, it is important to obtain all available records to help determine what may have contributed to his complications. **A hypospadias repair may fail because of an inadequate correction of chordee or an inadequate urethra, with a stricture, fistula, or diverticulum** (Winslow et al, 1986). **Many times, it is readily apparent from the records that not all aspects of the hypospadias deformity** (Fig. 33–18) (i.e., ventrally displaced meatus, ventral chordee, and some expression of inadequacy of ventral tissue fusion) **were addressed in the previous repairs.** Adults with urethral strictures are often seen who

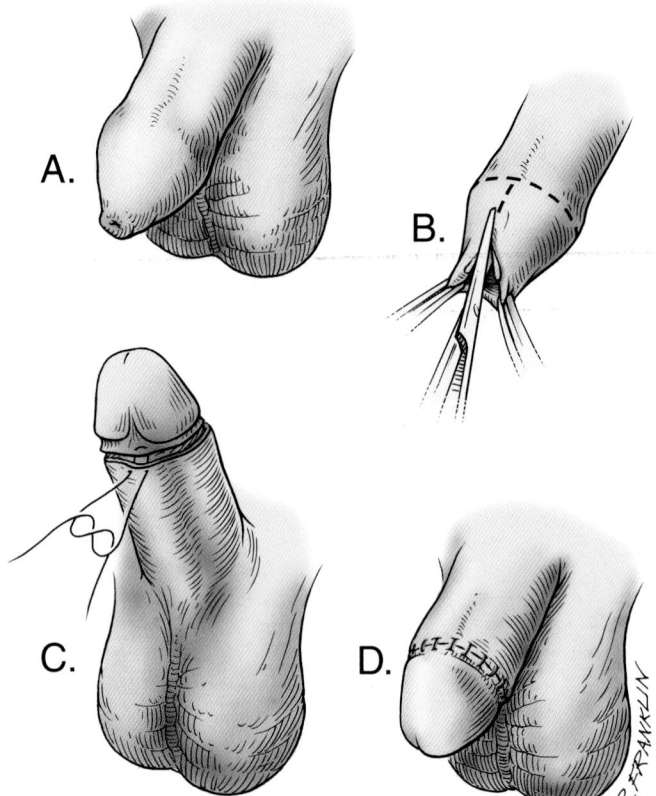

Figure 33–17. Circumcision in a patient with phimosis. **A,** Appearance before dorsal slit. **B,** Incision in the dorsal aspect of the foreskin, which has been drawn over the glans. The broken line indicates the point of incision for removal of the foreskin. **C,** Suture in the frenulum. **D,** Closure.

have had hypospadias surgery as children. Depending on the age of the patient and the preference of the treating urologist, a variety of different techniques may have been used to repair the original hypospadias. Many of these patients have persistent chordee and a subcoronal meatus. Adults have also been seen who have had long-standing evidence of urethral fistula. In addition, some patients may have clinical findings not related to hypospadias that should have been recognized previously, especially when hypospadias is part of an overlying intersex problem. In years past, problems associated with previous failures have been caused by errors in design, technique, or postoperative care (Devine CJ et al, 1978). **With more modern techniques available and with most hypospadias treated by surgeons with considerable experience, failures seem to be associated with perioperative infections or other factors that adversely affect wound healing.** Complex hypospadias repair failures are currently encountered with much less frequency, and most that are encountered are in patients who had previous procedures more than 15 to 20 years ago. Truly, their complications resulted not from poorly designed surgery at the time but rather from the "state of the art" at the time.

Evaluation of a failed hypospadias repair includes retrograde urethrography, voiding cystourethrography, and cystoscopy. In an older patient, a reliable preoperative assessment of residual chordee can be made on the basis of the history and photographs taken at home. In younger patients,

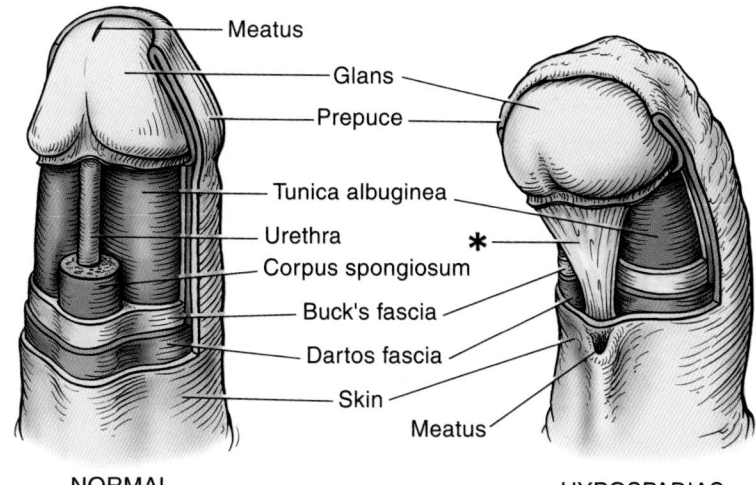

Figure 33-18. Anatomy of the normal penis *(left)* and with hypospadias *(right)*. The fan-shaped band, which is the splayed corpus spongiosum *(asterisk)*, is tissue that can contribute in some patients to chordee. Hypospadias is a defect that can involve all of the structures on the ventrum of the penis from skin to ventral corpora cavernosa. (From Devine CJ Jr, Horton EC: Bent penis. Semin Urol 1987;5:252.)

NORMAL   HYPOSPADIAS

complete evaluation of more complex situations with use of anesthesia may be necessary.

In the adult patient, a detailed discussion must occur regarding the positive and negative aspects of the various approaches. Patients who were initially operated on before the late 1970s probably underwent either a graft or some form of repair using almost exclusively ventral tissue. Some of these patients still have the remnants of a dorsal hood or enough dorsal skin for a dorsal transverse penile skin island type of reconstruction to be performed.

We believe that surgical correction of complex cases requires an aggressive approach by the surgeon (Secrest et al, 1993). All residual dysgenetic and scarred tissue causing chordee must be excised and the penis straightened, with employment of various techniques as they are necessary. All the fibrotic tissue around the neourethra must be excised. If the urethra is inadequate, it too must be excised. The most difficult cases clearly present a challenge to the reconstructive surgeon. The techniques for the release of chordee and repair of urethral strictures are discussed later in this chapter. In particular, we have found the dorsal transverse penile skin island flap repair, the buccal epithelial onlay graft procedure, and the staged graft techniques especially useful for this group of complicated redo hypospadias patients.

Residual Genital Abnormality in Patients with Closed or Diverted Exstrophy

General

Residual genital defects in men who have had exstrophy repaired as children can cause functional, aesthetic, and psychological problems. The effects of these problems are compounded in men who have undergone urinary diversion and who must wear stomal appliances, although with the improvement of continent diversions, this is less of a factor. Except in the most severe forms of bladder exstrophy or cloacal exstrophy when the penis or the halves of the bifid penis are truly inadequate, successful reconstruction is possible. Even then, if normal testes are present, the success of newer techniques of

phallic construction (see subsequent discussion) should lend support to consideration of the option of raising such a child as a boy, possibly preserving his reproductive potential through puberty. In these very difficult cases, we think that the parents must be presented with both options, gender reassignment versus eventual phalloplasty. Remarkable progress has been made in the treatment of difficult cases (Johnston, 1975; Hendren, 1979; Jeffs, 1979; Snyder, 1990; Perovic et al, 1992; Mitchell and Bagli, 1996) as well as in techniques of primary closure. However, many patients need further genital surgery as they experience the hypertrophic growth spurt of the penis associated with puberty.

The goals of reconstructive surgery in male patients with exstrophy or epispadias are to produce a dangling penis with erectile bodies of satisfactory length and shape to allow sexual function and to construct a urethra that serves as a conduit for the passage of urine and ejaculate. However, experience has shown that in the diverted exstrophy patient with only a bladder remnant, construction of a urethra that is essentially defunctionalized is difficult. These urethras all eventually seem to fibrose and stenose. The bladder neck remnant thus becomes a cyst that is often colonized. Bouts of virulent epididymitis or the formation of what is really a bladder neck remnant abscess begin to occur. We have now seen two patients who developed carcinoma of the prostate in a bladder neck remnant. The diagnosis in these patients was difficult and the resultant surgery even more difficult. Neither patient did well from the standpoint of treatment of the carcinoma. Both were seen before the aggressive use and better understanding of prostate-specific antigen.

Many patients who have undergone surgery as children do not present for correction of inadequacies of the external genitalia until after they have completed puberty and realize that their situation has not improved and is not likely to improve. Some have been in sexual situations and have encountered problems. We employ a systematic approach to accomplishing the reconstruction necessary to correct the anatomic defects in these patients (Devine CJ et al, 1980; Winslow et al, 1988). Surgery is undertaken in a sequential fashion beginning with the simplest procedure that will achieve the desired functional result.

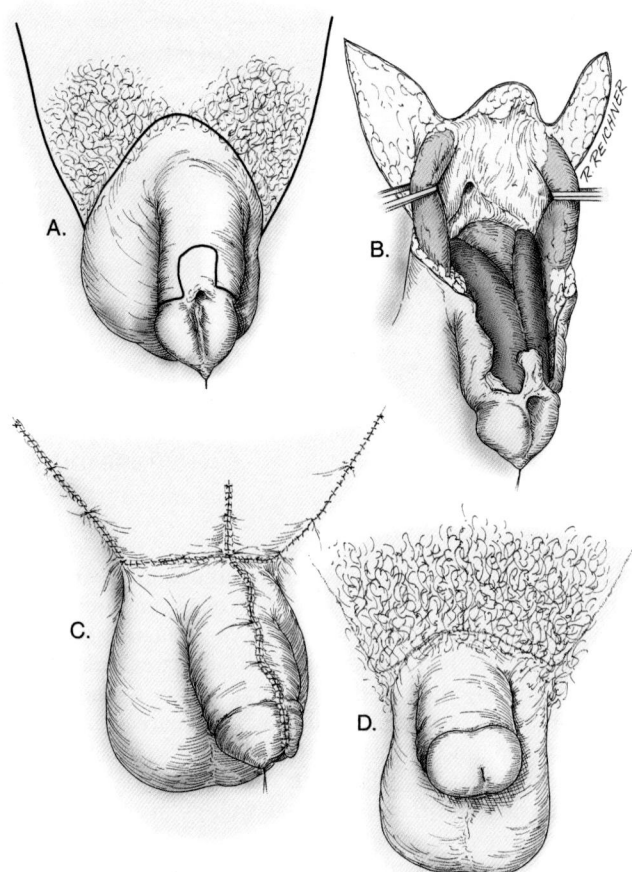

Figure 33–19. **A,** Diagram illustrates development of the superiorly based W flap for exposure of the penile shaft in exstrophy and correction of the abnormal distribution of the pubic hair. **B,** The flap is developed, and the structures of the cord are mobilized and retracted laterally. A midline incision in the skin exposes the penile shaft. **C,** At completion of the repair, the penile skin is closed, and transposition of the limbs of the W to the midline has placed the pubic hair above the base of the penis. **D,** After healing, the scars are hidden in the escutcheon of the incision. (**A** to **D,** from Winslow BH, et al: Epispadias and exstrophy of the bladder. In Mustarde JC, Jackson IT, eds: Plastic Surgery in Infancy and Childhood, 3rd ed. New York, Churchill Livingstone, 1988:527.)

Lower abdominal wall scarring can be corrected or defects can be closed by fashioning peripenile flaps that are shaped like a W (Fig. 33–19). In many patients, there may be wide diastasis recti that is really a ventral hernia. Anchoring of meshes or Gore-Tex can be difficult, and in several cases we have resorted to a fibular bone flap to reconstruct the continuity of the pubis, allowing effective closure of the abdominal hernia.

Surgical Technique

Correction of Chordee. Correction of residual curvature of the penis can be done by a number of methods. In the patient who has undergone multiple operations, curvature can often be caused by the tethering effect of scarred superficial tissues or in some cases a scarred urethra. Since the application of newer techniques that transpose the urethra to the ventrum, at the time of primary closure, dorsal curvature secondary to a scarred dorsal urethra is fortunately not often seen.

Excision of ellipses of the tunica albuginea from the convex (i.e., ventral) aspect of the corporal bodies with approximation of the cut edges is often applicable (Fig. 33–20A). This technique tends to shorten the length of what is already a short penis but is useful for the patient who has a well-functioning urethra that should be preserved (Winslow et al, 1986).

Koff and Eakins (1984) described inward corporal rotation to correct chordee. After mobilization of the ventral aspects of the corporal bodies, several deep midline polydioxanone sutures are placed to rotate the corporal bodies inward, attaching them in the midline (Fig. 33–20B). If artificial erection now shows the penis to be straight, the tunica of each corporal body is incised and joined by suturing the respective edges together to ensure persistence of the rotation.

One can also lengthen the dorsal aspect of the corpora cavernosa by graft inlays (i.e., dermis, tunica vaginalis, and vein) (Fig. 33–21). We avoid the use of synthetic grafts in these circumstances, although their use has not been rigorously examined. During artificial erection, the dorsal aspect of each of the corporal bodies is marked at the point of maximal concavity. Incisions at these marks extend from the medial midline of the corporal bodies to the lateral midline, thus allowing the tunica to elongate, leaving the vascular erectile tissue exposed.

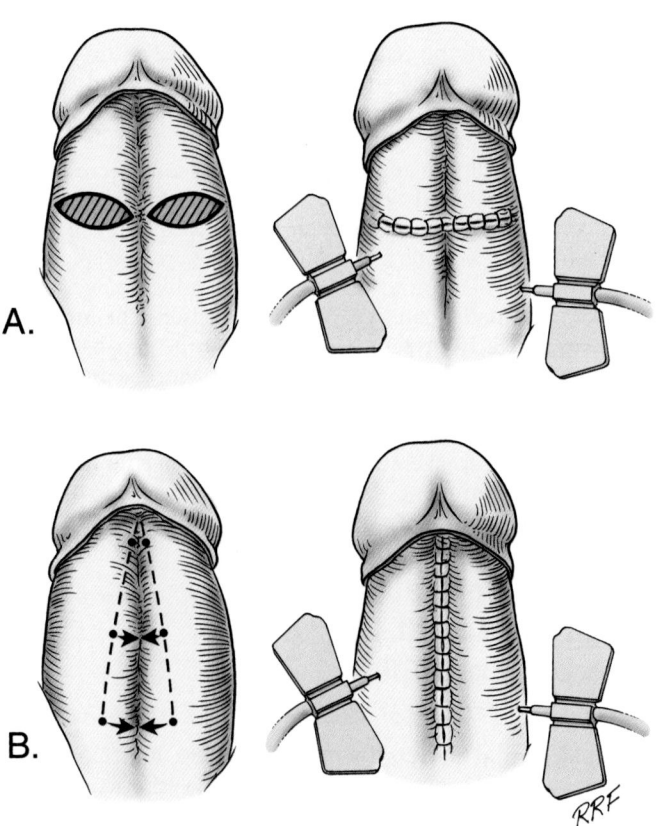

Figure 33–20. **A,** Nesbit-type ellipses are excised from the ventral aspect of the two erectile bodies. Closure of these can straighten chordee. **B,** Koff's procedure. The corporal bodies are rotated to the midline and tacked in place. If this maneuver corrects the chordee, a longitudinal incision is made in the tunica and the rotation is fixed with absorbable monofilament sutures. (**A** and **B,** from Winslow BH, et al: Epispadias and exstrophy of the bladder. In Mustarde JC, Jackson IT, eds: Plastic Surgery in Infancy and Childhood, 3rd ed. New York, Churchill Livingstone, 1988:527.)

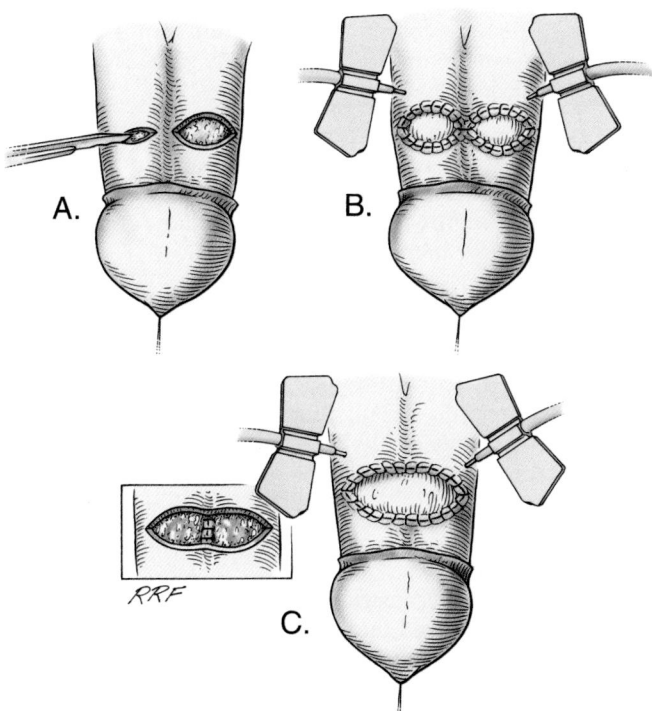

Figure 33–21. Correction of chordee with a dermal graft. **A,** Transverse incisions are made in the dorsal aspect of the corporal bodies. A lenticular dermal graft is placed in each of these defects (**B**), or the medial ends of the incision are sewn together with absorbable monofilament sutures and the conjoined defect is closed with a simple graft (**C**). (**A** to **C,** from Winslow BH, et al: Epispadias and exstrophy of the bladder. In Mustarde JC, Jackson IT, eds: Plastic Surgery in Infancy and Childhood, 3rd ed. New York, Churchill Livingstone, 1988:527.)

To preserve the increased length, the defects are patched with graft inlays. We can use lenticular grafts, each individually placed in the defects in the corpora cavernosa. In most cases, however, the medial aspects of the incisions are approximated and then the merged defect is covered with a single graft. Once the penis is straight, the task of urethral construction can be undertaken.

Urethral Construction. Graft-graft interfaces must be avoided because of the potential for interference with take in the area where the grafts are coapted. If a graft has been used to straighten the penis and it appears that a graft will be necessary for urethral reconstruction, it may be advisable to proceed with urethral construction at another stage. We never construct the urethra with a tubed graft if it can be avoided. At this point, the first step of a grafted first-stage reconstruction would be done on the ventrum. If it is preferable to complete urethral reconstruction in one stage, this may be possible by one of the following techniques.

A flap of ventral penile skin can be tubed to form a urethra. The flap can be passed to the dorsum or left on the ventrum. Passing the flap to the dorsum may be a compromise that allows better closure of the penile skin.

If a tubed graft is the only option, it can be brought to the ventral aspect of the penis by passing it between the corporal bodies at their base, keeping it well away from the dermal grafts.

For patients with epispadias and for patients with exstrophy who still have sufficient penile skin, we prefer the skin from the ventrum of the penis for urethral construction. However, redundancy of the penile skin is usually not present, and thus urethral construction often requires grafting techniques. As with all urethral reconstruction, the graft options include penile or preputial skin, bladder epithelium, and buccal mucosa. In reality, it is probably not advisable to diminish the closed exstrophy bladder compliance and volume by harvesting a bladder epithelial graft. In addition, in the case of the cloacal exstrophy bladder, scarring may make harvesting of such a graft extremely difficult. Likewise, penile skin is usually at a premium, leaving the buccal mucosal graft, at the time of this writing, the most likely option for graft urethral construction. In some patients presenting for secondary exstrophy reconstruction, the midline abdominal skin is not scarred or hirsute, and the tumble-tube technique described by Snyder (1990) may be helpful.

If a patient has undergone previous urinary diversion, the construction of a urethra may not be necessary and coverage of the penis completes the procedure. However, if these patients have a remnant of the bladder neck, a sinus must be created to allow the escape of prostatic secretions and ejaculate. Failure to create such a sinus track allows these fluids to collect in what becomes rather sizable suprapubic cysts. The sinus may be placed in the abdominal wall above the base of the penis, or if there is a posterior urethral remnant that can be formed into a tube, it can be brought out between the corpora cavernosa to open in the skin below the penis. As mentioned, the previously held opinion that one could accomplish a defunctionalized island reconstruction to the sinus, and it would stay open, has not withstood the test of time.

In exstrophy, as part of the midline abnormality, the hair-bearing skin of the escutcheon is lateral to the penis and scrotum, as already mentioned earlier (see Fig. 33–19). Usually, there is no umbilicus, as the cord enters from the upper edge of the exstrophic bladder patch. When it is present, the umbilicus is usually caudally displaced and prone to hernia formation. In some centers, the umbilical stump is dissected from the "dome" of the bladder patch and transposed through the abdominal wall to the normal anatomic location. As they mature, these children then have a true umbilicus. The W flaps transpose the skin, making the escutcheon appear more anatomically correct, but more important, there is a contouring of the suprapubic area. A large amount of dead space is often created by the elevation of these flaps. The interface between the flaps must be drained with small suction drains. In some cases, it is helpful to fill the space at the base of the penis with a vertical inferior rectus abdominis muscle flap. This option must be carefully evaluated; in some circumstances, transposition of the flap could further weaken the lower abdominal wall and increase the complexity of the ventral hernias that these patients not uncommonly have.

PENETRATING TRAUMA TO THE PENIS

Penetrating injuries of the penis can involve the urethra, the corporal bodies, or both. Our choice in managing the acute injury is exploration and attempted immediate anatomic repair, perhaps needing to place a suprapubic tube should

KEY POINTS: SELECTED PROCESSES

■ Urethral hemangioma is a rare condition and usually persistent. It can offer a significant challenge to the surgeon. All reported cases of urethral hemangioma have been benign, and management depends on the size and location of the lesion.

■ Reiter's syndrome is characterized by a classic triad of arthritis, conjunctivitis, and urethritis. Urethral involvement is usually mild, self-limited, and a minor portion of the disease.

■ Lichen sclerosus was referred to in the past as balanitis xerotica obliterans. Diagnosis is made through biopsy. Lichen sclerosus is thought to be possibly premalignant for the development of squamous cell carcinoma of the glans. It is the most common cause of meatal stenosis. Management of patients with lichen sclerosus–related stricture is complex, and results to date are less than optimal. The management is determined by the desire of the patient and the need for functional reconstruction.

■ Amyloidosis is a rare disease of the urethra and should be considered in the evaluation of any patient with a urethral mass. Patients present with hematuria, dysuria, or urethral obstruction.

■ A urethrocutaneous fistula is a track lined with epithelium that leads from the urethra to the skin. It may be a complication of urethral surgery or develop secondary to periurethral infection associated with inflammatory strictures or treatment of a urethral growth. Treatment of the urethral fistula must be directed not only to the defect but also to the underlying process that led to its development.

■ A congenital urethral diverticulum is a transitional cell epithelium-lined pouch that is the result of either a distention of a segment of the urethra or the attachment of a structure to the urethra by a narrow neck. In males, congenital anterior urethral diverticulum may result from incomplete development of the urethra or may possibly be the result of straddle trauma that led to an intracorporal spongiosal hematoma. Congenital diverticulum in the prostatic urethra is a remnant of the müllerian duct.

■ Paraphimosis is a painful swelling of the foreskin distal to a phimotic ring. It occurs when the foreskin has been retracted and not reduced. Edema then forms in the distal skin.

■ Urethral meatal stenosis in the young boy appears to be a consequence of circumcision. The circumcision allows the development of ammoniacal meatitis, which then can heal with a membrane across the ventral portion of the meatus. Controversy continues about whether neonatal circumcision should or should not be performed. If it is going to be performed, an adequate circumcision needs to be done. The most common complication of neonatal circumcision, in the authors' opinion, is the fact that it is inadequately done.

■ A patient with failed hypospadias repair can be complex. Many are victims of the technology of the time when they had their initial reconstruction. When the urethra is involved, all should be evaluated as if they have urethral stricture disease.

■ Advanced techniques for the reconstruction of exstrophy-epispadias complex have led to much better functional results and less need for secondary exstrophy reconstruction. Secondary exstrophy reconstruction is aimed at the area of the escutcheon, the dorsal base of the penis, the penile shaft, the urethra, and the penoscrotal junction.

extensive urethral reconstruction be required. With bullet trauma, the velocity and the construction of the projectile are important factors. Small "slow" bullet injuries of the urethra can be successfully reconstructed primarily; however, larger high-velocity wounds may require diversion and delayed reconstruction. Some projectiles are designed to fragment and even if "low velocity" can cause considerable adjacent tissue damage. Later reconstruction is directed at urethral stricture, if it occurs after the initial injury, or curvature of the penis secondary to damage of the corporal bodies, or both. Fistulas that result from penetrating trauma to the penis are usually treatable by primary closure with interposition of superficial tissue layers between the urethra and the skin. Large fistulas may require more complex tissue transfer and in many ways become more of a problem of urethral reconstruction as for stricture. The principles are discussed elsewhere in the chapter. Recent military actions, in which injury is due to blasts with shrapnel and high-velocity nonfragmenting projectiles, have redefined the thinking on mechanisms surrounding penetrating trauma. For example, it has been learned that high-velocity projectiles can truly penetrate peripheral structures with little cavitation effect, not the effect previously noted with wounds to the abdomen and chest.

Amputation of the Penis

Amputation is the ultimate penetrating penile injury. **If the patient presents acutely with the amputated distal part of his penis, microvascular replantation is the favored approach** (Fig. 33–22). If there is no microvascular surgeon at the center where the patient presents, he should be transferred. The amputated portion of the penis should be cleaned, wrapped in a sponge soaked in sterile saline, and placed in a sterile zipper-sealed plastic bag. This is kept in ice slush, and replantation can be accomplished as long as 18 hours after amputation. Often, the amputation is self-inflicted, usually during an acute psychotic break. This should not preclude replantation unless the patient adamantly refuses such treatment. Even then, with court order or the agreement of two or more surgeons, replantation may be undertaken. Current legal opinion regarding a patient's right of refusal is remarkably

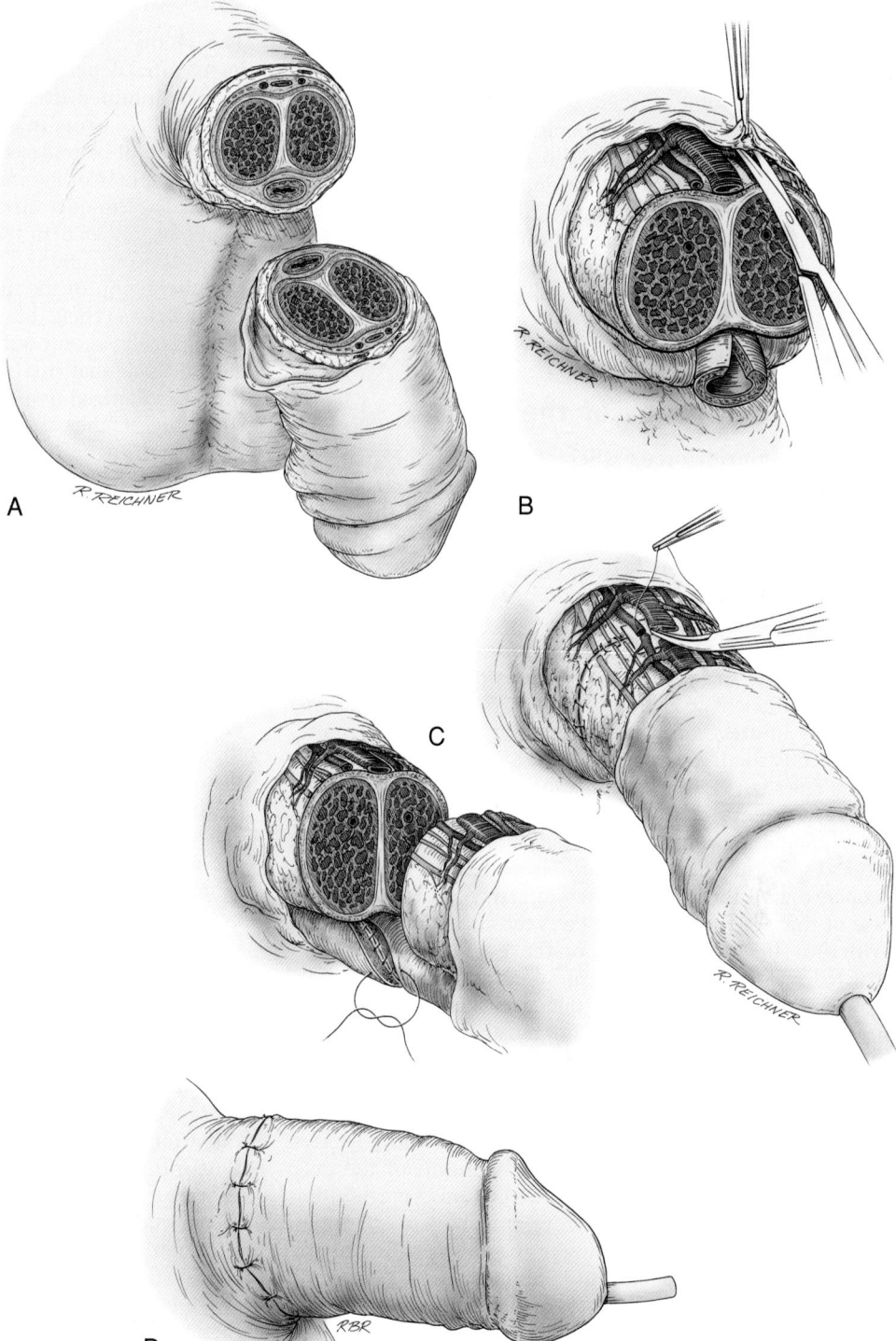

Figure 33–22. Technique of microscopic replantation after amputation of the penis. **A,** The typical appearance of a penile amputation injury. **B,** The urethra, corpora cavernosa, and dorsal neurovascular structures are exposed and minimally débrided. **C,** A two-layer spatulated urethral anastomosis is completed. Microvascular coaptation of the dorsal vein, dorsal artery, and dorsal nerves is accomplished. **D,** Coverage is accomplished with the native skin. If the patient is circumcised, the sleeve of skin between the amputation injury and the old circumcision scar should not be discarded. Should chronic edema develop, revision can be accomplished at a later date. Note: diversion is by way of a suprapubic cystostomy tube. The reconstructed urethra is stented. (**A** to **D,** from Jordan GH, Gilbert DA: Management of amputation injuries of the male genitalia. Urol Clin North Am 1989;16:359-367.)

unhelpful in clarifying circumstances in which a patient refuses treatment but may not really be capable of true informed consent. Applying for a court order may be the safest method for obtaining consent. **The patient's condition or other circumstances may prevent his transfer for microvascular replantation. If so, replantation by the technique described by McRoberts and colleagues** (1968) **should be carried out. This and other series show that a high degree of** success can be expected after replantation without microvascular reanastomosis (Chapple et al, 2004; Morey et al, 2004).

If the patient presents with the distal part having been disposed of or otherwise unavailable, the wound should be closed. The penis has often been stretched out during the amputation, and an excess of skin has been removed, leaving a length of intact but denuded shaft structures proximal to the

SECTION VII

amputation wound. We close the corporal bodies with 4-0 or 5-0 polydioxanone suture, widely spatulate the urethral meatus, and immediately cover the penile shaft with a split-thickness skin graft. Others bury the shaft beneath the skin of the scrotum. In some of these patients, primary grafting of the stump allows a functional penis. However, many require phallic construction or penile reconstruction later.

A number of sophisticated techniques for reconstruction of the traumatized penis are available. The forearm flaps have become the mainstay of penile reconstructive procedures (see subsequent discussion). The initial stage of reconstruction of the amputated penis consists of mobilization of the penile and urethral stumps.

Degloving Injuries of the Penis

Degloving injuries occur when the skin of the penis or scrotum is trapped and stripped from the deeper structures, exposing the uninjured corpora cavernosa and the testes. The tear is deep to the elastic dartos fascia. Bleeding is usually not a problem because there are not many large vessels in this space. The appearance of the "bare" testes and penile shaft, however, is impressive.

When the patient presents, the wounds should be dressed in sterile saline-soaked bandages. A delay of approximately 24 hours is sufficient to define the extent of the damage. Most degloving injuries can then be managed acutely with immediate reconstruction by the application of split-thickness skin grafts. The shaft is covered with a sheet graft of split-thickness skin. The testes are sutured together in the midline, fixed in their anatomically correct position, and covered with a meshed split-thickness skin graft. The parietal tunica vaginalis is opened, and the graft is placed directly on the testes. After take of this graft, the meshing gives the appearance of rugae. With time, the effect of gravity on the testes causes the reconstructed scrotum to become pendulous and sometimes even redundant. In this repair, split-thickness skin grafts are more successful than full-thickness skin grafts because the host bed is less than optimal after a degloving injury. Although split-thickness grafts cannot be employed for single-stage urethroplasty because of contraction, contraction has not been a problem with such grafts applied to the penile shaft or testes. Adequate shaft sensation is achieved by means of the deep structures beneath the graft. Should the testis be avulsed as part of the injury, replantation is usually not an option because the process of stretching of the vessels before breaking leads to an unpredictable intimal injury.

Some surgeons bury the shaft of the penis in a subcutaneous tunnel on the abdomen and bury the testes in subcutaneous thigh pouches. McDougal (1983) has described a technique to mobilize the buried testes with the overlying thigh skin, combining scrotal reconstruction with testicular replacement (Fig. 33–23). In patients so managed, this is a good way of transposing the testes and overlying tissues to an anatomically correct location. When we have managed patients who have been previously treated acutely with the placement of the testes and penis in subcutaneous tunnels, we have mobilized the testes and the penile shaft from their tunnels and immediately applied grafts of split-thickness skin, as already discussed (Morey et al, 2004).

Genital Burns

The ability to reconstruct the damage caused by genital burns often depends on how well the normal structures have been maintained after the acute injury. Careful débridement is the rule in acute management of genital burns. Corporal tissue cannot be replaced with transferred tissue. The physiologic functions of genital tissues cannot be accurately duplicated. The unique vascularity of genital tissue allows less aggressive rather than more aggressive débridement.

Devastating urethral injuries occur with many burns. Reconstruction of the urethra is dependent on the nature of the injuries. When the urethra has been nearly obliterated, there usually is not sufficient uninvolved, nonhirsute local genital tissue that can be transferred for urethral reconstruction. Vascularized tissue must be imported to support reconstruction of the urethra with graft techniques. In many patients, the penis has become incarcerated in contracted scar tissue after the acute injury is healed. Successful transposition of a gracilis musculocutaneous flap introduces compliant vascular tissue and skin into the area, allowing release of the penile shaft. Subsequently, the penile shaft can be covered with a split-thickness skin graft. In some patients, the genital scarring is so severe that microvascular transfer of a free flap is necessary to replace the penile shaft.

For many patients, reconstruction requires a number of stages. In several of our patients, the urethra has been obliterated literally from the entry of the membranous urethra into the bulbospongiosus to the tip of the penis. A perineal urethrostomy has been required while transfer of vascular tissues to the area of the perineum and penis was accomplished. When these tissues are in place, subsequent reconstruction of the urethra can be undertaken with meshed split-thickness skin grafts or buccal mucosal grafts. For coverage of large perineal or groin defects, the posterior thigh flap offers excellent bulky, sensate tissue.

Radiation Trauma

Radiation trauma to the penis occurs in two subsets of patients: patients in whom radiation has been used therapeutically for a lesion on the penis and those in whom radiation to the pelvis has caused chronic lymphedema. Therapeutic radiation can produce chronic suppurative gangrene. In most cases, these lesions are not amenable to reconstruction and are best managed by partial penectomy and later reconstruction, when the patient is proved to be cancer free. Also, we have treated several patients who developed tissue atrophy and further fibrosis after radiation therapy for Peyronie's disease. Delivered at near-tumoricidal doses, this radiation made dermal graft repair much more difficult.

In patients who have had pelvic irradiation, the genitalia usually have one or more of the following: lymphedema, cellulitis, weeping of fluid, or lymphangiectasia. If cellulitis is part of the problem, prolonged treatment (i.e., for months) should be considered before reconstruction. We have in fact had several patients with recurrent cellulitis who had prolonged antibiotic therapy (we use ciprofloxacin); not only did their cellulitis become quiescent, but the lymphedema resolved significantly.

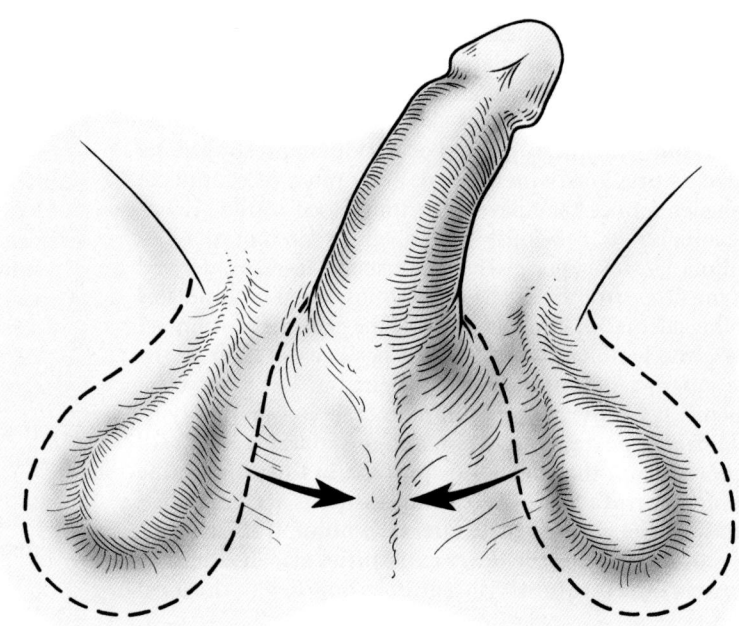

A

Figure 33–23. Technique of elevation and transposition of testes from thigh pouches. **A,** Testes in thigh pouches with a random superiorly based flap outlined. **B,** Flaps and testes are transposed to the correct anatomic area, and the lateral defects are covered with a skin graft. In some cases, primary closure of the thigh defects is possible. (**A** and **B,** From McDougal WS: Scrotal reconstruction using thigh pedicle flaps. J Urol 1983;129:757-759.)

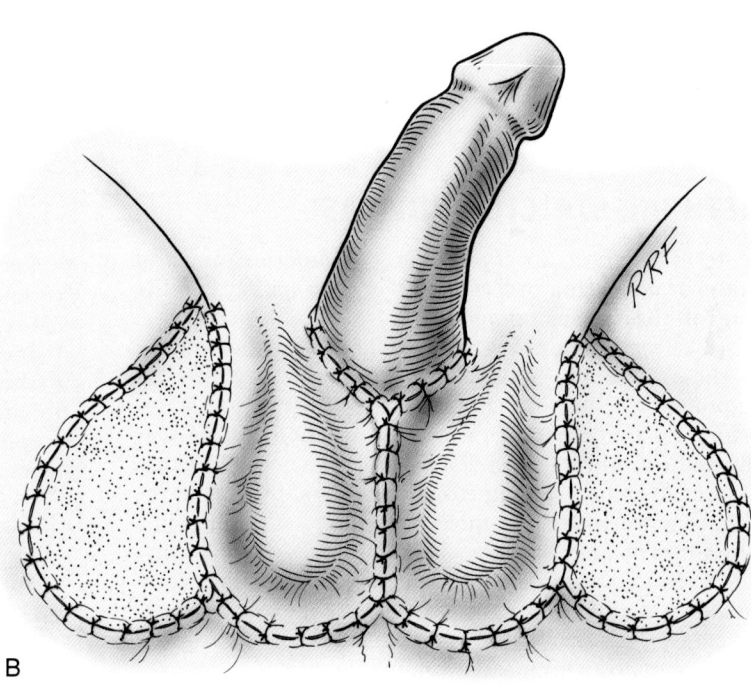

B

    The genitalia of patients with lymphedema can be readily reconstructed. Lymphedema of the penis involves the tissues of the dartos fascia and the dermal layer of the skin. In the penis, the lymphedematous tissue can be excised by removing the dartos fascia and skin, dissecting in the layer immediately superficial to Buck's fascia. In the scrotum, Colles' fascia–tunica dartos and skin of the scrotum must be removed. When the lymphedematous tissue has been excised, the testes are free, and, as in a degloving injury, they must be fixed in the midline in an anatomically correct position. The scrotal skin peripheral to the edema is often normal and can be advanced to cover the testes. The shaft of the penis should be covered with a split-thickness skin graft. If the scrotum cannot be closed, a meshed split-thickness skin graft is used to cover the testes, as described previously. Grafts provide optimal reconstruction in these patients. Not uncommonly, these patients have hydroceles; the parietal tunica vaginalis must be excised, and grafting can be done directly onto the visceral tunica vaginalis of the testes. If there are hydroceles, the process often is "systemic" and not local. In these cases, reconstructing the lateral scrotal skin is seldom effective.

Unlike the full-thickness skin graft, split-thickness skin carries little of the reticular dermis and hence few of the lymphatic channels. Reaccumulation of lymphedema will occur within a full-thickness skin graft and can recur in a thick split-thickness graft. Local skin flaps should be avoided as previously mentioned. They often reaccumulate lymphedema once they have been transposed to the area of the genitalia. As previously noted, grafts do not develop sensation. However, good sensation usually develops, derived from the deep structures. The glans almost never accumulates disabling edema, and the sensation of the glans remains intact because the lymphedematous tissue has been excised in the plane superficial to Buck's fascia, sparing the dorsal nerves of the penis. It is observed that in many cases of genital lymphedema, the posterior scrotum and the lateral scrotal wall are spared from the edematous process; in those cases, the bulk of the scrotum is excised, and closure is accomplished with use of the posterior and lateral scrotum. If the edematous process involves the lower extremities also, it is best to reconstruct the scrotum with a graft as opposed to the local tissues.

Direct radiation to the penis can cause urethral injury. However, it is unusual for the urethra to be injured without damage to adjacent structures. Often, because of the vascularity of the corpus spongiosum, minimal débridement can be accomplished, leaving the patient with a fistula that can be reconstructed at a later date. The success of such reconstruction depends on the damage that the radiation has done to the adjacent structures.

URETHRAL STRICTURE DISEASE

The term *urethral stricture* refers to anterior urethral disease, or a scarring process involving the spongy erectile tissue of the corpus spongiosum (spongiofibrosis) (Fig. 33–24). The spongy erectile tissue of the corpus spongiosum underlies the urethral epithelium, and in some cases, the scarring process extends through the tissues of the corpus spongiosum and into adjacent tissues. Contraction of this scar reduces the urethral lumen. For example, if a normal urethra measures 30 French, its diameter is 10 mm and the area of the lumen is approximately 78 mm². If scarring has resulted in a urethra that measures 15 French, the lumen is only 55 mm², or 29% reduced. It is therefore evident that scar contraction caused by anterior urethral stricture disease can for a while be markedly asymptomatic but as the lumen is further reduced can be associated with marked voiding symptoms.

In contrast, posterior urethral "strictures" are not included in the common definition of urethral stricture. Posterior urethral stricture is an obliterative process in the posterior urethra that has resulted in fibrosis and is generally the effect of distraction in that area caused by either trauma or radical prostatectomy. Although the distraction defect can be lengthy in some cases, the actual process involving the tissues of the urethra is usually confined. By consensus of the World Health Organization conference, the term *stricture* is limited to the anterior urethra; distraction defects are those processes of the membranous urethra associated with pelvic fracture and other narrowing of the posterior urethra, urethral contractures, or stenosis (Bhargava et al, 2004).

KEY POINTS: TRAUMA TO THE GENITALIA

- Penetrating injuries to the penis can involve the urethra, the corporal bodies, or both.

- With regard to bullet injuries of the urethra, the velocity of the projectile must be considered. Recent military actions have shown, however, that high-speed projectiles can pass through superficial structures with relatively little cavitation effect and hence less propagation of energy to the adjacent tissues.

- If the patient presents acutely with the amputated distal part of his penis, microvascular replantation is the favored approach. If the patient's condition or other circumstances prevent his transfer for microvascular replantation, replantation by the technique described by McRoberts should be carried out and can yield excellent results.

- Degloving injuries to the penis occur when the penis or scrotal skin is trapped and stripped from the deeper structures. Bleeding is usually not a problem. The tissues must be allowed to demarcate; acute reconstruction with grafts can be done.

- The damage caused by genital burns depends on how well the normal structures have been maintained after the acute injury. The unique vascular qualities of the penis allow careful repeated débridement as opposed to aggressive débridement.

- Radiation trauma to the penis occurs in two potential subsets: patients in whom radiation has been used therapeutically for a lesion on the penis and those in whom radiation to the pelvis has caused chronic lymphedema. The patient with genital lymphedema can be readily reconstructed by either a split-thickness skin graft or, in select cases, the lateral margins and the posterior margins of the scrotum.

Urethral Anatomy

Although urethral anatomy is described in the earlier section on anatomy, it is useful to re-emphasize key anatomic points. The bulbous urethra is eccentrically placed in relation to the corpus spongiosum and is much closer to the dorsum of the penile structures (Fig. 33–25). As one moves distally, the pendulous or penile urethra becomes more centrally placed within the corpus spongiosum.

The genital skin has a dual (proximal and distal) and bilateral blood supply, forming a fasciocutaneous system (see Fig. 33–9A). The corpus spongiosum receives blood from the common penile artery, the terminal branch of the internal pudendal artery (see Fig. 33–11). The corpus spongiosum also has a dual blood supply—a proximal blood supply and a retrograde blood supply by way of the dorsal arteries as they arborize in the glans penis.

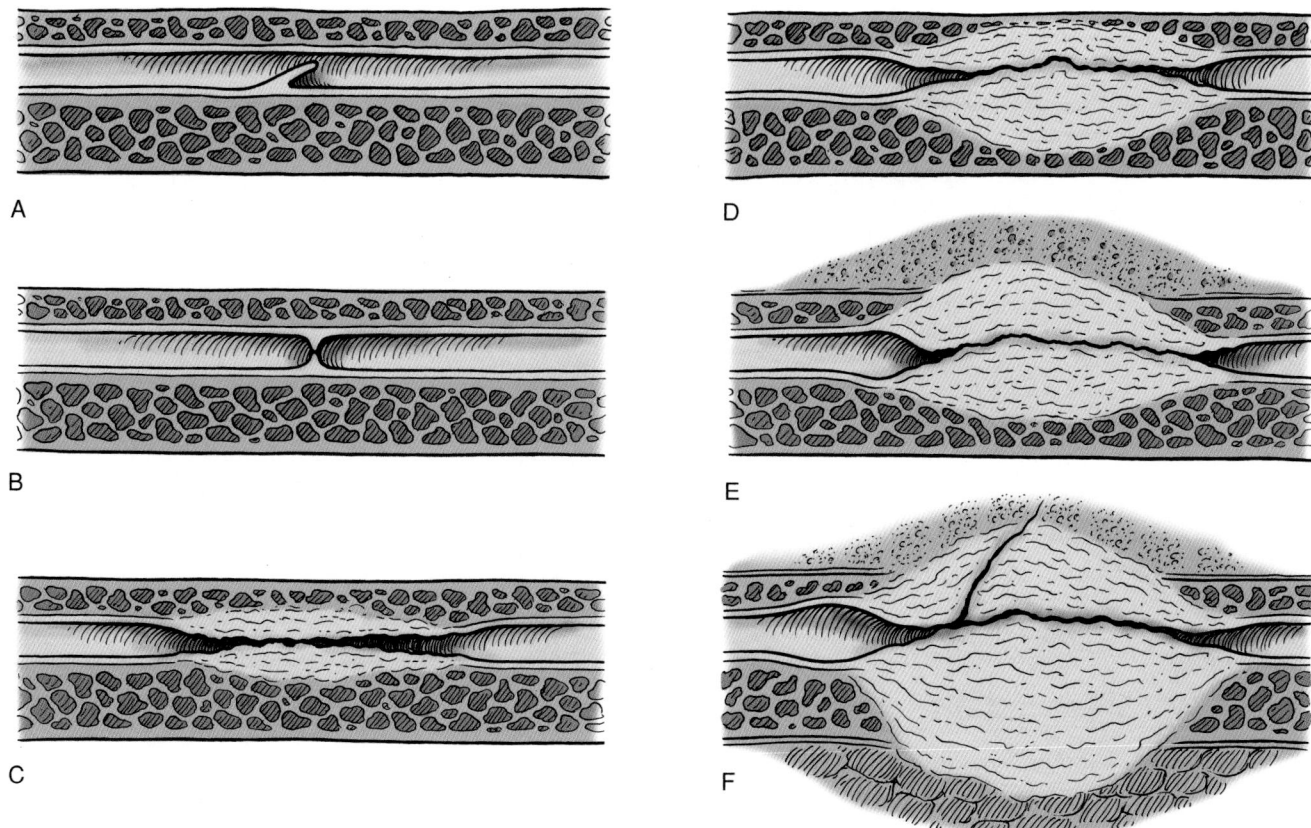

Figure 33–24. The anatomy of anterior urethral strictures includes, in most cases, underlying spongiofibrosis. **A,** Mucosal fold. **B,** Iris constriction. **C,** Full-thickness involvement with minimal fibrosis in the spongy tissue. **D,** Full-thickness spongiofibrosis. **E,** Inflammation and fibrosis involving tissues outside the corpus spongiosum. **F,** Complex stricture complicated by a fistula. This can proceed to the formation of an abscess, or the fistula may open to the skin or the rectum. (**A** to **F,** from Jordan GH: Management of anterior urethral stricture disease. Probl Urol 1987;1:199-225.)

Etiology

Any process that injures the urethral epithelium or the underlying corpus spongiosum to the point that healing results in a scar can cause an anterior urethral stricture. Today, most urethral strictures are the result of trauma (usually straddle trauma). This trauma to the urethra often goes unrecognized until the patient presents with voiding symptoms resulting from the obstruction of the stricture or scar. In most straddle trauma, the injury to the bulbous urethra is readily reconstructable (Park and McAninch, 2004). Unfortunately, iatrogenic trauma to the urethra still exists, but with the development of small endoscopes and the limitation of indications for cystoscopy in boys, we see fewer iatrogenic strictures today than in the past. The place of idiopathic ure-throrrhagia with regard to strictures in children is not clear; some question whether it may be a cause of strictures in young boys irrespective of the child's having undergone an endo-scopic procedure (Rourke et al, 2003). We are, however, seeing an increase in strictures associated with lichen sclerosus, and those strictures clearly behave much more like inflammatory strictures than traumatically induced isolated scars. Finally, posterior urethral distraction injuries, traumatic by definition, result in "strictures" that are associated with extensive fibrosis interposed between the distracted ends of the urethra.

On the other hand, inflammatory strictures associated with gonorrhea were the most commonly seen in the past and are less common now. With the advent of prompt and effective antibiotic treatment, gonococcal urethritis now progresses less often to gonococcal urethral strictures. The place of *Chlamydia* and *Ureaplasma urealyticum* (i.e., nonspecific urethritis) in the development of anterior urethral strictures is not clear. To date, no clear association between nonspecific urethritis and the development of anterior urethral stricture has been established.

There is, as mentioned earlier, a definite association between the development of an inflammatory stricture and lichen sclerosus–balanitis xerotica obliterans (LS-BXO). LS-BXO usually begins with inflammation of the glans and inevitably causes meatal stenosis, if not a true stricture of the fossa navicularis. The cause of this distal penile skin and ure-thral inflammation is not known. Literature suggests the possibility that bacterial infection is the cause of the resultant skin changes. There is some evidence to suggest that the progression of the stricture eventually to involve the anterior urethra extensively may be due to high-pressure voiding that causes intravasation of urine into the glands of Littre, inflammation of these glands, and, perhaps, microabscesses and deep spongiofibrosis. Whether the urethral changes and eventual fibrosis are also related to bacterial injury has not, to our

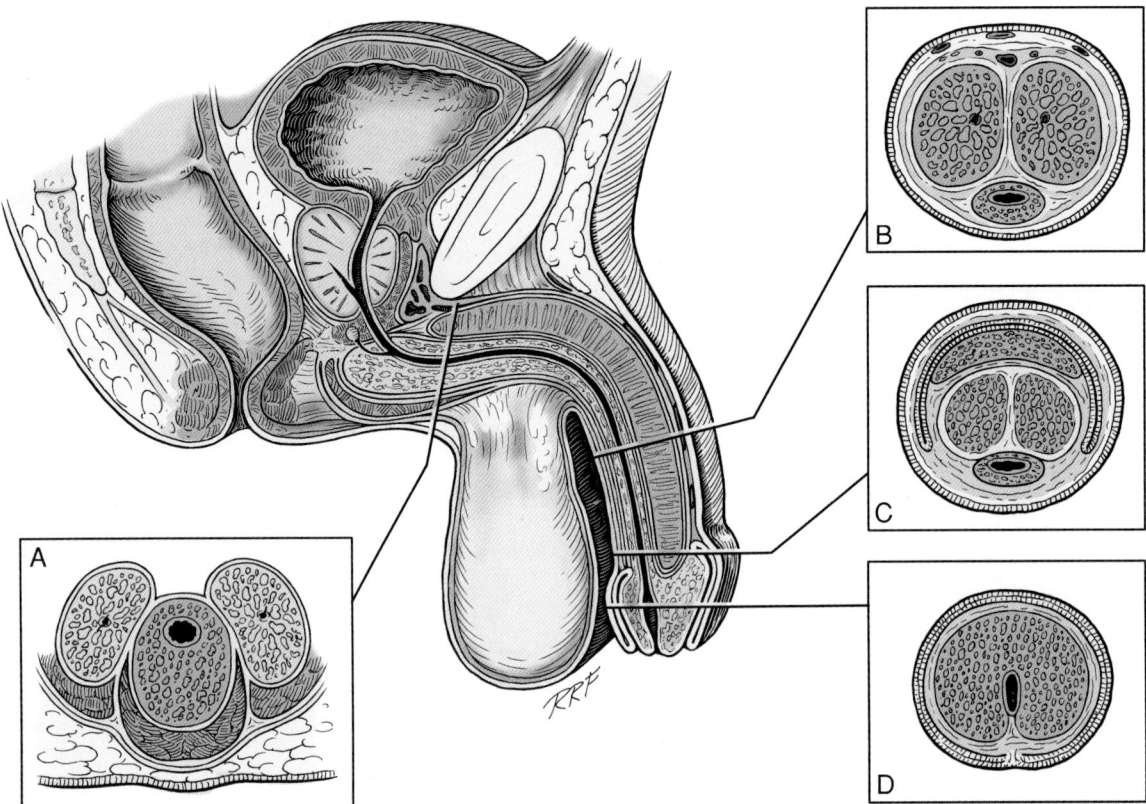

Figure 33–25. Diagrammatic cross sections of the anterior urethra. **A,** The bulbous urethra. The urethra is eccentrically placed in the corpus spongiosum. Proximally, the corpora cavernosa have split into individual crura, with the urethra lying against the triangular ligament. **B,** In the shaft of the penis, the urethra is more centrally placed with relation to the corpus spongiosum, and the corpora cavernosa are intimately fused, separated only by septal fibers. **C,** At the coronal margin, the urethra remains relatively centrally placed, and the corpora cavernosa are fused, again separated by septal fibers. The spongy tissue of the corpus spongiosum has become incorporated as the deep tissues of the glans. **D,** The fossa navicularis widens somewhat in caliber and is totally surrounded by the spongy erectile tissue of the glans penis. The urethra here is relatively ventrally placed in relation to the body of the corpus spongiosum. (**A** to **D,** from Jordan GH: Complications of interventional techniques of urethral stricture disease: Direct visual internal urethrotomy, stents and laser. In Carson C, ed: Topics in Clinical Urology: Complications of Interventional Techniques. New York, Igaku-Shoin, 1996:86-94.)

knowledge, been well defined. Although the use of antibiotics seems in these patients to limit obstructive voiding symptoms, to our knowledge the literature does not show resolution of the stricture process with the use of antibiotics.

What is known as a congenital stricture is an entity that is difficult to understand. If, in embryologic development, a stricture is found at a natural place where a fusion of structures occurs (i.e., the posterior and anterior urethra), a congenital stricture might be a reasonable assumption. However, the term *congenital stricture* is used by some to define a stricture for which there is no identifiable cause. We propose, however, that it is reasonable to define a stricture as congenital only if it is not an inflammatory stricture, it is a short-length stricture, and it is not associated with a history of or potential for urethral trauma. This then limits the term *congenital stricture* to strictures of the anterior urethra found in infants before they attempt erect ambulation. So defined, congenital strictures will clearly be the rarest encountered.

Diagnosis and Evaluation

Patients who have urethral strictures most often present with obstructive voiding symptoms or urinary tract infections such as prostatitis and epididymitis. Some patients also present with urinary retention. However, on close inquiry, most of these patients are found to have tolerated notable voiding obstructive symptoms for a long time before progressing to complete obstruction.

Not uncommonly, when a patient cannot void, an attempt is made to pass a urethral catheter. If the catheter does not pass, the nature of the obstruction is determined by dynamic retrograde urethrography. Thus, most cases are managed with acute dilation, and clearly there are many instances in which this is not the best course for the patient. When there is doubt, we determine the nature of the stricture when possible, and not uncommonly we place a suprapubic cystostomy catheter to treat the acute situation and allow time for a more appropriate treatment plan to be devised. The practice of blind passage of filiforms and blind dilation without knowledge of the anatomy of the urethral stricture is condemned. Although detailed imaging is not always available, flexible endoscopy is almost universally available in the United States. At the least, the stricture can be visualized and a guide wire passed under direct vision through the lumen.

For an appropriate treatment plan to be devised, it is important to determine the location, length, depth, and density of the stricture (spongiofibrosis). The length and

location of the stricture can be determined with radiography, urethroscopy, and ultrasonography. The depth and density of the scar in the spongy tissue can be deduced from the physical examination, the appearance of the urethra in contrast-enhanced studies, and the amount of elasticity noted on urethroscopy. The depth and density of fibrosis are difficult to determine objectively. The absolute length of spongiofibrosis may not be evident on ultrasound evaluation. Ultrasound examination clearly can augment contrast-enhanced studies and is accurate in determining the length of narrow-caliber annularity (Morey and McAninch, 1996a). Contrast studies of the urethra are best carried out by or under the direct supervision of the surgeon responsible for treatment of the patient.

In 1979, McCallum and Colapinto described the use of dynamic radiographic studies and emphasized the need for these studies to be dynamic as opposed to static (Fig. 33–26). At our center, imaging includes dynamic studies that are accomplished during retrograde injection of contrast material and while the patient is voiding. Even with gentle technique, extravasation during retrograde urethrography is possible in patients in whom the urethra is markedly inflamed. For this reason, contrast studies should be carried out with contrast material that is suitable for intravenous injection and used either directly from the bottle or diluted according to the manufacturer's guidelines. Contrast materials that have been thickened with lubricating jelly or anesthetic gels can be a source of problems and offer little with regard to enhancement of radiographic studies, nor do they make the studies more comfortable. Real-time ultrasound evaluation of the urethra after it has been filled with a lubricating jelly or saline has been described by Morey and McAninch (1996a, 1996b). It is a misconception, however, that ultrasonography always directly visualizes the spongiofibrosis. However, Morey and McAninch (1996a, 1996b) believe that ultrasonography of the bulbous urethra possibly more accurately determines the length of the stricture, which could be important in considering an anastomotic repair. If the patient is not in steep lateral oblique position for retrograde urethrography, the length of the stricture will be underestimated. Finally, it should be understood that during contrast-enhanced urethrography, more than one projection may be necessary to visualize the stricture. Magnetic resonance is also being explored as an adjunct to the evaluation of urethral stricture as well as pelvic fracture urethral distraction defects. In our experience, the use of magnetic resonance for routine strictures or pelvic fracture urethral distraction defects is not beneficial. In the case of urethral tumors, we have found magnetic resonance to be invaluable. The experiences of others is commensurate with ours (Pavlica et al, 2003).

Endoscopic examination may be necessary after the contrast studies. The flexible cystoscope has simplified this evaluation, and when local anesthesia is used, there is little discomfort associated with it. The scope can be passed to the stricture, and many times it is not necessary to pass it beyond that level. In addition, it is not always necessary and usually not beneficial to dilate the stricture at the time of the initial endoscopic evaluation. Pediatric endoscopic equipment has proved to be extremely valuable for examination of the urethra proximal to a narrow-caliber area without the need to dilate the narrowest area. In the patient who cannot void and

has a suprapubic tube, combined contrast studies with endoscopy are helpful in defining the stricture anatomy (Fig. 33–27).

It is imperative, however, to completely evaluate the urethra proximal and distal to the stricture with endoscopy and bougienage during surgery to ensure that all the involved urethra is included in the reconstruction. Whereas hydraulic pressure generated by voiding may keep segments proximal to the stricture patent, unless these segments are included in the repair, they are at risk for contraction after obstruction of the narrow-caliber segment is relieved with reconstruction. For this reason, any abnormal areas of the urethra that are proximal to a narrow-caliber segment of the stricture must be treated with suspicion. If the lumen does not appear to demonstrate evidence of diminished compliance, we presume that area to be uninvolved in active stricture disease. However, coning down of the urethra suggests its involvement in the scar.

In some patients, the urethra proximal to a narrow area may remain confusing with regard to its potential for continued constriction after reconstruction. In select patients, we have found it useful to place a suprapubic tube to defunctionalize the urethra. After 6 to 8 weeks, if there is going to be constriction of an area that was hydrodilated with voiding, the tendency for that constriction to occur should become apparent.

Treatment

Although the treatment of urethral stricture disease dates to the foundations of our specialty, significant progress made during the last 50 years allows many of the most complex strictures to be reliably reconstructed in one stage. In the past, a concept known as the reconstructive ladder was used as a treatment guideline for urethral strictures. That concept was based on the principle that the simplest procedure should always be attempted first, and sometimes repeated after failure, before moving on to more complex approaches. This approach is considered archaic in modern urethral reconstruction.

Both the patient and the physician must have a good understanding of the goal of treatment before the treatment choice is made. To this end, treatment options should be discussed with the patient, with care taken to emphasize the anticipated outcome with regard to "cure." Some patients may prefer stricture management and choose to have periodic dilations in the office, at home, or in the hospital rather than undergo technically detailed open surgery. Others may have cure as a goal and choose surgical management; many surgical procedures today have short- and mid-term results approaching long-term success rates of more than 90% to 95% for many strictures.

Dilation

Urethral dilation is the oldest and simplest treatment of urethral stricture disease, and for the patient with an epithelial stricture without spongiofibrosis, it may be curative. The goal of this treatment, a concept that is frequently forgotten, is to stretch the scar without producing more scarring. If bleeding occurs during dilation, the stricture has been torn rather than stretched, further injuring the involved area.

SECTION VII

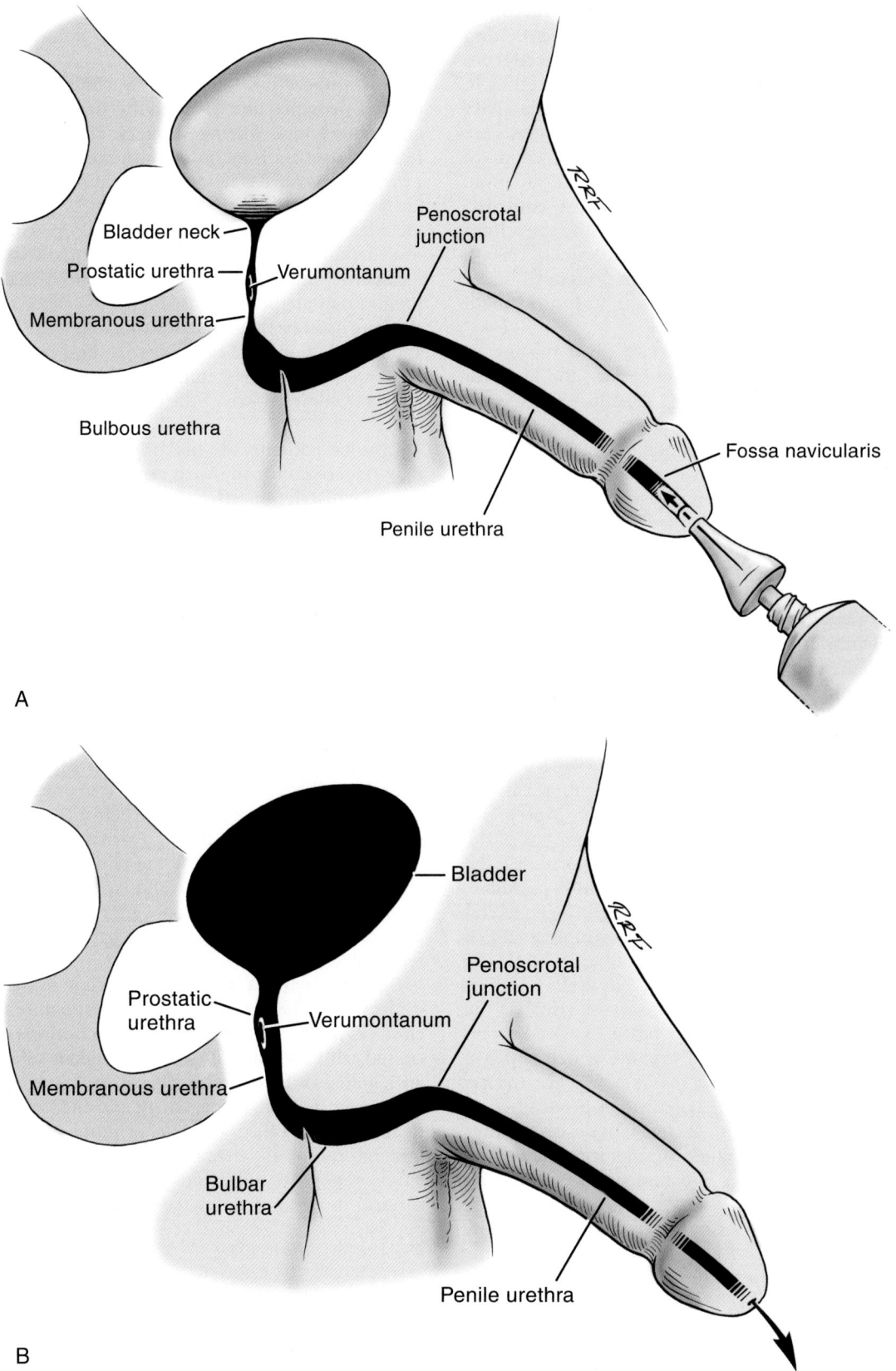

A

B

Figure 33–26. **A,** Representation of a dynamic retrograde urethrogram with the criteria of McCallum illustrated. **B,** Representation of a dynamic voiding urethrogram with the criteria of McCallum illustrated. (**A** and **B,** modified from McCallum RW: The adult male urethra. Radiol Clin North Am 1979;17:227-244.)

Continued

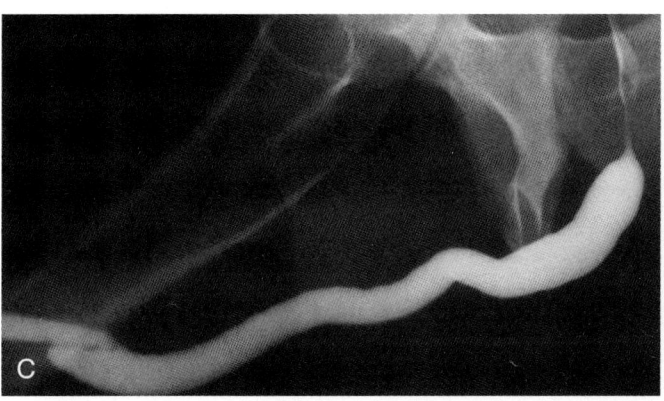
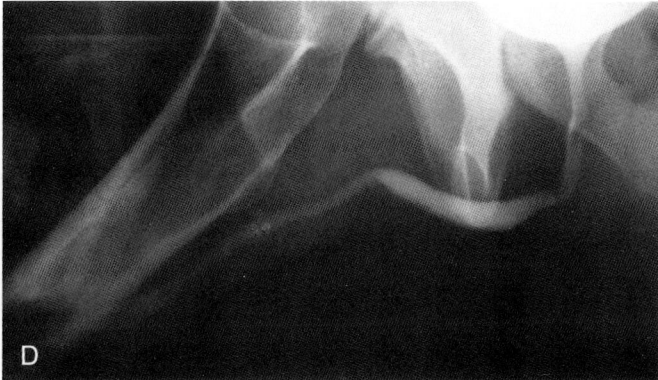

Figure 33–26, cont'd.   **C**, A normal retrograde urethrogram. **D**, A normal voiding urethrogram.

KEY POINTS: URETHRAL STRICTURE

- The term *urethral stricture* refers to anterior urethral disease and is a scarring process that involves the epithelium as well as the spongy erectile tissue of the corpus spongiosum. Contraction of the scar reduces the urethral lumen. In contrast, posterior urethral strictures are more correctly referred to as pelvic fracture urethral distraction defects; strictures of the prostatic urethra or bladder neck are properly referred to as contractures or stenoses.

- The anterior urethra is invested by the corpus spongiosum and as it proceeds proximally is eccentrically placed in relation to the corpus spongiosum. The genital skin has a dual and bilateral blood supply, forming a fasciocutaneous vascular system. The vascularity of the corpus spongiosum is based on the common penile artery.

- In general, most anterior urethral strictures are the result of trauma. Inflammatory strictures associated with gonorrhea are rarely seen; however, strictures associated with lichen sclerosus clearly behave like inflammatory strictures.

- Patients who have urethral strictures most often present with obstructive voiding symptoms or urinary tract infections such as prostatitis and epididymitis. Those patients who present with urinary retention, on close inquiry, have tolerated notable voiding obstructive symptoms for a long time.

- For an appropriate treatment plan to be devised, it is important to determine the length, location, depth, and density of the spongiofibrosis. This can be done with a combination of contrast-enhanced studies, endoscopy, and selective ultrasonography. It is imperative to completely evaluate the urethra proximal and distal to the stricture with endoscopy. A pediatric cystoscope is useful.

The least traumatic method to stretch the urethra is to use soft techniques over multiple treatment sessions. We believe that the safest method of urethral dilation currently available involves the use of urethral balloon dilating catheters. These catheters may be attached to a filiform tip or passed over a guide wire or may come with an integral coudé tip. For initial dilation, we favor the use of balloons placed over wires that have been passed through the stricture under endoscopic control.

Internal Urethrotomy

Internal urethrotomy refers to any procedure that opens the stricture by incising it transurethrally. The urethrotomy procedure involves incision through the scar to healthy tissue to allow the scar to expand (release of scar contracture) **and the lumen to heal enlarged.** The goal is for the resultant larger luminal caliber to be maintained after healing.

With epithelial apposition, wound healing occurs by primary intention. Internal urethrotomy does not provide an epithelial approximation but rather aims to separate the scarred epithelium so that the healing occurs by secondary intention. In healing by secondary intention, epithelialization progresses from the wound edges. As it progresses from the wound edge, epithelialization slows. In an effort to aid epithelialization, nature invokes the forces of wound contraction, not to be confused with scar contraction. Wound contraction closes the wound defect and limits the size of the area that requires epithelialization, hastening the healing of the surface defect. In the case of internal urethrotomy, however, wound contraction merely tries to reapproximate the edges of the scar, putting a race into effect. If epithelialization progresses completely before wound contraction significantly narrows the lumen, the internal urethrotomy may be a success. If wound contraction significantly narrows the lumen before completion of epithelialization, the stricture has recurred.

Many surgeons have learned to perform internal urethrotomy by making a single incision at the 12-o'clock position. This location might be questioned, however, on the basis of the location of the urethra within the corpus spongiosum (see Fig. 33–25). On examination of a cross section of the corpus spongiosum, it can be seen that the thinnest portion of the anterior aspect is from 10-o'clock to 2-o'clock. The distance between the anterior wall of the urethra and the corpora

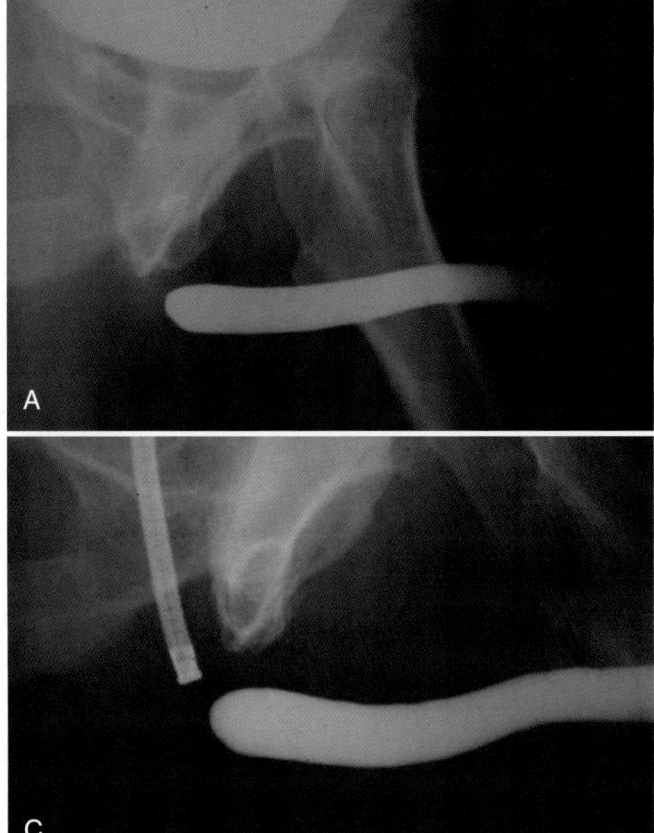

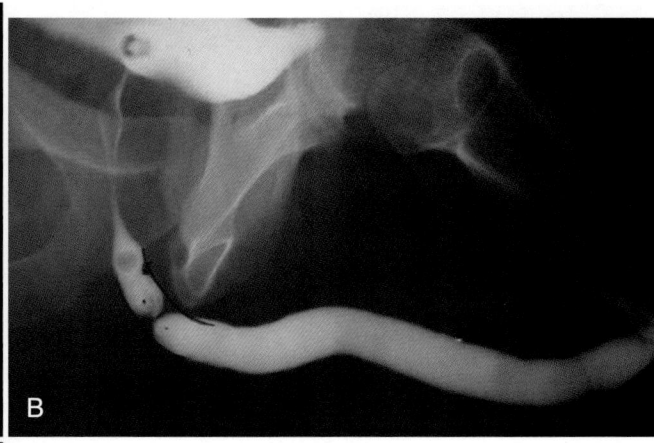

Figure 33-27. A series of radiographs demonstrating the usefulness of the combination of contrast enhancement with endoscopy. **A,** A retrograde urethrogram shows a totally obliterative process involving the proximal bulbous urethra. **B,** The patient was successful in relaxing to void; however, there is suggestion of a wide-caliber annular area proximal to the obliterative process of the bulbous urethra. **C,** Endoscopy through the suprapubic cystostomy tube clarifies the anatomy of the proximal urethra and demonstrates the length of the obliterative process.

cavernosa is likewise short in the bulbous urethra, and a single 12-o'clock cut could rapidly penetrate the corpus spongiosum and extend into the triangular ligament; although it might not enter the corpora cavernosa, a deep cut could enter the intracrural space. Distally, although the anterior aspect of the corpus spongiosum is thicker, on the other hand, a deep incision in the more distal aspects of the anterior urethra will certainly enter the corpora cavernosa, and these incisions have been associated with erectile dysfunction thought to be due to local cavernosal veno-occlusive dysfunction. Vigorous incisions at 10-o'clock and 2-o'clock in the bulbous urethra risk the same problem. If deep spongiofibrosis is present, stricture cure is impossible by internal urethrotomy, and these deep incisions are therefore unnecessary.

The most common complication of internal urethrotomy is recurrence of stricture. Less commonly noted complications of internal urethrotomy include bleeding (almost always associated with erections immediately after the procedure) and extravasation of irrigation fluid into the perispongiosal tissues. These complications are rare today, however, because of the less frequent use of aggressive internal urethrotomy as a treatment modality for urethral strictures. Normal saline should be used as the irrigant when direct visual internal urethrotomy is performed.

A major problem with assessing the success rates of internal urethrotomy is that the nature of the strictures that have been treated with internal urethrotomy has been poorly reported. In addition, the literature is not clear regarding the goal of internal urethrotomy. For many, an internal urethrot-

omy is successful if it offers temporary relief. Therefore, in many cases, internal urethrotomy has been reported as successful despite the fact that it has been associated with eventual stricture recurrence. A report published by Santucci and McAninch (2001) using actuarial techniques shows the curative success rate of internal urethrotomy to be approximately 20%. Evaluations by Pansadoro and Emiliozzi (1996) and others show the curative success rate of direct visual internal urethrotomy to be approximately 30% to 35%. Their analysis also shows that there is virtually no increase in success rate with a second internal urethrotomy. **The data show that strictures at the bulbous urethra that are less than 1.5 cm in length and not associated with dense, deep spongiofibrosis (i.e., straddle injuries) can be managed with internal urethrotomy with a 74% moderately long-term success rate.** Pansadoro's study did not have any long-term successes for treated strictures outside the bulbous urethra. The variables associated with success of internal urethrotomy have been verified by other studies (Heyns et al, 1998). A number of studies now show that the success of reconstruction is diminished by multiple prior urethral dilations and internal urethrotomy (Stone et al, 1983; Albers et al, 1996; Heyns et al, 1998; Boccon-Gibod, 2005).

Because of this dismal success rate, several techniques have been employed to oppose the process of wound contraction and to prevent stricture recurrence. One method is to leave an indwelling Foley catheter for as long as 6 weeks after urethrotomy, in the hope that the urethra will mold around the catheter as it heals. Studies have shown, however, that the failure rate of long-term catheterization after internal ure-throtomy is similar to that seen with 3 to 7 days of catheterization, and even 6 weeks is not sufficient time to oppose the forces of wound contraction.

Another technique used to oppose the forces of wound contraction after internal urethrotomy is home self-catheterization or home urethral obturation. After internal urethrotomy, patients generally have an indwelling catheter placed for a period of 3 to 5 days. When the catheter is removed, the patient is begun on a urethral obturation regimen. Most regimens require more frequent catheterizations early in the recovery period, with a tapering schedule during the next 3 to 6 months. Anecdotally, many have reported an improved cure rate with self-catheterization in combination with internal urethrotomy. It has been our experience, however, that the stricture inevitably recurs when the patient stops self-obturation, regardless of how long it has been used. That being understood, this can effectively manage the problems when it is combined with a urethral dilating regimen in the properly motivated patient.

Urethral stents (removable or permanently implantable) are another modality used in opposing the forces of wound contraction after internal urethrotomy or dilation. Removable urethral stents are designed to prevent the process of epithelialization from incorporating the stent into the urethral wall and are left in place for as long as 6 months to 1 year before they are removed. The greatest experience with these removable stents comes from Israel (Yachia and Beyar, 1991), and centers there report good success in small series. The Memokath is currently in studies in the United States. It is a removable stent made of nitinol.

The majority of experience with permanently implantable stents comes from Europe and the United Kingdom. Milroy (1993) has reported a success rate of 84% at 4.5 years with use of the permanently implantable UroLume (Rousseau et al, 1987; Sigwart et al, 1987; Milroy et al, 1988, 1989; Sarramon et al, 1990; Ashken et al, 1991; Krah et al, 1992; Sneller and Bosch, 1992; Verhamme et al, 1993; Badlani et al, 1995; Milroy and Allen, 1996; Jordan, 1997; Tillem et al, 1997; Brandes and McAninch, 1998; Shah et al, 2003). The UroLume, made of an alloy, is designed to be incorporated into the wall of the urethra and corpus spongiosum. Available data show that the stent is best employed for relatively short strictures of the bulbous urethra associated with minimal spongiofibrosis. However, these are the strictures that are most successfully reconstructed with open techniques that offer better long-term success rates. The North American Study Group 11-year data have been published (Shah et al, 2003). Of 179 patients originally enrolled in the North American Study, 24 patients completed 11 years of follow-up. The overall success rate for all patients enrolled at 11 years is less than 30% (Shah et al, 2003). A 10-year follow-up study from the Netherlands (De Vocht et al, 2003) reported results thought to "weaken the optimistic early results"; of 15 patients implanted, only 2 were satisfied with their stent at 10 years.

Permanently implantable stents are associated with some unique complications. The stents must be **placed only in the bulbous urethra,** and when they are placed beyond the area of the scrotal urethra, placement has been associated with pain on sitting and intercourse. Some patients (particularly young patients) **complain of perineal pain,** often with vigorous

activity, even after implantation of the stent in the deep bulbous urethra. In addition, **longer, bulbous strictures require two stents that are overlapped.** These **stents can migrate** away from each other, leaving a gap between them where recurrence of stricture is inevitable. When this occurs, the stricture recurrence is excised and a third stent is placed to span the gap.

There are also **specific contraindications to the use of the UroLume.** Patients who have undergone **prior substitution urethral reconstruction,** particularly where skin has been incorporated into the urethra, have been shown to be poor candidates for implantation with the UroLume stent because contact of the stent with the skin is associated with a virulent hypertrophic reaction. These patients experience postvoid dribbling, and the hypertrophic reaction can be so severe in some cases that functional recurrence of the stricture results. Another subset of patients shown to be **poor candidates for the UroLume are those with strictures associated with deep spongiofibrosis.** Patients who fall into this category are **those who have had urethral distraction injuries and straddle injuries associated with deep fibrosis.** As of this writing, the UroLume is approved by the U.S. Food and Drug Administration. The product insert clearly contraindicates use of the UroLume in patients with pelvic fracture urethral distraction defects. Many greeted the arrival of the UroLume as a panacea. Experience is accumulating not only with use of the UroLume but also with misuse of the device, and its use should therefore be approached with the utmost caution. Some centers in Europe are now advocating use of the UroLume only in patients who are older than 50 years or who have other significant medical problems that make the option of lengthy open urethral reconstruction less appealing. At our center, we have seen teenagers implanted, many patients implanted for pelvic fracture urethral distraction, patients with stents palpable on the shaft of the penis, and patients with both prostatic stents and urethral stents—all absolute contraindications. We have seen patients with as many as six stents in place, and although the maximal number of stents is not absolutely defined, if the first stent does not work, it is probably wise to refer the patient for reconstruction, which is possible with acceptable results (86% with mean follow-up of 25 months) (Barbagli et al, 1999). Placement of more stents, except when two stents were originally placed and then migrate from each other, is probably futile. However, in carefully selected elderly patients, the UroLume can be life changing for the patients, with minimal morbidity associated with the implantation procedure.

Lasers

Types of lasers that have been used for the treatment of urethral stricture disease include carbon dioxide, argon, KTP, Nd:YAG, holmium:YAG, and excimer lasers. The ideal laser for use in the treatment of urethral stricture disease is one that totally vaporizes tissue, exhibits negligible peripheral tissue destruction, is not absorbed by water, and is easily propagated along a fiber. Although the carbon dioxide laser appears to be ideally suited, it must be used with a gas cystoscope, which carries the potential threat of a carbon dioxide embolus.

For both the argon and the Nd:YAG lasers, the predominant mode of action is thermal necrosis, which leads to a significant potential for peripheral tissue injury rather than vaporization.

The Nd:YAG laser has also been used with a bare fiber in the contact mode. A bare fiber carries with it a risk of forward scatter. When it is used in the contact mode, the YAG energy is transferred to a sapphire tip. Advocates of the use of a contact laser suggest that it obliterates the scar by vaporization; however, results with use of these fibers are no better than those with direct cold-knife visual internal urethrotomy.

A KTP laser is essentially an Nd:YAG laser that has passed through a KTP crystal, resulting in a reduced depth of penetration. A KTP laser urethrotomy is accomplished by passing the fiber over the scar tissue to make urethrotomy cuts. The holmium:YAG laser has properties similar to the KTP laser, and like the KTP laser, it provides both direct contact cutting and vaporization with minimal forward scatter. Experience with the holmium:YAG laser is accumulating; anecdotally, it may have a place in the management of some strictures, in particular strictures that are relatively isolated and short.

The excimer laser is a true vaporizing laser that has little forward scatter or peripheral tissue necrosis associated with it. Little experience with this laser has been reported, but future investigation is clearly warranted.

To date, the results of laser urethrotomy are mixed. With the advent of new lasers and experience with them, however, future data may show better results.

Open Reconstruction

Excision and Reanastomosis. It has now been demonstrated with certainty that the most dependable technique of anterior urethral reconstruction is the complete excision of the area of fibrosis, with a primary reanastomosis of the normal ends of the anterior urethra (Fig. 33–28). The best results are achieved when **the following technical points are observed: the area of fibrosis is totally excised; the urethral anastomosis is widely spatulated, creating a large ovoid anastomosis; and the anastomosis is tension free.**

The **success of this procedure relies on vigorous mobilization of the corpus spongiosum.** With vigorous mobilization, dissection of Buck's fascia to improve compliance, development of the intracrural space, and detachment of the bulbospongiosus from the perineal body, significant lengths of stricture can be excised and reanastomosed. Strictures of 1 to 2 cm are generally easily excised with reanastomosis. In some cases, strictures as long as 3 to 5 cm can be totally excised and a primary reanastomosis of the anterior urethra performed. For very proximal short-length bulbous strictures, tension-free anastomosis can be facilitated by the dissection of the membranous urethra (Fig. 33–29). As a rule, the closer the stricture is to the membranous urethra, the longer it can be and still be reconstructed with anastomotic techniques. For many proximal strictures, a single-layer anastomosis is preferable. When the length of stricture precludes total excision of fibrosis with primary anastomosis, tissue transfer is required. Morey published a series of patients who had stricture excision with anastomosis for strictures up to 5 cm. He makes the point that the younger patient has more compliant tissue, thus allowing the limits to be stretched (Kizer and Morey, 2005).

Morey also reported an interesting variant of excision with anastomosis for anterior stricture. In that case report, a patient had two independent areas of stricture apparently separated by totally normal urethra and corpus spongiosum. The authors excised both areas of stricture independently with

respective anastomosis of each site. Although this case was successful, we think that the authors' considerable experience allowed them to achieve a successful result, and a safer reconstruction with use of onlay or augmented onlay might have been better (DeCastro et al, 2002).

Four grafts that have been successfully used for primary urethral reconstruction are the full-thickness skin graft, the bladder epithelial graft, the buccal mucosal graft, and the rectal mucosal graft. Split-thickness skin grafts have been used for staged anterior urethral reconstruction. The characteristics and microvascularity of some of those grafts are discussed earlier in this chapter in the section "Principles of Reconstructive Surgery."

In years past, graft reconstruction of the urethra was almost abandoned in favor of flap reconstruction techniques. However, since the late 1990s, there has been a resurgence of interest in the use of grafts and specifically the use of buccal mucosal grafts (Hellstrom et al, 1996; Weinberg et al, 2002; Barbagli et al, 2003; Elliott et al, 2003; Bhargava and Chapple, 2004; Kellner et al, 2004; Xu et al, 2004; Dubey et al, 2005). **Grafts have been shown to be most successfully employed in the area of the bulbous urethra where the urethra is invested by the bulk of the ischiocavernosus muscles. However, the use of grafts elsewhere than the bulbous urethra and, in some cases, tubed reconstruction are reported in increasing numbers.** The grafts can be applied to the ventrum of the urethra; however, a ventral urethrotomy seems to be of advantage only if one contemplates the use of the spongioplasty maneuver (Fig. 33–30A). The spongioplasty procedure requires that the corpus spongiosum adjacent to the area of the stricture be relatively normal and free of fibrosis. There are data to support superiority of results with the dorsal onlay technique and other reports showing no difference in success. We preferred in the past to use lateral graft onlay (Fig. 33–30B) or dorsal graft onlay (Fig. 33–30C). Placement of the urethrostomy laterally allows one to expose the urethra while cutting through the corpus spongiosum, where it is relatively thinner, thus limiting bleeding and maximizing exposure. In addition, in the bulbous urethra, the graft can be sutured to the underlying muscle bed in the hope of improving graft host bed immobilization and approximation.

The Monseur (1980) urethral reconstruction was applied in only a few select centers. In this technique, the urethrostomy was made through the stricture on the dorsal wall. The edges of the stricture were then sutured open to the underlying triangular ligament or corpora cavernosa, or both. Barbagli and associates (1995) have modified the Monseur technique (Fig. 33–31). In that modification, the urethrostomy is through the stricture on the dorsal wall. In the area of the urethrostomy, a graft is then applied, spread fixed to the triangular ligament or corpora cavernosa, or both. In turn, the edges of the stricturotomy are then sutured to the edges of the graft as well as to the adjacent structures. The results of this technique are excellent. The ventral and dorsal graft onlay techniques can both be used with stricture excision and strip anastomosis (augmented anastomotic procedure) (Fig. 33–32).

Another option is the two-staged application of a mesh split-thickness skin graft, buccal mucosal graft, or posterior auricular full-thickness skin graft. In the first stage of the staged graft procedure, a medium-thickness split-thickness

Text continued on p. 1067.

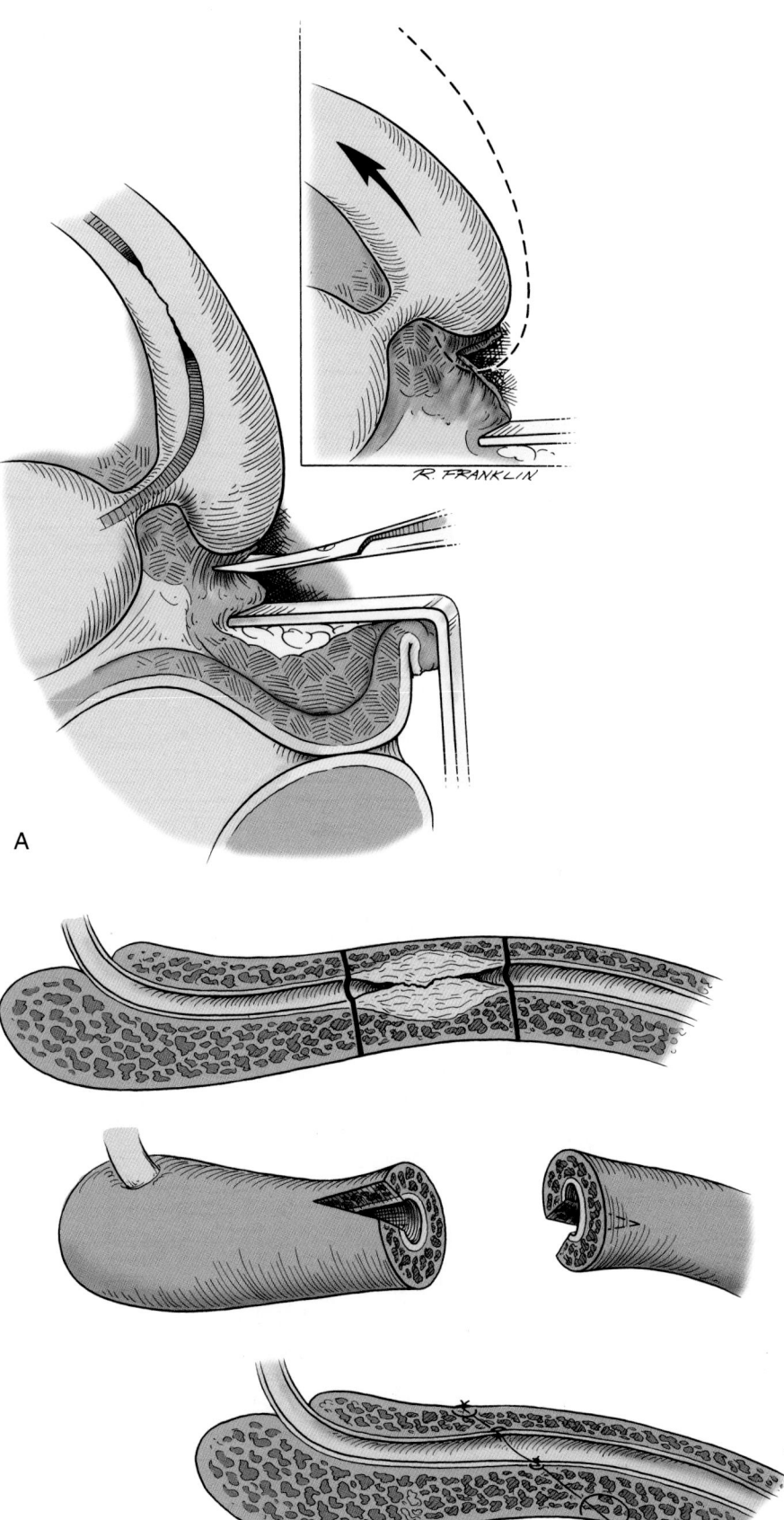

Figure 33–28. Techniques for excision and primary reanastomosis of anterior urethral stricture. **A,** The bulbospongiosus is released from its attachment to the perineal body. The arteries to the bulb are not divided. This technique allows the urethra to be mobilized distally. This technique combined with development of the intracrural space can shorten the path of the urethra by approximately 1 to 1.5 cm. **B,** Technique of a primary spatulated anastomosis after excision of an anterior urethral stricture. (**A** and **B,** from Jordan GH: Principles of plastic surgery. In Droller MJ, ed: Surgical Management of Urologic Disease: An Anatomic Approach. Philadelphia, Mosby–Year Book, 1992:1218-1237.)

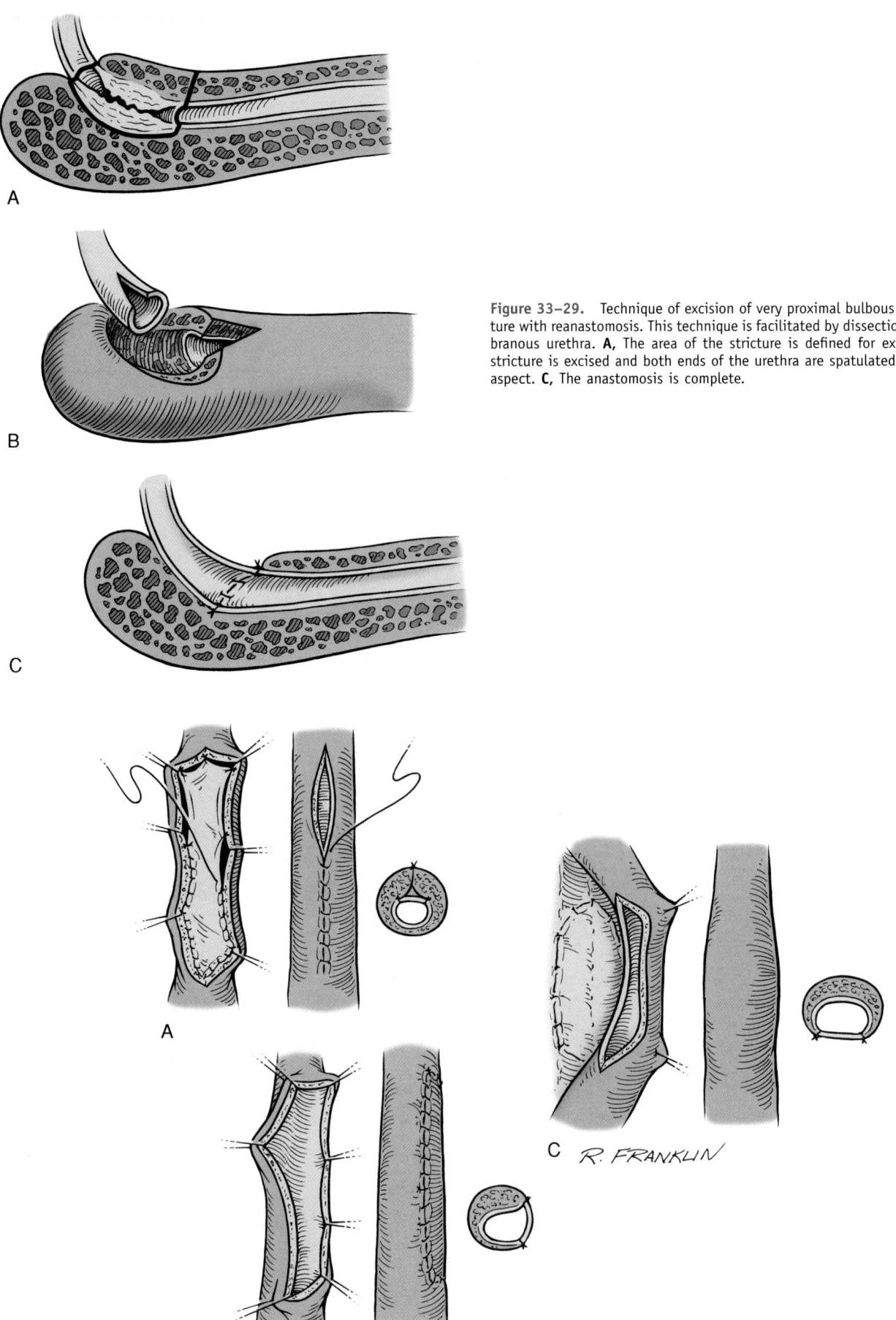

Figure 33–29. Technique of excision of very proximal bulbous urethral stricture with reanastomosis. This technique is facilitated by dissection of the membranous urethra. **A,** The area of the stricture is defined for excision. **B,** The stricture is excised and both ends of the urethra are spatulated on the dorsal aspect. **C,** The anastomosis is complete.

Figure 33–30. Diagram of various techniques of graft onlay. **A,** Ventral onlay with spongioplasty. **B,** Lateral onlay with quilting to the ischiocavernosus muscle. **C,** Dorsal onlay with spread fixation of the graft.

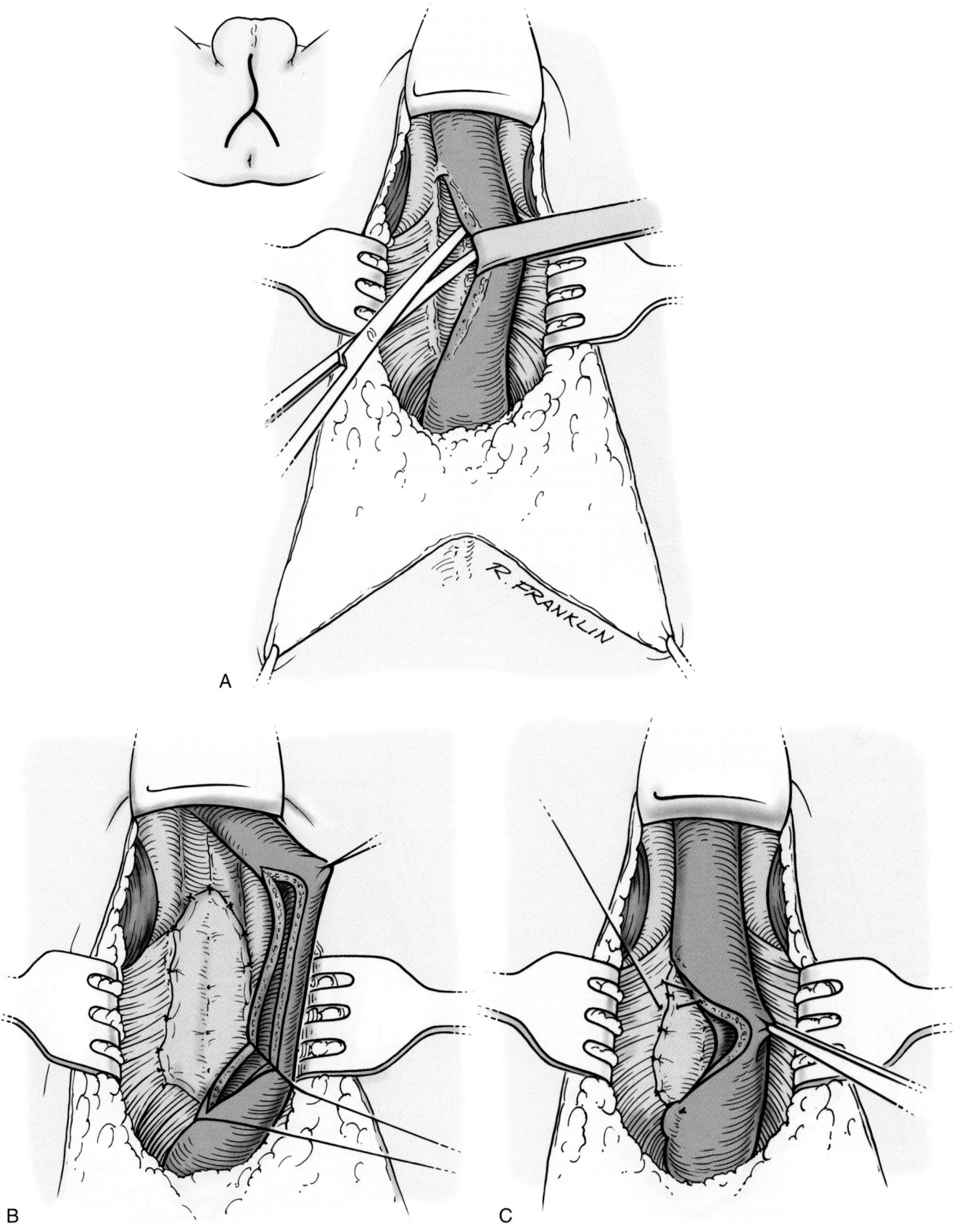

Figure 33–31. Technique of dorsal graft onlay popularized by Barbagli. **A,** The corpus spongiosum is detached from the triangular ligament and corpora cavernosa. **B,** A dorsal urethrostomy is performed. The graft is spread fixed to the corpora cavernosa. Note the pie-crusting incision. **C,** The edges of the stricturotomy are then sutured to the graft as well as to the corpora cavernosa.

SECTION VII

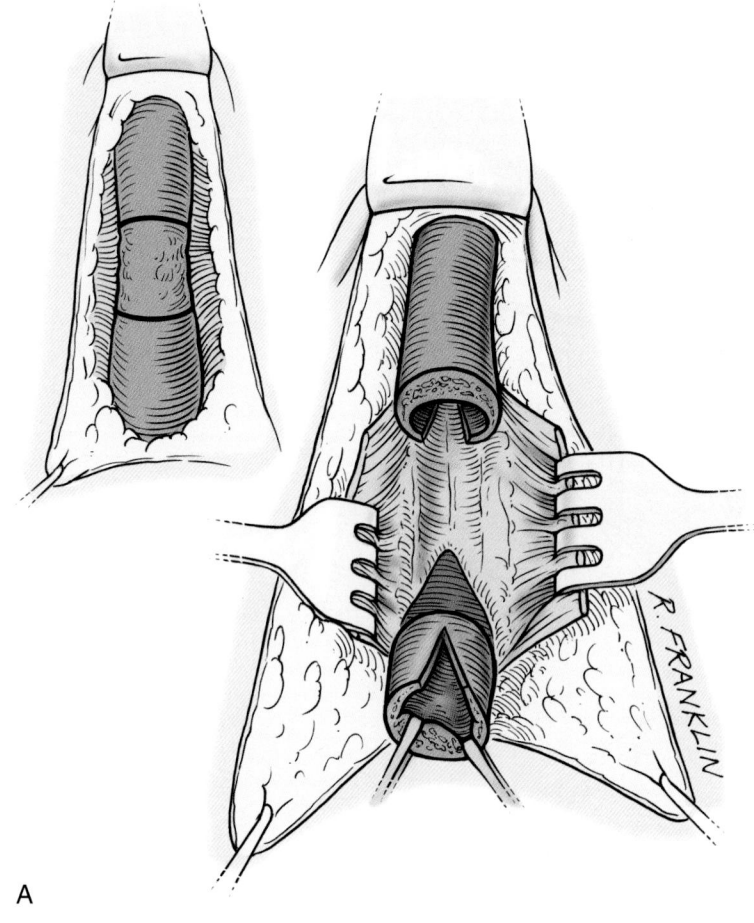

Figure 33–32. Technique of augmented anastomosis with graft onlay. **A,** The corpus spongiosum is detached from the triangular ligament and the corpora cavernosa. The area of spongiofibrosis is identified and marked, and the area of narrowest caliber stricture is excised. The urethral ends are then spatulated on the dorsum. **B,** A two-layer floor strip anastomosis is performed and the graft is spread fixed to the corpora cavernosa. Note the piecrusting incisions and the mattress sutures. **C,** The edges of the stricturotomy are then sutured to the graft as well as to the corpora cavernosa.

A

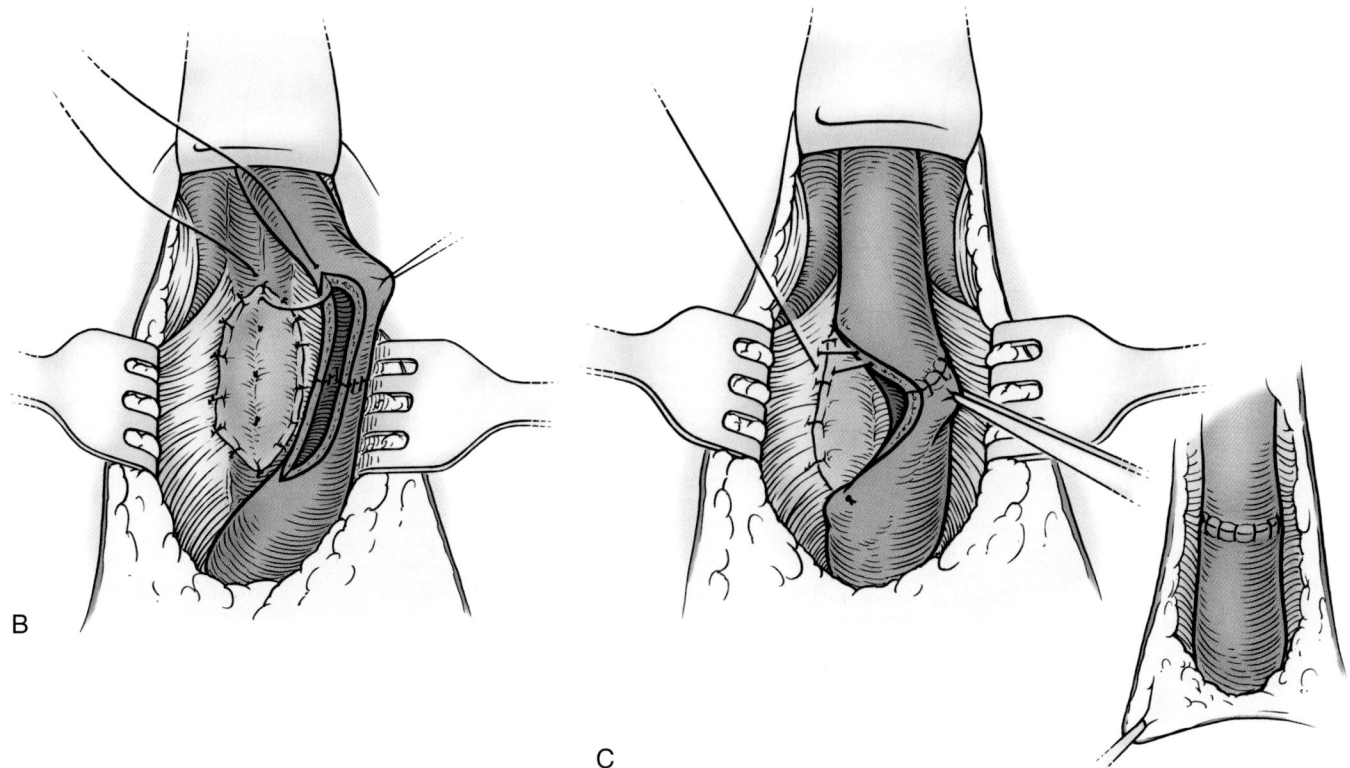

B

C

skin graft, a buccal mucosal graft, or a Wolff graft is placed over the dartos fascia. If the graft is placed immediately onto the tunica albuginea or corpora cavernosa, the inability to mobilize the graft makes second-stage tubularization difficult. However, there is an advantage to having at least a midline strip of the graft adherent to the corpora cavernosa. At a later date, second-stage surgery is performed to tubularize the graft. Whereas Schreiter and Noll (1989), who first described the procedure of mesh split-thickness skin graft, often proceed to the second stage within 3 to 4 months, we wait 12 months between the first- and second-stage surgeries if a split-thickness skin graft is used. This procedure has been found useful for select cases in both the United States and Europe. In the United States, its use has mostly been confined to the most difficult cases, however, with single-stage reconstruction still applied to the majority. As already mentioned, staged graft techniques have been effectively used in the complicated hypospadias patient. Staged buccal graft operations have been successfully employed in the LS-BXO patients with midterm follow-up. In addition, in the complicated hypospadias patient, staged buccal grafts and posterior auricular skin grafts have been successfully employed.

A number of applications of genital skin islands, mobilized on either the dartos fascia of the penis or the tunica dartos of the scrotum, have been proposed for the repair of urethral stricture disease. In the past, these "flap operations" were considered to be separate procedures. We suggest that all these procedures are really different applications of a single concept, proposed by the microinjection studies of Quartey (1983). Skin islands can be viewed as passengers on fascial flaps, and the design of flaps for urethral reconstruction can be paralleled to the design of flaps for reconstruction in general.

There are **three important considerations for the use of flaps in urethral reconstruction: the nature of the flap tissue, the vasculature of the flap, and the mechanics of flap transfer.** The skin must be nonhirsute for urethral reconstruction. **In addition, for donor site consideration, it is most convenient to use the areas of redundant nonhirsute genital skin.**

If the redundancy is dorsal, the skin island can be oriented transversely and mobilized on the dorsal dartos fascia after the techniques described by Duckett and Standoli in 1984 (Fig. 33–33). If there is redundancy of the ventral skin, the skin island can be mobilized as a ventral longitudinal island. These islands can be either vigorously mobilized on a ventrolaterally oriented dartos fascial flap for transposition to the perineum or less vigorously mobilized and transposed and inverted into a pendulous urethral stricture defect (Fig. 33–34). Ventral islands can be oriented transversely (Fig. 33–35) as well as longitudinally (Fig. 33–36). Longer skin islands can be mobilized by orienting the island both ventrally and transversely at the distal extent. This "hockey stick" orientation allows islands as long as 7 to 9 cm (Fig. 33–37).

Where there is general redundancy to the penile skin, the islands can be oriented circumferentially. These "circular skin islands" are mobilized on the entire penile dartos fascia, and the mechanics of transposition suggest that they are most efficient when they are ventrally based, with the pedicle split dorsally. In some cases, circular skin islands as long as 15 cm can be obtained. The so-called Q flap circular island design can provide even longer islands, sometimes necessary for complex

Text continued on p. 1073.

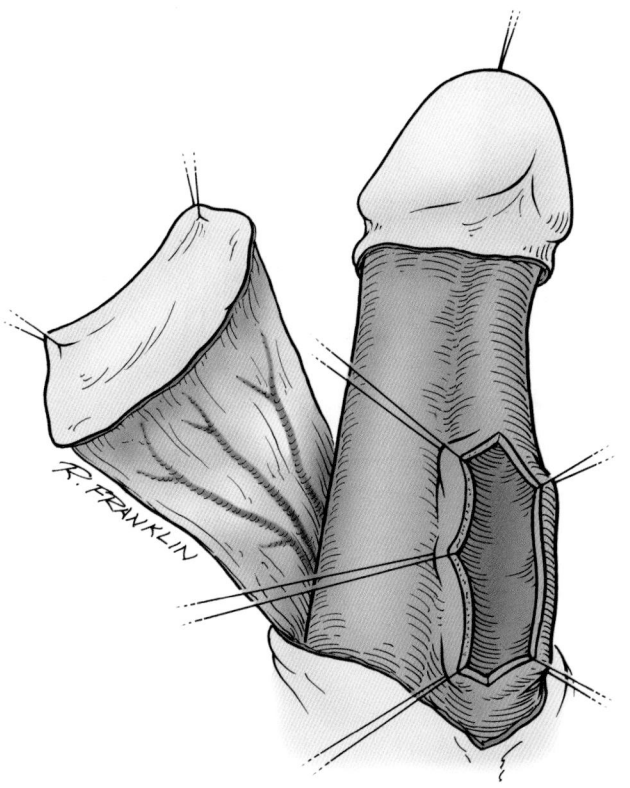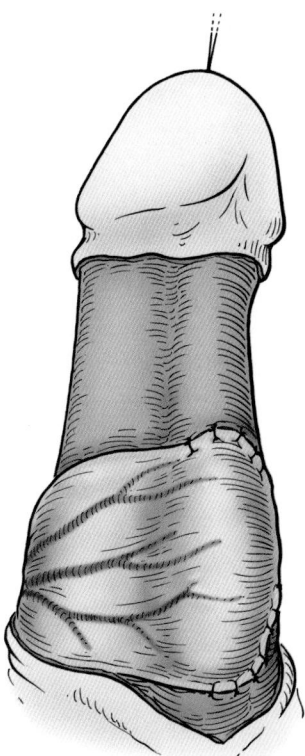

Figure 33–33. A dorsal transverse island of penile skin applied to a stricture of the urethra. The flap has been elevated on the dartos fascia, and a lateral incision has been made into the urethra. The flap is secured in place *(right)*. (From Jordan GH: Management of anterior urethral stricture disease. In Webster GD, ed: Problems in Urology. Philadelphia, JB Lippincott, 1987:217.)

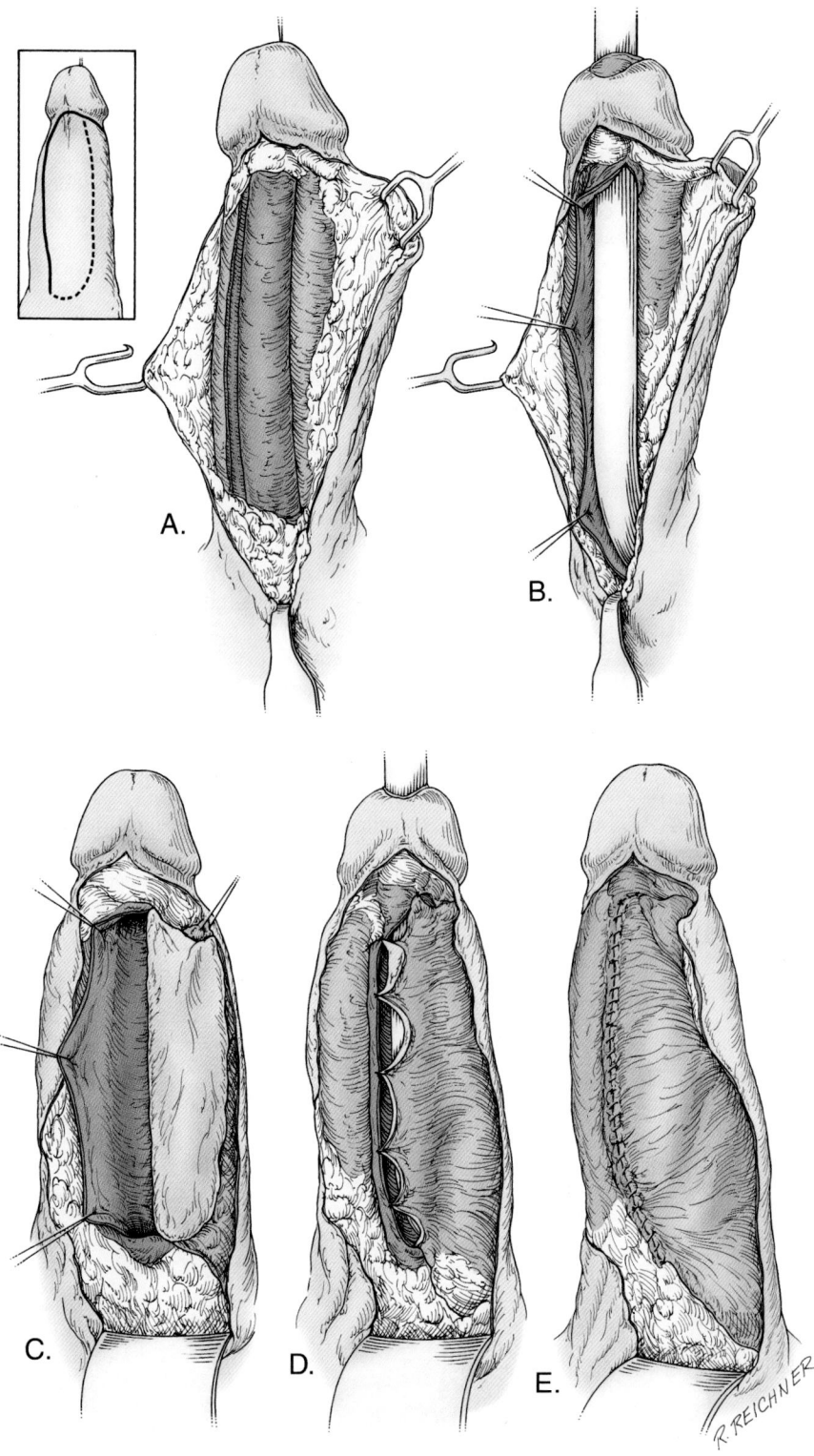

Figure 33–34. Penile longitudinal skin island. The incisions to be made to mobilize the flap are demonstrated in the inset. The heavy line is the primary incision made full thickness through the dartos fascia and superficial Buck's fascia lateral to the corpus spongiosum. **A,** Dissection elevates the dartos fascial flap well past the corpus spongiosum in the midline. **B,** A lateral urethrostomy placed to face the flap has opened the entire length of the stricture. **C,** The skin paddle of the flap has been developed by making the incision outlined by the dotted line *(inset)* and undermining the skin lateral to it. The medial edge of the flap has been fixed to the edge of the stricturotomy. **D,** The flap is inverted into the defect. **E,** A watertight subepithelial suture line has been completed with a running absorbable monofilament suture. The skin will be closed with subcutaneous sutures and interrupted cutaneous sutures. (**A** to **E,** from Jordan GH: Management of anterior urethral stricture disease. In Webster GD, ed: Problems in Urology. Philadelphia, JB Lippincott, 1987:214.)

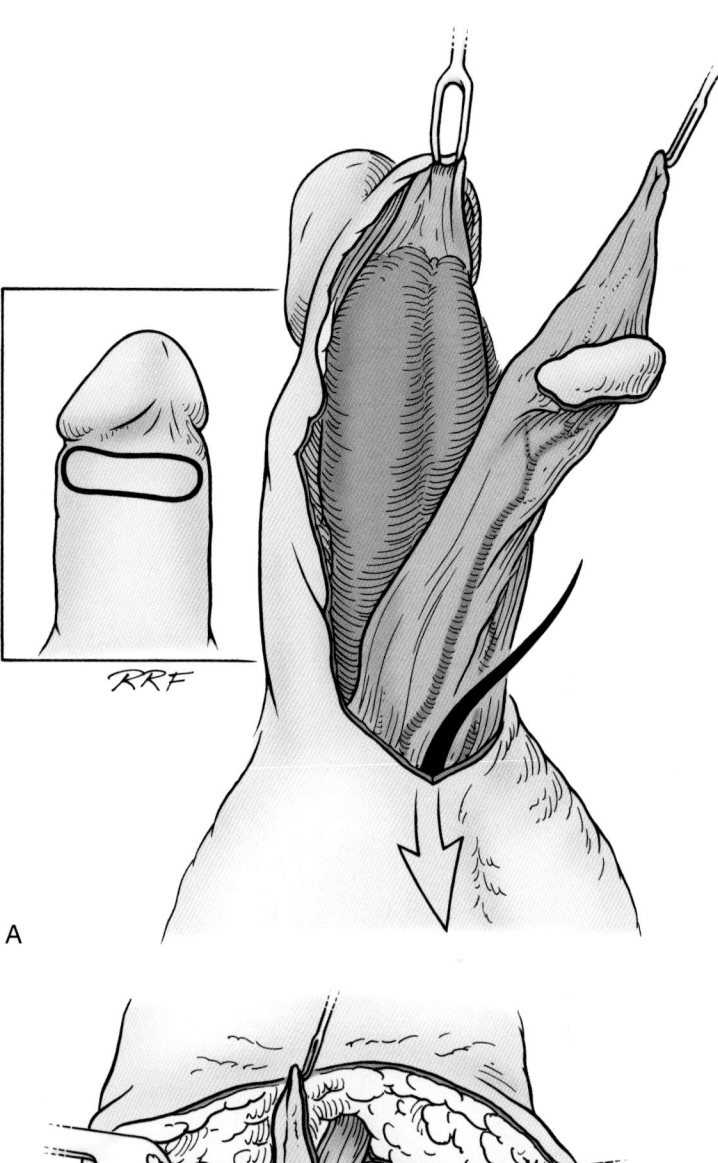

Figure 33–35. A ventral transverse skin island is elevated on the penile dartos fascia, inverted to the area of the perineum where flap onlay is accomplished. **A,** The skin island is elevated on the dartos fascia. **B,** The appearance of the flap transposed to the area of the perineum for onlay in a proximal bulbous urethral stricture.

A

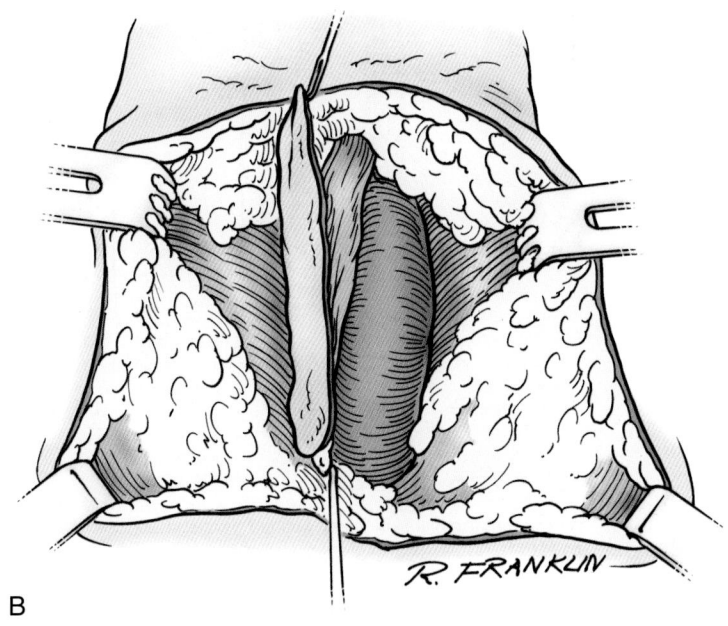

B

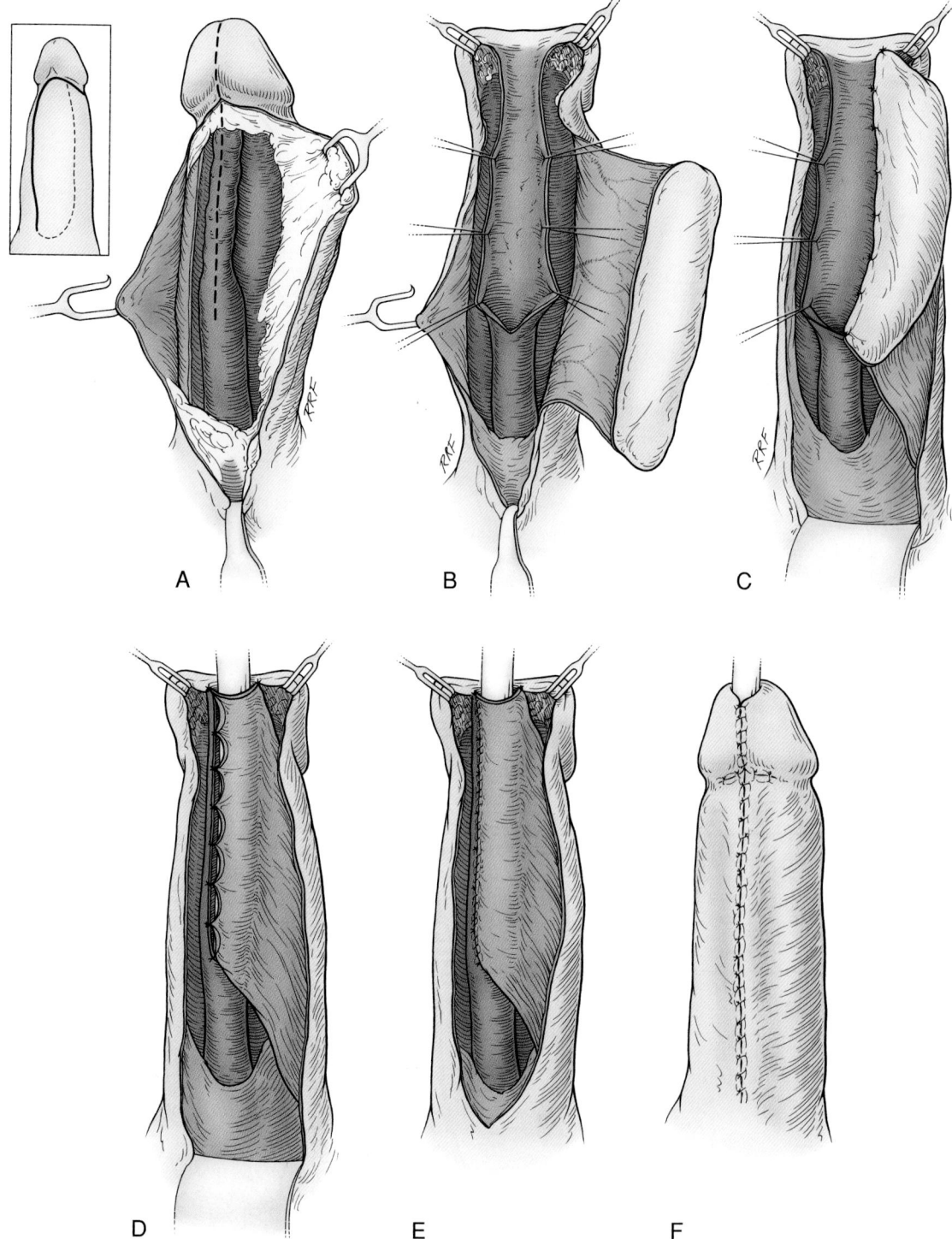

A

B

C

D

E

F

Figure 33–36.　Ventral longitudinal skin island applied for distal urethral stricture disease extending to the meatus. In this case, the flap is elevated more aggressively on the dartos fascia, allowing inversion of the skin island into the defect with advancement to the meatus. **A,** The corpus spongiosum is exposed. **B,** Urethrostomy is performed; the skin island is elevated on the dartos fascia. **C,** The skin island onlay is being accomplished. **D,** The flap is inverted with the contralateral suture line tacked. **E,** The skin island onlay is complete. **F,** The appearance of the ventrum of the closed penis. For transposition to the perineum, the flap is further elevated, with the flap and pedicle passed "beneath" to the scrotum. (From Jordan GH: Reconstruction of the meatus–fossa navicularis using flap techniques. In Schreiter F, ed: Plastic-Reconstructive Surgery in Urology. Stuttgart, Georg Thieme, 1999:338-344).

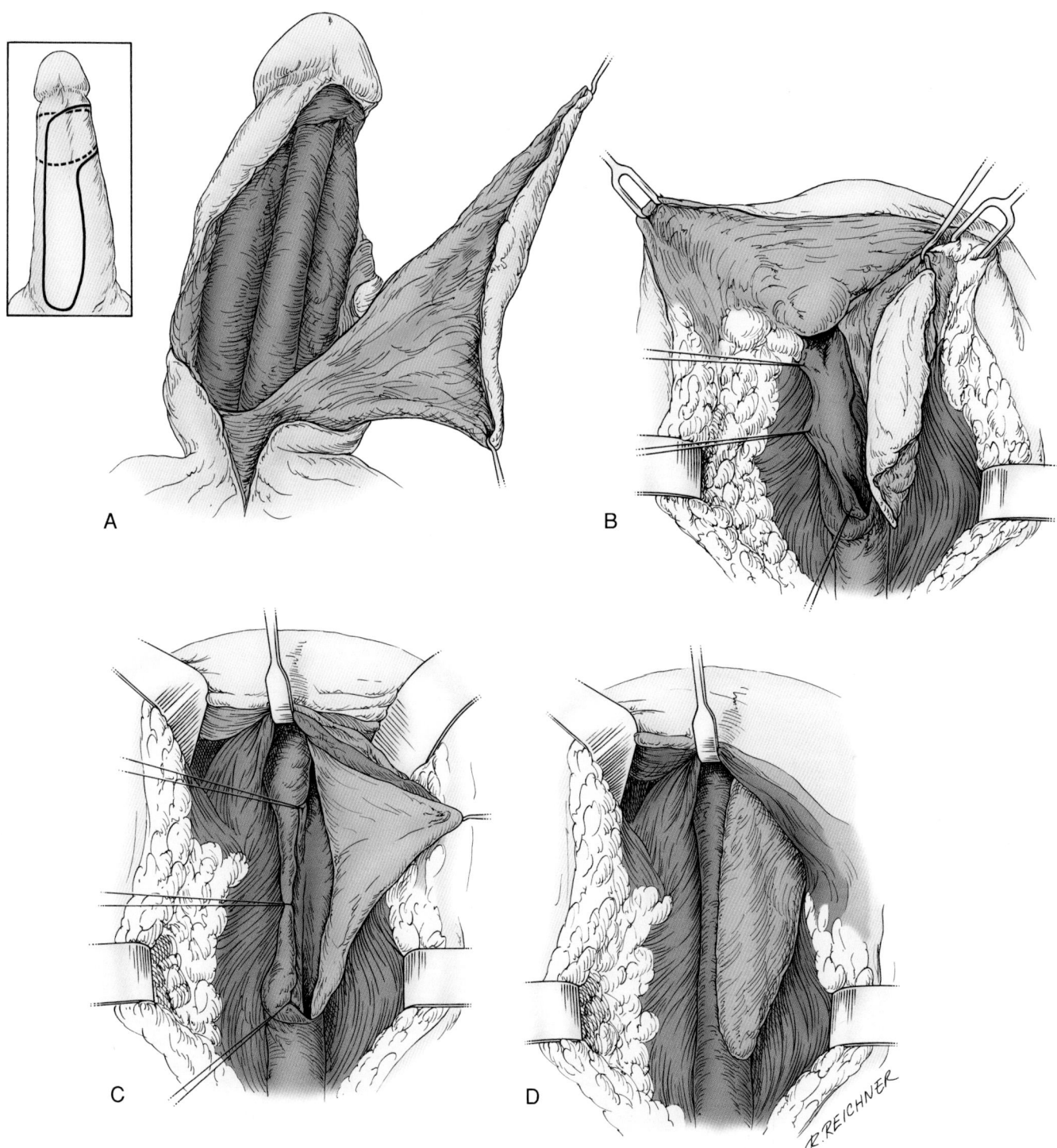

Figure 33–37.   Ventral skin island for long bulbous stricture. The skin paddle of the flap is developed on the ventral midline of the penis and can be extended around the penile shaft at its distal end. **A,** The paddle of the flap has been incised and its pedicle elevated. This pedicle includes Buck's fascia and dartos fascia, denuding the tunica of the corpus spongiosum and the corpora cavernosa. The pedicle (the dartos fascia bilaterally) is based on the superficial external pudendal vessels and the internal pudendal vessels in the scrotum. Development of this pedicle allows the flap to be moved to any area of the urethra. **B,** The flap has been passed through a tunnel beneath the scrotum developed by dissection along the corpus spongiosum. A laterally placed urethrostomy has opened the urethral stricture. **C,** The deep edge of the flap is secured by the suture techniques previously described. **D,** Anastomosis of the flap has been completed. The pedicle can be seen extending beneath the scrotum. (**A** to **D,** from Jordan GH, McCraw JB: Tissue transfer techniques for genitourinary surgery, Part III. AUA Update Series 1988;7.)

SECTION VII

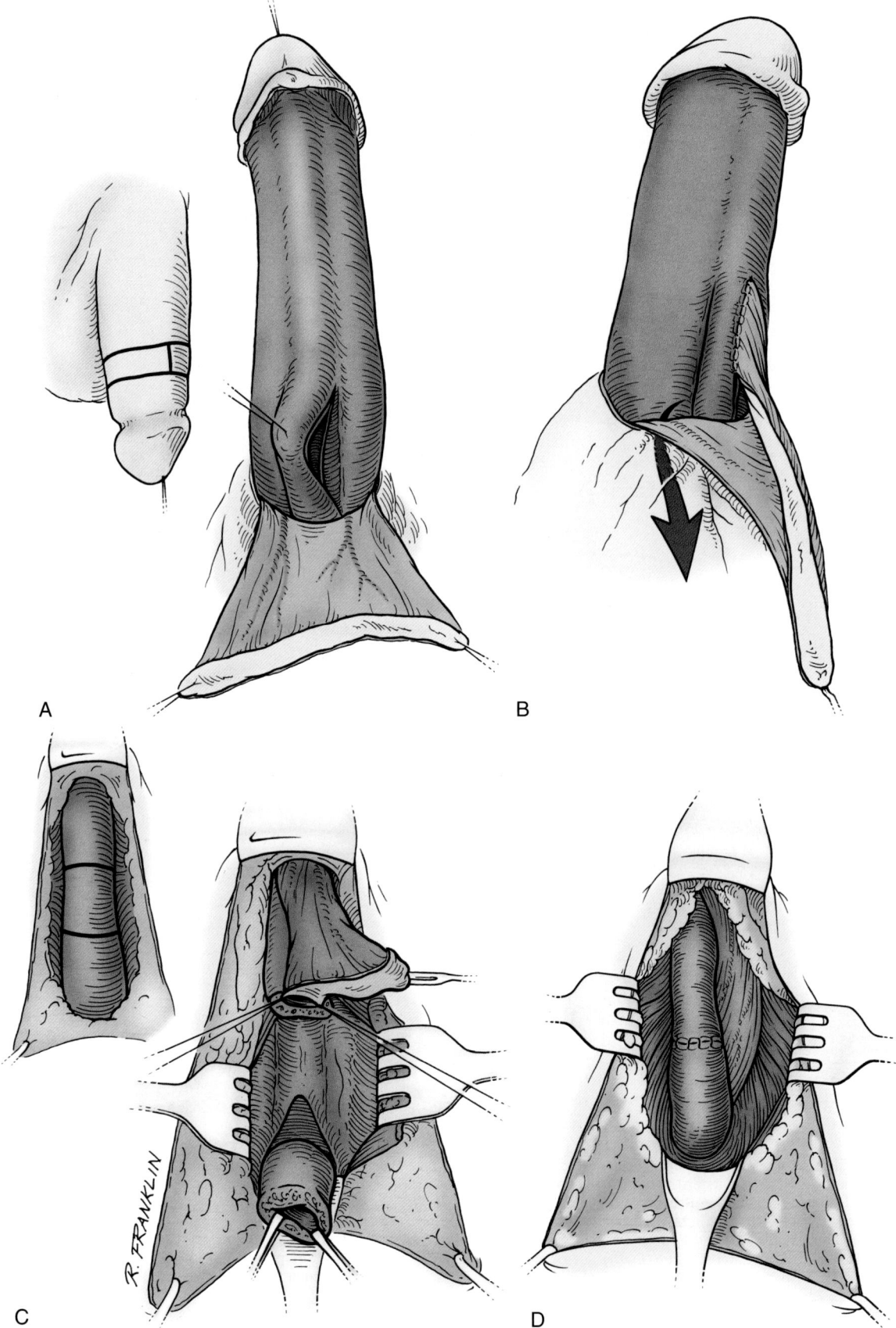

A

B

C

D

R. FRANKLIN

Figure 33–38.   Illustration of reconstruction in a patient with a long anterior urethral stricture with a relatively short narrow-caliber section (technique of augmented anastomosis with circular skin island). **A,** A circular skin island is elevated on the dartos fascia. The patient is positioned flat on the table. **B,** The skin island onlay is begun, the rest of the flap is placed into the perineal dissection, and the penis is closed; the patient is then repositioned in the lithotomy position. **C,** The flap is retrieved through the perineal dissection. The narrow-caliber section is excised, and the urethra is spatulated on the dorsum. **D,** The onlay is completed, and the floor strip anastomosis is closed.   *Continued*

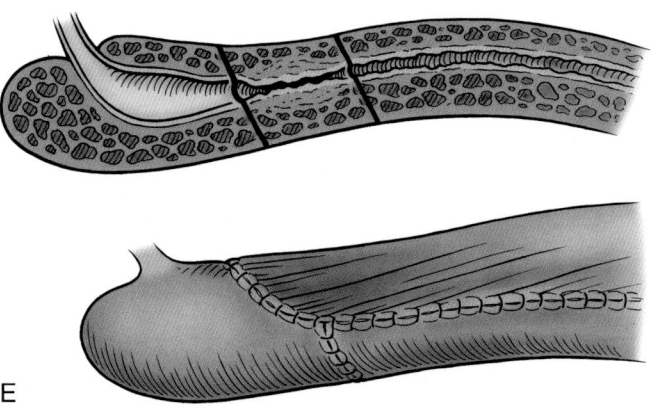

E

Figure 33–38, cont'd. **E,** Schematic of the surgery. (**A** to **E,** from Stack RS, Schlossberg SM, Jordan GH: Reconstruction of anterior urethral strictures by the technique of excision and primary anastomosis. Atlas Urol Clin North Am 1997;5:11-21.)

long-length anterior urethral reconstruction (Morey et al, 2000).

Many times, it is beneficial to combine the excision of the stricture with a skin island onlay (Fig. 33–38) **or a graft onlay** (see Fig. 33–32, augmented anastomosis). We have found that **segments of very narrow caliber (nearly or totally obliterating) are difficult to deal with.** These segments can often be completely excised; a roof or floor strip anastomosis

of the urethra is performed, and the remaining urethrotomy defect is filled with either a graft or a skin island onlay. In some patients, there are relatively large nonhirsute areas of the scrotal skin that can be elevated on the tunica dartos of the scrotum. This flap has in the past been maligned in the literature. However, we and others have large experience with these flaps and in select cases have had very good results. The fascial flap must be based laterally, and so oriented, these flaps have been shown to be extremely reliable. Because the tunica dartos has a significant muscle component, the skin island must be carefully tailored. If these skin islands are correctly tailored at the outset, they are not attended with diverticular development as some have believed they were in the past. We now have used these flaps in more than 80 patients with excellent results and good long-term follow-up (>12 years at this writing). Scrotal skin islands are not our first choice; however, for difficult cases, they remain a reasonable option.

These procedures using skin islands oriented on the penile dartos fascia have also been useful for reconstruction of the fossa navicularis (De Sy, 1984; Jordan, 1987; Armenakas et al, 1998). In the past, meatal strictures and strictures of the fossa navicularis were managed with repeated dilations or sequential meatotomies. Because these meatotomies were seldom successful in the long term, techniques were developed that allowed the spatulation of random penile skin flaps into the meatotomy defects (Fig. 33–39). These procedures function-

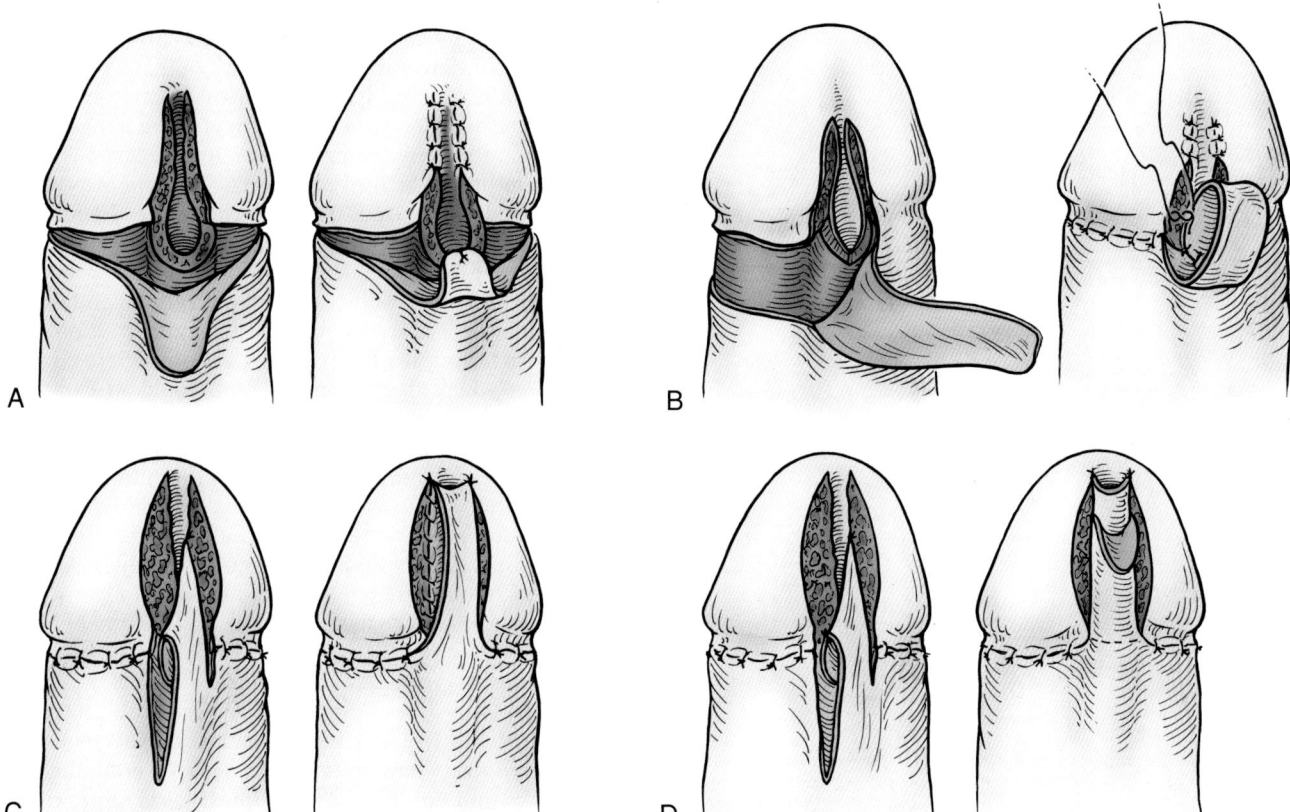

A B C D

Figure 33–39. Collage of techniques for reconstruction of the fossa navicularis and meatus. **A,** Technique after Blandy in which a random penile skin island is advanced into a meatotomy defect. **B,** Technique after Cohney in which a transversely oriented random flap is advanced into the meatotomy defect. **C,** Technique after Brannen in which a midline random flap is advanced into the meatotomy defect. This technique was an attempt to improve the cosmetic result of prior procedures. **D,** Technique after De Sy in which a ventral longitudinal skin island is advanced into the meatotomy defect. The skin island is developed by deepithelialization of a portion of the longitudinal flap. (After Jordan GH: Management of anterior urethral stricture disease. Probl Urol 1987;1:199-225.)

ally improved the results; however, the cosmetic appearance of the penis was less than optimal. With the use of skin islands elevated on the dartos fascia, excellent functional as well as cosmetic results became the norm. Again, the design of these islands must take into consideration the location of hair on the shaft of the penis as well as the mechanics of flap transfer (i.e., transposition versus advancement) (Fig. 33–40; see also Fig. 33–39D). In addition, full-thickness skin has been used to reconstruct the fossa navicularis, but when they can be avoided, skin grafts are not thought to be appropriate for reconstruction in cases of LS-BXO. As already mentioned, there is question about the use of skin islands in general in patients with LS-BXO.

The literature has made it clear that onlay procedures (graft or flap) are attended with a higher success rate than tubularized grafts or tubularized skin islands. Tubularized grafts and skin islands should therefore be avoided, if possible. When tubularized segments cannot be avoided, the length of these segments can be limited by combining aggressive mobilization and excision. Without question, tubularized flaps provide better results than tubularized grafts. Where extremely long segments of the anterior urethra

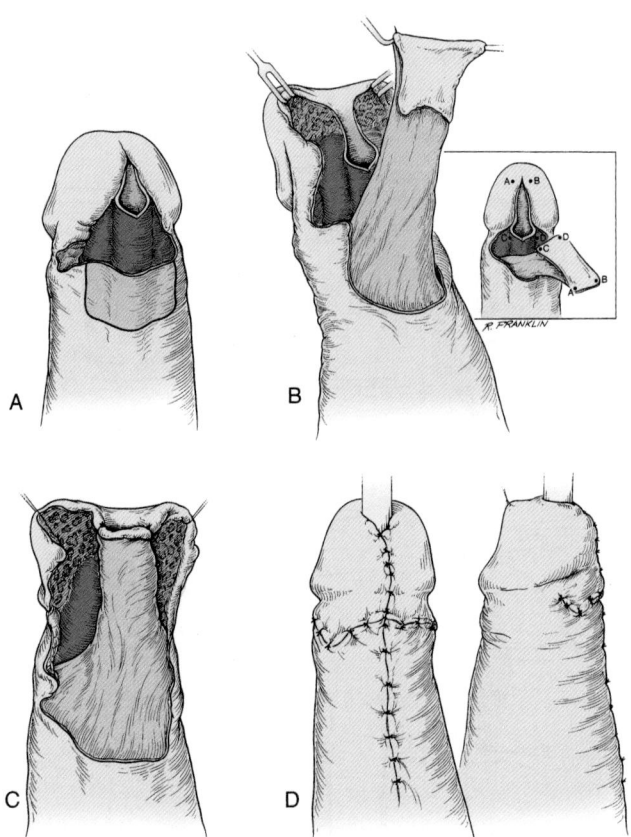

Figure 33–40. Technique of reconstruction of the fossa navicularis after Jordan. **A,** The ventral corpus spongiosum is exposed and the urethra opened ventrally through the area of stenosis. A transverse ventral skin island is outlined on the distal penile skin. **B,** The skin island is elevated on the ventral dartos fascia. **C,** The skin island is transposed and inverted into the meatotomy defect *(inset).* **D,** The appearance of the penis closed after the procedure. (**A** to **C,** from Jordan GH: Reconstruction of the fossa navicularis. J Urol 1987;138:1210. **D,** from Jordan GH: Reconstruction of the meatus–fossa navicularis using flap techniques. In Schreiter F, ed: Plastic-Reconstructive Surgery in Urology. Stuttgart, Georg Thieme, 1999:338-344.)

require reconstruction, a flap can be used distally and augmented by graft onlay proximally (Wessells et al, 1997). Where tubed reconstruction is required, the combination of a graft spread fixed to reestablish the "urethral plate" with flap onlay, in a small series with only short follow-up, seems perhaps to be better than tubed flap reconstruction even when it is employed in the onlay-tube-onlay configuration (Morey, 2001).

A flap procedure that can be used as an alternative to the split-thickness skin grafts when nonhirsute skin is unavailable is the epilated midline genital skin island. Like the split-thickness skin graft, this procedure must be viewed as a staged procedure, with the epilations being the initial stage or stages. Epilation can be accomplished with either a narrow-gauge needle and monopolar cautery or epilation needles and machines. The interval between the epilations must be 6 to 8 weeks, and urethral reconstruction cannot be accomplished until 10 to 12 weeks after the last epilation. The actual stricture repair involves elevation of the midline skin island, based on both the dartos fascia of the penis and the tunica dartos of the scrotum. As with nonhirsute scrotal skin islands in general, the importance of meticulous tailoring of the scrotal portion of the island cannot be overemphasized.

Mundy (1994) **analyzed a large series of urethral reconstructions. His data show that when follow-up is limited to 1 year, the success rate with tissue transfer clusters at about 95%. With longer follow-up, however, there is a deterioration over time. With excision and primary anastomosis, the success seen at 1 year seems to be durable, however, and does not appear to deteriorate with time.** We have reported our long-term data for excision and primary anastomosis with anterior urethral stenosis in 220 patients with a mean follow-up of 44 months; three recurrences were noted, two within the first 6 months and a third at 4 years. The rate of postoperative erectile dysfunction is 2%, with the severe straddle population being at increased risk. **Wessells, in a meta-analysis of graft onlay procedures compared with flap procedures, showed equivalent results for graft operations and flap procedures** (Wessells and McAninch, 1998), and graft onlay procedures are technically far easier to perform. There clearly are some cases where flap reconstruction would be expected to provide superior results (i.e., radiation strictures, patients with multiple operations, pendulous strictures). However, with the increased knowledge gained by the enthusiastic application of graft reconstruction, there is currently a redefined paradigm for anterior reconstruction. Whereas grafts have been used successfully for all segments of the anterior urethra, many think that flaps are best suited for distal reconstruction and grafts for proximal reconstruction, all other variables equivalent (Greenwell et al, 1999).

The issue of postoperative erectile dysfunction must be discussed. Our rates for anterior urethral anastomotic reconstruction are quoted earlier. **In an analysis by Coursey, 200 urethroplasty patients were studied. Overall, the rate of erectile dysfunction after urethroplasty was approximately equal to that with circumcision. However, longer segment reconstructions did have a higher risk of postoperative erectile dysfunction, although in many, over time, the patient's erectile function improved** (Coursey et al, 2001).

Special mention must be made regarding reconstruction for strictures associated with LS-BXO. With the advent of flap

KEY POINTS: TREATMENT OF URETHRAL STRICTURE

- In the treatment of urethral stricture disease, both the patient and the physician must have a good understanding of the goals of treatment before the treatment choice is made.

- Urethral dilation is the oldest and simplest treatment of urethral stricture disease. However, the goal of dilation is to stretch the scar atraumatically. Dilation is seldom used curatively.

- Internal urethrotomy refers to any procedure that opens the stricture by incising it transurethrally. The factors that contribute to success of internal urethrotomy have been defined as follows: internal urethrotomy should be reserved for strictures of the bulbous urethra; the stricture should be less than 1.5 cm in length; and the stricture should not be associated with dense deep spongiofibrosis. Repeated dilation and internal urethrotomies have been shown in a number of studies to diminish the success rate of eventual open urethral reconstruction.

- Urethral stents can be either removable or permanently implantable. The UroLume is the Food and Drug Administration–approved permanently implantable stent. The long-term data have not held up to the original enthusiasm for use of the UroLume. The greatest experience with explantable urethral stents comes from Europe. The concept of these stents is different in that they are designed to prevent epithelial incorporation.

- A number of lasers have been used for anterior urethral strictures. To date, the results of laser urethrotomy are mixed.

- Excision with primary anastomosis has proved to be the "gold standard" form of repair for anterior urethral strictures. In years past, excision with primary anastomosis was thought to be a relatively limited procedure and applicable only for strictures less than 1.5 to 2 cm. However, with better understanding of the anatomy, longer and longer strictures have been successfully addressed with excision and primary anastomosis.

- Admittedly there are strictures that require tissue transfer, and grafts and flaps have been successfully employed. A meta-analysis by Wessells has shown that the results of graft reconstruction and flap reconstruction are equivalent. Clearly, the complexity of flap procedures is greater than that of graft procedures. The concept of augmented anastomosis can be used with both graft and flap onlay and is thought, in many cases, to provide better results than just pure onlay. When flaps are employed for urethral reconstruction, conceptually all become one operation with multidimensional application.

techniques, many centers embraced these techniques for these strictures. However, analysis of results of these patients from several large centers has shown a very high recurrence rate. Because of that, these centers adjusted by applying staged graft techniques. Interestingly, staged graft techniques using skin grafts again had a very high recurrence rate on a number of analyses. **It is theorized that because LS-BXO is a skin condition, the use of skin as a flap, single-stage graft, or staged graft does not preclude involvement of the skin with the inflammatory process. Thus, a number of centers believe that for reconstruction of strictures associated with LS-BXO, staged buccal graft techniques should be employed.** Short follow-up suggests better success with this approach. Long-term follow-up is not available. At the time of this writing, this center has completed a cursory assessment of our series of patients with LS-BXO–associated strictures who underwent reconstruction with flap–skin island techniques and skin graft. Preliminary results at our center are not as dismal as those from other centers, but the success rate is clearly far less (approximately 60%) than for strictures not associated with LS-BXO.

DISTRACTION INJURIES OF THE URETHRA

Urethral distraction injuries are the result of blunt pelvic trauma and accompany about 10% of pelvic fracture injuries. Although it is possible to totally disrupt the urethra with a straddle injury, these injuries most commonly involve only the bulbous urethra. However, the ensuing spongiofibrosis can be associated with complete obliteration of the urethra. **Distraction injuries are for all intents unique to the membranous urethra.** Pelvic fracture distraction injuries of the membranous urethra have been compared with plucking an apple (prostate) off its stem (the membranous urethra). This analogy implies that the injury most frequently occurs at the apex of the prostate. Experience shows that this is not the case, however, and the most frequent point of distraction is at the departure of the membranous urethra from the bulbospongiosus (Andrich and Mundy, 2001; Mouraviev and Santucci, 2005). The distraction can, however, involve all or any portion of the membranous urethra between the departure of the bulbospongiosus and the apex of the prostate. In the postpubescent male, the injury seldom involves the prostatic urethra. In the prepubescent male, in whom the prostatic urethra is more fragile, the injury can extend into that area.

Many injuries appear not to totally distract the entire circumference of the urethra. Instead, a strip of epithelium is left intact. In these patients, the placement of an aligning catheter may allow the urethra to heal virtually unscarred or with an easily managed stricture. Because of flexible endoscopy equipment, the placement of an aligning catheter is relatively straightforward. If distraction is complete, the catheter then serves to align the obliterated urethral ends, and reconstruction is facilitated. Because of the ready availability of flexible cystoscopes, some centers are now acutely evaluating these injuries only with endoscopy. Those enthusiastic for this approach believe that not only can the injury be completely evaluated but the entire process, including the placement of an aligning catheter, is expedited (Kielb et al, 2001). **Aligning catheters are just what the name implies, a guide, not a mechanism for placing traction on the bladder and prostate.** Aligning catheters also seem to act as a drain as the pelvic hematoma liquefies, and perhaps the presence of the catheter may allow more rapid and complete resolution of the process (Rehman et al, 1998; Mouraviev et al, 2005).

Evaluation

As with the repair of any stricture, it is important to define the precise anatomy of the distraction defect before treatment is undertaken; this includes the depth, density, length, and location. In pelvic fracture urethral distraction defects, the depth and density of fibrosis are predictable. Although the location of the distraction injury has been demonstrated to be an important factor in continence after reconstruction, this information should be a factor only in counseling of patients before the reconstruction and not in the treatment approach. The length of the defect is an important consideration and must be determined as precisely as possible.

Contrast studies are a first-line tool for the evaluation of distraction defects. A cystogram outlines the bladder and provides information about rostral displacement of the proximal urethra. A lack of contrast material in the posterior urethra gives some information, albeit inconclusive, about the integrity of the bladder neck.

When the patient is successful in relaxing to void and the cystogram outlines the posterior urethra, a simultaneous retrograde urethrogram nicely outlines the length of the distraction defect. However, this situation is the exception rather than the rule, and retrograde urethrography is most useful for determining whether the anterior urethra is normal. If the anterior urethra is normal, **it has been our experience, as well as that of others, that a successful anastomotic repair is ensured.** In fact, a primary anastomosis has been shown to be possible even with some involvement of the anterior urethra. Even in cases of prior failed posterior urethral reconstruction, primary anastomotic repair is often feasible, although the failure rate is slightly higher in these cases (Chapple and Pang, 1999; Flynn et al, 2003; Koraitim, 2003; Shenfeld et al, 2004). **Thus, primary anastomosis is unquestionably the goal in all these patients until it is proved impossible to perform.**

When the proximal urethra is not visualized on a simultaneous cystogram with urethrogram, endoscopy through the suprapubic tract in combination with retrograde urethrography can be used to outline the defect. After the endoscopic appearance of the bladder neck is assessed, the flexible endoscope can be advanced through the bladder neck and into the posterior urethra to the level of the obstruction. **The appearance of the bladder neck on contrast studies or on antegrade endoscopy does not accurately predict the ultimate function of the bladder neck after urethral reconstruction** (Iselin and Webster, 1999). A simultaneous retrograde urethrogram will then outline the anterior urethra, with the space not visualized representing the distraction defect.

Some have also advocated magnetic resonance imaging for the evaluation of patients with distraction injuries. We have had little experience with this modality for that purpose; however, we have not found the information obtained on the few studies that we have done to be very useful. In these cases, there was the question of bone interposition into the distraction defect, and magnetic resonance imaging nicely outlined that. We evaluated a case in which the prostatic urethra appeared obliterated. On magnetic resonance imaging, one could easily see that the prostate was not only distracted from the membranous urethra but also distracted from the bladder. This information was essential to planning of subsequent reconstruction in this case. It would seem intuitively obvious that the length of distraction as determined would be helpful in determining the precise approach and steps necessary for reconstruction. However, the literature is not clear on this matter (Andrich et al, 2003; Koraitim, 2004), and it is our experience that the surgeon must be prepared to exercise all options of reconstruction in virtually all such cases.

Repair

The timetable for the reconstruction of distraction defects is determined by the type and extent of associated injuries. If possible, it is desirable to proceed within 4 to 6 months after trauma. However, orthopedic injuries of the lower extremities often necessitate a delay in proceeding with urethral reconstruction (Brandes and Borrelli, 2001).

In the majority of cases, distraction injuries are not long, and the resultant obliteration is amenable to a technically straightforward mobilization of the corpus spongiosum with a primary anastomotic technique. The classic reconstruction consists of a spatulated anastomosis of the proximal anterior urethra to the apical prostatic urethra. Experience has demonstrated, however, that anastomosis of the proximal anterior urethra to any segment of the posterior urethra (apical, prostatic, or below) **can be successfully accomplished by a widely spatulated anastomosis in which optimal epithelial apposition is achieved.** About 10% of distraction injuries are associated with more complex injuries and can be associated with fistulas (most commonly urethral rectal fistulas). Reconstruction of these injuries is technically more demanding.

Several series support the concept that the bulk of distraction injuries, even the most difficult cases, can be managed by the perineal approach (Koraitim, 1997; Flynn et al, 2003). In fact, a transpubic or an abdominal-perineal approach, as pioneered by Waterhouse and colleagues (1973), in the authors' experience is not necessary for the reconstruction of distraction injuries. In addition, pubectomy can be associated with long-term sequelae that include shortening of the penis, destabilization of erection, and destabilization of the pelvis, resulting in a chronic pain syndrome with exercise. However, there are authors who continue to rely heavily on the transpubic approach (Koraitim, 1997; Das et al, 2004).

Alternatively, the above-and-below approach does have merit when concomitant surgery is planned in the region of the bladder neck. We have found and Iselin and Webster (1999) have reported that the competence of the bladder neck is difficult to assess accurately before the reestablishment of urethral continuity. In the past, great reliance was placed on whether the bladder neck was closed or open on cystography. We now know, however, that contrast material can opacify the prostatic urethra when the bladder neck is more than adequately competent for continence. Similarly, confidence has been placed in the appearance of the bladder neck on endoscopic examination through the suprapubic tube. Again, even when an obvious scar is noted to involve the bladder neck, follow-up of these patients after the urethral reconstruction establishes continuity of the urethra and finds many patients with more than adequate continence. Still other patients are believed to have incontinence due to scar incarceration of the bladder neck, caused by the extensive fibrosis left behind by resolution of the hematoma. In our experience, however, this is an infrequent occurrence, and the appearance of the bladder neck by any modality available is not predictive of continence. Therefore, it is currently our practice to reestablish the continuity of the urethra and, when there are concerns about continence, forewarn the patient before the urethral reconstruction. If these patients find that they experience less than adequate continence postoperatively, the problem is addressed in a subsequent procedure (Bhargava et al, 2004).

At the time of reconstruction, before the patient is placed in the lithotomy position, endoscopy is performed through the meatus and again through the suprapubic tube sinus. Endoscopy on the table is designed to ensure that there is no concomitant vesicolithiasis. This endoscopy is performed with a rigid endoscope, which is manipulated through the suprapubic tube sinus and the bladder neck and positioned against the area of total obliteration. On gentle manipulation of the endoscope, if the impulse of the endoscope tip is felt on the patient's perineum, the impulse will be palpable at the time the perineum is opened and an instrument is manipulated through the bladder neck during reconstruction. If the impulse is not palpable perineally at this time, it may not be palpable during dissection, and in those cases, we create a temporary vesicostomy. This allows us to position an instrument reliably through the bladder neck because the vesicostomy allows the surgeon to palpably identify the bladder neck before instrumentation of the posterior urethra. This maneuver has eliminated the occurrence of false passages with use of a sound such as the Haygrove staff through the suprapubic site and also has eliminated the occurrence of misanastomosis of the anterior urethra to sites other than the apical proximal urethra.

We prefer the use of the exaggerated lithotomy position for the perineal approach (Fig. 33–41). This position is safe and provides optimal exposure to the area of the membranous and apical prostatic urethra (Angermeier and Jordan, 1994). A custom Skytron table, modified to allow the exaggerated lithotomy position, and a Stille-Scandia table, designed to place patients in the lithotomy position, are our preferences. The legs are carefully positioned in the Allen- or Guardian-style stirrups. Care is taken to avoid pressure on the lateral aspects of the lower extremities and calf muscles (Fig. 33–42). The patient's hips are elevated into position by raising the buttocks portion of the operating table. The boots are positioned to avoid stretch injuries of the common peroneal nerves (Fig. 33–43).

After the patient is correctly positioned, the perineal approach to reconstruction begins with an incision and dissection anterior to the transverse perinei musculature (anterior perineal triangle). This is in contrast to the approach posterior to the transverse perinei musculature (posterior anal triangle), useful for perineal prostatectomy. We use a λ-shaped incision (Fig. 33–44) that is carried sharply down to the midline fusion of the ischiocavernosus musculature (Fig. 33–44A), then beneath the scrotum, to expose the uninvested portion of the corpus spongiosum. We then place a self-retaining ring retractor.

The fusion of the ischiocavernosus musculature is divided, and the musculature is cleanly dissected from the corpus spongiosum and bulbospongiosum (Fig. 33–44B to D). The corpus spongiosum is detached from the triangular ligament and corpora cavernosa (Fig. 33–44E), the bulbospongiosum is detached from the perineal body, and the dissection is carried farther down to the infrapubic space. Posterior detachment of the bulbospongiosum is carried anteriorly, and the dissection is eventually carried through the area of fibrosis (Fig. 33–44F).

In some cases, the proximal blood supply is encountered and must be controlled. We have found that these arteries are easily controlled with a sharp tip hemostat and monopolar cautery. Suture ligature should be avoided in the case of the arteries to the bulbospongiosum because of their proximity to the nerves as they are coursing into the corpora cavernosa.

We then divide the triangular ligament and vigorously develop the intracrural space down to the pubis (Fig. 33–45). If the dorsal vein is encountered, it is ligated and divided. It is important to make sure that the arteries were not rolled into the intracrural space when the tissues were dislocated during trauma. It is not uncommon to see the penetration of the cavernosal arteries or the dorsal arteries, or both, into this space. If there is doubt about the nature of the vessels encountered, Doppler sonography should be used. When the pubis is exposed, the periosteal elevator can be gently introduced onto the retropubic surface, releasing and allowing the descent of the tissues from beneath the pubis.

We then introduce a Haygrove staff into the suprapubic sinus and through the bladder neck to the distal limits of the posterior urethra (Fig. 33–44G and H). The impulse is palpated, and the fibrosis is resected until normal tissue planes are encountered. The tissue is submitted for histologic examination. The tip of the Haygrove staff is eventually concealed only by the normal urethral epithelium, at which point we open the epithelium and control it with either a skin hook or a stitch. We then perform endoscopy to ensure that the urethrotomy is at the distal limits of the posterior urethra. If a tension-free anastomosis is not thought possible, we mobilize the corpus spongiosum beneath the scrotum from its attachment to the corpora cavernosa. Aggressive mobilization of the corpus spongiosum is the last maneuver undertaken because it is thought to have possible ill effects on the retrograde blood supply, which in the pelvic fracture patient may be tenuous. Meticulous detachment of the investment of Buck's fascia from the corpus spongiosum increases the compliance of the corpus and limits the need for aggressive mobilization.

It is important to try to avoid the creation of chordee during the repair of a distraction injury. To prevent chordee, the attachment cannot be carried beyond the area of the penoscrotal attachment. It is warranted in some cases, however, to preoperatively counsel patients that they may have some chordee after aggressive mobilization that results in a primary anastomotic repair. Primary anastomotic repairs carry success rates in the high 90% range. If a technique of tissue transfer

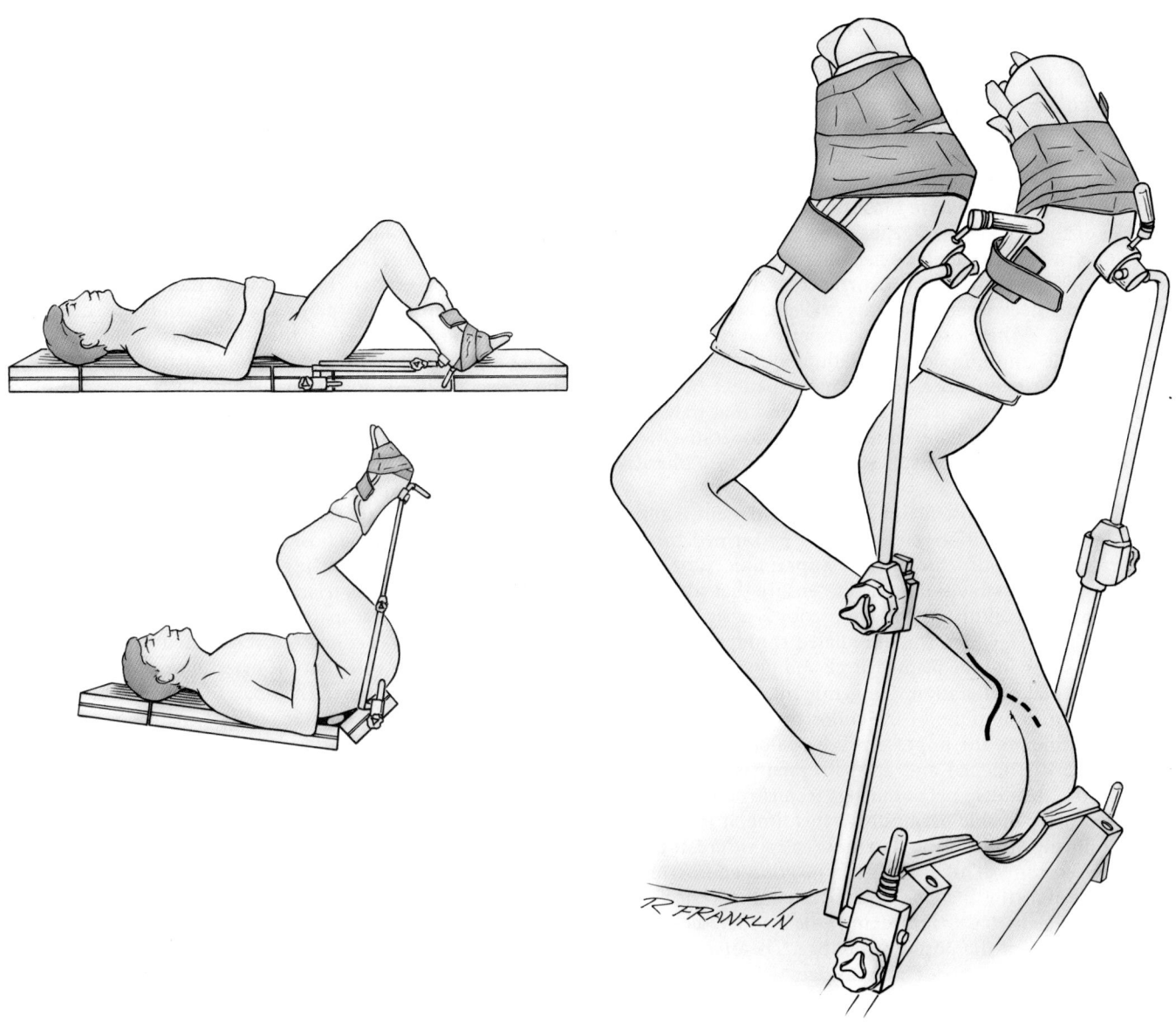

Figure 33–41. Patient placed in an exaggerated lithotomy position. The hips have been rotated into position by elevation of the buttocks portion of a specially modified table. The legs are suspended from boot-style stirrups with as little flexion of the hips and knees as allowed by the design of the stirrups. (From Angermeier KW, Jordan GH: Complications of the exaggerated lithotomy position: A review of 177 cases. J Urol 1994;151:866-868.)

is needed, the long-term cure rates may eventually only be in the mid 80% range. Most of these patients are young. Successful, durable reconstruction is of paramount importance. If chordee results, it is most often mild and not disabling sexually; in our and other surgeons' minds, it is probably a fair trade for optimizing the urethral reconstruction. Development of the intracrural space, mobilization of the corpus spongiosum, infrapubectomy, and, if needed, rerouting of the corpus spongiosum shorten the course that the corpus spongiosum must traverse and allow reconstruction without attendant chordee.

The proximal urethrotomy is spatulated so that it accepts at least a 32 French bougie à boule, and 10 to 12 anastomotic sutures are placed and tagged to allow identification of their position in the proximal anastomosis. We have used a combi-

nation of 3-0 Monocryl and 3-0 polydioxanone sutures for this purpose. Special needles are not required for the placement of these sutures. However, a Heaney needle driver and a Ravitch needle driver can be useful in difficult cases. A lighted sucker is also beneficial at this point in the procedure.

After spatulation of the proximal urethrotomy and placement of the sutures, we spatulate the proximal portion of the anterior urethra. The spatulation is continued until the urethrotomy accepts a 30 to 32 French bougie à boule, and the anastomotic sutures are placed in their respective locations. Before seating the anastomosis, we introduce a soft silicone (Silastic) ribbed urethral stenting catheter through the anastomosis under direct vision. The wound is then copiously irrigated to reduce the clot around the area of the anastomosis, and the anastomosis is seated.

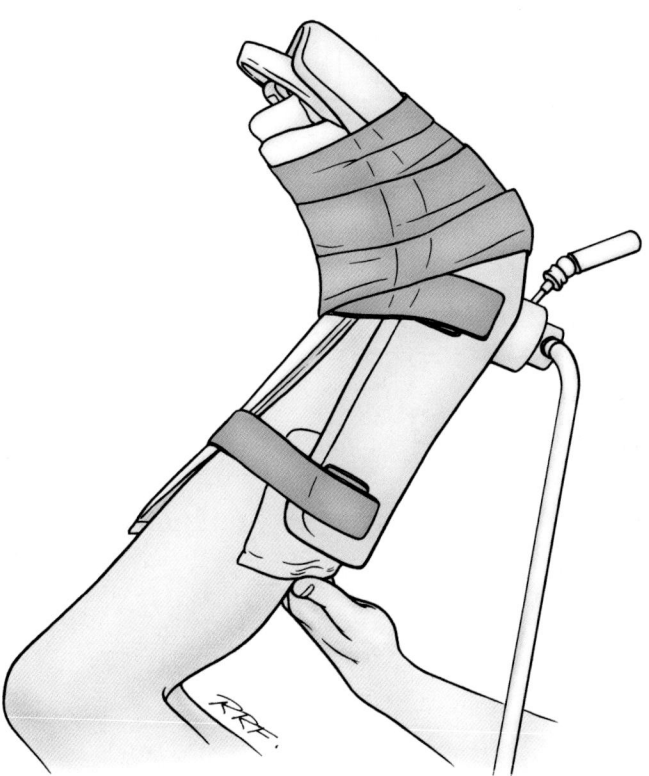

Figure 33–42. Positioning of feet and lower legs in boot-style stirrups. Note that there is absolutely no pressure on the calves and that the feet hang in the stirrups. (From Jordan GH: Management of anterior urethral stricture disease. Probl Urol 1987;1:199-225.)

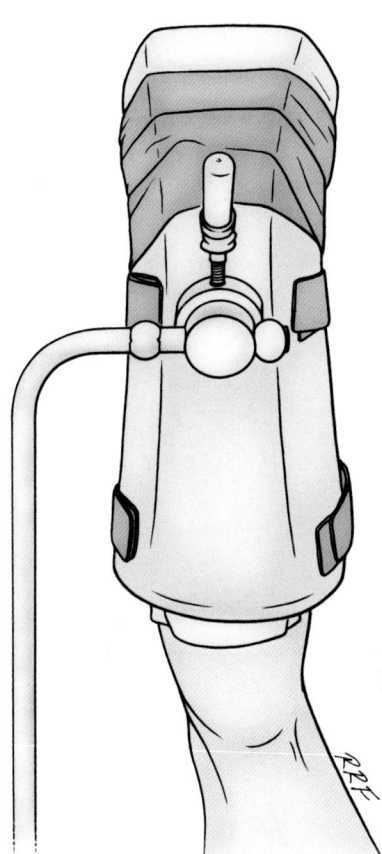

Figure 33–43. Legs are suspended without any internal rotation of the feet in the stirrups. This position is believed to lessen the potential for neurapraxia injuries associated with prolonged positioning. (From Angermeier KW, Jordan GH: Complications of the exaggerated lithotomy position: A review of 177 cases. J Urol 1994;151:866-868.)

Next, we reattach the corpus spongiosum to the corpora cavernosa and the bulbospongiosum to the perineal body. We then place a small suction drain deep to the closure of the ischiocavernosus musculature and Colles' fascia and a second one superficial to that closure and beneath the subcutaneous closure.

In those cases in which the proximal urethra is significantly distracted in a rostral direction, the surgeon must be prepared to perform infrapubectomy (Fig. 33–46) or corporal rerouting, or both (Fig. 33–47). The performance of the infrapubectomy, along with the development of the intercrural space, allows exposure of the apical prostatic urethra. When the prostatic urethra remains rostrally displaced, the impulse of the sound or instrument placed through the cystostomy tract into the bladder neck is often not readily apparent. In these situations, it is comforting to be able to palpate the bladder neck and the properly placed sound before embarking on a dissection beneath the pubis. In addition, if the rostral distraction is significant, the path of the anterior urethra over the hilum of the penis into the infrapubectomy often does not allow a tension-free anastomosis, and the infrapubectomy can be continued beneath one side of the corpora cavernosa, allowing rerouting of the corpus spongiosum (see Fig. 33–47).

Postoperative Management

We use a small soft silicone (Silastic) stenting catheter. Urine is diverted by way of the suprapubic cystostomy, and the urethral catheter is plugged and serves as a stent only. After the

reconstruction, patients are initially kept at bed rest for 24 to 48 hours and then ambulated and discharged with the suprapubic catheter and stenting urethral catheter in place. They are also discharged on a regimen of oxybutynin and a suppressive antibiotic. The drains are removed as drainage allows.

A voiding trial with contrast material is performed between 15 and 28 days postoperatively. Patients are directed to stop taking oxybutynin 24 hours before the voiding trial. In anastomoses that are technically straightforward, the trial is performed at 21 days, and in those cases with more rostral distraction of the proximal urethra, the trial is delayed for 3 to 5 days longer. The trial involves removing the urethral catheter, filling the patient's bladder with contrast material, and instructing him to void. We do not use pericatheter retrograde urethrography for the evaluation of patients who have undergone urethral reconstruction. The voiding film is examined to ensure that there is not extravasation and that the reanastomosis appears widely patent. A urine culture specimen is also obtained, and the suprapubic catheter is plugged. The patient is allowed to void through the urethra for 5 to 7 days, and the suprapubic catheter is then removed. Patients remain on the suppressive antibiotic regimen until they are tube free and a culture and a sensitivity test are performed. At that time, they are prescribed a short regimen of culture-specific antibiotic.

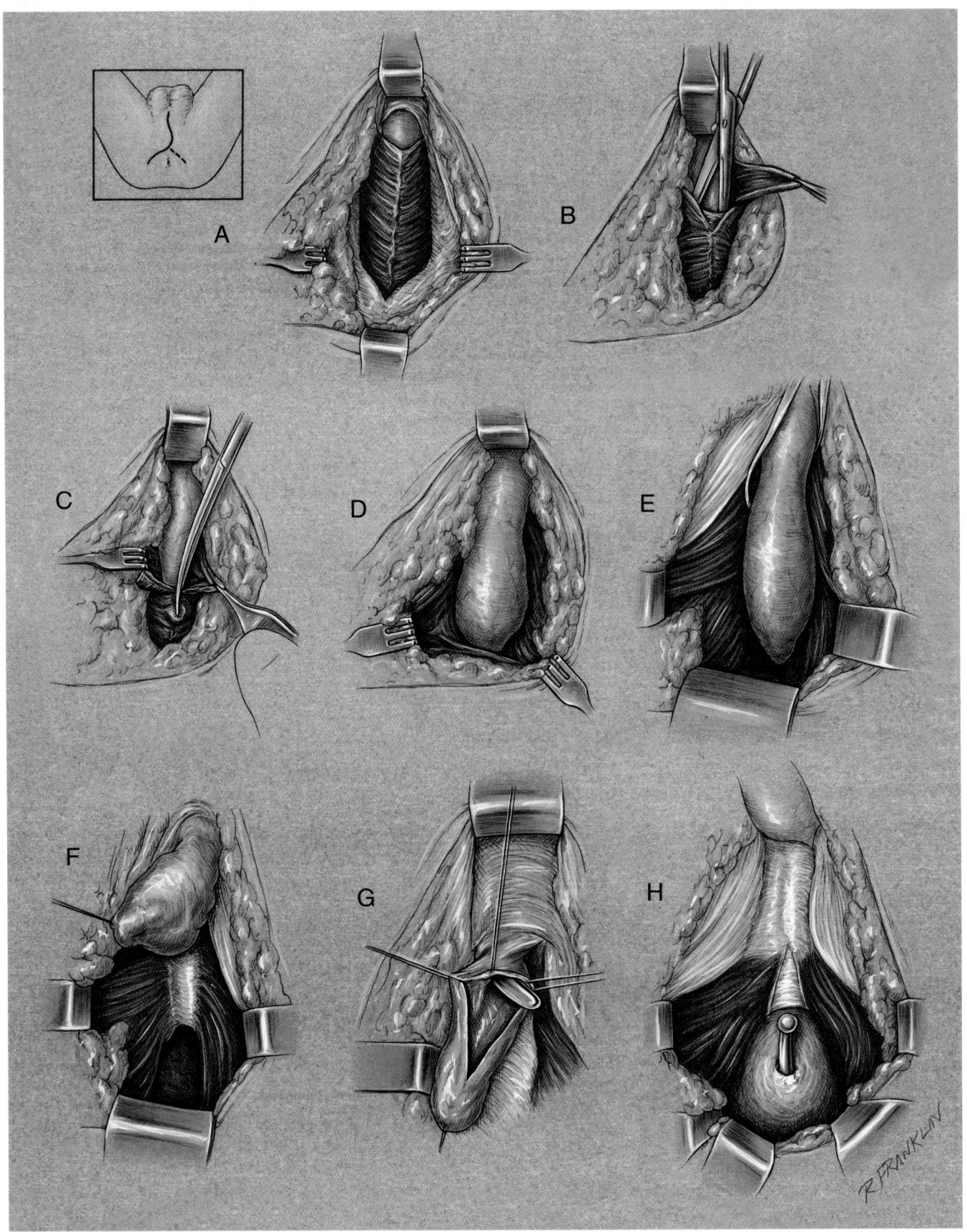

Figure 33–44. Diagram of a perineal repair of a membranous urethral stricture. A λ incision extends from the midline of the scrotum to the ischial tuberosities. **A,** Colles' fascia has been opened to expose the midline fusion of the ischiocavernosus muscles and the tunica of the corpus spongiosum distal to the edge of the muscles. **B,** The scissors are introduced to develop the space between the muscle and the bulb of the urethra. **C,** An incision is made in the midline with the scissors, exposing the length of the bulb. **D,** The ischiocavernosus muscle is retracted to expose the full length of the bulb. **E,** The self-retaining retractor is placed to expose the inferior fascia of the genitourinary diaphragm. The bulb of the corpus spongiosum (bulbospongiosum) can now be mobilized to gain access to the fibrosed area of the urethra. **F,** The fibrosed urethra is incised, freeing the bulb. **G,** The anterior urethra is opened to make an adequate lumen. **H,** The Haygrove staff has been passed through the suprapubic cystostomy. Resection of the fibrotic distraction defect has allowed it to pass into the perineum.

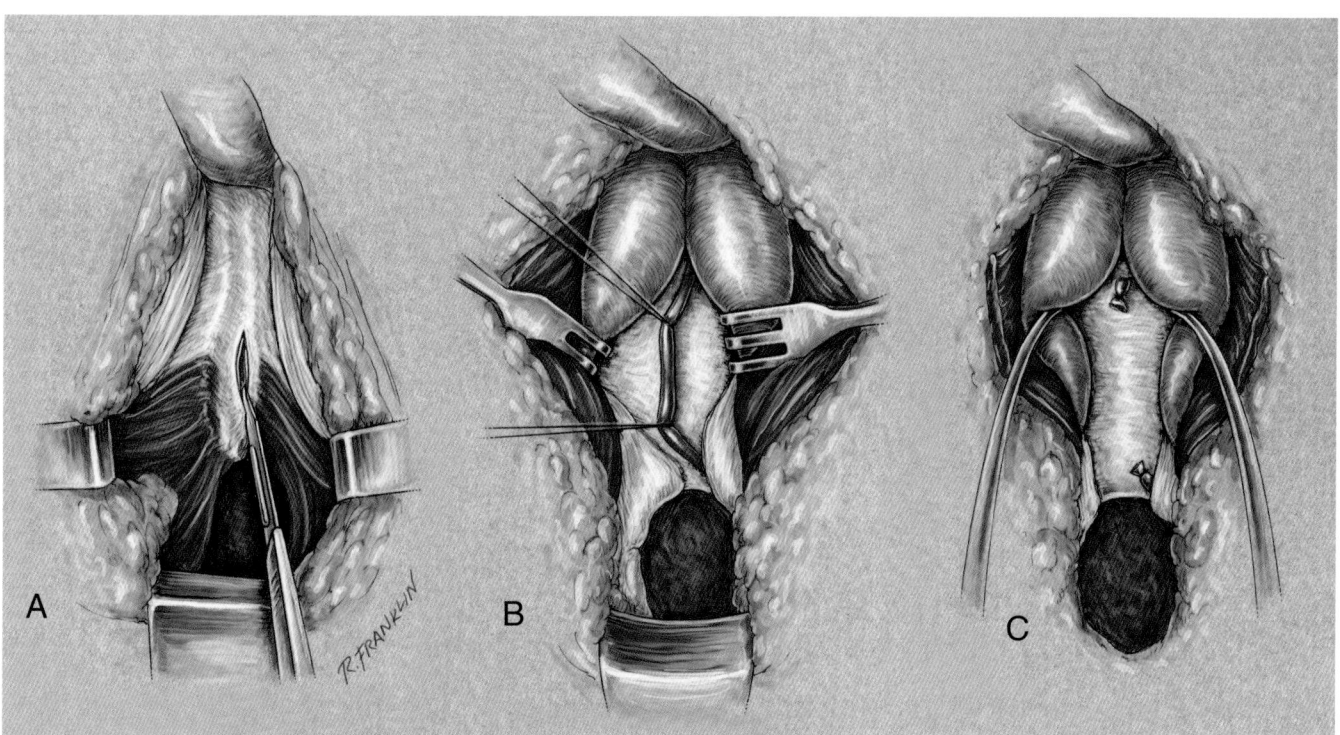

Figure 33–45. Division of the triangular ligament and development of the intracrural space. When the prostatic urethra is displaced and the arc that the urethra must traverse needs to be shortened, that length can be shortened by incision of the triangular ligament (**A**). **B,** Incision and mobilization of the perichondrium and periosteum of the symphysis pubis to allow placement of retractors without trauma to the erectile bodies. Lateral displacement of the crura will expose the dorsal vein of the penis; after careful identification, the vein can be ligated and divided. **C,** Completion of the dissection affords additional exposure for resection of the fibrosis that surrounds the apex of the prostate and the proximal end of the disrupted urethra. (**A** to **C,** from Jordan GH: Reconstruction of the meatus–fossa navicularis using flap techniques. In Schreiter F, ed: Plastic-Reconstructive Surgery in Urology. Stuttgart, Georg Thieme, 1999:338-344.)

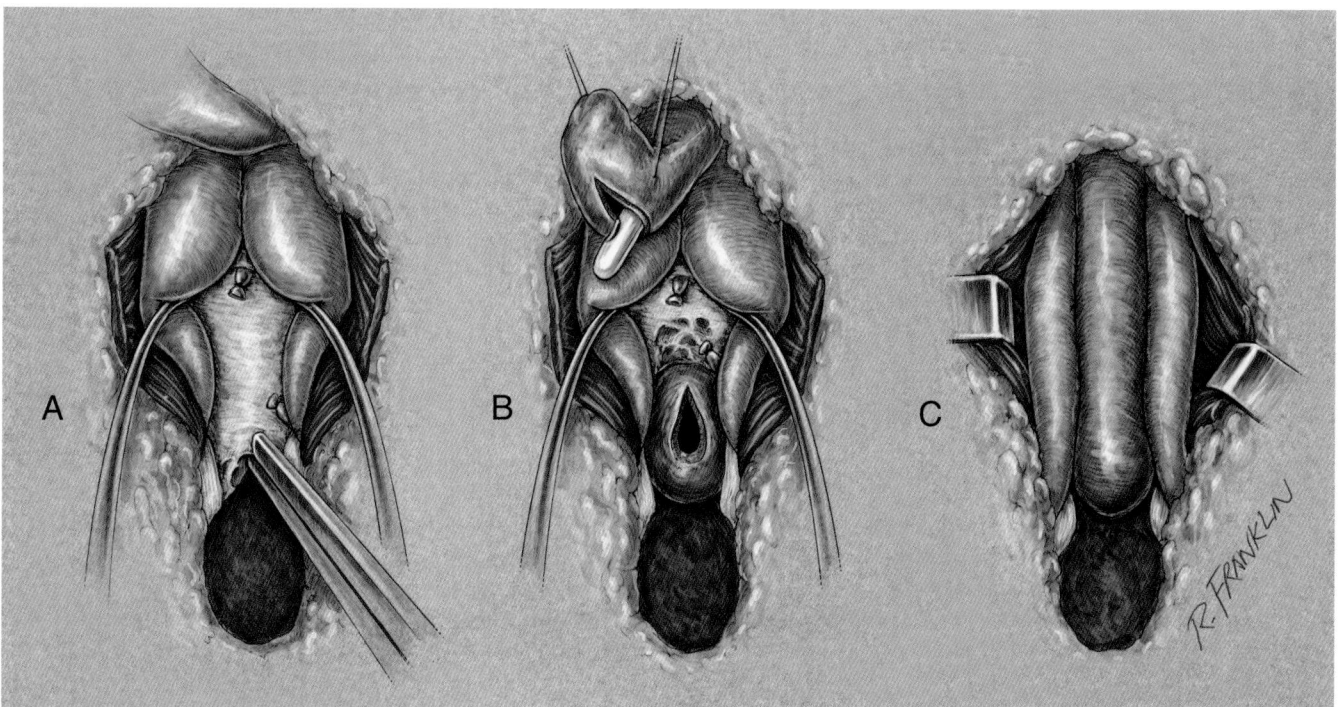

Figure 33–46. Infrapubectomy. If the prostate is elevated behind the symphysis pubis (**A**), the inferior aspect of the symphysis is resected with a Kerrison rongeur. As much of the bone can be removed as necessary (**B**) to afford a simple approximation of the ends of the urethra (**C**).

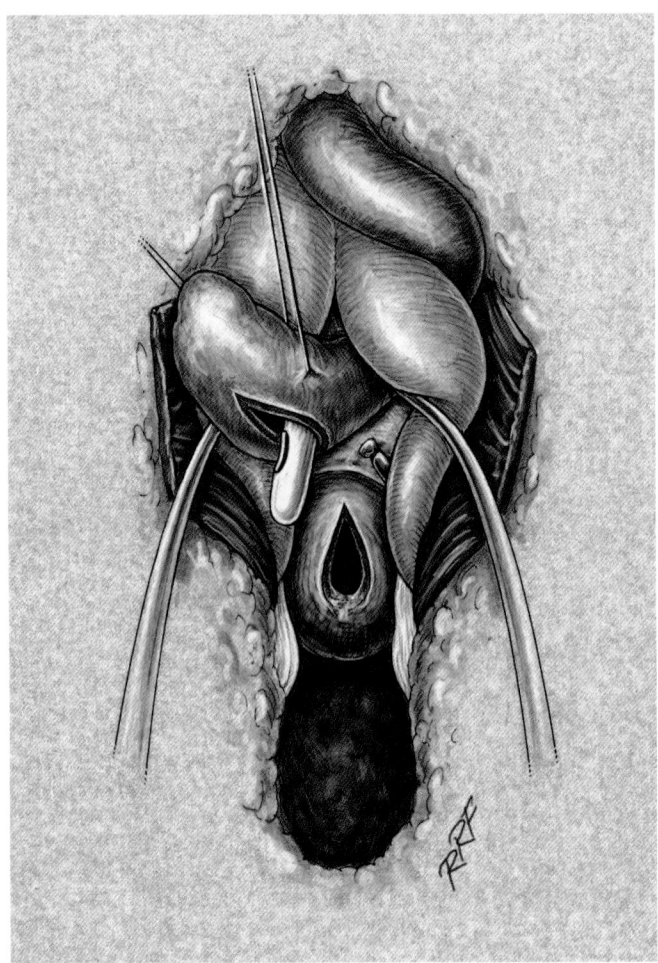

Figure 33–47. Resection of the pubis and rerouting of the urethra around the crus. When the prostate is markedly displaced, it may be necessary to expand the infrapubectomy. Sometimes, despite separation of the crura to the full extent possible, the two ends of the urethra do not meet when they are brought directly through the crus. It is necessary to bring the urethra lateral to one of the crura to make up this length.

At approximately 6 months postoperatively and again at 1 year later, the patients are evaluated with a flexible endoscope. At that time, we consider the reconstruction to be mature, and it should be widely patent. In the absence of the reappearance of symptoms, we refer further follow-ups to the referring urologist.

We have almost completely replaced postoperative retrograde studies with flexible endoscopy. We have not found flow studies to be valuable in observing these patients and have found in many cases (anterior urethral reconstruction) that retrograde urethrography is more confusing than helpful.

With the use of the techniques discussed or similar techniques, curative rates for reconstruction of posterior urethral distraction injuries are in the high 90% range. Failures are not, in large centers, due to technical problems (i.e., anastomotic restenosis). In general, failures are indicative of ischemia of the proximal corpus spongiosum with ensuing stenosis of the mobilized corpus spongiosum. This occurs because with mobilization, the corpus spongiosum, in essence, becomes a flap with the vascular pedicle being the retrograde vascularity from the arborization of the dorsal arteries through the glans (Fig. 33–48).

We have studied this phenomenon in our trauma patients and have now arrived at conclusions that we believe allow us to predict the patients at risk for this ischemic atrophy phenomenon. Initially, we used pudendal angiography to study all our trauma patients who seemed to be at risk for bilateral deep internal pudendal artery injury at the time of trauma. These were patients who had evidence of injury to the dorsal penile nerves, patients in whom reconstruction at other centers had failed, patients with lateral impact pelvic fractures, and patients whose pelvic fractures were of the "windswept" variety (Brandes and Borrelli, 2001). We found that many patients had evidence of either unilateral or bilateral pudendal artery lesions but that most had evidence of vascular reconstitution. **Patients with an intact pudendal artery on one side often were potent and were reliably cured with reconstruction. Patients with only reconstituted vessels, either unilateral or bilateral, never were potent but were reliably reconstructed.** We found that these patients were optimal candidates for corporal arterial revascularization to improve potency. Because we noted this relationship to potency, we began looking at our patients with duplex ultrasonography. We found that patients with normal pudendal arteries, either unilateral or bilateral, demonstrated normal arterial parameters on duplex evaluation. Those with only reconstituted arteries, either bilateral or unilateral, never had normal arterial parameters on duplex ultrasonography.

This now allows us to proceed to pudendal angiography only in those patients with abnormal arterial parameters on duplex ultrasonography; the patients with normal findings on ultrasonography predictably do well with reconstruction. Our data also show that patients do well with reconstruction if they have at least one side that is reconstituted, and those patients at risk for ischemic stenosis are only those with bilateral complete obstruction of the internal pudendal vessels. In such a patient, we now perform corporal arterial revascularization to augment the vascularity and, with that accomplished, then proceed to urethral reconstruction (Jordan, 2005). In many cases of pelvic fracture urethral distraction defects, erectile dysfunction is a consequence of the injury, although clearly in some patients, erectile dysfunction results from the reconstructive surgery. We think that the incidence of injury to the pudendal arteries is drastically underreported and underrecognized. We thus, along with others, believe that in many of these cases, the cause of erectile dysfunction is vascular (Brandes and Borrelli, 2001). However, others think that in most, the cause is neurologic (Shenfeld et al, 2003).

Summary

Using the maneuvers outlined, we have found that virtually all distraction injuries can be reconstructed by way of a perineal approach with an anastomotic technique. Although the above-and-below approach is used when concomitant bladder neck surgery is performed, the inability to accurately identify those patients has led us to perform bladder neck surgery at a second setting. We have therefore abandoned a transpubic approach as applied to posterior urethral distraction injuries.

Although we favor primary reconstruction of posterior urethral distraction injuries, others choose to manage these

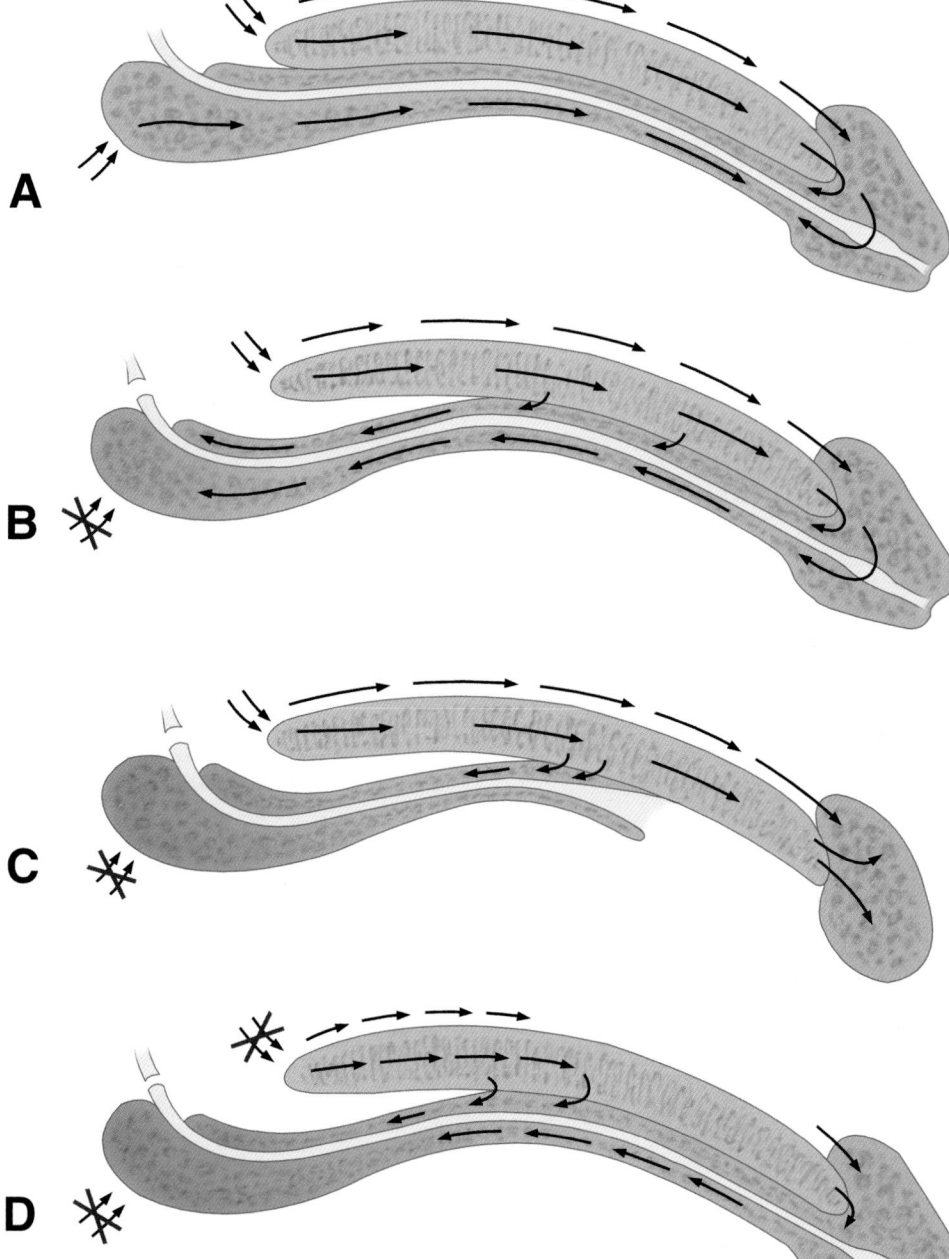

Figure 33–48. Diagrammatic representation of the deep vasculature of the penis. **A,** In the normal situation, via the common penile artery, flow is directed to the tip of the penis with arborization into the spongy erectile tissue of the glans penis. This provides retrograde flow into the corpus spongiosum. If the arteries of the bulb are intact, there is also antegrade arterial flow to the corpus spongiosum. **B,** With interruption of the arteries to the bulb and mobilization of the corpus spongiosum, all flow to the corpus spongiosum is retrograde via the common penile arterial system. **C,** In the case of hypospadias, in which the distal corpus spongiosum may have been interrupted, with proximal mobilization of the corpus spongiosum and therefore division of the arteries to the bulb, even if the common penile circulation is intact to the tip of the penis, it may not adequately provide retrograde vascularity to the corpus spongiosum; hence, ischemic stenosis can ensue. **D,** In the case of injury to the common penile artery, with elevation of the proximal corpus spongiosum and division of the arteries to the bulb, blood flow to the proximal corpus spongiosum may not be adequate, leading to ischemic necrosis or ischemic stenosis.

injuries endoscopically. We have found that the endoscopic management of urethral distraction defects is not a simple procedure and must be undertaken only by a skilled and experienced surgeon. Many of these procedures can be categorized as a "cut-for-light" procedure. Although there are surgeons who report success, the majority of cut-for-light procedures are not done with sufficient precision to allow adequate realignment of the urethra. We have seen many disasters that have resulted from these procedures and in most cases condemn the use of these modalities. In addition, no cut-for-light series compares favorably, with regard to long-term success rates, with series from large centers that use primary anastomotic techniques (Levine and Wessells, 2001).

In 1989, Marshall described his method of using stereotactic techniques for endoscopic alignment of the ends of the urethra. He emphasized the length of time it takes to obtain precise alignment before undertaking the endoscopic portion of the procedure. In his procedure, he passes a wire through the aligned ends of the urethra, minimally dilating the channel, and widening it with transurethral resection. The scar is stabilized by a period of self-catheterization. A communication with Marshall has determined that he has limited the applications of this procedure and does not advocate it as a primary modality. Patients whose medical condition, age, or concomitant orthopedic injury prevents them from being placed in the exaggerated lithotomy position or reconstructed by way of a transpubic approach may be managed with this technique.

In children, the goals of surgery are the same as in adults. In our experience, most children can be reconstructed by the same perineal exposure as in adults. Exposure is clearly more difficult, but nonetheless perineal anastomosis can be done (Hafez et al, 2005). However, the posterior, sagittal transsphincteric approach has been proposed as a better approach in children (Mathews et al, 1998; Peña and Hong, 2004). We agree that the posterior approach is an elegant method of exposure; however, our observation is that with this approach, surgeons tend to resort to techniques of substitution reconstruction where primary anastomosis could be done and in our opinion is superior.

KEY POINTS: DISTRACTION INJURIES OF THE URETHRA

- Urethral distraction injuries are the result of blunt pelvic trauma and accompany about 10% of pelvic fracture injuries. Many injuries appear to not totally distract the entire circumference of the urethra; instead, a strip of epithelium can be left behind.

- The use of aligning catheters acutely is somewhat controversial, but most would agree that the aligning catheter at the very worst facilitates subsequent reconstruction and at best often leaves the patient with an endoscopically manageable stenosis.

- As with any stricture, it is important to define the precise anatomy. The combination of contrast-enhanced studies with endoscopy and selective magnetic resonance imaging are useful. The appearance of the bladder neck on contrast-enhanced studies or on antegrade endoscopy is not predictive of ultimate function of the bladder neck. Hence, simultaneous reconstruction of the bladder neck and the posterior urethra is for the most part not currently undertaken.

VESICOURETHRAL DISTRACTION DEFECTS

Enthusiastic use of radical prostatectomy has unfortunately led to an increasing experience with patients who have had total obliteration of their vesicourethral anastomosis. In some patients, there is distraction of the vesicourethral anastomosis with either a totally obliterating distraction defect or severe anastomotic stenosis. In addition, with the proposal that bladder tube interposition might enhance continence, a new entity, the stenotic or obliterated vesicourethral anastomosis due to ischemia of the bladder tube, is now encountered.

As with other defects, it is important to accurately determine the length of the defect. This can be accomplished by simultaneous cystography with retrograde urethrography, simultaneous retrograde urethrography and antegrade endoscopy through the suprapubic tube, or both (Fig. 33–49).

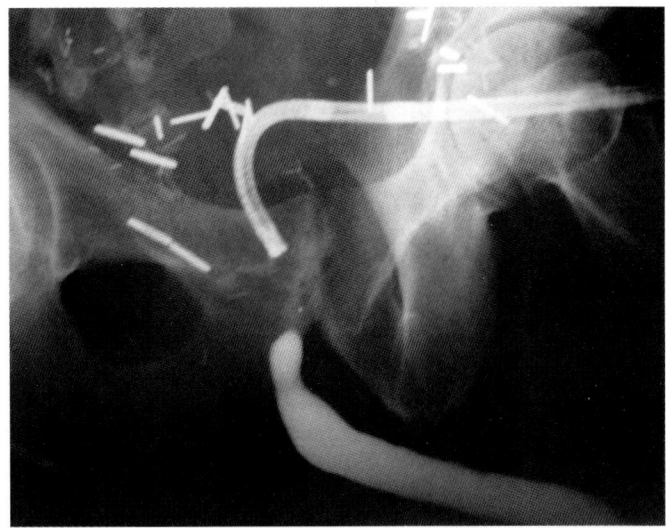

Figure 33–49. Radiograph shows results of simultaneous retrograde urethrography and antegrade endoscopy through a suprapubic tube in a patient after radical prostatectomy with vesicourethral distraction.

There are a number of options for the management of these complex patients. Many have other medical problems, and it has been our observation that many have thick and small bladders, possibly contributing to the difficulty with the initial surgery. The ever present issue of body habitus also must be considered and in our opinion contributes to problems with the initial anastomosis. An indwelling suprapubic tube must always be considered an option. In the individual who is significantly overweight, the results of aggressive reconstruction have not been good. The place for endoscopic techniques is covered later in this section; however, in the case of short-length distractions, we have had good success with aggressive incisions at the 3-o'clock and 9-o'clock positions followed in approximately 3 weeks with repeated incisions. Whether the holmium laser is better than the cold knife can be debated; the hot knife is not necessary. We were enthusiastic about the use of the green light laser, but currently available sheaths made that laser almost unusable in these cases. If one must "core through" to establish continuity, in our opinion endoscopic procedures have no place except as discussed later.

In some cases, a continent catheterizable bladder augmentation may indeed be a better operation than aggressive functional reconstruction; however, the very heavy patient makes construction of a functional catheter channel difficult. Diversion must also be entertained, and in patients in whom functional reconstruction is not an obvious choice, it then becomes a primary option.

If functional reconstruction is deemed possible, we think it is a reasonable choice and our technique is as follows. We place the patients in a low lithotomy position and use an abdominal-perineal combined approach. We make a lower midline incision, exposing the bladder and dissecting it from the lateral sidewall and further mobilizing the anterior bladder from beneath the pubis as aggressively as can be safely undertaken from above. We then open the peritoneum and develop the retrovesical space, again taking care to complete the dissection as safely as can be accomplished from above.

A second surgeon then begins the perineal dissection by a curvilinear perineal incision like that used for a radical perineal prostatectomy. The dissection is posterior to the transverse perinei musculature (posterior anal triangle) and carried along the anterior rectal wall to the area where fibrosis is encountered from the prior radical prostatectomy dissection. The impulse of the perineal surgeon's digits can usually be felt adjacent and lateral to the area of fibrosis and distraction at this point. In addition, the abdominal surgeon places a finger at the limits of the retrovesical dissection from above to provide another palpable landmark and to ensure a safe dissection anterior to the rectal wall and posterior to the bladder and trigone. The perineal dissection is then joined to the abdominal dissection, and the rectal wall is completely peeled off of the area of fibrosis associated with the distraction defect. We then place drains between the rectum and the distraction defect, encircling the area of fibrosis.

The dissection beneath the pubis is made easier by the excision of an ellipse of the rim of the superior pubic ramus. Total pubectomy is not required. The partial pubectomy can be performed with the reciprocating attachment of the Aesculap surgical drilling device; this makes placement of the sutures technically straightforward and improves the exposure for the dissection and resection of the distraction fibrosis.

At this point, the bladder is opened and the area of the bladder neck is determined. A sound is placed and advanced to the area of obliteration. This allows us to completely resect the well-defined area of fibrosis. The urethral stump is exposed and opened, and the site of the neobladder neck, having been identified, is opened. We marsupialize the bladder epithelium as described by Walsh (1985), place anastomotic sutures in the urethral stump, and pass a stenting catheter.

Before the vesicourethral anastomosis is seated, the omentum is mobilized and placed between the posterior wall of the anastomosis and the anterior rectal wall (Fig. 33–50). We then seat the anastomosis and wrap the omentum around the area of anastomosis, tagging it into place. The lateral vesical spaces are drained with closed-suction drains, and a suprapubic tube is left in place when the vesicostomy is closed.

Postoperative care is the same as for a radical prostatectomy. The patients are discharged when their drainage and ambulation allow and their diet has been resumed. We evaluate the patients 4 to 6 weeks postoperatively, with the stenting urethral catheter removed and the bladder filled by way of the suprapubic tube.

Because one attempt has failed in these patients, we generally are conservative with the timing of a voiding trial. In some cases, voiding trials are being done at 2 to 3 weeks, thus being more commensurate with current practice after radical prostatectomy.

In most of these cases, although it is a Foley catheter, the stenting urethral catheter does not have the balloon inflated. The catheter is positioned and held in place by a monofilament suture looped to an abdominal wall button. When there may be tension on the anastomosis, it can be performed in association with Vest-type sutures, although to date we have not had to do this.

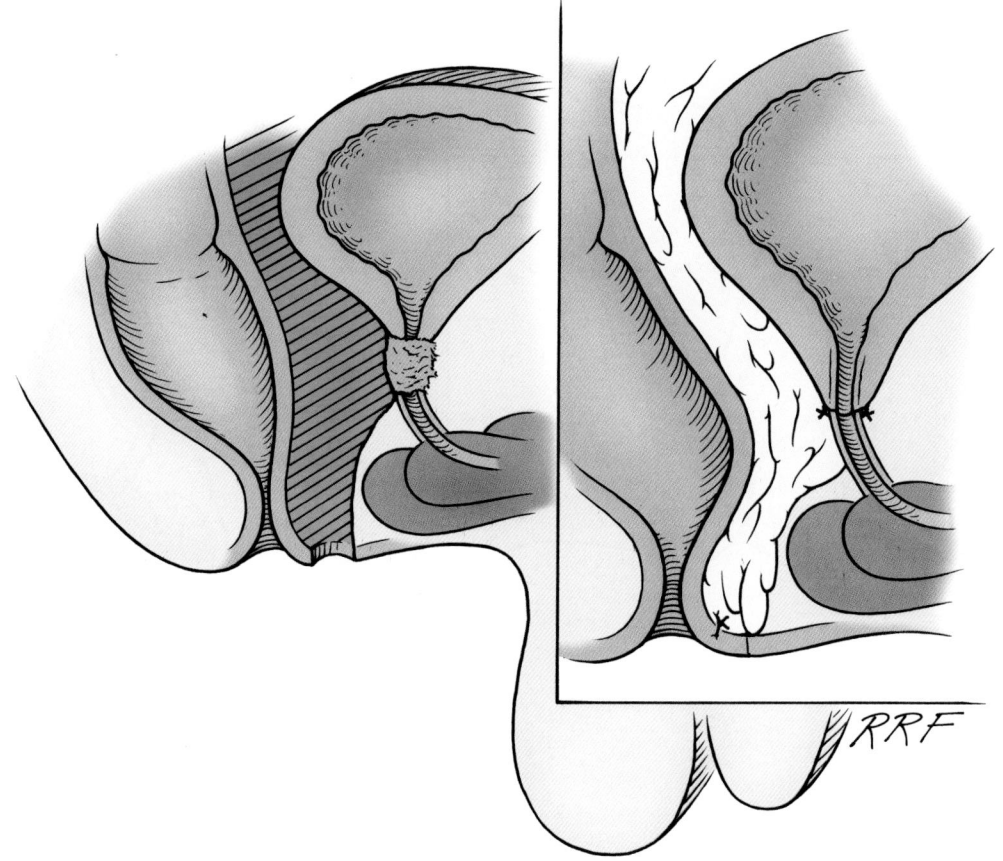

Figure 33–50. Reconstruction for vesicourethral distraction. Exposure is gained using an abdominal-perineal approach. The perineal dissection is through the posterior perineal triangle. The area of the distraction defect is dissected from the rectum and then isolated. The area of fibrosis is resected. A primary anastomosis of the bladder to the membranous urethra is performed. Omentum is placed to surround the reanastomosis.

Our series continues to grow and we continue to have excellent success in reconstruction. We have some patients who deem their continence adequate for their lifestyle; in the others, we have been successful with the placement of an artificial sphincter.

Others have proposed a different approach to these very difficult cases. Elliott and Boone, in patients in whom multiple attempts at dilation or incision of these vesicourethral anastomotic stenoses have failed, propose an incision with placement of the UroLume endoprosthesis followed at an interval by the placement of an artificial sphincter. They initially described nine men treated with this approach; seven of the men were satisfied with the results of their treatment at 17.5 months of mean follow-up (Elliott and Boone, 2001). Others (Kaplan, 2004; Anger et al, 2005) have proposed slight modifications of this approach and are also reporting adequate patency and continence in these patients.

COMPLEX FISTULAS OF THE POSTERIOR URETHRA

The increase in the performance of radical prostatectomy has also led to an increased incidence of vesicorectal or vesicourethrorectal fistulas. In most cases, these are small and managed by a transperineal, transanal-transsphincteric, or posterior approach. However, some cases are complex, with the fistulas associated with large granulated cavities. The **problem is magnified when radiation (brachytherapy, external beam therapy, or both) is part of the equation.** With radiation fistulas, a number of centers have gone to diversion with ileal conduit or bowel pouch as opposed to functional reconstruction. These cases have also been managed with the approach described earlier for vesicourethral distraction problems (Fig. 33–51). The omentum, however, serves an even more important purpose in these cases. In addition, with the increasing application of "minimally invasive" modalities for carcinoma of the prostate (i.e., brachytherapy, combined brachytherapy with external beam irradiation, higher dose external beam irradiation, and cryotherapy), the magnitude of complexity of these problems of prostatic urethral fistulas, granulated cavities, and severe rectal injury continues to increase. We have tried to approach these problems aggressively, with preservation of function, where possible.

In many of these cases, salvage prostatectomy can be combined with rectosigmoid resection. In some cases, we have successfully reanastomosed the bladder to the membranous urethra. Preservation of continence has been mixed. Where vesicourethral anastomosis is not possible, a urachal-peritoneal flap combined with a rectus abdominis muscle flap is used to bolster the closed bladder neck and to keep the closed bladder neck from sticking to the back of the pubis. The bladder is augmented, and a continent catheterizable channel is developed. In some cases, the continuity of the colon cannot be reestablished, and a colostomy is performed as distally on the descending portion of the colon as possible. Whenever

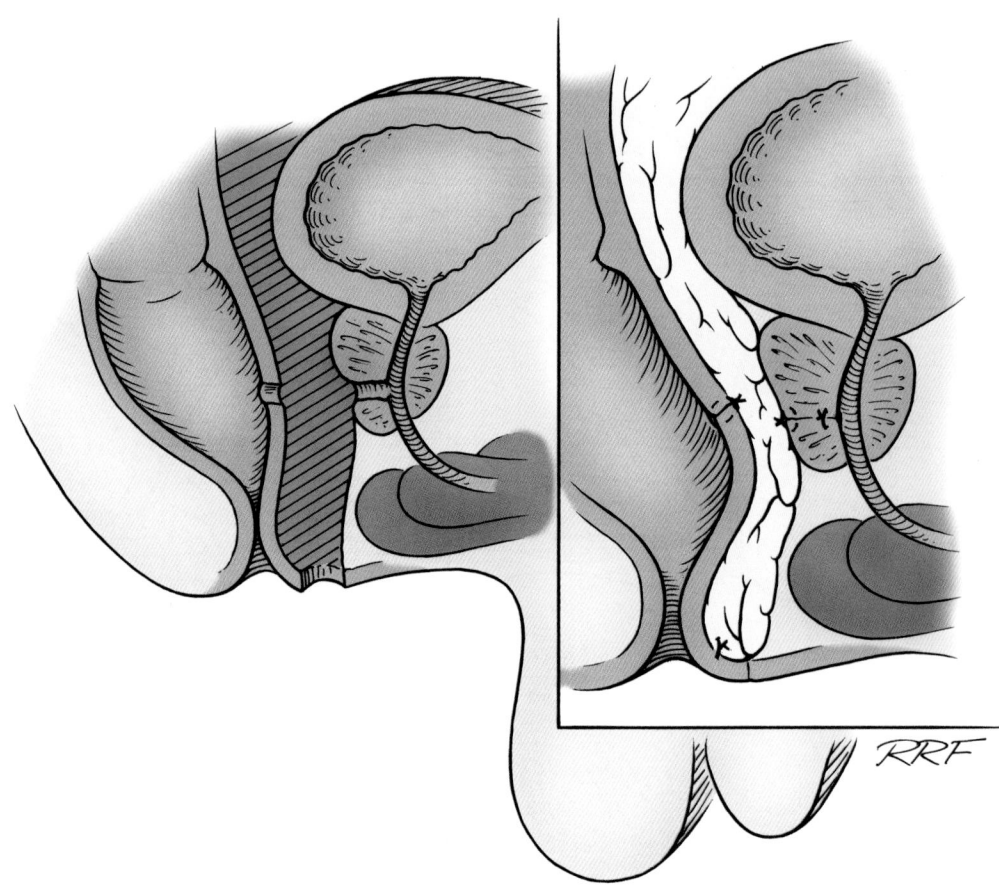

Figure 33–51. Diagram illustrating a complex fistula between the prostatic urethra and the rectum. Simple fistulas can be addressed through a transperineal or transanal-transsphincteric posterior approach with great facility. However, complex cases associated with radiotherapy or large granulated cavities require a different approach. A combined abdominal-perineal exposure with repair of the fistulas as possible and interposition of omentum, rectus abdominis muscle flap, and peritoneal urachal flap have been used.

continuity of the colon can be reestablished, a J-pouch coloanal anastomosis is done. Omentum is used to envelop the rectal closure or to separate the rectal closure from the vesicourethral anastomosis. The combined abdominal-perineal approach that was previously described provides excellent safe exposure for management of these complex situations. The morbidity of this approach has been acceptable.

One must be careful in addressing the irradiated bowel. We had a patient who did well with his surgery for continent catheterizable augmentation and bowel closure, but when his colostomy was reversed, he developed an overwhelming colitis and refistula, with an eventual septic death. Another patient had a breakdown of his bladder neck closure and to date remains with a large vesicoabdominal fistula. Thus, it cannot be overemphasized that these cases must be individualized. When they go well, they go wonderfully well; when they do not, they become a disaster for the patient, the patient's family, and the surgeons involved.

KEY POINTS: VESICOURETHRAL DISTRACTION DEFECTS AND COMPLEX FISTULAS OF THE POSTERIOR URETHRA

- Vesicourethral distraction defects are an unfortunate complication of radical prostatectomy.

- There are a number of options for management of these complex patients. An indwelling suprapubic tube must always be considered an option, long term. Likewise, in some cases, a continent catheterizable bladder augmentation may indeed be a better operation than aggressive functional reconstruction. If functional reconstruction is deemed reasonable, we have employed an above-and-below technique, in which laparotomy is combined with a posterior perineal triangle dissection.

- The interposition of omentum has been used both for distraction defects and for complex fistulas. This approach allows safe mobilization of the rectum from the area of the distraction scar or from the fistula site.

- When radiation is added to the equation, the complexity of reconstruction is magnified. The effects of radiation must be allowed to settle; tissue interposition is the rule, and in many cases functional reconstruction is not possible. Some think that diversion, in the case of the irradiated patient, is the safest and best option.

CURVATURES OF THE PENIS

Normal elasticity and compliance of all tissue layers of the penis are critical for erectile function, tumescence, and rigidity. Tissues must expand in all dimensions as the penis engorges with blood; eventually, the tissues of the tunica albuginea and the septal fibers of the corpora cavernosa are stretched to the limits of their compliance, and tumescence is converted to rigidity. In the normal penis, the tissues are symmetrically elastic and the erection is straight. In curvature of the penis, there is relative asymmetry of one aspect of the erect penis. In some cases, this arises from diminished compliance of one aspect of the tunica albuginea or outright foreshortening of one aspect of the erectile bodies.

The term *chordee* means curvature, but it is commonly used as if it refers to the tissues causing the curvature. This misuse of the term is seen in the statement "the chordee was resected"; properly phrased, "the chordee can be corrected by resecting the inelastic tissues that are causing the chordee."

Curvatures of the penis can be congenital or acquired. Some confusion also exists in common usage of the term *congenital curvature of the penis*. The terms *congenital curvature of the penis* and *chordee without hypospadias* have often been used interchangeably. We prefer to reserve the term *chordee without hypospadias* for those patients in whom the meatus is properly located on the tip of the glans penis, yet a ventral curvature is associated with abnormalities of the ventral fascial tissues or corpus spongiosum, or both. It has long been recognized that hypospadias is a condition that is associated in some males with either a diminutive penis or a micropenis. Although a small penis is not diagnostic of hypospadias, it is highly unusual for a patient with hypospadias to have an exceptionally large erect penis. In contrast, other congenital curvatures of the penis (ventral, lateral, or dorsal) are inevitably associated with the finding of a large erect penis. Because the trauma that results in acquired curvature is virtually always associated with intercourse, the occurrence of acquired curvature is nil before the onset of puberty. We have seen some patients in whom there was a history of trauma during vigorous masturbation, but these patients are the exception. Like congenital curvatures of the penis, acquired curvatures may be dorsal, lateral, ventral, or complex.

Types of Congenital Curvature of the Penis

The urethra begins as an epithelial groove in the midline of the ventral surface of the developing penis. As the groove extends, it deepens, with the edges eventually meeting to fuse into a tube. Fusion begins proximally and progresses distally. During normal development, the fusion of the urethral tube eventually reaches the tip of the glans penis. Proliferating mesenchyma surrounds the tube, separating it from the skin, and differentiates to form the corpus spongiosum, Buck's fascia, dartos fascia, and overlying ventral skin of the penis. Fetal development of the penis is regulated by testosterone, produced by the fetal testis, which is converted by 5α-reductase to dihydrotestosterone. Dihydrotestosterone acts directly on cells with androgen receptors and on all layers of the male external genitalia. This embryologic process explains the development of the anterior urethra that is unique to males.

Maturation of these tissues into normal structures depends on the same growth factors that control the formation of the urethra. Even though urethral development has progressed normally, mesenchymal tissue development in the penis may be deficient or abnormal and result in dysgenetic and inelastic fascial layers. In unpublished data, Galloway and associates (El-Galley et al, 1997) have shown that at least in hypospadias, there is a deficiency of growth factors in the ventral penile skin. To the authors' knowledge, to date there are no data that show the same factor deficiencies for the deeper tissues.

In 1973, C. J. Devine Jr. and Horton proposed a typing of the various congenital curvatures. In type I congenital curvature, the urethral meatus is at the tip of the glans. None of the surrounding layers are normally formed, however, and the epithelial urethra is associated with malfusion of the corpus spongiosum and all the tissues superficial to the urethra. Skin coverage of the epithelial tube is present. In type II, a dysgenetic band of fibrous tissue thought to be derived from the mesenchyma, which would have produced Buck's fascia and the dartos fascia, lies beneath and lateral to the urethra. However, the urethra is contained within a normally developed and fused corpus spongiosum.

In type III, the urethra, corpus spongiosum, and Buck's fascia are all normally developed and ventrally fused. However, there is a short area of inelastic tissue in the dartos layer of the penis that causes a relatively sharp bend. Abnormal development of the dartos fascia is frequently associated with complex curvatures. With extensive involvement, the inelastic dartos can be sufficient to restrain the penis and conceal the penile shaft. In many of these cases, there would appear to be abnormal prominence of the mons fat pad. These stigmata are thought to be associated with an abnormality in the proper progression of virilization during fetal development.

In type IV, although the urethra, corpus spongiosum, and fascial layers are normally developed, there is relative shortness or inelasticity of one aspect of the tunica albuginea of the corpora cavernosa. Experience has shown that most patients whose congenital curvature is type IV seem to actually demonstrate evidence of a hypercompliance of the tunica albuginea. In these patients, the flaccid penis is normal in size and not necessarily impressively large, whereas the erect penis is large. The tunica albuginea of the corpora cavernosa is required to expand through a wide range, and if there is asymmetry in the compliance of the tunica, curvature occurs. It is not uncommon for patients with type IV curvature to have noticed curvature before puberty; but as they traverse puberty, an increase in the curvature is noted because of the penile hypertrophic growth spurt that occurs during this time.

Type V congenital curvature is also known as the congenital short urethra. This implies that there has been correct fusion of all elements of the penis (i.e., tunica albuginea, urethral epithelium, corpus spongiosum, Buck's fascia, dartos fascia, and ventral skin). However, during erection, the correctly fused urethra and corpus spongiosum are not long or compliant enough to match the compliance of the other ventral tissue layers.

If type V congenital curvature exists at all, it occurs so rarely that when it is encountered, one should doubt the findings. Whereas discussion of the condition in the past has centered on the best location to "cut the urethra" during the repair, on the rare occasions when this condition is encountered, it is our belief that it should be diagnosed and treated only by the most experienced surgeons. In general, if the urethral meatus has developed to the tip of the glans, the urethra should not be divided to correct ventral curvature of the penis. Although

there will obviously be extremely rare exceptions to this bold statement, if those exceptions are encountered, their existence should still be questioned.

The congenital curvature types I, II, and III represent forms of the hypospadias anomaly, and we prefer to refer to them collectively under the term *chordee without hypospadias.* **This term implies that although the meatus is not improperly placed, curvature is due to inappropriate fetal development of the ventral penile structures. We prefer to refer to the type IV anomaly as congenital curvature of the penis.** If a patient has findings of hypercompliance of the corpora cavernosa and a ventral curvature, the patient is diagnosed as having congenital ventral curvature of the penis; and if the hypercompliance causes a lateral curvature, it is referred to as congenital lateral curvature of the penis (left or right). Although, as mentioned, **the type V anomaly is so rarely encountered that it deserves its own diagnosis, we believe its correction is best discussed with types I, II, and III, under the category of chordee without hypospadias.**

Chordee Without Hypospadias in Young Men

Patients with chordee without hypospadias usually present with either ventral curvature or ventral curvature associated with torsion (complex curvature). These young men do not typically have a greater than average stretched penile length (13.1 cm) (Schonfeld and Beebe, 1942) and will have noted curvature throughout life. If prepubescent, they have obvious curvature with erection; if postpubescent, they may offer a history of increasing curvature as they pass through puberty.

In many cases, there are abnormalities of the ventral penile skin. These might consist of either an element of hooded preputial skin or a high insertion of the penoscrotal junction. Although the patients have fusion of the preputial skin, there is also often a wrinkled appearance dorsally that we now recognize to be a form of the classic hooded preputial skin. In addition, in many cases, the tissues on the ventrum of the penis seem inelastic as the patient's penis is examined on stretch. This palpable inelasticity on the ventral penis consists of dysgenetic tissue, which can replace the Buck's and dartos fascia layers; and in some cases, there is an element of inelasticity of the tunica itself.

During surgical exploration, C. J. Devine Jr. and Pepe obtained tissue from these patients for evaluation of 5α-reductase levels. Those data suggested a deficiency of the enzyme in the ventral dysgenetic tissue. The values were inconclusive at the time and the study was discontinued. Galloway and associates (El-Galley et al, 1997) also looked for growth factor deficiency in tissues of males with hypospadias and found a correlation. To our knowledge, however, a growth factor analysis has not been undertaken in patients with chordee without hypospadias.

An important part of the preoperative evaluation is the submission of instant or digital photographs of the erect penis, taken by the patient, documenting the curvature. The photographs are especially helpful in differentiating between the patients we refer to as having chordee without hypospadias and those with congenital curvatures of the penis. In a patient who has chordee without hypospadias, the photograph reveals an erect penis commensurate with the size of the detumesced penis; whereas in the congenital curvature patient, the erect penis is noticeably large.

Many of our patients are also evaluated preoperatively by our sex therapy colleague. Because of their congenital anomaly, these patients often become relatively reclusive and have poor self-images and genital images. For a successful surgical outcome, it is important to address the psychological aspects of the condition as an integral part of the treatment.

Corrective surgery for chordee without hypospadias is highly successful, and in almost all cases, an effective correction can be accomplished with a single operation (Devine et al, 1991). In some cases, the penis has been straightened by excision of all the dysgenetic tissues from the ventral side of the penis and wide mobilization of the corpus spongiosum from the glans penis into the perineum.

Even in patients with obvious abnormalities of the corpus spongiosum (i.e., poor ventral fusion or frank bifid corpus spongiosum), wide mobilization usually reveals that it is not the corpus spongiosum that remains as the ventral limiting factor. In most patients, the penis remains curved because of the inelasticity of the ventral aspect of the corpora cavernosa themselves. Furthermore, in an occasional patient, the corpus spongiosum becomes atretic distal on the shaft, and the urethra itself is only an epithelium-lined tube. Even in these patients, it is usually not found that with wide mobilization of the epithelial distal portion and elevation of the proximal corpus spongiosum, the corpus spongiosum or the epithelial tube is limiting the ventral erection. If the epithelial tube has served as an adequate urethra (i.e., it is not stenotic), the morbidity of urethral division and subsequent need for urethral reconstruction must be considered before such a procedure is undertaken. Because the evolution of hypospadias repairs accomplished by wide mobilization of the corpus spongiosum and epithelial and corpus spongiosal elements distal to the meatus has allowed onlay procedures, the morbidities of urethral division must be strongly considered and, we believe, usually avoided.

In children, after mobilization and excision of the dysgenetic tissues, the residual chordee can usually be corrected by making a longitudinal incision, with a sharp blade, in the ventral midline of the corpora cavernosa while an artificial erection is maintained. The incision (midline ventral septotomy) can often be extended between the corporal bodies for a significant distance, allowing the edges of the ventral tunica to move laterally. The penis will noticeably straighten with erection.

If this maneuver is not sufficient, the dorsal neurovascular structures can be mobilized in concert with Buck's fascia, and a small ellipse or ellipses of dorsal tunica albuginea can be excised and closed with watertight plicating sutures. Caution is important, however, when the dorsal neurovascular structures are mobilized; with poor development of the ventral structures, which occurs in some patients, the arborization of the dorsal arteries provides the dominant vascularity to the glans.

Congenital Curvatures of the Penis

Patients with congenital curvature of the penis can have ventral, lateral (which is most often to the left), or, **unusually, dorsal curvature. Photographs of the erect penis demonstrate a smooth curvature that generally involves the entire pendulous portion of the penile shaft.**

Patients usually present as otherwise healthy young men between the ages of 18 and 30 years. Many of these patients have noticed curvature before passing through puberty but have presumed it to be normal. With puberty, however, they discover that the curvature is not normal, or they become sexually active and discover that the curvature impedes their efforts; or they notice increasing curvature as they pass through puberty, and this, in their minds, clearly would preclude sexual intercourse. On occasion, a patient waits until he is older than 30 years to deal with the anomaly, and even less often, a younger adolescent presents who is able to discuss his genitalia with his parents.

Our surgical approach to patients with a congenital ventral curvature is illustrated in Figure 33–52. Most of our patients have been circumcised and the patterns of venous and lymphatic drainage of the skin established with that procedure. In circumcised patients, we make an incision through the circumcision scar, which in many cases is displaced well down on the penile shaft. Even with relatively significant displacement of the circumcision scar on the shaft of the penis, however, the reincision should be through the circumcision scar. The penis is then degloved by dissection of the layer immediately superficial to the superficial lamina of Buck's fascia.

An artificial erection is obtained with normal saline. A high-pressure, high-volume pump is useful for this purpose. We do not routinely recommend a tourniquet device because constricting devices can conceal the proximal limits of the curvature. This is of most significance in cases of ventral curvatures, which frequently extend proximally. On occasion, some element of perineal pressure is initially required, but these are patients with normal erectile function, and their venous occlusive function is normal. We also do not use pharmacologic agents to induce erection, although there are some centers that favor this approach.

The artificial erection demonstrates the character of the curvature and the location of maximal curvature. In patients with ventral curvature, there may be some illusion of thickening of the dartos and Buck's fascia, and in those patients, the fibrous tissue is mobilized and completely excised. The corpus spongiosum is detached from the corpora cavernosa and mobilized from the glans to the penoscrotal junction.

After these tissues are excised, the artificial erection is repeated, and an occasional patient is found to have been completely straightened. Most patients, however, suffer from a differential elasticity between the dorsal and the ventral aspects of the corporal bodies, and although the curvature may have been lessened, it persists unless further procedures are done to straighten the penis.

In the adult patient with persistent curvature, there are two options for surgical correction: (1) to lengthen the ventral aspect of the penis by making transverse incisions in the ventral tunica and placing an autologous tissue graft (we currently use the small intestinal submucosal graft at our institution); and (2) to shorten the dorsal aspect of the penis by elevating the neurovascular bundle, excising an ellipse or ellipses from the dorsum of the tunica albuginea, and closing the defects in watertight fashion (Nesbitt [1965] procedure).

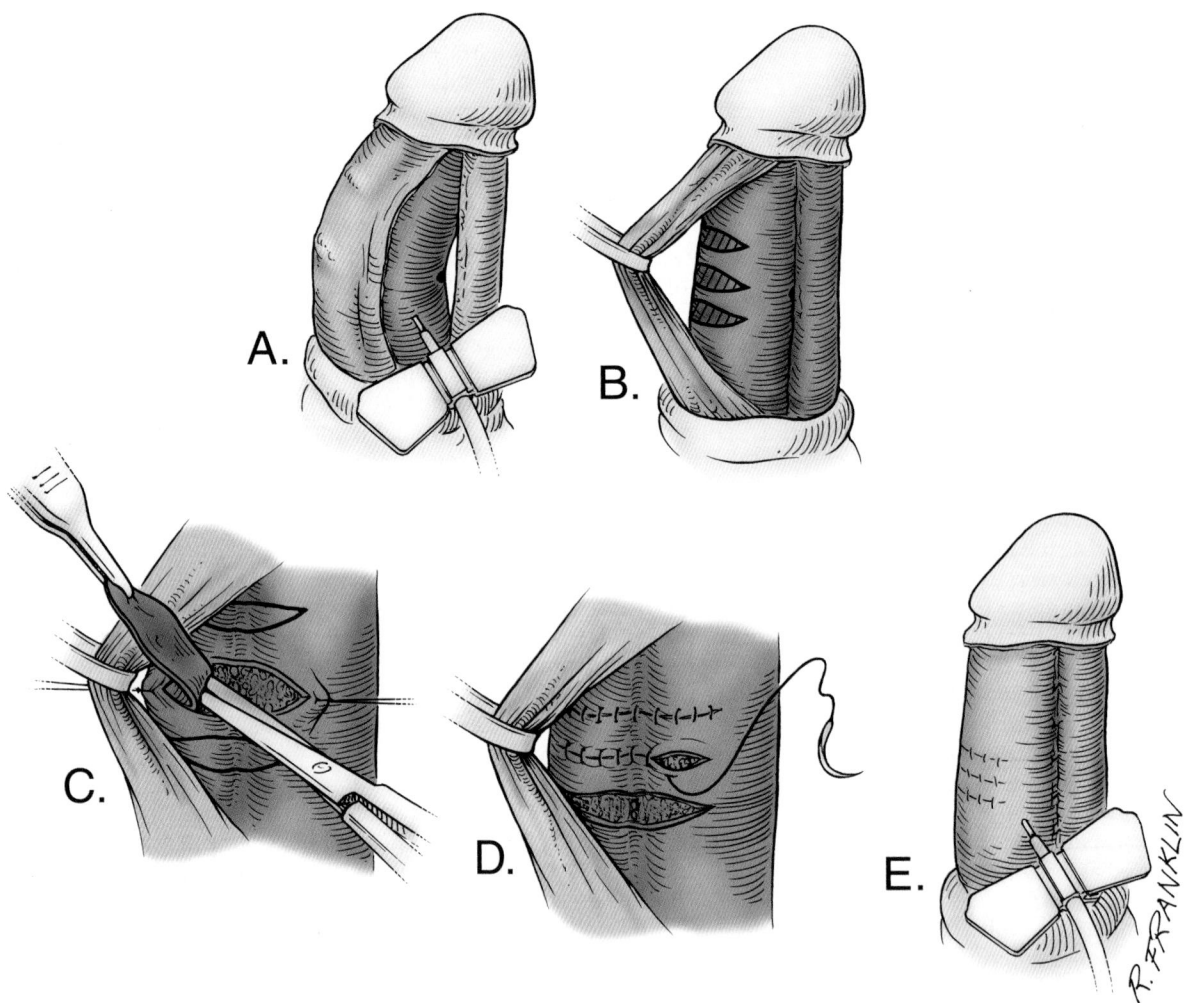

Figure 33–52. Surgery for congenital curvature of the penis. **A,** A circumcising incision has been made and the urethra mobilized by resection of the dartos fascia and Buck's fascia. The needle is in place for an artificial erection. The erection shows continuing chordee. The elastic urethra is not the cause of this curvature. The point of maximal concavity has been marked. **B,** Ellipses of tissue are outlined opposite the point of maximal concavity. **C,** Excision of the ellipses of the tunica. Note the tips of the septal strands in the midline. **D,** Closure of the edges of the incisions. **E,** Artificial erection revealing a straight penis. When the bend is more complex, ellipses must be excised in other locations.

Because the size of the erect penis is usually not a problem in these cases of congenital curvature, we have chosen the second option and are strenuously against ventral grafting. The recovery period after this procedure is much shorter, and the variabilities of graft take do not have to be considered. In addition, when a graft is used, there is always the possibility, although uncommon, of the development of graft-induced veno-occlusive dysfunction. In a 2000 consensus conference sanctioned by the World Health Organization, the committee on Peyronie's disease and congenital curvature of the penis agreed that the majority if not all of the cases in men with the classic finding of congenital curvature of the penis were best managed with a plication or corporoplasty technique and not grafting techniques (Jardin et al, 2000). This consensus was reiterated at the next World Health Organization conference. It is therefore preferable to shorten the longer aspect of the penis in patients with congenital curvature. However, if the patient falls into the category of chordee without hypospadias and shortness of the penis is an issue, we selectively use inci-sions with grafts to correct the curvature (Devine CJ and Horton, 1975).

After the decision has been made to proceed with excisions of ellipses of dorsal tunica, Buck's fascia can be elevated, in concert with the dorsal neurovascular structures, by beginning just lateral to the corpus spongiosum and carrying the dissection dorsally across the midline. Alternatively, the tunica can be exposed by excising the deep dorsal vein of the penis and opening the inner lamina of Buck's fascia. Elevation of the neurovascular structures is done by dissecting from the dorsal midline laterally around to the corpus spongiosum and from the coronal margin to the penopubic junction, thus limiting the effects of stretching the dorsal structures with exposure of the dorsum of the penis.

An artificial erection is obtained to plan the proposed ellipse excisions. We prefer to use several small ellipses rather than try to correct the curvature with one large ellipse. The first ellipse is usually positioned at the point of maximal concavity. The edges of the planned ellipse are then apposed with

Prolene suture. The artificial erection is repeated to assess the effects of that excision. If there is good straightening in that area of the shaft, the incisions are again well marked, the plicating sutures are removed, and the ellipses of tunica are made with a sharp scalpel blade. By dissection in the space of Smith and removal of only an ellipse of tunica, the ellipses are carefully excised to avoid damage to the underlying erectile tissue or can be merely closed under the reapproximated edge of the defect in the tunica albuginea. The edge of the ellipse is reapproximated with a combination of interrupted 4-0 polydioxanone sutures and a watertight running 4-0 polydioxanone suture.

After closure, we repeat the artificial erection to assess the results of the first ellipse with the others. A final artificial erection should demonstrate the penis to be perfectly straight. In cases of ventral curvature, or when complex curvatures are associated with an element of ventral curvature, a minimal degree of dorsal curvature after correction is acceptable. In most cases, as the sutures dissolve, the penis either remains minimally dorsiflexed or becomes perfectly straight.

Buck's fascia is closed. Two small suction drains are placed superficial to Buck's fascia but deep to the dartos fascia. We then replace the skin sleeve, with its edges apposed with interrupted small Vicryl or Monocryl sutures. In all patients, we place a small Foley catheter, which is removed on the first postoperative day. The two small suction drains are also removed at 12 to 24 hours. Depending on the amount of edema and drainage, patients are discharged from the hospital on the evening of the first or early the second postoperative day.

A congenital lateral curvature of the penis is often associated with some complexity of curvature; patients frequently notice lateral curvature in association with a ventral or, less commonly, a dorsal curvature. However, some patients present with only lateral curvature, with the right side larger than the left, and curvature to the left.

In some cases, a repair of the lateral curvature can be approached through a small incision at the point of maximal curvature. Laterally placed incisions on the penile shaft are not cosmetically optimal. We prefer, however, a degloving incision after exposure of the deep penile structures; the point of maximal concavity is then marked. Prolene sutures are placed, and an artificial erection is again performed. The size of the ellipse is then assessed, and the ellipse is excised and closed as discussed earlier.

As mentioned, however, most cases of lateral curvature are associated with complex curvatures. In these patients, the correction of the curvature is similar to that described for patients with ventral curvature, by a circumcising incision with the skin reflected. In contrast to a ventral curvature, however, with a lateral curvature, the entire dorsal neurovascular bundle does not need to be reflected; therefore, it is seldom required, nor is it considered beneficial, to excise the deep dorsal vein in approaching the dorsum of the penis. The postoperative care is the same as described for a ventral curvature.

For the uncommon patient with a congenital dorsal curvature of the penis, the repair is best accomplished by mobilizing the lateral aspect of the corpus spongiosum to allow small ellipses lateral to the midline to be positioned on the ventrum of the penis, by the technique described before. Again, postoperative care is as described for a ventral curvature.

Although described as a method for plication for curvature associated with Peyronie's disease, corporoplasty, the procedure described by Yachia (1993), is also useful for the correction of congenital curvatures. The procedure essentially consists of longitudinal incisions in the tunica albuginea with transverse closure. Thus, the "long side" is plicated without the need for excision; however, the plication is durable in that the tunica is opened and closed with a resulting scar, rather than reliance only on the strength of sutures as originally described by Nesbit (1965). With this technique, closure is done with absorbable monofilament suture.

Acquired Curvatures of the Penis

Acquired curvatures of the penis inevitably follow trauma to the penis. Many of these cases are associated with Peyronie's disease, also believed to be associated with trauma to the penis during intercourse. An occasional patient also presents who has had vigorous internal urethrotomy, with the incision extended outside the urethra and corpus spongiosum and involving the tunica of the corporal bodies, causing scarring that is significant enough to be associated with curvature.

Acquired Curvatures of the Penis That Are Not Peyronie's Disease

When a young man presents with an acquired curvature of the penis, one must always consider Peyronie's disease. However, many will not have true Peyronie's disease. These patients on close questioning reveal a history of minimal lateral curvature of the penis and a clear memory of a lateral buckling injury that occurred during intercourse. In some cases, the patient remembers hearing a "snap" and notices immediate detumescence and significant ecchymosis of the penis. These patients are often referred with a diagnosis of Peyronie's disease, but a diagnosis of curvature secondary to penile fracture is more accurate. Because of the noticeable events associated with fracture of the penis, many patients present acutely, and reconstruction can be accomplished at that time.

On occasion, however, a patient or his initial care physician ignores the stigmata of the trauma (often described as "minimal" by patients), and the patient presents with a noticeable lateral scar that causes both indentation of the lateral aspect of the penis and, in some cases, curvature. Patients who had preexisting lateral curvature may actually notice that their penis has been straightened by the trauma, but they are disturbed by the concavity caused by the scar. In others, the small linear scar causes a significant lateral curvature.

Another group of patients presents after a similar buckling trauma to the penis but without associated detumescence or ecchymosis. These patients report noticing that their erections were painful for a period after the trauma, and then a nodule developed in the lateral aspect of the penis. Eventually, they present with a lateral linear scar that has led to curvature and indentation at the site. We refer to this injury as a subclinical fracture of the penis.

The lesion of a subclinical fracture of the penis is believed to be due to the disruption of the outer longitudinal layer of the tunica albuginea during the buckling trauma. The inner, circular layer is not disrupted, however, and maintains the blood-tight continuity of the corpus spongiosum. Another

possible scenario is that both layers of the tunica albuginea are disrupted but the overlying Buck's fascia maintains its integrity. There are also patients who notice a pop with intercourse and a period of pain with erections, followed by curvature of the penis—usually dorsal. These patients probably tear the septal insertion completely. These patients clearly behave more like Peyronie's disease patients.

Patients usually have normal erectile function after subclinical or clinical fracture of the penis; there appears not to be an association with concomitant global cavernosal veno-occlusive dysfunction. However, the association of cavernosal veno-occlusive dysfunction and trauma of the penis continues to be seen, and some patients have significant problems with erectile dysfunction after fracture-type injuries of the penis. These injuries are not associated with shortening of the penis. In most cases, it is the lack of erectile dysfunction and penile shortening that help distinguish these patients from Peyronie's disease patients. If a detailed history leads one to suspect blighted erectile function, an evaluation of erectile function should be accomplished before proceeding with surgery. At our institution, we evaluate these patients with duplex ultrasonography and selectively with dynamic infusion cavernosometry and cavernosography.

Although foreshortening of the penis is not a characteristic of either the injury itself or the resulting scar in either of these injuries, these patients are not thought to be best treated by approaching the opposite aspect of the scar and excising an ellipse of the tunica. This would result in bilateral scars, which would cause bilateral indentations of the penis, and although the penis would have been straightened by the correction, most patients are upset by the cosmetic and functional result of a near-circumferential indentation of the penis. Instead, we excise the scar and place a graft to replace the corporotomy defect caused by the scar excision. Because these scars are on the lateral aspect of the penis, minimal mobilization of Buck's fascia, associated dorsal neurovascular structures, and corpus spongiosum is required at the site.

The results of the surgical correction described have been extremely effective. All such patients treated at the authors' institution have been successfully corrected with a single operation.

TOTAL PENILE RECONSTRUCTION
General

The principal techniques of penile reconstruction were originally developed for treatment of trauma patients, and in many cases these patients were victims of war injuries. In 1936, Bogaraz described a technique for phallic construction in a series of war-injured patients, and in 1944, Frumkin followed with a series from the Soviet Union. Aware of the work in the Soviet Union, Gillies and Harrison (1948) reported on a series of patients in whom they had accomplished penile reconstruction while stationed at a major hospital in the outskirts of London during World War II. In this series, there were a number of patients with a complete absence of the penis.

Initially, all procedures for phallic construction involved delayed formation and transfer of tubed abdominal flaps. These tubes were produced from random flaps of skin and

because of their size were based on a tenuous blood supply. To allow new vascular patterns to become established in the transferred tissue, they were formed in stages, with a "delay" between the stages. In the "tube-within-a-tube" design, the inner tube allowed the placement of a baculum during intercourse, and the outer tube provided skin coverage. Patients voided through a proximal urethrostomy. This continued to be the "state-of-the-art" phallic construction and penile reconstruction until 1972, when Orticochea described total reconstruction of the penis using the gracilis musculocutaneous flap.

In 1978, Puckett and Montie reported a series in which they constructed the penis with a tubed groin flap. In the early cases in this series, the flap was transferred in delayed fashion to the area of the penile stump. Later in the series, a microvascular free transfer technique was employed.

In 1984, Chang and Hwang popularized the forearm flap, based on the radial artery, for phallic reconstruction. Biemer (1988) reported a modification of the forearm flap, which was also based on the radial artery; and in 1990, Farrow and associates reported their "cricket bat" modification of the radial forearm flap. **Today, forearm flaps are the most commonly employed method for total phallic construction and penile reconstruction.**

The forearm flap is usually harvested from the nondominant forearm. Preoperatively, the Allen test is used to screen patients carefully for arterial insufficiency. This test involves palpation of the radial and ulnar arteries in the wrist, with the patient making a tight fist to express blood from his hand. As he opens his hand, the fingers are pale, but if palmar circulation is normal and both arteries are patent, the fingers turn pink when one of the arteries is released. If, on the basis of either the Allen test or the patient's history, there is any doubt about the integrity of the radial and ulnar arteries or the palmar arch, upper extremity angiography is performed.

As described, the forearm flap is a fasciocutaneous flap vascularized by the radial artery; however, the ulnar artery also vascularizes the forearm fascia and most of the forearm skin. The radial artery arises as a continuation of the brachial artery and proximally lies beneath the belly of the brachioradial is muscle, becoming more superficial at the wrist. The ulnar artery is also a continuation of the brachial artery and vascularizes a similar area of skin and underlying adipose tissue. The vascularity of the overlying skin is achieved by way of the underlying (antebrachial) fascia, which is the superficial fascia investing the musculature of the forearm.

The forearm flap can be elevated and transferred on the superficial fascia. The lateral and medial antebrachial cutaneous nerves appear proximally beneath the fascia. The cephalic, basilic, and medial antebrachial veins are also included in the flap and constitute a portion of the venous drainage. In some patients, the vena comitans is the dominant venous drainage system. At the time of flap transfer, it is imperative to assess both the venous comitans and the superficial veins to determine which is the dominant system in the individual patient.

The various modifications of the forearm flap do not represent changes in the technique of flap elevation; rather, they are modifications in the design of the skin island and the relative position of the urethral paddle in relation to the skin that will eventually become shaft coverage. Each of these modifications has advantages in different situations.

In the forearm flap as described by Chang and Hwang (1984) (Fig. 33–53*A*), the shaft is covered with the radial aspect of the skin paddle. A deepithelialized strip is made, and a second skin island, on the ulnar aspect of the skin paddle, is tubed to form the urethra. The urethral tube is then rolled within the tube of skin to form a tube-within-a-tube design. In the white population, this flap has demonstrated a tendency to lead to ischemic stenosis of the lateral paddle, where the urethra is constructed.

In the cricket bat modification (Fig. 33–53*B*), the urethral tube extends distally, closely overlying either the radial or the ulnar artery. We have experience with elevation of the cricket bat modification on both arteries. Proximal to the urethral strip, a broader portion of the skin paddle provides coverage of the shaft. The urethral portion is tubed and transposed by inverting it into the center of the shaft portion of the skin paddle. The advantage of this modification lies in centering the urethral portion over the respective artery, in contrast to the Chinese design, in which the ulnar aspect is far distal from the radial artery, with the potential for ischemic stenosis or loss of that portion. The cricket bat modification has been useful in trauma patients, particularly in those who have a significant stump of erectile bodies and urethra left after the injury.

The modification by Biemer (1988) also centers the urethral portion of the flap over the artery (Fig. 33-53*C*). As described by Biemer, the flap is elevated on the radial artery and includes a vascularized piece of the radial bone intended to provide rigidity to the new penis. The inclusion of cartilage and bone has not been universally successful, however, and rigidity in these flaps is obtainable by the use of either an externally applied or internally implanted prosthesis. If the bone is not

elevated, the Biemer flap design can be elevated on either the radial or the ulnar artery. At our center, we most often elevate the flap on the ulnar artery, in a modification of the Biemer design.

Modifications of the Biemer design also include the glans construction technique that was originally described by Puckett and Montie (1978). In the original Biemer design, a central strip becomes the urethra, and lateral to that strip, two deepithelialized portions and two lateral islands (lateral aspects of that skin paddle) are fused dorsally and ventrally to cover the shaft. With the modification of Puckett and colleagues (1982), a large island is left distally and flared back over the tip of the tubed flaps, creating the illusion of a glans penis. The Biemer design, especially when it is combined with Puckett's design for glanular construction, offers the best cosmetic results.

There are several disadvantages to the use of a forearm flap for phallic construction. The major disadvantage of forearm flaps, which yield an unsightly scar, is the obvious donor site deformity. We have reconstructed the donor site with full-thickness skin grafts taken from the area of the inguinal crease, and the cosmetic result is far superior to that obtained when the donor site is reconstructed with split-thickness skin (even thick split-thickness skin). A second disadvantage lies in the possibility of the development of cold intolerance in the hand of the donor side. Early in our experience with the forearm flap, we reconstructed the radial artery with an interposition vein graft. We have since abandoned this procedure in the majority of our series and have not seen cold intolerance in our patients. Another disadvantage occurs in both male and virilized transgender patients when the forearm skin is hirsute, as the hair can be problematic if it is included in the portion of the flap used for urethral construction. In such patients, we try to identify the potential for the problem and refer them for epilation before surgery.

Sadove and McRoberts proposed the use of the fibular osteocutaneous flap for phallic construction. The fibula is elevated on the periosteal vessel along with the overlying skin paddle. As described by them, urethral reconstruction is by tubed graft techniques, and their procedure had a 100% urethral complication rate. The center from Munich has proposed use of this flap with a prefabricated urethra. They place a tubed graft initially in the center of the paddle while it is still on the leg, then elevate the flap later and attach the urethra. The presumption that these tubed grafted urethras would behave differently escapes the authors; however, the surgeons in Munich propose it as better. An obvious compromise, which might be better, is to prefabricate an open "urethral plate" with a sheet graft at the first stage; then, at the second stage, the urethral plate is closed along with flap elevation. We have limited experience with this flap as just described and think it appropriate only for cases in which the forearm is not usable. The technique of urethral construction is merely an application of the staged, graft reconstruction. The graft could be split-thickness skin; it is unlikely one could use buccal graft. However, with a number of centers proposing the use of cultured buccal graft, in time that might be a wonderful solution and then raises the possibility of "epilating" the forearm flap (urethral portion) by first replacing the proposed urethral strip with buccal mucosa at a stage preceding the true phallic construction procedure.

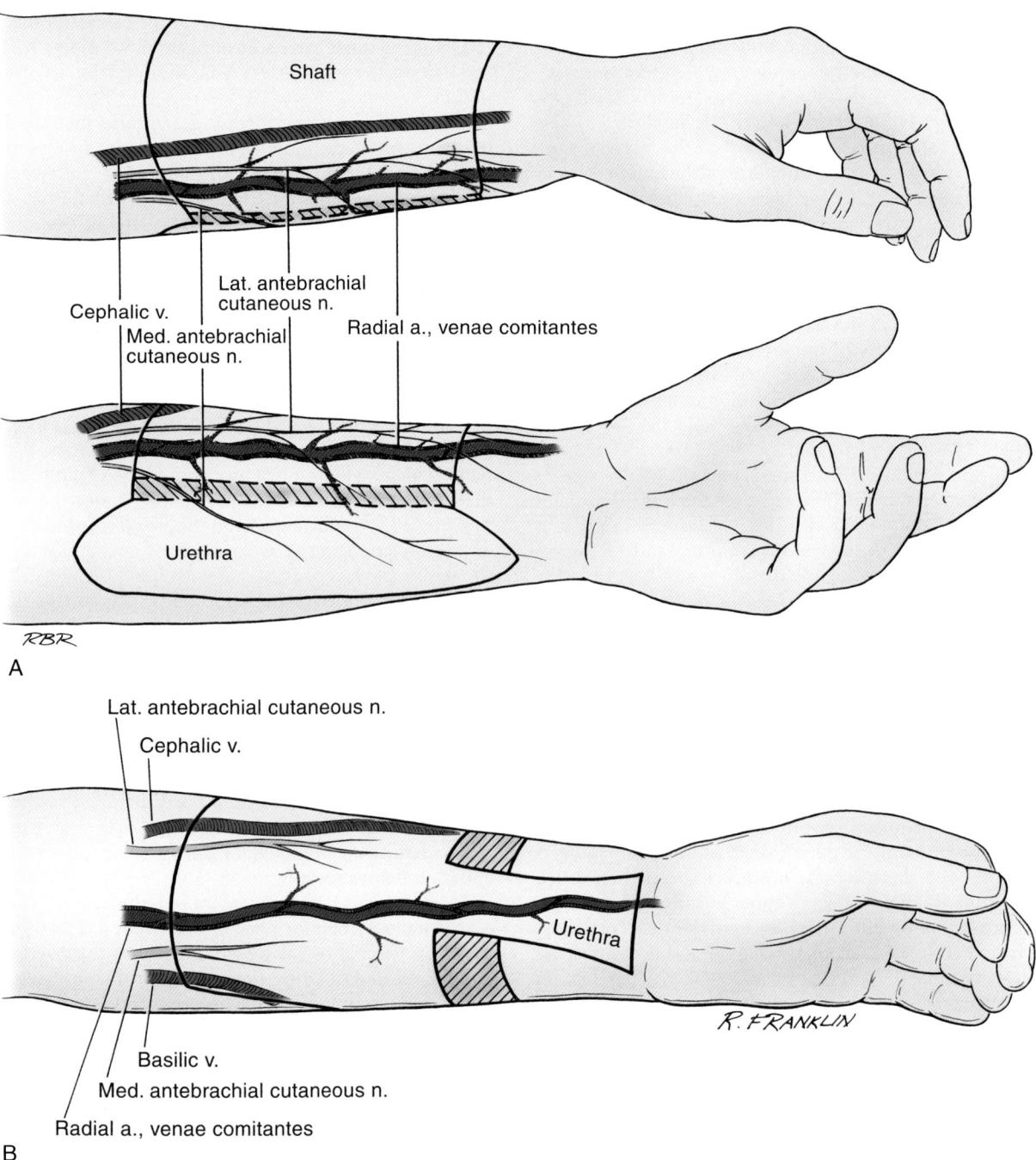

Figure 33–53. Variations of the forearm flap for phallic construction. **A,** The Chang "Chinese" flap based on the radial artery. Notice that the skin island has two separate paddles. An ulnar "urethral" paddle is separated from the shaft coverage paddle by a deepithelialized strip. **B,** The "cricket bat" modification of the radial forearm flap proposed by Farrow and Boyd. The urethral portion extends centered over the artery. The shaft coverage portion is on the proximal forearm. The deepithelialized areas *(crosshatched)* add bulk to the glans. The urethral portion is flipped into the middle of the flap and tubularized.

Continued

For patients who only need vascularized tissue to cover the shaft of the penis, we have used the upper lateral arm flap. This is a fasciocutaneous flap, and its cutaneous vascular territory is centered on the radial collateral artery. The skin of the lateral upper arm is thin, with little subcutaneous adiposity. To mark the location of the lateral intramuscular septum and the course of the superior radial collateral artery, we draw a line joining the insertion of the deltoid with the lateral epicondyle. We begin the dissection posteriorly, elevating the superficial fascia until the posterior lateral portion of the intramuscular septum has been identified. A potential disadvantage of this flap lies in the fact that the entire venous drainage is dependent on the vena comitans, and although superficial veins do traverse the flap, none of them seems to

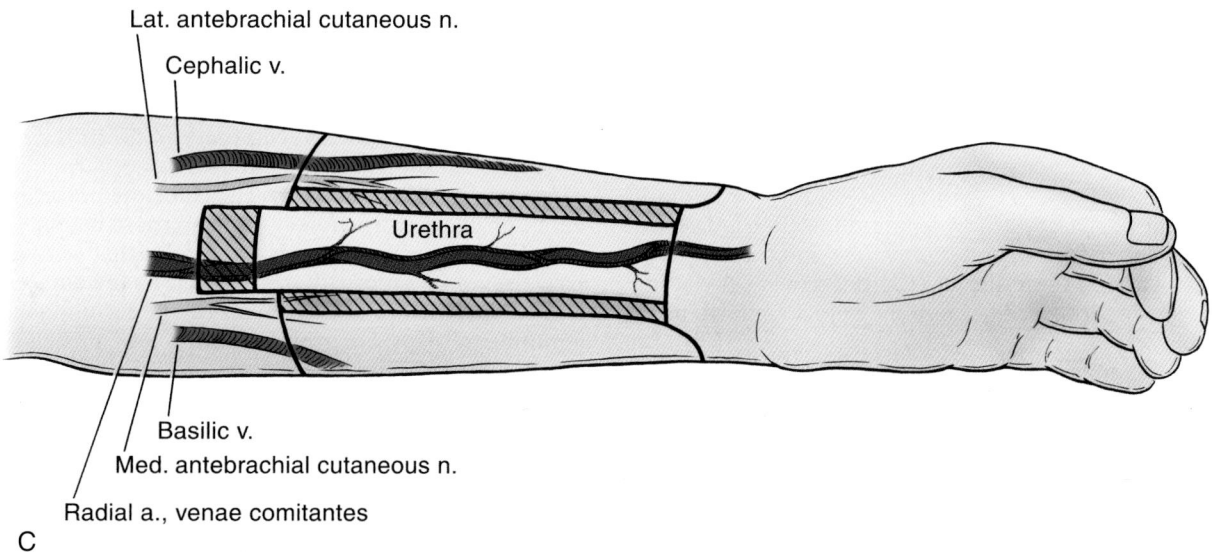

Lat. antebrachial cutaneous n.

Cephalic v.

Urethra

Basilic v.

Med. antebrachial cutaneous n.

Radial a., venae comitantes

C

Figure 33–53, cont'd. **C,** Modification of the forearm flap as proposed by Biemer (1988). The urethral paddle is a midline strip separated by the two lateral paddles by a deepithelialized strip. The lateral paddles are tubularized, with the urethral paddle tubularized in the center.

provide significant venous drainage. Although this is disquieting, we have found the flap to be completely reliable thus far, with no losses due to venous insufficiency.

This flap has also been used for total phallic construction. For this purpose, the flap is expanded by tissue expander and elevated across the elbow, and the distal flap is elevated on the recurrent radial artery. As with the forearm flap, the donor site of an upper lateral arm flap can be disfiguring. However, because the scar is on the upper arm, it is more easily concealed beneath a shirtsleeve than a scar in the forearm. All the flaps described allow microneurosurgical coaptation of the flap cutaneous nerves with recipient nerves. With total phallic construction, the cutaneous nerves can be attached either to the dorsal nerves of the penis or to the dorsal nerves of the clitoris in the transsexual patient. When these nerves are not available, the nerves can be coapted to the pudendal nerve, which in most patients requires an interposition graft. These nerves are thought to provide the best restoration of erogenous cutaneous sensibility. We have also coapted the flap's cutaneous nerves to the ilioinguinal nerves, which provide sensation to the inner aspect of the thigh and the lateral aspect of the scrotum, and have achieved a reasonable degree of erogenous sensibility.

In most patients, the deep inferior epigastric vessels are the recipient vasculature for flap transfer. These vessels are medial branches of the iliac system and lie on the dorsal aspect of the rectus abdominis muscle. The artery usually remains deep to the muscle, although an early penetration of the artery into the muscle can be observed in some patients. The artery classically bifurcates at the level of the umbilicus and is generally accompanied by two or more venae comitantes. These vessels have been elevated by several methods, and Lund and colleagues (1995) described their elevation for penile revascularization with laparoscopic techniques. When the deep inferior epigastric vessels are used, it is often necessary to also include a saphenous vein for further venous runoff.

In some patients, however, these vessels are not available, and we have used a saphenous interposition graft to the superficial femoral artery. With use of this technique, we mobilize the saphenous vein well down the upper aspect of the thigh and then attach the vein to the femoral artery, making a temporary arteriovenous fistula. The fistula is divided, with the saphenous vein becoming the venous runoff and the interposition graft providing the arterial inflow. This system of recipient vessels is greatly inferior to a direct arterial anastomosis. Because of this, in a few patients we have divided the profunda femoris vessel and vigorously dissected it from its other branches. We have then done an end-to-end (artery-to-artery) anastomosis of the ulnar artery to the profunda femoris. However, the long-term consequences to the patient of dividing the profunda femoris are not clear. Immediate reconstruction of the profunda does not appear to be advantageous, as the dissection required to mobilize the profunda femoris to become a recipient vessel requires the division of a number of proximal branches, and these would not be reconstructed with an immediate reconstruction of the profunda femoris. Mention of this as a potential means of "creating" recipient vessels is not to recommend the procedure, as the procedure may be determined to have unacceptable long-term consequences. Another option in extreme cases is to use the superficial femoral, which could be reconstructed with a vein interposition. When the "classic" recipient vessels are not available, these other methods may be acceptable. However, we strenuously caution concerning their use, as the long-term consequences are not known.

In the latter part of our series, we included the routine transfer of gracilis muscle to cover the area of the urethral anastomosis, increasing the vascularity to that area and significantly altering the incidence of anastomotic fistula and stricture formation. We have also elevated a bipedicled flap from the area of the penile shaft base, which is transposed beneath the phallic flap. This flap provides increased bulk and some modicum of scrotal construction, and when it is combined with the gracilis muscle, its thickness provides excellent coverage for the juncture of the flap with the base of the neoscrotum. Mobilization of a tunica dartos flap with tunica vaginalis pedicle, or a Martius flap in the transgender patient, may obviate the necessity to elevate and transpose a gracilis muscle flap.

During the phallic construction procedure, urine is diverted by means of a suprapubic cystostomy tube, and the urethra is stented with a No. 14 soft silicone (Silastic) catheter. A voiding study is usually performed between the third and fourth postoperative week.

Rigidity for intercourse in the patient with phallic construction is usually achieved by either an externally applied or a permanently implanted prosthesis. Prosthetic implantation is never undertaken until 1 year after phallic construction, as protective sensibility must be demonstrated in the flap. When the flap is transferred, it is, by definition, rendered insensate. At about 3 to 4 months after reconstruction, however, as nerve regeneration occurs, sensation becomes noticeable. In addition, before prosthetic implantation is undertaken, the urethra must be patent and proved to be durable.

At our center, we now have a large series of patients with internally implanted devices. We have implanted both hydraulic and articulated prostheses encased in Gore-Tex neocorpora. These devices are anchored to the ischial tuberosity and the pubis by anchoring the neocorpora to these bone structures. In most patients, we implant two cylinders or rods. Early in our series, we had problems with hematoma and seroma formation and subsequent infection. However, since modifying our antibiotic regimen and including the routine use of suction drains with the implant procedure, we have had excellent success with implantation. We currently place the antibiotic-coated (InhibiZone) AMS 700CXR.*

We also have implanted testicular prostheses in a number of patients. In patients in whom we have used a hydraulic device, we implanted the pump in one neohemiscrotum and a testicular prosthesis in the opposite one. At present, patients are implanted on the basis of enrollment in clinical trials.

Reconstruction after Trauma

In many ways, the problems of trauma patients are more challenging to solve than are those of patients who require total phallic construction. We have treated a large number of patients who have had devastating injuries to the penis after complicated prosthetic surgery or surgery to correct penile curvatures of Peyronie's disease. The goal in these patients is to preserve the penile structures and function as much as possible yet correct the deficiencies that are imposed on the patient by the trauma.

Acutely, urine must be diverted, necrotic tissue must be carefully débrided, and any foreign bodies that may have been implanted must be removed. Vigorous acute wound management stabilizes the wounds and allows active granulation to

progress. In all trauma patients, an attempt should be made to save as many of the penile structures as possible.

Approximately 3 to 6 weeks after trauma, primary reconstruction can be undertaken, although we have elected to wait 4 to 6 months in some patients, depending on the situation. When significant adjacent tissue loss has occurred, the adjacent areas must be well reconstructed before proceeding with either phallic construction or penile reconstruction.

In the trauma patient, it is imperative that well-vascularized tissues be eventually transposed to the adjacent area, and reconstruction of these areas can be accomplished with a number of flaps. For groin reconstruction, the tensor fascia lata flap has been useful. The rectus femoris flap, characteristically long and large, can be transposed to the area of the lower abdomen and has been an extremely useful flap for inguinal and lower abdominal reconstruction. The gracilis muscle is an excellent flap for reconstruction of the perineum and the groin. Alternatively, the posterior thigh flap can be used for reconstruction of the groin and perineum and, in some cases, transposed to the lowermost portion of the lower abdomen. The rectus abdominis flap is a useful flap and can be elevated with a vertical or transverse skin paddle. In addition, the flap can be transposed to either the ipsilateral or contralateral side. Care must be taken in the patient who has had lower abdominal external beam irradiation.

Variations of the flap designs described for complete phallic construction have been successfully applied in select patients for penile reconstruction. An example is seen in one patient who suffered an injury to his penis from a shotgun blast. The blast injured a large portion of the patient's right corpus cavernosum, and the majority of the penile skin was either destroyed or used for urethral reconstruction. In this patient, a flap based on the Chinese design was elevated. However, because the urethral reconstruction was accomplished with a penile skin island, the ulnar portion of the flap was not needed for that purpose. Therefore, the ulnar portion was deepithelialized and tubularized to form bulk and a new right corporal body. This patient is now sexually active, and the bulk of the tube's dermal section gives adequate support to his penis for intercourse.

Another patient required only distal urethral construction and glans reconstruction. For this patient, we based a flap on the Biemer design to construct a glans. The proximal portions of the flap were deepithelialized, allowing fixation of the neoglans on the tips of the corporal bodies, and an excellent functional and cosmetic result was achieved for this patient. The versatility of free flap technology allows the solution of complex issues with reasonably acceptable functional and cosmetic results.

FEMALE-TO-MALE TRANSSEXUALISM

Female-to-male transsexual patients present a unique challenge, and no patient should be considered for definitive reassignment surgery without having undergone complex screening and evaluation by a team consisting of mental health professionals as well as surgeons who are skilled in undertaking transgender surgery. It is imperative that an ongoing, stable, therapeutic relationship be established between the patient and a mental health professional at the time of definitive gender reassignment surgery. At our

---

*American Medical Systems, Inc., 10700 Bren Road West, Minnetonka, MN 55343; 952-930-6000.

institution, the Harry Benjamin criteria (Ramsey, 1996) are strictly adhered to, and surgery is accomplished by a team of urologists, plastic surgeons, and gynecologists.

In most patients, the first stage of female-to-male transsexual surgery consists of bilateral salpingo-oophorectomy, hysterectomy, vaginectomy, and urethral lengthening with colpocleisis. Even in the virginal patient, our surgeons have become skilled at accomplishing a hysterectomy and bilateral salpingo-oophorectomy by way of transvaginal surgery. We perform a vaginectomy at the same operation, leaving the anterior vaginal wall to be transposed as a random flap to lengthen the female urethra and allow colpocleisis. Lengthening of the female urethra brings the base of the native urethra up to what will be the base of the phallic flap; along with the transfer of gracilis muscle, it has significantly altered our surgical results with regard to urethral anastomotic fistula and stricture. Urine is diverted with a suprapubic tube, and a voiding trial is performed in approximately 21 days. Patients are generally in the hospital for 2 to 3 days and return 3 to 4 months later for phallic construction.

For phallic construction in the transsexual patient, we elevate a bipedicled flap of skin, as already described, from the area where the phallic structure will be implanted and transpose it to the undersurface of the neopenis. The patient is generally in the hospital for a period of 10 to 14 days after total phallic construction, and a voiding trial with contrast material is done at about 28 days postoperatively. After 1 year, when erogenous sensibility is demonstrated and the urethra is proved to be durable, prosthetic implantation is considered.

KEY POINTS: TOTAL PENILE RECONSTRUCTION

■ The principal techniques of penile reconstruction were originally developed for treatment of victims of war injuries. Initially, all of the procedures involved delayed tissue transfer. In 1978, Puckett and Montie reported a series of phallic reconstructions in which a groin flap was transferred by microvascular free transfer techniques to the area of the penis. The phallus was insensible, but that represented the first free flap reconstruction for phallic construction. In 1984, Chang and Hwang popularized use of the forearm flap. That flap has been modified by a number of individuals.

■ Our preference is to use an ulnar forearm flap with a combined Puckett modification of the flap and Biemer modification of the glans. These flaps allow sensible phallic construction that lets the patient stand to void and permits eventual prosthetic implantation as the phallus has both protective and erogenous sensibility.

■ The techniques employed in the transsexual patient are not different from those in the trauma patient. Often, the shapes of the skin paddles must be tailored to the individual patient.

SUGGESTED READINGS

Aboseif SR, Breza J, Lue TF, Tanagho EA: Penile venous drainage in erectile dysfunction: Anatomical, radiological and functional considerations. Br J Urol 1989;64:183-190.

Akporiaye LE, Jordan GH, Devine CJ Jr: Balanitis xerotica obliterans (BXO). AUA Update Series 1997;16:166-167.

Chapple CR, Pang D: Contemporary management of urethral trauma and the post-traumatic stricture. Curr Opin Urol 1999;9:253-260.

Chapple C, Barbagli G, Jordan G, et al: Consensus statement on urethral trauma. BJU Int 2004;93:1195-1202.

Coursey JW, Morey AF, McAninch JW, et al: Erectile function after anterior urethroplasty. J Urol 2001;166:2273-2276.

Devine CJ Jr, Blackley SK, Horton CE, Gilbert DA: The surgical treatment of chordee without hypospadias in men. J Urol 1991;146:325-329.

Fichtner J, Filipas D, Fisch M, et al: Long-term outcome of ventral buccal mucosa onlay graft urethroplasty for urethral stricture repair. Urology 2004;64:648-650.

Heyns CF, Steenkamp JW, de Kock ML, Whitaker P: Treatment of male urethral strictures: Is repeated dilation or internal urethrotomy useful? J Urol 1998;160:356-358.

Iselin CE, Webster GD: The significance of the open bladder neck associated with pelvic fracture urethral distraction defects. J Urol 1999;162:34-51.

Jordan GH: The application of tissue transfer techniques in urologic surgery. In Webster G, Kirby R, King L, et al, eds: Reconstructive Urology. Oxford, Blackwell Scientific, 1993:143-169.

Levine J, Wessells H: Comparison of open and endoscopic treatment of posttraumatic posterior urethral strictures. World J Surg 2001;25:1597-1601.

McCallum RW, Colapinto V: The role of urethrography in urethral disease. Part I. Accurate radiological localization of the membranous urethra and distal sphincters in normal male subjects. J Urol 1979;122:607-611.

McCallum RW, Colapinto V: The role of urethrography in urethral disease. Part II. Indications for transsphincter urethroplasty in patients with primary bulbous strictures. J Urol 1979;122:612-618.

McRoberts JW, Chapman WH, Answell JS: Primary anastomosis of the traumatically amputated penis: Case report and summary of literature. J Urol 1968;100:751-754.

Morey AF, Metro MJ, Carney KJ, et al: Consensus on genitourinary trauma: External genitalia. BJU Int 2004;94:507-515.

Pansadoro V, Emiliozzi P: Internal urethrotomy in the management of anterior urethral strictures: Long-term followup. J Urol 1996;156:73-75.

Quartey JK: One stage penile/preputial cutaneous island flap urethroplasty for urethral stricture: A preliminary report. J Urol 1983;129:284-287.

Rourke KF, McCammon KA, Sumfest JM, et al: Open reconstruction of pediatric and adolescent urethral strictures: Long-term follow-up. J Urol 2003;169:1818-1821; discussion 1821.

Webster GD, Mathes GL, Selli C: Prostatomembranous urethral injuries: A review of the literature and a rational approach to their management. J Urol 1983;130:898-902.

Surgery of the Scrotum and Seminal Vesicles

JAY I. SANDLOW, MD • HOWARD N. WINFIELD, MD •
MARC GOLDSTEIN, MD

SCROTUM

SEMINAL VESICLES

SCROTUM
Surgical Anatomy

The scrotal contents are unique in their accessibility for physical examination, imaging modalities, and surgical intervention. **The success of surgery for male infertility and scrotal disorders is predicated on selection of the correct operation and most appropriate surgical approach.** The details of the history and careful physical examination, followed by confirmatory, judiciously selected laboratory and imaging procedures, are presented in Chapter 19, "Male Infertility." When surgical intervention for diagnostic or therapeutic purposes is indicated, a thorough understanding of the anatomy and physiology of the male reproductive system (see Chapter 2, "Anatomy of the Lower Urinary Tract and Male Genitalia," and Chapter 18, "Male Reproductive Physiology") is requisite for planning and carrying out a surgical procedure with the highest probability of success and the lowest morbidity. The blood supply of major scrotal organs is summarized in Table 34–1.

Preparation

Before scrotal surgery, the patient should be completely shaved, preferably in the operating room. **Previous studies have demonstrated the improved postoperative infection rate with shaving in the operating room compared with before surgery** (Alexander et al, 1983). Furthermore, although the infection rate for scrotal surgery is typically low (between 0% and 10%), it has been recommended that patients undergoing scrotal surgery receive preoperative antibiotics; the scrotum is an area that may be considered "clean-contaminated" because of its proximity to the perineum (Kiddoo et al, 2004). It is the authors' opinion that other than for vasectomy and other percutaneous procedures, patients undergoing open scrotal surgery should receive

antibiotics, such as a first-generation cephalosporin, just before surgery. Topical antibiotic irrigation with neomycin or kanamycin solution, initiated as soon as the incision is made and continued intermittently throughout the procedure, may be as effective as systemic administration of antibiotics (O'Connor and Goldstein, 2002).

Postoperative Care

Although there are no standard methods for postoperative care after scrotal surgery, several authors have suggested various ways of preventing edema, hematoma, and infection. These range from compressive scrotal dressings (Manson and MacDonald, 1987) to suturing of the scrotum to the abdominal wall (Oesterling, 1990). **The opinion of the authors is that any method that provides compression and elevation of the scrotum will prevent significant postoperative complications, but none will supercede the need for meticulous hemostasis at the end of the procedure.** There are currently no data available for the routine use of postoperative antibiotics, but there is typically no indication for their routine use.

Vasectomy

Vasectomy is a safe and effective method of permanent contraception (Schwingl and Guess, 2000). **In the United States, it is employed by nearly 11% of all married couples and performed on approximately 500,000 men per year, more than any other urologic surgical procedure.** Impressive as these numbers may seem, far fewer vasectomies are performed worldwide than female sterilizations by tubal ligation (Rowlands and Hannaford, 2003). This is in spite of the fact that vasectomy is less expensive and associated with much less morbidity and mortality than tubal ligation. Some men fear pain and complications, whereas others falsely equate vasectomy with castration or loss of masculinity.

The procedure should be performed in a warm room and with warm preparation solution to relax the scrotum. Shaving should be performed in the room just before preparation, thus reducing the chance of infection. The decision to use a single midline incision versus bilateral incisions is left to the surgeon. However, it is the authors' opinion that bilateral incisions

Table 34–1. Blood Supply to Testis, Epididymis, and Vas Deferens

Testis
Testicular (internal spermatic) artery from aorta (main blood supply)
Deferential artery from internal iliac (hypogastric) artery–superior vesical artery
Cremasteric (external spermatic) artery from inferior epigastric artery

Epididymis
Superior epididymal artery derived from testicular artery
Inferior epididymal artery derived from vasal (deferential) artery

Vas deferens
Seminal vesicle end: deferential artery
Testicular end: deferential artery and inferior epididymal artery

are superior for several reasons. First, there is no chance of dividing the same side twice as there is with a single midline incision (although this situation can be avoided by gently pulling on the vas and asking the patient to identify which side is being manipulated). Second, it is much easier to divide the vas far from the testis with bilateral incisions. This may help prevent post-vasectomy congestive pain (see later). Finally, the longer the testicular vasal remnant, the greater the likelihood of a successful vasectomy reversal (if desired) (Witt et al, 1994). Although this should not necessarily be a consideration in performing vasectomy, leaving a longer testicular remnant does nothing to lessen the chances of a successful vasectomy outcome.

Local Anesthesia

Vasectomy is typically performed as an outpatient procedure with use of local anesthetics. Some physicians also give sedatives, such as diazepam, orally 1 hour before the procedure to relax the patient. The choice of local anesthetic is determined by the surgeon, although the authors prefer a mixture of 1% plain lidocaine and 0.5% bupivacaine in a 1:1 ratio. The vas deferens is separated from the spermatic cord vessels and manipulated to a superficial position under the scrotal skin. The vas is firmly trapped between the middle finger, the index finger, and the thumb of the left hand. A small superficial skin wheal is raised with a 1.5-inch 25-gauge needle. The needle is then advanced within the perivasal sheath, and a small amount of local anesthetic is injected around the vas without moving the needle in and out. This produces a vasal nerve block and minimizes edema at the actual vasectomy site (Li et al, 1991). The contralateral vas deferens may be anesthetized at the same time or just before that side is addressed. **Avoidance of multiple punctures and excess needle movement minimizes the risk of hematoma.**

Conventional Incisional Technique

After adequate anesthesia is induced, 1-cm bilateral transverse incisions are carried down through the vas sheath until bare vas is exposed. The vas is delivered, and the deferential artery, veins, and accompanying nerves are dissected free of the vas and spared. A small segment is removed, and the ends are occluded by one of the techniques described later in this section. Suture closure of the scrotal wounds is optional. Fluff gauze dressings are held in place by a snug-fitting athletic supporter.

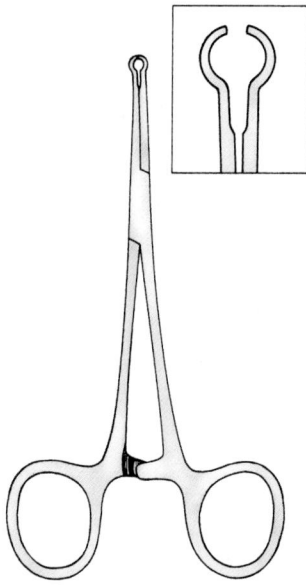

Figure 34–1. Ring-tipped vas deferens fixation clamp. Cantilevered design prevents injury to the scrotal skin. (From Li S, Goldstein M, Zhu J, Huber D: The no-scalpel vasectomy. J Urol 1991;145:341-344.)

No-Scalpel Vasectomy

An elegant method for gaining access to the vas deferens through a single tiny puncture hole was developed in China in 1974 (Li, 1976) and introduced to the United States in 1985 (Li et al, 1991). **This method eliminates the incision, results in fewer hematomas and infections, and leaves a much smaller wound than by conventional methods of accessing the vas deferens for vasectomy** (Sokal et al, 1999).

In the original description, a vasal nerve block is performed as described previously. The ring-tipped fixation clamp (Fig. 34–1) is grasped with the right hand and opened while pressing downward, stretching the scrotal skin tightly over the vas and locking the vas within the clamp. The ring clamp is placed in the left hand and the trapped vas is elevated with the left index finger, tightening the scrotal skin over the vas (Fig. 34–2). **A sharp-pointed, curved mosquito hemostat (Fig. 34–3) (introduced through the same needle puncture hole used for anesthesia) punctures the scrotal skin, vas sheath, and vas wall with one blade of the clamp** (Fig. 34–4).

In an alternative method, particularly if the scrotum is thick or tight, after mobilization and anesthetization of the vas, the skin is punctured first with the sharp, curved hemostat and spread until the vertical slitlike opening is just large enough to introduce the ringed clamp. The ringed clamp is introduced into the opening, the vas is grasped and brought up to the opening, and the surgeon proceeds as described before.

At this point, the surrounding layers are stripped, thus exposing the bare vas. This may be accomplished by using the blades of the sharp hemostat, spreading all layers until the bare vas can be visualized. By using the right blade of the hemostat, the vas wall is skewered from inside the lumen out at a 45-degree angle and the dissecting clamp is rotated laterally 180 degrees. Alternatively, a scalpel can be used to incise the vasal fascia. **The vas is delivered through the**

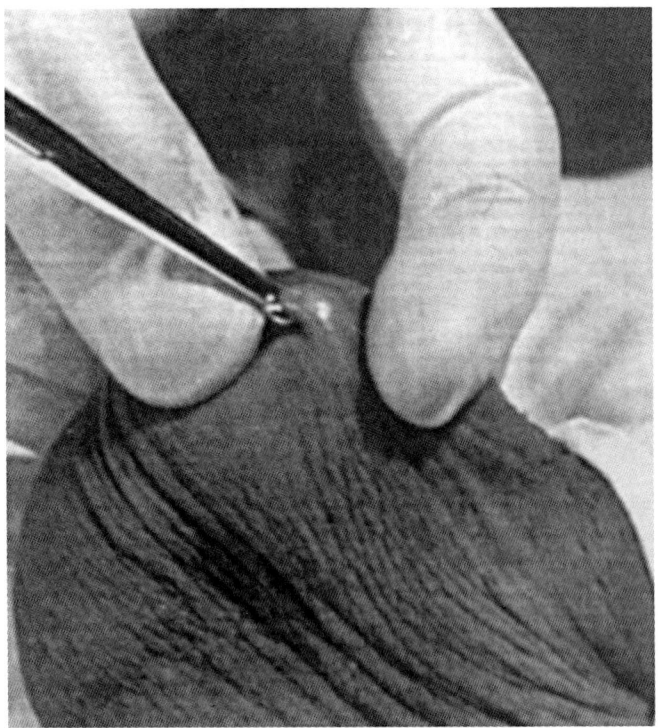

Figure 34–2. Vas fixed in the ring clamp. The scrotal skin is tightly stretched over the most prominent portion of the vas. (From Li S, Goldstein M, Zhu J, Huber D: The no-scalpel vasectomy. J Urol 1991;145:341-344.)

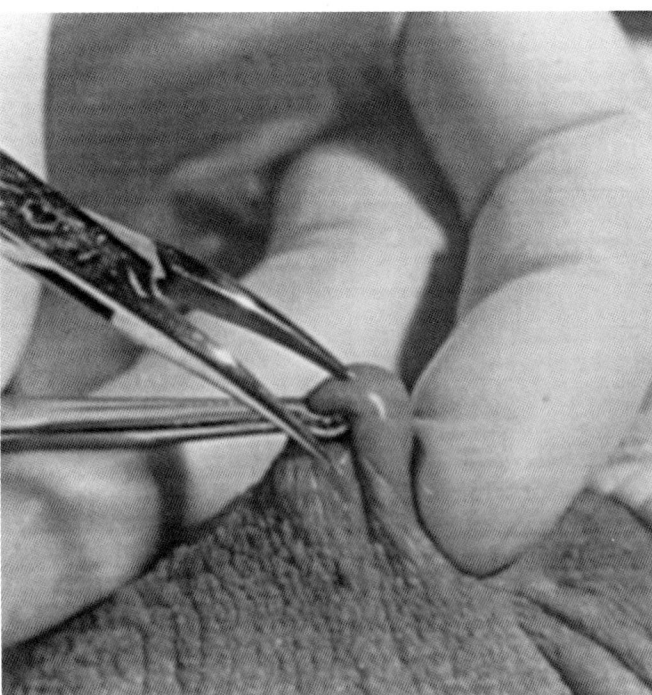

Figure 34–4. Puncture of the skin, vas sheath, and wall into the lumen. (From Li S, Goldstein M, Zhu J, Huber D: The no-scalpel vasectomy. J Urol 1991;145:341-344.)

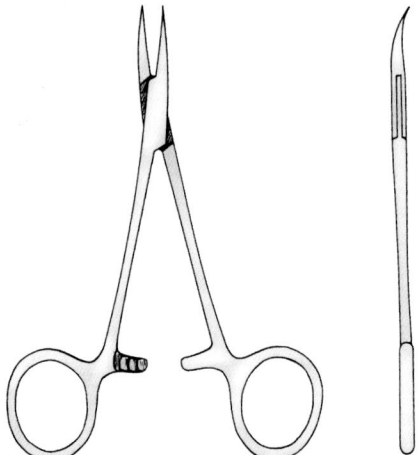

Figure 34–3. Sharp, curved mosquito hemostat. (From Li S, Goldstein M, Zhu J, Huber D: The no-scalpel vasectomy. J Urol 1991;145:341-344.)

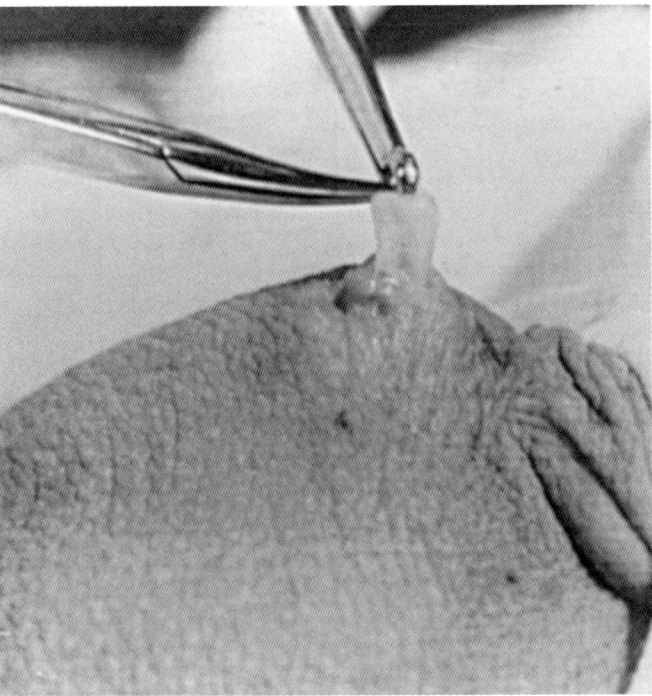

Figure 34–5. Delivery of the clean vas. (From Li S, Goldstein M, Huber D: The no-scalpel vasectomy. J Urol 1991;145:341-344.)

puncture hole while the ringed fixation clamp is released (Fig 34–5). **The ring clamp is used to secure the delivered vas.** The sharp hemostat is used to clean the vasal vessels away from the vas, yielding a clean segment at least 2 cm in length (Fig 34–6).

The vas is then divided, and occlusion is effected by one of the techniques described later in this section. **Many authors advocate closing the fascia over one end of the cut vas (fascial interposition) to reduce the likelihood of recanalization** (Sokal et al, 2004a, 2004b).

After checking for bleeding, the authors use a small hemostat to tag the vasal ends to inspect for any bleeding before

returning the vas to the scrotum. The contralateral vas is then approached in an identical fashion. **After both vasa are returned to the scrotum, the puncture hole is pinched for a minute and inspected for bleeding.** The puncture hole contracts and is virtually invisible. Antibiotic ointment is applied

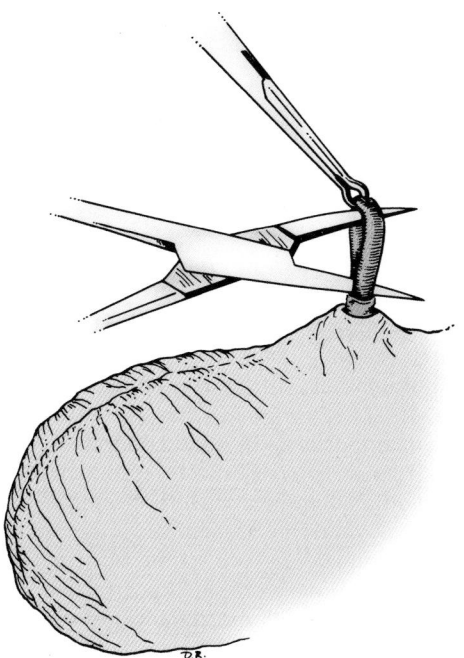

Figure 34–6. Segment cleaned. (From Li S, Goldstein M, Zhu J, Huber D: The no-scalpel vasectomy. J Urol 1991;145:341-344.)

to the site, and sterile fluff dressings are held in place with a snug-fitting athletic supporter.

Most urologists insist on removal of a segment of vas for pathologic verification, primarily for medicolegal reasons. Even from the legal point of view, a pathologist's report confirming the presence of vas in the vasectomy specimen offers little or no protection from litigation. **Documented counseling, diligent follow-up to obtain at least one azoospermic semen specimen postoperatively, and careful selection of appropriate candidates for vasectomy in the first place provide the best protection from malpractice suits.**

Studies in the United States and China (Li et al, 1991) as well as a large controlled study carried out in Thailand (Nirapathpongporn et al, 1990) comparing no-scalpel with conventional vasectomy have clearly shown that the no-scalpel technique results in a significantly reduced incidence of hematoma, infection, and pain. In addition, the no-scalpel vasectomy is performed in about 40% less time. Although this method of vasectomy appears deceptively simple, it is more difficult to learn than conventional vasectomy and requires intensive hands-on training. Its use, however, may enhance the popularity of vasectomy and make it a more significant part of the urologist's practice.

Percutaneous Vasectomy

The Chinese have performed more than 500,000 truly percutaneous vasectomies (and an equal number of vasographies) by chemical occlusion with a combination of cyanoacrylate and phenol (Ban, 1980; Li, 1980; Tao, 1980). After fixation of the vas with the same ring clamp described earlier, the scrotal skin and vas wall are punctured with a 22-gauge needle and the lumen is cannulated with a 24-gauge blunt needle. The needle's position within the vas lumen is confirmed by a series of ingenious tests, with final confirmation obtained by injec-

tion of Congo red into the abdominal side of the right vas deferens and methylene blue into the left vas. Injection of 20 μL of two parts phenol mixed with one part N-butyl-2-cyanoacrylate mixture through the 24-gauge blunt-tipped needle occludes the lumen. The patient voids at the termination of the procedure. Excretion of red urine means the left side was missed, and blue urine means the right side was missed; brown urine means both sides were successfully cannulated. Pharmacologic tests of the cyanoacrylate-phenol mixture in China have demonstrated no toxicity or carcinogenesis. However, these chemicals are not approved by the U.S. Food and Drug Administration for use in the United States. Furthermore, gaining percutaneous access to the 300-μm-diameter lumen of the vas is a feat requiring great skill and considerable training.

High-frequency ultrasonography has been used for percutaneous vasectomy (Roberts et al, 2002a) and epididymal occlusion (Roberts et al, 2002b) in dogs. Occlusion is unreliable, and skin burns are problematic. To date, it does not appear that this will be a feasible method of vasectomy.

Methods of Vasal Occlusion and Vasectomy Failure (Table 34–2)

The technique employed for occlusion of the vasal lumens determines the incidence of recanalization. Suture ligature, still the most common method employed worldwide, may result in necrosis and sloughing of the cut end distal to the ligature. If this occurs on the testicular end of the cut vas, a sperm granuloma will result. If both ends slough, recanalization is more likely to occur. The incidence of vasectomy failure ranges from 1% to 5% when ligatures alone are used for occlusion.

When the vasa are sealed with two medium hemoclips on each end, failure rates are reduced to less than 1% (Moss, 1974; Bennett, 1976). The wider diameter of hemoclips compared with sutures more evenly distributes pressure on the vasal wall, resulting in less necrosis and sloughing.

Intraluminal occlusion with needle electrocautery, or battery-driven thermal cautery set at a power sufficient to destroy mucosa but not high enough to cause transmural destruction of the vas, reduces recanalization rates to less than 0.5% (Schmidt, 1987; Barone et al, 2004). At least 1 cm of lumen should be cauterized in each direction. Thermal wires should be rotated to cauterize the entire mucosal surface.

Interposition of fascia between the cut ends, folding back of the vasal ends, and securing one end within the dartos muscle are techniques that have been advocated with the intent of reducing vasectomy failure rates (Esho and Cass, 1978; Sokal et al, 2004b).

Open-Ended Vasectomy

Since the late 1960s, attempts have been made to develop reversible methods of vasectomy. Most of these efforts focused on the use of mechanical valves that could be opened and closed. Unfortunately, these attempts have not been successful because of the damage to the epididymis that occurs after long-term obstruction.

There is some evidence that leakage of sperm at the vasectomy site prevents this pressure-induced damage and may increase the chances of successful reversal when accurate microsurgical vasovasostomy is performed (Silber, 1977). **If the testicular end of the vas deferens is not sealed (open-ended technique), a sperm granuloma forms at the vasectomy site and damage to the epididymis is reduced.** Early experience with this technique resulted in an unacceptably high incidence of vasectomy failure, varying from 7% to 50% (Shapiro and Silber, 1979; Goldstein, 1983). Better methods of sealing and burying the abdominal end of the vas reduce the failure rate of open-ended vasectomy to about 4%. This is still a substantially higher incidence of failure than that obtained with the closed occlusion techniques described earlier. **Because recanalization after vasectomy is invariably associated with sperm granuloma formation, it is likely that open-ended vasectomy will always be associated with higher failure rates** unless extraordinary efforts are made to widely separate the vasal ends or very long lengths of vas are destroyed on the seminal vesicle side. These measures, however, would either unduly complicate the performance of vasectomy or, paradoxically, make it less reversible.

Postoperative Semen Analysis

No technique of vasal occlusion, short of removing the entire scrotal vas, is 100% effective (Maatman et al, 1997). **There is no absolute standard of care when it comes to declaring a patient sterile.** Follow-up semen analysis at least 2 to 3 months after vasectomy, with the goal of obtaining at least one and preferably two absolutely azoospermic specimens 4 to 6 weeks apart, is recommended (Barone et al, 2003). However, it is rare that a patient will return for further semen analyses once he has become azoospermic (Belker et al, 1990). **If any motile sperm are found in the ejaculate 3 months after vasectomy, the procedure should be repeated.** If rare non-motile sperm are found, contraception may be cautiously discontinued; recent evidence demonstrates that these men will ultimately become azoospermic (Aradhya et al, 2005). Rare complete sperm in a spun semen analysis pellet are found in 10% of semen specimens at a mean of 10 years after vasectomy (Lemack and Goldstein, 1996).

Complications

Hematoma and Infection. Hematoma is the most common complication of vasectomy, with an average incidence of 2% (range, 0.09% to 29%) (Kendrick et al, 1987). Infection is relatively uncommon with the no-scalpel technique, although older series report rates from 12% to 38% (Appell and Evans, 1980; Randall et al, 1983, 1985). **The experience of the vasectomist is the single most important factor relating to complications** (Kendrick et al, 1987). The hematoma rate was significantly higher among physicians performing 1 to 10 vasectomies (4.6%) than among those performing 11 to 50 vasectomies (2.4%) or more than 50 vasectomies (1.6%) per year. A similar relationship was seen for hospitalization rate.

Sperm Granuloma. Sperm granulomas form when sperm leak from the testicular end of the vas. Sperm are highly antigenic, and an intense inflammatory reaction occurs when sperm escape outside the reproductive epithelium. Sperm granulomas are rarely symptomatic. The presence or absence of a sperm granuloma at the vasectomy site seems to be of importance in modulating the local effects of chronic obstruction on the male reproductive tract. The sperm granuloma's complex network of epithelialized channels provides an additional absorptive surface that helps vent the high intraluminal pressure in the obstructed excurrent ducts. Numerous animal studies have correlated the presence or absence of sperm granuloma at the vasectomy site with the degree of epididymal and testicular damage. Species that always develop granulomas after vasectomy have minimal damage to the seminiferous tubules. Some studies of men undergoing vasectomy reversal have revealed somewhat higher success rates in men who have a sperm granuloma at the vasectomy site (Silber, 1977), whereas another large study has not (Belker et al, 1991).

Although sperm granulomas at the vasectomy site are present microscopically in 10% to 30% of men undergoing reversal, it is likely, given enough time, that virtually all men develop sperm granulomas at the vasectomy site, the epididymis, or the rete testis.

Long-term Effects

Long-term effects of vasectomy in humans include vasitis nodosa, chronic testicular or epididymal pain, alterations in testicular function, chronic epididymal obstruction, postulated systemic effects of vasectomy, and, possibly, increased incidence of prostate cancer (Choe and Kirkemo, 1996). Although vasitis nodosa has been reported in up to 66% of vasectomy specimens in men undergoing vasectomy reversal (Freund et al, 1989), this entity does not appear to be associated with pain or significant medical sequelae.

In humans, **micropuncture studies have revealed that the markedly increased pressures that occur on the testicular side of the vas as well as in the epididymis after vasectomy are not transmitted to the seminiferous tubules** (Johnson and Howards, 1975). Therefore, little disruption of spermatogenesis is expected in humans. Biopsies up to 15 years after vasectomy show the testes to be essentially normal by light microscopy. Electron microscopic studies, however, have revealed thickening of the basal lamina and scattered areas of disrupted spermatogenesis in portions of the biopsy specimens (Jarow et al, 1985). Chronic orchialgia or epididymal pain after vasectomy occurs in perhaps 1 in 1000 patients (McConaghy et al, 1996). In some cases, vasectomy reversal or, alternatively, an open-ended vasectomy as described previously might be considered. The brunt of pressure-induced damage after vasectomy falls on the epididymis and efferent ductules. These structures become markedly distended and then adapt to reabsorb large volumes of testicular fluid and sperm products. When pain and tenderness are localized in the epididymis, total epididymectomy relieves pain in 95% of men (Selikowitz and Schned, 1985) (see "Epididymectomy").

Systemic effects of vasectomy have been postulated. **Vasectomy disrupts the blood-testis barrier, resulting in detectable levels of serum antisperm antibodies in 60% to 80% of men** (Lepow and Crozier, 1979; Fuchs and Alexander, 1983). Some studies suggest that the antibody titers diminish 2 years or more after vasectomy. Others suggest that these antibody titers persist. However, neither circulating immune complexes nor deposits are increased after vasectomy in man (Witkin et al, 1982). **Studies in animals and man have failed to find any association between antisperm antibodies and immune complex–mediated diseases such as lupus erythematosus, scleroderma, rheumatoid arthritis, and myasthenia gravis** (Massey et al, 1984). Although one study in cynomolgus monkeys found more frequent and extensive atherosclerosis of the major vessels in previously vasectomized monkeys fed a high-cholesterol diet (Alexander and Clarkson, 1978), no evidence of excess cardiovascular disease (Walker et al, 1981a), illness requiring hospitalization (Walker et al, 1981b; Petitti et al, 1982), or biochemical alterations (Smith and Paulson, 1980) has been found in more than 15 reports (12 employing matched controls) examining thousands of men (Schuman et al, 1993).

Major among the controversies is the possible link between vasectomy and prostate cancer. Studies have found an increased risk of prostate cancer in men who had a vasectomy 20 years previously (Giovannucci et al, 1993a, 1993b). **However, two large-scale cohort studies evaluated men from a wide range of socioeconomic strata and did not find a link between vasectomy and prostate cancer.** Another study of vasectomy sequelae found no increased incidence of cancer or other diseases (Schuman et al, 1993). However, despite this evidence, many urologists have changed the way they practice and counsel vasectomized men to be screened earlier (Sandlow and Kreder, 1996).

The most likely explanation for the increased diagnosis of prostate cancer in vasectomized men is detection bias. Vasectomized men are more likely to visit a urologist and therefore are more likely to have cancer diagnosed earlier. Furthermore, men who choose to undergo vasectomy may be more likely to seek health care, increasing their opportunity for prostate cancer detection. **A multidisciplinary National Institutes of Health panel concluded that the epidemiologic associations between vasectomy and prostate cancer are weak. It recommended no change in clinical or public health practice and said that screening for prostate cancer should not be any different for vasectomized men** (Healy, 1993). Nevertheless, men seeking vasectomy should be informed of these and other related studies and counseled about the controversies.

Surgery of the Epididymis

Detailed knowledge of epididymal anatomy and physiology (presented in Chapter 2, "Anatomy of the Lower Urinary Tract and Male Genitalia," and Chapter 18, "Male Reproductive

KEY POINTS: VASECTOMY

■ Adequate counseling is the keystone to successful vasectomy.

■ No technique is 100% effective in rendering the patient sterile.

■ Open-ended vasectomy theoretically has a lower chance of post-vasectomy pain, but failure rates are potentially higher because of recanalization.

■ Long-term effects of vasectomy do not appear to be serious, although the true incidence of post-vasectomy pain is currently unknown.

Physiology") is essential before undertaking surgery of this delicate but important structure. **Because the corpus and cauda epididymis is a single tubule with a very small diameter, injury or occlusion of a tubule anywhere along its length will lead to total obstruction of outflow at that level.** For these reasons, **magnification, with loupes for macrodissection and with the operating microscope for anastomosis, for excision of epididymal cysts or spermatoceles is essential for performing all epididymal surgery.**

Fortunately, the epididymis is blessed with a rich blood supply derived from the testicular vessels superiorly and the deferential vessels inferiorly. **Because of the extensive interconnections between these branches, either the testicular or the deferential branches (but not both) to the epididymis may be divided without compromise of epididymal viability.** Conversely, because the epididymal branches of the testicular artery are medial to and separate from the main testicular artery and veins, surgical procedures may be performed on the epididymis without compromise of testicular blood supply.

Epididymectomy

Epididymectomy may be indicated in men with chronic infection or abscess of the epididymis unresponsive to antibiotic therapy. Men with AIDS may develop cytomegalovirus infection of the epididymis requiring epididymectomy (Randazzo et al, 1986). Chronic unremitting epididymal pain after vasectomy may be relieved by total epididymectomy (Selikowitz and Schned, 1985). All patients should be counseled preoperatively that the procedure may impair their fertility or, in the case of bilateral epididymectomy, render them sterile.

Surgical Technique. Through a vertical median raphe or transverse scrotal incision, the testis is delivered. The vas deferens is isolated at the junction of its straight and convoluted regions and doubly ligated and divided with the deferential vessels included. The convoluted vas is then dissected free of its attachments to the epididymal tunica and traced to the vasoepididymal junction (Fig. 34–7). The tunica vaginalis is opened, and dissection is continued in the plane between the epididymis and the testis (Fig. 34–8).

Use of loupes or an operating microscope (2.5×) and elevation of the epididymis with an encircling Penrose drain, with transillumination of the mesentery between the testis and the epididymis, allow better visualization of the epididymal blood supply. This maneuver prevents injury to the spermatic cord vessels, which are encountered at the junction of the middle and upper thirds of the testis, entering medial to the epididymis. In addition, the use of a Doppler microprobe helps identify the testicular blood supply. This can be helpful in the case of large epididymal masses, such as spermatoceles.

The efferent ducts, located superior to the testicular vascular pedicle, are ligated with an absorbable suture, and the epididymectomy specimen is removed. The edges of the tunica vaginalis along the base of the resected epididymis should be oversewn with a continuous absorbable suture for hemostasis. The dartos is loosely closed with absorbable sutures, and the skin is closed with an absorbable suture as well.

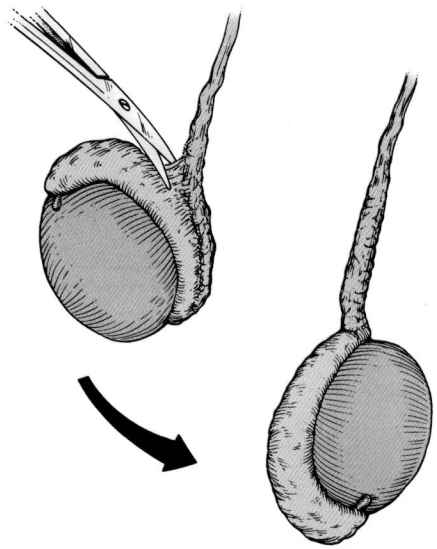

Figure 34–7. Convoluted vas dissected off the epididymal tunica.

Spermatocelectomy

A spermatocele is the epididymal equivalent of a berry aneurysm; it may occur anywhere in the epididymis but is more common in the caput region. It is exceedingly common, increasing in frequency with age, and identified incidentally in up to 30% of men undergoing high-resolution scrotal ultrasonography. **Intervention for spermatocele is rarely indicated. A spermatocele is usually painless and does not obstruct the epididymal tubule from which it arises. Resection of the spermatocele may cause epididymal obstruction.** Spermatocelectomy is indicated when the spermatocele is associated with unremitting pain or has grown to an uncomfortably large size. By definition, a spermatocele contains sperm. Puncture with a 30-gauge needle and identification of sperm in the aspirated fluid confirm the diagnosis.

Surgical Technique. The testis is delivered through a median raphe or transverse scrotal incision and the tunica vaginalis opened. The spermatocele is dissected free of the epididymis with use of the operating microscope to avoid inadvertent injury to epididymal tubules. The attachment of the spermatocele to the epididymis is ligated with 6-0 nylon or monofilament absorbable suture to prevent extravasation of sperm and granuloma formation. The tunica vaginalis is reapproximated with a continuous 5-0 Vicryl suture, and the dartos and the skin are closed in separate layers.

Complications and Adverse Effects of Spermatocelectomy. Complications are uncommon but may include bleeding, re-formation of spermatocele, testicular atrophy (secondary to vascular injury), and vasal or epididymal obstruction (Kiddoo et al, 2004; Zahalsky et al, 2004). Although complication rates may be as high as 20%, this is typically for the less serious events, such as infection or swelling. Use of a postoperative drain did not have an impact on outcome (Kiddoo et al, 2004).

Excision of spermatoceles can cause epididymal obstruction; one study reported epididymis in the surgical specimen in 17% of patients (Zahalsky et al, 2004). **Thus, all patients should be counseled about this possibility and, if necessary, offered either delayed repair or sperm cryopreservation (in the case of bilateral lesions).**

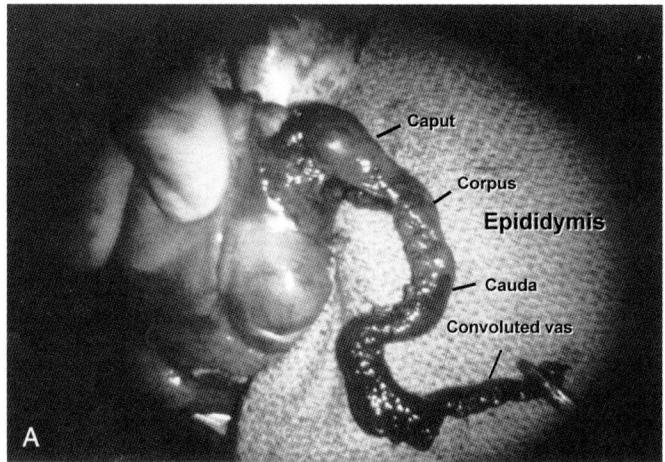

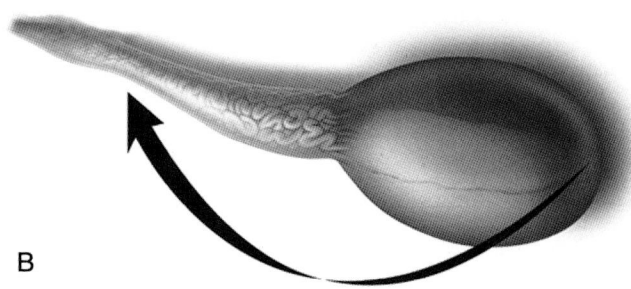

Figure 34–8. **A** and **B,** Entire vasoepididymal complex is dissected to the caput.

Excision of Epididymal Tumors and Cysts

Most nontransilluminable epididymal masses are benign adenomatoid tumors. Malignant epididymal tumors are exceedingly rare. As with any potentially malignant testicular mass, they should be managed by inguinal exploration, clamping of the cord, and delivery of the testis. If malignancy of the mass is uncertain, the field should be isolated and cooled with slush ice before the tunica vaginalis is opened for direct inspection and biopsy. This modification of Chevassu's maneuver is particularly useful for exploration of epididymal tumors, which are usually benign, and prevents needless orchiectomy (Goldstein and Waterhouse, 1983). If malignant neoplasia has been excluded, the epididymal tumor or cyst is excised in a fashion identical to that employed for a spermatocele.

Hydrocelectomy

Inguinal Approach. High-resolution scrotal ultrasonography should be performed in all men with hydrocele. An inguinal approach to hydrocelectomy is indicated when sonography or palpation suggests an intratesticular mass. The surgical approach is identical to that employed for radical orchiectomy. A modification of the Chevassu maneuver is employed (Goldstein and Waterhouse, 1983). The cord is doubly occluded with rubber-shod clamps, the hydrocele is delivered, and the gubernaculum is ligated and divided before the sac is opened. The field is isolated and the testis cooled with slush ice after the sac is opened. This technique allows inspection of the testis and epididymis and biopsy of suspicious areas without compromising a good cancer operation (Hopps and Goldstein, 2002). If no malignant disease is found, needless orchiectomy is avoided. Hydrocelectomy is then performed by one of the techniques described later in this section.

Scrotal Approach. Scrotal hydrocelectomy may be safely performed when ultrasonographic examination of the testis is normal. Under these circumstances, either a transverse incision within the scrotal folds and between the scrotal vessels or a median raphe incision results in minimal bleeding and a virtually invisible postoperative scar.

Methods of Repair. If surgical repair is employed, the hydrocele sac is exposed, dissected, and delivered intact. It is opened in an avascular area anteriorly, away from the testis, epididymis, vas deferens, and cord structures. If indicated, samples of hydrocele fluid are collected for cultures and cytologic studies. **Large hydroceles can severely distort the normal anatomic relationships.** The internal spermatic vessels and vas deferens are encircled with Penrose drains for positive identification and their courses traced to avoid injury to these structures. The opening in the sac is enlarged with a Bovie cautery in a direction away from the testis, epididymis, vessels, and vas. The testis and epididymis are inspected for masses, evidence of epididymitis, or dilated epididymal tubules suggestive of obstruction. The margins of the epididymis may be difficult to clearly identify. In large longstanding hydroceles, the epididymis may be splayed out far from the testis. The convoluted portion of the vas deferens may be distorted and splayed out within the layers of the hydrocele sac. **Magnification with loupes or an operating**

microscope is sometimes useful in positively identifying the margins of the epididymis.

After all the key structures within and adjacent to the hydrocele sac are inspected and identified, repair is accomplished by one of the techniques described next.

Excisional Techniques. **Excisional techniques are most certain to result in permanent elimination of the hydrocele.** Excision is performed for long-standing hydroceles with thick-walled sacs and for multiloculated hydroceles. After simple excision of the hydrocele sac, leaving a one-finger-breadth margin to avoid injury to the epididymis, the edges are oversewn with a 4-0 chromic catgut baseball stitch (Fig. 34–9). When large, thin, floppy sacs are excised, the Jaboulay (1902) bottleneck operation, in which the sac edges are sewn together behind the cord (Fig. 34–10), reduces the chance of recurrence caused by reapposition of the edges of the hydrocele sac. When the bottleneck operation is employed, the sac margins should be left 1 cm wider to prevent constriction of the cord. If necessary, a Penrose drain is brought out through the dependent portion of the hemiscrotum and fixed in place with a 2-0 silk suture and safety pin. The dartos is closed with a continuous absorbable suture, and the skin is closed with a subcuticular absorbable suture. Fluff dressings are stuffed inside a snug-fitting scrotal supporter.

Plication Techniques. **Plication operations (Lord, 1964) can be employed for thin sacs but are not suitable for multiloculated hydroceles or long-standing thick-walled hydroceles because plication will leave a large bundle of residual tissue within the scrotum.** Because the sac is not dissected, plication is quick and relatively bloodless.

The sac is opened and the cut edges are cauterized or oversewn for hemostasis. The testis is delivered, and the sac is

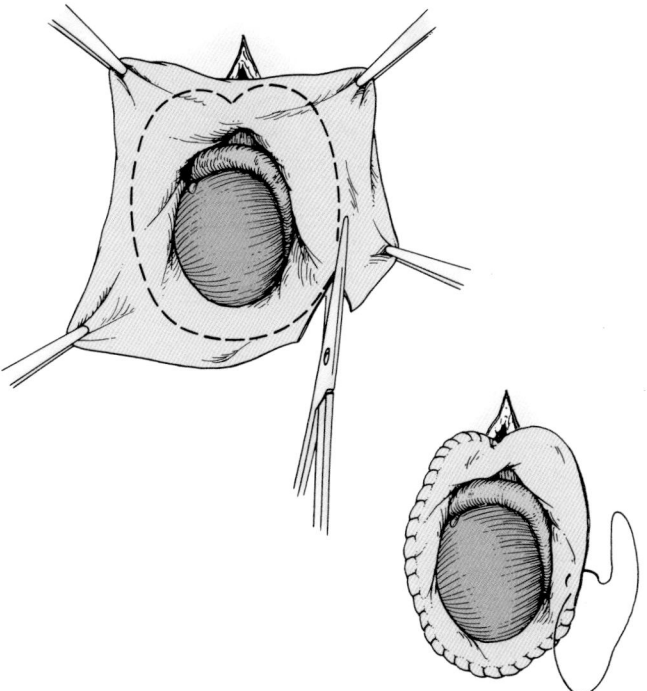

Figure 34–9. Simple excision of the thick-walled hydrocele sac and oversewn edges.

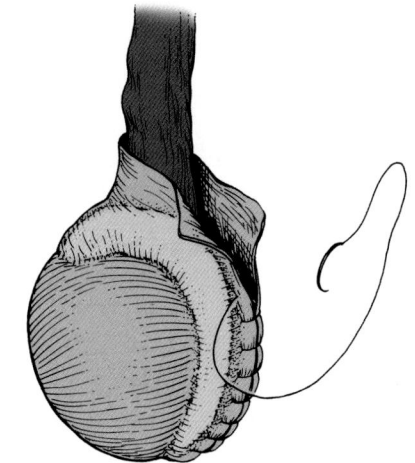

Figure 34–10. Jaboulay's bottleneck technique for excision of thin, floppy sacs.

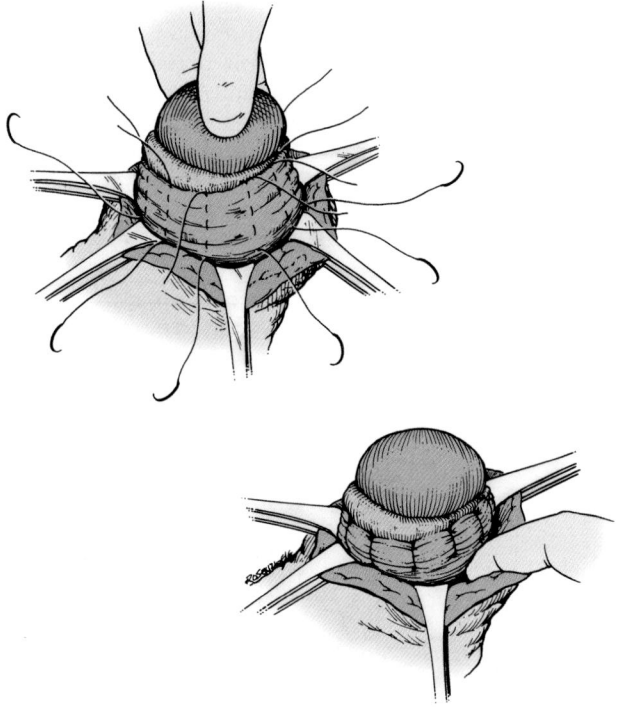

Figure 34–11. Lord's plication technique.

inverted. Beginning one fingerbreadth away from the testis and epididymis, 8 to 12 catgut sutures are placed radially to plicate the sac (Fig. 34–11). Drains are not necessary. Closure is performed as described earlier.

Sclerotherapy. Sclerotherapy has also been used with some success in the treatment of hydrocele. Several different techniques and sclerosants have been used with varying success. The steps common to most of these are aspiration of the hydrocele fluid and instillation of local anesthesia, followed by instillation of the sclerosant for a time. Some authors drain the sclerosant; others allow it to be reabsorbed. Sclerotherapy with tetracycline derivatives or other irritating agents, such as 95% alcohol, may result in epididymal obstruction (Nash,

1980; Osegbe, 1991; Ross and Flom, 1991). It can be associated with substantial postoperative pain, and recurrence is not uncommon (Thomson and Odell, 1979; Osegbe, 1991). When a hydrocele recurs after sclerotherapy, it is usually multiloculated and more difficult to repair. **Sclerotherapy is most useful in older men in whom fertility is no longer an issue** (Sigurdsson et al, 1994).

Complications. Hematoma is the most common complication of hydrocelectomy. When excision techniques are employed, the incidence of hematoma can be minimized by meticulously oversewing all raw edges of the sac and draining the scrotum when necessary (Kiddoo et al, 2004). The use of a drain does not appear to change the incidence of complications, although use of a drain may be judicious in select patients.

In men desiring future fertility, the primary dangers associated with hydrocelectomy operations are injury to the epididymis or the vas deferens (Zahalsky et al, 2004). In some large hydroceles, the anatomy can be extremely distorted. The epididymis may not be identifiable. The vas deferens, especially in its convoluted portion, may be splayed out within the hydrocele layers. Regardless of the approach to hydrocelectomy, the vas deferens and the epididymis should be positively identified to avoid injury to these structures. The internal spermatic vessels should also be positively identified and encircled with a Penrose drain to prevent injury during excision of the hydrocele sac.

KEY POINTS: SCROTAL SURGERY

- Indications for surgery of the epididymis and hydrocele vary, but men of reproductive age should be approached with caution.

- Preoperative imaging with scrotal ultrasonography is almost always indicated.

- Hematoma is the most common complication in scrotal surgery, and extra precautions should be taken to avoid this.

Orchiopexy in Adults

An undescended testis sometimes escapes detection until adulthood. If the contralateral testis is normal, these men are likely to be fertile. If both testes are truly undescended, infertility is very likely, with most of the patients being azoospermic (Hadziselimovic, 2002). In the past, bilateral orchiectomy was often recommended in adults with undescended testes because of the substantially increased risk of testis tumors (Martin and Menck, 1975). Orchiectomy, however, condemns these men to absolute sterility and a lifetime of hormone replacement therapy. **Bilateral orchiopexy in adults can result in induction of spermatogenesis and pregnancy** (Shin et al, 1997). It also preserves testicular hormonal function.

The technique of orchiopexy in adults is identical to that employed for children. Even with a normal contralateral testis, orchiopexy is worthwhile to bring down a unilateral undescended testis to a scrotal location, if possible, where it can be examined. Leydig cell function in the undescended testis can be retained. Even a solitary cryptorchid testis, when it is properly placed in the scrotum, can provide enough testosterone to obviate the need for hormone replacement. Although the goal of orchiopexy in adults is to achieve a scrotal testis, an inguinal or subcutaneous location that permits examination is acceptable. When orchiopexy is performed in adults, regular self-examination is mandatory and yearly sonography may be considered. When fertility is no longer an issue, some authors recommend orchiectomy. In the past, the maximal age at which orchiectomy was performed, compared with observation, was typically 32 years (Farrer et al, 1985). However, with improvements in the outcome of patients with testicular cancer as well as a decline in perioperative mortality, the current recommendation is now 50 years of age (Oh, 2002).

Retractile Testes in Adults

Retractile testes in boys are usually not surgically repaired if the testes can be manually manipulated to stay down into the scrotum either in the office or under anesthesia. **The fate of persistently retractile testes in adults is unknown.** A subset of men with retractile testes will be infertile (Caucci et al, 1997). The semen analyses of these men often demonstrate a typical stress pattern similar to that of men with varicoceles. These men, however, do not have palpable varicoceles. They all have at least one testis that retracts out of the scrotum and into the abdomen and remains there for an hour or more a day, and frequently both testes do. In some men, these testes remain in the abdomen virtually all the time, except in a warm shower or under anesthesia. It is likely that these testes will suffer from impaired temperature regulation and impaired spermatogenesis. Scrotal orchiopexy can improve the semen quality and fertility of some of these men.

When scrotal orchiopexy is performed for retractile testis, a dartos pouch operation should be performed. Simple suture orchiopexy of the tunica albuginea of the testis to the dartos, such as is performed sometimes to prevent torsion, will not prevent retraction of these testes into the groin. Construction of a dartos pouch will keep the testis well down into the scrotum and permanently prevent retraction. This is also the most reliable and safest technique for the prevention of testicular torsion (Redman and Barthold, 1995).

Orchiopexy for Intermittent Torsion

Men with chronic intermittent torsion have a history of episodes of sudden onset of testicular pain, as in acute testicular torsion. The pain is often associated with nausea. They may also observe that the testis is elevated and transverse-lying with a variable degree of scrotal enlargement from edema. However, the pain with intermittent torsion spontaneously disappears after a few minutes to a few hours. In men with a recurrent history of this type of pain, scrotal orchiopexy as described earlier is usually curative. Prophylactic orchiopexy of the contralateral testis is recommended at the same sitting.

Torsion is uncommon in adults. A history of sudden-onset intermittent testicular pain often accompanied by nausea is suggestive of torsion. A high transverse-lying testis associated with these symptoms supports the diagnosis. The differential diagnoses include epididymitis and testis tumor. A scrotal sonogram with color Doppler and/or radionuclide scintigraphy can accurately confirm the diagnosis. Orchiopexy should be done bilaterally. A two- or three-stitch (nonabsorbable) orchiopexy under direct vision is recommended. Care is taken to avoid injury to or ligation of subtunical vessels. Alternatively, a dartos pouch orchiopexy, although more difficult to perform, is a highly effective approach that eliminates the need to place sutures in the tunica albuginea.

Chronic Orchialgia

Chronic orchialgia is defined as intermittent or constant scrotal pain, which may be unilateral, bilateral, or bilaterally alternating, lasting longer than 3 months (Davis et al, 1990; Costabile et al, 1991). Chronic testicular pain has a variety of potential causes. **All men with chronic orchialgia should have a high-resolution scrotal ultrasound examination with color flow Doppler study** to completely evaluate the scrotal contents and to rule out any underlying pathologic process, such as a testicular tumor. Successful treatment requires identification of the cause so that specific therapy can be instituted.

Chronic Epididymitis

A persistently tender, indurated epididymis, especially one associated with a positive semen or urine culture after adequate cleaning of the genital skin, suggests chronic epididymitis. Therapy should be instituted with specific antibiotics according to the results of the cultures. Sitz baths and nonsteroidal anti-inflammatory agents should also be prescribed. **Diagnostic epididymal puncture should never be performed in men desiring fertility because of the high risk of epididymal obstruction.**

Recurrent urinary tract infections, especially if they are associated with urethral strictures, may cause infected urine to reflux up the ejaculatory ducts and result in epididymitis. Treatment of the stricture and appropriate antibiotics are indicated.

For chronic epididymitis unresponsive to conservative measures such as antibiotics, anti-inflammatory agents, and sitz baths, total epididymectomy, as described earlier, is curative and appropriate, especially for men in whom fertility is no longer an issue.

Varicocele

Large varicoceles can cause a persistent, aching discomfort often described by patients as a heavy sensation or a sensation of increased heat in the scrotum. This is almost always relieved when patients are in the supine position because the varicocele will collapse. **Patients presenting with typical varicocele pain along with a clearly palpable large varicocele that collapses in the supine position will usually respond to microsurgical varicocelectomy** (Peterson et al, 1998). Small varicoceles rarely cause significant discomfort and therefore are typically not a cause of chronic orchialgia. A trial of nonsteroidal anti-inflammatories, with subsequent decrease or disappearance of discomfort, may provide reassurance that surgical repair will alleviate the pain.

Post–Hernia Repair Orchialgia

Chronic testicular pain after hernia repair may be associated with nerve entrapment injuries (Starling et al, 1987). These usually resolve with conservative therapy. If they do not, inguinal exploration and removal of any non-absorbable suture materials may result in relief. Mesh repairs can result in nerve entrapment either from the mesh itself (Uzzo et al, 1999) or from the sutures used to sew the mesh in. Sewing the mesh in with absorbable sutures, which will eventually dissolve, reduces the likelihood of post–hernia repair discomfort.

Post-Vasectomy Pain Syndrome

Post-vasectomy chronic orchialgia is disappointingly common and difficult to treat (McConaghy et al, 1996; Christiansen and Sandlow, 2003). Although early pain lasting a few weeks is fairly common after vasectomy (present in up to 30% of men), **long-term pain requiring some kind of interventional or surgical therapy probably occurs in approximately 1 in 1000 vasectomized men.** Causes of post-vasectomy pain syndrome are chronic congestive epididymitis and sperm granuloma.

Chronic Congestive Epididymitis. After vasectomy, testicular sperm and fluid continue to be produced at nearly the same rate as before vasectomy. The brunt of the pressure buildup after vasectomy is borne by the epididymis, which becomes markedly distended. Although most men are completely asymptomatic from this distention, some men develop chronic, dull, aching pain occasionally exacerbated by ejaculation. For these men, a conservative course of therapy, including nonsteroidal anti-inflammatory agents and sitz baths, should be instituted for a minimum of 3 months. If there is still no relief, spermatic cord blocks or the employment of local intralesional steroids by a pain management specialist can offer relief. **If none of these methods alleviates the pain, either vasectomy reversal or a total epididymectomy is indicated.** Because most of these pain syndromes present within only a few months or years after vasectomy, most of these men will require only a vasovasostomy, which, in experienced hands, has up to a 99% patency rate and more than a 70% chance of relieving the pain. The disadvantage of this is that the patient will then require other forms of contraception (Nangia et al, 2000). Another alternative is open-ended vasectomy, although this may lead to other complications, such as recanalization, symptomatic sperm granulomas, and late scarring with return of pain.

Epididymectomy may be considered in severe cases (West et al, 2000). Obviously, epididymectomy renders the vasectomy completely irreversible, and the procedure may also jeopardize the blood supply of the testis, causing ischemic atrophy. The results of this invasive procedure for chronic epididymitis are not entirely satisfactory, however, because 30% to 90% of these patients have persistent scrotal pain (Padmore et al, 1996); some patients eventually proceed to removal of the ipsilateral testis. In addition, a significant proportion of these patients have histologically normal epididymides. **The etiology of chronic intrascrotal pain in these patients is uncertain.** This further highlights the importance of careful selection of patients and adequate preoperative counseling.

Sperm Granuloma. A sperm granuloma forms when sperm leak from the testicular end of the vas. Sperm are highly antigenic and normally not exposed to the body's immune system. Sperm have unique sperm surface antigens. **When the immune system sees sperm outside the normal protective lining of the male reproductive tract, an inflammatory reaction ensues.** The resulting sperm granuloma consists of multiple epithelialized channels filled with sperm and macrophages.

Sperm granulomas can grow up to 2 cm in diameter and can be tender to the touch (Schmidt, 1979). Most sperm granulomas will eventually decrease in size and are usually asymptomatic. The use of intraluminal cautery instead of ligatures during vasectomy can prevent sperm granulomas. Sperm granulomas are easily palpable on the testicular end of the vas after vasectomy. If they are exquisitely tender and palpation duplicates the pain that the patient feels, removal of the granuloma with intraluminal cautery of the vas will usually relieve the pain. **When chronic post-vasectomy pain is localized to the granuloma, excision and occlusion of the vasa with intraluminal cautery usually relieve the pain and prevent recurrence** (Schmidt, 1979). Conversely, men with post-vasectomy congestive epididymitis may be relieved of their pain by open-ended vasectomy designed to purposefully produce a pressure-relieving sperm granuloma. If the granuloma recurs, excision of the granuloma and microsurgical vasovasostomy with a leakproof anastomosis will permanently alleviate the pain.

Chronic Orchialgia of Undetermined Etiology

The underlying etiology of chronic orchialgia may not always be obvious. Lower urinary tract symptoms, distal ureteral stone, occult hernia, irritable bowel syndrome, and referred pain are some of the possible causes of the symptoms. **Even when no specific cause can be found, conservative therapy, including nonsteroidal anti-inflammatory agents, sitz baths, and scrotal support for a period of 3 to 6 months, is indicated.**

Not infrequently, conservative management, including pharmacologic therapy, local anesthesia, and even psychological and behavioral therapy, may fail in these patients. Microsurgical total denervation of the spermatic cord is a measure with reported success in 80% of cases in several small series (Levine et al, 1996; Cadeddu et al, 1999). Denervation is performed by mobilization of the spermatic cord, as in varicocelectomy, with preservation of the vasal vessels, testicular artery, and one or two lymphatics while the rest of the cord is transected (Fig. 34–12). Some authors advocate preservation of the vas deferens as well (Cadeddu et al, 1999). However, if fertility is not an issue, it is recommended that the vas be divided to obliterate the sympathetic fibers that innervate the testis and may be responsible for some of the patient's symptoms (Levine et al, 1996). The goal of the procedure is to denervate the testis by transection of all the nerve fibers of the genitofemoral nerve. Under the operating microscope, spermatic nerves appear as 0.2- to 1-mm-diameter almost transparent structures that can be distinguished from lymphatics by characteristic transverse white striations.

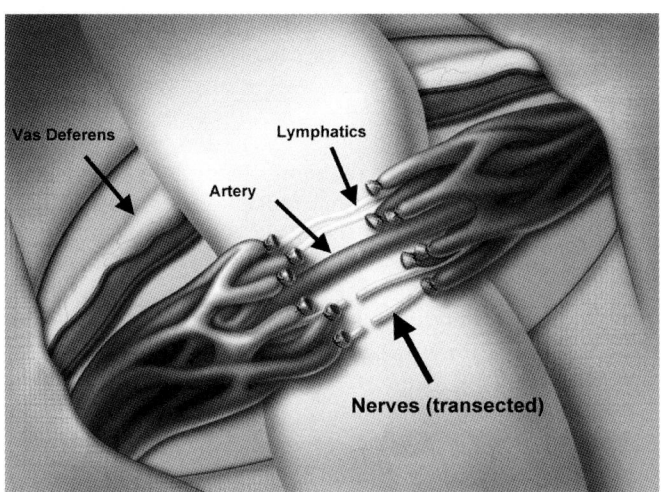

Figure 34–12. Microsurgical denervation. The goal is to transect all branches of the genitofemoral nerve while preserving the vas deferens, vasal vessels, testicular artery, and lymphatics.

KEY POINTS: TESTICULAR PAIN

- ■ Chronic testicular pain, regardless of etiology, is an indication for scrotal ultrasound examination.

- ■ Testicular pain caused by varicocele, epididymitis, and post–hernia repair nerve entrapment is typically treated successfully with directed therapy.

- ■ Chronic testicular pain of unknown etiology is less successfully treated. Multimodality therapy includes medical, psychological, and, if necessary, surgical treatment.

SEMINAL VESICLES

The seminal vesicles were first described by Fallopius in 1561 (Brewster, 1985) as paired male organs. Primary disease within the seminal vesicles is rare, but secondary lesions are more common. In the past, insufficient imaging methods led to infrequent definition of either primary or secondary seminal vesicle disease. The use of ultrasonography, computed tomography (CT), and magnetic resonance imaging (MRI) has improved diagnostic visibility and facilitated the diagnosis and treatment of seminal vesicle disease. The necessity of surgical intervention is rare but includes congenital cysts with infection or obstruction causing infertility, ureteral ectopy into a seminal vesicle with resultant obstruction or dysplasia of the ipsilateral kidney, and primary tumors, either benign or malignant. Surgical access to the seminal vesicles is mostly through routes familiar to the urologic surgeon, but surgery on the seminal vesicles alone (without adjacent organ removal) is a unique challenge.

Embryology

Normal Development. An understanding of the normal embryologic development of the seminal vesicles is necessary for the diagnosis and treatment of diseases involving these structures. The seminal vesicle, a strictly male organ (no female homolog), develops as a dorsolateral bulbous swelling of the distal mesonephric duct at approximately 12 fetal weeks (Arey, 1965; Brewster, 1985). Initially, the cloaca is subdivided by downward growth of the urorectal septum into the posterior anal canal and the anterior urogenital sinus (Fig. 34–13A). The division is completed around the seventh week. The mesonephric duct (wolffian duct) is thus included in an area called the vesicourethral canal within the urogenital sinus. The ureter is a bud originating from the mesonephric duct at 4 weeks that eventually attains a separate opening into the bladder by absorption and cranial migration (Fig. 34–13B). The mesonephric duct becomes the vas deferens, which normally drains into the urethra at the ejaculatory duct where it is surrounded by the prostatic glands. Separate symmetrical buds extend from the distal mesonephric duct just proximal to the ejaculatory duct at approximately 12 weeks to form the seminal vesicles (Fig. 34–13C).

Embryologic Abnormalities. Developmental anomalies form by alteration of this orderly process. If the ureteral bud arises too far cranially on the mesonephric duct, it will be absorbed late. This results in failure to meet the metanephric blastema, thus leading to renal dysplasia or agenesis and causing the ureter to enter ectopically anywhere along the vas deferens or posterior urethra (Tanagho, 1976; MacDonald, 1986). **Gordon and Kessler (1972) showed that 50% of ectopic ureters in males enter the posterior urethra, whereas 30% join the seminal vesicle. The remainder enter the vas deferens or the ejaculatory ducts.** Because formation of the seminal vesicles occurs at week 12 of embryogenesis, an alteration in ureteral bud development from the mesonephric duct may have an impact on formation of the seminal vesicles. There is an association between absence of the seminal vesicle and ipsilateral renal anomalies. This is discussed later.

Physiology

The physiologic role of the seminal vesicle is not entirely known; however, the secreted fluid is important in the motility and metabolism of ejaculated sperm. **The secretions from the seminal vesicle contribute approximately 50% to 80% of the ejaculate volume, with an average volume of 2.5 mL and a pH in the neutral to alkaline range.** Seminal vesicle secretions primarily contain carbohydrates such as fructose, a necessary component for sperm motility, and prostaglandins E, A, B, and F as well as a coagulation factor (Tauber et al, 1975, 1976). A 52-kD protein, semenogelin 1, has been identified. It is postulated that this is a sperm motility inhibitor and is cleaved by a proteolytic enzyme, prostate-specific antigen, after ejaculation (Robert and Gagnon, 1999).

Anatomy

General Description. The normal adult seminal vesicle is 5 to 10 cm in length and 3 to 5 cm in diameter. The volume capacity of the seminal vesicle averages 13 mL. The right gland is slightly larger than the left in one third of men, but the size of both decreases with advancing age (Redman, 1987). There are three major anatomic types; the most common type

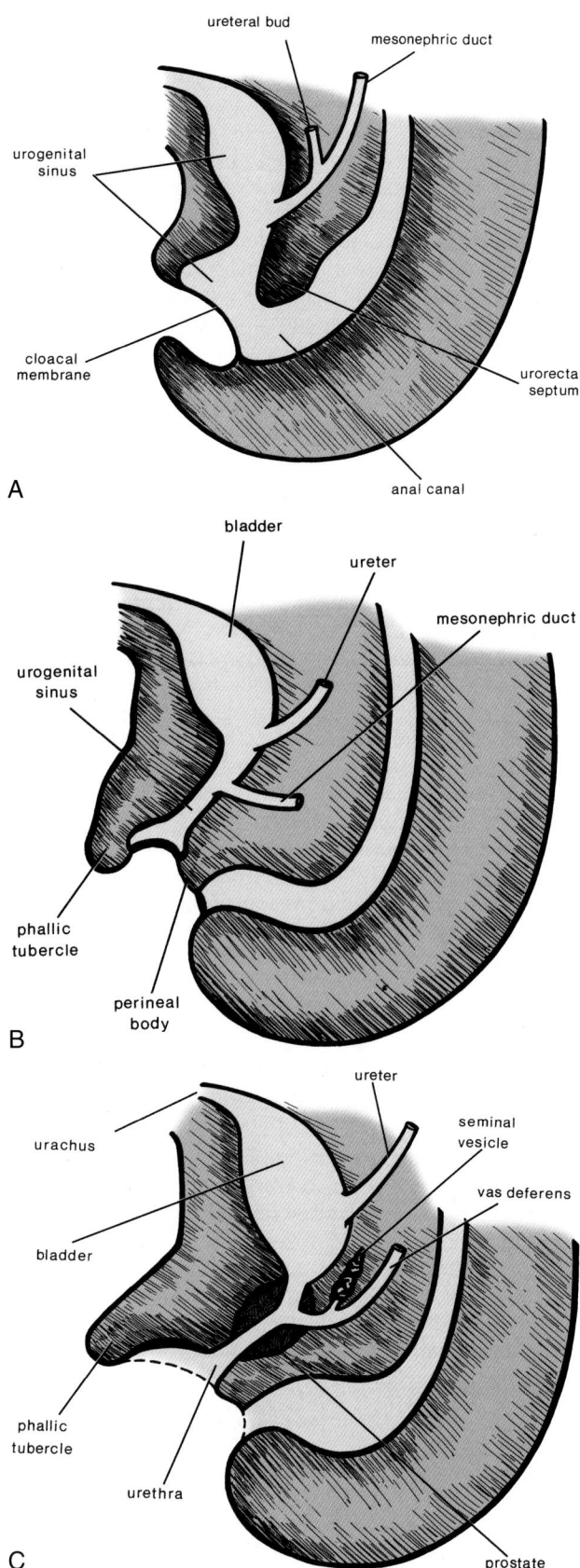

Figure 34–13. Intrauterine (fetal) development of the seminal vesicles. **A,** Fifth week. **B,** Eighth week. **C,** Thirteenth week. (Redrawn from Langman J: Medical Embryology, 4th ed. Baltimore, Williams & Wilkins, 1981:242-243.)

contains one central canal with minimal tortuosity and only a few side branches (Aboul-Azm, 1979). The major canal of the seminal vesicle empties into the ejaculatory duct (average length of 2.2 cm) at the terminal portion of the vas deferens within the prostate. On histologic evaluation, the ejaculatory ducts are a continuation of the seminal vesicles. However, the thick muscle wall of the seminal vesicle is not present within the ejaculatory duct. Normal ejaculatory duct luminal and wall dimensions are remarkably uniform among men. Statistically, a luminal diameter of more than 2.3 mm defines a dilated system (Nguyen et al, 1996).

Vasculature and Innervation. The blood supply to the seminal vesicle is from the vesiculodeferential artery, a branch of the umbilical artery (Braithwaite, 1952). On occasion, the inferior vesicle artery provides a communicating vessel. Venous drainage is from the vesiculodeferential veins and the inferior vesical plexus. The seminal vesicles are innervated by the pelvic nerve and the hypogastric nerve. The hypogastric nerve sends both adrenergic and cholinergic fibers to the seminal vesicles (Mawhinney and Tarry, 1991). Lymphatic drainage is through the internal iliac nodes.

Diagnosis

The diagnosis of seminal vesicle neoplasms can be difficult because they often do not cause symptoms until late in their course. General symptoms that may occur include urinary retention, dysuria, hematuria, and hematospermia. A mass is often palpable above the prostate and is usually not tender. Transrectal ultrasonography (TRUS) is usually the next step in diagnosis and may be accompanied by needle aspiration or biopsy for diagnosis. CT or MRI would then be appropriate to stage the tumor. Because prostate cancer may be mistaken for primary seminal vesicle cancer, serum prostate-specific antigen and prostatic acid phosphatase determinations as well as tissue immunohistochemical stains for both enzymes help define the prostate as the site of primary disease. Malignant neoplasms of the seminal vesicles and interestingly of the epididymis are exceedingly rare.

Physical Examination and Laboratory Testing

Physical diagnosis and vasography were once the only diagnostic tools available for studying the seminal vesicle. TRUS, CT, and MRI have each added substantially to examination and diagnosis of pathologic conditions of the seminal vesicle.

The normal seminal vesicle and adjacent ducts are not palpable in the normal male. On rectal examination, the area directly craniad to the base of the prostate where the seminal vesicles reside is soft and nondescript. The seminal vesicles lie anterior to the surrounding relatively thick and inelastic two layers of Denonvilliers' fascia, but no anatomic detail of the vesicles or ducts is usually appreciated by palpation even if the glands are asymmetrical. The area immediately above the prostate on rectal examination may be enlarged and relatively compressible in the presence of a seminal vesicle cyst or solid and firm if there is a seminal vesicle tumor. These lesions may compress the bladder base anteriorly instead and thus may not be readily palpable. Secondary involvement of the seminal vesicle from prostate or bladder disease is palpated as hard areas above the prostate but may not be absolutely definable on physical examination.

Laboratory examination of seminal vesicle fluid requires obtaining a semen sample and testing directly for exclusively seminal vesicle excretions, such as fructose, and indirectly by measuring the volume and observing liquefaction of the semen sample. **A low semen volume and a lack of both fructose and liquefaction imply either absent seminal vesicles or ejaculatory duct obstruction.** Although the terminal portion of the ejaculate originates from the seminal vesicles, split ejaculate bacterial culture specimens are more likely contaminated by multiple other sites along the lower urinary tract and thus are not useful for localizing the site of infection (Stamey, 1980). TRUS-guided perineal aspiration cultures and abscess drainage have been successful, however (Lee et al, 1986).

Ultrasonography

Ultrasonography, by either the transabdominal or the transrectal (preferred) route, has become one of the most accurate methods of evaluating the seminal vesicle. The advent of probes with high resolution at short focal lengths has allowed rapid, noninvasive, inexpensive, and accurate seminal vesicle examination in an outpatient setting.

The normal seminal vesicle on TRUS is an elongated, flat, paired structure between the rectum and the bladder just superior to the prostate (Fig. 34–14). The seminal vesicle appears predominantly symmetrical and is smooth with apparent saccularity. The center of the seminal vesicle is echopenic, with occasional areas of increased echogenicity relating to luminal folds within the vesicle itself (Carter et al, 1989). The ampulla of the vas can usually be seen, particularly near the prostate, as a tortuous tube on sagittal scans. The ejaculatory duct may also be seen within the substance of the prostate. The verumontanum is characteristically seen as a

more densely echoic structure in the midline at the termination of the ejaculatory ducts. Although sagittal images are best for examining the length of seminal vesicles and adjacent ductular anatomy, transaxial scans are best for detecting symmetry and volume. TRUS of the seminal vesicles does not require any special preparation, although a half-full bladder allows easier differentiation of the vesicles and adjacent structures.

Abnormal findings on TRUS include seminal vesicle aplasia, atrophy, obstruction, and cyst formation. Aplasia and atrophy are commonly associated with infertility in up to 2.5% of infertile men (Carter et al, 1989). TRUS-guided seminal vesiculography is a technique that couples ultrasonography with radiography to evaluate male factor infertility secondary to obstruction. Seminal vesiculography helps image the distal male reproductive tract (vas deferens, seminal vesicles, ejaculatory ducts) and has been found to be an improvement over standard vasography (Jones et al, 1997). Findings consistent with obstruction include anteroposterior diameter of more than 15 mm, length longer than 35 mm, and large anechoic areas containing sperm on aspiration (Jarow, 1996; Colpi et al, 1997).

Cysts, although rare, may be congenital and associated with an ipsilateral ectopic ureter or an aplastic kidney, or they may be acquired as a result of obstruction after transurethral prostatectomy. However, in one study, 5% of men screened for prostate cancer were found to have asymptomatic cystic dilation of the seminal vesicles (Wessels et al, 1992). The majority of patients with a seminal vesicle cyst are asymptomatic; however, they may present with urinary tract symptoms including dysuria, painful ejaculation, hematospermia, and recurrent epididymitis. Ultrasonography reveals these cystic lesions to be anechoic masses within the substance of the seminal vesicle or larger anechoic saccular lesions that might rise out of the pelvis and displace the bladder and other pelvic structures (Steers and Corriere, 1986). Ultrasonography can be used to guide needle placement for drainage or contrast

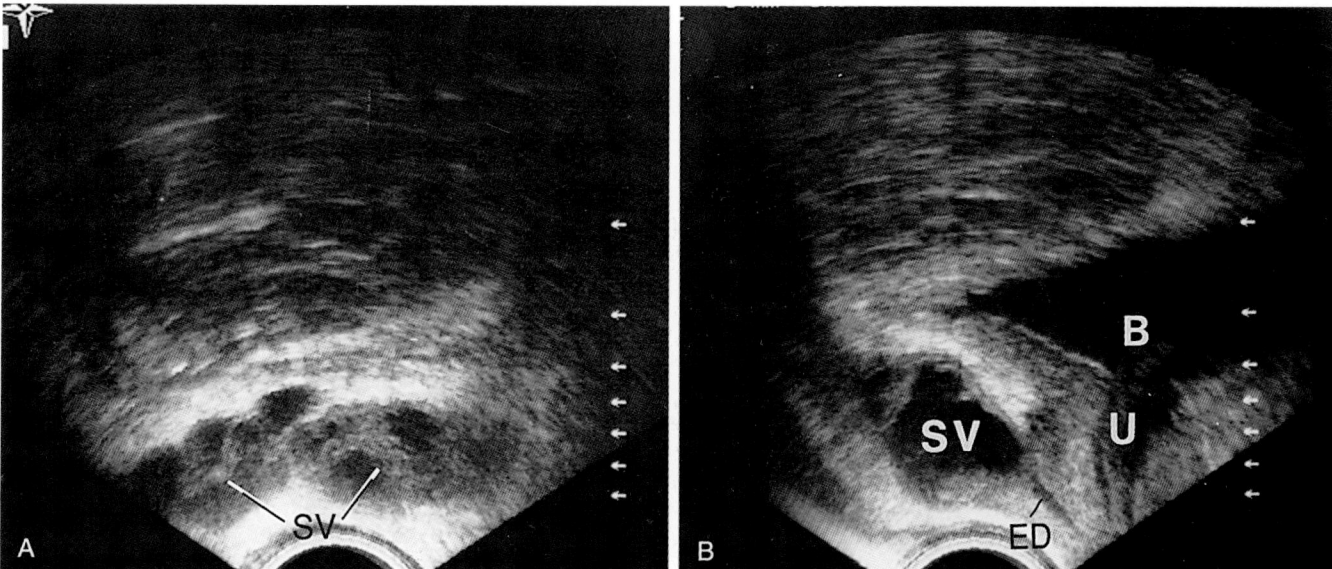

Figure 34–14. Transrectal ultrasound examination of normal seminal vesicles. **A,** Transverse view. **B,** Sagittal view. B, bladder; ED, ejaculatory duct; SV, seminal vesicle; U, urethra.

studies to more fully delineate the lesion (Shabsigh et al, 1989). Ultrasonography has also been used to attempt to differentiate inflammatory conditions of the seminal vesicle; however, other than calcifications with chronic bilharziasis, TRUS findings in patients with chronic prostatourethritis or prostatodynia are relatively nonspecific (Littrup et al, 1988).

Sonographic findings of a tumor within the seminal vesicle depend on whether the tumor is primary or secondary. Primary tumors are usually unilateral, whereas secondary tumors more likely involve both seminal vesicles and may be difficult to distinguish as to their origin (i.e., from the rectum, bladder, or prostate). The TRUS image of a solid tumor is isoechoic to the prostate but relatively hyperechoic with respect to the normal seminal vesicle. There are no image characteristics indicative of benign versus malignant or primary versus secondary tumors, except that primary tumors are commonly unilateral and tend not to be contiguous with the prostate, whereas prostate cancer invading the seminal vesicle may be at the base of both seminal vesicles and contiguous with the prostate tumor. Specimens obtained by ultrasound-guided transrectal or perineal aspiration or core biopsy can be useful for pathologic diagnosis of a seminal vesicle neoplasm.

Computed Tomography

CT is a considerable improvement over conventional radiography for evaluation of the pelvis. Evaluation of seminal vesicle disease by CT, however, has not been systematically studied. Silverman and colleagues (1985) reviewed a group of 50 patients with normal seminal vesicles by CT and determined a mean length of 3.1 cm, width of 1.5 cm, and overall area of 3.6 cm. The volume tended to decrease with age, and the shape varied from ovoid (70%) to tubular (20%) to rounded (10%). The seminal vesicles were symmetrical in 67% of those studied. **The seminal vesicles themselves are medium contrast structures (similar to muscle) routinely seen directly below the bladder.** The surrounding Denonvilliers' fascia is not discernible on CT. Goldstein and Schlossberg (1988) studied CT in patients who had absent vas deferens and found that not all had absent seminal vesicles; they concluded that CT is accurate for detection of the presence of seminal vesicles. CT has been used to detect congenital anomalies, and perhaps this may be its best use in seminal vesicle diagnosis (Fig. 34–15). Cystic structures have CT attenuation numbers (Hounsfield units) from 0 to 10, like most clear fluid-filled structures, although the density may be higher secondary to debris, pus, or hemorrhage.

Tumor within the seminal vesicle is readily seen on CT as an enlarged vesicle with a higher CT attenuation number in the area of the tumor mass than in normal seminal vesicle and with a normal bladder and prostate (Fig. 34–16). The lesion may be cystic, however, as a result of tumor necrosis (King et al, 1989). CT cannot distinguish between benign and malignant tumors and cannot routinely distinguish between primary and secondary tumors, although tissue planes are usually obliterated by secondary tumors invading from prostate or rectum (Sussman et al, 1986). Inflammatory masses in the seminal vesicles, such as tuberculosis or old bacterial abscesses, can be calcified (Patel and Wilbur, 1987; Schwartz et al, 1988; Birnbaum et al, 1990) and thus distinguished from tumors, although a history of infection and related symptoms can usually be elicited. A long-term history

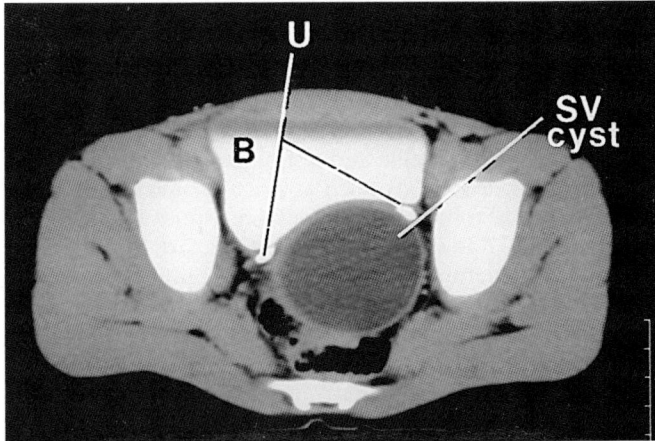

Figure 34–15. CT scan of seminal vesicle cyst (SV cyst). B, bladder; U, ureters.

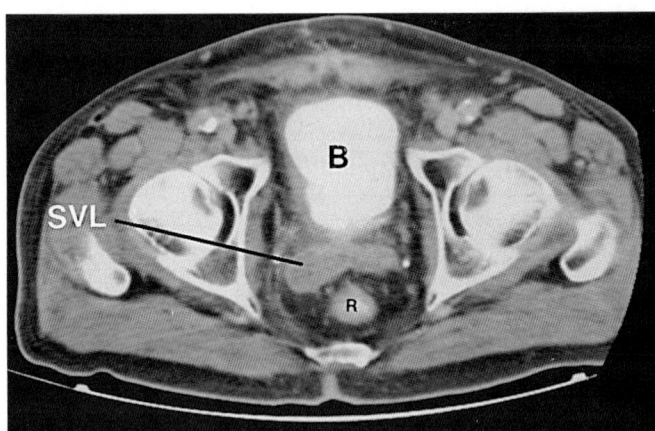

Figure 34–16. CT scan of seminal vesicle lymphoma (SVL). B, bladder; R, rectum.

of diabetes mellitus has also been associated with seminal vesicle calcification (King et al, 1989).

Magnetic Resonance Imaging

Although MRI is not, in general, more sensitive than CT or ultrasonography for diagnosis, the anatomic relationships are more clearly seen, multiplanar imaging is readily available, and the minimal amount of fat in the pelvis and the characteristics of the magnetic resonance phenomenon (T1- and T2-weighted images) allow more definitive diagnosis of cystic lesions and more accurate staging of solid neoplasms in the pelvis. Normally, the anatomic relationships of the seminal vesicles are similar to those shown on CT except that on T1-weighted images, seminal vesicles are of low signal intensity, which increases substantially on T2-weighted images (Fig. 34–17). This is thought to be secondary to the secretions present in the ductular lumen of the seminal vesicle. The surrounding Denonvilliers' fascia is of low intensity on both T1- and T2-weighted images. In general, on T2-weighted images, signal intensity is lower than that of fat in prepubertal children, similar to or higher than that of fat in adults, and similar to or lower than that of fat in patients older than 70 years. Endocrine therapy and radiation therapy influence the size

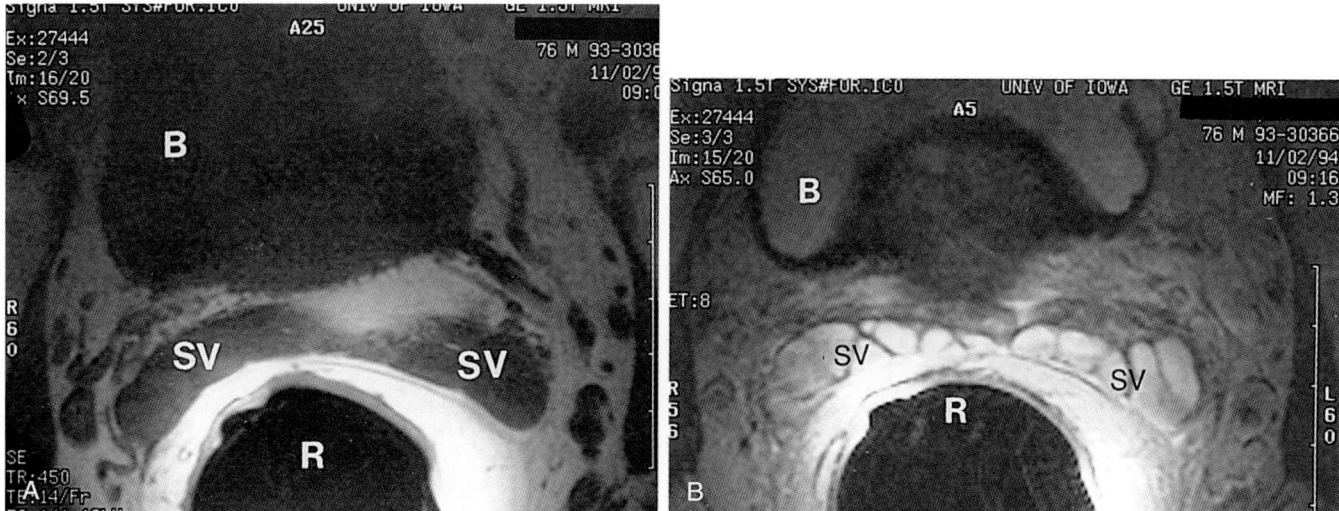

Figure 34–17. Transaxial MRI of normal seminal vesicles (SV) with endorectal coil. **A,** T1-weighted image. **B,** T2-weighted image. B, bladder; R, rectum.

and intensity of the seminal vesicles (Secaf et al, 1991). Seminal vesicle cysts are similar to cysts in other locations in that the T1-weighted image is of low intensity but the T2-weighted image is that of a unilocular smooth wall with uniform high intensity and a well-defined margin (Gevenois et al, 1990; Hihara et al, 1993). Hemorrhagic cysts have high signal intensity on both T1- and T2-weighted images (Sue et al, 1989). Seminal vesiculitis shows decreased signal intensity on the T1-weighted image, whereas T2-weighted image intensity is higher than that of both fat and the normal seminal vesicle.

MRI of seminal vesicle tumors shows a heterogeneous mass with a medium intensity on T1-weighted image and a heterogeneous intensity on T2-weighted image. There has been no systematic MRI study of seminal vesicle tumors, and MRI cannot distinguish between benign and malignant solid masses within the seminal vesicle.

Patients with a suspected seminal vesicle abnormality or mass felt on rectal examination should first have TRUS. If the mass is solid and noncystic, a transperineal or TRUS-guided biopsy is a reasonable next step. If the tumor is confirmed, a CT scan should be done next for staging purposes; MRI is necessary only to confirm the hemorrhagic nature of the mass or to more definitively stage the extent of the mass to contiguous organs within the pelvis. Definitive treatment of most seminal vesicle lesions, however, can be appropriately determined without MRI.

Vasography

Vasography, accomplished either by transurethral injection of contrast material at the seminal colliculus or by surgical exposure of the scrotal vas followed by injection of contrast material, was once the preferred means to image the seminal vesicles (Fig. 34–18). Transurethral routes of injection were often unsuccessful owing to the length of time, special equipment, and expertise required. Antegrade injection through the surgically exposed vas is highly successful, particularly in evaluating duct obstruction in azoospermic individuals or those with prior surgical trauma (Al-Omari et al, 1985). Vasography

does not, however, provide accurate demonstration of the pathologic condition of the seminal vesicles in patients with vesiculitis, cysts, or tumors (Dunnick et al, 1982; King et al, 1989). Direct transrectal needle seminal vesiculography has also been reported as a method for diagnosis or drug delivery but is not recommended for routine cases (Meyer et al, 1979; Fuse et al, 1988).

Pathology

Congenital Lesions

Agenesis of the Seminal Vesicles. Unilateral agenesis of the seminal vesicles is not uncommon, with an incidence of 0.6% to 1%. It may be associated with unilateral absence of the vas deferens as well as ipsilateral renal anomalies (Fig. 34–19). This is thought to result from an embryologic insult before the separation of the ureteral bud from the mesonephric duct, which typically occurs at 7 weeks' gestation. It is thought that if the insult occurs after 7 weeks' gestation, the seminal vesicle anomaly may not be associated with renal agenesis (Hall and Oates, 1993). The frequency of associated renal anomalies varies, but in one series, 79% of patients with absence of a seminal vesicle or vas deferens had ipsilateral renal agenesis, 12% had ipsilateral renal abnormalities, and only 9% had normal kidneys bilaterally (Donohue and Fauver, 1989).

Bilateral absence of the seminal vesicles is frequently found in association with congenital bilateral absence of the vas deferens. This is commonly associated with a mutation of the cystic fibrosis transmembrane receptor. Seventy percent to 80% of men with bilateral absence of the vas deferens or seminal vesicles are carriers of the genetic mutation associated with cystic fibrosis (Anguiano et al, 1994; Chillon et al, 1995). Conversely, 80% to 95% of men with cystic fibrosis have bilateral absence of the vas deferens or seminal vesicles (Holsclaw et al, 1971; Boat et al, 1989). In men who have genitourinary anomalies with congenital bilateral absence of the vas deferens or seminal vesicle agenesis, the incidence of cystic fibrosis transmembrane receptor mutation is extremely low (de la

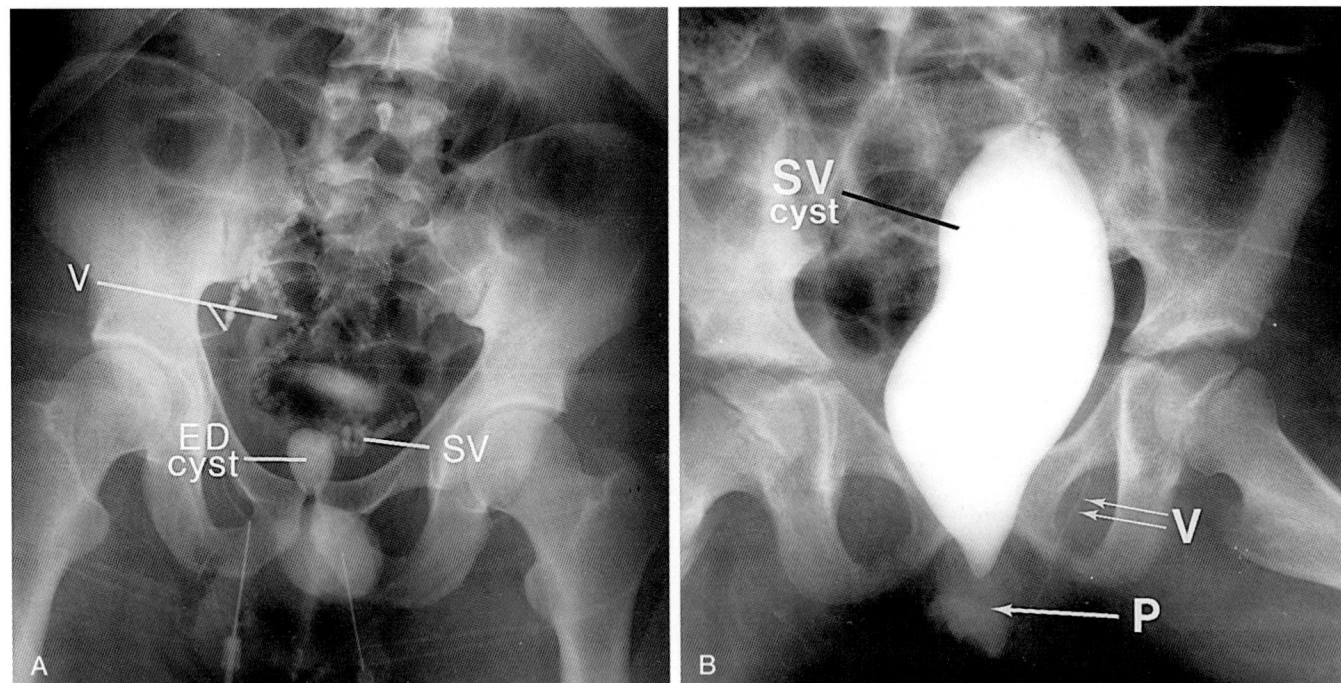

Figure 34–18. Vasograms of patients with ejaculatory duct–seminal vesicle cysts. **A,** Bilateral vasogram of a patient with right ejaculatory duct obstruction. **B,** Vasogram showing seminal vesicle cyst in the patient from Figure 34–16. ED, ejaculatory duct; P, prostate; SV, seminal vesicle; V, vas deferens.

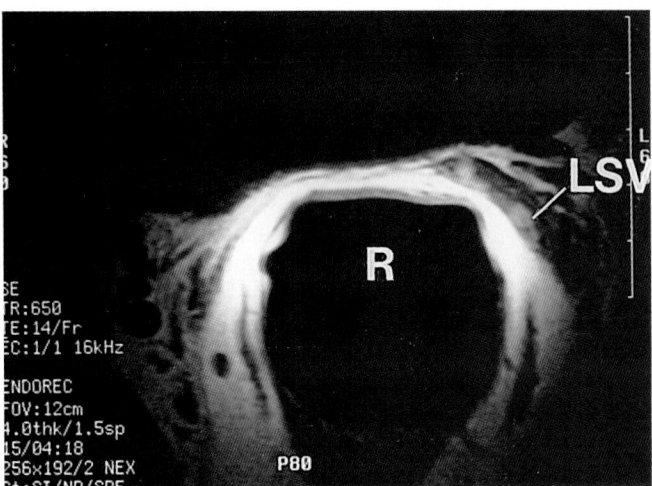

Figure 34–19. Transaxial T1-weighted endorectal magnetic resonance image of absent right seminal vesicle. LSV, left seminal vesicle; R, rectum.

Taille et al, 1998). However, lack of a vas deferens does not necessarily imply an absent seminal vesicle unless the ipsilateral ureter is also not present (Goldstein and Schlossberg, 1988). Seminal vesicle agenesis requires no treatment.

Obstruction of the Seminal Vesicles. Whereas absence of the seminal vesicles may be asymptomatic, obstruction is frequently associated with symptoms. Unilateral obstruction may be due to entrance of an ectopic ureter, leading to infection of the obstructed organ. The kidney associated with the ectopic ureter is frequently dysplastic. Obstruction may also be due to local invasion of bladder or prostate cancer

(Fig. 34–20). Bilateral obstruction (Fig. 34–21) is frequently associated with infertility (Donohue and Fauver, 1989; Hall and Oates, 1993). Several authors have described diagnosis of obstruction with TRUS and aspiration or injection of the seminal vesicles (Jones et al, 1997; Orhan et al, 1999; Seifman et al, 1999). This is covered in further detail in Chapter 19.

Infection

Vesiculitis. Infection of the seminal vesicles is an uncommon problem in the United States. In less developed countries, tuberculosis and schistosomiasis remain common causes of seminal vesicle masses, abscesses, and calcification. Chronic bacterial vesiculitis is rare and difficult to diagnose; however, transrectal or perineal needle aspiration for diagnosis or treatment of abscesses has been successful. **Bacterial infections are commonly due to colonic flora and are thought to be secondary to bacterial prostatitis.** In the distant past, bilateral seminal vesiculectomy was used for treatment of infections of the seminal vesicle, but today, selected systemic antibiotics are usually curative, obviating surgery (Gutierrez et al, 1994). On occasion, chronic bacterial seminal vesiculitis may require surgical removal to eliminate symptoms and to prevent recurrent septicemia. Any of the surgical approaches to be described subsequently would be appropriate (Indudhara et al, 1991).

Abscess. Abscesses of the seminal vesicles usually have an unknown etiology, although predisposing factors include diabetes mellitus, chronic indwelling catheter, and endoscopic manipulation. Signs and symptoms vary but are typically related to inflammation. Conservative drainage through a percutaneous route is occasionally successful, but most abscesses of the seminal vesicles require open drainage (Gutierrez et al, 1994; Kore et al, 1994). Imaging of the abscess

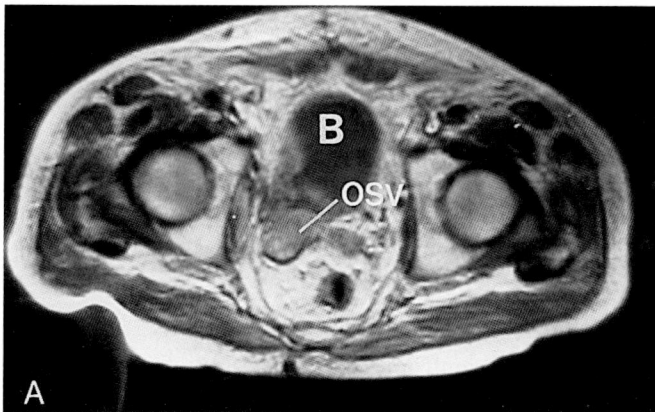

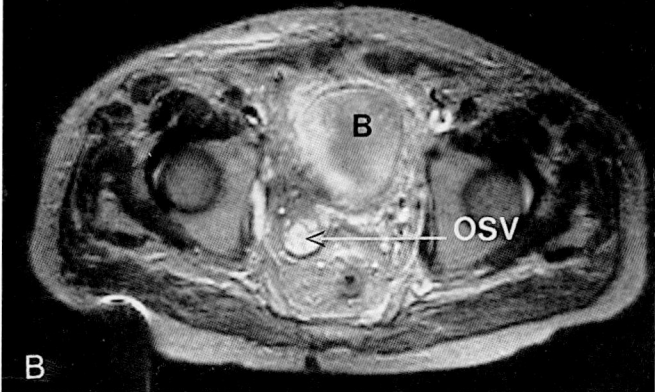

Figure 34–20. MRI of an obstructed right seminal vesicle (OSV) as a result of invasive bladder cancer. B, bladder. **A,** Transaxial T1-weighted image. **B,** Transaxial T2-weighted image.

is best accomplished with MRI because of the high fluid content of the seminal vesicles. In contrast to the normal hypointense T1-weighted image, inflammation results in a less intense image. The normally hyperintense signal found on a T2-weighted image is increased further with inflammation. The systemic administration of gadolinium or diethylenetri-aminepentaacetic acid offers better enhancement and visualization (Chandra et al, 1991; Doringer et al, 1991).

Calculi. Stones within the seminal vesicles are usually related to obstruction, infection, or both (Li, 1991; Wilkinson, 1993). Patients usually present with either pain or infection related to the stone, although hematospermia or infertility can be the presenting complaint. Treatment requires removal of the stone, usually through an open vesiculectomy. Adjuvant treatment with antibiotics may be necessary, particularly in cases of systemic infection.

Masses. Most masses within the seminal vesicles are not neoplastic. Tumors of the seminal vesicles are extremely rare. Benign primary tumors are the most common, including papillary adenoma, cystadenoma, fibroma, and leiomyoma (Mostofi and Price, 1973; Lundhus et al, 1984; Narayana, 1985; Mazur et al, 1987; Bullock, 1988). Simple cysts of the seminal vesicle are seen not uncommonly and may be associated with other genitourinary anomalies, such as ipsilateral renal agenesis or malformation (Lynch and Flannigan, 1992; Sheih et al, 1993).

Seminal Vesicle Cysts

Cysts of the seminal vesicles (see Fig. 34–21) **may be either congenital or acquired** (King et al, 1991) and are thought to be due to obstruction of the ejaculatory duct (Heaney et al,

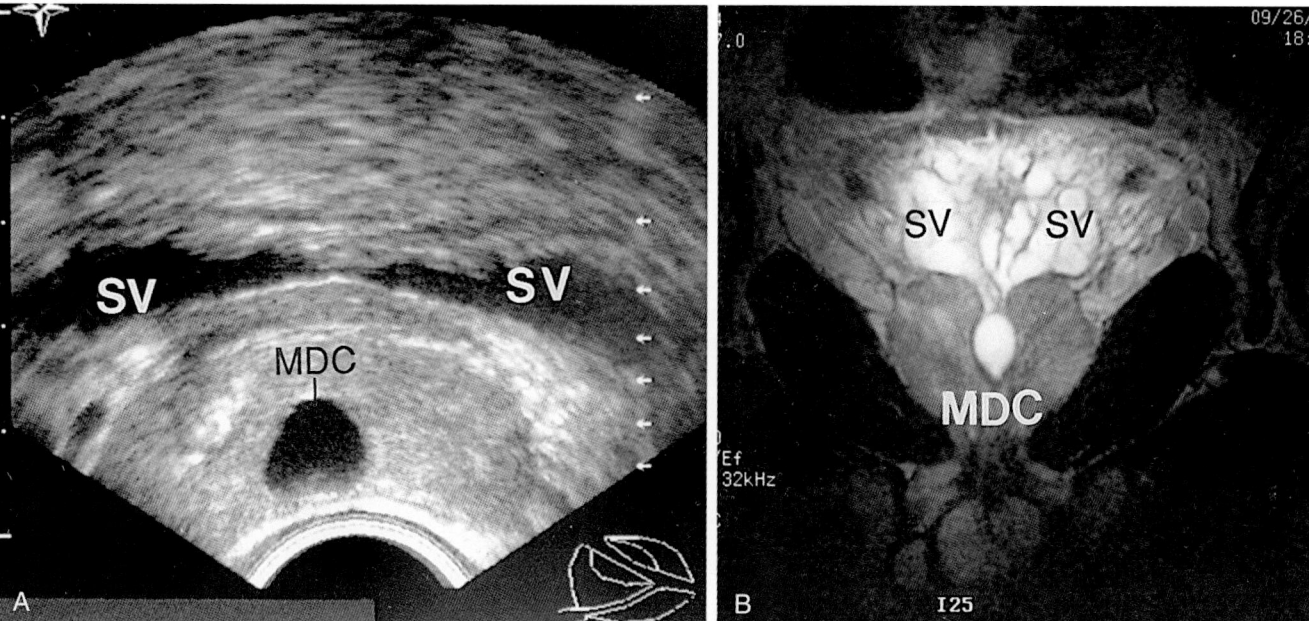

Figure 34–21. A, Transrectal ultrasound examination of patient with seminal vesicle obstruction because of müllerian duct cyst. **B,** T2-weighted magnetic resonance image of same patient. MDC, müllerian duct cyst; SV, seminal vesicle.

1987; Conn et al, 1992). Numerous authors have reported an association between seminal vesicle cysts and other abnormalities, including renal agenesis (Kimchi and Wiesenfeld, 1963; Roehrborn et al, 1986), infertility (Nazli et al, 1994), hematospermia (Mayersak and Viviano, 1992; Wang et al, 1993), and genitourinary infection (Beeby, 1974; Roehrborn et al, 1986; Lynch and Flannigan, 1992).

Others have reported an association between seminal vesicle cysts and adult polycystic kidney disease (Alpern et al, 1991; Hihara et al, 1993; Hendry et al, 1998). In contrast to typical benign cysts, some think that the pathogenesis of these cysts associated with polycystic kidney disease is a general defect in the basement membrane of multiple organs, including the seminal vesicles. One report cited the presence of seminal vesicle cysts in 60% of patients with polycystic kidney disease (Danaci et al, 1998). These authors, as well as others, recommend that all patients with cysts of the seminal vesicles have imaging of the kidneys to rule out polycystic kidney disease (Alpern et al, 1991; Danaci et al, 1998; Hendry et al, 1998).

Unless these cystic lesions are symptomatic, treatment is not usually necessary (Surya et al, 1988). If the lesion causes symptoms, percutaneous transperineal drainage of the cysts with TRUS guidance can be successful (Kirkali et al, 1991; Wang et al, 1993); if not, open or laparoscopic surgical excision may be necessary. If an ectopic ureter is present, a nephroureterectomy, including removal of the seminal vesicle, should be curative.

Benign Tumors

Papillary Adenoma or Cystadenoma. This may mimic a simple seminal vesicle cyst in its presentation and imaging. It generally occurs in middle-aged men and involves one side; only one case of bilateral involvement has been reported (Mazur et al, 1987). Some think that it originates from embryologic remnants (Tock et al, 1991; Mazzucchelli et al, 1992; Ranschaert et al, 1992). Open surgical removal is the treatment of choice because preoperative diagnosis is rarely made.

Amyloid of the Seminal Vesicles. Subepithelial deposits of amyloid in the seminal vesicles have been reported in 4% to 17% of male autopsies, with an incidence up to 20% in men older than 76 years (Pitkanen et al, 1983; Ramchandani et al, 1993). Because of increased incidence in the older population, it is frequently concomitant with other conditions, such as bladder or prostate cancer. Therefore, it is possible to misinterpret enlargement of the seminal vesicles from senile amyloidosis as carcinomatous invasion. MRI of the pelvis can usually distinguish tumor invasion, although not with complete accuracy (Kaji et al, 1992). In contrast to senile amyloidosis, the systemic form of amyloidosis may involve multiple organ systems with amyloid deposits in the blood vessels and muscle cells as opposed to the subepithelium (Coyne and Kealy, 1993). If patients are asymptomatic, no treatment is necessary.

Malignant Tumors

The main difficulty encountered with seminal vesicle neoplasms is determining that they are, in fact, primary within the seminal vesicles. Indeed, it is more common for carcinoma of the bladder, adenocarcinoma of the prostate, lymphoma, or rectal carcinoma to secondarily involve the seminal vesicle (Mostofi and Price, 1973; Jakse et al, 1987; Ro et al, 1987).

Very few primary tumors of the seminal vesicles have been reported. This is due in part to the paucity of symptoms and the lack of detection on physical examination for small, benign tumors; it was also once due to the lack of diagnostic imaging capable of accurately depicting the seminal vesicles. It is surprising that a tumor arising from an analog similar to that of the prostate and responding to similar hormonal influences has so few recognized pathologic conditions. Perhaps the extremely low proliferative activity of seminal vesicle epithelium partly accounts for this (Meyer et al, 1982).

Adenocarcinoma. Primary seminal vesicle adenocarcinoma occurs in patients older than 50 years. The tumor usually extends locally into prostate and bladder or rectum; commonly, there is prostatic or ureteral obstruction. Pathologic examination reveals a mucin-producing papillary or anaplastic carcinoma that may also contain lipofuscin in a patient with no other pelvic primary tumor. Serum levels of markers for prostate cancer (prostate-specific antigen, prostatic acid phosphatase) are normal, and serum carcinoembryonic antigen is elevated (Mostofi and Price, 1973; Benson et al, 1984; Tanaka et al, 1987; Chinoy and Kulkarni, 1993). Positive staining for cancer antigen 125 has been reported and may be useful to distinguish this from other adenocarcinomas, such as that of the prostate or bladder (Ohmori et al, 1994; Ormsby et al, 2000).

Sarcoma. Sarcomas of the seminal vesicles have been reported by various authors and are extremely rare. They are usually diagnosed late in the course of the disease. There are no distinguishing features except for biopsy findings (Benson et al, 1984; Chiou et al, 1985; Schned et al, 1986; Tanaka et al, 1987; Davis et al, 1988; Kawahara et al, 1988). These include leiomyosarcoma (Amirkhan, 1994) and angiosarcoma (Lamont et al, 1991) as well as müllerian adenosarcoma-like tumor (Laurila et al, 1992). These all display aggressive behavior. Treatment is similar to that for carcinoma; radical extirpation yields varying results.

Other Pathologic Processes

Other pathologic processes include hydatid cyst (Kuyumcuoglu et al, 1991) and carcinoid (Soyer et al, 1991). Other primary malignant tumors of the seminal vesicles that have been reported include cystosarcoma phyllodes (Fain, 1993) and primary seminoma (Adachi et al, 1991). Hydatid disease affecting the seminal vesicles can cause hematospermia, infertility, infection, or pain. Carcinoid of the seminal vesicle appears homogeneous with intense enhancement on CT. On MRI, hypointense images are demonstrated on both T1- and T2-weighted images, with T2-weighted images demonstrating heterogeneity (Soyer et al, 1991).

Treatment

If a solid lesion identified in the seminal vesicle shows no evidence of local spread and is benign on biopsy, treatment depends on symptoms. If the patient is asymptomatic, close follow-up consisting of repeated rectal examination and

TRUS to determine subsequent growth of the tumor is reasonable, although it may be difficult to be totally certain the tumor is not malignant. If the mass enlarges or if the patient has symptoms referable to the mass, simple seminal vesiculectomy is advisable. This may be accomplished through one of several routes described in the following.

If the mass is large and solid and demonstrates questionable margins, or if the biopsy specimen shows malignant columnar or poorly differentiated carcinoma cells, the treatment of choice is different. **Because fewer than 10 cases of primary tumors of the seminal vesicles have been treated at any one institution, it is difficult to define optimal treatment with any degree of certainty. Radical excision,** which usually includes a cystoprostatectomy with pelvic lymphadenectomy, **is the treatment of choice unless the tumor is extremely small.** This recommendation is based on the extensive nature of the majority of the cancers when they are detected. The excision may include the rectum (total pelvic exenteration) if it is thought to be invading the surrounding structures. Adjuvant therapy has no proven efficacy, although the only long-term survivors in the literature received radical surgery with subsequent pelvic radiation therapy or androgen deprivation therapy. No chemotherapeutic regimen is known to be efficacious.

Surgery

Surgical approaches to the seminal vesicle have varied considerably since the first seminal vesicle was removed by Ullmann in 1889 (de Assis, 1952). Large series (up to 700 by one surgeon) of seminal vesiculectomies have been described—most for tuberculosis or suspected inflammation. **Today, seminal vesiculectomy is rarely necessary.** The most useful open surgical methods include transperineal, similar to radical perineal prostatectomy; transvesical, achieved by incision through the posterior bladder wall; paravesical; retrovesical; and transcoccygeal. During the last decade, the laparoscopic or robotically assisted approach to benign seminal vesicle lesions has been found to be remarkably direct and associated with much less postoperative morbidity in comparison to the open surgical approach (Carmignani et al, 1995; Ikari et al, 1999; McDougall et al, 2001).

The choice of surgical approach, of course, depends partly on the characteristics of the lesion to be treated but probably more on the experience and expertise of the surgeon. **For the most part, congenital lesions require an abdominal approach so that the ipsilateral kidney can be dealt with concomitantly,** if necessary. Such lesions may be dealt with by laparoscopic or open surgical intervention. Benign lesions may be approached perineally; however, the risk of impotence is high even if a nerve-sparing approach is attempted. **A laparoscopic approach, in skilled hands, may be the simplest and least invasive approach.** Larger benign tumors or cysts are best handled by an anterior abdominal approach, although a transcoccygeal method may be as useful. Again, the transperitoneal or retroperitoneal laparoscopic approach has great merit for such lesions. **Patients with malignant disease require radical extirpation,** which commonly includes cystoprostato–seminal vesiculectomy and pelvic lymphadenectomy. This operation is no different from a routine procedure for bladder cancer and thus is not described here.

Indications. Most surgeries on seminal vesicles are in conjunction with radical surgical treatment of pelvic neoplasms, such as bladder, prostate, or urethral cancer and, occasionally, rectal cancer. The indications and surgical principles for treatment of these conditions are detailed in other chapters in this book.

Treatments of conditions of the seminal vesicles alone are limited to transperineal or transvesical aspiration of seminal vesicle cysts or abscesses, transurethral unroofing of seminal vesicle cysts or abscesses, laparoscopic or robotic dissection, and open resection of one or both seminal vesicles.

Preoperative Preparation. Preoperative preparation for laparoscopic, robotic, or open seminal vesicle surgery depends on the extent of the pathologic process and the planned incision. Transperineal, transcoccygeal, and transvesical approaches should be prefaced by a complete bowel preparation. The authors use a mechanical preparation with GoLYTELY orally the evening before surgery, followed by the standard antibiotic bowel regimen. This is in anticipation of the uncommon but not unlikely possibility of a rectal laceration. A similar bowel preparation should also be considered if the laparoscopic or robotic surgical route is planned. A prophylactic systemic antibiotic of choice is administered perioperatively (i.e., immediately before surgery and two doses following). Some method to prevent phlebothrombosis in the legs, such as use of intermittent compression stockings during and immediately after surgery, is advisable.

The blood loss expected from seminal vesicle surgery depends on the surgical approach used and the pathologic process anticipated. For the laparoscopic or robotic approach, patients are typed and screened for blood products as hemorrhage is unlikely and the expected condition is benign. One or two units at least should be prepared for the open anterior approach or perineal and transcoccygeal approaches as the anticipated condition may be malignant, requiring more extensive dissection and possible radical prostatectomy or cystectomy. Preoperative autologous blood donation may be considered.

Open Surgical Techniques

Indications for an open technique are uncommon; however, we include the following descriptions for historical interest as well as completeness of this chapter.

Patients with chronic seminal vesiculitis or a small benign tumor of the seminal vesicle can have a seminal vesiculectomy through the perineal route, similar to a radical perineal prostatectomy. Large benign tumors or cysts require removal through either an anterior incision or a transcoccygeal approach because the perineal route limits the ability to reach more than a few centimeters craniad to the bladder neck or to physically remove large masses through the relatively small opening.

Patients with an ectopic ureter into a seminal vesicle cyst require an anterior approach so that the kidney, ureter, and seminal vesicle can be removed completely. We prefer a midline incision so that the kidney and ureter can be approached transperitoneally after mobilization of the colon. The ureter can then be followed and dissected from the bladder in a paravesical approach, similar to performing a nephroureterectomy for urothelial cancer.

Transperineal Approach. **The transperineal approach follows the standard positioning and incision described for a radical perineal prostatectomy.** To find the seminal vesicles above the prostate, the rectal wall needs to be dissected free and released higher on the base of the prostate and seminal vesicles than is usually necessary for initiation of radical prostatectomy. The incision in Denonvilliers' fascia is then made either transversely, just above the level of the base of the seminal vesicles on the prostate (Fig. 34–22), or vertically, if an attempt is being made to save the neurovascular bundles responsible for potency (Weldon and Tavel, 1988). In this latter case, Denonvilliers' fascia is carefully dissected laterally away from the underlying seminal vesicle and ampulla of the vas so as not to tear the longitudinal tissue carrying the neurovascular bundle. The dissection at the base of the seminal vesicle may be enhanced by posterior traction on a Lowsley tractor placed through the urethra into the bladder, thus elevating the prostate and putting tension on Denonvilliers' fascia. The two ampullae of the vas deferens should easily be dissected directly above the prostate and just under Denonvilliers' fascia. They are somewhat friable but can be clipped with metal clips (not placed too tightly) if necessary. In the case of a simple seminal vesicle cyst or small adenoma, the vas can be spared, and the dissection then proceeds to the vesicle of concern. If the reason for surgery is cancer or recurrent infection, a wider resection, including the ampulla of the vas, may be advisable. If the diagnosis is benign, the dissection can begin directly on the seminal vesicle.

There is usually an easily dissected plane that can be found along the seminal vesicle, surrounding retroperitoneal tissue, and Denonvilliers' fascia. After dissection around the seminal vesicle at the base of the prostate, it is usually possible to pass a right-angle clamp around the seminal vesicle and use an absorbable 2-0 suture to ligate the stump of the seminal vesicle directly on the prostate. A second tie or clip on the distal seminal vesicle will keep the secretions from obscuring the field after the vesicle is cut across, which is the next step. Although some surgeons may prefer to attempt to dissect out the seminal vesicle completely before ligating its entry into the prostate, this makes the operation more difficult and lengthy and serves no useful purpose when the seminal vesicle is being removed for a benign condition. Once the seminal vesicle has been ligated and cut across at the base, an Allis clamp can be used on the cut edge to put countertraction on the seminal vesicle so that spreading dissection with Metzenbaum scissors can free the seminal vesicle from the surrounding tissue. The vascular pedicle is usually encountered within 1 cm of the distal tip, and after it is ligated with metal clips and cut across, the organ can be removed. The wound is then closed in layers exactly as outlined for a radical perineal prostatectomy. A Penrose drain is left in the bed of the seminal vesicle and removed within 24 hours if no drainage is noted.

The perineal approach is extremely well tolerated by patients and affords them minimal blood loss, early ambulation, and minimal postoperative pain. Because there is no urethral anastomosis, patients may be ready for discharge within 24 to 48 hours. Intraoperative complications primarily entail inadvertent rectal wall laceration, although it is possible to lacerate the trigone area of the bladder or the ipsilateral ureter during deep dissection of the distal tip of the seminal vesicle. If an adequate bowel preparation has been given preoperatively and no gross fecal contamination is seen, a two-layer closure of the rectum with a running mucosal layer of 3-0 absorbable suture and a submucosal layer of interrupted 4-0 silk is usually sufficient. Anal dilation before the patient is awakened may be useful. A large laceration or fecal contamination should cause consideration of a temporary colostomy, although such a measure has not been necessary in our experience. If a bladder injury is noted, it should be closed in two layers with absorbable suture as in any bladder incision and a urethral catheter left indwelling for 7 to 10 days postoperatively. If a ureteral injury occurs, an attempt to place a self-retaining (double-J) catheter should be made and the ureter then repaired with absorbable suture. If the ureter cannot be catheterized, flexible cystoscopy and retrograde placement of a ureteral stent should be performed on the table with the stent left in place for 10 to 14 days postoperatively.

Transvesical Approach. **The transvesical approach to the seminal vesicle has been described by numerous authors** (Walker and Bowles, 1968; Politano et al, 1975). A midline extraperitoneal suprapubic incision is made up to the umbilicus, and the rectus muscles are separated on the midline. Retzius' space is opened by downward displacement of the transverse fascia on the pubis, and an Omni retractor is placed to expose the anterior bladder wall. Care is taken during this

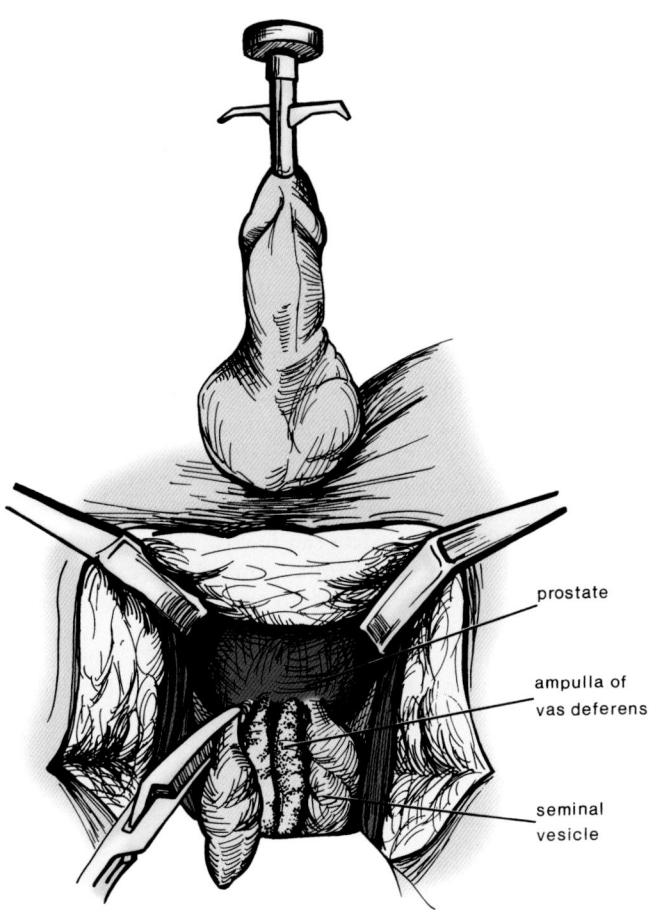

prostate

ampulla of
vas deferens

seminal
vesicle

Figure 34–22. Transperineal approach to seminal vesiculectomy. (Redrawn from Hinman F Jr: Atlas of Urologic Surgery. Philadelphia, WB Saunders, 1989:381.)

dissection to not injure the epigastric vessels on either side of the pubis. The bladder is opened longitudinally approximately 7 to 10 cm, ending 2 to 3 cm away from the bladder neck. Moist 4 × 8 sponges are placed on the bladder wall laterally and at the dome of the bladder, and specialized blades are placed to put the open bladder on stretch. Although it is not absolutely necessary, it is preferable to place long 8 French feeding tubes in the ureters at this point for definition of the orifices and to help with identification of the subtrigonal ureters to prevent their injury later in the dissection.

With a Bovie cutting stylet, a vertical incision is made through the trigone on the posterior midline approximately 5 cm in length (Fig. 34–23A). Alternatively, a transverse incision just above the bladder neck can be used, but it is not preferred (Fig. 34–23B). The vertical incision is deepened through the bladder muscle, and the ampullae of the vas should be recognized directly beneath the bladder neck. They can be dissected by scissors down to their entrance into the prostate and then either ligated and divided or left intact, depending on the pathologic process, as described in the perineal approach. Just lateral to the ampullae on the prostate base, the seminal vesicles should be identified and the plane surrounding them entered easily unless there has been prior inflammatory disease. The seminal vesicles should be encircled and dissected completely free. Metal clips should be placed on the vascular pedicle and a 2-0 chromic tie on the distal end at the prostate. A clip is placed across the proximal end of the vas to prevent seminal vesicle contents from obscuring the field, and then the vesicle is transected and removed. If there is a moderate-sized cyst, the dissection is more involved but is usually made simple because the perivesical plane is usually more pronounced. The plane may be difficult to establish if there was prior vesiculitis, and in this instance the ureteral catheters are a welcome safeguard—care must be taken not to dissect completely through Denonvilliers' fascia posteriorly and into the rectum. The posterior bladder incision is then closed with a running 2-0 absorbable suture in the muscle layer followed by a running 4-0 absorbable suture in the mucosal layer. The ureteral stents and 4 × 8 sponges are removed, a 20 French urethral catheter is placed, and the anterior bladder wall is closed as the posterior wall was. Suprapubic tube placement is an option but is not necessary. A suction drain is placed through a separate stab incision and positioned in the prevesical space away from the suture line. The drain is left for 2 or 3 days and then removed when the drainage has proved not to be urine and is less than 50 mL/day. The urethral catheter is removed in 5 to 7 days. Early ambulation is the rule, and the patient is usually discharged within 3 to 5 days after surgery.

This approach is more prone to blood loss and ureteral injury than the perineal approach, but a rectal laceration is much less likely. These complications are handled as described previously.

Paravesical Approach. The paravesical incision is used in children, when there is a large unilateral cyst that lies lateral to and above the bladder, and when nephroureterectomy is required. A midline or Pfannenstiel's extraperitoneal suprapubic incision is made. The bladder is finger dissected away from the lateral pelvic sidewall on the affected side. The vas deferens is identified, placed on tension, and dissected down

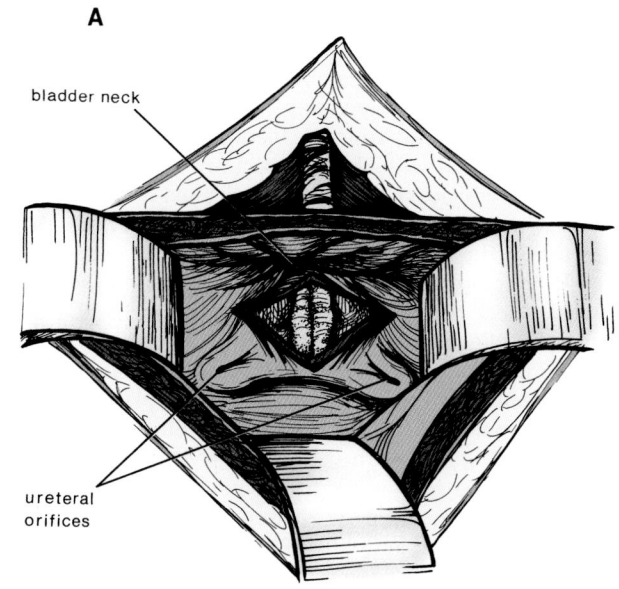

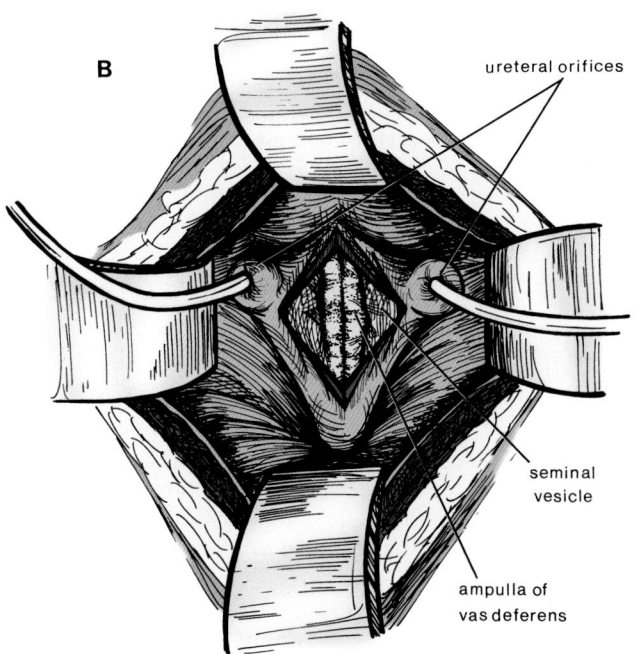

Figure 34–23. Transvesical approach to seminal vesiculectomy. **A,** Vertical incision between the ureteral orifices. **B,** Transverse incision 2 cm superior to the bladder neck below the ureteral orifices. (Redrawn from Hinman F Jr: Atlas of Urologic Surgery. Philadelphia, WB Saunders, 1989:382.)

toward the base of the bladder. If the seminal vesicle mass is distended, it should be visible rather quickly as the vas comes close to the bladder posteriorly. Placement of a catheter in the bladder to empty it usually allows the plane between the bladder and the cyst to be readily identified. The plane is incised with scissors, and the seminal vesicle cyst is carefully dissected away sharply. When the tip of the cyst is clearly identified, a 1-0 chromic suture is placed into it to provide traction, making further dissection easier.

The ureter crosses the vas and must be identified to prevent its injury. In addition, the superior vesical artery and perhaps the inferior vesical artery may be sacrificed to gain access to the base of the seminal vesicle. This will cause no harm and should be done without major concern. As the dissection proceeds, the bladder is progressively rolled over medially, and the mass is dissected away from the bladder laterally. The plane is easily maintained with sharp dissection. Any vessels feeding the seminal vesicles should be suture ligated or metal clipped.

As the prostate is approached, caution must be used to stay directly on the mass so as not to injure the neurovascular bundle lying just lateral to the seminal vesicle. At the prostate base, the neck of the seminal vesicle is encircled and ligated with a 2-0 absorbable suture. A clamp is placed across just distal to the tie, and the seminal vesicle is severed. There may be no need to clip the vas. A suction drain is placed in the bed of the seminal vesicle and brought out through a separate stab incision. The wound is then closed in layers.

Postoperative care is as previously described, except with this approach, the drain can be removed within 24 hours if there is no drainage, and the urethral catheter can be removed within 24 hours. The patient may be discharged within 2 or 3 days. Complications include ureteral injury and excessive blood loss. If the principles outlined earlier are followed, these are unlikely events.

Retrovesical Approach. The retrovesical approach should be considered in patients requiring bilateral excision of small seminal vesicle cysts or benign masses (de Assis, 1952). A midline suprapubic incision is made into the peritoneal space. A catheter is placed, and the urine is evacuated. The reflection of the peritoneum over the rectum at the posterior bladder wall is incised transversely, with care taken not to incise into the rectum (Fig. 34–24A). The bladder is peeled back from the rectum progressively with sharp dissection until the ampullae of the vasa and the tips of the seminal vesicles come into view (Fig. 34–24B). The seminal vesicles are dissected down to the base of the prostate, much as described in the transvesical approach, and the neck of the seminal vesicle is ligated and divided bilaterally. The ampullae are usually not taken unless necessary (Fig. 34–24C). A suction drain is left in the area posterior to the bladder and brought out as before.

Postoperative care is as described for a paravesical resection. Complications include rectal injury, bladder laceration, and hemorrhage. In this situation, a rectal injury would be within the peritoneum well above the levator ani muscles. After a two-layer closure as before, strong consideration should be given to placement of omentum over the closure between the bladder base and the rectum as well as to a temporary colostomy.

Transcoccygeal Approach. The transcoccygeal approach may not be familiar to most urologic surgeons and is unlikely to be a common choice because of fear of rectal injury and impotence. **In individuals for whom the perineal or supine position may be difficult to maintain or who have had multiple suprapubic or perineal surgeries, the transcoccygeal approach may be useful.**

The patient is placed on the table, ventral side down (prone) and in a relative jackknife position (Kreager and Jordan, 1965). The incision is made in an L shape from midway on the sacrum (10 cm from the tip of the coccyx) and angled at the tip of the coccyx down the gluteal cleft within 3 cm of the anus (Fig. 34–25A). The incision is carried down to the lateral side

of the coccyx, which is dissected free from the underlying rectum and eventually totally removed (Fig. 34–25B). The gluteus maximus muscle layers are moved aside, and the rectosigmoid is encountered and dissected carefully from the underside of the sacrum. With careful dissection, the lateral wall of the rectum on the side of the lesion is dissected medially from the levator ani muscle and surrounding tissue until the prostate is encountered (Fig. 34–25C). It is possible that the neurovascular bundle will be recognized from this approach; if the dissection is unilateral, injury may be of little consequence. Once the prostate is palpated, dissection of the tissue directly superior to the base on the midline should reveal the ampulla of the vas and, lateral to it, the seminal vesicle (Fig. 34–25D). If difficulty is encountered in dissecting the rectum away from the prostate, a finger in the anus via an O'Connor sheath will allow the correct plane to be determined. Dissection and removal of the seminal vesicles should follow the principles outlined previously. A Penrose drain should be left in the area, exiting through a separate stab incision at closure. The rectum should be carefully scrutinized; if injury is found, it is closed in two layers as previously described. The wound is closed in layers as well.

Postoperative care does not differ from that previously described; as in the perineal approach, the patient should have a rapid and easy recovery. The drain should be removed within 2 or 3 days if there is no drainage.

Laparoscopic Technique

Most laparoscopic surgery performed on seminal vesicles has been in conjunction with radical prostatectomy. The procedure was originally described by Kavoussi and colleagues (1993). After completion of a laparoscopic pelvic lymph node dissection for prostate cancer, the seminal vesicles are laparoscopically mobilized to facilitate subsequent radical perineal prostatectomy. It is known that dissection of the ampulla of the vas and seminal vesicles is a challenging part of a perineal prostatectomy, and thus prior mobilization of these structures made this easier. Its application for benign seminal vesicle disease is limited to case reports or small series (Carmignani et al, 1995; Ikari et al, 1999; McDougall et al, 2001).

Preparation of the Patient. Patients are placed supine with the arms carefully padded and tucked in by the sides. Access to the perineum is usually not necessary for benign seminal vesicle disease, whereas if a laparoscopic or robotic prostatectomy will be performed in addition, the legs are abducted but left straight with the use of an operating table that allows a split-leg arrangement (Fig. 34–26A). If possible, the low lithotomy position is avoided to minimize the risk of lower extremity thrombosis or neuromuscular injury. Patients are carefully strapped to the operating table with wide cloth tape across the chest and thighs as steep Trendelenburg position (approximately 20 degrees) is required for deep pelvic laparoscopic visualization. After the patient is prepared and draped, a Foley catheter is inserted into the bladder under sterile conditions. An orogastric tube placed in the stomach is optional.

Transperitoneal Approach. A transperitoneal approach is preferred for benign seminal vesicle lesions. After establishment of a suitable pneumoperitoneum up to 15 mm Hg with the Veress needle placed at the inferior or superior umbilical crease, four laparoscopic ports are usually adequate for

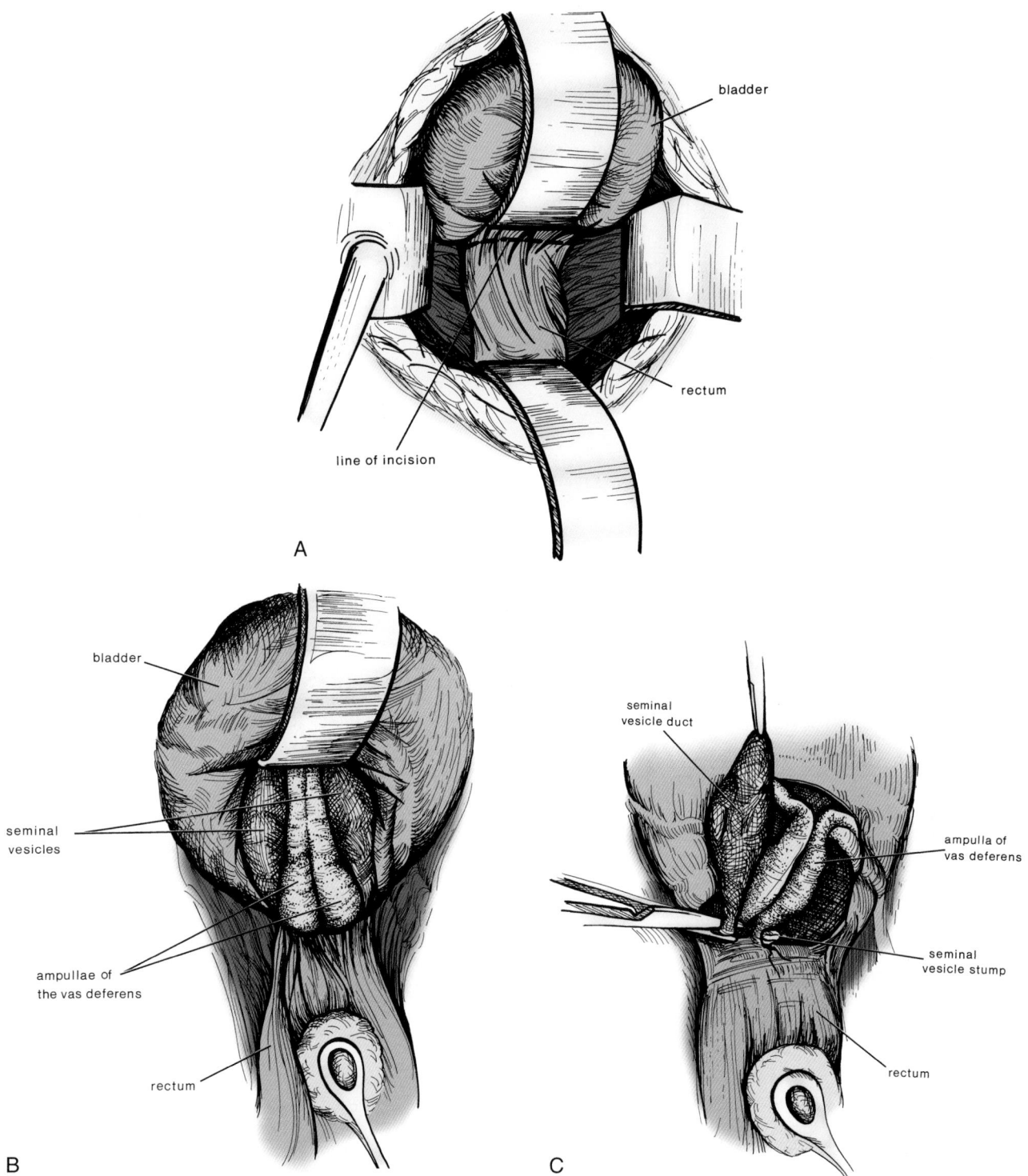

Figure 34–24. Retrovesical approach to seminal vesiculectomy. **A,** Incision line between base of bladder and peritoneal reflection over the rectum. **B,** Caudal dissection reveals the ampullae of the vas deferens on the midline and seminal vesicles immediately lateral to them. **C,** The duct of the seminal vesicle is ligated and transected. (Redrawn from Hinman F Jr: Atlas of Urologic Surgery. Philadelphia, WB Saunders, 1989:379-380.)

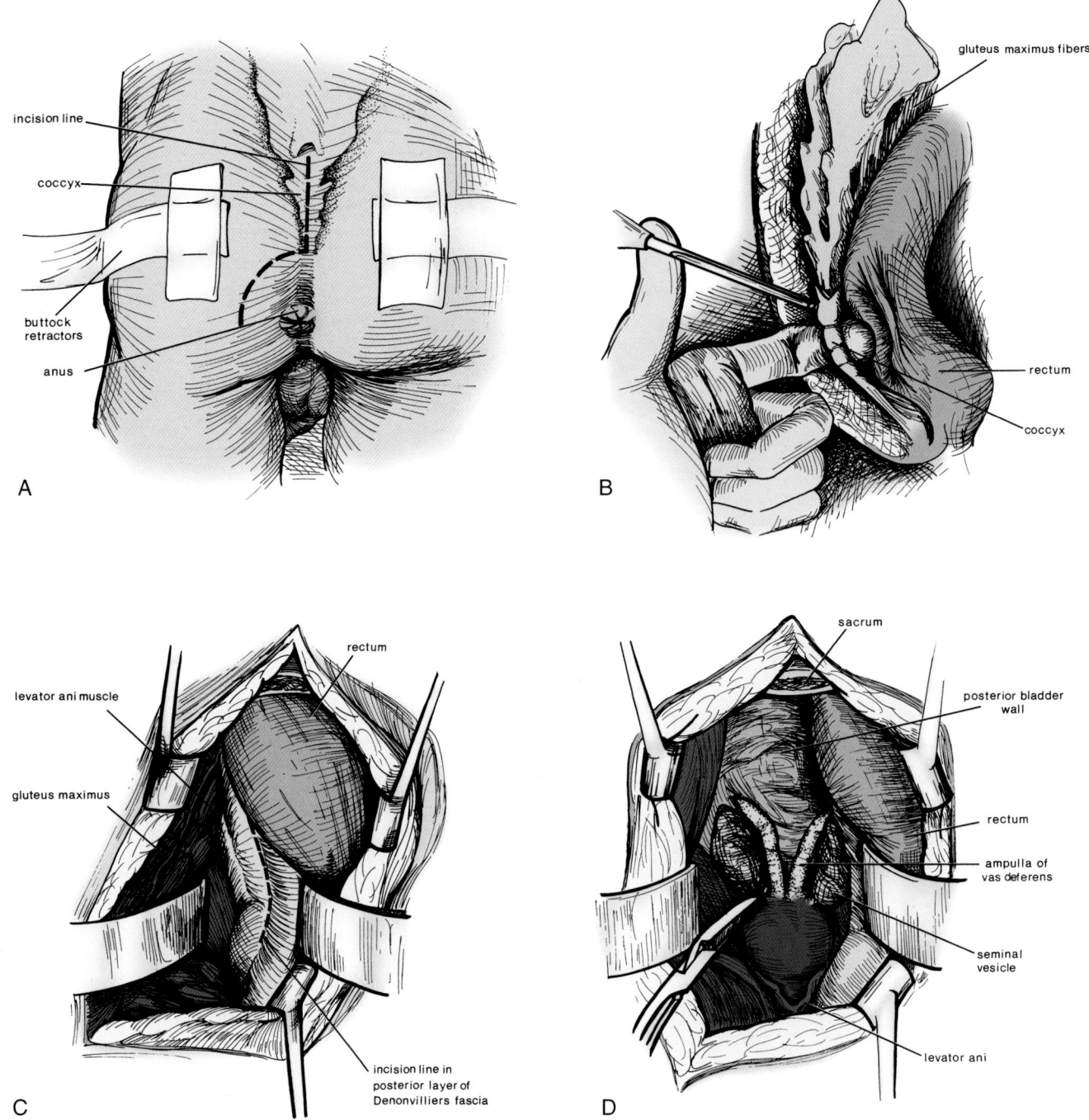

Figure 34–25. Transcoccygeal seminal vesiculectomy. **A,** Incision line over the lower sacrum on coccyx surrounding the anus. **B,** Dissection of the coccyx. **C,** Incision of Denonvilliers' fascia after the rectum has been displaced. **D,** Exposure of the prostate and seminal vesicles. (Redrawn from Hinman F Jr: Atlas of Urologic Surgery. Philadelphia, WB Saunders, 1989:385-388.)

excision of seminal vesicle benign disease. These ports, varying from 5 to 12 mm in size, may be placed in a diamond shape (Fig. 34–26B) or horseshoe arrangement (Fig. 34–26C). With the patient in steep Trendelenburg, the peritoneum just anterior to the rectum in the rectovesical pouch (pouch of Douglas) is incised transversely between the two obliterated umbilical ligaments (Fig. 34–27). Large seminal vesicle cysts are usually easily visualized, and the dissection is carried close

to the seminal vesicles to avoid injury to surrounding viscera and the neurovascular bundle. Use of bipolar coagulation is highly recommended over monopolar energy to minimize injury to these surrounding structures. The dissection can be completed with laparoscopic scissors and curved graspers by blunt and sharp dissection. **The main arterial branch to the tip of the seminal vesicle is easily handled with bipolar coagulation, but a laparoscopic clip is also a good choice.** The

Figure 34–26. **A,** Positioning of the patient for laparoscopic seminal vesicle dissection. **B,** Diamond configuration of laparoscopic ports. **C,** Inverted U-shaped configuration of laparoscopic ports in obese patients. (From Winfield HN: Laparoscopic pelvic lymph node dissection for urological pelvic malignancies. Atlas Urol Clin North Am 1993;1:33-47.)

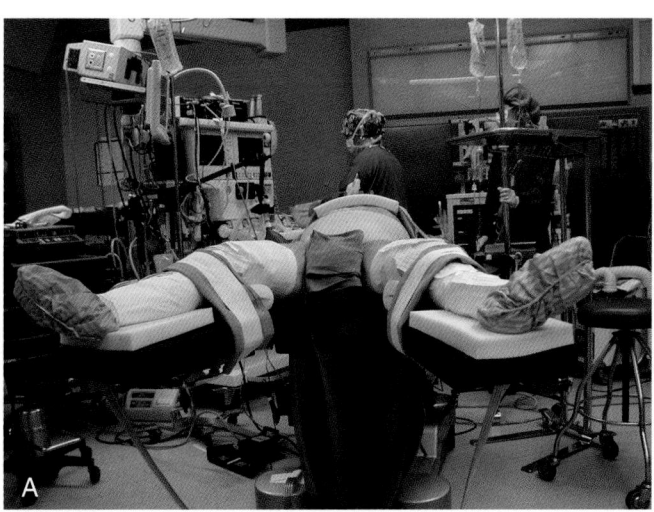

A

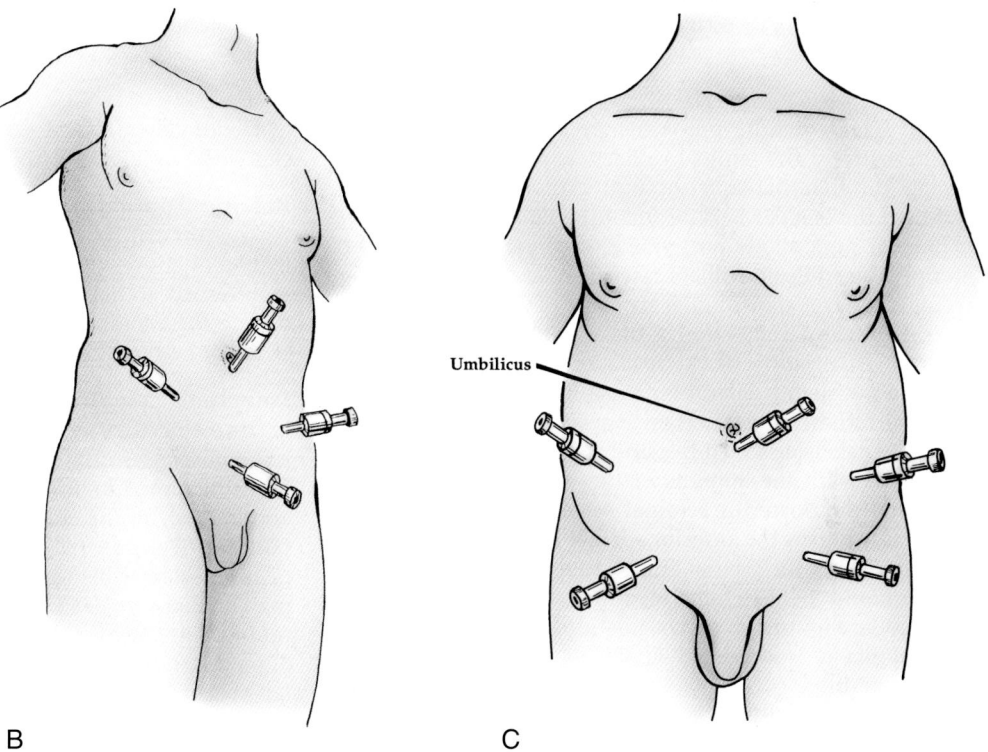

Umbilicus

B

C

seminal vesicle should be dissected caudally down to its juncture with the ampulla of vas and then clipped en bloc. With completion of the dissection, the specimen is placed in an entrapment device* or Endocatch bag† and extracted through one of the larger laparoscopic ports. Large cysts may be aspirated before extraction to minimize the specimen size, obviating the need to enlarge the incision. Inspection is performed to ensure hemostasis and surrounding visceral integrity, and then the laparoscopic ports are closed in the usual fashion.

In select cases, a concomitant ipsilateral nephroureterectomy may be required should an atrophic kidney have an ectopic ureter draining into the seminal vesicle. It is recommended that the laparoscopic nephroureterectomy be performed before the seminal vesicle dissection. Thus, the patient begins the procedure in a modified lateral decubitus position, and then the operating table is rotated to bring the patient into a relative supine and Trendelenburg direction. The operative details of laparoscopic nephrectomy for benign disease are described in Chapter 51.

If the seminal vesicles are being excised in conjunction with laparoscopic or robotic radical prostatectomy, this posterior access may be transperitoneal as described before (Guillonneau and Vallancien, 1999; Guillonneau et al, 2000).

*LapSac, Cook Urological Inc., Spencer, Ind.
†U.S. Surgical, Tyco Healthcare, Norwalk, Conn.

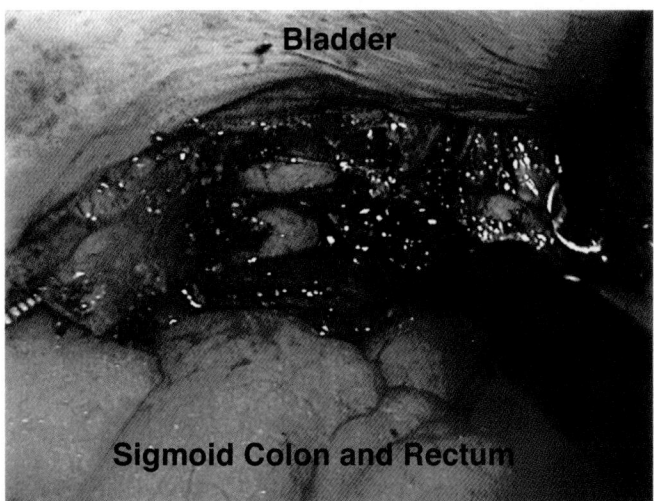

Figure 34–27. Laparoscopic incision through posterior peritoneum in rectovesical pouch (pouch of Douglas).

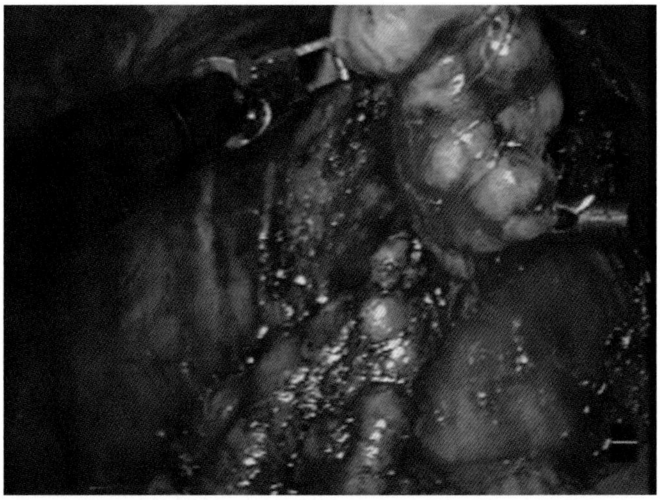

Figure 34–28. Dissected seminal vesicles during robotically assisted radical retropubic prostatectomy. (Courtesy of Thomas E. Ahlering, MD.)

Further details of this approach may be found in Chapter 99. Alternatively, the seminal vesicles may be approached by incising through the anterior and posterior walls of the urethra at the bladder neck. Cranial retraction of the posterior bladder neck allows posterior dissection, whereupon the anterior layer of Denonvilliers' fascia is now exposed. Incising through this layer allows initial exposure of the ampulla of the vas. Isolation and transection of the ampulla of the vas allows excellent visualization of the ipsilateral seminal vesicle just posterior and slightly lateral. As these structures are included with the radical prostatectomy specimen, the tip of the seminal vesicle is dissected free and the body is freed back to its junction with the ampulla of the vas (Fig. 34–28). **It is noted that the posterior seminal vesicle plane is relatively bloodless, whereas the anterior surface is more vascular and adherent.** Again, the arterial branch to the tips of the seminal vesicle should be carefully identified and managed with laparoscopic clips or bipolar coagulation. The seminal vesicles and ampulla of vas remain attached to the prostate and extracted en bloc.

A laparoscopic retrograde approach to the seminal vesicles has also been reported in conjunction with radical prostatectomy. Such an approach would require prior transection of the dorsal venous complex and urethra below the apex of the prostate. This technique would more closely mimic the open radical retropubic prostatectomy approach as described in Chapter 97.

Retroperitoneoscopic Approach. A retroperitoneoscopic approach to the seminal vesicles in conjunction with radical prostatectomy was first described by Raboy and colleagues (1997), who performed a single procedure. This approach gained increasing attention by other centers by 2001 (Bollens et al, 2001; Stolzenburg et al, 2003).

The preperitoneal space is established through a 1.5-cm paraumbilical incision. A balloon trocar is introduced in the preperitoneal space and inflated under direct vision. The details of this approach are described in detail in Chapter 7. Once the prostate and bladder neck are exposed, the bladder neck is transected as described previously. The anterior layer

of Denonvilliers' fascia is incised, exposing the seminal vesicles with ampulla of vas.

Robotic Approach. Surgery of the seminal vesicles with laparoscopic or robotic assistance has usually been performed in conjunction with radical prostatectomy. The technique, with respect to port placement and approach, is almost identical to the standard laparoscopic route described (Menon et al, 2003; Lee et al, 2004).

Potential Complications. Although the transperitoneal laparoscopic-robotic or retroperitoneoscopic approach to the seminal vesicles offers improved visualization, the proximity to bladder, rectum, ureter, and neurovascular bundle must be appreciated by the surgeon. Transperitoneal incision in the pouch of Douglas that is too anterior may lead to perforation of the posterior bladder wall. A subtle hint that the surgeon may be dissecting too anterior is the appearance of detrusor musculature, which is vascular and tends to bleed easily. Should a hole be made in the bladder, it can be repaired laparoscopically or robotically without undue difficulty.

Similarly, the rectal wall may be incised at any point in the seminal vesicle mobilization. Assuming the patient has received a satisfactory bowel preparation, such rectal lacerations may be laparoscopically or robotically repaired in two layers. The anal sphincter is dilated at the termination of the procedure, and the patient's diet is advanced slowly. Electrocautery must be used judiciously close to the rectum. Use of precise bipolar coagulation is recommended.

The distal ureter runs close to the tip of the seminal vesicle. Any tubular structure that is lateral to the seminal vesicle may be the vas arching upward to the internal ring but also could be the ureter. The surgeon may easily become disoriented as to which ampulla of the vas is being dissected, leading to shifting of the dissection too far lateral and possibly injuring or transecting the ureter. Injection of intravenous methylene blue quickly confirms the ureteral injury. Should this unfortunate complication occur, the ureter could possibly be repaired by laparoscopic or robotic suturing. However, a ureterovesical reimplantation may be required and necessitate open surgical conversion. Placement of a double-J ureteral stent after repair is wise, and a pelvic drain is strongly advised in the presence of any bladder, rectal, or ureteral injury that may have occurred during the course of laparoscopic or robotic seminal vesicle dissection.

Finally, the neurovascular bundle is just lateral to the tips of the seminal vesicles. Injury to this structure will impair erectile function and cause a serious problem, especially to the potent patient who may be undergoing seminal vesicle excision for benign disease.

Although data are limited for laparoscopic and robotic excision of benign seminal vesicle disease alone, this approach appears to afford superb visualization with minimal postoperative morbidity and shorter hospitalization compared with the open surgical alternatives (Carmignani et al, 1995; Ikari et al, 1999; McDougall et al, 2001). To date, there are no case reports of laparoscopic excision of primary seminal vesicle carcinoma. In most cases, the seminal vesicle is excised laparoscopically or robotically in conjunction with radical prostatectomy or cystoprostatectomy.

Endoscopic Treatment

Transurethral Resection. If the cyst or abscess is adjacent to the prostate (not in the middle or distal end of the seminal vesicle), it may be possible to unroof the cavity with a deep transurethral resection into the prostatic substance just distal to the bladder neck at the 5-o'clock or 7-o'clock position (Frye and Loughlin, 1988; de Lichtenberg and Hvidt, 1989). However, urinary reflux, with resultant postvoid dribbling, and infection are potential complications (Goluboff et al, 1995). Several groups have reported on endoscopic treatment of seminal vesicle abscesses with use of semirigid ureteroscopes (Razvi and Denstedt, 1995; Shimada and Yoshida, 1996; Okubo et al, 1998). Another report detailed drainage of a seminal vesicle cyst cystoscopically with an incision by a Collins knife (Gonzalez and Dalton, 1998).

Endoscopic Stone Removal. Seminal vesicle stones are extremely rare, although isolated cases have been reported. Seminal vesicle endoscopic stone removal is feasible in select cases that can accept a small-caliber ureteroscope (Ozgok et al, 2005).

Medical-Radiologic Treatment

Small seminal vesicle cysts obstructing ejaculatory ducts or causing local symptoms should undergo an initial attempt at transperineal or TRUS-guided aspiration. If this is not successful because the cyst reaccumulates, consideration could be given to reaspiration with injection of a sclerosing solution such as tetracycline. Similarly, an abscess in the seminal vesicle could be aspirated for culture and drained, perhaps even with a short-term indwelling catheter through a transperineal or transvesical percutaneous route by TRUS or CT guidance (Frye and Loughlin, 1988; Shabsigh et al, 1989; Gutierrez et al, 1994). Direct irrigation of the cavity and subsequent antibiotic injection may be curative (Fox et al, 1988; Fuse et al, 1988).

Conclusion

The seminal vesicles are difficult organs to access, but they fortunately have a small number of primary pathologic conditions. There are very few reasons to operate solely on the seminal vesicles, but when the indications are appropriate, the approach and surgical principles are not particularly different from those of other pelvic conditions more frequently encountered by the urologic surgeon. Today, the laparoscopically or robotically assisted routes offer a minimally invasive approach to these areas, thus decreasing the overall morbidity to the patient.

Laparoscopic Varicocelectomy

A varicocele is an abnormal chronic dilation of the pampiniform plexus that constitutes the primary drainage of the testicle. Approximately 15% of men develop varicoceles, the majority of which (80% to 90%) appear on the left side (Saypol, 1981). Conventional explanation of the pathophysiologic process is that incompetent venous valves and increased resistance within the left gonadal vein—due to its drainage into the left renal vein—result in pooling of blood in the pampiniform plexus (Saypol, 1981; Pryor and Howards, 1987). Several approaches, including surgical and radiologic techniques, are currently used to treat varicoceles. Since the first laparoscopic varix ligation by a single-trocar technique was reported in 1988 (Sanchez de Badajoz, 1988), extensive experience with reasonable follow-up has been reported (Donovan and Winfield, 1992; Jarow et al, 1993).

Diagnosis and Indications

Varicoceles are usually identified on physical examination and generally graded with respect to size or appearance. Subclinical varicoceles are detected by imaging modalities such as Doppler sonography, radionuclide angiography, and venography. These studies, particularly color Doppler sonography, help identify contralateral varices or recurrence in follow-up (Petros et al, 1991).

Varix ligation is indicated only in patients with a clinically apparent varicocele and male factor infertility, adolescent testicular growth retardation, or scrotal pain not attributable to another pathologic process. Treatment of patients with subclinical varices remains controversial.

In addition to laparoscopy, surgical options include retroperitoneal, inguinal, and subinguinal procedures (Palomo, 1949; Marmar et al, 1985; Goldstein et al, 1992). The primary nonsurgical alternative is transvenous embolization or sclerosis (Wheatley et al, 1991). A previous failed retroperitoneal varix ligation and a history of multiple abdominal surgeries that preclude safe trocar insertion are contraindications to laparoscopic ligation.

Surgical Technique

After induction of general anesthesia and placement of an orogastric tube and Foley catheter, the patient is positioned supine with the abdomen and genitals prepared widely. The Trendelenburg position facilitates bowel retraction with exposure of the pelvis and spermatic vessels.

The procedure is performed with three transperitoneal ports. The first (10/11 mm) is placed at the inferior margin of the umbilicus after insufflation with a Veress needle or by use of the Hasson technique. The next two ports, both 3 to 5 mm, are positioned so instruments can easily reach the site of varix ligation, 3 to 5 cm cephalad to the internal ring. In general,

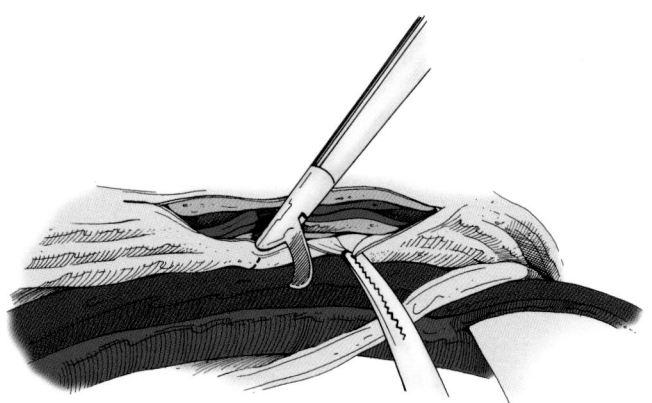

Figure 34–29. Peritoneal T incision bisects the peritoneal flap that is first elevated by sweeping the spermatic vessels from the underlying surface. (From Donovan JF, Sanchez de Badajoz E: Laparoscopic varix ligation. In Graham SD, ed: Glenn's Urologic Surgery, 5th ed. Philadelphia, Lippincott-Raven, 1998:1019.)

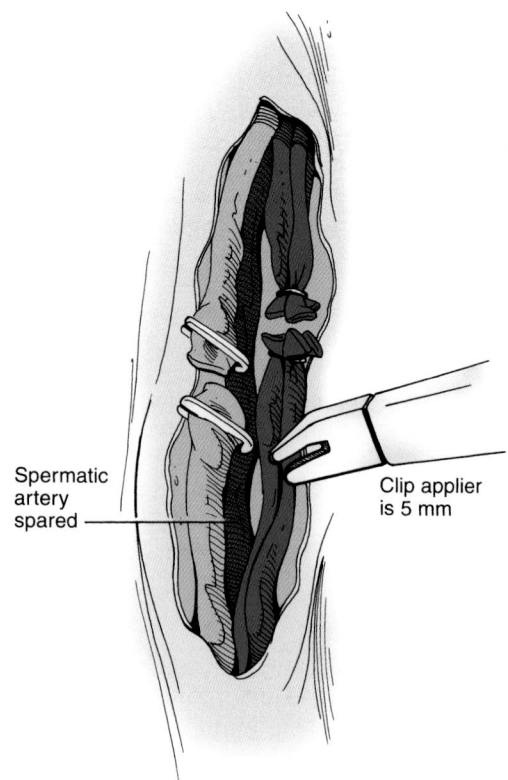

Figure 34–30. On completion of the procedure, only the spermatic artery remains intact. All veins are ligated and divided by either clip or suture. (From Donovan JF, Sanchez de Badajoz E: Laparoscopic varix ligation. In Graham SD, ed: Glenn's Urologic Surgery, 5th ed. Philadelphia, Lippincott-Raven, 1998:1019.)

they are placed in each lower quadrant just below the umbilicus and lateral to the rectus muscles.

In addition to a curved dissector and curved scissors, a 5-mm laparoscopic Doppler probe may be considered to assist with identification and isolation of the spermatic artery or arteries (Loughlin and Brooks, 1992; Donovan and Sanchez de Badajoz, 1998). A 3- to 5-cm incision through the posterior peritoneum is made lateral and parallel to the spermatic vessels a few centimeters cephalad to the internal inguinal ring. A second perpendicular incision through the medial peritoneal flap results in a T incision that provides easy access to the spermatic veins (Fig. 34–29). The entire spermatic vascular bundle is then bluntly mobilized and isolated. In general, three to eight veins and one artery (located posterior and medial to the veins) are identified. **The artery is identified with the laparoscopic Doppler probe or by inspection for pulsation. Once its location is confirmed, each vein is clipped (5-mm clip applier) or ligated and divided so that only the artery remains** (Fig. 34–30). Before the abdomen is exited, the insufflation pressure is lowered to 5 mm Hg to confirm hemostasis. Scrotal emphysema often occurs and should be expressed back into the peritoneum and vented through a trocar-sheath before closure of the port site.

Results

Laparoscopic varicocelectomy is generally an outpatient procedure, although a few patients may require overnight hospitalization to recover from the general anesthetic. In a series of 82 patients and 115 laparoscopic varix ligations, Kwon and associates (1996) reported a mean operative time of 102 minutes and preservation of the spermatic artery in 95% of cases. Equally important, the recurrence rate (or persistence) of a varicocele was 1.8%, and the rates of major and minor complications were only 1.2% and 8.5%, respectively. Similarly, Jarow and colleagues (1993) reported a persistent varicocele rate of 1%, a spermatic artery preservation rate of 80%, and a complication rate of 4%.

The role of laparoscopic varicocelectomy remains controversial (Donovan, 1994; Jarow, 1994). **Since inguinal or subinguinal approaches can be performed under local anesthesia with equal efficacy, morbidity, and convalescence and at a reduced cost compared with laparoscopy, the final role of laparoscopic varix ligation is unresolved** (Enquist et al, 1994; Jarow, 1994). However, results of these alternative techniques are optimized by use of the operating microscope (Goldstein et al, 1992; Jarow, 1994), which is not readily available to many urologists. For surgeons skilled at laparoscopy, the effectiveness and low complication rate of laparoscopic varicocelectomy support its continued use in urologic practice, especially in the case of bilateral varicocele.

Acknowledgment

The authors wish to acknowledge Dr. Richard D. Williams for all of his assistance in the preparation of this chapter as well as previous versions. We would also like to thank Ms. Kristina Greiner for her editorial expertise.

SUGGESTED READINGS

Aboul-Azm TE: Anatomy of the human seminal vesicles and ejaculatory ducts. Arch Androl 1979;3:287-292.

Alpern MB, Dorfman, RE, Gross BH, et al: Seminal vesicle cysts: Association with adult polycystic kidney disease. Radiology 1991;180:79-80.

Anguiano A, Oates RD, Amos JA, et al: Congenital bilateral absence of the vas deferens: A primarily genital form of cystic fibrosis. JAMA 1994;267:1794-1797.

Aradhya KW, Best K, Sokal DC: Recent developments in vasectomy. BMJ 2005;330:296-299.

Brewster SF: The development and differentiation of human seminal vesicles. J Anat 1985;143:45-55.

Carter SS, Shinohara K, Lipshultz LI: Transrectal ultrasonography in disorders of the seminal vesicles and ejaculatory ducts. Urol Clin North Am 1989;16:773-790.

Davis BE, Noble MJ, Weigel JW, et al: Analysis and management of chronic testicular pain. J Urol 1990;143:936-939.

Guillonneau B, Vallancien G: Laparoscopic radical prostatectomy: The Montsouris experience. J Urol 2000;163:418-422.

Healy B: From the National Institutes of Health. Does vasectomy cause prostate cancer? JAMA 1993;269:2620.

Kavoussi LR, Schuessler WW, Vancaillie TG, et al: Laparoscopic approach to the seminal vesicles. J Urol 1993;150:417-419.

Kiddoo DA, Wollin TA, Mador DR: A population based assessment of complications following outpatient hydrocelectomy and spermatocelectomy. J Urol 2004;171:746-748.

Li S, Goldstein M, Zhu J, Huber D: The no-scalpel vasectomy. J Urol 1991;145:341-344.

Sokal D, Irsula B, Chen-Mok M, et al: A comparison of vas occlusion techniques: Cautery more effective than ligation and excision with fascial interposition. BMC Urol 2004;4:12.

INDEX

Note: Page numbers followed by the letter f refer to figures; those followed by t refer to tables.

Cystectomy *(Continued)*
    and urinary diversion, 2523-2527. *See also* Urinary diversion, laparoscopic-assisted.
    retained male urethra after, 1015-1018
        considerations in, 1015
        total urethrectomy for
            after cutaneous division, 1015, 1016f-1017f
            after orthotopic division, 1018
    salvage, for metastatic bladder cancer, 2478
    simple, 2501-2503
        complications of, 2503
        indications for, 2501
        postoperative management of, 2502-2503
        surgical technique of, 2501-2502, 2501f, 2502f
    supratrigonal, for painful bladder syndrome/interstitial cystitis, 366-367
    urethral recurrence after, in females, 1021-1022
Cysteinyl leukotriene D4 receptor antagonist, for painful bladder syndrome/interstitial cystitis, 360t, 361
Cystic fibrosis, male infertility in, 611
Cystic fibrosis transmembrane conductance regulator *(CFTR)* gene. *See CFTR* gene.
Cystic nephroma, 1580, 1581f
    multiloculated, 3339-3343, 3340f. *See also* Multilocular cyst.
    in children, 3899
Cystine calculi, 1385-1386, 1385f, 1406, 1406f, 1425f
Cystinuria, 107, 1406, 1406f
    genetics of, 1385-1386
    in children, 3223
    treatment of, 1424
Cystitis
    after renal transplantation, 1321
    chronic, bladder cancer associated with, 2415
    clinical presentation of, 255, 255f
    complicated, 258-259
        host factors in, 258t
        treatment of, 259, 259t
    definition of, 224
    diagnosis of, 255-256
    differential diagnosis of, 256
    in children, 3234-3236, 3235f
        eosinophilic, 3582
        inflammatory hemorrhagic, 3263
        interstitial, 3263-3264
    interstitial. *See also* Painful bladder syndrome/interstitial cystitis.
        antibiotics causing, 338-339
        bladder cancer associated with, 335
        feline, 337-338
        gynecologic problems mimicking, 351
        ICDB Study Eligibility Criteria for, 332, 333t
        in children, 3263-3264
        NIDDK diagnostic criteria for, 332, 332t
        prostatitis and, 309-310
        sacral neuromodulation for, 2156-2157
    management of
        antibiotics in, 256-257, 256t
        cost of therapy in, 257
        duration of therapy in, 257
        follow-up in, 257
    signs and symptoms of, 238
    uncomplicated, 254-258
Cystitis glandularis, in pelvic lipomatosis, 1217

Cystocele. *See also* Vagina, prolapse of.
    leak point pressure measurement in, 2007, 2240-2241, 2242f
    sling procedures for, 2236-2237
Cystography, in vesicoureteral reflux, 4332-4333, 4334f
Cystolitholapexy, for bladder calculi, 2668-2669
Cystolithotomy, for bladder calculi, 2669
Cystolysis, 2290-2291
Cystometrography. *See also* Cystometry.
    bladder capacity in, 1992-1993
    bladder compliance in, 1993, 1993f
    bladder emptying in, 1995
    bladder sensation in, 1993, 1994t
    bladder storage in, 1993, 1993f, 1995, 1995f
    in benign prostatic hyperplasia, 2772
    phases of, 1992
        fill rate of, 1991-1992
    pitfalls in, 1995
    pressure measurement in, 1991
    special testing in, 1995
    studies in, 1991-1995
Cystometry. *See also* Cystometrography.
    for painful bladder syndrome/interstitial cystitis, 352-353, 352f, 353f
    potassium chloride in, 354
    types of, 1992
Cystometry Sensation Scale, 2084t
Cystometry transducers, 1988
Cystoplasty
    augmentation. *See also* Bladder augmentation.
        artificial sphincter placement with, 2402
        for bladder filling/storage disorders, 2291
        for genitourinary tuberculosis, 446
        for incontinence, 2073-2074
        for painful bladder syndrome/interstitial cystitis, 367
    in children, 3672-3691
        alkalosis after, 3682
        alternative(s) to, 3687-3691
            autoaugmentation as, 3688-3690, 3689f
            bladder regeneration as, 3690-3691
            seromuscular enteroplasty as, 3690, 3691f
            ureteroplasty as, 3687-3688, 3688f
        bladder calculi after, 3684
        bladder compliance after, 3680-3681, 3681f
        cecocystoplasty in, 3675
        decreasing necessity for, 3691
        delayed growth after, 3682
        delayed spontaneous bladder perforation after, 3684-3686, 3685f
        gastrocystoplasty in
            antrum technique of, 3678
            body technique of, 3678-3679, 3678f
        gastrointestinal effects of, 3680
        hematuria-dysuria syndrome after, 3682-3683
        ileocecocystoplasty in
            appendix in, 3675
            ileocecal valve in, 3675, 3677
            technique of, 3675, 3675f, 3676f, 3677
        ileocystoplasty in, 3673-3675, 3674f
        intestinal segment choice for, 3686-3687
        intestinal segment management in, 3673
        intestinal segment mucus production after, 3683
        metabolic complications of, 3681-3682
        native bladder management in, 3672-3673, 3673f
        postoperative management of, 3679
        pregnancy following, 3686

Cystoplasty *(Continued)*
        results and complications of, 3679-3687
        sigmoid cystoplasty in, 3677, 3677f
        tumor formation after, 3684
        urinary tract infection after, 3683-3684
    laparoscopic approach to, 2544, 2545f, 2546f
    reduction, 2299
        for prune-belly syndrome, 3491
    sigmoid, in children, 3677, 3677f
    substitution, for painful bladder syndrome/interstitial cystitis, 367
Cystosarcoma phyllodes, of seminal vesicles, 1116
Cystoscopic incision, of ureterocele, 3407-3408, 3407f, 3408f
Cystoscopy
    antibiotic prophylaxis for, 252
    flexible, 166, 167, 168f, 1515
    in benign prostatic hyperplasia, 2769
    in bladder cancer, 2437-2438
        non–muscle-invasive, 2454, 2454f, 2455f
        surveillance, 2463
    in genitourinary tuberculosis, 443
    in pelvic lipomatosis, 1218-1219
    in pelvic organ prolapse, 2209-2210
    in urothelial tumors, 1645
    in vesicoureteral reflux, 4351
    in vesicouterine fistula, 2345, 2345f, 2346f
    in vesicovaginal fistula, 2327-2328, 2328f
    preoperative, for urinary tract reconstruction, in children, 3661
    rigid, 167, 167f, 1515
Cystostomy
    Stamey percutaneous, 164, 165f
    suprapubic, for urethral injury, 2659
Cystourethrectomy, for painful bladder syndrome/interstitial cystitis, 367
Cystourethrography, 116
    of detrusor-sphincter dyssynergia, 2022f, 2023f
    static, 116, 117f
    voiding, 116, 118, 119f, 120f
        of anterior urethral valves, 3600f, 3601f
        of bladder diverticula, 2362f, 2364
            in children, 3579f, 3580
        of bladder duplication, 3581f
        of congenital megacystis, 3574, 3575f
        of ectopic kidney, 3279, 3280f
        of ectopic ureter, 3392, 3392f
        of patent urachus, in children, 3577, 3578f
        of pediatric urologic patient, 3213
        of posterior urethral valves, 3589-3590, 3591f
        of prune-belly syndrome, 3484, 3484f
        of urethral diverticula, 2379-2380, 2380f, 2381f
        of urethrovaginal fistula, 2348, 2348f
        of urinary tract infections, 243
            pediatric, 3254-3255, 3255f
        of vesicovaginal fistula, 2328-2329, 2328f, 2329f
    preoperative, of hypospadias, 3711
Cystourethroscopy, 166-169
    equipment for, 167-168, 167f-169f
    indications for, 166-167
    of urethral diverticula, 2378-2379, 2379f
    patient preparation for, 167
    technique of, 168-169
    video-cystoscopy unit for, 168, 169f
Cytogenetic abnormalities, in chromophilic renal cell carcinoma, 1594-1595

Fetus (Continued)
  diagnostic findings in, 3176-3178, 3177f,
    3177t, 3179f, 3180f
  incidence of, 3186
  interventions for, 3187-3189, 3187t, 3188f
  management of, 3186-3189
  pathophysiology of, 3185-3186
  postnatal evaluation and management of,
    3189-3194, 3190t
  vesicoureteral reflux in, 4324
Fever
  filarial, 456
  in children
    bacterial infections and, 3206, 3206t
    management of, 3206
    urinary tract infection and, 3198, 3203
      management of, 3261
  in early graft dysfunction, 1318, 1319t
  in urinary tract infection, 240-241
  patient history of, 88
Fexofenadine, for Peyronie's disease, 827
Fibrin glue, in laparoscopy, 193
Fibroblast growth factor, 2708-2709
  in activation of angiogenesis, 542
  in benign prostatic hyperplasia, 2731-2732,
    2731f
  properties of, 2706t
Fibroepithelial polyps, 431, 433
  in children, 3900
  of upper urinary tract, abnormal urothelium
    in, 1643
  percutaneous treatment of, 1556-1557
Fibroid. See Leiomyoma.
Fibroma
  ovarian, ureteral obstruction due to, 1221
  renal medullary, 1582
Fibromuscular hyperplasia, of renal artery,
  1157t, 1161
Fibromyalgia, painful bladder
  syndrome/interstitial cystitis and, 336
Fibroplasia, of renal artery
  intimal, 1157t, 1159, 1159f, 1160f
  medial, 1157t, 1159-1160, 1160f
  perimedial, 1157t, 1160-1161, 1160f, 1161f
Fibrosis
  associated with intracavernous injection
    therapy, 781
  cavernosal, penile prosthesis for, 798-800,
    799f, 800f
  in urinary tract obstruction
    cellular and molecular changes leading to,
      1204
    congenital, 3169-3171, 3170f
  initiation of, angiotensin II in, 1204
  pelvic, as contraindication to laparoscopy,
    174-175
  renal, experimental treatment approaches to,
    1205-1206
  retroperitoneal. See Retroperitoneal fibrosis.
Fibrous dysplasia, percutaneous transluminal
  angioplasty for, 1181-1182, 1181t, 1182f
Fibular osteocutaneous flap. See also Flap(s).
  in penile reconstruction, 1093
Field theory, of epithelial spread, of urothelial
  tumors, 1641
Filariasis, lymphatic, 455-458
  clinical manifestations of, 456-457
  diagnosis of, 457
  early infection in, 456
  late infection in, 456, 456f
  pathogenesis of, 455-456
  pathology of, 455-456
  prevention of, 458
  treatment of, 457-458

Filiform catheter, 163, 165f
Filmy penile adhesions, after circumcision, 3748
Filtration fraction, in renal blood flow, 1131
Finasteride
  erectile dysfunction caused by, 745
  for benign prostatic hyperplasia, 2788-2792,
    2789f, 2791f
    dosage of, 2788t
    efficacy of, 2790t
    vs. combination therapy, 2793, 2795t
  for lowering PSA levels, 2916
  for prostate cancer, prophylactic, 2869-2870,
    2870t
  for prostatitis, clinical trial data on, 322-323,
    327t
Finasteride Study Group, 741
Fine-needle aspiration biopsy
  of inguinal lymph nodes, in penile cancer, 980
  of prostate, 2891
  of renal cell carcinoma, disease staging with,
    1603
  of renal cysts, 1772
  of renal tumors, 1571-1572
  of testicular sperm, 658
  of testis, sperm retrieval through, 701, 703,
    705-706, 705f-707f
FISH (fluorescent in situ hybridization), in
  diagnosis of oncology, 548
Fistula(s)
  arteriovenous
    delayed bleeding due to, following
      percutaneous procedures, 1546, 1546f
    renal, 1189-1190, 1189f, 3297
  complex, of posterior urethra, reconstructive
    surgery for, 1086-1087, 1086f
  due to intestinal anastomosis, 2549
  due to ureterointestinal anastomosis, 2556t,
    2562
  pancreatic, after radical nephrectomy, 1719
  pyeloenteric, 2353
  pyelovascular, 2357
  rectourethral, after cryotherapy, 3050
  renovascular, 2357
  ureteroenteric, 2353
  ureterovaginal, 2341-2345
    diagnosis of, 2341-2343, 2342f-2344f
    etiology and presentation of, 2341, 2342t
    management of, 2343-2345
  ureterovascular, 2357-2359, 2358t
  urethral, congenital, 3757-3758
  urethrocutaneous, 1042-1043, 1043f
    after hypospadias repair, 3739
  urethrorectal (rectourethral), 2353-2357
    etiology and presentation of, 2354-2355,
      2354f, 2355f
    management of, 2355-2357, 2356f
  urethrovaginal, 2347-2351
    diagnosis of, 2348, 2348f, 2349f
    etiology and presentation of, 2347-2348,
      2347f, 2348f
    management of, 2348-2351, 2350f
  urinary tract, 2322-2359
    after partial nephrectomy, 1730
    cutaneous, 2359
    general considerations in, 2322-2323
    repair of, 2322-2323, 2323t
    urethrocutaneous, 2359
  uroenteric, 2351-2357
  urogynecologic, 2323-2351
  urovascular, 2357-2359
  vesicoenteric, 2351-2353
    diagnosis of, 2352
    etiology and presentation of, 2351, 2351t
    management of, 2352-2353

Fistula(s) (Continued)
  vesicouterine, 2345-2347
    diagnosis of, 2345-2346, 2345f-2346f
    etiology and presentation of, 2345
    management of, 2346-2347
  vesicovaginal, 2323-2340, 2323f. See also
    Vesicovaginal fistula.
Fixed particle growth theory, of crystal
  formation, 1367-1368
Flank incisions, in renal surgery, 1691-1694,
  1691f-1695f
Flank muscles, lateral, 8-9, 9t, 10f
Flank pain
  in urinary tract infection, 240-241
  ureteropelvic junction obstruction and, in
    children, 3363, 3364f
Flap(s)
  axial, 1026, 1027f
  Boari. See Boari flap.
  in correction of Peyronie's disease, H-shaped,
    833, 835f, 836, 836f
  in hypospadias repair, 3725, 3726f-3727f
    onlay island, 3725-3726, 3728, 3728f-
      3729f
    one-stage, 3729, 3731
    split prepuce in-situ technique of, 3725,
      3728, 3730f-3731f, 3743
    reoperative, 3740-3741
    subcutaneous (dartos), 3716, 3716f
    tissue (fasciocutaneous), 3716-3717
    transverse preputial island, 3731-3732,
      3732f-3733f, 3734
  in penile reconstruction
    bipedicled, 1095-1096
    fibular osteocutaneous, 1093
    forearm, 1092-1093
      disadvantages of, 1093
      modifications of, 1093, 1094f, 1095f
    upper arm, 1094-1095
  in pyeloplasty techniques, 1243-1245, 1245f
  in reconstructive surgery, 1026, 1026f, 1027f,
    1028
  in urethral diverticula repair, 2387f, 2388
  in urethral stricture repair, 1067, 1067f-1073f,
    1073
  in urethrovaginal fistula repair, 2349, 2351
  in vesicovaginal fistula repair, 2332, 2340
    splitting of, 2333-2335, 2334f, 2335f
  island, 1026, 1027f, 1028
  musculocutaneous, 1026, 1027f
  onlay island, in hypospadias repair, 3725-
    3726, 3728, 3728f-3729f
    one-stage, 3729, 3731
    split prepuce in-situ technique of, 3725,
      3728, 3730f-3731f, 3742
  peninsular, 1026, 1027f
  random, 1026, 1026f
  skin island, 1028
    in urethral stricture repair, 1072f-1074f,
      1073-1075
  skin paddle, 1028
  subcutaneous (dartos), in hypospadias repair,
    3716, 3716f
  tissue (fasciocutaneous)
    in hypospadias repair, 3716-3717
    in reoperative hypospadias repair, 3740-
      3741
  transverse preputial island, in hypospadias
    repair, 3731-3732, 3732f-3733f, 3734
Flavoxate
  for incontinence, in elderly, 2317t
  for overactive bladder/detrusor overactivity,
    2093t, 2103
Floating ball electrode, in laparoscopy, 191-192

Hypospadias (*Continued*)
  distal, 3722-3725. *See also* Hypospadias, repair of, distal procedure in.
  middle, 3725-3729. *See also* Hypospadias, repair of, middle procedure in.
  proximal, 3729-3738. *See also* Hypospadias, repair of, proximal procedure in.
  proximal procedure in, 3729-3738
    one-stage, 3729-3734
      onlay techniques for, 3729-3731
      other, 3734, 3735f
      tubularization techniques for, 3731-3732, 3732f-3733f, 3734
    two-stage, 3734, 3735-3738, 3736f-3737f
    free-graft for neourethral formation in, 3734, 3736-3738, 3738f
  radiologic evaluation for, 3711
  reoperative
    general principles of, 3740
    specific techniques in, 3740-3741
  sexual function after, 3742
  suture technique in, 3719
  timing of (age at), 3718
  urethroplasty in, 3715-3718
    neourethral coverage in, 3716, 3716f, 3717f, 3718
    neourethral formation in, 3715-3716
  uroflow after, 3742
  syndromes associated with, 3709, 3710t
Hypospadias cripples, 3740
Hypospermatogenesis, 634
Hypothalamic-pituitary axis, in males, aging of, 580
Hypothalamic-pituitary-gonadal axis, normal, in testicular descent, 3766
Hypothalamus
  in male reproductive axis, 577-578
  involved in sexual function, 726t
  steroid feedback on, 578-579
Hypothermia
  anesthesia-related, in laparoscopy, 211
  induction of, intraoperative renal ischemia and, 1690-1691
Hypothyroidism, erectile dysfunction associated with, 740
Hypoxia, perinatal, functional response to, 3161
Hypoxis rooperi (South African star grass), for benign prostatic hyperplasia, 2800
Hysterectomy
  ureteral injury caused by, 1283
  vesicovaginal fistula following, 2323, 2323f, 2324f, 2326
Hysteresis, 1902
Hysterosalpingography, in evaluation of fertility, 612
HZV (herpes zoster virus), infection with, voiding dysfunction caused by, 2033

I

Ice water test, 1995
Idiopathic hypercalciuria, 1374, 1402, 1402t
Idiopathic hyperoxaluria, 1378-1379
Idiopathic hypocitraturia, 1404
Idiotope, of antigen-binding site, 478
Ifosfamide, for nonseminomatous germ cell tumors, 923
IgA nephropathy (Berger's disease)
  after renal transplantation, 1298
  end-stage renal disease and, 1346
  hematuria in, 99-100
  in children, 3226-3227
Ileal bladder substitute, Studer, for orthotopic urinary diversion, 2635, 2636f

Ileal conduit
  in conduit urinary diversion
    complications of, 2566, 2566f, 2566t
      long-term, 2614t
    preparation for, 2564
    procedure in, 2564, 2565f, 2566
    in laparoscopic-assisted urinary diversion, 2523-2524, 2524f-2526f
Ileal neobladder
  for orthotopic urinary diversion
    Hautmann, 2635, 2635f
    T pouch, 2638, 2639f-2640f, 2640
  orthotopic, in laparoscopic-assisted urinary diversion, 2524, 2527f
Ileal neovagina, creation of, 3836-3837, 3837f, 3838f
Ileal pouch, vesical, for orthotopic urinary diversion, 2634
Ileal reservoir (Kock pouch)
  for continent urinary diversion, 2589, 2590f-2591f
  for orthotopic urinary diversion, 2636, 2637f
Ileal union, delayed, after osteotomy, in exstrophy patient, 3516
Ileal ureteral substitution, for ureteral stricture, 1266, 1267f
  laparoscopic, 1266-1267
Ileal valve, intussuscepted, 2561-2562, 2561f
Ileal vesicostomy, 2570
Ileal-ileal stapled anastomosis, end-to-end, 2544, 2544f
Ileocecal conduit, in conduit urinary diversion, 2568
  complications of, 2569
Ileocecal valves
  for continent urinary diversion, in children, 3696
  in ileocecocystoplasty, 3675, 3677
  intussuscepted, 2561, 2561f
  loss of, conduit urinary diversion and, 2575
Ileocecocystoplasty, in children
  appendix in, 3675
  ileocecal valve in, 3675, 3677
  technique of, 3675, 3675f, 3676f, 3677
Ileocolonic anastomosis
  stapled, with circular stapling device, 2543-2544, 2543f
  sutured
    end-to-end, 2542, 2542f
    end-to-side, 2541-2542, 2541f, 2542f
Ileocolonic (Le Bag) pouch, for orthotopic urinary diversion, 2641-2642, 2642f
Ileocystoplasty, in children, 3673-3675, 3674f
Ileostomy, loop end, 2553, 2553f
Ileum
  anatomy of, 2534
  intussuscepted terminal, right colon pouches with, for continent urinary diversion, 2596
  reinforced nipple valves of, for antireflux surgery, in children, 3662
  selection of, for urinary diversion, 2536
Iliac artery
  aneurysm of
    as contraindication to laparoscopy, 175
    ureteral obstruction due to, 1222-1223, 1222f
  external, 46, 48t, 50f
  internal (hypogastric), 46, 48t, 50f, 51
  preureteral, 3420, 3421f
Iliac crest, 38, 39f
Iliac lymph nodes, 52, 52f
Iliac spine, 38, 39f

Iliac vein
  common, 11f, 13, 14f
  external, 52
  internal (hypogastric), 11f, 13, 51, 52
Iliacus muscle, 9, 9f, 9t
Iliococcygeus ligament suspension, in apical vaginal prolapse repair, 2227-2228, 2228t
Iliococcygeus muscle, 44, 46f, 2191, 2191f
Iliohypogastric nerve, 18, 18f, 52, 53t
Ilioinguinal lymphadenectomy, for penile cancer, 982
  radical, 1006-1008, 1006f-1010f, 1011
Ilioinguinal nerve, 18, 18f, 43, 43f, 52, 53t, 73
Iliorenal bypass, 1743-1744, 1743f
Ilium, 38, 39f
Illness(es), patient history of
  present, 81-88
  previous, 88
Imaging, in staging of prostate cancer, 2930
Imaging modalities. *See specific modality.*
Imidazole, 469
Imipramine
  for incontinence, 2072
    in elderly, 2317t
  for overactive bladder/detrusor overactivity, 2093t, 2104
    contraindications to, 2105
  for retrograde ejaculation, 648
  for stress incontinence, 2075, 2111
    in elderly, 2318
Imiprem, for pediatric urinary tract infections, 3248t
Imiquimod cream, for genital warts, 381
Immobilization techniques, in bladder exstrophy repair, 3515, 3515f, 3516f
  complications of, 3515-3516
Immotile cilia syndrome, 611, 623
Immune function, laparoscopic surgery and, 202-203
Immune homeostasis, role of chemokines in, 494-495
Immune modulators, for prostatitis, 322
Immune status, in pediatric urinary tract infection, 3239
Immune system
  adhesion molecules and lymphocyte trafficking in, 492-494, 493f, 493t
  apoptosis in, 488-490, 489f
  cell populations in, 475-478, 476t, 478f
  cell signal transduction in, 482-484, 482f
  cell surface activation of, 479f, 480f
  chemokines and leukocyte recruitment in, 494-495, 494t
  complement and, 474, 474f
  infections affecting, 500-502, 502t
  lymphocyte tolerance in, 490-492
  lymphoid tissue and organs in, 475, 475f
  phagocytosis and, 474
  prostatic, alterations in, 308-309
  T cell activation and effector function in, 484-488, 485f-487f, 486t
  tumor immunology and, 495-500, 496t, 498f
Immune tolerance, in renal cell carcinoma, 1588-1589
Immune-based strategies, with HAART, for HIV infection, 403-404
Immunity
  active, 502
  adaptive, 473
  cell-mediated responses to, 475
  humoral responses to, 475
  initiation of, 478
  innate, 473
    complement in, 474, 474f

Injection therapy (*Continued*)
  calcium hydroxyapatite, 2286
  dextranomer microspheres, 2286
  Durasphere and Durasphere Exp, 2274, 2275f
    efficacy of, 2282
  ethylene vinyl alcohol, 2274-2275
    efficacy of, 2282
  future of, 2285-2287
  GAX-collagen, 2274
    adverse effects of, 2284t
    efficacy of, 2282-2283
    safety of, 2285
  historical chronology of, 2273
  hyaluronic acid, 2286
  Hylagel Uro, 2286
  implantable balloons, 2286-2287
  polytetrafluoroethylene, 2273-2274
    efficacy of, 2281
    safety of, 2284-2285
  silicone polymers, 2275
    efficacy of, 2281-2282
  intraurethral technique of, 2275-2280
    in children, 2280
    in females, 2277-2280, 2278f, 2279f
    in males, 2276-2277, 2276f
  patient selection for, 2272-2273
  postoperative care following, 2280
  safety of, 2284-2285
  for late-onset hypogonadism, testosterone in, 857, 858t
  for tissue engineering, 567-569, 568f
  with bulking agents, for bladder neck reconstruction, in children, 3665-3666
Injury. *See* Trauma; *at anatomic site; specific injury.*
INK4, G₁S checkpoint and, 523
Innervation. *See* Nerve(s); *under anatomy.*
Innominate bones, 38, 39f
Innovations, in percutaneous nephrostomy, 1563
Insemination, intrauterine. *See also* Assisted reproductive techniques (ARTs).
  natural cycle of, 651
INSL3 gene, in testicular descent, 3145
INSL3 hormone, in testicular descent, 3769
Instillation therapy, for urothelial tumors, 1681, 1681f
Institute of Medicine (IOM) report, on androgen therapy, 860, 860t
Instrumentation. *See also* Equipment.
  for laparoscopic surgery, 189-197. *See also* Laparoscopic surgery, instrumentation in.
    extraperitoneal space development with, 181-189
    in children, 3916-3917
  for percutaneous nephrolithotomy, in children, 3909-3911, 3910f
  for robotic-assisted laparoscopic prostatectomy, 2986t
  for transurethral needle ablation of prostate, 2810, 2811f
  for ureteroscopy, 1508-1514, 1511t. *See also* Ureteroscopy, instrumentation for.
    in children, 3907, 3908t
  for vasectomy reversal, 666-667, 667f
Insufflant system, for pneumoperitoneum, 178-179
  choice of, 199-200
Insulin-like growth factor(s)
  cancer and, 537
  in benign prostatic hyperplasia, 2731, 2731f
Insulin-like growth factor receptor, in renal cell carcinoma, 1590

Insulin-like growth factor-1, 2710-2711
  for tubal regeneration, in acute tubular necrosis, 1337
  in prostate cancer, epidemiologic studies of, 2861
  properties of, 2706t
  role of, in compensatory renal growth, 1206-1207
Insulin-like growth factor-2, 2710-2711
  properties of, 2706t
Integral theory, of stress incontinence, 2052-2053
Integrins, 539-540, 2695
  in activation of leukocytes, 492-493, 493t
Intensity-modulated radiotherapy, for prostate cancer, 3018-3020, 3018f, 3019f
Intercellular communication, in male sexual function, 737
Interferon(s)
  as inhibitors of angiogenesis, 544
  for non–muscle-invasive bladder cancer, 2457
    BCG with, 2461
  for Peyronie's disease, 828
Interferon-alpha
  for penile cancer, 988-989
  for renal cell carcinoma, 1623, 1624t, 1626-1627, 1626f, 1627t
    cytoreductive nephrectomy with, 1624-1625, 1624t
    interleukin-2 with, 1629
Interferon-gamma
  in benign prostatic hyperplasia, 2733
  in tumor regression, 499
  source and activity of, 486t
Intergroup Rhabdomyosarcoma Study Group
  clinical staging of, 3879t
  grouping classification of, 3879t
Interlabial mass(es), 3841-3846
  hymenal skin tags as, 3843, 3843f, 3844f
  imperforate hymen as, 3843-3844, 3844f
  introital cysts as, 3842-3843, 3842f, 3843f
  labial adhesions as, 3841-3842, 3842f
  prolapsed ureterocele as, 3845, 3845f
  prolapsed urethra as, 3844-3845, 3845f
  urethral polyp as, 3845-3846, 3846f
  vaginal rhabdomyosarcoma as, 3846, 3846f
Interleukin(s)
  in benign prostatic hyperplasia, 2733
  source and activity of, 486t
Interleukin-2
  for renal cell carcinoma, 1623, 1624t, 1626f, 1627-1628, 1628t
    cytoreductive nephrectomy with, 1625
    interferon-alpha with, 1629
  in allograft rejection, 1315
  in tumor regression, 499
Interleukin-10, in suppression of tumor immunity, 498
Intermesenteric nerve, to testis, 581
Intermittency, urinary, 84
Intermittent therapy, self-start, for recurrent urinary tract infections, 264-265
International Consultation on Sexual Medicine (ICSM) recommendations, for erectile dysfunction, 750-751, 751f, 752f
International Continence Society (ICS)
  classification
    of incontinence, 2046-2047
    of voiding dysfunction, 1980-1981, 1981t
International Continence Society (ICS) criteria, for filling rates during cystometry, 1991
International Continence Society (ICS)
  Cystometry Terms, 1994t

International Continence Society (ICS)
  definition
    of incontinence, 2046, 2082
    of overactive bladder, 2079
    of painful bladder syndrome, 332
    of urgency, 333
International Continence Society (ICS)
  provisional nomogram, for outflow obstruction, 1999-2000, 1999f, 2000f
International Continence Society (ICS)
  standards, minimal, 1988t
International Index of Erectile Function (IIEF) questionnaire, 751-752, 753f
International Prostate Symptom Score (IPSS), 85-86, 85t, 2768-2769
International Reflux Study in Children, 3239
International Society of Paediatric Oncology, rhabdomyosarcoma clinical trials conducted by, 3894-3895, 3895f
Interpersonal process, in quality of health care, 148
Intersex condition(s)
  evaluation of, before hypospadias repair, 3711
  hypospadias and, 3709
  laparoscopic examination of, in children, 3914-3915, 3914t
  surgical reconstruction of, 3853-3864
    current operative techniques in, 3855-3862, 3857f
    for high vaginal confluence with or without clitoral hypertrophy, 3858-3859, 3859f-3861f
    for low vaginal confluence with clitoral hypertrophy, 3856-3858, 3858f
    initial management, timing, and principles in, 3853-3855, 3854f-3856f
    results of, 3863-3864
    urogenital mobilization in, total or partial, 3859-3862, 3861f-3864f
Interstitial cell(s), of bladder, 1929-1930, 1930f
Interstitial cell tumors, testicular, 925-927, 926t. *See also* Leydig cell tumor(s).
Interstitial cystitis. *See also* Painful bladder syndrome/interstitial cystitis.
  antibiotics causing, 338-339
  bladder cancer associated with, 335
  feline, 337-338
  gynecologic problems mimicking, 351
  ICDB Study Eligibility Criteria for, 332, 333t
  in children, 3263-3264
  NIDDK diagnostic criteria for, 332, 332t
  prostatitis and, 309-310
  sacral neuromodulation for, 2156-2157
Interstitial Cystitis Association (ICA)
  recommendations, of foods to avoid, in painful bladder syndrome/interstitial cystitis, 359t
Interstitial Cystitis Database (ICDB) Study Eligibility Criteria, for interstitial cystitis, 332, 333t
Interstitial laser, for benign prostatic hyperplasia, 2823
  clinical results of, 2826-2827
Interstitial nephritis, in acute renal failure, 1328-1329, 1328t
Interstitium, of testis, 581, 581f, 584-585, 585f-587f, 587
Intertrigo, candidal, 424, 424f
Intervertebral disks, disease of, voiding dysfunction with, 2012t, 2031
Intestinal anastomosis, 2539-2551
  complication(s) of, 2549-2551, 2550t
    bowel obstruction as, 2549-2550, 2550t, 2551f

Mortality rates *(Continued)*
 positive biopsies and, in low-risk and
 favorable intermediate-risk patients,
 3009, 3009f-3011f
 pretreatment risk groups and, 3007, 3008f
 worldwide, 2855-2856
 for renal bypass surgery, 1749
 for renal replacement therapy, 1355
 for transurethral resection of prostate, 2837-
 2838
 for urothelial tumors, 1638
 prenatal, bacteriuria and, 291
Mosquito hemostat, in vasectomy, 1099, 1100f
Motility
 intestinal, with pneumoperitoneum, 201
 sperm
 defects in, 621-623, 621f, 622f
 maturation and, 601-602, 601f
 reference range for, 618
Motor activity, in conduit urinary diversion,
 2577-2578
Motor unit action potential, neurophysiologic
 studies of, 2003-2004, 2004f
MPB chemotherapy regimen, for penile cancer,
 988t
MRA. *See* Magnetic resonance angiography
 (MRA).
MRI. *See* Magnetic resonance imaging (MRI).
MRU. *See* Magnetic resonance urography
 (MRU).
MSR1 gene, in hereditary prostate cancer, 518
Mucinous adenocarcinoma, of prostate, 2880
Mucormycosis, 466
Mucus, production of, by intestinal segments
 used in augmentation cystoplasty, 3683
Müllerian aplasia, 3833. *See also* Mayer-
 Rokitansky-Küster-Hauser syndrome.
Müllerian duct, differentiation of, 3805, 3806f,
 3831
Müllerian duct syndrome, persistent, 3826-3827
Müllerian-inhibiting substance (MIS), 3137
 fetal secretion of, 3761-3762
 in gonadal differentiation, 2679
 in sexual differentiation, 3804, 3805, 3806f
 in testicular descent, 3145, 3767-3768
 properties of, 2706t
 Sertoli cell secretion of, 3144-3145
Multichannel urodynamic monitoring, 2004-
 2005, 2004f. *See also* Urodynamic
 evaluation.
 of incontinent patient, 2064-2068
 filling/storage phase in, 2065-2067, 2065f-
 2067f
 indications for, 2065t
 voiding/emptying phase in, 2068
Multichannel videourodynamic monitoring, of
 incontinent patient, 2068-2069, 2069f
Multicystic dysplastic kidney, 3334-3339, 3335f
 bunch of grapes appearance of, 3334, 3335f
 characteristics of, 3314t
 clinical features of, 3335-3336
 etiology of, 3334-3335
 evaluation of, 3337
 genes active in, 3334
 histopathology of, 3336-3337, 3336f
 hydronephrotic form of, 3334, 3335f
 hypertension in, 3337, 3339
 in horseshoe kidney, 3336, 3336f
 in utero diagnosis of, 3336
 involution in, 3336
 prenatal diagnosis of, 3182-3183, 3183f
 differential diagnosis in, 3183, 3184f
 postnatal evaluation and management with,
 3193-3194

Multicystic dysplastic kidney *(Continued)*
 solid cystic form of, 3334, 3335f
 treatment and prognosis of, 3337-3339, 3660t
 vesicoureteral reflux in, 4344
 Wilms' tumors associated with, 3337
Multicystic kidney tumor, benign adenomatous,
 3341
Multidrug regimens, for hormone-refractory
 prostate cancer, clinical trials of, 3106,
 3107t, 3108
Multidrug resistance (MDR) proteins, in renal
 cell carcinoma, 1589, 1626
Multilocular cyst
 benign, 3339-3343, 3340f
 characteristics of, 3314t
 clinical features of, 3340
 evaluation of, 3341, 3343
 histopathology of, 3340-3341, 3342f
 treatment of, 3343
 solitary, in children, 3899
Multimodal therapy, for metastatic renal cell
 carcinoma, 1631-1632, 1631f
Multiple endocrine neoplasia (MEN)
 pheochromocytoma associated with, 1861,
 1862t
 type I, 516t
 type II, 515t
Multiple malformation syndromes, with renal
 cysts, 3329-3339, 3330t. *See also specific
 disorder.*
Multiple punctures, for percutaneous
 nephrolithotomy, 1490-1491, 1491f
Multiple sclerosis
 sacral neuromodulation for, 2156
 voiding dysfunction in, 2012t, 2019-2020
Multiple system atrophy
 voiding dysfunction in, 2012t, 2018-2019
 vs. Parkinson's disease, 2019
Multisystemic disease, syndromes associated
 with, 3200t
Mumps orchitis, infertility due to, 643
Muscarinic receptors
 in bladder contraction, 2091-2093
 location of, 2092
 pharmacologically defined, 2092
 uropharmacology of, 1949-1951, 1949f,
 1950t
 selectivity of, 1951
Muscle(s). *See also named muscle.*
 abdominal wall
 anterior, 40, 41f, 42f
 posterior, 3, 6f-9f, 8, 9t
 pelvic, 43-44, 46f, 47f, 2191-2194, 2191f-2194f
 renal pelvic, urothelial tumor invasion of,
 1640
 smooth. *See* Smooth muscle.
 striated. *See* Striated muscle.
 urethral, 1935-1937
 fiber types of, 1936-1937
Muscle hypertrophy, in ureteral obstruction,
 1911, 1911f
Muscle precursor cells, injectable, for urinary
 incontinence, 568-569
Muscle relaxants
 affecting lower urinary tract function, 3628t
 for prostatitis, 322
Muscular dystrophy, voiding dysfunction in,
 2042-2043
Musculocutaneous flap(s), 1026, 1027f. *See also*
 Flap(s).
Mutagenesis, xenografts and, 545-546
Mutation(s)
 carcinogenesis and, 513, 513f
 of oncogenes, relevance of, 514

Mutation(s) *(Continued)*
 somatic, associated with prostate cancer
 initiation and progression, 2865-2867
Myasthenia gravis, voiding dysfunction in, 2041
MYC oncogene, 513
Mycobacteria, in urinary tract, 228
Mycobacterium tuberculosis, 436, 440. *See also*
 Tuberculosis.
 transmission of, 441
Mycophenolate mofetil, as immunosuppressant,
 1316, 1316f, 1316t
Mycoplasma genitalium
 in genital tract, 384
 in urethritis, 625
 testing for, 626
Mycoplasma hominis
 in genital tract, 384
 in painful bladder syndrome/interstitial
 cystitis, 339
 in semen cultures, 625-626
Mycosis fungoides, 430, 431f
Myelitis, acute transverse, voiding dysfunction
 in, 2029
Myelodysplasia, 3628-3640
 assessment of, in neonate, 3630-3631
 bowel function and, 3640
 detrusor leak point pressure in, 2005
 familial risk of, 3629t
 neurologic findings in, 3634-3635, 3635f,
 3636f
 pathogenesis of, 3629-3630, 3629f, 3630t
 recommendations for, 3632-3634, 3634f
 sexuality and, 3639-3640
 surveillance of infants with, 3635t
 urinary continence and, management of,
 3636-3639, 3638f
 urodynamic findings in, 3631-3632, 3632f,
 3633f
 vesicoureteral reflux with, management of,
 3635-3636, 3637f
Myelolipoma, adrenal, 1839-1840, 1840f
Myelomeningocele, 3629, 3629f. *See also*
 Myelodysplasia.
 bowel emptying regimen for, 3640
 closure of, 3629-3630
 imaging of, 3634, 3635f
 spinal level of, 3630t
 voiding dysfunction with, 2029-2030
Myelopathy
 cervical, voiding dysfunction in, 2028-2029
 schistosomal, voiding dysfunction in, 2036-
 2037
Myoblastoma, granular cell, of bladder, 2445
Myocardial infarction, after renal
 transplantation, 1324
MyoD gene, in rhabdomyosarcoma, 3879
Myofascial trigger point release, for prostatitis,
 323-324
Myogenic failure, in valve patients, 3597
Myogenic hypothesis, of detrusor overactivity,
 2080
Myoid cell(s), peritubular, function of, 588
Myoplasty
 bladder, 2299-2300
 for functional sphincter reconstruction, 2294
Myosin, of smooth muscle, 1891, 1898, 1899f
Myotomy, closure of, in laparoscopic antireflux
 surgery, 4366
Myotonic dystrophy, infertility in, 643

N

Nalidixic acid, for pediatric urinary tract
 infections, 3248t
 prophylactic, 3252

Protein(s) (Continued)
  β-inhibin, 2723-2724
  kallikrein 1, 2719t, 2720
  kallikrein 2, 2719t, 2720
  kallikrein 11, 2720
  lactate dehydrogenase, 2724
  leucine aminopeptidase, 2724
  microseminoprotein, 2723-2724
  prostate stem cell antigen, 2722-2723
  prostate-specific antigen, 2718-2720, 2719t
  prostate-specific membrane antigen, 2719t,
      2721-2722
  prostate-specific protein 94, 2723-2724
  prostatic acid phosphatase, 2723
  semenogelins I and II, 2721
  seminal vesicle secretory proteins, 2724-
      2725
  transferrin, 2724
  transglutaminases, 2720-2721
  intake of, in acute renal failure, 1338
  renal reabsorption of, in proximal convoluted
      tubules, 1140
  restriction of
    for nephrolithiasis, 1412-1413
    in chronic renal failure, 1350
  secretory, of seminal vesicles, 2724-2725
  synthesis of, 512
Protein kinase A, in male sexual function, 734
Protein kinase C, activation of, 483
Protein kinase G, in male sexual function, 735
  cross-activation of, 736
Protein-polyubiquitin complex, destruction of,
      512
Proteinuria
  detection of, 101-102
  evaluation of, 102-103, 103f
  glomerular, 101
  in acute interstitial nephritis, 1328
  in children, 3219-3221
    evaluation of, 3220, 3221f
    investigation of, 3220-3221
    quantitation of urinary protein in, 3219
  in chronic renal failure, 1348
  nephrotic-range, definition of, 3225
  overflow, 101
  pathophysiology of, 101
  patient history of, 100-103, 103f
  persistent, 102-103
  tubular, 101
Proteomics, in diagnosis of oncology, 549
Proton beam therapy, for prostate cancer, 3020-
      3021, 3020f
Proto-oncogene(s). See also Oncogene(s).
  conversion of, to oncogene, 514
Proximal procedure, in hypospadias repair,
      3729-3738
  one-stage, 3729-3734
    onlay techniques for, 3729-3731
    other, 3734, 3735f
    tubularization techniques for, 3731-3732,
        3732f-3733f, 3734
  two-stage, 3734, 3735-3738, 3736f-3737f
    free-graft for neourethral formation in,
        3734, 3736-3738, 3738f
Prune-belly syndrome, 3208, 3482-3496
  abdominal wall defect in, 3486, 3486f
    reconstruction of, 3493
  accessory sex organs in, 3484
  antenatal detection of, 3574
  anterior urethra in, 3484-3485, 3485f
    surgical repair of, 3491, 3491f, 3492f
  bladder in, 3484, 3484f
  cardiac anomalies in, 3485t, 3486
  clinical features of, 3483-3487

Prune-belly syndrome (Continued)
  embryology of, 3482
  evaluation of, 3489
  extragenitourinary anomalies in, 3485-3487,
      3485t
  female, 3488-3489
  gastrointestinal anomalies in, 3485t, 3487
  genetics of, 3482
  genitourinary anomalies in, 3483-3485, 3483f-
      3485f
  incidence of, 3482
  incomplete, 3488
  kidneys in, 3483, 3483f
  long-term outlook for, 3493, 3496
  management of, 3489-3493
    abdominal wall reconstruction in, 3493
    anterior urethral reconstruction in, 3491,
        3491f, 3492f
    controversies of, in category II disease, 3490
    cutaneous vesicostomy in, 3490
    Ehrlich technique in, 3493
    internal urethrotomy in, 3490-3491
    Monfort technique in, 3493, 3494f-3496f
    orchidopexy in, 3492-3493
      Fowler-Stephens, 3492-3493
      transabdominal, 3492, 3493f
    Randolph technique in, 3493
    reduction cystoplasty in, 3491
    supravesical urinary diversion in, 3490
    surgical, 3490-3493
    ureteral reconstruction in, 3491
  megalourethra in, 3485, 3485f
    surgical repair of, 3491, 3492f
  orthopedic anomalies in, 3485t, 3487
  prenatal diagnosis of, 3487-3488, 3487f
  presentation of, 3487-3489
    adult, 3488
    neonatal, 3488
  prostate in, 3484
  pulmonary anomalies in, 3485t, 3486-3487
  renal hypodysplasia associated with, 3313
  spectrum of disease in, 3488, 3488t
Pruritus
  in atopic dermatitis, 408
  in scabies, 425
PSA. See Prostate-specific antigen (PSA).
Pseudoaneurysm(s). See also Aneurysm(s).
  delayed bleeding due to, following
      percutaneous procedures, 1546, 1546f
  embolization of, 1546-1547, 1547f
Pseudo-Cushing's syndrome, 1832
Pseudodyssynergia, 2015, 2018
Pseudoephedrine
  for retrograde ejaculation, 648
  for stress incontinence, 2109
  in elderly, 2318
Pseudoepitheliomatous, keratotic, and
      micaceous balanitis, of male genitalia, 429,
      429f
Pseudoepitheliomatous micaceous growth, of
      penis, 960
Pseudoexstrophy, in adult male, 3550, 3551f
Pseudohermaphroditism, 3816-3827
  dysgenetic male, 3812-3813
  female, 3816-3821
    congenital adrenal hyperplasia in, 3816-
        3820, 3817f, 3818f
    secondary to maternal androgens,
        progestins, and tumors, 3820-3821
  male, 3821-3827
    androgen receptor and postreceptor defects
        in, 3823-3825
    17α-hydroxylase deficiency in, 3822
    3β-hydroxysteroid deficiency in, 3821-3822

Pseudohermaphroditism (Continued)
    17β-hydroxysteroid oxidoreductase
        deficiency in, 3822-3823
    Leydig cell aplasia in, 3821
    17,20-lyase deficiency in, 3822
    persistent müllerian duct syndrome in,
        3826-3827
    5α-reductase deficiency in, 3825-3826,
        3825f, 3826f
    StAR deficiency in, 3821
    syndrome of complete androgen
        insensitivity in, 3823-3824
    syndrome of partial androgen resistance in,
        3824-3825
    testosterone biosynthesis disorders in,
        3821-3823
Pseudomembranous enterocolitis, antibiotic
      bowel preparation causing, 2539
Pseudo-obstruction, due to intestinal
      anastomosis, 2550-2551
Pseudosarcoma, of bladder, 2418
Pseudotumor, of kidney, 3302, 3302f
PSMA. See Prostate-specific membrane antigen
      (PSMA).
Psoas muscle, 9, 9f, 9t
Psoas muscle hitch
  for lower ureteral injuries, 1288
  for ureteral stricture, 1261, 1262f, 1263f
    laparoscopic, 1261
  in children, 3662, 3663f
  in redo ureteral reimplantation, 4362, 4362f
  ureteroneocystostomy with
    indications for, 1667
    technique of, 1667-1668, 1669f-1671f, 1671
Psoriasis, of male genitalia, 410-411, 411f
Psychological support, for prostatitis, 324
Psychological therapy, for premature ejaculation,
      785
Psychometric validation, of HRQOL
      instruments, 152-154, 152t, 153f
Psychosexual issues, after hypospadias repair,
      3742
Psychosexual sexual differentiation, 3805, 3808
Psychosexual therapy, for erectile dysfunction,
      770-771
Psychosocial history
  of erectile dysfunction, 755-756, 755t
  of female sexual health concerns, 865-866
Psychotropic agents, erectile dysfunction caused
      by, 743-745
Psychotypic sexual differentiation, 3805, 3806f,
      3807f
PT-141, for erectile dysfunction, intranasal
      administration of, 782-783
PTA. See Percutaneous transluminal angioplasty
      (PTA).
PTEN gene, 535-536
  alterations in, 535
  in prostate cancer, 2866
PTEN/MMAC tumor suppressor gene, 535
PTH. See Parathyroid hormone (PTH).
Puberty
  delayed, in 46,XY complete gonadal
      dysgenesis, 3813
  factors affecting, 580
Pubic diastasis, partial recurrence of, after
      osteotomy, in exstrophy patient, 3516
Pubic rami, straddle fractures of, 2658, 2658f
Pubic tubercle, 38, 39f
Pubis, 38, 39f
Pubococcygeus muscle, 44, 46f, 2191, 2191f,
      2192
Puboprostatic ligament, division of, in radical
      retropubic prostatectomy, 2961, 2961f

Renal transplantation *(Continued)*
donor for
cadaver, 1296, 1303, 1305-1306
biopsy grading system in, 1305, 1305t
criteria for, 1303, 1305
goals of resuscitation in, 1305-1306
midline incisions in, 1306, 1307f-1308f
recipient selection for, 1308-1309
selection of, 1303, 1305-1306
living, 1296
evaluation of, 1302f
imaging techniques for, 1301t
selection of, 1301, 1303
nephrectomy in, 1301, 1303, 1304f-1305f
selection and preparation of, 1301-1303
for acquired renal cystic disease, 3354, 3355f
for end-stage renal disease, 1295-1296
in children, 1296
for valve patients, 3599
history of, 1296-1297
kidney graft in
early dysfunction of, 1318, 1319t
expanded criteria donor and, 1303, 1305
candidates for, 1309
definition of, 1303
preparation of, 1309, 1309f, 1310f
preservation of
cellular injury and, 1306
clinical, 1306-1308
cold storage in, 1306
rejection of, 1314-1317, 1315f-1317f, 1317t, 1318t
percutaneous nephrolithotomy after, 1498
postoperative care following, 1312-1314
autocoagulation in, 1314
fluid and electrolyte management in, 1312-1313
tube and drain management in, 1313-1314
preoperative assessment in, 1309
primary, survival rates for, 1296t
recipients of
active malignancy in, 1298-1299
cadaver kidney for, allocation of, 1308-1309
compliance issues in, 1299
infection in, 1298
kidney disease recurrence in, 1297-1298
operation for, 1309-1310, 1309t, 1311f, 1312
perioperative morbidity and mortality in, 1299
preliminary screening of, 1297, 1298f
selection and preparation of, 1297-1301
unsuitable conditions for technical success in, 1299-1301, 1299t, 1300t
rejection in, 1314-1317
classification of, 1315-1316
histocompatibility in, 1314-1315, 1315f, 1315t
immunosuppression in, 1316-1317, 1316f, 1317f, 1317t, 1318t
timing of, 1296
urinary tract reconstruction in, 1310, 1313f-1314f
vascular anastomoses in, 1310, 1311f, 1312
waiting lists for, 1296
Renal tubular acidosis, 1153-1154
calcium stone formation associated with, 1380-1381
causes of, 1404t
in children, 3154-3155, 3155f, 3228-3229
in infants, 3154-3155, 3155f
management of, 1422

Renal tubular acidosis *(Continued)*
type 1, 1380, 1381f, 1403-1404, 1404f, 1404t
type 2, 1381
type 4, 1381
Renal tubular cells, in urinary sediment, 107
Renal tubule(s). *See also* Nephron(s).
atrophy and cell death in, mechanisms leading to, 1205
collecting. *See also* Renal collecting system.
cortical, 1144-1145, 1145f, 1146f
medullary, 1145-1146
distal, 31, 33f
disorders of, in children, 3228-3229
function of, 1144
function of, 1138-1148, 1144-1148
basic, 1138, 1139f
congenital urinary tract obstruction and, 3172
effects of ureteral obstruction on, 1200
in infant and child, 3154-3156, 3155f
organization of, 1138, 1139f
proximal, 31, 33f
disorders of, in children, 3228
function of, 1138-1141, 1140f, 1141f
Renal tumor(s), 1567-1636
ablative therapy for, 1810-1818
cryoablation as, 1811-1814. *See also* Cryoablation.
high-intensity focused ultrasonography as, 1817-1818
interstitial laser coagulation as, 1817
microwave ablation as, 1816-1817
radiofrequency ablation as, 1814-1816. *See also* Radiofrequency ablation.
radiosurgery as, 1818
rationale in, 1810-1811
success of, 1811
benign, 1575-1582
adenomas as, 1575-1576, 1576f
angiomyolipoma as, 1578-1580, 1579f
cystic nephroma as, 1580, 1581f
cysts as. *See* Renal cyst(s).
distinctive features of, 1583
leiomyoma as, 1582
lipoma as, 1582
medullary fibroma as, 1582
mixed epithelial stomal tumor as, 1581-1582
oncocytoma as, 1577-1578, 1577f
reninoma as, 1582
classification of, 1568-1569, 1568t
pathologic, 1569t
radiographic, 1570t
simplified, 1569t
CT scan of, 1571, 1571f, 1572f
fine-needle aspiration of, 1571-1572
functioning, reduced, 3159-3160
historical considerations in, 1567-1568
hypernephroid, 1567
malignant, 1582-1636. *See also* Renal cell carcinoma.
carcinoids as, 1635-1636
in children, 3885-3900. *See also specific tumor, e.g.,* Wilms' tumor.
leiomyosarcoma as, 1633, 1633f
leukemia as, 1634-1635
liposarcoma as, 1634
lymphoma as, 1634-1635, 1634t
metastases of, 1635
osteogenic sarcoma as, 1634
peripheral neuroectodermal tumor as, 1636
sarcomas as, 1632-1634, 1633f
small cell carcinoma as, 1636

Renal tumor(s) *(Continued)*
MR imaging of, 1571, 1573f
prenatal diagnosis of, 3185
radiographic evaluation of, 1569, 1570f-1574f, 1571-1575
reduction of, in chronic renal failure, 1342
Renal vascular tone, control of, 1134, 1134t
vasoconstrictors in, 1134-1135, 1134f, 1134t
vasodilators in, 1134t, 1135
Renal vein(s), 11f, 13-14, 14f, 29, 30f
extension of, in renal transplantation, 1309, 1309f
injuries to, repair of, 1279, 1280f, 1281
lacerations of, nephrostomy causing, 1544-1545, 1545f
renin levels in, renovascular hypertension and, 1169-1170
thrombosis of, in neonates, 3196
Renin
in renin-angiotensin-aldosterone system, 1161-1162
renal vein levels of, in renovascular hypertension, 1169-1170
secretion of
barorecptor mechanism in, 1162
macula densa mechanism in, 1162
neural control in, 1162
Renin-angiotensin system
changes in, congenital urinary tract obstruction and, 3172
in kidney development, 3135
in male sexual function, 728
in renal development, 3157-3158, 3158f
Renin-angiotensin-aldosterone system
activation and inhibition of, factors in, 1826-1827, 1826f, 1827f
CNS, 1163
gonadal, 1163
physiology of, 1161-1164
angiotensin II in, 1162-1163
angiotensin II receptor subtypes in, 1163-1164
angiotensin-converting enzyme in, 1162
angiotensinogen in, 1161
barorecptor mechanism in, 1162
endocrine/paraendocrine mechanisms in, 1162
intracellular mechanisms in, 1162
macula densa mechanism in, 1162
neural mechanism in, 1162
renin in, 1161-1162
Reninoma, 1582
Renography, radionuclide. *See* Scintigraphy, renographic.
Renorrhaphy, technique of, 1279, 1280f
Renovascular fistula, 2357
Renovascular hypertension, 1156-1174
clinical features of, 1166-1167
definition of, 1157
diagnosis of, 1168-1173
captopril renography in, 1170
captopril test in, 1169
computed tomography angiography in, 1172
contrast arteriography in, 1172-1173
cost-effective approach to, 1173
duplex ultrasonography in, 1170-1171
intravenous urography in, 1169
magnetic resonance angiography in, 1171-1172
peripheral plasma renin activity in, 1169
renal vein renin analysis on, 1169-1170
experimental
human correlates in, 1165
one-kidney, one-clip model in, 1164-1165

Seminal vesicles *(Continued)*
  innervation of, 1110
  magnetic resonance imaging of, 1112-1113,
    1113f
  obstruction of, 1114, 1115f
  pain in, patient history of, 82-83
  pathology of, 1113-1116
    congenital lesions in, 1113-1114, 1114f,
      1115f
    infectious, 1114-1115
    masses in
      cystic, 1115-1116, 1115f
        medical-radiologic treatment of, 1125
      solid tumors in, 1116
    treatment of, 1116-1126. *See also* Seminal
      vesicles, surgical approaches to.
  physical examination of, 1110-1111
  physiology of, 1109
  secretions from, 1109
  secretory proteins of, 2724-2725
  sparing of, in radical retropubic
    prostatectomy, 2975-2976
  surgical approaches to, 1117-1126
    anterior, 1117
    endoscopic, 1125
    indications for, 1117
    laparoscopic technique in, 1120, 1122-1125.
      See also Laparoscopic surgery, of
      seminal vesicles.
    open techniques in, 1117-1120
    paravesical, 1119-1120
    preoperative preparation for, 1117
    retrovesical, 1120, 1121f
    transcoccygeal, 1120, 1122f
    transperitoneal, 1118, 1118f
    transvesical, 1118-1119, 1119f
  tumors of, 1115
    benign, 1116
    diagnosis of, 1110
    malignant, 1116
  ultrasonography of, 1111-1112, 1111f
  vasography of, 1113, 1114f
Seminal vesiculectomy, 1117. *See also* Seminal
  vesicles, surgical approaches to.
Seminal vesiculitis, 326-327
Seminal vesiculography, 710, 711f
Seminiferous tubules
  degeneration of, 3809
  dysgenesis of, 3808-3809. *See also* Klinefelter's
    syndrome.
  epithelium of, 592
  function of, 587
  peritubular tissue surrounding, 587-588, 588f
  structure of, 581
Seminoma(s)
  anaplastic, 895
  from cryptorchid testis, 3773
  histologic classification of, 893, 894t
  histopathologic characteristics of, 894
  incidence, pathology, and presentation of,
    897t
  risk of, in complete androgen insensitivity
    syndrome, 3824
  spermatocytic, 895
  treatment of, 909-913
    algorithm in, 910f
    for stage I disease, 909-911, 910f, 911t
      surveillance studies after, 911-912, 911t
    for stage IIA and stage IIB disease, 910f,
      912
    for stage IIC and stage III disease, 910f,
      912, 913t
      postchemotherapy residual mass after,
        912-913

Seminoma(s) *(Continued)*
  typical, 894-895
  vs. nonseminomatous germ cell tumors, 956-
    957
Senior-Loken syndrome, 3327
  characteristics of, 3314t
Sensorium, altered, conduit urinary diversion
  causing, 2573
Sensory nerves, role of, in ureteral function,
  1906
Sentinel lymph node(s), biopsy of, in penile
  cancer, 979, 1003-1005, 1004f
Sepsis
  bacteriology of, 288
  BCG, 447
  characteristics of, 287t
  definition of, 287
  dental, treatment of, prior to renal
    transplantation, 1298
  due to intestinal anastomosis, 2549
  in neonate, 3196
  management of, 288-289
  percutaneous nephrostomy causing, 1548
Septic shock
  bacterial cell wall components in, 287-288
  bacteriology of, 288
  biologic effects of, 288
  clinical presentation of, 288
  definition of, 287
  diagnosis of, 288
  pathophysiology of, 287
Sequelae, delayed, in locally advanced prostate
  cancer, treatment of, 3067-3068
Serenoa repens (saw palmetto berry)
  for benign prostatic hyperplasia, 2799, 2799t
    dosage of, 2800t
  for prostatitis, 323
Seromuscular enteroplasty, in children, 3690,
  3691f
Serotonin
  effect of
    on male sexual function, 729-730
    on ureteral function, 1918-1919
  uropharmacology of, 1957
Sertoli cell(s), 3136
  characteristics of, 588
  differentiation of, 3803-3804
  germ cells associated with, 588, 589f, 591-592,
    591f
  in spermatogenesis, 579-580
  müllerian-inhibiting substance secretion by,
    3804, 3805
  precursors of, 579
  secretion of müllerian-inhibiting substance
    by, 3144-3145
  secretory products of, 588-589
Sertoli cell tumor(s), 637, 927-928
  in children, 3901, 3904
  treatment of, 926t, 927
Sertoli cell–only syndrome
  infertility in, 642-643
  pure vs. acquired, 643t
Sertraline, for premature ejaculation, 785,
  786t
Serum biomarkers. *See also* Tumor marker(s).
  for prostate cancer, molecular biology of,
    2909-2910
Serum tests, for pediatric urinary tract
  infections, 3245
Sex
  chromosomal, 3799-3801, 3800f-3802f
  determination of, *SRY* gene in, 3146-3147,
    3146f
  fetal, determination of, 3178, 3180f, 3573

Sex accessory gland(s). *See also* Bulbourethral
  glands; Prostate, Seminal vesicles.
  embryonic development of, 2678-2679
  in prune-belly syndrome, 3484
  secretions of, spermatozoal function and, 604-
    606
Sex cord–mesenchymal tumor(s), 925-928, 926t.
  See also specific tumor.
Sex hormone(s)
  fluctuations in, germ cell tumors due to, 901
  synthesis of, 1825, 1825f
Sex hormone–binding globulin, 767
  assessment of, in females, 872
Sex maturity stages, in boys, Tanner
  classification of, 3745, 3746t
Sex reversal syndrome, 639
Sex steroids. *See also specific steroid.*
  average plasma levels of, in males, 2686t
  uropharmacology of, 1956
Sextant biopsy, TRUS-guided, of prostate, 2890
Sexual abuse, of children, evaluation of, 3199,
  3203, 3210
Sexual activity
  preoperative documentation of, in
    vesicovaginal fistula repair, 2332-2333
  prostate cancer associated with, 2862
  urinary tract infection and, in adolescents,
    3240
Sexual arousal
  in females, disorders of, 864
  in males
    benign prostatic hyperplasia and, 2744,
      2744f
    disorders of. *See specific disorder.*
    neural activation during, imaging of, 726-
      728
    release of neurotransmitters in, 723, 723f
    visual, brain activation with, 727t
Sexual aversion disorder, in females, 864
Sexual behaviors, HIV infection associated with,
  388
Sexual desire
  in hypogonadal men, 859
  problems with, in females, 864
Sexual differentiation, 3799-3829. *See also*
  Genitalia; Gonad(s).
  abnormal, 3808-3827, 3808t
    evaluation and management of, 3827-3829,
      3828f
    gender assignment in, 3829
    gonadal disorders in, 3808-3816
    gonadal dysgenesis syndromes as, 3809-
      3814. *See also specific syndrome.*
    hermaphroditism as, 3815-3816, 3815f
    Mayer-Rokitansky-Küster-Hauser
      syndrome as, 3827
    pseudohermaphroditism as, 3816-3827. *See*
      also Pseudohermaphroditism.
    seminiferous tubule dysgenesis as, 3808-
      3809
    testicular regression as, 3814-3815
    vanishing testes as, 3814-3815
    XX maleness as, 3809
  molecular mechanism of, 3146-3148, 3146f
  müllerian-inhibiting substance in, 2679, 3761-
    3762
  normal, 3799-3808
    chromosomal sex and, 3799-3801, 3800f-
      3802f
    genes involved in, 3802-3803, 3802f
    gonadal function in, 3804-3805, 3805f
    gonadal stage of, 3803-3804, 3803f
    psychosexual, 3805, 3808
    psychotypic, 3805, 3806f, 3807f

Transverse preputial island flap. *See also* Flap(s).
  in hypospadias repair, 3731-3732, 3732f-3733f, 3734
Transverse resection, in partial nephrectomy, 1724-1725, 1727f
Transversus abdominis muscle, 8-9, 9t, 10f
Transvesical infiltration, of pelvic plexus, 2291
Trapped penis, 3750f, 3751
  resulting from circumcision, 3750f
Trauma. *See also at anatomic site; specific type of injury.*
  germ cell tumors due to, 901
  ulcerative, to genitalia, 418-419
Tray agglutination test, for antisperm antibodies, 624t
Trazodone, for erectile dysfunction, 782
Tremor, in early graft dysfunction, 1318
Treponema pallidum, in syphilis, 375. *See also* Syphilis.
Trestle stent, 2806
Triage, of pediatric urologic patient, 3198-3204, 3199t
  emergent evaluations in, 3198-3200, 3200t-3201t, 3202t, 3203, 3203t
  routine evaluations in, 3203-3204
  semi-urgent evaluations in, 3203
  urgent evaluations in, 3203
Triamterene calculi, 1389
Triazoles, 469
Trichlormethiazide
  for absorptive hypercalciuria, 1418
  for calcium oxalate stone prevention, 1421t
  for calcium oxalate stones, 1421t
Trichloroacetic acid, for genital warts, 381
Trichloroethylene, exposure to, renal cell carcinoma associated with, 1584
Trichomonas, in prostatitis, 307
Trichomonas vaginalis, 380
  in urinary sediment, 109, 109f
Trichomoniasis, 380
Trichomycosis axillaris, of male genitalia, 423-424, 424f
Tricyclic antidepressants. *See also* Antidepressants; *specific agent.*
  erectile dysfunction caused by, 744
  for urethral sphincter dysfunction, in children, 3620
Trigone, 59f, 60, 60f
  formation of, 3132-3133, 3134f
Trigonosigmoidostomy, in exstrophy patient, 3537-3538
Trimethoprim, for pediatric urinary tract infections, prophylactic, 3250t, 3252
Trimethoprim-sulfamethoxazole
  for cystitis, 256-257, 256t
  for urinary tract infections, 245, 245t, 246t, 247t
    in children, 3248t
    prophylactic, 3250t, 3251, 3251t
  low-dose prophylactic, for recurrent urinary tract infections, 262t, 263
  prophylactic, for vesicoureteral reflux, 4348
Trimetrexate, for bladder cancer, metastatic, 2478
Trisphosphate, in ureteral smooth muscle contraction, 1901, 1902f
Trocar(s)
  blind insertion of, 180
    complications related to, 206-209, 207t, 208f
  closure of, in hand-assisted laparoscopic nephrectomy, 1798

Trocar(s) *(Continued)*
  configuration of, in robotic-assisted laparoscopic radical prostatectomy, 2986f, 2988-2989, 2989f
  placement of
    in laparoscopic antireflux surgery, 4366
    in laparoscopic nephrectomy, 1762, 1764f, 1765f
      hand-assisted, 1791, 1792f-1796f
      retroperitoneal approach, 1788-1789, 1789f, 1790f
      transperitoneal approach, 1781
    initial, 187
    secondary, 187-189, 188f, 189f
      complications related to, 209-210, 209f, 210f
  recurrence of, after laparoscopic surgery, 1779, 1779f, 1780t, 1781, 1781t
  technology of, 185-187, 186f
  types of, 185, 185f
Tropical pulmonary eosinophilia, in filariasis, 457
Tropical spastic paraparesis, voiding dysfunction in, 2035-2036
Tropomyosin, of smooth muscle, 1898
Troponin, of smooth muscle, 1898
Trospium
  for incontinence, in elderly, 2316, 2317t
  for overactive bladder/detrusor overactivity, 2093t, 2095-2096
TRUS. *See* Transrectal ultrasonography (TRUS).
TSC1 gene, in tuberous sclerosis, 3306, 3330, 3331, 3899
TSC2 gene, in tuberous sclerosis, 1599, 3306, 3330, 3331, 3899
TSH (thyroid-stimulating hormone), secretion of, 578
Tuberculin reaction, CDC definition of, 440, 441t
Tuberculin test, for genitourinary tuberculosis, 440, 441t
Tuberculosis, 436-447
  arteriography of, 443
  biopsy in, 443
  clinical features of, 437-438, 440
  computed tomography of, 442, 443f
  cystoscopy of, 443
  development of, 437
  diagnosis of, 440-441
  epidemiology of, 436-437
  history of, 436
  immunology of, 437
  incidence of, 436-437, 437t
  intravenous urography of, 441-442, 442f
  magnetic resonance imaging of, 443
  microbiology of, 440
  multidrug-resistant, 444
  of bladder, 438, 439f
  of epididymis, 438, 440
  of kidney, 438, 438f
    in AIDS patients, 396
  of penis, 440
  of prostate, 440
  of testis, 440
  of ureter, 438, 439f, 440f
  of urethra, 440
  pathogenesis of, 437
  pathology of, 437-438, 438f-440f, 440
  percutaneous antegrade pyelography of, 443
  radiography of, 437f, 441
  retrograde pyelography of, 443
  transmission of, 437

Tuberculosis *(Continued)*
  treatment of
    antituberculous drugs in, 443-444, 445t
    excision of diseased tissue in, 444-446
    intravesical BCG therapy in, 447
    medical, regimens in, 444
    reconstructive surgery in, 446-447
    surgical, 444-447
    vaccine prospects in, 447
  tuberculin test for, 440, 441t
  ultrasonography of, 442-443
  urine examination in, 440-441
Tuberous sclerosis, 3329-3332, 3330t
  angiomyolipoma in, 1578, 1579f, 1580, 3331
  characteristics of, 3314t
  clinical features of, 3331-3332
  evaluation of, 3331
  genes responsible for, 3306
  genetics of, 3330-3331
  histopathology of, 3331
  pheochromocytoma associated with, 1861
  renal angiomyolipoma with, 3899-3900, 3900f
  renal cell carcinoma associated with, 3332
    screening for, 1599
  renal cysts in, 3329, 3329f, 3330t, 3331-3332, 3331f
Tubo-ovarian abscess, ureteral obstruction due to, 1220
Tubular interstitial disease, in chronic renal failure, 1346-1347
Tubularization techniques, of hypospadias repair, 3722-3723, 3724f, 3725, 3729, 3731-3732, 3732f-3733f, 3734
Tubularized flap technique, dismembered, of laparoscopic pyeloplasty, 1253
Tubularized incised plate (TIP) urethroplasty, in hypospadias repair, 3722, 3724f, 3725
Tubulogenesis, cell-cell interactions in, 3130-3131, 3130f
Tubuloglomerular feedback, 3172
  in glomerular filtration rate, 1132
TUIP. *See* Transurethral incision of prostate (TUIP).
Tumor(s). *See also named tumor and at anatomic site.*
  formation of, after augmentation cystoplasty, 3684
Tumor biology, of renal cell carcinoma, 1588-1591
Tumor DNA, somatic mutations in, 2865-2867
Tumor immunology, 495-500
  adoptive cell therapy in, 499
  allogeneic bone marrow transplantation in, 500
  antigens in, 495-496, 496t
  cancer vaccines in, 499-500
  cytokines and interferons in, 499
  immunotherapy in, 499-500
  mechanism(s) of tumor escape in, 497-498, 498f
    impaired antigen presentation as, 497
    induction of apoptosis of T cells as, 498-499
    secretion of immunosuppressive products as, 497-498, 498f
  mechanisms of tumor evasion in, 496-497
  monoclonal antibodies in, 500
  role of NK cells in, 496
  role of T cells in, 495
Tumor marker(s). *See also specific tumor marker.*
  clinical applications of, 907
  combination of, 2430
  histologic subtype prediction with, 907-908
  monitoring response of, 907